2 0 0 3

ICD•9•CM

Professional for Physicians
Volumes 1 and 2

International Classification of Diseases
9th Revision
Clinical Modification

Sixth Edition

Effective October 1, 2002–September 30, 2003

Edited by:
Anita C. Hart, RHIA, CCS, CCS-P
Catherine A. Hopkins, CPC

St. Anthony Publishing/Medicode

Additional copies may be ordered from:

Your local bookstore
or
1-800-INGENIX (464-3649)

IPP ISBN 1-56329-872-4

DISCLAIMER

American Academy of Professional Coders (AAPC)
Continuing Education Units Credits: 5 CEUs
Contact AAPC directly for credits: 1.800.626.CODE

St. Anthony Publishing/Medicode

2525 Lake Park Boulevard • Salt Lake City, UT 84120
11410 Isaac Newton Square • Reston, VA 20190

St. Anthony Publishing/Medicode

Dear Ingenix Customer:

St. Anthony Publishing and Medicode joined their expertise and after intense research involving real-world coders developed a new and innovative code book. Your *2003 ICD-9-CM Professional for Physicians, Volumes 1 & 2,* 'is the result of this effort. Designed by coders for coders, we are certain you will find the new page design and intuitive symbols will improve coding accuracy and efficiency.

The codes contained in this book are the official code set issued by the U.S. Department of Health and Human Services, effective October 1, 2002 through September 30, 2003.

Your new *2003 ICD-9-CM Professional for Physicians, Volumes 1 and 2,* features:

- New! ICD-9-CM convention — Code, if applicable any causal condition first
- fiscal year 2003 official ICD-9-CM codes
- summary of code changes for 2003
- symbols indicating code changes and pages are dated to indicate when the changes occurred
- clinically-oriented illustrations and comprehensive definitions
- check fourth- and fifth-digit symbols in the index and tabular sections
- age and sex edit symbols

.......PLUS the accuracy and quality you expect from the leaders!

We appreciate your choosing Ingenix/St. Anthony Publishing/Medicode/ to meet your coding needs. If you have any questions or comments concerning your *2003 ICD-9-CM Professional for Physicians, Volumes 1 and 2,* please do not hesitate to call our customer service department. The toll free number is 1.800.INGENIX (464-3649).

Note: The ICD-9-CM Coordination and Maintenance Committee has undertaken the task of completely revising the official coding guidelines. At the time of press the guidelines had not yet been finalized. The new guidelines build upon the current set and therefore, the guidance provided by the current set is still valid. Release of the revised guidelines is expected before the effective date of October 1, 2002. We have created a web site specifically to provide you with the revised guidelines once they are released. You will be able to log on to www.ingenixonline.com/I9guidelines toward the end of September to view and print the new ICD-9-CM official coding guidelines.

Cordially

Elizabeth Boudrie

Elizabeth Boudrie
Vice President, Regulatory Services

2003 Publications

2003 ICD-9-CM Code Books for Physicians Volumes 1 & 2

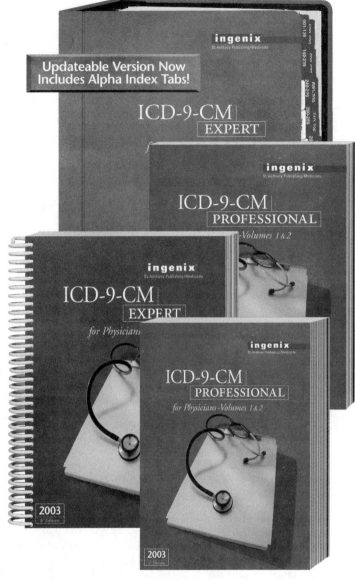

ICD-9-CM Professional for Physicians, Vols. 1 & 2

Softbound
ISBN: 1-56329-872-4   Item No. 3650 **$64.95**
Available: September 2002

Compact
ISBN: 1-56329-873-2   Item No. 3661 **$64.95**
Available: September 2002

ICD-9-CM Expert for Physicians, Vols. 1 & 2

Spiral
ISBN: 1-56329-874-0   Item No. 3652 **$84.95**
Available: September 2002

Updateable Binder
ISBN: 1-56329-875-9   Item No. 3534 **$144.95**

Our page design, featuring intuitive symbols, exclusive color-coding, and additional resources provides a new approach to pertinent coding and reimbursement information. New codes and changes to the ICD-9-CM make our 2003 code books a must buy! Order today and keep current on all changes!

Professional and Expert Editions of ICD-9-CM for Physicians Feature:

- New and Revised Code Symbols
- Fourth-and Fifth-digit Requirement Alerts
- Complete Official Coding Guidelines
- Age and Sex Edits
- Clinically Oriented Definitions and Illustrations
- Medicare as Secondary Payer Indicators

- Manifestation Code Alerts
- "Other" and "Unspecified" Diagnosis Alerts
- Symbols Identifying V Codes Designated for only Primary or only Secondary Diagnosis Use

Expert **Editions Also Include These Enhancements:**

- Special Reports Via E-mail.
- Code Tables--Complex coding issues are simplified in coding tables, as developed for I-9 Express
- Valid Three-digit Category List

The *Expert* Updateable Binder Subscriptions Feature:

- Money Saving Update Service
- Three Updates per Year [October (full text), January and July]

Call Toll-Free 1.877.INGENIX (464.3649) or Shop Online at www.IngenixOnline.com

Also Available from your Medical Bookstore or Distributor

060102

St. Anthony Publishing/Medicode

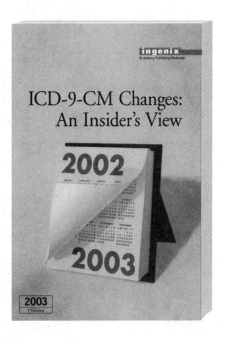

NEW!
CPT® Changes 2003: An Insider's View

7" x 10" Perfect Bound

The American Medical Association and Ingenix Publishing present *CPT® Changes 2003: An Insider's View*, a must-have resource for Physicians' Current Procedural Terminology (CPT®) Professional users! This book serves as a reference tool to understanding each of the CPT® code changes found in CPT® 2003.

In both books you'll find:

- **Every new, revised and deleted code change**—Listed along with a detailed rationale for the change. Index changes, convention changes and instructional note changes are also explained.

- **Organized by ICD-9-CM and CPT® code section and code number**—Includes a separate section that discusses index changes.

- **Illustrated**—Helps orient you to change in code.

- **Clinical Examples/Diagnostic or Procedural Descriptions**—Helps you understand the practical application of the code.

CPT is a registered trademark of the American Medical Association

NEW!
ICD-9-CM Changes 2003: An Insider's View

7" x 10" Perfect Bound
Item No. 4951 **$54.95**
Available: November 2002

A must have resource for ICD-9-CM users! *ICD-9-CM Changes 2003: An Insider's View* serves as a reference tool to understanding each of the ICD-9-CM code changes found in ICD-9-CM 2003.

CPT® Changes for 2003:
- 204 New Codes
- 23 Deleted Codes
- 203 Revised Codes
- Place of Service section added to appendices

ICD-9-CM Changes for 2003:
- 163 New Diagnosis Codes
- 23 Revised Diagnosis Codes
- 25 New Procedure Codes
- 3 Revised Procedure Codes
- New chapter on New Technology and Medical Services in Volume 3
- Changes to conventions and to the index

Call Toll-Free 1.877.INGENIX (1.877.464.3649) or Shop Online at www.IngenixOnLine.com

Also Available from your Medical Bookstore or Distributor   020606

St. Anthony Publishing/Medicode

The Best CPT® Reference in the Industry!

2003 CPT® Expert

Spiral bound
ISBN: 1-56329-855-4   Item No. 4529 **$84.95**

Compact
ISBN: 1-56329-856-2   Item No. 4508 **$74.95**
Available: December 2002

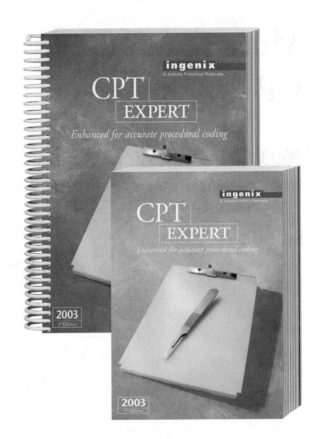

If you are not using the current information , your Medicare claims will be rejected! In 2002, there were more changes in *Physicians' Current Procedural Terminology* (CPT®) codes than ever. Be ready this year for what is expected to be another significant year in CPT® code revisions. With full descriptions, *CPT® Expert* will help you interpret these changes and speed reimbursement. Order today to see for yourself!

Features and Benefits Include:

- **Comprehensive**—Includes EVERY CPT® code with FULL descriptions

- **Exclusive**—Complete index helps you find codes quickly

- **Exclusive**—Color keys and icons revealing Correct Coding Initiative Comprehensive codes, Medicare, CLIA and other common coding rules

- **Exclusive**—Code-specific definitions, rules, and tips compiled from the *Medicare Carriers Manual and Coverage Issues Manual*, and other sources speed reimbursement

- **Illustrated**—Detailed illustrations orient you to the procedures

Publisher's Note: CPT Expert is not a replacement for the American Medical Association's CPT 2003 Standard and Professional code books.

CPT is a registered trademark of the American Medical Association

Call Toll-Free 1.877.INGENIX (464.3649) or Shop Online at www.IngenixOnLine.com
Also Available from your Medical Bookstore or Distributor
060102

St. Anthony Publishing/Medicode

More than 400 CPT® Changes

2003 CPT® Professional Edition

ISBN: 1-57947-303-2   Item No. 4382 **$79.95**
Available: November 2002

Standard Edition

ISBN: 1-57947-302-4   Item No. 4379 **$54.95**
Available: November 2002

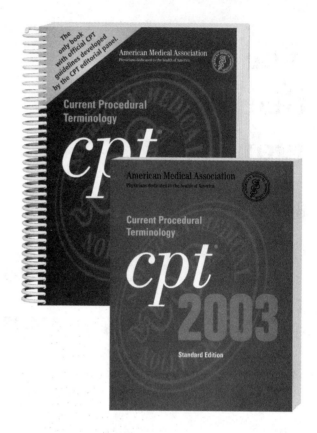

It's imperative your office or facility have the latest CPT codes. These AMA-published code books are comprehensive, informative, easy-to-use, and available in two formats. Don't risk rejected claims, delayed payments or even charges of fraud and abuse. Make sure you have the latest official CPT on the market in your office.

CPT Standard — Softbound and economical

- **More than 400 changes!**—Stay current. Numerous code changes will impact code accuracy and claims submission.

- **Category III "Emerging Technology" subsections**—Learn the latest of these new code sets

- **Comprehensive Index**—Find the codes you need.

- **Easy-to-use Tabs**—Preprinted tabs speed usage

Professional Spiral — **All the features of the** *Standard* **edition, plus:**

- **Deleted Codes with Strikeout**—Helps you code claims from 2002

- **Illustrations**—More than130 procedural and anatomical illustrations

- **Easy identification**—Color-coded keys make identifying section headings, coding changes and coding alerts easier

- **Spiral Binding** — Easy-to-Use spiral binding helps you look up what you need to know.

CPT is a registered trademark of the American Medical Association

St. Anthony Publishing/Medicode

Numerous Code Changes Expected in 2003!

2003 HCPCS Level II Code Books

2003 HCPCS Level II Professional
ISBN: 1-56329-857-0   Item No. 4520 **$64.95**
Available: December 2002

2003 HCPCS Level II Expert

Spiral bound
ISBN: 1-56329-858-9   Item No. 4521 **$84.95**

Compact
1-56329-859-7   Item No. 4522 **$74.95**

NEW! Updateable
1-5639-922-4   Item No. 4524 **$134.95**
Available: December 2002

H CPCS is an evolving and dynamic code set. You simply cannot afford to miss a year. 2003 code changes will be driven by:

■ Elimination of private payer local codes

■ Migration of local Medicare codes to national codes

■ New technologies, new devices, and new drugs with new code assignments

In the *HCPCS Professional* You'll Find:

• **Complete**—Includes all HCPCS codes and modifiers, including deleted codes for 2003

• **Easy-to-use**—Easy-to-understand color-keyed bars, icons, and tabs help you know which codes are governed by what Medicare and coding rules

• **Organized Format**—It's easy to find what you need in the detailed, cross-referenced index

• **EXCLUSIVE**—ASC designation and flagged quantity codes to speed reimbursement

• HCPCS codes deleted before 2003

• Appendix of payers who accept HCPCS Level II codes

• **Table of Drugs and Their Codes**—Ease submitting bills

• *Medicare Carriers Manual and Coverage Issues Manual* **references and Excerpts**—Help indicate which drugs and service are not reimbursed

The *HCPCS Expert* Includes All the Exclusive features of the *Professional,* Plus:

• **Medicare and National Fees for HCPCS codes**

• **E-mail Special Reports**—Know the latest changes when they happen

• **Choice of Formats**—8.5" x 11" Spiral Bound , 6" x 9" Compact, and NEW 8.5" x 11" Binder, updateable

The only updateable book to help you to keep current with dynamic HCPCS changes.

• 3 updates a year, February, April and July

• Easily remove page for photocopying

• Add program memos and other documents easily

ingenix
St. Anthony Publishing/Medicode

The Expert Coding Solution

Encoder Pro

Item No. D4178   Subscriptions Start at **$499.95**

CALL TODAY FOR A FREE DEMO ON CD-ROM!

Available: October 2002

The best only gets better. Ingenix CodeLogic™ search technology now gives you intuitive results for even faster coding. More search terms! Faster results! Larger reference library to support every level of code selection.

Encoder Pro gives users a complete code and reference library at their fingertips. Complete with Sticky Notes, Bookmarks, and Notepad features, Encoder Pro provides a customizable user experience, with annotations and icons for powerful medical coding!

- **Ingenix CodeLogic™ Search Engine.** Searches simultaneously across all three code sets. Employs built-in spell-check, abbreviations, and narrow functions for finding the right codes fast.

- **"Code Book" Navigation.** Gives users the familiarity they'll need to use Encoder Pro exclusively for all medical coding needs.

- **Surgical Cross Codes.** Help the user verify the right match among code sets.

- **Notepad, Bookmarks, and Sticky Notes.** Make the most out of code searches and allow for a customizable experience.

- **CCI Unbundling Edits.** Up-to-date Medicare NCCI edits for comprehensive unbundling rules.

- **Lay Descriptions, Annotations, and Icons.** Help improve Physicians Current Procedural Terminolgy (CPT™), ICD-9-CM, and HCPCS Level II code selection.

- **Continuing Education Units (CEUs).** Earn 8 CEUs through AAPC.

REQUIREMENTS	
Local Deployment Recommended Hardware	**ASP Deployment Recommended Hardware**
• 256 MB of RAM	• 128 MB of RAM
• 800X600 SVGA	• 800X600 SVGA
• PIII 800 MHZ	• PII 233 MHZ
• 125 MB Disk Space	• 60 MB Disk Space
	• Requires High-speed Internet Access

CPT is a registered trademark of the American Medical Association

Call Toll-Free 1.877.INGENIX (464.3649) or Shop Online at www.IngenixOnline.com

Also Available from your Medical Bookstore or Distributor

060102

St. Anthony Publishing/Medicode

E/M Coding Made Easy

Evaluation and Management Coding and Documentation Guide

ISBN: 1-56329-896-1   Item No. 3018 **$129.95**

Available: December 2002

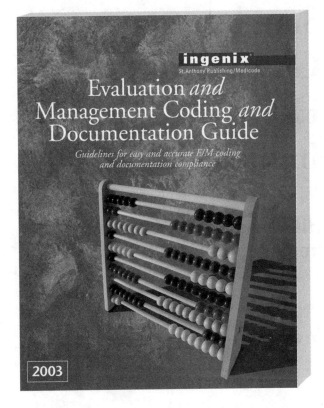

This comprehensive guide to CMS's (formerly HCFA) E/M (evaluation/management services) guidelines provides instructions for correctly documenting to a specific level of E/M service.

- **Real-life Clinical Case Studies Updated for 2003.** Illustrate how to apply the guidelines in everyday situations. Use them to train your staff.

- **Documentation Templates.** Templates provided on disk aid in the documentation process and help to eliminate common mistakes.

- **2003 Physicians' Current Procedural Terminology (CPT®) Code Changes.** Updated with the latest CPT® codes for 2003.

- **Self-audit Forms.** Create a checklist of important documentation needed to support the appropriate level of E/M service.

- **1995, 1995, and 2000 E/M Guidelines.** Prepare the user for the transition to the stricter documentation requirements ahead. Allow users to see the impact of these stricter guidelines.

- **Handy E/M Fast Finder.** A portable reference, organized by place of service and illustrated with tables. Practitioners can take E/M Fast Finder with them into the exam room.

- **Real-life Audit Scenarios.** Help you uncover areas of risk in your own organization so you can fix problems now—not after fines or penalties.

- **Continuing Education Units (CEUs).** Earn 5 CEUs through AAPC.

CPT is a registered trademark of the American Medical Association

Call Toll-Free 1.877.INGENIX (464.3649) or Shop Online at www.IngenixOnline.com

Also Available from your Medical Bookstore or Distributor

060102

Step-by-step Guidance for HIPAA Implementation

HIPAA Assessment and Implementation Manual

ISBN: 1-56329-924-0   Item No. 3183 **$229.95**

Available: June 2002

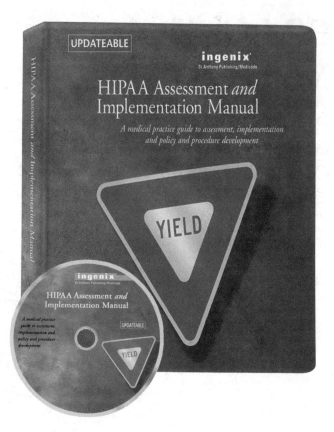

HIPAA Assessment and Implementation Manual is designed to help users put into effect HIPAA provisions using an easy and systematic process. This manual is designed to assist the user with assessing the impact of HIPAA on business as well as helping establish a HIPAA project plan. *HIPAA Assessment and Implementation Manual* also contains valuable information helping you evaluate business associates and current contracts, integrate HIPAA compliance into current structures, and develop policies and procedures.

- **Assessment and Implementation Guidance for Each Provision.** Each provision has a separate chapter dedicated to focusing on issues specific to that provision, allowing users to perform comprehensive and accurate assessments that lead to successful implementation.

- **Easy-to-use and Printable Templates.** The templates contained in this manual are designed to help the user assess current HIPAA readiness and transfer their findings into an action plan.

- **Free Updates.** These updates help keep you up to date with changes to HIPAA policies as they occur and alert you to additional changes under consideration.

- **Policy and Procedure Development Guidance and Templates.** Each provision chapter has guidelines for developing effective policies and procedures.

- **Guidance for Evaluating Business Associates.** Know what defines a business associate and what such associates are accountable for.

- **HIPAA Compliance Integration.** Helps you to incorporate HIPAA compliance efforts into your current compliance structure.

- **Free "E" Book Included.** Forms, templates, and official regulations included for easy lookup and printing.

Call Toll-Free 1.877.INGENIX (464.3649) or Shop Online at www.IngenixOnline.com
Also Available from your Medical Bookstore or Distributor

060102

St. Anthony Publishing/Medicode

Up-to-date Medicare Reimbursement Information

Medicare Part B Correct Coding and Fee Guide

ISBN: 1-56329-711-6   Item No. 3024 **$279.95**

Available: Now

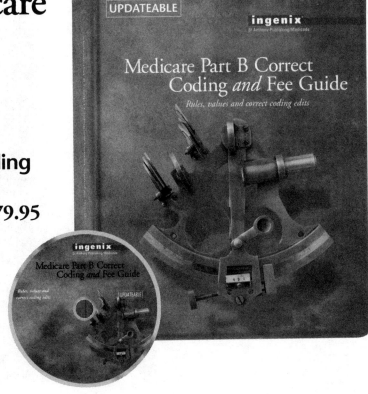

The most comprehensive and current manual of rules, payment restrictions, and claim submission edits, *Medicare Part B Correct Coding and Fee Guide* is critical for correctly reporting Part B procedures and services.

- **Free Updates for One Full Year.** Updates help you stay current as CMS implements changes.

- **Free Medicare Reimbursement Pro CD-ROM Updated Quarterly.** Easily calculate payments, determine NCCI edits, and more for both facility and physician office settings based on your geographic area.

- **Medicare Physician Fee Schedule.** Includes status indicators, global periods, supply codes, and more to help you correctly bill and project payment.

- **Complete RVUs and GPCIs.** So you can adjust fees for your geographic area, evaluate managed care contracts, and check code selection and sequencing for each service.

- **Current NCCI Edits with Policy Icons.** Help you understand the policy that determines the edit.

- **Transition Practice Expense RVU Adjustments.** Help you calculate your payments quickly and accurately according to your setting.

- **Overview of CMS's (formerly HCFA) Campaign Against Fraud and Abuse.** Know what the OIG is looking for.

- **National Average Payment.** Allows you to gauge individual pricing standards against national Medicare standards.

- **Continuing Education Units (CEUs).** Earn 5 CEUs from AAPC.

ingenix
St. Anthony Publishing/Medicode

Get Every Part B Dollar You're Entitled To…and Stay Compliant!

Complete Guide to Part B Billing and Compliance

ISBN: 1-56329-709-4   Item No. 3023 **$249.95**

Available: Now

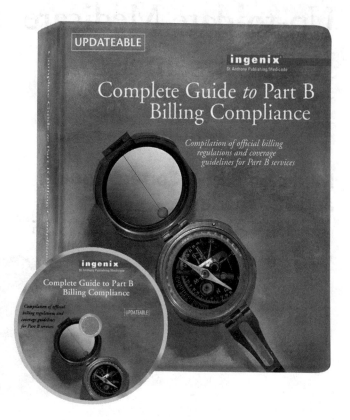

The most comprehensive, updateable compilation of billing regulations and coverage guidelines for Part B services, the *Complete Guide to Part B Billing and Compliance* clearly explains what you can and cannot bill for, how to bill for covered services, appropriate documentation to attach to claims, information that must be documented in medical records, correct codes and applicable modifiers to use, and how to prevent billing errors.

- **Free E Book.** Complete guide on CD-ROM, including the official resources used to produce the book.

- **Topics Organized Alphabetically.** Get fast answers to Medicare coverage and policy issues by topic.

- **Fraud Alerts.** Keep users informed about billing practices under government scrutiny.

- **Billing Compliance Sections.** Educate providers regarding official government guidelines for compliance by providing a chapter describing compliance regulations, legislative timelines, and CMS's (formerly HCFA) past and present fraud and abuse initiatives.

- **HCFA-1500 Form Instructions.** Show users how to fill out the HCFA-1500 form completely and accurately to ensure proper Medicare claim submission.

- **Cross-referenced Billing Topics Connected to the HCFA-1500 Form.** Users get a better understanding of similar billing topics and how to properly code for accurate, timely reimbursement.

- **Updates for One Year.** Users are informed when federal policies and regulations are revised by CMS.

- **Continuing Education Units (CEUs).** Earn 5 CEUs through AAPC.

2003 Publications

NEW!

A New Coder's Training System

These comprehensive education modules help beginning and advanced coders in the office, the facility, or the classroom. Designed to allow you to understand and master the skills needed to be an effective coder, each module includes a CD containing a student workbook and a teacher's guide, along with a three-month subscription to the popular *Code It Fast* look-up program.

All Books Include:

- **Student Workbook on CD**—Student workbook helps you convert information in the book to hands-on experience

- **Teacher's Guide on CD**—Teacher's guide helps instructors and managers tutor and challenge their students

- **Three-month Code It Fast CD**—*Code it Fast* look-up CD includes the latest ICD-9-CM, HCPCS, and CPT® codes

- **Complex Coding Scenarios**—Complex coding scenarios help assure fast and accurate physician reimbursement through example

NEW! Ingenix Coding Lab: Medical Billing Basics

Complete Foundation for Coding and Billing—Broad overview of coding, payers, and the reimbursement process for the entry-level coder or billing professional

ISBN: 1-56329-921-6   Item No. 5772 **$74.95**

Available: December 2002

NEW! Ingenix Coding Lab: Physician Offices

Complete Foundation for Physician Coding and Billing—Broad overview of physician reimbursement process for the coder or billing professional

ISBN: 1-56329-908-9   Item No. 3268 **$74.95**

Available: December 2002

NEW! Ingenix Coding Lab: Facilities and Ancillary Services

Complete Foundation for Facility Coding and Billing—Broad overview of facility reimbursement process for the coder or billing professional

ISBN: 1-56329-920-8   Item No. 3227 **$99.95**

Available: December 2002

CPT is a registered trademark of the American Medical Association

Call Toll-Free 1.877.INGENIX (464.3649) or Shop Online at www.IngenixOnLine.com

Also Available from your Medical Bookstore or Distributor   060102

4 Easy Ways to Order

CALL toll-free
1.800.INGENIX
(464.3649)
and mention the
Source Code: FOBA3

SHOP on line at
www.IngenixOnline.com

MAIL this form with
payment and/or purchase
order to:
PO Box 27116
Salt Lake City, UT 84127-0116

FAX this order form with
credit card information and /or
purchase order to 801.982.4033

100% Money Back Guarantee

If our merchandise* ever fails
to meet your expectations,
please contact our Customer
Service Department toll-free at
1.800.INGENIX (464.3649)
for an immediate response.
We will resolve any
concern without hesitation.

*Software: Credit will be
granted for unopened
packages only.

| Shipping and Handling ||
No. of Items	Fee
1	$9.95
2-4	$11.95
5-7	$14.95
8-10	$19.95
11+	Call

PUBLICATION ORDER AND FAX FORM

FOBA3

Customer No._____   Contact No._____

Purchase Order No._____   Source Code_____
(Attach copy of Purchase Order)

Contact Name _____   Title_____

Company_____

Address _____
(no P.O. Boxes, please)

City_____ State_____ Zip_____

Phone (_____)_____ Fax (_____)_____
(in case we have questions about your order)

IMPORTANT: E-MAIL REQUIRED FOR ORDER CONFIRMATION AND SELECT PRODUCT DELIVERY.

E-mail _____

❑ YES, I WANT TO RECEIVE SPECIAL REPORTS AND INFORMATION VIA E-MAIL.
❑ YES, I WANT TO RECEIVE NEW PRODUCT ANNOUNCEMENTS VIA E-MAIL.

Item #	Qty	Item Description	Price	Total
~~4025~~	~~1~~	~~(SAMPLE) DRG Guidebook~~	~~$89.95~~	~~$89.95~~
			Sub Total	
	TX, UT, OH, and VA residents please add applicable sales tax			
	Shipping & handling (see chart)			
	(11 plus items, foreign and Canadian orders, please call for shipping costs)			
	Total enclosed			

Payment Options

❑ Check enclosed. (Make payable to Ingenix, Inc.)

❑ Charge my: ❑ MasterCard ❑ VISA ❑ AMEX ❑ Discover

Card # | | | | | | | | | | | | | | | | | | | Exp. Date: | | | |
                                                                    MM   YR

❑ Bill Me P.O.#_____

Signature _____

Preface

ICD-9-CM for Physicians has been designed with the physician office coder in mind. The most recent official government versions of volumes 1 and 2 have been combined to provide physicians and their office staff with an ICD-9-CM book that is easy to use.

In addition, our technical experts have drawn upon their extensive hands-on experience to enhance the government's official version with valuable features essential to correct coding and reimbursement. With these enhancements, physician office coders will increase the efficiency and timeliness of claim submission for both Medicare and other third-party payers.

As you review the content, you'll find the following:

- All the official ICD-9-CM codes, indexes, notes, footnotes and symbols
- Complete official coding guidelines
- Our exclusive color coding, symbols, and footnotes that alert coders to coding and reimbursement issues. Medicare outpatient code edits, such as invalid fourth or fifth digit for diagnosis codes and circumstances under which Medicare may be secondary payer (MSP), are identified.
- Illustrations and clinically oriented definitions to aid in correct code assignment
- Symbols identifying new codes and text revisions; pages are dated to indicate when the changes were made
- Exclusive QuickFlip Color Tabs for quick, easy location of terms and codes in the index and tabular list

USE OF OFFICIAL SOURCES

This *ICD-9-CM for Physicians* contains the official U.S. Department of Health and Human Services, ICD-9-CM codes, effective for the current year.

The color coding, footnotes and symbols, which identify coding and reimbursement issues, are derived from official federal government sources, including the Medicare Outpatient Code Editor as well as the knowledge of our technical experts.

In addition to the editors, the following people have contributed to this book:

Kerrie Hornsby, Desktop Publishing Manger
Stacy Perry, Desktop Publishing Manager
Paul Driscoll, Illustrator
Sheri Bernard, Director of Essential Regulatory Products
Lynn Speirs, Managing Editor

IMPORTANT INFORMATION ABOUT YOUR SUBSCRIPTION SERVICE

If you have purchased the updateable *ICD-9-CM for Physicians*, your subscription includes an updating service throughout the year to keep the code book current and accurate. Whenever CMS issues changes or corrections to the ICD-9-CM codes, We will issue an update to the book. In July you will receive a list of all new, revised, and invalid codes for the upcoming year.

TECHNICAL EDITORS

Anita C. Hart, RHIA, CCS, CCS-P
Product Manager, Ingenix, Inc, Reston, VA

Ms. Hart's experience includes fifteen years conducting and publishing research in clinical medicine and human genetics for Yale University, Massachusetts General Hospital, and Massachusetts Institute of Technology. In addition, Ms. Hart has supervised medical records management, health information management, coding and reimbursement, and worker's compensation issues as the office manager for a physical therapy rehabilitation clinic. Ms. Hart is an expert in physician and facility coding, reimbursement systems, and compliance issues. Ms. Hart developed the *Complete Coding Tutor*, an advanced self-study guide for ICD-9-CM, CPT, and HCPCS Level II coding and served as technical consultant for numerous other publications for hospital and physician practices. Currrently, Ms. Hart is the Product Manager for the ICD-9-CM and DRG product lines.

Catherine A. Hopkins, CPC
Technical Consultant, Ingenix, Inc., Reston, VA

Ms. Hopkins has 17 years of experience in the healthcare field. Her experience includes six years as office manager and senior coding specialist for a large multi-specialty practice. Ms. Hopkins has written several coding manuals and newsletters and has taught seminars on CPT, HCPCS, and ICD-9-CM coding. She also serves as technical support for various software products.

WHAT TO DO IF YOU HAVE QUESTIONS

If you have any questions about your subscription, call our customer service department toll free at (800) INGENIX (464.3649).

If you have comments on the content of the code book, please address them in writing to:

Product Manager, Ingenix, Inc.
11410 Isaac Newton Square, Reston, VA 20190
Tel no.: (800) INGENIX (464.3649)
Fax no.: (801) 982-4033

ADDITIONAL COPIES

Contact the customer service order department toll free at (800) INGENIX (464-3649).

Introduction

HISTORY AND FUTURE OF ICD•9

The International Classification of Diseases, Ninth Revision, Clinical Modification (ICD-9-CM) is based on the official version of the World Health Organization's Ninth Revision, International Classification of Diseases (ICD-9). ICD-9-CM classifies morbidity and mortality information for statistical purposes, indexing of hospital records by disease and operations, data storage, and retrieval.

This modification of ICD-9 supplants the Eighth Revision International Classification of Diseases, Adapted for Use in the United States (ICDA-8) and the Hospital Adaptation of ICDA (H-ICDA).

The concept of extending the International Classification of Diseases for use in hospital indexing was originally developed in response to a need for a more efficient basis for storage and retrieval of diagnostic data. In 1950, the U.S. Public Health Service and the Veterans Administration began independent tests of the International Classification of Diseases for hospital indexing purposes. The following year, the Columbia Presbyterian Medical Center in New York City adopted the International Classification of Diseases, Sixth Revision, with some modifications for use in its medical record department. A few years later, the Commission on Professional and Hospital Activities (CPHA) in Ann Arbor, Mich., adopted the International Classification of Diseases with similar modifications for use in hospitals participating in the Professional Activity Study.

The problem of adapting ICD for indexing hospital records was addressed by the U.S. National Committee on Vital and Health Statistics through its subcommittee on hospital statistics. The subcommittee reviewed the modifications made by the various users of ICD and proposed that uniform changes be made. This was done by a small working party.

In view of the growing interest in the use of the International Classification of Diseases for hospital indexing, a study was undertaken in 1956 by the American Hospital Association and the American Medical Record Association (then the American Association of Medical Record Librarians) of the relative efficiencies of coding systems for diagnostic indexing. This study indicated the International Classification of Diseases provided a suitable and efficient framework for indexing hospital records. The major users of the International Classification of Diseases for hospital indexing purposes then consolidated their experiences, and an adaptation was first published in December 1959. A revision was issued in 1962 and the first "Classification of Operations and Treatments" was included.

In 1966, the international conference for revising the International Classification of Diseases noted the eighth revision of ICD had been constructed with hospital indexing in mind and considered the revised classification suitable, in itself, for hospital use in some countries. However, it was recognized that the basic classification might provide inadequate detail for diagnostic indexing in other countries. A group of consultants was asked to study the eighth revision of ICD (ICD-8) for applicability to various users in the United States. This group recommended that further detail be provided for coding of hospital and morbidity data. The American Hospital Association was requested to develop the needed adaptation proposals. This was done by an advisory committee (the Advisory Committee to the Central Office on ICDA). In 1968 the United States Public Health Service published the product, Eighth Revision International Classification of Diseases, Adapted for Use in the United States. This became commonly known as ICDA-8, and beginning in 1968 it served as the basis for coding diagnostic data for both official morbidity and mortality statistics in the United States.

In 1968, the CPHA published the Hospital Adaptation of ICDA (H-ICDA) based on both the original ICD-8 and ICDA-8. In 1973, CPHA published a revision of H-ICDA, referred to as H-ICDA-2. Hospitals throughout the United States were divided in their use of these classifications until January 1979, when ICD-9-CM was made the single classification intended primarily for use in the United States, replacing these earlier related, but somewhat dissimilar, classifications.

Physicians have been required by law to submit diagnosis codes for Medicare reimbursement since the passage of the Medicare Catastrophic Coverage Act of 1988. This act requires physician offices to include the appropriate diagnosis codes when billing for services provided to Medicare beneficiaries on or after April 1, 1989. The Centers for Medicare and Medicaid Services (CMS) designated ICD-9-CM as the coding system physicians must use.

In 1993 the World Health Organization published the newest version of International Classification of Diseases, Tenth Revision, ICD-10. This version contains the greatest number of changes in the history of ICD. There are more codes (5,500 more than ICD-9) to allow more specific reporting of diseases and newly recognized conditions. ICD-10 consists of three volumes; tabular list (volume I), instructions (volume 2) and the alphabetic index (volume 3). It contains 21 chapters including two supplementary ones. The codes are alphanumeric (A00–T98, V01–Y98 and Z00–Z99). Currently ICD-10 is being used in some European countries with implementation expected after the year 2000 in the United States.

ICD-9-CM BACKGROUND

In February 1977, a steering committee was convened by the National Center for Health Statistics to provide advice and counsel in developing a clinical modification of ICD-9. The organizations represented on the steering committee included the following:

• American Association of Health Data Systems

- American Hospital Association
- American Medical Record Association
- Association for Health Records
- Council on Clinical Classifications
- Centers for Medicare and Medicaid Services (formerly known as Health Care Financing Administration), Department of Health and Human Services
- WHO Center for Classification of Diseases for North America, sponsored by the National Center for Health Statistics, Department of Health and Human Services

The Council on Clinical Classifications was sponsored by the following:

- American Academy of Pediatrics
- American College of Obstetricians and Gynecologists
- American College of Physicians
- American College of Surgeons
- American Psychiatric Association
- Commission on Professional and Hospital Activities

The steering committee met periodically in 1977. Clinical guidance and technical input were provided by task forces on classification from the Council on Clinical Classification's sponsoring organizations.

ICD-9-CM is a clinical modification of the World Health Organization's ICD-9. The term "clinical" is used to emphasize the modification's intent: to serve as a useful tool to classify morbidity data for indexing medical records, medical care review, and ambulatory and other medical care programs, as well as for basic health statistics. To describe the clinical picture of the patient, the codes must be more precise than those needed only for statistical groupings and trend analysis.

CHARACTERISTICS OF ICD-9-CM
ICD-9-CM far exceeds its predecessors in the number of codes provided. The disease classification has been expanded to include health-related conditions and to provide greater specificity at the fifth-digit level of detail. These fifth digits are not optional; they are intended for use in recording the information substantiated in the clinical record.

Volume I (tabular list) of ICD-9-CM contains five appendices:

Appendix A:	Morphology of Neoplasms
Appendix B:	Glossary of Mental Disorders
Appendix C:	Classification of Drugs by American Hospital Formulary Service List Number and Their ICD-9-CM Equivalents
Appendix D:	Classification of Industrial Accidents According to Agency
Appendix E:	List of Three-Digit Categories

These appendices are included as a reference to provide further information about the patient's clinical picture, to further define a diagnostic statement, to aid in classifying new drugs or to reference three-digit categories.

Volume 2 (alphabetic index) of ICD-9-CM contains many diagnostic terms that do not appear in volume I since the index includes most diagnostic terms currently in use.

THE DISEASE CLASSIFICATION
ICD-9-CM is totally compatible with its parent system, ICD-9, thus meeting the need for comparability of morbidity and mortality statistics at the international level. A few fourth-digit codes were created in existing three-digit rubrics only when the necessary detail could not be accommodated by the use of a fifth-digit subclassification. To ensure that each rubric of ICD-9-CM collapses back to its ICD-9 counterpart the following specifications governed the ICD-9-CM disease classification:

Specifications for the tabular list:

1. Three-digit rubrics and their contents are unchanged from ICD-9.
2. The sequence of three-digit rubrics is unchanged from ICD-9.
3. Three-digit rubrics are not added to the main body of the classification.
4. Unsubdivided three-digit rubrics are subdivided where necessary to
   - add clinical detail
   - isolate terms for clinical accuracy
5. The modification in ICD-9-CM is accomplished by adding a fifth digit to existing ICD-9 rubrics, except as noted under #7 below.
6. The optional dual classification in ICD-9 is modified.
   - Duplicate rubrics are deleted:
     - four-digit manifestation categories duplicating etiology entries
     - manifestation inclusion terms duplicating etiology entries
   - Manifestations of disease are identified, to the extent possible, by creating five-digit codes in the etiology rubrics.
   - When the manifestation of a disease cannot be included in the etiology rubrics, provision for its identification is made by retaining the ICD-9 rubrics used for classifying manifestations of disease.
7. The format of ICD-9-CM is revised from that used in ICD-9.
   - American spelling of medical terms is used.
   - Inclusion terms are indented beneath the titles of codes.
   - Codes not to be used for primary tabulation of disease are printed in italics with the notation, "code first underlying disease."

Specifications for the alphabetic index:

1. The format of the alphabetic index follows that of ICD-9.
2. When two codes are required to indicate etiology and manifestation, the manifestation code appears in brackets (e.g., diabetic cataract 250.5 [366.41]).

How to Use the ICD•9•CM for Physicians (Volumes 1 & 2)

This *ICD-9-CM for Physicians* is based on the official version of the International Classification of Diseases, Ninth Revision, Clinical Modification, Sixth Edition, issued by the U.S. Department of Health and Human Services. Annual code changes are implemented by the government and are effective Oct. 1 and valid through Sept. 30 of the following year.

To accommodate the coder's approach to coding, the alphabetic index (Volume 2) has been placed before the tabular list (Volume 1). This allows the user to locate the term in the index, then confirm the accuracy of the code in the tabular list.

10 STEPS TO CORRECT CODING

To code accurately, it is necessary to have a working knowledge of medical terminology and to understand the characteristics, terminology and conventions of ICD-9-CM. Transforming descriptions of diseases, injuries, conditions and procedures into numerical designations (coding) is a complex activity and should not be undertaken without proper training.

Originally, coding allowed retrieval of medical information by diagnoses and operations for medical research, education and administration. Coding today is used to describe the medical necessity of a procedure which then facilitates payment of health services, to evaluate utilization patterns and to study the appropriateness of health care costs. Coding provides the basis for epidemiological studies and research into the quality of health care. Incorrect or inaccurate coding can lead to investigations of fraud and abuse. Therefore, coding must be performed correctly and consistently to produce meaningful statistics to aid in planning for the health needs of the nation.

Follow the steps below to code correctly:

Step 1: Identify the reason for the visit (e.g., sign, symptom, diagnosis, condition to be coded).

Physicians describe the patient's condition using terminology that includes specific diagnoses as well as symptoms, problems or reasons for the encounter. If symptoms are present but a definitive diagnosis has not yet been determined, code the symptoms. Do not code conditions that are referred to as "rule out," "suspected," "probable" or "questionable."

Step 2: Always consult the Alphabetic Index, Volume 2, before turning to the tabular list.

The most critical rule is to begin a code search in the index. Never turn first to the Tabular List (Volume 1), as this will lead to coding errors and less specificity in code assignments. To prevent coding errors, use both the Alphabetic Index and the tabular list when locating and assigning a code.

Step 3: Locate the main entry term.

The Alphabetic Index is arranged by condition. Conditions may be expressed as nouns, adjectives and eponyms. Some conditions have multiple entries under their synonyms. Main terms are identified using boldface type.

Step 4: Read and interpret any notes listed with the main term

Notes are identified using italicized type.

Step 5: Review entries for modifiers

Nonessential modifiers are in parentheses. These parenthetical terms are supplementary words or explanatory information that may either be present or absent in the diagnostic statement and do not affect code assignment.

Step 6: Interpret abbreviations, cross-references, symbols and brackets

Cross-references used are "*see*," "*see* category" or "*see* also." The abbreviation NEC may follow main terms or subterms. NEC (not elsewhere classified) indicates that there is no specific code for the condition even though the medical documentation may be very specific. The ✓5ᵗʰ box indicates the code requires a fifth digit. If the appropriate fifth digits are not found in the index, in a box beneath the main term, you MUST refer to the tabular list. Italicized brackets [ ], are used to enclose a second code number that must be used with the code immediately preceding it and in that sequence.

Step 7: Choose a tentative code and locate it in the tabular list.

Be guided by any inclusion or exclusion terms, notes or other instructions, such as "*code first*" and "use additional code," that would direct the use of a different or additional code from that selected in the index for a particular diagnosis, condition or disease.

Step 8: Determine whether the code is at the highest level of specificity.

Assign three-digit codes (category codes) if there are no four-digit codes within the code category. Assign four-digit codes (subcategory codes) if there are no five-digit codes for that category. Assign five-digit codes (fifth-digit subclassification codes) for those categories where they are available.

Step 9: **Consult the color coding and reimbursement prompts, including the age, sex and Medicare as secondary payer edits. Refer to the key at the bottom of the page for definitions of colors and symbols.**

Step 10: Assign the code.

ORGANIZATION

Introduction
The introductory material in this book includes the history and future of ICD-9-CM as well as an overview of the classification system

Official ICD-9-CM Conventions
This section provides a full explanation of all the official footnotes, symbols, instructional notes, and conventions found in the official government version

Additional Conventions
Exclusive color-coding, symbols, and notations have been included in the *ICD-9-CM for Physicians*, *Volumes 1 and 2*, to alert coders to important coding and reimbursement issues. This section provides a full explanation of the additional conventions used throughout this book.

Synopsis of Code Changes
This section includes a complete listing of all code changes for the current year.

Coding Guidelines
Included in this book are the official ICD-9-CM coding guidelines as approved by the four cooperating parties of the ICD-9-CM Coordination and Maintenance Committee. Failure to comply with these official coding guidelines may result in denied or delayed claims.

Disease Classification: Alphabetic Index to Diseases
The Alphabetic Index to Diseases is separated by tabs labeled with the letters of the alphabet, contains diagnostic terms for illnesses, injuries and reasons for encounters with health care professionals. Both the Table of Drugs and Chemicals and the Alphabetic Index to External Causes of Injury and Poisoning are easily located with the tabs in this section.

Disease Classification: Tabular List of Diseases
The Tabular List of Diseases arranges the ICD-9-CM codes and descriptors numerically. Tabs divide this section into chapters, identified by the code range on the tab.

The tabular list includes two supplementary classifications:

- V Codes—Supplementary Classification of Factors Influencing Health Status and Contact with Health Services (V01–V83)
- E Codes—Supplementary Classification of External Causes of Injury and Poisoning (E800–E999)

ICD-9-CM includes five official appendixes.

- Appendix A   Morphology of Neoplasms
- Appendix B   Glossary of Mental Disorders
- Appendix C   Classification of Drugs by AHFS List
- Appendix D   Classification of Industrial Accidents According to Agency
- Appendix E   List of Three-digit Categories

Resources
Listed below are the exclusive resources found ONLY in the *ICD-9-CM Expert for Physicians, Volumes 1 & 2.*

Code Tables
Exclusive coding tables covering abortion, burns, complications, diabetes, hernia, pregnancy, and others are provided to simplify those complex coding issues.

Valid Three-digit Code Table
ICD-9-CM is composed of codes with either 3, 4, or 5 digits. A code is invalid if it has not been coded to the full number of digits required for that code. There are a certain number codes that are valid for reporting as three digit codes. A list of these valid three-digit code is included as a convenient reference when auditing claims.

ICD-9-CM Official Conventions

ICD-9-CM FOOTNOTES, SYMBOLS, INSTRUCTIONAL NOTES AND CONVENTIONS

This *ICD-9-CM for Physicians* preserves all the footnotes, symbols, instructional notes and conventions found in the government's official version. Accurate coding depends upon understanding the meaning of these elements.

The following appear in the disease tabular list, unless otherwise noted.

OFFICIAL GOVERNMENT SYMBOLS

§ The section mark preceding a code denotes a footnote on the page. This symbol is used only in the Tabular List of Diseases.

ICD-9-CM CONVENTIONS USED IN THE TABULAR LIST

In addition to the symbols and footnotes above, the ICD-9-CM disease tabular has certain abbreviations, punctuation, symbols and other conventions. Our *ICD-9-CM for Physicians* preserves these conventions. Proper use of the conventions will lead to efficient and accurate coding.

Abbreviations

NEC Not elsewhere classifiable

This abbreviation is used when the ICD-9-CM system does not provide a code specific for the patient's condition.

NOS Not otherwise specified

This abbreviation is the equivalent of 'unspecified' and is used only when the coder lacks the information necessary to code to a more specific four-digit subcategory.

[ ] Brackets enclose synonyms, alternative terminology or explanatory phrases:

482.2 Pneumonia due to Hemophilus influenzae [H. influenzae]

Brackets that appear beneath a code indicate the fifth digits that are considered valid fifth digits for the code. This convention is applied for those instances in ICD-9-CM where not all common fifth digits are considered valid for each subcategory within a category.

715.0 Osteoarthrosis, generalized
[0,4,9]

Generalized arthrosis can only be assigned in cases for which the degenerative joint disease involves multiple joints. Therefore, this code is considered for arthrosis in the sites described as unspecified, hand (which consists of multiple joints), or multiple sites. Therefore, only fifth digits 0, 4, and 9 are valid with subcategory 715.0.

( ) Parentheses enclose supplementary words, called nonessential modifiers, that may be present in the narrative description of a disease without affecting the code assignment:

198.4 Other parts of nervous system
    Meninges (cerebral) (spinal)

: Colons are used in the tabular list after an incomplete term that needs one or more of the modifiers that follow in order to make it assignable to a given category:

021.1 Enteric tularemia
    Tularemia:
        cryptogenic
        intestinal
        typhoidal

} Braces enclose a series of terms, each of which is modified by the statement appearing to the right of the brace:

560.2 Volvulus

Knotting
Strangulation } of intestine, bowel, or
Torsion } colon
Twist

OTHER CONVENTIONS

Boldface Boldface type is used for all codes and titles in the tabular list.

Italicized Italicized type is used for all exclusion notes and to identify codes that should not be used for describing the primary diagnosis.

INSTRUCTIONAL NOTES

These notes appear only in the Tabular List of Diseases

Includes An includes note further defines or clarifies the content of the chapter, subchapter, category, subcategory or subclassification. The includes note in the example below applies only to category 461.

Excludes Terms following the word "*Excludes*" are not classified to the chapter, subchapter, category, subcategory or specific subclassification code under which it is found. The note also may provide the location of the excluded diagnosis. Excludes notes are italicized.

2003 Ingenix, Inc.

461   Acute sinusitis

    INCLUDES   abscess
                empyema
                infection   acute, of sinus
                inflammation   (accessory)
                suppuration   (nasal)

    EXCLUDES   *chronic or unspecified sinusitis
                (473.0-473.9)*

Use additional code:

This instruction signals the coder that an additional code should be used if the information is available to provide a more complete picture of that diagnosis.

330   Cerebral degenerations usually manifest in childhood

    Use additional code to identify
    associated mental retardation

Code first underlying disease:

This instruction is used in those categories not intended for primary tabulation of disease. These codes, called manifestation codes, may never be used alone or indicated as the primary diagnosis (i.e., sequenced first). They must always be preceded by another code.

The code and its descriptor appear in italics in the tabular list. The instruction "*Code first underlying disease*" is usually followed by the code or codes for the most common underlying disease (etiology). Record the code for the etiology or origin of the disease, and then record the italicized manifestation code in the next position.

590.81   Pyelitis or pyelonephritis in diseases classified elsewhere

    Code first underlying disease as:
    tuberculosis (016.0)

Code, if applicable, any causal condition first:

A code with this note may be principal if no causal condition is applicable or known.

590.0   Chronic pyelonephritis

    Chronic pyelitis
    Chronic pyonephrosis
    Code, if applicable, any causal condition
    first

Omit code

"*Omit code*" is used to instruct the coder that no code is to be assigned. When this instruction is found in the Alphabetic Index to Diseases the medical term should not be coded as a diagnosis.

Metaplasia
    cervix—*omit code*

Additional Conventions

SYMBOLS AND NOTATIONS

New and Revised Text Symbols

● A bullet at a code or line of text indicates that that the entry is new.

▲ A triangle in the Tabular List indicates that the code title is revised. In the Alphabetic Index the triangle indicates that a code has changed.

►◄ These symbols appear at the beginning and at the end of a section of new or revised text.

When these symbols appear on a page there will be a date on the lower outside corner of the page indicating the date of the change, (e.g., October 2001).

Additional Digits Required

✓4ᵗʰ This symbol indicates that the code requires a fourth digit.

✓5ᵗʰ This symbol indicates that a code requires a fifth digit.

Age and Sex Edit Symbols

The age edits below address OCE edits and are used to detect inconsistencies between the patient's age and diagnosis. They appear in the Tabular List of Diseases to the right of the code description.

Newborn Age: 0

These diagnoses are intended for newborns and neonates and the patient's age must be 0 years

Pediatric Age: 0-17

These diagnoses are intended for children and the patient's age must between 0 and 17 years

Maternity Age: 12-55

These diagnoses are intended for the patients between the age of 12 and 55 years

Adult Age 15-124

These diagnoses are intended for the patients between the age of 15 and 124 years.

The sex symbols below address OCE edits and are used to detect inconsistencies between the patient's sex and diagnosis. They appear in the Tabular List of Diseases to the right of the code description:

♂ **Male diagnosis only**

This symbol appears to the right of the code description. This reference appears in the disease tabular list.

♀ **Female diagnosis only**

This symbol appears to the right of the code description. This reference appears in the disease tabular list.

COLOR CODING

To alert the coder to Medicare outpatient code edits and other important reimbursement issues, color bars have been added over the code descriptors in the tabular list. Some codes carry more than one color.

Carriers use the Medicare Outpatient Code Editor (OCE) to examine claims for coding and billing accuracy and completeness. Color codes in this book signify Medicare code edits for E codes and manifestation codes as a primary diagnosis, Medicare secondary payer alerts and when a more specific diagnosis or code should be used.

Manifestation Code

These codes will appear in italic type as well as with a blue color bar over the code title. A manifestation code is not allowed to be reported as a primary diagnosis because each describes a manifestation of some other underlying disease, not the disease itself. This is also referred to as mandatory multiple coding. Code the underlying disease first. A Code first underlying disease instructional note will appear with underlying disease codes identified. In the Alphabetic Index these codes are listed as the secondary code in slanted bracket with the code for the underlying disease listed first.

Other Specified Code

These codes will appear with a gray color bar over the code title. Use these codes when the documentation indicates a specified diagnosis, but the ICD-9-CM system does not have a specific code that describes the diagnosis. These codes are may be stated as "Other" or "Not elsewhere classified (NEC)."

Unspecified Code

These codes will have a yellow color bar over the code title. Use these codes when the neither the diagnostic statement nor the documentation provides enough information to assign a more specified diagnosis code. These codes may be stated as "Unspecified" or "Not otherwise specified (NOS)." Note: Do not assign these codes when a more specific diagnosis has been determined.

OTHER NOTATIONS

DEF: This symbol indicates a definition of disease or procedure term. The definition will appear in blue type in the Disease Tabular Lists.

MSP This identifies specific trauma codes that alert the carrier that another carrier should be billed first and Medicare billed second if payment from the first payer does not equal or exceed the amount Medicare would pay.

PDx This symbol identifies a V code that can only be used as a primary diagnosis

SDx This symbol identifies a V code that can only be used as a secondary diagnosis

Note: A V code without a symbol may be used as either a primary or secondary diagnosis

2001 Ingenix, Inc.

Summary of Code Changes

DISEASE TABULAR LIST (VOLUME 1)

038   Excludes term added
- 040.82   Toxic shock syndrome
  Use additional code note added

062.8   Excludes note added

066.3   Includes term deleted
- 066.4   West Nile fever
  Includes notes added

256.2   Use additional code note added
  Excludes term deleted

256.3   Use additional code note revised

277.00   Includes note added
- 277.02   Cystic fibrosis with pulmonary manifestations
  Includes note added
  Use additional code note added
- 277.03   Cystic fibrosis with gastrointestinal manifestations
  Excludes note added
- 277.09   Cystic fibrosis with other manifestations

277.7   Use additional code note revised

337.3   Use additional code note revised

357.8   Includes note deleted
- 357.81   Chronic inflammatory demyelinating polyneuritis
- 357.82   Critical illness polyneuropathy
  Includes note added
- 357.89   Other inflammatory and toxic neuropathy
- 359.81   Critical illness myopathy
  Includes note added
- 359.89   Other myopathies
- 365.83   Aqueous misdirection
  Includes note added

368.6   Includes term deleted

402   Use additional code note added
▲ 402.00   Hypertensive heart disease, malignant, without congestive heart failure
▲ 402.01   Hypertensive heart disease, malignant, with ~~congestive~~ heart failure
▲ 402.10   Hypertensive heart disease, benign, without ~~congestive~~ heart failure
▲ 402.11   Hypertensive heart disease, benign, with ~~congestive~~ heart failure
▲ 402.90   Hypertensive heart disease, unspecified, without ~~congestive~~ heart failure
▲ 402.91   Hypertensive heart disease, unspecified, with ~~congestive~~ heart failure

404   Use additional code note added
  Fifth-digit code definitions revised

0   without mention of ~~congestive~~ heart failure or renal failure
1   with ~~congestive~~ heart failure
2   with ~~congestive~~ heart failure and renal failure

▲ 404.00   Hypertensive heart and renal disease, malignant, without mention of ~~congestive~~ heart failure or renal failure
▲ 404.01   Hypertensive heart and renal disease, malignant, with ~~congestive~~ heart failure
▲ 404.03   Hypertensive heart and renal disease, malignant, with ~~congestive~~ heart failure and renal failure
▲ 404.10   Hypertensive heart and renal disease, benign, without mention of ~~congestive~~ heart failure or renal failure
▲ 404.11   Hypertensive heart and renal disease, benign, with ~~congestive~~ heart failure
▲ 404.13   Hypertensive heart and renal disease, benign, with ~~congestive~~ heart failure and renal failure
▲ 404.90   Hypertensive heart and renal disease, unspecified, without mention of ~~congestive~~ heart failure or renal failure
▲ 404.91   Hypertensive heart and renal disease, unspecified, with ~~congestive~~ heart failure
▲ 404.93   Hypertensive heart and renal disease, unspecified, with ~~congestive~~ heart failure and renal failure

411.81   Excludes terms revised
- 414.06   Coronary atherosclerosis of coronary artery of transplanted heart
▲ 414.1   Aneurysm ▶and dissection◀ of heart
▲ 414.10   ▶Aneurysm◀ of heart (wall)
▲ 414.11   ▶Aneurysm◀ of coronary vessels
- 414.12   Dissection of coronary artery
▲ 414.19   Other ▶aneurysm of heart◀

427.89   Excludes terms added

428   Excludes term deleted
  Code, if applicable, note added
▲ 428.0   Congestive heart failure, ▶unspecified◀
  Excludes note added
- 428.2   Systolic heart failure
  Excludes note added
- 428.20   Systolic heart failure, unspecified
- 428.21   Systolic heart failure, acute
- 428.22   Systolic heart failure, chronic
- 428.23   Systolic heart failure, acute on chronic

- 428.3   Diastolic heart failure
  Excludes note added
- 428.30   Diastolic heart failure, unspecified
- 428.31   Diastolic heart failure, acute
- 428.32   Diastolic heart failure, chronic
- 428.33   Diastolic heart failure, acute on chronic
- 428.4   Combined systolic and diastolic heart failure
- 428.40   Combined systolic and diastolic heart failure, unspecified
- 428.41   Combined systolic and diastolic heart failure, acute
- 428.42   Combined systolic and diastolic heart failure, chronic
- 428.43   Combined systolic and diastolic heart failure, acute on chronic

(430-438)   Cerebrovascular Disease section
  Excludes term added

436   Excludes term added
- 438.6   Late effects of cerebrovascular disease, alterations of sensations
  Use additional code note added
- 438.7   Late effects of cerebrovascular disease, disturbances of vision
  Use additional code note added
- 438.83   Other late effects of cerebrovascular disease, facial weakness
  Includes term added
- 438.84   Other late effects of cerebrovascular disease, ataxia
- 438.85   Other late effects of cerebrovascular disease, vertigo

440   Excludes term added
440.8   Excludes term revised
441.0   Includes note deleted
- 443.2   Other arterial dissection
  Excludes note added
- 443.21   Dissection of carotid artery
- 443.22   Dissection of iliac artery
- 443.23   Dissection of renal artery
- 443.24   Dissection of vertebral artery
- 443.29   Dissection of other artery

444   Excludes term added
- 445   Atheroembolism
  Includes note added
- 445.0   Atheroembolism, of extermities
- 445.01   Atheroembolism, upper extermity
- 445.02   Atheroembolism, lower extremity
- 445.8   Atheroembolism, of other sites
- 445.81   Atheroembolism, kidney
  Use additional code note added
- 445.89   Atheroembolism, other site

447.6   Excludes term revised
- 454.8   Varicose veins of the lower extremities, with other

---

▶◀ Revised Text   ● New Code   ▲ Revised Code Title

	complications	
	Includes note added	
▲ 454.9	Varicose veins of lower extremities, ~~without mention of ulcer or inflammation~~ ▶asmyptomatic varicose veins◀ Includes term added	
459.1	Includes note added Excludes note added	
● 459.10	Postphlebetic syndrome without complications Includes note added	
● 459.11	Postphlebetic syndrome with ulcer	
● 459.12	Postphlebetic syndrome with inflammation	
● 459.13	Postphlebetic syndrome with ulcer and inflammation	
● 459.19	Postphlebetic syndrome with other complication	
● 459.3	Chronic venous hypertension (idiopathic) Includes note added Excludes note added	
● 459.30	Chronic venous hypertension without complications Includes note added	
● 459.31	Chronic venous hypertension with ulcer	
● 459.32	Chronic venous hypertension with inflammation	
● 459.33	Chronic venous hypertension with ulcer and inflammation	
● 459.39	Chronic venous hypertension with other complication	
491.2	Includes term deleted	
491.20	Includes term deleted	
491.21	Includes term deleted	
493.2	Includes term added Excludes term deleted	
518.81	Excludes term revised	
518.82	Excludes term revised	
● 537.84	Dieulafoy lesion (hemorrhagic) of stomach and duodenum	
● 569.86	Dieulafoy lesion (hemorrhagic) of intestine	
577.8	Excludes term revised	
590.0	Code first note deleted Code, if applicable, note added	
593.7	Use additional code note deleted	
599.0	Excludes term added	
602.3	Includes terms revised Excludes terms revised	
622.1	Includes terms added	
▲ 627.2	▶Symptomatic◀ menopausal or female climacteric states	
▲ 627.4	▶Symptomatic◀ states associated with artificial menopause	
629.0	Excludes term revised	
● 633.00	Abdominal pregnancy without intrauterine pregnancy	
● 633.01	Abdominal pregnancy with intrauterine pregnancy	
● 633.10	Tubal pregnancy without intrauterine pregnancy	
● 633.11	Tubal pregnancy with intrauterine pregnancy	

● 633.20	Ovarian pregnancy without intrauterine pregnancy	
● 633.21	Ovarian pregnancy with intrauterine pregnancy	
● 633.80	Other ectopic pregnancy without intrauterine pregnancy	
● 633.81	Other ectopic pregnancy with intrauterine pregnancy	
● 633.90	Unspecified ectopic pregnancy without intrauterine pregnancy	
● 633.91	Unspecified ectopic pregnancy with intrauterine pregnancy	
646.6	Includes term revised	
647.1	Excludes note added	
707.1	Code first note revised Code, if applicable, terms added	
710	Use additional code note deleted	
710.1	Use additional code note added	
718.7	Excludes terms deleted Excludes terms added	
723.5	Excludes term added	
730.1	Includes term deleted	
733.4	Excludes term deleted	
● 747.83	Persistent fetal circulation Includes note added	
751.7	Excludes term revised	
753.0	Code first note deleted	
753.15	Code first note deleted	
(764-779)	Other conditions originating in the perinatal period section Fifth-digit subclassification instructions revised	
▲ 765	Disorders relating to short gestation and low birthweight	
765.0	Instructional note revised Use additional code note added	
765.1	Instrucitonal note revised Use additional code note added	
● 765.2	Disorders relating to short gestation and low birthweight, weeks of gestation	
● 765.20	Unspecified weeks of gestation	
● 765.21	Less than 24 completed weeks of gestation	
● 765.22	24 completed weeks of gestation	
● 765.23	25-26 completed weeks of gestation	
● 765.24	27-28 completed weeks of gestation	
● 765.25	29-30 completed weeks of gestation	
● 765.26	31-32 completed weeks of gestation	
● 765.27	33-34 completed weeks of gestation	
● 765.28	35-36 completed weeks of gestation	
● 765.29	37 or more completed weeks of gestation	
770.8	Includes note deleted	
● 770.81	Primary apnea of newborn Includes note added	
● 770.82	Other apnea of newborn Includes note added	
● 770.83	Cyanotic attacks of newborn	
● 770.84	Respiratory failure of newborn Excludes note added	

● 770.89	Other respiratory problems after birth	
771.8	Includes note deleted Use additional code note added	
● 771.81	Septicemia [sepsis] of newborn	
● 771.82	Urinary tract infection of newborn	
● 771.83	Bacteremia of newborn	
● 771.89	Other infections specific to the perinatal period Includes note added	
774.5	Code first term revised	
● 779.81	Neonatal bradycardia Excludes note added	
● 779.82	Neonatal tachycardia Excludes note added	
● 779.89	Other specified conditions originating in the perinatal period	
780.9	Includes note deleted	
● 780.91	Fussy infant (baby)	
● 780.92	Excessive crying of infant (baby)	
● 780.99	Other general symptoms Includes note added	
● 781.93	Ocular torticollis	
782.5	Excludes note revised	
785.0	Excludes note added	
786.03	Excludes term added	
786.09	Excludes terms revised	
788.3	Code first note deleted Code, if applicable, note added	
790.7	Excludes term added	
795.0	Includes note deleted Excludes note added	
● 795.00	Nonspecific abnormal Papanicolaou smear of cervix, unspecified	
● 795.01	Atypical squamous cell changes of undetermined significance favor benign (ASCUS favor benign) Includes note added	
● 795.02	Atypical squamous cell changes of undetermined significance favor dysplasia (ASCUS favor dysplasia) Includes note added	
● 795.09	Other nonspecific abnormal Papanicolaou smear of cervix Includes note added	
● 795.31	Nonspecific positive findings for anthrax Includes term added	
● 795.39	Other nonspecific positive culture findings	
799.1	Excludes terms revised	
(800-829)	Fractures section Instructional note revised	
● 813.45	Torus fracture of radius	
● 823.4	Fracture of tibia and fibula, torus fracture	
959.01	Excludes term added	
991.6	Excludes term revised	
995.0	Code first note deleted	
● 995.9	Systemic inflammatory response syndrome (SIRS)	

▶◀ Revised Text   ● New Code   ▲ Revised Code Title

2001 Ingenix, Inc.

- 995.90 Systemic inflammatory response syndrome, unspecified
  Includes note added
- 995.91 Systemic inflammatory response syndrome due to infectious process without organ dysfunction
- 995.92 Systemic inflammatory response syndrome due to infectious process with organ dysfunction
  Includes note added
  Use additional code note added
- 995.93 Systemic inflammatory response syndrome due to non-infectious process without organ dysfunction
- 995.94 Systemic inflammatory response syndrome due to non-infectious process with organ dysfunction
  Use additional code note added
- 996.72 Excludes note revised
- 998.31 Disruption of internal operation wound
- 998.32 Disruption of external operation wound
  Includes note added
- V01.81 Contact with or exposure to anthrax
- V01.89 Contact with or exposure to other communicable diseases
- V13.21 Personal history of pre-term labor
  Excludes note added
- V13.29 Personal history of other genital system and obstetric disorders
- V23.41 Pregnancy with history of pre-term labor
- V23.49 Pregnancy with other poor obstetric history
- V46.2 Other dependence on machines, supplemental oxygen
  Includes note added
- ▲ V49.81 ▶Asymptomatic◀ postmenopausal status (age-related) (natural)
- V54.0 Excludes term revised
- V54.1 Aftercare for healing traumatic fracture
- V54.10 Aftercare for healing traumatic fracture of arm, unspecified
- V54.11 Aftercare for healing traumatic fracture of upper arm
- V54.12 Aftercare for healing traumatic fracture of lower arm
- V54.13 Aftercare for healing traumatic fracture of hip
- V54.14 Aftercare for healing traumatic fracture of leg, unspecified
- V54.15 Aftercare for healing traumatic fracture of upper leg
  Excludes note added
- V54.16 Aftercare for healing traumatic fracture of lower leg
- V54.17 Aftercare for healing traumatic fracture of vertebrae
- V54.19 Aftercare for healing traumatic fracture of other bone
- V54.2 Aftercare for healing pathologic fracture

- V54.20 Aftercare for healing pathologic fracture of arm, unspecified
- V54.21 Aftercare for healing pathologic fracture of upper arm
- V54.22 Aftercare for healing pathologic fracture of lower arm
- V54.23 Aftercare for healing pathologic fracture of hip
- V54.24 Aftercare for healing pathologic fracture of leg, unspecified
- V54.25 Aftercare for healing pathologic fracture of upper leg
  Excludes note added
- V54.26 Aftercare for healing pathologic fracture of lower leg
- V54.27 Aftercare for healing pathologic fracture of vertebrae
- V54.29 Aftercare for healing pathologic fracture of other bone
- V54.8 Includes note deleted
- V54.81 Aftercare following joint replacement
  Use additional code note added
- V54.89 Other orthopedic aftercare
  Includes note added
- V58.4 Instructional note added
- V58.42 Aftercare following surgery for neoplasm
  Includes note added
- V58.43 Aftercare following surgery for injury and trauma
  Includes note added
  Excludes note added
- V58.7 Aftercare following surgery to specified body systems, not elsewhere classified
  Instructional note added
- V58.71 Aftercare following surgery of the sense organs, NEC
  Includes note added
- V58.72 Aftercare following surgery of the nervous system, NEC
  Includes note added
  Excludes note added
- V58.73 Aftercare following surgery of the circulatory system, NEC
  Includes note added
- V58.74 Aftercare following surgery of the respiratory system, NEC
  Includes note added
- V58.75 Aftercare following surgery of the teeth, oral cavity and digestive system, NEC
  Includes note added
- V58.76 Aftercare following surgery of the genitourinary system, NEC
  Includes note added
  Excludes note added
- V58.77 Aftercare following surgery of the skin and subcutaneous tissue, NEC
  Includes note added
- V58.78 Aftercare following surgery of the musculoskeletal system, NEC
  Includes note added
- V58.83 Use additional code note added
- ▲ V71.8 Observation ▶and evaluation◀ for other specified suspected conditions

- V71.82 Observation and evaluation for suspected exposure to anthrax
- V71.83 Observation and evaluation for suspected exposure to other biological agent
- V83.8 Other genetic carrier status
- V83.81 Cystic fibrosis gene carrier
- V83.89 Other genetic carrier status
- E885.0 Fall from (nonmotorized) scooter
- E922.5 Accident caused by firearm, and air gun missle, paintball gun
- E955.7 Suicide and self-inflicted injury by firearms, air guns and explosives, paintball gun
- E960-E969 Homicide and injury purposely inflicted by other persons section
  Excludes term added
- (E979) Terrorism (E979) new section
- E979 Terrorism
  Instructional note added
- E979.0 Terrorism involving explosion of marine weapons
  Includes note added
- E979.1 Terrorism involving destruction of aircraft
  Includes note added
- E979.2 Terrorism involving other explosions and fragments
  Includes note added
- E979.3 Terrorism involving fires, conflagration and hot substances
  Includes note added
- E979.4 Terrorism involving firearms
  Includes note added
- E979.5 Terrorism involving nuclear weapons
  Includes note added
- E979.6 Terrorism involving biological weapons
  Includes note added
- E979.7 Terrorism involving chemical weapons
  Includes note added
- E979.8 Terrorism involving other means
  Includes note added
- E979.9 Terrorism, secondary effects
  Instructional note added
  Excludes note added
- E985.7 Injury by paintball gun, undetermined whether accidentally or purposely inflicted
- ▲ E999 Late effect of injury due to war operations wand terrorismx
  Instructional note revised
- E999.0 Late effect of injury due to war operations
- E999.1 Late effect of injury due to terrorism

Coding Guidelines

OFFICIAL ICD-9-CM GUIDELINES FOR CODING AND REPORTING

The Public Health Service and the Centers for Medicare and Medicaid (formerly know as Health Care Financing Administration) of the U.S. Department of Health and Human Services present the following guidelines for coding and reporting using the International Classification of Diseases, 9th Revision, Clinical Modification (ICD-9-CM). These guidelines should be used as a companion document to the official versions of the ICD-9-CM.

These guidelines for coding and reporting have been developed and approved by the cooperating parties for ICD-9-CM: American Hospital Association, American Health Information Management Association, Center for Medicare and Medicaid Services and the National Center for Health Statistics. These guidelines previously appeared in the Coding Clinic for ICD-9-CM, published by the American Hospital Association.

These guidelines have been developed to assist the user in coding and reporting in situations where the ICD-9-CM manual does not provide direction. Coding and sequencing instructions in the three ICD-9-CM manuals take precedence over any guidelines.

These guidelines are not exhaustive. The cooperating parties are continuing to conduct review of these guidelines and develop new guidelines as needed. Users of the ICD-9-CM should be aware that only guidelines approved by the cooperating parties are official. Revision of these guidelines and new guidelines will be published by the U.S. Department of Health and Human Services when they are approved by the cooperating parties.

OUTPATIENT SERVICES

(Hospital-Based and Physician Office)

Table of Contents

INPATIENT SERVICES

Table of Contents

Coding Guidelines

Coding Guidelines—Outpatient

OFFICIAL GUIDELINES FOR CODING AND REPORTING OUTPATIENT SERVICES (HOSPITAL-BASED AND PHYSICIAN OFFICE)

Introduction

These revised coding guidelines for outpatient diagnoses have been approved for use by hospitals/physicians in coding and reporting hospital-based outpatient services and physician office visits.

The terms encounter and visit are often used interchangeably in describing outpatient service contacts and, therefore, appear together in these guidelines without distinguishing one from the other.

Coding guidelines for outpatient and physician reporting of diagnoses will vary in a number of instances from those for inpatient diagnoses, recognizing that:

The Uniform Hospital Discharge Data Set (UHDDS) definition of principal diagnosis applies only to inpatients in acute, short-term, general hospitals.

Coding guidelines for inconclusive diagnoses (probable, suspected, rule out, etc.) were developed for inpatient reporting and do not apply to outpatients.

Diagnoses often are not established at the time of the initial encounter/visit. It may take two or more visits before the diagnosis is confirmed.

The most critical rule involves beginning the search for the correct code assignment through the Alphabetic Index. Never begin searching initially in the Tabular List as this will lead to coding errors.

Basic Coding Guidelines for Outpatient Services

A.   Code Range

The appropriate code or codes from 001.0 through V82.9 must be used to identify diagnoses, symptoms, conditions, problems, complaints, or other reason(s) for the encounter/visit.

B.   Accurate Reporting

For accurate reporting of ICD-9-CM diagnosis codes, the documentation should describe the patient's condition, using terminology which includes specific diagnoses as well as symptoms, problems, or reasons for the encounter. There are ICD-9-CM codes to describe all of these.

C.   Code Selection

The selection of codes 001.0 through 999.9 will frequently be used to describe the reason for the encounter. These codes are from the section of ICD-9-CM for the classification of diseases and injuries (e.g. infectious and parasitic diseases; neoplasms; symptoms, signs, and ill-defined conditions, etc.).

D.   Symptoms, Signs and Ill-defined Conditions

Codes that describe symptoms and signs, as opposed to diagnoses, are acceptable for reporting purposes when an established diagnosis has not been diagnosed (confirmed) by the physician. Chapter 16 of ICD-9-CM, Symptoms, Signs, and Ill-defined conditions (codes 780.0 - 799.9) contain many, but not all codes for symptoms.

E.   Circumstances other than Disease or Injury

ICD-9-CM provides codes to deal with encounters for circumstances other than a disease or injury. The Supplementary Classification of factors Influencing Health Status and Contact with Health Services (V01.0- V82.9) is provided to deal with occasions when circumstances other than a disease or injury are recorded as diagnosis or problems. The V codes should be used for encounters of this type. For example, the correct code for a cancer patient who is seen solely for radiotherapy is V58.0, radiotherapy session.

Example:

Discharge diagnosis: Open-angle glaucoma

Reason for visit code: 365.10

Discharge diagnosis: Follow-up examination after surgery

Reason for visit code: V67.0

F.   Code Specificity

ICD-9-CM is composed of codes with either 3, 4, or 5 digits. Codes with 3 digits are included in ICD-9-CM as the heading of a category of codes that may be further subdivided by the use of fourth and/or fifth digits which provide greater specificity. A code is invalid if it has not been coded to the full number of digits required for that code.

- Assign three-digit codes only if there are no four-digit codes within that code category.
- Assign four-digit codes only if there is no fifth-digit subclassification for that subcategory.
- Assign the fifth-digit subclassification code for those subcategories where it exists.

Example:

Diagnosis: Acute tonsillitis

Correct code: 463

Diagnosis: Benign neoplasm of colon

Incorrect code: 211

Correct code: 211.3

G.   Code Sequence

List first the ICD-9-CM code for the diagnosis, condition, problem, or other reason for encounter/visit shown in the medical record to be chiefly responsible for the services provided. List additional codes that describe any coexisting conditions.

H.   Uncertain Diagnosis

Do not code diagnoses documented as "probable", "suspected," "questionable," "rule out," or working diagnosis. Rather, code the condition(s) to the highest degree of certainty for that encounter/visit, such as symptoms, signs, abnormal test results, or other reason for the visit.

Coders should be aware that this is contrary to the coding practices used by health information management departments for coding the diagnoses of hospital inpatients. For inpatient coding, all discharge diagnoses listed as "probable," "suspected," "questionable" or "rule out" would be coded as if the condition existed. Further, coding symptoms for inpatients is generally unacceptable, particularly when there is an established diagnosis. A requirement that conditions listed as "probable," "suspected," "questionable" or "rule out" be coded in the outpatient setting as if the condition existed would lead to significant over-reporting of conditions. Therefore codes for symptoms and signs are appropriate and acceptable for hospital outpatient reporting.

Example:

Reason for visit: Chest pain, code 786.50

Discharge diagnosis: Rule out angina, code 413.9

Correct code: 786.50

Comment: Do not code angina as if it were established; code the reason for the visit.

I.   Chronic Disease

Chronic diseases treated on an ongoing basis may be coded and reported as many times as the patient receives treatment and care for the condition(s).

Example:

History of illness: Patient is seen for monthly lumbar epidural block with steroid injection.

Discharge diagnosis: Chronic low back pain, code 724.2

Comment: Report code 724.2, low back pain, for each visit during which the patient receives lumbar-block treatment, regardless of the number or frequency of visits.

J.   Coexisting Conditions

Code all documented conditions that coexist at the time of the encounter/visit, and require or affect patient care treatment or management. Do not code conditions that were previously treated and no longer exist. However, history codes (V10- V19) may be used as secondary codes if the historical condition or family history has an impact on current care or influences treatment.

Coders are advised to exercise care in identifying (a) conditions presently existing, (b) conditions no longer existing, (c) residuals (late effects) of conditions no longer existing, and (d) certain postoperative status conditions that require consideration in managing patient care and that warrant coding. Some physicians add to the list of conditions currently being treated any previous surgery or conditions that no longer exist to provide easy reference of the patient's history for recapitulation in the ongoing care of the patient. These conditions should not be coded unless they require or affect patient care treatment or management.

Example:

Chief complaint: Uncontrolled diabetes mellitus, 250.02

Review of systems: Patient has congestive heart failure (428.0) and is curently on Lasix.

Medical history: Patient is status three months post right inguinal herniorrherapy for incarcerated inguinal hernia.

Comment: First code "uncontrolled diabetes mellitus" as the reason for the visit, followed by "congestive heart failure" as a coexisting condition. Do not code the incarcerated inguinal hernia; it was treated successfully.

Code sequence: 250.02, 428.0

K. Ancillary Diagnostic Services

For patients receiving diagnostic services only during an encounter/visit, sequence first the diagnosis, condition, problem, or other reason for encounter/visit shown in the medical record to be chiefly responsible for the outpatient services provided during the encounter/visit. Codes for other diagnoses (e.g., chronic conditions) may be sequenced as additional diagnoses.

Example:

Chief complaint: Hematuria, code 599.7

Laboratory studies: Intravenous pyelogram, code V72.5

History of illness: Patient was referred to hospital outpatient clinic for intravenous pyelogram only. Will provide patient's physician with the results.

Code sequence: 599.7

L. Ancillary Therapeutic Services

For patients receiving therapeutic services only during an encounter/visit, sequence first the diagnosis, condition, problem, or other reason for encounter/visit shown in the medical record to be chiefly responsible for the outpatient services provided during the encounter/visit. Codes for other diagnoses (e.g., chronic conditions) may be sequenced as additional diagnoses.

Example:

Chief complaint: Chronic renal failure, code 585

Procedure performed: Hemodialysis, code V56.0

History of illness: Patient is being seen for hemodialysis treatment.

Code sequence: 585

NOTE: The appropriate V code can be listed first for patients receiving the following (the diagnosis or problem for which the service is being performed should be listed second):

•   chemotherapy
•   radiation therapy
•   rehabilitation.

Example:

Chief complaint: Trigone bladder cancer, code 188.0

Procedure performed: Chemotherapy infusion, code V58.1

History of illness: Patient is being seen for second course of five chemotherapy infusions.

Code sequence: V58.1, 188.0

M. [Guideline M-deleted in the official guidelines]

N. Preoperative Evaluations

For patient's receiving preoperative evaluations only, sequence a code from category V72.8, Other specified examinations, to describe the pre-op consultations. Assign a code for the condition to describe the reason for the surgery as an additional diagnosis. Code also any findings related to the pre-op evaluation.

Example:

Chief complaint: Rhegmatogenous retinal detachment in left eye, code 361.00

Procedure performed: Preoperative cardiovascular examination, V72.81

History of illness: Patient is being seen for preoperative cardiovascular examination, due to history of myocardial infarction 1 year ago. Patient is scheduled for a repair of his retinal detachment next week.

Code sequence: V72.81, 361.00

O. Ambulatory Surgery

For ambulatory surgery, code the diagnosis for which the surgery was performed. If the postoperative diagnosis is known to be different from the preoperative diagnosis at the time the diagnosis is confirmed, select the postoperative diagnosis for coding, since it is the most definitive.

Example:

Preoperative diagnosis: Breast mass, code 611.72

Postoperative diagnosis: Fibrocystic breast disease, code 610.3

Comment: Code 610.3 as the reason for the visit because it is the postoperative diagnosis.

OFFICIAL GUIDELINES FOR CODING AND REPORTING INPATIENT SERVICES

1. GENERAL INPATIENT CODING GUIDELINES

   1.1. Use of Both Alphabetic Index and Tabular List

   A. Use both the Alphabetic Index and the Tabular List when locating and assigning a code. Reliance on only the Alphabetic Index or the Tabular List leads to errors in code assignments and less specificity in code selection.

   B. Locate each term in the Alphabetic Index and verify the code selected in the Tabular List. Read and be guided by instructional notations that appear in both the Alphabetic Index and the Tabular List.

   1.2. Level of Specificity in Coding

   Diagnostic and procedure codes are to be used at their highest level of specificity:

   - Assign three-digit codes only if there are no four-digit codes within that code category.

   - Assign four-digit codes only if there is no fifth-digit subclassification for that category.

   - Assign the fifth-digit subclassification code for those categories where it exists.

   1.3. Other (NEC) and Unspecified (NOS) Code Titles

   Codes labeled "other specified" (NEC—not elsewhere classified) or "unspecified" (NOS—not otherwise specified) are used only when neither the diagnostic statement nor a thorough review of the medical record provides adequate information to permit assignment of a more specific code.

   - Use the code assignment for "other" or NEC when the information at hand specifies a condition but no separate code for that condition is provided.

   - Use "unspecified" (NOS) when the information at hand does not permit either a more specific or "other" code assignment.

   - When the Alphabetic Index assigns a code to a category labeled "other (NEC)" or to a category labeled "unspecified (NOS)", refer to the Tabular List and review the titles and inclusion terms in the subdivisions under that particular three-digit category (or subdivision under the four-digit code) to determine if the information at hand can be appropriately assigned to a more specific code.

   1.4. Acute and Chronic Conditions

   If the same condition is described as both acute (subacute) and chronic and separate subentries exist in the Alphabetic Index at the same indentation level, code both and sequence the acute (subacute) code first.

   1.5. Combination Code

   A single code used to classify two diagnoses or a diagnosis with an associated secondary process (manifestation) or an associated complication is called a combination code. Combination codes are identified by referring to subterm entries in the Alphabetic Index and by reading the inclusion and exclusion notes in the Tabular List.

   Assign only the combination code when that code fully identifies the diagnostic conditions involved or when the Alphabetic Index so directs. Multiple coding should not be used when the classification provides a combination code that clearly identifies all of the elements documented in the diagnosis. When the combination code lacks necessary specificity in describing the manifestation or complication, an additional code may be used as a secondary code.

   1.6. Multiple Coding of Diagnoses

   Multiple coding is required for certain conditions not subject to the rules for combination codes.

   Instruction for conditions that require multiple coding appear in the Alphabetic Index and the Tabular List.

   A. Alphabetic Index: Codes for both etiology and manifestation of a disease appear following the subentry term, with the second code in brackets. Assign both codes in the same sequence in which they appear in the Alphabetic Index.

   B. Tabular List: Instructional terms, such as "Code first...," "Use additional code for any...," and "Note...," indicate when to use more than one code.

   - "Code first underlying disease" - Assign the codes for both the manifestation and underlying cause. The codes for manifestations cannot be used (designated) as principal diagnosis.

   - "Use additional code, to identify manifestation, as ..." - Assign also the code that identifies the manifestation, such as, but not limited to, the examples listed. The codes for manifestations cannot be used (designated) as principal diagnosis.

   C. Apply multiple coding instructions throughout the classification where appropriate, whether or not multiple coding directions appear in the Alphabetic Index or the Tabular List. Avoid indiscriminate multiple coding or irrelevant information, such as symptoms or signs characteristic of the diagnosis.

1.7. Late Effect

A late effect is the residual effect (condition produced) after the acute phase of an illness or injury has terminated. There is no time limit on when a late effect code can be used. The residual may be apparent early, such as in cerebrovascular accident cases, or it may occur months or years later, such as that due to a previous injury.

Coding of late effects requires two codes:

- The residual condition or nature of the late effect
- The cause of the late effect

The residual condition or nature of the late effect is sequenced first, followed by the cause of the late effect, except in those few instances where the code for late effect is followed by a manifestation code identified in the Tabular List and title or the late effect code has been expanded (at the fourth and fifth-digit levels) to include the manifestation(s).

The code for the acute phase of an illness or injury that led to the late effect is never used with a code for the cause of the late effect.

A. Late Effects of Cerebrovascular Disease

Category 438 is used to indicate conditions classifiable to categories 430-437 as the causes of late effects (neurologic deficits), themselves classified elsewhere. These "late effects" include neurologic deficits that persist after initial onset of conditions classifiable to 430-437. The neurologic deficits caused by cerebrovascular disease may be present from the onset or may arise at any time after the onset of the condition classifiable to 430–437.

- Codes from category 438 may be assigned on a health care record with codes from 430–437, if the patient has a current CVA and deficits from an old CVA.
- Assign code V12.59 (and not a code from category 438) as an additional code for history of cerebrovascular disease when no neurologic deficits are present.

1.8. Uncertain Diagnosis

If the diagnosis documented at the time of discharge is qualified as "probable", "suspected", "likely", "questionable", "possible", or "still to be ruled out", code the condition as if it existed or was established. The bases for this guidelines are the diagnostic workup, arrangements for further workup or observation, and initial therapeutic approach that correspond most closely with the established diagnosis.

1.9. Impending or Threatened Condition

Code any condition described at the time of discharge as "impending" or "threatened" as follows:

If it did occur, code as confirmed diagnosis.

If it did not occur, reference the Alphabetic Index to determine if the condition has a subentry term for "impending" or "threatened" and also reference main term entries for Impending and for Threatened.

- If the subterms are listed, assign the given code.
- If the subterms are not listed, code the existing forerunner condition(s) and not the condition described as impending or threatened.

2. SELECTION OF PRINCIPAL DIAGNOSIS

The circumstances of inpatient admission always govern the selection of principal diagnosis. The principal diagnosis is defined in the Uniform Hospital Discharge Data Set (UHDDS) as "that condition established after study to be chiefly responsible for occasioning the admission of the patient to the hospital for care".

In determining principal diagnosis the coding directives in the ICD-9-CM manuals, Volumes I, II, and III, take precedence over all other guidelines.

The importance of consistent, complete documentation in the medical record cannot be overemphasized. Without such documentation the application of all coding guidelines is a difficult, if not impossible, task.

2.1. Codes for symptoms, signs, and ill-defined conditions

Codes for symptoms, signs, and ill-defined conditions from Chapter 16 are not to be used as principal diagnosis when a related definitive diagnosis has been established.

2.2. Codes in brackets

Codes in brackets in the Alphabetic Index can never be sequenced as principal diagnosis. Coding directives require that the codes in brackets be sequenced in the order as they appear in the Alphabetic Index.

2.3. Acute and chronic conditions

If the same condition is described as both acute (subacute) and chronic and separate subentries exist in the Alphabetic Index at the same indentation level, code both and sequence the acute (subacute) code first.

2.4. Two or more interrelated conditions, each potentially meeting the definition for principal diagnosis

When there are two or more interrelated conditions (such as diseases in the same ICD-9-CM chapter or manifestations characteristically associated with a certain disease) potentially meeting the definition of principal diagnosis, either condition may be sequenced first, unless the circumstances of the admission, the therapy provided, the Tabular List, or the Alphabetic Index indicate otherwise.

2.5. Two or more diagnoses that equally meet the definition for principal diagnosis

In the unusual instance when two or more diagnoses equally meet the criteria for principal diagnosis as determined by the circumstances of admission, diagnostic workup and/or therapy provided, and the Alphabetic Index, Tabular List, or another coding guidelines does not provide sequencing direction, any one of the diagnoses may be sequenced first.

2.6. Two or more comparative or contrasting conditions

In those rare instances when two or more contrasting or comparative diagnoses are documented as "either/or" (or similar terminology), they are coded as if the diagnoses were confirmed and the diagnoses are sequenced according to the circumstances of the admission. If no further determination can be made as to which diagnosis should be principal, either diagnosis may be sequenced first.

2.7. A symptom(s) followed by contrasting/comparative diagnoses

When a symptom(s) is followed by contrasting/comparative diagnoses, the symptom code is sequenced first. All the contrasting/comparative diagnoses should be coded as suspected conditions.

2.8. Codes from the V71.0-V71.9 series, Observation and evaluation for suspected conditions

Codes from the V71.0-V71.9 series are assigned as principal diagnoses for encounters or admissions to evaluate the patient's condition when there is some evidence to suggest the existence of an abnormal condition or following an accident or other incident that ordinarily results in a health problem, and where no supporting evidence for the suspected condition is found and no treatment is currently required. The fact that the patient may be scheduled for continuing observation in the office/clinic setting following discharge does not limit the use of this category.

2.9. Original treatment plan not carried out

Sequence as the principal diagnosis the condition which after study occasioned the admission to the hospital, even though treatment may not have been carried out due to unforeseen circumstances.

2.10. Residual condition or nature of late effect

The residual condition or nature of the late effect is sequenced first, followed by the late

effect code for the cause of the residual condition, except in a few instances where the Alphabetic Index or Tabular List directs otherwise.

2.11. Multiple burns

Sequence first the code that reflects the highest degree of burn when more than one burn is present. (See also Burns guideline 8.3)

2.12. Multiple injuries

When multiple injuries exist, the code for the most severe injury as determined by the attending physician is sequenced first.

2.13. Neoplasms

A. If the treatment is directed at the malignancy, designate the malignancy as the principal diagnosis, except when the purpose of the encounter or hospital admission is for radiotherapy session(s), V58.0, or for chemotherapy session(s), V58.1, in which instance the malignancy is coded and sequenced second.

B. When a patient is admitted for the purpose of radiotherapy or chemotherapy and develops complications such as uncontrolled nausea and vomiting or dehydration, the principal diagnosis is Encounter for radiotherapy, V58.0, or Encounter for chemotherapy, V58.1.

C. When an episode of inpatient care involves surgical removal of a primary site or secondary site malignancy followed by adjunct chemotherapy or radiotherapy, code the malignancy as the principal diagnosis, using codes in the 140-198 series or where appropriate in the 200-203 series.

D. When the reason for admission is to determine the extent of the malignancy, or for a procedure such as paracentesis or thoracentesis, the primary malignancy or appropriate metastatic site is designated as the principal diagnosis, even though chemotherapy or radiotherapy is administered.

E. When the primary malignancy has been previously excised or eradicated from its site and there is not adjunct treatment directed to that site and no evidence of any remaining malignancy at the primary site, use the appropriate code from the V10 series to indicate the former site of primary malignancy. Any mention of extension, invasion, or metastasis to a nearby structure or organ or to a distant site is coded as a secondary malignant neoplasm to that site and may be the principal diagnosis in the absence of the primary site.

F. When a patient is admitted because of a primary neoplasm with metastasis and treatment is directed toward the secondary site only, the secondary neoplasm is designated as the principal diagnosis even though the primary malignancy is still present.

G. Symptoms, signs, and ill-defined conditions listed in Chapter 16 characteristic of, or associated with, an existing primary or secondary site malignancy cannot be used to replace the malignancy as principal diagnosis, regardless of the number of admissions or encounters for treatment and care of the neoplasm.

H. Coding and sequencing of complications associated with the malignant neoplasm or with the therapy thereof are subject to the following guidelines:

- When admission is for management of an anemia associated with the malignancy, and the treatment is only for anemia, the anemia is designated at the principal diagnosis and is followed by the appropriate code(s) for the malignancy.

- When the admission is for management of an anemia associated with chemotherapy or radiotherapy and the only treatment is for the anemia, the anemia is designated as the principal diagnosis followed by the appropriate code(s) for the malignancy.

- When the admission is for management of dehydration due to the malignancy or the therapy, or a combination of both, and only the dehydration is being treated (intravenous rehydration), the dehydration is designated as the principal diagnosis, followed by the code(s) for the malignancy.

- When the admission is for treatment of a complication resulting from a surgical procedure performed for the treatment of an intestinal malignancy, designate the complication as the principal diagnosis if treatment is directed at resolving the complication.

2.14. Poisoning

When coding a poisoning or reaction to the improper use of a medication (e.g., wrong dose, wrong substance, wrong route of administration) the poisoning code is sequenced first, followed by a code for the manifestation. If there is also a diagnosis of

drug abuse or dependence to the substance, the abuse or dependence is coded as an additional code.

2.15. Complications of surgery and other medical care

When the admission is for treatment of a complication resulting from surgery or other medical care, the complication code is sequenced as the principal diagnosis. If the complication is classified to the 996-999 series, an additional code for the specific complication may be assigned.

2.16. Complication of pregnancy

When a patient is admitted because of a condition that is either a complication pregnancy or that is complicating the pregnancy, the code for the obstetric complication is the principal diagnosis. An additional code may be assigned as needed to provide specificity.

3. REPORTING OTHER (ADDITIONAL) DIAGNOSES

A joint effort between the attending physician and coder is essential to achieve complete and accurate documentation, code assignment, and reporting of diagnoses and procedures.

These guidelines have been developed and approved by the Cooperating Parties to assure both the physician and the coder in identifying those diagnoses that are to be reported in addition to the principal diagnosis. Hospitals may record other diagnoses as needed for internal data use.

The UHDDS definitions are used by acute care short-term hospitals to report inpatient data elements in a standardized manner. These data elements and their definitions can be found in the July 31, 1985, Federal Register (Vol. 50, No, 147), pp. 31038-40.

The UHDDS item #11-b defines Other Diagnoses as "all conditions that coexist at the time of admission, that develop subsequently, or that affect the treatment received and/or the length of stay. Diagnoses that relate to an earlier episode which have no bearing on the current hospital stay are to be excluded".

General Rule

For reporting purposes the definition for "other diagnoses" is interpreted as additional conditions that affect patient care in terms of requiring:

- clinical evaluation; or
- therapeutic treatment; or
- diagnostic procedures; or
- extended length of hospital stay; or
- increased nursing care and/or monitoring.

The following guidelines are to be applied in designating "other diagnoses" when neither the Alphabetic Index nor the Tabular List in ICD-9-CM provide direction.

The listing of the diagnoses on the attestation statement is the responsibility of the attending physician.

3.1. Previous conditions

If the physician has included a diagnosis in the final diagnostic statement, such as the discharge summary or the face sheet, it should ordinarily be coded. Some physicians include in the diagnostic statement resolved conditions or diagnoses and status-post procedures from previous admission that have no bearing on the current stay. Such conditions are not to be reported and are coded only if required by hospital policy.

However, history codes (V10-V19) may be used as secondary codes if the historical condition or family history has an impact on current care or influences treatment.

3.2. Diagnoses not listed in the final diagnostic statement

When the physician has documented what appears to be a current diagnosis in the body of the record, but has not included the diagnosis in the final diagnostic statement, the physician should be asked whether the diagnosis should be added.

3.3. Conditions that are an integral part of a disease process

Conditions that are integral to the disease process should not be assigned as additional codes.

3.4. Conditions that are not an integral part of a disease process

Additional conditions that may not be associated routinely with a disease process should be coded when present.

3.5. Abnormal findings

Abnormal findings (laboratory, x-ray, pathologic, and other diagnostic results) are not coded and reported unless the physician indicates their clinical significance. If the findings are outside the normal range and the physician has ordered other tests to evaluate the condition or prescribed treatment, it is appropriate to ask the physician whether the diagnosis should be added.

4. HYPERTENSION

4.1. Hypertension, Essential, or NOS

Assign hypertension (arterial) (essential) (primary) (systemic) (NOS) to category code 401 with the appropriate fourth digit to indicate malignant (.0), benign (.1), or unspecified (.9). Do not use either .0 malignant or .1 benign unless medical record documentation supports such a designation.

4.2. Hypertension with Heart Disease

Certain heart conditions (425.8, 428, 429.0-429.3, 429.8, 429.9) are assigned to a code

from category 402 when a causal relationship is stated (due to hypertension) or implied (hypertensive). Use only the code from category 402.

The same heart conditions (425.8, 428, 429.0-429.3, 429.8, 429.9) with hypertension, but without a stated casual relationship, are coded separately. Sequence according to the circumstances of the admission.

4.3. Hypertensive Renal Disease with Chronic Renal Failure

Assign codes from category 403, Hypertensive renal disease, when conditions classified to categories 585-587 are present. Unlike hypertension with heart disease, ICD-9-CM presumes a cause-and-effect relationship and classifies renal failure with hypertension as hypertensive renal disease.

4.4. Hypertensive Heart and Renal Disease

Assign codes from combination category 404, Hypertensive heart and renal disease, when both hypertensive renal disease and hypertensive heart disease are stated in the diagnosis. Assume a relationship between the hypertension and the renal disease, whether or not the condition is so designated.

4.5. Hypertensive Cerebrovascular Disease.

First assign codes from 430-438, Cerebrovascular disease, then the appropriate hypertension code from categories 401-405.

4.6. Hypertensive Retinopathy

Two codes are necessary to identify the condition. First assign the code from subcategory 362.11, Hypertensive retinopathy, then the appropriate code from categories 401-405 to indicate the type of hypertension.

4.7. Hypertension, Secondary

Two codes are required: one to identify the underlying condition and one from category 405 to identify the hypertension. Sequencing of codes is determined by the reason for admission to the hospital.

4.8. Hypertension, Transient

Assign code 796.2, Elevated blood pressure reading without diagnosis of hypertension, unless patient has an established diagnosis of hypertension. Assign code 642.3x for transient hypertension of pregnancy.

4.9. Hypertension, Controlled

Assign appropriate code from categories 401-405. This diagnostic statement usually refers to an existing state of hypertension under control by therapy.

4.10. Hypertension, Uncontrolled

Uncontrolled hypertension may refer to untreated hypertension or hypertension not responding to current therapeutic regimen. In either case. assign the appropriate code from categories 401-405 to designate the stage and type of hypertension. Code to the type of hypertension.

4.11. Elevated Blood Pressure

For a statement of elevated blood pressure without further specificity, assign code 796.2, Elevated blood pressure reading without diagnosis of hypertension, rather than a code from category 401.

5. OBSTETRICS

Introduction

These guidelines have been developed and approved by the Cooperating Parties in conjunction with the Editorial Advisory Board of Coding Clinic and the American College of Obstetricians and Gynecologists, to assist the coder in coding and reporting obstetric cases. Where feasible, previously published advice has been incorporated. Some advice in these new guidelines may supersede previous advice. The guidelines are provided for reporting purposes. Health care facilities may record additional diagnoses as needed for internal data needs.

5.1. General Rules

A. Obstetric cases require codes from chapter 11, codes in the range 630-677, Complications of Pregnancy, Childbirth, and the Puerperium. Should the physician document that the pregnancy is incidental to the encounter then code V22.2 should be used in place of any chapter 11 codes. It is the physician's responsibility to state that the condition being treated is not affecting the pregnancy.

B. Chapter 11 codes have sequencing priority over codes from other chapters. Additional codes from other chapters may be used in conjunction with chapter 11 codes to further specify conditions.

C. Chapter 11 codes are to be used only on the maternal record, never on the record of the newborn.

D. An outcome of delivery code, V27.0-V27.9, should be included on every maternal record when a delivery has occurred. These codes are not to be used on subsequent records or on the newborn record.

5.2. Selection of Principal Diagnosis

A. The circumstances of the encounter govern the selection of the principal diagnosis.

B. In episodes when no delivery occurs the principal diagnosis should correspond to the principal complication of the pregnancy which necessitated the encounter. Should more than one complication exist, all of which are treated or monitored, any of the complications codes may be sequenced first.

C. When a delivery occurs the principal diagnosis should correspond to the main circumstances or complication of the delivery. In cases of cesarean deliveries, the principal diagnosis should correspond to the reason the cesarean was performed, unless the reason for admission was unrelated to the condition resulting in the cesarean delivery.

D. For routine prenatal visits when no complications are present codes V22.0, Supervision of normal first pregnancy, and V22.1, Supervision of other normal pregnancy, should be used as principal diagnoses. These codes should not be used in conjunction with chapter 11 codes.

E. For prenatal outpatient visits for patients with high-risk pregnancies, a code from category V23, Supervision of high-risk pregnancy, should be used as the principal diagnosis. Secondary chapter 11 codes may be used in conjunction with these codes if appropriate. A thorough review of any pertinent excludes note is necessary to be certain that these V codes are being used properly.

5.3. Chapter 11 Fifth-digits

A. Categories 640-648, 651-676 have required fifth-digits which indicate whether the encounter is antepartum, postpartum and whether a delivery has also occurred.

B. The fifth-digits which are appropriate for each code number are listed in brackets under each code. The fifth-digits on each code should all be consistent with each other. That is, should a delivery occur all of the fifth-digits should indicate the delivery.

5.4. Fetal Conditions Affecting the Management of the Mother.

Codes from category 655, Known or suspected fetal abnormality affecting management of the mother, and category 656, Other fetal and placental problems affecting the management of the mother, are assigned only when the fetal condition is actually responsible for modifying the management of the mother, i.e., by requiring diagnostic studies, additional observation, special care, or termination of pregnancy. The fact that the fetal condition exists does not justify assigning a code from this series to the mother's record.

5.5. Normal Delivery, 650

A. Code 650 is for use in cases when a woman is admitted for a full-term normal delivery and delivers a single, healthy infant without any complications antepartum, during the delivery, or postpartum during the delivery episode.

B. 650 may be used if the patient had a complications at some point during her pregnancy but the complication is not present at the time of the admission for delivery.

C. Code 650 is always a principal diagnosis. It is not to be used if any other code from chapter 11 is needed to describe a current complication of the antenatal, delivery, or perinatal period. Additional codes from other chapters may be used with code 650 if they are not related to or are in any way complicating the pregnancy.

D. V27.0, Single liveborn, is the only outcome of delivery code appropriate for use with 650.

5.6. Procedure Codes

A. In cases of cesarean delivery, the selection of the principal diagnosis should correspond to the reason the cesarean delivery was performed unless the reason for admission was unrelated to the condition resulting in the cesarean delivery.

B. A delivery procedure code should not be used for a woman who has delivered prior to admission to the hospital. Any postpartum repairs should be coded.

5.7. The Postpartum Period

A. The postpartum period begins immediately after delivery and continues for 6 weeks following delivery.

B. A postpartum complication is any complication occurring within the 6 week period.

C. Chapter 11 codes may also be used to describe pregnancy-related complications after the 6 week period should the physician document that a condition is pregnancy related.

D. Postpartum complications that occur during the same admission as the delivery are identified with a fifth digit of "2". Subsequent admissions for postpartum complications should identified with a fifth digit of "4".

E. When the mother delivers outside the hospital prior to admission and is admitted for routine postpartum care and no complications are noted, code V24.0, Postpartum care and

examination immediately after delivery, should be assigned as the principal diagnosis.

5.8. Abortions

A. Fifth-digits are required for abortion categories 634-637. Fifth-digit 1, incomplete, indicates that all of the products of conception have not been expelled from the uterus. Fifth-digit 2, complete, indicates that all products of conception have been expelled from the uterus prior to the episode of care.

B. A code from categories 640-648 and 651-657 may be used as additional codes with an abortion code to indicate the complication leading to the abortion.

Fifth digit 3 is assigned with codes from these categories when used with an abortion code because the other fifth digits will not apply. Codes from the 660-669 series are not to be used for complications of abortion.

C. Code 639 is to be used for all complications following abortion. Code 639 cannot be assigned with codes from categories 634-638.

D. Abortion with Liveborn Fetus. When an attempted termination of pregnancy results in a liveborn fetus assign code 644.21, Early onset of delivery, with an appropriate code from category V27, Outcome of Delivery. The procedure code for the attempted termination of pregnancy should also be assigned.

E. Retained Products of Conception following an abortion. Subsequent admissions for retained products of conception following a spontaneous or legally induced abortion are assigned the appropriate code from category 634, Spontaneous abortion, or legally induced abortion, with a fifth digit of "1" (incomplete). This advice is appropriate even when the patient was discharged previously with a discharge diagnosis of complete abortion.

5.9. Code 677, Late effect of complication of pregnancy, childbirth, and the puerperium

A. Code 677, Late effect of complication of pregnancy, childbirth, and the puerperium is for use in those cases when an initial complication of a pregnancy develops a sequelae requiring care or treatment at a future date.

B. This code may be used at any time after the initial postpartum period.

C. This code, like all late effect codes, is to be sequenced following the code describing the sequelae of the complication.

6. NEWBORN GUIDELINES

Definition

The newborn period is defined as beginning at birth and lasting through the 28th day following birth.

The following guidelines are provided for reporting purposes. Hospitals may record other diagnoses as needed for internal data use.

General Rule

All clinically significant conditions noted on routine newborn examination should be coded. A condition is clinically significant if it requires:

- clinical evaluation; or
- therapeutic treatment; or
- diagnostic procedures; or
- extended length of hospital stay; or
- increased nursing care and/or monitoring; or
- has implications for future health care needs.

Note: The newborn guidelines listed above are the same as the general coding guidelines for "other diagnoses," except for the final bullet regarding implications for future health care needs. Whether or not a condition is clinically significant can only be determined by the physician.

6.1. Use of Codes V30-V39

When coding the birth of an infant, assign a code from categories V30-V39, according to the type of birth. A code from this series is assigned as a principal diagnosis, and assigned only once to a newborn at the time of birth.

6.2. Newborn Transfers

If the newborn is transferred to another institution, the V30 series is not used.

6.3. Use of Category V29

A. Assign a code from category V29, Observation and evaluation of newborns and infants for suspected conditions not found, to identify those instances when a healthy newborn is evaluated for a suspected condition that is determined after study not to be present. Do not use a code from category V29 when the patient has identified signs or symptoms of a suspected problem; in such cases, code the sign or symptom.

B. A V29 code is to be used as a secondary code after the V30, Outcome of delivery, code. It may also be assigned as a principal code for readmissions or encounters when the V30 code no longer applies. It is for use only for healthy newborns and infants for which no condition after study is found to be present.

6.4. Maternal Causes of Perinatal Morbidity

Codes from categories 760-763, Maternal causes of perinatal morbidity and mortality, are assigned only when the maternal condition has actually affected the fetus or newborn. The fact that the mother has an associated medical condition or experiences some complication of pregnancy, labor or delivery does not justify the routine assignment of codes from these categories to the newborn record.

6.5. Congenital Anomalies

Assign an appropriate code from categories 740-759, Congenital Anomalies, when a specific abnormality is diagnosed for an infant. Such abnormalities may occur as a set of symptoms or multiple malformations. A code should be assigned for each presenting manifestation of the syndrome if the syndrome is not specifically indexed in ICD-9-CM.

6.6. Coding of Other (Additional) Diagnoses

A. Assign codes for conditions that require treatment or further investigation, prolong the length of stay, or require resource utilization.

B. Assign codes for conditions that have been specified by the physician as having implications for future health care needs.

NOTE: This guideline should not be used for adult patients.

C. Assign a code for Newborn conditions originating in the perinatal period (categories 760-779), as well as complications arising during the current episode of care classified in other chapters, only if the diagnoses have been documented by the responsible physician at the time of transfer or discharge as having affected the fetus or newborn.

D. Insignificant conditions or signs or symptoms that resolve without treatment are not coded.

6.7. Prematurity and Fetal Growth Retardation

Codes from categories 764 and 765 should not be assigned based solely on recorded birthweight or estimated gestational age, but upon the attending physician's clinical assessment of maturity of the infant.

NOTE: Since physicians may utilize different criteria in determining prematurity, do not code the diagnosis of prematurity unless the physician documents this condition.

7. SEPTICEMIA AND SEPTIC SHOCK

When the diagnosis of septicemia with shock or the diagnosis of general sepsis with septic shock is documented, code and list the septicemia first and report the septic shock code as a secondary condition. The septicemia code assignment should identify the type of bacteria if it is known.

Sepsis and septic shock associated with abortion, ectopic pregnancy, and molar pregnancy are classified to category codes in Chapter 11 (630-639).

Negative or inconclusive blood cultures do not preclude a diagnosis of septicemia in patients with clinical evidence of the condition.

8. TRAUMA

8.1. Coding for Multiple Injuries

When coding multiple injuries such as fracture of tibia and fibula, assign separate codes for each injury unless a combination code is provided, in which case the combination code is assigned. Multiple injury codes are provided in ICD-9-CM, but should not be assigned unless information for a more specific code is not available.

A. The code for the most serious injury, as determined by the physician, is sequenced first.

B. Superficial injuries such as abrasions or contusions are not coded when associated with more severe injuries of the same site.

C. When a primary injury results in minor damage to peripheral nerves or blood vessels, the primary injury is sequenced first with additional code(s) from categories 950-957, Injury to nerves and spinal cord, and/or 900-904, Injury to blood vessels. When the primary injury is to the blood vessels or nerves, that injury should be sequenced first.

8.2. Coding for Multiple Fractures

The principle of multiple coding of injuries should be followed in coding multiple fractures. Multiple fractures of specified sites are coded individually by site in accordance with both the provisions within categories 800-829 and the level of detail furnished by medical record content. Combination categories for multiple fractures are provided for use when there is insufficient detail in the medical record (such as trauma cases transferred to another hospital), when the reporting form limits the number of codes that can be used in reporting pertinent clinical data, or when there is insufficient specificity at the fourth-digit or fifth-digit level. More specific guidelines are as follows:

A. Multiple fractures of same limb classifiable to the same three-digit or four-digit category are coded to that category.

B. Multiple unilateral or bilateral fractures of same bone(s) but classified to different fourth-digit subdivisions (bone part) within the same three-digit category are coded individually by site.

C. Multiple fracture categories 819 and 828 classify bilateral fractures of both upper limbs (819) and both lower limbs (828), but without any detail at the fourth-digit level other than open and closed type of fractures.

D. Multiple fractures are sequenced in accordance with the severity of the fracture and the physician should be asked to list the fracture diagnoses in the order of severity.

8.3. Current Burns and Encounters for Late Effects of Burns

Current burns (940-948) are classified by depth, extent and, if desired, by agent (E code). By depth burns are classified as first degree (erythema), second degree (blistering), and third degree (full-thickness involvement).

A. All burns are coded with the highest degree of burn sequenced first.

B. Classify burns of the same local site (three-digit category level, (940-947) but of different degrees to the subcategory identifying the highest degree recorded in the diagnosis.

C. Non-healing burns are coded as acute burns. Necrosis of burned skin should be coded as a non-healed burn.

D. Assign code 958.3, Posttraumatic wound infection, not elsewhere classified, as an additional code for any documented infected burn site.

E. When coding multiple burns, assign separate codes for each burn site. Category 946 Burns of Multiple specified sites, should only be used if the location of the burns are not documented. Category 949, Burn, unspecified, is extremely vague and should rarely be used.

F. Assign codes from category 948, Burns classified according to extent of body surface involved, when the site of the burn is not specified or when there is a need for additional data. It is advisable to use category 948 as additional coding when needed to provide data for evaluating burn mortality, such as that needed by burn units. It is also advisable to use category 948 as an additional code for reporting purposes when there is mention of a third-degree burn involving 20 percent or more of the body surface. In assigning a code from category 948:

- Four-digit codes are used to identify the percentage of total body surface involved in a burn (all degree).

- Fifth-digits are assigned to identify the percentage of body surface involved in third-degree burn.

- Fifth-digit zero (0) is assigned when less than 10 percent or when no body surface is involved in a third-degree burn.

Category 948 is based on the classic "rule of nines" in estimating body surface involved: head and neck are assigned nine percent, each arm nine percent, each leg 18 percent, the anterior trunk 18 percent, posterior trunk 18 percent, and genitalia one percent. Physicians may change these percentage assignments where necessary to accommodate infants and children who have proportionately larger heads than adults and patients who have large buttocks, thighs, or abdomen that involve burns.

G. Encounters for the treatment of the late effects of burns (i.e., scars or joint contractures) should be coded to the residual condition (sequelae) followed by the appropriate late effect code (906.5-906.9). A late effect E code may also be used, if desired.

H. When appropriate, both a sequelae with a late effect code, and a current burn code may be assigned on the same record.

8.4. Debridement of Wound, Infection, or Burn

A. For coding purposes, excisional debridement, 86.22, is assigned only when the procedure is performed by a physician.

B. For coding purposes, nonexcisional debridement performed by the physician or nonphysician health care professional is assigned to 86.28. Any "excisional" type procedure performed by a nonphysician is assigned to 86.   28.

9. ADVERSE EFFECTS AND POISONING

The properties of certain drugs, medicinal and biological substances or combinations of such substances, may cause toxic reactions. The occurrence of drug toxicity is classified in ICD-9-CM as follows:

9.1. Adverse Effect

When the drug was correctly prescribed and properly administered, code the reaction plus the appropriate code from the E930-E949 series.

Adverse effects of therapeutic substances correctly prescribed and properly administered (toxicity, synergistic reaction, side effect, and idiosyncratic reaction) may be due to (1) differences among patients, such as age, sex, disease, and genetic factors, and (2) drug-related factors, such as type of drug, route of administration, duration of therapy, dosage, and bioavailability.

Codes from the E930-E949 series must be used to identify the causative substance for an adverse effect of drug, medicinal and biological substances, correctly prescribed and properly administered. The effect, such as tachycardia, delirium, gastrointestinal hemorrhaging, vomiting, hypokalemia, hepatitis, renal failure, or respiratory failure, is coded and followed by the appropriate code from the E930-E949 series.

9.2. Poisoning

Poisoning when an error was made in drug prescription or in the administration of the drug by physician, nurse, patient, or other person, use the appropriate code from the 960-979 series. If an overdose of a drug was intentionally taken or administered and resulted in drug toxicity, it would be coded as a poisoning (960-979 series). If a nonprescribed drug or medicinal agent was taken in combination with a correctly prescribed and properly administered drug, any drug toxicity or other reaction resulting from the interaction of the two drugs would be classified as a poisoning.

10. HUMAN IMMUNODEFICIENCY VIRUS (HIV) INFECTIONS

10.1. Code only confirmed cases of HIV infection/illness.

This is an exception to guideline 1.8 which states "If the diagnosis documented at the time of discharge is qualified as 'probable,' 'suspected,' 'likely,' 'questionable,' 'possible,' or 'still to be ruled out,' code the condition as if it existed or was established..."

In this context, "confirmation" does not require documentation of positive serology or culture for HIV; the physician's diagnostic statement that the patient is HIV positive, or has an HIV-related illness is sufficient.

10.2. Selection of HIV code

042 Human Immunodeficiency Virus [HIV] Disease

Patients with an HIV-related illness should be coded to 042, Human Immunodeficiency Virus [HIV] Disease.

V08 Asymptomatic Human Immunodeficiency Virus [HIV] Infection

Patients with physician-documented asymptomatic HIV infections who have never had an HIV-related illness should be coded to V08, Asymptomatic Human Immunodeficiency Virus [HIV] Infection.

795.71   Nonspecific Serologic Evidence of Human Immunodeficiency Virus [HIV]

Code 795.71, Nonspecific serologic evidence of human immunodeficiency virus [HIV], should be used for patients (including infants) with inconclusive HIV test results.

10.3. Previously diagnosed HIV-related illness

Patients with any known prior diagnosis of an HIV-related illness should be coded to 042. Once a patient had developed an HIV-related illness, the patient should always be assigned code 042 on every subsequent admission. Patients previously diagnosed with any HIV illness (042) should never be assigned to 795.71 or V 08.

10.4. Sequencing

The sequencing of diagnoses for patients with HIV-related illnesses follows guideline 2 for selection of principal diagnosis. That is, the circumstances of admission govern the selection of principal diagnosis, "that condition established after study to be chiefly responsible for occasioning the admission of the patient to the hospital for care."

Patients who are admitted for an HIV-related illness should be assigned a minimum of two codes: first assign code 042 to identify the HIV disease and then sequence additional codes to identify the other diagnoses. If a patient is admitted for an HIV-related condition, the principal diagnosis should be 042, followed by additional diagnosis codes for all reported HIV-related conditions.

If a patient with HIV disease is admitted for an unrelated condition (such as a traumatic injury), the code for the unrelated condition (e.g., the nature of injury code) should be the principal diagnosis. Other diagnoses would be 042 followed by additional diagnosis codes for all reported HIV-related conditions.

Whether the patient is newly diagnosed or has had previous admissions for HIV conditions (or has expired) is irrelevant to the sequencing decision.

10.5. HIV Infection in Pregnancy, Childbirth and the Puerperium

During pregnancy, childbirth or the puerperium, a patient admitted because of an HIV-related illness should receive a principal diagnosis of 647.6X, Other specified infectious and parasitic diseases in the mother classifiable elsewhere, but complicating the pregnancy, childbirth or the puerperium, followed by 042 and the code(s) for the HIV-related illness(es). This is an exception to the sequencing rule found in 10.4 above.

Patients with asymptomatic HIV infection status admitted during pregnancy, childbirth, or the puerperium should receive codes of 647.6X and V08.

10.6. Asymptomatic HIV Infection

V08 Asymptomatic human immunodeficiency virus [HIV] infection, is to be applied when the patient without any documentation of symptoms is listed as being "HIV positive," "known HIV," "HIV test positive," or similar terminology. Do not use this code if the term "AIDS" is used or if the patient is treated for any HIV-related illness or is described as having any condition(s) resulting from his/her HIV positive status; use 042 in these cases.

10.7. Inconclusive Laboratory Test for HIV

Patients with inconclusive HIV serology, but no definitive diagnosis or manifestations of the illness may be assigned code 795.71.Inconclusive serologic test for Human Immunodeficiency Virus [HIV]

10.8. Testing for HIV

If the patient is asymptomatic but wishes to know his/her HIV status, use code V73.89, Screening for other specified viral disease. Use code V69.8, Other problems related to lifestyle, as a secondary code if an asymptomatic patient is in a known high-risk group for HIV. Should a patient with signs or symptoms or illness, or a confirmed HIV related diagnosis be tested for HIV code the signs and symptoms or the diagnosis. An additional counseling code V65.44 may be used if counseling is provided during the encounter for the test.

When the patient returns to be informed of his/her HIV test results use code V65.44, HIV counseling, if the results of the test are negative. If the results are positive but the patient is asymptomatic use code V08, Asymptomatic HIV infection. If the results are positive and the patient is symptomatic use code 042, HIV infection, with codes for the HIV related symptoms or diagnosis. The HIV counseling code may also be used if counseling is provided for patients with positive test results.

11. GUIDELINES FOR CODING EXTERNAL CAUSES OF INJURIES, POISONINGS AND ADVERSE EFFECTS OF DRUGS (E Codes)

Introduction

These guidelines are provided for those who are currently collecting E codes in order that there will be standardization in the process. If your institution plans to begin collecting E codes, these guidelines are to be applied. The use of E codes are supplemental to the application of basic ICD-9-CM codes. E codes are never to be recorded as principal diagnosis (first listed in the outpatient setting) and are not required for reporting to the Health Care Financing Administration.

Injuries are a major cause of mortality, morbidity and disability. In the United States, the care of patients who suffer intentional and unintentional injuries and poisonings contributes significantly to the increase in medical care costs. External causes of injury and poisoning codes (E codes) are intended to provide data for injury research and evaluation of injury prevention strategies. E codes capture how the injury or poisoning happened (cause), the intent (unintentional or accidental; or intentional, such as suicide or assault), and the place where the event occurred. Some major categories of E codes include:

- transport accidents
- poisoning and adverse effects of drugs, medicinal substances and biologicals
- accidental falls
- accidents caused by fire and flames
- accidents due to natural and environmental factors
- late effects of accidents, assaults or self injury
- assaults or purposely inflicted injury
- suicide or self inflicted injury

These guidelines apply for the coding and collection of E code from records in hospitals, outpatient clinics, emergency departments, other ambulatory care settings and physician offices except when other specific guidelines apply. (See Reporting Diagnostic Guidelines for Hospital-based Outpatient Services/Reporting Requirements for Physician Billing.)

11.1. General E Code Coding Guidelines

A. An E code may be used with any code in the range of 001-V83.89 which indicates an injury, poisoning, or adverse effect due to an external cause.

B. Assign the appropriate E-code for all initial treatments of an injury, poisoning, or adverse effect of drugs.

C. Use a late effect E code for subsequent visits when a late effect of the initial injury or poisoning is being treated. There is no late effect E code for adverse effects of drugs.

D. Use the full range of E codes to completely describe the cause, the intent and the place of occurrence, if applicable, for all injuries, poisonings, and adverse effects of drugs.

E. Assign as many E codes as necessary to fully explain each cause. If only one E code can be recorded, assign the E code most related to the principal diagnosis.

F. The selection of the appropriate E code is guided by the Index to External Causes which is located after the alphabetical index to diseases and by Inclusion and Exclusion notes in the Tabular List.

G. An E code can never be a principal (first listed) diagnosis.

11.2. Place of Occurrence Guideline

Use an additional code from category E849 to indicate the Place of Occurrence for injuries and poisonings. The Place of Occurrence describes the place where the event occurred and not the patient's activity at the time of the event.

Do not use E849.9 if the place of occurrence is not stated.

11.3. Poisonings and Adverse Effects of Drugs, Medicinal and Biological Substances Guidelines

A. Do not code directly from the Table of Drugs and Chemicals. Always refer back to the Tabular List.

B. Use as many codes as necessary to describe completely all drugs, medicinal or biological substances.

C. If the same E code would describe the causative agent for more than one adverse reaction, assign the code only once.

D. If two or more drugs, medicinal or biological substances are reported, code each individually unless the combination code is listed in the Table of Drugs and Chemicals. In that case, assign the E code for the combination.

E. When a reaction results from the interaction of a drug(s) and alcohol, use poisoning codes and E codes for both.

F. If the reporting format limits the number of E codes that can be used in reporting clinical data, code the one most related to the principal diagnosis. Include at least one from each category (cause, intent, place) if possible.

- If there are different fourth digit codes in the same three digit category, use the code for "Other specified" of that category. If there is no "Other specified" code in that category, use the appropriate "Unspecified" code in that category.

- If the codes are in different three digit categories, assign the appropriate E code for other multiple drugs and medicinal substances.

11.4. Multiple Cause E Code Coding Guidelines

If two or more events cause separate injuries, an E code should be assigned for each cause. The first listed E code will be selected in the following order:

- E codes for child and adult abuse take priority over all other E code—see Child and Adult abuse guidelines
- E codes for cataclysmic events take priority over all other E codes except child and adult abuse
- E codes for transport accidents take priority over all other E codes except cataclysmic events and child and adult abuse

The first listed E code should correspond to the cause of the most serious diagnosis due to an assault, accident, or self-harm, following the order of hierarchy listed above.

11.5. Child and Adult Abuse Guideline

A. When the cause of an injury or neglect is intentional child or adult abuse, the first listed E code should be assigned from categories E960-E968, Homicide and injury purposely inflicted by other persons, (except category E967). An E code from category E967, Child and adult battering and other maltreatment, should be added as an additional code to identify the perpetrator, if known.

B. In cases of neglect when the intent is determined to be accidental E code E904.0, Abandonment or neglect of infant and helpless person, should be the first listed E code.

11.6. Unknown or Suspected Intent Guideline

A. If the intent (accident, self-harm, assault) of the cause of an injury or poisoning is unknown or unspecified, code the intent as undetermined E980-E989.

B. If the intent (accident, self-harm, assault) of the cause of an injury or poisoning is questionable, probable or suspected, code the intent as undetermined E980-E989.

11.7. Undetermined Cause

When the intent of an injury or poisoning is known, but the cause is unknown, use codes: E928.9, Unspecified accident, E958.9, Suicide and self-inflicted injury by unspecified means, and E968.9, Assault by unspecified means.

These E codes should rarely be used as the documentation in the medical record, in both the inpatient and outpatient settings, should normally provide sufficient detail to determine the cause of the injury.

11.8. Late Effects of External Cause Guidelines

A. Late effect E codes exist for injuries and poisonings but not for adverse effects of drugs, misadventures and surgical complications.

B. A late effect E code (E929, E959, E969, E977, E989, or E999) should be used with any report of a late effect or sequela resulting from a previous injury or poisoning (905-909).

C. A late effect E code should nev er be used with a related current nature of injury code.

11.9. Misadventures and Complications of Care Guidelines

A. Assign a code in the range of E870-E876 if misadventures are stated by the physician.

B. Assign a code in the range of E878-E879 if the physician attributes an abnormal reaction or later complication to a surgical or medical procedure, but does not mention misadventure at the time of the procedure as the cause of the reaction.

A

AAV (disease) (illness) (infection) — *see* Human immunodeficiency virus (disease) (illness) (infection)

Abactio — *see* Abortion, induced

Abactus venter — *see* Abortion, induced

Abarognosis 781.99

Abasia (-astasia) 307.9
  atactica 781.3
  choreic 781.3
  hysterical 300.11
  paroxysmal trepidant 781.3
  spastic 781.3
  trembling 781.3
  trepidans 781.3

Abderhalden-Kaufmann-Lignac syndrome (cystinosis) 270.0

Abdomen, abdominal — *see also* condition
  accordion 306.4
  acute 789.0 ✔5ᵗʰ
    angina 557.1
  burst 868.00
  convulsive equivalent (*see also* Epilepsy) 345.5 ✔5ᵗʰ
  heart 746.87
  muscle deficiency syndrome 756.79
  obstipum 756.79

Abdominalgia 789.0 ✔5ᵗʰ
  periodic 277.3

Abduction contracture, hip or other joint — *see* Contraction, joint

Abercrombie's syndrome (amyloid degeneration) 277.3

Aberrant (congenital) — *see also* Malposition, congenital
  adrenal gland 759.1
  blood vessel NEC 747.60
    arteriovenous NEC 747.60
    cerebrovascular 747.81
    gastrointestinal 747.61
    lower limb 747.64
    renal 747.62
    spinal 747.82
    upper limb 747.63
  breast 757.6
  endocrine gland NEC 759.2
  gastrointestinal vessel (peripheral) 747.61
  hepatic duct 751.69
  lower limb vessel (peripheral) 747.64
  pancreas 751.7
  parathyroid gland 759.2
  peripheral vascular vessel NEC 747.60
  pituitary gland (pharyngeal) 759.2
  renal blood vessel 747.62
  sebaceous glands, mucous membrane, mouth 750.26
  spinal vessel 747.82
  spleen 759.0
  testis (descent) 752.51
  thymus gland 759.2
  thyroid gland 759.2
  upper limb vessel (perpipheral) 747.63

Aberratio
  lactis 757.6
  testis 752.51

Aberration — *see also* Anomaly
  chromosome — *see* Anomaly, chromosome(s)
  distantial 368.9
  mental (*see also* Disorder, mental, nonpsychotic) 300.9

Abetalipoproteinemia 272.5

Abionarce 780.79

Abiotrophy 799.8

Ablatio
  placentae — *see* Placenta, ablatio
  retinae (*see also* Detachment, retina) 361.9

Ablation
  pituitary (gland) (with hypofunction) 253.7
  placenta — *see* Placenta, ablatio
  uterus 621.8

Ablepharia, ablepharon, ablephary 743.62

Ablepsia — *see* Blindness

Ablepsy — *see* Blindness

Ablutomania 300.3

Abnormal, abnormality, abnormalities — *see also* Anomaly
  acid-base balance 276.4
    fetus or newborn — *see* Distress, fetal
  adaptation curve, dark 368.63
  alveolar ridge 525.9
  amnion 658.9 ✔5ᵗʰ
    affecting fetus or newborn 762.9
  anatomical relationship NEC 759.9
  apertures, congenital, diaphragm 756.6
  auditory perception NEC 388.40
  autosomes NEC 758.5
    13 758.1
    18 758.2
    21 or 22 758.0
    D₁ 758.1
    E₃ 758.2
    G 758.0
  ballistocardiogram 794.39
  basal metabolic rate (BMR) 794.7
  biosynthesis, testicular androgen 257.2
  blood level (of)
    cobalt 790.6
    copper 790.6
    iron 790.6
    lithium 790.6
    magnesium 790.6
    mineral 790.6
    zinc 790.6
  blood pressure
    elevated (without diagnosis of hypertension) 796.2
    low (*see also* Hypotension) 458.9
      reading (incidental) (isolated) (nonspecific) 796.3
  bowel sounds 787.5
  breathing behavior — *see* Respiration
  caloric test 794.19
  cervix (acquired) NEC 622.9
    congenital 752.40
    in pregnancy or childbirth 654.6 ✔5ᵗʰ
      causing obstructed labor 660.2 ✔5ᵗʰ
        affecting fetus or newborn 763.1
  chemistry, blood NEC 790.6
  chest sounds 786.7
  chorion 658.9 ✔5ᵗʰ
    affecting fetus or newborn 762.9
  chromosomal NEC 758.89
    analysis, nonspecific result 795.2
    autosomes (*see also* Abnormal, autosomes NEC) 758.5
    fetal, (suspected) affecting management of pregnancy 655.1 ✔5ᵗʰ
    sex 758.81
  clinical findings NEC 796.4
  communication — *see* Fistula
  configuration of pupils 379.49
  coronary
    artery 746.85
    vein 746.9
  cortisol-binding globulin 255.8
  course, Eustachian tube 744.24
  dentofacial NEC 524.9
    functional 524.5
    specified type NEC 524.8
  development, developmental NEC 759.9
    bone 756.9
    central nervous system 742.9
  direction, teeth 524.3
  Dynia (*see also* Defect, coagulation) 286.9
  Ebstein 746.2
  echocardiogram 793.2
  echoencephalogram 794.01
  echogram NEC — *see* Findings, abnormal, structure
  electrocardiogram (ECG) (EKG) 794.31
  electroencephalogram (EEG) 794.02
  electromyogram (EMG) 794.17
    ocular 794.14
  electro-oculogram (EOG) 794.12
  electroretinogram (ERG) 794.11
  erythrocytes 289.9
    congenital, with perinatal jaundice 282.9 [774.0]
  Eustachian valve 746.9
  excitability under minor stress 301.9

Abnormal, abnormality, abnormalities — *see also* Anomaly — *continued*
  fat distribution 782.9
  feces 787.7
  fetal heart rate — *see* Distress, fetal
  fetus NEC
    affecting management of pregnancy — *see* Pregnancy, management affected by, fetal
    causing disproportion 653.7 ✔5ᵗʰ
      affecting fetus or newborn 763.1
      causing obstructed labor 660.1 ✔5ᵗʰ
        affecting fetus or newborn 763.1
    findings without manifest disease — *see* Findings, abnormal
  fluid
    amniotic 792.3
    cerebrospinal 792.0
    peritoneal 792.9
    pleural 792.9
    synovial 792.9
    vaginal 792.9
  forces of labor NEC 661.9 ✔5ᵗʰ
    affecting fetus or newborn 763.7
  form, teeth 520.2
  function studies
    auditory 794.15
    bladder 794.9
    brain 794.00
    cardiovascular 794.30
    endocrine NEC 794.6
    kidney 794.4
    liver 794.8
    nervous system
      central 794.00
      peripheral 794.19
    oculomotor 794.14
    pancreas 794.9
    placenta 794.9
    pulmonary 794.2
    retina 794.11
    special senses 794.19
    spleen 794.9
    thyroid 794.5
    vestibular 794.16
  gait 781.2
    hysterical 300.11
  gastrin secretion 251.5
  globulin
    cortisol-binding 255.8
    thyroid-binding 246.8
  glucagon secretion 251.4
  glucose tolerance test 790.2
    in pregnancy, childbirth, or puerperium 648.8 ✔5ᵗʰ
      fetus or newborn 775.0
  gravitational (G) forces or states 994.9
  hair NEC 704.2
  hard tissue formation in pulp 522.3
  head movement 781.0
  heart
    rate
      fetus, affecting liveborn infant
        before the onset of labor 763.81
        during labor 763.82
        unspecified as to time of onset 763.83
      intrauterine
        before the onset of labor 763.81
        during labor 763.82
        unspecified as to time of onset 763.83
      newborn
        before the onset of labor 763.81
        during labor 763.82
        unspecified as to time of onset 763.83
    shadow 793.2
    sounds NEC 785.3
  hemoglobin (*see also* Disease, hemoglobin) 282.7
    trait — *see* Trait, hemoglobin, abnormal
  hemorrhage, uterus — *see* Hemorrhage, uterus
  histology NEC 795.4
  increase
    in
      appetite 783.6
      development 783.9
  involuntary movement 781.0
  jaw closure 524.5

AAV — Abnormal

Abnormal, abnormality, abnormalities — *see also* Anomaly — *continued*
karyotype 795.2
knee jerk 796.1
labor NEC 661.9 ✓5ᵗʰ
   affecting fetus or newborn 763.7
laboratory findings — *see* Findings, abnormal
length, organ or site, congenital — *see* Distortion
loss of height 781.91
loss of weight 783.21
lung shadow 793.1
mammogram 793.80
   microcalcification 793.81
Mantoux test 795.5
membranes (fetal)
   affecting fetus or newborn 762.9
   complicating pregnancy 658.8 ✓5ᵗʰ
menstruation — *see* Menstruation
metabolism (*see also* condition) 783.9
movement 781.0
   disorder NEC 333.90
      specified NEC 333.99
   head 781.0
   involuntary 781.0
   specified type NEC 333.99
muscle contraction, localized 728.85
myoglobin (Aberdeen) (Annapolis) 289.9
narrowness, eyelid 743.62
optokinetic response 379.57
organs or tissues of pelvis NEC
   in pregnancy or childbirth 654.9 ✓5ᵗʰ
      affecting fetus or newborn 763.89
      causing obstructed labor 660.2 ✓5ᵗʰ
         affecting fetus or newborn 763.1
origin — *see* Malposition, congenital
palmar creases 757.2
Papanicolaou (smear)
   cervix 795.00 ▲
      atypical squamous cell changes of undetermined significance ●
      favor benign (ASCUS favor benign) 795.01 ●
      favor dysplasia (ASCUS favor dysplasia) 795.02 ●
      nonspecific finding NEC 795.09 ●
   other site 795.1
parturition
   affecting fetus or newborn 763.9
   mother — *see* Delivery, complicated
pelvis (bony) — *see* Deformity, pelvis
percussion, chest 786.7
periods (grossly) (*see also* Menstruation) 626.9
phonocardiogram 794.39
placenta — *see* Placenta, abnormal
plantar reflex 796.1
plasma protein — *see* Deficiency, plasma, protein
pleural folds 748.8
position — *see also* Malposition
   gravid uterus 654.4 ✓5ᵗʰ
      causing obstructed labor 660.2 ✓5ᵗʰ
      affecting fetus or newborn 763.1
posture NEC 781.92
presentation (fetus) — *see* Presentation, fetus, abnormal
product of conception NEC 631
puberty — *see* Puberty
pulmonary
   artery 747.3
   function, newborn 770.89 ▲
   test results 794.2
   ventilation, newborn 770.89 ▲
      hyperventilation 786.01
pulsations in neck 785.1
pupil reflexes 379.40
quality of milk 676.8 ✓5ᵗʰ
radiological examination 793.9
   abdomen NEC 793.6
   biliary tract 793.3
   breast 793.89
      mammogram NOS 793.80
      mammographic microcalcification 793.81
   gastrointestinal tract 793.4
   genitourinary organs 793.5
   head 793.0
   intrathoracic organ NEC 793.2

Abnormal, abnormality, abnormalities — *see also* Anomaly — *continued*
radiological examination — *continued*
   lung (field) 793.1
   musculoskeletal system 793.7
   retroperitoneum 793.6
   skin and subcutaneous tissue 793.9
   skull 793.0
red blood cells 790.09
   morphology 790.09
   volume 790.09
reflex NEC 796.1
renal function test 794.4
respiration signs — *see* Respiration
response to nerve stimulation 794.10
retinal correspondence 368.34
rhythm, heart — *see also* Arrhythmia
   fetus — *see* Distress, fetal
saliva 792.4
scan
   brain 794.09
   kidney 794.4
   liver 794.8
   lung 794.2
   thyroid 794.5
secretion
   gastrin 251.5
   glucagon 251.4
semen 792.2
serum level (of)
   acid phosphatase 790.5
   alkaline phosphatase 790.5
   amylase 790.5
   enzymes NEC 790.5
   lipase 790.5
shape
   cornea 743.41
   gallbladder 751.69
   gravid uterus 654.4 ✓5ᵗʰ
      affecting fetus or newborn 763.89
      causing obstructed labor 660.2 ✓5ᵗʰ
         affecting fetus or newborn 763.1
   head (*see also* Anomaly, skull) 756.0
   organ or site, congenital NEC — *see* Distortion
sinus venosus 747.40
size
   fetus, complicating delivery 653.5 ✓5ᵗʰ
      causing obstructed labor 660.1 ✓5ᵗʰ
   gallbladder 751.69
   head (*see also* Anomaly, skull) 756.0
   organ or site, congenital NEC — *see* Distortion
   teeth 520.2
skin and appendages, congenital NEC 757.9
soft parts of pelvis — *see* Abnormal, organs or tissues of pelvis
spermatozoa 792.2
sputum (amount) (color) (excessive) (odor) (purulent) 786.4
stool NEC 787.7
   bloody 578.1
      occult 792.1
   bulky 787.7
   color (dark) (light) 792.1
   content (fat) (mucus) (pus) 792.1
   occult blood 792.1
synchondrosis 756.9
test results without manifest disease — *see* Findings, abnormal
thebesian valve 746.9
thermography — *see* Findings, abnormal, structure
threshold, cones or rods (eye) 368.63
thyroid-binding globulin 246.8
thyroid product 246.8
toxicology (findings) NEC 796.0
tracheal cartilage (congenital) 748.3
transport protein 273.8
ultrasound results — *see* Findings, abnormal, structure
umbilical cord
   affecting fetus or newborn 762.6
   complicating delivery 663.9 ✓5ᵗʰ
   specified NEC 663.8 ✓5ᵗʰ
union
   cricoid cartilage and thyroid cartilage 748.3
   larynx and trachea 748.3

Abnormal, abnormality, abnormalities — *see also* Anomaly — *continued*
union — *continued*
   thyroid cartilage and hyoid bone 748.3
urination NEC 788.69
   psychogenic 306.53
   stream
      intermittent 788.61
      slowing 788.62
      splitting 788.61
      weak 788.62
urine (constituents) NEC 791.9
uterine hemorrhage (*see also* Hemorrhage, uterus) 626.9
   climacteric 627.0
   postmenopausal 627.1
vagina (acquired) (congenital)
   in pregnancy or childbirth 654.7 ✓5ᵗʰ
      affecting fetus or newborn 763.89
      causing obstructed labor 660.2 ✓5ᵗʰ
         affecting fetus or newborn 763.1
vascular sounds 785.9
vectorcardiogram 794.39
visually evoked potential (VEP) 794.13
vulva (acquired) (congenital)
   in pregnancy or childbirth 654.8 ✓5ᵗʰ
      affecting fetus or newborn 763.89
      causing obstructed labor 660.2 ✓5ᵗʰ
         affecting fetus or newborn 763.1
weight
   gain 783.1
      of pregnancy 646.1 ✓5ᵗʰ
         with hypertension — *see* Toxemia, of pregnancy
   loss 783.21
x-ray examination — *see* Abnormal, radiological examination

Abnormally formed uterus — *see* Anomaly, uterus

Abnormity (any organ or part) — *see* Anomaly

ABO
hemolytic disease 773.1
incompatibility reaction 999.6

Abocclusion 524.2

Abolition, language 784.69

Aborter, habitual or recurrent NEC
without current pregnancy 629.9
current abortion (*see also* Abortion, spontaneous) 634.9 ✓5ᵗʰ
   affecting fetus or newborn 761.8
observation in current pregnancy 646.3 ✓5ᵗʰ

Abortion (complete) (incomplete) (inevitable) (with retained products of conception) 637.9 ✓5ᵗʰ

> *Note* — *Use the following fifth-digit subclassification with categories 634–637:*
>
> 0   unspecified
> 1   incomplete
> 2   complete

with
   complication(s) (any) following previous abortion — *see* category 639 ✓4ᵗʰ
   damage to pelvic organ (laceration) (rupture) (tear) 637.2 ✓5ᵗʰ
   embolism (air) (amniotic fluid) (blood clot) (pulmonary) (pyemic) (septic) (soap) 637.6 ✓5ᵗʰ
   genital tract and pelvic infection 637.0 ✓5ᵗʰ
   hemorrhage, delayed or excessive 637.1 ✓5ᵗʰ
   metabolic disorder 637.4 ✓5ᵗʰ
   renal failure (acute) 637.3 ✓5ᵗʰ
   sepsis (genital tract) (pelvic organ) 637.0 ✓5ᵗʰ
      urinary tract 637.7 ✓5ᵗʰ
   shock (postoperative) (septic) 637.5 ✓5ᵗʰ
   specified complication NEC 637.7 ✓5ᵗʰ
   toxemia 637.3 ✓5ᵗʰ
   unspecified complication(s) 637.8 ✓5ᵗʰ
   urinary tract infection 637.7 ✓5ᵗʰ
accidental — *see* Abortion, spontaneous
artificial — *see* Abortion, induced
attempted (failed) — *see* Abortion, failed
criminal — *see* Abortion, illegal
early — *see* Abortion, spontaneous
elective — *see* Abortion, legal

Abortion — *continued*
  failed (legal) 638.9
    with
      damage to pelvic organ (laceration)
        (rupture) (tear) 638.2
      embolism (air) (amniotic fluid) (blood clot)
        (pulmonary) (pyemic) (septic) (soap)
        638.6
      genital tract and pelvic infection 638.0
      hemorrhage, delayed or excessive 638.1
      metabolic disorder 638.4
      renal failure (acute) 638.3
      sepsis (genital tract) (pelvic organ) 638.0
        urinary tract 638.7
      shock (postoperative) (septic) 638.5
      specified complication NEC 638.7
      toxemia 638.3
      unspecified complication(s) 638.8
      urinary tract infection 638.7
  fetal indication — *see* Abortion, legal
  fetus 779.6
  following threatened abortion — *see* Abortion,
    by type
  habitual or recurrent (care during pregnancy)
    646.3 ✓5ᵗʰ
    with current abortion (*see also* Abortion,
      spontaneous) 634.9 ✓5ᵗʰ
    affecting fetus or newborn 761.8
    without current pregnancy 629.9
  homicidal — *see* Abortion, illegal
  illegal 636.9 ✓5ᵗʰ
    with
      damage to pelvic organ (laceration)
        (rupture) (tear) 636.2 ✓5ᵗʰ
      embolism (air) (amniotic fluid) (blood clot)
        (pulmonary) (pyemic) (septic) (soap)
        636.6 ✓5ᵗʰ
      genital tract and pelvic infection
        636.0 ✓5ᵗʰ
      hemorrhage, delayed or excessive
        636.1 ✓5ᵗʰ
      metabolic disorder 636.4 ✓5ᵗʰ
      renal failure 636.3 ✓5ᵗʰ
      sepsis (genital tract) (pelvic organ)
        636.0 ✓5ᵗʰ
        urinary tract 636.7 ✓5ᵗʰ
      shock (postoperative) (septic) 636.5 ✓5ᵗʰ
      specified complication NEC 636.7 ✓5ᵗʰ
      toxemia 636.3 ✓5ᵗʰ
      unspecified complication(s) 636.8 ✓5ᵗʰ
      urinary tract infection 636.7 ✓5ᵗʰ
  fetus 779.6
  induced 637.9 ✓5ᵗʰ
    illegal — *see* Abortion, illegal
    legal indications — *see* Abortion, legal
    medical indications — *see* Abortion, legal
    therapeutic — *see* Abortion, legal
  late — *see* Abortion, spontaneous
  legal (legal indication) (medical indication)
    (under medical supervision) 635.9 ✓5ᵗʰ
    with
      damage to pelvic organ (laceration)
        (rupture) (tear) 635.2 ✓5ᵗʰ
      embolism (air) (amniotic fluid) (blood clot)
        (pulmonary) (pyemic) (septic) (soap)
        635.6 ✓5ᵗʰ
      genital tract and pelvic infection
        635.0 ✓5ᵗʰ
      hemorrhage, delayed or excessive
        635.1 ✓5ᵗʰ
      metabolic disorder 635.4 ✓5ᵗʰ
      renal failure (acute) 635.3 ✓5ᵗʰ
      sepsis (genital tract) (pelvic organ)
        635.0 ✓5ᵗʰ
        urinary tract 635.7 ✓5ᵗʰ
      shock (postoperative) (septic) 635.5 ✓5ᵗʰ
      specified complication NEC 635.7 ✓5ᵗʰ
      toxemia 635.3 ✓5ᵗʰ
      unspecified complication(s) 635.8 ✓5ᵗʰ
      urinary tract infection 635.7 ✓5ᵗʰ
  fetus 779.6
  medical indication — *see* Abortion, legal
  mental hygiene problem — *see* Abortion, legal
  missed 632
  operative — *see* Abortion, legal
  psychiatric indication — *see* Abortion, legal

Abortion — *continued*
  recurrent — *see* Abortion, spontaneous
  self-induced — *see* Abortion, illegal
  septic — *see* Abortion, by type, with sepsis
  spontaneous 634.9 ✓5ᵗʰ
    with
      damage to pelvic organ (laceration)
        (rupture) (tear) 634.2 ✓5ᵗʰ
      embolism (air) (amniotic fluid) (blood clot)
        (pulmonary) (pyemic) (septic) (soap)
        634.6 ✓5ᵗʰ
      genital tract and pelvic infection
        634.0 ✓5ᵗʰ
      hemorrhage, delayed or excessive
        634.1 ✓5ᵗʰ
      metabolic disorder 634.4 ✓5ᵗʰ
      renal failure 634.3 ✓5ᵗʰ
      sepsis (genital tract) (pelvic organ)
        634.0 ✓5ᵗʰ
        urinary tract 634.7 ✓5ᵗʰ
      shock (postoperative) (septic) 634.5 ✓5ᵗʰ
      specified complication NEC 634.7 ✓5ᵗʰ
      toxemia 634.3 ✓5ᵗʰ
      unspecified complication(s) 634.8 ✓5ᵗʰ
      urinary tract infection 634.7 ✓5ᵗʰ
  fetus 761.8
  threatened 640.0 ✓5ᵗʰ
    affecting fetus or newborn 762.1
  surgical — *see* Abortion, legal
  therapeutic — *see* Abortion, legal
  threatened 640.0 ✓5ᵗʰ
    affecting fetus or newborn 762.1
  tubal — *see* Pregnancy, tubal
  voluntary — *see* Abortion, legal

Abortus fever 023.9

Aboulomania 301.6

Abrachia 755.20

Abrachiatism 755.20

Abrachiocephalia 759.89

Abrachiocephalus 759.89

Abrami's disease (acquired hemolytic jaundice)
  283.9

Abramov-Fiedler myocarditis (acute isolated
  myocarditis) 422.91

Abrasion — *see also* Injury, superficial, by site
  cornea 918.1
  dental 521.2
  teeth, tooth (dentifrice) (habitual) (hard tissues)
    (occupational) (ritual) (traditional) (wedge
    defect) 521.2

Abrikossov's tumor (M9580/0) — *see also*
  Neoplasm, connective tissue, benign
  malignant (M9580/3) — *see* Neoplasm,
    connective tissue, malignant

Abrism 988.8

Abruption, placenta — *see* Placenta, abruptio

Abruptio placentae — *see* Placenta, abruptio

Abscess (acute) (chronic) (infectional)
    (lymphangitic) (metastatic) (multiple)
    (pyogenic) (septic) (with lymphangitis) (*see
    also* Cellulitis) 682.9
  abdomen, abdominal
    cavity — *see* Abscess, peritoneum
    wall 682.2
  abdominopelvic — *see* Abscess, peritoneum
  accessory sinus (chronic) (*see also* Sinusitis)
    473.9
  adrenal (capsule) (gland) 255.8
  alveolar 522.5
    with sinus 522.7
  amebic 006.3
    bladder 006.8
    brain (with liver or lung abscess) 006.5
    liver (without mention of brain or lung
      abscess) 006.3
      with
        brain abscess (and lung abscess)
          006.5
        lung abscess 006.4
    lung (with liver abscess) 006.4
      with brain abscess 006.5
    seminal vesicle 006.8
    specified site NEC 006.8
    spleen 006.8

Abscess (*see also* Cellulitis) — *continued*
  anaerobic 040.0
  ankle 682.6
  anorectal 566
  antecubital space 682.3
  antrum (chronic) (Highmore) (*see also* Sinusitis,
    maxillary) 473.0
  anus 566
  apical (tooth) 522.5
    with sinus (alveolar) 522.7
  appendix 540.1
  areola (acute) (chronic) (nonpuerperal) 611.0
    puerperal, postpartum 675.1 ✓5ᵗʰ
  arm (any part, above wrist) 682.3
  artery (wall) 447.2
  atheromatous 447.2
  auditory canal (external) 380.10
  auricle (ear) (staphylococcal) (streptococcal)
    380.10
  axilla, axillary (region) 682.3
    lymph gland or node 683
  back (any part) 682.2
  Bartholin's gland 616.3
    with
      abortion — *see* Abortion, by type, with
        sepsis
      ectopic pregnancy (*see also* categories
        633.0-633.9) 639.0
      molar pregnancy (*see also* categories 630-
        632) 639.0
    complicating pregnancy or puerperium
      646.6 ✓5ᵗʰ
    following
      abortion 639.0
      ectopic or molar pregnancy 639.0
  bartholinian 616.3
  Bezold's 383.01
  bile, biliary, duct or tract (*see also*
    Cholecystitis) 576.8
  bilharziasis 120.1
  bladder (wall) 595.89
    amebic 006.8
  bone (subperiosteal) (*see also* Osteomyelitis)
    730.0 ✓5ᵗʰ
    accessory sinus (chronic) (*see also* Sinusitis)
      473.9
    acute 730.0 ✓5ᵗʰ
    chronic or old 730.1 ✓5ᵗʰ
    jaw (lower) (upper) 526.4
    mastoid — *see* Mastoiditis, acute
    petrous (*see also* Petrositis) 383.20
    spinal (tuberculous) (*see also* Tuberculosis)
      015.0 ✓5ᵗʰ [730.88]
      nontuberculous 730.08
  bowel 569.5
  brain (any part) 324.0
    amebic (with liver or lung abscess) 006.5
    cystic 324.0
    late effect — *see* category 326
    otogenic 324.0
    tuberculous (*see also* Tuberculosis)
      013.3 ✓5ᵗʰ
  breast (acute) (chronic) (nonpuerperal) 611.0
    newborn 771.5
    puerperal, postpartum 675.1 ✓5ᵗʰ
    tuberculous (*see also* Tuberculosis)
      017.9 ✓5ᵗʰ
  broad ligament (chronic) (*see also* Disease,
    pelvis, inflammatory) 614.4
    acute 614.3
  Brodie's (chronic) (localized) (*see also*
    Osteomyelitis) 730.1 ✓5ᵗʰ
  bronchus 519.1
  buccal cavity 528.3
  bulbourethral gland 597.0
  bursa 727.89
    pharyngeal 478.29
  buttock 682.5
  canaliculus, breast 611.0
  canthus 372.20
  cartilage 733.99
  cecum 569.5
    with appendicitis 540.1
  cerebellum, cerebellar 324.0
    late effect — *see* category 326
  cerebral (embolic) 324.0
    late effect — *see* category 326

▲

●

✓4ᵗʰ Fourth-digit Required   ✓5ᵗʰ Fifth-digit Required   ►◄ Revised Text   ● New Line   ▲ Revised Code

Abscess (*see also* Cellulitis) — *continued*
 cervical (neck region) 682.1
  lymph gland or node 683
  stump (*see also* Cervicitis) 616.0
 cervix (stump) (uteri) (*see also* Cervicitis) 616.0
 cheek, external 682.0
  inner 528.3
 chest 510.9
  with fistula 510.0
  wall 682.2
 chin 682.0
 choroid 363.00
 ciliary body 364.3
 circumtonsillar 475
 cold (tuberculous) — *see also* Tuberculosis,
   abscess
  articular — *see* Tuberculosis, joint
 colon (wall) 569.5
 colostomy or enterostomy 569.61
 conjunctiva 372.00
 connective tissue NEC 682.9
 cornea 370.55
  with ulcer 370.00
 corpus
  cavernosum 607.2
  luteum (*see also* Salpingo-oophoritis) 614.2
 Cowper's gland 597.0
 cranium 324.0
 cul-de-sac (Douglas') (posterior) (*see also*
   Disease, pelvis, inflammatory) 614.4
  acute 614.3
 dental 522.5
  with sinus (alveolar) 522.7
 dentoalveolar 522.5
  with sinus (alveolar) 522.7
 diaphragm, diaphragmatic — *see* Abscess,
   peritoneum
 digit NEC 681.9
 Douglas' cul-de-sac or pouch (*see also* Disease,
   pelvis, inflammatory) 614.4
  acute 614.3
 Dubois' 090.5
 ductless gland 259.8
 ear
  acute 382.00
  external 380.10
  inner 386.30
  middle — *see* Otitis media
 elbow 682.3
 endamebic — *see* Abscess, amebic
 entamebic — *see* Abscess, amebic
 enterostomy 569.61
 epididymis 604.0
 epidural 324.9
  brain 324.0
  late effect — *see* category 326
  spinal cord 324.1
 epiglottis 478.79
 epiploon, epiploic — *see* Abscess, peritoneum
 erysipelatous (*see also* Erysipelas) 035
 esophagus 530.19
 ethmoid (bone) (chronic) (sinus) (*see also*
   Sinusitis, ethmoidal) 473.2
 external auditory canal 380.10
 extradural 324.9
  brain 324.0
  late effect — *see* category 326
  spinal cord 324.1
 extraperitoneal — *see* Abscess, peritoneum
 eye 360.00
 eyelid 373.13
 face (any part, except eye) 682.0
 fallopian tube (*see also* Salpingo-oophoritis)
   614.2
 fascia 728.89
 fauces 478.29
 fecal 569.5
 femoral (region) 682.6
 filaria, filarial (*see also* Infestation, filarial)
   125.9
 finger (any) (intrathecal) (periosteal)
   (subcutaneous) (subcuticular) 681.00
 fistulous NEC 682.9
 flank 682.2
 foot (except toe) 682.7
 forearm 682.3
 forehead 682.0

Abscess (*see also* Cellulitis) — *continued*
 frontal (sinus) (chronic) (*see also* Sinusitis,
   frontal) 473.1
 gallbladder (*see also* Cholecystitis, acute) 575.0
 gastric 535.0 ☑5ᵗʰ
 genital organ or tract NEC
  female 616.9
   with
    abortion — *see* Abortion, by type, with
      sepsis
    ectopic pregnancy (*see also* categories
      633.0-633.9) 639.0
    molar pregnancy (*see also* categories
      630-632) 639.0
   following
    abortion 639.0
    ectopic or molar pregnancy 639.0
   puerperal, postpartum, childbirth 670
     ☑5ᵗʰ
  male 608.4
 genitourinary system, tuberculous (*see also*
   Tuberculosis) 016.9 ☑5ᵗʰ
 gingival 523.3
 gland, glandular (lymph) (acute) NEC 683
 glottis 478.79
 gluteal (region) 682.5
 gonorrheal NEC (*see also* Gonococcus) 098.0
 groin 682.2
 gum 523.3
 hand (except finger or thumb) 682.4
 head (except face) 682.8
 heart 429.89
 heel 682.7
 helminthic (*see also* Infestation, by specific
   parasite) 128.9
 hepatic 572.0
  amebic (*see also* Abscess, liver, amebic)
    006.3
  duct 576.8
 hip 682.6
  tuberculous (active) (*see also* Tuberculosis)
    015.1 ☑5ᵗʰ
 ileocecal 540.1
 ileostomy (bud) 569.61
 iliac (region) 682.2
  fossa 540.1
 iliopsoas (tuberculous) (*see also* Tuberculosis)
   015.0 ☑5ᵗʰ *[730.88]*
  nontuberculous 728.89
 infraclavicular (fossa) 682.3
 inguinal (region) 682.2
  lymph gland or node 683
 intersphincteric (anus) 566
 intestine, intestinal 569.5
  rectal 566
 intra-abdominal (*see also* Abscess, peritoneum)
   567.2
  postoperative 998.59
 intracranial 324.0
  late effect — *see* category 326
 intramammary — *see* Abscess, breast
 intramastoid (*see also* Mastoiditis, acute)
   383.00
 intraorbital 376.01
 intraperitoneal — *see* Abscess, peritoneum
 intraspinal 324.1
  late effect — *see* category 326
 intratonsillar 475
 iris 364.3
 ischiorectal 566
 jaw (bone) (lower) (upper) 526.4
  skin 682.0
 joint (*see also* Arthritis, pyogenic) 711.0 ☑5ᵗʰ
  vertebral (tuberculous) (*see also*
    Tuberculosis) 015.0 ☑5ᵗʰ *[730.88]*
  nontuberculous 724.8
 kidney 590.2
  with
   abortion — *see* Abortion, by type, with
     urinary tract infection
   calculus 592.0
   ectopic pregnancy (*see also* categories
     633.0-633.9) 639.8
   molar pregnancy (*see also* categories 630-
     632) 639.8

Abscess (*see also* Cellulitis) — *continued*
 kidney — *continued*
  complicating pregnancy or puerperium
    646.6 ☑5ᵗʰ
   affecting fetus or newborn 760.1
  following
   abortion 639.8
   ectopic or molar pregnancy 639.8
 knee 682.6
  joint 711.06
  tuberculous (active) (*see also* Tuberculosis)
    015.2 ☑5ᵗʰ
 labium (majus) (minus) 616.4
  complicating pregnancy, childbirth, or
    puerperium 646.6 ☑5ᵗʰ
 lacrimal (passages) (sac) (*see also*
   Dacryocystitis) 375.30
  caruncle 375.30
  gland (*see also* Dacryoadenitis) 375.00
 lacunar 597.0
 larynx 478.79
 lateral (alveolar) 522.5
  with sinus 522.7
 leg, except foot 682.6
 lens 360.00
 lid 373.13
 lingual 529.0
  tonsil 475
 lip 528.5
 Littre's gland 597.0
 liver 572.0
  amebic 006.3
   with
    brain abscess (and lung abscess)
      006.5
    lung abscess 006.4
  due to Entamoeba histolytica 006.3
  dysenteric (*see also* Abscess, liver, amebic)
    006.3
  pyogenic 572.0
  tropical (*see also* Abscess, liver, amebic)
    006.3
 loin (region) 682.2
 lumbar (tuberculous) (*see also* Tuberculosis)
   015.0 ☑5ᵗʰ *[730.88]*
  nontuberculous 682.2
 lung (miliary) (putrid) 513.0
  amebic (with liver abscess) 006.4
   with brain abscess 006.5
 lymph, lymphatic, gland or node (acute) 683
  any site, except mesenteric 683
  mesentery 289.2
 lymphangitic, acute — *see* Cellulitis
 malar 526.4
 mammary gland — *see* Abscess, breast
 marginal (anus) 566
 mastoid (process) (*see also* Mastoiditis, acute)
   383.00
  subperiosteal 383.01
 maxilla, maxillary 526.4
  molar (tooth) 522.5
   with sinus 522.7
  premolar 522.5
  sinus (chronic) (*see also* Sinusitis, maxillary)
    473.0
 mediastinum 513.1
 meibomian gland 373.12
 meninges (*see also* Meningitis) 320.9
 mesentery, mesenteric — *see* Abscess,
   peritoneum
 mesosalpinx (*see also* Salpingo-oophoritis)
   614.2
 milk 675.1 ☑5ᵗʰ
 Monro's (psoriasis) 696.1
 mons pubis 682.2
 mouth (floor) 528.3
 multiple sites NEC 682.9
 mural 682.2
 muscle 728.89
 myocardium 422.92
 nabothian (follicle) (*see also* Cervicitis) 616.0
 nail (chronic) (with lymphangitis) 681.9
  finger 681.02
  toe 681.11
 nasal (fossa) (septum) 478.1
  sinus (chronic) (*see also* Sinusitis) 473.9
 nasopharyngeal 478.29

Abscess (*see also* Cellulitis) — *continued*
nates 682.5
navel 682.2
  newborn NEC 771.4
neck (region) 682.1
  lymph gland or node 683
nephritic (*see also* Abscess, kidney) 590.2
nipple 611.0
  puerperal, postpartum 675.0 ✓5ᵗʰ
nose (septum) 478.1
  external 682.0
omentum — *see* Abscess, peritoneum
operative wound 998.59
orbit, orbital 376.01
ossifluent — *see* Abscess, bone
ovary, ovarian (corpus luteum) (*see also*
  Salpingo-oophoritis) 614.2
oviduct (*see also* Salpingo-oophoritis) 614.2
palate (soft) 528.3
  hard 526.4
palmar (space) 682.4
pancreas (duct) 577.0
paradontal 523.3
parafrenal 607.2
parametric, parametrium (chronic) (*see also*
  Disease, pelvis, inflammatory) 614.4
  acute 614.3
paranephric 590.2
parapancreatic 577.0
parapharyngeal 478.22
pararectal 566
parasinus (*see also* Sinusitis) 473.9
parauterine (*see also* Disease, pelvis,
  inflammatory) 614.4
  acute 614.3
paravaginal (*see also* Vaginitis) 616.10
parietal region 682.8
parodontal 523.3
parotid (duct) (gland) 527.3
  region 528.3
parumbilical 682.2
  newborn 771.4
pectoral (region) 682.2
pelvirectal — *see* Abscess, peritoneum
pelvis, pelvic
  female (chronic) (*see also* Disease, pelvis,
    inflammatory) 614.4
    acute 614.3
  male, peritoneal (cellular tissue) — *see*
    Abscess, peritoneum
  tuberculous (*see also* Tuberculosis)
    016.9 ✓5ᵗʰ
penis 607.2
  gonococcal (acute) 098.0
    chronic or duration of 2 months or over
      098.2
perianal 566
periapical 522.5
  with sinus (alveolar) 522.7
periappendiceal 540.1
pericardial 420.99
pericecal 540.1
pericemental 523.3
pericholecystic (*see also* Cholecystitis, acute)
  575.0
pericoronal 523.3
peridental 523.3
perigastric 535.0 ✓5ᵗʰ
perimetric (*see also* Disease, pelvis,
  inflammatory) 614.4
  acute 614.3
perinephric, perinephritic (*see also* Abscess,
  kidney) 590.2
perineum, perineal (superficial) 682.2
  deep (with urethral involvement) 597.0
  urethra 597.0
periodontal (parietal) 523.3
  apical 522.5
periosteum, periosteal (*see also* Periostitis)
  730.3 ✓5ᵗʰ
  with osteomyelitis (*see also* Osteomyelitis)
    730.2 ✓5ᵗʰ
    acute or subacute 730.0 ✓5ᵗʰ
    chronic or old 730.1 ✓5ᵗʰ
peripleuritic 510.9
  with fistula 510.0
periproctic 566
periprostatic 601.2

Abscess (*see also* Cellulitis) — *continued*
perirectal (staphylococcal) 566
perirenal (tissue) (*see also* Abscess, kidney)
  590.2
perisinuous (nose) (*see also* Sinusitis) 473.9
peritoneum, peritoneal (perforated) (ruptured)
  567.2
  with
    abortion — *see* Abortion, by type, with
      sepsis
    appendicitis 540.1
    ectopic pregnancy (*see also* categories
      633.0-633.9) 639.0
    molar pregnancy (*see also* categories 630-
      632) 639.0
  following
    abortion 639.0
    ectopic or molar pregnancy 639.0
  pelvic, female (*see also* Disease, pelvis,
    inflammatory) 614.4
    acute 614.3
  postoperative 998.59
  puerperal, postpartum, childbirth 670 ✓4ᵗʰ
  tuberculous (*see also* Tuberculosis)
    014.0 ✓5ᵗʰ
peritonsillar 475
perityphlic 540.1
periureteral 593.89
periurethral 597.0
  gonococcal (acute) 098.0
    chronic or duration of 2 months or over
      098.2
periuterine (*see also* Disease, pelvis,
  inflammatory) 614.4
  acute 614.3
perivesical 595.89
pernicious NEC 682.9
petrous bone — *see* Petrositis
phagedenic NEC 682.9
  chancroid 099.0
pharynx, pharyngeal (lateral) 478.29
phlegmonous NEC 682.9
pilonidal 685.0
pituitary (gland) 253.8
pleura 510.9
  with fistula 510.0
popliteal 682.6
postanal 566
postcecal 540.1
postlaryngeal 478.79
postnasal 478.1
postpharyngeal 478.24
posttonsillar 475
posttyphoid 002.0
Pott's (*see also* Tuberculosis) 015.0 ✓5ᵗʰ
  [730.88]
pouch of Douglas (chronic) (*see also* Disease,
  pelvis, inflammatory) 614.4
premammary — *see* Abscess, breast
prepatellar 682.6
prostate (*see also* Prostatitis) 601.2
  gonococcal (acute) 098.12
    chronic or duration of 2 months or over
      098.32
psoas (tuberculous) (*see also* Tuberculosis)
  015.0 ✓5ᵗʰ [730.88]
  nontuberculous 728.89
pterygopalatine fossa 682.8
pubis 682.2
puerperal — Puerperal, abscess, by site
pulmonary — *see* Abscess, lung
pulp, pulpal (dental) 522.0
  finger 681.01
  toe 681.10
pyemic — *see* Septicemia
pyloric valve 535.0 ✓5ᵗʰ
rectovaginal septum 569.5
rectovesical 595.89
rectum 566
regional NEC 682.9
renal (*see also* Abscess, kidney) 590.2
retina 363.00
retrobulbar 376.01
retrocecal — *see* Abscess, peritoneum
retrolaryngeal 478.79
retromammary — *see* Abscess, breast
retroperineal 682.2

Abscess (*see also* Cellulitis) — *continued*
retroperitoneal — *see* Abscess, peritoneum
retropharyngeal 478.24
  tuberculous (*see also* Tuberculosis)
    012.8 ✓5ᵗʰ
retrorectal 566
retrouterine (*see also* Disease, pelvis,
  inflammatory) 614.4
  acute 614.3
retrovesical 595.89
root, tooth 522.5
  with sinus (alveolar) 522.7
round ligament (*see also* Disease, pelvis,
  inflammatory) 614.4
  acute 614.3
rupture (spontaneous) NEC 682.9
sacrum (tuberculous) (*see also* Tuberculosis)
  015.0 ✓5ᵗʰ [730.88]
  nontuberculous 730.08
salivary duct or gland 527.3
scalp (any part) 682.8
scapular 730.01
sclera 379.09
scrofulous (*see also* Tuberculosis) 017.2 ✓5ᵗʰ
scrotum 608.4
seminal vesicle 608.0
  amebic 006.8
septal, dental 522.5
  with sinus (alveolar) 522.7
septum (nasal) 478.1
serous (*see also* Periostitis) 730.3 ✓5ᵗʰ
shoulder 682.3
side 682.2
sigmoid 569.5
sinus (accessory) (chronic) (nasal) (*see also*
  Sinusitis) 473.9
  intracranial venous (any) 324.0
  late effect — *see* category 326
Skene's duct or gland 597.0
skin NEC 682.9
  tuberculous (primary) (*see also*
    Tuberculosis) 017.0 ✓5ᵗʰ
sloughing NEC 682.9
specified site NEC 682.8
  amebic 006.8
spermatic cord 608.4
sphenoidal (sinus) (*see also* Sinusitis,
  sphenoidal) 473.3
spinal
  cord (any part) (staphylococcal) 324.1
    tuberculous (*see also* Tuberculosis) 013.5
      ✓5ᵗʰ
  epidural 324.1
spine (column) (tuberculous) (*see also*
  Tuberculosis) 015.0 ✓5ᵗʰ [730.88]
  nontuberculous 730.08
spleen 289.59
  amebic 006.8
staphylococcal NEC 682.9
stitch 998.59
stomach (wall) 535.0 ✓5ᵗʰ
strumous (tuberculous) (*see also* Tuberculosis)
  017.2 ✓5ᵗʰ
subarachnoid 324.9
  brain 324.0
  cerebral 324.0
  late effect — *see* category 326
  spinal cord 324.1
subareolar — *see also* Abscess, breast
  puerperal, postpartum 675.1 ✓5ᵗʰ
subcecal 540.1
subcutaneous NEC 682.9
subdiaphragmatic — *see* Abscess, peritoneum
subdorsal 682.2
subdural 324.9
  brain 324.0
  late effect — *see* category 326
  spinal cord 324.1
subgaleal 682.8
subhepatic — *see* Abscess, peritoneum
sublingual 528.3
  gland 527.3
submammary — *see* Abscess, breast
submandibular (region) (space) (triangle) 682.0
  gland 527.3
submaxillary (region) 682.0
  gland 527.3

Abscess (see also Cellulitis) — continued
  submental (pyogenic) 682.0
    gland 527.3
  subpectoral 682.2
  subperiosteal — see Abscess, bone
  subperitoneal — see Abscess, peritoneum
  subphrenic — see also Abscess, peritoneum
    postoperative 998.59
  subscapular 682.2
  subungual 681.9
  suburethral 597.0
  sudoriparous 705.89
  suppurative NEC 682.9
  supraclavicular (fossa) 682.3
  suprahepatic — see Abscess, peritoneum
  suprapelvic (see also Disease, pelvis,
      inflammatory) 614.4
    acute 614.3
  suprapubic 682.2
  suprarenal (capsule) (gland) 255.8
  sweat gland 705.89
  syphilitic 095.8
  teeth, tooth (root) 522.5
    with sinus (alveolar) 522.7
    supporting structures NEC 523.3
  temple 682.0
  temporal region 682.0
  temporosphenoidal 324.0
    late effect — see category 326
  tendon (sheath) 727.89
  testicle — see Orchitis
  thecal 728.89
  thigh (acquired) 682.6
  thorax 510.9
    with fistula 510.0
  throat 478.29
  thumb (intrathecal) (periosteal) (subcutaneous)
      (subcuticular) 681.00
  thymus (gland) 254.1
  thyroid (gland) 245.0
  toe (any) (intrathecal) (periosteal)
      (subcutaneous) (subcuticular) 681.10
  tongue (staphylococcal) 529.0
  tonsil(s) (lingual) 475
  tonsillopharyngeal 475
  tooth, teeth (root) 522.5
    with sinus (alveolar) 522.7
    supporting structure NEC 523.3
  trachea 478.9
  trunk 682.2
  tubal (see also Salpingo-oophoritis) 614.2
  tuberculous — see Tuberculosis, abscess
  tubo-ovarian (see also Salpingo-oophoritis)
      614.2
  tunica vaginalis 608.4
  umbilicus NEC 682.2
    newborn 771.4
  upper arm 682.3
  upper respiratory 478.9
  urachus 682.2
  urethra (gland) 597.0
  urinary 597.0
  uterus, uterine (wall) (see also Endometritis)
      615.9
    ligament (see also Disease, pelvis,
        inflammatory) 614.4
      acute 614.3
    neck (see also Cervicitis) 616.0
  uvula 528.3
  vagina (wall) (see also Vaginitis) 616.10
  vaginorectal (see also Vaginitis) 616.10
  vas deferens 608.4
  vermiform appendix 540.1
  vertebra (column) (tuberculous) (see also
      Tuberculosis) 015.0 ✓5ᵗʰ [730.88]
    nontuberculous 730.0 ✓5ᵗʰ
  vesical 595.89
  vesicouterine pouch (see also Disease, pelvis,
      inflammatory) 614.4
  vitreous (humor) (pneumococcal) 360.04
  vocal cord 478.5
  von Bezold's 383.01
  vulva 616.4
    complicating pregnancy, childbirth, or
        puerperium 646.6 ✓5ᵗʰ
  vulvovaginal gland (see also Vaginitis) 616.3
  web-space 682.4
  wrist 682.4

Absence (organ or part) (complete or partial)
  acoustic nerve 742.8
  adrenal (gland) (congenital) 759.1
    acquired V45.79
  albumin (blood) 273.8
  alimentary tract (complete) (congenital) (partial)
      751.8
    lower 751.5
    upper 750.8
  alpha-fucosidase 271.8
  alveolar process (acquired) 525.8
    congenital 750.26
  anus, anal (canal) (congenital) 751.2
  aorta (congenital) 747.22
  aortic valve (congenital) 746.89
  appendix, congenital 751.2
  arm (acquired) V49.60
    above elbow V49.66
    below elbow V49.65
    congenital (see also Deformity, reduction,
        upper limb) 755.20
      lower — see Absence, forearm, congenital
      upper (complete) (partial) (with absence of
          distal elements, incomplete) 755.24
        with
          complete absence of distal elements
              755.21
            forearm (incomplete) 755.23
  artery (congenital) (peripheral) NEC (see also
      Anomaly, peripheral vascular system)
      747.60
    brain 747.81
      cerebral 747.81
    coronary 746.85
    pulmonary 747.3
    umbilical 747.5
  atrial septum 745.69
  auditory canal (congenital) (external) 744.01
  auricle (ear) (with stenosis or atresia of
      auditory canal), congenital 744.01
  bile, biliary duct (common) or passage
      (congenital) 751.61
  bladder (acquired) V45.74
    congenital 753.8
  bone (congenital) NEC 756.9
    marrow 284.9
      acquired (secondary) 284.8
      congenital 284.0
      hereditary 284.0
      idiopathic 284.9
    skull 756.0
  bowel sounds 787.5
  brain 740.0
    specified part 742.2
  breast(s) (acquired) V45.71
    congenital 757.6
  broad ligament (congenital) 752.19
  bronchus (congenital) 748.3
  calvarium, calvaria (skull) 756.0
  canaliculus lacrimalis, congenital 743.65
  carpal(s) (congenital) (complete) (partial) (with
      absence of distal elements, incomplete)
      (see also Deformity, reduction, upper
      limb) 755.28
    with complete absence of distal elements
        755.21
  cartilage 756.9
  caudal spine 756.13
  cecum (acquired) (postoperative)
      (posttraumatic) V45.72
    congenital 751.2
  cementum 520.4
  cerebellum (congenital) (vermis) 742.2
  cervix (acquired) (uteri) V45.77
    congenital 752.49
  chin, congenital 744.89
  cilia (congenital) 743.63
    acquired 374.89
  circulatory system, part NEC 747.89
  clavicle 755.51
  clitoris (congenital) 752.49
  coccyx, congenital 756.13
  cold sense (see also Disturbance, sensation)
      782.0
  colon (acquired) (postoperative) V45.72
    congenital 751.2

Absence — continued
  congenital
    lumen — see Atresia
    organ or site NEC — see Agenesis
    septum — see Imperfect, closure
  corpus callosum (congenital) 742.2
  cricoid cartilage 748.3
  diaphragm (congenital) (with hernia) 756.6
    with obstruction 756.6
  digestive organ(s) or tract, congenital (complete)
      (partial) 751.8
    acquired V45.79
    lower 751.5
    upper 750.8
  ductus arteriosus 747.89
  duodenum (acquired) (postoperative) V45.72
    congenital 751.1
  ear, congenital 744.09
    acquired V45.79
    auricle 744.01
    external 744.01
    inner 744.05
    lobe, lobule 744.21
    middle, except ossicles 744.03
      ossicles 744.04
    ossicles 744.04
  ejaculatory duct (congenital) 752.8
  endocrine gland NEC (congenital) 759.2
  epididymis (congenital) 752.8
    acquired V45.77
  epiglottis, congenital 748.3
  epileptic (atonic) (typical) (see also Epilepsy)
      345.0 ✓5ᵗʰ
  erythrocyte 284.9
  erythropoiesis 284.9
    congenital 284.0
  esophagus (congenital) 750.3
  Eustachian tube (congenital) 744.24
  extremity (acquired)
    congenital (see also Deformity, reduction)
        755.4
    lower V49.70
    upper V49.60
  extrinsic muscle, eye 743.69
  eye (acquired) V45.78
    adnexa (congenital) 743.69
    congenital 743.00
    muscle (congenital) 743.69
  eyelid (fold), congenital 743.62
    acquired 374.89
  face
    bones NEC 756.0
    specified part NEC 744.89
  fallopian tube(s) (acquired) V45.77
    congenital 752.19
  femur, congenital (complete) (partial) (with
      absence of distal elements, incomplete)
      (see also Deformity, reduction, lower
      limb) 755.34
    with
      complete absence of distal elements
          755.31
        tibia and fibula (incomplete) 755.33
  fibrin 790.92
  fibrinogen (congenital) 286.3
    acquired 286.6
  fibula, congenital (complete) (partial) (with
      absence of distal elements, incomplete)
      (see also Deformity, reduction, lower
      limb) 755.37
    with
      complete absence of distal elements
          755.31
        tibia 755.35
          with
            complete absence of distal elements
                755.31
              femur (incomplete) 755.33
                with complete absence of distal
                    elements 755.31
  finger (acquired) V49.62
    congenital (complete) (partial) (see also
        Deformity, reduction, upper limb)
        755.29
      meaning all fingers (complete) (partial)
          755.21
      transverse 755.21

✓4ᵗʰ Fourth-digit Required   ✓5ᵗʰ Fifth-digit Required   ▶◀ Revised Text   ● New Line   ▲ Revised Code

Absence — *continued*
  fissures of lungs (congenital) 748.5
  foot (acquired) V49.73
    congenital (complete) 755.31
  forearm (acquired) V49.65
    congenital (complete) (partial) (with absence
      of distal elements, incomplete) (*see
      also* Deformity, reduction, upper limb)
      755.25
      with
        complete absence of distal elements
          (hand and fingers) 755.21
        humerus (incomplete) 755.23
  fovea centralis 743.55
  fucosidase 271.8
  gallbladder (acquired) V45.79
    congenital 751.69
  gamma globulin (blood) 279.00
  genital organs
    acquired V45.77
    congenital
      female 752.8
        external 752.49
        internal NEC 752.8
      male 752.8
        penis 752.69
  genitourinary organs, congenital NEC 752.8
  glottis 748.3
  gonadal, congenital NEC 758.6
  hair (congenital) 757.4
    acquired — *see* Alopecia
  hand (acquired) V49.63
    congenital (complete) (*see also* Deformity,
      reduction, upper limb) 755.21
  heart (congenital) 759.89
    acquired — *see* Status, organ replacement
  heat sense (*see also* Disturbance, sensation)
    782.0
  humerus, congenital (complete) (partial) (with
    absence of distal elements, incomplete)
    (*see also* Deformity, reduction, upper
    limb) 755.24
    with
      complete absence of distal elements
        755.21
      radius and ulna (incomplete) 755.23
  hymen (congenital) 752.49
  ileum (acquired) (postoperative) (posttraumatic)
    V45.72
    congenital 751.1
  immunoglobulin, isolated NEC 279.03
    IgA 279.01
    IgG 279.03
    IgM 279.02
  incus (acquired) 385.24
    congenital 744.04
  internal ear (congenital) 744.05
  intestine (acquired) (small) V45.72
    congenital 751.1
      large 751.2
    large V45.72
      congenital 751.2
  iris (congenital) 743.45
  jaw — *see* Absence, mandible
  jejunum (acquired) V45.72
    congenital 751.1
  joint, congenital NEC 755.8
  kidney(s) (acquired) V45.73
    congenital 753.0
  labium (congenital) (majus) (minus) 752.49
  labyrinth, membranous 744.05
  lacrimal apparatus (congenital) 743.65
  larynx (congenital) 748.3
  leg (acquired) V49.70
    above knee V49.76
    below knee V49.75
    congenital (partial) (unilateral) (*see also*
      Deformity, reduction, lower limb)
      755.31
      lower (complete) (partial) (with absence of
        distal elements, incomplete) 755.35
        with
          complete absence of distal elements
            (foot and toes) 755.31
          thigh (incomplete) 755.33
            with complete absence of distal
              elements 755.31

Absence — *continued*
  leg — *continued*
    congenital — *continued*
      upper — *see* Absence, femur
  lens (congenital) 743.35
    acquired 379.31
  ligament, broad (congenital) 752.19
  limb (acquired)
    congenital (complete) (partial) (*see also*
      Deformity, reduction) 755.4
      lower 755.30
        complete 755.31
        incomplete 755.32
        longitudinal — *see* Deficiency, lower
          limb, longitudinal
        transverse 755.31
      upper 755.20
        complete 755.21
        incomplete 755.22
        longitudinal — *see* Deficiency, upper
          limb, longitudinal
        transverse 755.21
    lower NEC V49.70
    upper NEC V49.60
  lip 750.26
  liver (congenital) (lobe) 751.69
  lumbar (congenital) (vertebra) 756.13
    isthmus 756.11
    pars articularis 756.11
  lumen — *see* Atresia
  lung (bilateral) (congenital) (fissure) (lobe)
    (unilateral) 748.5
    acquired (any part) V45.76
  mandible (congenital) 524.09
  maxilla (congenital) 524.09
  menstruation 626.0
  metacarpal(s), congenital (complete) (partial)
    (with absence of distal elements,
    incomplete) (*see also* Deformity,
    reduction, upper limb) 755.28
    with all fingers, complete 755.21
  metatarsal(s), congenital (complete) (partial)
    (with absence of distal elements,
    incomplete) (*see also* Deformity,
    reduction, lower limb) 755.38
    with complete absence of distal elements
      755.31
  muscle (congenital) (pectoral) 756.81
    ocular 743.69
  musculoskeletal system (congenital) NEC 756.9
  nail(s) (congenital) 757.5
  neck, part 744.89
  nerve 742.8
  nervous system, part NEC 742.8
  neutrophil 288.0
  nipple (congenital) 757.6
  nose (congenital) 748.1
    acquired 738.0
  nuclear 742.8
  ocular muscle (congenital) 743.69
  organ
    of Corti (congenital) 744.05
    or site
      acquired V45.79
      congenital NEC 759.89
  osseous meatus (ear) 744.03
  ovary (acquired) V45.77
    congenital 752.0
  oviduct (acquired) V45.77
    congenital 752.19
  pancreas (congenital) 751.7
    acquired (postoperative) (posttraumatic)
      V45.79
  parathyroid gland (congenital) 759.2
  parotid gland(s) (congenital) 750.21
  patella, congenital 755.64
  pelvic girdle (congenital) 755.69
  penis (congenital) 752.69
    acquired V45.77
  pericardium (congenital) 746.89
  perineal body (congenital) 756.81
  phalange(s), congenital 755.4
    lower limb (complete) (intercalary) (partial)
      (terminal) (*see also* Deformity,
      reduction, lower limb) 755.39
      meaning all toes (complete) (partial)
        755.31

Absence — *continued*
  phalange(s), congenital — *continued*
    lower limb (*see also* Deformity, reduction,
      lower limb) — *continued*
      transverse 755.31
    upper limb (complete) (intercalary) (partial)
      (terminal) (*see also* Deformity,
      reduction, upper limb) 755.29
      meaning all digits (complete) (partial)
        755.21
      transverse 755.21
  pituitary gland (congenital) 759.2
  postoperative — *see* Absence, by site, acquired
  prostate (congenital) 752.8
    acquired V45.77
  pulmonary
    artery 747.3
    trunk 747.3
    valve (congenital) 746.01
    vein 747.49
  punctum lacrimale (congenital) 743.65
  radius, congenital (complete) (partial) (with
    absence of distal elements, incomplete)
    755.26
    with
      complete absence of distal elements
        755.21
      ulna 755.25
        with
          complete absence of distal elements
            755.21
          humerus (incomplete) 755.23
  ray, congenital 755.4
    lower limb (complete) (partial) (*see also*
      Deformity, reduction, lower limb)
      755.38
      meaning all rays 755.31
      transverse 755.31
    upper limb (complete) (partial) (*see also*
      Deformity, reduction, upper limb)
      755.28
      meaning all rays 755.21
      transverse 755.21
  rectum (congenital) 751.2
    acquired V45.79
  red cell 284.9
    acquired (secondary) 284.8
    congenital 284.0
    hereditary 284.0
    idiopathic 284.9
  respiratory organ (congenital) NEC 748.9
  rib (acquired) 738.3
    congenital 756.3
  roof of orbit (congenital) 742.0
  round ligament (congenital) 752.8
  sacrum, congenital 756.13
  salivary gland(s) (congenital) 750.21
  scapula 755.59
  scrotum, congenital 752.8
  seminal tract or duct (congenital) 752.8
    acquired V45.77
  septum (congenital) — *see also* Imperfect,
    closure, septum
    atrial 745.69
      and ventricular 745.7
    between aorta and pulmonary artery 745.0
    ventricular 745.3
      and atrial 745.7
  sex chromosomes 758.81
  shoulder girdle, congenital (complete) (partial)
    755.59
  skin (congenital) 757.39
  skull bone 756.0
    with
      anencephalus 740.0
      encephalocele 742.0
      hydrocephalus 742.3
        with spina bifida (*see also* Spina
          bifida) 741.0 ✓5ᵗʰ
      microcephalus 742.1
  spermatic cord (congenital) 752.8
  spinal cord 742.59
  spine, congenital 756.13
  spleen (congenital) 759.0
    acquired V45.79
  sternum, congenital 756.3

Absence — *continued*
stomach (acquired) (partial) (postoperative) V45.75
  with postgastric surgery syndrome 564.2
  congenital 750.7
submaxillary gland(s) (congenital) 750.21
superior vena cava (congenital) 747.49
tarsal(s), congenital (complete) (partial) (with absence of distal elements, incomplete) (*see also* Deformity, reduction, lower limb) 755.38
teeth, tooth (congenital) 520.0
  with abnormal spacing 524.3
  acquired 525.10
    with malocclusion 524.3
    due to
      caries 525.13
      extraction 525.10
      periodontal disease 525.12
      trauma 525.11
tendon (congenital) 756.81
testis (congenital) 752.8
  acquired V45.77
thigh (acquired) 736.89
thumb (acquired) V49.61
  congenital 755.29
thymus gland (congenital) 759.2
thyroid (gland) (surgical) 246.8
  with hypothyroidism 244.0
  cartilage, congenital 748.3
  congenital 243
tibia, congenital (complete) (partial) (with absence of distal elements, incomplete) (*see also* Deformity, reduction, lower limb) 755.36
  with
    complete absence of distal elements 755.31
    fibula 755.35
      with
        complete absence of distal elements 755.31
        femur (incomplete) 755.33
          with complete absence of distal elements 755.31
toe (acquired) V49.72
  congenital (complete) (partial) 755.39
    meaning all toes 755.31
    transverse 755.31
  great V49.71
tongue (congenital) 750.11
tooth, teeth, (congenital) 520.0
  with abnormal spacing 524.3
  acquired 525.10
    with malocclusion 524.3
    due to
      caries 525.13
      extraction 525.10
      periodontal disease 525.12
      trauma 525.11
trachea (cartilage) (congenital) (rings) 748.3
transverse aortic arch (congenital) 747.21
tricuspid valve 746.1
ulna, congenital (complete) (partial) (with absence of distal elements, incomplete) (*see also* Deformity, reduction, upper limb) 755.27
  with
    complete absence of distal elements 755.21
    radius 755.25
      with
        complete absence of distal elements 755.21
        humerus (incomplete) 755.23
umbilical artery (congenital) 747.5
ureter (congenital) 753.4
  acquired V45.74
urethra, congenital 753.8
  acquired V45.74
urinary system, part NEC, congenital 753.8
  acquired V45.74
uterus (acquired) V45.77
  congenital 752.3
uvula (congenital) 750.26
vagina, congenital 752.49
  acquired V45.77

Absence — *continued*
vas deferens (congenital) 752.8
  acquired V45.77
vein (congenital) (peripheral) NEC (*see also* Anomaly, peripheral vascular system) 747.60
  brain 747.81
  great 747.49
  portal 747.49
  pulmonary 747.49
vena cava (congenital) (inferior) (superior) 747.49
ventral horn cell 742.59
ventricular septum 745.3
vermis of cerebellum 742.2
vertebra, congenital 756.13
vulva, congenital 752.49
Absentia epileptica (*see also* Epilepsy) 345.0 ✓5ᵗʰ
Absinthemia (*see also* Dependence) 304.6 ✓5ᵗʰ
Absinthism (*see also* Dependence) 304.6 ✓5ᵗʰ
Absorbent system disease 459.89
Absorption
alcohol, through placenta or breast milk 760.71
antibiotics, through placenta or breast milk 760.74
anti-infective, through placenta or breast milk 760.74
chemical NEC 989.9
  specified chemical or substance — *see* Table of Drugs and Chemicals
  through placenta or breast milk (fetus or newborn) 760.70
    alcohol 760.71
    anti-infective agents 760.74
    cocaine 760.75
    "crack" 760.75
    diethylstilbestrol [DES] 760.76
    hallucinogenic agents 760.73
    medicinal agents NEC 760.79
    narcotics 760.72
    obstetric anesthetic or analgesic drug 763.5
    specified agent NEC 760.79
    suspected, affecting management of pregnancy 655.5 ✓5ᵗʰ
cocaine, through placenta or breast milk 760.75
drug NEC (*see also* Reaction, drug)
  through placenta or breast milk (fetus or newborn) 760.70
    alcohol 760.71
  through placenta or breast milk (fetus or newborn) — *continued*
    anti-infective agents 760.74
    cocaine 760.75
    "crack" 760.75
    diethylstilbestrol [DES] 760.76
    hallucinogenic agents 760.73
    medicinal agents NEC 760.79
    narcotics 760.72
    obstetric anesthetic or analgesic drug 763.5
    specified agent NEC 760.79
    suspected, affecting management of pregnancy 655.5 ✓5ᵗʰ
fat, disturbance 579.8
hallucinogenic agents, through placenta or breast milk 760.73
immune sera, through placenta or breast milk 760.79
lactose defect 271.3
medicinal agents NEC, through placenta or breast milk 760.79
narcotics, through placenta or breast milk 760.72
noxious substance, — *see* Absorption, chemical
protein, disturbance 579.8
pus or septic, general — *see* Septicemia
quinine, through placenta or breast milk 760.74
toxic substance, — *see* Absorption, chemical
uremic — *see* Uremia
Abstinence symptoms or syndrome
alcohol 291.81
drug 292.0

Abt-Letterer-Siwe syndrome (acute histiocytosis X) (M9722/3) 202.5 ✓5ᵗʰ
Abulia 799.8
Abulomania 301.6
Abuse
adult 995.80
  emotional 995.82
  multiple forms 995.85
  neglect (nutritional) 995.84
  physical 995.81
  psychological 995.82
  sexual 995.83
alcohol (*see also* Alcoholism) 305.0 ✓5ᵗʰ
  dependent 303.9 ✓5ᵗʰ
  non-dependent 305.0 ✓5ᵗʰ
child 995.50
  counseling
    perpetrator
      non-parent V62.83
      parent V61.22
    victim V61.21
  emotional 995.51
  multiple forms 995.59
  neglect (nutritional) 995.52
  psychological 995.51
  physical 995.54
    shaken infant syndrome 995.55
  sexual 995.53
drugs, nondependent 305.9 ✓5ᵗʰ

> *Note* — *Use the following fifth-digit subclassification with the following codes: 305.0, 305.2-305.9:*
>
> | | | | |
> |---|---|---|---|
> | 0 | unspecified | 2 | episodic |
> | 1 | continuous | 3 | in remission |

  amphetamine type 305.7 ✓5ᵗʰ
  antidepressants 305.8 ✓5ᵗʰ
  barbiturates 305.4 ✓5ᵗʰ
  caffeine 305.9 ✓5ᵗʰ
  cannabis 305.2 ✓5ᵗʰ
  cocaine type 305.6 ✓5ᵗʰ
  hallucinogens 305.3 ✓5ᵗʰ
  hashish 305.2 ✓5ᵗʰ
  LSD 305.3 ✓5ᵗʰ
  marijuana 305.2 ✓5ᵗʰ
  mixed 305.9 ✓5ᵗʰ
  morphine type 305.5 ✓5ᵗʰ
  opioid type 305.5 ✓5ᵗʰ
  phencyclidine (PCP) 305.9 ✓5ᵗʰ
  specified NEC 305.9 ✓5ᵗʰ
  tranquilizers 305.4 ✓5ᵗʰ
spouse 995.80
tobacco 305.1
Acalcerosis 275.40
Acalcicosis 275.40
Acalculia 784.69
developmental 315.1
Acanthocheilonemiasis 125.4
Acanthocytosis 272.5
Acanthokeratodermia 701.1
Acantholysis 701.8
bullosa 757.39
Acanthoma (benign) (M8070/0) — *see also* Neoplasm, by site, benign
malignant (M8070/3) — *see* Neoplasm, by site, malignant
Acanthosis (acquired) (nigricans) 701.2
adult 701.2
benign (congenital) 757.39
congenital 757.39
glycogenic
  esophagus 530.89
juvenile 701.2
tongue 529.8
Acanthrocytosis 272.5
Acapnia 276.3
Acarbia 276.2
Acardia 759.89
Acardiacus amorphus 759.89
Acardiotrophia 429.1
Acardius 759.89

Acariasis 133.9
  sarcoptic 133.0
Acaridiasis 133.9
Acarinosis 133.9
Acariosis 133.9
Acarodermatitis 133.9
  urticarioides 133.9
Acarophobia 300.29
Acatalasemia 277.8
Acatalasia 277.8
Acatamathesia 784.69
Acataphasia 784.5
Acathisia 781.0
  due to drugs 333.99
Acceleration, accelerated
  atrioventricular conduction 426.7
  idioventricular rhythm 427.89
Accessory (congenital)
  adrenal gland 759.1
  anus 751.5
  appendix 751.5
  atrioventricular conduction 426.7
  auditory ossicles 744.04
  auricle (ear) 744.1
  autosome(s) NEC 758.5
    21 or 22 758.0
  biliary duct or passage 751.69
  bladder 753.8
  blood vessels (peripheral) (congenital) NEC (see
      also Anomaly, peripheral vascular
      system) 747.60
    cerebral 747.81
    coronary 746.85
  bone NEC 756.9
    foot 755.67
  breast tissue, axilla 757.6
  carpal bones 755.56
  cecum 751.5
  cervix 752.49
  chromosome(s) NEC 758.5
    13-15 758.1
    16-18 758.2
    21 or 22 758.0
    autosome(s) NEC 758.5
    D_1 758.1
    E_3 758.2
    G 758.0
    sex 758.81
  coronary artery 746.85
  cusp(s), heart valve NEC 746.89
    pulmonary 746.09
  cystic duct 751.69
  digits 755.00
  ear (auricle) (lobe) 744.1
  endocrine gland NEC 759.2
  external os 752.49
  eyelid 743.62
  eye muscle 743.69
  face bone(s) 756.0
  fallopian tube (fimbria) (ostium) 752.19
  fingers 755.01
  foreskin 605
  frontonasal process 756.0
  gallbladder 751.69
  genital organ(s)
    female 752.8
      external 752.49
      internal NEC 752.8
    male NEC 752.8
      penis 752.69
  genitourinary organs NEC 752.8
  heart 746.89
    valve NEC 746.89
      pulmonary 746.09
  hepatic ducts 751.69
  hymen 752.49
  intestine (large) (small) 751.5
  kidney 753.3
  lacrimal canal 743.65
  leaflet, heart valve NEC 746.89
    pulmonary 746.09
  ligament, broad 752.19
  liver (duct) 751.69
  lobule (ear) 744.1
  lung (lobe) 748.69

Accessory — continued
  muscle 756.82
  navicular of carpus 755.56
  nervous system, part NEC 742.8
  nipple 757.6
  nose 748.1
  organ or site NEC — see Anomaly, specified
      type NEC
  ovary 752.0
  oviduct 752.19
  pancreas 751.7
  parathyroid gland 759.2
  parotid gland (and duct) 750.22
  pituitary gland 759.2
  placental lobe — see Placenta, abnormal
  preauricular appendage 744.1
  prepuce 605
  renal arteries (multiple) 747.62
  rib 756.3
    cervical 756.2
  roots (teeth) 520.2
  salivary gland 750.22
  sesamoids 755.8
  sinus — see condition
  skin tags 757.39
  spleen 759.0
  sternum 756.3
  submaxillary gland 750.22
  tarsal bones 755.67
  teeth, tooth 520.1
    causing crowding 524.3
  tendon 756.89
  thumb 755.01
  thymus gland 759.2
  thyroid gland 759.2
  toes 755.02
  tongue 750.13
  tragus 744.1
  ureter 753.4
  urethra 753.8
  urinary organ or tract NEC 753.8
  uterus 752.2
  vagina 752.49
  valve, heart NEC 746.89
    pulmonary 746.09
  vertebra 756.19
  vocal cords 748.3
  vulva 752.49
Accident, accidental — see also condition
  birth NEC 767.9
  cardiovascular (see also Disease,
      cardiovascular) 429.2
  cerebral (see also Disease, cerebrovascular,
      acute) 436
  cerebrovascular (current) (CVA) (see also
      Disease, cerebrovascular, acute) 436
    healed or old V12.59
    impending 435.9
    late effect — see Late effect(s) (of)
        cerebrovascular disease
    postoperative 997.02   ●
  coronary (see also Infarct, myocardium)
      410.9 ✓5th
  craniovascular (see also Disease,
      cerebrovascular, acute) 436
  during pregnancy, to mother
      affecting fetus or newborn 760.5
  heart, cardiac (see also Infarct, myocardium)
      410.9 ✓5th
  intrauterine 779.89   ▲
  vascular — see Disease, cerebrovascular, acute
Accommodation
  disorder of 367.51
    drug-induced 367.89
    toxic 367.89
  insufficiency of 367.4
  paralysis of 367.51
    hysterical 300.11
  spasm of 367.53
Accouchement — see Delivery
Accreta placenta (without hemorrhage) 667.0 ✓5th
  with hemorrhage 666.0 ✓5th
Accretio cordis (nonrheumatic) 423.1
Accretions on teeth 523.6
Accumulation secretion, prostate 602.8
Acephalia, acephalism, acephaly 740.0

Acephalic 740.0
Acephalobrachia 759.89
Acephalocardia 759.89
Acephalocardius 759.89
Acephalochiria 759.89
Acephalochirus 759.89
Acephalogaster 759.89
Acephalostomus 759.89
Acephalothorax 759.89
Acephalus 740.0
Acetonemia 790.6
  diabetic 250.1 ✓5th
Acetonglycosuria 982.8
Acetonuria 791.6
Achalasia 530.0
  cardia 530.0
  digestive organs congenital NEC 751.8
  esophagus 530.0
  pelvirectal 751.3
  psychogenic 306.4
  pylorus 750.5
  sphincteral NEC 564.89
Achard-Thiers syndrome (adrenogenital) 255.2
Ache(s) — see Pain
Acheilia 750.26
Acheiria 755.21
Achillobursitis 726.71
Achillodynia 726.71
Achlorhydria, achlorhydric 536.0
  anemia 280.9
  diarrhea 536.0
  neurogenic 536.0
  postvagotomy 564.2
  psychogenic 306.4
  secondary to vagotomy 564.2
Achloroblepsia 368.52
Achloropsia 368.52
Acholia 575.8
Acholuric jaundice (familial) (splenomegalic) (see
      also Spherocytosis) 282.0
  acquired 283.9
Achondroplasia 756.4
Achrestic anemia 281.8
Achroacytosis, lacrimal gland 375.00
  tuberculous (see also Tuberculosis) 017.3 ✓5th
Achroma, cutis 709.00
Achromate (congenital) 368.54
Achromatopia 368.54
Achromatopsia (congenital) 368.54
Achromia
  congenital 270.2
  parasitica 111.0
  unguium 703.8
Achylia
  gastrica 536.8
    neurogenic 536.3
    psychogenic 306.4
  pancreatica 577.1
Achylosis 536.8
Acid
  burn — see also Burn, by site
    from swallowing acid — see Burn, internal
        organs
  deficiency
    amide nicotinic 265.2
    amino 270.9
    ascorbic 267
    folic 266.2
    nicotinic (amide) 265.2
    pantothenic 266.2
  intoxication 276.2
  peptic disease 536.8
  stomach 536.8
    psychogenic 306.4
Acidemia 276.2
  arginosuccinic 270.6
  fetal
    affecting management of pregnancy
        656.3 ✓5th
    before onset of labor, in liveborn infant
        768.2

Acidemia — *continued*
  fetal — *continued*
    during labor, in liveborn infant 768.3
    intrauterine — *see* Distress, fetal 656.3 ✓5ᵗʰ
    unspecified as to time of onset, in liveborn
      infant 768.4
  pipecolic 270.7
Acidity, gastric (high) (low) 536.8
  psychogenic 306.4
Acidocytopenia 288.0
Acidocytosis 288.3
Acidopenia 288.0
Acidosis 276.2 ✓5ᵗʰ
  diabetic 250.1 ✓5ᵗʰ
  fetal, affecting management of pregnancy
    756.8 ✓5ᵗʰ
  fetal, affecting newborn 768.9
  kidney tubular 588.8
  lactic 276.2
  metabolic NEC 276.2
    with respiratory acidosis 276.4
    late, of newborn 775.7
  renal
    hyperchloremic 588.8
    tubular (distal) (proximal) 588.8
  respiratory 276.2
    complicated by
      metabolic acidosis 276.4
      metabolic alkalosis 276.4
Aciduria 791.9
  arginosuccinic 270.6
  beta-aminoisobutyric (BAIB) 277.2
  glycolic 271.8
  methylmalonic 270.3
    with glycinemia 270.7
  organic 270.9
  orotic (congenital) (hereditary) (pyrimidine
    deficiency) 281.4
Acladiosis 111.8
  skin 111.8
Aclasis
  diaphyseal 756.4
  tarsoepiphyseal 756.59
Acleistocardia 745.5
Aclusion 524.4
Acmesthesia 782.0
Acne (pustular) (vulgaris) 706.1
  agminata (*see also* Tuberculosis) 017.0 ✓5ᵗʰ
  artificialis 706.1
  atrophica 706.0
  cachecticorum (Hebra) 706.1
  conglobata 706.1
  conjunctiva 706.1
  cystic 706.1
  decalvans 704.09
  erythematosa 695.3
  eyelid 706.1
  frontalis 706.0
  indurata 706.1
  keloid 706.1
  lupoid 706.0
  necrotic, necrotica 706.0
    miliaris 704.8
  nodular 706.1
  occupational 706.1
  papulosa 706.1
  rodens 706.0
  rosacea 695.3
  scorbutica 267
  scrofulosorum (Bazin) (*see also* Tuberculosis)
    017.0 ✓5ᵗʰ
  summer 692.72
  tropical 706.1
  varioliformis 706.0
Acneiform drug eruptions 692.3
Acnitis (primary) (*see also* Tuberculosis)
  017.0 ✓5ᵗʰ
Acomia 704.00
Acontractile bladder 344.61
Aconuresis (*see also* Incontinence) 788.30
Acosta's disease 993.2
Acousma 780.1
Acoustic — *see* condition
Acousticophobia 300.29

Acquired — *see* condition
Acquired immune deficiency syndrome — *see*
  Human immunodeficiency virus (disease)
  (illness) (infection)
Acquired immunodeficiency syndrome — *see*
  Human immunodeficiency virus (disease)
  (illness) (infection)
Acragnosis 781.99
Acrania 740.0
Acroagnosis 781.99
Acroasphyxia, chronic 443.89
Acrobrachycephaly 756.0
Acrobystiolith 608.89
Acrobystitis 607.2
Acrocephalopolysyndactyly 755.55
Acrocephalosyndactyly 755.55
Acrocephaly 756.0
Acrochondrohyperplasia 759.82
Acrocyanosis 443.89
  newborn 770.83
Acrodermatitis 686.8
  atrophicans (chronica) 701.8
  continua (Hallopeau) 696.1
  enteropathica 686.8
  Hallopeau's 696.1
  perstans 696.1
  pustulosa continua 696.1
  recalcitrant pustular 696.1
Acrodynia 985.0
Acrodysplasia 755.55
Acrohyperhidrosis 780.8
Acrokeratosis verruciformis 757.39
Acromastitis 611.0
Acromegaly, acromegalia (skin) 253.0
Acromelalgia 443.89
Acromicria acromikria 756.59
Acronyx 703.0
Acropachy, thyroid (*see also* Thyrotoxicosis)
  242.9 ✓5ᵗʰ
Acropachyderma 757.39
Acroparesthesia 443.89
  simple (Schultz's type) 443.89
  vasomotor (Nothnagel's type) 443.89
Acropathy thyroid (*see also* Thyrotoxicosis)
  242.9 ✓5ᵗʰ
Acrophobia 300.29
Acroposthitis 607.2
Acroscleriasis (*see also* Scleroderma) 710.1
Acroscleroderma (*see also* Scleroderma) 710.1
Acrosclerosis (*see also* Scleroderma) 710.1
Acrosphacelus 785.4
Acrosphenosyndactylia 755.55
Acrospiroma, eccrine (M8402/0) — *see*
  Neoplasm, skin, benign
Acrostealgia 732.9
Acrosyndactyly (*see also* Syndactylism) 755.10
Acrotrophodynia 991.4
Actinic — *see also* condition
  cheilitis (due to sun) 692.72
    chronic NEC 692.74
    due to radiation, except from sun 692.82
  conjunctivitis 370.24
  dermatitis (due to sun) (*see also* Dermatitis,
    actinic 692.70
  due to
    roentgen rays or radioactive substance
      692.82
    ultraviolet radiation, except from sun
      692.82
      sun NEC 692.70
  elastosis solare 692.74
  granuloma 692.73
  keratitis 370.24
  ophthalmia 370.24
  reticuloid 692.73
Actinobacillosis, general 027.8
Actinobacillus
  lignieresii 027.8
  mallei 024
  muris 026.1

Actinocutitis NEC (*see also* Dermatitis, actinic)
  692.70
Actinodermatitis NEC (*see also* Dermatitis,
  actinic) 692.70
Actinomyces
  israelii (infection) — *see* Actinomycosis
  muris-ratti (infection) 026.1
Actinomycosis, actinomycotic 039.9
  with
    pneumonia 039.1
  abdominal 039.2
  cervicofacial 039.3
  cutaneous 039.0
  pulmonary 039.1
  specified site NEC 039.8
  thoracic 039.1
Actinoneuritis 357.89 ▲
Action, heart
  disorder 427.9
    postoperative 997.1
  irregular 427.9
    postoperative 997.1
    psychogenic 306.2
Active — *see* condition
Activity decrease, functional 780.99 ▲
Acute — *see also* condition
  abdomen NEC 789.0 ✓5ᵗʰ
  gallbladder (*see also* Cholecystitis, acute) 575.0
Acyanoblepsia 368.53
Acyanopsia 368.53
Acystia 753.8
Acystinervia — *see* Neurogenic, bladder
Acystineuria — *see* Neurogenic, bladder
Adactylia, adactyly (congenital) 755.4
  lower limb (complete) (intercalary) (partial)
    (terminal) (*see also* Deformity, reduction,
    lower limb) 755.39
    meaning all digits (complete) (partial) 755.31
    transverse (complete) (partial) 755.31
  upper limb (complete) (intercalary) (partial)
    (terminal) (*see also* Deformity, reduction,
    upper limb) 755.29
    meaning all digits (complete) (partial) 755.21
    transverse (complete) (partial) 755.21
Adair-Dighton syndrome (brittle bones and blue
  sclera, deafness) 756.51
Adamantinoblastoma (M9310/0) — *see*
  Ameloblastoma
Adamantinoma (M9310/0) — *see* Ameloblastoma
Adamantoblastoma (M9310/0) — *see*
  Ameloblastoma
Adams-Stokes (-Morgagni) disease or syndrome
  (syncope with heart block) 426.9
Adaptation reaction (*see also* Reaction,
  adjustment) 309.9
Addiction — *see also* Dependence
  absinthe 304.6 ✓5ᵗʰ
  alcoholic (ethyl) (methyl) (wood) 303.9 ✓5ᵗʰ
    complicating pregnancy, childbirth, or
      puerperium 648.4 ✓5ᵗʰ
      affecting fetus or newborn 760.71
    suspected damage to fetus affecting
      management of pregnancy 655.4 ✓5ᵗʰ
  drug (*see also* Dependence) 304.9 ✓5ᵗʰ
  ethyl alcohol 303.9 ✓5ᵗʰ
  heroin 304.0 ✓5ᵗʰ
  hospital 301.51
  methyl alcohol 303.9 ✓5ᵗʰ
  methylated spirit 303.9 ✓5ᵗʰ
  morphine (-like substances) 304.0 ✓5ᵗʰ
  nicotine 305.1
  opium 304.0 ✓5ᵗʰ
  tobacco 305.1
  wine 303.9 ✓5ᵗʰ
Addison's
  anemia (pernicious) 281.0
  disease (bronze) (primary adrenal insufficiency)
    255.4
    tuberculous (*see also* Tuberculosis)
      017.6 ✓5ᵗʰ
  keloid (morphea) 701.0
  melanoderma (adrenal cortical hypofunction)
    255.4

Addison-Biermer anemia (pernicious) 281.0

Addison-Gull disease — *see* Xanthoma

Addisonian crisis or melanosis (acute adrenocortical insufficiency) 255.4

Additional — *see also* Accessory
chromosome(s) 758.5
　13-15 758.1
　16-18 758.2
　21 758.0
　autosome(s) NEC 758.5
　sex 758.81

Adduction contracture, hip or other joint — *see* Contraction, joint

Adenasthenia gastrica 536.0

Aden fever 061

Adenitis (*see also* Lymphadenitis) 289.3
acute, unspecified site 683
　epidemic infectious 075
axillary 289.3
　acute 683
　chronic or subacute 289.1
Bartholin's gland 616.8
bulbourethral gland (*see also* Urethritis) 597.89
cervical 289.3
　acute 683
　chronic or subacute 289.1
chancroid (Ducrey's bacillus) 099.0
chronic (any lymph node, except mesenteric) 289.1
　mesenteric 289.2
Cowper's gland (*see also* Urethritis) 597.89
epidemic, acute 075
gangrenous 683
gonorrheal NEC 098.89
groin 289.3
　acute 683
　chronic or subacute 289.1
infectious 075
inguinal (region) 289.3
　acute 683
　chronic or subacute 289.1
lymph gland or node, except mesenteric 289.3
　acute 683
　chronic or subacute 289.1
　mesenteric (acute) (chronic) (nonspecific) (subacute) 289.2
mesenteric (acute) (chronic) (nonspecific) (subacute) 289.2
　due to Pasteurella multocida (P. septica) 027.2
parotid gland (suppurative) 527.2
phlegmonous 683
salivary duct or gland (any) (recurring) (suppurative) 527.2
scrofulous (*see also* Tuberculosis) 017.2 ✓5ᵗʰ
septic 289.3
Skene's duct or gland (*see also* Urethritis) 597.89
strumous, tuberculous (*see also* Tuberculosis) 017.2 ✓5ᵗʰ
subacute, unspecified site 289.1
sublingual gland (suppurative) 527.2
submandibular gland (suppurative) 527.2
submaxillary gland (suppurative) 527.2
suppurative 683
tuberculous — *see* Tuberculosis, lymph gland
urethral gland (*see also* Urethritis) 597.89
venereal NEC 099.8
Wharton's duct (suppurative) 527.2

Adenoacanthoma (M8570/3) — *see* Neoplasm, by site, malignant

Adenoameloblastoma (M9300/0) 213.1
upper jaw (bone) 213.0

Adenocarcinoma (M8140/3) — *see also* Neoplasm, by site, malignant

> *Note* — *The following list of adjectival modifiers is not exhaustive. A description of adenocarcinoma that does not appear in this list should be coded in the same manner as carcinoma with that description. Thus, "mixed acidophil-basophil adenocarcinoma," should be coded in the same manner as "mixed acidophil-basophil carcinoma," which appears in the list under "Carcinoma."*
>
> *Except where otherwise indicated, the morphological varieties of adenocarcinoma in the list should be coded by site as for "Neoplasm, malignant."*

with
　apocrine metaplasia (M8573/3)
　cartilaginous (and osseous) metaplasia (M8571/3)
　osseous (and cartilaginous) metaplasia (M8571/3)
　spindle cell metaplasia (M8572/3)
　squamous metaplasia (M8570/3)
acidophil (M8280/3)
　specified site — *see* Neoplasm, by site, malignant
　unspecified site 194.3
acinar (M8550/3)
acinic cell (M8550/3)
adrenal cortical (M8370/3) 194.0
alveolar (M8251/3)
　and
　　epidermoid carcinoma, mixed (M8560/3)
　　squamous cell carcinoma, mixed (M8560/3)
apocrine (M8401/3)
　breast — *see* Neoplasm, breast, malignant
　specified site NEC — *see* Neoplasm, skin, malignant
　unspecified site 173.9
basophil (M8300/3)
　specified site — *see* Neoplasm, by site, malignant
　unspecified site 194.3
bile duct type (M8160/3)
　liver 155.1
　specified site NEC — *see* Neoplasm, by site, malignant
　unspecified site 155.1
bronchiolar (M8250/3) — *see* Neoplasm, lung, malignant
ceruminous (M8420/3) 173.2
chromophobe (M8270/3)
　specified site — *see* Neoplasm, by site, malignant
　unspecified site 194.3
clear cell (mesonephroid type) (M8310/3)
colloid (M8480/3)
cylindroid type (M8200/3)
diffuse type (M8145/3)
　specified site — *see* Neoplasm, by site, malignant
　unspecified site 151.9
duct (infiltrating) (M8500/3)
　with Paget's disease (M8541/3) — *see* Neoplasm, breast, malignant
　specified site — *see* Neoplasm, by site, malignant
　unspecified site 174.9
embryonal (M9070/3)
endometrioid (M8380/3) — *see* Neoplasm, by site, malignant
eosinophil (M8280/3)
　specified site — *see* Neoplasm, by site malignant
　unspecified site 194.3
follicular (M8330/3)
　and papillary (M8340/3) 193
　moderately differentiated type (M8332/3) 193
　pure follicle type (M8331/3) 193
　specified site — *see* Neoplasm, by site, malignant
　trabecular type (M8332/3) 193
　unspecified type 193
　well differentiated type (M8331/3) 193
gelatinous (M8480/3)

Adenocarcinoma — *see also* Neoplasm, by site, malignant — *continued*
granular cell (M8320/3)
Hürthle cell (M8290/3) 193
in
　adenomatous
　　polyp (M8210/3)
　　polyposis coli (M8220/3) 153.9
　polypoid adenoma (M8210/3)
　tubular adenoma (M8210/3)
　villous adenoma (M8261/3)
infiltrating duct (M8500/3)
　with Paget's disease (M8541/3) — *see* Neoplasm, breast, malignant
　specified site — *see* Neoplasm, by site, malignant
　unspecified site 174.9
inflammatory (M8530/3)
　specified site — *see* Neoplasm, by site, malignant
　unspecified site 174.9
in situ (M8140/2) — *see* Neoplasm, by site, in situ
intestinal type (M8144/3)
　specified site — *see* Neoplasm, by site, malignant
　unspecified site 151.9
intraductal (noninfiltrating) (M8500/2)
　papillary (M8503/2)
　　specified site — *see* Neoplasm, by site, in situ
　　unspecified site 233.0
　specified site — *see* Neoplasm, by site, in situ
　unspecified site 233.0
islet cell (M8150/3)
　and exocrine, mixed (M8154/3)
　　specified site — *see* Neoplasm, by site, malignant
　　unspecified site 157.9
　pancreas 157.4
　specified site NEC — *see* Neoplasm, by site, malignant
　unspecified site 157.4
lobular (M8520/3)
　specified site — *see* Neoplasm, by site, malignant
　unspecified site 174.9
medullary (M8510/3)
mesonephric (M9110/3)
mixed cell (M8323/3)
mucinous (M8480/3)
mucin-producing (M8481/3)
mucoid (M8480/3) — *see also* Neoplasm, by site, malignant
　cell (M8300/3)
　　specified site — *see* Neoplasm, by site, malignant
　　unspecified site 194.3
nonencapsulated sclerosing (M8350/3) 193
oncocytic (M8290/3)
oxyphilic (M8290/3)
papillary (M8260/3)
　and follicular (M8340/3) 193
　intraductal (noninfiltrating) (M8503/2)
　　specified site — *see* Neoplasm, by site, in situ
　　unspecified site 233.0
　serous (M8460/3)
　　specified site — *see* Neoplasm, by site, malignant
　　unspecified site 183.0
papillocystic (M8450/3)
　specified site — *see* Neoplasm, by site, malignant
　unspecified site 183.0
pseudomucinous (M8470/3)
　specified site — *see* Neoplasm, by site, malignant
　unspecified site 183.0
renal cell (M8312/3) 189.0
sebaceous (M8410/3)
serous (M8441/3) — *see also* Neoplasm, by site, malignant
　papillary
　　specified site — *see* Neoplasm, by site malignant

Adenocarcinoma — *see also* Neoplasm, by site, malignant — *continued*
  serous — *see also* Neoplasm, by site, malignant — *continued*
    papillary — *continued*
      unspecified site 183.0
  signet ring cell (M8490/3)
  superficial spreading (M8143/3)
  sweat gland (M8400/3) — *see* Neoplasm, skin, malignant
  trabecular (M8190/3)
  tubular (M8211/3)
  villous (M8262/3)
  water-clear cell (M8322/3) 194.1

Adenofibroma (M9013/0)
  clear cell (M8313/0) — *see* Neoplasm, by site, benign
  endometrioid (M8381/0) 220
    borderline malignancy (M8381/1) 236.2
    malignant (M8381/3) 183.0
  mucinous (M9015/0)
    specified site — *see* Neoplasm, by site, benign
    unspecified site 220
  prostate 600.2
  serous (M9014/0)
    specified site — *see* Neoplasm, by site, benign
    unspecified site 220
  specified site — *see* Neoplasm, by site, benign
  unspecified site 220

Adenofibrosis
  breast 610.2
  endometrioid 617.0

Adenoiditis 474.01
  acute 463
  chronic 474.01
    with chronic tonsillitis 474.02

Adenoids (congenital) (of nasal fossa) 474.9
  hypertrophy 474.12
  vegetations 474.2

Adenolipomatosis (symmetrical) 272.8

Adenolymphoma (M8561/0)
  specified site — *see* Neoplasm, by site, benign
  unspecified 210.2

Adenoma (sessile) (M8140/0) — *see also* Neoplasm, by site, benign

> *Note* — Except where otherwise indicated, the morphological varieties of adenoma in the list below should be coded by site as for "Neoplasm, benign."

  acidophil (M8280/0)
    specified site — *see* Neoplasm, by site, benign
    unspecified site 227.3
  acinar (cell) (M8550/0)
  acinic cell (M8550/0)
  adrenal (cortex) (cortical) (functioning) (M8370/0) 227.0
    clear cell type (M8373/0) 227.0
    compact cell type (M8371/0) 227.0
    glomerulosa cell type (M8374/0) 227.0
    heavily pigmented variant (M8372/0) 227.0
    mixed cell type (M8375/0) 227.0
  alpha cell (M8152/0)
    pancreas 211.7
    specified site NEC — *see* Neoplasm, by site, benign
    unspecified site 211.7
  alveolar (M8251/0)
  apocrine (M8401/0)
    breast 217
    specified site NEC — *see* Neoplasm, skin, benign
    unspecified site 216.9
  basal cell (M8147/0)
  basophil (M8300/0)
    specified site — *see* Neoplasm, by site, benign
    unspecified site 227.3
  beta cell (M8151/0)
    pancreas 211.7

Adenoma — *see also* Neoplasm, by site, benign — *continued*
  beta cell — *continued*
    specified site NEC — *see* Neoplasm, by site, benign
    unspecified site 211.7
  bile duct (M8160/0) 211.5
  black (M8372/0) 227.0
  bronchial (M8140/1) 235.7
    carcinoid type (M8240/3) — *see* Neoplasm, lung, malignant
    cylindroid type (M8200/3) — *see* Neoplasm, lung, malignant
  ceruminous (M8420/0) 216.2
  chief cell (M8321/0) 227.1
  chromophobe (M8270/0)
    specified site — *see* Neoplasm, by site, benign
    unspecified site 227.3
  clear cell (M8310/0)
  colloid (M8334/0)
    specified site — *see* Neoplasm, by site, benign
    unspecified site 226
  cylindroid type, bronchus (M8200/3) — *see* Neoplasm, lung, malignant
  duct (M8503/0)
  embryonal (M8191/0)
  endocrine, multiple (M8360/1)
    single specified site — *see* Neoplasm, by site, uncertain behavior
    two or more specified sites 237.4
    unspecified site 237.4
  endometrioid (M8380/0) — *see also* Neoplasm, by site, benign
    borderline malignancy (M8380/1) — *see* Neoplasm, by site, uncertain behavior
  eosinophil (M8280/0)
    specified site — *see* Neoplasm, by site, benign
    unspecified site 227.3
  fetal (M8333/0)
    specified site — *see* Neoplasm, by site, benign
    unspecified site 226
  follicular (M8330/0)
    specified site — *see* Neoplasm, by site, benign
    unspecified site 226
  hepatocellular (M8170/0) 211.5
  Hürthle cell (M8290/0) 226
  intracystic papillary (M8504/0)
  islet cell (functioning) (M8150/0)
    pancreas 211.7
    specified site NEC — *see* Neoplasm, by site, benign
    unspecified site 211.7
  liver cell (M8170/0) 211.5
  macrofollicular (M8334/0)
    specified site NEC — *see* Neoplasm, by site, benign
    unspecified site 226
  malignant, malignum (M8140/3) — *see* Neoplasm, by site, malignant
  mesonephric (M9110/0)
  microfollicular (M8333/0)
    specified site — *see* Neoplasm, by site, benign
    unspecified site 226
  mixed cell (M8323/0)
  monomorphic (M8146/0)
  mucinous (M8480/0)
  mucoid cell (M8300/0)
    specified site — *see* Neoplasm, by site, benign
    unspecified site 227.3
  multiple endocrine (M8360/1)
    single specified site — *see* Neoplasm, by site, uncertain behavior
    two or more specified sites 237.4
    unspecified site 237.4
  nipple (M8506/0) 217
  oncocytic (M8290/0)
  oxyphilic (M8290/0)
  papillary (M8260/0) — *see also* Neoplasm, by site, benign
    intracystic (M8504/0)
  papillotubular (M8263/0)

Adenoma — *see also* Neoplasm, by site, benign — *continued*
  Pick's tubular (M8640/0)
    specified site — *see* Neoplasm, by site, benign
    unspecified site
      female 220
      male 222.0
  pleomorphic (M8940/0)
  polypoid (M8210/0)
  prostate (benign) 600.2
  rete cell 222.0
  sebaceous, sebaceum (gland) (senile) (M8410/0) — *see also* Neoplasm, skin, benign
    disseminata 759.5
  Sertoli cell (M8640/0)
    specified site — *see* Neoplasm, by site, benign
    unspecified site
      female 220
      male 222.0
  skin appendage (M8390/0) — *see* Neoplasm, skin, benign
  sudoriferous gland (M8400/0) — *see* Neoplasm, skin, benign
  sweat gland or duct (M8400/0) — *see* Neoplasm, skin, benign
  testicular (M8640/0)
    specified site — *see* Neoplasm, by site, benign
    unspecified site
      female 220
      male 222.0
  thyroid 226
  trabecular (M8190/0)
  tubular (M8211/0) — *see also* Neoplasm, by site, benign
    papillary (M8460/3)
    Pick's (M8640/0)
      specified site — *see* Neoplasm, by site, benign
      unspecified site
        female 220
        male 222.0
  tubulovillous (M8263/0)
  villoglandular (M8263/0)
  villous (M8261/1) — *see* Neoplasm, by site, uncertain behavior
  water-clear cell (M8322/0) 227.1
  wolffian duct (M9110/0)

Adenomatosis (M8220/0)
  endocrine (multiple) (M8360/1)
    single specified site — *see* Neoplasm, by site, uncertain behavior
    two or more specified sites 237.4
    unspecified site 237.4
  erosive of nipple (M8506/0) 217
  pluriendocrine — *see* Adenomatosis, endocrine
  pulmonary (M8250/1) 235.7
    malignant (M8250/3) — *see* Neoplasm, lung, malignant
  specified site — *see* Neoplasm, by site, benign
  unspecified site 211.3

Adenomatous
  cyst, thyroid (gland) — *see* Goiter, nodular
  goiter (nontoxic) (*see also* Goiter, nodular) 241.9
    toxic or with hyperthyroidism 242.3 ✔5ᵗʰ

Adenomyoma (M8932/0) — *see also* Neoplasm, by site, benign
  prostate 600.2

Adenomyometritis 617.0

Adenomyosis (uterus) (internal) 617.0

Adenopathy (lymph gland) 785.6
  inguinal 785.6
  mediastinal 785.6
  mesentery 785.6
  syphilitic (secondary) 091.4
  tracheobronchial 785.6
    tuberculous (*see also* Tuberculosis) 012.1 ✔5ᵗʰ
      primary, progressive 010.8 ✔5ᵗʰ
  tuberculous (*see also* Tuberculosis, lymph gland) 017.2 ✔5ᵗʰ
    tracheobronchial 012.1 ✔5ᵗʰ
      primary, progressive 010.8 ✔5ᵗʰ

Adenopharyngitis 462

Adenophlegmon 683

Adenosalpingitis 614.1

Adenosarcoma (M8960/3) 189.0

Adenosclerosis 289.3

Adenosis
  breast (sclerosing) 610.2
  vagina, congenital 752.49

Adentia (complete) (partial) (see also Absence, teeth) 520.0

Adherent
  labium (minus) 624.4
  pericardium (nonrheumatic) 423.1
    rheumatic 393
  placenta 667.0 ☑5ᵗʰ
    with hemorrhage 666.0 ☑5ᵗʰ
  prepuce 605
  scar (skin) NEC 709.2
  tendon in scar 709.2

Adhesion(s), adhesive (postinfectional) (postoperative)
  abdominal (wall) (see also Adhesions, peritoneum) 568.0
  amnion to fetus 658.8 ☑5ᵗʰ
    affecting fetus or newborn 762.8
  appendix 543.9
  arachnoiditis — see Meningitis
  auditory tube (Eustachian) 381.89
  bands — see also Adhesions, peritoneum
    cervix 622.3
    uterus 621.5
  bile duct (any) 576.8
  bladder (sphincter) 596.8
  bowel (see also Adhesions, peritoneum) 568.0
  cardiac 423.1
    rheumatic 398.99
  cecum (see also Adhesions, peritoneum) 568.0
  cervicovaginal 622.3
    congenital 752.49
    postpartal 674.8 ☑5ᵗʰ
      old 622.3
  cervix 622.3
  clitoris 624.4
  colon (see also Adhesions, peritoneum) 568.0
  common duct 576.8
  congenital — see also Anomaly, specified type NEC
    fingers (see also Syndactylism, fingers) 755.11
    labium (majus) (minus) 752.49
    omental, anomalous 751.4
    ovary 752.0
    peritoneal 751.4
    toes (see also Syndactylism, toes) 755.13
    tongue (to gum or roof of mouth) 750.12
  conjunctiva (acquired) (localized) 372.62
    congenital 743.63
    extensive 372.63
  cornea — see Opacity, cornea
  cystic duct 575.8
  diaphragm (see also Adhesions, peritoneum) 568.0
  due to foreign body — see Foreign body
  duodenum (see also Adhesions, peritoneum) 568.0
    with obstruction 537.3
  ear, middle — see Adhesions, middle ear
  epididymis 608.89
  epidural — see Adhesions, meninges
  epiglottis 478.79
  Eustachian tube 381.89
  eyelid 374.46
    postoperative 997.99
      surgically created V45.69
  gallbladder (see also Disease, gallbladder) 575.8
  globe 360.89
  heart 423.1
    rheumatic 398.99
  ileocecal (coil) (see also Adhesions, peritoneum) 568.0
  ileum (see also Adhesions, peritoneum) 568.0
  intestine (postoperative) (see also Adhesions, peritoneum) 568.0

Adhesion(s), adhesive — continued
  intestine (see also Adhesions, peritoneum) — continued
    with obstruction 560.81
      with hernia — see also Hernia, by site, with obstruction
        gangrenous — see Hernia, by site, with gangrene
  intra-abdominal (see also Adhesions, peritoneum) 568.0
  iris 364.70
    to corneal graft 996.79
  joint (see also Ankylosis) 718.5 ☑5ᵗʰ
  kidney 593.89
  labium (majus) (minus), congenital 752.49
  liver 572.8
  lung 511.0
  mediastinum 519.3
  meninges 349.2
    cerebral (any) 349.2
      congenital 742.4
    congenital 742.8
    spinal (any) 349.2
      congenital 742.59
    tuberculous (cerebral) (spinal) (see also Tuberculosis, meninges) 013.0 ☑5ᵗʰ
  mesenteric (see also Adhesions, peritoneum) 568.0
  middle ear (fibrous) 385.10
    drum head 385.19
      to
        incus 385.11
        promontorium 385.13
        stapes 385.12
    specified NEC 385.19
  nasal (septum) (to turbinates) 478.1
  nerve NEC 355.9
    spinal 355.9
      root 724.9
        cervical NEC 723.4
        lumbar NEC 724.4
        lumbosacral 724.4
        thoracic 724.4
  ocular muscle 378.60
  omentum (see also Adhesions, peritoneum) 568.0
  organ or site, congenital NEC — see Anomaly, specified type NEC
  ovary 614.6
    congenital (to cecum, kidney, or omentum) 752.0
  parauterine 614.6
  parovarian 614.6
  pelvic (peritoneal)
    female (postoperative) (postinfection) 614.6
    male (postoperative) (postinfection) (see also Adhesions, peritoneum) 568.0
    postpartal (old) 614.6
    tuberculous (see also Tuberculosis) 016.9 ☑5ᵗʰ
  penis to scrotum (congenital) 752.69
  periappendiceal (see also Adhesions, peritoneum) 568.0
  pericardium (nonrheumatic) 423.1
    rheumatic 393
    tuberculous (see also Tuberculosis) 017.9 ☑5ᵗʰ [420.0]
  pericholecystic 575.8
  perigastric (see also Adhesions, peritoneum) 568.0
  periovarian 614.6
  periprostatic 602.8
  perirectal (see also Adhesions, peritoneum) 568.0
  perirenal 593.89
  peritoneum, peritoneal (fibrous) (postoperative) 568.0
    with obstruction (intestinal) 560.81
      with hernia — see also Hernia, by site, with obstruction
        gangrenous — see Hernia, by site, with gangrene
      duodenum 537.3
    congenital 751.4
    female (postoperative) (postinfective) 614.6
    pelvic, female 614.6
    pelvic, male 568.0
    postpartal, pelvic 614.6

Adhesion(s), adhesive — continued
  peritoneum, peritoneal — continued
    to uterus 614.6
  peritubal 614.6
  periureteral 593.89
  periuterine 621.5
  perivesical 596.8
  perivesicular (seminal vesicle) 608.89
  pleura, pleuritic 511.0
    tuberculous (see also Tuberculosis, pleura) 012.0 ☑5ᵗʰ
  pleuropericardial 511.0
  postoperative (gastrointestinal tract) (see also Adhesions, peritoneum) 568.0
    eyelid 997.99
      surgically created V45.69
    pelvic female 614.9
    pelvic male 568.0
    urethra 598.2
  postpartal, old 624.4
  preputial, prepuce 605
  pulmonary 511.0
  pylorus (see also Adhesions, peritoneum) 568.0
  Rosenmüller's fossa 478.29
  sciatic nerve 355.0
  seminal vesicle 608.89
  shoulder (joint) 726.0
  sigmoid flexure (see also Adhesions, peritoneum) 568.0
  spermatic cord (acquired) 608.89
    congenital 752.8
  spinal canal 349.2
    nerve 355.9
      root 724.9
        cervical NEC 723.4
        lumbar NEC 724.4
        lumbosacral 724.4
        thoracic 724.4
  stomach (see also Adhesions, peritoneum) 568.0
  subscapular 726.2
  tendonitis 726.90
    shoulder 726.0
  testicle 608.89
  tongue (congenital) (to gum or roof of mouth) 750.12
    acquired 529.8
  trachea 519.1
  tubo-ovarian 614.6
  tunica vaginalis 608.89
  ureter 593.89
  uterus 621.5
    to abdominal wall 614.6
      in pregnancy or childbirth 654.4 ☑5ᵗʰ
        affecting fetus or newborn 763.89
  vagina (chronic) (postoperative) (postradiation) 623.2
  vaginitis (congenital) 752.49
  vesical 596.8
  vitreous 379.29

Adie (-Holmes) syndrome (tonic pupillary reaction) 379.46

Adiponecrosis neonatorum 778.1

Adiposa dolorosa 272.8

Adiposalgia 272.8

Adiposis
  cerebralis 253.8
  dolorosa 272.8
  tuberosa simplex 272.8

Adiposity 278.00
  heart (see also Degeneration, myocardial) 429.1
  localized 278.1

Adiposogenital dystrophy 253.8

Adjustment
  prosthesis or other device — see Fitting of
  reaction — see Reaction, adjustment

Administration, prophylactic
  antibiotics V07.39
  antitoxin, any V07.2
  antivenin V07.2
  chemotherapeutic agent NEC V07.39
  chemotherapy V07.39
  diphtheria antitoxin V07.2
  fluoride V07.31
  gamma globulin V07.2
  immune sera (gamma globulin) V07.2

Administration — Admission

Administration, prophylactic — *continued*
  passive immunization agent V07.2
  RhoGAM V07.2
Admission (encounter)
  as organ donor — *see* Donor
  by mistake V68.9
  for
    adequacy testing (for)
      hemodialysis V56.31
      peritoneal dialysis V56.32
    adjustment (of)
      artificial
        arm (complete) (partial) V52.0
        eye V52.2
        leg (complete) (partial) V52.1
      brain neuropacemaker V53.02
      breast
        implant V52.4
        prosthesis V52.4
      cardiac device V53.39
        defibrillator, automatic implantable
          V53.32
        pacemaker V53.31
          carotid sinus V53.39
      catheter
        non-vascular V58.82
        vascular V58.81
      cerebral ventricle (communicating) shunt
        V53.01
      colostomy belt V55.3
      contact lenses V53.1
      cystostomy device V53.6
      dental prosthesis V52.3
      device NEC V53.9
        abdominal V53.5
        cardiac V53.39
          defibrillator, automatic implantable
            V53.32
          pacemaker V53.31
        carotid sinus V53.39
        cerebral ventricle (communicating)
          shunt V53.01
        intrauterine contraceptive V25.1
        nervous system V53.09
        orthodontic V53.4
        prosthetic V52.9
          breast V52.4
          dental V52.3
          eye V52.2
          specified type NEC V52.8
        special senses V53.09
        substitution
          auditory V53.09
          nervous system V53.09
          visual V53.09
        urinary V53.6
      dialysis catheter
        extracorporeal V56.1
        peritoneal V56.2
      diaphragm (contraceptive) V25.02
      hearing aid V53.2
      ileostomy device V55.2
      intestinal appliance or device NEC V53.5
      intrauterine contraceptive device V25.1
      neuropacemaker (brain) (peripheral nerve)
        (spinal cord) V53.02
      orthodontic device V53.4
      orthopedic (device) V53.7
        brace V53.7
        cast V53.7
        shoes V53.7
      pacemaker
        brain V53.02
        cardiac V53.31
        carotid sinus V53.39
        peripheral nerve V53.02
        spinal cord V53.02
      prosthesis V52.9
        arm (complete) (partial) V52.0
        breast V52.4
        dental V52.3
        eye V52.2
        leg (complete) (partial) V52.1
        specified type NEC V52.8
      spectacles V53.1
      wheelchair V53.8

Admission — *continued*
  for — *continued*
    adoption referral or proceedings V68.89
    aftercare (*see also* Aftercare) V58.9
      cardiac pacemaker V53.31
      chemotherapy V58.1
      dialysis
        extracorporeal (renal) V56.0
        peritoneal V56.8
        renal V56.0
      fracture (*see also* Aftercare, fracture)
        V54.9
      medical NEC V58.89
      orthopedic V54.9
        specified care NEC V54.89 ▲
      pacemaker device
        brain V53.02
        cardiac V53.31
        carotid sinus V53.39
        nervous system V53.02
        spinal cord V53.02
      postoperative NEC V58.49
        wound closure, planned V58.41
      postpartum
        immediately after delivery V24.0
        routine follow-up V24.2
      postradiation V58.0
      radiation therapy V58.0
      removal of
        non-vascular catheter V58.82
        vascular catheter V58.81
      specified NEC V58.89
      surgical NEC V58.49
        wound closure, planned V58.41
    artificial insemination V26.1
    attention to artificial opening (of) V55.9
      artificial vagina V55.7
      colostomy V55.3
      cystostomy V55.5
      enterostomy V55.4
      gastrostomy V55.1
      ileostomy V55.2
      jejunostomy V55.4
      nephrostomy V55.6
      specified site NEC V55.8
        intestinal tract V55.4
        urinary tract V55.6
      tracheostomy V55.0
      ureterostomy V55.6
      urethrostomy V55.6
    battery replacement
      cardiac pacemaker V53.31
    boarding V65.0
    breast
      augmentation or reduction V50.1
      removal, prophylactic V50.41
    change of
      cardiac pacemaker (battery) V53.31
      carotid sinus pacemaker V53.39
      catheter in artificial opening — *see*
        Attention to, artificial, opening
      dressing V58.3
      fixation device
        external V54.89 ▲
        internal V54.0
      Kirschner wire V54.89 ▲
      neuropacemaker device (brain)
        (peripheral nerve) (spinal cord)
        V53.02
      pacemaker device
        brain V53.02
        cardiac V53.31
        carotid sinus V53.39
        nervous system V53.02
      plaster cast V54.89
      splint, external V54.89 ▲
      Steinmann pin V54.89 ▲
      surgical dressing V58.3
      traction device V54.89 ▲
    checkup only V70.0
    chemotherapy V58.1
    circumcision, ritual or routine (in absence of
      medical indication) V50.2
    clinical research investigation (control)
      (normal comparison) (participant)
      V70.7

Admission — *continued*
  for — *continued*
    closure of artificial opening — *see* Attention
      to, artificial, opening
    contraceptive
      counseling V25.09
      management V25.9
        specified type NEC V25.8
    convalescence following V66.9
      chemotherapy V66.2
      psychotherapy V66.3
      radiotherapy V66.1
      surgery V66.0
      treatment (for) V66.5
        combined V66.6
        fracture V66.4
        mental disorder NEC V66.3
        specified condition NEC V66.5
    cosmetic surgery NEC V50.1
      following healed injury or operation V51
    counseling (*see also* Counseling) V65.40
      without complaint or sickness V65.49
      contraceptive management V25.09
      dietary V65.3
      exercise V65.41
      for
        nonattending third party V65.1
        victim of abuse
          child V61.21
          partner or spouse V61.11
      genetic V26.3
      gonorrhea V65.45
      HIV V65.44
      human immunodeficiency virus V65.44
      injury prevention V65.43
      procreative management V26.4
      sexually transmitted disease NEC V65.45
        HIV V65.44
      specified reason NEC V65.49
      substance use and abuse V65.42
      syphilis V65.45
      victim of abuse
        child V61.21
        partner or spouse V61.11
    desensitization to allergens V07.1
    dialysis V56.0
      catheter
        fitting and adjustment
          extracorporeal V56.1
          peritoneal V56.2
        removal or replacement
          extracorporeal V56.1
          peritoneal V56.2
      extracorporeal (renal) V56.0
      peritoneal V56.8
      renal V56.0
    dietary surveillance and counseling V65.3
    drug monitoring, therapeutic V58.83
    ear piercing V50.3
    elective surgery V50.9
      breast
        augmentation or reduction V50.1
        removal, prophylactic V50.41
      circumcision, ritual or routine (in
        absence of medical indication)
        V50.2
      cosmetic NEC V50.1
        following healed injury or operation
        V51
      ear piercing V50.3
      face-lift V50.1
      hair transplant V50.0
      plastic
        cosmetic NEC V50.1
        following healed injury or operation
        V51
      prophylactic organ removal V50.49
        breast V50.41
        ovary V50.42
      repair of scarred tissue (following healed
        injury or operation) V51
      specified type NEC V50.8
    end-of-life care V66.7
    examination (*see also* Examination) V70.9
      administrative purpose NEC V70.3
      adoption V70.3

✔4ᵗʰ Fourth-digit Required   ✔5ᵗʰ Fifth-digit Required   ▶◀ Revised Text   ● New Line   ▲ Revised Code

Admission — *continued*
  for — *continued*
    examination (*see also* Examination) —
      continued
      allergy V72.7
      at health care facility V70.0
      athletic team V70.3
      camp V70.3
      cardiovascular, preoperative V72.81
      clinical research investigation (control)
        (participant) V70.7
      dental V72.2
      developmental testing (child) (infant)
        V20.2
      donor (potential) V70.8
      driver's license V70.3
      ear V72.1
      employment V70.5
      eye V72.0
      follow-up (routine) — *see* Examination,
        follow-up
      for admission to
        old age home V70.3
        school V70.3
      general V70.9
        specified reason NEC V70.8
      gynecological V72.3
      health supervision (child) (infant) V20.2
      hearing V72.1
      immigration V70.3
      insurance certification V70.3
      laboratory V72.6
      marriage license V70.3
      medical (general) (*see also* Examination,
        medical) V70.9
      medicolegal reasons V70.4
      naturalization V70.3
      pelvic (annual) (periodic) V72.3
      postpartum checkup V24.2
      pregnancy (possible) (unconfirmed) V72.4
      preoperative V72.84
        cardiovascular V72.81
        respiratory V72.82
        specified NEC V72.83
      prison V70.3
      psychiatric (general) V70.2
        requested by authority V70.1
      radiological NEC V72.5
      respiratory, preoperative V72.82
      school V70.3
      screening — *see* Screening
      skin hypersensitivity V72.7
      specified type NEC V72.85
      sport competition V70.3
      vision V72.0
      well baby and child care V20.2
    exercise therapy V57.1
    face-lift, cosmetic reason V50.1
    fitting (of)
      artificial
        arm (complete) (partial) V52.0
        eye V52.2
        leg (complete) (partial) V52.1
      biliary drainage tube V58.82
      brain neuropacemaker V53.02
      breast V52.4
        implant V52.4
        prosthesis V52.4
      cardiac pacemaker V53.31
      catheter
        non-vascular V58.82
        vascular V58.81
      cerebral ventricle (communicating) shunt
        V53.01
      chest tube V58.82
      colostomy belt V55.2
      contact lenses V53.1
      cystostomy device V53.6
      dental prosthesis V52.3
      device NEC V53.9
        abdominal V53.5
        cerebral ventricle (communicating)
          shunt V53.01
        intrauterine contraceptive V25.1
        nervous system V53.09
        orthodontic V53.4

Admission — *continued*
  for — *continued*
    fitting — *continued*
      device NEC — *continued*
        prosthetic V52.9
          breast V52.4
          dental V52.3
          eye V52.2
        special senses V53.09
        substitution
          auditory V53.09
          nervous system V53.09
          visual V53.09
      diaphragm (contraceptive) V25.02
      fistula (sinus tract) drainage tube V58.82
      hearing aid V53.2
      ileostomy device V55.2
      intestinal appliance or device NEC V53.5
      intrauterine contraceptive device V25.1
      neuropacemaker (brain) (peripheral nerve)
        (spinal cord) V53.02
      orthodontic device V53.4
      orthopedic (device) V53.7
        brace V53.7
        cast V53.7
        shoes V53.7
      pacemaker
        brain V53.02
        cardiac V53.31
        carotid sinus V53.39
        spinal cord V53.02
      pleural drainage tube V58.82
      prosthesis V52.9
        arm (complete) (partial) V52.0
        breast V52.4
        dental V52.3
        eye V52.2
        leg (complete) (partial) V52.1
        specified type NEC V52.8
      spectacles V53.1
      wheelchair V53.8
    follow-up examination (routine) (following)
      V67.9
      cancer chemotherapy V67.2
      chemotherapy V67.2
      high-risk medication NEC V67.51
      injury NEC V67.59
      psychiatric V67.3
      psychotherapy V67.3
      radiotherapy V67.1
      specified surgery NEC V67.09
      surgery V67.00
        vaginal pap smear V67.01
      treatment (for) V67.9
        combined V67.6
        fracture V67.4
        involving high-risk medication NEC
          V67.51
        mental disorder V67.3
        specified NEC V67.59
    hair transplant, for cosmetic reason V50.0
    health advice, education, or instruction
      V65.4
    hospice care V66.7
    insertion (of)
      subdermal implantable contraceptive
        V25.5
    intrauterine device
      insertion V25.1
      management V25.42
    investigation to determine further
      disposition V63.8
    isolation V07.0
    issue of
      medical certificate NEC V68.0
      repeat prescription NEC V68.1
        contraceptive device NEC V25.49
    kidney dialysis V56.0
    mental health evaluation V70.2
      requested by authority V70.1
    nonmedical reason NEC V68.89
    nursing care evaluation V63.8
    observation (without need for further
      medical care) (*see also* Observation)
      V71.9
      accident V71.4

Admission — *continued*
  for — *continued*
    observation (*see also* Observation) —
      continued
      alleged rape or seduction V71.5
      criminal assault V71.6
      following accident V71.4
        at work V71.3
      foreign body ingestion V71.89
      growth and development variations,
        childhood V21.0
      inflicted injury NEC V71.6
      ingestion of deleterious agent or foreign
        body V71.89
      injury V71.6
      malignant neoplasm V71.1
      mental disorder V71.09
      newborn — *see* Observation, suspected,
        condition, newborn
      rape V71.5
      specified NEC V71.89
      suspected disorder V71.9
        abuse V71.81
        accident V71.4
          at work V71.3
        benign neoplasm V71.89
        cardiovascular V71.7
        exposure   ●
          anthrax V71.82   ●
          biological agent NEC V71.83   ●
        heart V71.7
        inflicted injury NEC V71.6
        malignant neoplasm V71.1
        mental NEC V71.09
        neglect V71.81
        specified condition NEC V71.89
        tuberculosis V71.2
      tuberculosis V71.2
    occupational therapy V57.21
    organ transplant, donor — *see* Donor
    ovary, ovarian removal, prophylactic V50.42
    palliative care V66.7
    Papanicolaou smear
      cervix V76.2
        for suspected malignant neoplasm
          V76.2
          no disease found V71.1
        routine, as part of gynecological
          examination V72.3
      vaginal V76.47
        following hysterectomy for malignant
          condition V67.01
    passage of sounds or bougie in artificial
      opening — *see* Attention to, artificial,
      opening
    paternity testing V70.4
    peritoneal dialysis V56.32
    physical therapy NEC V57.1
    plastic surgery
      cosmetic NEC V50.1
      following healed injury or operation V51
    postmenopausal hormone replacement
      therapy V07.4
    postpartum observation
      immediately after delivery V24.0
      routine follow-up V24.2
    poststerilization (for restoration) V26.0
    procreative management V26.9
      specified type NEC V26.8
    prophylactic
      administration of
        antibiotics V07.39
        antitoxin, any V07.2
        antivenin V07.2
        chemotherapeutic agent NEC V07.39
        chemotherapy NEC V07.39
        diphtheria antitoxin V07.2
        fluoride V07.31
        gamma globulin V07.2
        immune sera (gamma globulin) V07.2
        RhoGAM V07.2
        tetanus antitoxin V07.2
      breathing exercises V57.0
      chemotherapy NEC V07.39
        fluoride V07.31
      measure V07.9
        specified type NEC V07.8

Admission — *continued*
for — *continued*
prophylactic — *continued*
organ removal V50.49
breast V50.41
ovary V50.42
psychiatric examination (general) V70.2
requested by authority V70.1
radiation management V58.0
radiotherapy V58.0
reforming of artificial opening — *see*
Attention to, artificial, opening
rehabilitation V57.9
multiple types V57.89
occupational V57.21
orthoptic V57.4
orthotic V57.81
physical NEC V57.1
specified type NEC V57.89
speech V57.3
vocational V57.22
removal of
cardiac pacemaker V53.31
cast (plaster) V54.89 ▲
catheter from artificial opening — *see*
Attention to, artificial, opening
cerebral ventricle (communicating) shunt
V53.01
cystostomy catheter V55.5
device
cerebral ventricle (communicating)
shunt V53.01
fixation
external V54.89 ▲
internal V54.0
intrauterine contraceptive V25.42
traction, external V54.89 ▲
dressing V58.3
fixation device
external V54.89 ▲
internal V54.0
intrauterine contraceptive device V25.42
Kirschner wire V54.89 ▲
neuropacemaker (brain) (peripheral nerve)
(spinal cord) V53.02
orthopedic fixation device
external V54.89 ▲
internal V54.0
pacemaker device
brain V53.02
cardiac V53.31
carotid sinus V53.39
nervous system V53.02
plaster cast V54.89 ▲
plate (fracture) V54.0
rod V54.0
screw (fracture) V54.0
splint, traction V54.89 ▲
Steinmann pin V54.89 ▲
subdermal implantable contraceptive
V25.43
surgical dressing V58.3
sutures V58.3
traction device, external V54.89 ▲
ureteral stent V53.6
repair of scarred tissue (following healed
injury or operation) V51
reprogramming of cardiac pacemaker
V53.31
restoration of organ continuity
(poststerilization) (tuboplasty)
(vasoplasty) V26.0
sensitivity test — *see also* Test, skin
allergy NEC V72.7
bacterial disease NEC V74.9
Dick V74.8
Kveim V82.89
Mantoux V74.1
mycotic infection NEC V75.4
parasitic disease NEC V75.8
Schick V74.3
Schultz-Charlton V74.8
social service (agency) referral or evaluation
V63.8
speech therapy V57.3
sterilization V25.2

Admission — *continued*
for — *continued*
suspected disorder (ruled out) (without need
for further care) — *see* Observation
terminal care V66.7
tests only — *see* Test
therapeutic drug monitoring V58.83
therapy
blood transfusion, without reported
diagnosis V58.2
breathing exercises V57.0
chemotherapy V58.1
prophylactic NEC V07.39
fluoride V07.31
dialysis (intermittent) (treatment)
extracorporeal V56.0
peritoneal V56.8
renal V56.0
specified type NEC V56.8
exercise (remedial) NEC V57.1
breathing V57.0
long-term (current) drug use NEC V58.69
antibiotics V58.62
anticoagulant V58.61
occupational V57.21
orthoptic V57.4
physical NEC V57.1
radiation V58.0
speech V57.3
vocational V57.22
toilet or cleaning
of artificial opening — *see* Attention to,
artificial, opening
of non-vascular catheter V58.82
of vascular catheter V58.81
tubal ligation V25.2
tuboplasty for previous sterilization V26.0
vaccination, prophylactic (against)
arthropod-borne virus, viral NEC V05.1
disease NEC V05.1
encephalitis V05.0
Bacille Calmette Guérin (BCG) V03.2
BCG V03.2
chickenpox V05.4
cholera alone V03.0
with typhoid-paratyphoid (cholera +
TAB) V06.0
common cold V04.7
dengue V05.1
diphtheria alone V03.5
diphtheria-tetanus [Td] without pertussis
V06.5
diphtheria-tetanus-pertussis (DTP) V06.1
with
poliomyelitis (DTP + polio) V06.3
typhoid-paratyphoid (DTP + TAB)
V06.2
disease (single) NEC V05.9
bacterial NEC V03.9
specified type NEC V03.89
combinations NEC V06.9
specified type NEC V06.8
specified type NEC V05.8
encephalitis, viral, arthropod-borne V05.0
Hemophilus infuenzae, type B [Hib]
V03.81
hepatitis, viral V05.3
immune sera (gamma globulin) V07.2
influenza V04.8
with
Streptococcus pneumoniae
[pneumococcus] V06.6
Leishmaniasis V05.2
measles alone V04.2
measles-mumps-rubella (MMR) V06.4
mumps alone V04.6
with measles and rubella (MMR) V06.4
not done because of contraindication
V64.0
pertussis alone V03.6
plague V03.3
pneumonia V03.82
poliomyelitis V04.0
with diphtheria-tetanus-pertussis
(DTP+ polio) V06.3
rabies V04.5

Admission — *continued*
for — *continued*
vaccination, prophylactic — *continued*
rubella alone V04.3
with measles and mumps (MMR)
V06.4
smallpox V04.1
specified type NEC V05.8
Streptococcus pneumoniae
[pneumococcus] V03.82
with
influenza V06.6
tetanus toxoid alone V03.7
with diphtheria [Td] V06.5
and pertussis (DTP) V06.1
tuberculosis (BCG) V03.2
tularemia V03.4
typhoid alone V03.1
with diphtheria-tetanus-pertussis (TAB
+ DTP) V06.2
typhoid-paratyphoid alone (TAB) V03.1
typhus V05.8
varicella (chicken pox) V05.4
viral encephalitis, arthropod-borne V05.0
viral hepatitis V05.3
yellow fever V04.4
vasectomy V25.2
vasoplasty for previous sterilization V26.0
vision examination V72.0
vocational therapy V57.22
waiting period for admission to other facility
V63.2
undergoing social agency investigation
V63.8
well baby and child care V20.2
x-ray of chest
for suspected tuberculosis V71.2
routine V72.5

Adnexitis (suppurative) (*see also* Salpingo-
oophoritis) 614.2
Adolescence NEC V21.2
Adoption
agency referral V68.89
examination V70.3
held for V68.89
Adrenal gland — *see* condition
Adrenalism 255.9
tuberculous (*see also* Tuberculosis) 017.6 ✓5ᵗʰ
Adrenalitis, adrenitis 255.8
meningococcal hemorrhagic 036.3
Adrenarche, precocious 259.1
Adrenocortical syndrome 255.2
Adrenogenital syndrome (acquired) (congenital)
255.2
iatrogenic, fetus or newborn 760.79
Adventitious bursa — *see* Bursitis
Adynamia (episodica) (hereditary) (periodic) 359.3
Adynamic
ileus or intestine (*see also* Ileus) 560.1
ureter 753.22
Aeration lung, imperfect, newborn 770.5
Aerobullosis 993.3
Aerocele — *see* Embolism, air
Aerodermectasia
subcutaneous (traumatic) 958.7
surgical 998.81
surgical 998.81
Aerodontalgia 993.2
Aeroembolism 993.3
Aerogenes capsulatus infection (*see also*
Gangrene, gas) 040.0
Aero-otitis media 993.0
Aerophagy, aerophagia 306.4
psychogenic 306.4
Aerosinusitis 993.1
Aerotitis 993.0
Affection, affections — *see also* Disease
sacroiliac (joint), old 724.6
shoulder region NEC 726.2
Afibrinogenemia 286.3
acquired 286.6
congenital 286.3

Afibrinogenemia — *continued*
  postpartum 666.3 ✓5ᵗʰ
African
  sleeping sickness 086.5
  tick fever 087.1
  trypanosomiasis 086.5
    Gambian 086.3
    Rhodesian 086.4
Aftercare V58.9
  artificial openings — *see* Attention to, artificial, opening
  blood transfusion without reported diagnosis V58.2
  breathing exercise V57.0
  cardiac device V53.39
    defibrillator, automatic implantable V53.32
    pacemaker V53.31
      carotid sinus V53.39
  carotid sinus pacemaker V53.39
  cerebral ventricle (communicating) shunt V53.01
  chemotherapy session (adjunctive) (maintenance) V58.1
  defibrillator, automatic implantable cardiac V53.32
  exercise (remedial) (therapeutic) V57.1
    breathing V57.0
  extracorporeal dialysis (intermittent) (treatment) V56.0
  following surgery NEC V58.49
    for
      injury V58.43 ●
      neoplasm V58.42 ●
      trauma V58.43 ●
    joint replacement V54.81 ●
    of
      circulatory system V58.73 ●
      digestive system V58.75 ●
      genital organs V58.76 ●
      genitourinary system V58.76 ●
      musculoskeletal system V58.78 ●
      nervous system V58.72 ●
      oral cavity V58.75 ●
      respiratory system V58.74 ●
      sense organs V58.71 ●
      skin V58.77 ●
      subcutaneous tissue V58.77 ●
      teeth V58.75 ●
      urinary system V58.76 ●
    wound closure, planned V58.41
  fracture V54.9
    healing V54.89 ●
      pathologic
        arm V54.20 ●
          lower V54.22 ●
          upper V54.21 ●
        hip V54.23 ●
        leg V54.24 ●
          lower V54.26 ●
          upper V54.25 ●
        specified site NEC V54.29 ●
        vertebrae V54.27 ●
      traumatic
        arm V54.10 ●
          lower V54.12 ●
          upper V54.11 ●
        hip V54.13 ●
        leg V54.14 ●
          lower V54.16 ●
          upper V54.15 ●
        specified site NEC V54.19 ●
        vertebrae V54.17 ●
    removal of
      external fixation device V54.89 ▲
      internal fixation device V54.0
    specified care NEC V54.89 ▲
  gait training V57.1
    for use of artificial limb(s) V57.81
  involving
    dialysis (intermittent) (treatment)
      extracorporeal V56.0
      peritoneal V56.8
      renal V56.0
    gait training V57.1
      for use of artificial limb(s) V57.81
    orthoptic training V57.4

Aftercare — *continued*
  involving — *continued*
    orthotic training V57.81
    radiotherapy session V58.0
    removal of
      dressings V58.3
      fixation device
        external V54.89 ▲
        internal V54.0
      fracture plate V54.0
      pins V54.0
      plaster cast V54.89 ▲
      rods V54.0
      screws V54.0
      surgical dressings V58.3
      sutures V58.3
      traction device, external V54.89 ▲
    neuropacemaker (brain) (peripheral nerve) (spinal cord) V53.02
    occupational therapy V57.21
    orthodontic V58.5
    orthopedic V54.9
      change of external fixation or traction device V54.89 ▲
      following joint replacement V54.81 ●
      removal of fixation device
        external V54.89 ▲
        internal V54.0
      specified care NEC V54.89 ▲
    orthoptic training V57.4
    orthotic training V57.81
    pacemaker
      brain V53.02
      cardiac V53.31
      carotid sinus V53.39
      peripheral nerve V53.02
      spinal cord V53.02
    peritoneal dialysis (intermittent) (treatment) V56.8
    physical therapy NEC V57.1
      breathing exercises V57.0
    radiotherapy session V58.0
    rehabilitation procedure V57.9
      breathing exercises V57.0
      multiple types V57.89
      occupational V57.21
      orthoptic V57.4
      orthotic V57.81
      physical therapy NEC V57.1
      remedial exercises V57.1
      specified type NEC V57.89
      speech V57.3
      therapeutic exercises V57.1
      vocational V57.22
    renal dialysis (intermittent) (treatment) V56.0
    specified type NEC V58.89
      removal of non-vascular catheter V58.82
      removal of vascular catheter V58.81
    speech therapy V57.3
    vocational rehabilitation V57.22
After-cataract 366.50
  obscuring vision 366.53
  specified type, not obscuring vision 366.52
Agalactia 676.4 ✓5ᵗʰ
Agammaglobulinemia 279.00
  with lymphopenia 279.2
  acquired (primary) (secondary) 279.06
  Bruton's X-linked 279.04
  infantile sex-linked (Bruton's) (congenital) 279.04
  Swiss-type 279.2
Aganglionosis (bowel) (colon) 751.3
AGCUS (atypical glandular cell changes of undetermined significance) ●
  favor benign 795.01 ●
  favor dysplasia 795.02 ●
Age (old) (*see also* Senile) 797
Agenesis — *see also* Absence, by site, congenital
  acoustic nerve 742.8
  adrenal (gland) 759.1
  alimentary tract (complete) (partial) NEC 751.8
    lower 751.2
    upper 750.8
  anus, anal (canal) 751.2
  aorta 747.22
  appendix 751.2

Agenesis — *see also* Absence, by site, congenital — *continued*
  arm (complete) (partial) (*see also* Deformity, reduction, upper limb) 755.20
  artery (peripheral) NEC (*see also* Anomaly, peripheral vascular system) 747.60
    brain 747.81
    coronary 746.85
    pulmonary 747.3
    umbilical 747.5
  auditory (canal) (external) 744.01
  auricle (ear) 744.01
  bile, biliary duct or passage 751.61
  bone NEC 756.9
  brain 740.0
    specified part 742.2
  breast 757.6
  bronchus 748.3
  canaliculus lacrimalis 743.65
  carpus NEC (*see also* Deformity, reduction, upper limb) 755.28
  cartilage 756.9
  cecum 751.2
  cerebellum 742.2
  cervix 752.49
  chin 744.89
  cilia 743.63
  circulatory system, part NEC 747.89
  clavicle 755.51
  clitoris 752.49
  coccyx 756.13
  colon 751.2
  corpus callosum 742.2
  cricoid cartilage 748.3
  diaphragm (with hernia) 756.6
  digestive organ(s), or tract (complete) (partial) NEC 751.8
    lower 751.2
    upper 750.8
  ductus arteriosus 747.89
  duodenum 751.1
  ear NEC 744.09
    auricle 744.01
    lobe 744.21
  ejaculatory duct 752.8
  endocrine (gland) NEC 759.2
  epiglottis 748.3
  esophagus 750.3
  Eustachian tube 744.24
  extrinsic muscle, eye 743.69
  eye 743.00
    adnexa 743.69
  eyelid (fold) 743.62
  face
    bones NEC 756.0
    specified part NEC 744.89
  fallopian tube 752.19
  femur NEC (*see also* Absence, femur, congenital) 755.34
  fibula NEC (*see also* Absence, fibula, congenital) 755.37
  finger NEC (*see also* Absence, finger, congenital) 755.29
  foot (complete) (*see also* Deformity, reduction, lower limb) 755.31
  gallbladder 751.69
  gastric 750.8
  genitalia, genital (organ)
    female 752.8
      external 752.49
      internal NEC 752.8
    male 752.8
      penis 752.69
  glottis 748.3
  gonadal 758.6
  hair 757.4
  hand (complete) (*see also* Deformity, reduction, upper limb) 755.21
  heart 746.89
    valve NEC 746.89
      aortic 746.89
      mitral 746.89
      pulmonary 746.01
  hepatic 751.69
  humerus NEC (*see also* Absence, humerus, congenital) 755.24
  hymen 752.49
  ileum 751.1

✓4ᵗʰ Fourth-digit Required   ✓5ᵗʰ Fifth-digit Required   ▶◀ Revised Text   ● New Line   ▲ Revised Code

Albuminuria, albuminuric — *continued*
  Bence-Jones 791.0
  cardiac 785.9
  complicating pregnancy, childbirth, or
      puerperium 646.2 ✓5ᵗʰ
    with hypertension — *see* Toxemia, of
        pregnancy
    affecting fetus or newborn 760.1
  cyclic 593.6
  gestational 646.2 ✓5ᵗʰ
  gravidarum 646.2 ✓5ᵗʰ
    with hypertension — *see* Toxemia, of
        pregnancy
    affecting fetus or newborn 760.1
  heart 785.9
  idiopathic 593.6
  orthostatic 593.6
  postural 593.6
  pre-eclamptic (mild) 642.4 ✓5ᵗʰ
    affecting fetus or newborn 760.0
    severe 642.5 ✓5ᵗʰ
      affecting fetus or newborn 760.0
  recurrent physiologic 593.6
  scarlatinal 034.1
Albumosuria 791.0
  Bence-Jones 791.0
  myelopathic (M9730/3) 203.0 ✓5ᵗʰ
Alcaptonuria 270.2
Alcohol, alcoholic
  abstinence 291.81
  acute intoxication 305.0 ✓5ᵗʰ
    with dependence 303.0 ✓5ᵗʰ
  addiction (*see also* Alcoholism) 303.9 ✓5ᵗʰ
    maternal
      with suspected fetal damage affecting
          management of pregnancy
          655.4 ✓5ᵗʰ
      affecting fetus or newborn 760.71
  amnestic disorder, persisting 291.1
  anxiety 291.89
  brain syndrome, chronic 291.2
  cardiopathy 425.5
  chronic (*see also* Alcoholism) 303.9 ✓5ᵗʰ
  cirrhosis (liver) 571.2
  delirium 291.0
    acute 291.0
    chronic 291.1
    tremens 291.0
    withdrawal 291.0
  dementia NEC 291.2
  deterioration 291.2
  drunkenness (simple) 305.0 ✓5ᵗʰ
  hallucinosis (acute) 291.3
  insanity 291.9
  intoxication (acute) 305.0 ✓5ᵗʰ
    with dependence 303.0 ✓5ᵗʰ
    pathological 291.4
  jealousy 291.5
  Korsakoff's, Korsakov's, Korsakow's 291.1
  liver NEC 571.3
    acute 571.1
    chronic 571.2
  mania (acute) (chronic) 291.9
  mood 291.89
  paranoia 291.5
  paranoid (type) psychosis 291.5
  pellagra 265.2
  poisoning, accidental (acute) NEC 980.9
    specified type of alcohol — *see* Table of
        Drugs and Chemicals
  psychosis (*see also* Psychosis, alcoholic) 291.9
    Korsakoff's, Korsakov's, Korsakow's 291.1
    polyneuritic 291.1
      with
        delusions 291.5
        hallucinations 291.3
  withdrawal symptoms, syndrome NEC 291.81
    delirium 291.0
    hallucinosis 291.3

Alcoholism 303.9 ✓5ᵗʰ

> *Note* — *Use the following fifth-digit*
> *subclassification with category 303:*
>
> 0   *unspecified*
> 1   *continuous*
> 2   *episodic*
> 3   *in remission*

  with psychosis (*see also* Psychosis, alcoholic)
      291.9
  acute 303.0 ✓5ᵗʰ
  chronic 303.9 ✓5ᵗʰ
    with psychosis 291.9
  complicating pregnancy, childbirth, or
      puerperium 648.4 ✓5ᵗʰ
    affecting fetus or newborn 760.71
  history V11.3
  Korsakoff's, Korsakov's, Korsakow's 291.1
  suspected damage to fetus affecting
      management of pregnancy 655.4 ✓5ᵗʰ
Alder's anomaly or syndrome (leukocyte
    granulation anomaly) 288.2
Alder-Reilly anomaly (leukocyte granulation)
    288.2
Aldosteronism (primary) (secondary) 255.1
  congenital 255.1
Aldosteronoma (M8370/1) 237.2
Aldrich (-Wiskott) syndrome (eczema-
    thrombocytopenia) 279.12
Aleppo boil 085.1
Aleukemic — *see* condition
Aleukia
  congenital 288.0
  hemorrhagica 284.9
    acquired (secondary) 284.8
    congenital 284.0
    idiopathic 284.9
  splenica 289.4
Alexia (congenital) (developmental) 315.01
  secondary to organic lesion 784.61
Algoneurodystrophy 733.7
Algophobia 300.29
Alibert's disease (mycosis fungoides) (M9700/3)
    202.1 ✓5ᵗʰ
Alibert-Bazin disease (M9700/3) 202.1 ✓5ᵗʰ
Alice in Wonderland syndrome 293.89
Alienation, mental (*see also* Psychosis) 298.9
Alkalemia 276.3
Alkalosis 276.3
  metabolic 276.3
    with respiratory acidosis 276.4
  respiratory 276.3
Alkaptonuria 270.2
Allen-Masters syndrome 620.6
Allergic bronchopulmonary aspergillosis 518.6
Allergy, allergic (reaction) 995.3
  air-borne substance (*see also* Fever, hay) 477.9
    specified allergen NEC 477.8
  alveolitis (extrinsic) 495.9
    due to
      Aspergillus clavatus 495.4
      cryptostroma corticale 495.6
      organisms (fungal, thermophilic
          actinomycete, other) growing in
          ventilation (air conditioning
          systems) 495.7
    specified type NEC 495.8
  anaphylactic shock 999.4
    due to food — *see* Anaphylactic shock, due
        to, food
  angioneurotic edema 995.1
  animal (dander) (epidermal) (hair) 477.8
  arthritis (*see also* Arthritis, allergic) 716.2 ✓5ᵗʰ
  asthma — *see* Asthma
  bee sting (anaphylactic shock) 989.5
  biological — *see* Allergy, drug
  bronchial asthma — *see* Asthma
  conjunctivitis (eczematous) 372.14
  dander (animal) 477.8
  dandruff 477.8
  dermatitis (venenata) — *see* Dermatitis

Allergy, allergic — *continued*
  diathesis V15.09
  drug, medicinal substance, and biological (any)
      (correct medicinal substance properly
      administered) (external) (internal) 995.2
    wrong substance given or taken NEC 977.9
      specified drug or substance — *see* Table
          of Drugs and Chemicals
  dust (house) (stock) 477.8
  eczema — *see* Eczema
  endophthalmitis 360.19
  epidermal (animal) 477.8
  feathers 477.8
  food (any) (ingested) 693.1
    atopic 691.8
    in contact with skin 692.5
  gastritis 535.4 ✓5ᵗʰ
  gastroenteritis 558.3
  gastrointestinal 558.3
  grain 477.0
  grass (pollen) 477.0
    asthma (*see also* Asthma) 493.0 ✓5ᵗʰ
    hay fever 477.0
  hair (animal) 477.8
  hay fever (grass) (pollen) (ragweed) (tree) (*see
      also* Fever, hay) 477.9
  history (of) V15.09
    to
      eggs V15.03
      food additives V15.05
      insect bite V15.06
      latex V15.07
      milk products V15.02
      nuts V15.05
        peanuts V15.01
      radiographic dye V15.08
      seafood V15.04
      specified food NEC V15.05
      spider bite V15.06
  horse serum — *see* Allergy, serum
  inhalant 477.9
    dust 477.8
    pollen 477.0
    specified allergen other than pollen 477.8
  kapok 477.8
  medicine — *see* Allergy, drug
  migraine 346.2 ✓5ᵗʰ
  pannus 370.62
  pneumonia 518.3
  pollen (any) (hay fever) 477.0
    asthma (*see also* Asthma) 493.0 ✓5ᵗʰ
  primrose 477.0
  primula 477.0
  purpura 287.0
  ragweed (pollen) (Senecio jacobae) 477.0
    asthma (*see also* Asthma) 493.0 ✓5ᵗʰ
    hay fever 477.0
  respiratory (*see also* Allergy, inhalant) 477.9
    due to
      drug — *see* Allergy, drug
      food — *see* Allergy, food
  rhinitis (*see also* Fever, hay) 477.9
    due to food 477.1
  rose 477.0
  Senecio jacobae 477.0
  serum (prophylactic) (therapeutic) 999.5
    anaphylactic shock 999.4
  shock (anaphylactic) (due to adverse effect of
      correct medicinal substance properly
      administered) 995.0
    food — *see* Anaphylactic shock, due to, food
    from serum or immunization 999.5
      anaphylactic 999.4
  sinusitis (*see also* Fever, hay) 477.9
  skin reaction 692.9
    specified substance — *see* Dermatitis, due
        to
  tree (any) (hay fever) (pollen) 477.0
    asthma (*see also* Asthma) 493.0 ✓5ᵗʰ
  upper respiratory (*see also* Fever, hay) 477.9
  urethritis 597.89
  urticaria 708.0
  vaccine — *see* Allergy, serum
Allescheriosis 117.6
Alligator skin disease (ichthyosis congenita)
    757.1
  acquired 701.1

Albuminuria — Alligator skin disease

Allocheiria, allochiria (see also Disturbance, sensation) 782.0
Almeida's disease (Brazilian blastomycosis) 116.1
Alopecia (atrophicans) (pregnancy) (premature) (senile) 704.00
  adnata 757.4
  areata 704.01
  celsi 704.01
  cicatrisata 704.09
  circumscripta 704.01
  congenital, congenitalis 757.4
  disseminata 704.01
  effluvium (telogen) 704.02
  febrile 704.09
  generalisata 704.09
  hereditaria 704.09
  marginalis 704.01
  mucinosa 704.09
  postinfectional 704.09
  seborrheica 704.09
  specific 091.82
  syphilitic (secondary) 091.82
  telogen effluvium 704.02
  totalis 704.09
  toxica 704.09
  universalis 704.09
  x-ray 704.09
Alpers' disease 330.8
Alpha-lipoproteinemia 272.4
Alpha thalassemia 282.4
Alphos 696.1
Alpine sickness 993.2
Alport's syndrome (hereditary hematurianephropathy-deafness) 759.89
Alteration (of), altered
  awareness 780.09
    transient 780.02
  consciousness 780.09
    persistent vegetative state 780.03
    transient 780.02
  mental status 780.99   ▲
Alternaria (infection) 118
Alternating — see condition
Altitude, high (effects) — see Effect, adverse, high altitude
Aluminosis (of lung) 503
Alvarez syndrome (transient cerebral ischemia) 435.9
Alveolar capillary block syndrome 516.3
Alveolitis
  allergic (extrinsic) 495.9
    due to organisms (fungal, thermophilic actinomycete, other) growing in ventilation (air conditioning systems) 495.7
    specified type NEC 495.8
  due to
    Aspergillus clavatus 495.4
    Cryptostroma corticale 495.6
  fibrosing (chronic) (cryptogenic) (lung) 516.3
    idiopathic 516.3
    rheumatoid 714.81
  jaw 526.5
    sicca dolorosa 526.5
Alveolus, alveolar — see condition
Alymphocytosis (pure) 279.2
Alymphoplasia, thymic 279.2
Alzheimer's
  dementia (senile)
    with behavioral disturbance 331.0 [294.11]
    without behavioral disturbance 331.0 [294.10]
  disease or sclerosis 331.0
    with dementia — see Alzheimer's, dementia
Amastia (see also Absence, breast) 611.8
Amaurosis (acquired) (congenital) (see also Blindness) 369.00
  fugax 362.34
  hysterical 300.11
  Leber's (congenital) 362.76
  tobacco 377.34
  uremic — see Uremia

Amaurotic familial idiocy (infantile) (juvenile) (late) 330.1
Ambisexual 752.7
Amblyopia (acquired) (congenital) (partial) 368.00
  color 368.59
    acquired 368.55
  deprivation 368.02
  ex anopsia 368.00
  hysterical 300.11
  nocturnal 368.60
    vitamin A deficiency 264.5
  refractive 368.03
  strabismic 368.01
  suppression 368.01
  tobacco 377.34
  toxic NEC 377.34
  uremic — see Uremia
Ameba, amebic (histolytica) — see also Amebiasis
  abscess 006.3
    bladder 006.8
    brain (with liver and lung abscess) 006.5
    liver 006.3
      with
        brain abscess (and lung abscess) 006.5
        lung abscess 006.4
    lung (with liver abscess) 006.4
      with brain abscess 006.5
    seminal vesicle 006.8
    spleen 006.8
  carrier (suspected of) V02.2
  meningoencephalitis
    due to Naegleria (gruberi) 136.2
    primary 136.2
Amebiasis NEC 006.9
  with
    brain abscess (with liver or lung abscess) 006.5
    liver abscess (without mention of brain or lung abscess) 006.3
    lung abscess (with liver abscess) 006.4
      with brain abscess 006.5
  acute 006.0
  bladder 006.8
  chronic 006.1
  cutaneous 006.6
  cutis 006.6
  due to organism other than Entamoeba histolytica 007.8
  hepatic (see also Abscess, liver, amebic) 006.3
  nondysenteric 006.2
  seminal vesicle 006.8
  specified
    organism NEC 007.8
    site NEC 006.8
Ameboma 006.8
Amelia 755.4
  lower limb 755.31
  upper limb 755.21
Ameloblastoma (M9310/0) 213.1
  jaw (bone) (lower) 213.1
    upper 213.0
  long bones (M9261/3) — see Neoplasm, bone, malignant
  malignant (M9310/3) 170.1
    jaw (bone) (lower) 170.1
      upper 170.0
  mandible 213.1
  tibial (M9261/3) 170.7
Amelogenesis imperfecta 520.5
  nonhereditaria (segmentalis) 520.4
Amenorrhea (primary) (secondary) 626.0
  due to ovarian dysfunction 256.8
  hyperhormonal 256.8
Amentia (see also Retardation, mental) 319
  Meynert's (nonalcoholic) 294.0
    alcoholic 291.1
  nevoid 759.6
American
  leishmaniasis 085.5
  mountain tick fever 066.1
  trypanosomiasis — see Trypanosomiasis, American
Ametropia (see also Disorder, accommodation) 367.9

Amianthosis 501
Amimia 784.69
Amino acid
  deficiency 270.9
    anemia 281.4
  metabolic disorder (see also Disorder, amino acid) 270.9
Aminoaciduria 270.9
  imidazole 270.5
Amnesia (retrograde) 780.99   ▲
  auditory 784.69
    developmental 315.31
    secondary to organic lesion 784.69
  hysterical or dissociative type 300.12
  psychogenic 300.12
  transient global 437.7
Amnestic (confabulatory) syndrome 294.0
  alcohol induced 291.1
  drug-induced 292.83
  posttraumatic 294.0
Amniocentesis screening (for) V28.2
  alphafetoprotein level, raised V28.1
  chromosomal anomalies V28.0
Amnion, amniotic — see also condition
  nodosum 658.8 ✔5ᵗʰ
Amnionitis (complicating pregnancy) 658.4 ✔5ᵗʰ
  affecting fetus or newborn 762.7
Amoral trends 301.7
Amotio retinae (see also Detachment, retina) 361.9
Ampulla
  lower esophagus 530.89
  phrenic 530.89
Amputation
  any part of fetus, to facilitate delivery 763.89
  cervix (supravaginal) (uteri) 622.8
    in pregnancy or childbirth 654.6 ✔5ᵗʰ
      affecting fetus or newborn 763.89
  clitoris — see Wound, open, clitoris
  congenital
    lower limb 755.31
    upper limb 755.21
  neuroma (traumatic) — see also Injury, nerve, by site
    surgical complication (late) 997.61
  penis — see Amputation, traumatic, penis
  status (without complication) — see Absence, by site, acquired
  stump (surgical) (posttraumatic)
    abnormal, painful, or with complication (late) 997.60
    healed or old NEC — see also Absence, by site, acquired
      lower V49.70
      upper V49.60
  traumatic (complete) (partial)

> Note — "Complicated" includes traumatic amputation with delayed healing, delayed treatment, foreign body, or infection.

    arm 887.4
      at or above elbow 887.2
        complicated 887.3
      below elbow 887.0
        complicated 887.1
      both (bilateral) (any level(s)) 887.6
        complicated 887.7
      complicated 887.5
    finger(s) (one or both hands) 886.0
      with thumb(s) 885.0
        complicated 885.1
      complicated 886.1
    foot (except toe(s) only) 896.0
      and other leg 897.6
        complicated 897.7
      both (bilateral) 896.2
        complicated 896.3
      complicated 896.1
      toe(s) only (one or both feet) 895.0
        complicated 895.1
    genital organ(s) (external) NEC 878.8
      complicated 878.9
    hand (except finger(s) only) 887.0
      and other arm 887.6

Amputation — *continued*
  traumatic — *continued*
    hand — *continued*
      and other arm — *continued*
        complicated 887.7
        both (bilateral) 887.6
          complicated 887.7
        complicated 887.1
        finger(s) (one or both hands) 886.0
          with thumb(s) 885.0
            complicated 885.1
          complicated 886.1
        thumb(s) (with fingers of either hand) 885.0
          complicated 885.1
    head 874.9
    late effect — *see* Late, effects (of), amputation
    leg 897.4
      and other foot 897.6
        complicated 897.7
      at or above knee 897.2
        complicated 897.3
      below knee 897.0
        complicated 897.1
      both (bilateral) 897.6
        complicated 897.7
      complicated 897.5
    lower limb(s) except toe(s) — *see* Amputation, traumatic, leg
    nose — *see* Wound, open, nose
    penis 878.0
      complicated 878.1
    sites other than limbs — *see* Wound, open, by site
    thumb(s) (with finger(s) of either hand) 885.0
      complicated 885.1
    toe(s) (one or both feet) 895.0
      complicated 895.1
    upper limb(s) — *see* Amputation, traumatic, arm

Amputee (bilateral) (old) — *see also* Absence, by site, acquired V49.70

Amusia 784.69
  developmental 315.39
  secondary to organic lesion 784.69

Amyelencephalus 740.0

Amyelia 742.59

Amygdalitis — *see* Tonsillitis

Amygdalolith 474.8

Amyloid disease or degeneration 277.3
  heart 277.3 [425.7]

Amyloidosis (familial) (general) (generalized) (genetic) (primary) (secondary) 277.3
  with lung involvement 277.3 [517.8]
  heart 277.3 [425.7]
  nephropathic 277.3 [583.81]
  neuropathic (Portuguese) (Swiss) 277.3 [357.4]
  pulmonary 277.3 [517.8]
  systemic, inherited 277.3

Amylopectinosis (brancher enzyme deficiency) 271.0

Amylophagia 307.52

Amyoplasia, congenita 756.89

Amyotonia 728.2
  congenita 358.8

Amyotrophia, amyotrophy, amyotrophic 728.2
  congenita 756.89
  diabetic 250.6 ☑5ᵗʰ [358.1]
  lateral sclerosis (syndrome) 335.20
  neuralgic 353.5
  sclerosis (lateral) 335.20
  spinal progressive 335.21

Anacidity, gastric 536.0
  psychogenic 306.4

Anaerosis of newborn 768.9   ▲

Analbuminemia 273.8

Analgesia (*see also* Anesthesia) 782.0

Analphalipoproteinemia 272.5

Anaphylactic shock or reaction (correct substance properly administered) 995.0
  due to
    food 995.60
      additives 995.66
      crustaceans 995.62
      eggs 995.68
      fish 995.65
      fruits 995.63
      milk products 995.67
      nuts (tree) 995.64
      peanuts 995.61
      seeds 995.64
      specified NEC 995.69
      tree nuts 995.64
      vegetables 995.63
    immunization 999.4
    overdose or wrong substance given or taken 977.9
      specified drug — *see* Table of Drugs and Chemicals
    serum 999.4
  following sting(s) 989.5
  purpura 287.0
  serum 999.4

Anaphylactoid shock or reaction — *see* Anaphylactic shock

Anaphylaxis — *see* Anaphylactic shock

Anaplasia, cervix 622.1

Anarthria 784.5

Anarthritic rheumatoid disease 446.5

Anasarca 782.3
  cardiac (*see also* Failure, heart) 428.0
  fetus or newborn 778.0
  lung 514
  nutritional 262
  pulmonary 514
  renal (*see also* Nephrosis) 581.9

Anaspadias 752.62

Anastomosis
  aneurysmal — *see* Aneurysm
  arteriovenous, congenital NEC (*see also* Anomaly, arteriovenous) 747.60
    ruptured, of brain (*see also* Hemorrhage, subarachnoid) 430
  intestinal 569.89
    complicated NEC 997.4
      involving urinary tract 997.5
  retinal and choroidal vessels 743.58
    acquired 362.17

Anatomical narrow angle (glaucoma) 365.02

Ancylostoma (infection) (infestation) 126.9
  americanus 126.1
  braziliense 126.2
  caninum 126.8
  ceylanicum 126.3
  duodenale 126.0
  Necator americanus 126.1

Ancylostomiasis (intestinal) 126.9
  Ancylostoma
    americanus 126.1
    caninum 126.8
    ceylanicum 126.3
    duodenale 126.0
  braziliense 126.2
  Necator americanus 126.1

Anders' disease or syndrome (adiposis tuberosa simplex) 272.8

Andersen's glycogen storage disease 271.0

Anderson's disease 272.7

Andes disease 993.2

Andrews' disease (bacterid) 686.8

Androblastoma (M8630/1)
  benign (M8630/0)
    specified site — *see* Neoplasm, by site, benign
    unspecified site
      female 220
      male 222.0
  malignant (M8630/3)
    specified site — *see* Neoplasm, by site, malignant
    unspecified site
      female 183.0

Androblastoma — *continued*
  malignant — *continued*
    unspecified site — *continued*
      male 186.9
    specified site — *see* Neoplasm, by site, uncertain behavior
  tubular (M8640/0)
    with lipid storage (M8641/0)
      specified site — *see* Neoplasm, by site, benign
      unspecified site
        female 220
        male 222.0
    specified site — *see* Neoplasm, by site, benign
    unspecified site
      female 220
      male 222.0
  unspecified site
    female 236.2
    male 236.4

Android pelvis 755.69
  with disproportion (fetopelvic) 653.3 ☑5ᵗʰ
    affecting fetus or newborn 763.1
    causing obstructed labor 660.1 ☑5ᵗʰ
      affecting fetus or newborn 763.1

Anectasis, pulmonary (newborn or fetus) 770.5

Anemia 285.9
  with
    disorder of
      anaerobic glycolysis 282.3
      pentose phosphate pathway 282.2
    koilonychia 280.9
  6-phosphogluconic dehydrogenase deficiency 282.2
  achlorhydric 280.9
  achrestic 281.8
  Addison's (pernicious) 281.0
  Addison-Biermer (pernicious) 281.0
  agranulocytic 288.0
  amino acid deficiency 281.4
  aplastic 284.9
    acquired (secondary) 284.8
    congenital 284.0
    constitutional 284.0
    due to
      chronic systemic disease 284.8
      drugs 284.8
      infection 284.8
      radiation 284.8
    idiopathic 284.9
    myxedema 244.9
    of or complicating pregnancy 648.2 ☑5ᵗʰ
    red cell (acquired) (pure) (with thymoma) 284.8
      congenital 284.0
    specified type NEC 284.8
    toxic (paralytic) 284.8
  aregenerative 284.9
    congenital 284.0
  asiderotic 280.9
  atypical (primary) 285.9
  autohemolysis of Selwyn and Dacie (type I) 282.2
  autoimmune hemolytic 283.0
  Baghdad Spring 282.2
  Balantidium coli 007.0
  Biermer's (pernicious) 281.0
  blood loss (chronic) 280.0
    acute 285.1
  bothriocephalus 123.4
  brickmakers' (*see also* Ancylostomiasis) 126.9
  cerebral 437.8
  childhood 285.9
  chlorotic 280.9
  chronica congenita aregenerativa 284.0
  chronic simple 281.9
  combined system disease NEC 281.0 [336.2]
    due to dietary deficiency 281.1 [336.2]
  complicating pregnancy or childbirth 648.2 ☑5ᵗʰ
  congenital (following fetal blood loss) 776.5
    aplastic 284.0
    due to isoimmunization NEC 773.2
    Heinz-body 282.7
    hereditary hemolytic NEC 282.9
    nonspherocytic
      Type I 282.2

Anemia — *continued*
  congenital — *continued*
    nonspherocytic — *continued*
      Type II 282.3
    pernicious 281.0
    spherocytic (*see also* Spherocytosis) 282.0
  Cooley's (erythroblastic) 282.4
  crescent — *see* Disease, sickle-cell
  cytogenic 281.0
  Dacie's (nonspherocytic)
    type I 282.2
    type II 282.3
  Davidson's (refractory) 284.9
  deficiency 281.9
    2, 3 diphosphoglycurate mutase 282.3
    2, 3 PG 282.3
    6-PGD 282.2
    6-phosphogluronic dehydrogenase 282.2
    amino acid 281.4
    combined B_{12} and folate 281.3
    enzyme, drug-induced (hemolytic) 282.2
    erythrocytic glutathione 282.2
    folate 281.2
      dietary 281.2
      drug-induced 281.2
    folic acid 281.2
      dietary 281.2
      drug-induced 281.2
    G-6-PD 282.2
    GGS-R 282.2
    glucose-6-phosphate dehydrogenase (G-6-PD) 282.2
    glucose-phosphate isomerase 282.3
    glutathione peroxidase 282.2
    glutathione reductase 282.2
    glyceraldehyde phosphate dehydrogenase 282.3
    GPI 282.3
    G SH 282.2
    hexokinase 282.3
    iron (Fe) 280.9
      specified NEC 280.8
    nutritional 281.9
      with
        poor iron absorption 280.9
        specified deficiency NEC 281.8
      due to inadequate dietary iron intake 280.1
      specified type NEC 281.8
    of or complicating pregnancy 648.2 ✔5ᵗʰ
    pentose phosphate pathway 282.2
    PFK 282.3
    phosphofructo-aldolase 282.3
    phosphofructokinase 282.3
    phosphoglycerate kinase 282.3
    PK 282.3
    protein 281.4
    pyruvate kinase (PK) 282.3
    TPI 282.3
    triosephosphate isomerase 282.3
    vitamin B_{12} NEC 281.1
      dietary 281.1
      pernicious 281.0
  Diamond-Blackfan (congenital hypoplastic) 284.0
  dibothriocephalus 123.4
  dimorphic 281.9
  diphasic 281.8
  diphtheritic 032.89
  Diphyllobothrium 123.4
  drepanocytic (*see also* Disease, sickle-cell) 282.60
  due to
    blood loss (chronic) 280.0
      acute 285.1
    defect of Embden-Meyerhof pathway glycolysis 282.3
    disorder of glutathione metabolism 282.2
    fetal blood loss 776.5
    fish tapeworm (D. latum) infestation 123.4
    glutathione metabolism disorder 282.2
    hemorrhage (chronic) 280.0
      acute 285.1
    hexose monophosphate (HMP) shunt deficiency 282.2
    impaired absorption 280.9

Anemia — *continued*
  due to — *continued*
    loss of blood (chronic) 280.0
      acute 285.1
    myxedema 244.9
    Necator americanus 126.1
    prematurity 776.6
    selective vitamin B_{12} malabsorption with proteinuria 281.1
  Dyke-Young type (secondary) (symptomatic) 283.9
  dyserythropoietic (congenital) (types I, II, III) 285.8
  dyshemopoietic (congenital) 285.8
  Egypt (*see also* Ancylostomiasis) 126.9
  elliptocytosis (*see also* Elliptocytosis) 282.1
  enzyme deficiency, drug-induced 282.2
  epidemic (*see also* Ancylostomiasis) 126.9
  erythroblastic
    familial 282.4
    fetus or newborn (*see also* Disease, hemolytic) 773.2
    late 773.5
  erythrocytic glutathione deficiency 282.2
  essential 285.9
  Faber's (achlorhydric anemia) 280.9
  factitious (self-induced blood letting) 280.0
  familial erythroblastic (microcytic) 282.4
  Fanconi's (congenital pancytopenia) 284.0
  favism 282.2
  fetal, following blood loss 776.5
  fetus or newborn
    due to
      ABO
        antibodies 773.1
        incompatibility, maternal/fetal 773.1
        isoimmunization 773.1
      Rh
        antibodies 773.0
        incompatibility, maternal/fetal 773.0
        isoimmunization 773.0
    following fetal blood loss 776.5
  fish tapeworm (D. latum) infestation 123.4
  folate (folic acid) deficiency 281.2
    dietary 281.2
    drug-induced 281.2
  folate malabsorption, congenital 281.2
  folic acid deficiency 281.2
    dietary 281.2
    drug-induced 281.2
  G-6-PD 282.2
  general 285.9
  glucose-6-phosphate dehydrogenase deficiency 282.2
  glutathione-reductase deficiency 282.2
  goat's milk 281.2
  granulocytic 288.0
  Heinz-body, congenital 282.7
  hemoglobin deficiency 285.9
  hemolytic 283.9
    acquired 283.9
      with hemoglobinuria NEC 283.2
      autoimmune (cold type) (idiopathic) (primary) (secondary) (symptomatic) (warm type) 283.0
      due to
        cold reactive antibodies 283.0
        drug exposure 283.0
        warm reactive antibodies 283.0
      fragmentation 283.19
      idiopathic (chronic) 283.9
      infectious 283.19
        autoimmune 283.0
      non-autoimmune NEC 283.10
      toxic 283.19
      traumatic cardiac 283.19
    acute 283.9
      due to enzyme deficiency NEC 282.3
      fetus or newborn (*see also* Disease, hemolytic) 773.2
      late 773.5
      Lederer's (acquired infectious hemolytic anemia) 283.19
    autoimmune (acquired) 283.0
    chronic 282.9
      idiopathic 283.9
    cold type (secondary) (symptomatic) 283.0

Anemia — *continued*
  hemolytic — *continued*
    congenital (spherocytic) (*see also* Spherocytosis) 282.0
      nonspherocytic — *see* Anemia, hemolytic, nonspherocytic, congenital
    drug-induced 283.0
      enzyme deficiency 282.2
    due to
      cardiac conditions 283.19
      drugs 283.0
      enzyme deficiency NEC 282.3
        drug-induced 282.2
      presence of shunt or other internal prosthetic device 283.19
      thrombotic thrombocytopenic purpura 446.6
    elliptocytotic (*see also* Elliptocytosis) 282.1
    familial 282.9
    hereditary 282.9
      due to enzyme deficiency NEC 282.3
      specified NEC 282.8
    idiopathic (chronic) 283.9
    infectious (acquired) 283.19
    mechanical 283.19
    microangiopathic 283.19
    non-autoimmune NEC 283.10
    nonspherocytic
      congenital or hereditary NEC 282.3
        glucose-6-phosphate dehydrogenase deficiency 282.2
        pyruvate kinase (PK) deficiency 282.3
        type I 282.2
        type II 282.3
      type I 282.2
      type II 282.3
    of or complicating pregnancy 648.2 ✔5ᵗʰ
    resulting from presence of shunt or other internal prosthetic device 283.19
    secondary 283.19
      autoimmune 283.0
    sickle-cell — *see* Disease, sickle-cell
    Stransky-Regala type (Hb-E) (*see also* Disease, hemoglobin) 282.7
    symptomatic 283.19
      autoimmune 283.0
    toxic (acquired) 283.19
    uremic (adult) (child) 283.11
    warm type (secondary) (symptomatic) 283.0
  hemorrhagic (chronic) 280.0
    acute 285.1
  HEMPAS 285.8
  hereditary erythroblast multinuclearity-positive acidified serum test 285.8
  Herrick's (hemoglobin S disease) 282.61
  hexokinase deficiency 282.3
  high A_2 282.4
  hookworm (*see also* Ancylostomiasis) 126.9
  hypochromic (idiopathic) (microcytic) (normoblastic) 280.9
    with iron loading 285.0
    due to blood loss (chronic) 280.0
      acute 285.1
    familial sex linked 285.0
    pyridoxine-responsive 285.0
  hypoplasia, red blood cells 284.8
    congenital or familial 284.0
  hypoplastic (idiopathic) 284.9
    congenital 284.0
    familial 284.0
    of childhood 284.0
  idiopathic 285.9
    hemolytic, chronic 283.9
  in
    chronic illness NEC 285.29
    end-stage renal disease 285.21
    neoplastic disease 285.22
  infantile 285.9
  infective, infectional 285.9
  intertropical (*see also* Ancylostomiasis) 126.9
  iron (Fe) deficiency 280.9
    due to blood loss (chronic) 280.0
      acute 285.1
    of or complicating pregnancy 648.2 ✔5ᵗʰ
    specified NEC 280.8
  Jaksch's (pseudoleukemia infantum) 285.8

☑4ᵗʰ Fourth-digit Required   ☑5ᵗʰ Fifth-digit Required   ►◄ Revised Text   ● New Line   ▲ Revised Code

Aneurysm — *continued*
brain — *continued*
arteriovenous 747.81
acquired 437.3
ruptured (*see also* Hemorrhage, subarachnoid) 430
ruptured (*see also* Hemorrhage, subarachnoid) 430
berry (congenital) (ruptured) (*see also* Hemorrhage, subarachnoid) 430
congenital 747.81
ruptured (*see also* Hemorrhage, subarachnoid) 430
meninges 437.3
ruptured (*see also* Hemorrhage, subarachnoid) 430
miliary (congenital) (ruptured) (*see also* Hemorrhage, subarachnoid) 430
mycotic 421.0
ruptured (*see also* Hemorrhage, subarachnoid) 430
nonruptured 437.3
ruptured (*See also* Hemorrhage, subarachnoid) 430
syphilitic (hemorrhage) 094.87
syphilitic 094.87
traumatic — *see* Injury, intracranial
cardiac (false) (*see also* Aneurysm, heart) 414.10
carotid artery (common) (external) 442.81
internal (intracranial portion) 437.3
extracranial portion 442.81
ruptured into brain (*see also* Hemorrhage, subarachnoid) 430
syphilitic 093.89
intracranial 094.87
cavernous sinus (*see also* Aneurysm, brain) 437.3
arteriovenous 747.81
ruptured (*see also* Hemorrhage, subarachnoid) 430
congenital 747.81
ruptured (*see also* Hemorrhage, subarachnoid) 430
celiac 442.84
central nervous system, syphilitic 094.89
cerebral — *see* Aneurysm, brain
chest — *see* Aneurysm, thorax
circle of Willis (*see also* Aneurysm, brain) 437.3
congenital 747.81
ruptured (*see also* Hemorrhage, subarachnoid) 430
ruptured (*see also* Hemorrhage, subarachnoid) 430
common iliac artery 442.2
congenital (peripheral) NEC 747.60
brain 747.81
ruptured (*see also* Hemorrhage, subarachnoid) 430
cerebral — *see* Aneurysm, brain, congenital
coronary 746.85
gastrointestinal 747.61
lower limb 747.64
pulmonary 747.3
renal 747.62
retina 743.58
specified site NEC 747.89
spinal 747.82
upper limb 747.63
conjunctiva 372.74
conus arteriosus (*see also* Aneurysm, heart) 414.10
coronary (arteriosclerotic) (artery) (vein) (*see also* Aneurysm, heart) 414.11
arteriovenous 746.85
congenital 746.85
syphilitic 093.89
cylindrical 441.9
ruptured 441.5
syphilitic 093.9
dissecting 442.9
aorta (any part) 441.00
abdominal 441.02
thoracic 441.01
thoracoabdominal 441.03
syphilitic 093.9

Aneurysm — *continued*
ductus arteriosus 747.0
embolic — *see* Embolism, artery
endocardial, infective (any valve) 421.0
femoral 442.3
gastroduodenal 442.84
gastroepiploic 442.84
heart (chronic or with a stated duration of over 8 weeks) (infectional) (wall) 414.10
acute or with a stated duration of 8 weeks or less (*see also* Infarct, myocardium) 410.9 ☑5ᵗʰ
congenital 746.89
valve — *see* Endocarditis
hepatic 442.84
iliac (common) 442.2
infective (any valve) 421.0
innominate (nonsyphilitic) 442.89
syphilitic 093.89
interauricular septum (*see also* Aneurysm, heart) 414.10
interventricular septum (*see also* Aneurysm, heart) 414.10
intracranial — *see* Aneurysm, brain
intrathoracic (nonsyphilitic) 441.2
ruptured 441.1
syphilitic 093.0
jugular vein 453.8
lower extremity 442.3
lung (pulmonary artery) 417.1
malignant 093.9
mediastinal (nonsyphilitic) 442.89
syphilitic 093.89
miliary (congenital) (ruptured) (*see also* Hemorrhage, subarachnoid) 430
mitral (heart) (valve) 424.0
mural (arteriovenous) (heart) (*see also* Aneurysm, heart) 414.10
mycotic, any site 421.0
ruptured, brain (*see also* Hemorrhage, subarachnoid) 430
myocardium (*see also* Aneurysm, heart) 414.10
neck 442.81
pancreaticoduodenal 442.84
patent ductus arteriosus 747.0
peripheral NEC 442.89
congenital NEC (*see also* Aneurysm, congenital) 747.60
popliteal 442.3
pulmonary 417.1
arteriovenous 747.3
acquired 417.0
syphilitic 093.89
valve (heart) (*see also* Endocarditis, pulmonary) 424.3
racemose 442.9
congenital (peripheral) NEC 747.60
radial 442.0
Rasmussen's (*see also* Tuberculosis) 011.2 ☑5ᵗʰ
renal 442.1
retinal (acquired) 362.17
congenital 743.58
diabetic 250.5 ☑5ᵗʰ [362.01]
sinus, aortic (of Valsalva) 747.29
specified site NEC 442.89
spinal (cord) 442.89
congenital 747.82
syphilitic (hemorrhage) 094.89
spleen, splenic 442.83
subclavian 442.82
syphilitic 093.89
superior mesenteric 442.84
syphilitic 093.9
aorta 093.0
central nervous system 094.89
congenital 090.5
spine, spinal 094.89
thoracoabdominal 441.7
ruptured 441.6
thorax, thoracic (arch) (nonsyphilitic) 441.2
dissecting 441.0 ☑5ᵗʰ
ruptured 441.1
syphilitic 093.0
traumatic (complication) (early) — *see* Injury, blood vessel, by site
tricuspid (heart) (valve) — *see* Endocarditis, tricuspid
ulnar 442.0

Aneurysm — *continued*
upper extremity 442.0
valve, valvular — *see* Endocarditis
venous 456.8
congenital NEC (*see also* Aneurysm, congenital) 747.60
ventricle (arteriovenous) (*see also* Aneurysm, heart) 414.10
visceral artery NEC 442.84

Angiectasis 459.89

Angiectopia 459.9

Angiitis 447.6
allergic granulomatous 446.4
hypersensitivity 446.20
Goodpasture's syndrome 446.21
specified NEC 446.29
necrotizing 446.0
Wegener's (necrotizing respiratory granulomatosis) 446.4

Angina (attack) (cardiac) (chest) (effort) (heart) (pectoris) (syndrome) (vasomotor) 413.9
abdominal 557.1
agranulocytic 288.0
aphthous 074.0
catarrhal 462
crescendo 411.1
croupous 464.4
cruris 443.9
due to atherosclerosis NEC (*see also* Arteriosclerosis, extremities) 440.20
decubitus 413.0
diphtheritic (membranous) 032.0
erysipelatous 034.0
erythematous 462
exudative, chronic 476.0
faucium 478.29
gangrenous 462
diphtheritic 032.0
infectious 462
initial 411.1
intestinal 557.1
ludovici 528.3
Ludwig's 528.3
malignant 462
diphtheritic 032.0
membranous 464.4
diphtheritic 032.0
mesenteric 557.1
monocytic 075
nocturnal 413.0
phlegmonous 475
diphtheritic 032.0
preinfarctional 411.1
Prinzmetal's 413.1
progressive 411.1
pseudomembranous 101
psychogenic 306.2
pultaceous, diphtheritic 032.0
scarlatinal 034.1
septic 034.0
simple 462
stable NEC 413.9
staphylococcal 462
streptococcal 034.0
stridulous, diphtheritic 032.3
syphilitic 093.9
congenital 090.5
tonsil 475
trachealis 464.4
unstable 411.1
variant 413.1
Vincent's 101

Angioblastoma (M9161/1) — *see* Neoplasm, connective tissue, uncertain behavior

Angiocholecystitis (*see also* Cholecystitis, acute) 575.0

Angiocholitis (*see also* Cholecystitis, acute) 576.1

Angiodysgensis spinalis 336.1

Angiodysplasia (intestinalis) (intestine) 569.84
with hemorrhage 569.85
duodenum 537.82
with hemorrhage 537.83
stomach 537.82
with hemorrhage 537.83

☑4ᵗʰ Fourth-digit Required ☑5ᵗʰ Fifth-digit Required ▶◀ Revised Text ● New Line ▲ Revised Code

Angioedema (allergic) (any site) (with urticaria) 995.1
  hereditary 277.6
Angioendothelioma (M9130/1) — *see also*
  Neoplasm, by site, uncertain behavior
  benign (M9130/0) (*see also* Hemangioma, by site) 228.00
  bone (M9260/3) — *see* Neoplasm, bone, malignant
  Ewing's (M9260/3) — *see* Neoplasm, bone, malignant
  nervous system (M9130/0) 228.09
Angiofibroma (M9160/0) — *see also* Neoplasm, by site, benign
  juvenile (M9160/0) 210.7
    specified site — *see* Neoplasm, by site, benign
    unspecified site 210.7
Angiohemophilia (A) (B) 286.4
Angioid streaks (choroid) (retina) 363.43
Angiokeratoma (M9141/0) — *see also* Neoplasm, skin, benign
  corporis diffusum 272.7
Angiokeratosis
  diffuse 272.7
Angioleiomyoma (M8894/0) — *see* Neoplasm, connective tissue, benign
Angioleucitis 683
Angiolipoma (M8861/0) (*see also* Lipoma, by site) 214.9
  infiltrating (M8861/1) — *see* Neoplasm, connective tissue, uncertain behavior
Angioma (M9120/0) (*see also* Hemangioma, by site) 228.00
  capillary 448.1
  hemorrhagicum hereditaria 448.0
  malignant (M9120/3) — *see* Neoplasm, connective tissue, malignant
  pigmentosum et atrophicum 757.33
  placenta — *see* Placenta, abnormal
  plexiform (M9131/0) — *see* Hemangioma, by site
  senile 448.1
  serpiginosum 709.1
  spider 448.1
  stellate 448.1
Angiomatosis 757.32
  bacillary 083.8
  corporis diffusum universale 272.7
  cutaneocerebral 759.6
  encephalocutaneous 759.6
  encephalofacial 759.6
  encephalotrigeminal 759.6
  hemorrhagic familial 448.0
  hereditary familial 448.0
  heredofamilial 448.0
  meningo-oculofacial 759.6
  multiple sites 228.09
  neuro-oculocutaneous 759.6
  retina (Hippel's disease) 759.6
  retinocerebellosa 759.6
  retinocerebral 759.6
  systemic 228.09
Angiomyolipoma (M8860/0)
  specified site — *see* Neoplasm, connective tissue, benign
  unspecified site 223.0
Angiomyoliposarcoma (M8860/3) — *see* Neoplasm, connective tissue, malignant
Angiomyoma (M8894/0) — *see* Neoplasm, connective tissue, benign
Angiomyosarcoma (M8894/3) — *see* Neoplasm, connective tissue, malignant
Angioneurosis 306.2
Angioneurotic edema (allergic) (any site) (with urticaria) 995.1
  hereditary 277.6
Angiopathia, angiopathy 459.9
  diabetic (peripheral) 250.7 ✔5ᵗʰ [443.81]
  peripheral 443.9
    diabetic 250.7 ✔5ᵗʰ [443.81]
    specified type NEC 443.89
  retinae syphilitica 093.89

Angiopathia, angiopathy — *continued*
  retinalis (juvenilis) 362.18
    background 362.10
    diabetic 250.5 ✔5ᵗʰ [362.01]
    proliferative 362.29
    tuberculous (*see also* Tuberculosis) 017.3 ✔5ᵗʰ [362.18]
Angiosarcoma (M9120/3) — *see* Neoplasm, connective tissue, malignant
Angiosclerosis — *see* Arteriosclerosis
Angioscotoma, enlarged 368.42
Angiospasm 443.9
  brachial plexus 353.0
  cerebral 435.9
  cervical plexus 353.2
  nerve
    arm 354.9
      axillary 353.0
      median 354.1
      ulnar 354.2
    autonomic (*see also* Neuropathy, peripheral, autonomic) 337.9
    axillary 353.0
    leg 355.8
      plantar 355.6
    lower extremity — *see* Angiospasm, nerve, leg
    median 354.1
    peripheral NEC 355.9
    spinal NEC 355.9
    sympathetic (*see also* Neuropathy, peripheral, autonomic) 337.9
    ulnar 354.2
    upper extremity — *see* Angiospasm, nerve, arm
  peripheral NEC 443.9
  traumatic 443.9
    foot 443.9
    leg 443.9
  vessel 443.9
Angiospastic disease or edema 443.9
Anguillulosis 127.2
Angulation
  cecum (*see also* Obstruction, intestine) 560.9
  coccyx (acquired) 738.6
    congenital 756.19
  femur (acquired) 736.39
    congenital 755.69
  intestine (large) (small) (*see also* Obstruction, intestine) 560.9
  sacrum (acquired) 738.5
    congenital 756.19
  sigmoid (flexure) (*see also* Obstruction, intestine) 560.9
  spine (*see also* Curvature, spine) 737.9
  tibia (acquired) 736.89
    congenital 755.69
  ureter 593.3
  wrist (acquired) 736.09
    congenital 755.59
Angulus infectiosus 686.8
Anhedonia 302.72
Anhidrosis (lid) (neurogenic) (thermogenic) 705.0
Anhydration 276.5
  with
    hypernatremia 276.0
    hyponatremia 276.1
Anhydremia 276.5
  with
    hypernatremia 276.0
    hyponatremia 276.1
Anidrosis 705.0
Aniridia (congenital) 743.45
Anisakiasis (infection) (infestation) 127.1
Anisakis larva infestation 127.1
Aniseikonia 367.32
Anisocoria (pupil) 379.41
  congenital 743.46
Anisocytosis 790.09
Anisometropia (congenital) 367.31
Ankle — *see* condition
Ankyloblepharon (acquired) (eyelid) 374.46
  filiforme (adnatum) (congenital) 743.62

Ankyloblepharon — *continued*
  total 743.62
Ankylodactly (*see also* Syndactylism) 755.10
Ankyloglossia 750.0
Ankylosis (fibrous) (osseous) 718.50
  ankle 718.57
  any joint, produced by surgical fusion V45.4
  cricoarytenoid (cartilage) (joint) (larynx) 478.79
  dental 521.6
  ear ossicle NEC 385.22
    malleus 385.21
  elbow 718.52
  finger 718.54
  hip 718.55
  incostapedial joint (infectional) 385.22
  joint, produced by surgical fusion NEC V45.4
  knee 718.56
  lumbosacral (joint) 724.6
  malleus 385.21
  multiple sites 718.59
  postoperative (status) V45.4
  sacroiliac (joint) 724.6
  shoulder 718.51
  specified site NEC 718.58
  spine NEC 724.9
  surgical V45.4
  teeth, tooth (hard tissues) 521.6
  temporomandibular joint 524.61
  wrist 718.53
Ankylostoma — *see* Ancylostoma
Ankylostomiasis (intestinal) — *see* Ancylostomiasis
Ankylurethria (*see also* Stricture, urethra) 598.9
Annular — *see also* condition
  detachment, cervix 622.8
  organ or site, congenital NEC — *see* Distortion
  pancreas (congenital) 751.7
Anodontia (complete) (partial) (vera) 520.0
  with abnormal spacing 524.3
  acquired 525.10
    causing malocclusion 524.3
    due to
      caries 525.13
      extraction 525.10
      periodontal disease 525.12
      trauma 525.11
Anomaly, anomalous (congenital) (unspecified type) 759.9
  abdomen 759.9
  abdominal wall 756.70
  acoustic nerve 742.9
  adrenal (gland) 759.1
  Alder (-Reilly) (leukocyte granulation) 288.2
  alimentary tract 751.9
    lower 751.5
    specified type NEC 751.8
    upper (any part, except tongue) 750.9
      tongue 750.10
        specified type NEC 750.19
  alveolar ridge (process) 525.8
  ankle (joint) 755.69
  anus, anal (canal) 751.5
  aorta, aortic 747.20
    arch 747.21
    coarctation (postductal) (preductal) 747.10
    cusp or valve NEC 746.9
    septum 745.0
    specified type NEC 747.29
  aorticopulmonary septum 745.0
  apertures, diaphragm 756.6
  appendix 751.5
  aqueduct of Sylvius 742.3
    with spina bifida (*see also* Spina bifida) 741.0 ✔5ᵗʰ
  arm 755.50
    reduction (*see also* Deformity, reduction, upper limb) 755.20
  arteriovenous (congenital) (peripheral) NEC 747.60
    brain 747.81
    cerebral 747.81
    coronary 746.85
    gastrointestinal 747.61
    lower limb 747.64
    renal 747.62
    specified site NEC 747.69

Angioedema — Anomaly

Anomaly, anomalous — *continued*
  arteriovenous — *continued*
    spinal 747.82
    upper limb 747.63
  artery (*see also* Anomaly, peripheral vascular
    system) NEC 747.60
    brain 747.81
    cerebral 747.81
    coronary 746.85
    eye 743.9
    pulmonary 747.3
    renal 747.62
    retina 743.9
    umbilical 747.5
  arytenoepiglottic folds 748.3
  atrial
    bands 746.9
    folds 746.9
    septa 745.5
  atrioventricular
    canal 745.69
    common 745.69
    conduction 426.7
    excitation 426.7
    septum 745.4
  atrium — *see* Anomaly, atrial
  auditory canal 744.3
    specified type NEC 744.29
      with hearing impairment 744.02
  auricle
    ear 744.3
      causing impairment of hearing 744.02
    heart 746.9
      septum 745.5
  autosomes, autosomal NEC 758.5
  Axenfeld's 743.44
  back 759.9
  band
    atrial 746.9
    heart 746.9
    ventricular 746.9
  Bartholin's duct 750.9
  biliary duct or passage 751.60
    atresia 751.61
  bladder (neck) (sphincter) (trigone) 753.9
    specified type NEC 753.8
  blood vessel 747.9
    artery — *see* Anomaly, artery
    peripheral vascular — *see* Anomaly,
      peripheral vascular system
    vein — *see* Anomaly, vein
  bone NEC 756.9
    ankle 755.69
    arm 755.50
    chest 756.3
    cranium 756.0
    face 756.0
    finger 755.50
    foot 755.67
    forearm 755.50
    frontal 756.0
    head 756.0
    hip 755.63
    leg 755.60
    lumbosacral 756.10
    nose 748.1
    pelvic girdle 755.60
    rachitic 756.4
    rib 756.3
    shoulder girdle 755.50
    skull 756.0
      with
        anencephalus 740.0
        encephalocele 742.0
        hydrocephalus 742.3
          with spina bifida (*see also* Spina
            bifida) 741.0 ✓5ᵗʰ
        microcephalus 742.1
    toe 755.66
  brain 742.9
    multiple 742.4
    reduction 742.2
    specified type NEC 742.4
    vessel 747.81
  branchial cleft NEC 744.49
    cyst 744.42
    fistula 744.41

Anomaly, anomalous — *continued*
  branchial cleft NEC — *continued*
    persistent 744.41
    sinus (external) (internal) 744.41
  breast 757.9
  broad ligament 752.10
    specified type NEC 752.19
  bronchus 748.3
  bulbar septum 745.0
  bulbus cordis 745.9
    persistent (in left ventricle) 745.8
  bursa 756.9
  canal of Nuck 752.9
  canthus 743.9
  capillary NEC (*see also* Anomaly, peripheral
    vascular system) 747.60
  cardiac 746.9
    septal closure 745.9
      acquired 429.71
    valve NEC 746.9
      pulmonary 746.00
      specified type NEC 746.89
  cardiovascular system 746.9
    complicating pregnancy, childbirth, or
      puerperium 648.5 ✓5ᵗʰ
  carpus 755.50
  cartilage, trachea 748.3
  cartilaginous 756.9
  caruncle, lacrimal, lachrymal 743.9
  cascade stomach 750.7
  cauda equina 742.59
  cecum 751.5
  cerebral — *see also* Anomaly, brain vessels
    747.81
  cerebrovascular system 747.81
  cervix (uterus) 752.40
    with doubling of vagina and uterus 752.2
    in pregnancy or childbirth 654.6 ✓5ᵗʰ
      affecting fetus or newborn 763.89
      causing obstructed labor 660.2 ✓5ᵗʰ
        affecting fetus or newborn 763.1
  Chédiak-Higashi (-Steinbrinck) (congenital
    gigantism of peroxidase granules) 288.2
  cheek 744.9
  chest (wall) 756.3
  chin 744.9
    specified type NEC 744.89
  chordae tendineae 746.9
  choroid 743.9
    plexus 742.9
  chromosomes, chromosomal 758.9
    13 (13-15) 758.1
    18 (16-18) 758.2
    21 or 22 758.0
    autosomes NEC (*see also* Abnormality,
      autosomes) 758.5
    deletion 758.3
    Christchurch 758.3
    D₁ 758.1
    E₃ 758.2
    G 758.0
    mitochondrial 758.9
    mosaics 758.89
    sex 758.81
      complement, XO 758.6
      complement, XXX 758.81
      complement, XXY 758.7
      complement, XYY 758.81
      gonadal dysgenesis 758.6
      Klinefelter's 758.7
      Turner's 758.6
    trisomy 21 758.0
  cilia 743.9
  circulatory system 747.9
    specified type NEC 747.89
  clavicle 755.51
  clitoris 752.40
  coccyx 756.10
  colon 751.5
  common duct 751.60
  communication
    coronary artery 746.85
    left ventricle with right atrium 745.4
  concha (ear) 744.3
  connection
    renal vessels with kidney 747.62
    total pulmonary venous 747.41

Anomaly, anomalous — *continued*
  connective tissue 756.9
    specified type NEC 756.89
  cornea 743.9
    shape 743.41
    size 743.41
    specified type NEC 743.49
  coronary
    artery 746.85
    vein 746.89
  cranium — *see* Anomaly, skull
  cricoid cartilage 748.3
  cushion, endocardial 745.60
    specified type NEC 745.69
  cystic duct 751.60
  dental arch relationship 524.2
  dentition 520.6
  dentofacial NEC 524.9
    functional 524.5
    specified type NEC 524.8
  dermatoglyphic 757.2
  Descemet's membrane 743.9
    specified type NEC 743.49
  development
    cervix 752.40
    vagina 752.40
    vulva 752.40
  diaphragm, diaphragmatic (apertures) NEC
    756.6
  digestive organ(s) or system 751.9
    lower 751.5
    specified type NEC 751.8
    upper 750.9
  distribution, coronary artery 746.85
  ductus
    arteriosus 747.0
    Botalli 747.0
  duodenum 751.5
  dura 742.9
    brain 742.4
    spinal cord 742.59
  ear 744.9
    causing impairment of hearing 744.00
      specified type NEC 744.09
    external 744.3
      causing impairment of hearing 744.02
      specified type NEC 744.29
    inner (causing impairment of hearing)
      744.05
    middle, except ossicles (causing impairment
      of hearing) 744.03
      ossicles 744.04
    ossicles 744.04
    prominent auricle 744.29
    specified type NEC 744.29
      with hearing impairment 744.09
  Ebstein's (heart) 746.2
    tricuspid valve 746.2
  ectodermal 757.9
  Eisenmenger's (ventricular septal defect) 745.4
  ejaculatory duct 752.9
    specified type NEC 752.8
  elbow (joint) 755.50
  endocardial cushion 745.60
    specified type NEC 745.69
  endocrine gland NEC 759.2
  epididymis 752.9
  epiglottis 748.3
  esophagus 750.9
    specified type NEC 750.4
  Eustachian tube 744.3
    specified type NEC 744.24
  eye (any part) 743.9
    adnexa 743.9
      specified type NEC 743.69
    anophthalmos 743.00
    anterior
      chamber and related structures 743.9
        angle 743.9
          specified type NEC 743.44
        specified type NEC 743.44
      segment 743.9
        combined 743.48
        multiple 743.48
        specified type NEC 743.49
    cataract (*see also* Cataract) 743.30
    glaucoma (*see also* Buphthalmia) 743.20

Anomaly, anomalous — *continued*
 eye — *continued*
  lid 743.9
   specified type NEC 743.63
  microphthalmos (*see also* Microphthalmos)
    743.10
  posterior segment 743.9
   specified type NEC 743.59
   vascular 743.58
   vitreous 743.9
    specified type NEC 743.51
  ptosis (eyelid) 743.61
  retina 743.9
   specified type NEC 743.59
  sclera 743.9
   specified type NEC 743.47
  specified type NEC 743.8
 eyebrow 744.89
 eyelid 743.9
  specified type NEC 743.63
 face (any part) 744.9
  bone(s) 756.0
  specified type NEC 744.89
 fallopian tube 752.10
  specified type NEC 752.19
 fascia 756.9
  specified type NEC 756.89
 femur 755.60
 fibula 755.60
 finger 755.50
  supernumerary 755.01
  webbed (*see also* Syndactylism, fingers)
    755.11
 fixation, intestine 751.4
 flexion (joint) 755.9
  hip or thigh (*see also* Dislocation, hip,
    congenital) 754.30
 folds, heart 746.9
 foot 755.67
 foramen
  Botalli 745.5
  ovale 745.5
 forearm 755.50
 forehead (*see also* Anomaly, skull) 756.0
 form, teeth 520.2
 fovea centralis 743.9
 frontal bone (*see also* Anomaly, skull) 756.0
 gallbladder 751.60
 Gartner's duct 752.11
 gastrointestinal tract 751.9
  specified type NEC 751.8
  vessel 747.61
 genitalia, genital organ(s) or system
  female 752.9
   external 752.40
    specified type NEC 752.49
   internal NEC 752.9
  male (external and internal) 752.9
   epispadias 752.62
   hidden penis 752.65
   hydrocele, congenital 778.6
   hypospadias 752.61
   micropenis 752.64
   testis, undescended 752.51
    retractile 752.52
  specified type NEC 752.8
 genitourinary NEC 752.9
 Gerbode 745.4
 globe (eye) 743.9
 glottis 748.3
 granulation or granulocyte, genetic 288.2
  constitutional 288.2
  leukocyte 288.2
 gum 750.9
 gyri 742.9
 hair 757.9
  specified type NEC 757.4
 hand 755.50
 hard tissue formation in pulp 522.3
 head (*see also* Anomaly, skull) 756.0
 heart 746.9
  auricle 746.9
  bands 746.9
  fibroelastosis cordis 425.3
  folds 746.9
  malposition 746.87
  maternal, affecting fetus or newborn 760.3

Anomaly, anomalous — *continued*
 heart — *continued*
  obstructive NEC 746.84
  patent ductus arteriosus (Botalli) 747.0
  septum 745.9
   acquired 429.71
   aortic 745.0
   aorticopulmonary 745.0
   atrial 745.5
   auricular 745.5
   between aorta and pulmonary artery
     745.0
   endocardial cushion type 745.60
    specified type NEC 745.69
   interatrial 745.5
   interventricular 745.4
    with pulmonary stenosis or atresia,
     dextraposition of aorta, and
     hypertrophy of right ventricle
     745.2
    acquired 429.71
   specified type NEC 745.8
   ventricular 745.4
    with pulmonary stenosis or atresia,
     dextraposition of aorta, and
     hypertrophy of right ventricle
     745.2
    acquired 429.71
  specified type NEC 746.89
  tetralogy of Fallot 745.2
  valve NEC 746.9
   aortic 746.9
    atresia 746.89
    bicuspid valve 746.4
    insufficiency 746.4
    specified type NEC 746.89
    stenosis 746.3
     subaortic 746.81
     supravalvular 747.22
   mitral 746.9
    atresia 746.89
    insufficiency 746.6
    specified type NEC 746.89
    stenosis 746.5
   pulmonary 746.00
    atresia 746.01
    insufficiency 746.09
    stenosis 746.02
     infundibular 746.83
     subvalvular 746.83
   tricuspid 746.9
    atresia 746.1
    stenosis 746.1
  ventricle 746.9
 heel 755.67
 Hegglin's 288.2
 hemianencephaly 740.0
 hemicephaly 740.0
 hemicrania 740.0
 hepatic duct 751.60
 hip (joint) 755.63
 hourglass
  bladder 753.8
  gallbladder 751.69
  stomach 750.7
 humerus 755.50
 hymen 752.40
 hypersegmentation of neutrophils, hereditary
   288.2
 hypophyseal 759.2
 ileocecal (coil) (valve) 751.5
 ileum (intestine) 751.5
 ilium 755.60
 integument 757.9
  specified type NEC 757.8
 intervertebral cartilage or disc 756.10
 intestine (large) (small) 751.5
  fixational type 751.4
 iris 743.9
  specified type NEC 743.46
 ischium 755.60
 jaw NEC 524.9
  closure 524.5
  size (major) NEC 524.00
  specified type NEC 524.8
 jaw-cranial base relationship 524.10
  specified NEC 524.19

Anomaly, anomalous — *continued*
 jejunum 751.5
 joint 755.9
  hip
   dislocation (*see also* Dislocation, hip,
     congenital) 754.30
   predislocation (*see also* Subluxation,
     congenital, hip) 754.32
   preluxation (*see also* Subluxation,
     congenital, hip) 754.32
   subluxation (*see also* Subluxation,
     congenital, hip) 754.32
  lumbosacral 756.10
   spondylolisthesis 756.12
   spondylosis 756.11
  multiple arthrogryposis 754.89
  sacroiliac 755.69
 Jordan's 288.2
 kidney(s) (calyx) (pelvis) 753.9
  vessel 747.62
 Klippel-Feil (brevicollis) 756.16
 knee (joint) 755.64
 labium (majus) (minus) 752.40
 labyrinth, membranous (causing impairment of
   hearing) 744.05
 lacrimal
  apparatus, duct or passage 743.9
   specified type NEC 743.65
  gland 743.9
   specified type NEC 743.64
 Langdon Down (mongolism) 758.0
 larynx, laryngeal (muscle) 748.3
  web, webbed 748.2
 leg (lower) (upper) 755.60
  reduction NEC (*see also* Deformity,
    reduction, lower limb) 755.30
 lens 743.9
  shape 743.36
  specified type NEC 743.39
 leukocytes, genetic 288.2
  granulation (constitutional) 288.2
 lid (fold) 743.9
 ligament 756.9
  broad 752.10
  round 752.9
 limb, except reduction deformity 755.9
  lower 755.60
   reduction deformity (*see also* Deformity,
     reduction, lower limb) 755.30
   specified type NEC 755.69
  upper 755.50
   reduction deformity (*see also* Deformity,
     reduction, upper limb) 755.20
   specified type NEC 755.59
 lip 750.9
  harelip (*see also* Cleft, lip) 749.10
  specified type NEC 750.26
 liver (duct) 751.60
  atresia 751.69
 lower extremity 755.60
  vessel 747.64
 lumbosacral (joint) (region) 756.10
 lung (fissure) (lobe) NEC 748.60
  agenesis 748.5
  specified type NEC 748.69
 lymphatic system 759.9
 Madelung's (radius) 755.54
 mandible 524.9
  size NEC 524.00
 maxilla 524.9
  size NEC 524.00
 May (-Hegglin) 288.2
 meatus urinarius 753.9
  specified type NEC 753.8
 meningeal bands or folds, constriction of 742.8
 meninges 742.9
  brain 742.4
  spinal 742.59
 meningocele (*see also* Spina bifida) 741.9 ✓5ᵗʰ
 mesentery 751.9
 metacarpus 755.50
 metatarsus 755.67
 middle ear, except ossicles (causing impairment
   of hearing) 744.03
  ossicles 744.04
 mitral (leaflets) (valve) 746.9
  atresia 746.89

✓4ᵗʰ Fourth-digit Required   ✓5ᵗʰ Fifth-digit Required   ►◄ Revised Text   ● New Line   ▲ Revised Code

Anomaly, anomalous — *continued*
  mitral — *continued*
    insufficiency 746.6
      specified type NEC 746.89
    stenosis 746.5
  mouth 750.9
    specified type NEC 750.26
  multiple NEC 759.7
    specified type NEC 759.89
  muscle 756.9
    eye 743.9
      specified type NEC 743.69
    specified type NEC 756.89
  musculoskeletal system, except limbs 756.9
    specified type NEC 756.9
  nail 757.9
    specified type NEC 757.5
  narrowness, eyelid 743.62
  nasal sinus or septum 748.1
  neck (any part) 744.9
    specified type NEC 744.89
  nerve 742.9
    acoustic 742.9
      specified type NEC 742.8
    optic 742.9
      specified type NEC 742.8
    specified type NEC 742.8
  nervous system NEC 742.9
    brain 742.9
      specified type NEC 742.4
    specified type NEC 742.8
  neurological 742.9
  nipple 757.9
  nonteratogenic NEC 754.89
  nose, nasal (bone) (cartilage) (septum) (sinus)
      748.1
  ocular muscle 743.9
  omphalomesenteric duct 751.0
  opening, pulmonary veins 747.49
  optic
    disc 743.9
      specified type NEC 743.57
    nerve 742.9
  opticociliary vessels 743.9
  orbit (eye) 743.9
    specified type NEC 743.66
  organ
    of Corti (causing impairment of hearing)
        744.05
    or site 759.9
      specified type NEC 759.89
  origin
    both great arteries from same ventricle
        745.11
    coronary artery 746.85
    innominate artery 747.69
    left coronary artery from pulmonary artery
        746.85
    pulmonary artery 747.3
    renal vessels 747.62
    subclavian artery (left) (right) 747.21
  osseous meatus (ear) 744.03
  ovary 752.0
  oviduct 752.10
  palate (hard) (soft) 750.9
    cleft (*see also* Cleft, palate) 749.00
  pancreas (duct) 751.7
  papillary muscles 746.9
  parathyroid gland 759.2
  paraurethral ducts 753.9
  parotid (gland) 750.9
  patella 755.64
  Pelger-Huët (hereditary hyposegmentation)
      288.2
  pelvic girdle 755.60
    specified type NEC 755.69
  pelvis (bony) 755.60
    complicating delivery 653.0 ✓5ᵗʰ
    rachitic 268.1
      fetal 756.4
  penis (glans) 752.69
  pericardium 746.89
  peripheral vascular system NEC 747.60
    gastrointestinal 747.61
    lower limb 747.64
    renal 747.62
    specified site NEC 747.69

Anomaly, anomalous — *continued*
  peripheral vascular system NEC — *continued*
    spinal 747.82
    upper limb 747.63
  Peter's 743.44
  pharynx 750.9
    branchial cleft 744.41
    specified type NEC 750.29
  Pierre Robin 756.0
  pigmentation NEC 709.00
    congenital 757.33
  pituitary (gland) 759.2
  pleural folds 748.8
  portal vein 747.40
  position tooth, teeth 524.3
  preauricular sinus 744.46
  prepuce 752.9
  prostate 752.9
  pulmonary 748.60
    artery 747.3
    circulation 747.3
    specified type NEC 748.69
    valve 746.00
      atresia 746.01
      insufficiency 746.09
      specified type NEC 746.09
      stenosis 746.02
        infundibular 746.83
        subvalvular 746.83
    vein 747.40
    venous
      connection 747.49
        partial 747.42
        total 747.41
      return 747.49
        partial 747.42
        total (TAPVR) (complete)
            (subdiaphragmatic)
            (supradiaphrag-matic) 747.41
  pupil 743.9
  pylorus 750.9
    hypertrophy 750.5
    stenosis 750.5
  rachitic, fetal 756.4
  radius 755.50
  rectovaginal (septum) 752.40
  rectum 751.5
  refraction 367.9
  renal 753.9
    vessel 747.62
  respiratory system 748.9
    specified type NEC 748.8
  rib 756.3
    cervical 756.2
  Rieger's 743.44
  rings, trachea 748.3
  rotation — *see also* Malrotation
    hip or thigh (*see also* Subluxation,
        congenital, hip) 754.32
  round ligament 752.9
  sacroiliac (joint) 755.69
  sacrum 756.10
  saddle
    back 754.2
    nose 754.0
      syphilitic 090.5
  salivary gland or duct 750.9
    specified type NEC 750.26
  scapula 755.50
  sclera 743.9
    specified type NEC 743.47
  scrotum 752.9
  sebaceous gland 757.9
  seminal duct or tract 752.9
  sense organs 742.9
    specified type NEC 742.8
  septum
    heart — *see* Anomaly, heart, septum
    nasal 748.1
  sex chromosomes NEC (*see also* Anomaly,
      chromosomes) 758.81
  shoulder (girdle) (joint) 755.50
    specified type NEC 755.59
  sigmoid (flexure) 751.5
  sinus of Valsalva 747.29
  site NEC 759.9
  skeleton generalized NEC 756.50

Anomaly, anomalous — *continued*
  skin (appendage) 757.9
    specified type NEC 757.39
  skull (bone) 756.0
    with
      anencephalus 740.0
      encephalocele 742.0
      hydrocephalus 742.3
        with spina bifida (*see also* Spina
            bifida) 741.0 ✓5ᵗʰ
      microcephalus 742.1
  specified type NEC
    adrenal (gland) 759.1
    alimentary tract (complete) (partial) 751.8
      lower 751.5
      upper 750.8
    ankle 755.69
    anus, anal (canal) 751.5
    aorta, aortic 747.29
      arch 747.21
    appendix 751.5
    arm 755.59
    artery (peripheral) NEC (*see also* Anomaly,
        peripheral vascular system) 747.60
      brain 747.81
      coronary 746.85
      eye 743.58
      pulmonary 747.3
      retinal 743.58
      umbilical 747.5
    auditory canal 744.29
      causing impairment of hearing 744.02
    bile duct or passage 751.69
    bladder 753.8
      neck 753.8
    bone(s) 756.9
      arm 755.59
      face 756.0
      leg 755.69
      pelvic girdle 755.69
      shoulder girdle 755.59
      skull 756.0
        with
          anencephalus 740.0
          encephalocele 742.0
          hydrocephalus 742.3
            with spina bifida (*see also* Spina
                bifida) 741.0 ✓5ᵗʰ
          microcephalus 742.1
    brain 742.4
    breast 757.6
    broad ligament 752.19
    bronchus 748.3
    canal of Nuck 752.8
    cardiac septal closure 745.8
    carpus 755.59
    cartilaginous 756.9
    cecum 751.5
    cervix 752.49
    chest (wall) 756.3
    chin 744.89
    ciliary body 743.46
    circulatory system 747.89
    clavicle 755.51
    clitoris 752.49
    coccyx 756.19
    colon 751.5
    common duct 751.69
    connective tissue 756.89
    cricoid cartilage 748.3
    cystic duct 751.69
    diaphragm 756.6
    digestive organ(s) or tract 751.8
      lower 751.5
      upper 750.8
    duodenum 751.5
    ear 744.29
      auricle 744.29
        causing impairment of hearing 744.02
      causing impairment of hearing 744.09
      inner (causing impairment of hearing)
          744.05
      middle, except ossicles 744.03
        ossicles 744.04
    ejaculatory duct 752.8
    endocrine 759.2
    epiglottis 748.3

✓4ᵗʰ Fourth-digit Required   ✓5ᵗʰ Fifth-digit Required   ▶◀ Revised Text   ● New Line   ▲ Revised Code

Anomaly, anomalous — *continued*
  specified type NEC — *continued*
    esophagus 750.4
    Eustachian tube 744.24
    eye 743.8
      lid 743.63
      muscle 743.69
    face 744.89
      bone(s) 756.0
    fallopian tube 752.19
    fascia 756.89
    femur 755.69
    fibula 755.69
    finger 755.59
    foot 755.67
    fovea centralis 743.55
    gallbladder 751.69
    Gartner's duct 752.8
    gastrointestinal tract 751.8
    genitalia, genital organ(s)
      female 752.8
        external 752.49
        internal NEC 752.8
      male 752.8
        penis 752.69
    genitourinary tract NEC 752.8
    glottis 748.3
    hair 757.4
    hand 755.59
    heart 746.89
      valve NEC 746.89
        pulmonary 746.09
    hepatic duct 751.69
    hydatid of Morgagni 752.8
    hymen 752.49
    integument 757.8
    intestine (large) (small) 751.5
      fixational type 751.4
    iris 743.46
    jejunum 751.5
    joint 755.8
    kidney 753.3
    knee 755.64
    labium (majus) (minus) 752.49
    labyrinth, membranous 744.05
    larynx 748.3
    leg 755.69
    lens 743.39
    limb, except reduction deformity 755.8
      lower 755.69
        reduction deformity (*see also*
          Deformity, reduction, lower limb)
          755.30
      upper 755.59
        reduction deformity (*see also*
          Deformity, reduction, upper
          limb) 755.20
    lip 750.26
    liver 751.69
    lung (fissure) (lobe) 748.69
    meatus urinarius 753.8
    metacarpus 755.59
    mouth 750.26
    muscle 756.89
      eye 743.69
    musculoskeletal system, except limbs 756.9
    nail 757.5
    neck 744.89
    nerve 742.8
      acoustic 742.8
      optic 742.8
    nervous system 742.8
    nipple 757.6
    nose 748.1
    organ NEC 759.89
      of Corti 744.05
    osseous meatus (ear) 744.03
    ovary 752.0
    oviduct 752.19
    pancreas 751.7
    parathyroid 759.2
    patella 755.64
    pelvic girdle 755.69
    penis 752.69
    pericardium 746.89

Anomaly, anomalous — *continued*
  specified type NEC — *continued*
    peripheral vascular system NEC (*see also*
      Anomaly, peripheral vascular system)
      747.60
    pharynx 750.29
    pituitary 759.2
    prostate 752.8
    radius 755.59
    rectum 751.5
    respiratory system 748.8
    rib 756.3
    round ligament 752.8
    sacrum 756.19
    salivary duct or gland 750.26
    scapula 755.59
    sclera 743.47
    scrotum 752.8
    seminal duct or tract 752.8
    shoulder girdle 755.59
    site NEC 759.89
    skin 757.39
    skull (bone(s)) 756.0
      with
        anencephalus 740.0
        encephalocele 742.0
        hydrocephalus 742.3
          with spina bifida (*see also* Spina
            bifida) 741.0 ☑5ᵗʰ
        microcephalus 742.1
    specified organ or site NEC 759.89
    spermatic cord 752.8
    spinal cord 742.59
    spine 756.19
    spleen 759.0
    sternum 756.3
    stomach 750.7
    tarsus 755.67
    tendon 756.89
    testis 752.8
    thorax (wall) 756.3
    thymus 759.2
    thyroid (gland) 759.2
      cartilage 748.3
    tibia 755.69
    toe 755.66
    tongue 750.19
    trachea (cartilage) 748.3
    ulna 755.59
    urachus 753.7
    ureter 753.4
      obstructive 753.29
    urethra 753.8
      obstructive 753.6
    urinary tract 753.8
    uterus 752.3
    uvula 750.26
    vagina 752.49
    vascular NEC (*see also* Anomaly, peripheral
      vascular system) 747.60
      brain 747.81
    vas deferens 752.8
    vein(s) (peripheral) NEC (*see also* Anomaly,
      peripheral vascular system) 747.60
      brain 747.81
      great 747.49
      portal 747.49
      pulmonary 747.49
    vena cava (inferior) (superior) 747.49
    vertebra 756.19
    vulva 752.49
  spermatic cord 752.9
  spine, spinal 756.10
    column 756.10
    cord 742.9
      meningocele (*see also* Spina bifida)
        741.9 ☑5ᵗʰ
      specified type NEC 742.59
      spina bifida (*see also* Spina bifida)
        741.9 ☑5ᵗʰ
      vessel 747.82
    meninges 742.59
    nerve root 742.9
  spleen 759.0
  Sprengel's 755.52
  sternum 756.3

Anomaly, anomalous — *continued*
  stomach 750.9
    specified type NEC 750.7
  submaxillary gland 750.9
  superior vena cava 747.40
  talipes — *see* Talipes
  tarsus 755.67
    with complete absence of distal elements
      755.31
  teeth, tooth NEC 520.9
    position 524.3
    spacing 524.3
  tendon 756.9
    specified type NEC 756.89
  termination
    coronary artery 746.85
  testis 752.9
  thebesian valve 746.9
  thigh 755.60
    flexion (*see also* Subluxation, congenital,
      hip) 754.32
  thorax (wall) 756.3
  throat 750.9
  thumb 755.50
    supernumerary 755.01
  thymus gland 759.2
  thyroid (gland) 759.2
    cartilage 748.3
  tibia 755.60
    saber 090.5
  toe 755.66
    supernumerary 755.02
    webbed (*see also* Syndactylism, toes) 755.13
  tongue 750.10
    specified type NEC 750.19
  trachea, tracheal 748.3
    cartilage 748.3
    rings 748.3
  tragus 744.3
  transverse aortic arch 747.21
  trichromata 368.59
  trichromatopsia 368.59
  tricuspid (leaflet) (valve) 746.9
    atresia 746.1
    Ebstein's 746.2
    specified type NEC 746.89
    stenosis 746.1
  trunk 759.9
  Uhl's (hypoplasia of myocardium, right
    ventricle) 746.84
  ulna 755.50
  umbilicus 759.9
    artery 747.5
  union, trachea with larynx 748.3
  unspecified site 759.9
  upper extremity 755.50
    vessel 747.63
  urachus 753.7
    specified type NEC 753.7
  ureter 753.9
    obstructive 753.20
    specified type NEC 753.4
      obstructive 753.29
  urethra (valve) 753.9
    obstructive 753.6
    specified type NEC 753.8
  urinary tract or system (any part, except
    urachus) 753.9
    specified type NEC 753.8
    urachus 753.7
  uterus 752.3
    with only one functioning horn 752.3
    in pregnancy or childbirth 654.0 ☑5ᵗʰ
      affecting fetus or newborn 763.89
      causing obstructed labor 660.2 ☑5ᵗʰ
        affecting fetus or newborn 763.1
  uvula 750.9
  vagina 752.40
  valleculae 748.3
  valve (heart) NEC 746.9
    formation, ureter 753.29
    pulmonary 746.00
    specified type NEC 746.89
  vascular NEC (*see also* Anomaly, peripheral
    vascular system) 747.60
    ring 747.21
  vas deferens 752.9

Anomaly, anomalous — *continued*
 vein(s) (peripheral) NEC (*see also* Anomaly,
  peripheral vascular system) 747.60
  brain 747.81
  cerebral 747.81
  coronary 746.89
  great 747.40
   specified type NEC 747.49
  portal 747.40
  pulmonary 747.40
  retina 743.9
 vena cava (inferior) (superior) 747.40
 venous return (pulmonary) 747.49
  partial 747.42
  total 747.41
 ventricle, ventricular (heart) 746.9
  bands 746.9
  folds 746.9
  septa 745.4
 vertebra 756.10
 vesicourethral orifice 753.9
 vessels NEC (*see also* Anomaly, peripheral
  vascular system) 747.60
  optic papilla 743.9
 vitelline duct 751.0
 vitreous humor 743.9
  specified type NEC 743.51
 vulva 752.40
 wrist (joint) 755.50
Anomia 784.69
Anonychia 757.5
 acquired 703.8
Anophthalmos, anophthalmus (clinical)
 (congenital) (globe) 743.00
 acquired V45.78
Anopsia (altitudinal) (quadrant) 368.46
Anorchia 752.8
Anorchism, anorchidism 752.8
Anorexia 783.0
 hysterical 300.11
 nervosa 307.1
Anosmia (*see also* Disturbance, sensation) 781.1
 hysterical 300.11
 postinfectional 478.9
 psychogenic 306.7
 traumatic 951.8
Anosognosia 780.99   ▲
Anosphrasia 781.1
Anosteoplasia 756.50
Anotia 744.09
Anovulatory cycle 628.0
Anoxemia 799.0
 newborn 768.9   ▲
Anoxia 799.0
 altitude 993.2
 cerebral 348.1
  with
   abortion — *see* Abortion, by type, with
    specified complication NEC
   ectopic pregnancy (*see also* categories
    633.0-633.9) 639.8
   molar pregnancy (*see also* categories 630-
    632) 639.8
  complicating
   delivery (cesarean) (instrumental)
    669.4 ✓5ᵗʰ
   ectopic or molar pregnancy 639.8
   obstetric anesthesia or sedation
    668.2 ✓5ᵗʰ
  during or resulting from a procedure 997.01
  following
   abortion 639.8
   ectopic or molar pregnancy 639.8
  newborn (*see also* Distress, fetal, liveborn
   infant) 768.9
 due to drowning 994.1
 fetal, affecting newborn 768.9   ▲
 heart — *see* Insufficiency, coronary
 high altitude 993.2
 intrauterine
  fetal death (before onset of labor) 768.0
   during labor 768.1
  liveborn infant — *see* Distress, fetal,
   liveborn infant

Anoxia — *continued*
 myocardial — *see* Insufficiency, coronary
 newborn 768.9
  mild or moderate 768.6
  severe 768.5
 pathological 799.0
Anteflexion — *see* Anteversion
Antenatal
 care, normal pregnancy V22.1
  first V22.0
 screening (for) V28.9
  based on amniocentesis NEC V28.2
   chromosomal anomalies V28.0
   raised alphafetoprotein levels V28.1
  chromosomal anomalies V28.0
  fetal growth retardation using ultrasonics
   V28.4
  isoimmunization V28.5
  malformations using ultrasonics V28.3
  raised alphafetoprotein levels in amniotic
   fluid V28.1
  specified condition NEC V28.8
  Streptococcus B V28.6
Antepartum — *see* condition
Anterior — *see also* condition
 spinal artery compression syndrome 721.1
Antero-occlusion 524.2
Anteversion
 cervix (*see also* Anteversion, uterus) 621.6
 femur (neck), congenital 755.63
 uterus, uterine (cervix) (postinfectional)
  (postpartal, old) 621.6
  congenital 752.3
  in pregnancy or childbirth 654.4 ✓5ᵗʰ
   affecting fetus or newborn 763.89
   causing obstructed labor 660.2 ✓5ᵗʰ
    affecting fetus or newborn 763.1
Anthracosilicosis (occupational) 500
Anthracosis (lung) (occupational) 500
 lingua 529.3
Anthrax 022.9
 with pneumonia 022.1 *[484.5]*
 colitis 022.2
 cutaneous 022.0
 gastrointestinal 022.2
 intestinal 022.2
 pulmonary 022.1
 respiratory 022.1
 septicemia 022.3
 specified manifestation NEC 022.8
Anthropoid pelvis 755.69
 with disproportion (fetopelvic) 653.2 ✓5ᵗʰ
  affecting fetus or newborn 763.1
  causing obstructed labor 660.1 ✓5ᵗʰ
   affecting fetus or newborn 763.1
Anthropophobia 300.29
Antibioma, breast 611.0
Antibodies
 maternal (blood group) (*see also*
  Incompatibility) 656.2 ✓5ᵗʰ
  anti-D, cord blood 656.1 ✓5ᵗʰ
  fetus or newborn 773.0
Antibody deficiency syndrome
 agammaglobulinemic 279.00
 congenital 279.04
 hypogammaglobulinemic 279.00
Anticoagulant, circulating (*see also* Circulating
 anticoagulants) 286.5
Antimongolism syndrome 758.3
Antimonial cholera 985.4
Antisocial personality 301.7
Antithrombinemia (*see also* Circulating
 anticoagulants) 286.5
Antithromboplastinemia (*see also* Circulating
 anticoagulants) 286.5
Antithromboplastinogenemia (*see also*
 Circulating anticoagulants) 286.5
Antitoxin complication or reaction — *see*
 Complications, vaccination
Anton (-Babinski) syndrome
 (hemiasomatognosia) 307.9
Antritis (chronic) 473.0
 acute 461.0

Antrum, antral — *see* condition
Anuria 788.5
 with
  abortion — *see* Abortion, by type, with renal
   failure
  ectopic pregnancy (*see also* categories
   633.0-633.9) 639.3
  molar pregnancy (*see also* categories 630-
   632) 639.3
 calculus (impacted) (recurrent) 592.9
  kidney 592.0
  ureter 592.1
 congenital 753.3
 due to a procedure 997.5
 following
  abortion 639.3
  ectopic or molar pregnancy 639.3
 newborn 753.3
 postrenal 593.4
 puerperal, postpartum, childbirth 669.3 ✓5ᵗʰ
 specified as due to a procedure 997.5
 sulfonamide
  correct substance properly administered
   788.5
  overdose or wrong substance given or taken
   961.0
 traumatic (following crushing) 958.5
Anus, anal — *see* condition
Anusitis 569.49
Anxiety (neurosis) (reaction) (state) 300.00
 alcohol-induced 291.89
 depression 300.4
 drug-induced 292.89
 due to or associated with physical condition
  293.84
 generalized 300.02
 hysteria 300.20
 in
  acute stress reaction 308.0
  transient adjustment reaction 309.24
 panic type 300.01
 separation, abnormal 309.21
 syndrome (organic) (transient) 293.84
Aorta, aortic — *see* condition
Aortectasia 441.9
Aortitis (nonsyphilitic) 447.6
 arteriosclerotic 440.0
 calcific 447.6
 Döhle-Heller 093.1
 luetic 093.1
 rheumatic (*see also* Endocarditis, acute,
  rheumatic) 391.1
 rheumatoid — *see* Arthritis, rheumatoid
 specific 093.1
 syphilitic 093.1
  congenital 090.5
Apethetic thyroid storm (*see also* Thyrotoxicosis)
 242.9 ✓5ᵗʰ
Apepsia 536.8
 achlorhydric 536.0
 psychogenic 306.4
Aperistalsis, esophagus 530.0
Apert's syndrome (acrocephalosyndactyly) 755.55
Apert-Gallais syndrome (adrenogenital) 255.2
Apertognathia 524.2
Aphagia 787.2
 psychogenic 307.1
Aphakia (acquired) (bilateral) (postoperative)
 (unilateral) 379.31
 congenital 743.35
Aphalangia (congenital) 755.4
 lower limb (complete) (intercalary) (partial)
  (terminal) 755.39
  meaning all digits (complete) (partial) 755.31
  transverse 755.31
 upper limb (complete) (intercalary) (partial)
  (terminal) 755.29
  meaning all digits (complete) (partial) 755.21
  transverse 755.21

Aphasia (amnestic) (ataxic) (auditory) (Broca's) (choreatic) (classic) (expressive) (global) (ideational) (ideokinetic) (ideomotor) (jargon) (motor) (nominal) (receptive) (semantic) (sensory) (syntactic) (verbal) (visual) (Wernicke's) 784.3
  developmental 315.31
  syphilis, tertiary 094.89
  uremic — *see* Uremia

Aphemia 784.3
  uremic — *see* Uremia

Aphonia 784.41
  clericorum 784.49
  hysterical 300.11
  organic 784.41
  psychogenic 306.1

Aphthae, aphthous — *see also* condition
  Bednar's 528.2
  cachectic 529.0
  epizootic 078.4
  fever 078.4
  oral 528.2
  stomatitis 528.2
  thrush 112.0
  ulcer (oral) (recurrent) 528.2
    genital organ(s) NEC
      female 629.8
      male 608.89
    larynx 478.79

Apical — *see* condition

Aplasia — *see also* Agenesis
  alveolar process (acquired) 525.8
    congenital 750.26
  aorta (congenital) 747.22
  aortic valve (congenital) 746.89
  axialis extracorticalis (congenital) 330.0
  bone marrow (myeloid) 284.9
    acquired (secondary) 284.8
    congenital 284.0
    idiopathic 284.9
  brain 740.0
    specified part 742.2
  breast 757.6
  bronchus 748.3
  cementum 520.4
  cerebellar 742.2
  congenital pure red cell 284.0
  corpus callosum 742.2
  erythrocyte 284.8
    congenital 284.0
  extracortical axial 330.0
  eye (congenital) 743.00
  fovea centralis (congenital) 743.55
  germinal (cell) 606.0
  iris 743.45
  labyrinth, membranous 744.05
  limb (congenital) 755.4
    lower NEC 755.30
    upper NEC 755.20
  lung (bilateral) (congenital) (unilateral) 748.5
  nervous system NEC 742.8
  nuclear 742.8
  ovary 752.0
  Pelizaeus-Merzbacher 330.0
  prostate (congenital) 752.8
  red cell (pure) (with thymoma) 284.8
    acquired (secondary) 284.8
    congenital 284.0
    hereditary 284.0
    of infants 284.0
    primary 284.0
  round ligament (congenital) 752.8
  salivary gland 750.21
  skin (congenital) 757.39
  spinal cord 742.59
  spleen 759.0
  testis (congenital) 752.8
  thymic, with immunodeficiency 279.2
  thyroid 243
  uterus 752.3
  ventral horn cell 742.59

Apleuria 756.3

Apnea, apneic (spells) 786.03
  newborn, neonatorum 770.81 ▲
    essential 770.81 ●

Apnea, apneic — *continued*
  newborn, neonatorum — *continued*
    obstructive 770.82 ●
    primary 770.81 ●
    sleep 770.81 ●
    specified NEC 770.82 ●
  psychogenic 306.1
  sleep NEC 780.57
    with
      hypersomnia 780.53
      hyposomnia 780.51
      insomnia 780.51
      sleep disturbance NEC 780.57

Apneumatosis newborn 770.4

Apodia 755.31

Apophysitis (bone) (*see also* Osteochondrosis) 732.9
  calcaneus 732.5
  juvenile 732.6

Apoplectiform convulsions (*see also* Disease, cerebrovascular, acute) 436

Apoplexia, apoplexy, apoplectic (*see also* Disease, cerebrovascular, acute) 436
  abdominal 569.89
  adrenal 036.3
  attack 436
  basilar (*see also* Disease, cerebrovascular, acute) 436
  brain (*see also* Disease, cerebrovascular, acute) 436
  bulbar (*see also* Disease, cerebrovascular, acute) 436
  capillary (*see also* Disease, cerebrovascular, acute) 436
  cardiac (*see also* Infarct, myocardium) 410.9 ✔5ᵗʰ
  cerebral (*see also* Disease, cerebrovascular acute) 436
  chorea (*see also* Disease, cerebrovascular, acute) 436
  congestive (*see also* Disease, cerebrovascular, acute) 436
    newborn 767.4
  embolic (*see also* Embolism, brain) 434.1 ✔5ᵗʰ
  fetus 767.0
  fit (*see also* Disease, cerebrovascular, acute) 436
  healed or old V12.59
  heart (auricle) (ventricle) (*see also* Infarct, myocardium) 410.9 ✔5ᵗʰ
  heat 992.0
  hemiplegia (*see also* Disease, cerebrovascular, acute) 436
  hemorrhagic (stroke) (*see also* Hemorrhage, brain) 432.9
  ingravescent (*see also* Disease, cerebrovascular, acute) 436
  late effect — *see* Late effect(s) (of) cerebrovascular disease
  lung — *see* Embolism, pulmonary
  meninges, hemorrhagic (*see also* Hemorrhage subarachnoid) 430
  neonatorum 767.0
  newborn 767.0
  pancreatitis 577.0
  placenta 641.2 ✔5ᵗʰ
  progressive (*see also* Disease, cerebrovascular, acute) 436
  pulmonary (artery) (vein) — *see* Embolism, pulmonary
  sanguineous (*see also* Disease, cerebrovascular, acute) 436
  seizure (*see also* Disease, cerebrovascular, acute) 436
  serous (*see also* Disease, cerebrovascular, acute) 436
  spleen 289.59
  stroke (*see also* Disease, cerebrovascular, acute) 436
  thrombotic (*see also* Thrombosis, brain) 434.0 ✔5ᵗʰ
  uremic — *see* Uremia
  uteroplacental 641.2 ✔5ᵗʰ

Appendage
  fallopian tube (cyst of Morgagni) 752.11
  intestine (epiploic) 751.5

Appendage — *continued*
  preauricular 744.1
  testicular (organ of Morgagni) 752.8

Appendicitis 541
  with
    perforation, peritonitis (generalized), or rupture 540.0
      with peritoneal abscess 540.1
    peritoneal abscess 540.1
  acute (catarrhal) (fulminating) (gangrenous) (inflammatory) (obstructive) (retrocecal) (suppurative) 540.9
    with
      perforation, peritonitis, or rupture 540.0
        with peritoneal abscess 540.1
      peritoneal abscess 540.1
  amebic 006.8
  chronic (recurrent) 542
  exacerbation — *see* Appendicitis, acute
  fulminating — *see* Appendicitis, acute
  gangrenous — *see* Appendicitis, acute
  healed (obliterative) 542
  interval 542
  neurogenic 542
  obstructive 542
  pneumococcal 541
  recurrent 542
  relapsing 542
  retrocecal 541
  subacute (adhesive) 542
  subsiding 542
  suppurative — *see* Appendicitis, acute
  tuberculous (*see also* Tuberculosis) 014.8 ✔5ᵗʰ

Appendiclausis 543.9

Appendicolithiasis 543.9

Appendicopathia oxyurica 127.4

Appendix, appendicular — *see also* condition
  Morgagni (male) 752.8
    fallopian tube 752.11

Appetite
  depraved 307.52
  excessive 783.6
    psychogenic 307.51
  lack or loss (*see also* Anorexia) 783.0
    nonorganic origin 307.59
  perverted 307.52
    hysterical 300.11

Apprehension, apprehensiveness (abnormal) (state) 300.00
  specified type NEC 300.09

Approximal wear 521.1

Apraxia (classic) (ideational) (ideokinetic) (ideomotor) (motor) 784.69
  oculomotor, congenital 379.51
  verbal 784.69

Aptyalism 527.7

Aqueous misdirection 365.83 ●

Arabicum elephantiasis (*see also* Infestation, filarial) 125.9

Arachnidism 989.5

Arachnitis — *see* Meningitis

Arachnodactyly 759.82

Arachnoidism 989.5

Arachnoiditis (acute) (adhesive) (basic) (brain) (cerebrospinal) (chiasmal) (chronic) (spinal) (*see also* Meningitis) 322.9
  meningococcal (chronic) 036.0
  syphilitic 094.2
  tuberculous (*see also* Tuberculosis meninges) 013.0 ✔5ᵗʰ

Araneism 989.5

Arboencephalitis, Australian 062.4

Arborization block (heart) 426.6

Arbor virus, arbovirus (infection) NEC 066.9

ARC 042

Arches — *see* condition

Arcuatus uterus 752.3

Arcus (cornea)
  juvenilis 743.43
    interfering with vision 743.42
  senilis 371.41

Arc-welders' lung 503

✔4ᵗʰ Fourth-digit Required   ✔5ᵗʰ Fifth-digit Required   ▶◀ Revised Text   ● New Line   ▲ Revised Code

Arc-welders' syndrome (photokeratitis) 370.24
Areflexia 796.1
Areola — *see* condition
Argentaffinoma (M8241/1) — *see also* Neoplasm, by site, uncertain behavior
  benign (M8241/0) — *see* Neoplasm, by site, benign
  malignant (M8241/3) — *see* Neoplasm, by site, malignant
  syndrome 259.2
Argentinian hemorrhagic fever 078.7
Arginosuccinicaciduria 270.6
Argonz-Del Castillo syndrome (nonpuerperal galactorrhea and amenorrhea) 253.1
Argyll-Robertson phenomenon, pupil, or syndrome (syphilitic) 094.89
  atypical 379.45
  nonluetic 379.45
  nonsyphilitic 379.45
  reversed 379.45
Argyria, argyriasis NEC 985.8
  conjunctiva 372.55
  cornea 371.16
  from drug or medicinal agent
    correct substance properly administered 709.09
    overdose or wrong substance given or taken 961.2
Arhinencephaly 742.2
Arias-Stella phenomenon 621.3
Ariboflavinosis 266.0
Arizona enteritis 008.1
Arm — *see* condition
Armenian disease 277.3
Arnold-Chiari obstruction or syndrome (*see also* Spina bifida) 741.0 ✓5ᵗʰ
  type I 348.4
  type II (*see also* Spina bifida) 741.0 ✓5ᵗʰ
  type III 742.0
  type IV 742.2
Arrest, arrested
  active phase of labor 661.1 ✓5ᵗʰ
    affecting fetus or newborn 763.7
  any plane in pelvis
    complicating delivery 660.1 ✓5ᵗʰ
      affecting fetus or newborn 763.1
  bone marrow (*see also* Anemia, aplastic) 284.9
  cardiac 427.5
    with
      abortion — *see* Abortion, by type, with specified complication NEC
      ectopic pregnancy (*see also* categories 633.0-633.9) 639.8
      molar pregnancy (*see also* categories 630-632) 639.8
    complicating
      anesthesia
        correct substance properly administered 427.5
        obstetric 668.1 ✓5ᵗʰ
        overdose or wrong substance given 968.4
          specified anesthetic — *see* Table of Drugs and Chemicals
      delivery (cesarean) (instrumental) 669.4 ✓5ᵗʰ
      ectopic or molar pregnancy 639.8
      surgery (nontherapeutic) (therapeutic) 997.1
    fetus or newborn 779.89 ▲
    following
      abortion 639.8
      ectopic or molar pregnancy 639.8
    postoperative (immediate) 997.1
      long-term effect of cardiac surgery 429.4
  cardiorespiratory (*see also* Arrest, cardiac) 427.5
  deep transverse 660.3 ✓5ᵗʰ
    affecting fetus or newborn 763.1
  development or growth
    bone 733.91
    child 783.40

Arrest, arrested — *continued*
  development or growth — *continued*
    fetus 764.9 ✓5ᵗʰ
      affecting management of pregnancy 656.5 ✓5ᵗʰ
    tracheal rings 748.3
    epiphyseal 733.91
    granulopoiesis 288.0
    heart — *see* Arrest, cardiac
    respiratory 799.1
      newborn 770.89 ▲
    sinus 426.6
    transverse (deep) 660.3 ✓5ᵗʰ
      affecting fetus or newborn 763.1
Arrhenoblastoma (M8630/1)
  benign (M8630/0)
    specified site — *see* Neoplasm, by site, benign
    unspecified site
      female 220
      male 222.0
  malignant (M8630/3)
    specified site — *see* Neoplasm, by site, malignant
    unspecified site
      female 183.0
      male 186.9
  specified site — *see* Neoplasm, by site, uncertain behavior
  unspecified site
    female 236.2
    male 236.4
Arrhinencephaly 742.2
  due to
    trisomy 13 (13-15) 758.1
    trisomy 18 (16-18) 758.2
Arrhythmia (auricle) (cardiac) (cordis) (gallop rhythm) (juvenile) (nodal) (reflex) (sinus) (supraventricular) (transitory) (ventricle) 427.9
  bigeminal rhythm 427.89
  block 426.9
  bradycardia 427.89
  contractions, premature 427.60
  coronary sinus 427.89
  ectopic 427.89
  extrasystolic 427.60
  postoperative 997.1
  psychogenic 306.2
  vagal 780.2
Arrillaga-Ayerza syndrome (pulmonary artery sclerosis with pulmonary hypertension) 416.0
Arsenical
  dermatitis 692.4
  keratosis 692.4
  pigmentation 985.1
    from drug or medicinal agent
      correct substance properly administered 709.09
      overdose or wrong substance given or taken 961.1
Arsenism 985.1
  from drug or medicinal agent
    correct substance properly administered 692.4
    overdose or wrong substance given or taken 961.1
Arterial — *see* condition
Arteriectasis 447.8
Arteriofibrosis — *see* Arteriosclerosis
Arteriolar sclerosis — *see* Arteriosclerosis
Arteriolith — *see* Arteriosclerosis
Arteriolitis 447.6
  necrotizing, kidney 447.5
  renal — *see* Hypertension, kidney
Arteriolosclerosis — *see* Arteriosclerosis
Arterionephrosclerosis (*see also* Hypertension, kidney) 403.90
Arteriopathy 447.9
Arteriosclerosis, arteriosclerotic (artery) (deformans) (diffuse) (disease) (endarteritis) (general) (obliterans) (obliterative) (occlusive) (senile) (with calcification) 440.9

Arteriosclerosis, arteriosclerotic — *continued*
  with
    gangrene 440.24
    psychosis (*see also* Psychosis, arteriosclerotic) 290.40
    ulceration 440.23
  aorta 440.0
  arteries of extremities — *see* Arteriosclerosis, extremities
  basilar (artery) (*see also* Occlusion, artery, basilar) 433.0 ✓5ᵗʰ
  brain 437.0
  bypass graft
    coronary artery 414.05
      autologous artery (gastroepiploic) (internal mammary) 414.04
      autologous vein 414.02
      nonautologous biological 414.03
    extremity 440.30
      autologous vein 440.31
      nonautologous biological 440.32
  cardiac — *see* Arteriosclerosis, coronary
  cardiopathy — *see* Arteriosclerosis, coronary
  cardiorenal (*see also* Hypertension, cardiorenal) 404.90
  cardiovascular (*see also* Disease, cardiovascular) 429.2
  carotid (artery) (common) (internal) (*see also* Occlusion, artery, carotid) 433.1 ✓5ᵗʰ
  central nervous system 437.0
  cerebral 437.0
    late effect — *see* Late effect(s) (of) cerebrovascular disease
  cerebrospinal 437.0
  cerebrovascular 437.0
  coronary (artery) 414.00
    graft — *see* Arteriosclerosis, bypass graft
    native artery 414.01
    of transplanted heart 414.06 ●
  extremities (native artery) NEC 440.20
    bypass graft 440.30
      autologous vein 440.31
      nonautologous biological 440.32
    claudication (intermittent) 440.21
    and
      gangrene 440.24
      rest pain 440.22
        and
          gangrene 440.24
          ulceration 440.23
            and gangrene 440.24
        ulceration 440.23
          and gangrene 440.24
    gangrene 440.24
    rest pain 440.22
      and
        gangrene 440.24
        ulceration 440.23
          and gangrene 440.24
    specified site NEC 440.29
    ulceration 440.23
      and gangrene 440.24
  heart (disease) — *see also* Arteriosclerosis, coronary
    valve 424.99
      aortic 424.1
      mitral 424.0
      pulmonary 424.3
      tricuspid 424.2
  kidney (*see also* Hypertension, kidney) 403.90
  labyrinth, labyrinthine 388.00
  medial NEC 440.20
  mesentery (artery) 557.1
  Mönckeberg's 440.20
  myocarditis 429.0
  nephrosclerosis (*see also* Hypertension, kidney) 403.90
  peripheral (of extremities) — *see* Arteriosclerosis, extremities
  precerebral 433.9 ✓5ᵗʰ
    specified artery NEC 433.8 ✓5ᵗʰ
  pulmonary (idiopathic) 416.0
  renal (*see also* Hypertension, kidney) 403.90
    arterioles (*see also* Hypertension, kidney) 403.90
    artery 440.1
  retinal (vascular) 440.8 [362.13]

Arteriosclerosis, arteriosclerotic — *continued*
  specified artery NEC 440.8
    with gangrene 440.8 [785.4]
  spinal (cord) 437.0
  vertebral (artery) (*see also* Occlusion, artery,
    vertebral) 433.2 ✓5th
Arteriospasm 443.9
Arteriovenous — *see* condition
Arteritis 447.6
  allergic (*see also* Angiitis, hypersensitivity)
    446.20
  aorta (nonsyphilitic) 447.6
    syphilitic 093.1
  aortic arch 446.7
  brachiocephalica 446.7
  brain 437.4
    syphilitic 094.89
  branchial 446.7
  cerebral 437.4
    late effect — *see* Late effect(s) (of)
      cerebrovascular disease
    syphilitic 094.89
  coronary (artery) — *see also* Arteriosclerosis,
    coronary
    rheumatic 391.9
      chronic 398.99
    syphilitic 093.89
  cranial (left) (right) 446.5
  deformans — *see* Arteriosclerosis
  giant cell 446.5
  necrosing or necrotizing 446.0
  nodosa 446.0
  obliterans — *see also* Arteriosclerosis
    subclaviocarotica 446.7
  pulmonary 417.8
  retina 362.18
  rheumatic — *see* Fever, rheumatic
  senile — *see* Arteriosclerosis
  suppurative 447.2
  syphilitic (general) 093.89
    brain 094.89
    coronary 093.89
    spinal 094.89
  temporal 446.5
  young female, syndrome 446.7
Artery, arterial — *see* condition
Arthralgia (*see also* Pain, joint) 719.4 ✓5th
  allergic (*see also* Pain, joint) 719.4 ✓5th
  in caisson disease 993.3
  psychogenic 307.89
  rubella 056.71
  Salmonella 003.23
  temporomandibular joint 524.62
Arthritis, arthritic (acute) (chronic) (subacute)
  716.9 ✓5th
  meaning Osteoarthritis — *see* Osteoarthrosis

> *Note* — Use the following fifth-digit
> subclassification with categories 711-712,
> 715-716:
>
>   0   *site unspecified*
>   1   *shoulder region*
>   2   *upper arm*
>   3   *forearm*
>   4   *hand*
>   5   *pelvic region and thigh*
>   6   *lower leg*
>   7   *ankle and foot*
>   8   *other specified sites*
>   9   *multiple sites*

  allergic 716.2 ✓5th
  ankylosing (crippling) (spine) 720.0
    sites other than spine 716.9 ✓5th
  atrophic 714.0
    spine 720.9
  back (*see also* Arthritis, spine) 721.90
  Bechterew's (ankylosing spondylitis) 720.0
  blennorrhagic 098.50
  cervical, cervicodorsal (*see also* Spondylosis,
    cervical) 721.0
  Charcôt's 094.0 [713.5]
    diabetic 250.6 ✓5th [713.5]
    syringomyelic 336.0 [713.5]

Arthritis, arthritic — *continued*
  Charcôt's — *continued*
    tabetic 094.0 [713.5]
  chylous (*see also* Filariasis) 125.9 [711.7] ✓5th
  climacteric NEC 716.3 ✓5th
  coccyx 721.8
  cricoarytenoid 478.79
  crystal (-induced) — *see* Arthritis, due to
    crystals
  deformans (*see also* Osteoarthrosis) 715.9 ✓5th
    spine 721.90
      with myelopathy 721.91
  degenerative (*see also* Osteoarthrosis)
    715.9 ✓5th
    idiopathic 715.09
    polyarticular 715.09
    spine 721.90
      with myelopathy 721.91
  dermatoarthritis, lipoid 272.8 [713.0]
  due to or associated with
    acromegaly 253.0 [713.0]
    actinomycosis 039.8 [711.4] ✓5th
    amyloidosis 277.3 [713.7]
    bacterial disease NEC 040.89 [711.4] ✓5th
    Behçet's syndrome 136.1 [711.2] ✓5th
    blastomycosis 116.0 [711.6] ✓5th
    brucellosis (*see also* Brucellosis)
      023.9 [711.4] ✓5th
    caisson disease 993.3
    coccidioidomycosis 114.3 [711.6] ✓5th
    coliform (Escherichia coli) 711.0 ✓5th
    colitis, ulcerative (*see also* Colitis, ulcerative)
      556.9 [713.1]
    cowpox 051.0 [711.5] ✓5th
    crystals — *see also* Gout
      dicalcium phosphate 275.49 [712.1]
      pyrophosphate 275.49 [712.2]
      specified NEC 275.49 [712.8]
    dermatoarthritis, lipoid 272.8 [713.0]
    dermatological disorder NEC 709.9 [713.3]
    diabetes 250.6 ✓5th [713.5]
    diphtheria 032.89 [711.4] ✓5th
    dracontiasis 125.7 [711.7] ✓5th
    dysentery 009.0 [711.3] ✓5th
    endocrine disorder NEC 259.9 [713.0]
    enteritis NEC 009.1 [711.3] ✓5th
      infectious (*see also* Enteritis, infectious)
        009.0 [711.3] ✓5th
        specified organism NEC 008.8
          [711.3] ✓5th
      regional (*see also* Enteritis, regional)
        555.9 [713.1]
      specified organism NEC 008.8 [711.3] ✓5th
    epiphyseal slip, nontraumatic (old)
      716.8 ✓5th
    erysipelas 035 [711.4] ✓5th
    erythema
      epidemic 026.1
      multiforme 695.1 [713.3]
      nodosum 695.2 [713.3]
    Escherichia coli 711.0 ✓5th
    filariasis NEC 125.9 [711.7] ✓5th
    gastrointestinal condition NEC 569.9 [713.1]
    glanders 024 [711.4] ✓5th
    Gonococcus 098.50
    gout 274.0
    H. influenzae 711.0 ✓5th
    helminthiasis NEC 128.9 [711.7] ✓5th
    hematological disorder NEC 289.9 [713.2]
    hemochromatosis 275.0 [713.0]
    hemoglobinopathy NEC (*see also* Disease,
      hemoglobin) 282.7 [713.2]
    hemophilia (*see also* Hemophilia) 286.0
      [713.2]
    Hemophilus influenzae (H. influenzae)
      711.0 ✓5th
    Henoch (-Schönlein) purpura 287.0 [713.6]
    histoplasmosis NEC (*see also*
      Histoplasmosis) 115.99 [711.6] ✓5th
    hyperparathyroidism 252.0 [713.0]
    hypersensitivity reaction NEC 995.3 [713.6]
    hypogammaglobulinemia (*see also*
      Hypogamma-globulinemia) 279.00
      [713.0]
    hypothyroidism NEC 244.9 [713.0]
    infection (*see also* Arthritis, infectious)
      711.9 ✓5th

Arthritis, arthritic — *continued*
  due to or associated with — *continued*
    infectious disease NEC 136.9 [711.8] ✓5th
    leprosy (*see also* Leprosy) 030.9 [711.4] ✓5th
    leukemia NEC (M9800/3) 208.9 ✓5th [713.2]
    lipoid dermatoarthritis 272.8 [713.0]
    Lyme disease 088.81 [711.8] ✓5th
    Mediterranean fever, familial 277.3 [713.7]
    meningococcal infection 036.82
    metabolic disorder NEC 277.9 [713.0]
    multiple myelomatosis (M9730/3) 203.0 ✓5th
      [713.2]
    mumps 072.79 [711.5] ✓5th
    mycobacteria 031.8 [711.4] ✓5th
    mycosis NEC 117.9 [711.6] ✓5th
    neurological disorder NEC 349.9 [713.5]
    ochronosis 270.2 [713.0]
    O'Nyong Nyong 066.3 [711.5] ✓5th
    parasitic disease NEC 136.9 [711.8] ✓5th
    paratyphoid fever (*see also* Fever,
      paratyphoid) 002.9 [711.3] ✓5th
    Pneumococcus 711.0 ✓5th
    poliomyelitis (*see also* Poliomyelitis)
      045.9 ✓5th [711.5] ✓5th
    Pseudomonas 711.0 ✓5th
    psoriasis 696.0
    pyogenic organism (E. coli) (H. influenzae)
      (Pseudomonas) (Streptococcus)
      711.0 ✓5th
    rat-bite fever 026.1 [711.4] ✓5th
    regional enteritis (*see also* Enteritis,
      regional) 555.9 [713.1]
    Reiter's disease 099.3 [711.1] ✓5th
    respiratory disorder NEC 519.9 [713.4]
    reticulosis, malignant (M9720/3) 202.3 ✓5th
      [713.2]
    rubella 056.71
    salmonellosis 003.23
    sarcoidosis 135 [713.7]
    serum sickness 999.5 [713.6]
    Staphylococcus 711.0 ✓5th
    Streptococcus 711.0 ✓5th
    syphilis (*see also* Syphilis) 094.0 [711.4] ✓5th
    syringomyelia 336.0 [713.5]
    thalassemia 282.4 [713.2]
    tuberculosis (*see also* Tuberculosis,
      arthritis) 015.9 ✓5th [711.4] ✓5th
    typhoid fever 002.0 [711.3] ✓5th
    ulcerative colitis (*see also* Colitis, ulcerative)
      556.9 [713.1]
    urethritis
      nongonococcal (*see also* Urethritis,
        nongonococcal) 099.40 [711.1] ✓5th
      nonspecific (*see also* Urethritis,
        nongonococcal) 099.40 [711.1] ✓5th
      Reiter's 099.3 [711.1] ✓5th
    viral disease NEC 079.99 [711.5] ✓5th
  erythema epidemic 026.1
  gonococcal 098.50
  gouty (acute) 274.0
  hypertrophic (*see also* Osteoarthrosis)
    715.9 ✓5th
    spine 721.90
      with myelopathy 721.91
  idiopathic, blennorrheal 099.3
  in caisson disease 993.3 [713.8]
  infectious or infective (acute) (chronic)
    (subacute) NEC 711.9 ✓5th
    nonpyogenic 711.9 ✓5th
    spine 720.9
  inflammatory NEC 714.9
  juvenile rheumatoid (chronic) (polyarticular)
    714.30
    acute 714.31
    monoarticular 714.33
    pauciarticular 714.32
  lumbar (*see also* Spondylosis, lumbar) 721.3
  meningococcal 036.82
  menopausal NEC 716.3 ✓5th
  migratory — *see* Fever, rheumatic
  neuropathic (Charcôt's) 094.0 [713.5]
    diabetic 250.6 ✓5th [713.5]
    nonsyphilitic NEC 349.9 [713.5]
    syringomyelic 336.0 [713.5]
    tabetic 094.0 [713.5]
  nodosa (*see also* Osteoarthrosis) 715.9 ✓5th
    spine 721.90
      with myelopathy 721.91

Arthritis, arthritic — *continued*
nonpyogenic NEC 716.9 ✓5th
  spine 721.90
    with myelopathy 721.91
ochronotic 270.2 *[713.0]*
palindromic (see also Rheumatism,
  palindromic) 719.3 ✓5th
pneumococcal 711.0 ✓5th
postdysenteric 009.0 *[711.3]* ✓5th
postrheumatic, chronic (Jaccoud's) 714.4
primary progressive 714.0
  spine 720.9
proliferative 714.0
  spine 720.0
psoriatic 696.0
purulent 711.0 ✓5th
pyogenic or pyemic 711.0 ✓5th
rheumatic 714.0
  acute or subacute — see Fever, rheumatic
  chronic 714.0
  spine 720.9
rheumatoid (nodular) 714.0
  with
    splenoadenomegaly and leukopenia 714.1
    visceral or systemic involvement 714.2
  aortitis 714.89
  carditis 714.2
  heart disease 714.2
  juvenile (chronic) (polyarticular) 714.30
    acute 714.31
    monoarticular 714.33
    pauciarticular 714.32
  spine 720.0
rubella 056.71
sacral, sacroiliac, sacrococcygeal (see also
  Spondylosis, sacral) 721.3
scorbutic 267
senile or senescent (see also Osteoarthrosis)
  715.9 ✓5th
  spine 721.90
    with myelopathy 721.91
septic 711.0 ✓5th
serum (nontherapeutic) (therapeutic) 999.5
  [713.6]
specified form NEC 716.8 ✓5th
spine 721.90
  with myelopathy 721.91
  atrophic 720.9
  degenerative 721.90
    with myelopathy 721.91
  hypertrophic (with deformity) 721.90
    with myelopathy 721.91
  infectious or infective NEC 720.9
  Marie-Strümpell 720.0
  nonpyogenic 721.90
    with myelopathy 721.91
  pyogenic 720.9
  rheumatoid 720.0
  traumatic (old) 721.7
  tuberculous (see also Tuberculosis)
    015.0 ✓5th *[720.81]*
staphylococcal 711.0 ✓5th
streptococcal 711.0 ✓5th
suppurative 711.0 ✓5th
syphilitic 094.0 *[713.5]*
  congenital 090.49 *[713.5]*
syphilitica deformans (Charcôt) 094.0 *[713.5]*
temporomandibular joint 524.69
thoracic (see also Spondylosis, thoracic) 721.2
toxic of menopause 716.3 ✓5th
transient 716.4 ✓5th
traumatic (chronic) (old) (post) 716.1 ✓5th
  current injury — see nature of injury
tuberculous (see also Tuberculosis, arthritis)
  015.9 ✓5th *[711.4]* ✓5th
urethritica 099.3 *[711.1]* ✓5th
urica, uratic 274.0
venereal 099.3 *[711.1]* ✓5th
vertebral (see also Arthritis, spine) 721.90
villous 716.8 ✓5th
von Bechterew's 720.0
Arthrocele (see also Effusion, joint) 719.0 ✓5th
Arthrochondritis — see Arthritis
Arthrodesis status V45.4
Arthrodynia (see also Pain, joint) 719.4 ✓5th
  psychogenic 307.89

Arthrodysplasia 755.9
Arthrofibrosis, joint (see also Ankylosis)
  718.5 ✓5th
Arthrogryposis 728.3
  multiplex, congenita 754.89
Arthrokatadysis 715.35
Arthrolithiasis 274.0
Arthro-onychodysplasia 756.89
Arthro-osteo-onychodysplasia 756.89
Arthropathy (see also Arthritis) 716.9 ✓5th

> Note — Use the following fifth-digit
> subclassification with categories 711-712,
> 716:
>
> 0   site unspecified
> 1   shoulder region
> 2   upper arm
> 3   forearm
> 4   hand
> 5   pelvic region and thigh
> 6   lower leg
> 7   ankle and foot
> 8   other specified sites
> 9   multiple sites

Behçets 136.1 *[711.2]* ✓5th
Charcôt's 094.0 *[713.5]*
  diabetic 250.6 ✓5th *[713.5]*
  syringomyelic 336.0 *[713.5]*
  tabetic 094.0 *[713.5]*
crystal (-induced) — see Arthritis, due to
  crystals
gouty 274.0
neurogenic, neuropathic (Charcôt's) (tabetic)
  094.0 *[713.5]*
  diabetic 250.6 ✓5th *[713.5]*
  nonsyphilitic NEC 349.9 *[713.5]*
  syringomyelic 336.0 *[713.5]*
postdysenteric NEC 009.0 *[711.3]* ✓5th
postrheumatic, chronic (Jaccoud's) 714.4
psoriatic 696.0
pulmonary 731.2
specified NEC 716.8 ✓5th
syringomyelia 336.0 *[713.5]*
tabes dorsalis 094.0 *[713.5]*
tabetic 094.0 *[713.5]*
transient 716.4 ✓5th
traumatic 716.1 ✓5th
uric acid 274.0
Arthophyte (see also Loose, body, joint) 718.1 ✓5th
Arthrophytis 719.80
  ankle 719.87
  elbow 719.82
  foot 719.87
  hand 719.84
  hip 719.85
  knee 719.86
  multiple sites 719.89
  pelvic region 719.85
  shoulder (region) 719.81
  specified site NEC 719.88
  wrist 719.83
Arthropyosis (see also Arthritis, pyogenic)
  711.0 ✓5th
Arthrosis (deformans) (degenerative) (see also
  Osteoarthrosis) 715.9 ✓5th
  Charcôt's 094.0 *[713.5]*
  polyarticular 715.09
  spine (see also Spondylosis) 721.90
Arthus' phenomenon 995.2
  due to
    correct substance properly administered
      995.2
    overdose or wrong substance given or taken
      977.9
      specified drug — see Table of Drugs and
        Chemicals
    serum 999.5
Articular — see also condition
  disc disorder (reducing or non-reducing)
    524.63
  spondylolisthesis 756.12

Artificial
  device (prosthetic) — see Fitting, device
  insemination V26.1
  menopause (states) (symptoms) (syndrome)
    627.4
  opening status (functioning) (without
    complication) V44.9
    anus (colostomy) V44.3
    colostomy V44.3
    cystostomy V44.50
      appendico-vesicostomy V44.52
      cutaneous-vesicostomy V44.51
      specified type NEC V44.59
    enterostomy V44.4
    gastrostomy V44.1
    ileostomy V44.2
    intestinal tract NEC V44.4
    jejunostomy V44.4
    nephrostomy V44.6
    specified site NEC V44.8
    tracheostomy V44.0
    ureterostomy V44.6
    urethrostomy V44.6
    urinary tract NEC V44.6
    vagina V44.7
  vagina status V44.7
ARV (disease) (illness) (infection) — see Human
  immunodeficiency virus (disease) (illness)
  (infection)
Arytenoid — see condition
Asbestosis (occupational) 501
Asboe-Hansen's disease (incontinentia
  pigmenti) 757.33
Ascariasis (intestinal) (lung) 127.0
Ascaridiasis 127.0
Ascaris 127.0
  lumbricoides (infestation) 127.0
  pneumonia 127.0
Ascending — see condition
Aschoff's bodies (see also Myocarditis,
  rheumatic) 398.0
Ascites 789.5
  abdominal NEC 789.5
  cancerous (M80000/6) 197.6
  cardiac 428.0
  chylous (nonfilarial) 457.8
    filarial (see also Infestation, filarial) 125.9
  congenital 778.0
  due to S. japonicum 120.2
  fetal, causing fetopelvic disproportion 653.7 ✓5th
  heart 428.0
  joint (see also Effusion, joint) 719.0 ✓5th
  malignant (M8000/6) 197.6
  pseudochylous 789.5
  syphilitic 095.2
  tuberculous (see also Tuberculosis) 014.0 ✓5th
Ascorbic acid (vitamin C) **deficiency** (scurvy) 267
ASCUS (atypical squamous cell changes of ●
  undetermined significance) ●
  favor benign 795.01 ●
  favor dysplasia 795.02 ●
ASCVD (arteriosclerotic cardiovascular disease)
  429.2
Aseptic — see condition
Asherman's syndrome 621.5
Asialia 527.7
Asiatic cholera (see also Cholera) 001.9
Asocial personality or trends 301.7
Asomatognosia 781.8
Aspergillosis 117.3
  with pneumonia 117.3 *[484.6]*
  allergic bronchopulmonary 518.6
  nonsyphilitic NEC 117.3
Aspergillus (flavus) (fumigatus) (infection)
  (terreus) 117.3
Aspermatogenesis 606.0
Aspermia (testis) 606.0
Asphyxia, asphyxiation (by) 799.0
  antenatal — see Distress, fetal
  bedclothes 994.7
  birth (see also Ashpyxia, newborn) 768.9
  bunny bag 994.7
  carbon monoxide 986

✓4th Fourth-digit Required   ✓5th Fifth-digit Required   ►◄ Revised Text   ● New Line   ▲ Revised Code

Asphyxia, asphyxiation — *continued*
  caul (*see also* Asphyxia, newborn)
  cave-in 994.7
    crushing — *see* Injury, internal,
      intrathoracic organs
  constriction 994.7
  crushing — *see* Injury, internal, intrathoracic
    organs
  drowning 994.1
  fetal, affecting newborn 768.9   ▲
  food or foreign body (in larynx) 933.1
    bronchioles 934.8
    bronchus (main) 934.1
    lung 934.8
    nasopharynx 933.0
    nose, nasal passages 932
    pharynx 933.0
    respiratory tract 934.9
      specified part NEC 934.8
    throat 933.0
    trachea 934.0
  gas, fumes, or vapor NEC 987.9
    specified — *see* Table of Drugs and
      Chemicals
  gravitational changes 994.7
  hanging 994.7
  inhalation — *see* Inhalation
  intrauterine
    fetal death (before onset of labor) 768.0
      during labor 768.1
    liveborn infant — *see* Distress, fetal,
      liveborn infant
  local 443.0
  mechanical 994.7
    during birth (*see also* Distress, fetal)
      768.9   ▲
  mucus 933.1
    bronchus (main) 934.1
    larynx 933.1
    lung 934.8
    nasal passages 932
    newborn 770.1
    pharynx 933.0
    respiratory tract 934.9
      specfied part NEC 934.8
    throat 933.0
    trachea 934.0
    vaginal (fetus or newborn) 770.1
  newborn 768.9
    blue 768.6
    livida 768.6
    mild or moderate 768.6
    pallida 768.5
    severe 768.5
    white 768.5
  pathological 799.0
  plastic bag 994.7
  postnatal (*see also* Asphyxia, newborn) 768.9
    mechanical 994.7
  pressure 994.7
  reticularis 782.61
  strangulation 994.7
  submersion 994.1
  traumatic NEC — *see* Injury, internal,
    intrathoracic organs
  vomiting, vomitus — *see* Asphyxia, food or
    foreign body
Aspiration
  acid pulmonary (syndrome) 997.3
    obstetric 668.0 ☑5ᵗʰ
  amniotic fluid 770.1
  bronchitis 507.0
  contents of birth canal 770.1
  fetal pneumonitis 770.1
  food, foreign body, or gasoline (with
    asphyxiation) — *see* Asphyxia, food or
    foreign body
  meconium 770.1
  mucus 933.1
    into
      bronchus (main) 934.1
      lung 934.8
      respiratory tract 934.9
        specified part NEC 934.8
      trachea 934.0
    newborn 770.1
    vaginal (fetus or newborn) 770.1

Aspiration — *continued*
  newborn 770.1
  pneumonia 507.0
  pneumonitis 507.0
    fetus or newborn 770.1
    obstetric 668.0 ☑5ᵗʰ
  syndrome of newborn (massive) (meconium)
    770.1
  vernix caseosa 770.1
Asplenia 759.0
  with mesocardia 746.87
Assam fever 085.0
Assimilation, pelvis
  with disproportion 653.2 ☑5ᵗʰ
    affecting fetus or newborn 763.1
    causing obstructed labor 660.1 ☑5ᵗʰ
      affecting fetus or newborn 763.1
Assmann's focus (*see also* Tuberculosis)
  011.0 ☑5ᵗʰ
Astasia (-asbasia) 307.9
  hysterical 300.11
Asteatosis 706.8
  cutis 706.8
Astereognosis 780.99   ▲
Asterixis 781.3
  in liver disease 572.8
Asteroid hyalitis 379.22
Asthenia, asthenic 780.79
  cardiac (*see also* Failure, heart) 428.9
    psychogenic 306.2
  cardiovascular (*see also* Failure, heart) 428.9
    psychogenic 306.2
  heart (*see also* Failure, heart) 428.9
    psychogenic 306.2
  hysterical 300.11
  myocardial (*see also* Failure, heart) 428.9
    psychogenic 306.2
  nervous 300.5
  neurocirculatory 306.2
  neurotic 300.5
  psychogenic 300.5
  psychoneurotic 300.5
  psychophysiologic 300.5
  reaction, psychoneurotic 300.5
  senile 797
  Stiller's 780.79
  tropical anhidrotic 705.1
Asthenopia 368.13
  accommodative 367.4
  hysterical (muscular) 300.11
  psychogenic 306.7
Asthenospermia 792.2
Asthma, asthmatic (bronchial) (catarrh)
  (spasmodic) 493.9 ☑5ᵗʰ

> *Note* — *Use the following fifth-digit*
> *subclassification with category 493:*
>
> 0   *without mention of status*
>   *asthmaticus or acute exacerbation*
>   *or unspecified*
> 1   *with status asthmaticus*
> 2   *with acute exacerbation*

  with
    chronic obstructive pulmonary disease
      (COPD) 493.2 ☑5ᵗʰ
    hay fever 493.0 ☑5ᵗʰ
    rhinitis, allergic 493.0 ☑5ᵗʰ
  allergic 493.9 ☑5ᵗʰ
    stated cause (external allergen) 493.0 ☑5ᵗʰ
  atopic 493.0 ☑5ᵗʰ
  cardiac (*see also* Failure, ventricular, left) 428.1
  cardiobronchial (*see also* Failure, ventricular,
    left) 428.1
  cardiorenal (*see also* Hypertension, cardiorenal)
    404.90
  childhood 493.0 ☑5ᵗʰ
  colliers' 500
  croup 493.9 ☑5ᵗʰ
  detergent 507.8
  due to
    detergent 507.8
    inhalation of fumes 506.3
    internal immunological process 493.0 ☑5ᵗʰ
  endogenous (intrinsic) 493.1 ☑5ᵗʰ

Asthma, asthmatic — *continued*
  eosinophilic 518.3
  exogenous (cosmetics) (dander or dust) (drugs)
    (dust) (feathers) (food) (hay) (platinum)
    (pollen) 493.0 ☑5ᵗʰ
  extrinsic 493.0 ☑5ᵗʰ
  grinders' 502
  hay 493.0 ☑5ᵗʰ
  heart (*see also* Failure, ventricular, left) 428.1
  IgE 493.0 ☑5ᵗʰ
  infective 493.1 ☑5ᵗʰ
  intrinsic 493.1 ☑5ᵗʰ
  Kopp's 254.8
  late-onset 493.1 ☑5ᵗʰ
  meat-wrappers' 506.9
  Millar's (laryngismus stridulus) 478.75
  millstone makers' 502
  miners' 500
  Monday morning 504
  New Orleans (epidemic) 493.0 ☑5ᵗʰ
  platinum 493.0 ☑5ᵗʰ
  pneumoconiotic (occupational) NEC 505
  potters' 502
  psychogenic 316 [*493.9*] ☑5ᵗʰ
  pulmonary eosinophilic 518.3
  red cedar 495.8
  Rostan's (*see also* Failure, ventricular, left)
    428.1
  sandblasters' 502
  sequoiosis 495.8
  stonemasons' 502
  thymic 254.8
  tuberculous (*see also* Tuberculosis, pulmonary)
    011.9 ☑5ᵗʰ
  Wichmann's (laryngismus stridulus) 478.75
  wood 495.8
Astigmatism (compound) (congenital) 367.20
  irregular 367.22
  regular 367.21
Astroblastoma (M9430/3)
  nose 748.1
  specified site — *see* Neoplasm, by site,
    malignant
  unspecified site 191.9
Astrocytoma (cystic) (M9400/3)
  anaplastic type (M9401/3)
    specified site — *see* Neoplasm, by site,
      malignant
    unspecified site 191.9
  fibrillary (M9420/3)
    specified site — *see* Neoplasm, by site,
      malignant
    unspecified site 191.9
  fibrous (M9420/3)
    specified site — *see* Neoplasm, by site,
      malignant
    unspecified site 191.9
  gemistocytic (M9411/3)
    specified site — *see* Neoplasm, by site,
      malignant
    unspecified site 191.9
  juvenile (M9421/3)
    specified site — *see* Neoplasm, by site,
      malignant
    unspecified site 191.9
  nose 748.1
  pilocytic (M9421/3)
    specified site — *see* Neoplasm, by site,
      malignant
    unspecified site 191.9
  piloid (M9421/3)
    specified site — *see* Neoplasm, by site,
      malignant
    unspecified site 191.9
  protoplasmic (M9410/3)
    specified site — *see* Neoplasm, by site,
      malignant
    unspecified site 191.9
  specified site — *see* Neoplasm, by site,
    malignant
  subependymal (M9383/1) 237.5
    giant cell (M9384/1) 237.5
  unspecified site 191.9
Astroglioma (M9400/3)
  nose 748.1
  specified site — *see* Neoplasm, by site,
    malignant
  unspecified site 191.9

Asymbolia 784.60

Asymmetrical breathing 786.09

Asymmetry — *see also* Distortion
  chest 786.9
  face 754.0
  jaw NEC 524.12
    maxillary 524.11
  pelvis with disproportion 653.0 ✓5ᵗʰ
    affecting fetus or newborn 763.1
    causing obstructed labor 660.1 ✓5ᵗʰ
      affecting fetus or newborn 763.1

Asynergia 781.3

Asynergy 781.3
  ventricular 429.89

Asystole (heart) (*see also* Arrest, cardiac) 427.5

Ataxia, ataxy, ataxic 781.3
  acute 781.3
  brain 331.89
  cerebellar 334.3
    hereditary (Marie's) 334.2
    in
      alcoholism 303.9 ✓5ᵗʰ [334.4]
      myxedema (*see also* Myxedema) 244.9
        [334.4]
      neoplastic disease NEC 239.9 [334.4]
  cerebral 331.89
  family, familial 334.2
    cerebral (Marie's) 334.2
    spinal (Friedreich's) 334.0
  Friedreich's (heredofamilial) (spinal) 334.0
  frontal lobe 781.3
  gait 781.2
    hysterical 300.11
  general 781.3
  hereditary NEC 334.2
    cerebellar 334.2
    spastic 334.1
    spinal 334.0
  heredofamilial (Marie's) 334.2
  hysterical 300.11
  locomotor (progressive) 094.0
    diabetic 250.6 ✓5ᵗʰ [337.1]
  Marie's (cerebellar) (heredofamilial) 334.2
  nonorganic origin 307.9
  partial 094.0
  postchickenpox 052.7
  progressive locomotor 094.0
  psychogenic 307.9
  Sanger-Brown's 334.2
  spastic 094.0
    hereditary 334.1
    syphilitic 094.0
  spinal
    hereditary 334.0
    progressive locomotor 094.0
  telangiectasia 334.8

Ataxia-telangiectasia 334.8

Atelectasis (absorption collapse) (complete)
  (compression) (massive) (partial)
  (postinfective) (pressure collapse)
  (pulmonary) (relaxation) 518.0
  newborn (congenital) (partial) 770.5
    primary 770.4
  primary 770.4
  tuberculous (*see also* Tuberculosis, pulmonary)
    011.9 ✓5ᵗʰ

Ateleiosis, ateliosis 253.3

Atelia — *see* Distortion

Ateliosis 253.3

Atelocardia 746.9

Atelomyelia 742.59

Athelia 757.6

Atheroembolism
  extremity ●
    lower 445.02 ●
    upper 445.01 ●
  kidney 445.81 ●
  specified site NEC 445.89 ●

Atheroma, atheromatous (*see also*
  Arteriosclerosis) 440.9
  aorta, aortic 440.0
    valve (*see also* Endocarditis, aortic) 424.1
  artery — *see* Arteriosclerosis

Atheroma, atheromatous (*see also*
  Arteriosclerosis) — *continued*
  basilar (artery) (*see also* Occlusion, artery,
    basilar) 433.0 ✓5ᵗʰ
  carotid (artery) (common) (internal) (*see also*
    Occlusion, artery, carotid) 433.1 ✓5ᵗʰ
  cerebral (arteries) 437.0
  coronary (artery) — *see* Arteriosclerosis,
    coronary
  degeneration — *see* Arteriosclerosis
  heart, cardiac — *see* Arteriosclerosis, coronary
  mitral (valve) 424.0
  myocardium, myocardial — *see*
    Arteriosclerosis, coronary
  pulmonary valve (heart) (*see also* Endocarditis,
    pulmonary) 424.3
  skin 706.2
  tricuspid (heart) (valve) 424.2
  valve, valvular — *see* Endocarditis
  vertebral (artery) (*see also* Occlusion, artery,
    vertebral) 433.2 ✓5ᵗʰ

Atheromatosis — *see also* Arteriosclerosis
  arterial, congenital 272.8

Atherosclerosis — *see* Arteriosclerosis

Athetosis (acquired) 781.0
  bilateral 333.7
  congenital (bilateral) 333.7
  double 333.7
  unilateral 781.0

Athlete's
  foot 110.4
  heart 429.3

Athletic team examination V70.3

Athrepsia 261

Athyrea (acquired) (*see also* Hypothyroidism)
  244.9
  congenital 243

Athyreosis (congenital) 243
  acquired — *see* Hypothyroidism

Athyroidism (acquired) (*see also* Hypothyroidism)
  244.9
  congenital 243

Atmospheric pyrexia 992.0

Atonia, atony, atonic
  abdominal wall 728.2
  bladder (sphincter) 596.4
    neurogenic NEC 596.54
      with cauda equina syndrome 344.61
  capillary 448.9
  cecum 564.89
    psychogenic 306.4
  colon 564.89
    psychogenic 306.4
  congenital 779.89
  dyspepsia 536.3
    psychogenic 306.4
  intestine 564.89
    psychogenic 306.4
  stomach 536.3
    neurotic or psychogenic 306.4
    psychogenic 306.4
  uterus 666.1 ✓5ᵗʰ
    affecting fetus or newborn 763.7
  vesical 596.4

Atopy NEC V15.09

Atransferrinemia, congenital 273.8

Atresia, atretic (congenital) 759.89
  alimentary organ or tract NEC 751.8
    lower 751.2
    upper 750.8
  ani, anus, anal (canal) 751.2
  aorta 747.22
    with hypoplasia of ascending aorta and
      defective development of left ventricle
      (with mitral valve atresia) 746.7
    arch 747.11
    ring 747.21
  aortic (orifice) (valve) 746.89
    arch 747.11
  aqueduct of Sylvius 742.3
    with spina bifida (*see also* Spina bifida)
      741.0 ✓5ᵗʰ
  artery NEC (*see also* Atresia, blood vessel)
    747.60
    cerebral 747.81

Atresia, atretic — *continued*
  artery NEC (*see also* Atresia, blood vessel) —
    continued
    coronary 746.85
    eye 743.58
    pulmonary 747.3
    umbilical 747.5
  auditory canal (external) 744.02
  bile, biliary duct (common) or passage 751.61
    acquired (*see also* Obstruction, biliary)
      576.2
  bladder (neck) 753.6
  blood vessel (peripheral) NEC 747.60
    cerebral 747.81
    gastrointestinal 747.61
    lower limb 747.64
    pulmonary artery 747.3
    renal 747.62
    spinal 747.82
    upper limb 747.63
  bronchus 748.3
  canal, ear 744.02
  cardiac
    valve 746.89
      aortic 746.89
      mitral 746.89
      pulmonary 746.01
      tricuspid 746.1
  cecum 751.2
  cervix (acquired) 622.4
    congenital 752.49
    in pregnancy or childbirth 654.6 ✓5ᵗʰ
      affecting fetus or newborn 763.89
      causing obstructed labor 660.2 ✓5ᵗʰ
        affecting fetus or newborn 763.1
  choana 748.0
  colon 751.2
  cystic duct 751.61
    acquired 575.8
      with obstruction (*see also* Obstruction,
        gallbladder) 575.2
  digestive organs NEC 751.8
  duodenum 751.1
  ear canal 744.02
  ejaculatory duct 752.8
  epiglottis 748.3
  esophagus 750.3
  Eustachian tube 744.24
  fallopian tube (acquired) 628.2
    congenital 752.19
  follicular cyst 620.0
  foramen of
    Luschka 742.3
      with spina bifida (*see also* Spina bifida)
        741.0 ✓5ᵗʰ
    Magendie 742.3
      with spina bifida (*see also* Spina bifida)
        741.0 ✓5ᵗʰ
  gallbladder 751.69
  genital organ
    external
      female 752.49
      male NEC 752.8
        penis 752.69
    internal
      female 752.8
      male 752.8
  glottis 748.3
  gullet 750.3
  heart
    valve NEC 746.89
      aortic 746.89
      mitral 746.89
      pulmonary 746.01
      tricuspid 746.1
  hymen 752.42
    acquired 623.3
    postinfective 623.3
  ileum 751.1
  intestine (small) 751.1
    large 751.2
  iris, filtration angle (*see also* Buphthalmia)
    743.20
  jejunum 751.1
  kidney 753.3
  lacrimal, apparatus 743.65
    acquired — *see* Stenosis, lacrimal

Atresia, atretic — *continued*
  larynx 748.3
  ligament, broad 752.19
  lung 748.5
  meatus urinarius 753.6
  mitral valve 746.89
    with atresia or hypoplasia of aortic orifice or
      valve, with hypoplasia of ascending
      aorta and defective development of left
      ventricle 746.7
  nares (anterior) (posterior) 748.0
  nasolacrimal duct 743.65
  nasopharynx 748.8
  nose, nostril 748.0
    acquired 738.0
  organ or site NEC — *see* Anomaly, specified
      type NEC
  osseous meatus (ear) 744.03
  oviduct (acquired) 628.2
    congenital 752.19
  parotid duct 750.23
    acquired 527.8
  pulmonary (artery) 747.3
    valve 746.01
    vein 747.49
  pulmonic 746.01
  pupil 743.46
  rectum 751.2
  salivary duct or gland 750.23
    acquired 527.8
  sublingual duct 750.23
    acquired 527.8
  submaxillary duct or gland 750.23
    acquired 527.8
  trachea 748.3
  tricuspid valve 746.1
  ureter 753.29
  ureteropelvic junction 753.21
  ureterovesical orifice 753.22
  urethra (valvular) 753.6
  urinary tract NEC 753.29
  uterus 752.3
    acquired 621.8
  vagina (acquired) 623.2
    congenital 752.49
    postgonococcal (old) 098.2
    postinfectional 623.2
    senile 623.2
  vascular NEC (*see also* Atresia, blood vessel)
      747.60
    cerebral 747.81
  vas deferens 752.8
  vein NEC (*see also* Atresia, blood vessel) 747.60
    cardiac 746.89
    great 747.49
    portal 747.49
    pulmonary 747.49
  vena cava (inferior) (superior) 747.49
  vesicourethral orifice 753.6
  vulva 752.49
    acquired 624.8

Atrichia, atrichosis 704.00
  congenital (universal) 757.4

Atrioventricularis commune 745.69

Atrophia — *see also* Atrophy
  alba 709.09
  cutis 701.8
    idiopathica progressiva 701.8
    senilis 701.8
  dermatological, diffuse (idiopathic) 701.8
  flava hepatis (acuta) (subacuta) (*see also*
      Necrosis, liver) 570
  gyrata of choroid and retina (central) 363.54
    generalized 363.57
  senilis 797
    dermatological 701.8
  unguium 703.8
    congenita 757.5

Atrophoderma, atrophodermia 701.9
  diffusum (idiopathic) 701.8
  maculatum 701.3
    et striatum 701.3
      due to syphilis 095.8
    syphilitic 091.3
  neuriticum 701.8
  pigmentosum 757.33
  reticulatum symmetricum faciei 701.8

Atrophoderma, atrophodermia — *continued*
  senile 701.8
  symmetrical 701.8
  vermiculata 701.8

Atrophy, atrophic
  adrenal (autoimmune) (capsule) (cortex) (gland)
      255.4
    with hypofunction 255.4
  alveolar process or ridge (edentulous) 525.2
  appendix 543.9
  Aran-Duchenne muscular 335.21
  arm 728.2
  arteriosclerotic — *see* Arteriosclerosis
  arthritis 714.0
    spine 720.9
  bile duct (any) 576.8
  bladder 596.8
  blanche (of Milian) 701.3
  bone (senile) 733.99
    due to
      disuse 733.7
      infection 733.99
      tabes dorsalis (neurogenic) 094.0
    posttraumatic 733.99
  brain (cortex) (progressive) 331.9
    with dementia 290.10
    Alzheimer's 331.0
      with dementia — *see* Alzheimer's,
        dementia
    circumscribed (Pick's) 331.1
      with dementia
        with behavioral disturbance 331.1
          [294.11]
        without behavioral disturbance 331.1
          [294.10]
    congenital 742.4
    hereditary 331.9
    senile 331.2
  breast 611.4
    puerperal, postpartum 676.3 ✓5ᵗʰ
  buccal cavity 528.9
  cardiac (brown) (senile) (*see also* Degeneration,
      myocardial) 429.1
  cartilage (infectional) (joint) 733.99
  cast, plaster of Paris 728.2
  cerebellar — *see* Atrophy, brain
  cerebral — *see* Atrophy, brain
  cervix (endometrium) (mucosa) (myometrium)
      (senile) (uteri) 622.8
    menopausal 627.8
  Charcôt-Marie-Tooth 356.1
  choroid 363.40
    diffuse secondary 363.42
    hereditary (*see also* Dystrophy, choroid)
        363.50
      gyrate
        central 363.54
        diffuse 363.57
        generalized 363.57
    senile 363.41
  ciliary body 364.57
  colloid, degenerative 701.3
  conjunctiva (senile) 372.89
  corpus cavernosum 607.89
  cortical (*see also* Atrophy, brain) 331.9
  Cruveilhier's 335.21
  cystic duct 576.8
  dacryosialadenopathy 710.2
  degenerative
    colloid 701.3
    senile 701.3
  Déjérine-Thomas 333.0
  diffuse idiopathic, dermatological 701.8
  disuse
    bone 733.7
    muscle 728.2
  Duchenne-Aran 335.21
  ear 388.9
  edentulous alveolar ridge 525.2
  emphysema, lung 492.8
  endometrium (senile) 621.8
    cervix 622.8
  enteric 569.89
  epididymis 608.3
  eyeball, cause unknown 360.41
  eyelid (senile) 374.50
  facial (skin) 701.9

Atrophy, atrophic — *continued*
  facioscapulohumeral (Landouzy-Déjérine) 359.1
  fallopian tube (senile), acquired 620.3
  fatty, thymus (gland) 254.8
  gallbladder 575.8
  gastric 537.89
  gastritis (chronic) 535.1 ✓5ᵗʰ
  gastrointestinal 569.89
  genital organ, male 608.89
  glandular 289.3
  globe (phthisis bulbi) 360.41
  gum 523.2
  hair 704.2
  heart (brown) (senile) (*see also* Degeneration,
      myocardial) 429.1
  hemifacial 754.0
    Romberg 349.89
  hydronephrosis 591
  infantile 261
    paralysis, acute (*see also* Poliomyelits, with
        paralysis) 045.1 ✓5ᵗʰ
  intestine 569.89
  iris (generalized) (postinfectional) (sector
      shaped) 364.59
    essential 364.51
    progressive 364.51
    sphincter 364.54
  kidney (senile) (*see also* Sclerosis, renal) 587
    with hypertension (*see also* Hypertension,
        kidney) 403.90
    congenital 753.0
    hydronephrotic 591
    infantile 753.0
  lacrimal apparatus (primary) 375.13
    secondary 375.14
  Landouzy-Déjérine 359.1
  laryngitis, infection 476.0
  larynx 478.79
  Leber's optic 377.16
  lip 528.5
  liver (acute) (subacute) (*see also* Necrosis, liver)
      570
    chronic (yellow) 571.8
    yellow (congenital) 570
      with
        abortion — *see* Abortion, by type, with
          specified complication NEC
        ectopic pregnancy (*see also* categories
          633.0-633.9) 639.8
        molar pregnancy (*see also* categories
          630-632) 639.8
    chronic 571.8
    complicating pregnancy 646.7 ✓5ᵗʰ
    following
      abortion 639.8
      ectopic or molar pregnancy 639.8
    from injection, inoculation or transfusion
        (onset within 8 months after
        administration) — *see* Hepatitis,
        viral
    healed 571.5
    obstetric 646.7 ✓5ᵗʰ
    postabortal 639.8
    postimmunization — *see* Hepatitis, viral
    posttransfusion — *see* Hepatitis, viral
    puerperal, postpartum 674.8 ✓5ᵗʰ
  lung (senile) 518.89
    congenital 748.69
  macular (dermatological) 701.3
    syphilitic, skin 091.3
      striated 095.8
  muscle, muscular 728.2
    disuse 728.2
    Duchenne-Aran 335.21
    extremity (lower) (upper) 728.2
    familial spinal 335.11
    general 728.2
    idiopathic 728.2
    infantile spinal 335.0
    myelopathic (progressive) 335.10
    myotonic 359.2
    neuritic 356.1
    neuropathic (peroneal) (progressive) 356.1
    peroneal 356.1
    primary (idiopathic) 728.2
    progressive (familial) (hereditary) (pure)
        335.21

Atrophy, atrophic — *continued*
  muscle, muscular — *continued*
    progressive — *continued*
      adult (spinal) 335.19
      infantile (spinal) 335.0
      juvenile (spinal) 335.11
      spinal 335.10
        adult 335.19
        Aran-Duchenne 335.10
        hereditary or familial 335.11
        infantile 335.0
    pseudohypertrophic 359.1
    spinal (progressive) 335.10
      adult 335.19
      Aran-Duchenne 335.21
      familial 335.11
      hereditary 335.11
      infantile 335.0
      juvenile 335.11
    syphilitic 095.6
  myocardium (*see also* Degeneration, myocardial) 429.1
  myometrium (senile) 621.8
    cervix 622.8
  myotatic 728.2
  myotonia 359.2
  nail 703.8
    congenital 757.5
  nasopharynx 472.2
  nerve — *see also* Disorder, nerve
    abducens 378.54
    accessory 352.4
    acoustic or auditory 388.5
    cranial 352.9
      first (olfactory) 352.0
      second (optic) (*see also* Atrophy, optic nerve) 377.10
      third (oculomotor)(partial) 378.51
        total 378.52
      fourth (trochlear) 378.53
      fifth (trigeminal) 350.8
      sixth (abducens) 378.54
      seventh (facial) 351.8
      eighth (auditory) 388.5
      ninth (glossopharyngeal) 352.2
      tenth (pneumogastric) (vagus) 352.3
      eleventh (accessory) 352.4
      twelfth (hypoglossal) 352.5
    facial 351.8
    glossopharyngeal 352.2
    hypoglossal 352.5
    oculomotor (partial) 378.51
      total 378.52
    olfactory 352.0
    peripheral 355.9
    pneumogastric 352.3
    trigeminal 350.8
    trochlear 378.53
    vagus (pneumogastric) 352.3
  nervous system, congenital 742.8
  neuritic (*see also* Disorder, nerve) 355.9
  neurogenic NEC 355.9
    bone
      tabetic 094.0
  nutritional 261
  old age 797
  olivopontocerebellar 333.0
  optic nerve (ascending) (descending) (infectional) (nonfamilial) (papillomacular bundle) (postretinal) (secondary NEC) (simple) 377.10
    associated with retinal dystrophy 377.13
    dominant hereditary 377.16
    glaucomatous 377.14
    hereditary (dominant) (Leber's) 377.16
    Leber's (hereditary) 377.16
    partial 377.15
    postinflammatory 377.12
    primary 377.11
    syphilitic 094.84
      congenital 090.49
      tabes dorsalis 094.0
  orbit 376.45
  ovary (senile), acquired 620.3
  oviduct (senile), acquired 620.3
  palsy, diffuse 335.20
  pancreas (duct) (senile) 577.8

Atrophy, atrophic — *continued*
  papillary muscle 429.81
  paralysis 355.9
  parotid gland 527.0
  patches skin 701.3
    senile 701.8
  penis 607.89
  pharyngitis 472.1
  pharynx 478.29
  pluriglandular 258.8
  polyarthritis 714.0
  prostate 602.2
  pseudohypertrophic 359.1
  renal (*see also* Sclerosis, renal) 587
  reticulata 701.8
  retina (*see also* Degeneration, retina) 362.60
    hereditary (*see also* Dystrophy, retina) 362.70
  rhinitis 472.0
  salivary duct or gland 527.0
  scar NEC 709.2
  sclerosis, lobar (of brain) 331.0
    with dementia
      with behavioral disturbance 331.1 [294.11]
      without behavioral disturbance 331.1 [294.10]
  scrotum 608.89
  seminal vesicle 608.89
  senile 797
    degenerative, of skin 701.3
  skin (patches) (senile) 701.8
  spermatic cord 608.89
  spinal (cord) 336.8
    acute 336.8
    muscular (chronic) 335.10
      adult 335.19
      familial 335.11
      juvenile 335.10
    paralysis 335.10
      acute (*see also* Poliomyelitis, with paralysis) 045.1
  spine (column) 733.99
  spleen (senile) 289.59
  spots (skin) 701.3
    senile 701.8
  stomach 537.89
  striate and macular 701.3
    syphilitic 095.8
  subcutaneous 701.9
    due to injection 999.9
  sublingual gland 527.0
  submaxillary gland 527.0
  Sudeck's 733.7
  suprarenal (autoimmune) (capsule) (gland) 255.4
    with hypofunction 255.4
  tarso-orbital fascia, congenital 743.66
  testis 608.3
  thenar, partial 354.0
  throat 478.29
  thymus (fat) 254.8
  thyroid (gland) 246.8
    with
      cretinism 243
      myxedema 244.9
    congenital 243
  tongue (senile) 529.8
    papillae 529.4
    smooth 529.4
  trachea 519.1
  tunica vaginalis 608.89
  turbinate 733.99
  tympanic membrane (nonflaccid) 384.82
    flaccid 384.81
  ulcer (*see also* Ulcer, skin) 707.9
  upper respiratory tract 478.9
  uterus, uterine (acquired) (senile) 621.8
    cervix 622.8
    due to radiation (intended effect) 621.8
  vagina (senile) 627.3
  vascular 459.89
  vas deferens 608.89
  vertebra (senile) 733.99
  vulva (primary) (senile) 624.1
  Werdnig-Hoffmann 335.0

Atrophy, atrophic — *continued*
  yellow (acute) (congenital) (liver) (subacute) (*see also* Necrosis, liver) 570
    chronic 571.8
    resulting from administration of blood, plasma, serum, or other biological substance (within 8 months of administration) — *see* Hepatitis, viral

Attack
  akinetic (*see also* Epilepsy) 345.0 ✔5ᵗʰ
  angina — *see* Angina
  apoplectic (*see also* Disease, cerebrovascular, acute) 436
  benign shuddering 333.93
  bilious — *see* Vomiting
  cataleptic 300.11
  cerebral (*see also* Disease, cerebrovascular, acute) 436
  coronary (*see also* Infarct, myocardium) 410.9 ✔5ᵗʰ
  cyanotic, newborn 770.83 ▲
  epileptic (*see also* Epilepsy) 345.9 ✔5ᵗʰ
  epileptiform 780.39
  heart (*see also* Infarct, myocardium) 410.9 ✔5ᵗʰ
  hemiplegia (*see also* Disease, cerebrovascular, acute) 436
  hysterical 300.11
  jacksonian (*see also* Epilepsy) 345.5 ✔5ᵗʰ
  myocardium, myocardial (*see also* Infarct, myocardium) 410.9 ✔5ᵗʰ
  myoclonic (*see also* Epilepsy) 345.1 ✔5ᵗʰ
  panic 300.01
  paralysis (*see also* Disease, cerebrovascular, acute) 436
  paroxysmal 780.39
  psychomotor (*see also* Epilepsy) 345.4 ✔5ᵗʰ
  salaam (*see also* Epilepsy) 345.6 ✔5ᵗʰ
  schizophreniform (*see also* Schizophrenia) 295.4 ✔5ᵗʰ
  sensory and motor 780.39
  syncope 780.2
  toxic, cerebral 780.39
  transient ischemic (TIA) 435.9
  unconsciousness 780.2
    hysterical 300.11
  vasomotor 780.2
  vasovagal (idiopathic) (paroxysmal) 780.2

Attention to
  artificial opening (of) V55.9
    digestive tract NEC V55.4
    specified site NEC V55.8
    urinary tract NEC V55.6
    vagina V55.7
  colostomy V55.3
  cystostomy V55.5
  gastrostomy V55.1
  ileostomy V55.2
  jejunostomy V55.4
  nephrostomy V55.6
  surgical dressings V58.3
  sutures V58.3
  tracheostomy V55.0
  ureterostomy V55.6
  urethrostomy V55.6

Attrition
  gum 523.2
  teeth (excessive) (hard tissues) 521.1

Atypical — *see also* condition
  distribution, vessel (congenital) (peripheral) NEC 747.60
  endometrium 621.9
  glandular cell changes of undetermined significance ●
    favor benign (AGCUS favor benign) 795.01 ●
    favor dysplasia (AGCUS favor dysplasia) 795.02 ●
  kidney 593.89
  squamous cell changes of undetermined significance ●
    favor benign (ASCUS favor benign) 795.01 ●
    favor dysplasia (ASCUS favor dysplasia) 795.02 ●

Atypism, cervix 622.1

Audible tinnitus (*see also* Tinnitus) 388.30

✔4ᵗʰ Fourth-digit Required   ✔5ᵗʰ Fifth-digit Required   ►◄ Revised Text   ● New Line   ▲ Revised Code

Auditory — see condition
Audry's syndrome (acropachyderma) 757.39
Aujeszky's disease 078.89
Aura, jacksonian (see also Epilepsy) 345.5 ✓5th
Aurantiasis, cutis 278.3
Auricle, auricular — see condition
Auriculotemporal syndrome 350.8
Australian
  Q fever 083.0
  X disease 062.4
Autism, autistic (child) (infantile) 299.0 ✓5th
Autodigestion 799.8
Autoerythrocyte sensitization 287.2
Autographism 708.3
Autoimmune
  cold sensitivity 283.0
  disease NEC 279.4
  hemolytic anemia 283.0
  thyroiditis 245.2
Autoinfection, septic — see Septicemia
Autointoxication 799.8
Automatism 348.8
  epileptic (see also Epilepsy) 345.4 ✓5th
  paroxysmal, idiopathic (see also Epilepsy) 345.4 ✓5th
Autonomic, autonomous
  bladder 596.54
    neurogenic NEC 596.54
      with cauda equina 344.61
  dysreflexia 337.3
  faciocephalalgia (see also Neuropathy, peripheral, autonomic) 337.9
  hysterical seizure 300.11
  imbalance (see also Neuropathy, peripheral, autonomic) 337.9
Autophony 388.40
Autosensitivity, erythrocyte 287.2
Autotopagnosia 780.99 ▲
Autotoxemia 799.8
Autumn — see condition
Avellis' syndrome 344.89
Aviators
  disease or sickness (see also Effect, adverse, high altitude) 993.2
  ear 993.0
  effort syndrome 306.2
Avitaminosis (multiple NEC) (see also Deficiency, vitamin) 269.2
  A 264.9
  B 266.9
    with
      beriberi 265.0
      pellagra 265.2
  B₁ 265.1
  B₂ 266.0
  B₆ 266.1
  B₁₂ 266.2
  C (with scurvy) 267
  D 268.9
    with
      osteomalacia 268.2
      rickets 268.0
  E 269.1
  G 266.0
  H 269.1
  K 269.0
  multiple 269.2
  nicotinic acid 265.2
  P 269.1
Avulsion (traumatic) 879.8
  blood vessel — see Injury, blood vessel, by site
  cartilage — see also Dislocation, by site
    knee, current (see also Tear, meniscus) 836.2
    symphyseal (inner), complicating delivery 665.6 ✓5th
  complicated 879.9
  diaphragm — see Injury, internal, diaphragm
  ear — see Wound, open, ear
  epiphysis of bone — see Fracture, by site
  external site other than limb — see Wound, open, by site
  eye 871.3

Avulsion — continued
  fingernail — see Wound, open, finger
  fracture — see Fracture, by site
  genital organs, external — see Wound, open, genital organs
  head (intracranial) NEC — see also Injury, intracranial, with open intracranial wound
    complete 874.9
    external site NEC 873.8
      complicated 873.9
  internal organ or site — see Injury, internal, by site
  joint — see also Dislocation, by site
    capsule — see Sprain, by site
  ligament — see Sprain, by site
  limb — see also Amputation, traumatic, by site
    skin and subcutaneous tissue — see Wound, open, by site
  muscle — see Sprain, by site
  nerve (root) — see Injury, nerve, by site
  scalp — see Wound, open, scalp
  skin and subcutaneous tissue — see Wound, open, by site
  symphyseal cartilage (inner), complicating delivery 665.6 ✓5th
  tendon — see also Sprain, by site
    with open wound — see Wound, open, by site
  toenail — see Wound, open, toe(s)
  tooth 873.63
    complicated 873.73
Awareness of heart beat 785.1
Axe grinders' disease 502
Axenfeld's anomaly or syndrome 743.44
Axilla, axillary — see also condition
  breast 757.6
Axonotmesis — see Injury, nerve, by site
Ayala's disease 756.89
Ayerza's disease or syndrome (pulmonary artery sclerosis with pulmonary hypertension) 416.0
Azoospermia 606.0
Azotemia 790.6
  meaning uremia (see also Uremia) 586
Aztec ear 744.29
Azorean disease (of the nervous system) 334.8
Azygos lobe, lung (fissure) 748.69

B

Baader's syndrome (erythema multiforme exudativum) 695.1
Baastrup's syndrome 721.5
Babesiasis 088.82
Babesiosis 088.82
Babington's disease (familial hemorrhagic telangiectasia) 448.0
Babinski's syndrome (cardiovascular syphilis) 093.89
Babinski-Fröhlich syndrome (adiposogenital dystrophy) 253.8
Babinski-Nageotte syndrome 344.89
Bacillary — see condition
Bacilluria 791.9
  asymptomatic, in pregnancy or puerperium 646.5 ✓5th
  tuberculous (see also Tuberculosis) 016.9 ✓5th
Bacillus — see also Infection, bacillus
  abortus infection 023.1
  anthracis infection 022.9
  coli
    infection 041.4
      generalized 038.42
      intestinal 008.00
    pyemia 038.42
    septicemia 038.42
  Flexner's 004.1
  fusiformis infestation 101
  mallei infection 024
  Shiga's 004.0
  suipestifer infection (see also Infection, Salmonella) 003.9

Back — see condition
Backache (postural) 724.5
  psychogenic 307.89
  sacroiliac 724.6
Backflow (pyelovenous) (see also Disease, renal) 593.9
Backknee (see also Genu, recurvatum) 736.5
Bacteremia 790.7
  with
    sepsis — see Septicemia
  during
    labor 659.3 ✓5th
    pregnancy 647.8 ✓5th
  newborn 771.83 ▲
Bacteria
  in blood (see also Bacteremia) 790.7
  in urine (see also Bacteriuria) 599.0
Bacterial — see condition
Bactericholia (see also Cholecystitis, acute) 575.0
Bacterid, bacteride (Andrews' pustular) 686.8
Bacteriuria, bacteruria 791.9
  with
    urinary tract infection 599.0
  asymptomatic 791.9
    in pregnancy or puerperium 646.5 ✓5th
      affecting fetus or newborn 760.1
Bad
  breath 784.9
  heart — see Disease, heart
  trip (see also Abuse, drugs, nondependent) 305.3 ✓5th
Baehr-Schiffrin disease (thrombotic thrombocytopenic purpura) 446.6
Baelz's disease (cheilitis glandularis apostematosa) 528.5
Baerensprung's disease (eczema marginatum) 110.3
Bagassosis (occupational) 495.1
Baghdad boil 085.1
Bagratuni's syndrome (temporal arteritis) 446.5
Baker's
  cyst (knee) 727.51
    tuberculous (see also Tuberculosis) 015.2 ✓5th
  itch 692.82
Bakwin-Krida syndrome (craniometaphyseal dysplasia) 756.89
Balanitis (circinata) (gangraenosa) (infectious) (vulgaris) 607.1
  amebic 006.8
  candidal 112.2
  chlamydial 099.53
  due to Ducrey's bacillus 099.0
  erosiva circinata et gangraenosa 607.1
  gangrenous 607.1
  gonococcal (acute) 098.0
    chronic or duration of 2 months or over 098.2
  nongonococcal 607.1
  phagedenic 607.1
  venereal NEC 099.8
  xerotica obliterans 607.81
Balanoposthitis 607.1
  chlamydial 099.53
  gonococcal (acute) 098.0
    chronic or duration of 2 months or over 098.2
  ulcerative NEC 099.8
Balanorrhagia — see Balanitis
Balantidiasis 007.0
Balantidiosis 007.0
Balbuties, balbutio 307.0
Bald
  patches on scalp 704.00
  tongue 529.4
Baldness (see also Alopecia) 704.00
Balfour's disease (chloroma) 205.3 ✓5th
Balint's syndrome (psychic paralysis of visual fixation) 368.16
Balkan grippe 083.0

Ball
  food 938
  hair 938
Ballantyne (-Runge) syndrome (postmaturity) 766.2
Balloon disease (*see also* Effect, adverse, high altitude) 993.2
Ballooning posterior leaflet syndrome 424.0
Baló's disease or concentric sclerosis 341.1
Bamberger's disease (hypertrophic pulmonary osteoarthropathy) 731.2
Bamberger-Marie disease (hypertrophic pulmonary osteoarthropathy) 731.2
Bamboo spine 720.0
Bancroft's filariasis 125.0
Band(s)
  adhesive (*see also* Adhesions, peritoneum) 568.0
  amniotic 658.8 ✓5ᵗʰ
    affecting fetus or newborn 762.8
  anomalous or congenital — *see also* Anomaly, specified type NEC
    atrial 746.9
    heart 746.9
    intestine 751.4
    omentum 751.4
    ventricular 746.9
  cervix 622.3
  gallbladder (congenital) 751.69
  intestinal (adhesive) (*see also* Adhesions, peritoneum) 568.0
    congenital 751.4
  obstructive (*see also* Obstruction, intestine) 560.81
  periappendiceal (congenital) 751.4
  peritoneal (adhesive) (*see also* Adhesions, peritoneum) 568.0
    with intestinal obstruction 560.81
    congenital 751.4
  uterus 621.5
  vagina 623.2
Bandl's ring (contraction)
  complicating delivery 661.4 ✓5ᵗʰ
    affecting fetus or newborn 763.7
Bang's disease (Brucella abortus) 023.1
Bangkok hemorrhagic fever 065.4
Bannister's disease 995.1
Bantam-Albright-Martin disease (pseudohypoparathyroidism) 275.49
Banti's disease or syndrome (with cirrhosis) (with portal hypertension) — *see* Cirrhosis, liver
Bar
  calcaneocuboid 755.67
  calcaneonavicular 755.67
  cubonavicular 755.67
  prostate 600.9
  talocalcaneal 755.67
Baragnosis 780.99 ▲
Barasheh, barashek 266.2
Barcoo disease or rot (*see also* Ulcer, skin) 707.9
Bard-Pic syndrome (carcinoma, head of pancreas) 157.0
Bärensprung's disease (eczema marginatum) 110.3
Baritosis 503
Barium lung disease 503
Barlow's syndrome (meaning mitral valve prolapse) 424.0
Barlow (-Möller) disease or syndrome (meaning infantile scurvy) 267
Barodontalgia 993.2
Baron Münchausen syndrome 301.51
Barosinusitis 993.1
Barotitis 993.0
Barotrauma 993.2
  odontalgia 993.2
  otitic 993.0
  sinus 993.1
Barraquer's disease or syndrome (progressive lipodystrophy) 272.6

Barré-Guillain syndrome 357.0
Barré-Liéou syndrome (posterior cervical sympathetic) 723.2
Barrel chest 738.3
Barrett's syndrome or ulcer (chronic peptic ulcer of esophagus) 530.2
Bársony-Polgár syndrome (corkscrew esophagus) 530.5
Bársony-Teschendorf syndrome (corkscrew esophagus) 530.5
Bartholin's
  adenitis (*see also* Bartholinitis) 616.8
  gland — *see* condition
Bartholinitis (suppurating) 616.8
  gonococcal (acute) 098.0
    chronic or duration of 2 months or over 098.2
Bartonellosis 088.0
Bartter's syndrome (secondary hyperaldosteronism with juxtaglomerular hyperplasia) 255.1
Basal — *see* condition
Basan's (hidrotic) ectodermal dysplasia 757.31
Baseball finger 842.13
Basedow's disease or syndrome (exophthalmic goiter) 242.0 ✓5ᵗʰ
Basic — *see* condition
Basilar — *see* condition
Bason's (hidrotic) ectodermal dysplasia 757.31
Basopenia 288.0
Basophilia 288.8
Basophilism (corticoadrenal) (Cushing's) (pituitary) (thymic) 255.0
Bassen-Kornzweig syndrome (abetalipoproteinemia) 272.5
Bat ear 744.29
Bateman's
  disease 078.0
  purpura (senile) 287.2
Bathing cramp 994.1
Bathophobia 300.23
Batten's disease, retina 330.1 [362.71]
Batten-Mayou disease 330.1 [362.71]
Batten-Steinert syndrome 359.2
Battered
  adult (syndrome) 995.81
  baby or child (syndrome) 995.54
  spouse (syndrome) 995.81
Battey mycobacterium infection 031.0
Battledore placenta — *see* Placenta, abnormal
Battle exhaustion (*see also* Reaction, stress, acute) 308.9
Baumgarten-Cruveilhier (cirrhosis) disease, or syndrome 571.5
Bauxite
  fibrosis (of lung) 503
  workers' disease 503
Bayle's disease (dementia paralytica) 094.1
Bazin's disease (primary) (*see also* Tuberculosis) 017.1 ✓5ᵗʰ
Beach ear 380.12
Beaded hair (congenital) 757.4
Beard's disease (neurasthenia) 300.5
Bearn-Kunkel (-Slater) syndrome (lupoid hepatitis) 571.49
Beat
  elbow 727.2
  hand 727.2
  knee 727.2
Beats
  ectopic 427.60
  escaped, heart 427.60
    postoperative 997.1
  premature (nodal) 427.60
    atrial 427.61
    auricular 427.61
    postoperative 997.1
    specified type NEC 427.69

Beats — *continued*
  premature (nodal) — *continued*
    supraventricular 427.61
    ventricular 427.69
Beau's
  disease or syndrome (*see also* Degeneration, myocardial) 429.1
  lines (transverse furrows on fingernails) 703.8
Bechterew's disease (ankylosing spondylitis) 720.0
Bechterew-Strümpell-Marie syndrome (ankylosing spondylitis) 720.0
Beck's syndrome (anterior spinal artery occlusion) 433.8 ✓5ᵗʰ
Becker's
  disease (idiopathic mural endomyocardial disease) 425.2
  dystrophy 359.1
Beckwith (-Wiedemann) syndrome 759.89
Bedclothes, asphyxiation or suffocation by 994.7
Bednar's aphthae 528.2
Bedsore 707.0
  with gangrene 707.0 [785.4]
Bedwetting (*see also* Enuresis) 788.36
Beer-drinkers' heart (disease) 425.5
Bee sting (with allergic or anaphylactic shock) 989.5
Begbie's disease (exophthalmic goiter) 242.0 ✓5ᵗʰ
Behavior disorder, disturbance — *see also* Disturbance, conduct
  antisocial, without manifest psychiatric disorder
    adolescent V71.02
    adult V71.01
    child V71.02
  dyssocial, without manifest psychiatric disorder
    adolescent V71.02
    adult V71.01
    child V71.02
  high risk — *see* Problem
Behçet's syndrome 136.1
Behr's disease 362.50
Beigel's disease or morbus (white piedra) 111.2
Bejel 104.0
Bekhterev's disease (ankylosing spondylitis) 720.0
Bekhterev-Strümpell-Marie syndrome (ankylosing spondylitis) 720.0
Belching (*see also* Eructation) 787.3
Bell's
  disease (*see also* Psychosis, affective) 296.0 ✓5ᵗʰ
  mania (*see also* Psychosis, affective) 296.0 ✓5ᵗʰ
  palsy, paralysis 351.0
    infant 767.5
    newborn 767.5
    syphilitic 094.89
  spasm 351.0
Bence-Jones albuminuria, albuminosuria, or proteinuria 791.0
Bends 993.3
Benedikt's syndrome (paralysis) 344.89
Benign — *see also* condition
  cellular changes, cervix 795.09 ●
  prostate
    hyperplasia 600.0
    neoplasm 222.2
Bennett's
  disease (leukemia) 208.9 ✓5ᵗʰ
  fracture (closed) 815.01
    open 815.11
Benson's disease 379.22
Bent
  back (hysterical) 300.11
  nose 738.0
    congenital 754.0
Bereavement V62.82
  as adjustment reaction 309.0
Berger's paresthesia (lower limb) 782.0
Bergeron's disease (hysteroepilepsy) 300.11

✓4ᵗʰ Fourth-digit Required   ✓5ᵗʰ Fifth-digit Required   ▶◀ Revised Text   ● New Line   ▲ Revised Code

Beriberi (acute) (atrophic) (chronic) (dry)
(subacute) (wet) 265.0
with polyneuropathy 265.0 *[357.4]*
heart (disease) 265.0 *[425.7]*
leprosy 030.1
neuritis 265.0 *[357.4]*
Berlin's disease or edema (traumatic) 921.3
Berloque dermatitis 692.72
Bernard-Horner syndrome (*see also* Neuropathy,
peripheral, autonomic) 337.9
Bernard-Sergent syndrome (acute adrenocortical
insufficiency) 255.4
Bernard-Soulier disease or thrombopathy 287.1
Bernhardt's disease or paresthesia 355.1
Bernhardt-Roth disease or syndrome
(paresthesia) 355.1
Bernheim's syndrome (*see also* Failure, heart)
428.0
Bertielliasis 123.8
Bertolotti's syndrome (sacralization of fifth
lumbar vertebra) 756.15
Berylliosis (acute) (chronic) (lung) (occupational)
503
Besnier's
lupus pernio 135
prurigo (atopic dermatitis) (infantile eczema)
691.8
Besnier-Boeck disease or sarcoid 135
Besnier-Boeck-Schaumann disease (sarcoidosis)
135
Best's disease 362.76
Bestiality 302.1
**Beta-adrenergic hyperdynamic circulatory
state** 429.82
Beta-aminoisobutyric aciduria 277.2
Beta-mercaptolactate-cysteine disulfiduria
270.0
Beta thalassemia (major) (minor) (mixed) 282.4
Beurmann's disease (sporotrichosis) 117.1
Bezoar 938
intestine 936
stomach 935.2
Bezold's abscess (*see also* Mastoiditis) 383.01
Bianchi's syndrome (aphasia-apraxia-alexia)
784.69
Bicornuate or bicornis uterus 752.3
in pregnancy or childbirth 654.0 ☑5ᵗʰ
with obstructed labor 660.2 ☑5ᵗʰ
affecting fetus or newborn 763.1
affecting fetus or newborn 763.89
Bicuspid aortic valve 746.4
Biedl-Bardet syndrome 759.89
Bielschowsky's disease 330.1
Bielschowsky-Jansky
amaurotic familial idiocy 330.1
disease 330.1
Biemond's syndrome (obesity, polydactyly, and
mental retardation) 759.89
Biermer's anemia or disease (pernicious anemia)
281.0
Biett's disease 695.4
Bifid (congenital) — *see also* Imperfect, closure
apex, heart 746.89
clitoris 752.49
epiglottis 748.3
kidney 753.3
nose 748.1
patella 755.64
scrotum 752.8
toe 755.66
tongue 750.13
ureter 753.4
uterus 752.3
uvula 749.02
with cleft lip (*see also* Cleft, palate, with cleft
lip) 749.20
Biforis uterus (suprasimplex) 752.3
Bifurcation (congenital) — *see also* Imperfect,
closure
gallbladder 751.69
kidney pelvis 753.3

Bifurcation — *see also* Imperfect, closure —
continued
renal pelvis 753.3
rib 756.3
tongue 750.13
trachea 748.3
ureter 753.4
urethra 753.8
uvula 749.02
with cleft lip (*see also* Cleft, palate, with cleft
lip) 749.20
vertebra 756.19
Bigeminal pulse 427.89
Bigeminy 427.89
Big spleen syndrome 289.4
Bilateral — *see* condition
Bile duct — *see* condition
Bile pigments in urine 791.4
Bilharziasis (*see also* Schistosomiasis) 120.9
chyluria 120.0
cutaneous 120.3
galacturia 120.0
hematochyluria 120.0
intestinal 120.1
lipemia 120.9
lipuria 120.0
Oriental 120.2
piarhemia 120.9
pulmonary 120.2
tropical hematuria 120.0
vesical 120.0
Biliary — *see* condition
Bilious (attack) — *see also* Vomiting
fever, hemoglobinuric 084.8
Bilirubinuria 791.4
Biliuria 791.4
Billroth's disease
meningocele (*see also* Spina bifida) 741.9 ☑5ᵗʰ
Bilobate placenta — *see* Placenta, abnormal
Bilocular
heart 745.7
stomach 536.8
Bing-Horton syndrome (histamine cephalgia)
346.2 ☑5ᵗʰ
Binswanger's disease or dementia 290.12
Biörck (-Thorson) syndrome (malignant
carcinoid) 259.2
Biparta, bipartite — *see also* Imperfect, closure
carpal scaphoid 755.59
patella 755.64
placenta — *see* Placenta, abnormal
vagina 752.49
Bird
face 756.0
fanciers' lung or disease 495.2
Bird's disease (oxaluria) 271.8
Birth
abnormal fetus or newborn 763.9
accident, fetus or newborn — *see* Birth, injury
complications in mother — *see* Delivery,
complicated
compression during NEC 767.9
defect — *see* Anomaly
delayed, fetus 763.9
difficult NEC, affecting fetus or newborn 763.9
dry, affecting fetus or newborn 761.1
forced, NEC, affecting fetus or newborn 763.89
forceps, affecting fetus or newborn 763.2
hematoma of sternomastoid 767.8
immature 765.1 ☑5ᵗʰ
extremely 765.0 ☑5ᵗʰ
inattention, after or at 995.52
induced, affecting fetus or newborn 763.89
infant — *see* Newborn
injury NEC 767.9
adrenal gland 767.8
basal ganglia 767.0
brachial plexus (paralysis) 767.6
brain (compression) (pressure) 767.0
cerebellum 767.0
cerebral hemorrhage 767.0
conjunctiva 767.8
eye 767.8

Birth — *continued*
injury NEC — *continued*
fracture
bone, any except clavicle or spine 767.3
clavicle 767.2
femur 767.3
humerus 767.3
long bone 767.3
radius and ulna 767.3
skeleton NEC 767.3
skull 767.3
spine 767.4
tibia and fibula 767.3
hematoma 767.8
liver (subcapsular) 767.8
mastoid 767.8
skull 767.1
sternomastoid 767.8
testes 767.8
vulva 767.8
intracranial (edema) 767.0
laceration
brain 767.0
by scalpel 767.8
peripheral nerve 767.7
liver 767.8
meninges
brain 767.0
spinal cord 767.4
nerves (cranial, peripheral) 767.7
brachial plexus 767.6
facial 767.5
paralysis 767.7
brachial plexus 767.6
Erb (-Duchenne) 767.6
facial nerve 767.5
Klumpke (-Déjérine) 767.6
radial nerve 767.6
spinal (cord) (hemorrhage) (laceration)
(rupture) 767.4
rupture
intracranial 767.0
liver 767.8
spinal cord 767.4
spleen 767.8
viscera 767.8
scalp 767.1
scalpel wound 767.8
skeleton NEC 767.3
specified NEC 767.8
spinal cord 767.4
spleen 767.8
subdural hemorrhage 767.0
tentorial, tear 767.0
testes 767.8
vulva 767.8
instrumental, NEC, affecting fetus or newborn
763.2
lack of care, after or at 995.52
multiple
affected by maternal complications of
pregnancy 761.5
healthy liveborn — *see* Newborn, multiple
neglect, after or at 995.52
newborn — *see* Newborn
palsy or paralysis NEC 767.7
precipitate, fetus or newborn 763.6
premature (infant) 765.1 ☑5ᵗʰ
prolonged, affecting fetus or newborn 763.9
retarded, fetus or newborn 763.9
shock, newborn 779.89   ▲
strangulation or suffocation
due to aspiration of amniotic fluid 770.1
mechanical 767.8
trauma NEC 767.9
triplet
affected by maternal complications of
pregnancy 761.5
healthy liveborn — *see* Newborn, multiple
twin
affected by maternal complications of
pregnancy 761.5
healthy liveborn — *see* Newborn, twin
ventouse, affecting fetus or newborn 763.3
Birthmark 757.32
Bisalbuminemia 273.8

Beriberi — Bisalbuminemia

Biskra button 085.1

Bite(s)
with intact skin surface — *see* Contusion
animal — *see* Wound, open, by site
    intact skin surface — *see* Contusion
centipede 989.5
chigger 133.8
fire ant 989.5
flea — *see* Injury, superficial, by site
human (open wound) — *see also* Wound, open,
    by site
    intact skin surface — *see* Contusion
insect
    nonvenomous — *see* Injury, superficial, by
        site
    venomous 989.5
mad dog (death from) 071
poisonous 989.5
red bug 133.8
reptile 989.5
    nonvenomous — *see* Wound, open, by site
snake 989.5
    nonvenomous — *see* Wound, open, by site
spider (venomous) 989.5
    nonvenomous — *see* Injury, superficial, by
        site
venomous 989.5

Biting
cheek or lip 528.9
nail 307.9

Black
death 020.9
eye NEC 921.0
hairy tongue 529.3
lung disease 500

Blackfan-Diamond anemia or syndrome
    (congenital hypoplastic anemia) 284.0

Blackhead 706.1

Blackout 780.2

Blackwater fever 084.8

Bladder — *see* condition

Blast
blindness 921.3
concussion — *see* Blast, injury
injury 869.0
    with open wound into cavity 869.1
    abdomen or thorax — *see* Injury, internal,
        by site
    brain (*see also* Concussion, brain) 850.9
        with skull fracture — *see* Fracture, skull
    ear (acoustic nerve trauma) 951.5
        with perforation, tympanic membrane —
            see Wound, open, ear, drum
    lung (*see also* Injury, internal, lung) 861.20
    otitic (explosive) 388.11

Blastomycosis, blastomycotic (chronic)
    (cutaneous) (disseminated) (lung)
    (pulmonary) (systemic) 116.0
Brazilian 116.1
European 117.5
keloidal 116.2
North American 116.0
primary pulmonary 116.0
South American 116.1

Bleb(s) 709.8
emphysematous (bullous) (diffuse) (lung)
    (ruptured) (solitary) 492.0
filtering, eye (postglaucoma) (status) V45.69
    with complication 997.99
    postcataract extraction (complication)
        997.99
lung (ruptured) 492.0
    congenital 770.5
subpleural (emphysematous) 492.0

Bleeder (familial) (hereditary) (*see also* Defect,
    coagulation) 286.9
nonfamilial 286.9

Bleeding (*see also* Hemorrhage) 459.0
anal 569.3
anovulatory 628.0
atonic, following delivery 666.1 ✔5ᵗʰ
capillary 448.9
due to subinvolution 621.1
    puerperal 666.2 ✔5ᵗʰ
ear 388.69

Bleeding (*see also* Hemorrhage) — *continued*
excessive, associated with menopausal onset
    627.0
familial (*see also* Defect, coagulation) 286.9
following intercourse 626.7
gastrointestinal 578.9
gums 523.8
hemorrhoids — *see* Hemorrhoids, bleeding
intermenstrual
    irregular 626.6
    regular 626.5
intraoperative 998.11
irregular NEC 626.4
menopausal 627.0
mouth 528.9
nipple 611.79
nose 784.7
ovulation 626.5
postclimacteric 627.1
postcoital 626.7
postmenopausal 627.1
    following induced menopause 627.4
postoperative 998.11
preclimacteric 627.0
puberty 626.3
    excessive, with onset of menstrual periods
        626.3
rectum, rectal 569.3
tendencies (*see also* Defect, coagulation) 286.9
throat 784.8
umbilical stump 772.3
umbilicus 789.9
unrelated to menstrual cycle 626.6
uterus, uterine 626.9
    climacteric 627.0
    dysfunctional 626.8
    functional 626.8
    unrelated to menstrual cycle 626.6
vagina, vaginal 623.8
    functional 626.8
vicarious 625.8

Blennorrhagia, blennorrhagic — *see* Blennorrhea

Blennorrhea (acute) 098.0
adultorum 098.40
alveolaris 523.4
chronic or duration of 2 months or over 098.2
gonococcal (neonatorum) 098.40
inclusion (neonatal) (newborn) 771.6
neonatorum 098.40

Blepharelosis (*see also* Entropion) 374.00

Blepharitis (eyelid) 373.00
angularis 373.01
ciliaris 373.00
    with ulcer 373.01
marginal 373.00
    with ulcer 373.01
scrofulous (*see also* Tuberculosis) 017.3 ✔5ᵗʰ
    [373.00]
squamous 373.02
ulcerative 373.01

Blepharochalasis 374.34
congenital 743.62

Blepharoclonus 333.81

Blepharoconjunctivitis (*see also* Conjunctivitis)
    372.20
angular 372.21
contact 372.22

Blepharophimosis (eyelid) 374.46
congenital 743.62

Blepharoplegia 374.89

Blepharoptosis 374.30
congenital 743.61

Blepharopyorrhea 098.49

Blepharospasm 333.81

Blessig's cyst 362.62

Blighted ovum 631

Blind
bronchus (congenital) 748.3
eye — *see also* Blindness
    hypertensive 360.42
    hypotensive 360.41
loop syndrome (postoperative) 579.2
sac, fallopian tube (congenital) 752.19
spot, enlarged 368.42
tract or tube (congenital) NEC — *see* Atresia

Blindness (acquired) (congenital) (both eyes)
    369.00
blast 921.3
    with nerve injury — *see* Injury, nerve, optic
Bright's — *see* Uremia
color (congenital) 368.59
    acquired 368.55
    blue 368.53
    green 368.52
    red 368.51
    total 368.54
concussion 950.9
cortical 377.75
day 368.10   ▲
    acquired 368.10   ▲
    congenital 368.10   ▲
    hereditary 368.10   ▲
    specified type NEC 368.10   ▲
due to
    injury NEC 950.9
    refractive error — *see* Error, refractive
eclipse (total) 363.31
emotional 300.11
hysterical 300.11
legal (both eyes) (USA definition) 369.4
    with impairment of better (less impaired) eye
        near-total 369.02
            with
                lesser eye impairment 369.02
                    near-total 369.04
                    total 369.03
        profound 369.05
            with
                lesser eye impairment 369.05
                    near-total 369.07
                    profound 369.08
                    total 369.06
        severe 369.21
            with
                lesser eye impairment 369.21
                    blind 369.11
                    near-total 369.13
                    profound 369.14
                    severe 369.22
                    total 369.12
        total
            with lesser eye impairment
                total 369.01
mind 784.69
moderate
    both eyes 369.25
        with impairment of lesser eye (specified
            as)
            blind, not further specified 369.15
            low vision, not further specified 369.23
            near-total 369.17
            profound 369.18
            severe 369.24
            total 369.16
    one eye 369.74
        with vision of other eye (specified as)
            near-normal 369.75
            normal 369.76
near-total
    both eyes 369.04
        with impairment of lesser eye (specified
            as)
            blind, not further specified 369.02
            total 369.03
    one eye 369.64
        with vision of other eye (specified as)
            near-normal 369.65
            normal 369.66
night 368.60
    acquired 368.62
    congenital (Japanese) 368.61
    hereditary 368.61
    specified type NEC 368.69
    vitamin A deficiency 264.5
nocturnal — *see* Blindness, night
one eye 369.60
    with low vision of other eye 369.10
profound
    both eyes 369.08
        with impairment of lesser eye (specified
            as)
            blind, not further specified 369.05

✔4ᵗʰ Fourth-digit Required   ✔5ᵗʰ Fifth-digit Required   ▶◀ Revised Text   ● New Line   ▲ Revised Code

Blindness — *continued*
  profound — *continued*
    both eyes — *continued*
      with impairment of lesser eye (specified as) — *continued*
        near-total 369.07
        total 369.06
    one eye 369.67
      with vision of other eye (specified as)
        near-normal 369.68
        normal 369.69
  psychic 784.69
  severe
    both eyes 369.22
      with impairment of lesser eye (specified as)
        blind, not further specified 369.11
        low vision, not further specified 369.21
        near-total 369.13
        profound 369.14
        total 369.12
    one eye 369.71
      with vision of other eye (specified as)
        near-normal 369.72
        normal 369.73
  snow 370.24
  sun 363.31
  temporary 368.12
  total
    both eyes 369.01
    one eye 369.61
      with vision of other eye (specified as)
        near-normal 369.62
        normal 369.63
  transient 368.12
  traumatic NEC 950.9
  word (developmental) 315.01
    acquired 784.61
    secondary to organic lesion 784.61
Blister — *see also* Injury, superficial, by site
  beetle dermatitis 692.89
  due to burn — *see* Burn, by site, second degree
  fever 054.9
  multiple, skin, nontraumatic 709.8
Bloating 787.3
Bloch-Siemens syndrome (incontinentia pigmenti) 757.33
Bloch-Stauffer dyshormonal dermatosis 757.33
Bloch-Sulzberger disease or syndrome (incontinentia pigmenti) (melanoblastosis) 757.33
Block
  alveolar capillary 516.3
  arborization (heart) 426.6
  arrhythmic 426.9
  atrioventricular (AV) (incomplete) (partial) 426.10
    with
      2:1 atrioventricular response block 426.13
      atrioventricular dissociation 426.0
    first degree (incomplete) 426.11
    second degree (Mobitz type I) 426.13
      Mobitz (type) II 426.12
    third degree 426.0
    complete 426.0
      congenital 746.86
    congenital 746.86
    Mobitz (incomplete)
      type I (Wenckebach's) 426.13
      type II 426.12
    partial 426.13
  auriculoventricular (*see also* Block, atrioventricular) 426.10
    complete 426.0
      congenital 746.86
    congenital 746.86
  bifascicular (cardiac) 426.53
  bundle branch (complete) (false) (incomplete) 426.50
    bilateral 426.53
    left (complete) (main stem) 426.3
      with right bundle branch block 426.53

Block — *continued*
  bundle branch — *continued*
    left — *continued*
      anterior fascicular 426.2
        with
          posterior fascicular block 426.3
          right bundle branch block 426.52
      hemiblock 426.2
      incomplete 426.2
        with right bundle branch block 426.53
      posterior fascicular 426.2
        with
          anterior fascicular block 426.3
          right bundle branch block 426.51
    right 426.4
      with
        left bundle branch block (incomplete) (main stem) 426.53
        left fascicular block 426.53
          anterior 426.52
          posterior 426.51
    Wilson's type 426.4
  cardiac 426.9
  conduction 426.9
    complete 426.0
  Eustachian tube (*see also* Obstruction, Eustachian tube) 381.60
  fascicular (left anterior) (left posterior) 426.2
  foramen Magendie (acquired) 331.3
    congenital 742.3
      with spina bifida (*see also* Spina bifida) 741.0 ✓5ᵗʰ
  heart 426.9
    first degree (atrioventricular) 426.11
    second degree (atrioventricular) 426.13
    third degree (atrioventricular) 426.0
    bundle branch (complete) (false) (incomplete) 426.50
      bilateral 426.53
      left (*see also* Block, bundle branch, left) 426.3
      right (*see also* Block, bundle branch, right) 426.4
    complete (atrioventricular) 426.0
    congenital 746.86
    incomplete 426.13
    intra-atrial 426.6
    intraventricular NEC 426.6
    sinoatrial 426.6
    specified type NEC 426.6
  hepatic vein 453.0
  intraventricular (diffuse) (myofibrillar) 426.6
    bundle branch (complete) (false) (incomplete) 426.50
      bilateral 426.53
      left (*see also* Block, bundle branch, left) 426.3
      right (*see also* Block, bundle branch, right) 426.4
  kidney (*see also* Disease, renal) 593.9
    postcystoscopic 997.5
  myocardial (*see also* Block, heart) 426.9
  nodal 426.10
  optic nerve 377.49
  organ or site (congenital) NEC — *see* Atresia
  parietal 426.6
  peri-infarction 426.6
  portal (vein) 452
  sinoatrial 426.6
  sinoauricular 426.6
  spinal cord 336.9
  trifascicular 426.54
  tubal 628.2
  vein NEC 453.9
Blocq's disease or syndrome (astasia-abasia) 307.9
Blood
  constituents, abnormal NEC 790.6
  disease 289.9
    specified NEC 289.8
  donor V59.01
    other blood components V59.09
    stem cells V59.02
    whole blood V59.01

Blood — *continued*
  dyscrasia 289.9
    with
      abortion — *see* Abortion, by type, with hemorrhage, delayed or excessive
      ectopic pregnancy (*see also* categories 633.0-633.9) 639.1
      molar pregnancy (*see also* categories 630-632) 639.1
    fetus or newborn NEC 776.9
    following
      abortion 639.1
      ectopic or molar pregnancy 639.1
    puerperal, postpartum 666.3 ✓5ᵗʰ
  flukes NEC (*see also* Infestation, Schistosoma) 120.9
  in
    feces (*see also* Melena) 578.1
      occult 792.1
    urine (*see also* Hematuria) 599.7
  mole 631
  occult 792.1
  poisoning (*see also* Septicemia) 038.9
  pressure
    decreased, due to shock following injury 958.4
    fluctuating 796.4
    high (*see also* Hypertension) 401.9
      incidental reading (isolated) (nonspecific), without diagnosis of hypertension 796.2
    low (*see also* Hypotension) 458.9
      incidental reading (isolated) (nonspecific), without diagnosis of hypotension 796.3
  spitting (*see also* Hemoptysis) 786.3
  staining cornea 371.12
  transfusion
    without reported diagnosis V58.2
    donor V59.01
      stem cells V59.02
    reaction or complication — *see* Complications, transfusion
  tumor — *see* Hematoma
  vessel rupture — *see* Hemorrhage
  vomiting (*see also* Hematemesis) 578.0
Blood-forming organ disease 289.9
Bloodgood's disease 610.1
Bloodshot eye 379.93
Bloom (-Machacek) (-Torre) syndrome 757.39
Blotch, palpebral 372.55
Blount's disease (tibia vara) 732.4
Blount-Barber syndrome (tibia vara) 732.4
Blue
  baby 746.9
  bloater 491.20
    with acute bronchitis or exacerbation 491.21
  diaper syndrome 270.0
  disease 746.9
  dome cyst 610.0
  drum syndrome 381.02
  sclera 743.47
    with fragility of bone and deafness 756.51
  toe syndrome — *see* Atherosclerosis
Blueness (*see also* Cyanosis) 782.5
Blurring, visual 368.8
Blushing (abnormal) (excessive) 782.62
Boarder, hospital V65.0
  infant V65.0
Bockhart's impetigo (superficial folliculitis) 704.8
Bodechtel-Guttmann disease (subacute sclerosing panencephalitis) 046.2
Boder-Sedgwick syndrome (ataxia-telangiectasia) 334.8
Body, bodies
  Aschoff (*see also* Myocarditis, rheumatic) 398.0
  asteroid, vitreous 379.22
  choroid, colloid (degenerative) 362.57
    hereditary 362.77
  cytoid (retina) 362.82
  drusen (retina) (*see also* Drusen) 362.57
    optic disc 377.21
  fibrin, pleura 511.0

Body — Breath

Body, bodies — *continued*
   foreign — *see* Foreign body
   Hassall-Henle 371.41
   loose
      joint (*see also* Loose, body, joint) 718.1 ✓5ᵗʰ
         knee 717.6
      knee 717.6
      sheath, tendon 727.82
      Mallory's 034.1
      Mooser 081.0
      Negri 071
      rice (joint) (*see also* Loose, body, joint) 718.1 ✓5ᵗʰ
         knee 717.6
      rocking 307.3
Boeck's
   disease (sarcoidosis) 135
   lupoid (miliary) 135
   sarcoid 135
Boerhaave's syndrome (spontaneous esophageal rupture) 530.4
Boggy
   cervix 622.8
   uterus 621.8
Boil (*see also* Carbuncle) 680.9
   abdominal wall 680.2
   Aleppo 085.1
   ankle 680.6
   anus 680.5
   arm (any part, above wrist) 680.3
   auditory canal, external 680.0
   axilla 680.3
   back (any part) 680.2
   Baghdad 085.1
   breast 680.2
   buttock 680.5
   chest wall 680.2
   corpus cavernosum 607.2
   Delhi 085.1
   ear (any part) 680.0
   eyelid 373.13
   face (any part, except eye) 680.0
   finger (any) 680.4
   flank 680.2
   foot (any part) 680.7
   forearm 680.3
   Gafsa 085.1
   genital organ, male 608.4
   gluteal (region) 680.5
   groin 680.2
   hand (any part) 680.4
   head (any part, except face) 680.8
   heel 680.7
   hip 680.6
   knee 680.6
   labia 616.4
   lacrimal (*see also* Dacryocystitis) 375.30
      gland (*see also* Dacryoadenitis) 375.00
      passages (duct) (sac) (*see also* Dacryocystitis) 375.30
   leg, any part except foot 680.6
   multiple sites 680.9
   natal 085.1
   neck 680.1
   nose (external) (septum) 680.0
   orbit, orbital 376.01
   partes posteriores 680.5
   pectoral region 680.2
   penis 607.2
   perineum 680.2
   pinna 680.0
   scalp (any part) 680.8
   scrotum 608.4
   seminal vesicle 608.0
   shoulder 680.3
   skin NEC 680.9
   specified site NEC 680.8
   spermatic cord 608.4
   temple (region) 680.0
   testis 608.4
   thigh 680.6
   thumb 680.4
   toe (any) 680.7
   tropical 085.1
   trunk 680.2
   tunica vaginalis 608.4
   umbilicus 680.2

Boil (*see also* Carbuncle) — *continued*
   upper arm 680.3
   vas deferens 608.4
   vulva 616.4
   wrist 680.4
Bold hives (*see also* Urticaria) 708.9
Bolivian hemorrhagic fever 078.7
Bombé, iris 364.74
Bomford-Rhoads anemia (refractory) 284.9
Bone — *see* condition
Bonnevie-Ullrich syndrome 758.6
Bonnier's syndrome 386.19
Bonvale Dam fever 780.79
Bony block of joint 718.80
   ankle 718.87
   elbow 718.82
   foot 718.87
   hand 718.84
   hip 718.85
   knee 718.86
   multiple sites 718.89
   pelvic region 718.85
   shoulder (region) 718.81
   specified site NEC 718.88
   wrist 718.83
Borderline
   intellectual functioning V62.89
   pelvis 653.1 ✓5ᵗʰ
      with obstruction during labor 660.1 ✓5ᵗʰ
         affecting fetus or newborn 763.1
   psychosis (*see also* Schizophrenia) 295.5 ✓5ᵗʰ
      of childhood (*see also* Psychosis, childhood) 299.8 ✓5ᵗʰ
   schizophrenia (*see also* Schizophrenia) 295.5 ✓5ᵗʰ
Borna disease 062.9
Bornholm disease (epidemic pleurodynia) 074.1
Borrelia vincentii (mouth) (pharynx) (tonsils) 101
Bostock's catarrh (*see also* Fever, hay) 477.9
Boston exanthem 048
Botalli, ductus (patent) (persistent) 747.0
Bothriocephalus latus infestation 123.4
Botulism 005.1
Bouba (*see also* Yaws) 102.9
Bouffée délirante 298.3
Bouillaud's disease or syndrome (rheumatic heart disease) 391.9
Bourneville's disease (tuberous sclerosis) 759.5
Boutonneuse fever 082.1
Boutonniere
   deformity (finger) 736.21
   hand (intrinsic) 736.21
Bouveret (-Hoffmann) disease or syndrome (paroxysmal tachycardia) 427.2
Bovine heart — *see* Hypertrophy, cardiac
Bowel — *see* condition
Bowen's
   dermatosis (precancerous) (M8081/2) — *see* Neoplasm, skin, in situ
   disease (M8081/2) — *see* Neoplasm, skin, in situ
   epithelioma (M8081/2) — *see* Neoplasm, skin, in situ
   type
      epidermoid carcinoma in situ (M8081/2) — *see* Neoplasm, skin, in situ
      intraepidermal squamous cell carcinoma (M8081/2) — *see* Neoplasm, skin, in situ
Bowing
   femur 736.89
      congenital 754.42
   fibula 736.89
      congenital 754.43
   forearm 736.09
      away from midline (cubitus valgus) 736.01
      toward midline (cubitus varus) 736.02
   leg(s), long bones, congenital 754.44
   radius 736.09
      away from midline (cubitus valgus) 736.01
      toward midline (cubitus varus) 736.02

Bowing — *continued*
   tibia 736.89
      congenital 754.43
Bowleg(s) 736.42
   congenital 754.44
   rachitic 268.1
Boyd's dysentery 004.2
Brachial — *see* condition
Brachman-de Lange syndrome (Amsterdam dwarf, mental retardation, and brachycephaly) 759.89
Brachycardia 427.89
Brachycephaly 756.0
Brachymorphism and ectopia lentis 759.89
Bradley's disease (epidemic vomiting) 078.82
Bradycardia 427.89
   chronic (sinus) 427.81
   newborn 779.81
   nodal 427.89
   postoperative 997.1
   reflex 337.0
   sinoatrial 427.89
      with paroxysmal tachyarrhythmia or tachycardia 427.81
         chronic 427.81
   sinus 427.89
      with paroxysmal tachyarrhythmia or tachycardia 427.81
         chronic 427.81
      persistent 427.81
      severe 427.81
   tachycardia syndrome 427.81
   vagal 427.89
Bradypnea 786.09
Brailsford's disease 732.3
   radial head 732.3
   tarsal scaphoid 732.5
Brailsford-Morquio disease or syndrome (mucopolysac-charidosis IV) 277.5
Brain — *see also* condition
   death 348.8
   syndrome (acute) (chronic) (nonpsychotic) (organic) (with neurotic reaction) (with behavioral reaction) (*see also* Syndrome, brain) 310.9
      with
         presenile brain disease 290.10
         psychosis, psychotic reaction (*see also* Psychosis, organic) 294.9
      congenital (*see also* Retardation, mental) 319
Branched-chain amino-acid disease 270.3
Branchial — *see* condition
Branchopulmonitis — *see* Pneumonia, broncho-
Brandt's syndrome (acrodermatitis enteropathica) 686.8
Brash (water) 787.1
Brass-founders', ague 985.8
Bravais-Jacksonian epilepsy (*see also* Epilepsy) 345.5 ✓5ᵗʰ
Braxton Hicks contractions 644.1 ✓5ᵗʰ
Braziers' disease 985.8
Brazilian
   blastomycosis 116.1
   leishmaniasis 085.5
Break
   cardiorenal — *see* Hypertension, cardiorenal
   retina (*see also* Defect, retina) 361.30
Breakbone fever 061
Breakdown
   device, implant, or graft — *see* Complications, mechanical
   nervous (*see also* Disorder, mental, nonpsychotic) 300.9
   perineum 674.2 ✓5ᵗʰ
Breast — *see* condition
Breast feeding difficulties 676.8 ✓5ᵗʰ
Breath
   foul 784.9
   holder, child 312.81
   holding spells 786.9
   shortness 786.05

▲

Breathing
asymmetrical 786.09
bronchial 786.09
exercises V57.0
labored 786.09
mouth 784.9
periodic 786.09
tic 307.20

Breathlessness 786.09

Breda's disease (see also Yaws) 102.9

Breech
delivery, affecting fetus or newborn 763.0
extraction, affecting fetus or newborn 763.0
presentation (buttocks) (complete) (frank) 652.2 ✓5ᵗʰ
with successful version 652.1 ✓5ᵗʰ
before labor, affecting fetus or newborn 761.7
during labor, affecting fetus or newborn 763.0

Breisky's disease (kraurosis vulvae) 624.0

Brennemann's syndrome (acute mesenteric lymphadenitis) 289.2

Brenner's
tumor (benign) (M9000/0) 220
borderline malignancy (M9000/1) 236.2
malignant (M9000/3) 183.0
proliferating (M9000/1) 236.2

Bretonneau's disease (diphtheritic malignant angina) 032.0

Breus' mole 631

Brevicollis 756.16

Bricklayers' itch 692.89

Brickmakers' anemia 126.9

Bridge
myocardial 746.85

Bright's
blindness — see Uremia
disease (see also Nephritis) 583.9
arteriosclerotic (see also Hypertension, kidney) 403.90

Brill's disease (recrudescent typhus) 081.1
flea-borne 081.0
louse-borne 081.1

Brill-Symmers disease (follicular lymphoma) (M9690/3) 202.0 ✓5ᵗʰ

Brill-Zinsser disease (recrudescent typhus) 081.1

Brinton's disease (linitis plastica) (M8142/3) 151.9

Brion-Kayser disease (see also Fever, paratyphoid) 002.9

Briquet's disorder or syndrome 300.81

Brissaud's
infantilism (infantile myxedema) 244.9
motor-verbal tic 307.23

Brissaud-Meige syndrome (infantile myxedema) 244.9

Brittle
bones (congenital) 756.51
nails 703.8
congenital 757.5

Broad — see also condition
beta disease 272.2
ligament laceration syndrome 620.6

Brock's syndrome (atelectasis due to enlarged lymph nodes) 518.0

Brocq's disease 691.8
atopic (diffuse) neurodermatitis 691.8
lichen simplex chronicus 698.3
parakeratosis psoriasiformis 696.2
parapsoriasis 696.2

Brocq-Duhring disease (dermatitis herpetiformis) 694.0

Brodie's
abscess (localized) (chronic) (see also Osteomyelitis) 730.1 ✓5ᵗʰ
disease (joint) (see also Osteomyelitis) 730.1 ✓5ᵗʰ

Broken
arches 734
congenital 755.67

Broken — continued
back — see Fracture, vertebra, by site
bone — see Fracture, by site
compensation — see Disease, heart
implant or internal device — see listing under Complications, mechanical
neck — see Fracture, vertebra, cervical
nose 802.0
open 802.1
tooth, teeth 873.63
complicated 873.73

Bromhidrosis 705.89

Bromidism, bromism
acute 967.3
correct substance properly administered 349.82
overdose or wrong substance given or taken 967.3
chronic (see also Dependence) 304.1 ✓5ᵗʰ

Bromidrosiphobia 300.23

Bromidrosis 705.89

Bronchi, bronchial — see condition

Bronchiectasis (cylindrical) (diffuse) (fusiform) (localized) (moniliform) (postinfectious) (recurrent) (saccular) 494.0
with acute exacerbation 494.1
congenital 748.61
tuberculosis (see also Tuberculosis) 011.5 ✓5ᵗʰ

Bronchiolectasis — see Bronchiectasis

Bronchiolitis (acute) (infectious) (subacute) 466.19
with
bronchospasm or obstruction 466.19
influenza, flu, or grippe 487.1
catarrhal (acute) (subacute) 466.19
chemical 506.0
chronic 506.4
chronic (obliterative) 491.8
due to external agent — see Bronchitis, acute, due to
fibrosa obliterans 491.8
influenzal 487.1
obliterans 491.8
with organizing pneumonia (B.O.O.P.) 516.8
status post lung transplant 996.84
obliterative (chronic) (diffuse) (subacute) 491.8
due to fumes or vapors 506.4
respiratory syncytial virus 466.11
vesicular — see Pneumonia, broncho-

Bronchitis (diffuse) (hypostatic) (infectious) (inflammatory) (simple) 490
with
emphysema — see Emphysema
influenza, flu, or grippe 487.1
obstruction airway, chronic 491.20
with acute exacerbation 491.21
tracheitis 490
acute or subacute 466.0
with bronchospasm or obstruction 466.0
chronic 491.8
acute or subacute 466.0
with
bronchospasm 466.0
chronic
bronchitis (obstructive) 491.21
obstructive pulmonary disease (COPD) 491.21
obstruction 466.0
tracheitis 466.0
chemical (due to fumes or vapors) 506.0
due to
fumes or vapors 506.0
radiation 508.8
allergic (acute) (see also Asthma) 493.9 ✓5ᵗʰ
arachidic 934.1
aspiration 507.0
due to fumes or vapors 506.0
asthmatic (acute) 493.90
with
acute exacerbation 493.92
status asthmaticus 493.91
chronic 493.2 ✓5ᵗʰ ▲
capillary 466.19
with bronchospasm or obstruction 466.19

Bronchitis — continued
capillary — continued
chronic 491.8
caseous (see also Tuberculosis) 011.3 ✓5ᵗʰ
Castellani's 104.8
catarrhal 490
acute — see Bronchitis, acute
chronic 491.0
chemical (acute) (subacute) 506.0
chronic 506.4
due to fumes or vapors (acute) (subacute) 506.0
chronic 506.4
chronic 491.9
with
tracheitis (chronic) 491.8
asthmatic 493.2 ✓5ᵗʰ ▲
catarrhal 491.0
chemical (due to fumes and vapors) 506.4
due to
fumes or vapors (chemical) (inhalation) 506.4
radiation 508.8
tobacco smoking 491.0
mucopurulent 491.1
obstructive 491.20
with acute bronchitis or acute exacerbation 491.21
purulent 491.1
simple 491.0
specified type NEC 491.8
croupous 466.0
with bronchospasm or obstruction 466.0
due to fumes or vapors 506.0
emphysematous 491.20
with acute bronchitis or acute exacerbation 491.21
exudative 466.0
fetid (chronic) (recurrent) 491.1
fibrinous, acute or subacute 466.0
with bronchospasm or obstruction 466.0
grippal 487.1
influenzal 487.1
membranous, acute or subacute 466.0
with bronchospasm or obstruction 466.0
moulders' 502
mucopurulent (chronic) (recurrent) 491.1
acute or subacute 466.0
non-obstructive 491.0
obliterans 491.8
obstructive (chronic) 491.20
with acute bronchitis or acute exacerbation 491.21
pituitous 491.1
plastic (inflammatory) 466.0
pneumococcal, acute or subacute 466.0
with bronchospasm or obstruction 466.0
pseudomembranous 466.0
purulent (chronic) (recurrent) 491.1
acute or subacute 466.0
with bronchospasm or obstruction 466.0
putrid 491.1
scrofulous (see also Tuberculosis) 011.3 ✓5ᵗʰ
senile 491.9
septic, acute or subacute 466.0
with bronchospasm or obstruction 466.0
smokers' 491.0
spirochetal 104.8
suffocative, acute or subacute 466.0
summer (see also Asthma) 493.9 ✓5ᵗʰ
suppurative (chronic) 491.1
acute or subacute 466.0
tuberculous (see also Tuberculosis) 011.3 ✓5ᵗʰ
ulcerative 491.8
Vincent's 101
Vincent's 101
viral, acute or subacute 466.0

Bronchoalveolitis 485

Bronchoaspergillosis 117.3

Bronchocele
meaning
dilatation of bronchus 519.1
goiter 240.9

Bronchogenic carcinoma 162.9

Bronchohemisporosis 117.9

Broncholithiasis 518.89
  tuberculous (see also Tuberculosis) 011.3 ✓5ᵗʰ
Bronchomalacia 748.3
Bronchomoniliasis 112.89
Bronchomycosis 112.89
Bronchonocardiosis 039.1
Bronchopleuropneumonia — see Pneumonia,
  broncho-
Bronchopneumonia — see Pneumonia, broncho-
Bronchopneumonitis — see Pneumonia,
  broncho-
Bronchopulmonary — see condition
Bronchorrhagia 786.3
  newborn 770.3
  tuberculous (see also Tuberculosis) 011.3 ✓5ᵗʰ
Bronchorrhea (chronic) (purulent) 491.0
  acute 466.0
Bronchospasm 519.1
  with
    asthma — see Asthma
    bronchiolitis
      due to respiratory syncytial virus 466.11
    bronchitis — see Bronchitis
    chronic obstructive pulmonary disease
      (COPD) 496
    emphysema — see Emphysema
    due to external agent — see Condition,
      respiratory, acute, due to
Bronchospirochetosis 104.8
Bronchostenosis 519.1
Bronchus — see condition
Bronze, bronzed
  diabetes 275.0
  disease (Addison's) (skin) 255.4
    tuberculous (see also Tuberculosis)
      017.6 ✓5ᵗʰ
Brooke's disease or tumor (M8100/0) — see
  Neoplasm, skin, benign
Brown's tendon sheath syndrome 378.61
Brown enamel of teeth (hereditary) 520.5
Brown-Séquard's paralysis (syndrome) 344.89
Brow presentation complicating delivery
  652.4 ✓5ᵗʰ
Brucella, brucellosis (infection) 023.9
  abortus 023.1
  canis 023.3
  dermatitis, skin 023.9
  melitensis 023.0
  mixed 023.8
  suis 023.2
Bruck's disease 733.99
Bruck-de Lange disease or syndrome
  (Amsterdam dwarf, mental retardation, and
  brachycephaly) 759.89
Brugada syndrome 746.89
Brugsch's syndrome (acropachyderma) 757.39
Brug's filariasis 125.1
Bruhl's disease (splenic anemia with fever) 285.8
Bruise (skin surface intact) — see also Contusion
  with
    fracture — see Fracture, by site
    open wound — see Wound, open, by site
  internal organ (abdomen, chest, or pelvis) —
    see Injury, internal, by site
  umbilical cord 663.6 ✓5ᵗʰ
    affecting fetus or newborn 762.6
Bruit 785.9
  arterial (abdominal) (carotid) 785.9
  supraclavicular 785.9
Brushburn — see Injury, superficial, by site
Bruton's X-linked agammaglobulinemia 279.04
Bruxism 306.8
Bubbly lung syndrome 770.7
Bubo 289.3
  blennorrhagic 098.89
  chancroidal 099.0
  climatic 099.1
  due to Hemophilus ducreyi 099.0
  gonococcal 098.89
  indolent NEC 099.8
  inguinal NEC 099.8

Bubo — continued
  inguinal NEC — continued
    chancroidal 099.0
    climatic 099.1
    due to H. ducreyi 099.0
  scrofulous (see also Tuberculosis) 017.2 ✓5ᵗʰ
  soft chancre 099.0
  suppurating 683
  syphilitic 091.0
    congenital 090.0
  tropical 099.1
  venereal NEC 099.8
  virulent 099.0
Bubonic plague 020.0
Bubonocele — see Hernia, inguinal
Buccal — see condition
Buchanan's disease (juvenile osteochondrosis of
  iliac crest) 732.1
Buchem's syndrome (hyperostosis corticalis)
  733.3
Buchman's disease (osteochondrosis, juvenile)
  732.1
Bucket handle fracture (semilunar cartilage) (see
  also Tear, meniscus) 836.2
Budd-Chiari syndrome (hepatic vein thrombosis)
  453.0
Budgerigar-fanciers' disease or lung 495.2
Büdinger-Ludloff-Läwen disease 717.89
Buerger's disease (thromboangiitis obliterans)
  443.1
Bulbar — see condition
Bulbus cordis 745.9
  persistent (in left ventricle) 745.8
Bulging fontanels (congenital) 756.0
Bulimia 783.6
  nonorganic origin 307.51
Bulky uterus 621.2
Bulla(e) 709.8
  lung (emphysematous) (solitary) 492.0
Bullet wound — see also Wound, open, by site
  fracture — see Fracture, by site, open
  internal organ (abdomen, chest, or pelvis) —
    see Injury, internal, by site, with open
    wound
  intracranial — see Laceration, brain, with open
    wound
Bullis fever 082.8
Bullying (see also Disturbance, conduct)
  312.0 ✓5ᵗʰ
Bundle
  branch block (complete) (false) (incomplete)
    426.50
    bilateral 426.53
    left (see also Block, bundle branch, left)
      426.3
      hemiblock 426.2
    right (see also Block, bundle branch, right)
      426.4
  of His — see condition
  of Kent syndrome (anomalous atrioventricular
    excitation) 426.7
Bungpagga 040.81
Bunion 727.1
Bunionette 727.1
Bunyamwera fever 066.3
Buphthalmia, buphthalmos (congenital) 743.20
  associated with
    keratoglobus, congenital 743.22
    megalocornea 743.22
    ocular anomalies NEC 743.22
  isolated 743.21
  simple 743.21
Bürger-Grütz disease or syndrome (essential
  familial hyperlipemia) 272.3
Buried roots 525.3
Burke's syndrome 577.8
Burkitt's
  tumor (M9750/3) 200.2 ✓5ᵗʰ
  type malignant, lymphoma, lymphoblastic, or
    undifferentiated (M9750/3) 200.2 ✓5ᵗʰ

Burn (acid) (cathode ray) (caustic) (chemical)
  (electric heating appliance) (electricity) (fire)
  (flame) (hot liquid or object) (irradiation)
  (lime) (radiation) (steam) (thermal) (x-ray)
  949.0

Note — Use the following fifth-digit
subclassification with category 948 to
indicate the percent of body surface with
third degree burn:

0	Less than 10% or unspecified
1	10–19%
2	20–29%
3	30–39%
4	40–49%
5	50–59%
6	60–69%
7	70–79%
8	80–89%
9	90% or more of body surface

  with
    blisters — see Burn, by site, second degree
    erythema — see Burn, by site, first degree
    skin loss (epidermal) — see also Burn, by
      site, second degree
      full thickness — see also Burn, by site,
        third degree
        with necrosis of underlying tissues —
          see Burn, by site, third degree,
          deep
  first degree — see Burn, by site, first degree
  second degree — see Burn, by site, second
    degree
  third degree — see Burn, by site, third degree
    deep — see Burn, by site, third degree, deep
  abdomen, abdominal (muscle) (wall) 942.03
    with
      trunk — see Burn, trunk, multiple sites
    first degree 942.13
    second degree 942.23
    third degree 942.33
      deep 942.43
        with loss of body part 942.53
  ankle 945.03
    with
      lower limb(s) — see Burn, leg, multiple
        sites
    first degree 945.13
    second degree 945.23
    third degree 945.33
      deep 945.43
        with loss of body part 945.53
  anus — see Burn, trunk, specified site NEC
  arm(s) 943.00
    first degree 943.10
    second degree 943.20
    third degree 943.30
      deep 943.40
        with loss of body part 943.50
    lower — see Burn, forearm(s)
    multiple sites, except hand(s) or wrist(s)
      943.09
      first degree 943.19
      second degree 943.29
      third degree 943.39
        deep 943.49
          with loss of body part 943.59
    upper 943.03
      first degree 943.13
      second degree 943.23
      third degree 943.33
        deep 943.43
          with loss of body part 943.53
  auditory canal (external) — see Burn, ear
  auricle (ear) — see Burn, ear
  axilla 943.04
    with
      upper limb(s) except hand(s) or wrist(s) —
        see Burn, arm(s), multiple sites
    first degree 943.14
    second degree 943.24
    third degree 943.34
      deep 943.44
        with loss of body part 943.54

Burn — *continued*
back 942.04
with
trunk — *see* Burn, trunk, multiple sites
first degree 942.14
second degree 942.24
third degree 942.34
deep 942.44
with loss of body part 942.54
biceps
brachii — *see* Burn, arm(s), upper
femoris — *see* Burn, thigh
breast(s) 942.01
with
trunk — *see* Burn, trunk, multiple sites
first degree 942.11
second degree 942.21
third degree 942.31
deep 942.41
with loss of body part 942.51
brow — *see* Burn, forehead
buttock(s) — *see* Burn, back
canthus (eye) 940.1
chemical 940.0
cervix (uteri) 947.4
cheek (cutaneous) 941.07
with
face or head — *see* Burn, head, multiple sites
first degree 941.17
second degree 941.27
third degree 941.37
deep 941.47
with loss of body part 941.57
chest wall (anterior) 942.02
with
trunk — *see* Burn, trunk, multiple sites
first degree 942.12
second degree 942.22
third degree 942.32
deep 942.42
with loss of body part 942.52
chin 941.04
with
face or head — *see* Burn, head, multiple sites
first degree 941.14
second degree 941.24
third degree 941.34
deep 941.44
with loss of body part 941.54
clitoris — *see* Burn, genitourinary organs, external
colon 947.3
conjunctiva (and cornea) 940.4
chemical
acid 940.3
alkaline 940.2
cornea (and conjunctiva) 940.4
chemical
acid 940.3
alkaline 940.2
costal region — *see* Burn, chest wall
due to ingested chemical agent — *see* Burn, internal organs
ear (auricle) (canal) (drum) (external) 941.01
with
face or head — *see* Burn, head, multiple sites
first degree 941.11
second degree 941.21
third degree 941.31
deep 941.41
with loss of a body part 941.51
elbow 943.02
with
hand(s) and wrist(s) — *see* Burn, multiple specified sites
upper limb(s) except hand(s) or wrist(s) — *see also* Burn, arm(s), multiple sites
first degree 943.12
second degree 943.22
third degree 943.32
deep 943.42
with loss of body part 943.52

Burn — *continued*
electricity, electric current — *See* Burn, by site
entire body — *see* Burn, multiple, specified sites
epididymis — *see* Burn, genitourinary organs, external
epigastric region — *see* Burn, abdomen
epiglottis 947.1
esophagus 947.2
extent (percent of body surface)
less than 10 percent 948.0 ✓5ᵗʰ
10-19 percent 948.1 ✓5ᵗʰ
20-29 percent 948.2 ✓5ᵗʰ
30-39 percent 948.3 ✓5ᵗʰ
40-49 percent 948.4 ✓5ᵗʰ
50-59 percent 948.5 ✓5ᵗʰ
60-69 percent 948.6 ✓5ᵗʰ
70-79 percent 948.7 ✓5ᵗʰ
80-89 percent 948.8 ✓5ᵗʰ
90 percent or more 948.9 ✓5ᵗʰ
extremity
lower — *see* Burn, leg
upper — *see* Burn, arm(s)
eye(s) (and adnexa) (only) 940.9
with
face, head, or neck 941.02
first degree 941.12
second degree 941.22
third degree 941.32
deep 941.42
with loss of body part 941.52
other sites (classifiable to more than one category in 940-945) — *see* Burn, multiple, specified sites
resulting rupture and destruction of eyeball 940.5
specified part — *see* Burn, by site
eyeball — *see also* Burn, eye with resulting rupture and destruction of eyeball 940.5
eyelid(s) 940.1
chemical 940.0
face — *see* Burn, head
finger (nail) (subungual) 944.01
with
hand(s) — *see* Burn, hand(s), multiple sites
other sites — *see* Burn, multiple, specified sites
thumb 944.04
first degree 944.14
second degree 944.24
third degree 944.34
deep 944.44
with loss of body part 944.54
first degree 944.11
second degree 944.21
third degree 944.31
deep 944.41
with loss of body part 944.51
multiple (digits) 944.03
with thumb — *see* Burn, finger, with thumb
first degree 944.13
second degree 944.23
third degree 944.33
deep 944.43
with loss of body part 944.53
flank — *see* Burn, abdomen
foot 945.02
with
lower limb(s) — *see* Burn, leg, multiple sites
first degree 945.12
second degree 945.22
third degree 945.32
deep 945.42
with loss of body part 945.52
forearm(s) 943.01
with
upper limb(s) except hand(s) or wrist(s) — *see* Burn, arm(s), multiple sites
first degree 943.11
second degree 943.21
third degree 943.31
deep 943.41
with loss of body part 943.51

Burn — *continued*
forehead 941.07
with
face or head — *see* Burn, head, multiple sites
first degree 941.17
second degree 941.27
third degree 941.37
deep 941.47
with loss of body part 941.57
fourth degree — *see* Burn, by site, third degree, deep
friction — *see* Injury, superficial, by site
from swallowing caustic or corrosive substance NEC — *see* Burn, internal organs
full thickness — *see* Burn, by site, third degree
gastrointestinal tract 947.3
genitourinary organs
external 942.05
with
trunk — *see* Burn, trunk, multiple sites
first degree 942.15
second degree 942.25
third degree 942.35
deep 942.45
with loss of body part 942.55
internal 947.8
globe (eye) — *see* Burn, eyeball
groin — *see* Burn, abdomen
gum 947.0
hand(s) (phalanges) (and wrist) 944.00
first degree 944.10
second degree 944.20
third degree 944.30
deep 944.40
with loss of body part 944.50
back (dorsal surface) 944.06
first degree 944.16
second degree 944.26
third degree 944.36
deep 944.46
with loss of body part 944.56
multiple sites 944.08
first degree 944.18
second degree 944.28
third degree 944.38
deep 944.48
with loss of body part 944.58
head (and face) 941.00
eye(s) only 940.9
specified part — *see* Burn, by site
first degree 941.10
second degree 941.20
third degree 941.30
deep 941.40
with loss of body part 941.50
multiple sites 941.09
with eyes — *see* Burn, eyes, with face, head, or neck
first degree 941.19
second degree 941.29
third degree 941.39
deep 941.49
with loss of body part 941.59
heel — *see* Burn, foot
hip — *see* Burn, trunk, specified site NEC
iliac region — *see* Burn, trunk, specified site NEC
infected 958.3
inhalation (*see also* Burn, internal organs) 947.9
internal organs 947.9
from caustic or corrosive substance (swallowing) NEC 947.9
specified NEC (*see also* Burn, by site) 947.8
interscapular region — *see* Burn, back
intestine (large) (small) 947.3
iris — *see* Burn, eyeball
knee 945.05
with
lower limb(s) — *see* Burn, leg, multiple sites
first degree 945.15
second degree 945.25

Burn — Burn

Burn

Burn — *continued*
  knee — *continued*
    third degree 945.35
      deep 945.45
        with loss of body part 945.55
  labium (majorus) (minus) — *see* Burn, genitourinary organs, external
  lacrimal apparatus, duct, gland, or sac 940.1
    chemical 940.0
  larynx 947.1
  late effect — *see* Late, effects (of), burn
  leg 945.00
    first degree 945.10
    second degree 945.20
    third degree 945.30
      deep 945.40
        with loss of body part 945.50
    lower 945.04
      with other part(s) of lower limb(s) — *see* Burn, leg, multiple sites
      first degree 945.14
      second degree 945.24
      third degree 945.34
        deep 945.44
          with loss of body part 945.54
    multiple sites 945.09
      first degree 945.19
      second degree 945.29
      third degree 945.39
        deep 945.49
          with loss of body part 945.59
    upper — *see* Burn, thigh
  lightning — *see* Burn, by site
  limb(s)
    lower (including foot or toe(s)) — *see* Burn, leg
    upper (except wrist and hand) — *see* Burn, arm(s)
  lip(s) 941.03
    with
      face or head — *see* Burn, head, multiple sites
    first degree 941.13
    second degree 941.23
    third degree 941.33
      deep 941.43
        with loss of body part 941.53
  lumbar region — *see* Burn, back
  lung 947.1
  malar region — *see* Burn, cheek
  mastoid region — *see* Burn, scalp
  membrane, tympanic — *see* Burn, ear
  midthoracic region — *see* Burn, chest wall
  mouth 947.0
  multiple (*see also* Burn, unspecified) 949.0
    specified sites classifiable to more than one category in 940-945 946.0
      first degree 946.1
      second degree 946.2
      third degree 946.3
        deep 946.4
          with loss of body part 946.5
  muscle, abdominal — *see* Burn, abdomen
  nasal (septum) — *see* Burn, nose
  neck 941.08
    with
      face or head — *see* Burn, head, multiple sites
    first degree 941.18
    second degree 941.28
    third degree 941.38
      deep 941.48
        with loss of body part 941.58
  nose (septum) 941.05
    with
      face or head — *see* Burn, head, multiple sites
    first degree 941.15
    second degree 941.25
    third degree 941.35
      deep 941.45
        with loss of body part 941.55
  occipital region — *see* Burn, scalp
  orbit region 940.1
    chemical 940.0
  oronasopharynx 947.0
  palate 947.0

Burn — *continued*
  palm(s) 944.05
    with
      hand(s) and wrist(s) — *see* Burn, hand(s), multiple sites
    first degree 944.15
    second degree 944.25
    third degree 944.35
      deep 944.45
        with loss of a body part 944.55
  parietal region — *see* Burn, scalp
  penis — *see* Burn, genitourinary organs, external
  perineum — *see* Burn, genitourinary organs, external
  periocular area 940.1
    chemical 940.0
  pharynx 947.0
  pleura 947.1
  popliteal space — *see* Burn, knee
  prepuce — *see* Burn, genitourinary organs, external
  pubic region — *see* Burn, genitourinary organs, external
  pudenda — *see* Burn, genitourinary organs, external
  rectum 947.3
  sac, lacrimal 940.1
    chemical 940.0
  sacral region — *see* Burn, back
  salivary (ducts) (glands) 947.0
  scalp 941.06
    with
      face or neck — *see* Burn, head, multiple sites
    first degree 941.16
    second degree 941.26
    third degree 941.36
      deep 941.46
        with loss of body part 941.56
  scapular region 943.06
    with
      upper limb(s), except hand(s) or wrist(s) — *see* Burn, arm(s), multiple sites
    first degree 943.16
    second degree 943.26
    third degree 943.36
      deep 943.46
        with loss of body part 943.56
  sclera — *see* Burn, eyeball
  scrotum — *see* Burn, genitourinary organs, external
  septum, nasal — *see* Burn, nose
  shoulder(s) 943.05
    with
      hand(s) and wrist(s) — *see* Burn, multiple, specified sites
      upper limb(s), except hand(s) or wrist(s) — *see* Burn, arm(s), multiple sites
    first degree 943.15
    second degree 943.25
    third degree 943.35
      deep 943.45
        with loss of body part 943.55
  skin NEC (*see also* Burn, unspecified) 949.0
  skull — *see* Burn, head
  small intestine 947.3
  sternal region — *see* Burn, chest wall
  stomach 947.3
  subconjunctival — *see* Burn, conjunctiva
  subcutaneous — *see* Burn, by site, third degree
  submaxillary region — *see* Burn, head
  submental region — *see* Burn, chin
  sun — *see* Sunburn
  supraclavicular fossa — *see* Burn, neck
  supraorbital — *see* Burn, forehead
  temple — *see* Burn, scalp
  temporal region — *see* Burn, scalp
  testicle — *see* Burn, genitourinary organs, external
  testis — *see* Burn, genitourinary organs, external
  thigh 945.06
    with
      lower limb(s) — *see* Burn, leg, multiple sites

Burn — *continued*
  thigh — *continued*
    first degree 945.16
    second degree 945.26
    third degree 945.36
      deep 945.46
        with loss of body part 945.56
  thorax (external) — *see* Burn, chest wall
  throat 947.0
  thumb(s) (nail) (subungual) 944.02
    with
      finger(s) — *see* Burn, finger, with other sites, thumb
      hand(s) and wrist(s) — *see* Burn, hand(s), multiple sites
    first degree 944.12
    second degree 944.22
    third degree 944.32
      deep 944.42
        with loss of body part 944.52
  toe (nail) (subungual) 945.01
    with
      lower limb(s) — *see* Burn, leg, multiple sites
    first degree 945.11
    second degree 945.21
    third degree 945.31
      deep 945.41
        with loss of body part 945.51
  tongue 947.0
  tonsil 947.0
  trachea 947.1
  trunk 942.00
    first degree 942.10
    second degree 942.20
    third degree 942.30
      deep 942.40
        with loss of body part 942.50
    multiple sites 942.09
      first degree 942.19
      second degree 942.29
      third degree 942.39
        deep 942.49
          with loss of body part 942.59
    specified site NEC 942.09
      first degree 942.19
      second degree 942.29
      third degree 942.39
        deep 942.49
          with loss of body part 942.59
  tunica vaginalis — *see* Burn, genitourinary organs, external
  tympanic membrane — *see* Burn, ear
  tympanum — *see* Burn, ear
  ultraviolet 692.82
  unspecified site (multiple) 949.0
    with extent of body surface involved specified
      less than 10 percent 948.0 √5ᵗʰ
      10-19 percent 948.1 √5ᵗʰ
      20-29 percent 948.2 √5ᵗʰ
      30-39 percent 948.3 √5ᵗʰ
      40-49 percent 948.4 √5ᵗʰ
      50-59 percent 948.5 √5ᵗʰ
      60-69 percent 948.6 √5ᵗʰ
      70-79 percent 948.7 √5ᵗʰ
      80-89 percent 948.8 √5ᵗʰ
      90 percent or more 948.9 √5ᵗʰ
    first degree 949.1
    second degree 949.2
    third degree 949.3
      deep 949.4
        with loss of body part 949.5
  uterus 947.4
  uvula 947.0
  vagina 947.4
  vulva — *see* Burn, genitourinary organs, external
  wrist(s) 944.07
    with
      hand(s) — *see* Burn, hand(s), multiple sites
    first degree 944.17
    second degree 944.27
    third degree 944.37
      deep 944.47
        with loss of body part 944.57

√4ᵗʰ Fourth-digit Required   √5ᵗʰ Fifth-digit Required   ►◄ Revised Text   ● New Line   ▲ Revised Code

Burnett's syndrome (milk-alkali) 999.9
Burnier's syndrome (hypophyseal dwarfism) 253.3
Burning
feet syndrome 266.2
sensation (*see also* Disturbance, sensation) 782.0
tongue 529.6
Burns' disease (osteochondrosis, lower ulna) 732.3
Bursa — *see also* condition
pharynx 478.29
Bursitis NEC 727.3
Achilles tendon 726.71
adhesive 726.90
shoulder 726.0
ankle 726.79
buttock 726.5
calcaneal 726.79
collateral ligament
fibular 726.63
tibial 726.62
Duplay's 726.2
elbow 726.33
finger 726.8
foot 726.79
gonococcal 098.52
hand 726.4
hip 726.5
infrapatellar 726.69
ischiogluteal 726.5
knee 726.60
occupational NEC 727.2
olecranon 726.33
pes anserinus 726.61
pharyngeal 478.29
popliteal 727.51
prepatellar 726.65
radiohumeral 727.3
scapulohumeral 726.19
adhesive 726.0
shoulder 726.10
adhesive 726.0
subacromial 726.19
adhesive 726.0
subcoracoid 726.19
subdeltoid 726.19
adhesive 726.0
subpatellar 726.69
syphilitic 095.7
Thornwaldt's, Tornwaldt's (pharyngeal) 478.29
toe 726.79
trochanteric area 726.5
wrist 726.4
Burst stitches or sutures (complication of surgery) ▶(external)◀ 998.32 ▲
internal 998.31 ●
Buruli ulcer 031.1
Bury's disease (erythema elevatum diutinum) 695.89
Buschke's disease or scleredema (adultorum) 710.1
Busquet's disease (osteoperiostitis) (*see also* Osteomyelitis) 730.1 ✔5ᵗʰ
Busse-Buschke disease (cryptococcosis) 117.5
Buttock — *see* condition
Button
Biskra 085.1
Delhi 085.1
oriental 085.1
Buttonhole hand (intrinsic) 736.21
Bwamba fever (encephalitis) 066.3
Byssinosis (occupational) 504
Bywaters' syndrome 958.5

C

Cacergasia 300.9
Cachexia 799.4
cancerous (M8000/3) 199.1
cardiac — *see* Disease, heart

Cachexia — *continued*
dehydration 276.5
with
hypernatremia 276.0
hyponatremia 276.1
due to malnutrition 261
exophthalmic 242.0 ✔5ᵗʰ
heart — *see* Disease, heart
hypophyseal 253.2
hypopituitary 253.2
lead 984.9
specified type of lead — *see* Table of Drugs and Chemicals
malaria 084.9
malignant (M8000/3) 199.1
marsh 084.9
nervous 300.5
old age 797
pachydermic — *see* Hypothyroidism
paludal 084.9
pituitary (postpartum) 253.2
renal (*see also* Disease, renal) 593.9
saturnine 984.9
specified type of lead — *see* Table of Drugs and Chemicals
senile 797
Simmonds' (pituitary cachexia) 253.2
splenica 289.59
strumipriva (*see also* Hypothyroidism) 244.9
tuberculous NEC (*see also* Tuberculosis) 011.9 ✔5ᵗʰ
Café au lait spots 709.09
Caffey's disease or syndrome (infantile cortical hyperostosis) 756.59
Caisson disease 993.3
Caked breast (puerperal, postpartum) 676.2 ✔5ᵗʰ
Cake kidney 753.3
Calabar swelling 125.2
Calcaneal spur 726.73
Calcaneoapophysitis 732.5
Calcaneonavicular bar 755.67
Calcareous — *see* condition
Calcicosis (occupational) 502
Calciferol (vitamin D) deficiency 268.9
with
osteomalacia 268.2
rickets (*see also* Rickets) 268.0
Calcification
adrenal (capsule) (gland) 255.4
tuberculous (*see also* Tuberculosis) 017.6 ✔5ᵗʰ
aorta 440.0
artery (annular) — *see* Arteriosclerosis
auricle (ear) 380.89
bladder 596.8
due to S. hematobium 120.0
brain (cortex) — *see* Calcification, cerebral
bronchus 519.1
bursa 727.82
cardiac (*see also* Degeneration, myocardial) 429.1
cartilage (postinfectional) 733.99
cerebral (cortex) 348.8
artery 437.0
cervix (uteri) 622.8
choroid plexus 349.2
conjunctiva 372.54
corpora cavernosa (penis) 607.89
cortex (brain) — *see* Calcification, cerebral
dental pulp (nodular) 522.2
dentinal papilla 520.4
disc, intervertebral 722.90
cervical, cervicothoracic 722.91
lumbar, lumbosacral 722.93
thoracic, thoracolumbar 722.92
fallopian tube 620.8
falx cerebri — *see* Calcification, cerebral
fascia 728.89
gallbladder 575.8
general 275.40
heart (*see also* Degeneration, myocardial) 429.1
valve — *see* Endocarditis
intervertebral cartilage or disc (postinfectional) 722.90
cervical, cervicothoracic 722.91

Calcification — *continued*
intervertebral cartilage or disc — *continued*
lumbar, lumbosacral 722.93
thoracic, thoracolumbar 722.92
intracranial — *see* Calcification, cerebral
intraspinal ligament 728.89
joint 719.80
ankle 719.87
elbow 719.82
foot 719.87
hand 719.84
hip 719.85
knee 719.86
multiple sites 719.89
pelvic region 719.85
shoulder (region) 719.81
specified site NEC 719.88
wrist 719.83
kidney 593.89
tuberculous (*see also* Tuberculosis) 016.0 ✔5ᵗʰ
larynx (senile) 478.79
lens 366.8
ligament 728.89
intraspinal 728.89
knee (medial collateral) 717.89
lung 518.89
active 518.89
postinfectional 518.89
tuberculous (*see also* Tuberculosis, pulmonary) 011.9 ✔5ᵗʰ
lymph gland or node (postinfectional) 289.3
tuberculous (*see also* Tuberculosis, lymph gland) 017.2 ✔5ᵗʰ
massive (paraplegic) 728.10
medial NEC (*see also* Arteriosclerosis, extremities) 440.20
meninges (cerebral) 349.2
metastatic 275.40
Mönckeberg's — *see* Arteriosclerosis
muscle 728.10
heterotopic, postoperative 728.13
myocardium, myocardial (*see also* Degeneration, myocardial) 429.1
ovary 620.8
pancreas 577.8
penis 607.89
periarticular 728.89
pericardium (*see also* Pericarditis) 423.8
pineal gland 259.8
pleura 511.0
postinfectional 518.89
tuberculous (*see also* Tuberculosis, pleura) 012.0 ✔5ᵗʰ
pulp (dental) (nodular) 522.2
renal 593.89
Rider's bone 733.99
sclera 379.16
semilunar cartilage 717.89
spleen 289.59
subcutaneous 709.3
suprarenal (capsule) (gland) 255.4
tendon (sheath) 727.82
with bursitis, synovitis or tenosynovitis 727.82
trachea 519.1
ureter 593.89
uterus 621.8
vitreous 379.29
Calcified — *see also* Calcification
hematoma NEC 959.9
Calcinosis (generalized) (interstitial) (tumoral) (universalis) 275.49
circumscripta 709.3
cutis 709.3
intervertebralis 275.49 [722.90]
Raynaud's
phenomenonsclerodactylytelangiectasis (CRST) 710.1
Calcium
blood
high (*see also* Hypercalcemia) 275.42
low (*see also* Hypocalcemia) 275.41
deposits — *see also* Calcification, by site
in bursa 727.82

Calcium — continued
deposits — see also Calcification, by site — continued
in tendon (sheath) 727.82
with bursitis, synovitis or tenosynovitis 727.82
salts or soaps in vitreous 379.22
Calciuria 791.9
Calculi — see Calculus
Calculosis, intrahepatic — see Choledocholithiasis
Calculus, calculi, calculous 592.9
ampulla of Vater — see Choledocholithiasis
anuria (impacted) (recurrent) 592.0
appendix 543.9
bile duct (any) — see Choledocholithiasis
biliary — see Cholelithiasis
bilirubin, multiple — see Cholelithiasis
bladder (encysted) (impacted) (urinary) 594.1
diverticulum 594.0
bronchus 518.89
calyx (kidney) (renal) 592.0
congenital 753.3
cholesterol (pure) (solitary) — see Cholelithiasis
common duct (bile) — see Choledocholithiasis
conjunctiva 372.54
cystic 594.1
duct — see Cholelithiasis
dental 523.6
subgingival 523.6
supragingival 523.6
epididymis 608.89
gallbladder — see also Cholelithiasis
congenital 751.69
hepatic (duct) — see Choledocholithiasis
intestine (impaction) (obstruction) 560.39
kidney (impacted) (multiple) (pelvis) (recurrent) (staghorn) 592.0
congenital 753.3
lacrimal (passages) 375.57
liver (impacted) — see Choledocholithiasis
lung 518.89
nephritic (impacted) (recurrent) 592.0
nose 478.1
pancreas (duct) 577.8
parotid gland 527.5
pelvis, encysted 592.0
prostate 602.0
pulmonary 518.89
renal (impacted) (recurrent) 592.0
congenital 753.3
salivary (duct) (gland) 527.5
seminal vesicle 608.89
staghorn 592.0
Stensen's duct 527.5
sublingual duct or gland 527.5
congenital 750.26
submaxillary duct, gland, or region 527.5
suburethral 594.8
tonsil 474.8
tooth, teeth 523.6
tunica vaginalis 608.89
ureter (impacted) (recurrent) 592.1
urethra (impacted) 594.2
urinary (duct) (impacted) (passage) (tract) 592.9
lower tract NEC 594.9
specified site 594.8
vagina 623.8
vesical (impacted) 594.1
Wharton's duct 527.5
Caliectasis 593.89
California
disease 114.0
encephalitis 062.5
Caligo cornea 371.03
Callositas, callosity (infected) 700
Callus (infected) 700
bone 726.91
excessive, following fracture — see also Late, effect (of), fracture
Calvé (-Perthes) disease (osteochondrosis, femoral capital) 732.1
Calvities (see also Alopecia) 704.00
Cameroon fever (see also Malaria) 084.6
Camptocormia 300.11

Camptodactyly (congenital) 755.59
Camurati-Engelmann disease (diaphyseal sclerosis) 756.59
Canal — see condition
Canaliculitis (lacrimal) (acute) 375.31
Actinomyces 039.8
chronic 375.41
Canavan's disease 330.0
Cancer (M8000/3) — see also Neoplasm, by site, malignant

Note — The term "cancer" when modified by an adjective or adjectival phrase indicating a morphological type should be coded in the same manner as "carcinoma" with that adjective or phrase. Thus, "squamous-cell cancer" should be coded in the same manner as "squamous-cell carcinoma," which appears in the list under "Carcinoma."

bile duct type (M8160/3), liver 155.1
hepatocellular (M8170/3) 155.0
Cancerous (M8000/3) — see Neoplasm, by site, malignant
Cancerphobia 300.29
Cancrum oris 528.1
Candidiasis, candidal 112.9
with pneumonia 112.4
balanitis 112.2
congenital 771.7
disseminated 112.5
endocarditis 112.81
esophagus 112.84
intertrigo 112.3
intestine 112.85
lung 112.4
meningitis 112.83
mouth 112.0
nails 112.3
neonatal 771.7
onychia 112.3
otitis externa 112.82
otomycosis 112.82
paronychia 112.3
perionyxis 112.3
pneumonia 112.4
pneumonitis 112.4
skin 112.3
specified site NEC 112.89
systemic 112.5
urogenital site NEC 112.2
vagina 112.1
vulva 112.1
vulvovaginitis 112.1
Candidiosis — see Candidiasis
Candiru infection or infestation 136.8
Canities (premature) 704.3
congenital 757.4
Canker (mouth) (sore) 528.2
rash 034.1
Cannabinosis 504
Canton fever 081.9
Cap
cradle 690.11
Capillariasis 127.5
Capillary — see condition
Caplan's syndrome 714.81
Caplan-Colinet syndrome 714.81
Capsule — see condition
Capsulitis (joint) 726.90
adhesive (shoulder) 726.0
hip 726.5
knee 726.60
labyrinthine 387.8
thyroid 245.9
wrist 726.4
Caput
crepitus 756.0
medusae 456.8
succedaneum 767.1
Carapata disease 087.1
Carate — see Pinta

Carboxyhemoglobinemia 986
Carbuncle 680.9
abdominal wall 680.2
ankle 680.6
anus 680.5
arm (any part, above wrist) 680.3
auditory canal, external 680.0
axilla 680.3
back (any part) 680.2
breast 680.2
buttock 680.5
chest wall 680.2
corpus cavernosum 607.2
ear (any part) (external) 680.0
eyelid 373.13
face (any part except eye) 680.0
finger (any) 680.4
flank 680.2
foot (any part) 680.7
forearm 680.3
genital organ (male) 608.4
gluteal (region) 680.5
groin 680.2
hand (any part) 680.4
head (any part except face) 680.8
heel 680.7
hip 680.6
kidney (see also Abscess, kidney) 590.2
knee 680.6
labia 616.4
lacrimal
gland (see also Dacryoadenitis) 375.00
passages (duct) (sac) (see also Dacryocystitis) 375.30
leg, any part except foot 680.6
lower extremity, any part except foot 680.6
malignant 022.0
multiple sites 680.9
neck 680.1
nose (external) (septum) 680.0
orbit, orbital 376.01
partes posteriores 680.5
pectoral region 680.2
penis 607.2
perineum 680.2
pinna 680.0
scalp (any part) 680.8
scrotum 608.4
seminal vesicle 608.0
shoulder 680.3
skin NEC 680.9
specified site NEC 680.8
spermatic cord 608.4
temple (region) 680.0
testis 608.4
thigh 680.6
thumb 680.4
toe (any) 680.7
trunk 680.2
tunica vaginalis 608.4
umbilicus 680.2
upper arm 680.3
urethra 597.0
vas deferens 608.4
vulva 616.4
wrist 680.4
Carbunculus (see also Carbuncle) 680.9
Carcinoid (tumor) (M8240/1) — see also Neoplasm, by site, uncertain behavior
and struma ovarii (M9091/1) 236.2
argentaffin (M8241/1) — see Neoplasm, by site, uncertain behavior
malignant (M8241/3) — see Neoplasm, by site, malignant
benign (M9091/0) 220
composite (M8244/3) — see Neoplasm, by site, malignant
goblet cell (M8243/3) — see Neoplasm, by site, malignant
malignant (M8240/3) — see Neoplasm, by site, malignant
nonargentaffin (M8242/1) — see also Neoplasm, by site, uncertain behavior
malignant (M8242/3) — see Neoplasm, by site, malignant
strumal (M9091/1) 236.2
syndrome (intestinal) (metastatic) 259.2

Carcinoid — *see also* Neoplasm, by site,
uncertain behavior — *continued*
type bronchial adenoma (M8240/3) — *see*
Neoplasm, lung, malignant
Carcinoidosis 259.2
Carcinoma (M8010/3) — *see also* Neoplasm, by
site, malignant

> Note — *Except where otherwise indicated,
> the morphological varieties of carcinoma in
> the list below should be coded by site as for
> "Neoplasm, malignant."*

with
apocrine metaplasia (M8573/3)
cartilaginous (and osseous) metaplasia
(M8571/3)
osseous (and cartilaginous) metaplasia
(M8571/3)
productive fibrosis (M8141/3)
spindle cell metaplasia (M8572/3)
squamous metaplasia (M8570/3)
acidophil (M8280/3)
specified site — *see* Neoplasm, by site,
malignant
unspecified site 194.3
acidophil-basophil, mixed (M8281/3)
specified site — *see* Neoplasm, by site,
malignant
unspecified site 194.3
acinar (cell) (M8550/3)
acinic cell (M8550/3)
adenocystic (M8200/3)
adenoid
cystic (M8200/3)
squamous cell (M8075/3)
adenosquamous (M8560/3)
adnexal (skin) (M8390/3) — *see* Neoplasm,
skin, malignant
adrenal cortical (M8370/3) 194.0
alveolar (M8251/3)
cell (M8250/3) — *see* Neoplasm, lung,
malignant
anaplastic type (M8021/3)
apocrine (M8401/3)
breast — *see* Neoplasm, breast, malignant
specified site NEC — *see* Neoplasm, skin,
malignant
unspecified site 173.9
basal cell (pigmented) (M8090/3) — *see also*
Neoplasm, skin, malignant
fibro-epithelial type (M8093/3) — *see*
Neoplasm, skin, malignant
morphea type (M8092/3) — *see* Neoplasm,
skin, malignant
multicentric (M8091/3) — *see* Neoplasm,
skin, malignant
basaloid (M8123/3)
basal-squamous cell, mixed (M8094/3) — *see*
Neoplasm, skin, malignant
basophil (M8300/3)
specified site — *see* Neoplasm, by site,
malignant
unspecified site 194.3
basophil-acidophil, mixed (M8281/3)
specified site — *see* Neoplasm, by site,
malignant
unspecified site 194.3
basosquamous (M8094/3) — *see* Neoplasm,
skin, malignant
bile duct type (M8160/3)
and hepatocellular, mixed (M8180/3) 155.0
liver 155.1
specified site NEC — *see* Neoplasm, by site,
malignant
unspecified site 155.1
branchial or branchiogenic 146.8
bronchial or bronchogenic — *see* Neoplasm,
lung, malignant
bronchiolar (terminal) (M8250/3) — *see*
Neoplasm, lung, malignant
bronchiolo-alveolar (M8250/3) — *see*
Neoplasm, lung, malignant
bronchogenic (epidermoid) 162.9
C cell (M8510/3)
specified site — *see* Neoplasm, by site,
malignant
unspecified site 193

Carcinoma — *see also* Neoplasm, by site,
malignant — *continued*
ceruminous (M8420/3) 173.2
chorionic (M9100/3)
specified site — *see* Neoplasm, by site,
malignant
unspecified site
female 181
male 186.9
chromophobe (M8270/3)
specified site — *see* Neoplasm, by site,
malignant
unspecified site 194.3
clear cell (mesonephroid type) (M8310/3)
cloacogenic (M8124/3)
specified site — *see* Neoplasm, by site,
malignant
unspecified site 154.8
colloid (M8480/3)
cribriform (M8201/3)
cylindroid type (M8200/3)
diffuse type (M8145/3)
specified site — *see* Neoplasm, by site,
malignant
unspecified site 151.9
duct (cell) (M8500/3)
with Paget's disease (M8541/3) — *see*
Neoplasm, breast, malignant
infiltrating (M8500/3)
specified site — *see* Neoplasm, by site,
malignant
unspecified site 174.9
ductal (M8500/3)
ductular, infiltrating (M8521/3)
embryonal (M9070/3)
and teratoma, mixed (M9081/3)
combined with choriocarcinoma (M9101/3)
— *see* Neoplasm, by site, malignant
infantile type (M9071/3)
liver 155.0
polyembryonal type (M9072/3)
endometrioid (M8380/3)
eosinophil (M8280/3)
specified site — *see* Neoplasm, by site,
malignant
unspecified site 194.3
epidermoid (M8070/3) — *see also* Carcinoma,
squamous cell
and adenocarcinoma, mixed (M8560/3)
in situ, Bowen's type (M8081/2) — *see*
Neoplasm, skin, in situ
intradermal — *see* Neoplasm, skin, in situ
fibroepithelial type basal cell (M8093/3) — *see*
Neoplasm, skin, malignant
follicular (M8330/3)
and papillary (mixed) (M8340/3) 193
moderately differentiated type (M8332/3)
193
pure follicle type (M8331/3) 193
specified site — *see* Neoplasm, by site,
malignant
trabecular type (M8332/3) 193
unspecified site 193
well differentiated type (M8331/3) 193
gelatinous (M8480/3)
giant cell (M8031/3)
and spindle cell (M8030/3)
granular cell (M8320/3)
granulosa cell (M8620/3) 183.0
hepatic cell (M8170/3) 155.0
hepatocellular (M8170/3) 155.0
and bile duct, mixed (M8180/3) 155.0
hepatocholangiolitic (M8180/3) 155.0
Hürthle cell (thyroid) 193
hypernephroid (M8311/3)
in
adenomatous
polyp (M8210/3)
polyposis coli (M8220/3) 153.9
pleomorphic adenoma (M8940/3)
polypoid adenoma (M8210/3)
situ (M8010/3) — *see* Carcinoma, in situ
tubular adenoma (M8210/3)
villous adenoma (M8261/3)
infiltrating duct (M8500/3)
with Paget's disease (M8541/3) — *see*
Neoplasm, breast, malignant

Carcinoma — *see also* Neoplasm, by site,
malignant — *continued*
infiltrating duct — *continued*
specified site — *see* Neoplasm, by site,
malignant
unspecified site 174.9
inflammatory (M8530/3)
specified site — *see* Neoplasm, by site,
malignant
unspecified site 174.9
in situ (M8010/2) — *see also* Neoplasm, by
site, in situ
epidermoid (M8070/2) — *see also* Neoplasm,
by site, in situ
with questionable stromal invasion
(M8076/2)
specified site — *see* Neoplasm, by site,
in situ
unspecified site 233.1
Bowen's type (M8081/2) — *see*
Neoplasm, skin, in situ
intraductal (M8500/2)
specified site — *see* Neoplasm, by site, in
situ
unspecified site 233.0
lobular (M8520/2)
specified site — *see* Neoplasm, by site, in
situ
unspecified site 233.0
papillary (M8050/2) — *see* Neoplasm, by
site, in situ
squamous cell (M8070/2) — *see also*
Neoplasm, by site, in situ
with questionable stromal invasion
(M8076/2)
specified site — *see* Neoplasm, by site,
in situ
unspecified site 233.1
transitional cell (M8120/2) — *see* Neoplasm,
by site, in situ
intestinal type (M8144/3)
specified site — *see* Neoplasm, by site,
malignant
unspecified site 151.9
intraductal (noninfiltrating) (M8500/2)
papillary (M8503/2)
specified site — *see* Neoplasm, by site, in
situ
unspecified site 233.0
specified site — *see* Neoplasm, by site, in
situ
unspecified site 233.0
intraepidermal (M8070/2) — *see also*
Neoplasm, skin, in situ
squamous cell, Bowen's type (M8081/2) —
see Neoplasm, skin, in situ
intraepithelial (M8010/2) — *see also* Neoplasm,
by site, in situ
squamous cell (M8072/2) — *see* Neoplasm,
by site, in situ
intraosseous (M9270/3) 170.1
upper jaw (bone) 170.0
islet cell (M8150/3)
and exocrine, mixed (M8154/3)
specified site — *see* Neoplasm, by site,
malignant
unspecified site 157.9
pancreas 157.4
specified site NEC — *see* Neoplasm, by site,
malignant
unspecified site 157.4
juvenile, breast (M8502/3) — *see* Neoplasm,
breast, malignant
Kulchitsky's cell (carcinoid tumor of intestine)
259.2
large cell (M8012/3)
squamous cell, nonkeratinizing type
(M8072/3)
Leydig cell (testis) (M8650/3)
specified site — *see* Neoplasm, by site,
malignant
unspecified site 186.9
female 183.0
male 186.9
liver cell (M8170/3) 155.0

Carcinoma — see also Neoplasm, by site,
   malignant — continued
   lobular (infiltrating) (M8520/3)
      non-infiltrating (M8520/3)
         specified site — see Neoplasm, by site, in
            situ
         unspecified site 233.0
      specified site — see Neoplasm, by site,
         malignant
      unspecified site 174.9
   lymphoepithelial (M8082/3)
   medullary (M8510/3)
      with
         amyloid stroma (M8511/3)
            specified site — see Neoplasm, by site,
               malignant
            unspecified site 193
         lymphoid stroma (M8512/3)
            specified site — see Neoplasm, by site,
               malignant
            unspecified site 174.9
   mesometanephric (M9110/3)
   mesonephric (M9110/3)
   metastatic (M8010/6) — see Metastasis, cancer
   metatypical (M8095/3) — see Neoplasm, skin,
      malignant
   morphea type basal cell (M8092/3) — see
      Neoplasm, skin, malignant
   mucinous (M8480/3)
   mucin-producing (M8481/3)
   mucin-secreting (M8481/3)
   mucoepidermoid (M8430/3)
   mucoid (M8480/3)
      cell (M8300/3)
         specified site — see Neoplasm, by site,
            malignant
         unspecified site 194.3
   mucous (M8480/3)
   nonencapsulated sclerosing (M8350/3) 193
   noninfiltrating
      intracystic (M8504/2) — see Neoplasm, by
         site, in situ
      intraductal (M8500/2)
         papillary (M8503/2)
            specified site — see Neoplasm, by site,
               in situ
            unspecified site 233.0
         specified site — see Neoplasm, by site, in
            situ
         unspecified site 233.0
      lobular (M8520/2)
         specified site — see Neoplasm, by site, in
            situ
         unspecified site 233.0
   oat cell (M8042/3)
      specified site — see Neoplasm, by site,
         malignant
      unspecified site 162.9
   odontogenic (M9270/3) 170.1
      upper jaw (bone) 170.0
   onocytic (M8290/3)
   oxyphilic (M8290/3)
   papillary (M8050/3)
      and follicular (mixed) (M8340/3) 193
      epidermoid (M8052/3)
      intraductal (noninfiltrating) (M8503/2)
         specified site — see Neoplasm, by site, in
            situ
         unspecified site 233.0
      serous (M8460/3)
         specified site — see Neoplasm, by site,
            malignant
         surface (M8461/3)
            specified site — see Neoplasm, by site,
               malignant
            unspecified site 183.0
         unspecified site 183.0
      squamous cell (M8052/3)
      transitional cell (M8130/3)
   papillocystic (M8450/3)
      specified site — see Neoplasm, by site,
         malignant
      unspecified site 183.0
   parafollicular cell (M8510/3)
      specified site — see Neoplasm, by site,
         malignant
      unspecified site 193

Carcinoma — see also Neoplasm, by site,
   malignant — continued
   pleomorphic (M8022/3)
   polygonal cell (M8034/3)
   prickle cell (M8070/3)
   pseudoglandular, squamous cell (M8075/3)
   pseudomucinous (M8470/3)
      specified site — see Neoplasm, by site,
         malignant
      unspecified site 183.0
   pseudosarcomatous (M8033/3)
   regaud type (M8082/3) — see Neoplasm,
      nasopharynx, malignant
   renal cell (M8312/3) 189.0
   reserve cell (M8041/3)
   round cell (M8041/3)
   Schmincke (M8082/3) — see Neoplasm,
      nasopharynx, malignant
   Schneiderian (M8121/3)
      specified site — see Neoplasm, by site,
         malignant
      unspecified site 160.0
   scirrhous (M8141/3)
   sebaceous (M8410/3) — see Neoplasm, skin,
      malignant
   secondary (M8010/6) — see Neoplasm, by site,
      malignant, secondary
   secretory, breast (M8502/3) — see Neoplasm,
      breast, malignant
   serous (M8441/3)
      papillary (M8460/3)
         specified site — see Neoplasm, by site,
            malignant
         unspecified site 183.0
      surface, papillary (M8461/3)
         specified site — see Neoplasm, by site,
            malignant
         unspecified site 183.0
   Sertoli cell (M8640/3)
      specified site — see Neoplasm, by site,
         malignant
      unspecified site 186.9
   signet ring cell (M8490/3)
      metastatic (M8490/6) — see Neoplasm, by
         site, secondary
   simplex (M8231/3)
   skin appendage (M8390/3) — see Neoplasm,
      skin, malignant
   small cell (M8041/3)
      fusiform cell type (M8043/3)
      squamous cell, non-keratinizing type
         (M8073/3)
   solid (M8230/3)
      with amyloid stroma (M8511/3)
         specified site — see Neoplasm, by site,
            malignant
         unspecified site 193
   spheroidal cell (M8035/3)
   spindle cell (M8032/3)
      and giant cell (M8030/3)
   spinous cell (M8070/3)
   squamous (cell) (M8070/3)
      adenoid type (M8075/3)
      and adenocarcinoma, mixed (M8560/3)
      intraepidermal, Bowen's type — see
         Neoplasm, skin, in situ
      keratinizing type (large cell) (M8071/3)
      large cell, non-keratinizing type (M8072/3)
      microinvasive (M8076/3)
         specified site — see Neoplasm, by site,
            malignant
         unspecified site 180.9
      non-keratinizing type (M8072/3)
      papillary (M8052/3)
      pseudoglandular (M8075/3)
      small cell, non-keratinizing type (M8073/3)
      spindle cell type (M8074/3)
      verrucous (M805l/3)
   superficial spreading (M8143/3)
   sweat gland (M8400/3) — see Neoplasm, skin,
      malignant
   theca cell (M8600/3) 183.0
   thymic (M8580/3) 164.0
   trabecular (M8190/3)
   transitional (cell) (M8120/3)
      papillary (M8130/3)
      spindle cell type (M8122/3)

Carcinoma — see also Neoplasm, by site,
   malignant — continued
   tubular (M8211/3)
   undifferentiated type (M8020/3)
   urothelial (M8120/3)
   ventriculi 151.9
   verrucous (epidermoid) (squamous cell)
      (M8051/3)
   villous (M8262/3)
   water-clear cell (M8322/3) 194.1
   wolffian duct (M9110/3)
Carcinomaphobia 300.29
Carcinomatosis
   peritonei (M8010/6) 197.6
   specified site NEC (M8010/3) — see Neoplasm,
      by site, malignant
   unspecified site (M8010/6) 199.0
Carcinosarcoma (M8980/3) — see also Neoplasm,
   by site, malignant
   embryonal type (M8981/3) — see Neoplasm, by
      site, malignant
Cardia, cardial — see condition
Cardiac — see also condition
   death — see Disease, heart
   device
      defibrillator, automatic implantable V45.02
      in situ NEC V45.00
      pacemaker
         cardiac
            fitting or adjustment V53.31
            in situ V45.01
         carotid sinus
            fitting or adjustment V53.39
            in situ V45.09
   pacemaker — see Cardiac, device, pacemaker
   tamponade 423.9
Cardialgia (see also Pain, precordial) 786.51
Cardiectasis — see Hypertrophy, cardiac
Cardiochalasia 530.81
Cardiomalacia (see also Degeneration,
   myocardial) 429.1
Cardiomegalia glycogenica diffusa 271.0
Cardiomegaly (see also Hypertrophy, cardiac)
   429.3
   congenital 746.89
   glycogen 271.0
   hypertensive (see also Hypertension, heart)
      402.90
   idiopathic 429.3
Cardiomyoliposis (see also Degeneration,
   myocardial) 429.1
Cardiomyopathy (congestive) (constrictive)
   (familial) (infiltrative) (obstructive)
   (restrictive) (sporadic) 425.4
   alcoholic 425.5
   amyloid 277.3 [425.7]
   beriberi 265.0 [425.7]
   cobalt-beer 425.5
   congenital 425.3
   due to
      amyloidosis 277.3 [425.7]
      beriberi 265.0 [425.7]
      cardiac glycogenosis 271.0 [425.7]
      Chagas' disease 086.0
      Friedreich's ataxia 334.0 [425.8]
      hypertension —see Hypertension, with,
         heart involvement
      mucopolysaccharidosis 277.5 [425.7]
      myotonia atrophica 359.2 [425.8]
      progressive muscular dystrophy 359.1
         [425.8]
      sarcoidosis 135 [425.8]
   glycogen storage 271.0 [425.7]
   hypertensive — see Hypertension, with, heart
      involvement
   hypertrophic
      nonobstructive 425.4
      obstructive 425.1
         congenital 746.84
   idiopathic (concentric) 425.4
   in
      Chagas' disease 086.0
      sarcoidosis 135 [425.8]
   ischemic 414.8

Cardiomyopathy — *continued*
metabolic NEC 277.9 *[425.7]*
amyloid 277.3 *[425.7]*
thyrotoxic (*see also* Thyrotoxicosis)
242.9 ✓5ᵗʰ *[425.7]*
thyrotoxicosis (*see also* Thyrotoxicosis)
242.9 ✓5ᵗʰ *[425.7]*
nutritional 269.9 *[425.7]*
beriberi 265.0 *[425.7]*
obscure of Africa 425.2
postpartum 674.8 ✓5ᵗʰ
primary 425.4
secondary 425.9
thyrotoxic (*see also* Thyrotoxicosis) 242.9 ✓5ᵗʰ
[425.7]
toxic NEC 425.9
tuberculous (*see also* Tuberculosis) 017.9 ✓5ᵗʰ
[425.8]
Cardionephritis — *see* Hypertension, cardiorenal
Cardionephropathy — *see* Hypertension,
cardiorenal
Cardionephrosis — *see* Hypertension, cardiorenal
Cardioneurosis 306.2
Cardiopathia nigra 416.0
Cardiopathy (*see also* Disease, heart) 429.9
hypertensive (*see also* Hypertension, heart)
402.90
idiopathic 425.4
mucopolysaccharidosis 277.5 *[425.7]*
Cardiopericarditis (*see also* Pericarditis) 423.9
Cardiophobia 300.29
Cardioptosis 746.87
Cardiorenal — *see* condition
Cardiorrhexis (*see also* Infarct, myocardium)
410.9 ✓5ᵗʰ
Cardiosclerosis — *see* Arteriosclerosis, coronary
Cardiosis — *see* Disease, heart
Cardiospasm (esophagus) (reflex) (stomach) 530.0
congenital 750.7
Cardiostenosis — *see* Disease, heart
Cardiosymphysis 423.1
Cardiothyrotoxicosis — *see* Hyperthyroidism
Cardiovascular — *see* condition
Carditis (acute) (bacterial) (chronic) (subacute)
429.89
Coxsackie 074.20
hypertensive (*see also* Hypertension, heart)
402.90
meningococcal 036.40
rheumatic — *see* Disease, heart, rheumatic
rheumatoid 714.2
Care (of)
child (routine) V20.1
convalescent following V66.9
chemotherapy V66.2
medical NEC V66.5
psychotherapy V66.3
radiotherapy V66.1
surgery V66.0
surgical NEC V66.0
treatment (for) V66.5
combined V66.6
fracture V66.4
mental disorder NEC V66.3
specified type NEC V66.5
end-of-life V66.7
family member (handicapped) (sick)
creating problem for family V61.49
provided away from home for holiday relief
V60.5
unavailable, due to
absence (person rendering care) (sufferer)
V60.4
inability (any reason) of person rendering
care V60.4
holiday relief V60.5
hospice V66.7
lack of (at or after birth) (infant) (child) 995.52
adult 995.84
lactation of mother V24.1
palliative V66.7
postpartum
immediately after delivery V24.0
routine follow-up V24.2

Care (of) — *continued*
prenatal V22.1
first pregnancy V22.0
high risk pregnancy V23.9
specified problem NEC V23.89
terminal V66.7
unavailable, due to
absence of person rendering care V60.4
inability (any reason) of person rendering
care V60.4
well baby V20.1
Caries (bone) (*see also* Tuberculosis, bone)
015.9 ✓5ᵗʰ *[730.8]* ✓5ᵗʰ
arrested 521.04
cementum 521.03
cerebrospinal (tuberculous) 015.0 ✓5ᵗʰ *[730.88]*
dental (acute) (chronic) (incipient) (infected)
521.09
with pulp exposure 521.03
extending to
dentine 521.02
pulp 521.03
other specified NEC 521.09
dentin (acute) (chronic) 521.02
enamel (acute) (chronic) (incipient) 521.01
external meatus 380.89
hip (*see also* Tuberculosis) 015.1 ✓5ᵗʰ *[730.85]*
knee 015.2 ✓5ᵗʰ *[730.86]*
labyrinth 386.8
limb NEC 015.7 ✓5ᵗʰ *[730.88]*
mastoid (chronic) (process) 383.1
middle ear 385.89
nose 015.7 ✓5ᵗʰ *[730.88]*
orbit 015.7 ✓5ᵗʰ *[730.88]*
ossicle 385.24
petrous bone 383.20
sacrum (tuberculous) 015.0 ✓5ᵗʰ *[730.88]*
spine, spinal (column) (tuberculous) 015.0 ✓5ᵗʰ
[730.88]
syphilitic 095.5
congenital 090.0 *[730.8]* ✓5ᵗʰ
teeth (internal) 521.00
initial 521.01
vertebra (column) (tuberculous) 015.0 ✓5ᵗʰ
[730.88]
Carini's syndrome (ichthyosis congenita) 757.1
Carious teeth 521.00
Carneous mole 631
Carnosinemia 270.5
Carotid body or sinus syndrome 337.0
Carotidynia 337.0
Carotinemia (dietary) 278.3
Carotinosis (cutis) (skin) 278.3
Carpal tunnel syndrome 354.0
Carpenter's syndrome 759.89
Carpopedal spasm (*see also* Tetany) 781.7
Carpoptosis 736.05
Carrier (suspected) **of**
amebiasis V02.2
bacterial disease (meningococcal,
staphylococcal, streptococcal) NEC
V02.59
cholera V02.0
cystic fibrosis gene V83.81 ●
defective gene V83.89 ▲
diphtheria V02.4
dysentery (bacillary) V02.3
amebic V02.2
Endamoeba histolytica V02.2
gastrointestinal pathogens NEC V02.3
genetic defect V83.89 ▲
gonorrhea V02.7
group B streptococcus V02.51
HAA (hepatitis Australian-antigen) V02.61
hemophilia A (asymptomatic) V83.01
symptomatic V83.02
hepatitis V02.60
Australian-antigen (HAA) V02.61
B V02.61
C V02.62
serum V02.61
specified type NEC V02.69
viral V02.60
infective organism NEC V02.9
malaria V02.9

Carrier (suspected) **of** — *continued*
paratyphoid V02.3
Salmonella V02.3
typhosa V02.1
serum hepatitis V02.61
Shigella V02.3
Staphylococcus NEC V02.59
Streptococcus NEC V02.52
group B V02.51
typhoid V02.1
venereal disease NEC V02.8
Carrión's disease (Bartonellosis) 088.0
Car sickness 994.6
Carter's
relapsing fever (Asiatic) 087.0
Cartilage — *see* condition
Caruncle (inflamed)
abscess, lacrimal (*see also* Dacryocystitis)
375.30
conjunctiva 372.00
acute 372.00
eyelid 373.00
labium (majus) (minus) 616.8
lacrimal 375.30
urethra (benign) 599.3
vagina (wall) 616.8
Cascade stomach 537.6
Caseation lymphatic gland (*see also*
Tuberculosis) 017.2 ✓5ᵗʰ
Caseous
bronchitis — *see* Tuberculosis, pulmonary
meningitis 013.0 ✓5ᵗʰ
pneumonia — *see* Tuberculosis, pulmonary
Cassidy (-Scholte) syndrome (malignant
carcinoid) 259.2
Castellani's bronchitis 104.8
Castleman's tumor or lymphoma (mediastinal
lymph node hyperplasia) 785.6
Castration, traumatic 878.2
complicated 878.3
Casts in urine 791.7
Cat's ear 744.29
Catalepsy 300.11
catatonic (acute) (*see also* Schizophrenia)
295.2 ✓5ᵗʰ
hysterical 300.11
schizophrenic (*see also* Schizophrenia)
295.2 ✓5ᵗʰ
Cataphasia 307.0
Cataplexy (idiopathic) 347
Cataract (anterior cortical) (anterior polar) (black)
(capsular) (central) (cortical) (hypermature)
(immature) (incipient) (mature) 366.9
anterior
and posterior axial embryonal 743.33
pyramidal 743.31
subcapsular polar
infantile, juvenile, or presenile 366.01
senile 366.13
associated with
calcinosis 275.40 *[366.42]*
craniofacial dysostosis 756.0 *[366.44]*
galactosemia 271.1 *[366.44]*
hypoparathyroidism 252.1 *[366.42]*
myotonic disorders 359.2 *[366.43]*
neovascularization 366.33
blue dot 743.39
cerulean 743.39
complicated NEC 366.30
congenital 743.30
capsular or subcapsular 743.31
cortical 743.32
nuclear 743.33
specified type NEC 743.39
total or subtotal 743.34
zonular 743.32
coronary (congenital) 743.39
acquired 366.12
cupuliform 366.14
diabetic 250.5 ✓5ᵗʰ *[366.41]*
drug-induced 366.45
due to
chalcosis 360.24 *[366.34]*

Cataract — *continued*
 due to — *continued*
   chronic choroiditis (*see also* Choroiditis)
    363.20 *[366.32]*
   degenerative myopia 360.21 *[366.34]*
   glaucoma (*see also* Glaucoma) 365.9
    [366.31]
   infection, intraocular NEC 366.32
   inflammatory ocular disorder NEC 366.32
   iridocyclitis, chronic 364.10 *[366.33]*
   pigmentary retinal dystrophy 362.74
    [366.34]
   radiation 366.46
 electric 366.46
 glassblowers' 366.46
 heat ray 366.46
 heterochromic 366.33
 in eye disease NEC 366.30
 infantile (*see also* Cataract, juvenile) 366.00
 intumescent 366.12
 irradiational 366.46
 juvenile 366.00
   anterior subcapsular polar 366.01
   combined forms 366.09
   cortical 366.03
   lamellar 366.03
   nuclear 366.04
   posterior subcapsular polar 366.02
   specified NEC 366.09
   zonular 366.03
 lamellar 743.32
   infantile, juvenile, or presenile 366.03
 morgagnian 366.18
 myotonic 359.2 *[366.43]*
 myxedema 244.9 *[366.44]*
 nuclear 366.16
 posterior, polar (capsular) 743.31
   infantile, juvenile, or presenile 366.02
   senile 366.14
 presenile (*see also* Cataract, juvenile) 366.00
 punctate
   acquired 366.12
   congenital 743.39
 secondary (membrane) 366.50
   obscuring vision 366.53
   specified type, not obscuring vision 366.52
 senile 366.10
   anterior subcapsular polar 366.13
   combined forms 366.19
   cortical 366.15
   hypermature 366.18
   immature 366.12
   incipient 366.12
   mature 366.17
   nuclear 366.16
   posterior subcapsular polar 366.14
   specified NEC 366.19
   total or subtotal 366.17
 snowflake 250.5 ✔5ᵗʰ *[366.41]*
 specified NEC 366.8
 subtotal (senile) 366.17
   congenital 743.34
 sunflower 360.24 *[366.34]*
 tetanic NEC 252.1 *[366.42]*
 total (mature) (senile) 366.17
   congenital 743.34
   localized 366.21
   traumatic 366.22
 toxic 366.45
 traumatic 366.20
   partially resolved 366.23
   total 366.22
 zonular (perinuclear) 743.32
   infantile, juvenile, or presenile 366.03
Cataracta 366.10
 brunescens 366.16
 cerulea 743.39
 complicata 366.30
 congenita 743.30
 coralliformis 743.39
 coronaria (congenital) 743.39
   acquired 366.12
 diabetic 250.5 ✔5ᵗʰ *[366.41]*
 floriformis 360.24 *[366.34]*
 membranacea
   accreta 366.50
   congenita 743.39
 nigra 366.16

Catarrh, catarrhal (inflammation) (*see also*
   condition) 460
 acute 460
 asthma, asthmatic (*see also* Asthma) 493.9 ✔5ᵗʰ
 Bostock's (*see also* Fever, hay) 477.9
 bowel — *see* Enteritis
 bronchial 490
   acute 466.0
   chronic 491.0
   subacute 466.0
 cervix, cervical (canal) (uteri) — *see* Cervicitis
 chest (*see also* Bronchitis) 490
 chronic 472.0
 congestion 472.0
 conjunctivitis 372.03
 due to syphilis 095.9
   congenital 090.0
 enteric — *see* Enteritis
 epidemic 487.1
 Eustachian 381.50
 eye (acute) (vernal) 372.03
 fauces (*see also* Pharyngitis) 462
 febrile 460
 fibrinous acute 466.0
 gastroenteric — *see* Enteritis
 gastrointestinal — *see* Enteritis
 gingivitis 523.0
 hay (*see also* Fever, hay) 477.9
 infectious 460
 intestinal — *see* Enteritis
 larynx (*see also* Laryngitis, chronic) 476.0
 liver 070.1
   with hepatic coma 070.0
 lung (*see also* Bronchitis) 490
   acute 466.0
   chronic 491.0
 middle ear (chronic) — *see* Otitis media,
   chronic
 mouth 528.0
 nasal (chronic) (*see also* Rhinitis) 472.0
   acute 460
 nasobronchial 472.2
 nasopharyngeal (chronic) 472.2
   acute 460
 nose — *see* Catarrh, nasal
 ophthalmia 372.03
 pneumococcal, acute 466.0
 pulmonary (*see also* Bronchitis) 490
   acute 466.0
   chronic 491.0
 spring (eye) 372.13
 suffocating (*see also* Asthma) 493.9 ✔5ᵗʰ
 summer (hay) (*see also* Fever, hay) 477.9
 throat 472.1
 tracheitis 464.10
   with obstruction 464.11
 tubotympanal 381.4
   acute (*see also* Otitis media, acute,
    nonsuppurative) 381.00
   chronic 381.10
 vasomotor (*see also* Fever, hay) 477.9
 vesical (bladder) — *see* Cystitis
Catarrhus aestivus (*see also* Fever, hay) 477.9
Catastrophe, cerebral (*see also* Disease,
   cerebrovascular, acute) 436
Catatonia, catatonic (acute) 781.99
 with
   affective psychosis — *see* Psychosis,
    affective
 agitation 295.2 ✔5ᵗʰ
 Churg-Strauss syndrome 446.4
 dementia (praecox) 295.2 ✔5ᵗʰ
 due to or associated with physical condition
   293.89
 excitation 295.2 ✔5ᵗʰ
 excited type 295.2 ✔5ᵗʰ
 schizophrenia 295.2 ✔5ᵗʰ
 stupor 295.2 ✔5ᵗʰ
Cat-scratch — *see also* Injury, superficial disease
   or fever 078.3
Cauda equina — *see also* condition
 syndrome 344.60
Cauliflower ear 738.7
Caul over face 768.9

Causalgia 355.9
 lower limb 355.71
 upper limb 354.4
Cause
 external, general effects NEC 994.9
 not stated 799.9
 unknown 799.9
Caustic burn — *see also* Burn, by site
 from swallowing caustic or corrosive substance
   — *see* Burn, internal organs
Cavare's disease (familial periodic paralysis)
   359.3
Cave-in, injury
 crushing (severe) (*see also* Crush, by site)
   869.1
 suffocation 994.7
Cavernitis (penis) 607.2
 lymph vessel — *see* Lymphangioma
Cavernositis 607.2
Cavernous — *see* condition
Cavitation of lung (*see also* Tuberculosis)
   011.2 ✔5ᵗʰ
 nontuberculous 518.89
 primary, progressive 010.8 ✔5ᵗʰ
Cavity
 lung — *see* Cavitation of lung
 optic papilla 743.57
 pulmonary — *see* Cavitation of lung
 teeth 521.00
 vitreous (humor) 379.21
Cavovarus foot, congenital 754.59
Cavus foot (congenital) 754.71
 acquired 736.73
Cazenave's
 disease (pemphigus) NEC 694.4
 lupus (erythematosus) 695.4
Cecitis — *see* Appendicitis
Cecocele — *see* Hernia
Cecum — *see* condition
Celiac
 artery compression syndrome 447.4
 disease 579.0
 infantilism 579.0
Cell, cellular — *see also* condition
 anterior chamber (eye) (positive aqueous ray)
   364.04
Cellulitis (diffuse) (with lymphangitis) (*see also*
   Abscess) 682.9
 abdominal wall 682.2
 anaerobic (*see also* Gas gangrene) 040.0
 ankle 682.6
 anus 566
 areola 611.0
 arm (any part, above wrist) 682.3
 auditory canal (external) 380.10
 axilla 682.3
 back (any part) 682.2
 breast 611.0
   postpartum 675.1 ✔5ᵗʰ
 broad ligament (*see also* Disease, pelvis,
   inflammatory) 614.4
   acute 614.3
 buttock 682.5
 cervical (neck region) 682.1
 cervix (uteri) (*see also* Cervicitis) 616.0
 cheek, external 682.0
   internal 528.3
 chest wall 682.2
 chronic NEC 682.9
 corpus cavernosum 607.2
 digit 681.9
 Douglas' cul-de-sac or pouch (chronic) (*see also*
   Disease, pelvis, inflammatory) 614.4
   acute 614.3
 drainage site (following operation) 998.59
 ear, external 380.10
 enterostomy 569.61
 erysipelar (*see also* Erysipelas) 035
 eyelid 373.13
 face (any part, except eye) 682.0
 finger (intrathecal) (periosteal) (subcutaneous)
   (subcuticular) 681.00
 flank 682.2
 foot (except toe) 682.7

Cellulitis (*see also* Abscess) — *continued*
  forearm 682.3
  gangrenous (*see also* Gangrene) 785.4
  genital organ NEC
      female — *see* Abscess, genital organ, female
      male 608.4
  glottis 478.71
  gluteal (region) 682.5
  gonococcal NEC 098.0
  groin 682.2
  hand (except finger or thumb) 682.4
  head (except face) NEC 682.8
  heel 682.7
  hip 682.6
  jaw (region) 682.0
  knee 682.6
  labium (majus) (minus) (*see also* Vulvitis) 616.10
  larynx 478.71
  leg, except foot 682.6
  lip 528.5
  mammary gland 611.0
  mouth (floor) 528.3
  multiple sites NEC 682.9
  nasopharynx 478.21
  navel 682.2
      newborn NEC 771.4
  neck (region) 682.1
  nipple 611.0
  nose 478.1
      external 682.0
  orbit, orbital 376.01
  palate (soft) 528.3
  pectoral (region) 682.2
  pelvis, pelvic
      with
          abortion — *see* Abortion, by type, with sepsis
          ectopic pregnancy (*see also* categories 633.0— 633.9) 639.0
          molar pregnancy (*see also* categories 630— 632) 639.0
      female (*see also* Disease, pelvis, inflammatory) 614.4
          acute 614.3
      following
          abortion 639.0
          ectopic or molar pregnancy 639.0
      male (*see also* Abscess, peritoneum) 567.2
      puerperal, postpartum, childbirth 670 ☑4ᵗʰ
  penis 607.2
  perineal, perineum 682.2
  perirectal 566
  peritonsillar 475
  periurethral 597.0
  periuterine (*see also* Disease, pelvis, inflammatory) 614.4
      acute 614.3
  pharynx 478.21
  phlegmonous NEC 682.9
  rectum 566
  retromammary 611.0
  retroperitoneal (*see also* Peritonitis) 567.2
  round ligament (*see also* Disease, pelvis, inflammatory) 614.4
      acute 614.3
  scalp (any part) 682.8
      dissecting 704.8
  scrotum 608.4
  septic NEC 682.9
  shoulder 682.3
  specified sites NEC 682.8
  spermatic cord 608.4
  submandibular (region) (space) (triangle) 682.0
      gland 527.3
  submaxillary 528.3
      gland 527.3
  submental (pyogenic) 682.0
      gland 527.3
  suppurative NEC 682.9
  testis 608.4
  thigh 682.6
  thumb (intrathecal) (periosteal) (subcutaneous) (subcuticular) 681.00
  toe (intrathecal) (periosteal) (subcutaneous) (subcuticular) 681.10

Cellulitis (*see also* Abscess) — *continued*
  tonsil 475
  trunk 682.2
  tuberculous (primary) (*see also* Tuberculosis) 017.0 ☑5ᵗʰ
  tunica vaginalis 608.4
  umbilical 682.2
      newborn NEC 771.4
  vaccinal 999.3
  vagina — *see* Vaginitis
  vas deferens 608.4
  vocal cords 478.5
  vulva (*see also* Vulvitis) 616.10
  wrist 682.4
Cementoblastoma, benign (M9273/0) 213.1
  upper jaw (bone) 213.0
Cementoma (M9273/0) 213.1
  gigantiform (M9276/0) 213.1
      upper jaw (bone) 213.0
  upper jaw (bone) 213.0
Cementoperiostitis 523.4
Cephalgia, cephalagia (*see also* Headache) 784.0
  histamine 346.2 ☑5ᵗʰ
  nonorganic origin 307.81
  psychogenic 307.81
  tension 307.81
Cephalhematocele, cephalematocele
  due to birth injury 767.1
  fetus or newborn 767.1
  traumatic (*see also* Contusion, head) 920
Cephalhematoma, cephalematoma (calcified)
  due to birth injury 767.1
  fetus or newborn 767.1
  traumatic (*see also* Contusion, head) 920
Cephalic — *see* condition
Cephalitis — *see* Encephalitis
Cephalocele 742.0
Cephaloma — *see* Neoplasm, by site, malignant
Cephalomenia 625.8
Cephalopelvic — *see* condition
Cercomoniasis 007.3
Cerebellitis — *see* Encephalitis
Cerebellum (cerebellar) — *see* condition
Cerebral — *see* condition
Cerebritis — *see* Encephalitis
Cerebrohepatorenal syndrome 759.89
Cerebromacular degeneration 330.1
Cerebromalacia (*see also* Softening, brain) 434.9 ☑5ᵗʰ
Cerebrosidosis 272.7
Cerebrospasticity — *see* Palsy, cerebral
Cerebrospinal — *see* condition
Cerebrum — *see* condition
Ceroid storage disease 272.7
Cerumen (accumulation) (impacted) 380.4
Cervical — *see also* condition
  auricle 744.43
  rib 756.2
Cervicalgia 723.1
Cervicitis (acute) (chronic) (nonvenereal) (subacute) (with erosion or ectropion) 616.0
  with
      abortion — *see* Abortion, by type, with sepsis
      ectopic pregnancy (*see also* categories 633.0-633.9) 639.0
      molar pregnancy (*see also* categories 630-632) 639.0
      ulceration 616.0
  chlamydial 099.53
  complicating pregnancy or puerperium 646.6 ☑5ᵗʰ
      affecting fetus or newborn 760.8
  following
      abortion 639.0
      ectopic or molar pregnancy 639.0
  gonococcal (acute) 098.15
      chronic or duration of 2 months or more 098.35
  senile (atrophic) 616.0
  syphilitic 095.8
  trichomonal 131.09

Cervicitis — *continued*
  tuberculous (*see also* Tuberculosis) 016.7 ☑5ᵗʰ
Cervicoaural fistula 744.49
Cervicocolpitis (emphysematosa) (*see also* Cervicitis) 616.0
Cervix — *see* condition
Cesarean delivery, operation or section NEC 669.7 ☑5ᵗʰ
  affecting fetus or newborn 763.4
  post mortem, affecting fetus or newborn 761.6
  previous, affecting management of pregnancy 654.2 ☑5ᵗʰ
Céstan's syndrome 344.89
Céstan-Chenais paralysis 344.89
Céstan-Raymond syndrome 433.8 ☑5ᵗʰ
Cestode infestation NEC 123.9
  specified type NEC 123.8
Cestodiasis 123.9
Chabert's disease 022.9
Chacaleh 266.2
Chafing 709.8
Chagas' disease (*see also* Trypanosomiasis, American) 086.2
  with heart involvement 086.0
Chagres fever 084.0
Chalasia (cardiac sphincter) 530.81
Chalazion 373.2
Chalazoderma 757.39
Chalcosis 360.24
  cornea 371.15
  crystalline lens 360.24 [366.34]
  retina 360.24
Chalicosis (occupational) (pulmonum) 502
Chancre (any genital site) (hard) (indurated) (infecting) (primary) (recurrent) 091.0
  congenital 090.0
  conjunctiva 091.2
  Ducrey's 099.0
  extragenital 091.2
  eyelid 091.2
  Hunterian 091.0
  lip (syphilis) 091.2
  mixed 099.8
  nipple 091.2
  Nisbet's 099.0
  of
      carate 103.0
      pinta 103.0
      yaws 102.0
  palate, soft 091.2
  phagedenic 099.0
  Ricord's 091.0
  Rollet's (syphilitic) 091.0
  seronegative 091.0
  seropositive 091.0
  simple 099.0
  soft 099.0
      bubo 099.0
  urethra 091.0
  yaws 102.0
Chancriform syndrome 114.1
Chancroid 099.0
  anus 099.0
  penis (Ducrey's bacillus) 099.0
  perineum 099.0
  rectum 099.0
  scrotum 099.0
  urethra 099.0
  vulva 099.0
Chandipura fever 066.8
Chandler's disease (osteochondritis dissecans, hip) 732.7
Change(s) (of) — *see also* Removal of
  arteriosclerotic — *see* Arteriosclerosis
  battery
      cardiac pacemaker V53.31
  bone 733.90
      diabetic 250.8 ☑5ᵗʰ [731.8]
      in disease, unknown cause 733.90
  bowel habits 787.99

Change(s) (of) — *see also* Removal of — *continued*
  cardiorenal (vascular) (*see also* Hypertension, cardiorenal) 404.90
  cardiovascular — *see* Disease, cardiovascular
  circulatory 459.9
  cognitive or personality change of other type, nonpsychotic 310.1
  color, teeth, tooth
    during formation 520.8
    posteruptive 521.7
  contraceptive device V25.42
  cornea, corneal
    degenerative NEC 371.40
    membrane NEC 371.30
    senile 371.41
  coronary (*see also* Ischemia, heart) 414.9
  degenerative
    chamber angle (anterior) (iris) 364.56
    ciliary body 364.57
    spine or vertebra (*see also* Spondylosis) 721.90
  dental pulp, regressive 522.2
  dressing V58.3
  fixation device V54.89 ▲
    external V54.89 ▲
    internal V54.0
  heart — *see also* Disease, heart
  hip joint 718.95
  hyperplastic larynx 478.79
  hypertrophic
    nasal sinus (*see also* Sinusitis) 473.9
    turbinate, nasal 478.0
    upper respiratory tract 478.9
  inflammatory — *see* Inflammation
  joint (*see also* Derangement, joint) 718.90
    sacroiliac 724.6
  Kirschner wire V54.89 ▲
  knee 717.9
  macular, congenital 743.55
  malignant (M—— /3) — *see also* Neoplasm, by site, malignant

> Note — for malignant change occurring in a neoplasm, use the appropriate M code with behavior digit /3 e.g., malignant change in uterine fibroid — M8890/3. For malignant change occurring in a nonneoplastic condition (e.g., gastric ulcer) use the M code M8000/3.

  mental (status) NEC 780.99 ▲
    due to or associated with physical condition — *see* Syndrome, brain
  myocardium, myocardial — *see* Degeneration, myocardial
  of life (*see also* Menopause) 627.2
  pacemaker battery (cardiac) V53.31
  peripheral nerve 355.9
  personality (nonpsychotic) NEC 310.1
  plaster cast V54.89 ▲
  refractive, transient 367.81
  regressive, dental pulp 522.2
  retina 362.9
    myopic (degenerative) (malignant) 360.21
    vascular appearance 362.13
  sacroiliac joint 724.6
  scleral 379.19
    degenerative 379.16
  senile (*see also* Senility) 797
  sensory (*see also* Disturbance, sensation) 782.0
  skin texture 782.8
  spinal cord 336.9
  splint, external V54.89 ▲
  subdermal implantable contraceptive V25.5
  suture V58.3
  traction device V54.89 ▲
  trophic 355.9
    arm NEC 354.9
    leg NEC 355.8
    lower extremity NEC 355.8
    upper extremity NEC 354.9
  vascular 459.9
  vasomotor 443.9
  voice 784.49
    psychogenic 306.1

Changing sleep-work schedule, affecting sleep 307.45

Changuinola fever 066.0

Chapping skin 709.8

Character
  depressive 301.12

Charcôt's
  arthropathy 094.0 [713.5]
  cirrhosis — *see* Cirrhosis, biliary
  disease 094.0
    spinal cord 094.0
  fever (biliary) (hepatic) (intermittent) — *see* Choledocholithiasis
  joint (disease) 094.0 [713.5]
    diabetic 250.6 ✓5ᵗʰ [713.5]
    syringomyelic 336.0 [713.5]
  syndrome (intermittent claudication) 443.9
    due to atherosclerosis 440.21

Charcôt-Marie-Tooth disease, paralysis, or syndrome 356.1

Charleyhorse (quadriceps) 843.8
  muscle, except quadriceps — *see* Sprain, by site

Charlouis' disease (*see also* Yaws) 102.9

Chauffeur's fracture — *see* Fracture, ulna, lower end

Cheadle (-Möller) (-Barlow) disease or syndrome (infantile scurvy) 267

Checking (of)
  contraceptive device (intrauterine) V25.42
  device
    fixation V54.89
      external V54.89 ▲
      internal V54.0
    traction V54.89 ▲
    Kirschner wire V54.89 ▲
    plaster cast V54.89 ▲
    splint, external V54.89 ▲

Checkup
  following treatment — *see* Examination
  health V70.0
  infant (not sick) V20.2
  pregnancy (normal) V22.1
    first V22.0
    high risk pregnancy V23.9
      specified problem NEC V23.89

Chédiak-Higashi (-Steinbrinck) anomaly, disease, or syndrome (congenital gigantism of peroxidase granules) 288.2

Cheek — *see* condition
  biting 528.9

Cheese itch 133.8

Cheese washers' lung 495.8

Cheilitis 528.5
  actinic (due to sun) 692.72
    chronic NEC 692.72
      due to radiation, except from sun 692.82
    due to radiation, except from sun 692.82
  acute 528.5
  angular 528.5
  catarrhal 528.5
  chronic 528.5
  exfoliative 528.5
  gangrenous 528.5
  glandularis apostematosa 528.5
  granulomatosa 351.8
  infectional 528.5
  membranous 528.5
  Miescher's 351.8
  suppurative 528.5
  ulcerative 528.5
  vesicular 528.5

Cheilodynia 528.5

Cheilopalatoschisis (*see also* Cleft, palate, with cleft lip) 749.20

Cheilophagia 528.9

Cheiloschisis (*see also* Cleft, lip) 749.10

Cheilosis 528.5
  with pellagra 265.2
  angular 528.5
  due to
    dietary deficiency 266.0
    vitamin deficiency 266.0

Cheiromegaly 729.89

Cheiropompholyx 705.81

Cheloid (*see also* Keloid) 701.4

Chemical burn — *see also* Burn, by site
  from swallowing chemical — *see* Burn, internal organs

Chemodectoma (M8693/1) — *see* Paraganglioma, nonchromaffin

Chemoprophylaxis NEC V07.39

Chemosis, conjunctiva 372.73

Chemotherapy
  convalescence V66.2
  encounter (for) V58.1
  maintenance V58.1
  prophylactic NEC V07.39
    fluoride V07.31

Cherubism 526.89

Chest — *see* condition

Cheyne-Stokes respiration (periodic) 786.04

Chiari's
  disease or syndrome (hepatic vein thrombosis) 453.0
  malformation
    type I 348.4
    type II (*see also* Spina bifida) 741.0 ✓5ᵗʰ
    type III 742.0
    type IV 742.2
  network 746.89

Chiari-Frommel syndrome 676.6 ✓5ᵗʰ

Chicago disease (North American blastomycosis) 116.0

Chickenpox (*see also* Varicella) 052.9
  vaccination and inoculation (prophylactic) V05.4

Chiclero ulcer 085.4

Chiggers 133.8

Chignon 111.2
  fetus or newborn (from vacuum extraction) 767.1

Chigoe disease 134.1

Chikungunya fever 066.3

Chilaiditi's syndrome (subphrenic displacement, colon) 751.4

Chilblains 991.5
  lupus 991.5

Child
  behavior causing concern V61.20

Childbed fever 670 ✓4ᵗʰ

Childbirth — *see also* Delivery
  puerperal complications — *see* Puerperal

Childhood, period of rapid growth V21.0

Chill(s) 780.99 ▲
  with fever 780.6
  congestive 780.99 ▲
    in malarial regions 084.6
  septic — *see* Septicemia
  urethral 599.84

Chilomastigiasis 007.8

Chin — *see* condition

Chinese dysentery 004.9

Chiropractic dislocation (*see also* Lesion, nonallopathic, by site) 739.9

Chitral fever 066.0

Chlamydia, chlamydial — *see* condition

Chloasma 709.09
  cachecticorum 709.09
  eyelid 374.52
    congenital 757.33
    hyperthyroid 242.0 ✓5ᵗʰ
  gravidarum 646.8 ✓5ᵗʰ
  idiopathic 709.09
  skin 709.09
  symptomatic 709.09

Chloroma (M9930/3) 205.3 ✓5ᵗʰ

Chlorosis 280.9
  Egyptian (*see also* Ancylostomiasis) 126.9
  miners' (*see also* Ancylostomiasis) 126.9

Chlorotic anemia 280.9

Chocolate cyst (ovary) 617.1

Choked
  disk or disc — *see* Papilledema
  on food, phlegm, or vomitus NEC (*see also* Asphyxia, food) 933.1
  phlegm 933.1

Choked — *continued*
  while vomiting NEC (*see also* Asphyxia, food) 933.1
Chokes (resulting from bends) 993.3
Choking sensation 784.9
Cholangiectasis (*see also* Disease, gallbladder) 575.8
Cholangiocarcinoma (M8160/3)
  and hepatocellular carcinoma, combined (M8180/3) 155.0
  liver 155.1
  specified site NEC — *see* Neoplasm, by site, malignant
  unspecified site 155.1
Cholangiohepatitis 575.8
  due to fluke infestation 121.1
Cholangiohepatoma (M8180/3) 155.0
Cholangiolitis (acute) (chronic) (extrahepatic) (gangrenous) 576.1
  intrahepatic 575.8
  paratyphoidal (*see also* Fever, paratyphoid) 002.9
  typhoidal 002.0
Cholangioma (M8160/0) 211.5
  malignant — *see* Cholangiocarcinoma
Cholangitis (acute) (ascending) (catarrhal) (chronic) (infective) (malignant) (primary) (recurrent) (sclerosing) (secondary) (stenosing) (suppurative) 576.1
  chronic nonsuppurative destructive 571.6
  nonsuppurative destructive (chronic) 571.6
Cholecystdocholithiasis — *see* Choledocholithiasis
Cholecystitis 575.10
  with
    calculus, stones in
      bile duct (common) (hepatic) — *see* Choledocholithiasis
      gallbladder — *see* Cholelithiasis
  acute 575.0
  acute and chronic 575.12
  chronic 575.11
  emphysematous (acute) (*see also* Cholecystitis, acute) 575.0
  gangrenous (*see also* Cholecystitis, acute) 575.0
  paratyphoidal, current (*see also* Fever, paratyphoid) 002.9
  suppurative (*see also* Cholecystitis, acute) 575.0
  typhoidal 002.0
Choledochitis (suppurative) 576.1
Choledocholith — *see* Choledocholithiasis
Choledocholithiasis 574.5 ✓5ᵗʰ

> *Note* — Use the following fifth-digit subclassification with category 574:
>
> 0   *without mention of obstruction*
> 1   *with obstruction*

  with
    cholecystitis 574.4 ✓5ᵗʰ
      acute 574.3 ✓5ᵗʰ
      chronic 574.4 ✓5ᵗʰ
    cholelithiasis 574.9 ✓5ᵗʰ
      with
        cholecystitis 574.7 ✓5ᵗʰ
          acute 574.6 ✓5ᵗʰ
            and chronic 574.8 ✓5ᵗʰ
        chronic 574.7 ✓5ᵗʰ
Cholelithiasis (impacted) (multiple) 574.2 ✓5ᵗʰ

> *Note* — Use the following fifth-digit subclassification with category 574:
>
> 0   *without mention of obstruction*
> 1   *with obstruction*

  with
    cholecystitis 574.1 ✓5ᵗʰ
      acute 574.0 ✓5ᵗʰ
      chronic 574.1 ✓5ᵗʰ

Cholelithiasis — *continued*
  with — *continued*
    choledocholithiasis 574.9 ✓5ᵗʰ
      with
        cholecystitis 574.7 ✓5ᵗʰ
          acute 574.6 ✓5ᵗʰ
            and chronic 574.8 ✓5ᵗʰ
        chronic cholecystitis 574.7 ✓5ᵗʰ
Cholemia (*see also* Jaundice) 782.4
  familial 277.4
  Gilbert's (familial nonhemolytic) 277.4
Cholemic gallstone — *see* Cholelithiasis
Choleperitoneum, choleperitonitis (*see also* Disease, gallbladder) 567.8
Cholera (algid) (Asiatic) (asphyctic) (epidemic) (gravis) (Indian) (malignant) (morbus) (pestilential) (spasmodic) 001.9
  antimonial 985.4
  carrier (suspected) of V02.0
  classical 001.0
  contact V01.0
  due to
    Vibrio
      cholerae (Inaba, Ogawa, Hikojima serotypes) 001.0
      El Tor 001.1
  El Tor 001.1
  exposure to V01.0
  vaccination, prophylactic (against) V03.0
Cholerine (*see also* Cholera) 001.9
Cholestasis 576.8
Cholesteatoma (ear) 385.30
  attic (primary) 385.31
  diffuse 385.35
  external ear (canal) 380.21
  marginal (middle ear) 385.32
    with involvement of mastoid cavity 385.33
    secondary (with middle ear involvement) 385.33
  mastoid cavity 385.30
  middle ear (secondary) 385.32
    with involvement of mastoid cavity 385.33
  postmastoidectomy cavity (recurrent) 383.32
  primary 385.31
  recurrent, postmastoidectomy cavity 383.32
  secondary (middle ear) 385.32
    with involvement of mastoid cavity 385.33
Cholesteatosis (middle ear) (*see also* Cholesteatoma) 385.30
  diffuse 385.35
Cholesteremia 272.0
Cholesterin
  granuloma, middle ear 385.82
  in vitreous 379.22
Cholesterol
  deposit
    retina 362.82
    vitreous 379.22
  imbibition of gallbladder (*see also* Disease, gallbladder) 575.6
Cholesterolemia 272.0
  essential 272.0
  familial 272.0
  hereditary 272.0
Cholesterosis, cholesterolosis (gallbladder) 575.6
  with
    cholecystitis — *see* Cholecystitis
    cholelithiasis — *see* Cholelithiasis
  middle ear (*see also* Cholesteatoma) 385.30
Cholocolic fistula (*see also* Fistula, gallbladder) 575.5
Choluria 791.4
Chondritis (purulent) 733.99
  costal 733.6
    Tietze's 733.6
  patella, posttraumatic 717.7
  posttraumatica patellae 717.7
  tuberculous (active) (*see also* Tuberculosis) 015.9 ✓5ᵗʰ
    intervertebral 015.0 ✓5ᵗʰ [730.88]
Chondroangiopathia calcarea seu punctate 756.59

Chondroblastoma (M9230/0) — *see also* Neoplasm, bone, benign
  malignant (M9230/3) — *see* Neoplasm, bone, malignant
Chondrocalcinosis (articular) (crystal deposition) (dihydrate) (*see also* Arthritis, due to, crystals) 275.49 [712.3] ✓5ᵗʰ
  due to
    calcium pyrophosphate 275.49 [712.2] ✓5ᵗʰ
    dicalcium phosphate crystals 275.49 [712.1] ✓5ᵗʰ
    pyrophosphate crystals 275.49 [712.2] ✓5ᵗʰ
Chondrodermatitis nodularis helicis 380.00
Chondrodysplasia 756.4
  angiomatose 756.4
  calcificans congenita 756.59
  epiphysialis punctata 756.59
  hereditary deforming 756.4
Chondrodystrophia (fetalis) 756.4
  calcarea 756.4
  calcificans congenita 756.59
  fetalis hypoplastica 756.59
  hypoplastica calcinosa 756.59
  punctata 756.59
  tarda 277.5
Chondrodystrophy (familial) (hypoplastic) 756.4
Chondroectodermal dysplasia 756.55
Chondrolysis 733.99
Chondroma (M9220/0) — *see also* Neoplasm cartilage, benign
  juxtacortical (M9221/0) — *see* Neoplasm, bone, benign
  periosteal (M9221/0) — *see* Neoplasm, bone, benign
Chondromalacia 733.92
  epiglottis (congenital) 748.3
  generalized 733.92
  knee 717.7
  larynx (congenital) 748.3
  localized, except patella 733.92
  patella, patellae 717.7
  systemic 733.92
  tibial plateau 733.92
  trachea (congenital) 748.3
Chondromatosis (M9220/1) — *see* Neoplasm, cartilage, uncertain behavior
Chondromyxosarcoma (M9220/3) — *see* Neoplasm, cartilage, malignant
Chondro-osteodysplasia (Morquio- Brailsford type) 277.5
Chondro-osteodystrophy 277.5
Chondro-osteoma (M9210/0) — *see* Neoplasm, bone, benign
Chondropathia tuberosa 733.6
Chondrosarcoma (M9220/3) — *see also* Neoplasm, cartilage, malignant
  juxtacortical (M9221/3) — *see* Neoplasm, bone, malignant
  mesenchymal (M9240/3) — *see* Neoplasm, connective tissue, malignant
Chordae tendineae rupture (chronic) 429.5
Chordee (nonvenereal) 607.89
  congenital 752.63
  gonococcal 098.2
Chorditis (fibrinous) (nodosa) (tuberosa) 478.5
Chordoma (M9370/3) — *see* Neoplasm, by site, malignant
Chorea (gravis) (minor) (spasmodic) 333.5
  with
    heart involvement — *see* Chorea with rheumatic heart disease
    rheumatic heart disease (chronic, inactive, or quiescent) (conditions classifiable to 393-398) — *see also* Rheumatic heart condition involved
      active or acute (conditions classifiable to 391) 392.0
  acute — *see* Chorea, Sydenham's
  apoplectic (*see also* Disease, cerebrovascular, acute) 436
  chronic 333.4
  electric 049.8
  gravidarum — *see* Eclampsia, pregnancy

Chorea — *continued*
  habit 307.22
  hereditary 333.4
  Huntington's 333.4
  posthemiplegic 344.89
  pregnancy — *see* Eclampsia, pregnancy
  progressive 333.4
    chronic 333.4
    hereditary 333.4
  rheumatic (chronic) 392.9
    with heart disease or involvement — *see*
        Chorea, with rheumatic heart disease
  senile 333.5
  Sydenham's 392.9
    with heart involvement — *see* Chorea, with
        rheumatic heart disease
    nonrheumatic 333.5
  variabilis 307.23
Choreoathetosis (paroxysmal) 333.5
Chorioadenoma (destruens) (M9100/1) 236.1
Chorioamnionitis 658.4 ✓5ᵗʰ
  affecting fetus or newborn 762.7
Chorioangioma (M9120/0) 219.8
Choriocarcinoma (M9100/3)
  combined with
    embryonal carcinoma (M9101/3) — *see*
        Neoplasm, by site, malignant
    teratoma (M9101/3) — *see* Neoplasm, by
        site, malignant
  specified site — *see* Neoplasm, by site,
      malignant
  unspecified site
    female 181
    male 186.9
Chorioencephalitis, lymphocytic (acute) (serous)
  049.0
Chorioepithelioma (M9100/3) — *see*
  Choriocarcinoma
Choriomeningitis (acute) (benign) (lymphocytic)
  (serous) 049.0
Chorionepithelioma (M9100/3) — *see*
  Choriocarcinoma
Chorionitis (*see also* Scleroderma) 710.1
Chorioretinitis 363.20
  disseminated 363.10
    generalized 363.13
    in
      neurosyphilis 094.83
      secondary syphilis 091.51
    peripheral 363.12
    posterior pole 363.11
    tuberculous (*see also* Tuberculosis)
        017.3 ✓5ᵗʰ [363.13]
  due to
    histoplasmosis (*see also* Histoplasmosis)
        115.92
    toxoplasmosis (acquired) 130.2
      congenital (active) 771.2
  focal 363.00
    juxtapapillary 363.01
    peripheral 363.04
    posterior pole NEC 363.03
  juxtapapillaris, juxtapapillary 363.01
  progressive myopia (degeneration) 360.21
  syphilitic (secondary) 091.51
    congenital (early) 090.0 [363.13]
      late 090.5 [363.13]
    late 095.8 [363.13]
  tuberculous (*see also* Tuberculosis) 017.3 ✓5ᵗʰ
      [363.13]
Choristoma — *see* Neoplasm, by site, benign
Choroid — *see* condition
Choroideremia, choroidermia (initial stage) (late
  stage) (partial or total atrophy) 363.55
Choroiditis (*see also* Chorioretinitis) 363.20
  leprous 030.9 [363.13]
  senile guttate 363.41
  sympathetic 360.11
  syphilitic (secondary) 091.51
    congenital (early) 090.0 [363.13]
      late 090.5 [363.13]
    late 095.8 [363.13]
  Tay's 363.41
  tuberculous (*see also* Tuberculosis) 017.3 ✓5ᵗʰ
      [363.13]

Choroidopathy NEC 363.9
  degenerative (*see also* Degeneration, choroid)
      363.40
  hereditary (*see also* Dystrophy, choroid) 363.50
  specified type NEC 363.8
Choroidoretinitis — *see* Chorioretinitis
Choroidosis, central serous 362.41
Choroidretinopathy, serous 362.41
Christian's syndrome (chronic histiocytosis X)
  277.8
Christian-Weber disease (nodular nonsuppurative
  panniculitis) 729.30
Christmas disease 286.1
Chromaffinoma (M8700/0) — *see also* Neoplasm,
  by site, benign
  malignant (M8700/3) — *see* Neoplasm, by site,
      malignant
Chromatopsia 368.59
Chromhidrosis, chromidrosis 705.89
Chromoblastomycosis 117.2
Chromomycosis 117.2
Chromophytosis 111.0
Chromotrichomycosis 111.8
Chronic — *see* condition
Churg-Strauss syndrome 446.4
Chyle cyst, mesentery 457.8
Chylocele (nonfilarial) 457.8
  filarial (*see also* Infestation, filarial) 125.9
  tunica vaginalis (nonfilarial) 608.84
    filarial (*see also* Infestation, filarial) 125.9
Chylomicronemia (fasting) (with
  hyperprebetalipoproteinemia) 272.3
Chylopericardium (acute) 420.90
Chylothorax (nonfilarial) 457.8
  filarial (*see also* Infestation, filarial) 125.9
Chylous
  ascites 457.8
  cyst of peritoneum 457.8
  hydrocele 603.9
  hydrothorax (nonfilarial) 457.8
    filarial (*see also* Infestation, filarial) 125.9
Chyluria 791.1
  bilharziasis 120.0
  due to
    Brugia (malayi) 125.1
    Wuchereria (bancrofti) 125.0
      malayi 125.1
  filarial (*see also* Infestation, filarial) 125.9
  filariasis (*see also* Infestation, filarial) 125.9
  nonfilarial 791.1
Cicatricial (deformity) — *see* Cicatrix
Cicatrix (adherent) (contracted) (painful) (vicious)
  709.2
  adenoid 474.8
  alveolar process 525.8
  anus 569.49
  auricle 380.89
  bile duct (*see also* Disease, biliary) 576.8
  bladder 596.8
  bone 733.99
  brain 348.8
  cervix (postoperative) (postpartal) 622.3
    in pregnancy or childbirth 654.6 ✓5ᵗʰ
      causing obstructed labor 660.2 ✓5ᵗʰ
  chorioretinal 363.30
    disseminated 363.35
    macular 363.32
    peripheral 363.34
    posterior pole NEC 363.33
  choroid — *see* Cicatrix, chorioretinal
  common duct (*see also* Disease, biliary) 576.8
  congenital 757.39
  conjunctiva 372.64
  cornea 371.00
    tuberculous (*see also* Tuberculosis)
        017.3 ✓5ᵗʰ [371.05]
  duodenum (bulb) 537.3
  esophagus 530.3
  eyelid 374.46
    with
      ectropion — *see* Ectropion
      entropion — *see* Entropion
  hypopharynx 478.29

Cicatrix — *continued*
  knee, semilunar cartilage 717.5
  lacrimal
    canaliculi 375.53
    duct
      acquired 375.56
      neonatal 375.55
    punctum 375.52
    sac 375.54
  larynx 478.79
  limbus (cystoid) 372.64
  lung 518.89
  macular 363.32
    disseminated 363.35
    peripheral 363.34
  middle ear 385.89
  mouth 528.9
  muscle 728.89
  nasolacrimal duct
    acquired 375.56
    neonatal 375.55
  nasopharynx 478.29
  palate (soft) 528.9
  penis 607.89
  prostate 602.8
  rectum 569.49
  retina 363.30
    disseminated 363.35
    macular 363.32
    peripheral 363.34
    posterior pole NEC 363.33
  semilunar cartilage — *see* Derangement,
      meniscus
  seminal vesicle 608.89
  skin 709.2
    infected 686.8
    postinfectional 709.2
    tuberculous (*see also* Tuberculosis)
        017.0 ✓5ᵗʰ
  specified site NEC 709.2
  throat 478.29
  tongue 529.8
  tonsil (and adenoid) 474.8
  trachea 478.9
  tuberculous NEC (*see also* Tuberculosis)
      011.9 ✓5ᵗʰ
  ureter 593.89
  urethra 599.84
  uterus 621.8
  vagina 623.4
    in pregnancy or childbirth 654.7 ✓5ᵗʰ
      causing obstructed labor 660.2 ✓5ᵗʰ
  vocal cord 478.5
  wrist, constricting (annular) 709.2
CIN I [cervical intraepithelial neoplasia I] 622.1
CIN II [cervical intraepithelial neoplasia II] 622.1
CIN III [cervical intraepithelial neoplasia III] 233.1
Cinchonism
  correct substance properly administered 386.9
  overdose or wrong substance given or taken
      961.4
Circine herpes 110.5
Circle of Willis — *see* condition
Circular — *see also* condition
  hymen 752.49
Circulating anticoagulants 286.5
  following childbirth 666.3 ✓5ᵗʰ
  postpartum 666.3 ✓5ᵗʰ
Circulation
  collateral (venous), any site 459.89
  defective 459.9
    congenital 747.9
    lower extremity 459.89
  embryonic 747.9
  failure 799.8
    fetus or newborn 779.89   ▲
    peripheral 785.59
  fetal, persistent 747.83   ▲
  heart, incomplete 747.9
Circulatory system — *see* condition
Circulus senilis 371.41
Circumcision
  in absence of medical indication V50.2
  ritual V50.2
  routine V50.2

Chorea — Circumcision

Circumscribed — *see* condition
Circumvallata placenta — *see* Placenta, abnormal
Cirrhosis, cirrhotic 571.5
  with alcoholism 571.2
  alcoholic (liver) 571.2
  atrophic (of liver) — *see* Cirrhosis, portal
  Baumgarten-Cruveilhier 571.5
  biliary (cholangiolitic) (cholangitic) (cholestatic)
    (extrahepatic) (hypertrophic)
    (intrahepatic) (nonobstructive)
    (obstructive) (pericholangiolitic)
    (posthepatic) (primary) (secondary)
    (xanthomatous) 571.6
    due to
      clonorchiasis 121.1
      flukes 121.3
  brain 331.9
  capsular — *see* Cirrhosis, portal
  cardiac 571.5
    alcoholic 571.2
  central (liver) — *see* Cirrhosis, liver
  Charcôt's 571.6
  cholangiolitic — *see* Cirrhosis, biliary
  cholangitic — *see* Cirrhosis, biliary
  cholestatic — *see* Cirrhosis, biliary
  clitoris (hypertrophic) 624.2
  coarsely nodular 571.5
  congestive (liver) — *see* Cirrhosis, cardiac
  Cruveilhier-Baumgarten 571.5
  cryptogenic (of liver) 571.5
    alcoholic 571.2
  dietary (*see also* Cirrhosis, portal) 571.5
  due to
    bronzed diabetes 275.0
    congestive hepatomegaly — *see* Cirrhosis, cardiac
    cystic fibrosis 277.00
    hemochromatosis 275.0
    hepatolenticular degeneration 275.1
    passive congestion (chronic) — *see* Cirrhosis, cardiac
    Wilson's disease 275.1
    xanthomatosis 272.2
  extrahepatic (obstructive) — *see* Cirrhosis, biliary
  fatty 571.8
    alcoholic 571.0
  florid 571.2
  Glisson's — *see* Cirrhosis, portal
  Hanot's (hypertrophic) — *see* Cirrhosis, biliary
  hepatic — *see* Cirrhosis, liver
  hepatolienal — *see* Cirrhosis, liver
  hobnail — *see* Cirrhosis, portal
  hypertrophic — *see also* Cirrhosis, liver
    biliary — *see* Cirrhosis, biliary
    Hanot's — *see* Cirrhosis, biliary
  infectious NEC — *see* Cirrhosis, portal
  insular — *see* Cirrhosis, portal
  intrahepatic (obstructive) (primary) (secondary) — *see* Cirrhosis, biliary
  juvenile (*see also* Cirrhosis, portal) 571.5
  kidney (*see also* Sclerosis, renal) 587
  Laennec's (of liver) 571.2
    nonalcoholic 571.5
  liver (chronic) (hepatolienal) (hypertrophic) (nodular) (splenomegalic) (unilobar) 571.5
    with alcoholism 571.2
    alcoholic 571.2
    congenital (due to failure of obliteration of umbilical vein) 777.8
    cryptogenic 571.5
      alcoholic 571.2
    fatty 571.8
      alcoholic 571.0
    macronodular 571.5
      alcoholic 571.2
    micronodular 571.5
      alcoholic 571.2
    nodular, diffuse 571.5
      alcoholic 571.2
    pigmentary 275.0
    portal 571.5
      alcoholic 571.2
    postnecrotic 571.5
      alcoholic 571.2
    syphilitic 095.3

Cirrhosis, cirrhotic — *continued*
  lung (chronic) (*see also* Fibrosis, lung) 515
  macronodular (of liver) 571.5
    alcoholic 571.2
  malarial 084.9
  metabolic NEC 571.5
  micronodular (of liver) 571.5
    alcoholic 571.2
  monolobular — *see* Cirrhosis, portal
  multilobular — *see* Cirrhosis, portal
  nephritis (*see also* Sclerosis, renal) 587
  nodular — *see* Cirrhosis, liver
  nutritional (fatty) 571.5
  obstructive (biliary) (extrahepatic) (intrahepatic) — *see* Cirrhosis, biliary
  ovarian 620.8
  paludal 084.9
  pancreas (duct) 577.8
  pericholangiolitic — *see* Cirrhosis, biliary
  periportal — *see* Cirrhosis, portal
  pigment, pigmentary (of liver) 275.0
  portal (of liver) 571.5
    alcoholic 571.2
  posthepatitic (*see also* Cirrhosis, postnecrotic) 571.5
  postnecrotic (of liver) 571.5
    alcoholic 571.2
  primary (intrahepatic) — *see* Cirrhosis, biliary
  pulmonary (*see also* Fibrosis, lung) 515
  renal (*see also* Sclerosis, renal) 587
  septal (*see also* Cirrhosis, postnecrotic) 571.5
  spleen 289.51
  splenomegalic (of liver) — *see* Cirrhosis, liver
  stasis (liver) — *see* Cirrhosis, liver
  stomach 535.4 ✓5ᵗʰ
  Todd's (*see also* Cirrhosis, biliary) 571.6
  toxic (nodular) — *see* Cirrhosis, postnecrotic
  trabecular — *see* Cirrhosis, postnecrotic
  unilobar — *see* Cirrhosis, liver
  vascular (of liver) — *see* Cirrhosis, liver
  xanthomatous (biliary) (*see also* Cirrhosis, biliary) 571.6
    due to xanthomatosis (familial) (metabolic) (primary) 272.2
Cistern, subarachnoid 793.0
Citrullinemia 270.6
Citrullinuria 270.6
Ciuffini-Pancoast tumor (M8010/3) (carcinoma, pulmonary apex) 162.3
Civatte's disease or poikiloderma 709.09
Clam diggers' itch 120.3
Clap — *see* Gonorrhea
Clark's paralysis 343.9
Clarke-Hadfield syndrome (pancreatic infantilism) 577.8
Clastothrix 704.2
Claude's syndrome 352.6
Claude Bernard-Horner syndrome (*see also* Neuropathy, peripheral, autonomic) 337.9
Claudication, intermittent 443.9
  cerebral (artery) (*see also* Ischemia, cerebral, transient) 435.9
  due to atherosclerosis 440.21
  spinal cord (arteriosclerotic) 435.1
    syphilitic 094.89
  spinalis 435.1
  venous (axillary) 453.8
Claudicatio venosa intermittens 453.8
Claustrophobia 300.29
Clavus (infected) 700
Clawfoot (congenital) 754.71
  acquired 736.74
Clawhand (acquired) 736.06
  congenital 755.59
Clawtoe (congenital) 754.71
  acquired 735.5
Clay eating 307.52
Clay shovelers' fracture — *see* Fracture, vertebra, cervical
Cleansing of artificial opening (*see also* Attention to artificial opening) V55.9
Cleft (congenital) — *see also* Imperfect, closure
  alveolar process 525.8

Cleft — *see also* Imperfect, closure — *continued*
  branchial (persistent) 744.41
    cyst 744.42
  clitoris 752.49
  cricoid cartilage, posterior 748.3
  facial (*see also* Cleft, lip) 749.10
  lip 749.10
    with cleft palate 749.20
      bilateral (lip and palate) 749.24
        with unilateral lip or palate 749.25
        complete 749.23
        incomplete 749.24
      unilateral (lip and palate) 749.22
        with bilateral lip or palate 749.25
        complete 749.21
        incomplete 749.22
    bilateral 749.14
      with cleft palate, unilateral 749.25
      complete 749.13
      incomplete 749.14
    unilateral 749.12
      with cleft palate, bilateral 749.25
      complete 749.11
      incomplete 749.12
  nose 748.1
  palate 749.00
    with cleft lip 749.20
      bilateral (lip and palate) 749.24
        with unilateral lip or palate 749.25
        complete 749.23
        incomplete 749.24
      unilateral (lip and palate) 749.22
        with bilateral lip or palate 749.25
        complete 749.21
        incomplete 749.22
    bilateral 749.04
      with cleft lip, unilateral 749.25
      complete 749.03
      incomplete 749.04
    unilateral 749.02
      with cleft lip, bilateral 749.25
      complete 749.01
      incomplete 749.02
  penis 752.69
  posterior, cricoid cartilage 748.3
  scrotum 752.8
  sternum (congenital) 756.3
  thyroid cartilage (congenital) 748.3
  tongue 750.13
  uvula 749.02
    with cleft lip (*see also* Cleft, lip, with cleft palate) 749.20
  water 366.12
Cleft hand (congenital) 755.58
Cleidocranial dysostosis 755.59
Cleidotomy, fetal 763.89
Cleptomania 312.32
Clérambault's syndrome 297.8
  erotomania 302.89
Clergyman's sore throat 784.49
Click, clicking
  systolic syndrome 785.2
Clifford's syndrome (postmaturity) 766.2
Climacteric (*see also* Menopause) 627.2
  arthritis NEC (*see also* Arthritis, climacteric) 716.3 ✓5ᵗʰ
  depression (*see also* Psychosis, affective) 296.2 ✓5ᵗʰ
  disease 627.2
    recurrent episode 296.3 ✓5ᵗʰ
    single episode 296.2 ✓5ᵗʰ
  female (symptoms) 627.2
  male (symptoms) (syndrome) 608.89
  melancholia (*see also* Psychosis, affective) 296.2 ✓5ᵗʰ
    recurrent episode 296.3 ✓5ᵗʰ
    single episode 296.2 ✓5ᵗʰ
  paranoid state 297.2
  paraphrenia 297.2
  polyarthritis NEC 716.39
    male 608.89
  symptoms (female) 627.2
Clinical research investigation (control) (participant) V70.7
Clinodactyly 755.59

Colitis — *continued*
  mucous 564.9
    psychogenic 316 *[564.9]*
  necrotic 009.0
  polyposa (*see also* Colitis, ulcerative) 556.9
  protozoal NEC 007.9
  pseudomembranous 008.45
  pseudomucinous 564.9
  regional 555.1
  segmental 555.1
  septic (*see also* Enteritis, due to, specific
      organism) 009.0
  spastic 564.9
    psychogenic 316 *[564.9]*
  staphylococcus 008.41
    food 005.0
  thromboulcerative 557.0
  toxic 558.2
  transmural 555.1
  trichomonal 007.3
  tuberculous (ulcerative) 014.8 ✓5ᵗʰ
  ulcerative (chronic) (idiopathic) (nonspecific)
      556.9
    entero- 556.0
    fulminant 557.0
    ileo- 556.1
    left-sided 556.5
    procto- 556.2
    proctosigmoid 556.3
    psychogenic 316 *[556]* ✓4ᵗʰ
    specified NEC 556.8
    universal 556.6
Collagen disease NEC 710.9
  nonvascular 710.9
  vascular (allergic) (*see also* Angiitis,
      hypersensitivity) 446.20
Collagenosis (*see also* Collagen disease) 710.9
  cardiovascular 425.4
  mediastinal 519.3
Collapse 780.2
  adrenal 255.8
  cardiorenal (*see also* Hypertension, cardiorenal)
      404.90
  cardiorespiratory 785.51
    fetus or newborn 779.89   ▲
  cardiovascular (*see also* Disease, heart) 785.51
    fetus or newborn 779.89   ▲
  circulatory (peripheral) 785.59
    with
      abortion — *see* Abortion, by type, with
          shock
      ectopic pregnancy (*see also* categories
          633.0-633.9) 639.5
      molar pregnancy (*see also* categories 630-
          632) 639.5
    during or after labor and delivery 669.1 ✓5ᵗʰ
    fetus or newborn 779.89   ▲
    following
      abortion 639.5
      ectopic or molar pregnancy 639.5
    during or after labor and delivery 669.1 ✓5ᵗʰ
    fetus or newborn 779.89   ▲
  external ear canal 380.50
    secondary to
      inflammation 380.53
      surgery 380.52
      trauma 380.51
  general 780.2
  heart — *see* Disease, heart
  heat 992.1
  hysterical 300.11
  labyrinth, membranous (congenital) 744.05
  lung (massive) (*see also* Atelectasis) 518.0
    pressure, during labor 668.0 ✓5ᵗʰ
  myocardial — *see* Disease, heart
  nervous (*see also* Disorder, mental,
      nonpsychotic) 300.9
  neurocirculatory 306.2
  nose 738.0
  postoperative (cardiovascular) 998.0
  pulmonary (*see also* Atelectasis) 518.0
    fetus or newborn 770.5
      partial 770.5
      primary 770.4
  thorax 512.8
    iatrogenic 512.1
    postoperative 512.1

Collapse — *continued*
  trachea 519.1
  valvular — *see* Endocarditis
  vascular (peripheral) 785.59
    with
      abortion — *see* Abortion, by type, with
          shock
      ectopic pregnancy (*see also* categories
          633.0-633.9) 639.5
      molar pregnancy (*see also* categories 630-
          632) 639.5
    cerebral (*see also* Disease, cerebrovascular,
        acute) 436
    during or after labor and delivery 669.1 ✓5ᵗʰ
    fetus or newborn 779.89   ▲
    following
      abortion 639.5
      ectopic or molar pregnancy 639.5
  vasomotor 785.59
  vertebra 733.13
Collateral — *see also* condition
  circulation (venous) 459.89
  dilation, veins 459.89
Colles' fracture (closed) (reversed) (separation)
    813.41
  open 813.51
Collet's syndrome 352.6
Collet-Sicard syndrome 352.6
Colliculitis urethralis (*see also* Urethritis) 597.89
Colliers'
  asthma 500
  lung 500
  phthisis (*see also* Tuberculosis) 011.4 ✓5ᵗʰ
Collodion baby (ichthyosis congenita) 757.1
Colloid milium 709.3
Coloboma NEC 743.49
  choroid 743.59
  fundus 743.52
  iris 743.46
  lens 743.36
  lids 743.62
  optic disc (congenital) 743.57
    acquired 377.23
  retina 743.56
  sclera 743.47
Coloenteritis — *see* Enteritis
Colon — *see* condition
Coloptosis 569.89
Color
  amblyopia NEC 368.59
    acquired 368.55
  blindness NEC (congenital) 368.59
    acquired 368.55
Colostomy
  attention to V55.3
  fitting or adjustment V53.5
  malfunctioning 569.62
  status V44.3
Colpitis (*see also* Vaginitis) 616.10
Colpocele 618.6
Colpocystitis (*see also* Vaginitis) 616.10
Colporrhexis 665.4 ✓5ᵗʰ
Colpospasm 625.1
Column, spinal, vertebral — *see* condition
Coma 780.01
  apoplectic (*see also* Disease, cerebrovascular,
      acute) 436
  diabetic (with ketoacidosis) 250.3 ✓5ᵗʰ
    hyperosmolar 250.2 ✓5ᵗʰ
  eclamptic (*see also* Eclampsia) 780.39
  epileptic 345.3
  hepatic 572.2
  hyperglycemic 250.2 ✓5ᵗʰ
  hyperosmolar (diabetic) (nonketotic) 250.2 ✓5ᵗʰ
  hypoglycemic 251.0
    diabetic 250.3 ✓5ᵗʰ
  insulin 250.3 ✓5ᵗʰ
    hypersmolar 250.2 ✓5ᵗʰ
    non-diabetic 251.0
    organic hyperinsulinism 251.0
  Kussmaul's (diabetic) 250.3 ✓5ᵗʰ
  liver 572.2
  newborn 779.2

Coma — *continued*
  prediabetic 250.2 ✓5ᵗʰ
  uremic — *see* Uremia
Combat fatigue (*see also* Reaction, stress, acute)
    308.9
Combined — *see* condition
Comedo 706.1
Comedocarcinoma (M8501/3) — *see also*
    Neoplasm, breast, malignant
  noninfiltrating (M8501/2)
    specified site — *see* Neoplasm, by site, in
        situ
    unspecified site 233.0
Comedomastitis 610.4
Comedones 706.1
  lanugo 757.4
Comma bacillus, carrier (suspected) of V02.3
Comminuted fracture — *see* Fracture, by site
Common
  aortopulmonary trunk 745.0
  atrioventricular canal (defect) 745.69
  atrium 745.69
  cold (head) 460
    vaccination, prophylactic (against) V04.7
  truncus (arteriosus) 745.0
  ventricle 745.3
Commotio (current)
  cerebri (*see also* Concussion, brain) 850.9
    with skull fracture — *see* Fracture, skull, by
        site
  retinae 921.3
  spinalis — *see* Injury, spinal, by site
Commotion (current)
  brain (without skull fracture) (*see also*
      Concussion, brain) 850.9
    with skull fracture — *see* Fracture, skull, by
        site
  spinal cord — *see* Injury, spinal, by site
Communication
  abnormal — *see also* Fistula
    between
      base of aorta and pulmonary artery 745.0
      left ventricle and right atrium 745.4
      pericardial sac and pleural sac 748.8
      pulmonary artery and pulmonary vein
          747.3
    congenital, between uterus and anterior
        abdominal wall 752.3
      bladder 752.3
      intestine 752.3
      rectum 752.3
    left ventricular — right atrial 745.4
    pulmonary artery— pulmonary vein 747.3
Compensation
  broken — *see* Failure, heart
  failure — *see* Failure, heart
  neurosis, psychoneurosis 300.11
Complaint — *see also* Disease
  bowel, functional 564.9
    psychogenic 306.4
  intestine, functional 564.9
    psychogenic 306.4
  kidney (*see also* Disease, renal) 593.9
  liver 573.9
  miners' 500
Complete — *see* condition
Complex
  cardiorenal (*see also* Hypertension, cardiorenal)
      404.90
  castration 300.9
  Costen's 524.60
  ego-dystonic homosexuality 302.0
  Eisenmenger's (ventricular septal defect) 745.4
  homosexual, ego-dystonic 302.0
  hypersexual 302.89
  inferiority 301.9
  jumped process
    spine — *see* Dislocation, vertebra
  primary, tuberculosis (*see also* Tuberculosis)
      010.0 ✓5ᵗʰ
  Taussig-Bing (transposition, aorta and
      overriding pulmonary artery) 745.11

Complications

abortion NEC — *see* categories 634-639
accidental puncture or laceration during a
  procedure 998.2
amputation stump (late) (surgical) 997.60
  traumatic — *see* Amputation, traumatic
anastomosis (and bypass) NEC — *see also*
    Complications, due to (presence of) any
    device, implant, or graft classified to
    996.0-996.5 NEC
  hemorrhage NEC 998.11
  intestinal (internal) NEC 997.4
    involving urinary tract 997.5
  mechanical — *see* Complications,
    mechanical, graft
  urinary tract (involving intestinal tract)
    997.5
anesthesia, anesthetic NEC (*see also*
    Anesthesia, complication) 995.2
  in labor and delivery 668.9 ☑5ᵗʰ
    affecting fetus or newborn 763.5
    cardiac 668.1 ☑5ᵗʰ
    central nervous system 668.2 ☑5ᵗʰ
    pulmonary 668.0 ☑5ᵗʰ
    specified type NEC 668.8 ☑5ᵗʰ
aortocoronary (bypass) graft 996.03
  atherosclerosis — *see* Arteriosclerosis,
    coronary
  embolism 996.72
  occlusion NEC 996.72
  thrombus 996.72
arthroplasty 996.4
artificial opening
  cecostomy 569.60
  colostomy 569.60
  cystostomy 997.5
  enterostomy 569.60
  gastrostomy 536.40
  ileostomy 569.60
  jejunostomy 569.60
  nephrostomy 997.5
  tracheostomy 519.00
  ureterostomy 997.5
  urethrostomy 997.5
bile duct implant (prosthetic) NEC 996.79
  infection or inflammation 996.69
  mechanical 996.59
bleeding (intraoperative) (postoperative) 998.11
blood vessel graft 996.1
  aortocoronary 996.03
    atherosclerosis — *see* Arteriosclerosis,
      coronary
    embolism 996.72
    occlusion NEC 996.72
    thrombus 996.72
  atherosclerosis — *see* Arteriosclerosis,
    extremities
  embolism 996.74
  occlusion NEC 996.74
  thrombus 996.74
bone growth stimulator 996.78
  infection or inflammation 996.67
bone marrow transplant 996.85
breast implant (prosthetic) NEC 996.79
  infection or inflammation 996.69
  mechanical 996.54
bypass — *see also* Complications, anastomosis
  aortocoronary 996.03
    atherosclerosis — *see* Arteriosclerosis,
      coronary
    embolism 996.72
    occlusion NEC 996.72
    thrombus 996.72
  carotid artery 996.1
    atherosclerosis — *see* Arteriosclerosis,
      extremities
    embolism 996.74
    occlusion NEC 996.74
    thrombus 996.74
cardiac (*see also* Disease, heart) 429.9
  device, implant, or graft NEC 996.72
    infection or inflammation 996.61
    long-term effect 429.4
    mechanical (*see also* Complications,
      mechanical, by type) 996.00
      valve prosthesis 996.71
        infection or inflammation 996.61

Complications — *continued*
  cardiac (*see also* Disease, heart) — *continued*
    postoperative NEC 997.1
      long-term effect 429.4
  cardiorenal (*see also* Hypertension, cardiorenal)
    404.90
  carotid artery bypass graft 996.1
    atherosclerosis — *see* Arteriosclerosis,
      extremities
    embolism 996.74
    occlusion NEC 996.74
    thrombus 996.74
  cataract fragments in eye 998.82
  catheter device NEC — *see also* Complications,
    due to (presence of) any device, implant,
    or graft classified to 996.0-996.5 NEC
    mechanical — *see* Complications,
      mechanical, catheter
  cecostomy 569.60
  cesarean section wound 674.3 ☑5ᵗʰ
  chin implant (prosthetic) NEC 996.79
    infection or inflammation 996.69
    mechanical 996.59
  colostomy (enterostomy) 569.60
    specified type NEC 569.69
  contraceptive device, intrauterine NEC 996.76
    infection 996.65
    inflammation 996.65
    mechanical 996.32
  cord (umbilical) — *see* Complications, umbilical
    cord
  cornea
    due to
      contact lens 371.82
  coronary (artery) bypass (graft) NEC 996.03
    atherosclerosis — *see* Arterio-sclerosis,
      coronary
    embolism 996.72
    infection or inflammation 996.61
    mechanical 996.03
    occlusion NEC 996.72
    specified type NEC 996.72
    thrombus 996.72
  cystostomy 997.5
  delivery 669.9 ☑5ᵗʰ
    procedure (instrumental) (manual) (surgical)
      669.4 ☑5ᵗʰ
    specified type NEC 669.8 ☑5ᵗʰ
  dialysis (hemodialysis) (peritoneal) (renal) NEC
    999.9
    catheter NEC — *see also* Complications, due
      to (presence of) any device, implant or
      graft classified to 996.0-996.5 NEC
      infection or inflammation 996.62
        peritoneal 996.68
      mechanical 996.1
        peritoneal 996.56
  due to (presence of) any device, implant, or
    graft classified to 996.0-996.5 NEC
    996.70
    with infection or inflammation — *see*
      Complications, infection or
      inflammation, due to (presence of) any
      device, implant, or graft classified to
      996.0-996.5 NEC
    arterial NEC 996.74
      coronary NEC 996.03
        atherosclerosis — *see* Arteriosclerosis,
          coronary
        embolism 996.72
        occlusion NEC 996.72
        specified type NEC 996.72
        thrombus 996.72
      renal dialysis 996.73
    arteriovenous fistula or shunt NEC 996.74
    bone growth stimulator 996.78
    breast NEC 996.70
    cardiac NEC 996.72
      defibrillator 996.72
      pacemaker 996.72
      valve prosthesis 996.71
    catheter NEC 996.79
      spinal 996.75
      urinary, indwelling 996.76
      vascular NEC 996.74
        renal dialysis 996.73
      ventricular shunt 996.75

Complications — *continued*
  due to (presence of) any device, implant, or
    graft classified to 996.0-996.5 NEC —
    continued
    coronary (artery) bypass (graft) NEC 996.03
      atherosclerosis — *see* Arteriosclerosis,
        coronary
      embolism 996.72
      occlusion NEC 996.72
      thrombus 996.72
    electrodes
      brain 996.75
      heart 996.72
    gastrointestinal NEC 996.79
    genitourinary NEC 996.76
    heart valve prosthesis NEC 996.71
    infusion pump 996.74
    internal
      joint prosthesis 996.77
      orthopedic NEC 996.78
      specified type NEC 996.79
    intrauterine contraceptive device NEC
      996.76
    joint prosthesis, internal NEC 996.77
    mechanical — *see* Complications,
      mechanical
    nervous system NEC 996.75
    ocular lens NEC 996.79
    orbital NEC 996.79
    orthopedic NEC 996.78
      joint, internal 996.77
    renal dialysis 996.73
    specified type NEC 996.79
    urinary catheter, indwelling 996.76
    vascular NEC 996.74
    ventricular shunt 996.75
  during dialysis NEC 999.9
  ectopic or molar pregnancy NEC 639.9
  electroshock therapy NEC 999.9
  enterostomy 569.60
    specified type NEC 569.69
  external (fixation) device with internal
    component(s) NEC 996.78
    infection or inflammation 996.67
    mechanical 996.4
  extracorporeal circulation NEC 999.9
  eye implant (prosthetic) NEC 996.79
    infection or inflammation 996.69
    mechanical
      ocular lens 996.53
      orbital globe 996.59
  gastrointestinal, postoperative NEC (*see also*
    Complications, surgical procedures)
    997.4
  gastrostomy 536.40
    specified type NEC 536.49
  genitourinary device, implant or graft NEC
    996.76
    infection or inflammation 996.65
      urinary catheter, indwelling 996.64
    mechanical (*see also* Complications,
      mechanical, by type) 996.30
    specified NEC 996.39
  graft (bypass) (patch) NEC — *see also*
    Complications, due to (presence of) any
    device, implant, or graft classified to
    996.0-996.5 NEC
    bone marrow 996.85
    corneal NEC 996.79
      infection or inflammation 996.69
      rejection or reaction 996.51
    mechanical — *see* Complications,
      mechanical, graft
    organ (immune or nonimmune cause)
      (partial) (total) 996.80
      bone marrow 996.85
      heart 996.83
      intestines 996.87
      kidney 996.81
      liver 996.82
      lung 996.84
      pancreas 996.86
      specified NEC 996.89
    skin NEC 996.79
      infection or inflammation 996.69

Complications — *continued*
  graft (bypass) (patch) NEC — *see also*
      Complications, due to (presence of) any
      device, implant, or graft classified to
      996.0-996.5 NEC — *continued*
    skin NEC — *continued*
      rejection 996.52
        artificial 996.55
        decellularized allodermis 996.55
  heart — *see also* Disease, heart transplant
    (immune or nonimmune cause) 996.83
  hematoma (intraoperative) (postoperative)
    998.12
  hemorrhage (intraoperative) (postoperative)
    998.11
  hyperalimentation therapy NEC 999.9
  immunization (procedure) — *see*
    Complications, vaccination
  implant — *see also* Complications, due to
    (presence of) any device, implant, or graft
    classified to 996.0-996.5 NEC
    mechanical — *see* Complications,
      mechanical, implant
  infection and inflammation
    due to (presence of) any device, implant or
      graft classified to 996.0-996.5 NEC
      996.60
      arterial NEC 996.62
        coronary 996.61
        renal dialysis 996.62
      arteriovenous fistula or shunt 996.62
      bone growth stimulator 996.67
      breast 996.69
      cardiac 996.61
      catheter NEC 996.69
        peritoneal 996.68
        spinal 996.63
        urinary, indwelling 996.64
        vascular NEC 996.62
        ventricular shunt 996.63
      coronary artery bypass 996.61
      electrodes
        brain 996.63
        heart 996.61
      gastrointestinal NEC 996.69
      genitourinary NEC 996.65
        indwelling urinary catheter 996.64
      heart valve 996.61
      infusion pump 996.62
      intrauterine contraceptive device 996.65
      joint prosthesis, internal 996.66
      ocular lens 996.69
      orbital (implant) 996.69
      orthopedic NEC 996.67
        joint, internal 996.66
      specified type NEC 996.69
      urinary catheter, indwelling 996.64
      ventricular shunt 996.63
  infusion (procedure) 999.9
    blood — *see* Complications, transfusion
    infection NEC 999.3
    sepsis NEC 999.3
  inhalation therapy NEC 999.9
  injection (procedure) 999.9
    drug reaction (*see also* Reaction, drug) 995.2
    infection NEC 999.3
    sepsis NEC 999.3
    serum (prophylactic) (therapeutic) — *see*
      Complications, vaccination
    vaccine (any) — *see* Complications,
      vaccination
  inoculation (any) — *see* Complications,
    vaccination
  internal device (catheter) (electronic) (fixation)
    (prosthetic) NEC — *see also*
    Complications, due to (presence of) any
    device, implant, or graft classified to
    996.0-996.5 NEC
    mechanical — *see* Complications,
      mechanical
  intestinal transplant (immune or nonimmune
    cause) 996.87
  intraoperative bleeding or hemorrhage 998.11
  intrauterine contraceptive device 996.76 — *see*
    also Complications, contraceptive device
    with fetal damage affecting management of
      pregnancy 655.8 ☑5ᵗʰ

Complications — *continued*
  intrauterine contraceptive device 996.76 — *see*
    also Complications, contraceptive device
    — *continued*
    infection or inflammation 996.65
  jejunostomy 569.60
  kidney transplant (immune or nonimmune
    cause) 996.81
  labor 669.9 ☑5ᵗʰ
    specified condition NEC 669.8 ☑5ᵗʰ
  liver transplant (immune or nonimmune cause)
    996.82
  lumbar puncture 349.0
  mechanical.
    anastomosis — *see* Complications,
      mechanical, graft
    bypass — *see* Complications, mechanical,
      graft
    catheter NEC 996.59
      cardiac 996.09
      cystostomy 996.39
      dialysis (hemodialysis) 996.1
        peritoneal 996.56
      during a procedure 998.2
      urethral, indwelling 996.31
    colostomy 569.62
    device NEC 996.59
      balloon (counterpulsation), intra-aortic
        996.1
      cardiac 996.00
        automatic implantable defibrillator
          996.04
        long-term effect 429.4
        specified NEC 996.09
      contraceptive, intrauterine 996.32
      counterpulsation, intra-aortic 996.1
      fixation, external, with internal
        components 996.4
      fixation, internal (nail, rod, plate) 996.4
      genitourinary 996.30
        specified NEC 996.39
      nervous system 996.2
      orthopedic, internal 996.4
      prosthetic NEC 996.59
      umbrella, vena cava 996.1
      vascular 996.1
    dorsal column stimulator 996.2
    electrode NEC 996.59
      brain 996.2
      cardiac 996.01
      spinal column 996.2
    enterostomy 569.62
    fistula, arteriovenous, surgically created
      996.1
    gastrostomy 536.42
    graft NEC 996.52
      aortic (bifurcation) 996.1
      aortocoronary bypass 996.03
      blood vessel NEC 996.1
      bone 996.4
      cardiac 996.00
      carotid artery bypass 996.1
      cartilage 996.4
      corneal 996.51
      coronary bypass 996.03
      decellularized allodermis 996.55
      genitourinary 996.30
        specified NEC 996.39
      muscle 996.4
      nervous system 996.2
      organ (immune or nonimmune cause)
        996.80
        heart 996.83
        intestines 996.87
        kidney 996.81
        liver 996.82
        lung 996.84
        pancreas 996.86
        specified NEC 996.89
      orthopedic, internal 996.4
      peripheral nerve 996.2
      prosthetic NEC 996.59
      skin 996.52
        artificial 996.55
      specified NEC 996.59
      tendon 996.4

Complications — *continued*
  mechanical — *continued*
    graft NEC — *continued*
      tissue NEC 996.52
      tooth 996.59
      ureter, without mention of resection
        996.39
      vascular 996.1
    heart valve prosthesis 996.02
      long-term effect 429.4
    implant NEC 996.59
      cardiac 996.00
        automatic implantable defibrillator
          996.04
        long-term effect 429.4
        specified NEC 996.09
      electrode NEC 996.59
        brain 996.2
        cardiac 996.01
        spinal column 996.2
      genitourinary 996.30
      nervous system 996.2
      orthopedic, internal 996.4
      prosthetic NEC 996.59
        in
          bile duct 996.59
          breast 996.54
          chin 996.59
          eye
            ocular lens 996.53
            orbital globe 996.59
      vascular 996.1
    nonabsorbable surgical material 996.59
    pacemaker NEC 996.59
      brain 996.2
      cardiac 996.01
      nerve (phrenic) 996.2
    patch — *see* Complications, mechanical,
      graft
    prosthesis NEC 996.59
      bile duct 996.59
      breast 996.54
      chin 996.59
      ocular lens 996.53
      reconstruction, vas deferens 996.39
    reimplant NEC 996.59
      extremity (*see also* Complications,
        reattached, extremity) 996.90
      organ (*see also* Complications,
        transplant, organ, by site) 996.80
    repair — *see* Complications, mechanical,
      graft
    shunt NEC 996.59
      arteriovenous, surgically created 996.1
      ventricular (communicating) 996.2
    stent NEC 996.59
    tracheostomy 519.02
    vas deferens reconstruction 996.39
  medical care NEC 999.9
    cardiac NEC 997.1
    gastrointestinal NEC 997.4
    nervous system NEC 997.00
    peripheral vascular NEC 997.2
    respiratory NEC 997.3
    urinary NEC 997.5
    vascular
      mesenteric artery 997.71
      other vessels 997.79
      peripheral vessels 997.2
      renal artery 997.72
  nephrostomy 997.5
  nervous system
    device, implant, or graft NEC 349.1
      mechanical 996.2
    postoperative NEC 997.00
  obstetric 669.9 ☑5ᵗʰ
    procedure (instrumental) (manual) (surgical)
      669.4 ☑5ᵗʰ
    specified NEC 669.8 ☑5ᵗʰ
    surgical wound 674.3 ☑5ᵗʰ
  ocular lens implant NEC 996.79
    infection or inflammation 996.69
    mechanical 996.53
  organ transplant — *see* Complications,
    transplant, organ, by site

Complications — *continued*
orthopedic device, implant, or graft
internal (fixation) (nail) (plate) (rod) NEC
996.78
infection or inflammation 996.67
joint prosthesis 996.77
infection or inflammation 996.66
mechanical 996.4
pacemaker (cardiac) 996.72
infection or inflammation 996.61
mechanical 996.01
pancreas transplant (immune or nonimmune
cause) 996.86
perfusion NEC 999.9
perineal repair (obstetrical) 674.3 ✓5ᵗʰ
disruption 674.2 ✓5ᵗʰ
pessary (uterus) (vagina) — see Complications,
contraceptive device
phototherapy 990
postcystoscopic 997.5
postmastoidectomy NEC 383.30
postoperative — see Complications, surgical
procedures
pregnancy NEC 646.9 ✓5ᵗʰ
affecting fetus or newborn 761.9
prosthetic device, internal NEC — see also
Complications, due to (presence of) any
device, implant or graft classified to
996.0-996.5 NEC
mechanical NEC (see also Complications,
mechanical) 996.59
puerperium NEC (see also Puerperal) 674.9 ✓5ᵗʰ
puncture, spinal 349.0
pyelogram 997.5
radiation 990
radiotherapy 990
reattached
body part, except extremity 996.99
extremity (infection) (rejection) 996.90
arm(s) 996.94
digit(s) (hand) 996.93
foot 996.95
finger(s) 996.93
foot 996.95
forearm 996.91
hand 996.92
leg 996.96
lower NEC 996.96
toe(s) 996.95
upper NEC 996.94
reimplant NEC — see also Complications, to
(presence of) any device, implant, or graft
classified to 996.0-996.5 NEC
bone marrow 996.85
extremity (see also Complications,
reattached, extremity) 996.90
due to infection 996.90
mechanical — see Complications,
mechanical, reimplant
organ (immune or nonimmune cause)
(partial) (total) (see also Complications,
transplant, organ, by site) 996.80
renal allograft 996.81
renal dialysis — see Complications, dialysis
respiratory 519.9
device, implant or graft NEC 996.79
infection or inflammation 996.69
mechanical 996.59
distress syndrome, adult, following trauma
or surgery 518.5
insufficiency, acute, postoperative 518.5
postoperative NEC 997.3
therapy NEC 999.9
sedation during labor and delivery 668.9 ✓5ᵗʰ
affecting fetus or newborn 763.5
cardiac 668.1 ✓5ᵗʰ
central nervous system 668.2 ✓5ᵗʰ
pulmonary 668.0 ✓5ᵗʰ
specified type NEC 668.8 ✓5ᵗʰ
seroma (intraoperative) (postoperative)
(noninfected) 998.13
infected 998.51
shunt NEC — see also Complications, due to
(presence of) any device, implant, or graft
classified to 996.0-996.5 NEC
mechanical — see Complications,
mechanical, shunt

Complications — *continued*
specified body system NEC
device, implant, or graft NEC — see
Complications, due to (presence of)
any device, implant, or graft classified
to 996.0-996.5 NEC
postoperative NEC 997.99
spinal puncture or tap 349.0
stoma, external
gastrointestinal tract
colostomy 569.60
enterostomy 569.60
gastrostomy 536.40
urinary tract 997.5
surgical procedures 998.9
accidental puncture or laceration 998.2
amputation stump (late) 997.60
anastomosis — see Complications,
anastomosis
burst stitches or sutures ►(external)◄
998.32   ▲
internal 998.31   ●
cardiac 997.1
long-term effect following cardiac surgery
429.4
cataract fragments in eye 998.82
catheter device — see Complications,
catheter device
cecostomy malfunction 569.62
colostomy malfunction 569.62
cystostomy malfunction 997.5
dehiscence (of incision) ►(external)◄
998.32   ▲
internal 998.31   ●
dialysis NEC (see also Complications,
dialysis) 999.9
disruption
anastomosis (internal) — see
Complications, mechanical, graft
internal suture (line) 998.31   ▲
wound ►(external)◄ 998.32   ▲
internal 998.31   ●
dumping syndrome (postgastrectomy) 564.2
elephantiasis or lymphedema 997.99
postmastectomy 457.0
emphysema (surgical) 998.81
enterostomy malfunction 569.62
evisceration 998.32   ▲
fistula (persistent postoperative) 998.6
foreign body inadvertently left in wound
(sponge) (suture) (swab) 998.4
from nonabsorbable surgical material
(Dacron) (mesh) (permanent suture)
(reinforcing) (Teflon) — see
Complications, due to (presence of)
any device, implant, or graft classified
to 996.0-996.5 NEC
gastrointestinal NEC 997.4
gastrostomy malfunction 536.42
hematoma 998.12
hemorrhage 998.11
ileostomy malfunction 569.62
internal prosthetic device NEC (see also
Complications, internal device) 996.70
hemolytic anemia 283.19
infection or inflammation 996.60
malfunction — see Complications,
mechanical
mechanical complication — see
Complications, mechanical
thrombus 996.70
jejunostomy malfunction 569.62
nervous system NEC 997.00
obstruction, internal anastomosis — see
Complications, mechanical, graft
other body system NEC 997.99
peripheral vascular NEC 997.2
postcardiotomy syndrome 429.4
postcholecystectomy syndrome 576.0
postcommissurotomy syndrome 429.4
postgastrectomy dumping syndrome 564.2
postmastectomy lymphedema syndrome
457.0
postmastoidectomy 383.30
cholesteatoma, recurrent 383.32
cyst, mucosal 383.31
granulation 383.33

Complications — *continued*
surgical procedures — *continued*
postmastoidectomy — *continued*
inflammation, chronic 383.33
postvagotomy syndrome 564.2
postvalvulotomy syndrome 429.4
reattached extremity (infection) (rejection)
(see also Complications, reattached,
extremity) 996.90
respiratory NEC 997.3
seroma 998.13
shock (endotoxic) (hypovolemic) (septic)
998.0
shunt, prosthetic (thrombus) — see also
Complications, due to (presence of)
any device, implant, or graft classified
to 996.0-996.5 NEC
hemolytic anemia 283.19
specified complication NEC 998.89
stitch abscess 998.59
transplant — see Complications, graft
ureterostomy malfunction 997.5
urethrostomy malfunction 997.5
urinary NEC 997.5
vascular
mesenteric artery 997.71
other vessels 997.79
peripheral vessels 997.2
renal artery 997.72
wound infection 998.59
therapeutic misadventure NEC 999.9
surgical treatment 998.9
tracheostomy 519.00
transfusion (blood) (lymphocytes) (plasma) NEC
999.8
atrophy, liver, yellow, subacute (within 8
months of administration) — see
Hepatitis, viral
bone marrow 996.85
embolism
air 999.1
thrombus 999.2
hemolysis NEC 999.8
bone marrow 996.85
hepatitis (serum) (type B) (within 8 months
after administration) — see Hepatitis,
viral
incompatibility reaction (ABO) (blood group)
999.6
Rh (factor) 999.7
infection 999.3
jaundice (serum) (within 8 months after
administration) — see Hepatitis, viral
sepsis 999.3
shock or reaction NEC 999.8
bone marrow 996.85
subacute yellow atrophy of liver (within 8
months after administration) — see
Hepatitis, viral
thromboembolism 999.2
transplant NEC — see also Complications, due
to (presence of) any device, implant, or
graft classified to 996.0-996.5 NEC
bone marrow 996.85
organ (immune or nonimmune cause)
(partial) (total) 996.80
bone marrow 996.85
heart 996.83
intestines 996.87
kidney 996.81
liver 996.82
lung 996.84
pancreas 996.86
specified NEC 996.89
trauma NEC (early) 958.8
ultrasound therapy NEC 999.9
umbilical cord
affecting fetus or newborn 762.6
complicating delivery 663.9 ✓5ᵗʰ
affecting fetus or newborn 762.6
specified type NEC 663.8 ✓5ᵗʰ
urethral catheter NEC 996.76
infection or inflammation 996.64
mechanical 996.31
urinary, postoperative NEC 997.5
vaccination 999.9
anaphylaxis NEC 999.4

Complications — *continued*
vaccination — *continued*
  cellulitis 999.3
  encephalitis or encephalomyelitis 323.5
  hepatitis (serum) (type B) (within 8 months
    after administration) — *see* Hepatitis,
    viral
  infection (general) (local) NEC 999.3
  jaundice (serum) (within 8 months after
    administration) — *see* Hepatitis, viral
  meningitis 997.09 *[321.8]*
  myelitis 323.5
  protein sickness 999.5
  reaction (allergic) 999.5
    Herxheimer's 995.0
    serum 999.5
  sepsis 999.3
  serum intoxication, sickness, rash, or other
    serum reaction NEC 999.5
  shock (allergic) (anaphylactic) 999.4
  subacute yellow atrophy of liver (within 8
    months after administration) — *see*
    Hepatitis, viral
  vaccinia (generalized) 999.0
    localized 999.3
vascular
  device, implant, or graft NEC 996.74
    infection or inflammation 996.62
    mechanical NEC 996.1
      cardiac (*see also* Complications,
        mechanical, by type) 996.00
  following infusion, perfusion, or transfusion
    999.2
  postoperative NEC 997.2
    mesenteric artery 997.71
    other vessels 997.79
    peripheral vessels 997.2
    renal artery 997.72
  ventilation therapy NEC 999.9
Compound presentation, complicating delivery
  652.8 ✔5ᵗʰ
  causing obstructed labor 660.0 ✔5ᵗʰ
Compressed air disease 993.3
Compression
  with injury — *see* specific injury
  arm NEC 354.9
  artery 447.1
    celiac, syndrome 447.4
  brachial plexus 353.0
  brain (stem) 348.4
    due to
      contusion, brain — *see* Contusion, brain
      injury NEC — *see also* Hemorrhage,
        brain, traumatic
      birth — *see* Birth, injury, brain
      laceration, brain — *see* Laceration, brain
    osteopathic 739.0
  bronchus 519.1
  by cicatrix — *see* Cicatrix
  cardiac 423.9
  cauda equina 344.60
    with neurogenic bladder 344.61
  celiac (artery) (axis) 447.4
  cerebral — *see* Compression, brain
  cervical plexus 353.2
  cord (umbilical) — *see* Compression, umbilical
    cord
  cranial nerve 352.9
    second 377.49
    third (partial) 378.51
      total 378.52
    fourth 378.53
    fifth 350.8
    sixth 378.54
    seventh 351.8
  divers' squeeze 993.3
  duodenum (external) (*see also* Obstruction,
    duodenum) 537.3
  during birth 767.9
  esophagus 530.3
    congenital, external 750.3
  Eustachian tube 381.63
  facies (congenital) 754.0
  fracture — *see* Fracture, by site
  heart — *see* Disease, heart

Compression — *continued*
  intestine (*see also* Obstruction, intestine) 560.9
    with hernia — *see* Hernia, by site, with
      obstruction
  laryngeal nerve, recurrent 478.79
  leg NEC 355.8
  lower extremity NEC 355.8
  lumbosacral plexus 353.1
  lung 518.89
  lymphatic vessel 457.1
  medulla — *see* Compression, brain
  nerve NEC — *see also* Disorder, nerve
    arm NEC 354.9
    autonomic nervous system (*see also*
      Neuropathy, peripheral, autonomic)
      337.9
    axillary 353.0
    cranial NEC 352.9
    due to displacement of intervertebral disc
      722.2
      with myelopathy 722.70
      cervical 722.0
        with myelopathy 722.71
      lumbar, lumbosacral 722.10
        with myelopathy 722.73
      thoracic, thoracolumbar 722.11
        with myelopathy 722.72
    iliohypogastric 355.79
    ilioinguinal 355.79
    leg NEC 355.8
    lower extremity NEC 355.8
    median (in carpal tunnel) 354.0
    obturator 355.79
    optic 377.49
    plantar 355.6
    posterior tibial (in tarsal tunnel) 355.5
    root (by scar tissue) NEC 724.9
      cervical NEC 723.4
      lumbar NEC 724.4
      lumbosacral 724.4
      thoracic 724.4
    saphenous 355.79
    sciatic (acute) 355.0
    sympathetic 337.9
    traumatic — *see* Injury, nerve
    ulnar 354.2
    upper extremity NEC 354.9
  peripheral — *see* Compression, nerve
  spinal (cord) (old or nontraumatic) 336.9
    by displacement of intervertebral disc — *see*
      Displacement, intervertebral disc
    nerve
      root NEC 724.9
        postoperative 722.80
          cervical region 722.81
          lumbar region 722.83
          thoracic region 722.82
        traumatic — *see* Injury, nerve, spinal
      traumatic — *see* Injury, nerve, spinal
    spondylogenic 721.91
      cervical 721.1
      lumbar, lumbosacral 721.42
      thoracic 721.41
    traumatic — *see also* Injury, spinal, by site
      with fracture, vertebra — *see* Fracture,
        vertebra, by site, with spinal cord
        injury
  spondylogenic — *see* Compression, spinal cord,
    spondylogenic
  subcostal nerve (syndrome) 354.8
  sympathetic nerve NEC 337.9
  syndrome 958.5
  thorax 512.8
    iatrogenic 512.1
    postoperative 512.1
  trachea 519.1
    congenital 748.3
  ulnar nerve (by scar tissue) 354.2
  umbilical cord
    affecting fetus or newborn 762.5
      cord prolapsed 762.4
    complicating delivery 663.2 ✔5ᵗʰ
      cord around neck 663.1 ✔5ᵗʰ
      cord prolapsed 663.0 ✔5ᵗʰ
  upper extremity NEC 354.9
  ureter 593.3
  urethra — *see* Stricture, urethra

Compression — *continued*
  vein 459.2
  vena cava (inferior) (superior) 459.2
  vertebral NEC — *see* Compression, spinal
    (cord)
Compulsion, compulsive
  eating 307.51
  neurosis (obsessive) 300.3
  personality 301.4
  states (mixed) 300.3
  swearing 300.3
    in Gilles de la Tourette's syndrome 307.23
  tics and spasms 307.22
  water drinking NEC (syndrome) 307.9
Concato's disease (pericardial polyserositis) 423.2
  peritoneal 568.82
  pleural — *see* Pleurisy
Concavity, chest wall 738.3
Concealed
  hemorrhage NEC 459.0
  penis 752.65
Concentric fading 368.12
Concern (normal) about sick person in family
  V61.49
Concrescence (teeth) 520.2
Concretio cordis 423.1
  rheumatic 393
Concretion — *see also* Calculus
  appendicular 543.9
  canaliculus 375.57
  clitoris 624.8
  conjunctiva 372.54
  eyelid 374.56
  intestine (impaction) (obstruction) 560.39
  lacrimal (passages) 375.57
  prepuce (male) 605
    female (clitoris) 624.8
  salivary gland (any) 527.5
  seminal vesicle 608.89
  stomach 537.89
  tonsil 474.8
Concussion (current) 850.9
  with
    loss of consciousness 850.5
      brief (less than one hour) 850.1
      moderate (1-24 hours) 850.2
      prolonged (more than 24 hours) (with
        complete recovery) (with return to
        pre-existing conscious level) 850.3
        without return to pre-existing
          conscious level 850.4
    mental confusion or disorientation (without
      loss of consciousness) 850.0
      with loss of consciousness — *see*
        Concussion, with, loss of
        consciousness
    without loss of consciousness 850.0
  blast (air) (hydraulic) (immersion) (underwater)
    869.0
    with open wound into cavity 869.1
    abdomen or thorax — *see* Injury, internal,
      by site
    brain — *see* Concussion, brain
    ear (acoustic nerve trauma) 951.5
      with perforation, tympanic membrane —
        see Wound, open, ear drum
    thorax — *see* Injury, internal, intrathoracic
      organs NEC
  brain or cerebral (without skull fracture) 850.9
    with
      loss of consciousness 850.5
        brief (less than one hour) 850.1
        moderate (1-24 hours) 850.2
        prolonged (more than 24 hours) (with
          complete recovery) (with return
          to pre-existing conscious level)
          850.3
          without return to pre-existing
            conscious level 850.4
      mental confusion or disorientation
        (without loss of consciousness)
        850.0
        with loss of consciousness — *see*
          Concussion, brain, with, loss of
          consciousness

Concussion — *continued*
brain or cerebral — *continued*
with — *continued*
skull fracture — *see* Fracture, skull, by site
without loss of consciousness 850.0
cauda equina 952.4
cerebral — *see* Concussion, brain
conus medullaris (spine) 952.4
hydraulic — *see* Concussion, blast
internal organs — *see* Injury, internal, by site
labyrinth — *see* Injury, intracranial
ocular 921.3
osseous labyrinth — *see* Injury, intracranial
spinal (cord) — *see also* Injury, spinal, by site
due to
broken
back — *see* Fracture, vertebra, by site, with spinal cord injury
neck — *see* Fracture, vertebra, cervical, with spinal cord injury
fracture, fracture dislocation, or compression fracture of spine or vertebra — *see* Fracture, vertebra, by site, with spinal cord injury
syndrome 310.2
underwater blast — *see* Concussion, blast
Condition — *see also* Disease
psychiatric 298.9
respiratory NEC 519.9
acute or subacute NEC 519.9
due to
external agent 508.9
specified type NEC 508.8
fumes or vapors (chemical) (inhalation) 506.3
radiation 508.0
chronic NEC 519.9
due to
external agent 508.9
specified type NEC 508.8
fumes or vapors (chemical) (inhalation) 506.4
radiation 508.1
due to
external agent 508.9
specified type NEC 508.8
fumes or vapors (chemical) (inhalation) 506.9
Conduct disturbance (*see also* Disturbance, conduct) 312.9
adjustment reaction 309.3
hyperkinetic 314.2
Condyloma NEC 078.10
acuminatum 078.11
gonorrheal 098.0
latum 091.3
syphilitic 091.3
congenital 090.0
venereal, syphilitic 091.3
Confinement — *see* Delivery
Conflagration — *see also* Burn, by site
asphyxia (by inhalation of smoke, gases, fumes, or vapors) 987.9
specified agent — *see* Table of Drugs and Chemicals
Conflict
family V61.9
specified circumstance NEC V61.8
interpersonal NEC V62.81
marital V61.10
involving divorce or estrangement V61.0
parent-child V61.20
partner V61.10
Confluent — *see* condition
Confusion, confused (mental) (state) (*see also* State, confusional) 298.9
acute 293.0
epileptic 293.0
postoperative 293.9
psychogenic 298.2
reactive (from emotional stress, psychological trauma) 298.2
subacute 293.1
Congelation 991.9

Congenital — *see also* condition
aortic septum 747.29
intrinsic factor deficiency 281.0
malformation — *see* Anomaly
Congestion, congestive (chronic) (passive)
asphyxia, newborn 768.9
bladder 596.8
bowel 569.89
brain (*see also* Disease, cerebrovascular NEC) 437.8
malarial 084.9
breast 611.79
bronchi 519.1
bronchial tube 519.1
catarrhal 472.0
cerebral — *see* Congestion, brain
cerebrospinal — *see* Congestion, brain
chest 514
chill 780.99 ▲
malarial (*see also* Malaria) 084.6
circulatory NEC 459.9
conjunctiva 372.71
due to disturbance of circulation 459.9
duodenum 537.3
enteritis — *see* Enteritis
eye 372.71
fibrosis syndrome (pelvic) 625.5
gastroenteritis — *see* Enteritis
general 799.8
glottis 476.0
heart (*see also* Failure, heart) 428.0
hepatic 573.0
hypostatic (lung) 514
intestine 569.89
intracranial — *see* Congestion, brain
kidney 593.89
labyrinth 386.50
larynx 476.0
liver 573.0
lung 514
active or acute (*see also* Pneumonia) 486
congenital 770.0
chronic 514
hypostatic 514
idiopathic, acute 518.5
passive 514
malaria, malarial (brain) (fever) (*see also* Malaria) 084.6
medulla — *see* Congestion, brain
nasal 478.1
orbit, orbital 376.33
inflammatory (chronic) 376.10
acute 376.00
ovary 620.8
pancreas 577.8
pelvic, female 625.5
pleural 511.0
prostate (active) 602.1
pulmonary — *see* Congestion, lung
renal 593.89
retina 362.89
seminal vesicle 608.89
spinal cord 336.1
spleen 289.51
chronic 289.51
stomach 537.89
trachea 464.11
urethra 599.84
uterus 625.5
with subinvolution 621.1
viscera 799.8
Congestive — *see* Congestion
Conical
cervix 622.6
cornea 371.60
teeth 520.2
Conjoined twins 759.4
causing disproportion (fetopelvic) 653.7 ✓5ᵗʰ
Conjugal maladjustment V61.10
involving divorce or estrangement V61.0
Conjunctiva — *see* condition
Conjunctivitis (exposure) (infectious) (nondiphtheritic) (pneumococcal) (pustular) (staphylococcal) (streptococcal) NEC 372.30
actinic 370.24
acute 372.00

Conjunctivitis NEC — *continued*
acute — *continued*
atopic 372.05
contagious 372.03
follicular 372.02
hemorrhagic (viral) 077.4
adenoviral (acute) 077.3
allergic (chronic) 372.14
with hay fever 372.05
anaphylactic 372.05
angular 372.03
Apollo (viral) 077.4
atopic 372.05
blennorrhagic (neonatorum) 098.40
catarrhal 372.03
chemical 372.05
chlamydial 077.98
due to
Chlamydia trachomatis — *see* Trachoma
paratrachoma 077.0
chronic 372.10
allergic 372.14
follicular 372.12
simple 372.11
specified type NEC 372.14
vernal 372.13
diphtheritic 032.81
due to
dust 372.05
enterovirus type 70 077.4
erythema multiforme 695.1 [372.33]
filariasis (*see also* Filariasis) 125.9 [372.15]
mucocutaneous
disease NEC 372.33
leishmaniasis 085.5 [372.15]
Reiter's disease 099.3 [372.33]
syphilis 095.8 [372.10]
toxoplasmosis (acquired) 130.1
congenital (active) 771.2
trachoma — *see* Trachoma
dust 372.05
eczematous 370.31
epidemic 077.1
hemorrhagic 077.4
follicular (acute) 372.02
adenoviral (acute) 077.3
chronic 372.12
glare 370.24
gonococcal (neonatorum) 098.40
granular (trachomatous) 076.1
late effect 139.1
hemorrhagic (acute) (epidemic) 077.4
herpetic (simplex) 054.43
zoster 053.21
inclusion 077.0
infantile 771.6
influenzal 372.03
Koch-Weeks 372.03
light 372.05
medicamentosa 372.05
membranous 372.04
meningococcic 036.89
Morax-Axenfeld 372.02
mucopurulent NEC 372.03
neonatal 771.6
gonococcal 098.40
Newcastle's 077.8
nodosa 360.14
of Beal 077.3
parasitic 372.15
filariasis (*see also* Filariasis) 125.9 [372.15]
mucocutaneous leishmaniasis 085.5 [372.15]
Parinaud's 372.02
petrificans 372.39
phlyctenular 370.31
pseudomembranous 372.04
diphtheritic 032.81
purulent 372.03
Reiter's 099.3 [372.33]
rosacea 695.3 [372.31]
serous 372.01
viral 077.99
simple chronic 372.11
specified NEC 372.39
sunlamp 372.04
swimming pool 077.0

Conjunctivitis NEC — *continued*
  trachomatous (follicular) 076.1
    acute 076.0
    late effect 139.1
  traumatic NEC 372.39
  tuberculous (*see also* Tuberculosis) 017.3 ✓5ᵗʰ
    [370.31]
  tularemic 021.3
  tularensis 021.3
  vernal 372.13
    limbar 372.13 *[370.32]*
  viral 077.99
    acute hemorrhagic 077.4
    specified NEC 077.8
Conjunctivochalasis 372.81
Conjunctoblepharitis — *see* Conjunctivitis
Conn (-Louis) syndrome (primary aldosteronism)
  255.1
Connective tissue — *see* condition
Conradi (-Hünermann) syndrome or disease
  (chondrodysplasia calcificans congenita)
  756.59
Consanguinity V19.7
Consecutive — *see* condition
Consolidated lung (base) — *see* Pneumonia, lobar
Constipation 564.00
  atonic 564.09
  drug induced
    correct substance properly administered
      564.09
    overdose or wrong substance given or taken
      977.9
      specified drug — *see* Table of Drugs and
        Chemicals
  neurogenic 564.09
  other specified NEC 564.09
  outlet dysfunction 564.02
  psychogenic 306.4
  simple 564.00
  slow transit 564.01
  spastic 564.09
Constitutional — *see also* condition
  arterial hypotension (*see also* Hypotension)
    458.9
  obesity 278.00
    morbid 278.01
  psychopathic state 301.9
  short stature in childhood 783.43
  state, developmental V21.9
    specified development NEC V21.8
  substandard 301.6
Constitutionally substandard 301.6
Constriction
  anomalous, meningeal bands or folds 742.8
  aortic arch (congenital) 747.10
  asphyxiation or suffocation by 994.7
  bronchus 519.1
  canal, ear (*see also* Stricture, ear canal,
    acquired) 380.50
  duodenum 537.3
  gallbladder (*see also* Obstruction, gallbladder)
    575.2
    congenital 751.69
  intestine (*see also* Obstruction, intestine) 560.9
  larynx 478.74
    congenital 748.3
  meningeal bands or folds, anomalous 742.8
  organ or site, congenital NEC — *see* Atresia
  prepuce (congenital) 605
  pylorus 537.0
    adult hypertrophic 537.0
    congenital or infantile 750.5
    newborn 750.5
  ring (uterus) 661.4 ✓5ᵗʰ
    affecting fetus or newborn 763.7
  spastic — *see also* Spasm
    ureter 593.3
    urethra — *see* Stricture, urethra
  stomach 537.89
  ureter 593.3
  urethra — *see* Stricture, urethra
  visual field (functional) (peripheral) 368.45
Constrictive — *see* condition

Consultation
  medical — *see also* Counseling, medical
  specified reason NEC V65.8
  without complaint or sickness V65.9
    feared complaint unfounded V65.5
    specified reason NEC V65.8
Consumption — *see* Tuberculosis
Contact
  with
    AIDS virus V01.7
    anthrax V01.81   ●
    cholera V01.0
    communicable disease V01.9
      specified type NEC V01.89   ▲
      viral NEC V01.7
    German measles V01.4
    gonorrhea V01.6
    HIV V01.7
    human immunodeficiency virus V01.7
    parasitic disease NEC V01.89   ▲
    poliomyelitis V01.2
    rabies V01.5
    rubella V01.4
    smallpox V01.3
    syphilis V01.6
    tuberculosis V01.1
    venereal disease V01.6
    viral disease NEC V01.7
  dermatitis — *see* Dermatitis
Contamination, food (*see also* Poisoning, food)
  005.9
Contraception, contraceptive
  advice NEC V25.09
    family planning V25.09
    fitting of diaphragm V25.02
    prescribing or use of
      oral contraceptive agent V25.01
      specified agent NEC V25.02
  counseling NEC V25.09
    family planning V25.09
    fitting of diaphragm V25.02
    prescribing or use of
      oral contraceptive agent V25.01
      specified agent NEC V25.02
  device (in situ) V45.59
    causing menorrhagia 996.76
    checking V25.42
    complications 996.32
    insertion V25.1
    intrauterine V45.51
    reinsertion V25.42
    removal V25.42
    subdermal V45.52
  fitting of diaphragm V25.02
  insertion
    intrauterine contraceptive device V25.1
    subdermal implantable V25.5
  maintenance V25.40
    examination V25.40
      subdermal implantable V25.43
        intrauterine device V25.42
      oral contraceptive V25.41
      specified method NEC V25.49
    intrauterine device V25.42
    oral contraceptive V25.41
    specified method NEC V25.49
    subdermal implantable V25.43
  management NEC V25.49
  prescription
    oral contraceptive agent V25.01
      repeat V25.41
    specified agent NEC V25.02
      repeat V25.49
  sterilization V25.2
  surveillance V25.40
    intrauterine device V25.42
    oral contraceptive agent V25.41
      subdermal implantable V25.43
    specified method NEC V25.49
Contraction, contracture, contracted
  Achilles tendon (*see also* Short, tendon,
    Achilles) 727.81
  anus 564.89
  axilla 729.9
  bile duct (*see also* Disease, biliary) 576.8

Contraction, contracture, contracted —
  continued
  bladder 596.8
    neck or sphincter 596.0
  bowel (*see also* Obstruction, intestine) 560.9
  Braxton Hicks 644.1 ✓5ᵗʰ
  bronchus 519.1
  burn (old) — *see* Cicatrix
  cecum (*see also* Obstruction, intestine) 560.9
  cervix (*see also* Stricture, cervix) 622.4
    congenital 752.49
  cicatricial — *see* Cicatrix
  colon (*see also* Obstruction, intestine) 560.9
  conjunctiva trachomatous, active 076.1
    late effect 139.1
  Dupuytren's 728.6
  eyelid 374.41
  eye socket (after enucleation) 372.64
  face 729.9
  fascia (lata) (postural) 728.89
    Dupuytren's 728.6
    palmar 728.6
    plantar 728.71
  finger NEC 736.29
    congenital 755.59
    joint (*see also* Contraction, joint) 718.44
  flaccid, paralytic
    joint (*see also* Contraction, joint) 718.4 ✓5ᵗʰ
    muscle 728.85
      ocular 378.50
  gallbladder (*see also* Obstruction, gallbladder)
    575.2
  hamstring 728.89
    tendon 727.81
  heart valve — *see* Endocarditis
  Hicks' 644.1 ✓5ᵗʰ
  hip (*see also* Contraction, joint) 718.4 ✓5ᵗʰ
  hourglass
    bladder 596.8
      congenital 753.8
    gallbladder (*see also* Obstruction,
      gallbladder) 575.2
      congenital 751.69
    stomach 536.8
      congenital 750.7
      psychogenic 306.4
    uterus 661.4 ✓5ᵗʰ
      affecting fetus or newborn 763.7
  hysterical 300.11
  infantile (*see also* Epilepsy) 345.6 ✓5ᵗʰ
  internal os (*see also* Stricture, cervix) 622.4
  intestine (*see also* Obstruction, intestine) 560.9
  joint (abduction) (acquired) (adduction) (flexion)
    (rotation) 718.40
    ankle 718.47
    congenital NEC 755.8
      generalized or multiple 754.89
        lower limb joints 754.89
      hip (*see also* Subluxation, congenital, hip)
        754.32
      lower limb (including pelvic girdle) not
        involving hip 754.89
      upper limb (including shoulder girdle)
        755.59
    elbow 718.42
    foot 718.47
    hand 718.44
    hip 718.45
    hysterical 300.11
    knee 718.46
    multiple sites 718.49
    pelvic region 718.45
    shoulder (region) 718.41
    specified site NEC 718.48
    wrist 718.43
  kidney (granular) (secondary) (*see also*
    Sclerosis, renal) 587
    congenital 753.3
    hydronephritic 591
    pyelonephritic (*see also* Pyelitis, chronic)
      590.00
    tuberculous (*see also* Tuberculosis)
      016.0 ✓5ᵗʰ
  ligament 728.89
    congenital 756.89
  liver — *see* Cirrhosis, liver
  muscle (postinfectional) (postural) NEC 728.85

✓4ᵗʰ Fourth-digit Required   ✓5ᵗʰ Fifth-digit Required   ▶◀ Revised Text   ● New Line   ▲ Revised Code

Contraction — Contusion

Contraction, contracture, contracted —
continued
  muscle NEC — *continued*
    congenital 756.89
      sternocleidomastoid 754.1
    extraocular 378.60
    eye (extrinsic) (*see also* Strabismus) 378.9
      paralytic (*see also* Strabismus, paralytic)
        378.50
    flaccid 728.85
    hysterical 300.11
    ischemic (Volkmann's) 958.6
    paralytic 728.85
    posttraumatic 958.6
    psychogenic 306.0
      specified as conversion reaction 300.11
  myotonic 728.85
  neck (*see also* Torticollis) 723.5
    congenital 754.1
    psychogenic 306.0
  ocular muscle (*see also* Strabismus) 378.9
    paralytic (*see also* Strabismus, paralytic)
      378.50
  organ or site, congenital NEC — *see* Atresia
  outlet (pelvis) — *see* Contraction, pelvis
  palmar fascia 728.6
  paralytic
    joint (*see also* Contraction, joint) 718.4 ✓5ᵗʰ
    muscle 728.85
      ocular (*see also* Strabismus, paralytic)
        378.50
  pelvis (acquired) (general) 738.6
    affecting fetus or newborn 763.1
    complicating delivery 653.1 ✓5ᵗʰ
      causing obstructed labor 660.1 ✓5ᵗʰ
      generally contracted 653.1 ✓5ᵗʰ
        causing obstructed labor 660.1 ✓5ᵗʰ
      inlet 653.2 ✓5ᵗʰ
        causing obstructed labor 660.1 ✓5ᵗʰ
      midpelvic 653.8 ✓5ᵗʰ
        causing obstructed labor 660.1 ✓5ᵗʰ
      midplane 653.8 ✓5ᵗʰ
        causing obstructed labor 660.1 ✓5ᵗʰ
      outlet 653.3 ✓5ᵗʰ
        causing obstructed labor 660.1 ✓5ᵗʰ
  plantar fascia 728.71
  premature
    atrial 427.61
    auricular 427.61
    auriculoventricular 427.61
    heart (junctional) (nodal) 427.60
    supraventricular 427.61
    ventricular 427.69
  prostate 602.8
  pylorus (*see also* Pylorospasm) 537.81
  rectosigmoid (*see also* Obstruction, intestine)
    560.9
  rectum, rectal (sphincter) 564.89
    psychogenic 306.4
  ring (Bandl's) 661.4 ✓5ᵗʰ
    affecting fetus or newborn 763.7
  scar — *see* Cicatrix
  sigmoid (*see also* Obstruction, intestine) 560.9
  socket, eye 372.64
  spine (*see also* Curvature, spine) 737.9
  stomach 536.8
    hourglass 536.8
      congenital 750.7
      psychogenic 306.4
    psychogenic 306.4
  tendon (sheath) (*see also* Short, tendon) 727.81
  toe 735.8
  ureterovesical orifice (postinfectional) 593.3
  urethra 599.84
  uterus 621.8
    abnormal 661.9 ✓5ᵗʰ
      affecting fetus or newborn 763.7
    clonic, hourglass or tetanic 661.4 ✓5ᵗʰ
      affecting fetus or newborn 763.7
    dyscoordinate 661.4 ✓5ᵗʰ
      affecting fetus or newborn 763.7
    hourglass 661.4 ✓5ᵗʰ
      affecting fetus or newborn 763.7
    hypotonic NEC 661.2 ✓5ᵗʰ
      affecting fetus or newborn 763.7
    incoordinate 661.4 ✓5ᵗʰ
      affecting fetus or newborn 763.7

Contraction, contracture, contracted —
continued
  uterus — *continued*
    inefficient or poor 661.2 ✓5ᵗʰ
      affecting fetus or newborn 763.7
    irregular 661.2 ✓5ᵗʰ
      affecting fetus or newborn 763.7
    tetanic 661.4 ✓5ᵗʰ
      affecting fetus or newborn 763.7
  vagina (outlet) 623.2
  vesical 596.8
    neck or urethral orifice 596.0
  visual field, generalized 368.45
  Volkmann's (ischemic) 958.6

Contusion (skin surface intact) 924.9
  with
    crush injury — *see* Crush
    dislocation — *see* Dislocation, by site
    fracture — *see* Fracture, by site
    internal injury — *see also* Injury, internal,
      by site
      heart — *see* Contusion, cardiac
      kidney — *see* Contusion, kidney
      liver — *see* Contusion, liver
      lung — *see* Contusion, lung
      spleen — *see* Contusion, spleen
    intracranial injury — *see* Injury, intracranial
    nerve injury — *see* Injury, nerve
    open wound — *see* Wound, open, by site
  abdomen, abdominal (muscle) (wall) 922.2
    organ(s) NEC 868.00
  adnexa, eye NEC 921.9
  ankle 924.21
    with other parts of foot 924.20
  arm 923.9
    lower (with elbow) 923.10
    upper 923.03
      with shoulder or axillary region 923.09
  auditory canal (external) (meatus) (and other
    part(s) of neck, scalp, or face, except eye)
    920
  auricle, ear (and other part(s) of neck, scalp, or
    face except eye) 920
  axilla 923.02
    with shoulder or upper arm 923.09
  back 922.31
  bone NEC 924.9
  brain (cerebral) (membrane) (with hemorrhage)
    851.8 ✓5ᵗʰ

Note — Use the following fifth-digit
subclassification with categories 851-854:

0   *unspecified state of consciousness*
1   *with no loss of consciousness*
2   *with brief [less than one hour] loss*
     of consciousness
3   *with moderate [1-24 hours] loss of*
     consciousness
4   *with prolonged [more than 24 hours]*
     loss of consciousness and return to
     pre-existing conscious level
5   *with prolonged [more than 24 hours]*
     loss of consciousness, without
     return to pre-existing conscious level
     Use fifth-digit to designate when a patient
     is unconscious and dies before
     regaining consciousness, regardless
     of the duration of the loss of
     consciousness
6   *with loss of consciousness of*
     unspecified duration
9   *with concussion, unspecified*

    with
      open intracranial wound 851.9 ✓5ᵗʰ
      skull fracture — *see* Fracture, skull, by
        site
    cerebellum 851.4 ✓5ᵗʰ
      with open intracranial wound 851.5 ✓5ᵗʰ
    cortex 851.0 ✓5ᵗʰ
      with open intracranial wound 851.1 ✓5ᵗʰ
    occipital lobe 851.4 ✓5ᵗʰ
      with open intracranial wound 851.5 ✓5ᵗʰ

Contusion — *continued*
  brain — *continued*
    stem 851.4 ✓5ᵗʰ
      with open intracranial wound 851.5 ✓5ᵗʰ
  breast 922.0
  brow (and other part(s) of neck, scalp, or face,
    except eye) 920
  buttock 922.32
  canthus 921.1
  cardiac 861.01
    with open wound into thorax 861.11
  cauda equina (spine) 952.4
  cerebellum — *see* Contusion, brain, cerebellum
  cerebral — *see* Contusion, brain
  cheek(s) (and other part(s) of neck, scalp, or
    face, except eye) 920
  chest (wall) 922.1
  chin (and other part(s) of neck, scalp, or face,
    except eye) 920
  clitoris 922.4
  conjunctiva 921.1
  conus medullaris (spine) 952.4
  cornea 921.3
  corpus cavernosum 922.4
  cortex (brain) (cerebral) — *see* Contusion,
    brain, cortex
  costal region 922.1
  ear (and other part(s) of neck, scalp, or face
    except eye) 920
  elbow 923.11
    with forearm 923.10
  epididymis 922.4
  epigastric region 922.2
  eye NEC 921.9
  eyeball 921.3
  eyelid(s) (and periocular area) 921.1
  face (and neck, or scalp, any part except eye)
    920
  femoral triangle 922.2
  fetus or newborn 772.6
  finger(s) (nail) (subungual) 923.3
  flank 922.2
  foot (with ankle) (excluding toe(s)) 924.20
  forearm 923.10
  forehead (and other part(s) of neck, scalp, or
    face, except eye) 920
  genital organs, external 922.4
  globe (eye) 921.3
  groin 922.2
  gum(s) (and other part(s) of neck, scalp, or face,
    except eye) 920
  hand(s) (except fingers alone) 923.20
  head (any part, except eye) (and face) (and
    neck) 920
  heart — *see* Contusion, cardiac
  heel 924.20
  hip 924.01
    with thigh 924.00
  iliac region 922.2
  inguinal region 922.2
  internal organs (abdomen, chest, or pelvis) NEC
    — *see* Injury, internal, by site
  interscapular region 922.33
  iris (eye) 921.3
  kidney 866.01
    with open wound into cavity 866.11
  knee 924.11
    with lower leg 924.10
  labium (majus) (minus) 922.4
  lacrimal apparatus, gland, or sac 921.1
  larynx (and other part(s) of neck, scalp, or face,
    except eye) 920
  late effect — *see* Late, effects (of), contusion
  leg 924.5
    lower (with knee) 924.10
  lens 921.3
  lingual (and other part(s) of neck, scalp, or
    face, except eye) 920
  lip(s) (and other part(s) of neck, scalp, or face,
    except eye) 920
  liver 864.01
    with
      laceration — *see* Laceration, liver
      open wound into cavity 864.11
  lower extremity 924.5
    multiple sites 924.4
  lumbar region 922.31

✓4ᵗʰ Fourth-digit Required   ✓5ᵗʰ Fifth-digit Required   ▶◀ Revised Text   ● New Line   ▲ Revised Code

Contusion — continued

lung 861.21
  with open wound into thorax 861.31
malar region (and other part(s) of neck, scalp, or face, except eye) 920
mandibular joint (and other part(s) of neck, scalp, or face, except eye) 920
mastoid region (and other part(s) of neck, scalp. or face, except eye) 920
membrane, brain — see Contusion, brain
midthoracic region 922.1
mouth (and other part(s) of neck, scalp, or face, except eye) 920
multiple sites (not classifiable to same three-digit category) 924.8
  lower limb 924.4
  trunk 922.8
  upper limb 923.8
muscle NEC 924.9
myocardium — see Contusion, cardiac
nasal (septum) (and other part(s) of neck, scalp, or face, except eye) 920
neck (and scalp, or face any part, except eye) 920
nerve — see Injury, nerve, by site
nose (and other part(s) of neck, scalp, or face, except eye) 920
occipital region (scalp) (and neck or face, except eye) 920
  lobe — see Contusion, brain, occipital lobe
orbit (region) (tissues) 921.2
palate (soft) (and other part(s) of neck, scalp, or face, except eye) 920
parietal region (scalp) (and neck, or face, except eye) 920
  lobe — see Contusion, brain
penis 922.4
pericardium — see Contusion, cardiac
perineum 922.4
periocular area 921.1
pharynx (and other part(s) of neck, scalp, or face, except eye) 920
popliteal space (see also Contusion, knee) 924.11
prepuce 922.4
pubic region 922.4
pudenda 922.4
pulmonary — see Contusion, lung
quadriceps femoralis 924.00
rib cage 922.1
sacral region 922.32
salivary ducts or glands (and other part(s) of neck, scalp, or face, except eye) 920
scalp (and neck, or face any part, except eye) 920
scapular region 923.01
  with shoulder or upper arm 923.09
sclera (eye) 921.3
scrotum 922.4
shoulder 923.00
  with upper arm or axillar regions 923.09
skin NEC 924.9
skull 920
spermatic cord 922.4
spinal cord — see also Injury, spinal, by site
  cauda equina 952.4
  conus medullaris 952.4
spleen 865.01
  with open wound into cavity 865.11
sternal region 922.1
stomach — see Injury, internal, stomach
subconjunctival 921.1
subcutaneous NEC 924.9
submaxillary region (and other part(s) of neck, scalp, or face, except eye) 920
submental region (and other part(s) of neck, scalp, or face, except eye) 920
subperiosteal NEC 924.9
supraclavicular fossa (and other part(s) of neck, scalp, or face, except eye) 920
supraorbital (and other part(s) of neck, scalp, or face, except eye) 920
temple (region) (and other part(s) of neck, scalp, or face, except eye) 920
testis 922.4
thigh (and hip) 924.00

Contusion — continued

thorax 922.1
  organ — see Injury, internal, intrathoracic
throat (and other part(s) of neck, scalp, or face, except eye) 920
thumb(s) (nail) (subungual) 923.3
toe(s) (nail) (subungual) 924.3
tongue (and other part(s) of neck, scalp, or face, except eye) 920
trunk 922.9
  multiple sites 922.8
  specified site — see Contusion, by site
tunica vaginalis 922.4
tympanum (membrane) (and other part(s) of neck, scalp, or face, except eye) 920
upper extremity 923.9
  multiple sites 923.8
uvula (and other part(s) of neck, scalp, or face, except eye) 920
vagina 922.4
vocal cord(s) (and other part(s) of neck, scalp, or face, except eye) 920
vulva 922.4
wrist 923.21
  with hand(s), except finger(s) alone 923.20

Conus (any type) (congenital) 743.57
acquired 371.60
medullaris syndrome 336.8

Convalescence (following) V66.9
chemotherapy V66.2
medical NEC V66.5
psychotherapy V66.3
radiotherapy V66.1
surgery NEC V66.0
treatment (for) NEC V66.5
  combined V66.6
  fracture V66.4
  mental disorder NEC V66.3
  specified disorder NEC V66.5

Conversion
hysteria, hysterical, any type 300.11
laparoscopic surgical procedure to open procedure V64.4
neurosis, any 300.11
reaction, any 300.11

Converter, tuberculosis (test reaction) 795.5
Convulsions (idiopathic) 780.39
apoplectiform (see also Disease, cerebrovascular, acute) 436
brain 780.39
cerebral 780.39
cerebrospinal 780.39
due to trauma NEC — see Injury, intracranial
eclamptic (see also Eclampsia) 780.39
epileptic (see also Epilepsy) 345.9 ✓5ᵗʰ
epileptiform (see also Seizure, epileptiform) 780.39
epileptoid (see also Seizure, epileptiform) 780.39
ether
  anesthetic
    correct substance properly administered 780.39
    overdose or wrong substance given 968.2
  other specified type — see Table of Drugs and Chemicals
febrile 780.31
generalized 780.39
hysterical 300.11
infantile 780.39
  epilepsy — see Epilepsy
internal 780.39
jacksonian (see also Epilepsy) 345.5 ✓5ᵗʰ
myoclonic 333.2
newborn 779.0
paretic 094.1
pregnancy (nephritic) (uremic) — see Eclampsia, pregnancy
psychomotor (see also Epilepsy) 345.4 ✓5ᵗʰ
puerperal, postpartum — see Eclampsia, pregnancy
recurrent 780.39
  epileptic — see Epilepsy
reflex 781.0
repetitive 780.39
  epileptic — see Epilepsy

Convulsions — continued

salaam (see also Epilepsy) 345.6 ✓5ᵗʰ
scarlatinal 034.1
spasmodic 780.39
tetanus, tetanic (see also Tetanus) 037
thymic 254.8
uncinate 780.39
uremic 586
Convulsive — see also Convulsions
disorder or state 780.39
  epileptic — see Epilepsy
equivalent, abdominal (see also Epilepsy) 345.5 ✓5ᵗʰ
Cooke-Apert-Gallais syndrome (adrenogenital) 255.2
Cooley's anemia (erythroblastic) 282.4
Coolie itch 126.9
Cooper's
disease 610.1
hernia — see Hernia, Cooper's
Coordination disturbance 781.3
Copper wire arteries, retina 362.13
Copra itch 133.8
Coprolith 560.39
Coprophilia 302.89
Coproporphyria, hereditary 277.1
Coprostasis 560.39
with hernia — see also Hernia, by site, with obstruction
  gangrenous — see Hernia, by site, with gangrene
Cor
biloculare 745.7
bovinum — see Hypertrophy, cardiac
bovis — see also Hypertrophy, cardiac
pulmonale (chronic) 416.9
  acute 415.0
triatriatum, triatrium 746.82
triloculare 745.8
  biatriatum 745.3
  biventriculare 745.69
Corbus' disease 607.1
Cord — see also condition
around neck (tightly) (with compression)
  affecting fetus or newborn 762.5
  complicating delivery 663.1 ✓5ᵗʰ
    without compression 663.3 ✓5ᵗʰ
      affecting fetus or newborn 762.6
bladder NEC 344.61
  tabetic 094.0
prolapse
  affecting fetus or newborn 762.4
  complicating delivery 663.0 ✓5ᵗʰ
Cord's angiopathy (see also Tuberculosis) 017.3 ✓5ᵗʰ [362.18]
Cordis ectopia 746.87
Corditis (spermatic) 608.4
Corectopia 743.46
Cori type glycogen storage disease — see Disease, glycogen storage
Cork-handlers' disease or lung 495.3
Corkscrew esophagus 530.5
Corlett's pyosis (impetigo) 684
Corn (infected) 700
Cornea — see also condition
donor V59.5
guttata (dystrophy) 371.57
plana 743.41
Cornelia de Lange's syndrome (Amsterdam dwarf, mental retardation, and brachycephaly) 759.89
Cornual gestation or pregnancy — see Pregnancy, cornual
Cornu cutaneum 702.8
Coronary (artery) — see also condition
arising from aorta or pulmonary trunk 746.85
Corpora — see also condition
amylacea (prostate) 602.8
cavernosa — see condition
Corpulence (see also Obesity) 278.0 ✓5ᵗʰ
Corpus — see condition

Corrigan's disease — *see* Insufficiency, aortic

Corrosive burn — *see* Burn, by site

Corsican fever (*see also* Malaria) 084.6

Cortical — *see also* condition
  blindness 377.75
  necrosis, kidney (bilateral) 583.6

Corticoadrenal — *see* condition

Corticosexual syndrome 255.2

Coryza (acute) 460
  with grippe or influenza 487.1
  syphilitic 095.8
    congenital (chronic) 090.0

Costen's syndrome or complex 524.60

Costiveness (*see also* Constipation) 564.00

Costochondritis 733.6

Cotard's syndrome (paranoia) 297.1

Cot death 798.0

Cotungo's disease 724.3

Cough 786.2
  with hemorrhage (*see also* Hemoptysis) 786.3
  affected 786.2
  bronchial 786.2
    with grippe or influenza 487.1
  chronic 786.2
  epidemic 786.2
  functional 306.1
  hemorrhagic 786.3
  hysterical 300.11
  laryngeal, spasmodic 786.2
  nervous 786.2
  psychogenic 306.1
  smokers' 491.0
  tea tasters' 112.89

Counseling NEC V65.40
  without complaint or sickness V65.49
  abuse victim NEC V62.89
    child V61.21
    partner V61.11
    spouse V61.11
  child abuse, maltreatment, or neglect V61.21
  contraceptive NEC V25.09
    device (intrauterine) V25.02
    maintenance V25.40
      intrauterine contraceptive device V25.42
      oral contraceptive (pill) V25.41
      specified type NEC V25.49
      subdermal implantable V25.43
    management NEC V25.9
    oral contraceptive (pill) V25.01
    prescription NEC V25.02
      oral contraceptive (pill) V25.01
        repeat prescription V25.41
      repeat prescription V25.40
    subdermal implantable V25.43
    surveillance NEC V25.40
  dietary V65.3
  excercise V65.41
  explanation of
    investigation finding NEC V65.49
    medication NEC V65.49
  family planning V25.09
  for nonattending third party V65.1
  genetic V26.3
  gonorrhea V65.45
  health (advice) (education) (instruction) NEC
    V65.49
  HIV V65.44
  human immunodeficiency virus V65.44
  injury prevention V65.43
  marital V61.10
  medical (for) V65.9
    boarding school resident V60.6
    condition not demonstrated V65.5
    feared complaint and no disease found
      V65.5
    institutional resident V60.6
    on behalf of another V65.1
    person living alone V60.3
  parent-child conflict V61.20
    specified problem NEC V61.29
  partner abuse
    perpetrator V61.12
    victim V61.11

Counseling NEC — *continued*
  perpetrator of
    child abuse V62.83
      parental V61.22
    partner abuse V61.12
    spouse abuse V61.12
  procreative V65.49
  sex NEC V65.49
    transmitted disease NEC V65.45
      HIV V65.44
  specified reason NEC V65.49
  spousal abuse
    perpetrator V61.12
    victim V61.11
  substance use and abuse V65.42
  syphilis V65.45
  victim (of)
    abuse NEC V62.89
    child abuse V61.21
    partner abuse V61.11
    spousal abuse V61.11

Coupled rhythm 427.89

Couvelaire uterus (complicating delivery) — *see*
  Placenta, separation

Cowper's gland — *see* condition

Cowperitis (*see also* Urethritis) 597.89
  gonorrheal (acute) 098.0
    chronic or duration of 2 months or over
      098.2

Cowpox (abortive) 051.0
  due to vaccination 999.0
  eyelid 051.0 [373.5]
    postvaccination 999.0 [373.5]

Coxa
  plana 732.1
  valga (acquired) 736.31
    congenital 755.61
    late effect of rickets 268.1
  vara (acquired) 736.32
    congenital 755.62
    late effect of rickets 268.1

Coxae malum senilis 715.25

Coxalgia (nontuberculous) 719.45
  tuberculous (*see also* Tuberculosis) 015.1 ✓5ᵗʰ
    [730.85]

Coxalgic pelvis 736.30

Coxitis 716.65

Coxsackie (infection) (virus) 079.2
  central nervous system NEC 048
  endocarditis 074.22
  enteritis 008.67
  meningitis (aseptic) 047.0
  myocarditis 074.23
  pericarditis 074.21
  pharyngitis 074.0
  pleurodynia 074.1
  specific disease NEC 074.8

Crabs, meaning pubic lice 132.2

Crack baby 760.75

Cracked nipple 611.2
  puerperal, postpartum 676.1 ✓5ᵗʰ

Cradle cap 690.11

Craft neurosis 300.89

Craigiasis 007.8

Cramp(s) 729.82
  abdominal 789.0 ✓5ᵗʰ
  bathing 994.1
  colic 789.0 ✓5ᵗʰ
    psychogenic 306.4
  due to immersion 994.1
  extremity (lower) (upper) NEC 729.82
  fireman 992.2
  heat 992.2
  hysterical 300.11
  immersion 994.1
  intestinal 789.0 ✓5ᵗʰ
    psychogenic 306.4
  linotypist's 300.89
    organic 333.84
  muscle (extremity) (general) 729.82
    due to immersion 994.1
    hysterical 300.11
  occupational (hand) 300.89
    organic 333.84

Cramp(s) — *continued*
  psychogenic 307.89
  salt depletion 276.1
  stoker 992.2
  stomach 789.0 ✓5ᵗʰ
  telegraphers' 300.89
    organic 333.84
  typists' 300.89
    organic 333.84
  uterus 625.8
    menstrual 625.3
  writers' 333.84
    organic 333.84
    psychogenic 300.89

Cranial — *see* condition

Cranioclasis, fetal 763.89

Craniocleidodysostosis 755.59

Craniofenestria (skull) 756.0

Craniolacunia (skull) 756.0

Craniopagus 759.4

Craniopathy, metabolic 733.3

Craniopharyngeal — *see* condition

Craniopharyngioma (M9350/1) 237.0

Craniorachischisis (totalis) 740.1

Cranioschisis 756.0

Craniostenosis 756.0

Craniosynostosis 756.0

Craniotabes (cause unknown) 733.3
  rachitic 268.1
  syphilitic 090.5

Craniotomy, fetal 763.89

Cranium — *see* condition

Craw-craw 125.3

Creaking joint 719.60
  ankle 719.67
  elbow 719.62
  foot 719.67
  hand 719.64
  hip 719.65
  knee 719.66
  multiple sites 719.69
  pelvic region 719.65
  shoulder (region) 719.61
  specified site NEC 719.68
  wrist 719.63

Creeping
  eruption 126.9
  palsy 335.21
  paralysis 335.21

Crenated tongue 529.8

Creotoxism 005.9

Crepitus
  caput 756.0
  joint 719.60
    ankle 719.67
    elbow 719.62
    foot 719.67
    hand 719.64
    hip 719.65
    knee 719.66
    multiple sites 719.69
    pelvic region 719.65
    shoulder (region) 719.61
    specified site NEC 719.68
    wrist 719.63

Crescent or conus choroid, congenital 743.57

Cretin, cretinism (athyrotic) (congenital)
  (endemic) (metabolic) (nongoitrous)
  (sporadic) 243
  goitrous (sporadic) 246.1
  pelvis (dwarf type) (male type) 243
    with disproportion (fetopelvic) 653.1 ✓5ᵗʰ
      affecting fetus or newborn 763.1
      causing obstructed labor 660.1 ✓5ᵗʰ
        affecting fetus or newborn 763.1
  pituitary 253.3

Cretinoid degeneration 243

Creutzfeldt-Jakob disease (syndrome) 046.1
  with dementia
    with behavioral disturbance 046.1 [294.11]
    without behavioral disturbance 046.1
      [294.10]

▲

✓4ᵗʰ Fourth-digit Required   ✓5ᵗʰ Fifth-digit Required   ►◄ Revised Text   ● New Line   ▲ Revised Code

Crib death 798.0

Cribriform hymen 752.49

Cri-du-chat syndrome 758.3

Crigler-Najjar disease or syndrome (congenital hyperbilirubinemia) 277.4

Crimean hemorrhagic fever 065.0

Criminalism 301.7

Crisis
abdomen 789.0 ✓5ᵗʰ
addisonian (acute adrenocortical insufficiency) 255.4
adrenal (cortical) 255.4
asthmatic — *see* Asthma
brain, cerebral (*see also* Disease, cerebrovascular, acute) 436
celiac 579.0
Dietl's 593.4
emotional NEC 309.29
acute reaction to stress 308.0
adjustment reaction 309.9
specific to childhood and adolescence 313.9
gastric (tabetic) 094.0
glaucomatocyclitic 364.22
heart (*see also* Failure, heart) 428.9
hypertensive — *see* Hypertension
nitritoid
correct substance properly administered 458.2
overdose or wrong substance given or taken 961.1
oculogyric 378.87
psychogenic 306.7
Pel's 094.0
psychosexual identity 302.6
rectum 094.0
renal 593.81
sickle cell 282.62
stomach (tabetic) 094.0
tabetic 094.0
thyroid (*see also* Thyrotoxicosis) 242.9 ✓5ᵗʰ
thyrotoxic (*see also* Thyrotoxicosis) 242.9 ✓5ᵗʰ
vascular — *see* Disease, cerebrovascular, acute

Crocq's disease (acrocyanosis) 443.89

Crohn's disease (*see also* Enteritis, regional) 555.9

Cronkhite-Canada syndrome 211.3

Crooked septum, nasal 470

Cross
birth (of fetus) complicating delivery 652.3 ✓5ᵗʰ
with successful version 652.1 ✓5ᵗʰ
causing obstructed labor 660.0 ✓5ᵗʰ
bite, anterior or posterior 524.2
eye (*see also* Esotropia) 378.00

Crossed ectopia of kidney 753.3

Crossfoot 754.50

Croup, croupous (acute) (angina) (catarrhal) (infective) (inflammatory) (laryngeal) (membranous) (nondiphtheritic) (pseudomembranous) 464.4
asthmatic (*see also* Asthma) 493.9 ✓5ᵗʰ
bronchial 466.0
diphtheritic (membranous) 032.3
false 478.75
spasmodic 478.75
diphtheritic 032.3
stridulous 478.75
diphtheritic 032.3

Crouzon's disease (craniofacial dysostosis) 756.0

Crowding, teeth 524.3

CRST syndrome (cutaneous systemic sclerosis) 710.1

Cruchet's disease (encephalitis lethargica) 049.8

Cruelty in children (*see also* Disturbance, conduct) 312.9

Crural ulcer (*see also* Ulcer, lower extremity) 707.10

Crush, crushed, crushing (injury) 929.9
with
fracture — *see* Fracture, by site
abdomen 926.19
internal — *see* Injury, internal, abdomen
ankle 928.21
with other parts of foot 928.20

Crush, crushed, crushing — *continued*
arm 927.9
lower (and elbow) 927.10
upper 927.03
with shoulder or axillary region 927.09
axilla 927.02
with shoulder or upper arm 927.09
back 926.11
breast 926.19
buttock 926.12
cheek 925.1
chest — *see* Injury, internal, chest
ear 925.1
elbow 927.11
with forearm 927.10
face 925.1
finger(s) 927.3
with hand(s) 927.20
and wrist(s) 927.21
flank 926.19
foot, excluding toe(s) alone (with ankle) 928.20
forearm (and elbow) 927.10
genitalia, external (female) (male) 926.0
internal — *see* Injury, internal, genital organ NEC
hand, except finger(s) alone (and wrist) 927.20
head — *see* Fracture, skull, by site
heel 928.20
hip 928.01
with thigh 928.00
internal organ (abdomen, chest, or pelvis) — *see* Injury, internal, by site
knee 928.11
with leg, lower 928.10
labium (majus) (minus) 926.0
larynx 925.2
late effect — *see* Late, effects (of), crushing
leg 928.9
lower 928.10
and knee 928.11
upper 928.00
limb
lower 928.9
multiple sites 928.8
upper 927.9
multiple sites 927.8
multiple sites NEC 929.0
neck 925.2
nerve — *see* Injury, nerve, by site
nose 802.0
open 802.1
penis 926.0
pharynx 925.2
scalp 925.1
scapular region 927.01
with shoulder or upper arm 927.09
scrotum 926.0
shoulder 927.00
with upper arm or axillary region 927.09
skull or cranium — *see* Fracture, skull, by site
spinal cord — *see* Injury, spinal, by site
syndrome (complication of trauma) 958.5
testis 926.0
thigh (with hip) 928.00
throat 925.2
thumb(s) (and fingers) 927.3
toe(s) 928.3
with foot 928.20
and ankle 928.21
tonsil 925.2
trunk 926.9
chest — *see* Injury, internal, intrathoracic organs NEC
internal organ — *see* Injury, internal, by site
multiple sites 926.8
specified site NEC 926.19
vulva 926.0
wrist 927.21
with hand(s), except fingers alone 927.20

Crusta lactea 690.11

Crusts 782.8

Crutch paralysis 953.4

Cruveilhier's disease 335.21

Cruveilhier-Baumgarten cirrhosis, disease, or syndrome 571.5

Cruz-Chagas disease (*see also* Trypanosomiasis) 086.2

Cryoglobulinemia (mixed) 273.2

Crypt (anal) (rectal) 569.49

Cryptitis (anal) (rectal) 569.49

Cryptococcosis (European) (pulmonary) (systemic) 117.5

Cryptococcus 117.5
epidermicus 117.5
neoformans, infection by 117.5

Cryptopapillitis (anus) 569.49

Cryptophthalmos (eyelid) 743.06

Cryptorchid, cryptorchism, cryptorchidism 752.51

Cryptosporidiosis 007.4

Cryptotia 744.29

Crystallopathy
calcium pyrophosphate (*see also* Arthritis) 275.49 [712.2]
dicalcium phosphate (*see also* Arthritis) 275.49 [712.1]
gouty 274.0
pyrophosphate NEC (*see also* Arthritis) 275.49 [712.2]
uric acid 274.0

Crystalluria 791.9

Csillag's disease (lichen sclerosus or atrophicus) 701.0

Cuban itch 050.1

Cubitus
valgus (acquired) 736.01
congenital 755.59
late effect of rickets 268.1
varus (acquired) 736.02
congenital 755.59
late effect of rickets 268.1

Cultural deprivation V62.4

Cupping of optic disc 377.14

Curling's ulcer — *see* Ulcer, duodenum

Curling esophagus 530.5

Curschmann (-Batten) (-Steinert) disease or syndrome 359.2

Curvature
organ or site, congenital NEC — *see* Distortion
penis (lateral) 752.69
Pott's (spinal) (*see also* Tuberculosis) 015.0 ✓5ᵗʰ [737.43]
radius, idiopathic, progressive (congenital) 755.54
spine (acquired) (angular) (idiopathic) (incorrect) (postural) 737.9
congenital 754.2
due to or associated with
Charcôt-Marie-Tooth disease 356.1 [737.40]
mucopolysaccharidosis 277.5 [737.40]
neurofibromatosis 237.71 [737.40]
osteitis
deformans 731.0 [737.40]
fibrosa cystica 252.0 [737.40]
osteoporosis (*see also* Osteoporosis) 733.00 [737.40]
poliomyelitis (*see also* Poliomyelitis) 138 [737.40]
tuberculosis (Pott's curvature) (*see also* Tuberculosis) 015.0 ✓5ᵗʰ [737.43]
kyphoscoliotic (*see also* Kyphoscoliosis) 737.30
kyphotic (*see also* Kyphosis) 737.10
late effect of rickets 268.1 [737.40]
Pott's 015.0 ✓5ᵗʰ [737.40]
scoliotic (*see also* Scoliosis) 737.30
specified NEC 737.8
tuberculous 015.0 ✓5ᵗʰ [737.40]

Cushing's
basophilism, disease, or syndrome (iatrogenic) (idiopathic) (pituitary basophilism) (pituitary dependent) 255.0
ulcer — *see* Ulcer, peptic

Cushingoid due to steroid therapy
correct substance properly administered 255.0
overdose or wrong substance given or taken 962.0

Cut (external) — *see* Wound, open, by site

Cutaneous — *see also* condition
hemorrhage 782.7
horn (cheek) (eyelid) (mouth) 702.8
larva migrans 126.9

Cutis — *see also* condition
hyperelastic 756.83
acquired 701.8
laxa 756.83
senilis 701.8
marmorata 782.61
osteosis 709.3
pendula 756.83
acquired 701.8
rhomboidalis nuchae 701.8
verticis gyrata 757.39
acquired 701.8

Cyanopathy, newborn 770.83   ▲

Cyanosis 782.5
autotoxic 289.7
common atrioventricular canal 745.69
congenital 770.83   ▲
conjunctiva 372.71
due to
endocardial cushion defect 745.60
nonclosure, foramen botalli 745.5
patent foramen botalli 745.5
persistent foramen ovale 745.5
enterogenous 289.7
fetus or newborn 770.83   ▲
ostium primum defect 745.61
paroxysmal digital 443.0
retina, retinal 362.10

Cycle
anovulatory 628.0
menstrual, irregular 626.4

Cyclencephaly 759.89

Cyclical vomiting 536.2
psychogenic 306.4

Cyclitic membrane 364.74

Cyclitis (*see also* Iridocyclitis) 364.3
acute 364.00
primary 364.01
recurrent 364.02
chronic 364.10
in
sarcoidosis 135 *[364.11]*
tuberculosis (*see also* Tuberculosis)
017.3 ✔5ᵗʰ *[364.11]*
Fuchs' heterochromic 364.21
granulomatous 364.10
lens induced 364.23
nongranulomatous 364.00
posterior 363.21
primary 364.01
recurrent 364.02
secondary (noninfectious) 364.04
infectious 364.03
subacute 364.00
primary 364.01
recurrent 364.02

Cyclokeratitis — *see* Keratitis

Cyclophoria 378.44

Cyclopia, cyclops 759.89

Cycloplegia 367.51

Cyclospasm 367.53

Cyclosporiasis 007.5

Cyclothymia 301.13

Cyclothymic personality 301.13

Cyclotropia 378.33

Cyesis — *see* Pregnancy

Cylindroma (M8200/3) — *see also* Neoplasm, by
site, malignant
eccrine dermal (M8200/0) — *see* Neoplasm,
skin, benign
skin (M8200/0) — *see* Neoplasm, skin, benign

Cylindruria 791.7

Cyllosoma 759.89

Cynanche
diphtheritic 032.3
tonsillaris 475

Cynorexia 783.6

Cyphosis — *see* Kyphosis

Cyprus fever (*see also* Brucellosis) 023.9

Cyriax's syndrome (slipping rib) 733.99

Cyst (mucus) (retention) (serous) (simple)

> Note — In general, cysts are not neoplastic
> and are classified to the approriate category
> for disease of the specified anatomical site.
> This generalization does not apply to certain
> types of cysts which are neoplastic in nature,
> for example, dermoid, nor does it apply to
> cysts of certain structures, for example,
> branchial cleft, which are classified as
> developmental anomalies.
>
> The following listing includes some of the
> most frequently reported sites of cysts as
> well as qualifiers which indicate the type of
> cyst. The latter qualifiers usually are not
> repeated under the anatomical sites. Since
> the code assignment for a given site may
> vary depending upon the type of cyst, the
> coder should refer to the listings under the
> specified type of cyst before consideration is
> given to the site.

accessory, fallopian tube 752.11
adenoid (infected) 474.8
adrenal gland 255.8
congenital 759.1
air, lung 518.89
allantoic 753.7
alveolar process (jaw bone) 526.2
amnion, amniotic 658.8 ✔5ᵗʰ
anterior chamber (eye) 364.60
exudative 364.62
implantation (surgical) (traumatic) 364.61
parasitic 360.13
anterior nasopalatine 526.1
antrum 478.1
anus 569.49
apical (periodontal) (tooth) 522.8
appendix 543.9
arachnoid, brain 348.0
arytenoid 478.79
auricle 706.2
Baker's (knee) 727.51
tuberculous (*see also* Tuberculosis)
015.2 ✔5ᵗʰ
Bartholin's gland or duct 616.2
bile duct (*see also* Disease, biliary) 576.8
bladder (multiple) (trigone) 596.8
Blessig's 362.62
blood, endocardial (*see also* Endocarditis)
424.90
blue dome 610.0
bone (local) 733.20
aneurysmal 733.22
jaw 526.2
developmental (odontogenic) 526.0
fissural 526.1
latent 526.89
solitary 733.21
unicameral 733.21
brain 348.0
congenital 742.4
hydatid (*see also* Echinococcus) 122.9
third ventricle (colloid) 742.4
branchial (cleft) 744.42
branchiogenic 744.42
breast (benign) (blue dome) (pedunculated)
(solitary) (traumatic) 610.0
involution 610.4
sebaceous 610.8
broad ligament (benign) 620.8
embryonic 752.11
bronchogenic (mediastinal) (sequestration)
518.89
congenital 748.4
buccal 528.4
bulbourethral gland (Cowper's) 599.89
bursa, bursal 727.49
pharyngeal 478.26
calcifying odontogenic (M9301/0) 213.1
upper jaw (bone) 213.0
canal of Nuck (acquired) (serous) 629.1
congenital 752.41
canthus 372.75

Cyst — *continued*
carcinomatous (M8010/3) — *see* Neoplasm, by
site, malignant
cartilage (joint) — *see* Derangement, joint
cauda equina 336.8
cavum septi pellucidi NEC 348.0
celomic (pericardium) 746.89
cerebellopontine (angle) — *see* Cyst, brain
cerebellum — *see* Cyst, brain
cerebral — *see* Cyst, brain
cervical lateral 744.42
cervix 622.8
embryonal 752.41
nabothian (gland) 616.0
chamber, anterior (eye) 364.60
exudative 364.62
implantation (surgical) (traumatic) 364.61
parasitic 360.13
chiasmal, optic NEC (*see also* Lesion, chiasmal)
377.54
chocolate (ovary) 617.1
choledochal (congenital) 751.69
acquired 576.8
choledochus 751.69
chorion 658.8 ✔5ᵗʰ
choroid plexus 348.0
chyle, mesentery 457.8
ciliary body 364.60
exudative 364.64
implantation 364.61
primary 364.63
clitoris 624.8
coccyx (*see also* Cyst, bone) 733.20
colloid
third ventricle (brain) 742.4
thyroid gland — *see* Goiter
colon 569.89
common (bile) duct (*see also* Disease, biliary)
576.8
congenital NEC 759.89
adrenal glands 759.1
epiglottis 748.3
esophagus 750.4
fallopian tube 752.11
kidney 753.10
multiple 753.19
single 753.11
larynx 748.3
liver 751.62
lung 748.4
mediastinum 748.8
ovary 752.0
oviduct 752.11
pancreas 751.7
periurethral (tissue) 753.8
prepuce NEC 752.69
penis 752.69
sublingual 750.26
submaxillary gland 750.26
thymus (gland) 759.2
tongue 750.19
ureterovesical orifice 753.4
vulva 752.41
conjunctiva 372.75
cornea 371.23
corpora quadrigemina 348.0
corpus
albicans (ovary) 620.2
luteum (ruptured) 620.1
Cowper's gland (benign) (infected) 599.89
cranial meninges 348.0
craniobuccal pouch 253.8
craniopharyngeal pouch 253.8
cystic duct (*see also* Disease, gallbladder) 575.8
Cysticercus (any site) 123.1
Dandy-Walker 742.3
with spina bifida (*see also* Spina bifida)
741.0 ✔5ᵗʰ
dental 522.8
developmental 526.0
eruption 526.0
lateral periodontal 526.0
primordial (keratocyst) 526.0
root 522.8
dentigerous 526.0
mandible 526.0
maxilla 526.0

Cyst — *continued*
dermoid (M9084/0) — *see also* Neoplasm, by site, benign
  with malignant transformation (M9084/3) 183.0
  implantation
    external area or site (skin) NEC 709.8
    iris 364.61
    skin 709.8
    vagina 623.8
    vulva 624.8
  mouth 528.4
  oral soft tissue 528.4
  sacrococcygeal 685.1
    with abscess 685.0
developmental of ovary, ovarian 752.0
dura (cerebral) 348.0
  spinal 349.2
ear (external) 706.2
echinococcal (*see also* Echinococcus) 122.9
embryonal
  cervix uteri 752.41
  genitalia, female external 752.41
  uterus 752.3
  vagina 752.41
endometrial 621.8
  ectopic 617.9
endometrium (uterus) 621.8
  ectopic — *see* Endometriosis
enteric 751.5
enterogenous 751.5
epidermal (inclusion) (*see also* Cyst, skin) 706.2
epidermoid (inclusion) (*see also* Cyst, skin) 706.2
  mouth 528.4
  not of skin — *see* Cyst, by site
  oral soft tissue 528.4
epididymis 608.89
epiglottis 478.79
epiphysis cerebri 259.8
epithelial (inclusion) (*see also* Cyst, skin) 706.2
epoophoron 752.11
eruption 526.0
esophagus 530.89
ethmoid sinus 478.1
eye (retention) 379.8
  congenital 743.03
  posterior segment, congenital 743.54
eyebrow 706.2
eyelid (sebaceous) 374.84
  infected 373.13
  sweat glands or ducts 374.84
falciform ligament (inflammatory) 573.8
fallopian tube 620.8
female genital organs NEC 629.8
fimbrial (congenital) 752.11
fissural (oral region) 526.1
follicle (atretic) (graafian) (ovarian) 620.0
  nabothian (gland) 616.0
follicular (atretic) (ovarian) 620.0
  dentigerous 526.0
frontal sinus 478.1
gallbladder or duct 575.8
ganglion 727.43
Gartner's duct 752.11
gas, of mesentery 568.89
gingiva 523.8
gland of moll 374.84
globulomaxillary 526.1
graafian follicle 620.0
granulosal lutein 620.2
hemangiomatous (M9121/0) (*see also* Hemangioma) 228.00
hydatid (*see also* Echinococcus) 122.9
  fallopian tube (Morgagni) 752.11
  liver NEC 122.8
  lung NEC 122.9
  Morgagni 752.8
    fallopian tube 752.11
  specified site NEC 122.9
hymen 623.8
  embryonal 752.41
hypopharynx 478.26
hypophysis, hypophyseal (duct) (recurrent) 253.8
  cerebri 253.8

Cyst — *continued*
implantation (dermoid)
  anterior chamber (eye) 364.61
  external area or site (skin) NEC 709.8
  iris 364.61
  vagina 623.8
  vulva 624.8
incisor, incisive canal 526.1
inclusion (epidermal) (epithelial) (epidermoid) (mucous) (squamous) (*see also* Cyst, skin) 706.2
  not of skin — *see* Neoplasm, by site, benign
intestine (large) (small) 569.89
intracranial — *see* Cyst, brain
intraligamentous 728.89
  knee 717.89
intrasellar 253.8
iris (idiopathic) 364.60
  exudative 364.62
  implantation (surgical) (traumatic) 364.61
  miotic pupillary 364.55
  parasitic 360.13
Iwanoff's 362.62
jaw (bone) (aneurysmal) (extravasation) (hemorrhagic) (traumatic) 526.2
  developmental (odontogenic) 526.0
  fissural 526.1
keratin 706.2
kidney (congenital) 753.10
  acquired 593.2
  calyceal (*see also* Hydronephrosis) 591
  multiple 753.19
  pyelogenic (*see also* Hydronephrosis) 591
  simple 593.2
  single 753.11
  solitary (not congenital) 593.2
labium (majus) (minus) 624.8
  sebaceous 624.8
lacrimal
  apparatus 375.43
  gland or sac 375.12
larynx 478.79
lens 379.39
  congenital 743.39
lip (gland) 528.5
liver 573.8
  congenital 751.62
  hydatid (*see also* Echinococcus) 122.8
    granulosis 122.0
    multilocularis 122.5
lung 518.89
  congenital 748.4
  giant bullous 492.0
lutein 620.1
lymphangiomatous (M9173/0) 228.1
lymphoepithelial
  mouth 528.4
  oral soft tissue 528.4
macula 362.54
malignant (M8000/3) — *see* Neoplasm, by site, malignant
mammary gland (sweat gland) (*see also* Cyst, breast) 610.0
mandible 526.2
  dentigerous 526.0
  radicular 522.8
maxilla 526.2
  dentigerous 526.0
  radicular 522.8
median
  anterior maxillary 526.1
  palatal 526.1
mediastinum (congenital) 748.8
meibomian (gland) (retention) 373.2
  infected 373.12
membrane, brain 348.0
meninges (cerebral) 348.0
  spinal 349.2
meniscus knee 717.5
mesentery, mesenteric (gas) 568.89
  chyle 457.8
  gas 568.89
mesonephric duct 752.8
mesothelial
  peritoneum 568.89
  pleura (peritoneal) 569.89
milk 611.5

Cyst — *continued*
miotic pupillary (iris) 364.55
Morgagni (hydatid) 752.8
  fallopian tube 752.11
mouth 528.4
mullerian duct 752.8
multilocular (ovary) (M8000/1) 239.5
myometrium 621.8
nabothian (follicle) (ruptured) 616.0
nasal sinus 478.1
nasoalveolar 528.4
nasolabial 528.4
nasopalatine (duct) 526.1
  anterior 526.1
nasopharynx 478.26
neoplastic (M8000/1) — *see also* Neoplasm, by site, unspecified nature
  benign (M8000/0) — *see* Neoplasm, by site, benign
  uterus 621.8
nervous system — *see* Cyst, brain
neuroenteric 742.59
neuroepithelial ventricle 348.0
nipple 610.0
nose 478.1
  skin of 706.2
odontogenic, developmental 526.0
omentum (lesser) 568.89
  congenital 751.8
oral soft tissue (dermoid) (epidermoid) (lymphoepithelial) 528.4
ora serrata 361.19
orbit 376.81
ovary, ovarian (twisted) 620.2
  adherent 620.2
  chocolate 617.1
  corpus
    albicans 620.2
    luteum 620.1
  dermoid (M9084/0) 220
  developmental 752.0
  due to failure of involution NEC 620.2
  endometrial 617.1
  follicular (atretic) (graafian) (hemorrhagic) 620.0
  hemorrhagic 620.2
  in pregnancy or childbirth 654.4 ☑5ᵗʰ
    affecting fetus or newborn 763.89
    causing obstructed labor 660.2 ☑5ᵗʰ
      affecting fetus or newborn 763.1
  multilocular (M8000/1) 239.5
  pseudomucinous (M8470/0) 220
  retention 620.2
  serous 620.2
  theca lutein 620.2
  tuberculous (*see also* Tuberculosis) 016.6 ☑5ᵗʰ
  unspecified 620.2
oviduct 620.8
palatal papilla (jaw) 526.1
palate 526.1
  fissural 526.1
  median (fissural) 526.1
palatine, of papilla 526.1
pancreas, pancreatic 577.2
  congenital 751.7
  false 577.2
  hemorrhagic 577.2
  true 577.2
paranephric 593.2
para ovarian 752.11
paraphysis, cerebri 742.4
parasitic NEC 136.9
parathyroid (gland) 252.8
paratubal (fallopian) 620.8
paraurethral duct 599.89
paroophoron 752.11
parotid gland 527.6
  mucous extravasation or retention 527.6
parovarian 752.11
pars planus 364.60
  exudative 364.64
  primary 364.63

Cyst — *continued*
  pelvis, female
    in pregnancy or childbirth 654.4 ✔5ᵗʰ
      affecting fetus or newborn 763.89
      causing obstructed labor 660.2 ✔5ᵗʰ
        affecting fetus or newborn 763.1
  penis (sebaceous) 607.89
  periapical 522.8
  pericardial (congenital) 746.89
    acquired (secondary) 423.8
  pericoronal 526.0
  perineural (Tarlov's) 355.9
  periodontal 522.8
    lateral 526.0
  peripancreatic 577.2
  peripelvic (lymphatic) 593.2
  peritoneum 568.89
    chylous 457.8
  pharynx (wall) 478.26
  pilonidal (infected) (rectum) 685.1
    with abscess 685.0
    malignant (M9084/3) 173.5
  pituitary (duct) (gland) 253.8
  placenta (amniotic) — *see* Placenta, abnormal
  pleura 519.8
  popliteal 727.51
  porencephalic 742.4
    acquired 348.0
  postanal (infected) 685.1
    with abscess 685.0
  posterior segment of eye, congenital 743.54
  postmastoidectomy cavity 383.31
  preauricular 744.47
  prepuce 607.89
    congenital 752.69
  primordial (jaw) 526.0
  prostate 600.3
  pseudomucinous (ovary) (M8470/0) 220
  pudenda (sweat glands) 624.8
  pupillary, miotic 364.55
    sebaceous 624.8
  radicular (residual) 522.8
  radiculodental 522.8
  ranular 527.6
  Rathke's pouch 253.8
  rectum (epithelium) (mucous) 569.49
  renal — *see* Cyst, kidney
  residual (radicular) 522.8
  retention (ovary) 620.2
  retina 361.19
    macular 362.54
    parasitic 360.13
    primary 361.13
    secondary 361.14
  retroperitoneal 568.89
  sacrococcygeal (dermoid) 685.1
    with abscess 685.0
  salivary gland or duct 527.6
    mucous extravasation or retention 527.6
  Sampson's 617.1
  sclera 379.19
  scrotum (sebaceous) 706.2
    sweat glands 706.2
  sebaceous (duct) (gland) 706.2
    breast 610.8
    eyelid 374.84
    genital organ NEC
      female 629.8
      male 608.89
    scrotum 706.2
  semilunar cartilage (knee) (multiple) 717.5
  seminal vesicle 608.89
  serous (ovary) 620.2
  sinus (antral) (ethmoidal) (frontal) (maxillary)
      (nasal) (sphenoidal) 478.1
  Skene's gland 599.89
  skin (epidermal) (epidermoid, inclusion)
      (epithelial) (inclusion) (retention)
      (sebaceous) 706.2
    breast 610.8
    eyelid 374.84
    genital organ NEC
      female 629.8
      male 608.89
    neoplastic 216.3
    scrotum 706.2
  sweat gland or duct 705.89

Cyst — *continued*
  solitary
    bone 733.21
    kidney 593.2
  spermatic cord 608.89
  sphenoid sinus 478.1
  spinal meninges 349.2
  spine (*see also* Cyst, bone) 733.20
  spleen NEC 289.59
    congenital 759.0
    hydatid (*see also* Echinococcus) 122.9
  spring water (pericardium) 746.89
  subarachnoid 348.0
    intrasellar 793.0
  subdural (cerebral) 348.0
    spinal cord 349.2
  sublingual gland 527.6
    mucous extravasation or retention 527.6
  submaxillary gland 527.6
    mucous extravasation or retention 527.6
  suburethral 599.89
  suprarenal gland 255.8
  suprasellar — *see* Cyst, brain
  sweat gland or duct 705.89
  sympathetic nervous system 337.9
  synovial 727.40
    popliteal space 727.51
  Tarlov's 355.9
  tarsal 373.2
  tendon (sheath) 727.42
  testis 608.89
  theca-lutein (ovary) 620.2
  Thornwaldt's, Tornwaldt's 478.26
  thymus (gland) 254.8
  thyroglossal (duct) (infected) (persistent) 759.2
  thyroid (gland) 246.2
    adenomatous — *see* Goiter, nodular
    colloid (*see also* Goiter) 240.9
  thyrolingual duct (infected) (persistent) 759.2
  tongue (mucous) 529.8
  tonsil 474.8
  tooth (dental root) 522.8
  tubo-ovarian 620.8
    inflammatory 614.1
  tunica vaginalis 608.89
  turbinate (nose) (*see also* Cyst, bone) 733.20
  Tyson's gland (benign) (infected) 607.89
  umbilicus 759.89
  urachus 753.7
  ureter 593.89
  ureterovesical orifice 593.89
    congenital 753.4
  urethra 599.84
  urethral gland (Cowper's) 599.89
  uterine
    ligament 620.8
      embryonic 752.11
    tube 620.8
  uterus (body) (corpus) (recurrent) 621.8
    embryonal 752.3
  utricle (ear) 386.8
    prostatic 599.89
  utriculus masculinus 599.89
  vagina, vaginal (squamous cell) (wall) 623.8
    embryonal 752.41
    implantation 623.8
    inclusion 623.8
  vallecula, vallecular 478.79
  ventricle, neuroepithelial 348.0
  verumontanum 599.89
  vesical (orifice) 596.8
  vitreous humor 379.29
  vulva (sweat glands) 624.8
    congenital 752.41
    implantation 624.8
    inclusion 624.8
    sebaceous gland 624.8
  vulvovaginal gland 624.8
  wolffian 752.8

Cystadenocarcinoma (M8440/3) — *see also*
    Neoplasm, by site, malignant
  bile duct type (M8161/3) 155.1
  endometrioid (M8380/3) — *see* Neoplasm, by
      site, malignant

Cystadenocarcinoma — *see also* Neoplasm, by
    site, malignant — *continued*
  mucinous (M8470/3)
    papillary (M8471/3)
      specified site — *see* Neoplasm, by site,
          malignant
      unspecified site 183.0
    specified site — *see* Neoplasm, by site,
        malignant
    unspecified site 183.0
  papillary (M8450/3)
    mucinous (M8471/3)
      specified site — *see* Neoplasm, by site,
          malignant
      unspecified site 183.0
    pseudomucinous (M8471/3)
      specified site — *see* Neoplasm, by site,
          malignant
      unspecified site 183.0
    serous (M8460/3)
      specified site — *see* Neoplasm, by site,
          malignant
      unspecified site 183.0
    specified site — *see* Neoplasm, by site,
        malignant
    unspecified 183.0
  pseudomucinous (M8470/3)
    papillary (M8471/3)
      specified site — *see* Neoplasm, by site,
          malignant
      unspecified site 183.0
    specified site — *see* Neoplasm, by site,
        malignant
    unspecified site 183.0
  serous (M8441/3)
    papillary (M8460/3)
      specified site — *see* Neoplasm, by site,
          malignant
      unspecified site 183.0
    specified site — *see* Neoplasm, by site,
        malignant
    unspecified site 183.0

Cystadenofibroma (M9013/0)
  clear cell (M8313/0) — *see* Neoplasm, by site,
      benign
  endometrioid (M8381/0) 220
    borderline malignancy (M8381/1) 236.2
    malignant (M8381/3) 183.0
  mucinous (M9015/0)
    specified site — *see* Neoplasm, by site,
        benign
    unspecified site 220
  serous (M9014/0)
    specified site — *see* Neoplasm, by site,
        benign
    unspecified site 220
  specified site — *see* Neoplasm, by site, benign
  unspecified site 220

Cystadenoma (M8440/0) — *see also* Neoplasm,
    by site, benign
  bile duct (M8161/0) 211.5
  endometrioid (M8380/0) — *see also* Neoplasm,
      by site, benign
    borderline malignancy (M8380/1) — *see*
        Neoplasm, by site, uncertain behavior
    malignant (M8440/3) — *see* Neoplasm, by site,
        malignant
  mucinous (M8470/0)
    borderline malignancy (M8470/1)
      specified site — *see* Neoplasm, uncertain
          behavior
      unspecified site 236.2
    papillary (M8471/0)
      borderline malignancy (M8471/1)
        specified site — *see* Neoplasm, by site,
            uncertain behavior
        unspecified site 236.2
      specified site — *see* Neoplasm, by site,
          benign
      unspecified site 220
    specified site — *see* Neoplasm, by site,
        benign
    unspecified site 220
  papillary (M8450/0)
    borderline malignancy (M8450/1)
      specified site — *see* Neoplasm, by site,
          uncertain behavior

Cystadenoma — *see also* Neoplasm, by site, benign — *continued*
  papillary — *continued*
    borderline malignancy — *continued*
      unspecified site 236.2
    lymphomatosum (M8561/0) 210.2
    mucinous (M8471/0)
      borderline malignancy (M8471/1)
        specified site — *see* Neoplasm, by site, uncertain behavior
        unspecified site 236.2
      specified site — *see* Neoplasm, by site, benign
      unspecified site 220
    pseudomucinous (M8471/0)
      borderline malignancy (M8471/1)
        specified site — *see* Neoplasm, by site, uncertain behavior
        unspecified site 236.2
      specified site — *see* Neoplasm, by site, benign
      unspecified site 220
    serous (M8460/0)
      borderline malignancy (M8460/1)
        specified site — *see* Neoplasm, by site, uncertain behavior
        unspecified site 236.2
      specified site — *see* Neoplasm, by site, benign
      unspecified site 220
    specified site — *see* Neoplasm, by site, benign
    unspecified site 220
  pseudomucinous (M8470/0)
    borderline malignancy (M8470/1)
      specified site — *see* Neoplasm, by site, uncertain behavior
      unspecified site 236.2
    papillary (M8471/0)
      borderline malignancy (M8471/1)
        specified site — *see* Neoplasm, by site, uncertain behavior
        unspecified site 236.2
      specified site — *see* Neoplasm, by site, benign
      unspecified site 220
    specified site — *see* Neoplasm, by site, benign
    unspecified site 220
  serous (M8441/0)
    borderline malignancy (M8441/1)
      specified site — *see* Neoplasm, by site, uncertain behavior
      unspecified site 236.2
    papillary (M8460/0)
      borderline malignancy (M8460/1)
        specified site — *see* Neoplasm, by site, uncertain behavior
        unspecified site 236.2
      specified site — *see* Neoplasm, by site, benign
      unspecified site 220
    specified site — *see* Neoplasm, by site, benign
    unspecified site 220
  thyroid 226

Cystathioninemia 270.4

Cystathioninuria 270.4

Cystic — *see also* condition
  breast, chronic 610.1
  corpora lutea 620.1
  degeneration, congenital
    brain 742.4
    kidney 753.10
  disease
    breast, chronic 610.1
    kidney, congenital 753.10
      medullary 753.16
      multiple 753.19
      polycystic — *see* Polycystic, kidney
      single 753.11
      specified NEC 753.19
    liver, congenital 751.62
    lung 518.89
      congenital 748.4

Cystic — *see also* condition — *continued*
  disease — *continued*
    pancreas, congenital 751.7
    semilunar cartilage 717.5
  duct — *see* condition
  eyeball, congenital 743.03
  fibrosis (pancreas) 277.00
    with ●
      manifestations ●
        gastrointestinal 277.03 ●
        pulmonary 277.02 ●
        specified NEC 277.09 ●
      meconium ileus 277.01 ●
      pulmonary exacerbation 277.02 ●
  hygroma (M9173/0) 228.1
  kidney, congenital 753.10
    medullary 753.16
    multiple 753.19
    polycystic — *see* Polycystic, kidney
    single 753.11
    specified NEC 753.19
  liver, congenital 751.62
  lung 518.89
    congenital 748.4
  mass — *see* Cyst
  mastitis, chronic 610.1
  ovary 620.2
  pancreas, congenital 751.7

Cysticerciasis 123.1

Cysticercosis (mammary) (subretinal) 123.1

Cysticercus 123.1
  cellulosae infestation 123.1

Cystinosis (malignant) 270.0

Cystinuria 270.0

Cystitis (bacillary) (colli) (diffuse) (exudative) (hemorrhagic) (purulent) (recurrent) (septic) (suppurative) (ulcerative) 595.9
  with
    abortion — *see* Abortion, by type, with urinary tract infection
    ectopic pregnancy (*see also* categories 633.0-633.9) 639.8
    fibrosis 595.1
    leukoplakia 595.1
    malakoplakia 595.1
    metaplasia 595.1
    molar pregnancy (*see also* categories 630-632) 639.8
  actinomycotic 039.8 *[595.4]*
  acute 595.0
    of trigone 595.3
  allergic 595.89
  amebic 006.8 *[595.4]*
  bilharzial 120.9 *[595.4]*
  blennorrhagic (acute) 098.11
    chronic or duration of 2 months or more 098.31
  bullous 595.89
  calculous 594.1
  chlamydial 099.53
  chronic 595.2
    interstitial 595.1
    of trigone 595.3
  complicating pregnancy, childbirth, or puerperium 646.6 ☑5ᵗʰ
    affecting fetus or newborn 760.1
  cystic(a) 595.81
  diphtheritic 032.84
  echinococcal
    granulosus 122.3 *[595.4]*
    multilocularis 122.6 *[595.4]*
  emphysematous 595.89
  encysted 595.81
  follicular 595.3
  following
    abortion 639.8
    ectopic or molar pregnancy 639.8
  gangrenous 595.89
  glandularis 595.89
  gonococcal (acute) 098.11
    chronic or duration of 2 months or more 098.31
  incrusted 595.89
  interstitial 595.1
  irradiation 595.82
  irritation 595.89

Cystitis — *continued*
  malignant 595.89
  monilial 112.2
  of trigone 595.3
  panmural 595.1
  polyposa 595.89
  prostatic 601.3
  radiation 595.82
  Reiter's (abacterial) 099.3
  specified NEC 595.89
  subacute 595.2
  submucous 595.1
  syphilitic 095.8
  trichomoniasis 131.09
  tuberculous (*see also* Tuberculosis) 016.1 ☑5ᵗʰ
  ulcerative 595.1

Cystocele (-rectocele)
  female (without uterine prolapse) 618.0
    with uterine prolapse 618.4
      complete 618.3
      incomplete 618.2
  in pregnancy or childbirth 654.4 ☑5ᵗʰ
    affecting fetus or newborn 763.89
    causing obstructed labor 660.2 ☑5ᵗʰ
      affecting fetus or newborn 763.1
  male 596.8

Cystoid
  cicatrix limbus 372.64
  degeneration macula 362.53

Cystolithiasis 594.1

Cystoma (M8440/0) — *see also* Neoplasm, by site, benign
  endometrial, ovary 617.1
  mucinous (M8470/0)
    specified site — *see* Neoplasm, by site, benign
    unspecified site 220
  serous (M8441/0)
    specified site — *see* Neoplasm, by site, benign
    unspecified site 220
  simple (ovary) 620.2

Cystoplegia 596.53

Cystoptosis 596.8

Cystopyelitis (*see also* Pyelitis) 590.80

Cystorrhagia 596.8

Cystosarcoma phyllodes (M9020/1) 238.3
  benign (M9020/0) 217
  malignant (M9020/3) — *see* Neoplasm, breast, malignant

Cystostomy status V44.50
  appendico-vesicostomy V44.52
  cutaneous-vesicostomy V44.51
  specified type NEC V44.59
  with complication 997.5

Cystourethritis (*see also* Urethritis) 597.89

Cystourethrocele (*see also* Cystocele)
  female (without uterine prolapse) 618.0
    with uterine prolapse 618.4
      complete 618.3
      incomplete 618.2
  male 596.8

Cytomegalic inclusion disease 078.5
  congenital 771.1

Cytomycosis, reticuloendothelial (*see also* Histoplasmosis, American) 115.00

☑4ᵗʰ Fourth-digit Required   ☑5ᵗʰ Fifth-digit Required   ►◄ Revised Text   ● New Line   ▲ Revised Code

D

Daae (-Finsen) disease (epidemic pleurodynia) 074.1

Dabney's grip 074.1

Da Costa's syndrome (neurocirculatory asthenia) 306.2

Dacryoadenitis, dacryadenitis 375.00
  acute 375.01
  chronic 375.02

Dacryocystitis 375.30
  acute 375.32
  chronic 375.42
  neonatal 771.6
  phlegmonous 375.33
  syphilitic 095.8
    congenital 090.0
  trachomatous, active 076.1
    late effect 139.1
  tuberculous (see also Tuberculosis) 017.3 ✓5ᵗʰ

Dacryocystoblenorrhea 375.42

Dacryocystocele 375.43

Dacryolith, dacryolithiasis 375.57

Dacryoma 375.43

Dacryopericystitis (acute) (subacute) 375.32
  chronic 375.42

Dacryops 375.11

Dacryosialadenopathy, atrophic 710.2

Dacryostenosis 375.56
  congenital 743.65

Dactylitis 686.9
  bone (see also Osteomyelitis) 730.2 ✓5ᵗʰ
  sickle cell 282.61
  syphilitic 095.5
  tuberculous (see also Tuberculosis) 015.5 ✓5ᵗʰ

Dactylolysis opontana 136.0

Dactylosymphysis (see also Syndactylism) 755.10

Damage
  arteriosclerotic — see Arteriosclerosis
  brain 348.9
    anoxic, hypoxic 348.1
      during or resulting from a procedure 997.01
    child NEC 343.9
    due to birth injury 767.0
    minimal (child) (see also Hyperkinesia) 314.9
    newborn 767.0
  cardiac — see also Disease, heart
  cardiorenal (vascular) (see also Hypertension, cardiorenal) 404.90
  central nervous system — see Damage, brain
  cerebral NEC — see Damage, brain
  coccyx, complicating delivery 665.6 ✓5ᵗʰ
  coronary (see also Ischemia, heart) 414.9
  eye, birth injury 767.8
  heart — see also Disease, heart
    valve — see Endocarditis
  hypothalamus NEC 348.9
  liver 571.9
    alcoholic 571.3
  myocardium (see also Degeneration, myocardial) 429.1
  pelvic
    joint or ligament, during delivery 665.6 ✓5ᵗʰ
    organ NEC
      with
        abortion — see Abortion, by type, with damage to pelvic organs
        ectopic pregnancy (see also categories 633.0-633.9) 639.2
        molar pregnancy (see also categories 630-632) 639.2
      during delivery 665.5 ✓5ᵗʰ
      following
        abortion 639.2
        ectopic or molar pregnancy 639.2
  renal (see also Disease, renal) 593.9
  skin, solar 692.79
    acute 692.72
    chronic 692.74
  subendocardium, subendocardial (see also Degeneration, myocardial) 429.1
  vascular 459.9

Dameshek's syndrome (erythroblastic anemia) 282.4

Dana-Putnam syndrome (subacute combined sclerosis with pernicious anemia) 281.0 [336.2]

Danbolt (-Closs) syndrome (acrodermatitis enteropathica) 686.8

Dandruff 690.18

Dandy fever 061

Dandy-Walker deformity or syndrome (atresia, foramen of Magendie) 742.3
  with spina bifida (see also Spina bifida) 741.0 ✓5ᵗʰ

Dangle foot 736.79

Danielssen's disease (anesthetic leprosy) 030.1

Danlos' syndrome 756.83

Darier's disease (congenital) (keratosis follicularis) 757.39
  due to vitamin A deficiency 264.8
  meaning erythema annulare centrifugum 695.0

Darier-Roussy sarcoid 135

Darling's
  disease (see also Histoplasmosis, American) 115.00
  histoplasmosis (see also Histoplasmosis, American) 115.00

Dartre 054.9

Darwin's tubercle 744.29

Davidson's anemia (refractory) 284.9

Davies' disease 425.0

Davies-Colley syndrome (slipping rib) 733.99

Dawson's encephalitis 046.2

Day blindness (see also Blindness, day) 368.60

Dead
  fetus
    retained (in utero) 656.4 ✓5ᵗʰ
      early pregnancy (death before 22 completed weeks gestation) 632
      late (death after 22 completed weeks gestation) 656.4 ✓5ᵗʰ
    syndrome 641.3 ✓5ᵗʰ
  labyrinth 386.50
  ovum, retained 631

Deaf and dumb NEC 389.7

Deaf mutism (acquired) (congenital) NEC 389.7
  endemic 243
  hysterical 300.11
  syphilitic, congenital 090.0

Deafness (acquired) (bilateral) (both ears) (complete) (congenital) (hereditary) (middle ear) (partial) (unilateral) 389.9
  with blue sclera and fragility of bone 756.51
  auditory fatigue 389.9
  aviation 993.0
    nerve injury 951.5
  boilermakers' 951.5
  central 389.14
    with conductive hearing loss 389.2
  conductive (air) 389.00
    with sensorineural hearing loss 389.2
    combined types 389.08
    external ear 389.01
    inner ear 389.04
    middle ear 389.03
    multiple types 389.08
    tympanic membrane 389.02
  emotional (complete) 300.11
  functional (complete) 300.11
  high frequency 389.8
  hysterical (complete) 300.11
  injury 951.5
  low frequency 389.8
  mental 784.69
  mixed conductive and sensorineural 389.2
  nerve 389.12
    with conductive hearing loss 389.2
  neural 389.12
    with conductive hearing loss 389.2
  noise-induced 388.12
    nerve injury 951.5
  nonspeaking 389.7

Deafness — continued
  perceptive 389.10
    with conductive hearing loss 389.2
    central 389.14
    combined types 389.18
    multiple types 389.18
    neural 389.12
    sensory 389.11
  psychogenic (complete) 306.7
  sensorineural (see also Deafness, perceptive) 389.10
  sensory 389.11
    with conductive hearing loss 389.2
  specified type NEC 389.8
  sudden NEC 388.2
  syphilitic 094.89
  transient ischemic 388.02
  transmission — see Deafness, conductive
  traumatic 951.5
  word (secondary to organic lesion) 784.69
    developmental 315.31

Death
  after delivery (cause not stated) (sudden) 674.9 ✓5ᵗʰ
  anesthetic
    due to
      correct substance properly administered 995.4
      overdose or wrong substance given 968.4
        specified anesthetic — see Table of Drugs and Chemicals
    during delivery 668.9 ✓5ᵗʰ
  brain 348.8
  cardiac — see Disease, heart
  cause unknown 798.2
  cot (infant) 798.0
  crib (infant) 798.0
  fetus, fetal (cause not stated) (intrauterine) 779.9
    early, with retention (before 22 completed weeks gestation) 632
    from asphyxia or anoxia (before labor) 768.0
      during labor 768.1
    late, affecting management of pregnancy (after 22 completed weeks gestation) 656.4 ✓5ᵗʰ
  from pregnancy NEC 646.9 ✓5ᵗʰ
  instantaneous 798.1
  intrauterine (see also Death, fetus) 779.9
    complicating pregnancy 656.4 ✓5ᵗʰ
  maternal, affecting fetus or newborn 761.6
  neonatal NEC 779.9
  sudden (cause unknown) 798.1
    during delivery 669.9 ✓5ᵗʰ
      under anesthesia NEC 668.9 ✓5ᵗʰ
    infant, syndrome (SIDS) 798.0
    puerperal, during puerperium 674.9 ✓5ᵗʰ
  unattended (cause unknown) 798.9
  under anesthesia NEC
    due to
      correct substance properly administered 995.4
      overdose or wrong substance given 968.4
        specified anesthetic — see Table of Drugs and Chemicals
    during delivery 668.9 ✓5ᵗʰ
  violent 798.1

de Beurmann-Gougerot disease (sporotrichosis) 117.1

Debility (general) (infantile) (postinfectional) 799.3
  with nutritional difficulty 269.9
  congenital or neonatal NEC 779.9
  nervous 300.5
  old age 797
  senile 797

Débove's disease (splenomegaly) 789.2

Decalcification
  bone (see also Osteoporosis) 733.00
  teeth 521.8

Decapitation 874.9
  fetal (to facilitate delivery) 763.89

Decapsulation, kidney 593.89

Decay
  dental 521.00
  senile 797
  tooth, teeth 521.00

Decensus, uterus — *see* Prolapse, uterus
Deciduitis (acute)
  with
    abortion — *see* Abortion, by type, with
      sepsis
    ectopic pregnancy (*see also* categories
      633.0-633.9) 639.0
    molar pregnancy (*see also* categories 630-
      632) 639.0
  affecting fetus or newborn 760.8
  following
    abortion 639.0
    ectopic or molar pregnancy 639.0
  in pregnancy 646.6 ✓5ᵗʰ
  puerperal, postpartum 670 ✓4ᵗʰ
Deciduoma malignum (M9100/3) 181
Deciduous tooth (retained) 520.6
Decline (general) (*see also* Debility) 799.3
Decompensation
  cardiac (acute) (chronic) (*see also* Disease,
    heart) 429.9
    failure — *see* Failure, heart
  cardiorenal (*see also* Hypertension, cardiorenal)
    404.90
  cardiovascular (*see also* Disease,
    cardiovascular) 429.2
  heart (*see also* Disease, heart) 429.9
    failure — *see* Failure, heart
  hepatic 572.2
  myocardial (acute) (chronic) (*see also* Disease,
    heart) 429.9
    failure — *see* Failure, heart
  respiratory 519.9
Decompression sickness 993.3
Decrease, decreased
  blood
    platelets (*see also* Thrombocytopenia) 287.5
    pressure 796.3
      due to shock following
        injury 958.4
        operation 998.0
  cardiac reserve — *see* Disease, heart
  estrogen 256.39
    postablative 256.2
  fetal movements 655.7 ✓5ᵗʰ
  fragility of erythrocytes 289.8
  function
    adrenal (cortex) 255.4
      medulla 255.5
    ovary in hypopituitarism 253.4
    parenchyma of pancreas 577.8
    pituitary (gland) (lobe) (anterior) 253.2
      posterior (lobe) 253.8
  functional activity 780.99   ▲
  glucose 790.2
  haptoglobin (serum) NEC 273.8
  platelets (*see also* Thrombocytopenia) 287.5
  pulse pressure 785.9
  respiration due to shock following injury 958.4
  tear secretion NEC 375.15
  tolerance
    fat 579.8
    glucose 790.2
    salt and water 276.9
  vision NEC 369.9
Decubital gangrene 707.0 [785.4]
Decubiti (*see also* Decubitus) 707.0
Decubitus (ulcer) 707.0
  with gangrene 707.0 [785.4]
Deepening acetabulum 718.85
Defect, defective 759.9
  3-beta-hydroxysteroid dehydrogenase 255.2
  11-hydroxylase 255.2
  21-hydroxylase 255.2
  abdominal wall, congenital 756.70
  aorticopulmonary septum 745.0
  aortic septal 745.0
  atrial septal (ostium secundum type) 745.5
    acquired 429.71
    ostium primum type 745.61
    sinus venosus 745.8
  atrioventricular
    canal 745.69
    septum 745.4
      acquired 429.71

Defect, defective — *continued*
  atrium secundum 745.5
    acquired 429.71
  auricular septal 745.5
    acquired 429.71
  bilirubin excretion 277.4
  biosynthesis, testicular androgen 257.2
  bulbar septum 745.0
  butanol-insoluble iodide 246.1
  chromosome — *see* Anomaly, chromosome
  circulation (acquired) 459.9
    congenital 747.9
    newborn 747.9
  clotting NEC (*see also* Defect, coagulation)
    286.9
  coagulation (factor) (*see also* Deficiency,
    coagulation factor) 286.9
    with
      abortion — *see* Abortion, by type, with
        hemorrhage
      ectopic pregnancy (*see also* categories
        634-638) 639.1
      molar pregnancy (*see also* categories
        630-632) 639.1
    acquired (any) 286.7
    antepartum or intrapartum 641.3 ✓5ᵗʰ
      affecting fetus or newborn 762.1
    causing hemorrhage of pregnancy or delivery
      641.3 ✓5ᵗʰ
    due to
      liver disease 286.7
      vitamin K deficiency 286.7
    newborn, transient 776.3
    postpartum 666.3 ✓5ᵗʰ
    specified type NEC 286.3
  conduction (heart) 426.9
    bone (*see also* Deafness, conductive) 389.00
  congenital, organ or site NEC — *see also*
    Anomaly
    circulation 747.9
    Descemet's membrane 743.9
      specified type NEC 743.49
    diaphragm 756.6
    ectodermal 757.9
    esophagus 750.9
    pulmonic cusps — *see* Anomaly, heart valve
    respiratory system 748.9
      specified type NEC 748.8
  cushion endocardial 745.60
  dentin (hereditary) 520.5
  Descemet's membrane (congenital) 743.9
    acquired 371.30
    specific type NEC 743.49
  deutan 368.52
  developmental — *see also* Anomaly, by site
    cauda equina 742.59
    left ventricle 746.9
      with atresia or hypoplasia of aortic orifice
        or valve, with hypoplasia of
        ascending aorta 746.7
      in hypoplastic left heart syndrome 746.7
    testis 752.9
    vessel 747.9
  diaphragm
    with elevation, eventration, or hernia — *see*
      Hernia, diaphragm
    congenital 756.6
      with elevation, eventration, or hernia
        756.6
      gross (with elevation, eventration, or
        hernia) 756.6
  ectodermal, congenital 757.9
  Eisenmenger's (ventricular septal defect) 745.4
  endocardial cushion 745.60
    specified type NEC 745.69
  esophagus, congenital 750.9
  extensor retinaculum 728.9
  fibrin polymerization (*see also* Defect,
    coagulation) 286.3
  filling
    biliary tract 793.3
    bladder 793.5
    gallbladder 793.3
    kidney 793.5
    stomach 793.4
    ureter 793.5
  fossa ovalis 745.5

Defect, defective — *continued*
  gene, carrier (suspected) of V83.89   ▲
  Gerbode 745.4
  glaucomatous, without elevated tension 365.89
  Hageman (factor) (*see also* Defect, coagulation)
    286.3
  hearing (*see also* Deafness) 389.9
  high grade 317
  homogentisic acid 270.2
  interatrial septal 745.5
    acquired 429.71
  interauricular septal 745.5
    acquired 429.71
  interventricular septal 745.4
    with pulmonary stenosis or atresia,
      dextraposition of aorta, and
      hypertrophy of right ventricle 745.2
    acquired 429.71
    in tetralogy of Fallot 745.2
  iodide trapping 246.1
  iodotyrosine dehalogenase 246.1
  kynureninase 270.2
  learning, specific 315.2
  mental (*see also* Retardation, mental) 319
  osteochondral NEC 738.8
  ostium
    primum 745.61
    secundum 745.5
  pericardium 746.89
  peroxidase-binding 246.1
  placental blood supply — *see* Placenta,
    insufficiency
  platelet (qualitative) 287.1
    constitutional 286.4
  postural, spine 737.9
  protan 368.51
  pulmonic cusps, congenital 746.00
  renal pelvis 753.9
    obstructive 753.29
    specified type NEC 753.3
  respiratory system, congenital 748.9
    specified type NEC 748.8
  retina, retinal 361.30
    with detachment (*see also* Detachment,
      retina, with retinal defect) 361.00
    multiple 361.33
      with detachment 361.02
    nerve fiber bundle 362.85
    single 361.30
      with detachment 361.01
  septal (closure) (heart) NEC 745.9
    acquired 429.71
    atrial 745.5
    specified type NEC 745.8
  speech NEC 784.5
    developmental 315.39
    secondary to organic lesion 784.5
  Taussig-Bing (transposition, aorta and
    overriding pulmonary artery) 745.11
  teeth, wedge 521.2
  thyroid hormone synthesis 246.1
  tritan 368.53
  ureter 753.9
    obstructive 753.29
  vascular (acquired) (local) 459.9
    congenital (peripheral) NEC 747.60
      gastrointestinal 747.61
      lower limb 747.64
      renal 747.62
      specified NEC 747.69
      spinal 747.82
      upper limb 747.63
  ventricular septal 745.4
    with pulmonary stenosis or atresia,
      dextraposition of aorta, and
      hypertrophy of right ventricle 745.2
    acquired 429.71
    atrioventricular canal type 745.69
    between infundibulum and anterior portion
      745.4
    in tetralogy of Fallot 745.2
    isolated anterior 745.4
  vision NEC 369.9
  visual field 368.40
    arcuate 368.43
    heteronymous, bilateral 368.47
    homonymous, bilateral 368.46

■4ᵗʰ Fourth-digit Required   ■5ᵗʰ Fifth-digit Required   ▶◀ Revised Text   ● New Line   ▲ Revised Code

Defect, defective — *continued*
  visual field — *continued*
    localized NEC 368.44
    nasal step 368.44
    peripheral 368.44
    sector 368.43
  voice 784.40
  wedge, teeth (abrasion) 521.2
Defeminization syndrome 255.2
Deferentitis 608.4
  gonorrheal (acute) 098.14
    chronic or duration of 2 months or over 098.34
Defibrination syndrome (*see also* Fibrinolysis) 286.6
Deficiency, deficient
  3-beta-hydroxysteroid dehydrogenase 255.2
  6-phosphogluconic dehydrogenase (anemia) 282.2
  11-beta-hydroxylase 255.2
  17-alpha-hydroxylase 255.2
  18-hydroxysteroid dehydrogenase 255.2
  20-alpha-hydroxylase 255.2
  21-hydroxylase 255.2
  abdominal muscle syndrome 756.79
  accelerator globulin (Ac G) (blood) (*see also* Defect, coagulation) 286.3
  AC globulin (congenital) (*see also* Defect, coagulation) 286.3
    acquired 286.7
  activating factor (blood) (*see also,* Defect, coagulation) 286.3
  adenohypophyseal 253.2
  adenosine deaminase 277.2
  aldolase (hereditary) 271.2
  alpha-1-antitrypsin 277.6
  alpha-1-trypsin inhibitor 277.6
  alpha-fucosidase 271.8
  alpha-lipoprotein 272.5
  alpha-mannosidase 271.8
  amino acid 270.9
  anemia — *see* Anemia, deficiency
  aneurin 265.1
    with beriberi 265.0
  antibody NEC 279.00
  antidiuretic hormone 253.5
  antihemophilic
    factor (A) 286.0
      B 286.1
      C 286.2
    globulin (AHG) NEC 286.0
  antitrypsin 277.6
  argininosuccinate synthetase or lyase 270.6
  ascorbic acid (with scurvy) 267
  autoprothrombin
    I (*see also* Defect, coagulation) 286.3
    II 286.1
    C (*see also* Defect, coagulation) 286.3
  bile salt 579.8
  biotin 266.2
  biotinidase 277.6
  bradykinase-1 277.6
  brancher enzyme (amylopectinosis) 271.0
  calciferol 268.9
    with
      osteomalacia 268.2
      rickets (*see also* Rickets) 268.0
  calcium 275.40
    dietary 269.3
  calorie, severe 261
  carbamyl phosphate synthetase 270.6
  cardiac (*see also* Insufficiency, myocardial) 428.0
  carnitine palmityl transferase 791.3
  carotene 264.9
  Carr factor (*see also* Defect, coagulation) 286.9
  central nervous system 349.9
  ceruloplasmin 275.1
  cevitamic acid (with scurvy) 267
  choline 266.2
  Christmas factor 286.1
  chromium 269.3
  citrin 269.1
  clotting (blood) (*see also* Defect, coagulation) 286.9

Deficiency, deficient — *continued*
  coagulation factor NEC 286.9
    with
      abortion — *see* Abortion, by type, with hemorrhage
      ectopic pregnancy (*see also* categories 634-638) 639.1
      molar pregnancy (*see also* categories 630-632) 639.1
    acquired (any) 286.7
    antepartum or intrapartum 641.3 ✓5ᵗʰ
      affecting fetus or newborn 762.1
    due to
      liver disease 286.7
      vitamin K deficiency 286.7
    newborn, transient 776.3
    postpartum 666.3 ✓5ᵗʰ
    specified type NEC 286.3
  color vision (congenital) 368.59
    acquired 368.55
  combined, two or more coagulation factors (*see also* Defect, coagulation) 286.9
  complement factor NEC 279.8
  contact factor (*see also* Defect, coagulation) 286.3
  copper NEC 275.1
  corticoadrenal 255.4
  craniofacial axis 756.0
  cyanocobalamin (vitamin B₁₂) 266.2
  debrancher enzyme (limit dextrinosis) 271.0
  desmolase 255.2
  diet 269.9
  dihydrofolate reductase 281.2
  dihydropteridine reductase 270.1
  disaccharidase (intestinal) 271.3
  disease NEC 269.9
  ear(s) V48.8
  edema 262
  endocrine 259.9
  enzymes, circulating NEC (*see also* Deficiency, by specific enzyme) 277.6
  ergosterol 268.9
    with
      osteomalacia 268.2
      rickets (*see also* Rickets) 268.0
  erythrocytic glutathione (anemia) 282.2
  eyelid(s) V48.8
  factor (*See also* Defect, coagulation) 286.9
    I (congenital) (fibrinogen) 286.3
      antepartum or intrapartum 641.3 ✓5ᵗʰ
        affecting fetus or newborn 762.1
      newborn, transient 776.3
      postpartum 666.3 ✓5ᵗʰ
    II (congenital) (prothrombin) 286.3
    V (congenital) (labile) 286.3
    VII (congenital) (stable) 286.3
    VIII (congenital) (functional) 286.0
      with
        functional defect 286.0
        vascular defect 286.4
    IX (Christmas) (congenital) (functional) 286.1
    X (congenital) (Stuart-Prower) 286.3
    XI (congenital) (plasma thromboplastin antecedent) 286.2
    XII (congenital) (Hageman) 286.3
    XIII (congenital) (fibrin stabilizing) 286.3
    Hageman 286.3
    multiple (congenital) 286.9
      acquired 286.7
  fibrinase (*see also* Defect, coagulation) 286.3
  fibrinogen (congenital) (*see also* Defect, coagulation) 286.3
    acquired 286.6
  fibrin-stabilizing factor (congenital) (*see also* Defect, coagulation) 286.3
  finger — *see* Absence, finger
  fletcher factor (*see also* Defect, coagulation) 286.9
  fluorine 269.3
  folate, anemia 281.2
  folic acid (vitamin B₆) 266.2
    anemia 281.2
  fructokinase 271.2
  fructose-1, 6-diphosphate 271.2
  fructose-1-phosphate aldolase 271.2
  FSH (follicle-stimulating hormone) 253.4
  fucosidase 271.8

Deficiency, deficient — *continued*
  galactokinase 271.1
  galactose-1-phosphate uridyl transferase 271.1
  gamma globulin in blood 279.00
  glass factor (*see also* Defect, coagulation) 286.3
  glucocorticoid 255.4
  glucose-6-phosphatase 271.0
  glucose-6-phosphate dehydrogenase anemia 282.2
  glucuronyl transferase 277.4
  glutathione-reductase (anemia) 282.2
  glycogen synthetase 271.0
  growth hormone 253.3
  Hageman factor (congenital) (*see also* Defect, coagulation) 286.3
  head V48.0
  hemoglobin (*see also* Anemia) 285.9
  hepatophosphorylase 271.0
  hexose monophosphate (HMP) shunt 282.2
  HGH (human growth hormone) 253.3
  HG-PRT 277.2
  homogentisic acid oxidase 270.2
  hormone — *see also* Deficiency, by specific hormone
    anterior pituitary (isolated) (partial) NEC 253.4
      growth (human) 253.3
    follicle-stimulating 253.4
    growth (human) (isolated) 253.3
    human growth 253.3
    interstitial cell-stimulating 253.4
    luteinizing 253.4
    melanocyte-stimulating 253.4
    testicular 257.2
  human growth hormone 253.3
  humoral 279.00
    with
      hyper-IgM 279.05
        autosomal recessive 279.05
        X-linked 279.05
      increased IgM 279.05
    congenital hypogammaglobulinemia 279.04
    non-sex-linked 279.06
    selective immunoglobulin NEC 279.03
      IgA 279.01
      IgG 279.03
      IgM 279.02
        increased 279.05
    specified NEC 279.09
  hydroxylase 255.2
  hypoxanthine-guanine phosphoribosyltransferase (HG-PRT) 277.2
  ICSH (interstitial cell-stimulating hormone) 253.4
  immunity NEC 279.3
    cell-mediated 279.10
      with
        hyperimmunoglob-ulinemia 279.2
        thrombocytopenia and eczema 279.12
      specified NEC 279.19
    combined (severe) 279.2
      syndrome 279.2
    common variable 279.06
    humoral NEC 279.00
    IgA (secretory) 279.01
    IgG 279.03
    IgM 279.02
  immunoglobulin, selective NEC 279.03
    IgA 279.01
    IgG 279.03
    IgM 279.02
  inositol (B complex) 266.2
  interferon 279.4
  internal organ V47.0
  interstitial cell-stimulating hormone (ICSH) 253.4
  intrinsic factor (Castle's) (congenital) 281.0
  intrinsic (urethral) sphincter (ISD) 599.82
  invertase 271.3
  iodine 269.3
  iron, anemia 280.9
  labile factor (congenital) (*see also* Defect, coagulation) 286.3
    acquired 286.7
  lacrimal fluid (acquired) 375.15
    congenital 743.64
  lactase 271.3

✓4ᵗʰ Fourth-digit Required   ✓5ᵗʰ Fifth-digit Required   ▶◀ Revised Text   ● New Line   ▲ Revised Code

Deficiency, deficient — *continued*
Laki-Lorand factor (*see also* Defect, coagulation) 286.3
lecithin-cholesterol acyltranferase 272.5
LH (luteinizing hormone) 253.4
limb V49.0
lower V49.0
congenital (*see also* Deficiency, lower limb, congenital) 755.30
upper V49.0
congenital (*see also* Deficiency, upper limb, congenital) 755.20
lipocaic 577.8
lipoid (high-density) 272.5
lipoprotein (familial) (high density) 272.5
liver phosphorylase 271.0
lower limb V49.0
congenital 755.30
with complete absence of distal elements 755.31
longitudinal (complete) (partial) (with distal deficiencies, incomplete) 755.32
with complete absence of distal elements 755.31
combined femoral, tibial, fibular (incomplete) 755.33
femoral 755.34
fibular 755.37
metatarsal(s) 755.38
phalange(s) 755.39
meaning all digits 755.31
tarsal(s) 755.38
tibia 755.36
tibiofibular 755.35
transverse 755.31
luteinizing hormone (LH) 253.4
lysosomal alpha-1, 4 glucosidase 271.0
magnesium 275.2
mannosidase 271.8
melanocyte-stimulating hormone (MSH) 253.4
menadione (vitamin K) 269.0
newborn 776.0
mental (familial) (hereditary) (*see also* Retardation, mental) 319
mineral NEC 269.3
molybdenum 269.3
moral 301.7
multiple, syndrome 260
myocardial (*see also* Insufficiency myocardial) 428.0
myophosphorylase 271.0
NADH (DPNH)-methemoglobin-reductase (congenital) 289.7
NADH-diaphorase or reductase (congenital) 289.7
neck V48.1
niacin (amide) (-tryptophan) 265.2
nicotinamide 265.2
nicotinic acid (amide) 265.2
nose V48.8
number of teeth (*see also* Anodontia) 520.0
nutrition, nutritional 269.9
specified NEC 269.8
ornithine transcarbamylase 270.6
ovarian 256.39
oxygen (*see also* Anoxia) 799.0
pantothenic acid 266.2
parathyroid (gland) 252.1
phenylalanine hydroxylase 270.1
phosphofructokinase 271.2
phosphoglucomutase 271.0
phosphohexosisomerase 271.0
phosphorylase kinase, liver 271.0
pituitary (anterior) 253.2
posterior 253.5
placenta — *see* Placenta, insufficiency
plasma
cell 279.00
protein (paraproteinemia) (pyroglobulinemia) 273.8
gamma globulin 279.00
thrombosplastin
antecedent (PTA) 286.2
component (PTC) 286.1
platelet NEC 287.1
constitutional 286.4

Deficiency, deficient — *continued*
polyglandular 258.9
potassium (K) 276.8
proaccelerin (congenital) (*see also* Defect, congenital) 286.3
acquired 286.7
proconvertin factor (congenital) (*see also* Defect, coagulation) 286.3
acquired 286.7
prolactin 253.4
protein 260
anemia 281.4
plasma — *see* Deficiency, plasma protein
prothrombin (congenital) (*see also* Defect coagulation) 286.3
acquired 286.7
Prower factor (*see also* Defect, coagulation) 286.3
PRT 277.2
pseudocholinesterase 289.8
psychobiological 301.6
PTA 286.2
PTC 286.1
purine nucleoside phosphorylase 277.2
pyracin (alpha) (Beta) 266.1
pyridoxal 266.1
pyridoxamine 266.1
pyridoxine (derivatives) 266.1
pyruvate kinase (PK) 282.3
riboflavin (vitamin B_2) 266.0
saccadic eye movements 379.57
salivation 527.7
salt 276.1
secretion
ovary 256.39
salivary gland (any) 527.7
urine 788.5
selenium 269.3
serum
antitrypsin, familial 277.6
protein (congenital) 273.8
smooth pursuit movements (eye) 379.58
sodium (Na) 276.1
SPCA (*see also* Defect, coagulation) 286.3
specified NEC 269.8
stable factor (congenital) (*see also* Defect, coagulation) 286.3
acquired 286.7
Stuart (-Prower) factor (*see also* Defect, coagulation) 286.3
sucrase 271.3
sucrase-isomaltase 271.3
sulfite oxidase 270.0
syndrome, multiple 260
thiamine, thiaminic (chloride) 265.1
thrombokinase (*see also* Defect, coagulation) 286.3
newborn 776.0
thrombopoieten 287.3
thymolymphatic 279.2
thyroid (gland) 244.9
tocopherol 269.1
toe — *see* Absence, toe
tooth bud (*see also* Anodontia) 520.0
trunk V48.1
UDPG-glycogen transferase 271.0
upper limb V49.0
congenital 755.20
with complete absence of distal elements 755.21
longitudinal (complete) (partial) (with distal deficiencies, incomplete) 755.22
carpal(s) 755.28
combined humeral, radial, ulnar (incomplete) 755.23
humeral 755.24
metacarpal(s) 755.28
phalange(s) 755.29
meaning all digits 755.21
radial 755.26
radioulnar 755.25
ulnar 755.27
transverse (complete) (partial) 755.21
vascular 459.9
vasopressin 253.5
viosterol (*see also* Deficiency, calciferol) 268.9

Deficiency, deficient — *continued*
vitamin (multiple) NEC 269.2
A 264.9
with
Bitôt's spot 264.1
corneal 264.2
with corneal ulceration 264.3
keratomalacia 264.4
keratosis, follicular 264.8
night blindness 264.5
scar of cornea, xerophthalmic 264.6
specified manifestation NEC 264.8
ocular 264.7
xeroderma 264.8
xerophthalmia 264.7
xerosis
conjunctival 264.0
with Bitôt's spot 264.1
corneal 264.2
with corneal ulceraton 264.3
B (complex) NEC 266.9
with
beriberi 265.0
pellagra 265.2
specified type NEC 266.2
B_1 NEC 265.1
beriberi 265.0
B_2 266.0
B_6 266.1
B_{12} 266.2
B_9 (folic acid) 266.2
C (ascorbic acid) (with scurvy) 267
D (calciferol) (ergosterol) 268.9
with
osteomalacia 268.2
rickets (*see also* Rickets) 268.0
E 269.1
folic acid 266.2
G 266.0
H 266.2
K 269.0
of newborn 776.0
nicotinic acid 265.2
P 269.1
PP 265.2
specified NEC 269.1
zinc 269.3
Deficient — *see also* Deficiency
blink reflex 374.45
craniofacial axis 756.0
number of teeth (*see also* Anodontia) 520.0
secretion of urine 788.5
Deficit
neurologic NEC 781.99
due to
cerebrovascular lesion (*see also* Disease, cerebrovascular, acute) 436
late effect — *see* Late effect(s) (of) cerebrovascular disease
transient ischemic attack 435.9
oxygen 799.0
Deflection
radius 736.09
septum (acquired) (nasal) (nose) 470
spine — *see* Curvature, spine
turbinate (nose) 470
Defluvium
capillorum (*see also* Alopecia) 704.00
ciliorum 374.55
unguium 703.8
Deformity 738.9
abdomen, congential 759.9
abdominal wall
acquired 738.8
congenital 756.70
muscle deficiency syndrome 756.79
acquired (unspecified site) 738.9
specified site NEC 738.8
adrenal gland (congenital) 759.1
alimentary tract, congenital 751.9
lower 751.5
specified type NEC 751.8
upper (any part, except tongue) 750.9
specified type NEC 750.8
tongue 750.10
specified type NEC 750.19

Deformity — *continued*
ankle (joint) (acquired) 736.70
  abduction 718.47
  congenital 755.69
  contraction 718.47
  specified NEC 736.79   ●
anus (congenital) 751.5
  acquired 569.49
aorta (congenital) 747.20
  acquired 447.8
  arch 747.21
    acquired 447.8
  coarctation 747.10
aortic
  arch 747.21
    acquired 447.8
  cusp or valve (congenital) 746.9
    acquired (*see also* Endocarditis, aortic)
      424.1
  ring 747.21
appendix 751.5
arm (acquired) 736.89
  congenital 755.50
arteriovenous (congenital) (peripheral) NEC
  747.60
  gastrointestinal 747.61
  lower limb 747.64
  renal 747.62
  specified NEC 747.69
  spinal 747.82
  upper limb 747.63
artery (congenital) (peripheral) NEC (*see also*
  Deformity, vascular) 747.60
  acquired 447.8
  cerebral 747.81
  coronary (congenital) 746.85
    acquired (*see also* Ischemia, heart) 414.9
  retinal 743.9
  umbilical 747.5
atrial septal (congenital) (heart) 745.5
auditory canal (congenital) (external) (*see also*
  Deformity, ear) 744.3
  acquired 380.50
auricle
  ear (congenital) (*see also* Deformity, ear)
    744.3
    acquired 380.32
  heart (congenital) 746.9
back (acquired) — *see* Deformity, spine
Bartholin's duct (congenital) 750.9
bile duct (congenital) 751.60
  acquired 576.8
    with calculus, choledocholithiasis, or
      stones — *see* Choledocholithiasis
biliary duct or passage (congenital) 751.60
  acquired 576.8
    with calculus, choledocholithiasis, or
      stones — *see* Choledocholithiasis
bladder (neck) (spincter) (trigone) (acquired)
  596.8
  congenital 753.9
bone (acquired) NEC 738.9
  congenital 756.9
  turbinate 738.0
boutonniere (finger) 736.21
brain (congenital) 742.9
  acquired 348.8
  multiple 742.4
  reduction 742.2
  vessel (congenital) 747.81
breast (acquired) 611.8
  congenital 757.9
bronchus (congenital) 748.3
  acquired 519.1
bursa, congenital 756.9
canal of Nuck 752.9
canthus (congenital) 743.9
  acquired 374.89
capillary (acquired) 448.9
  congenital NEC (*see also* Deformity,
    vascular) 747.60
cardiac — *see* Deformity, heart
cardiovascular system (congenital) 746.9
caruncle, lacrimal (congenital) 743.9
  acquired 375.69
cascade, stomach 537.6
cecum (congenital) 751.5
  acquired 569.89

Deformity — *continued*
cerebral (congenital) 742.9
  acquired 348.8
cervix (acquired) (uterus) 622.8
  congenital 752.40
cheek (acquired) 738.19
  congenital 744.9
chest (wall) (acquired) 738.3
  congenital 754.89
  late effect of rickets 268.1
chin (acquired) 738.19
  congenital 744.9
choroid (congenital) 743.9
  acquired 363.8
  plexus (congenital) 742.9
    acquired 349.2
cicatricial — *see* Cicatrix
cilia (congenital) 743.9
  acquired 374.89
circulatory system (congenital) 747.9
clavicle (acquired) 738.8
  congenital 755.51
clitoris (congenital) 752.40
  acquired 624.8
clubfoot — *see* Clubfoot
coccyx (acquired) 738.6
  congenital 756.10
colon (congenital) 751.5
  acquired 569.89
concha (ear) (congenital) (*see also* Deformity,
  ear) 744.3
  acquired 380.32
congenital, organ or site not listed (*see also*
  Anomaly) 759.9
cornea (congenital) 743.9
  acquired 371.70
coronary artery (congenital) 746.85
  acquired (*see also* Ischemia, heart) 414.9
cranium (acquired) 738.19
  congenital (*see also* Deformity, skull,
    congenital) 756.0
cricoid cartilage (congenital) 748.3
  acquired 478.79
cystic duct (congenital) 751.60
  acquired 575.8
Dandy-Walker 742.3
  with spina bifida (*see also* Spina bifida)
    741.0 ✓5ᵗʰ
diaphragm (congenital) 756.6
  acquired 738.8
digestive organ(s) or system (congenital) NEC
  751.9
  specified type NEC 751.8
ductus arteriosus 747.0
duodenal bulb 537.89
duodenum (congenital) 751.5
  acquired 537.89
dura (congenital) 742.9
  brain 742.4
    acquired 349.2
  spinal 742.59
    acquired 349.2
ear (congenital) 744.3
  acquired 380.32
  auricle 744.3
    causing impairment of hearing 744.02
  causing impairment of hearing 744.00
  external 744.3
    causing impairment of hearing 744.02
  internal 744.05
  lobule 744.3
  middle 744.03
    ossicles 744.04
  ossicles 744.04
ectodermal (congenital) NEC 757.9
  specified type NEC 757.8
ejaculatory duct (congenital) 752.9
  acquired 608.89
elbow (joint) (acquired) 736.00
  congenital 755.50
  contraction 718.42
endocrine gland NEC 759.2
epididymis (congenital) 752.9
  acquired 608.89
  torsion 608.2
epiglottis (congenital) 748.3
  acquired 478.79

Deformity — *continued*
esophagus (congenital) 750.9
  acquired 530.89
Eustachian tube (congenital) NEC 744.3
  specified type NEC 744.24
extremity (acquired) 736.9
  congenital, except reduction deformity 755.9
    lower 755.60
    upper 755.50
  reduction — *see* Deformity, reduction
eye (congenital) 743.9
  acquired 379.8
  muscle 743.9
eyebrow (congenital) 744.89
eyelid (congenital) 743.9
  acquired 374.89
  specified type NEC 743.62
face (acquired) 738.19
  congenital (any part) 744.9
    due to intrauterine malposition and
      pressure 754.0
fallopian tube (congenital) 752.10
  acquired 620.8
femur (acquired) 736.89
  congenital 755.60
fetal
  with fetopelvic disproportion 653.7 ✓5ᵗʰ
    affecting fetus or newborn 763.1
  causing obstructed labor 660.1 ✓5ᵗʰ
    affecting fetus or newborn 763.1
  known or suspected, affecting management
    of pregnancy 655.9 ✓5ᵗʰ
finger (acquired) 736.20
  boutonniere type 736.21
  congenital 755.50
  flexion contracture 718.44
  swan neck 736.22
flexion (joint) (acquired) 736.9
  congenital NEC 755.9
  hip or thigh (acquired) 736.39
    congenital (*see also* Subluxation,
      congenital, hip) 754.32
foot (acquired) 736.70
  cavovarus 736.75
    congenital 754.59
  congenital NEC 754.70
    specified type NEC 754.79
  valgus (acquired) 736.79
    congenital 754.60
      specified type NEC 754.69
  varus (acquired) 736.79
    congenital 754.50
      specified type NEC 754.59
forearm (acquired) 736.00
  congenital 755.50
forehead (acquired) 738.19
  congenital (*see also* Deformity, skull,
    congenital) 756.0
frontal bone (acquired) 738.19
  congenital (*see also* Deformity, skull,
    congenital) 756.0
gallbladder (congenital) 751.60
  acquired 575.8
gastrointestinal tract (congenital) NEC 751.9
  acquired 569.89
  specified type NEC 751.8
genitalia, genital organ(s) or system NEC
  congenital 752.9
  female (congenital) 752.9
    acquired 629.8
    external 752.40
    internal 752.9
  male (congenital) 752.9
    acquired 608.89
globe (eye) (congenital) 743.9
  acquired 360.89
gum (congenital) 750.9
  acquired 523.9
gunstock 736.02
hand (acquired) 736.00
  claw 736.06
  congenital 755.50
  minus (and plus) (intrinsic) 736.09
  pill roller (intrinsic) 736.09
  plus (and minus) (intrinsic) 736.09
  swan neck (intrinsic) 736.09

✓4ᵗʰ Fourth-digit Required   ✓5ᵗʰ Fifth-digit Required   ►◄ Revised Text   ● New Line   ▲ Revised Code

Deformity — *continued*
- head (acquired) 738.10
  - congenital (*see also* Deformity, skull congenital) 756.0
  - specified NEC 738.19
- heart (congenital) 746.9
  - auricle (congenital) 746.9
  - septum 745.9
    - auricular 745.5
    - specified type NEC 745.8
    - ventricular 745.4
  - valve (congenital) NEC 746.9
    - acquired — *see* Endocarditis
    - pulmonary (congenital) 746.00
      - specified type NEC 746.89
  - ventricle (congenital) 746.9
- heel (acquired) 736.76
  - congenital 755.67
- hepatic duct (congenital) 751.60
  - acquired 576.8
    - with calculus, choledocholithiasis, or stones — *see* Choledocholithiasis
- hip (joint) (acquired) 736.30
  - congenital NEC 755.63
  - flexion 718.45
    - congenital (*see also* Subluxation, congenital, hip) 754.32
- hourglass — *see* Contraction, hourglass
- humerus (acquired) 736.89
  - congenital 755.50
- hymen (congenital) 752.40
- hypophyseal (congenital) 759.2
- ileocecal (coil) (valve) (congenital) 751.5
  - acquired 569.89
- ileum (intestine) (congenital) 751.5
  - acquired 569.89
- ilium (acquired) 738.6
  - congenital 755.60
- integument (congenital) 757.9
- intervertebral cartilage or disc (acquired) — *see also* Displacement, intervertebral disc
  - congenital 756.10
- intestine (large) (small) (congenital) 751.5
  - acquired 569.89
- iris (acquired) 364.75
  - congenital 743.9
  - prolapse 364.8
- ischium (acquired) 738.6
  - congenital 755.60
- jaw (acquired) (congenital) NEC 524.9
  - due to intrauterine malposition and pressure 754.0
- joint (acquired) NEC 738.8
  - congenital 755.9
  - contraction (abduction) (adduction) (extension) (flexion) — *see* Contraction, joint
- kidney(s) (calyx) (pelvis) (congenital) 753.9
  - acquired 593.89
  - vessel 747.62
    - acquired 459.9
- Klippel-Feil (brevicollis) 756.16
- knee (acquired) NEC 736.6
  - congenital 755.64
- labium (majus) (minus) (congenital) 752.40
  - acquired 624.8
- lacrimal apparatus or duct (congenital) 743.9
  - acquired 375.69
- larynx (muscle) (congenital) 748.3
  - acquired 478.79
  - web (glottic) (subglottic) 748.2
- leg (lower) (upper) (acquired) NEC 736.89
  - congenital 755.60
    - reduction — *see* Deformity, reduction, lower limb
- lens (congenital) 743.9
  - acquired 379.39
- lid (fold) (congenital) 743.9
  - acquired 374.89
- ligament (acquired) 728.9
  - congenital 756.9
- limb (acquired) 736.9
  - congenital, except reduction deformity 755.9
    - lower 755.60
      - reduction (*see also* Deformity, reduction, lower limb) 755.30

Deformity — *continued*
- limb — *continued*
  - congenital, except reduction deformity — *continued*
    - upper 755.50
      - reduction (*see also* Deformity, reduction, upper limb) 755.20
  - specified NEC 736.89
- lip (congenital) NEC 750.9
  - acquired 528.5
  - specified type NEC 750.26
- liver (congenital) 751.60
  - acquired 573.8
  - duct (congenital) 751.60
    - acquired 576.8
      - with calculus, choledocholithiasis, or stones — *see* Choledocholithiasis
- lower extremity — *see* Deformity, leg
- lumbosacral (joint) (region) (congenital) 756.10
  - acquired 738.5
- lung (congenital) 748.60
  - acquired 518.89
  - specified type NEC 748.69
- lymphatic system, congenital 759.9
- Madelung's (radius) 755.54
- maxilla (acquired) (congenital) 524.9
- meninges or membrane (congenital) 742.9
  - brain 742.4
    - acquired 349.2
  - spinal (cord) 742.59
    - acquired 349.2
- mesentery (congenital) 751.9
  - acquired 568.89
- metacarpus (acquired) 736.00
  - congenital 755.50
- metatarsus (acquired) 736.70
  - congenital 754.70
- middle ear, except ossicles (congenital) 744.03
  - ossicles 744.04
- mitral (leaflets) (valve) (congenital) 746.9
  - acquired — *see* Endocarditis, mitral
  - Ebstein's 746.89
  - parachute 746.5
  - specified type NEC 746.89
  - stenosis, congenital 746.5
- mouth (acquired) 528.9
  - congenital NEC 750.9
    - specified type NEC 750.26
- multiple, congenital NEC 759.7
  - specified type NEC 759.89
- muscle (acquired) 728.9
  - congenital 756.9
    - specified type NEC 756.89
    - sternocleidomastoid (due to intrauterine malposition and pressure) 754.1
- musculoskeletal system, congenital NEC 756.9
  - specified type NEC 756.9
- nail (acquired) 703.9
  - congenital 757.9
- nasal — *see* Deformity, nose
- neck (acquired) NEC 738.2
  - congenital (any part) 744.9
    - sternocleidomastoid 754.1
- nervous system (congenital) 742.9
- nipple (congenital) 757.9
  - acquired 611.8
- nose, nasal (cartilage) (acquired) 738.0
  - bone (turbinate) 738.0
  - congenital 748.1
    - bent 754.0
    - squashed 754.0
  - saddle 738.0
    - syphilitic 090.5
  - septum 470
    - congenital 748.1
  - sinus (wall) (congenital) 748.1
    - acquired 738.0
  - syphilitic (congenital) 090.5
    - late 095.8
- ocular muscle (congenital) 743.9
  - acquired 378.60
- opticociliary vessels (congenital) 743.9
- orbit (congenital) (eye) 743.9
  - acquired NEC 376.40
    - associated with craniofacial deformities 376.44

Deformity — *continued*
- orbit — *continued*
  - acquired NEC — *continued*
    - due to
      - bone disease 376.43
      - surgery 376.47
      - trauma 376.47
- organ of Corti (congenital) 744.05
- ovary (congenital) 752.0
  - acquired 620.8
- oviduct (congenital) 752.10
  - acquired 620.8
- palate (congenital) 750.9
  - acquired 526.89
  - cleft (congenital) (*see also* Cleft, palate) 749.00
  - hard, acquired 526.89
  - soft, acquired 528.9
- pancreas (congenital) 751.7
  - acquired 577.8
- parachute, mitral valve 746.5
- parathyroid (gland) 759.2
- parotid (gland) (congenital) 750.9
  - acquired 527.8
- patella (acquired) 736.6
  - congenital 755.64
- pelvis, pelvic (acquired) (bony) 738.6
  - with disproportion (fetopelvic) 653.0 ☑5ᵗʰ
    - affecting fetus or newborn 763.1
    - causing obstructed labor 660.1 ☑5ᵗʰ
      - affecting fetus or newborn 763.1
  - congenital 755.60
  - rachitic (late effect) 268.1
- penis (glans) (congenital) 752.9
  - acquired 607.89
- pericardium (congenital) 746.9
  - acquired — *see* Pericarditis
- pharynx (congenital) 750.9
  - acquired 478.29
- Pierre Robin (congenital) 756.0
- pinna (acquired) 380.32
  - congenital 744.3
- pituitary (congenital) 759.2
- pleural folds (congenital) 748.8
- portal vein (congenital) 747.40
- posture *see* Curvature, spine
- prepuce (congenital) 752.9
  - acquired 607.89
- prostate (congenital) 752.9
  - acquired 602.8
- pulmonary valve — *see* Endocarditis, pulmonary
- pupil (congenital) 743.9
  - acquired 364.75
- pylorus (congenital) 750.9
  - acquired 537.89
- rachitic (acquired), healed or old 268.1
- radius (acquired) 736.00
  - congenital 755.50
    - reduction — *see* Deformity, reduction, upper limb
- rectovaginal septum (congenital) 752.40
  - acquired 623.8
- rectum (congenital) 751.5
  - acquired 569.49
- reduction (extremity) (limb) 755.4
  - brain 742.2
  - lower limb 755.30
    - with complete absence of distal elements 755.31
    - longitudinal (complete) (partial) (with distal deficiencies, incomplete) 755.32
      - with complete absence of distal elements 755.31
      - combined femoral, tibial, fibular (incomplete) 755.33
      - femoral 755.34
      - fibular 755.37
      - metatarsal(s) 755.38
      - phalange(s) 755.39
        - meaning all digits 755.31
      - tarsal(s) 755.38
      - tibia 755.36
      - tibiofibular 755.35
    - transverse 755.31

Deformity — *continued*
  reduction — *continued*
    upper limb 755.20
      with complete absence of distal elements 755.21
      longitudinal (complete) (partial) (with distal deficiencies, incomplete) 755.22
        with complete absence of distal elements 755.21
        carpal(s) 755.28
        combined humeral, radial, ulnar (incomplete) 755.23
        humeral 755.24
        metacarpal(s) 755.28
        phalange(s) 755.29
          meaning all digits 755.21
        radial 755.26
        radioulnar 755.25
        ulnar 755.27
      transverse (complete) (partial) 755.21
  renal — *see* Deformity, kidney
  respiratory system (congenital) 748.9
    specified type NEC 748.8
  rib (acquired) 738.3
    congenital 756.3
      cervical 756.2
  rotation (joint) (acquired) 736.9
    congenital 755.9
    hip or thigh 736.39
      congenital (*see also* Subluxation, congenital, hip) 754.32
  sacroiliac joint (congenital) 755.69
    acquired 738.5
  sacrum (acquired) 738.5
    congenital 756.10
  saddle
    back 737.8
    nose 738.0
      syphilitic 090.5
  salivary gland or duct (congenital) 750.9
    acquired 527.8
  scapula (acquired) 736.89
    congenital 755.50
  scrotum (congenital) 752.9
    acquired 608.89
  sebaceous gland, acquired 706.8
  seminal tract or duct (congenital) 752.9
    acquired 608.89
  septum (nasal) (acquired) 470
    congenital 748.1
  shoulder (joint) (acquired) 736.89
    congenital 755.50
      specified type NEC 755.59
    contraction 718.41
  sigmoid (flexure) (congenital) 751.5
    acquired 569.89
  sinus of Valsalva 747.29
  skin (congenital) 757.9
    acquired NEC 709.8
  skull (acquired) 738.19
    congenital 756.0
      with
        anencephalus 740.0
        encephalocele 742.0
        hydrocephalus 742.3
          with spina bifida (*see also* Spina bifida) 741.0 ✓5ᵗʰ
        microcephalus 742.1
      due to intrauterine malposition and pressure 754.0
  soft parts, organs or tissues (of pelvis)
    in pregnancy or childbirth NEC 654.9 ✓5ᵗʰ
      affecting fetus or newborn 763.89
      causing obstructed labor 660.2 ✓5ᵗʰ
        affecting fetus or newborn 763.1
  spermatic cord (congenital) 752.9
    acquired 608.89
      torsion 608.2
  spinal
    column — *see* Deformity, spine
    cord (congenital) 742.9
      acquired 336.8
      vessel (congenital) 747.82
    nerve root (congenital) 742.9
      acquired 724.9

Deformity — *continued*
  spine (acquired) NEC 738.5
    congenital 756.10
      due to intrauterine malposition and pressure 754.2
    kyphoscoliotic (*see also* Kyphoscoliosis) 737.30
    kyphotic (*see also* Kyphosis) 737.10
    lordotic (*see also* Lordosis) 737.20
    rachitic 268.1
    scoliotic (*see also* Scoliosis) 737.30
  spleen
    acquired 289.59
    congenital 759.0
  Sprengel's (congenital) 755.52
  sternum (acquired) 738.3
    congenital 756.3
  stomach (congenital) 750.9
    acquired 537.89
  submaxillary gland (congenital) 750.9
    acquired 527.8
  swan neck (acquired)
    finger 736.22
    hand 736.09
  talipes — *see* Talipes
  teeth, tooth NEC 520.9
  testis (congenital) 752.9
    acquired 608.89
      torsion 608.2
  thigh (acquired) 736.89
    congenital 755.60
  thorax (acquired) (wall) 738.3
    congenital 754.89
    late effect of rickets 268.1
  thumb (acquired) 736.20
    congenital 755.50
  thymus (tissue) (congenital) 759.2
  thyroid (gland) (congenital) 759.2
    cartilage 748.3
      acquired 478.79
  tibia (acquired) 736.89
    congenital 755.60
    saber 090.5
  toe (acquired) 735.9
    congenital 755.66
    specified NEC 735.8
  tongue (congenital) 750.10
    acquired 529.8
  tooth, teeth NEC 520.9
  trachea (rings) (congenital) 748.3
    acquired 519.1
  transverse aortic arch (congenital) 747.21
  tricuspid (leaflets) (valve) (congenital) 746.9
    acquired — *see* Endocarditis, tricuspid
    atresia or stenosis 746.1
    specified type NEC 746.89
  trunk (acquired) 738.3
    congenital 759.9
  ulna (acquired) 736.00
    congenital 755.50
  upper extremity — *see* Deformity, arm
  urachus (congenital) 753.7
  ureter (opening) (congenital) 753.9
    acquired 593.89
  urethra (valve) (congenital) 753.9
    acquired 599.84
  urinary tract or system (congenital) 753.9
    urachus 753.7
  uterus (congenital) 752.3
    acquired 621.8
  uvula (congenital) 750.9
    acquired 528.9
  vagina (congenital) 752.40
    acquired 623.8
  valve, valvular (heart) (congenital) 746.9
    acquired — *see* Endocarditis
    pulmonary 746.00
    specified type NEC 746.89
  vascular (congenital) (peripheral) NEC 747.60
    acquired 459.9
  vas deferens (congenital) 752.9
    acquired 608.89
  vein (congenital) NEC (*see also* Deformity, vascular) 747.60
    brain 747.81
    coronary 746.9
    great 747.40

Deformity — *continued*
  vena cava (inferior) (superior) (congenital) 747.40
  vertebra — *see* Deformity, spine
  vesicourethral orifice (acquired) 596.8
    congenital NEC 753.9
      specified type NEC 753.8
  vessels of optic papilla (congenital) 743.9
  visual field (contraction) 368.45
  vitreous humor (congenital) 743.9
    acquired 379.29
  vulva (congenital) 752.40
    acquired 624.8
  wrist (joint) (acquired) 736.00
    congenital 755.50
    contraction 718.43
    valgus 736.03
      congenital 755.59
    varus 736.04
      congenital 755.59

Degeneration, degenerative
  adrenal (capsule) (gland) 255.8
    with hypofunction 255.4
    fatty 255.8
    hyaline 255.8
    infectional 255.8
    lardaceous 277.3
  amyloid (any site) (general) 277.3
  anterior cornua, spinal cord 336.8
  aorta, aortic 440.0
    fatty 447.8
    valve (heart) (*see also* Endocarditis, aortic) 424.1
  arteriovascular — *see* Arteriosclerosis
  artery, arterial (atheromatous) (calcareous) — *see also* Arteriosclerosis
    amyloid 277.3
    lardaceous 277.3
    medial NEC (*see also* Arteriosclerosis, extremities) 440.20
  articular cartilage NEC (*see also* Disorder, cartilage, articular) 718.0 ✓5ᵗʰ
    elbow 718.02
    knee 717.5
    patella 717.7
    shoulder 718.01
    spine (*see also* Spondylosis) 721.90
  atheromatous — *see* Arteriosclerosis
  bacony (any site) 277.3
  basal nuclei or ganglia NEC 333.0
  bone 733.90
  brachial plexus 353.0
  brain (cortical) (progressive) 331.9
    arteriosclerotic 437.0
    childhood 330.9
      specified type NEC 330.8
    congenital 742.4
    cystic 348.0
      congenital 742.4
    familial NEC 331.89
    grey matter 330.8
    heredofamilial NEC 331.89
    in
      alcoholism 303.9 ✓5ᵗʰ [331.7]
      beriberi 265.0 [331.7]
      cerebrovascular disease 437.9 [331.7]
      congenital hydrocephalus 742.3 [331.7]
        with spina bifida (*see also* Spina bifida) 741.0 ✓5ᵗʰ [331.7]
      Fabry's disease 272.7 [330.2]
      Gaucher's disease 272.7 [330.2]
      Hunter's disease or syndrome 277.5 [330.3]
      lipidosis
        cerebral 330.1
        generalized 272.7 [330.2]
      mucopolysaccharidosis 277.5 [330.3]
      myxedema (*see also* Myxedema) 244.9 [331.7]
      neoplastic disease NEC (M8000/1) 239.9 [331.7]
      Niemann-Pick disease 272.7 [330.2]
      sphingolipidosis 272.7 [330.2]
      vitamin B_{12} deficiency 266.2 [331.7]
    motor centers 331.89
    senile 331.2
    specified type NEC 331.89

✓4ᵗʰ Fourth-digit Required   ✓5ᵗʰ Fifth-digit Required   ▶◀ Revised Text   ● New Line   ▲ Revised Code

Degeneration — Degeneration

Degeneration, degenerative — *continued*
breast — *see* Disease, breast
Bruch's membrane 363.40
bundle of His 426.50
  left 426.3
  right 426.4
calcareous NEC 275.49
capillaries 448.9
  amyloid 277.3
  fatty 448.9
  lardaceous 277.3
cardiac (brown) (calcareous) (fatty) (fibrous)
  (hyaline) (mural) (muscular) (pigmentary)
  (senile) (with arteriosclerosis) (*see also*
  Degeneration, myocardial) 429.1
  valve, valvular — *see* Endocarditis
cardiorenal (*see also* Hypertension, cardiorenal)
  404.90
cardiovascular (*see also* Disease,
  cardiovascular) 429.2
  renal (*see also* Hypertension, cardiorenal)
    404.90
cartilage (joint) — *see* Derangement, joint
cerebellar NEC 334.9
  primary (hereditary) (sporadic) 334.2
cerebral — *see* Degeneration, brain
cerebromacular 330.1
cerebrovascular 437.1
  due to hypertension 437.2
  late effect — *see* Late effect(s) (of)
    cerbrovascular disease
cervical plexus 353.2
cervix 622.8
  due to radiation (intended effect) 622.8
    adverse effect or misadventure 622.8
changes, spine or vertebra (*see also*
  Spondylosis) 721.90
chitinous 277.3
chorioretinal 363.40
  congenital 743.53
  hereditary 363.50
choroid (colloid) (drusen) 363.40
  hereditary 363.50
  senile 363.41
    diffuse secondary 363.42
cochlear 386.8
collateral ligament (knee) (medial) 717.82
  lateral 717.81
combined (spinal cord) (subacute) 266.2 *[336.2]*
  with anemia (pernicious) 281.0 *[336.2]*
    due to dietary deficiency 281.1 *[336.2]*
    due to vitamin B$_{12}$ deficiency anemia
      (dietary) 281.1 *[336.2]*
conjunctiva 372.50
  amyloid 277.3 *[372.50]*
cornea 371.40
  calcerous 371.44
  familial (hereditary) (*see also* Dystrophy,
    cornea) 371.50
    macular 371.55
    reticular 371.54
  hyaline (of old scars) 371.41
  marginal (Terrien's) 371.48
  mosaic (shagreen) 371.41
  nodular 371.46
  peripheral 371.48
  senile 371.41
cortical (cerebellar) (parenchymatous) 334.2
  alcoholic 303.9 ✓5ᵗʰ *[334.4]*
  diffuse, due to arteriopathy 437.0
corticostriatal-spinal 334.8
cretinoid 243
cruciate ligament (knee) (posterior) 717.84
  anterior 717.83
cutis 709.3
  amyloid 277.3
dental pulp 522.2
disc disease — *see* Degeneration, intervertebral
  disc
dorsolateral (spinal cord) — *see* Degeration,
  combined
endocardial 424.90
extrapyramidal NEC 333.90
eye NEC 360.40
  macular (*see also* Degeneration, macula)
    362.50
    congenital 362.75
    hereditary 362.76

Degeneration, degenerative — *continued*
fatty (diffuse) (general) 272.8
  liver 571.8
    alcoholic 571.0
  localized site — *see* Degeneration, by site,
    fatty
  placenta — *see* Placenta, abnormal
globe (eye) NEC 360.40
  macular — *see* Degeneration, macula
grey matter 330.8
heart (brown) (calcareous) (fatty) (fibrous)
  (hyaline) (mural) (muscular) (pigmentary)
  (senile) (with arteriosclerosis) (*see also*
  Degeneration, myocardial) 429.1
  amyloid 277.3 *[425.7]*
  atheromatous — *see* Arteriosclerosis,
    coronary
  gouty 274.82
  hypertensive (*see also* Hypertension, heart)
    402.90
  ischemic 414.9
  valve, valvular — *see* Endocarditis
hepatolenticular (Wilson's) 275.1
hepatorenal 572.4
heredofamilial
  brain NEC 331.89
  spinal cord NEC 336.8
hyaline (diffuse) (generalized) 728.9
  localized — *see also* Degeneration, by site
    cornea 371.41
    keratitis 371.41
hypertensive vascular — *see* Hypertension
infrapatellar fat pad 729.31
internal semilunar cartilage 717.3
intervertebral disc 722.6
  with myelopathy 722.70
  cervical, cervicothoracic 722.4
    with myelopathy 722.71
  lumbar, lumbosacral 722.52
    with myelopathy 722.73
  thoracic, thoracolumbar 722.51
    with myelopathy 722.72
intestine 569.89
  amyloid 277.3
  lardaceous 277.3
iris (generalized) (*see also* Atrophy, iris) 364.59
  pigmentary 364.53
  pupillary margin 364.54
ischemic — *see* Ischemia
joint disease (*see also* Osteoarthrosis)
  715.9 ✓5ᵗʰ
  multiple sites 715.09
  spine (*see also* Spondylosis) 721.90
kidney (*see also* Sclerosis, renal 587
  amyloid 277.3 *[583.81]*
  cyst, cystic (multiple) (solitary) 593.2
    congenital (*see also* Cystic, disease,
      kidney) 753.10
  fatty 593.89
  fibrocystic (congenital) 753.19
  lardaceous 277.3 *[583.81]*
  polycystic (congenital) 753.12
    adult type (APKD) 753.13
    autosomal dominant 753.13
    autosomal recessive 753.14
    childhood type (CPKD) 753.14
    infantile type 753.14
  waxy 277.3 *[583.81]*
Kuhnt-Junius (retina) 362.52
labyrinth, osseous 386.8
lacrimal passages, cystic 375.12
lardaceous (any site) 277.3
lateral column (posterior), spinal cord (*see also*
  Degeneration, combined) 266.2 *[336.2]*
lattice 362.63
lens 366.9
  infantile, juvenile, or presenile 366.00
  senile 366.10
lenticular (familial) (progressive) (Wilson's) (with
  cirrhosis of liver) 275.1
  striate artery 437.0
lethal ball, prosthetic heart valve 996.02
ligament
  collateral (knee) (medial) 717.82
    lateral 717.81
  cruciate (knee) (posterior) 717.84
    anterior 717.83

Degeneration, degenerative — *continued*
liver (diffuse) 572.8
  amyloid 277.3
  congenital (cystic) 751.62
  cystic 572.8
    congenital 751.62
  fatty 571.8
    alcoholic 571.0
  hypertrophic 572.8
  lardaceous 277.3
  parenchymatous, acute or subacute (*see*
    also Necrosis, liver) 570
  pigmentary 572.8
  toxic (acute) 573.8
  waxy 277.3
lung 518.89
lymph gland 289.3
  hyaline 289.3
  lardaceous 277.3
macula (acquired) (senile) 362.50
  atrophic 362.51
  Best's 362.76
  congenital 362.75
  cystic 362.54
  cystoid 362.53
  disciform 362.52
  dry 362.51
  exudative 362.52
  familial pseudoinflammatory 362.77
  hereditary 362.76
  hole 362.54
  juvenile (Stargardt's) 362.75
  nonexudative 362.51
  pseudohole 362.54
  wet 362.52
medullary — *see* Degeneration, brain
membranous labyrinth, congenital (causing
  impairment of hearing) 744.05
meniscus — *see* Derangement, joint
microcystoid 362.62
mitral — *see* Insufficiency, mitral
Mönckeberg's (*see also* Arteriosclerosis,
  extremities) 440.20
moral 301.7
motor centers, senile 331.2
mural (*see also* Degeneration, myocardial)
  429.1
  heart, cardiac (*see also* Degeneration,
    myocardial) 429.1
  myocardium, myocardial (*see also*
    Degeneration, myocardial) 429.1
muscle 728.9
  fatty 728.9
  fibrous 728.9
  heart (*see also* Degeneration, myocardial)
    429.1
  hyaline 728.9
muscular progressive 728.2
myelin, central nervous system NEC 341.9
myocardium, myocardial (brown) (calcareous)
  (fatty) (fibrous) (hyaline) (mural)
  (muscular) (pigmentary) (senile) (with
  arteriosclerosis) 429.1
  with rheumatic fever (conditions classifiable
    to 390) 398.0
    active, acute, or subacute 391.2
      with chorea 392.0
    inactive or quiescent (with chorea) 398.0
  amyloid 277.3 *[425.7]*
  congenital 746.89
  fetus or newborn 779.89 ▲
  gouty 274.82
  hypertensive (*see also* Hypertension, heart)
    402.90
  ischemic 414.8
  rheumatic (*see also* Degeneration,
    myocardium, with rheumatic fever)
    398.0
  syphilitic 093.82
nasal sinus (mucosa) (*see also* Sinusitis) 473.9
  frontal 473.1
  maxillary 473.0
nerve — *see* Disorder, nerve
nervous system 349.89
  amyloid 277.3 *[357.4]*
  autonomic (*see also* Neuropathy, peripheral,
    autonomic) 337.9
  fatty 349.89

Degeneration, degenerative — *continued*
nervous system — *continued*
  peripheral autonomic NEC (*see also*
    Neuropathy, peripheral, autonomic)
    337.9
  nipple 611.9
  nose 478.1
  oculoacousticocerebral, congenital (progressive)
    743.8
  olivopontocerebellar (familial) (hereditary) 333.0
  osseous labyrinth 386.8
  ovary 620.8
    cystic 620.2
    microcystic 620.2
  pallidal, pigmentary (progressive) 333.0
  pancreas 577.8
    tuberculous (*see also* Tuberculosis)
      017.9 ✓5ᵗʰ
  papillary muscle 429.81
  paving stone 362.61
  penis 607.89
  peritoneum 568.89
  pigmentary (diffuse) (general)
    localized — *see* Degeneration, by site
    pallidal (progressive) 333.0
    secondary 362.65
  pineal gland 259.8
  pituitary (gland) 253.8
  placenta (fatty) (fibrinoid) (fibroid) — *see*
    Placenta, abnormal
  popliteal fat pad 729.31
  posterolateral (spinal cord) (*see also*
    Degeneration, combined) 266.2 [336.2]
  pulmonary valve (heart) (*see also* Endocarditis,
    pulmonary) 424.3
  pulp (tooth) 522.2
  pupillary margin 364.54
  renal (*see also* Sclerosis, renal) 587
    fibrocystic 753.19
    polycystic 753.12
      adult type (APKD) 753.13
      autosomal dominant 753.13
      autosomal recessive 753.14
      childhood type (CPKD) 753.14
      infantile type 753.14
  reticuloendothelial system 289.8
  retina (peripheral) 362.60
    with retinal defect (*see also* Detachment,
      retina, with retinal defect) 361.00
    cystic (senile) 362.50
    cystoid 362.53
    hereditary (*see also* Dystrophy, retina)
      362.70
      cerebroretinal 362.71
      congenital 362.75
      juvenile (Stargardt's) 362.75
      macula 362.76
    Kuhnt-Junius 362.52
    lattice 362.63
    macular (*see also* Degeneration, macula)
      362.50
    microcystoid 362.62
    palisade 362.63
    paving stone 362.61
    pigmentary (primary) 362.74
      secondary 362.65
    posterior pole (*see also* Degeneration,
      macula) 362.50
    secondary 362.66
    senile 362.60
      cystic 362.53
      reticular 362.64
  saccule, congenital (causing impairment of
    hearing) 744.05
  sacculocochlear 386.8
  senile 797
    brain 331.2
    cardiac, heart, or myocardium (*see also*
      Degeneration, myocardial) 429.1
    motor centers 331.2
    reticule 362.64
    retina, cystic 362.50
    vascular — *see* Arteriosclerosis
  silicone rubber poppet (prosthetic valve) 996.02
  sinus (cystic) (*see also* Sinusitis) 473.9
    polypoid 471.1

Degeneration, degenerative — *continued*
skin 709.3
  amyloid 277.3
  colloid 709.3
spinal (cord) 336.8
  amyloid 277.3
  column 733.90
  combined (subacute) (*see also* Degeneration,
    combined) 266.2 [336.2]
    with anemia (pernicious) 281.0 [336.2]
  dorsolateral (*see also* Degeneration,
    combined) 266.2 [336.2]
  familial NEC 336.8
  fatty 336.8
  funicular (*see also* Degeneration, combined)
    266.2 [336.2]
  heredofamilial NEC 336.8
  posterolateral (*see also* Degeneration,
    combined) 266.2 [336.2]
  subacute combined — *see* Degeneration,
    combined
  tuberculous (*see also* Tuberculosis)
    013.8 ✓5ᵗʰ
spine 733.90
spleen 289.59
  amyloid 277.3
  lardaceous 277.3
stomach 537.89
  lardaceous 277.3
strionigral 333.0
sudoriparous (cystic) 705.89
suprarenal (capsule) (gland) 255.8
  with hypofunction 255.4
sweat gland 705.89
synovial membrane (pulpy) 727.9
tapetoretinal 362.74
  adult or presenile form 362.50
testis (postinfectional) 608.89
thymus (gland) 254.8
  fatty 254.8
  lardaceous 277.3
thyroid (gland) 246.8
tricuspid (heart) (valve) *see* Endocarditis,
  tricuspid
tuberculous NEC (*see also* Tuberculosis)
  011.9 ✓5ᵗʰ
turbinate 733.90
uterus 621.8
  cystic 621.8
vascular (senile) — *see also* Arteriosclerosis
  hypertensive — *see* Hypertension
vitreoretinal (primary) 362.73
  secondary 362.66
vitreous humor (with infiltration) 379.21
wallerian NEC — *see* Disorder, nerve
waxy (any site) 277.3
Wilson's hepatolenticular 275.1

Deglutition
paralysis 784.9
  hysterical 300.11
pneumonia 507.0

Degos' disease or syndrome 447.8

**Degradation disorder, branched-chain amino
acid** 270.3

Dehiscence
anastomosis — *see* Complications, anastomosis
cesarean wound 674.1 ✓5ᵗʰ
episiotomy 674.2 ✓5ᵗʰ
operation wound 998.32 ▲
  internal 998.31 ●
perineal wound (postpartum) 674.2 ✓5ᵗʰ
postoperative 998.32 ▲
  abdomen 998.32 ▲
    internal 998.31 ●
  internal 998.31 ●
uterine wound 674.1 ✓5ᵗʰ

Dehydration (cachexia) 276.5
with
  hypernatremia 276.0 ●
  hyponatremia 276.1 ●
newborn 775.5

Deiters' nucleus syndrome 386.19

Déjérine's disease 356.0

Déjérine-Klumpke paralysis 767.6

Déjérine-Roussy syndrome 348.8

Déjérine-Sottas disease or neuropathy
(hypertrophic) 356.0

Déjérine-Thomas atrophy or syndrome 333.0

de Lange's syndrome (Amsterdam dwarf, mental
retardation, and brachycephaly) 759.89

Delay, delayed
adaptation, cones or rods 368.63
any plane in pelvis
  affecting fetus or newborn 763.1
  complicating delivery 660.1 ✓5ᵗʰ
birth or delivery NEC 662.1 ✓5ᵗʰ
  affecting fetus or newborn 763.89
  second twin, triplet, or multiple mate
    662.3 ✓5ᵗʰ
closure — *see also* Fistula
  cranial suture 756.0
  fontanel 756.0
coagulation NEC 790.92
conduction (cardiac) (ventricular) 426.9
delivery NEC 662.1 ✓5ᵗʰ
  second twin, triplet, etc. 662.3 ✓5ᵗʰ
  affecting fetus or newborn 763.89
development
  in childhood 783.40
    physiological 783.40
  intellectual NEC 315.9
  learning NEC 315.2
  reading 315.00
  sexual 259.0
  speech 315.39
    associated with hyperkinesis 314.1
  spelling 315.09
gastric emptying 536.8
menarche 256.39
  due to pituitary hypofunction 253.4
menstruation (cause unknown) 626.8
milestone in childhood 783.42
motility — *see* Hypomotility
passage of meconium (newborn) 777.1
primary respiration 768.9
puberty 259.0
sexual maturation, female 259.0

Del Castillo's syndrome (germinal aplasia) 606.0

Déleage's disease 359.89 ▲

Delhi (boil) (button) (sore) 085.1

Delinquency (juvenile) 312.9
group (*see also* Disturbance, conduct)
  312.2 ✓5ᵗʰ
neurotic 312.4

Delirium, delirious 780.09
acute (psychotic) 293.0
alcoholic 291.0
  acute 291.0
  chronic 291.1
alcoholicum 291.0
chronic (*see also* Psychosis) 293.89
  due to or associated with physical condition
    — *see* Psychosis, organic
drug-induced 292.81
eclamptic (*see also* Eclampsia) 780.39
exhaustion (*see also* Reaction, stress, acute)
  308.9
hysterical 300.11
in
  presenile dementia 290.11
  senile dementia 290.3
induced by drug 292.81
manic, maniacal (acute) (*see also* Psychosis,
  affective) 296.0 ✓5ᵗʰ
  recurrent episode 296.1 ✓5ᵗʰ
  single episode 296.0 ✓5ᵗʰ
puerperal 293.9
senile 290.3
subacute (psychotic) 293.1
thyroid (*see also* Thyrotoxicosis) 242.9 ✓5ᵗʰ
traumatic — *see also* Injury, intracranial
with
  lesion, spinal cord — *see* Injury, spinal,
    by site
  shock, spinal — *see* Injury, spinal, by site
tremens (impending) 291.0
uremic — *see* Uremia
withdrawal
  alcoholic (acute) 291.0
    chronic 291.1
  drug 292.0

Delivery

Note — Use the following fifth-digit subclassification with categories 640-648, 651-676:

  0   unspecified as to episode of care

  1   delivered, with or without mention of antepartum condition

  2   delivered, with mention of postpartum complication

  3   antepartum condition or complication

  4   postpartum condition or complication

breech (assisted) (spontaneous) 652.2 ✓5th
  affecting fetus or newborn 763.0
  extraction NEC 669.6 ✓5th
cesarean (for) 669.7 ✓5th
  abnormal
    cervix 654.6 ✓5th
    pelvic organs or tissues 654.9 ✓5th
    pelvis (bony) (major) NEC 653.0 ✓5th
    presentation or position 652.9 ✓5th
      in multiple gestation 652.6 ✓5th
    size, fetus 653.5 ✓5th
    soft parts (of pelvis) 654.9 ✓5th
    uterus, congenital 654.0 ✓5th
    vagina 654.7 ✓5th
    vulva 654.8 ✓5th
  abruptio placentae 641.2 ✓5th
  acromion presentation 652.8 ✓5th
  affecting fetus or newborn 763.4
  anteversion, cervix or uterus 654.4 ✓5th
  atony, uterus 666.1 ✓5th
  bicornis or bicornuate uterus 654.0 ✓5th
  breech presentation 652.2 ✓5th
  brow presentation 652.4 ✓5th
  cephalopelvic disproportion (normally formed fetus) 653.4 ✓5th
  chin presentation 652.4 ✓5th
  cicatrix of cervix 654.6 ✓5th
  contracted pelvis (general) 653.1 ✓5th
    inlet 653.2 ✓5th
    outlet 653.3 ✓5th
  cord presentation or prolapse 663.0 ✓5th
  cystocele 654.4 ✓5th
  deformity (acquired) (congenital)
    pelvic organs or tissues NEC 654.9 ✓5th
    pelvis (bony) NEC 653.0 ✓5th
  displacement, uterus NEC 654.4 ✓5th
  disproportion NEC 653.9 ✓5th
  distress
    fetal 656.8 ✓5th
    maternal 669.0 ✓5th
  eclampsia 642.6 ✓5th
  face presentation 652.4 ✓5th
  failed
    forceps 660.7 ✓5th
    trial of labor NEC 660.6 ✓5th
    vacuum extraction 660.7 ✓5th
    ventouse 660.7 ✓5th
  fetal deformity 653.7 ✓5th
  fetal-maternal hemorrhage 656.0 ✓5th
  fetus, fetal
    distress 656.8 ✓5th
    prematurity 656.8 ✓5th
  fibroid (tumor) (uterus) 654.1 ✓5th
  footling 652.8 ✓5th
    with successful version 652.1 ✓5th
  hemorrhage (antepartum) (intrapartum) NEC 641.9 ✓5th
  hydrocephalic fetus 653.6 ✓5th
  incarceration of uterus 654.3 ✓5th
  incoordinate uterine action 661.4 ✓5th
  inertia, uterus 661.2 ✓5th
    primary 661.0 ✓5th
    secondary 661.1 ✓5th
  lateroversion, uterus or cervix 654.4 ✓5th
  mal lie 652.9 ✓5th
  malposition
    fetus 652.9 ✓5th
      in multiple gestation 652.6 ✓5th
    pelvic organs or tissues NEC 654.9 ✓5th
    uterus NEC or cervix 654.4 ✓5th
  malpresentation NEC 652.9 ✓5th
    in multiple gestation 652.6 ✓5th

Delivery — continued
cesarean — continued
  maternal
    diabetes mellitus 648.0 ✓5th
    heart disease NEC 648.6 ✓5th
  meconium in liquor 656.8 ✓5th
    staining only 792.3
  oblique presentation 652.3 ✓5th
  oversize fetus 653.5 ✓5th
  pelvic tumor NEC 654.9 ✓5th
  placental insufficiency 656.5 ✓5th
  placenta previa 641.0 ✓5th
    with hemorrhage 641.1 ✓5th
  poor dilation, cervix 661.0 ✓5th
  preeclampsia 642.4 ✓5th
    severe 642.5 ✓5th
  previous
    cesarean delivery 654.2 ✓5th
    surgery (to)
      cervix 654.6 ✓5th
      gynecological NEC 654.9 ✓5th
      uterus NEC 654.9 ✓5th
        previous cesarean delivery 654.2 ✓5th
      vagina 654.7 ✓5th
  prolapse
    arm or hand 652.7 ✓5th
    uterus 654.4 ✓5th
  prolonged labor 662.1 ✓5th
  rectocele 654.4 ✓5th
  retroversion, uterus or cervix 654.3 ✓5th
  rigid
    cervix 654.6 ✓5th
    pelvic floor 654.4 ✓5th
    perineum 654.8 ✓5th
    vagina 654.7 ✓5th
    vulva 654.8 ✓5th
  sacculation, pregnant uterus 654.4 ✓5th
  scar(s)
    cervix 654.6 ✓5th
    cesarean delivery 654.2 ✓5th
    uterus NEC 654.9 ✓5th
      due to previous cesarean delivery 654.2 ✓5th
  Shirodkar suture in situ 654.5 ✓5th
  shoulder presentation 652.8 ✓5th
  stenosis or stricture, cervix 654.6 ✓5th
  transverse presentation or lie 652.3 ✓5th
  tumor, pelvic organs or tissues NEC 654.4 ✓5th
  umbilical cord presentation or prolapse 663.0 ✓5th
completely normal case — see category 650
complicated (by) NEC 669.9 ✓5th
  abdominal tumor, fetal 653.7 ✓5th
    causing obstructed labor 660.1 ✓5th
  abnormal, abnormality of
    cervix 654.6 ✓5th
      causing obstructed labor 660.2 ✓5th
    forces of labor 661.9 ✓5th
    formation of uterus 654.0 ✓5th
    pelvic organs or tissues 654.9 ✓5th
      causing obstructed labor 660.2 ✓5th
    pelvis (bony) (major) NEC 653.0 ✓5th
      causing obstructed labor 660.1 ✓5th
    presentation or position NEC 652.9 ✓5th
      causing obstructed labor 660.0 ✓5th
    size, fetus 653.5 ✓5th
      causing obstructed labor 660.1 ✓5th
    soft parts (of pelvis) 654.9 ✓5th
      causing obstructed labor 660.2 ✓5th
    uterine contractions NEC 661.9 ✓5th
    uterus (formation) 654.0 ✓5th
      causing obstructed labor 660.2 ✓5th
    vagina 654.7 ✓5th
      causing obstructed labor 660.2 ✓5th
  abnormally formed uterus (any type) (congenital) 654.0 ✓5th
    causing obstructed labor 660.2 ✓5th
  acromion presentation 652.8 ✓5th
    causing obstructed labor 660.0 ✓5th
  adherent placenta 667.0 ✓5th
    with hemorrhage 666.0 ✓5th
  adhesions, uterus (to abdominal wall) 654.4 ✓5th

Delivery — continued
complicated (by) NEC — continued
  advanced maternal age NEC 659.6 ✓5th
    multigravida 659.6 ✓5th
    primigravida 659.5 ✓5th
  air embolism 673.0 ✓5th
  amnionitis 658.4 ✓5th
  amniotic fluid embolism 673.1 ✓5th
  anesthetic death 668.9 ✓5th
  annular detachment, cervix 665.3 ✓5th
  antepartum hemorrhage — see Delivery, complicated, hemorrhage
  anteversion, cervix or uterus 654.4 ✓5th
    causing obstructed labor 660.2 ✓5th
  apoplexy 674.0 ✓5th
    placenta 641.2 ✓5th
  arrested active phase 661.1 ✓5th
  asymmetrical pelvis bone 653.0 ✓5th
    causing obstructed labor 660.1 ✓5th
  atony, uterus (hypotonic) (inertia) 666.1 ✓5th
    hypertonic 661.4 ✓5th
  Bandl's ring 661.4 ✓5th
  battledore placenta — see Placenta, abnormal
  bicornis or bicornuate uterus 654.0 ✓5th
    causing obstructed labor 660.2 ✓5th
  birth injury to mother NEC 665.9 ✓5th
  bleeding (see also Delivery, complicated, hemorrhage) 641.9 ✓5th
  breech presentation (assisted) (buttocks) (complete) (frank) (spontaneous) 652.2 ✓5th
    with successful version 652.1 ✓5th
  brow presentation 652.4 ✓5th
  cephalopelvic disproportion (normally formed fetus) 653.4 ✓5th
    causing obstructed labor 660.1 ✓5th
  cerebral hemorrhage 674.0 ✓5th
  cervical dystocia 661.0 ✓5th
  chin presentation 652.4 ✓5th
    causing obstructed labor 660.0 ✓5th
  cicatrix
    cervix 654.6 ✓5th
      causing obstructed labor 660.2 ✓5th
    vagina 654.7 ✓5th
      causing obstructed labor 660.2 ✓5th
  colporrhexis 665.4 ✓5th
    with perineal laceration 664.0 ✓5th
  compound presentation 652.8 ✓5th
    causing obstructed labor 660.0 ✓5th
  compression of cord (umbilical) 663.2 ✓5th
    around neck 663.1 ✓5th
    cord prolapsed 663.0 ✓5th
  contraction, contracted pelvis 653.1 ✓5th
    causing obstructed labor 660.1 ✓5th
    general 653.1 ✓5th
      causing obstructed labor 660.1 ✓5th
    inlet 653.2 ✓5th
      causing obstructed labor 660.1 ✓5th
    midpelvic 653.8 ✓5th
      causing obstructed labor 660.1 ✓5th
    midplane 653.8 ✓5th
      causing obstructed labor 660.1 ✓5th
    outlet 653.3 ✓5th
      causing obstructed labor 660.1 ✓5th
  contraction ring 661.4 ✓5th
  cord (umbilical) 663.9 ✓5th
    around neck, tightly or with compression 663.1 ✓5th
      without compression 663.3 ✓5th
    bruising 663.6 ✓5th
    complication NEC 663.9 ✓5th
      specified type NEC 663.8 ✓5th
    compression NEC 663.2 ✓5th
    entanglement NEC 663.3 ✓5th
      with compression 663.2 ✓5th
    forelying 663.0 ✓5th
    hematoma 663.6 ✓5th
    marginal attachment 663.8 ✓5th
    presentation 663.0 ✓5th
    prolapse (complete) (occult) (partial) 663.0 ✓5th
    short 663.4 ✓5th
    specified complication NEC 663.8 ✓5th
    thrombosis (vessels) 663.6 ✓5th
    vascular lesion 663.6 ✓5th

Delivery — *continued*
- complicated (by) NEC — *continued*
  - cord — *continued*
    - velamentous insertion 663.8 ✓5th
  - Couvelaire uterus 641.2 ✓5th
  - cretin pelvis (dwarf type) (male type) 653.1 ✓5th
    - causing obstructed labor 660.1 ✓5th
  - crossbirth 652.3 ✓5th
    - with successful version 652.1 ✓5th
    - causing obstructed labor 660.0 ✓5th
  - cyst (Gartner's duct) 654.7 ✓5th
  - cystocele 654.4 ✓5th
    - causing obstructed labor 660.2 ✓5th
  - death of fetus (near term) 656.4 ✓5th
    - early (before 22 completed weeks gestation) 632
  - deformity (acquired) (congenital)
    - fetus 653.7 ✓5th
      - causing obstructed labor 660.1 ✓5th
    - pelvic organs or tissues NEC 654.9 ✓5th
      - causing obstructed labor 660.2 ✓5th
    - pelvis (bony) NEC 653.0 ✓5th
      - causing obstructed labor 660.1 ✓5th
  - delay, delayed
    - delivery in multiple pregnancy 662.3 ✓5th
      - due to locked mates 660.5 ✓5th
    - following rupture of membranes (spontaneous) 658.2 ✓5th
      - artificial 658.3 ✓5th
  - depressed fetal heart tones 659.7 ✓5th
  - diastasis recti 665.8 ✓5th
  - dilation
    - bladder 654.4 ✓5th
      - causing obstructed labor 660.2 ✓5th
    - cervix, incomplete, poor or slow 661.0 ✓5th
  - diseased placenta 656.7 ✓5th
  - displacement uterus NEC 654.4 ✓5th
    - causing obstructed labor 660.2 ✓5th
  - disproportion NEC 653.9 ✓5th
    - causing obstructed labor 660.1 ✓5th
  - disruptio uteri — *see* Delivery, complicated, rupture, uterus
  - distress
    - fetal 656.8 ✓5th
    - maternal 669.0 ✓5th
  - double uterus (congenital) 654.0 ✓5th
    - causing obstructed labor 660.2 ✓5th
  - dropsy amnion 657 ✓4th
  - dysfunction, uterus 661.9 ✓5th
    - hypertonic 661.4 ✓5th
    - hypotonic 661.2 ✓5th
      - primary 661.0 ✓5th
      - secondary 661.1 ✓5th
    - incoordinate 661.4 ✓5th
  - dystocia
    - cervical 661.0 ✓5th
    - fetal — *see* Delivery, complicated, abnormal presentation
    - maternal — *see* Delivery, complicated, prolonged labor
    - pelvic — *see* Delivery, complicated, contraction pelvis
    - positional 652.8 ✓5th
    - shoulder girdle 660.4 ✓5th
  - eclampsia 642.6 ✓5th
  - ectopic kidney 654.4 ✓5th
    - causing obstructed labor 660.2 ✓5th
  - edema, cervix 654.6 ✓5th
    - causing obstructed labor 660.2 ✓5th
  - effusion, amniotic fluid 658.1 ✓5th
  - elderly multigravida 659.6 ✓5th
  - elderly primigravida 659.5 ✓5th
  - embolism (pulmonary) 673.2 ✓5th
    - air 673.0 ✓5th
    - amniotic fluid 673.1 ✓5th
    - blood clot 673.2 ✓5th
    - cerebral 674.0 ✓5th
    - fat 673.8 ✓5th
    - pyemic 673.3 ✓5th
    - septic 673.3 ✓5th
  - entanglement, umbilical cord 663.3 ✓5th
    - with compression 663.2 ✓5th
    - around neck (with compression) 663.1 ✓5th
  - eversion, cervix or uterus 665.2 ✓5th

Delivery — *continued*
- complicated (by) NEC — *continued*
  - excessive
    - fetal growth 653.5 ✓5th
      - causing obstructed labor 660.1 ✓5th
    - size of fetus 653.5 ✓5th
      - causing obstructed labor 660.1 ✓5th
  - face presentation 652.4 ✓5th
    - causing obstructed labor 660.0 ✓5th
    - to pubes 660.3 ✓5th
  - failure, fetal head to enter pelvic brim 652.5 ✓5th
    - causing obstructed labor 660.0 ✓5th
  - fetal
    - acid-base balance 656.8 ✓5th
    - death (near term) NEC 656.4 ✓5th
      - early (before 22 completed weeks gestation) 632
    - deformity 653.7 ✓5th
      - causing obstructed labor 660.1 ✓5th
    - distress 656.8 ✓5th
    - heart rate or rhythm 659.7 ✓5th
  - fetopelvic disproportion 653.4 ✓5th
    - causing obstructed labor 660.1 ✓5th
  - fever during labor 659.2 ✓5th
  - fibroid (tumor) (uterus) 654.1 ✓5th
    - causing obstructed labor 660.2 ✓5th
  - fibromyomata 654.1 ✓5th
    - causing obstructed labor 660.2 ✓5th
  - forelying umbilical cord 663.0 ✓5th
  - fracture of coccyx 665.6 ✓5th
  - hematoma 664.5 ✓5th
    - broad ligament 665.7 ✓5th
    - ischial spine 665.7 ✓5th
    - pelvic 665.7 ✓5th
    - perineum 664.5 ✓5th
    - soft tissues 665.7 ✓5th
    - subdural 674.0 ✓5th
    - umbilical cord 663.6 ✓5th
    - vagina 665.7 ✓5th
    - vulva or perineum 664.5 ✓5th
  - hemorrhage (uterine) (antepartum) (intrapartum) (pregnancy) 641.9 ✓5th
    - accidental 641.2 ✓5th
    - associated with
      - afibrinogenemia 641.3 ✓5th
      - coagulation defect 641.3 ✓5th
        - hyperfibrinolysis 641.3 ✓5th
        - hypofibrinogenemia 641.3 ✓5th
    - cerebral 674.0 ✓5th
    - due to
      - low-lying placenta 641.1 ✓5th
      - placenta previa 641.1 ✓5th
      - premature separation of placenta (normally implanted) 641.2 ✓5th
      - retained placenta 666.0 ✓5th
      - trauma 641.8 ✓5th
      - uterine leiomyoma 641.8 ✓5th
    - marginal sinus rupture 641.2 ✓5th
    - placenta NEC 641.9 ✓5th
    - postpartum (atonic) (immediate) (within 24 hours) 666.1 ✓5th
      - with retained or trapped placenta 666.0 ✓5th
      - delayed 666.2 ✓5th
      - secondary 666.2 ✓5th
      - third stage 666.0 ✓5th
  - hourglass contraction, uterus 661.4 ✓5th
  - hydramnios 657 ✓5th
  - hydrocephalic fetus 653.6 ✓5th
    - causing obstructed labor 660.1 ✓5th
  - hydrops fetalis 653.7 ✓5th
    - causing obstructed labor 660.1 ✓5th
  - hypertension — *see* Hypertension, complicating pregnancy
  - hypertonic uterine dysfunction 661.4 ✓5th
  - hypotonic uterine dysfunction 661.2 ✓5th
  - impacted shoulders 660.4 ✓5th
  - incarceration, uterus 654.3 ✓5th
    - causing obstructed labor 660.2 ✓5th
  - incomplete dilation (cervix) 661.0 ✓5th
  - incoordinate uterus 661.4 ✓5th
  - indication NEC 659.9 ✓5th
    - specified type NEC 659.8 ✓5th
  - inertia, uterus 661.2 ✓5th
    - hypertonic 661.4 ✓5th

Delivery — *continued*
- complicated (by) NEC — *continued*
  - inertia, uterus — *continued*
    - hypotonic 661.2 ✓5th
    - primary 661.0 ✓5th
    - secondary 661.1 ✓5th
  - infantile
    - genitalia 654.4 ✓5th
      - causing obstructed labor 660.2 ✓5th
    - uterus (os) 654.4 ✓5th
      - causing obstructed labor 660.2 ✓5th
  - injury (to mother) NEC 665.9 ✓5th
  - intrauterine fetal death (near term) NEC 656.4 ✓5th
    - early (before 22 completed weeks gestation) 632
  - inversion, uterus 665.2 ✓5th
  - kidney, ectopic 654.4 ✓5th
    - causing obstructed labor 660.2 ✓5th
  - knot (true), umbilical cord 663.2 ✓5th
  - labor, premature (before 37 completed weeks gestation) 644.2 ✓5th
  - laceration 664.9 ✓5th
    - anus (spincter) 664.2 ✓5th
      - with mucosa 664.3 ✓5th
    - bladder (urinary) 665.5 ✓5th
    - bowel 665.5 ✓5th
    - central 664.4 ✓5th
    - cervix (uteri) 665.3 ✓5th
    - fourchette 664.0 ✓5th
    - hymen 664.0 ✓5th
    - labia (majora) (minora) 664.0 ✓5th
    - pelvic
      - floor 664.1 ✓5th
      - organ NEC 665.5 ✓5th
    - perineum, perineal 664.4 ✓5th
      - first degree 664.0 ✓5th
      - second degree 664.1 ✓5th
      - third degree 664.2 ✓5th
      - fourth degree 664.3 ✓5th
      - central 664.4 ✓5th
      - extensive NEC 664.4 ✓5th
      - muscles 664.1 ✓5th
      - skin 664.0 ✓5th
      - slight 664.0 ✓5th
    - peritoneum 665.5 ✓5th
    - periurethral tissue 665.5 ✓5th
    - rectovaginal (septum) (without perineal laceration) 665.4 ✓5th
      - with perineum 664.2 ✓5th
        - with anal rectal mucosa 664.3 ✓5th
    - skin (perineum) 664.0 ✓5th
    - specified site or type NEC 664.8 ✓5th
    - sphincter ani 664.2 ✓5th
      - with mucosa 664.3 ✓5th
    - urethra 665.5 ✓5th
    - uterus 665.1 ✓5th
      - before labor 665.0 ✓5th
    - vagina, vaginal (deep) (high) (sulcus) (wall) (without perineal laceration) 665.4 ✓5th
      - with perineum 664.0 ✓5th
        - muscles, with perineum 664.1 ✓5th
    - vulva 664.0 ✓5th
  - lateroversion, uterus or cervix 654.4 ✓5th
    - causing obstructed labor 660.2 ✓5th
  - locked mates 660.5 ✓5th
  - low implantation of placenta — *see* Delivery, complicated, placenta, previa
  - mal lie 652.9 ✓5th
  - malposition
    - fetus NEC 652.9 ✓5th
      - causing obstructed labor 660.0 ✓5th
    - pelvic organs or tissues NEC 654.9 ✓5th
      - causing obstructed labor 660.2 ✓5th
    - placenta 641.1 ✓5th
      - without hemorrhage 641.0 ✓5th
    - uterus NEC or cervix 654.4 ✓5th
      - causing obstructed labor 660.2 ✓5th
  - malpresentation 652.9 ✓5th
    - causing obstructed labor 660.0 ✓5th
  - marginal sinus (bleeding) (rupture) 641.2 ✓5th
  - maternal hypotension syndrome 669.2 ✓5th
  - meconium in liquor 656.8 ✓5th

✓4th Fourth-digit Required   ✓5th Fifth-digit Required   ►◄ Revised Text   ● New Line   ▲ Revised Code

Delivery — Delivery

Delivery — *continued*
  complicated (by) NEC — *continued*
    membranes, retained — *see* Delivery,
      complicated, placenta, retained
    mentum presentation 652.4 ✓5th
      causing obstructed labor 660.0 ✓5th
    metrorrhagia (myopathia) — *see* Delivery,
      complicated, hemorrhage
    metrorrhexis — *see* Delivery, complicated,
      rupture, uterus
    multiparity (grand) 659.4 ✓5th
    myelomeningocele, fetus 653.7 ✓5th
      causing obstructed labor 660.1 ✓5th
    Nägele's pelvis 653.0 ✓5th
      causing obstructed labor 660.1 ✓5th
    nonengagement, fetal head 652.5 ✓5th
      causing obstructed labor 660.0 ✓5th
    oblique presentation 652.3 ✓5th
      causing obstructed labor 660.0 ✓5th
    obstetric
      shock 669.1 ✓5th
      trauma NEC 665.9 ✓5th
    obstructed labor 660.9 ✓5th
      due to
        abnormality pelvic organs or tissues
          (conditions classifiable to 654.0-
          654.9) 660.2 ✓5th
        deep transverse arrest 660.3 ✓5th
        impacted shoulders 660.4 ✓5th
        locked twins 660.5 ✓5th
        malposition and malpresentation of
          fetus (conditions classifiable to
          652.0-652.9) 660.0 ✓5th
        persistent occipitoposterior 660.3 ✓5th
        shoulder dystocia 660.4 ✓5th
    occult prolapse of umbilical cord 663.0 ✓5th
    oversize fetus 653.5 ✓5th
      causing obstructed labor 660.1 ✓5th
    pathological retraction ring, uterus
      661.4 ✓5th
    pelvic
      arrest (deep) (high) (of fetal head)
        (transverse) 660.3 ✓5th
      deformity (bone) — *see also* Deformity,
        pelvis, with disproportion
      soft tissue 654.9 ✓5th
        causing obstructed labor 660.2 ✓5th
      tumor NEC 654.9 ✓5th
        causing obstructed labor 660.2 ✓5th
    penetration, pregnant uterus by instrument
      665.1 ✓5th
    perforation — *see* Delivery, complicated,
      laceration
    persistent
      hymen 654.8 ✓5th
        causing obstructed labor 660.2 ✓5th
      occipitoposterior 660.3 ✓5th
    placenta, placental
      ablatio 641.2 ✓5th
      abnormality 656.7 ✓5th
        with hemorrhage 641.2 ✓5th
      abruptio 641.2 ✓5th
      accreta 667.0 ✓5th
        with hemorrhage 666.0 ✓5th
      adherent (without hemorrhage) 667.0 ✓5th
        with hemorrhage 666.0 ✓5th
      apoplexy 641.2 ✓5th
      battledore placenta — *see* Placenta,
        abnormal 663.8 ✓5th
      detachment (premature) 641.2 ✓5th
      disease 656.7 ✓5th
      hemorrhage NEC 641.9 ✓5th
      increta (without hemorrhage) 667.0 ✓5th
        with hemorrhage 666.0 ✓5th
      low (implantation) 641.0 ✓5th
        without hemorrhage 641.0 ✓5th
      malformation 656.7 ✓5th
        with hemorrhage 641.2 ✓5th
      malposition 641.1 ✓5th
        without hemorrhage 641.0 ✓5th
      marginal sinus rupture 641.2 ✓5th
      percreta 667.0 ✓5th
        with hemorrhage 666.0 ✓5th
      premature separation 641.2 ✓5th
      previa (central) (lateral) (marginal) partial)
        641.1 ✓5th

Delivery — *continued*
  complicated (by) NEC — *continued*
    placenta, placental — *continued*
      previa — *continued*
        without hemorrhage 641.0 ✓5th
      retained (with hemorrhage) 666.0 ✓5th
        without hemorrhage 667.0 ✓5th
      rupture of marginal sinus 641.2 ✓5th
      separation (premature) 641.2 ✓5th
      trapped 666.0 ✓5th
        without hemorrhage 667.0 ✓5th
      vicious insertion 641.1 ✓5th
    polyhydramnios 657 ✓4th
    polyp, cervix 654.6 ✓5th
      causing obstructed labor 660.2 ✓5th
    precipitate labor 661.3 ✓5th
    premature
      labor (before 37 completed weeks
        gestation) 644.2 ✓5th
      rupture, membranes 658.1 ✓5th
        delayed delivery following 658.2 ✓5th
    presenting umbilical cord 663.0 ✓5th
    previous
      cesarean delivery 654.2 ✓5th
      surgery
        cervix 654.6 ✓5th
          causing obstructed labor 660.2 ✓5th
        gynecological NEC 654.9 ✓5th
          causing obstructed labor 660.2 ✓5th
        perineum 654.8 ✓5th
        uterus NEC 654.9 ✓5th
          due to previous cesarean delivery
            654.2 ✓5th
        vagina 654.7 ✓5th
          causing obstructed labor 660.2 ✓5th
        vulva 654.8 ✓5th
    primary uterine inertia 661.0 ✓5th
    primipara, elderly or old 659.5 ✓5th
    prolapse
      arm or hand 652.7 ✓5th
        causing obstructed labor 660.0 ✓5th
      cord (umbilical) 663.0 ✓5th
      fetal extremity 652.8 ✓5th
      foot or leg 652.8 ✓5th
        causing obstructed labor 660.0 ✓5th
      umbilical cord (complete) (occult) (partial)
        663.0 ✓5th
      uterus 654.4 ✓5th
        causing obstructed labor 660.2 ✓5th
    prolonged labor 662.1 ✓5th
      first stage 662.0 ✓5th
      second stage 662.2 ✓5th
      active phase 661.2 ✓5th
      due to
        cervical dystocia 661.0 ✓5th
        contraction ring 661.4 ✓5th
        tetanic uterus 661.4 ✓5th
        uterine inertia 661.2 ✓5th
          primary 661.0 ✓5th
          secondary 661.1 ✓5th
      latent phase 661.0 ✓5th
    pyrexia during labor 659.2 ✓5th
    rachitic pelvis 653.2 ✓5th
      causing obstructed labor 660.1 ✓5th
    rectocele 654.4 ✓5th
      causing obstructed labor 660.2 ✓5th
    retained membranes or portions of placenta
      666.2 ✓5th
      without hemorrhage 667.1 ✓5th
    retarded (prolonged) birth 662.1 ✓5th
    retention secundines (with hemorrhage)
      666.2 ✓5th
      without hemorrhage 667.1 ✓5th
    retroversion, uterus or cervix 654.3 ✓5th
      causing obstructed labor 660.2 ✓5th
    rigid
      cervix 654.6 ✓5th
        causing obstructed labor 660.2 ✓5th
      pelvic floor 654.4 ✓5th
        causing obstructed labor 660.2 ✓5th
      perineum or vulva 654.8 ✓5th
        causing obstructed labor 660.2 ✓5th
      vagina 654.7 ✓5th
        causing obstructed labor 660.2 ✓5th
    Robert's pelvis 653.0 ✓5th
      causing obstructed labor 660.1 ✓5th

Delivery — *continued*
  complicated (by) NEC — *continued*
    rupture — *see also* Delivery, complicated,
      laceration
      bladder (urinary) 665.5 ✓5th
      cervix 665.3 ✓5th
      marginal sinus 641.2 ✓5th
      membranes, premature 658.1 ✓5th
      pelvic organ NEC 665.5 ✓5th
      perineum (without mention of other
        laceration) — *see* Delivery,
        complicated, laceration, perineum
      peritoneum 665.5 ✓5th
      urethra 665.5 ✓5th
      uterus (during labor) 665.1 ✓5th
        before labor 665.0 ✓5th
    sacculation, pregnant uterus 654.4 ✓5th
    sacral teratomas, fetal 653.7 ✓5th
      causing obstructed labor 660.1 ✓5th
    scar(s)
      cervix 654.6 ✓5th
        causing obstructed labor 660.2 ✓5th
      cesarean delivery 654.2 ✓5th
        causing obstructed labor 660.2 ✓5th
      perineum 654.8 ✓5th
        causing obstructed labor 660.2 ✓5th
      uterus NEC 654.9 ✓5th
        causing obstructed labor 660.2 ✓5th
        due to previous cesarean delivery
          654.2 ✓5th
      vagina 654.7 ✓5th
        causing obstructed labor 660.2 ✓5th
      vulva 654.8 ✓5th
        causing obstructed labor 660.2 ✓5th
    scoliotic pelvis 653.0 ✓5th
      causing obstructed labor 660.1 ✓5th
    secondary uterine inertia 661.1 ✓5th
    secundines, retained — *see* Delivery,
      complicated, placenta, retained
    separation
      placenta (premature) 641.2 ✓5th
      pubic bone 665.6 ✓5th
      symphysis pubis 665.6 ✓5th
    septate vagina 654.7 ✓5th
      causing obstructed labor 660.2 ✓5th
    shock (birth) (obstetric) (puerperal)
      669.1 ✓5th
    short cord syndrome 663.4 ✓5th
    shoulder
      girdle dystocia 660.4 ✓5th
      presentation 652.8 ✓5th
        causing obstructed labor 660.0 ✓5th
    Siamese twins 653.7 ✓5th
      causing obstructed labor 660.1 ✓5th
    slow slope active phase 661.2 ✓5th
    spasm
      cervix 661.4 ✓5th
      uterus 661.4 ✓5th
    spondylolisthesis, pelvis 653.3 ✓5th
      causing obstructed labor 660.1 ✓5th
    spondylolysis (lumbosacral) 653.3 ✓5th
      causing obstructed labor 660.1 ✓5th
    spondylosis 653.0 ✓5th
      causing obstructed labor 660.1 ✓5th
    stenosis or stricture
      cervix 654.6 ✓5th
        causing obstructed labor 660.2 ✓5th
      vagina 654.7 ✓5th
        causing obstructed labor 660.2 ✓5th
    sudden death, unknown cause 669.9 ✓5th
    tear (pelvic organ) (*see also* Delivery,
      complicated, laceration) 664.9 ✓5th
    teratomas, sacral, fetal 653.7 ✓5th
      causing obstructed labor 660.1 ✓5th
    tetanic uterus 661.4 ✓5th
    tipping pelvis 653.0 ✓5th
      causing obstructed labor 660.1 ✓5th
    transverse
      arrest (deep) 660.3 ✓5th
      presentation or lie 652.3 ✓5th
        with successful version 652.1 ✓5th
        causing obstructed labor 660.0 ✓5th
    trauma (obstetrical) NEC 665.9 ✓5th
    tumor
      abdominal, fetal 653.7 ✓5th
        causing obstructed labor 660.1 ✓5th

✓4th Fourth-digit Required   ✓5th Fifth-digit Required   ►◄ Revised Text   ● New Line   ▲ Revised Code

Delivery — *continued*
  complicated (by) NEC — *continued*
    tumor — *continued*
      pelvic organs or tissues NEC 654.9 ✓5ᵗʰ
        causing obstructed labor 660.2 ✓5ᵗʰ
      umbilical cord (*see also* Delivery,
          complicated, cord) 663.9 ✓5ᵗʰ
        around neck tightly, or with compression
            663.1 ✓5ᵗʰ
        entanglement NEC 663.3 ✓5ᵗʰ
          with compression 663.2 ✓5ᵗʰ
        prolapse (complete) (occult) (partial)
            663.0 ✓5ᵗʰ
      unstable lie 652.0 ✓5ᵗʰ
        causing obstructed labor 660.0 ✓5ᵗʰ
      uterine
        inertia (*see also* Delivery, complicated,
            inertia, uterus) 661.2 ✓5ᵗʰ
          spasm 661.4 ✓5ᵗʰ
      vasa previa 663.5 ✓5ᵗʰ
      velamentous insertion of cord 663.8 ✓5ᵗʰ
      young maternal age 659.8 ✓5ᵗʰ
  delayed NEC 662.1 ✓5ᵗʰ
    following rupture of membranes
        (spontaneous) 658.2 ✓5ᵗʰ
      artificial 658.3 ✓5ᵗʰ
    second twin, triplet, etc. 662.3 ✓5ᵗʰ
  difficult NEC 669.9 ✓5ᵗʰ
    previous, affecting management of
        pregnancy or childbirth V23.49   ▲
    specified type NEC 669.8 ✓5ᵗʰ
  early onset (spontaneous) 644.2 ✓5ᵗʰ
  footling 652.8 ✓5ᵗʰ
    with successful version 652.1 ✓5ᵗʰ
  forceps NEC 669.5 ✓5ᵗʰ
    affecting fetus or newborn 763.2
  missed (at or near term) 656.4 ✓5ᵗʰ
  multiple gestation NEC 651.9 ✓5ᵗʰ
    with fetal loss and retention of one or more
        fetus(es) 651.6 ✓5ᵗʰ
    specified type NEC 651.8 ✓5ᵗʰ
      with fetal loss and retention of one or
          more fetus(es) 651.6 ✓5ᵗʰ
  nonviable infant 656.4 ✓5ᵗʰ
  normal — *see* category 650
  precipitate 661.3 ✓5ᵗʰ
    affecting fetus or newborn 763.6
  premature NEC (before 37 completed weeks
      gestation) 644.2 ✓5ᵗʰ
    previous, affecting management of
        pregnancy V23.41   ▲
  quadruplet NEC 651.2 ✓5ᵗʰ
    with fetal loss and retention of one or more
        fetus(es) 651.5 ✓5ᵗʰ
  quintuplet NEC 651.8 ✓5ᵗʰ
    with fetal loss and retention of one or more
        fetus(es) 651.6 ✓5ᵗʰ
  sextuplet NEC 651.8 ✓5ᵗʰ
    with fetal loss and retention of one or more
        fetus(es) 651.6 ✓5ᵗʰ
  specified complication NEC 669.8 ✓5ᵗʰ
  stillbirth (near term) NEC 656.4 ✓5ᵗʰ
    early (before 22 completed weeks gestation)
        632
  term pregnancy (live birth) NEC — *see* category
      650
    stillbirth NEC 656.4 ✓5ᵗʰ
  threatened premature 644.2 ✓5ᵗʰ
  triplets NEC 651.1 ✓5ᵗʰ
    with fetal loss and retention of one or more
        fetus(es) 651.4 ✓5ᵗʰ
    delayed delivery (one or more mates)
        662.3 ✓5ᵗʰ
    locked mates 660.5 ✓5ᵗʰ
  twins NEC 651.0 ✓5ᵗʰ
    with fetal loss and retention of one fetus
        651.3 ✓5ᵗʰ
    delayed delivery (one or more mates)
        662.3 ✓5ᵗʰ
    locked mates 660.5 ✓5ᵗʰ
  uncomplicated — *see* category 650
  vacuum extractor NEC 669.5 ✓5ᵗʰ
    affecting fetus or newborn 763.3
  ventouse NEC 669.5 ✓5ᵗʰ
    affecting fetus or newborn 763.3
Dellen, cornea 371.41

Delusions (paranoid) 297.9
  grandiose 297.1
  parasitosis 300.29
  systematized 297.1
Dementia 294.8
  alcoholic (*see also* Psychosis, alcoholic) 291.2
  Alzheimer's — *see* Alzheimer's dementia
  arteriosclerotic (simple type) (uncomplicated)
      290.40
    with
      acute confusional state 290.41
      delirium 290.41
      delusional features 290.42
      depressive features 290.43
    depressed type 290.43
    paranoid type 290.42
  Binswanger's 290.12
  catatonic (acute) (*see also* Schizophrenia)
      295.2 ✓5ᵗʰ
  congenital (*see also* Retardation, mental) 319
  degenerative 290.9
    presenile-onset — *see* Dementia, presenile
    senile-onset — *see* Dementia, senile
  developmental (*see also* Schizophrenia)
      295.9 ✓5ᵗʰ
  dialysis 294.8
    transient 293.9
  due to or associated with condition(s) classified
      elsewhere
    Alzheimer's
      with behavioral disturbance
          331.0 [294.11]
      without behavioral disturbance
          331.0 [294.10]
    cerebral lipidoses
      with behavioral disturbance
          330.1 [294.11]
      without behavioral disturbance
          330.1 [294.10]
    epilepsy
      with behavioral disturbance
          345.9 ✓5ᵗʰ [294.11]
      without behavioral disturbance
          345.9 ✓5ᵗʰ [294.10]
    hepatolenticular degeneration
      with behavioral disturbance
          275.1 [294.11]
      without behavioral disturbance
          275.1 [294.10]
    HIV
      with behavioral disturbance 042 [294.11]
      without behavioral disturbance
          042 [294.10]
    Huntington's chorea
      with behavioral disturbance
          333.4 [294.11]
      without behavioral disturbance
          333.4 [294.10]
    Jakob-Cruetzfeldt disease
      with behavioral disturbance
          046.1 [294.11]
      without behavioral disturbance
          046.1 [294.10]
    multiple sclerosis
      with behavioral disturbance 340 [294.11]
      without behavioral disturbance
          340 [294.10]
    neurosyphilis
      with behavioral disturbance
          094.9 [294.11]
      without behavioral disturbance
          094.9 [294.10]
    Pelizaeus-Merzbacher disease
      with behavioral disturbance
          333.0 [294.11]
      without behavioral disturbance
          333.0 [294.10]
    Pick's disease
      with behavioral disturbance
          331.1 [294.11]
      without behavioral disturbance
          331.1 [294.10]
    polyarteritis nodosa
      with behavioral disturbance
          446.0 [294.11]

Dementia — *continued*
  due to or associated with condition(s) classified
      elsewhere — *continued*
    polyarteritis nodosa — *continued*
      without behavioral disturbance
          446.0 [294.10]
    syphilis
      with behavioral disturbance
          094.1 [294.11]
      without behavioral disturbance
          094.1 [294.10]
    Wilson's disease
      with behavioral disturbance
          275.1 [294.11]
      without behavioral disturbance
          275.1 [294.10]
  hebephrenic (acute) 295.1 ✓5ᵗʰ
  Heller's (infantile psychosis) (*see also*
      Psychosis, childhood) 299.1 ✓5ᵗʰ
  idiopathic 290.9
    presenile-onset — *see* Dementia, presenile
    senile-onset — *see* Dementia, senile
  in
    arteriosclerotic brain disease 290.40
    senility 290.0
  induced by drug 292.82
  infantile, infantilia (*see also* Psychosis,
      childhood) 299.0 ✓5ᵗʰ
  multi-infarct (cerebrovascular) (*see also*
      Dementia, arteriosclerotic) 290.40
  old age 290.0
  paralytica, paralytic 094.1
    juvenilis 090.40
    syphilitic 094.1
      congenital 090.40
    tabetic form 094.1
  paranoid (*see also* Schizophrenia) 295.3 ✓5ᵗʰ
  paraphrenic (*see also* Schizophrenia) 295.3 ✓5ᵗʰ
  paretic 094.1
  praecox (*see also* Schizophrenia) 295.9 ✓5ᵗʰ
  presenile 290.10
    with
      acute confusional state 290.11
      delirium 290.11
      delusional features 290.12
      depressive features 290.13
    depressed type 290.13
    paranoid type 290.12
    simple type 290.10
    uncomplicated 290.10
  primary (acute) (*see also* Schizophrenia)
      295.0 ✓5ᵗʰ
  progressive, syphilitic 094.1
  puerperal — *see* Psychosis, puerperal
  schizophrenic (*see also* Schizophrenia)
      295.9 ✓5ᵗʰ
  senile 290.0
    with
      acute confusional state 290.3
      delirium 290.3
      delusional features 290.20
      depressive features 290.21
    depressed type 290.21
    exhaustion 290.0
    paranoid type 290.20
  simple type (acute) (*see also* Schizophrenia)
      295.0 ✓5ᵗʰ
  simplex (acute) (*see also* Schizophrenia)
      295.0 ✓5ᵗʰ
  syphilitic 094.1
  uremic — *see* Uremia
  vascular 290.40
Demerol dependence (*see also* Dependence)
    304.0 ✓5ᵗʰ
Demineralization, ankle (*see also* Osteoporosis)
    733.00
Demodex folliculorum (infestation) 133.8
de Morgan's spots (senile angiomas) 448.1
Demyelinating
  polyneuritis, chronic inflammatory 357.81   ▲
Demyelination, demyelinization
  central nervous system 341.9
    specified NEC 341.8
  corpus callosum (central) 341.8
  global 340

Dengue (fever) 061
  sandfly 061
  vaccination, prophylactic (against) V05.1
  virus hemorrhagic fever 065.4

Dens
  evaginatus 520.2
  in dente 520.2
  invaginatus 520.2

Density
  increased, bone (disseminated) (generalized) (spotted) 733.99
  lung (nodular) 518.89

Dental — *see also* condition
  examination only V72.2

Dentia praecox 520.6

Denticles (in pulp) 522.2

Dentigerous cyst 526.0

Dentin
  irregular (in pulp) 522.3
  opalescent 520.5
  secondary (in pulp) 522.3
  sensitive 521.8

Dentinogenesis imperfecta 520.5

Dentinoma (M9271/0) 213.1
  upper jaw (bone) 213.0

Dentition 520.7
  abnormal 520.6
  anomaly 520.6
  delayed 520.6
  difficult 520.7
  disorder of 520.6
  precocious 520.6
  retarded 520.6

Denture sore (mouth) 528.9

Dependence

Note — Use the following fifth-digit subclassification with category 304:
  0   unspecified
  1   continuous
  2   episodic
  3   in remission

  with
    withdrawal symptoms
      alcohol 291.81
      drug 292.0
  14-hydroxy-dihydromorphinone 304.0 ✓5ᵗʰ
  absinthe 304.6 ✓5ᵗʰ
  acemorphan 304.0 ✓5ᵗʰ
  acetanilid(e) 304.6 ✓5ᵗʰ
  acetophenetidin 304.6 ✓5ᵗʰ
  acetorphine 304.0 ✓5ᵗʰ
  acetyldihydrocodeine 304.0 ✓5ᵗʰ
  acetyldihydrocodeinone 304.0 ✓5ᵗʰ
  Adalin 304.1 ✓5ᵗʰ
  Afghanistan black 304.3 ✓5ᵗʰ
  agrypnal 304.1 ✓5ᵗʰ
  alcohol, alcoholic (ethyl) (methyl) (wood) 303.9 ✓5ᵗʰ
    maternal, with suspected fetal damage affecting management of pregnancy 655.4 ✓5ᵗʰ
  allobarbitone 304.1 ✓5ᵗʰ
  allonal 304.1 ✓5ᵗʰ
  allylisopropylacetylurea 304.1 ✓5ᵗʰ
  alphaprodine (hydrochloride) 304.0 ✓5ᵗʰ
  Alurate 304.1 ✓5ᵗʰ
  Alvodine 304.0 ✓5ᵗʰ
  amethocaine 304.6 ✓5ᵗʰ
  amidone 304.0 ✓5ᵗʰ
  amidopyrine 304.6 ✓5ᵗʰ
  aminopyrine 304.6 ✓5ᵗʰ
  amobarbital 304.1 ✓5ᵗʰ
  amphetamine(s) (type) (drugs classifiable to 969.7) 304.4 ✓5ᵗʰ
  amylene hydrate 304.6 ✓5ᵗʰ
  amylobarbitone 304.1 ✓5ᵗʰ
  amylocaine 304.6 ✓5ᵗʰ
  Amytal (sodium) 304.1 ✓5ᵗʰ
  analgesic (drug) NEC 304.6 ✓5ᵗʰ
    synthetic with morphine-like effect 304.0 ✓5ᵗʰ

Dependence — *continued*
  anesthetic (agent) (drug) (gas) (general) (local) NEC 304.6 ✓5ᵗʰ
  Angel dust 304.6 ✓5ᵗʰ
  anileridine 304.0 ✓5ᵗʰ
  antipyrine 304.6 ✓5ᵗʰ
  aprobarbital 304.1 ✓5ᵗʰ
  aprobarbitone 304.1 ✓5ᵗʰ
  atropine 304.6 ✓5ᵗʰ
  Avertin (bromide) 304.6 ✓5ᵗʰ
  barbenyl 304.1 ✓5ᵗʰ
  barbital(s) 304.1 ✓5ᵗʰ
  barbitone 304.1 ✓5ᵗʰ
  barbiturate(s) (compounds) (drugs classifiable to 967.0) 304.1 ✓5ᵗʰ
  barbituric acid (and compounds) 304.1 ✓5ᵗʰ
  benzedrine 304.4 ✓5ᵗʰ
  benzylmorphine 304.0 ✓5ᵗʰ
  Beta-chlor 304.1 ✓5ᵗʰ
  bhang 304.3 ✓5ᵗʰ
  blue velvet 304.0 ✓5ᵗʰ
  Brevital 304.1 ✓5ᵗʰ
  bromal (hydrate) 304.1 ✓5ᵗʰ
  bromide(s) NEC 304.1 ✓5ᵗʰ
  bromine compounds NEC 304.1 ✓5ᵗʰ
  bromisovalum 304.1 ✓5ᵗʰ
  bromoform 304.1 ✓5ᵗʰ
  Bromo-seltzer 304.1 ✓5ᵗʰ
  bromural 304.1 ✓5ᵗʰ
  butabarbital (sodium) 304.1 ✓5ᵗʰ
  butabarpal 304.1 ✓5ᵗʰ
  butallylonal 304.1 ✓5ᵗʰ
  butethal 304.1 ✓5ᵗʰ
  buthalitone (sodium) 304.1 ✓5ᵗʰ
  Butisol 304.1 ✓5ᵗʰ
  butobarbitone 304.1 ✓5ᵗʰ
  butyl chloral (hydrate) 304.1 ✓5ᵗʰ
  caffeine 304.4 ✓5ᵗʰ
  cannabis (indica) (sativa) (resin) (derivatives) (type) 304.3 ✓5ᵗʰ
  carbamazepine 304.6 ✓5ᵗʰ
  Carbrital 304.1 ✓5ᵗʰ
  carbromal 304.1 ✓5ᵗʰ
  carisoprodol 304.6 ✓5ᵗʰ
  Catha (edulis) 304.4 ✓5ᵗʰ
  chloral (betaine) (hydrate) 304.1 ✓5ᵗʰ
  chloralamide 304.1 ✓5ᵗʰ
  chloralformamide 304.1 ✓5ᵗʰ
  chloralose 304.1 ✓5ᵗʰ
  chlordiazepoxide 304.1 ✓5ᵗʰ
  Chloretone 304.1 ✓5ᵗʰ
  chlorobutanol 304.1 ✓5ᵗʰ
  chlorodyne 304.1 ✓5ᵗʰ
  chloroform 304.6 ✓5ᵗʰ
  Cliradon 304.0 ✓5ᵗʰ
  coca (leaf) and derivatives 304.2 ✓5ᵗʰ
  cocaine 304.2 ✓5ᵗʰ
    hydrochloride 304.2 ✓5ᵗʰ
    salt (any) 304.2 ✓5ᵗʰ
  codeine 304.0 ✓5ᵗʰ
  combination of drugs (excluding morphine or opioid type drug) NEC 304.8 ✓5ᵗʰ
    morphine or opioid type drug with any other drug 304.7 ✓5ᵗʰ
  croton-chloral 304.1 ✓5ᵗʰ
  cyclobarbital 304.1 ✓5ᵗʰ
  cyclobarbitone 304.1 ✓5ᵗʰ
  dagga 304.3 ✓5ᵗʰ
  Delvinal 304.1 ✓5ᵗʰ
  Demerol 304.0 ✓5ᵗʰ
  desocodeine 304.0 ✓5ᵗʰ
  desomorphine 304.0 ✓5ᵗʰ
  desoxyephedrine 304.4 ✓5ᵗʰ
  DET 304.5 ✓5ᵗʰ
  dexamphetamine 304.4 ✓5ᵗʰ
  dexedrine 304.4 ✓5ᵗʰ
  dextromethorphan 304.0 ✓5ᵗʰ
  dextromoramide 304.0 ✓5ᵗʰ
  dextronorpseudoephedrine 304.4 ✓5ᵗʰ
  dextrorphan 304.0 ✓5ᵗʰ
  diacetylmorphine 304.0 ✓5ᵗʰ
  Dial 304.1 ✓5ᵗʰ
  diallylbarbituric acid 304.1 ✓5ᵗʰ
  diamorphine 304.0 ✓5ᵗʰ
  diazepam 304.1 ✓5ᵗʰ
  dibucaine 304.6 ✓5ᵗʰ
  dichloroethane 304.6 ✓5ᵗʰ
  diethyl barbituric acid 304.1 ✓5ᵗʰ

Dependence — *continued*
  diethylsulfone-diethylmethane 304.1 ✓5ᵗʰ
  difencloxazine 304.0 ✓5ᵗʰ
  dihydrocodeine 304.0 ✓5ᵗʰ
  dihydrocodeinone 304.0 ✓5ᵗʰ
  dihydrohydroxycodeinone 304.0 ✓5ᵗʰ
  dihydroisocodeine 304.0 ✓5ᵗʰ
  dihydromorphine 304.0 ✓5ᵗʰ
  dihydromorphinone 304.0 ✓5ᵗʰ
  dihydroxcodeinone 304.0 ✓5ᵗʰ
  Dilaudid 304.0 ✓5ᵗʰ
  dimenhydrinate 304.6 ✓5ᵗʰ
  dimethylmeperidine 304.0 ✓5ᵗʰ
  dimethyltriptamine 304.5 ✓5ᵗʰ
  Dionin 304.0 ✓5ᵗʰ
  diphenoxylate 304.6 ✓5ᵗʰ
  dipipanone 304.0 ✓5ᵗʰ
  d-lysergic acid diethylamide 304.5 ✓5ᵗʰ
  DMT 304.5 ✓5ᵗʰ
  Dolophine 304.0 ✓5ᵗʰ
  DOM 304.2 ✓5ᵗʰ
  Doriden 304.1 ✓5ᵗʰ
  dormiral 304.1 ✓5ᵗʰ
  Dormison 304.1 ✓5ᵗʰ
  Dromoran 304.0 ✓5ᵗʰ
  drug NEC 304.9 ✓5ᵗʰ
    analgesic NEC 304.6 ✓5ᵗʰ
    combination (excluding morphine or opioid type drug) NEC 304.8 ✓5ᵗʰ
      morphine or opioid type drug with any other drug 304.7 ✓5ᵗʰ
    complicating pregnancy, childbirth, or puerperium 648.3 ✓5ᵗʰ
      affecting fetus or newborn 779.5
    hallucinogenic 304.5 ✓5ᵗʰ
    hypnotic NEC 304.1 ✓5ᵗʰ
    narcotic NEC 304.9 ✓5ᵗʰ
    psychostimulant NEC 304.4 ✓5ᵗʰ
    sedative 304.1 ✓5ᵗʰ
    soporific NEC 304.1 ✓5ᵗʰ
    specified type NEC 304.6 ✓5ᵗʰ
    suspected damage to fetus affecting management of pregnancy 655.5 ✓5ᵗʰ
    synthetic, with morphine-like effect 304.0 ✓5ᵗʰ
    tranquilizing 304.1 ✓5ᵗʰ
  duboisine 304.6 ✓5ᵗʰ
  ectylurea 304.1 ✓5ᵗʰ
  Endocaine 304.6 ✓5ᵗʰ
  Equanil 304.1 ✓5ᵗʰ
  Eskabarb 304.1 ✓5ᵗʰ
  ethchlorvynol 304.1 ✓5ᵗʰ
  ether (ethyl) (liquid) (vapor) (vinyl) 304.6 ✓5ᵗʰ
  ethidene 304.6 ✓5ᵗʰ
  ethinamate 304.1 ✓5ᵗʰ
  ethoheptazine 304.6 ✓5ᵗʰ
  ethyl
    alcohol 303.9 ✓5ᵗʰ
    bromide 304.6 ✓5ᵗʰ
    carbamate 304.6 ✓5ᵗʰ
    chloride 304.6 ✓5ᵗʰ
    morphine 304.0 ✓5ᵗʰ
  ethylene (gas) 304.6 ✓5ᵗʰ
    dichloride 304.6 ✓5ᵗʰ
  ethylidene chloride 304.6 ✓5ᵗʰ
  etilfen 304.1 ✓5ᵗʰ
  etorphine 304.0 ✓5ᵗʰ
  etoval 304.1 ✓5ᵗʰ
  eucodal 304.0 ✓5ᵗʰ
  euneryl 304.1 ✓5ᵗʰ
  Evipal 304.1 ✓5ᵗʰ
  Evipan 304.1 ✓5ᵗʰ
  fentanyl 304.0 ✓5ᵗʰ
  ganja 304.3 ✓5ᵗʰ
  gardenal 304.1 ✓5ᵗʰ
  gardenpanyl 304.1 ✓5ᵗʰ
  gelsemine 304.6 ✓5ᵗʰ
  Gelsemium 304.6 ✓5ᵗʰ
  Gemonil 304.1 ✓5ᵗʰ
  glucochloral 304.1 ✓5ᵗʰ
  glue (airplane) (sniffing) 304.6 ✓5ᵗʰ
  glutethimide 304.1 ✓5ᵗʰ
  hallucinogenics 304.5 ✓5ᵗʰ
  hashish 304.3 ✓5ᵗʰ
  headache powder NEC 304.6 ✓5ᵗʰ
  Heavenly Blue 304.5 ✓5ᵗʰ
  hedonal 304.1 ✓5ᵗʰ
  hemp 304.3 ✓5ᵗʰ

Dependence — *continued*

heptabarbital 304.1 ✓5ᵗʰ
Heptalgin 304.0 ✓5ᵗʰ
heptobarbitone 304.1 ✓5ᵗʰ
heroin 304.0 ✓5ᵗʰ
　　salt (any) 304.0 ✓5ᵗʰ
hexethal (sodium) 304.1 ✓5ᵗʰ
hexobarbital 304.1 ✓5ᵗʰ
Hycodan 304.0 ✓5ᵗʰ
hydrocodone 304.0 ✓5ᵗʰ
hydromorphinol 304.0 ✓5ᵗʰ
hydromorphinone 304.0 ✓5ᵗʰ
hydromorphone 304.0 ✓5ᵗʰ
hydroxycodeine 304.0 ✓5ᵗʰ
hypnotic NEC 304.1 ✓5ᵗʰ
Indian hemp 304.3 ✓5ᵗʰ
intranarcon 304.1 ✓5ᵗʰ
Kemithal 304.1 ✓5ᵗʰ
ketobemidone 304.0 ✓5ᵗʰ
khat 304.4 ✓5ᵗʰ
kif 304.3 ✓5ᵗʰ
Lactuca (virosa) extract 304.1 ✓5ᵗʰ
lactucarium 304.1 ✓5ᵗʰ
laudanum 304.0 ✓5ᵗʰ
Lebanese red 304.3 ✓5ᵗʰ
Leritine 304.0 ✓5ᵗʰ
lettuce opium 304.1 ✓5ᵗʰ
Levanil 304.1 ✓5ᵗʰ
Levo-Dromoran 304.0 ✓5ᵗʰ
levo-iso-methadone 304.0 ✓5ᵗʰ
levorphanol 304.0 ✓5ᵗʰ
Librium 304.1 ✓5ᵗʰ
Lomotil 304.6 ✓5ᵗʰ
Lotusate 304.1 ✓5ᵗʰ
LSD (-25) (and derivatives) 304.5 ✓5ᵗʰ
Luminal 304.1 ✓5ᵗʰ
lysergic acid 304.5 ✓5ᵗʰ
　　amide 304.5 ✓5ᵗʰ
maconha 304.3 ✓5ᵗʰ
magic mushroom 304.5 ✓5ᵗʰ
marihuana 304.3 ✓5ᵗʰ
MDA (methylene dioxyamphetamine) 304.4 ✓5ᵗʰ
Mebaral 304.1 ✓5ᵗʰ
Medinal 304.1 ✓5ᵗʰ
Medomin 304.1 ✓5ᵗʰ
megahallucinogenics 304.5 ✓5ᵗʰ
meperidine 304.0 ✓5ᵗʰ
mephobarbital 304.1 ✓5ᵗʰ
meprobamate 304.1 ✓5ᵗʰ
mescaline 304.5 ✓5ᵗʰ
methadone 304.0 ✓5ᵗʰ
methamphetamine(s) 304.4 ✓5ᵗʰ
methaqualone 304.1 ✓5ᵗʰ
metharbital 304.1 ✓5ᵗʰ
methitural 304.1 ✓5ᵗʰ
methobarbitone 304.1 ✓5ᵗʰ
methohexital 304.1 ✓5ᵗʰ
methopholine 304.6 ✓5ᵗʰ
methyl
　　alcohol 303.9 ✓5ᵗʰ
　　bromide 304.6 ✓5ᵗʰ
　　morphine 304.0 ✓5ᵗʰ
　　sulfonal 304.1 ✓5ᵗʰ
methylated spirit 303.9 ✓5ᵗʰ
methylbutinol 304.6 ✓5ᵗʰ
methyldihydromorphinone 304.0 ✓5ᵗʰ
methylene
　　chloride 304.6 ✓5ᵗʰ
　　dichloride 304.6 ✓5ᵗʰ
　　dioxyamphetamine (MDA) 304.4 ✓5ᵗʰ
methylaparafynol 304.1 ✓5ᵗʰ
methylphenidate 304.4 ✓5ᵗʰ
methyprylone 304.1 ✓5ᵗʰ
metopon 304.0 ✓5ᵗʰ
Miltown 304.1 ✓5ᵗʰ
morning glory *seeds* 304.5 ✓5ᵗʰ
morphinan(s) 304.0 ✓5ᵗʰ
morphine (sulfate) (sulfite) (type) (drugs
　　classifiable to 965.00-965.09) 304.0 ✓5ᵗʰ
morphine or opioid type drug (drugs classifiable
　　to 965.00-965.09) with any other drug
　　304.7 ✓5ᵗʰ
morphinol(s) 304.0 ✓5ᵗʰ
morphinon 304.0 ✓5ᵗʰ
morpholinylethylmorphine 304.0 ✓5ᵗʰ
mylomid 304.1 ✓5ᵗʰ
myristicin 304.5 ✓5ᵗʰ
narcotic (drug) NEC 304.9 ✓5ᵗʰ

Dependence — *continued*

nealbarbital 304.1 ✓5ᵗʰ
nealbarbitone 304.1 ✓5ᵗʰ
Nembutal 304.1 ✓5ᵗʰ
Neonal 304.1 ✓5ᵗʰ
Neraval 304.1 ✓5ᵗʰ
Neravan 304.1 ✓5ᵗʰ
neurobarb 304.1 ✓5ᵗʰ
nicotine 305.1
Nisentil 304.0 ✓5ᵗʰ
nitrous oxide 304.6 ✓5ᵗʰ
Noctec 304.1 ✓5ᵗʰ
Noludar 304.1 ✓5ᵗʰ
nonbarbiturate sedatives and tranquilizers with
　　similar effect 304.1 ✓5ᵗʰ
noptil 304.1 ✓5ᵗʰ
normorphine 304.0 ✓5ᵗʰ
noscapine 304.0 ✓5ᵗʰ
Novocaine 304.6 ✓5ᵗʰ
Numorphan 304.0 ✓5ᵗʰ
nunol 304.1 ✓5ᵗʰ
Nupercaine 304.6 ✓5ᵗʰ
Oblivon 304.1 ✓5ᵗʰ
on
　　aspirator V46.0
　　hyperbaric chamber V46.8
　　iron lung V46.1
　　machine (enabling) V46.9
　　　　specified type NEC V46.8
　　Possum (Patient-Operated-Selector-
　　　　Mechanism) V46.8
　　renal dialysis machine V45.1
　　respirator V46.1
　　supplemental oxygen V46.2
opiate 304.0 ✓5ᵗʰ
opioids 304.0 ✓5ᵗʰ
opioid type drug 304.0 ✓5ᵗʰ
　　with any other drug 304.7 ✓5ᵗʰ
opium (alkaloids) (derivatives) (tincture)
　　304.0 ✓5ᵗʰ
ortal 304.1 ✓5ᵗʰ
Oxazepam 304.1 ✓5ᵗʰ
oxycodone 304.0 ✓5ᵗʰ
oxymorphone 304.0 ✓5ᵗʰ
Palfium 304.0 ✓5ᵗʰ
Panadol 304.6 ✓5ᵗʰ
pantopium 304.0 ✓5ᵗʰ
pantopon 304.0 ✓5ᵗʰ
papaverine 304.0 ✓5ᵗʰ
paracetamol 304.6 ✓5ᵗʰ
paracodin 304.0 ✓5ᵗʰ
paraldehyde 304.1 ✓5ᵗʰ
paregoric 304.0 ✓5ᵗʰ
Parzone 304.0 ✓5ᵗʰ
PCP (phencyclidine) 304.6 ✓5ᵗʰ
Pearly Gates 304.5 ✓5ᵗʰ
pentazocine 304.0 ✓5ᵗʰ
pentobarbital 304.1 ✓5ᵗʰ
pentobarbitone (sodium) 304.1 ✓5ᵗʰ
Pentothal 304.1 ✓5ᵗʰ
Percaine 304.6 ✓5ᵗʰ
Percodan 304.0 ✓5ᵗʰ
Perichlor 304.1 ✓5ᵗʰ
Pernocton 304.1 ✓5ᵗʰ
Pernoston 304.1 ✓5ᵗʰ
peronine 304.0 ✓5ᵗʰ
pethidine (hydrochloride) 304.0 ✓5ᵗʰ
petrichloral 304.1 ✓5ᵗʰ
peyote 304.5 ✓5ᵗʰ
Phanodron 304.1 ✓5ᵗʰ
phenacetin 304.6 ✓5ᵗʰ
phenadoxone 304.0 ✓5ᵗʰ
phenaglycodol 304.1 ✓5ᵗʰ
phenazocine 304.0 ✓5ᵗʰ
phencyclidine 304.6 ✓5ᵗʰ
phenmetrazine 304.4 ✓5ᵗʰ
phenobal 304.1 ✓5ᵗʰ
phenobarbital 304.1 ✓5ᵗʰ
phenobarbitone 304.1 ✓5ᵗʰ
phenomorphan 304.0 ✓5ᵗʰ
phenonyl 304.1 ✓5ᵗʰ
phenoperidine 304.0 ✓5ᵗʰ
pholcodine 304.0 ✓5ᵗʰ
piminodine 304.0 ✓5ᵗʰ
Pipadone 304.0 ✓5ᵗʰ
Pitkin's solution 304.6 ✓5ᵗʰ
Placidyl 304.1 ✓5ᵗʰ
polysubstance 304.8 ✓5ᵗʰ

Dependence — *continued*

Pontocaine 304.6 ✓5ᵗʰ
pot 304.3 ✓5ᵗʰ
potassium bromide 304.1 ✓5ᵗʰ
Preludin 304.4 ✓5ᵗʰ
Prinadol 304.0 ✓5ᵗʰ
probarbital 304.1 ✓5ᵗʰ
procaine 304.6 ✓5ᵗʰ
propanal 304.1 ✓5ᵗʰ
propoxyphene 304.6 ✓5ᵗʰ
psilocibin 304.5 ✓5ᵗʰ
psilocin 304.5 ✓5ᵗʰ
psilocybin 304.5 ✓5ᵗʰ
psilocyline 304.5 ✓5ᵗʰ
psilocyn 304.5 ✓5ᵗʰ
psychedelic agents 304.5 ✓5ᵗʰ
psychostimulant NEC 304.4 ✓5ᵗʰ
psychotomimetic agents 304.5 ✓5ᵗʰ
pyrahexyl 304.3 ✓5ᵗʰ
Pyramidon 304.6 ✓5ᵗʰ
quinalbarbitone 304.1 ✓5ᵗʰ
racemoramide 304.0 ✓5ᵗʰ
racemorphan 304.0 ✓5ᵗʰ
Rela 304.6 ✓5ᵗʰ
scopolamine 304.6 ✓5ᵗʰ
secobarbital 304.1 ✓5ᵗʰ
Seconal 304.1 ✓5ᵗʰ
sedative NEC 304.1 ✓5ᵗʰ
　　nonbarbiturate with barbiturate effect
　　　　304.1 ✓5ᵗʰ
Sedormid 304.1 ✓5ᵗʰ
sernyl 304.1 ✓5ᵗʰ
sodium bromide 304.1 ✓5ᵗʰ
Soma 304.6 ✓5ᵗʰ
Somnal 304.1 ✓5ᵗʰ
Somnos 304.1 ✓5ᵗʰ
Soneryl 304.1 ✓5ᵗʰ
soporific (drug) NEC 304.1 ✓5ᵗʰ
specified drug NEC 304.6 ✓5ᵗʰ
speed 304.4 ✓5ᵗʰ
spinocaine 304.6 ✓5ᵗʰ
Stovaine 304.6 ✓5ᵗʰ
STP 304.5 ✓5ᵗʰ
stramonium 304.6 ✓5ᵗʰ
Sulfonal 304.1 ✓5ᵗʰ
sulfonethylmethane 304.1 ✓5ᵗʰ
sulfonmethane 304.1 ✓5ᵗʰ
Surital 304.1 ✓5ᵗʰ
synthetic drug with morphine-like effect
　　304.0 ✓5ᵗʰ
talbutal 304.1 ✓5ᵗʰ
tetracaine 304.6 ✓5ᵗʰ
tetrahydrocannabinol 304.3 ✓5ᵗʰ
tetronal 304.1 ✓5ᵗʰ
THC 304.3 ✓5ᵗʰ
thebacon 304.0 ✓5ᵗʰ
thebaine 304.0 ✓5ᵗʰ
thiamil 304.1 ✓5ᵗʰ
thiamylal 304.1 ✓5ᵗʰ
thiopental 304.1 ✓5ᵗʰ
tobacco 305.1
toluene, toluol 304.6 ✓5ᵗʰ
tranquilizer NEC 304.1 ✓5ᵗʰ
　　nonbarbiturate with barbiturate effect
　　　　304.1 ✓5ᵗʰ
tribromacetaldehyde 304.6 ✓5ᵗʰ
tribromethanol 304.6 ✓5ᵗʰ
tribromomethane 304.6 ✓5ᵗʰ
trichloroethanol 304.6 ✓5ᵗʰ
trichoroethyl phosphate 304.1 ✓5ᵗʰ
triclofos 304.1 ✓5ᵗʰ
Trional 304.1 ✓5ᵗʰ
Tuinal 304.1 ✓5ᵗʰ
Turkish Green 304.3 ✓5ᵗʰ
urethan(e) 304.6 ✓5ᵗʰ
Valium 304.1 ✓5ᵗʰ
Valmid 304.1 ✓5ᵗʰ
veganin 304.0 ✓5ᵗʰ
veramon 304.1 ✓5ᵗʰ
Veronal 304.1 ✓5ᵗʰ
versidyne 304.6 ✓5ᵗʰ
vinbarbital 304.1 ✓5ᵗʰ
vinbarbitone 304.1 ✓5ᵗʰ
vinyl bitone 304.1 ✓5ᵗʰ
vitamin B_6 266.1
wine 303.9 ✓5ᵗʰ
Zactane 304.6 ✓5ᵗʰ

✓4ᵗʰ Fourth-digit Required　　　✓5ᵗʰ Fifth-digit Required　　　▶◀ Revised Text　　　● New Line　　　▲ Revised Code

Dependency — Dermatergosis

Dependency
passive 301.6
reactions 301.6
Depersonalization (episode, in neurotic state)
(neurotic) (syndrome) 300.6
Depletion
carbohydrates 271.9
complement factor 279.8
extracellular fluid 276.5
plasma 276.5
potassium 276.8
nephropathy 588.8
salt or sodium 276.1
causing heat exhaustion or prostration
992.4
nephropathy 593.9
volume 276.5
extracellular fluid 276.5
plasma 276.5
Deposit
argentous, cornea 371.16
bone, in Boeck's sarcoid 135
calcareous, calcium — see Calcification
cholesterol
retina 362.82
skin 709.3
vitreous (humor) 379.22
conjunctival 372.56
cornea, corneal NEC 371.10
argentous 371.16
in
cystinosis 270.0 [371.15]
mucopolysaccharidosis 277.5 [371.15]
crystalline, vitreous (humor) 379.22
hemosiderin, in old scars of cornea 371.11
metallic, in lens 366.45
skin 709.3
teeth, tooth (betel) (black) (green) (materia alba)
(orange) (soft) (tobacco) 523.6
urate, in kidney (see also Disease, renal) 593.9
Depraved appetite 307.52
Depression 311
acute (see also Psychosis, affective) 296.2 ✓5ᵗʰ
recurrent episode 296.3 ✓5ᵗʰ
single episode 296.2 ✓5ᵗʰ
agitated (see also Psychosis, affective)
296.2 ✓5ᵗʰ
recurrent episode 296.3 ✓5ᵗʰ
single episode 296.2 ✓5ᵗʰ
anaclitic 309.21
anxiety 300.4
arches 734
congenital 754.61
autogenous (see also Psychosis, affective)
296.2 ✓5ᵗʰ
recurrent episode 296.3 ✓5ᵗʰ
single episode 296.2 ✓5ᵗʰ
basal metabolic rate (BMR) 794.7
bone marrow 289.9
central nervous system 799.1
newborn 779.2
cerebral 331.9
newborn 779.2
cerebrovascular 437.8
newborn 779.2
chest wall 738.3
endogenous (see also Psychosis, affective)
296.2 ✓5ᵗʰ
recurrent episode 296.3 ✓5ᵗʰ
single episode 296.2 ✓5ᵗʰ
functional activity 780.99 ▲
hysterical 300.11
involutional, climacteric, or menopausal (see
also Psychosis, affective) 296.2 ✓5ᵗʰ
recurrent episode 296.3 ✓5ᵗʰ
single episode 296.2 ✓5ᵗʰ
manic (see also Psychosis, affective) 296.80
medullary 348.8
newborn 779.2
mental 300.4
metatarsal heads — see Depression, arches
metatarsus — see Depression, arches
monopolar (see also Psychosis, affective)
296.2 ✓5ᵗʰ
recurrent episode 296.3 ✓5ᵗʰ
single episode 296.2 ✓5ᵗʰ
nervous 300.4

Depression — continued
neurotic 300.4
nose 738.0
postpartum 648.4 ✓5ᵗʰ
psychogenic 300.4
reactive 298.0
psychoneurotic 300.4
psychotic (see also Psychosis, affective)
296.2 ✓5ᵗʰ
reactive 298.0
recurrent episode 296.3 ✓5ᵗʰ
single episode 296.2 ✓5ᵗʰ
reactive 300.4
neurotic 300.4
psychogenic 298.0
psychoneurotic 300.4
psychotic 298.0
recurrent 296.3 ✓5ᵗʰ
respiratory center 348.8
newborn 770.89
scapula 736.89
senile 290.21
situational (acute) (brief) 309.0
prolonged 309.1
skull 754.0
sternum 738.3
visual field 368.40 ▲
Depressive reaction — see also Reaction,
depressive
acute (transient) 309.0
with anxiety 309.28
prolonged 309.1
situational (acute) 309.0
prolonged 309.1
Deprivation
cultural V62.4
emotional V62.89
affecting
adult 995.82
infant or child 995.51
food 994.2
specific substance NEC 269.8
protein (familial) (kwashiorkor) 260
social V62.4
affecting
adult 995.82
infant or child 995.51
symptoms, syndrome
alcohol 291.81
drug 292.0
vitamins (see also Deficiency, vitamin) 269.2
water 994.3
de Quervain's
disease (tendon sheath) 727.04
thyroiditis (subacute granulomatous thyroiditis)
245.1
Derangement
ankle (internal) 718.97
current injury (see also Dislocation, ankle)
837.0
recurrent 718.37
cartilage (articular) NEC (see also Disorder,
cartilage, articular) 718.0 ✓5ᵗʰ
knee 717.9
recurrent 718.36
recurrent 718.3 ✓5ᵗʰ
collateral ligament (knee) (medial) (tibial)
717.82
current injury 844.1
lateral (fibular) 844.0
lateral (fibular) 717.81
current injury 844.0
cruciate ligament (knee) (posterior) 717.84
anterior 717.83
current injury 844.2
current injury 844.2
elbow (internal) 718.92
current injury (see also Dislocation, elbow)
832.00
recurrent 718.32
gastrointestinal 536.9
heart — see Disease, heart
hip (joint) (internal) (old) 718.95
current injury (see also Dislocation, hip)
835.00
recurrent 718.35

Derangement — continued
intervertebral disc — see Displacement,
intervertebral disc
joint (internal) 718.90
ankle 718.97
current injury — see also Dislocation, by
site
knee, meniscus or cartilage (see also
Tear, meniscus) 836.2
elbow 718.92
foot 718.97
hand 718.94
hip 718.95
knee 717.9
multiple sites 718.99
pelvic region 718.95
recurrent 718.30
ankle 718.37
elbow 718.32
foot 718.37
hand 718.34
hip 718.35
knee 718.36
multiple sites 718.39
pelvic region 718.35
shoulder (region) 718.31
specified site NEC 718.38
temporomandibular (old) 524.69
wrist 718.33
shoulder (region) 718.91
specified site NEC 718.98
spine NEC 724.9
temporomandibular 524.69
wrist 718.93
knee (cartilage) (internal) 717.9
current injury (see also Tear, meniscus)
836.2
ligament 717.89
capsular 717.85
collateral — see Derangement, collateral
ligament
cruciate — see Derangement, cruciate
ligament
specified NEC 717.85
recurrent 718.36
low back NEC 724.9
meniscus NEC (knee) 717.5
current injury (see also Tear, meniscus)
836.2
lateral 717.40
anterior horn 717.42
posterior horn 717.43
specified NEC 717.49
medial 717.3
anterior horn 717.1
posterior horn 717.2
recurrent 718.3 ✓5ᵗʰ
site other than knee — see Disorder,
cartilage, articular
mental (see also Psychosis) 298.9
rotator cuff (recurrent) (tear) 726.10
current 840.4
sacroiliac (old) 724.6
current — see Dislocation, sacroiliac
semilunar cartilage (knee) 717.5
current injury 836.2
lateral 836.1
medial 836.0
recurrent 718.3 ✓5ᵗʰ
shoulder (internal) 718.91
current injury (see also Dislocation,
shoulder) 831.00
recurrent 718.31
spine (recurrent) NEC 724.9
current — see Dislocation, spine
temporomandibular (internal) (joint) (old)
524.69
current — see Dislocation, jaw
Dercum's disease or syndrome (adiposis
dolorosa) 272.8
Derealization (neurotic) 300.6
Dermal — see condition
Dermaphytid — see Dermatophytosis
Dermatergosis — see Dermatitis

Dermatitis (allergic) (contact) (occupational)
    (venenata) 692.9
ab igne 692.82
acneiform 692.9
actinic (due to sun) 692.70
    acute 692.72
    chronic NEC 692.74
    other than from sun NEC 692.82
ambustionis
    due to
        burn or scald — *see* Burn, by site
        sunburn (*see also* Sunburn) 692.71
amebic 006.6
ammonia 691.0
anaphylactoid NEC 692.9
arsenical 692.4
artefacta 698.4
    psychogenic 316 [698.4]
asthmatic 691.8
atopic (allergic) (intrinsic) 691.8
    psychogenic 316 [691.8]
atrophicans 701.8
    diffusa 701.8
    maculosa 701.3
berlock, berloque 692.72
blastomycetic 116.0
blister beetle 692.89
Brucella NEC 023.9
bullosa 694.9
    striata pratensis 692.6
bullous 694.9
    mucosynechial, atrophic 694.60
        with ocular involvement 694.61
    seasonal 694.8
calorica
    due to
        burn or scald — *see* Burn, by site
        cold 692.89
        sunburn (*see also* Sunburn) 692.71
caterpillar 692.89
cercarial 120.3
combustionis
    due to
        burn or scald — *see* Burn, by site
        sunburn (*see also* Sunburn) 692.71
congelationis 991.5
contusiformis 695.2
diabetic 250.8 ☑5ᵗʰ
diaper 691.0
diphtheritica 032.85
due to
    acetone 692.2
    acids 692.4
    adhesive plaster 692.4
    alcohol (skin contact) (substances
        classifiable to 980.0-980.9) 692.4
        taken internally 693.8
    alkalis 692.4
    allergy NEC 692.9
    ammonia (household) (liquid) 692.4
    arnica 692.3
    arsenic 692.4
        taken internally 693.8
    blister beetle 692.89
    cantharides 692.3
    carbon disulphide 692.2
    caterpillar 692.89
    caustics 692.4
    cereal (ingested) 693.1
        contact with skin 692.5
    chemical(s) NEC 692.4
        internal 693.8
        irritant NEC 692.4
        taken internally 693.8
    chlorocompounds 692.2
    coffee (ingested) 693.1
        contact with skin 692.5
    cold weather 692.89
    cosmetics 692.81
    cyclohexanes 692.2
    deodorant 692.81
    detergents 692.0
    dichromate 692.4

Dermatitis — *continued*
due to — *continued*
    drugs and medicinals (correct substance
        properly administered) (internal use)
        693.0
        external (in contact with skin) 692.3
            wrong substance given or taken 976.9
            specified substance — *see* Table of
                Drugs and Chemicals
        wrong substance given or taken 977.9
            specified substance — *see* Table of
                Drugs and Chemicals
    dyes 692.89
        hair 692.89
    epidermophytosis — *see* Dermatophytosis
    esters 692.2
    external irritant NEC 692.9
        specified agent NEC 692.89
    eye shadow 692.81
    fish (ingested) 693.1
        contact with skin 692.5
    flour (ingested) 693.1
        contact with skin 692.5
    food (ingested) 693.1
        in contact with skin 692.5
    fruit (ingested) 693.1
        contact with skin 692.5
    fungicides 692.3
    furs 692.89
    glycols 692.2
    greases NEC 692.1
    hair dyes 692.89
    hot
        objects and materials — *see* Burn, by
            site
        weather or places 692.89
    hydrocarbons 692.2
    infrared rays, except from sun 692.82
        solar NEC (*see also* Dermatitis, due to,
            sun) 692.70
    ingested substance 693.9
        drugs and medicinals (*see also*
            Dermatitis, due to, drugs and
            medicinals) 693.0
        food 693.1
        specified substance NEC 693.8
    ingestion or injection of chemical 693.8
        drug (correct substance properly
            administered) 693.0
            wrong substance given or taken 977.9
                specified substance — *see* Table of
                    Drugs and Chemicals
    insecticides 692.4
    internal agent 693.9
        drugs and medicinals (*see also*
            Dermatitis, due to, drugs and
            medicinals) 693.0
        food (ingested) 693.1
            in contact with skin 692.5
        specified agent NEC 693.8
    iodine 692.3
    iodoform 692.3
    irradiation 692.82
    jewelry 692.83
    keratolytics 692.3
    ketones 692.2
    lacquer tree (Rhus verniciflua) 692.6
    light NEC (*see also* Dermatitis, due to, sun)
        692.70
        other 692.82
    low temperature 692.89
    mascara 692.81
    meat (ingested) 693.1
        contact with skin 692.5
    mercury, mercurials 692.3
    metals 692.83
    milk (ingested) 693.1
        contact with skin 692.5
    Neomycin 692.3
    nylon 692.4
    oils NEC 692.1
    paint solvent 692.2
    pediculocides 692.3
    petroleum products (substances classifiable
        to 981) 692.4
    phenol 692.3

Dermatitis — *continued*
due to — *continued*
    photosensitiveness, photosensitivity (sun)
        692.72
        other light 692.82
    plants NEC 692.6
    plasters, medicated (any) 692.3
    plastic 692.4
    poison
        ivy (Rhus toxicodendron) 692.6
        oak (Rhus diversiloba) 692.6
        plant or vine 692.6
        sumac (Rhus venenata) 692.6
        vine (Rhus radicans) 692.6
    preservatives 692.89
    primrose (primula) 692.6
    primula 692.6
    radiation 692.82
        sun NEC (*see also* Dermatitis, due to,
            sun) 692.70
        tanning bed 692.82
    radioactive substance 692.82
    radium 692.82
    ragweed (Senecio jacobae) 692.6
    Rhus (diversiloba) (radicans) (toxicodendron)
        (venenata) (verniciflua) 692.6
    rubber 692.4
    scabicides 692.3
    Senecio jacobae 692.6
    solar radiation — *see* Dermatitis, due to,
        sun
    solvents (any) (substances classifiable to
        982.0-982.8) 692.2
        chlorocompound group 692.2
        cyclohexane group 692.2
        ester group 692.2
        glycol group 692.2
        hydrocarbon group 692.2
        ketone group 692.2
        paint 692.2
    specified agent NEC 692.89
    sun 692.70
        acute 692.72
        chronic NEC 692.74
        specified NEC 692.79
    sunburn (*see also* Sunburn) 692.71
    sunshine NEC (*see also* Dermatitis, due to,
        sun) 692.70
    tanning bed 692.82
    tetrachlorethylene 692.2
    toluene 692.2
    topical medications 692.3
    turpentine 692.2
    ultraviolet rays, except from sun 692.82
        sun NEC (*see also* Dermatitis, due to,
            sun) 692.82
    vaccine or vaccination (correct substance
        properly administered) 693.0
        wrong substance given or taken
            bacterial vaccine 978.8
                specified — *see* Table of Drugs and
                    Chemicals
            other vaccines NEC 979.9
                specified — *see* Table of Drugs and
                    Chemicals
    varicose veins (*see also* Varicose, vein,
        inflamed or infected) 454.1
    x-rays 692.82
dyshydrotic 705.81
dysmenorrheica 625.8
eczematoid NEC 692.9
    infectious 690.8
eczematous NEC 692.9
epidemica 695.89
erysipelatosa 695.81
escharotica — *see* Burn, by site
exfoliativa, exfoliative 695.89
    generalized 695.89
    infantum 695.81
    neonatorum 695.81
eyelid 373.31
    allergic 373.32
    contact 373.32
    eczematous 373.31
    herpes (zoster) 053.20
        simplex 054.41

Dermatitis — *continued*
  eyelid — *continued*
    infective 373.5
      due to
        actinomycosis 039.3 *[373.5]*
        herpes
          simplex 054.41
          zoster 053.20
        impetigo 684 *[373.5]*
        leprosy (*see also* Leprosy)
          030.0 *[373.4]*
        lupus vulgaris (tuberculous) (*see also*
          Tuberculosis) 017.0 ☑5ᵗʰ *[373.4]*
        mycotic dermatitis (*see also*
          Dermatomycosis) 111.9 *[373.5]*
        vaccinia 051.0 *[373.5]*
        postvaccination 999.0 *[373.5]*
        yaws (*see also* Yaws) 102.9 *[373.4]*
  facta, factitia 698.4
    psychogenic 316 *[698.4]*
  ficta 698.4
    psychogenic 316 *[698.4]*
  flexural 691.8
  follicularis 704.8
  friction 709.8
  fungus 111.9
    specified type NEC 111.8
  gangrenosa, gangrenous (infantum) (*see also*
    Gangrene) 785.4
  gestationis 646.8 ☑5ᵗʰ
  gonococcal 098.89
  gouty 274.89
  harvest mite 133.8
  heat 692.89
  herpetiformis (bullous) (erythematous)
    (pustular) (vesicular) 694.0
    juvenile 694.2
    senile 694.5
  hiemalis 692.89
  hypostatic, hypostatica 454.1
    with ulcer 454.2
  impetiginous 684
  infantile (acute) (chronic) (intertriginous)
    (intrinsic) (seborrheic) 690.12
  infectiosa eczematoides 690.8
  infectious (staphylococcal) (streptococcal) 686.9
    eczematoid 690.8
  infective eczematoid 690.8
  Jacquet's (diaper dermatitis) 691.0
  leptus 133.8
  lichenified NEC 692.9
  lichenoid, chronic 701.0
  lichenoides purpurica pigmentosa 709.1
  meadow 692.6
  medicamentosa (correct substance properly
    administered) (internal use) (*see also*
    Dermatitis, due to, drugs, or medicinals)
    693.0
    due to contact with skin 692.3
  mite 133.8
  multiformis 694.0
    juvenile 694.2
    senile 694.5
  napkin 691.0
  neuro 698.3
  neurotica 694.0
  nummular NEC 692.9
  osteatosis, osteatotic 706.8
  papillaris capillitii 706.1
  pellagrous 265.2
  perioral 695.3
  perstans 696.1
  photosensitivity (sun) 692.72
    other light 692.82
  pigmented purpuric lichenoid 709.1
  polymorpha dolorosa 694.0
  primary irritant 692.9
  pruriginosa 694.0
  pruritic NEC 692.9
  psoriasiform nodularis 696.2
  psychogenic 316
  purulent 686.00
  pustular contagious 051.2
  pyococcal 686.00
  pyocyaneus 686.09
  pyogenica 686.00
  radiation 692.82

Dermatitis — *continued*
  repens 696.1
  Ritter's (exfoliativa) 695.81
  Schamberg's (progressive pigmentary
    dermatosis) 709.09
  schistosome 120.3
  seasonal bullous 694.8
  seborrheic 690.10
    infantile 690.12
  sensitization NEC 692.9
  septic (*see also* Septicemia) 686.00
    gonococcal 098.89
  solar, solare NEC (*see also* Dermatitis, due to,
    sun) 692.70
  stasis 459.81
    due to
      postphlebitic syndrome 459.12 ▲
        with ulcer 459.13 ●
      varicose veins — *see* Varicose
    ulcerated or with ulcer (varicose) 454.2
  sunburn (*see also* Sunburn) 692.71
  suppurative 686.00
  traumatic NEC 709.8
  trophoneurotica 694.0
  ultraviolet, except from sun 692.82
    due to sun NEC (*see also* Dermatitis, due to,
      sun) 692.70
  varicose 454.1
    with ulcer 454.2
  vegetans 686.8
  verrucosa 117.2
  xerotic 706.8

Dermatoarthritis, lipoid 272.8 *[713.0]*

Dermatochalasia, dermatochalasis 374.87

Dermatofibroma (lenticulare) (M8832/0) — *see
  also* Neoplasm, skin, benign
  protuberans (M8832/1) — *see* Neoplasm, skin,
    uncertain behavior

Dermatofibrosarcoma (protuberans) (M8832/3)
  — *see* Neoplasm, skin, malignant

Dermatographia 708.3

Dermatolysis (congenital) (exfoliativa) 757.39
  acquired 701.8
  eyelids 374.34
  palpebrarum 374.34
  senile 701.8

Dermatomegaly NEC 701.8

Dermatomucomyositis 710.3

Dermatomycosis 111.9
  furfuracea 111.0
  specified type NEC 111.8

Dermatomyositis (acute) (chronic) 710.3

Dermatoneuritis of children 985.0

Dermatophiliasis 134.1

Dermatophytide — *see* Dermatophytosis

Dermatophytosis (Epidermophyton) (infection)
  (microsporum) (tinea) (Trichophyton) 110.9
  beard 110.0
  body 110.5
  deep seated 110.6
  fingernails 110.1
  foot 110.4
  groin 110.3
  hand 110.2
  nail 110.1
  perianal (area) 110.3
  scalp 110.0
  scrotal 110.8
  specified site NEC 110.8
  toenails 110.1
  vulva 110.8

Dermatopolyneuritis 985.0

Dermatorrhexis 756.83
  acquired 701.8

Dermatosclerosis (*see also* Scleroderma) 710.1
  localized 701.0

Dermatosis 709.9
  Andrews' 686.8
  atopic 691.8
  Bowen's (M8081/2) — *see* Neoplasm, skin, in
    situ
  bullous 694.9
    specified type NEC 694.8
  erythematosquamous 690.8

Dermatosis — *continued*
  exfoliativa 695.89
  factitial 698.4
  gonococcal 098.89
  herpetiformis 694.0
    juvenile 694.2
    senile 694.5
  hysterical 300.11
  Linear IgA 694.8
  menstrual NEC 709.8
  neutrophilic, acute febrile 695.89
  occupational (*see also* Dermatitis) 692.9
  papulosa nigra 709.8
  pigmentary NEC 709.00
    progressive 709.09
    Schamberg's 709.09
    Siemens-Bloch 757.33
  progressive pigmentary 709.09
  psychogenic 316
  pustular subcorneal 694.1
  Schamberg's (progressive pigmentary) 709.09
  senile NEC 709.3
  Unna's (seborrheic dermatitis) 690.10

Dermographia 708.3

Dermographism 708.3

Dermoid (cyst) (M9084/0) — *see also* Neoplasm,
  by site, benign
  with malignant transformation (M9084/3)
    183.0

Dermopathy
  infiltrative, with throtoxicosis 242.0 ☑5ᵗʰ
  senile NEC 709.3

Dermophytosis — *see* Dermatophytosis

Descemet's membrane — *see* condition

Descemetocele 371.72

Descending — *see* condition

Descensus uteri (complete) (incomplete) (partial)
  (without vaginal wall prolapse) 618.1
  with mention of vaginal wall proplapse — *see*
    Prolapse, uterovaginal

Desensitization to allergens V07.1

Desert
  rheumatism 114.0
  sore (*see also* Ulcer, skin) 707.9

Desertion (child) (newborn) 995.52
  adult 995.84

Desmoid (extra-abdominal) (tumor) (M8821/1) —
  see also Neoplasm, connective tissue,
    uncertain behavior
  abdominal (M8822/1) — *see* Neoplasm,
    connective tissue, uncertain behavior

Despondency 300.4

Desquamative dermatitis NEC 695.89

Destruction
  articular facet (*see also* Derangement, joint)
    718.9 ☑5ᵗʰ
    vertebra 724.9
  bone 733.90
    syphilitic 095.5
  joint (*see also* Derangement, joint) 718.9 ☑5ᵗʰ
    sacroiliac 724.6
  kidney 593.89
  live fetus to facilitate birth NEC 763.89
  ossicles (ear) 385.24
  rectal sphincter 569.49
  septum (nasal) 478.1
  tuberculous NEC (*see also* Tuberculosis)
    011.9 ☑5ᵗʰ
  tympanic membrane 384.82
  tympanum 385.89
  vertebral disc — *see* Degeneration,
    intervertebral disc

Destructiveness (*see also* Disturbance, conduct)
  312.9
  adjustment reaction 309.3

Detachment
  cartilage — *see also* Sprain, by site
    knee — *see* Tear, meniscus
  cervix, annular 622.8
    complicating delivery 665.3 ☑5ᵗʰ
  choroid (old) (postinfectional) (simple)
    (spontaneous) 363.70
    hemorrhagic 363.72

Detachment — continued
choroid — continued
serous 363.71
knee, medial meniscus (old) 717.3
current injury 836.0
ligament — see Sprain, by site
placenta (premature) — see Placenta,
separation
retina (recent) 361.9
with retinal defect (rhegmatogenous) 361.00
giant tear 361.03
multiple 361.02
partial
with
giant tear 361.03
multiple defects 361.02
retinal dialysis (juvenile) 361.04
single defect 361.01
retinal dialysis (juvenile) 361.04
single 361.01
subtotal 361.05
total 361.05
delimited (old) (partial) 361.06
old
delimited 361.06
partial 361.06
total or subtotal 361.07
pigment epithelium (RPE) (serous) 362.42
exudative 362.42
hemorrhagic 362.43
rhegmatogenous (see also Detachment,
retina, with retinal defect) 361.00
serous (without retinal defect) 361.2
specified type NEC 361.89
traction (with vitreoretinal organization)
361.81
vitreous humor 379.21
Detergent asthma 507.8
Deterioration
epileptic
with behavioral disturbance 345.9 [294.11]
without behavioral disturbance
345.9 [294.10]
heart, cardiac (see also Degeneration,
myocardial) 429.1
mental (see also Psychosis) 298.9
myocardium, myocardial (see also
Degeneration, myocardial) 429.1
senile (simple) 797
transplanted organ — see Complications,
transplant, organ, by site
de Toni-Fanconi syndrome (cystinosis) 270.0
Deuteranomaly 368.52
Deuteranopia (anomalous trichromat) (complete)
(incomplete) 368.52
Deutschländer's disease — see Fracture, foot
Development
abnormal, bone 756.9
arrested 783.40
bone 733.91
child 783.40
due to malnutrition (protein-calorie) 263.2
fetus or newborn 764.9 ✓5ᵗʰ
tracheal rings (congenital) 748.3
defective, congenital — see also Anomaly
cauda equina 742.59
left ventricle 746.9
with atresia or hypoplasia of aortic orifice
or valve with hypoplasia of
ascending aorta 746.7
in hypoplastic left heart syndrome 746.7
delayed (see also Delay, development) 783.40
arithmetical skills 315.1
language (skills) 315.31
expressive 315.31
mixed receptive-expressive 315.32
learning skill, specified NEC 315.2
mixed skills 315.5
motor coordination 315.4
reading 315.00
specified
learning skill NEC 315.2
type NEC, except learning 315.8
speech 315.39
associated with hyperkinesia 314.1
phonological 315.39

Development — continued
delayed (see also Delay, development) —
continued
spelling 315.09
imperfect, congenital — see also Anomaly
heart 746.9
lungs 748.60
improper (fetus or newborn) 764.9 ✓5ᵗʰ
incomplete (fetus or newborn) 764.9 ✓5ᵗʰ
affecting management of pregnancy
656.5 ✓5ᵗʰ
bronchial tree 748.3
organ or site not listed — see Hypoplasia
respiratory system 748.9
sexual, precocious NEC 259.1
tardy, mental (see also Retardation, mental)
319
written expression 315.2
Developmental — see condition
Devergie's disease (pityriasis rubra pilaris) 696.4
Deviation
conjugate (eye) 378.87
palsy 378.81
spasm, spastic 378.82
esophagus 530.89
eye, skew 378.87
midline (jaw) (teeth) 524.2
specified site NEC — see Malposition
organ or site, congenital NEC — see
Malposition, congenital
septum (acquired) (nasal) 470
congenital 754.0
sexual 302.9
bestiality 302.9
coprophilia 302.89
ego-dystonic
homosexuality 302.0
lesbianism 302.0
erotomania 302.89
Clérambault's 297.8
exhibitionism (sexual) 302.4
fetishism 302.81
transvestic 302.3
frotteurism 302.89
homosexuality, ego-dystonic 302.0
pedophilic 302.2
lesbianism, ego-dystonic 302.0
masochism 302.83
narcissism 302.89
necrophilia 302.89
nymphomania 302.89
pederosis 302.2
pedophilia 302.2
sadism 302.84
sadomasochism 302.84
satyriasis 302.89
specified type NEC 302.89
transvestic fetishism 302.3
transvestism 302.3
voyeurism 302.82
zoophilia (erotica) 302.1
teeth, midline 524.2
trachea 519.1
ureter (congenital) 753.4
Devic's disease 341.0
Device
cerebral ventricle (communicating) in situ
V45.2
contraceptive — see Contraceptive, device
drainage, cerebrospinal fluid V45.2
Devil's
grip 074.1
pinches (purpura simplex) 287.2
Devitalized tooth 522.9
Devonshire colic 984.9
specified type of lead — see Table of Drugs and
Chemicals
Dextraposition, aorta 747.21
with ventricular septal defect, pulmonary
stenosis or atresia, and hypertrophy of
right ventricle 745.2
in tetralogy of Fallot 745.2
Dextratransposition, aorta 745.11
Dextrinosis, limit (debrancher enzyme deficiency)
271.0

Dextrocardia (corrected) (false) (isolated)
(secondary) (true) 746.87
with
complete transposition of viscera 759.3
situs inversus 759.3
Dextroversion, kidney (left) 753.3
Dhobie itch 110.3
Diabetes, diabetic (brittle) (congenital) (familial)
(mellitus) (severe) (slight) (without
complication) 250.0 ✓5ᵗʰ

> Note — Use the following fifth-digit
> subclassification with category 250:
>
> 0   type II [non-insulin dependent type]
>   [NIDDM type] [adult-onset type] or
>   unspecified type, not stated as
>   uncontrolled
>
> 1   type I [insulin dependent type]
>   [IDDM type] [juvenile type], not
>   stated as uncontrolled
>
> 2   type II [non-insulin dependent type]
>   [NIDDM type] [adult-onset type] or
>   unspecified type, uncontrolled
>
> 3   type I [insulin dependent type]
>   [IDDM] [juvenile type], uncontrolled

with
coma (with ketoacidosis) 250.3 ✓5ᵗʰ
hyperosmolar (nonketotic) 250.2 ✓5ᵗʰ
complication NEC 250.9 ✓5ᵗʰ
specified NEC 250.8 ✓5ᵗʰ
gangrene 250.7 ✓5ᵗʰ [785.4]
hyperosmolarity 250.2 ✓5ᵗʰ
ketosis, ketoacidosis 250.1 ✓5ᵗʰ
osteomyelitis 250.8 ✓5ᵗʰ [731.8]
specified manisfestations NEC 250.8 ✓5ᵗʰ
acetonemia 250.1 ✓5ᵗʰ
acidosis 250.1 ✓5ᵗʰ
amyotrophy 250.6 ✓5ᵗʰ [358.1]
angiopathy, peripheral 250.7 ✓5ᵗʰ [443.81]
asymptomatic 790.2
autonomic neuropathy (peripheral)
250.6 ✓5ᵗʰ [337.1]
bone change 250.8 ✓5ᵗʰ [731.8]
bronze, bronzed 275.0
cataract 250.5 ✓5ᵗʰ [366.41]
chemical 790.2
complicating pregnancy, childbirth, or
puerperium 648.8 ✓5ᵗʰ
coma (with ketoacidosis) 250.3 ✓5ᵗʰ
hyperglycemic 250.3 ✓5ᵗʰ
hyperosmolar (nonketotic) 250.2 ✓5ᵗʰ
hypoglycemic 250.3 ✓5ᵗʰ
insulin 250.3 ✓5ᵗʰ
complicating pregnancy, childbirth, or
puerperium (maternal) 648.0 ✓5ᵗʰ
affecting fetus or newborn 775.0
complication NEC 250.9 ✓5ᵗʰ
specified NEC 250.8 ✓5ᵗʰ
dorsal sclerosis 250.6 ✓5ᵗʰ [340] ✓5ᵗʰ
dwarfism-obesity syndrome 258.1
gangrene 250.7 ✓5ᵗʰ [785.4]
gastroparesis 250.6 ✓5ᵗʰ [536.3]
gestational 648.8 ✓5ᵗʰ
complicating pregnancy, childbirth, or
puerperium 648.8 ✓5ᵗʰ
glaucoma 250.5 ✓5ᵗʰ [365.44]
glomerulosclerosis (intercapillary)
250.4 ✓5ᵗʰ [581.81]
glycogenosis, secondary 250.8 ✓5ᵗʰ [259.8]
hemochromatosis 275.0
hyperosmolar coma 250.2 ✓5ᵗʰ
hyperosmolarity 250.2 ✓5ᵗʰ
hypertension-nephrosis syndrome
250.4 ✓5ᵗʰ [581.81]
hypoglycemia 250.8 ✓5ᵗʰ
hypoglycemic shock 250.8 ✓5ᵗʰ
insipidus 253.5
nephrogenic 588.1
pituitary 253.5
vasopressin-resistant 588.1
intercapillary glomerulosclerosis
250.4 ✓5ᵗʰ [581.81]
iritis 250.5 ✓5ᵗʰ [364.42]
ketosis, ketoacidosis 250.1 ✓5ᵗʰ

✓4ᵗʰ Fourth-digit Required   ✓5ᵗʰ Fifth-digit Required   ▶◀ Revised Text   ● New Line   ▲ Revised Code

Diabetes — Difficulty (vertical left margin)

Diabetes, diabetic — *continued*
  Kimmelstiel (-Wilson) disease or syndrome
    (intercapillary glomerulosclerosis)
    250.4 ✓5ᵗʰ *[581.81]*
  Lancereaux's (diabetes mellitus with marked
    emaciation) 250.8 ✓5ᵗʰ *[261]*
  latent (chemical) 790.2
    complicating pregnancy, childbirth, or
      puerperium 648. ✓5ᵗʰ
  lipoidosis 250.8 ✓5ᵗʰ *[272.7]*
  macular edema 250.5 ✓5ᵗʰ *[362.01]*
  maternal
    with manifest disease in the infant 775.1
    affecting fetus or newborn 775.0
  microaneurysms, retinal 250.5 ✓5ᵗʰ *[362.01]*
  mononeuropathy 250.6 ✓5ᵗʰ *[355.9]*
  neonatal, transient 775.1
  nephropathy 250.4 ✓5ᵗʰ *[583.81]*
  nephrosis (syndrome) 250.4 ✓5ᵗʰ *[581.81]*
  neuralgia 250.6 ✓5ᵗʰ *[357.2]*
  neuritis 250.6 ✓5ᵗʰ *[357.2]*
  neurogenic arthropathy 250.6 ✓5ᵗʰ *[713.5]*
  neuropathy 250.6 ✓5ᵗʰ *[357.2]*
  nonclinical 790.2
  osteomyelitis 250.8 ✓5ᵗʰ *[731.8]*
  peripheral autonomic neuropathy
    250.6 ✓5ᵗʰ *[337.1]*
  phosphate 275.3
  polyneuropathy 250.6 ✓5ᵗʰ *[357.2]*
  renal (true) 271.4
  retinal
    edema 250.5 ✓5ᵗʰ *[362.01]*
    hemorrhage 250.5 ✓5ᵗʰ *[362.01]*
    microaneurysms 250.5 ✓5ᵗʰ *[362.01]*
  retinitis 250.5 ✓5ᵗʰ *[362.01]*
  retinopathy 250.5 ✓5ᵗʰ *[362.01]*
    background 250.5 ✓5ᵗʰ *[362.01]*
    proliferative 250.5 ✓5ᵗʰ *[362.02]*
  steroid induced
    correct substance properly administered
      251.8
    overdose or wrong substance given or taken
      962.0
  stress 790.2
  subclinical 790.2
  subliminal 790.2
  sugar 250.0 ✓5ᵗʰ
  ulcer (skin) 250.8 ✓5ᵗʰ *[707.9]*
    lower extremity 250.8 ✓5ᵗʰ *[707.10]*
      ankle 250.8 *[707.13]*
      calf 250.8 *[707.12]*
      foot 250.8 *[707.15]*
      heel 250.8 *[707.14]*
      knee 250.8 *[707.19]*
      specified site NEC 250.8 *[707.19]*
      thigh 250.8 *[707.11]*
      toes 250.8 *[707.15]*
    specified site NEC 250.8 ✓5ᵗʰ *[707.8]*
  xanthoma 250.8 ✓5ᵗʰ *[272.2]*
Diacyclothrombopathia 287.1
Diagnosis deferred 799.9
Dialysis (intermittent) (treatment)
  anterior retinal (juvenile) (with detachment)
    361.04
  extracorporeal V56.0
  peritoneal V56.8
  renal V56.0
    status only V45.1
  specified type NEC V56.8
Diamond-Blackfan anemia or syndrome
  (congenital hypoplastic anemia) 284.0
Diamond-Gardener syndrome (autoerythrocyte
  sensitization) 287.2
Diaper rash 691.0
Diaphoresis (excessive) NEC 780.8
Diaphragm — *see* condition
Diaphragmalgia 786.52
Diaphragmitis 519.4
Diaphyseal aclasis 756.4
Diaphysitis 733.99

Diarrhea, diarrheal (acute) (autumn) (bilious)
  (bloody) (catarrhal) (choleraic) (chronic)
  (gravis) (green) (infantile) (lienteric)
  (noninfectious) (presumed noninfectious)
  (putrefactive) (secondary) (sporadic)
  (summer) (symptomatic) (thermic) 787.91
  achlorhydric 536.0
  allergic 558.3
  amebic (*see also* Amebiasis) 006.9
    with abscess — *see* Abscess, amebic
    acute 006.0
    chronic 006.1
    nondysenteric 006.2
  bacillary — *see* Dysentery, bacillary
  bacterial NEC 008.5
  balantidial — 007.0
  bile salt-induced 579.8
  cachectic NEC 787.91
  chilomastix 007.8
  choleriformis 001.1
  coccidial 007.2
  Cochin-China 579.1
    anguilluliasis 127.2
    psilosis 579.1
  Dientamoeba 007.8
  dietetic 787.91
  due to
    achylia gastrica 536.8
    Aerobacter aerogenes 008.2 ✓5ᵗʰ
    Bacillus coli — *see* Enteritis, E. coli
    bacteria NEC 008.5
    bile salts 579.8
    Capillaria
      hepatica 128.8
      philippinensis 127.5
    Clostridium perfringens (C) (F) 008.46
    Enterobacter aerogenes 008.2 ✓5ᵗʰ
    enterococci 008.49
    Escherichia coli — *see* Enteritis, E. coli
    Giardia lamblia 007.1
    Heterophyes heterophyes 121.6
    irritating foods 787.91
    Metagonimus yokogawai 121.5
    Necator americanus 126.1
    Paracolobactrum arizonae 008.1
    Paracolon bacillus NEC 008.47
      Arizona 008.1
    Proteus (bacillus) (mirabilis) (Morganii) 008.3
    Pseudomonas aeruginosa 008.42
    S. japonicum 120.2
    specified organism NEC 008.8
      bacterial 008.49
      viral NEC 008.69
    Staphylococcus 008.41
    Streptococcus 008.49
      anaerobic 008.46
    Strongyloides stercoralis 127.2
    Trichuris trichiuria 127.3
    virus NEC (*see also* Enteritis, viral) 008.69
  dysenteric 009.2
    due to specified organism NEC 008.8
  dyspeptic 787.91
  endemic 009.3
    due to specified organism NEC 008.8
  epidemic 009.2
    due to specified organism NEC 008.8
  fermentative 787.91
  flagellate 007.9
  Flexner's (ulcerative) 004.1
  functional 564.5
    following gastrointestinal surgery 564.4
    psychogenic 306.4
  giardial 007.1
  Giardia lamblia 007.1
  hill 579.1
  hyperperistalsis (nervous) 306.4
  infectious 009.2
    due to specified organism NEC 008.8
    presumed 009.3
  inflammatory 787.91
    due to specified organism NEC 008.8
  malarial (*see also* Malaria) 084.6
  mite 133.8
  mycotic 117.9
  nervous 306.4
  neurogenic 564.5
  parenteral NEC 009.2

Diarrhea, diarrheal — *continued*
  postgastrectomy 564.4
  postvagotomy 564.4
  prostaglandin induced 579.8
  protozoal NEC 007.9
  psychogenic 306.4
  septic 009.2
    due to specified organism NEC 008.8
  specified organism NEC 008.8
    bacterial 008.49
    viral NEC 008.69
  Staphylococcus 008.41
  Streptococcus 008.49
    anaerobic 008.46
  toxic 558.2
  travelers' 009.2
    due to specified organism NEC 008.8
  trichomonal 007.3
  tropical 579.1
  tuberculous 014.8 ✓5ᵗʰ
  ulcerative (chronic) (*see also* Colitis, ulcerative)
    556.9
  viral (*see also* Enteritis, viral) 008.8
  zymotic NEC 009.2
Diastasis
  cranial bones 733.99
    congenital 756.0
  joint (traumatic) — *see* Dislocation, by site
  muscle 728.84
    congenital 756.89
  recti (abdomen) 728.84
    complicating delivery 665.8 ✓5ᵗʰ
    congenital 756.79
Diastema, teeth, tooth 524.3
Diastematomyelia 742.51
Diathesis
  allergic V15.09
  bleeding (familial) 287.9
  cystine (familial) 270.0
  gouty 274.9
  hemorrhagic (familial) 287.9
    newborn NEC 776.0
  oxalic 271.8
  scrofulous (*see also* Tuberculosis) 017.2 ✓5ᵗʰ
  spasmophilic (*see also* Tetany) 781.7
  ulcer 536.9
  uric acid 274.9
Diaz's disease or osteochondrosis 732.5
Dibothriocephaliasis 123.4
  larval 123.5
Dibothriocephalus (infection) (infestation) (latus)
  123.4
  larval 123.5
Dicephalus 759.4
Dichotomy, teeth 520.2
Dichromat, dichromata (congenital) 368.59
Dichromatopsia (congenital) 368.59
Dichuchwa 104.0
Dicroceliasis 121.8
Didelphys, didelphic (*see also* Double uterus)
  752.2
Didymitis (*see also* Epididymitis) 604.90
Died — *see also* Death
  without
    medical attention (cause unknown) 798.9
    sign of disease 798.2
Dientamoeba diarrhea 007.8
Dietary
  inadequacy or deficiency 269.9
  surveillance and counseling V65.3
Dietl's crisis 593.4
Dieulafoy ▶lesion (hemorrhagic)◀
  of
    duodenum 537.84
    intestine 569.86
    stomach 537.84
Difficult
  birth, affecting fetus or newborn 763.9
  delivery NEC 669.9 ✓5ᵗʰ
Difficulty
  feeding 783.3
    breast 676.8 ✓5ᵗʰ

Difficulty — *continued*
feeding — *continued*
newborn 779.3
nonorganic (infant) NEC 307.59
mechanical, gastroduodenal stoma 537.89
reading 315.00
specific, spelling 315.09
swallowing (*see also* Dysphagia) 787.2
walking 719.7 ☑5ᵗʰ

Diffuse — *see* condition

Diffused ganglion 727.42

DiGeorge's syndrome (thymic hypoplasia) 279.11

Digestive — *see* condition

Di Guglielmo's disease or syndrome (M9841/3) 207.0 ☑5ᵗʰ

Diktyoma (M9051/3) — *see* Neoplasm, by site, malignant

Dilaceration, tooth 520.4

Dilatation
anus 564.89
venule — *see* Hemorrhoids
aorta (focal) (general) (*see also* Aneurysm, aorta) 441.9
congenital 747.29
infectional 093.0
ruptured 441.5
syphilitic 093.0
appendix (cystic) 543.9
artery 447.8
bile duct (common) (cystic) (congenital) 751.69
acquired 576.8
bladder (sphincter) 596.8
congenital 753.8
in pregnancy or childbirth 654.4 ☑5ᵗʰ
causing obstructed labor 660.2 ☑5ᵗʰ
affecting fetus or newborn 763.1
blood vessel 459.89
bronchus, bronchi 494.0
with acute exacerbation 494.1
calyx (due to obstruction) 593.89
capillaries 448.9
cardiac (acute) (chronic) (*see also* Hypertrophy, cardiac) 429.3
congenital 746.89
valve NEC 746.89
pulmonary 746.09
hypertensive (*see also* Hypertension, heart) 402.90
cavum septi pellucidi 742.4
cecum 564.89
psychogenic 306.4
cervix (uteri) — *see also* Incompetency, cervix
incomplete, poor, slow
affecting fetus or newborn 763.7
complicating delivery 661.0 ☑5ᵗʰ
affecting fetus or newborn 763.7
colon 564.7
congenital 751.3
due to mechanical obstruction 560.89
psychogenic 306.4
common bile duct (congenital) 751.69
acquired 576.8
with calculus, choledocholithiasis, or stones — *see* Choledocholithiasis
cystic duct 751.69
acquired (any bile duct) 575.8
duct, mammary 610.4
duodenum 564.89
esophagus 530.89
congenital 750.4
due to
achalasia 530.0
cardiospasm 530.0
Eustachian tube, congenital 744.24
fontanel 756.0
gallbladder 575.8
congenital 751.69
gastric 536.8
acute 536.1
psychogenic 306.4
heart (acute) (chronic) (*see also* Hypertrophy, cardiac) 429.3
congenital 746.89
hypertensive (*see also* Hypertension, heart) 402.90

Dilatation — *continued*
heart (*see also* Hypertrophy, cardiac) — *continued*
valve — *see also* Endocarditis
congenital 746.89
ileum 564.89
psychogenic 306.4
inguinal rings — *see* Hernia, inguinal
jejunum 564.89
psychogenic 306.4
kidney (calyx) (collecting structures) (cystic) (parenchyma) (pelvis) 593.89
lacrimal passages 375.69
lymphatic vessel 457.1
mammary duct 610.4
Meckel's diverticulum (congenital) 751.0
meningeal vessels, congenital 742.8
myocardium (acute) (chronic) (*see also* Hypertrophy, cardiac) 429.3
organ or site, congenital NEC — *see* Distortion
pancreatic duct 577.8
pelvis, kidney 593.89
pericardium — *see* Pericarditis
pharynx 478.29
prostate 602.8
pulmonary
artery (idiopathic) 417.8
congenital 747.3
valve, congenital 746.09
pupil 379.43
rectum 564.89
renal 593.89
saccule vestibularis, congenital 744.05
salivary gland (duct) 527.8
sphincter ani 564.89
stomach 536.8
acute 536.1
psychogenic 306.4
submaxillary duct 527.8
trachea, congenital 748.3
ureter (idiopathic) 593.89
congenital 753.20
due to obstruction 593.5
urethra (acquired) 599.84
vasomotor 443.9
vein 459.89
ventricular, ventricle (acute) (chronic) (*see also* Hypertrophy, cardiac) 429.3
cerebral, congenital 742.4
hypertensive (*see also* Hypertension, heart) 402.90
venule 459.89
anus — *see* Hemorrhoids
vesical orifice 596.8

Dilated, dilation — *see* Dilatation

Diminished
hearing (acuity) (*see also* Deafness) 389.9
pulse pressure 785.9
vision NEC 369.9
vital capacity 794.2

Diminuta taenia 123.6

Diminution, sense or sensation (cold) (heat) (tactile) (vibratory) (*see also* Disturbance, sensation) 782.0

Dimitri-Sturge-Weber disease (encephalocutaneous angiomatosis) 759.6

Dimple
parasacral 685.1
with abscess 685.0
pilonidal 685.1
with abscess 685.0
postanal 685.1
with abscess 685.0

Dioctophyma renale (infection) (infestation) 128.8

Dipetalonemiasis 125.4

Diphallus 752.69

Diphtheria, diphtheritic (gangrenous) (hemorrhagic) 032.9
carrier (suspected) of V02.4
cutaneous 032.85
cystitis 032.84
faucial 032.0
infection of wound 032.85
inoculation (anti) (not sick) V03.5
laryngeal 032.3
myocarditis 032.82

Diphtheria, diphtheritic — *continued*
nasal anterior 032.2
nasopharyngeal 032.1
neurological complication 032.89
peritonitis 032.83
specified site NEC 032.89

Diphyllobothriasis (intestine) 123.4
larval 123.5

Diplacusis 388.41

Diplegia (upper limbs) 344.2
brain or cerebral 437.8
congenital 343.0
facial 351.0
congenital 352.6
infantile or congenital (cerebral) (spastic) (spinal) 343.0
lower limbs 344.1
syphilitic, congenital 090.49

Diplococcus, diplococcal — *see* condition

Diplomyelia 742.59

Diplopia 368.2
refractive 368.15

Dipsomania (*see also* Alcoholism) 303.9 ☑5ᵗʰ
with psychosis (*see also* Psychosis, alcoholic) 291.9

Dipylidiasis 123.8
intestine 123.8

Direction, teeth, abnormal 524.3

Dirt-eating child 307.52

Disability
heart — *see* Disease, heart
learning NEC 315.2
special spelling 315.09

Disarticulation (*see also* Derangement, joint) 718.9 ☑5ᵗʰ
meaning
amputation
status — *see* Absence, by site
traumatic — *see* Amputation, traumatic
dislocation, traumatic or congenital — *see* Dislocation

Disaster, cerebrovascular (*see also* Disease, cerebrovascular, acute) 436

Discharge
anal NEC 787.99
breast (female) (male) 611.79
conjunctiva 372.89
continued locomotor idiopathic (*see also* Epilepsy) 345.5 ☑5ᵗʰ
diencephalic autonomic idiopathic (*see also* Epilepsy) 345.5 ☑5ᵗʰ
ear 388.60
blood 388.69
cerebrospinal fluid 388.61
excessive urine 788.42
eye 379.93
nasal 478.1
nipple 611.79
patterned motor idiopathic (*see also* Epilepsy) 345.5 ☑5ᵗʰ
penile 788.7
postnasal — *see* Sinusitis
sinus, from mediastinum 510.0
umbilicus 789.9
urethral 788.7
bloody 599.84
vaginal 623.5

Discitis 722.90
cervical, cervicothoracic 722.91
lumbar, lumbosacral 722.93
thoracic, thoracolumbar 722.92

Discogenic syndrome — *see* Displacement, intervertebral disc

Discoid
kidney 753.3
meniscus, congenital 717.5
semilunar cartilage 717.5

Discoloration
mouth 528.9
nails 703.8
teeth 521.7
due to
drugs 521.7

Discoloration — Disease

Discoloration — *continued*
  teeth — *continued*
    due to — *continued*
      metals (copper) (silver) 521.7
      pulpal bleeding 521.7
    during formation 520.8
    posteruptive 521.7
Discomfort
  chest 786.59
  visual 368.13
Discomycosis — *see* Actinomycosis
Discontinuity, ossicles, ossicular chain 385.23
Discrepancy
  leg length (acquired) 736.81
    congenital 755.30
  uterine size-date 646.8 ✓5ᵗʰ
Discrimination
  political V62.4
  racial V62.4
  religious V62.4
  sex V62.4   *
Disease, diseased — *see also* Syndrome
  Abrami's (acquired hemolytic jaundice) 283.9
  absorbent system 459.89
  accumulation — *see* Thesaurismosis
  acid-peptic 536.8
  Acosta's 993.2
  Adams-Stokes (-Morgagni) (syncope with heart
    block) 426.9
  Addison's (bronze) (primary adrenal
    insufficiency) 255.4
    anemia (pernicious) 281.0
    tuberculous (*see also* Tuberculosis)
      017.6 ✓5ᵗʰ
  Addison-Gull — *see* Xanthoma
  adenoids (and tonsils) (chronic) 474.9
  adrenal (gland) (capsule) (cortex) 255.9
    hyperfunction 255.3
    hypofunction 255.4
    specified type NEC 255.8
  ainhum (dactylolysis spontanea) 136.0
  akamushi (scrub typhus) 081.2
  Akureyri (epidemic neuromyasthenia) 049.8
  Albarrán's (colibacilluria) 791.9
  Albers-Schönberg's (marble bones) 756.52
  Albert's 726.71
  Albright (-Martin) (-Bantam) 275.49
  Alibert's (mycosis fungoides) (M9700/3)
    202.1 ✓5ᵗʰ
  Alibert-Bazin (M9700/3) 202.1 ✓5ᵗʰ
  alimentary canal 569.9
  alligator skin (ichthyosis congenita) 757.1
    acquired 701.1
  Almeida's (Brazilian blastomycosis) 116.1
  Alpers' 330.8
  alpine 993.2
  altitude 993.2
  alveoli, teeth 525.9
  Alzheimer's — *see* Alzheimer's
  amyloid (any site) 277.3
  anarthritic rheumatoid 446.5
  Anders' (adiposis tuberosa simplex) 272.8
  Andersen's (glycogenosis IV) 271.0
  Anderson's (angiokeratoma corporis diffusum)
    272.7
  Andes 993.2
  Andrews' (bacterid) 686.8
  angiospastic, angiospasmodic 443.9
    cerebral 435.9
      with transient neurologic deficit 435.9
    vein 459.89
  anterior
    chamber 364.9
    horn cell 335.9
      specified type NEC 335.8
  antral (chronic) 473.0
    acute 461.0
  anus NEC 569.49
  aorta (nonsyphilitic) 447.9
    syphilitic NEC 093.89
  aortic (heart) (valve) (*see also* Endocarditis,
    aortic) 424.1
  apollo 077.4
  aponeurosis 726.90
  appendix 543.9
  aqueous (chamber) 364.9

Disease, diseased — *see also* Syndrome —
    continued
  arc-welders' lung 503
  Armenian 277.3
  Arnold-Chiari (*see also* Spina bifida) 741.0 ✓5ᵗʰ
  arterial 447.9
    occlusive (*see also* Occlusion, by site)
      444.22
      with embolus or thrombus — *see*
        Occlusion, by site
      due to stricture or stenosis 447.1
    specified type NEC 447.8
  arteriocardiorenal (*see also* Hypertension,
    cardiorenal) 404.90
  arteriolar (generalized) (obliterative) 447.9
    specified type NEC 447.8
  arteriorenal — *see* Hypertension, kidney
  arteriosclerotic — *see also* Arteriosclerosis
    cardiovascular 429.2
    coronary — *see* Arteriosclerosis, coronary
    heart — *see* Arteriosclerosis, coronary
    vascular — *see* Arteriosclerosis
  artery 447.9
    cerebral 437.9
    coronary — *see* Arteriosclerosis, coronary
    specified type NEC 447.8
  arthropod-borne NEC 088.9
    specified type NEC 088.8
  Asboe-Hansen's (incontinentia pigmenti) 757.33
  atticoantral, chronic (with posterior or superior
    marginal perforation of ear drum) 382.2
  auditory canal, ear 380.9
  Aujeszky's 078.89
  auricle, ear NEC 380.30
  Australian X 062.4
  autoimmune NEC 279.4
    hemolytic (cold type) (warm type) 283.0
    parathyroid 252.1
    thyroid 245.2
  aviators' (*see also* Effect, adverse, high altitude)
    993.2
  ax(e)-grinders' 502
  Ayala's 756.89
  Ayerza's (pulmonary artery sclerosis with
    pulmonary hypertension) 416.0
  Azorean (of the nervous system) 334.8
  Babington's (familial hemorrhagic
    telangiectasia) 448.0
  back bone NEC 733.90
  bacterial NEC 040.89
    zoonotic NEC 027.9
    specified type NEC 027.8
  Baehr-Schiffrin (thrombotic thrombocytopenic
    purpura) 446.6
  Baelz's (cheilitis glandularis apostematosa)
    528.5
  Baerensprung's (eczema marginatum) 110.3
  Balfour's (chloroma) 205.3 ✓5ᵗʰ
  balloon (*see also* Effect, adverse, high altitude)
    993.2
  Baló's 341.1
  Bamberger (-Marie) (hypertrophic pulmonary
    osteoarthropathy) 731.2
  Bang's (Brucella abortus) 023.1
  Bannister's 995.1
  Banti's (with cirrhosis) (with portal
    hypertension) — *see* Cirrhosis, liver
  Barcoo (*see also* Ulcer, skin) 707.9
  barium lung 503
  Barlow (-Möller) (infantile scurvy) 267
  barometer makers' 985.0
  Barraquer (-Simons) (progressive lipodystrophy)
    272.6
  basal ganglia 333.90
    degenerative NEC 333.0
    specified NEC 333.89
  Basedow's (exophthalmic goiter) 242.0 ✓5ᵗʰ
  basement membrane NEC 583.89
    with
      pulmonary hemorrhage (Goodpasture's
        syndrome) 446.21 [583.81]
  Bateman's 078.0
    purpura (senile) 287.2
  Batten's 330.1 [362.71]
  Batten-Mayou (retina) 330.1 [362.71]
  Batten-Steinert 359.2
  Battey 031.0

Disease, diseased — *see also* Syndrome —
    continued
  Baumgarten-Cruveilhier (cirrhosis of liver)
    571.5
  bauxite-workers' 503
  Bayle's (dementia paralytica) 094.1
  Bazin's (primary) (*see also* Tuberculosis)
    017.1 ✓5ᵗʰ
  Beard's (neurasthenia) 300.5
  Beau's (*see also* Degeneration, myocardial)
    429.1
  Bechterew's (ankylosing spondylitis) 720.0
  Becker's (idiopathic mural endomyocardial
    disease) 425.2
  Begbie's (exophthalmic goiter) 242.0 ✓5ᵗʰ
  Behr's 362.50
  Beigel's (white piedra) 111.2
  Bekhterev's (ankylosing spondylitis) 720.0
  Bell's (*see also* Psychosis, affective) 296.0 ✓5ᵗʰ
  Bennett's (leukemia) 208.9 ✓5ᵗʰ
  Benson's 379.22
  Bergeron's (hysteroepilepsy) 300.11
  Berlin's 921.3
  Bernard-Soulier (thrombopathy) 287.1
  Bernhardt (-Roth) 355.1
  beryllium 503
  Besnier-Boeck (-Schaumann) (sarcoidosis) 135
  Best's 362.76
  Beurmann's (sporotrichosis) 117.1
  Bielschowsky (-Jansky) 330.1
  Biermer's (pernicious anemia) 281.0
  Biett's (discoid lupus erythematosus) 695.4
  bile duct (*see also* Disease, biliary) 576.9
  biliary (duct) (tract) 576.9
    with calculus, choledocholithiasis, or stones
      — *see* Choledocholithiasis
  Billroth's (meningocele) (*see also* Spina bifida)
    741.9 ✓5ᵗʰ
  Binswanger's 290.12
  Bird's (oxaluria) 271.8
  bird fanciers' 495.2
  black lung 500
  bladder 596.9
    specified NEC 596.8
  bleeder's 286.0
  Bloch-Sulzberger (incontinentia pigmenti)
    757.33
  Blocq's (astasia-abasia) 307.9
  blood (-forming organs) 289.9
    specified NEC 289.8
    vessel 459.9
  Bloodgood's 610.1
  Blount's (tibia vara) 732.4
  blue 746.9
  Bodechtel-Guttmann (subacute sclerosing
    panencephalitis) 046.2
  Boeck's (sarcoidosis) 135
  bone 733.90
    fibrocystic NEC 733.29
      jaw 526.2
    marrow 289.9
    Paget's (osteitis deformans) 731.0
    specified type NEC 733.99
    von Rechlinghausen's (osteitis fibrosa
      cystica) 252.0
  Bonfils' — *see* Disease, Hodgkin's
  Borna 062.9
  Bornholm (epidemic pleurodynia) 074.1
  Bostock's (*see also* Fever, hay) 477.9
  Bouchard's (myopathic dilatation of the
    stomach) 536.1
  Bouillaud's (rheumatic heart disease) 391.9
  Bourneville (-Brissaud) (tuberous sclerosis)
    759.5
  Bouveret (-Hoffmann) (paroxysmal tachycardia)
    427.2
  bowel 569.9
    functional 564.9
      psychogenic 306.4
  Bowen's (M8081/2) — *see* Neoplasm, skin, in
    situ
  Bozzolo's (multiple myeloma) (M973/3)
    203.0 ✓5ᵗʰ
  Bradley's (epidemic vomiting) 078.82
  Brailsford's 732.3
    radius, head 732.3
    tarsal, scaphoid 732.5

Disease, diseased — *see also* Syndrome —
continued
  Brailsford-Morquio (mucopolysaccharidosis IV)
    277.5
  brain 348.9
    Alzheimer's 331.0
      with dementia — *see* Alzheimer's,
        dementia
    arterial, artery 437.9
    arteriosclerotic 437.0
    congenital 742.9
    degenerative — *see* Degeneration, brain
    inflammatory — *see also* Encephalitis
      late effect — *see* category 326
    organic 348.9
      arteriosclerotic 437.0
    parasitic NEC 123.9
    Pick's 331.1
      with dementia
        with behavioral disturbance
          331.1 [294.11]
        without behavioral disturbance
          331.1 [294.10]
    senile 331.2
  brazier's 985.8
  breast 611.9
    cystic (chronic) 610.1
    fibrocystic 610.1
    inflammatory 611.0
    Paget's (M8540/3) 174.0
    puerperal, postpartum NEC 676.3 ✓5th
    specified NEC 611.8
  Breda's (*see also* Yaws) 102.9
  Breisky's (kraurosis vulvae) 624.0
  Bretonneau's (diphtheritic malignant angina)
    032.0
  Bright's (*see also* Nephritis) 583.9
    arteriosclerotic (*see also* Hypertension,
      kidney) 403.90
  Brill's (recrudescent typhus) 081.1
    flea-borne 081.0
    louse-borne 081.1
  Brill-Symmers (follicular lymphoma) (M9690/3)
    202.0 ✓5th
  Brill-Zinsser (recrudescent typhus) 081.1
  Brinton's (leather bottle stomach) (M8142/3)
    151.9
  Brion-Kayser (*see also* Fever, paratyphoid)
    002.9
  broad
    beta 272.2
    ligament, noninflammatory 620.9
      specified NEC 620.8
  Brocq's 691.8
    meaning
      atopic (diffuse) neurodermatitis 691.8
      dermatitis herpetiformis 694.0
      lichen simplex chronicus 698.3
      parapsoriasis 696.2
      prurigo 698.2
  Brocq-Duhring (dermatitis herpetiformis) 694.0
  Brodie's (joint) (*see also* Osteomyelitis)
    730.1 ✓5th
  bronchi 519.1
  bronchopulmonary 519.1
  bronze (Addison's) 255.4
    tuberculous (*see also* Tuberculosis)
      017.6 ✓5th
  Brown-Séquard 344.89
  Bruck's 733.99
  Bruck-de Lange (Amsterdam dwarf, mental
    retardation and brachycephaly) 759.89
  Bruhl's (splenic anemia with fever) 285.8
  Bruton's (X-linked agammaglobulinemia)
    279.04
  buccal cavity 528.9
  Buchanan's (juvenile osteochondrosis, iliac
    crest) 732.1
  Buchman's (osteochondrosis juvenile) 732.1
  Budgerigar-fanciers' 495.2
  Büdinger-Ludloff-Läwen 717.89
  Buerger's (thromboangiitis obliterans) 443.1
  Bürger-Grütz (essential familial hyperlipemia)
    272.3
  Burns' (lower ulna) 732.3
  bursa 727.9
  Bury's (erythema elevatum diutinum) 695.89

Disease, diseased — *see also* Syndrome —
continued
  Buschke's 710.1
  Busquet's (*see also* Osteomyelitis) 730.1 ✓5th
  Busse-Buschke (cryptococcosis) 117.5
  C_2 (*see also* Alcoholism) 303.9 ✓5th
  Caffey's (infantile cortical hyperostosis) 756.59
  caisson 993.3
  calculous 592.9
  California 114.0
  Calvé (-Perthes) (osteochondrosis, femoral
    capital) 732.1
  Camurati-Engelmann (diaphyseal sclerosis)
    756.59
  Canavan's 330.0
  capillaries 448.9
  Carapata 087.1
  cardiac — *see* Disease, heart
  cardiopulmonary, chronic 416.9
  cardiorenal (arteriosclerotic) (hepatic)
    (hypertensive) (vascular) (*see also*
    Hypertension, cardiorenal) 404.90
  cardiovascular (arteriosclerotic) 429.2
    congenital 746.9
    hypertensive (*see also* Hypertension, heart)
      402.90
      benign 402.10
      malignant 402.00
    renal (*see also* Hypertension, cardiorenal)
      404.90
    syphilitic (asymptomatic) 093.9
  carotid gland 259.8
  Carrión's (Bartonellosis) 088.0
  cartilage NEC 733.90
    specified NEC 733.99
  Castellani's 104.8
  cat-scratch 078.3
  Cavare's (familial periodic paralysis) 359.3
  Cazenave's (pemphigus) 694.4
  cecum 569.9
  celiac (adult) 579.0
    infantile 579.0
  cellular tissue NEC 709.9
  central core 359.0
  cerebellar, cerebellum — *see* Disease, brain
  cerebral (*see also* Disease, brain) 348.9
    arterial, artery 437.9
    degenerative — *see* Degeneration, brain
  cerebrospinal 349.9
  cerebrovascular NEC 437.9
    acute 436
      embolic — *see* Embolism, brain
      late effect — *see* Late effect(s) (of)
        cerebrovascular disease
      puerperal, postpartum, childbirth
        674.0 ✓5th
      thrombotic — *see* Thrombosis, brain
    arteriosclerotic 437.0
    embolic — *see* Embolism, brain
    ischemic, generalized NEC 437.1
    late effect — *see* Late effect(s) (of)
      cerebrovascular disease
    occlusive 437.1
    puerperal, postpartum, childbirth 674.0 ✓5th
    specified type NEC 437.8
    thrombotic — *see* Thrombosis, brain
  ceroid storage 272.7
  cervix (uteri)
    inflammatory 616.9
      specified NEC 616.8
    noninflammatory 622.9
      specified NEC 622.8
  Chabert's 022.9
  Chagas' (*see also* Trypanosomiasis, American)
    086.2
  Chandler's (osteochondritis dissecans, hip)
    732.7
  Charcots' (joint) 094.0 [713.5]
    spinal cord 094.0
  Charcôt-Marie-Tooth 356.1
  Charlouis' (*see also* Yaws) 102.9
  Cheadle (-Möller) (-Barlow) (infantile scurvy)
    267
  Chédiak-Steinbrinck (-Higashi) (congenital
    gigantism of peroxidase granules) 288.2
  cheek, inner 528.9
  chest 519.9

Disease, diseased — *see also* Syndrome —
continued
  Chiari's (hepatic vein thrombosis) 453.0
  Chicago (North American blastomycosis) 116.0
  chignon (white piedra) 111.2
  chigoe, chigo (jigger) 134.1
  childhood granulomatous 288.1
  Chinese liver fluke 121.1
  chlamydial NEC 078.88
  cholecystic (*see also* Disease, gallbladder) 575.9
  choroid 363.9
    degenerative (*see also* Degeneration, choroid)
      363.40
    hereditary (*see also* Dystrophy, choroid)
      363.50
    specified type NEC 363.8
  Christian's (chronic histiocytosis X) 277.8
  Christian-Weber (nodular nonsuppurative
    panniculitis) 729.30
  Christmas 286.1
  ciliary body 364.9
  circulatory (system) NEC 459.9
    chronic, maternal, affecting fetus or
      newborn 760.3
    specified NEC 459.89
    syphilitic 093.9
      congenital 090.5
  Civatte's (poikiloderma) 709.09
  climacteric 627.2
    male 608.89
  coagulation factor deficiency (congenital) (*see
    also* Defect, coagulation) 286.9
  Coats' 362.12
  coccidioidal pulmonary 114.5
    acute 114.0
    chronic 114.4
    primary 114.0
    residual 114.4
  Cockayne's (microcephaly and dwarfism)
    759.89
  Cogan's 370.52
  cold
    agglutinin 283.0
      or hemoglobinuria 283.0
        paroxysmal (cold) (nocturnal) 283.2
    hemagglutinin (chronic) 283.0
  collagen NEC 710.9
    nonvascular 710.9
    specified NEC 710.8
    vascular (allergic) (*see also* Angiitis,
      hypersensitivity) 446.20
  colon 569.9
    functional 564.9
      congenital 751.3
    ischemic 557.0
  combined system (of spinal cord) 266.2 [336.2]
    with anemia (pernicious) 281.0 [336.2]
  compressed air 993.3
  Concato's (pericardial polyserositis) 423.2
    peritoneal 568.82
    pleural — *see* Pleurisy
  congenital NEC 799.8
  conjunctiva 372.9
    chlamydial 077.98
      specified NEC 077.8
    specified type NEC 372.89
    viral 077.99
      specified NEC 077.8
  connective tissue, diffuse (*see also* Disease,
    collagen) 710.9
  Conor and Bruch's (boutonneuse fever) 082.1
  Conradi (-Hünermann) 756.59
  Cooley's (erythroblastic anemia) 282.4
  Cooper's 610.1
  Corbus' 607.1
  cork-handlers' 495.3
  cornea (*see also* Keratopathy) 371.9
  coronary (*see also* Ischemia, heart) 414.9
    congenital 746.85
    ostial, syphilitic 093.20
      aortic 093.22
      mitral 093.21
      pulmonary 093.24
      tricuspid 093.23
  Corrigan's — *see* Insufficiency, aortic
  Cotugno's 724.3
  Coxsackie (virus) NEC 074.8

Disease — Disease

Disease, diseased — *see also* Syndrome — *continued*
cranial nerve NEC 352.9
Creutzfeldt-Jakob 046.1
  with dementia
    with behavioral disturbance
      046.1 [294.11]
    without behavioral disturbance
      046.1 [294.10]
Crigler-Najjar (congenital hyperbilirubinemia)
  277.4
Crocq's (acrocyanosis) 443.89
Crohn's (intestine) (*see also* Enteritis, regional)
  555.9
Crouzon's (craniofacial dysostosis) 756.0
Cruchet's (encephalitis lethargica) 049.8
Cruveilhier's 335.21
Cruz-Chagas (*see also* Trypanosomiasis,
  American) 086.2
crystal deposition (*see also* Arthritis, due to,
  crystals) 712.9 ✓5ᵗʰ
Csillag's (lichen sclerosus et atrophicus) 701.0
Curschmann's 359.2
Cushing's (pituitary basophilism) 255.0
cystic
  breast (chronic) 610.1
  kidney, congenital (*see also* Cystic, disease,
    kidney) 753.10
  liver, congenital 751.62
  lung 518.89
    congenital 748.4
  pancreas 577.2
    congenital 751.7
  renal, congenital (*see also* Cystic, disease,
    kidney) 753.10
  semilunar cartilage 717.5
cysticercus 123.1
cystine storage (with renal sclerosis) 270.0
cytomegalic inclusion (generalized) 078.5
  with
    pneumonia 078.5 [484.1]
  congenital 771.1
Daae (-Finsen) (epidemic pleurodynia) 074.1
dancing 297.8
Danielssen's (anesthetic leprosy) 030.1
Darier's (congenital) (keratosis follicularis)
  757.39
  erythema annulare centrifugum 695.0
  vitamin A deficiency 264.8
Darling's (histoplasmosis) (*see also*
  Histoplasmosis, American) 115.00
Davies' 425.0
de Beurmann-Gougerot (sporotrichosis) 117.1
Débove's (splenomegaly) 789.2
deer fly (*see also* Tularemia) 021.9
deficiency 269.9
degenerative — *see also* Degeneration
  disc — *see* Degeneration, intervertebral disc
Degos' 447.8
Déjérine (-Sottas) 356.0
Déléage's 359.89 ▲
demyelinating, demyelinizating (brain stem)
  (central nervous system) 341.9
  multiple sclerosis 340
  specified NEC 341.8
de Quervain's (tendon sheath) 727.04
  thyroid (subacute granulomatous thyroiditis)
    245.1
Dercum's (adiposis dolorosa) 272.8
Deutschländer's — *see* Fracture, foot
Devergie's (pityriasis rubra pilaris) 696.4
Devic's 341.0
diaphorase deficiency 289.7
diaphragm 519.4
diarrheal, infectious 009.2
diatomaceous earth 502
Diaz's (osteochondrosis astragalus) 732.5
digestive system 569.9
Di Guglielmo's (erythemic myelosis) (M9841/3)
  207.0 ✓5ᵗʰ
Dimitri-Sturge-Weber (encephalocutaneous
  angiomatosis) 759.6
disc, degenerative — *see* Degeneration,
  intervertebral disc
discogenic (*see also* Disease, intervertebral
  disc) 722.90
diverticular — *see* Diverticula
Down's (mongolism) 758.0

Disease, diseased — *see also* Syndrome — *continued*
Dubini's (electric chorea) 049.8
Dubois' (thymus gland) 090.5
Duchenne's 094.0
  locomotor ataxia 094.0
  muscular dystrophy 359.1
  paralysis 335.22
  pseudohypertrophy, muscles 359.1
Duchenne-Griesinger 359.1
ductless glands 259.9
Duhring's (dermatitis herpetiformis) 694.0
Dukes (-Filatov) 057.8
duodenum NEC 537.9
  specified NEC 537.89
Duplay's 726.2
Dupré's (meningism) 781.6
Dupuytren's (muscle contracture) 728.6
Durand-Nicolas-Favre (climatic bubo) 099.1
Duroziez's (congenital mitral stenosis) 746.5
Dutton's (trypanosomiasis) 086.9
Eales' 362.18
ear (chronic) (inner) NEC 388.9
  middle 385.9
    adhesive (*see also* Adhesions, middle ear)
      385.10
    specified NEC 385.89
Eberth's (typhoid fever) 002.0
Ebstein's
  heart 746.2
  meaning diabetes 250.4 ✓5ᵗʰ [581.81]
Echinococcus (*see also* Echinococcus) 122.9
ECHO virus NEC 078.89
Economo's (encephalitis lethargica) 049.8
Eddowes' (brittle bones and blue sclera) 756.51
Edsall's 992.2
Eichstedt's (pityriasis versicolor) 111.0
Ellis-van Creveld (chondroectodermal
  dysplasia) 756.55
endocardium — *see* Endocarditis
endocrine glands or system NEC 259.9
  specified NEC 259.8
endomyocardial, idiopathic mural 425.2
Engel-von Recklinghausen (osteitis fibrosa
  cystica) 252.0
Engelmann's (diaphyseal sclerosis) 756.59
English (rickets) 268.0
Engman's (infectious eczematoid dermatitis)
  690.8
enteroviral, enterovirus NEC 078.89
  central nervous system NEC 048
epidemic NEC 136.9
epididymis 608.9
epigastric, functional 536.9
  psychogenic 306.4
Erb (-Landouzy) 359.1
Erb-Goldflam 358.0
Erichsen's (railway spine) 300.16
esophagus 530.9
  functional 530.5
  psychogenic 306.4
Eulenburg's (congenital paramyotonia) 359.2
Eustachian tube 381.9
Evans' (thrombocytopenic purpura) 287.3
external auditory canal 380.9
extrapyramidal NEC 333.90
eye 379.90
  anterior chamber 364.9
  inflammatory NEC 364.3
  muscle 378.9
eyeball 360.9
eyelid 374.9
eyeworm of Africa 125.2
Fabry's (angiokeratoma corporis diffusum)
  272.7
facial nerve (seventh) 351.9
  newborn 767.5
Fahr-Volhard (malignant nephrosclerosis)
  403.00
fallopian tube, noninflammatory 620.9
  specified NEC 620.8
familial periodic 277.3
  paralysis 359.3
Fanconi's (congenital pancytopenia) 284.0
Farber's (disseminated lipogranulomatosis)
  272.8
fascia 728.9
  inflammatory 728.9

Disease, diseased — *see also* Syndrome — *continued*
Fauchard's (periodontitis) 523.4
Favre-Durand-Nicolas (climatic bubo) 099.1
Favre-Racouchot (elastoidosis cutanea
  nodularis) 701.8
Fede's 529.0
Feer's 985.0
Felix's (juvenile osteochondrosis, hip) 732.1
Fenwick's (gastric atrophy) 537.89
Fernels' (aortic aneurysm) 441.9
fibrocaseous, of lung (*see also* Tuberculosis,
  pulmonary) 011.9 ✓5ᵗʰ
fibrocystic — *see also* Fibrocystic, disease
  newborn 277.01
Fiedler's (leptospiral jaundice) 100.0
fifth 057.0
Filatoff's (infectious mononucleosis) 075
Filatov's (infectious mononucleosis) 075
file-cutters' 984.9
  specified type of lead — *see* Table of Drugs
    and Chemicals
filterable virus NEC 078.89
fish skin 757.1
  acquired 701.1
Flajani (-Basedow) (exophthalmic goiter)
  242.0 ✓5ᵗʰ
Flatau-Schilder 341.1
flax-dressers' 504
Fleischner's 732.3
flint 502
fluke — *see* Infestation, fluke
Følling's (phenylketonuria) 270.1
foot and mouth 078.4
foot process 581.3
Forbes' (glycogenosis III) 271.0
Fordyce's (ectopic sebaceous glands) (mouth)
  750.26
Fordyce-Fox (apocrine miliaria) 705.82
Fothergill's
  meaning scarlatina anginosa 034.1
  neuralgia (*see also* Neuralgia, trigeminal)
    350.1
Fournier's 608.83
fourth 057.8
Fox (-Fordyce) (apocrine miliaria) 705.82
Francis' (*see also* Tularemia) 021.9
Franklin's (heavy chain) 273.2
Frei's (climatic bubo) 099.1
Freiberg's (flattening metarsal) 732.5
Friedländer's (endarteritis obliterans) — *see*
  Arteriosclerosis
Friedreich's
  combined systemic or ataxia 334.0
  facial hemihypertrophy 756.0
  myoclonia 333.2
Fröhlich's (adiposogenital dystrophy) 253.8
Frommel's 676.6 ✓5ᵗʰ
frontal sinus (chronic) 473.1
  acute 461.1
Fuller's earth 502
fungus, fungous NEC 117.9
Gaisböck's (polycythemia hypertonica) 289.0
gallbladder 575.9
  congenital 751.60
Gamna's (siderotic splenomegaly) 289.51
Gamstorp's (adynamia episodica hereditaria)
  359.3
Gandy-Nanta (siderotic splenomegaly) 289.51
gannister (occupational) 502
Garré's (*see also* Osteomyelitis) 730.1 ✓5ᵗʰ
gastric (*see also* Disease, stomach) 537.9
gastrointestinal (tract) 569.9
  amyloid 277.3
  functional 536.9
    psychogenic 306.4
Gaucher's (adult) (cerebroside lipidosis)
  (infantile) 272.7
Gayet's (superior hemorrhagic
  polioencephalitis) 265.1
Gee (-Herter) (-Heubner) (-Thaysen) (nontropical
  sprue) 579.0
generalized neoplastic (M8000/6) 199.0
genital organs NEC
  female 629.9
    specified NEC 629.8
  male 608.9
Gerhardt's (erythromelalgia) 443.89

Disease, diseased — *see also* Syndrome —
continued
Gerlier's (epidemic vertigo) 078.81
Gibert's (pityriasis rosea) 696.3
Gibney's (perispondylitis) 720.9
Gierke's (glycogenosis I) 271.0
Gilbert's (familial nonhemolytic jaundice) 277.4
Gilchrist's (North American blastomycosis)
116.0
Gilford (-Hutchinson) (progeria) 259.8
Gilles de la Tourette's (motor-verbal tic) 307.23
Giovannini's 117.9
gland (lymph) 289.9
Glanzmann's (hereditary hemorrhagic
thrombasthenia) 287.1
glassblowers' 527.1
Glénard's (enteroptosis) 569.89
Glisson's (*see also* Rickets) 268.0
glomerular
membranous, idiopathic 581.1
minimal change 581.3
glycogen storage (Andersen's) (Cori types 1-7)
(Forbes') (McArdle-Schmid-Pearson)
(Pompe's) (types I-VII) 271.0
cardiac 271.0 *[425.7]*
generalized 271.0
glucose-6-phosphatase deficiency 271.0
heart 271.0 *[425.7]*
hepatorenal 271.0
liver and kidneys 271.0
myocardium 271.0 *[425.7]*
von Gierke's (glycogenosis I) 271.0
Goldflam-Erb 358.0
Goldscheider's (epidermolysis bullosa) 757.39
Goldstein's (familial hemorrhagic telangiectasia)
448.0
gonococcal NEC 098.0
Goodall's (epidemic vomiting) 078.82
Gordon's (exudative enteropathy) 579.8
Gougerot's (trisymptomatic) 709.1
Gougerot-Carteaud (confluent reticulate
papillomatosis) 701.8
Gougerot-Hailey-Hailey (benign familial chronic
pemphigus) 757.39
graft-versus-host (bone marrow) 996.85
due to organ transplant NEC — *see*
Complications, transplant, organ
grain-handlers' 495.8
Grancher's (splenopneumonia) — *see*
Pneumonia
granulomatous (childhood) (chronic) 288.1
graphite lung 503
Graves' (exophthalmic goiter) 242.0 ✓5ᵗʰ
Greenfield's 330.0
green monkey 078.89
Griesinger's (*see also* Ancylostomiasis) 126.9
grinders' 502
Grisel's 723.5
Gruby's (tinea tonsurans) 110.0
Guertin's (electric chorea) 049.8
Guillain-Barré 357.0
Guinon's (motor-verbal tic) 307.23
Gull's (thyroid atrophy with myxedema) 244.8
Gull and Sutton's — *see* Hypertension, kidney
gum NEC 523.9
Günther's (congenital erythropoietic porphyria)
277.1
gynecological 629.9
specified NEC 629.8
H 270.0
Haas' 732.3
Habermann's (acute parapsoriasis varioliformis)
696.2
Haff 985.1
Hageman (congenital factor XII deficiency) (*see
also* Defect, congenital) 286.3
Haglund's (osteochondrosis os tibiale
externum) 732.5
Hagner's (hypertrophic pulmonary
osteoarthropathy) 731.2
Hailey-Hailey (benign familial chronic
pemphigus) 757.39
hair (follicles) NEC 704.9
specified type NEC 704.8
Hallervorden-Spatz 333.0
Halloopeau's (lichen sclerosus et atrophicus)
701.0

Disease, diseased — *see also* Syndrome —
continued
Hamman's (spontaneous mediastinal
emphysema) 518.1
hand, foot, and mouth 074.3
Hand-Schüller-Christian (chronic histiocytosis
X) 277.8
Hanot's — *see* Cirrhosis, biliary
Hansen's (leprosy) 030.9
benign form 030.1
malignant form 030.0
Harada's 363.22
Harley's (intermittent hemoglobinuria) 283.2
Hart's (pellagra-cerebellar ataxia renal
aminoaciduria) 270.0
Hartnup (pellagra-cerebellar ataxia renal
aminoaciduria) 270.0
Hashimoto's (struma lymphomatosa) 245.2
Hb — *see* Disease, hemoglobin
heart (organic) 429.9
with
acute pulmonary edema (*see also* Failure,
ventricular, left) 428.1
hypertensive 402.91
with renal failure 404.91
benign 402.11
with renal failure 404.11
malignant 402.01
with renal failure 404.01
kidney disease — *see* Hypertension,
cardiorenal
rheumatic fever (conditions classifiable to
390)
active 391.9
with chorea 392.0
inactive or quiescent (with chorea)
398.90
amyloid 277.3 *[425.7]*
aortic (valve) (*see also* Endocarditis, aortic)
424.1
arteriosclerotic or sclerotic (minimal) (senile)
— *see* Arteriosclerosis, coronary
artery — *see* Arteriosclerosis, coronary
atherosclerotic — *see* Arteriosclerosis,
coronary
beer drinkers' 425.5
beriberi 265.0 *[425.7]*
black 416.0
congenital NEC 746.9
cyanotic 746.9
maternal, affecting fetus or newborn
760.3
specified type NEC 746.89
congestive (*see also* Failure, heart) 428.0
coronary 414.9
cryptogenic 429.9
due to
amyloidosis 277.3 *[425.7]*
beriberi 265.0 *[425.7]*
cardiac glycogenosis 271.0 *[425.7]*
Friedreich's ataxia 334.0 *[425.8]*
gout 274.82
mucopolysaccharidosis 277.5 *[425.7]*
myotonia atrophica 359.2 *[425.8]*
progressive muscular dystrophy
359.1 *[425.8]*
sarcoidosis 135 *[425.8]*
fetal 746.9
inflammatory 746.89
fibroid (*see also* Myocarditis) 429.0
functional 427.9
postoperative 997.1
psychogenic 306.2
glycogen storage 271.0 *[425.7]*
gonococcal NEC 098.85
gouty 274.82
hypertensive (*see also* Hypertension, heart)
402.90
benign 402.10
malignant 402.00
hyperthyroid (*see also* Hyperthyroidism)
242.9 ✓5ᵗʰ *[425.7]*
incompletely diagnosed — *see* Disease, heart
ischemic (chronic) (*see also* Ischemia, heart)
414.9

Disease, diseased — *see also* Syndrome —
continued
heart — *continued*
ischemic (*see also* Ischemia, heart) —
continued
acute (*see also* Infarct, myocardium)
without myocardial infarction 411.89
with coronary (artery) occlusion
411.81
asymptomatic 412
diagnosed on ECG or other special
investigation but currently
presenting no symptoms 412
kyphoscoliotic 416.1
mitral (*see also* Endocarditis, mitral) 394.9
muscular (*see also* Degeneration,
myocardial) 429.1
postpartum 674.8 ✓5ᵗʰ
psychogenic (functional) 306.2
pulmonary (chronic) 416.9
acute 415.0
specified NEC 416.8
rheumatic (chronic) (inactive) (old)
(quiescent) (with chorea) 398.90
active or acute 391.9
with chorea (active) (rheumatic)
(Sydenham's) 392.0
specified type NEC 391.8
maternal, affecting fetus or newborn
760.3
rheumatoid — *see* Arthritis, rheumatoid
sclerotic — *see* Arteriosclerosis, coronary
senile (*see also* Myocarditis) 429.0
specified type NEC 429.89
syphilitic 093.89
aortic 093.1
aneurysm 093.0
asymptomatic 093.89
congenital 090.5
thyroid (gland) (*see also* Hyper-thyroidism)
242.9 ✓5ᵗʰ *[425.7]*
thyrotoxic (*see also* Thyrotoxicosis)
242.9 ✓5ᵗʰ *[425.7]*
tuberculous (*see also* Tuberculosis)
017.9 ✓5ᵗʰ *[425.8]*
valve, valvular (obstructive) (regurgitant) —
see also Endocarditis
congenital NEC (*see also* Anomaly, heart,
valve) 746.9
pulmonary 746.00
specified type NEC 746.89
vascular — *see* Disease, cardiovascular
heavy-chain (gamma G) 273.2
Heberden's 715.04
Hebra's
dermatitis exfoliativa 695.89
erythema multiforme exudativum 695.1
pityriasis
maculata et circinata 696.3
rubra 695.89
pilaris 696.4
prurigo 698.2
Heerfordt's (uveoparotitis) 135
Heidenhain's 290.10
with dementia 290.10
Heilmeyer-Schöner (M9842/3) 207.1 ✓5ᵗʰ
Heine-Medin (*see also* Poliomyelitis) 045.9 ✓5ᵗʰ
Heller's (*see also* Psychosis, childhood)
299.1 ✓5ᵗʰ
Heller-Döhle (syphilitic aortitis) 093.1
hematopoietic organs 289.9
hemoglobin (Hb) 282.7
with thalassemia 282.4
abnormal (mixed) NEC 282.7
with thalassemia 282.4
AS genotype 282.5
Bart's 282.7
C (Hb-C) 282.7
with other abnormal hemoglobin NEC
282.7
elliptocytosis 282.7
Hb-S 282.63
sickle-cell 282.63
thalassemia 282.4
constant spring 282.7

Disease, diseased — *see also* Syndrome —
  continued
  hemoglobin — *continued*
    D (Hb-D) 282.7
      with other abnormal hemoglobin NEC
        282.7
      Hb-S 282.69
      sickle-cell 282.69
      thalassemia 282.4
    E (Hb-E) 282.7
      with other abnormal hemoglobin NEC
        282.7
      Hb-S 282.69
      sickle-cell 282.69
      thalassemia 282.4
    elliptocytosis 282.7
    F (Hb-F) 282.7
    G (Hb-G) 282.7
    H (Hb-H) 282.4
    hereditary persistence, fetal (HPFH) ("Swiss
      variety") 282.7
    high fetal gene 282.7
    I thalassemia 282.4
    M 289.7
    S — see Disease, sickle-cell, Hb-S
    spherocytosis 282.7
    unstable, hemolytic 282.7
    Zurich (Hb-Zurich) 282.7
  hemolytic (fetus) (newborn) 773.2
    autoimmune (cold type) (warm type) 283.0
    due to or with
      incompatibility
        ABO (blood group) 773.1
        blood (group) (Duffy) (Kell) (Kidd)
          (Lewis) (M) (S) NEC 773.2
        Rh (blood group) (factor) 773.0
        Rh negative mother 773.0
    unstable hemoglobin 282.7
  hemorrhagic 287.9
    newborn 776.0
  Henoch (-Schönlein) (purpura nervosa) 287.0
  hepatic — *see* Disease, liver
  hepatolenticular 275.1
  heredodegenerative NEC
    brain 331.89
    spinal cord 336.8
  Hers' (glycogenosis VI) 271.0
  Herter (-Gee) (-Heubner) (nontropical sprue)
    579.0
  Herxheimer's (diffuse idiopathic cutaneous
    atrophy) 701.8
  Heubner's 094.89
  Heubner-Herter (nontropical sprue) 579.0
  high fetal gene or hemoglobin thalassemia
    282.4
  Hildenbrand's (typhus) 081.9
  hip (joint) NEC 719.95
    congenital 755.63
    suppurative 711.05
    tuberculous (*see also* Tuberculosis)
      015.1 ✓5ᵗʰ [730.85]
  Hippel's (retinocerebral angiomatosis) 759.6
  Hirschfield's (acute diabetes mellitus) (*see also*
    Diabetes) 250.0 ✓5ᵗʰ
  Hirschsprung's (congenital megacolon) 751.3
  His (-Werner) (trench fever) 083.1
  HIV 042
  Hodgkin's (M9650/3) 201.9 ✓5ᵗʰ

> *Note* — *Use the following fifth-digit*
> *subclassification with category 201:*
>
> 0   *unspecifed site*
> 1   *lymph nodes of head, face, and*
>   *neck*
> 2   *intrathoracic lymp nodes*
> 3   *intra-abdominal lymph nodes*
> 4   *lymph nodes of axilla and upper*
>   *limb*
> 5   *lymph nodes of inguinal region and*
>   *lower limb*
> 6   *intrapelvic lymph nodes*
> 7   *spleen*
> 8   *lymph nodes of multiple sites*

Disease, diseased — *see also* Syndrome —
  continued
  Hodgkin's — *continued*
    lymphocytic
      depletion (M9653/3) 201.7 ✓5ᵗʰ
        diffuse fibrosis (M9654/3) 201.7 ✓5ᵗʰ
        reticular type (M9655/3) 201.7 ✓5ᵗʰ
      predominance (M9651/3) 201.4 ✓5ᵗʰ
    lymphocytic-histiocytic predominance
      (M9651/3) 201.4 ✓5ᵗʰ
    mixed cellularity (M9652/3) 201.6 ✓5ᵗʰ
    nodular sclerosis (M9656/3) 201.5 ✓5ᵗʰ
      cellular phase (M9657/3) 201.5 ✓5ᵗʰ
  Hodgson's 441.9
    ruptured 441.5
  Hoffa (-Kastert) (liposynovitis prepatellaris)
    272.8
  Holla (*see also* Spherocytosis) 282.0
  homozygous-Hb-S 282.61
  hoof and mouth 078.4
  hookworm (*see also* Ancylostomiasis) 126.9
  Horton's (temporal arteritis) 446.5
  host-versus-graft (immune or nonimmune
    cause) 996.80
    bone marrow 996.85
    heart 996.83
    intestines 996.87
    kidney 996.81
    liver 996.82
    lung 996.84
    pancreas 996.86
    specified NEC 996.89
  HPFH (hereditary persistence of fetal
    hemoglobin) ("Swiss variety") 282.7
  Huchard's (continued arterial hypertension)
    401.9
  Huguier's (uterine fibroma) 218.9
  human immunodeficiency (virus) 042
  hunger 251.1
  Hunt's
    dyssynergia cerebellaris myoclonica 334.2
    herpetic geniculate ganglionitis 053.11
  Huntington's 333.4
  Huppert's (multiple myeloma) (M9730/3)
    203.0 ✓5ᵗʰ
  Hurler's (mucopolysaccharidosis I) 277.5
  Hutchinson's, meaning
    angioma serpiginosum 709.1
    cheiropompholyx 705.81
    prurigo estivalis 692.72
  Hutchinson-Boeck (sarcoidosis) 135
  Hutchinson-Gilford (progeria) 259.8
  hyaline (diffuse) (generalized) 728.9
    membrane (lung) (newborn) 769
  hydatid (*see also* Echinococcus) 122.9
  Hyde's (prurigo nodularis) 698.3
  hyperkinetic (*see also* Hyperkinesia) 314.9
    heart 429.82
  hypertensive (*see also* Hypertension) 401.9
  hypophysis 253.9
    hyperfunction 253.1
    hypofunction 253.2
  Iceland (epidemic neuromyasthenia) 049.8
  I cell 272.7
  ill-defined 799.8
  immunologic NEC 279.9
  immunoproliferative 203.8 ✓5ᵗʰ
  inclusion 078.5
    salivary gland 078.5
  infancy, early NEC 779.9
  infective NEC 136.9
  inguinal gland 289.9
  internal semilunar cartilage, cystic 717.5
  intervertebral disc 722.90
    with myelopathy 722.70
    cervical, cervicothoracic 722.91
      with myelopathy 722.71
    lumbar, lumbosacral 722.93
      with myelopathy 722.73
    thoracic, thoracolumbar 722.92
      with myelopathy 722.72
  intestine 569.9
    functional 564.9
      congenital 751.3
      psychogenic 306.4
    lardaceous 277.3

Disease, diseased — *see also* Syndrome —
  continued
  intestine — *continued*
    organic 569.9
    protozoal NEC 007.9
  iris 364.9
  iron
    metabolism 275.0
    storage 275.0
  Isambert's (*see also* Tuberculosis, larynx)
    012.3 ✓5ᵗʰ
  Iselin's (osteochondrosis, fifth metatarsal) 732.5
  Island (scrub typhus) 081.2
  itai-itai 985.5
  Jadassohn's (maculopapular erythroderma)
    696.2
  Jadassohn-Pellizari's (anetoderma) 701.3
  Jakob-Creutzfeldt 046.1
    with dementia
      with behavioral disturbance
        046.1 [294.11]
      without behavioral disturbance
        046.1 [294.10]
  Jaksch (-Luzet) (pseudoleukemia infantum)
    285.8
  Janet's 300.89
  Jansky-Bielschowsky 330.1
  jaw NEC 526.9
    fibrocystic 526.2
  Jensen's 363.05
  Jeune's (asphyxiating thoracic dystrophy) 756.4
  jigger 134.1
  Johnson-Stevens (erythema multiforme
    exudativum) 695.1
  joint NEC 719.9 ✓5ᵗʰ
    ankle 719.97
    Charcôt 094.0 [713.5]
    degenerative (*see also* Osteoarthrosis)
      715.9 ✓5ᵗʰ
      multiple 715.09
      spine (*see also* Spondylosis) 721.90
    elbow 719.92
    foot 719.97
    hand 719.94
    hip 719.95
    hypertrophic (chronic) (degenerative) (*see
      also* Osteoarthrosis) 715.9 ✓5ᵗʰ
      spine (*see also* Spondylosis) 721.90
    knee 719.96
    Luschka 721.90
    multiple sites 719.99
    pelvic region 719.95
    sacroiliac 724.6
    shoulder (region) 719.91
    specified site NEC 719.98
    spine NEC 724.9
      pseudarthrosis following fusion 733.82
      sacroiliac 724.6
    wrist 719.93
  Jourdain's (acute gingivitis) 523.0
  Jüngling's (sarcoidosis) 135
  Kahler (-Bozzolo) (multiple myeloma) (M9730/3)
    203.0 ✓5ᵗʰ
  Kalischer's 759.6
  Kaposi's 757.33
    lichen ruber 697.8
      acuminatus 696.4
      moniliformis 697.8
    xeroderma pigmentosum 757.33
  Kaschin-Beck (endemic polyarthritis) 716.00
    ankle 716.07
    arm 716.02
      lower (and wrist) 716.03
      upper (and elbow) 716.02
    foot (and ankle) 716.07
    forearm (and wrist) 716.03
    hand 716.04
    leg 716.06
      lower 716.06
      upper 716.05
    multiple sites 716.09
    pelvic region (hip) (thigh) 716.05
    shoulder region 716.01
    specified site NEC 716.08
  Katayama 120.2
  Kawasaki 446.1
  Kedani (scrub typhus) 081.2

Disease, diseased — *see also* Syndrome — *continued*

kidney (functional) (pelvis) (*see also* Disease, renal) 593.9
  cystic (congenital) 753.10
    multiple 753.19
    single 753.11
    specified NEC 753.19
  fibrocystic (congenital) 753.19
  in gout 274.10
  polycystic (congenital) 753.12
    adult type (APKD) 753.13
    autosomal dominant 753.13
    autosomal recessive 753.14
    childhood type (CPKD) 753.14
    infantile type 753.14
Kienböck's (carpal lunate) (wrist) 732.3
Kimmelstiel (-Wilson) (intercapillary glomerulosclerosis) 250.4 ✓5ᵗʰ [581.81]
Kinnier Wilson's (hepatolenticular degeneration) 275.1
kissing 075
Kleb's (*see also* Nephritis) 583.9
Klinger's 446.4
Klippel's 723.8
Klippel-Feil (brevicollis) 756.16
knight's 911.1
Köbner's (epidermolysis bullosa) 757.39
Koenig-Wichmann (pemphigus) 694.4
Köhler's
  first (osteoarthrosis juvenilis) 732.5
  second (Freiberg's infraction, metatarsal head) 732.5
  patellar 732.4
  tarsal navicular (bone) (osteoarthrosis juvenilis) 732.5
Köhler-Freiberg (infraction, metatarsal head) 732.5
Köhler-Mouchet (osteoarthrosis juvenilis) 732.5
Köhler-Pellegrini-Stieda (calcification, knee joint) 726.62
König's (osteochondritis dissecans) 732.7
Korsakoff's (nonalcoholic) 294.0
  alcoholic 291.1
Kostmann's (infantile genetic agranulocytosis) 288.0
Krabbe's 330.0
Kraepelin-Morel (*see also* Schizophrenia) 295.9 ✓5ᵗʰ
Kraft-Weber-Dimitri 759.6
Kufs' 330.1
Kugelberg-Welander 335.11
Kuhnt-Junius 362.52
Kümmell's (-Verneuil) (spondylitis) 721.7
Kundrat's (lymphosarcoma) 200.1 ✓5ᵗʰ
kuru 046.0
Kussmaul (-Meier) (polyarteritis nodosa) 446.0
Kyasanur Forest 065.2
Kyrle's (hyperkeratosis follicularis in cutem penetrans) 701.1
labia
  inflammatory 616.9
    specified NEC 616.8
  noninflammatory 624.9
    specified NEC 624.8
labyrinth, ear 386.8
lacrimal system (apparatus) (passages) 375.9
  gland 375.00
  specified NEC 375.89
Lafora's 333.2
Lagleyze-von Hippel (retinocerebral angiomatosis) 759.6
Lancereaux-Mathieu (leptospiral jaundice) 100.0
Landry's 357.0
Lane's 569.89
lardaceous (any site) 277.3
Larrey-Weil (leptospiral jaundice) 100.0
Larsen (-Johansson) (juvenile osteopathia patellae) 732.4
larynx 478.70
Lasègue's (persecution mania) 297.9
Leber's 377.16
Lederer's (acquired infectious hemolytic anemia) 283.19
Legg's (capital femoral osteochondrosis) 732.1

Disease, diseased — *see also* Syndrome — *continued*

Legg-Calvé-Perthes (capital femoral osteochondrosis) 732.1
Legg-Calvé-Waldenström (femoral capital osteochondrosis) 732.1
Legg-Perthes (femoral capital osteochrondosis) 732.1
Legionnaires' 482.84
Leigh's 330.8
Leiner's (exfoliative dermatitis) 695.89
Leloir's (lupus erythematosus) 695.4
Lenegre's 426.0
lens (eye) 379.39
Leriche's (osteoporosis, post-traumatic) 733.7
Letterer-Siwe (acute histiocytosis X) (M9722/3) 202.5 ✓5ᵗʰ
Lev's (acquired complete heart block) 426.0
Lewandowski's (*see also* Tuberculosis) 017.0 ✓5ᵗʰ
Lewandowski-Lutz (epidermodysplasia verruciformis) 078.19
Leyden's (periodic vomiting) 536.2
Libman-Sacks (verrucous endocarditis) 710.0 [424.91]
Lichtheim's (subacute combined sclerosis with pernicious anemia) 281.0 [336.2]
ligament 728.9
light chain 203.0 ✓5ᵗʰ
Lightwood's (renal tubular acidosis) 588.8
Lignac's (cystinosis) 270.0
Lindau's (retinocerebral angiomatosis) 759.6
Lindau-von Hippel (angiomatosis retinocerebellosa) 759.6
lip NEC 528.5
lipidosis 272.7
lipoid storage NEC 272.7
Lipschütz's 616.50
Little's — *see* Palsy, cerebral
liver 573.9
  alcoholic 571.3
    acute 571.1
    chronic 571.3
  chronic 571.9
    alcoholic 571.3
  cystic, congenital 751.62
  drug-induced 573.3
  due to
    chemicals 573.3
      fluorinated agents 573.3
      hypersensitivity drugs 573.3
      isoniazids 573.3
  fibrocystic (congenital) 751.62
  glycogen storage 271.0
  organic 573.9
  polycystic (congenital) 751.62
Lobo's (keloid blastomycosis) 116.2
Lobstein's (brittle bones and blue sclera) 756.51
locomotor system 334.9
Lorain's (pituitary dwarfism) 253.3
Lou Gehrig's 335.20
Lucas-Championnière (fibrinous bronchitis) 466.0
Ludwig's (submaxillary cellulitis) 528.3
luetic — *see* Syphilis
lumbosacral region 724.6
lung NEC 518.89
  black 500
  congenital 748.60
  cystic 518.89
    congenital 748.4
  fibroid (chronic) (*see also* Fibrosis, lung) 515
  fluke 121.2
    Oriental 121.2
  in
    amyloidosis 277.3 [517.8]
    polymyositis 710.4 [517.8]
    sarcoidosis 135 [517.8]
    Sjögren's syndrome 710.2 [517.8]
    syphilis 095.1
    systemic lupus erythematosus 710.0 [517.8]
    systemic sclerosis 710.1 [517.2]
  interstitial (chronic) 515
    acute 136.3
  nonspecific, chronic 496

Disease, diseased — *see also* Syndrome — *continued*

lung NEC — *continued*
  obstructive (chronic) (COPD) 496
    with
      acute exacerbation NEC 491.21
      alveolitis, allergic (*see also* Alveolitis, allergic) 495.9
      asthma (chronic) (obstructive) 493.2 ✓5ᵗʰ
      bronchiectasis 494.0
        with acute exacerbation 494.1
      bronchitis (chronic) 491.20
        with acute exacerbation 491.21
      emphysema NEC 492.8
    diffuse (with fibrosis) 496
  polycystic 518.89
    asthma (chronic) (obstructive) 493.2 ✓5ᵗʰ
    congenital 748.4
  purulent (cavitary) 513.0
  restrictive 518.89
  rheumatoid 714.81
    diffuse interstitial 714.81
  specified NEC 518.89
Lutembacher's (atrial septal defect with mitral stenosis) 745.5
Lutz-Miescher (elastosis perforans serpiginosa) 701.1
Lutz-Splendore-de Almeida (Brazilian blastomycosis) 116.1
Lyell's (toxic epidermal necrolysis) 695.1
  due to drug
    correct substance properly administered 695.1
    overdose or wrong substance given or taken 977.9
    specific drug — *see* Table of Drugs and Chemicals
Lyme 088.81
lymphatic (gland) (system) 289.9
  channel (noninfective) 457.9
  vessel (noninfective) 457.9
    specified NEC 457.8
lymphoproliferative (chronic) (M9970/1) 238.7
Machado-Joseph 334.8
Madelung's (lipomatosis) 272.8
Madura (actinomycotic) 039.9
  mycotic 117.4
Magitot's 526.4
Majocchi's (purpura annularis telangiectodes) 709.1
malarial (*see also* Malaria) 084.6
Malassez's (cystic) 608.89
Malibu 919.8
  infected 919.6
malignant (M8000/3) — *see also* Neoplasm, by site, malignant
  previous, affecting management of pregnancy V23.8 ✓5ᵗʰ
Manson's 120.1
maple bark 495.6
maple syrup (urine) 270.3
Marburg (virus) 078.89
Marchiafava (-Bignami) 341.8
Marfan's 090.49
  congenital syphilis 090.49
  meaning Marfan's syndrome 759.82
Marie-Bamberger (hypertrophic pulmonary osteoarthropathy) (secondary) 731.2
  primary or idiopathic (acropachyderma) 757.39
  pulmonary (hypertrophic osteoarthropathy) 731.2
Marie-Strümpell (ankylosing spondylitis) 720.0
Marion's (bladder neck obstruction) 596.0
Marsh's (exophthalmic goiter) 242.0 ✓5ᵗʰ
Martin's 715.27
mast cell 757.33
  systemic (M9741/3) 202.6 ✓5ᵗʰ
mastoid (*see also* Mastoiditis) 383.9
  process 385.9
maternal, unrelated to pregnancy NEC, affecting fetus or newborn 760.9
Mathieu's (leptospiral jaundice) 100.0
Mauclaire's 732.3
Mauriac's (erythema nodosum syphiliticum) 091.3 ✓5ᵗʰ

✓4ᵗʰ Fourth-digit Required   ✓5ᵗʰ Fifth-digit Required   ▶◀ Revised Text   ● New Line   ▲ Revised Code

Disease, diseased — *see also* Syndrome — *continued*
Maxcy's 081.0
McArdle (-Schmid-Pearson) (glycogenosis V) 271.0
mediastinum NEC 519.3
Medin's (*see also* Poliomyelitis) 045.9 ✓5ᵗʰ
Mediterranean (with hemoglobinopathy) 282.4
medullary center (idiopathic) (respiratory) 348.8
Meige's (chronic hereditary edema) 757.0
Meleda 757.39
Ménétrier's (hypertrophic gastritis) 535.2 ✓5ᵗʰ
Ménière's (active) 386.00
cochlear 386.02
cochleovestibular 386.01
inactive 386.04
in remission 386.04
vestibular 386.03
meningeal — *see* Meningitis
mental (*see also* Psychosis) 298.9
Merzbacher-Pelizaeus 330.0
mesenchymal 710.9
mesenteric embolic 557.0
metabolic NEC 277.9
metal polishers' 502
metastatic — *see* Metastasis
Mibelli's 757.39
microdrepanocytic 282.4
Miescher's 709.3
Mikulicz's (dryness of mouth, absent or decreased lacrimation) 527.1
Milkman (-Looser) (osteomalacia with pseudofractures) 268.2
Miller's (osteomalacia) 268.2
Mills' 335.29
Milroy's (chronic hereditary edema) 757.0
Minamata 985.0
Minor's 336.1
Minot's (hemorrhagic disease, newborn) 776.0
Minot-von Willebrand-Jürgens (angiohemophilia) 286.4
Mitchell's (erythromelalgia) 443.89
mitral — *see* Endocarditis, mitral
Mljet (mal de Meleda) 757.39
Möbius', Moebius' 346.8 ✓5ᵗʰ
Moeller's 267
Möller (-Barlow) (infantile scurvy) 267
Mönckeberg's (*see also* Arteriosclerosis, extremities) 440.20
Mondor's (thrombophlebitis of breast) 451.89
Monge's 993.2
Morel-Kraepelin (*see also* Schizophrenia) 295.9 ✓5ᵗʰ
Morgagni's (syndrome) (hyperostosis frontalis interna) 733.3
Morgagni-Adams-Stokes (syncope with heart block) 426.9
Morquio (-Brailsford) (-Ullrich) (mucopolysaccharidosis IV) 277.5
Morton's (with metatarsalgia) 355.6
Morvan's 336.0
motor neuron (bulbar) (mixed type) 335.20
Mouchet's (juvenile osteochondrosis, foot) 732.5
mouth 528.9
Moyamoya 437.5
Mucha (acute parapsoriasis varioliformis) 696.2
mu-chain 273.2
mucolipidosis (I) (II) (III) 272.7
Münchmeyer's (exostosis luxurians) 728.11
Murri's (intermittent hemoglobinuria) 283.2
muscle 359.9
inflammatory 728.9
ocular 378.9
musculoskeletal system 729.9
mushroom workers' 495.5
Myà's (congenital dilation, colon) 751.3
mycotic 117.9
myeloproliferative (chronic) (M9960/1) 238.7
myocardium, myocardial (*see also* Degeneration, myocardial) 429.1
hypertensive (*see also* Hypertension, heart) 402.90
primary (idiopathic) 425.4
myoneural 358.9
Naegeli's 287.1

Disease, diseased — *see also* Syndrome — *continued*
nail 703.9
specified type NEC 703.8
Nairobi sheep 066.1
nasal 478.1
cavity NEC 478.1
sinus (chronic) — *see* Sinusitis
navel (newborn) NEC 779.89 ▲
neoplastic, generalized (M8000/6) 199.0
nerve — *see* Disorder, nerve
nervous system (central) 349.9
autonomic, peripheral (*see also* Neuropathy, peripheral, autonomic) 337.9
congenital 742.9
inflammatory — *see* Encephalitis
parasympathetic (*see also* Neuropathy, peripheral, autonomic) 337.9
peripheral NEC 355.9
specified NEC 349.89
sympathetic (*see also* Neuropathy, peripheral, autonomic) 337.9
vegetative (*see also* Neuropathy, peripheral, autonomic) 337.9
Nettleship's (urticaria pigmentosa) 757.33
Neumann's (pemphigus vegetans) 694.4
neurologic (central) NEC (*see also* Disease, nervous system) 349.9
peripheral NEC 355.9
neuromuscular system NEC 358.9
Newcastle 077.8
Nicolas (-Durand) — Favre (climatic bubo) 099.1
Niemann-Pick (lipid histiocytosis) 272.7
nipple 611.9
Paget's (M8540/3) 174.0
Nishimoto (-Takeuchi) 437.5
nonarthropod-borne NEC 078.89
central nervous system NEC 049.9
enterovirus NEC 078.89
non-autoimmune hemolytic NEC 283.10
Nonne-Milroy-Meige (chronic hereditary edema) 757.0
Norrie's (congenital progressive oculoacousticocerebral degeneration) 743.8
nose 478.1
nucleus pulposus — *see* Disease, intervertebral disc
nutritional 269.9
maternal, affecting fetus or newborn 760.4
oasthouse, urine 270.2
obliterative vascular 447.1
Odelberg's (juvenile osteochondrosis) 732.1
Oguchi's (retina) 368.61
Ohara's (*see also* Tularemia) 021.9
Ollier's (chondrodysplasia) 756.4
Opitz's (congestive splenomegaly) 289.51
Oppenheim's 358.8
Oppenheim-Urbach (necrobiosis lipoidica diabeticorum) 250.8 ✓5ᵗʰ *[709.3]*
optic nerve NEC 377.49
orbit 376.9
specified NEC 376.89
Oriental liver fluke 121.1
Oriental lung fluke 121.2
Ormond's 593.4
Osgood's tibia (tubercle) 732.4
Osgood-Schlatter 732.4
Osler (-Vaquez) (polycythemia vera) (M9950/1) 238.4
Osler-Rendu (familial hemorrhagic telangiectasia) 448.0
osteofibrocystic 252.0
Otto's 715.35
outer ear 380.9
ovary (noninflammatory) NEC 620.9
cystic 620.2
polycystic 256.4
specified NEC 620.8
Owren's (congenital) (*see also* Defect, coagulation) 286.3
Paas' 756.59
Paget's (osteitis deformans) 731.0
with infiltrating duct carcinoma of the breast (M8541/3) — *see* Neoplasm, breast, malignant

Disease, diseased — *see also* Syndrome — *continued*
Paget's — *continued*
bone 731.0
osteosarcoma in (M9184/3) — *see* Neoplasm, bone, malignant
breast (M8540/3) 174.0
extramammary (M8542/3) — *see also* Neoplasm, skin, malignant
anus 154.3
skin 173.5
malignant (M8540/3)
breast 174.0
specified site NEC (M8542/3) — *see* Neoplasm, skin, malignant
unspecified site 174.0
mammary (M8540/3) 174.0
nipple (M8540/3) 174.0
palate (soft) 528.9
Paltauf-Sternberg 201.9 ✓5ᵗʰ
pancreas 577.9
cystic 577.2
congenital 751.7
fibrocystic 277.00
Panner's 732.3
capitellum humeri 732.3
head of humerus 732.3
tarsal navicular (bone) (osteochondrosis) 732.5
panvalvular — *see* Endocarditis, mitral
parametrium 629.9
parasitic NEC 136.9
cerebral NEC 123.9
intestinal NEC 129
mouth 112.0
skin NEC 134.9
specified type — *see* Infestation
tongue 112.0
parathyroid (gland) 252.9
specified NEC 252.8
Parkinson's 332.0
parodontal 523.9
Parrot's (syphilitic osteochondritis) 090.0
Parry's (exophthalmic goiter) 242.0 ✓5ᵗʰ
Parson's (exophthalmic goiter) 242.0 ✓5ᵗʰ
Pavy's 593.6
Paxton's (white piedra) 111.2
Payr's (splenic flexure syndrome) 569.89
pearl-workers' (chronic osteomyelitis) (*see also* Osteomyelitis) 730.1 ✓5ᵗʰ
Pel-Ebstein — *see* Disease, Hodgkin's
Pelizaeus-Merzbacher 330.0
with dementia
with behavioral disturbance 330.0 *[294.11]*
without behavioral disturbance 330.0 *[294.10]*
Pellegrini-Stieda (calcification, knee joint) 726.62
pelvis, pelvic
female NEC 629.9
specified NEC 629.8
gonococcal (acute) 098.19
chronic or duration of 2 months or over 098.39
infection (*see also* Disease, pelvis, inflammatory) 614.9
inflammatory (female) (PID) 614.9
with
abortion — *see* Abortion, by type, with sepsis
ectopic pregnancy (*see also* categories 633.0-633.9) 639.0
molar pregnancy (*see also* categories 630-632) 639.0
acute 614.3
chronic 614.4
complicating pregnancy 646.6 ✓5ᵗʰ
affecting fetus or newborn 760.8
following
abortion 639.0
ectopic or molar pregnancy 639.0
peritonitis (acute) 614.5
chronic NEC 614.7
puerperal, postpartum, childbirth 670 ✓4ᵗʰ
specified NEC 614.8

Disease, diseased — *see also* Syndrome — *continued*
pelvis, pelvic — *continued*
  organ, female NEC 629.9
    specified NEC 629.8
  peritoneum, female NEC 629.9
    specified NEC 629.8
penis 607.9
  inflammatory 607.2
peptic NEC 536.9
  acid 536.8
periapical tissues NEC 522.9
pericardium 423.9
  specified type NEC 423.8
perineum
  female
    inflammatory 616.9
      specified NEC 616.8
    noninflammatory 624.9
      specified NEC 624.8
  male (inflammatory) 682.2
periodic (familial) (Reimann's) NEC 277.3
  paralysis 359.3
periodontal NEC 523.9
  specified NEC 523.8
periosteum 733.90
peripheral
  arterial 443.9
  autonomic nervous system (*see also* Neuropathy, autonomic) 337.9
  nerve NEC (*see also* Neuropathy) 356.9
    multiple — *see* Polyneuropathy
  vascular 443.9
    specified type NEC 443.89
peritoneum 568.9
  pelvic, female 629.9
    specified NEC 629.8
Perrin-Ferraton (snapping hip) 719.65
persistent mucosal (middle ear) (with posterior or superior marginal perforation of ear drum) 382.2
Perthes' (capital femoral osteochondrosis) 732.1
Petit's (*see also* Hernia, lumbar) 553.8
Peutz-Jeghers 759.6
Peyronie's 607.89
Pfeiffer's (infectious mononucleosis) 075
pharynx 478.20
Phocas' 610.1
photochromogenic (acid-fast bacilli) (pulmonary) 031.0
  nonpulmonary 031.9
Pick's
  brain 331.1
    with dementia
      with behavioral disturbance 331.1 [294.11]
      without behavioral disturbance 331.1 [294.10]
  cerebral atrophy 331.1
    with dementia
      with behavioral disturbance 331.1 [294.11]
      without behavioral disturbance 331.1 [294.10]
  lipid histiocytosis 272.7
  liver (pericardial pseudocirrhosis of liver) 423.2
  pericardium (pericardial pseudocirrhosis of liver) 423.2
  polyserositis (pericardial pseudocirrhosis of liver) 423.2
Pierson's (osteochondrosis) 732.1
pigeon fanciers' or breeders' 495.2
pineal gland 259.8
pink 985.0
Pinkus' (lichen nitidus) 697.1
pinworm 127.4
pituitary (gland) 253.9
  hyperfunction 253.1
  hypofunction 253.2
pituitary snuff-takers' 495.8
placenta
  affecting fetus or newborn 762.2
  complicating pregnancy or childbirth 656.7 ✓5ᵗʰ
pleura (cavity) (*see also* Pleurisy) 511.0
Plummer's (toxic nodular goiter) 242.3 ✓5ᵗʰ

Disease, diseased — *see also* Syndrome — *continued*
pneumatic
  drill 994.9
  hammer 994.9
policeman's 729.2
Pollitzer's (hidradenitis suppurativa) 705.83
polycystic (congenital) 759.89
  kidney or renal 753.12
    adult type (APKD) 753.13
    autosomal dominant 753.13
    autosomal recessive 753.14
    childhood type (CPKD) 753.14
    infantile type 753.14
  liver or hepatic 751.62
  lung or pulmonary 518.89
    congenital 748.4
  ovary, ovaries 256.4
  spleen 759.0
Pompe's (glycogenosis II) 271.0
Poncet's (tuberculous rheumatism) (*see also* Tuberculosis) 015.9 ✓5ᵗʰ
Posada-Wernicke 114.9
Potain's (pulmonary edema) 514
Pott's (*see also* Tuberculosis) 015.0 ✓5ᵗʰ [730.88]
  osteomyelitis 015.0 ✓5ᵗʰ [730.88]
  paraplegia 015.0 ✓5ᵗʰ [730.88]
  spinal curvature 015.0 ✓5ᵗʰ [737.43]
  spondylitis 015.0 ✓5ᵗʰ [720.81]
Potter's 753.0
Poulet's 714.2
pregnancy NEC (*see also* Pregnancy) 646.9 ✓5ᵗʰ
Preiser's (osteoporosis) 733.09
Pringle's (tuberous sclerosis) 759.5
Profichet's 729.9
prostate 602.9
  specified type NEC 602.8
protozoal NEC 136.8
  intestine, intestinal NEC 007.9
pseudo-Hurler's (mucolipidosis III) 272.7
psychiatric (*see also* Psychosis) 298.9
psychotic (*see also* Psychosis) 298.9
Puente's (simple glandular cheilitis) 528.5
puerperal NEC (*see also* Puerperal) 674.9 ✓5ᵗʰ
pulmonary — *see also* Disease, lung
  amyloid 277.3 [517.8]
  artery 417.9
  circulation, circulatory 417.9
    specified NEC 417.8
  diffuse obstructive (chronic) 496
    with
      acute exacerbation NEC 491.21
      asthma (chronic) (obstructive) 493.2 ✓5ᵗʰ
  heart (chronic) 416.9
    specified NEC 416.8
  hypertensive (vascular) 416.0
    cardiovascular 416.0
  obstructive diffuse (chronic) 496
    with
      acute exacerbation NEC 491.21
      asthma (chronic) (obstructive) 493.2 ✓5ᵗʰ
      bronchitis (chronic) 491.20
        with acute exacerbation 491.21
  valve (*see also* Endocarditis, pulmonary) 424.3
pulp (dental) NEC 522.9
pulseless 446.7
Putnam's (subacute combined sclerosis with pernicious anemia) 281.0 [336.2]
Pyle (-Cohn) (craniometaphyseal dysplasia) 756.89
pyramidal tract 333.90
Quervain's
  tendon sheath 727.04
  thyroid (subacute granulomatous thyroiditis) 245.1
Quincke's — *see* Edema, angioneurotic
Quinquaud (acne decalvans) 704.09
rag sorters' 022.1
Raynaud's (paroxysmal digital cyanosis) 443.0
reactive airway — *see* Asthma
Recklinghausen's (M9540/1) 237.71
  bone (osteitis fibrosa cystica) 252.0
Recklinghausen-Applebaum (hemochromatosis) 275.0

Disease, diseased — *see also* Syndrome — *continued*
Reclus' (cystic) 610.1
rectum NEC 569.49
Refsum's (heredopathia atactica polyneuritiformis) 356.3
Reichmann's (gastrosuccorrhea) 536.8
Reimann's (periodic) 277.3
Reiter's 099.3
renal (functional) (pelvis) 593.9
  with
    edema (*see also* Nephrosis) 581.9
    exudative nephritis 583.89
    lesion of interstitial nephritis 583.89
    stated generalized cause — *see* Nephritis
  acute — *see* Nephritis, acute
  basement membrane NEC 583.89
    with
      pulmonary hemorrhage (Goodpasture's syndrome) 446.21 [583.81]
  chronic — *see* Nephritis, chronic
  complicating pregnancy or puerperium NEC 646.2 ✓5ᵗʰ
    with hypertension — *see* Toxemia, of pregnancy
    affecting fetus or newborn 760.1
  cystic, congenital (*see also* Cystic, disease, kidney) 753.10
  diabetic 250.4 ✓5ᵗʰ [583.81]
  due to
    amyloidosis 277.3 [583.81]
    diabetes mellitus 250.4 ✓5ᵗʰ [583.81]
    systemic lupus erythematosis 710.0 [583.81]
  end-stage 585
  exudative 583.89
  fibrocystic (congenital) 753.19
  gonococcal 098.19 [583.81]
  gouty 274.10
  hypertensive (*see also* Hypertension, kidney) 403.90
  immune complex NEC 583.89
  interstitial (diffuse) (focal) 583.89
  lupus 710.0 [583.81]
  maternal, affecting fetus or newborn 760.1
    hypertensive 760.0
  phosphate-losing (tubular) 588.0
  polycystic (congenital) 753.12
    adult type (APKD) 753.13
    autosomal dominant 753.13
    autosomal recessive 753.14
    childhood type (CPKD) 753.14
    infantile type 753.14
  specified lesion or cause NEC (*see also* Glomerulonephritis) 583.89
  subacute 581.9
  syphilitic 095.4
  tuberculous (*see also* Tuberculosis) 016.0 ✓5ᵗʰ [583.81]
  tubular (*see also* Nephrosis, tubular) 584.5
Rendu-Osler-Weber (familial hemorrhagic telangiectasia) 448.0
renovascular (arteriosclerotic) (*see also* Hypertension, kidney) 403.90
respiratory (tract) 519.9
  acute or subacute (upper) NEC 465.9
    due to fumes or vapors 506.3
    multiple sites NEC 465.8
    noninfectious 478.9
    streptococcal 034.0
  chronic 519.9
    arising in the perinatal period 770.7
    due to fumes or vapors 506.4
  due to
    aspiration of liquids or solids 508.9
    external agents NEC 508.9
      specified NEC 508.8
    fumes or vapors 506.9
      acute or subacute NEC 506.3
      chronic 506.4
  fetus or newborn NEC 770.9
  obstructive 496
  specified type NEC 519.8
  upper (acute) (infectious) NEC 465.9
    multiple sites NEC 465.8
    noninfectious NEC 478.9
    streptococcal 034.0

✓4ᵗʰ Fourth-digit Required   ✓5ᵗʰ Fifth-digit Required   ▶◀ Revised Text   ● New Line   ▲ Revised Code

Disease — Disease

Disease, diseased — *see also* Syndrome — *continued*
retina, retinal NEC 362.9
  Batten's or Batten-Mayou 330.1 *[362.71]*
  degeneration 362.89
  vascular lesion 362.17
rheumatic (*see also* Arthritis) 716.8 ☑5ᵗʰ
  heart — *see* Disease, heart, rheumatic
rheumatoid (heart) — *see* Arthritis, rheumatoid
rickettsial NEC 083.9
  specified type NEC 083.8
Riedel's (ligneous thyroiditis) 245.3
Riga (-Fede) (cachectic aphthae) 529.0
Riggs' (compound periodontitis) 523.4
Ritter's 695.81
Rivalta's (cervicofacial actinomycosis) 039.3
Robles' (onchocerciasis) 125.3 *[360.13]*
Roger's (congenital interventricular septal defect) 745.4
Rokitansky's (*see also* Necrosis, liver) 570
Romberg's 349.89
Rosenthal's (factor XI deficiency) 286.2
Rossbach's (hyperchlorhydria) 536.8
  psychogenic 306.4
Roth (-Bernhardt) 355.1
Runeberg's (progressive pernicious anemia) 281.0
Rust's (tuberculous spondylitis) (*see also* Tuberculosis) 015.0 ☑5ᵗʰ *[720.81]*
Rustitskii's (multiple myeloma) (M9730/3) 203.0 ☑5ᵗʰ
Ruysch's (Hirschsprung's disease) 751.3
Sachs (-Tay) 330.1
sacroiliac NEC 724.6
salivary gland or duct NEC 527.9
  inclusion 078.5
    streptococcal 034.0
  virus 078.5
Sander's (paranoia) 297.1
Sandhoff's 330.1
sandworm 126.9
Savill's (epidemic exfoliative dermatitis) 695.89
Schamberg's (progressive pigmentary dermatosis) 709.09
Schaumann's (sarcoidosis) 135
Schenck's (sporotrichosis) 117.1
Scheuermann's (osteochondrosis) 732.0
Schilder (-Flatau) 341.1
Schimmelbusch's 610.1
Schlatter's tibia (tubercle) 732.4
Schlatter-Osgood 732.4
Schmorl's 722.30
  cervical 722.39
  lumbar, lumbosacral 722.32
  specified region NEC 722.39
  thoracic, thoracolumbar 722.31
Scholz's 330.0
Schönlein (-Henoch) (purpura rheumatica) 287.0
Schottmüller's (*see also* Fever, paratyphoid) 002.9
Schüller-Christian (chronic histiocytosis X) 277.8
Schultz's (agranulocytosis) 288.0
Schwalbe-Ziehen-Oppenheimer 333.6
Schweninger-Buzzi (macular atrophy) 701.3
sclera 379.19
scrofulous (*see also* Tuberculosis) 017.2 ☑5ᵗʰ
scrotum 608.9
sebaceous glands NEC 706.9
Secretan's (posttraumatic edema) 782.3
semilunar cartilage, cystic 717.5
seminal vesicle 608.9
Senear-Usher (pemphigus erythematosus) 694.4
serum NEC 999.5
Sever's (osteochondrosis calcaneum) 732.5
Sézary's (reticulosis) (M9701/3) 202.2 ☑5ᵗʰ
Shaver's (bauxite pneumoconiosis) 503
Sheehan's (postpartum pituitary necrosis) 253.2
shimamushi (scrub typus) 081.2
shipyard 077.1
sickle cell 282.60
  with
    crisis 282.62
    Hb-S disease 282.61

Disease, diseased — *see also* Syndrome — *continued*
sickle cell — *continued*
  with — *continued*
    other abnormal hemoglobin (Hb-D) (Hb-E) (Hb-G) (Hb-J) (Hb-K) (Hb-O) (Hb-P) (high fetal gene) 282.69
  elliptocytosis 282.60
  Hb-C 282.63
  Hb-S 282.61
    with
      crisis 282.62
      Hb-C 282.63
      other abnormal hemoglobin (Hb-D) (Hb-E) (Hb-G) (Hb-J) (Hb-K) (Hb-O) (Hb-P) (high fetal gene) 282.69
  spherocytosis 282.60
  thalassemia 282.4
Siegal-Cattan-Mamou (periodic) 277.3
silo fillers' 506.9
Simian B 054.3
Simmonds' (pituitary cachexia) 253.2
Simons' (progressive lipodystrophy) 272.6
Sinding-Larsen (juvenile osteopathia patellae) 732.4
sinus — *see also* Sinusitis
  brain 437.9
  specified NEC 478.1
Sirkari's 085.0
sixth 057.8
Sjögren (-Gougerot) 710.2
  with lung involvement 710.2 *[517.8]*
Skevas-Zerfus 989.5
skin NEC 709.9
  due to metabolic disorder 277.9
  specified type NEC 709.8
sleeping 347
  meaning sleeping sickness (*see also* Trypanosomiasis) 086.5
small vessel 443.9
Smith-Strang (oasthouse urine) 270.2
Sneddon-Wilkinson (subcorneal pustular dermatosis) 694.1
South African creeping 133.8
Spencer's (epidemic vomiting) 078.82
Spielmeyer-Stock 330.1
Spielmeyer-Vogt 330.1
spine, spinal 733.90
  combined system (*see also* Degeneration, combined) 266.2 *[336.2]*
    with pernicious anemia 281.0 *[336.2]*
  cord NEC 336.9
    congenital 742.9
  demyelinating NEC 341.8
  joint (*see also* Disease, joint, spine) 724.9
  tuberculous 015.0 ☑5ᵗʰ *[730.8]* ☑5ᵗʰ
spinocerebellar 334.9
  specified NEC 334.8
spleen (organic) (postinfectional) 289.50
  amyloid 277.3
  lardaceous 277.3
  polycystic 759.0
  specified NEC 289.59
sponge divers' 989.5
Stanton's (melioidosis) 025
Stargardt's 362.75
Steinert's 359.2
Sternberg's — *see* Disease, Hodgkin's
Stevens-Johnson (erythema multiforme exudativum) 695.1
Sticker's (erythema infectiosum) 057.0
Stieda's (calcification, knee joint) 726.62
Still's (juvenile rheumatoid arthritis) 714.30
Stiller's (asthenia) 780.79
Stokes' (exophthalmic goiter) 242.0 ☑5ᵗʰ
Stokes-Adams (syncope with heart block) 426.9
Stokvis (-Talma) (enterogenous cyanosis) 289.7
stomach NEC (organic) 537.9
  functional 536.9
    psychogenic 306.4
  lardaceous 277.3
stonemasons' 502
storage
  glycogen (*see also* Disease, glycogen storage) 271.0
  lipid 272.7
  mucopolysaccharide 277.5

Disease, diseased — *see also* Syndrome — *continued*
striatopallidal system 333.90
  specified NEC 333.89
Strümpell-Marie (ankylosing spondylitis) 720.0
Stuart's (congenital factor X deficiency) (*see also* Defect, coagulation) 286.3
Stuart-Prower (congenital factor X deficiency) (*see also* Defect, coagulation) 286.3
Sturge (-Weber) (-Dimitri) (encephalocutaneous angiomatosis) 759.6
Stuttgart 100.89
Sudeck's 733.7
supporting structures of teeth NEC 525.9
suprarenal (gland) (capsule) 255.9
  hyperfunction 255.3
  hypofunction 255.4
Sutton's 709.09
Sutton and Gull's — *see* Hypertension, kidney
sweat glands NEC 705.9
  specified type NEC 705.89
sweating 078.2
Sweeley-Klionsky 272.4
Swift (-Feer) 985.0
swimming pool (bacillus) 031.1
swineherd's 100.89
Sylvest's (epidemic pleurodynia) 074.1
Symmers (follicular lymphoma) (M9690/3) 202.0 ☑5ᵗʰ
sympathetic nervous system (*see also* Neuropathy, peripheral, autonomic) 337.9
synovium 727.9
syphilitic — *see* Syphilis
systemic tissue mast cell (M9741/3) 202.6 ☑5ᵗʰ
Taenzer's 757.4
Takayasu's (pulseless) 446.7
Talma's 728.85
Tangier (familial high-density lipoprotein deficiency) 272.5
Tarral-Besnier (pityriasis rubra pilaris) 696.4
Tay-Sachs 330.1
Taylor's 701.8
tear duct 375.69
teeth, tooth 525.9
  hard tissues NEC 521.9
  pulp NEC 522.9
tendon 727.9
  inflammatory NEC 727.9
terminal vessel 443.9
testis 608.9
Thaysen-Gee (nontropical sprue) 579.0
Thomsen's 359.2
Thomson's (congenital poikiloderma) 757.33
Thornwaldt's, Tornwaldt's (pharyngeal bursitis) 478.29
throat 478.20
  septic 034.0
thromboembolic (*see also* Embolism) 444.9
thymus (gland) 254.9
  specified NEC 254.8
thyroid (gland) NEC 246.9
  heart (*see also* Hyperthyroidism) 242.9 ☑5ᵗʰ *[425.7]*
  lardaceous 277.3
  specified NEC 246.8
Tietze's 733.6
Tommaselli's
  correct substance properly administered 599.7
  overdose or wrong substance given or taken 961.4
tongue 529.9
tonsils, tonsillar (and adenoids) (chronic) 474.9
  specified NEC 474.8
tooth, teeth 525.9
  hard tissues NEC 521.9
  pulp NEC 522.9
Tornwaldt's (pharyngeal bursitis) 478.29
Tourette's 307.23
trachea 519.1
tricuspid — *see* Endocarditis, tricuspid
triglyceride-storage, type I, II, III 272.7
triple vessel (coronary arteries) — *see* Arteriosclerosis, coronary
trisymptomatic, Gourgerot's 709.1
trophoblastic (*see also* Hydatidiform mole) 630
  previous, affecting management of pregnancy V23.1

☑4ᵗʰ Fourth-digit Required   ☑5ᵗʰ Fifth-digit Required   ▶◀ Revised Text   ● New Line   ▲ Revised Code

Disease, diseased — *see also* Syndrome — *continued*
tsutsugamushi (scrub typhus) 081.2
tube (fallopian), noninflammatory 620.9
   specified NEC 620.8
tuberculous NEC (*see also* Tuberculosis) 011.9 ✓5ᵗʰ
tubo-ovarian
   inflammatory (*see also* Salpingo-oophoritis) 614.2
   noninflammatory 620.9
      specified NEC 620.8
tubotympanic, chronic (with anterior perforation of ear drum) 382.1
tympanum 385.9
Uhl's 746.84
umbilicus (newborn) NEC 779.89 ▲
Underwood's (sclerema neonatorum) 778.1
undiagnosed 799.9
Unna's (seborrheic dermatitis) 690.18
unstable hemoglobin hemolytic 282.7
Unverricht (-Lundborg) 333.2
Urbach-Oppenheim (necrobiosis lipoidica diabeticorum) 250.8 ✓5ᵗʰ [709.3]
Urbach-Wiethe (lipoid proteinosis) 272.8
ureter 593.9
urethra 599.9
   specified type NEC 599.84
urinary (tract) 599.9
   bladder 596.9
      specified NEC 596.8
   maternal, affecting fetus or newborn 760.1
Usher-Senear (pemphigus erythematosus) 694.4
uterus (organic) 621.9
   infective (*see also* Endometritis) 615.9
   inflammatory (*see also* Endometritis) 615.9
   noninflammatory 621.9
      specified type NEC 621.8
uveal tract
   anterior 364.9
   posterior 363.9
vagabonds' 132.1
vagina, vaginal
   inflammatory 616.9
      specified NEC 616.8
   noninflammatory 623.9
      specified NEC 623.8
Valsuani's (progressive pernicious anemia, puerperal) 648.2 ✓5ᵗʰ
   complicating pregnancy or puerperium 648.2 ✓5ᵗʰ
valve, valvular — *see* Endocarditis
van Bogaert-Nijssen (-Peiffer) 330.0
van Creveld-von Gierke (glycogenosis I) 271.0
van den Bergh's (enterogenous cyanosis) 289.7
van Neck's (juvenile osteochondrosis) 732.1
Vaquez (-Osler) (polycythemia vera) (M9950/1) 238.4
vascular 459.9
   arteriosclerotic — *see* Arteriosclerosis
   hypertensive — *see* Hypertension
   obliterative 447.1
      peripheral 443.9
   occlusive 459.9
   peripheral (occlusive) 443.9
      in diabetes mellitus 250.7 ✓5ᵗʰ [443.81]
      specified type NEC 443.89
vas deferens 608.9
vasomotor 443.9
vasopastic 443.9
vein 459.9
venereal 099.9
   chlamydial NEC 099.50
      anus 099.52
      bladder 099.53
      cervix 099.53
      epididymis 099.54
      genitourinary NEC 099.55
         lower 099.53
         specified NEC 099.54
      pelvic inflammatory disease 099.54
      perihepatic 099.56
      peritoneum 099.56
      pharynx 099.51
      rectum 099.52
      specified site NEC 099.54

Disease, diseased — *see also* Syndrome — *continued*
venereal — *continued*
   chlamydial NEC — *continued*
      testis 099.54
      vagina 099.53
      vulva 099.53
   fifth 099.1
   sixth 099.1
   complicating pregnancy, childbirth, or puerperium 647.2 ✓5ᵗʰ
   specified nature or type NEC 099.8
      chlamydial — *see* Disease, venereal, chlamydial
Verneuil's (syphilitic bursitis) 095.7
Verse's (calcinosis intervertebralis) 275.49 [722.90]
vertebra, vertebral NEC 733.90
   disc — *see* Disease, Intervertebral disc
vibration NEC 994.9
Vidal's (lichen simplex chronicus) 698.3
Vincent's (trench mouth) 101
Virchow's 733.99
virus (filterable) NEC 078.89
   arbovirus NEC 066.9
   arthropod-borne NEC 066.9
   central nervous system NEC 049.9
      specified type NEC 049.8
   complicating pregnancy, childbirth, or puerperium 647.6 ✓5ᵗʰ
   contact (with) V01.7
   exposure to V01.7
   Marburg 078.89
   maternal
      with fetal damage affecting management of pregnancy 655.3 ✓5ᵗʰ
   nonarthropod-borne NEC 078.89
      central nervous sytem NEC 049.9
      specified NEC 049.8
vitreous 379.29
vocal cords NEC 478.5
Vogt's (Cecile) 333.7
Vogt-Spielmeyer 330.1
Volhard-Fahr (malignant nephrosclerosis) 403.00
Volkmann's
   acquired 958.6
von Bechterew's (ankylosing spondylitis) 720.0
von Economo's (encephalitis lethargica) 049.8
von Eulenburg's (congenital paramyotonia) 359.2
von Gierke's (glycogenosis I) 271.0
von Graefe's 378.72
von Hippel's (retinocerebral angiomatosis) 759.6
von Hippel-Lindau (angiomatosis retinocerebellosa) 759.6
von Jaksch's (pseudoleukemia infantum) 285.8
von Recklinghausen's (M9540/1) 237.71
   bone (osteitis fibrosa cystica) 252.0
von Recklinghausen-Applebaum (hemochromatosis) 275.0
von Willebrand (-Jürgens) (angiohemophilia) 286.4
von Zambusch's (lichen sclerosus et atrophicus) 701.0
Voorhoeve's (dyschondroplasia) 756.4
Vrolik's (osteogenesis imperfecta) 756.51
vulva
   noninflammatory 624.9
      specified NEC 624.8
Wagner's (colloid milium) 709.3
Waldenström's (osteochondrosis capital femoral) 732.1
Wallgren's (obstruction of splenic vein with collateral circulation) 459.89
Wardrop's (with lymphangitis) 681.9
   finger 681.02
   toe 681.11
Wassilieff's (leptospiral jaundice) 100.0
wasting NEC 799.4
   due to malnutrition 261
   paralysis 335.21
Waterhouse-Friderichsen 036.3
waxy (any site) 277.3
Weber-Christian (nodular nonsuppurative panniculitis) 729.30

Disease, diseased — *see also* Syndrome — *continued*
Wegner's (syphilitic osteochondritis) 090.0
Weil's (leptospral jaundice) 100.0
   of lung 100.0
Weir Mitchell's (erythromelalgia) 443.89
Werdnig-Hoffmann 335.0
Werlhof's (*see also* Purpura, thrombocytopenic) 287.3
Wermer's 258.0
Werner's (progeria adultorum) 259.8
Werner-His (trench fever) 083.1
Werner-Schultz (agranulocytosis) 288.0
Wernicke's (superior hemorrhagic polioencephalitis) 265.1
Wernicke-Posadas 114.9
Whipple's (intestinal lipodystrophy) 040.2
whipworm 127.3
white
   blood cell 288.9
      specified NEC 288.8
   spot 701.0
White's (congenital) (keratosis follicularis) 757.39
Whitmore's (melioidosis) 025
Widal-Abrami (acquired hemolytic jaundice) 283.9
Wilkie's 557.1
Wilkinson-Sneddon (subcorneal pustular dermatosis) 694.1
Willis' (diabetes mellitus) (*see also* Diabetes) 250.0 ✓5ᵗʰ
Wilson's (hepatolenticular degeneration) 275.1
Wilson-Brocq (dermatitis exfoliativa) 695.89
winter vomiting 078.82
Wise's 696.2
Wohlfart-Kugelberg-Welander 335.11
Woillez's (acute idiopathic pulmonary congestion) 518.5
Wolman's (primary familial xanthomatosis) 272.7
wool-sorters' 022.1
Zagari's (xerostomia) 527.7
Zahorsky's (exanthem subitum) 057.8
Ziehen-Oppenheim 333.6
zoonotic, bacterial NEC 027.9
   specified type NEC 027.8

Disfigurement (due to scar) 709.2
head V48.6
limb V49.4
neck V48.7
trunk V48.7

Disgerminoma — *see* Dysgerminoma

Disinsertion, retina 361.04

Disintegration, complete, of the body 799.8
traumatic 869.1

Disk kidney 753.3

Dislocatable hip, congenital (*see also* Dislocation, hip, congenital) 754.30

Dislocation (articulation) (closed) (displacement) (simple) (subluxation) 839.8

> Note — "Closed" includes simple, complete, partial, uncomplicated, and unspecified dislocation.
>
> "Open" includes dislocation specified as infected or compound and dislocation with foreign body.
>
> "Chronic," "habitual," "old," or "recurrent" dislocations should be coded as indicated under the entry "Dislocation, recurrent," and "pathological" as indicated under the entry "Dislocation, pathological."
>
> For late effect of dislocation see Late, effect, dislocation.

with fracture — *see* Fracture, by site
acromioclavicular (joint) (closed) 831.04
   open 831.14
anatomical site (closed)
   specified NEC 839.69
      open 839.79
   unspecified or ill-defined 839.8
      open 839.9

Dislocation — continued
  ankle (scaphoid bone) (closed) 837.0
    open 837.1
  arm (closed) 839.8
    open 839.9
  astragalus (closed) 837.0
    open 837.1
  atlanto-axial (closed) 839.01
    open 839.11
  atlas (closed) 839.01
    open 839.11
  axis (closed) 839.02
    open 839.12
  back (closed) 839.8
    open 839.9
  Bell-Daly 723.8
  breast bone (closed) 839.61
    open 839.71
  capsule, joint — see Dislocation, by site
  carpal (bone) — see Dislocation, wrist
  carpometacarpal (joint) (closed) 833.04
    open 833.14
  cartilage (joint) — see also Dislocation, by site
    knee — see Tear, meniscus
  cervical, cervicodorsal, or cervicothoracic
      (spine) (vertebra) — see Dislocation,
      vertebra, cervical
  chiropractic (see also Lesion, nonallopathic)
      739.9
  chondrocostal — see Dislocation, costochondral
  chronic — see Dislocation, recurrent
  clavicle (closed) 831.04
    open 831.14
  coccyx (closed) 839.41
    open 839.51
  collar bone (closed) 831.04
    open 831.14
  compound (open) NEC 839.9
  congenital NEC 755.8
    hip (see also Dislocation, hip, congenital)
        754.30
    lens 743.37
    rib 756.3
    sacroiliac 755.69
    spine NEC 756.19
    vertebra 756.19
  coracoid (closed) 831.09
    open 831.19
  costal cartilage (closed) 839.69
    open 839.79
  costochondral (closed) 839.69
    open 839.79
  cricoarytenoid articulation (closed) 839.69
    open 839.79
  cricothyroid (cartilage) articulation (closed)
      839.69
    open 839.79
  dorsal vertebrae (closed) 839.21
    open 839.31
  ear ossicle 385.23
  elbow (closed) 832.00
    anterior (closed) 832.01
      open 832.11
    congenital 754.89
    divergent (closed) 832.09
      open 832.19
    lateral (closed) 832.04
      open 832.14
    medial (closed) 832.03
      open 832.13
    open 832.10
    posterior (closed) 832.02
      open 832.12
    recurrent 718.32
    specified type NEC 832.09
      open 832.19
  eye 360.81
    lateral 376.36
  eyeball 360.81
    lateral 376.36
  femur
    distal end (closed) 836.50
      anterior 836.52
        open 836.62
      lateral 836.53
        open 836.63

Dislocation — continued
  femur — continued
    distal end — continued
      medial 836.54
        open 836.64
      open 836.60
      posterior 836.51
        open 836.61
    proximal end (closed) 835.00
      anterior (pubic) 835.03
        open 835.13
      obturator 835.02
        open 835.12
      open 835.10
      posterior 835.01
        open 835.11
  fibula
    distal end (closed) 837.0
      open 837.1
    proximal end (closed) 836.59
      open 836.69
  finger(s) (phalanx) (thumb) (closed) 834.00
    interphalangeal (joint) 834.02
      open 834.12
    metacarpal (bone), distal end 834.01
      open 834.11
    metacarpophalangeal (joint) 834.01
      open 834.11
    open 834.10
    recurrent 718.34
  foot (closed) 838.00
    open 838.10
    recurrent 718.37
  forearm (closed) 839.8
    open 839.9
  fracture — see Fracture, by site
  glenoid (closed) 831.09
    open 831.19
  habitual — see Dislocation, recurrent
  hand (closed) 839.8
    open 839.9
  hip (closed) 835.00
    anterior 835.03
      obturator 835.02
        open 835.12
      open 835.13
    congenital (unilateral) 754.30
      with subluxation of other hip 754.35
      bilateral 754.31
    developmental 718.75
    open 835.10
    posterior 835.01
      open 835.11
    recurrent 718.35
  humerus (closed) 831.00
    distal end (see also Dislocation, elbow)
        832.00
    open 831.10
    proximal end (closed) 831.00
      anterior (subclavicular) (subcoracoid)
          (subglenoid) (closed) 831.01
        open 831.11
      inferior (closed) 831.03
        open 831.13
      open 831.10
      posterior (closed) 831.02
        open 831.12
  implant — see Complications, mechanical
  incus 385.23
  infracoracoid (closed) 831.01
    open 831.11
  innominate (pubic juntion) (sacral junction)
      (closed) 839.69
    acetabulum (see also Dislocation, hip)
        835.00
    open 839.79
  interphalangeal (joint)
    finger or hand (closed) 834.02
      open 834.12
    foot or toe (closed) 838.06
      open 838.16
  jaw (cartilage) (meniscus) (closed) 830.0
    open 830.1
    recurrent 524.69
  joint NEC (closed) 839.8
    developmental 718.7 ☑5ᵗʰ
    open 839.9

Dislocation — continued
  joint NEC — continued
    pathological — see Dislocation, pathological
    recurrent — see Dislocation, recurrent
  knee (closed) 836.50
    anterior 836.51
      open 836.61
    congenital (with genu recurvatum) 754.41
    habitual 718.36
    lateral 836.54
      open 836.64
    medial 836.53
      open 836.63
    old 718.36
    open 836.60
    posterior 836.52
      open 836.62
    recurrent 718.36
    rotatory 836.59
      open 836.69
  lacrimal gland 375.16
  leg (closed) 839.8
    open 839.9
  lens (crystalline) (complete) (partial) 379.32
    anterior 379.33
    congenital 743.37
    ocular implant 996.53
    posterior 379.34
    traumatic 921.3
  ligament — see Dislocation, by site
  lumbar (vertebrae) (closed) 839.20
    open 839.30
  lumbosacral (vertebrae) (closed) 839.20
    congenital 756.19
    open 839.30
  mandible (closed) 830.0
    open 830.1
  maxilla (inferior) (closed) 830.0
    open 830.1
  meniscus (knee) — see also Tear, meniscus
    other sites — see Dislocation, by site
  metacarpal (bone)
    distal end (closed) 834.01
      open 834.11
    proximal end (closed) 833.05
      open 833.15
  metacarpophalangeal (joint) (closed) 834.01
    open 834.11
  metatarsal (bone) (closed) 838.04
    open 838.14
  metatarsophalangeal (joint) (closed) 838.05
    open 838.15
  midcarpal (joint) (closed) 833.03
    open 833.13
  midtarsal (joint) (closed) 838.02
    open 838.12
  Monteggia's — see Dislocation, hip
  multiple locations (except fingers only or toes
      only) (closed) 839.8
    open 839.9
  navicular (bone) foot (closed) 837.0
    open 837.1
  neck (see also Dislocation, vertebra, cervical)
      839.00
  Nélaton's — see Dislocation, ankle
  nontraumatic (joint) — see Dislocation,
      pathological
  nose (closed) 839.69
    open 839.79
  not recurrent, not current injury — see
      Dislocation, pathological
  occiput from atlas (closed) 839.01
    open 839.11
  old — see Dislocation, recurrent
  open (compound) NEC 839.9
  ossicle, ear 385.23
  paralytic (flaccid) (spastic) — see Dislocation,
      pathological
  patella (closed) 836.3
    congenital 755.64
    open 836.4
  pathological NEC 718.20
    ankle 718.27
    elbow 718.22
    foot 718.27
    hand 718.24
    hip 718.25
    knee 718.26

☑4ᵗʰ Fourth-digit Required   ☑5ᵗʰ Fifth-digit Required   ▶◀ Revised Text   ● New Line   ▲ Revised Code

Dislocation — *continued*
　pathological NEC — *continued*
　　lumbosacral joint 724.6
　　multiple sites 718.29
　　pelvic region 718.25
　　sacroiliac 724.6
　　shoulder (region) 718.21
　　specified site NEC 718.28
　　spine 724.8
　　　sacroiliac 724.6
　　wrist 718.23
　pelvis (closed) 839.69
　　acetabulum (*see also* Dislocation, hip)
　　　835.00
　　open 839.79
　phalanx
　　foot or toe (closed) 838.09
　　　open 838.19
　　hand or finger (*see also* Dislocation, finger)
　　　834.00
　postpoliomyelitic — *see* Dislocation,
　　pathological
　prosthesis, internal — *see* Complications,
　　mechanical
　radiocarpal (joint) (closed) 833.02
　　open 833.12
　radioulnar (joint)
　　distal end (closed) 833.01
　　　open 833.11
　　proximal end (*see also* Dislocation, elbow)
　　　832.00
　radius
　　distal end (closed) 833.00
　　　open 833.10
　　proximal end (closed) 832.01
　　　open 832.11
　recurrent (*see also* Derangement, joint,
　　recurrent) 718.3 ✓5ᵗʰ
　　elbow 718.32
　　hip 718.35
　　joint NEC 718.38
　　knee 718.36
　　lumbosacral (joint) 724.6
　　patella 718.36
　　sacroiliac 724.6
　　shoulder 718.31
　　temporomandibular 524.69
　rib (cartilage) (closed) 839.69
　　congenital 756.3
　　open 839.79
　sacrococcygeal (closed) 839.42
　　open 839.52
　sacroiliac (joint) (ligament) (closed) 839.42
　　congenital 755.69
　　open 839.52
　　recurrent 724.6
　sacrum (closed) 839.42
　　open 839.52
　scaphoid (bone)
　　ankle or foot (closed) 837.0
　　　open 837.1
　　wrist (closed) (*see also* Dislocation, wrist)
　　　833.00
　　　open 833.10
　scapula (closed) 831.09
　　open 831.19
　semilunar cartilage, knee — *see* Tear, meniscus
　septal cartilage (nose) (closed) 839.69
　　open 839.79
　septum (nasal) (old) 470
　sesamoid bone — *see* Dislocation, by site
　shoulder (blade) (ligament) (closed) 831.00
　　anterior (subclavicular) (subcoracoid)
　　　(subglenoid) (closed) 831.01
　　　open 831.11
　　chronic 718.31
　　inferior 831.03
　　　open 831.13
　　open 831.10
　　posterior (closed) 831.02
　　　open 831.12
　　recurrent 718.31
　skull — *see* Injury, intracranial
　Smith's — *see* Dislocation, foot
　spine (articular process) (*see also* Dislocation,
　　vertebra) (closed) 839.40
　　atlanto-axial (closed) 839.01

Dislocation — *continued*
　spine (*see also* Dislocation, vertebra) —
　　continued
　　atlanto-axial — *continued*
　　　open 839.11
　　　recurrent 723.8
　　cervical, cervicodorsal, cervicothoracic
　　　(closed) (*see also* Dislocation,
　　　vertebrae, cervical) 839.00
　　　open 839.10
　　　recurrent 723.8
　　coccyx 839.41
　　　open 839.51
　　congenital 756.19
　　due to birth trauma 767.4
　　open 839.50
　　recurrent 724.9
　　sacroiliac 839.42
　　　recurrent 724.6
　　sacrum (sacrococcygeal) (sacroiliac) 839.42
　　　open 839.52
　spontaneous — *see* Dislocation, pathological
　sternoclavicular (joint) (closed) 839.61
　　open 839.71
　sternum (closed) 839.61
　　open 839.71
　subastragalar — *see* Dislocation, foot
　subglenoid (closed) 831.01
　　open 831.11
　symphysis
　　jaw (closed) 830.0
　　　open 830.1
　　mandibular (closed) 830.0
　　　open 830.1
　　pubis (closed) 839.69
　　　open 839.79
　tarsal (bone) (joint) 838.01
　　open 838.11
　tarsometatarsal (joint) 838.03
　　open 838.13
　temporomandibular (joint) (closed) 830.0
　　open 830.1
　　recurrent 524.69
　thigh
　　distal end (*see also* Dislocation, femur, distal
　　　end) 836.50
　　proximal end (*see also* Dislocation, hip)
　　　835.00
　thoracic (vertebrae) (closed) 839.21
　　open 839.31
　thumb(s) (*see also* Dislocation, finger) 834.00
　thyroid cartilage (closed) 839.69
　　open 839.79
　tibia
　　distal end (closed) 837.0
　　　open 837.1
　　proximal end (closed) 836.50
　　　anterior 836.51
　　　　open 836.61
　　　lateral 836.54
　　　　open 836.64
　　　medial 836.53
　　　　open 836.63
　　　open 836.60
　　　posterior 836.52
　　　　open 836.62
　　　rotatory 836.59
　　　　open 836.69
　tibiofibular
　　distal (closed) 837.0
　　　open 837.1
　　superior (closed) 836.59
　　　open 836.69
　toe(s) (closed) 838.09
　　open 838.19
　trachea (closed) 839.69
　　open 839.79
　ulna
　　distal end (closed) 833.09
　　　open 833.19
　　proximal end — *see* Dislocation, elbow
　vertebra (articular process) (body) (closed)
　　839.40
　　cervical, cervicodorsal or cervicothoracic
　　　(closed) 839.00
　　　first (atlas) 839.01
　　　　open 839.11

Dislocation — *continued*
　vertebra — *continued*
　　cervical, cervicodorsal or cervicothoracic —
　　　continued
　　　second (axis) 839.02
　　　　open 839.12
　　　third 839.03
　　　　open 839.13
　　　fourth 839.04
　　　　open 839.14
　　　fifth 839.05
　　　　open 839.15
　　　sixth 839.06
　　　　open 839.16
　　　seventh 839.07
　　　　open 839.17
　　　congential 756.19
　　　multiple sites 839.08
　　　　open 839.18
　　　open 839.10
　　congential 756.19
　　dorsal 839.21
　　　open 839.31
　　　recurrent 724.9
　　lumbar, lumbosacral 839.20
　　　open 839.30
　　open NEC 839.50
　　recurrent 724.9
　　specified region NEC 839.49
　　　open 839.59
　　thoracic 839.21
　　　open 839.31
　wrist (carpal bone) (scaphoid) (semilunar)
　　　(closed) 833.00
　　carpometacarpal (joint) 833.04
　　　open 833.14
　　metacarpal bone, proximal end 833.05
　　　open 833.15
　　midcarpal (joint) 833.03
　　　open 833.13
　　open 833.10
　　radiocarpal (joint) 833.02
　　　open 833.12
　　radioulnar (joint) 833.01
　　　open 833.11
　　recurrent 718.33
　　specified site NEC 833.09
　　　open 833.19
　　xiphoid cartilage (closed) 839.61
　　　open 839.71

Dislodgement
　artificial skin graft 996.55
　decellularized allodermis graft 996.55

Disobedience, hostile (covert) (overt) (*see also*
　Disturbance, conduct) 312.0 ✓5ᵗʰ

Disorder — *see also* Disease
　academic underachievement, childhood and
　　adolescence 313.83
　accommodation 367.51
　　drug-induced 367.89
　　toxic 367.89
　adjustment (*see also* Reaction, adjustment)
　　309.9
　adrenal (capsule) (cortex) (gland) 255.9
　　specified type NEC 255.8
　adrenogenital 255.2
　affective (*see also* Psychosis, affective) 296.90
　　atypical 296.81
　aggressive, unsocialized (*see also* Disturbance,
　　conduct) 312.0 ✓5ᵗʰ
　alcohol, alcoholic (*see also* Alcohol) 291.9
　allergic — *see* Allergy
　amnestic (*see also* Amnestic syndrome) 294.0
　amino acid (metabolic) (*see also* Disturbance,
　　metabolism, amino acid) 270.9
　　albinism 270.2
　　alkaptonuria 270.2
　　argininosuccinicaciduria 270.6
　　beta-amino-isobutyricaciduria 277.2
　　cystathioninuria 270.4
　　cystinosis 270.0
　　cystinuria 270.0
　　glycinuria 270.0
　　homocystinuria 270.4
　　imidazole 270.5
　　maple syrup (urine) disease 270.3

✓4ᵗʰ Fourth-digit Required　　✓5ᵗʰ Fifth-digit Required　　▶◀ Revised Text　　● New Line　　▲ Revised Code

Dislocation — Disorder

Disorder — *see also* Disease — *continued*
  amino acid (*see also* Disturbance, metabolism, amino acid) — *continued*
    neonatal, transitory 775.8
    oasthouse urine disease 270.2
    ochronosis 270.2
    phenylketonuria 270.1
    phenylpyruvic oligophrenia 270.1
    purine NEC 277.2
    pyrimidine NEC 277.2
    renal transport NEC 270.0
    specified type NEC 270.8
    transport NEC 270.0
      renal 270.0
    xanthinuria 277.2
  anaerobic glycolysis with anemia 282.3
  anxiety (*see also* Anxiety) 300.00
    due to or associated with physical condition 293.84
  arteriole 447.9
    specified type NEC 447.8
  artery 447.9
    specified type NEC 447.8
  articulation — *see* Disorder, joint
  Asperger's 299.8 ☑5ᵗʰ
  attachment of infancy 313.89
  attention deficit 314.00
    with hyperactivity 314.01
    predominantly
      combined hyperactive/inattentive 314.01
      hyperactive/impulsive 314.01
      inattentive 314.00
    residual type 314.8
  autoimmune NEC 279.4
    hemolytic (cold type) (warm type) 283.0
    parathyroid 252.1
    thyroid 245.2
  autistic 299.0 ☑5ᵗʰ
  avoidant, childhood or adolescence 313.21
  balance
    acid-base 276.9
      mixed (with hypercapnia) 276.4
    electrolyte 276.9
    fluid 276.9
  behavior NEC (*see also* Disturbance, conduct) 312.9
  bilirubin excretion 277.4
  bipolar (affective) (alternating) (type I) (*see also* Psychosis, affective) 296.7
    atypical 296.7
    currently
      depressed 296.5 ☑5ᵗʰ
      hypomanic 296.4 ☑5ᵗʰ
      manic 296.4 ☑5ᵗʰ
    mixed 296.6 ☑5ᵗʰ
    type II (recurrent major depressive episodes with hypomania) 296.89
  bladder 596.9
    functional NEC 596.59
    specified NEC 596.8
  bone NEC 733.90
    specified NEC 733.99
  brachial plexus 353.0
  branched-chain amino-acid degradation 270.3
  breast 611.9
    puerperal, postpartum 676.3 ☑5ᵗʰ
    specified NEC 611.8
  Briquet's 300.81
  bursa 727.9
    shoulder region 726.10
  carbohydrate metabolism, congenital 271.9
  cardiac, functional 427.9
    postoperative 997.1
    psychogenic 306.2
  cardiovascular, psychogenic 306.2
  cartilage NEC 733.90
    articular 718.00
      ankle 718.07
      elbow 718.02
      foot 718.07
      hand 718.04
      hip 718.05
      knee 717.9
      multiple sites 718.09
      pelvic region 718.05
      shoulder region 718.01

Disorder — *see also* Disease — *continued*
  cartilage NEC — *continued*
    articular — *continued*
      specified
        site NEC 718.08
        type NEC 733.99
      wrist 718.03
  catatonic — *see* Catatonia
  cervical region NEC 723.9
  cervical root (nerve) NEC 353.2
  character NEC (*see also* Disorder, personality) 301.9
  coagulation (factor) (*see also* Defect, coagulation) 286.9
    factor VIII (congenital) (functional) 286.0
    factor IX (congenital) (functional) 286.1
    neonatal, transitory 776.3
  coccyx 724.70
    specified NEC 724.79
  colon 569.9
    functional 564.9
      congenital 751.3
  cognitive 294.9
  conduct (*see also* Disturbance, conduct) 312.9
    adjustment reaction 309.3
    adolescent onset type 312.82
    childhood onset type 312.81
    compulsive 312.30
      specified type NEC 312.39
    hyperkinetic 314.2
    socialized (type) 312.20
      aggressive 312.23
      unaggressive 312.21
    specified NEC 312.89
  conduction, heart 426.9
    specified NEC 426.89
  convulsive (secondary) (*see also* Convulsions) 780.39
    due to injury at birth 767.0
    idiopathic 780.39
  coordination 781.3
  cornea NEC 371.89
    due to contact lens 371.82
  corticosteroid metabolism NEC 255.2
  cranial nerve — *see* Disorder, nerve, cranial
  cyclothymic 301.13
  degradation, branched-chain amino acid 270.3
  delusional 297.9
  dentition 520.6
  depressive NEC 311
    atypical 296.82
    major (*see also* Psychosis, affective) 296.2 ☑5ᵗʰ
      recurrent episode 296.3 ☑5ᵗʰ
      single episode 296.2 ☑5ᵗʰ
  development, specific 315.9
    associated with hyperkinesia 314.1
    language 315.31
    learning 315.2
      arithmetical 315.1
      reading 315.00
    mixed 315.5
    motor coordination 315.4
    specified type NEC 315.8
    speech 315.39
  diaphragm 519.4
  digestive 536.9
    fetus or newborn 777.9
    specified NEC 777.8
    psychogenic 306.4
  disintegrative (childhood) 299.1 ☑5ᵗʰ
  dissociative 300.14
    identity 300.14
  dysmorphic body 300.7
  dysthymic 300.4
  ear 388.9
    degenerative NEC 388.00
    external 380.9
      specified 380.89
    pinna 380.30
    specified type NEC 388.8
    vascular NEC 388.00
  eating NEC 307.50
  electrolyte NEC 276.9
    with
      abortion — *see* Abortion, by type, with metabolic disorder

Disorder — *see also* Disease — *continued*
  electrolyte NEC — *continued*
    with — *continued*
      ectopic pregnancy (*see also* categories 633.0-633.9) 639.4
      molar pregnancy (*see also* categories 630-632) 639.4
    acidosis 276.2
      metabolic 276.2
      respiratory 276.2
    alkalosis 276.3
      metabolic 276.3
      respiratory 276.3
    following
      abortion 639.4
      ectopic or molar pregnancy 639.4
    neonatal, transitory NEC 775.5
  emancipation as adjustment reaction 309.22
  emotional (*see also* Disorder, mental, nonpsychotic) V40.9
  endocrine 259.9
    specified type NEC 259.8
  esophagus 530.9
    functional 530.5
    psychogenic 306.4
  explosive
    intermittent 312.34
    isolated 312.35
  expressive language 315.31
  eye 379.90
    globe — *see* Disorder, globe
    ill-defined NEC 379.99
    limited duction NEC 378.63
    specified NEC 379.8
  eyelid 374.9
    degenerative 374.50
    sensory 374.44
    specified type NEC 374.89
    vascular 374.85
  factitious — *see* Illness, factitious
  factor, coagulation (*see also* Defect, coagulation) 286.9
    VIII (congenital) (functional) 286.0
    IX (congenital) (funcitonal) 286.1
  fascia 728.9
  feeding — *see* Feeding
  female sexual arousal 302.72
  fluid NEC 276.9
  gastric (functional) 536.9
    motility 536.8
    psychogenic 306.4
    secretion 536.8
  gastrointestinal (functional) NEC 536.9
    newborn (neonatal) 777.9
      specified NEC 777.8
    psychogenic 306.4
  gender (child) 302.6
    adult 302.85
  gender identity (childhood) 302.6
    adult-life 302.85
  genitourinary system, psychogenic 306.50
  globe 360.9
    degenerative 360.20
      specified NEC 360.29
    specified type NEC 360.89
  hearing — *see also* Deafness
    conductive type (air) (*see also* Deafness, conductive) 389.00
    mixed conductive and sensorineural 389.2
    nerve 389.12
    perceptive (*see also* Deafness, perceptive) 389.10
    sensorineural type NEC (*see also* Deafness, perceptive) 389.10
  heart action 427.9
    postoperative 997.1
  hematological, transient neonatal 776.9
    specified type NEC 776.8
  hematopoietic organs 289.9
  hemorrhagic NEC 287.9
    due to circulating anticoagulants 286.5
    specified type NEC 287.8
  hemostasis (*see also* Defect, coagulation) 286.9
  homosexual conflict 302.0
  hypomanic (chronic) 301.11

Disorder — see also Disease — continued
  identity
    childhood and adolescence 313.82
      gender 302.6
    gender 302.6
  immune mechanism (immunity) 279.9
    single complement (C-C) 279.8
    specified type NEC 279.8
  impulse control (see also Disturbance, conduct,
      compulsive) 312.30
  infant sialic acid storage 271.8
  integument, fetus or newborn 778.9
    specified type NEC 778.8
  interactional psychotic (childhood) (see also
      Psychosis, childhood) 299.1 ✓5ᵗʰ
  intermittent explosive 312.34
  intervertebral disc 722.90
    cervical, cervicothoracic 722.91
    lumbar, lumbosacral 722.93
    thoracic, thoracolumbar 722.92
  intestinal 569.9
    functional NEC 564.9
      congenital 751.3
      postoperative 564.4
    psychogenic 306.4
  introverted, of childhood and adolescence
      313.22
  iron, metabolism 275.0
  isolated explosive 312.35
  joint NEC 719.90
    ankle 719.97
    elbow 719.92
    foot 719.97
    hand 719.94
    hip 719.95
    knee 719.96
    multiple sites 719.99
    pelvic region 719.95
    psychogenic 306.0
    shoulder (region) 719.91
    specified site NEC 719.98
    temporomandibular 524.60
      specified NEC 524.69
    wrist 719.93
  kidney 593.9
    functional 588.9
      specified NEC 588.8
  labyrinth, labyrinthine 386.9
    specified type NEC 386.8
  lactation 676.9 ✓5ᵗʰ
  language (developmental) (expressive) 315.31
    mixed (receptive) (receptive-expressive)
        315.32
  ligament 728.9
  ligamentous attachments, peripheral — see
      also Enthesopathy
    spine 720.1
  limb NEC 729.9
    psychogenic 306.0
  lipid
    metabolism, congenital 272.9
    storage 272.7
  lipoprotein deficiency (familial) 272.5
  low back NEC 724.9
    psychogenic 306.0
  lumbosacral
    plexus 353.1
    root (nerve) NEC 353.4
  lymphoproliferative (chronic) NEC (M9970/1)
      238.7
  male erectile 302.72
    organic origin 607.84
  major depressive (see also Psychosis, affective)
      296.2 ✓5ᵗʰ
    recurrent episode 296.3 ✓5ᵗʰ
    single episode 296.2 ✓5ᵗʰ
  manic (see also Psychosis, affective) 296.0 ✓5ᵗʰ
    atypical 296.81
  meniscus NEC (see also Disorder, cartilage,
      articular) 718.0 ✓5ᵗʰ
  menopausal 627.9
    specified NEC 627.8
  menstrual 626.9
    psychogenic 306.52
    specified NEC 626.8
  mental (nonpsychotic) 300.9
    affecting management of pregnancy,
        childbirth, or puerperium 648.4 ✓5ᵗʰ

Disorder — see also Disease — continued
  mental — continued
    drug-induced 292.9
      hallucinogen persisting perception 292.89
      specified type NEC 292.89
    due to or associated with
      alcoholism 291.9
      drug consumption NEC 292.9
        specified type NEC 292.89
      physical condition NEC 293.9
    induced by drug 292.9
      specified type NEC 292.89
    neurotic (see also Neurosis) 300.9
    presenile 310.1
      psychotic NEC 290.10
    previous, affecting management of
        pregnancy V23.8 ✓5ᵗʰ
    psychoneurotic (see also Neurosis) 300.9
    psychotic (see also Psychosis) 298.9
      senile 290.20
    specific, following organic brain damage
        310.9
      cognitive or personality change of other
          type 310.1
      frontal lobe syndrome 310.0
      postconcussional syndrome 310.2
      specified type NEC 310.8
  metabolism NEC 277.9
    with
      abortion — see Abortion, by type with
          metabolic disorder
      ectopic pregnancy (see also categories
          633.0-633.9) 639.4
      molar pregnancy (see also categories 630-
          632) 639.4
    alkaptonuria 270.2
    amino acid (see also Disorder, amino acid)
        270.9
      specified type NEC 270.8
    ammonia 270.6
    arginine 270.6
    argininosuccinic acid 270.6
    basal 794.7
    bilirubin 277.4
    calcium 275.40
    carbohydrate 271.9
      specified type NEC 271.8
    cholesterol 272.9
    citrulline 270.6
    copper 275.1
    corticosteroid 255.2
    cystine storage 270.0
    cystinuria 270.0
    fat 272.9
    following
      abortion 639.4
      ectopic or molar pregnancy 639.4
    fructosemia 271.2
    fructosuria 271.2
    fucosidosis 271.8
    galactose-1-phosphate uridyl transferase
        271.1
    glutamine 270.7
    glycine 270.7
    glycogen storage NEC 271.0
      hepatorenal 271.0
    hemochromatosis 275.0
    in labor and delivery 669.0 ✓5ᵗʰ
    iron 275.0
    lactose 271.3
    lipid 272.9
      specified type NEC 272.8
      storage 272.7
    lipoprotein — see also Hyperlipemia
        deficiency (familial) 272.5
    lysine 270.7
    magnesium 275.2
    mannosidosis 271.8
    mineral 275.9
      specified type NEC 275.8
    mucopolysaccharide 277.5
    nitrogen 270.9
    ornithine 270.6
    oxalosis 271.8
    pentosuria 271.8
    phenylketonuria 270.1
    phosphate 275.3

Disorder — see also Disease — continued
  metabolism NEC — continued
    phosphorous 275.3
    plasma protein 273.9
      specified type NEC 273.8
    porphyrin 277.1
    purine 277.2
    pyrimidine 277.2
    serine 270.7
    sodium 276.9
    specified type NEC 277.8
    steroid 255.2
    threonine 270.7
    urea cycle 270.6
    xylose 271.8
  micturition NEC 788.69
    psychogenic 306.53
  misery and unhappiness, of childhood and
      adolescence 313.1
  mitral valve 424.0
  mood — see Psychosis, affective
  motor tic 307.20
    chronic 307.22
    transient, childhood 307.21
  movement NEC 333.90
    hysterical 300.11
    specified type NEC 333.99
    stereotypic 307.3
  mucopolysaccharide 277.5
  muscle 728.9
    psychogenic 306.0
    specified type NEC 728.3
  muscular attachments, peripheral — see also
      Enthesopathy
    spine 720.1
  musculoskeletal system NEC 729.9
    psychogenic 306.0
  myeloproliferative (chronic) NEC (M9960/1)
      238.7
  myoneural 358.9
    due to lead 358.2
    specified type NEC 358.8
    toxic 358.2
  myotonic 359.2
  neck region NEC 723.9
  nerve 349.9
    abducens NEC 378.54
    accessory 352.4
    acoustic 388.5
    auditory 388.5
    auriculotemporal 350.8
    axillary 353.0
    cerebral — see Disorder, nerve, cranial
    cranial 352.9
      first 352.0
      second 377.49
      third
        partial 378.51
        total 378.52
      fourth 378.53
      fifth 350.9
      sixth 378.54
      seventh NEC 351.9
      eighth 388.5
      ninth 352.2
      tenth 352.3
      eleventh 352.4
      twelfth 352.5
      multiple 352.6
    entrapment — see Neuropathy, entrapment
    facial 351.9
      specified NEC 351.8
    femoral 355.2
    glossopharyngeal NEC 352.2
    hypoglossal 352.5
    iliohypogastric 355.79
    ilioinguinal 355.79
    intercostal 353.8
    lateral
      cutaneous of thigh 355.1
      popliteal 355.3
    lower limb NEC 355.8
    medial, popliteal 355.4
    median NEC 354.1
    obturator 355.79

✓4ᵗʰ Fourth-digit Required   ✓5ᵗʰ Fifth-digit Required   ►◄ Revised Text   ● New Line   ▲ Revised Code

Disorder — *see also* Disease — *continued*
  nerve — *continued*
    oculomotor
      partial 378.51
      total 378.52
    olfactory 352.0
    optic 377.49
      ischemic 377.41
      nutritional 377.33
      toxic 377.34
    peroneal 355.3
    phrenic 354.8
    plantar 355.6
    pneumogastric 352.3
    posterior tibial 355.5
    radial 354.3
    recurrent laryngeal 352.3
    root 353.9
      specified NEC 353.8
    saphenous 355.79
    sciatic NEC 355.0
    specified NEC 355.9
      lower limb 355.79
      upper limb 354.8
    spinal 355.9
    sympathetic NEC 337.9
    trigeminal 350.9
      specified NEC 350.8
    trochlear 378.53
    ulnar 354.2
    upper limb NEC 354.9
    vagus 352.3
  nervous system NEC 349.9
    autonomic (peripheral) (*see also* Neuropathy, peripheral, autonomic) 337.9
    cranial 352.9
    parasympathetic (*see also* Neuropathy, peripheral, autonomic) 337.9
    specified type NEC 349.89
    sympathetic (*see also* Neuropathy, peripheral, autonomic) 337.9
    vegetative (*see also* Neuropathy, peripheral, autonomic) 337.9
  neurohypophysis NEC 253.6
  neurological NEC 781.99
    peripheral NEC 355.9
  neuromuscular NEC 358.9
    hereditary NEC 359.1
    specified NEC 358.8
    toxic 358.2
  neurotic 300.9
    specified type NEC 300.89
  neutrophil, polymorphonuclear (functional) 288.1
  obsessive-compulsive 300.3
  oppositional, childhood and adolescence 313.81
  optic
    chiasm 377.54
      associated with
        inflammatory disorders 377.54
        neoplasm NEC 377.52
          pituitary 377.51
        pituitary disorders 377.51
        vascular disorders 377.53
    nerve 377.49
    radiations 377.63
    tracts 377.63
  orbit 376.9
    specified NEC 376.89
  overanxious, of childhood and adolescence 313.0
  pancreas, internal secretion (other than diabetes mellitus) 251.9
    specified type NEC 251.8
  panic 300.01
    with agoraphobia 300.21
  papillary muscle NEC 429.81
  paranoid 297.9
    induced 297.3
    shared 297.3
  parathyroid 252.9
    specified type NEC 252.8
  paroxysmal, mixed 780.39
  pentose phosphate pathway with anemia 282.2
  personality 301.9
    affective 301.10
    aggressive 301.3

Disorder — *see also* Disease — *continued*
  personality — *continued*
    amoral 301.7
    anancastic, anankastic 301.4
    antisocial 301.7
    asocial 301.7
    asthenic 301.6
    boderline 301.83
    compulsive 301.4
    cyclothymic 301.13
    dependent-passive 301.6
    dyssocial 301.7
    emotional instability 301.59
    epileptoid 301.3
    explosive 301.3
    following organic brain damage 310.1
    histrionic 301.50
    hyperthymic 301.11
    hypomanic (chronic) 301.11
    hypothymic 301.12
    hysterical 301.50
    immature 301.89
    inadequate 301.6
    introverted 301.21
    labile 301.59
    moral deficiency 301.7
    obsessional 301.4
    obsessive (-compulsive) 301.4
    overconscientious 301.4
    paranoid 301.0
    passive (-dependent) 301.6
    passive-aggressive 301.84
    pathological NEC 301.9
    pseudosocial 301.7
    psychopathic 301.9
    schizoid 301.20
      introverted 301.21
      schizotypal 301.22
    schizotypal 301.22
    seductive 301.59
    type A 301.4
    unstable 301.59
  pervasive developmental, childhood-onset 299.8 ✓5ᵗʰ
  pigmentation, choroid (congenital) 743.53
  pinna 380.30
    specified type NEC 380.39
  pituitary, thalamic 253.9
    anterior NEC 253.4
    iatrogenic 253.7
    postablative 253.7
    specified NEC 253.8
  pityriasis-like NEC 696.8
  platelets (blood) 287.1
  polymorphonuclear neutrophils (functional) 288.1
  porphyrin metabolism 277.1
  postmenopausal 627.9
    specified type NEC 627.8
  posttraumatic stress 309.81
    acute 308.3
    brief 308.3
    chronic 309.81
  premenstrual dysphoric 625.4 ●
  psoriatic-like NEC 696.8
  psychic, with diseases classified elsewhere 316
  psychogenic NEC (*see also* condition) 300.9
    allergic NEC
      respiratory 306.1
    anxiety 300.00
      atypical 300.00
      generalized 300.02
    appetite 307.50
    articulation, joint 306.0
    asthenic 300.5
    blood 306.8
    cardiovascular (system) 306.2
    compulsive 300.3
    cutaneous 306.3
    depressive 300.4
    digestive (system) 306.4
    dysmenorrheic 306.52
    dyspneic 306.1
    eczematous 306.3
    endocrine (system) 306.6
    eye 306.7
    feeding 307.59
    functional NEC 306.9

Disorder — *see also* Disease — *continued*
  psychogenic NEC (*see also* condition) — *continued*
    gastric 306.4
    gastrointestinal (system) 306.4
    genitourinary (system) 306.50
    heart (function) (rhythm) 306.2
    hemic 306.8
    hyperventilatory 306.1
    hypochondriacal 300.7
    hysterical 300.10
    intestinal 306.4
    joint 306.0
    learning 315.2
    limb 306.0
    lymphatic (system) 306.8
    menstrual 306.52
    micturition 306.53
    monoplegic NEC 306.0
    motor 307.9
    muscle 306.0
    musculoskeletal 306.0
    neurocirculatory 306.2
    obsessive 300.3
    occupational 300.89
    organ or part of body NEC 306.9
    organs of special sense 306.7
    paralytic NEC 306.0
    phobic 300.20
    physical NEC 306.9
    pruritic 306.3
    rectal 306.4
    respiratory (system) 306.1
    rheumatic 306.0
    sexual (function) 302.70
      specified type NEC 302.79
    skin (allergic) (eczematous) (pruritic) 306.3
    sleep 307.40
      initiation or maintenance 307.41
        persistent 307.42
        transient 307.41
      specified type NEC 307.49
    specified part of body NEC 306.8
    stomach 306.4
  psychomotor NEC 307.9
    hysterical 300.11
  psychoneurotic (*see also* Neurosis) 300.9
    mixed NEC 300.89
  psychophysiologic (*see also* Disorder, psychosomatic) 306.9
  psychosexual identity (childhood) 302.6
    adult-life 302.85
  psychosomatic NEC 306.9
    allergic NEC
      respiratory 306.1
    articulation, joint 306.0
    cardiovascular (system) 306.2
    cutaneous 306.3
    digestive (system) 306.4
    dysmenorrheic 306.52
    dyspneic 306.1
    endocrine (system) 306.6
    eye 306.7
    gastric 306.4
    gastrointestinal (system) 306.4
    genitourinary (system) 306.50
    heart (functional) (rhythm) 306.2
    hyperventilatory 306.1
    intestinal 306.4
    joint 306.0
    limb 306.0
    lymphatic (system) 306.8
    menstrual 306.52
    micturition 306.53
    monoplegic NEC 306.0
    muscle 306.0
    musculoskeletal 306.0
    neurocirculatory 306.2
    organs of special sense 306.7
    paralytic NEC 306.0
    pruritic 306.3
    rectal 306.4
    respiratory (system) 306.1
    rheumatic 306.0
    sexual (function) 302.70
    specified type NEC 302.79
    skin 306.3
    specified part of body NEC 306.8

Disorder — *see also* Disease — *continued*
  psychosomatic NEC — *continued*
    stomach 306.4
  psychotic — *see* Psychosis
  purine metabolism NEC 277.2
  pyrimidine metabolism NEC 277.2
  reactive attachment (of infancy or early
    childhood) 313.89
  reading, developmental 315.00
  reflex 796.1
  renal function, impaired 588.9
    specified type NEC 588.8
  renal transport NEC 588.8
  respiration, respiratory NEC 519.9
    due to
      aspiration of liquids or solids 508.9
      inhalation of fumes or vapors 506.9
    psychogenic 306.1
  retina 362.9
    specified type NEC 362.89
  sacroiliac joint NEC 724.6
  sacrum 724.6
  schizo-affective (*see also* Schizophrenia)
    295.7 ☑5ᵗʰ
  schizoid, childhood or adolescence 313.22
  schizophreniform 295.4 ☑5ᵗʰ
  schizotypal personality 301.22
  secretion, thyrocalcitonin 246.0
  seizure 780.39
    recurrent 780.39
      epileptic — *see* Epilepsy
  sense of smell 781.1
    psychogenic 306.7
  separation anxiety 309.21
  sexual (*see also* Deviation, sexual) 302.9
    function, psychogenic 302.70
  shyness, of childhood and adolescence 313.21
  single complement (C-C) 279.8
  skin NEC 709.9
    fetus or newborn 778.9
      specified type 778.8
    psychogenic (allergic) (eczematous) (pruritic)
      306.3
    specified type NEC 709.8
    vascular 709.1
  sleep 780.50
    with apnea — *see* Apnea, sleep
    circadian rhythm 307.45
    initiation or maintenance (*see also*
      Insomnia) 780.52
      nonorganic origin (transient) 307.41
        persistent 307.42
    nonorganic origin 307.40
      specified type NEC 307.49
    specified NEC 780.59
  social, of childhood and adolescence 313.22
    specified NEC 780.59
  soft tissue 729.9
  somatization 300.81
  somatoform (atypical) (undifferentiated) 300.82
    severe 300.81
  speech NEC 784.5
    nonorganic origin 307.9
  spine NEC 724.9
    ligamentous or muscular attachments,
      peripheral 720.1
  steroid metabolism NEC 255.2
  stomach (functional) (*see also* Disorder, gastric)
    536.9
    psychogenic 306.4
  storage, iron 275.0
  stress (*see also* Reaction, stress, acute) 308.9
    posttraumatic
      acute 308.3
      brief 308.3
      chronic 309.81
  substitution 300.11
  suspected — *see* Observation
  synovium 727.9
  temperature regulation, fetus or newborn 778.4
  temporomandibular joint NEC 524.60
    specified NEC 524.69
  tendon 727.9
    shoulder region 726.10
  thoracic root (nerve) NEC 353.3
  thyrocalcitonin secretion 246.0

Disorder — *see also* Disease — *continued*
  thyroid (gland) NEC 246.9
    specified type NEC 246.8
  tic 307.20
    chronic (motor or vocal) 307.22
    motor-verbal 307.23
    organic origin 333.1
    transient of childhood 307.21
  tooth NEC 525.9
    development NEC 520.9
      specified type NEC 520.8
    eruption 520.6
      with abnormal position 524.3
    specified type NEC 525.8
  transport, carbohydrate 271.9
    specified type NEC 271.8
  tubular, phosphate-losing 588.0
  tympanic membrane 384.9
  unaggressive, unsocialized (*see also*
    Disturbance, conduct) 312.1 ☑5ᵗʰ
  undersocialized, unsocialized (*see also*
    Disturbance, conduct)
    aggressive (type) 312.0 ☑5ᵗʰ
    unaggressive (type) 312.1 ☑5ᵗʰ
  vision, visual NEC 368.9
    binocular NEC 368.30
    cortex 377.73
      associated with
        inflammatory disorders 377.73
        neoplasms 377.71
        vascular disorders 377.72
    pathway NEC 377.63
      associated with
        inflammatory disorders 377.63
        neoplasms 377.61
        vascular disorders 377.62
  wakefulness (*see also* Hypersomnia) 780.54
    nonorganic origin (transient) 307.43
      persistent 307.44
Disorganized globe 360.29
Displacement, displaced

> *Note* — For acquired displacement of bones,
> cartilage, joints, tendons, due to injury, see
> also Dislocation.
>
> Displacements at ages under one year
> should be considered congenital, provided
> there is no indication the condition was
> acquired after birth.

  acquired traumatic of bone, cartilage, joint,
    tendon NEC (without fracture) (*see also*
    Dislocation) 839.8
    with fracture — *see* Fracture, by site
  adrenal gland (congenital) 759.1
  appendix, retrocecal (congenital) 751.5
  auricle (congenital) 744.29
  bladder (acquired) 596.8
    congenital 753.8
  brachial plexus (congenital) 742.8
  brain stem, caudal 742.4
  canaliculus lacrimalis 743.65
  cardia, through esophageal hiatus 750.6
  cerebellum, caudal 742.4
  cervix (*see also* Malposition, uterus) 621.6
  colon (congenital) 751.4
  device, implant, or graft — *see* Complications,
    mechanical
  epithelium
    columnar of cervix 622.1
    cuboidal, beyond limits of external os
      (uterus) 752.49
  esophageal mucosa into cardia of stomach,
    congenital 750.4
  esophagus (acquired) 530.89
    congenital 750.4
  eyeball (acquired) (old) 376.36
    congenital 743.8
    current injury 871.3
    lateral 376.36
  fallopian tube (acquired) 620.4
    congenital 752.19
    opening (congenital) 752.19
  gallbladder (congenital) 751.69

Displacement, displaced — *continued*
  gastric mucosa 750.7
    into
      duodenum 750.7
      esophagus 750.7
      Meckel's diverticulum, congenital 750.7
  globe (acquired) (lateral) (old) 376.36
    current injury 871.3
  graft
    artificial skin graft 996.55
    decellularized allodermis graft 996.55
  heart (congenital) 746.87
    acquired 429.89
  hymen (congenital) (upward) 752.49
  internal prothesis NEC — *see* Complications,
    mechanical
  intervertebral disc (with neuritis, radiculitis,
    sciatica, or other pain) 722.2
    with myelopathy 722.70
    cervical, cervicodorsal, cervicothoracic 722.0
      with myelopathy 722.71
      due to major trauma — *see* Dislocation,
        vertebra, cervical
    due to major trauma — *see* Dislocation,
      vertebra
  intervertebral disc
    lumbar, lumbosacral 722.10
      with myelopathy 722.73
      due to major trauma — *see* Dislocation,
        vertebra, lumbar
    thoracic, thoracolumbar 722.11
      with myelopathy 722.72
      due to major trauma — *see* Dislocation,
        vertebra, thoracic
  intrauterine device 996.32
  kidney (acquired) 593.0
    congenital 753.3
  lacrimal apparatus or duct (congenital) 743.65
  macula (congenital) 743.55
  Meckel's diverticulum (congenital) 751.0
  nail (congenital) 757.5
    acquired 703.8
  opening of Wharton's duct in mouth 750.26
  organ or site, congenital NEC — *see*
    Malposition, congenital
  ovary (acquired) 620.4
    congenital 752.0
    free in peritoneal cavity (congenital) 752.0
    into hernial sac 620.4
  oviduct (acquired) 620.4
    congenital 752.19
  parathyroid (gland) 252.8
  parotid gland (congenital) 750.26
  punctum lacrimale (congenital) 743.65
  sacroiliac (congenital) (joint) 755.69
    current injury — *see* Dislocation, sacroiliac
    old 724.6
  spine (congenital) 756.19
  spleen, congenital 759.0
  stomach (congenital) 750.7
    acquired 537.89
  subglenoid (closed) 831.01
  sublingual duct (congenital) 750.26
  teeth, tooth 524.3
  tongue (congenital) (downward) 750.19
  trachea (congenital) 748.3
  ureter or ureteric opening or orifice (congenital)
    753.4
  uterine opening of oviducts or fallopian tubes
    752.19
  uterus, uterine (*see also* Malposition, uterus)
    621.6
    congenital 752.3
  ventricular septum 746.89
    with rudimentary ventricle 746.89
  xyphoid bone (process) 738.3
Disproportion 653.9 ☑5ᵗʰ
  affecting fetus or newborn 763.1
  caused by
    conjoined twins 653.7 ☑5ᵗʰ
    contraction, pelvis (general) 653.1 ☑5ᵗʰ
      inlet 653.2 ☑5ᵗʰ
      midpelvic 653.8 ☑5ᵗʰ
      midplane 653.8 ☑5ᵗʰ
      outlet 653.3 ☑5ᵗʰ
    fetal
      ascites 653.7 ☑5ᵗʰ
      hydrocephalus 653.6 ☑5ᵗʰ

Disproportion — *continued*
  caused by — *continued*
    fetal — *continued*
      hydrops 653.7 ✓5ᵗʰ
      meningomyelocele 653.7 ✓5ᵗʰ
      sacral teratoma 653.7 ✓5ᵗʰ
      tumor 653.7 ✓5ᵗʰ
    hydrocephalic fetus 653.6 ✓5ᵗʰ
    pelvis, pelvic, abnormality (bony) NEC
      653.0 ✓5ᵗʰ
    unusually large fetus 653.5 ✓5ᵗʰ
  causing obstructed labor 660.1 ✓5ᵗʰ
  cephalopelvic, normally formed fetus 653.4 ✓5ᵗʰ
    causing obstructed labor 660.1 ✓5ᵗʰ
  fetal NEC 653.5 ✓5ᵗʰ
    causing obstructed labor 660.1 ✓5ᵗʰ
  fetopelvic, normally formed fetus 653.4 ✓5ᵗʰ
    causing obstructed labor 660.1 ✓5ᵗʰ
  mixed maternal and fetal origin, normally
    formed fetus 653.4 ✓5ᵗʰ
  pelvis, pelvic (bony) NEC 653.1 ✓5ᵗʰ
    causing obstructed labor 660.1 ✓5ᵗʰ
  specified type NEC 653.8 ✓5ᵗʰ

Disruption
  cesarean wound 674.1 ✓5ᵗʰ
  family V61.0
  gastrointestinal anastomosis 997.4
  ligament(s) — *see also* Sprain
    knee
      current injury — *see* Dislocation knee
      old 717.89
        capsular 717.85
        collateral (medial) 717.82
          lateral 717.81
        cruciate (posterior) 717.84
          anterior 717.83
        specified site NEC 717.85
  marital V61.10
    involving divorce or estrangement V61.0
  operation wound ▶(external)◀ 998.32 ▲
    internal 998.31 ●
  organ transplant, anastomosis site — *see*
    Complications, transplant, organ, by site
  ossicles, ossicular chain 385.23
    traumatic — *see* Fracture, skull, base
  parenchyma
    liver (hepatic) — *see* Laceration, liver, major
    spleen — *see* Laceration, spleen,
      parenchyma, massive
  phase-shift, of 24-hour sleep-wake cycle
    780.55
    nonorganic origin 307.45
  sleep-wake cycle (24-hour) 780.55
    circadian rhythm 307.45
    nonorganic origin 307.45
  suture line (external) 998.32 ▲
    internal 998.31 ▲
  wound
    cesarean operation 674.1 ✓5ᵗʰ
    episiotomy 674.2 ✓5ᵗʰ
    operation 998.32 ▲
      cesarean 674.1 ✓5ᵗʰ
      internal 998.31 ●
    perineal (obstetric) 674.2 ✓5ᵗʰ
    uterine 674.1 ✓5ᵗʰ

Disruptio uteri — *see also* Rupture, uterus
  complicating delivery — *see* Delivery,
    complicated, rupture, uterus

Dissatisfaction with
  employment V62.2
  school environment V62.3

Dissecting — *see* condition

Dissection
  aorta 441.00
    abdominal 441.02
    thoracic 441.01
    thoracoabdominal 441.03
  artery, arterial ●
    carotid 443.21 ●
    coronary 414.12 ●
    iliac 443.22 ●
    renal 443.23 ●
    specified NEC 443.29 ●
    vertebral 443.24 ●
  vascular 459.9
  wound — *see* Wound, open, by site

Disseminated — *see* condition

Dissociated personality NEC 300.15

Dissociation
  auriculoventricular or atrioventricular (any
    degree) (AV) 426.89
    with heart block 426.0
  interference 426.89
  isorhythmic 426.89
  rhythm
    atrioventricular (AV) 426.89
    interference 426.89

Dissociative
  identity disorder 300.14
  reaction NEC 300.15

Dissolution, vertebra (*see also* Osteoporosis)
  733.00

Distention
  abdomen (gaseous) 787.3
  bladder 596.8
  cecum 569.89
  colon 569.89
  gallbladder 575.8
  gaseous (abdomen) 787.3
  intestine 569.89
  kidney 593.89
  liver 573.9
  seminal vesicle 608.89
  stomach 536.8
    acute 536.1
    psychogenic 306.4
  ureter 593.5
  uterus 621.8

Distichia, distichiasis (eyelid) 743.63

Distoma hepaticum infestation 121.3

Distomiasis 121.9
  bile passages 121.3
    due to Clonorchis sinensis 121.1
  hemic 120.9
  hepatic (liver) 121.3
    due to Clonorchis sinensis (clonorchiasis)
      121.1
  intestinal 121.4
  liver 121.3
    due to Clonorchis sinensis 121.1
  lung 121.2
  pulmonary 121.2

Distomolar (fourth molar) 520.1
  causing crowding 524.3

Disto-occlusion 524.2

Distortion (congenital)
  adrenal (gland) 759.1
  ankle (joint) 755.69
  anus 751.5
  aorta 747.29
  appendix 751.5
  arm 755.59
  artery (peripheral) NEC (*see also* Distortion,
    peripheral vascular system) 747.60
    cerebral 747.81
    coronary 746.85
    pulmonary 747.3
    retinal 743.58
    umbilical 747.5
  auditory canal 744.29
    causing impairment of hearing 744.02
  bile duct or passage 751.69
  bladder 753.8
  brain 742.4
  bronchus 748.3
  cecum 751.5
  cervix (uteri) 752.49
  chest (wall) 756.3
  clavicle 755.51
  clitoris 752.49
  coccyx 756.19
  colon 751.5
  common duct 751.69
  cornea 743.41
  cricoid cartilage 748.3
  cystic duct 751.69
  duodenum 751.5
  ear 744.29
    auricle 744.29
      causing impairment of hearing 744.02
    causing impairment of hearing 744.09
    external 744.29
      causing impairment of hearing 744.02

Distortion — *continued*
  ear — *continued*
    inner 744.05
    middle, except ossicles 744.03
      ossicles 744.04
    ossicles 744.04
  endocrine (gland) NEC 759.2
  epiglottis 748.3
  Eustachian tube 744.24
  eye 743.8
    adnexa 743.69
  face bone(s) 756.0
  fallopian tube 752.19
  femur 755.69
  fibula 755.69
  finger(s) 755.59
  foot 755.67
  gallbladder 751.69
  genitalia, genital organ(s)
    female 752.8
      external 752.49
      internal NEC 752.8
    male 752.8
      penis 752.69
  glottis 748.3
  gyri 742.4
  hand bone(s) 755.59
  heart (auricle) (ventricle) 746.89
    valve (cusp) 746.89
  hepatic duct 751.69
  humerus 755.59
  hymen 752.49
  ileum 751.5
  intestine (large) (small) 751.5
    with anomalous adhesions, fixation or
      malrotation 751.4
  jaw NEC 524.8
  jejunum 751.5
  kidney 753.3
  knee (joint) 755.64
  labium (majus) (minus) 752.49
  larynx 748.3
  leg 755.69
  lens 743.36
  liver 751.69
  lumbar spine 756.19
    with disproportion (fetopelvic) 653.0 ✓5ᵗʰ
      affecting fetus or newborn 763.1
      causing obstructed labor 660.1 ✓5ᵗʰ
  lumbosacral (joint) (region) 756.19
  lung (fissures) (lobe) 748.69
  nerve 742.8
  nose 748.1
  organ
    of Corti 744.05
    or site not listed — *see* Anomaly, specified
      type NEC
  ossicles, ear 744.04
  ovary 752.0
  oviduct 752.19
  pancreas 751.7
  parathyroid (gland) 759.2
  patella 755.64
  peripheral vascular system NEC 747.60
    gastrointestinal 747.61
    lower limb 747.64
    renal 747.62
    spinal 747.82
    upper limb 747.63
  pituitary (gland) 759.2
  radius 755.59
  rectum 751.5
  rib 756.3
  sacroiliac joint 755.69
  sacrum 756.19
  scapula 755.59
  shoulder girdle 755.59
  site not listed — *see* Anomaly, specified type
    NEC
  skull bone(s) 756.0
    with
      anencephalus 740.0
      encephalocele 742.0
      hydrocephalus 742.3
        with spina bifida (*see also* Spina
          bifida) 741.0 ✓5ᵗʰ
      microcephalus 742.1

✓4ᵗʰ Fourth-digit Required   ✓5ᵗʰ Fifth-digit Required   ▶◀ Revised Text   ● New Line   ▲ Revised Code

Disproportion — Distortion

Distortion — continued
spinal cord 742.59
spine 756.19
spleen 759.0
sternum 756.3
thorax (wall) 756.3
thymus (gland) 759.2
thyroid (gland) 759.2
cartilage 748.3
tibia 755.69
toe(s) 755.66
tongue 750.19
trachea (cartilage) 748.3
ulna 755.59
ureter 753.4
causing obstruction 753.20
urethra 753.8
causing obstruction 753.6
uterus 752.3
vagina 752.49
vein (peripheral) NEC (see also Distortion,
peripheral vascular system) 747.60
great 747.49
portal 747.49
pulmonary 747.49
vena cava (inferior) (superior) 747.49
vertebra 756.19
visual NEC 368.15
shape or size 368.14
vulva 752.49
wrist (bones) (joint) 755.59

Distress
abdomen 789.0 ✓5ᵗʰ
colon 789.0 ✓5ᵗʰ
emotional V40.9
epigastric 789.0 ✓5ᵗʰ
fetal (syndrome) 768.4
affecting management of pregnancy or
childbirth 656.8 ✓5ᵗʰ ▲
liveborn infant 768.4
first noted
before onset of labor 768.2
during labor or delivery 768.3
stillborn infant (death before onset of labor)
768.0
death during labor 768.1
gastrointestinal (functional) 536.9
psychogenic 306.4
intestinal (functional) NEC 564.9
psychogenic 306.4
intrauterine — see Distress, fetal
leg 729.5
maternal 669.0 ✓5ᵗʰ
mental V40.9
respiratory 786.09
acute (adult) 518.82
adult syndrome (following shock, surgery,
or trauma) 518.5
specified NEC 518.82
fetus or newborn 770.89 ▲
syndrome (idiopathic) (newborn) 769
stomach 536.9
psychogenic 306.4

Distribution vessel, atypical NEC 747.60
coronary artery 746.85
spinal 747.82

Districhiasis 704.2

Disturbance — see also Disease
absorption NEC 579.9
calcium 269.3
carbohydrate 579.8
fat 579.8
protein 579.8
specified type NEC 579.8
vitamin (see also Deficiency, vitamin) 269.2
acid-base equilibrium 276.9
activity and attention, simple, with
hyperkinesis 314.01
amino acid (metabolic) (see also Disorder,
amino acid) 270.9
imidazole 270.5
maple syrup (urine) disease 270.3
transport 270.0
assimilation, food 579.9
attention, simple 314.00
with hyperactivity 314.01

Disturbance — see also Disease — continued
auditory, nerve, except deafness 388.5
behavior (see also Disturbance, conduct) 312.9
blood clotting (hypoproteinemia) (mechanism)
(see also Defect, coagulation) 286.9
central nervous system NEC 349.9
cerebral nerve NEC 352.9
circulatory 459.9
conduct 312.9
adjustment reaction 309.3
adolescent onset type 312.82
childhood onset type 312.81

> *Note* — Use the following fifth-digit
> subclassification with categories
> 312.0–312.2:
>
> 0   unspecified
> 1   mild
> 2   moderate
> 3   severe

compulsive 312.30
intermittent explosive disorder 312.34
isolated explosive disorder 312.35
kleptomania 312.32
pathological gambling 312.31
pyromania 312.33
hyperkinetic 314.2
intermittent explosive 312.34
isolated explosive 312.35
mixed with emotions 312.4
socialized (type) 312.20
aggressive 312.23
unaggressive 312.21
specified type NEC 312.89
undersocialized, unsocialized
aggressive (type) 312.0 ✓5ᵗʰ
unaggressive (type) 312.1 ✓5ᵗʰ
coordination 781.3
cranial nerve NEC 352.9
deep sensibility — see Disturbance, sensation
digestive 536.9
psychogenic 306.4
electrolyte — see Imbalance, electrolyte
emotions specific to childhood and adolescence
313.9
with
academic underachievement 313.83
anxiety and fearfulness 313.0
elective mutism 313.23
identity disorder 313.82
jealousy 313.3
misery and unhappiness 313.1
oppositional disorder 313.81
overanxiousness 313.0
sensitivity 313.21
shyness 313.21
social withdrawal 313.22
withdrawal reaction 313.22
involving relationship problems 313.3
mixed 313.89
specified type NEC 313.89
endocrine (gland) 259.9
neonatal, transitory 775.9
specified NEC 775.8
equilibrium 780.4
feeding (elderly) (infant) 783.3
newborn 779.3
nonorganic origin NEC 307.59
psychogenic NEC 307.59
fructose metabolism 271.2
gait 781.2
hysterical 300.11
gastric (functional) 536.9
motility 536.8
psychogenic 306.4
secretion 536.8
gastrointestinal (functional) 536.9
psychogenic 306.4
habit, child 307.9
hearing, except deafness 388.40
heart, functional (conditions classifiable to 426,
427, 428)
due to presence of (cardiac) prosthesis 429.4
postoperative (immediate) 997.1
long-term effect of cardiac surgery 429.4

Disturbance — see also Disease — continued
heart, functional — continued
psychogenic 306.2
hormone 259.9
innervation uterus, sympathetic,
parasympathetic 621.8
keratinization NEC
gingiva 523.1
lip 528.5
oral (mucosa) (soft tissue) 528.7
tongue 528.7
labyrinth, labyrinthine (vestibule) 386.9
learning, specific NEC 315.2
memory (see also Amnesia) 780.99 ▲
mild, following organic brain
damage 310.1
mental (see also Disorder, mental) 300.9
associated with diseases classified elsewhere
316
metabolism (acquired) (congenital) (see also
Disorder, metabolism) 277.9
with
abortion — see Abortion, by type, with
metabolic disorder
ectopic pregnancy (see also categories
633.0-633.9) 639.4
molar pregnancy (see also categories 630-
632) 639.4
amino acid (see also Disorder, amino acid)
270.9
aromatic NEC 270.2
branched-chain 270.3
specified type NEC 270.8
straight-chain NEC 270.7
sulfur-bearing 270.4
transport 270.0
ammonia 270.6
arginine 270.6
argininosuccinic acid 270.6
carbohydrate NEC 271.9
cholesterol 272.9
citrulline 270.6
cystathionine 270.4
fat 272.9
following
abortion 639.4
ectopic or molar pregnancy 639.4
general 277.9
carbohydrate 271.9
iron 275.0
phosphate 275.3
sodium 276.9
glutamine 270.7
glycine 270.7
histidine 270.5
homocystine 270.4
in labor or delivery 669.0 ✓5ᵗʰ
iron 275.0
isoleucine 270.3
leucine 270.3
lipoid 272.9
specified type NEC 272.8
lysine 270.7
methionine 270.4
neonatal, transitory 775.9
specified type NEC 775.8
nitrogen 788.9
ornithine 270.6
phosphate 275.3
phosphatides 272.7
serine 270.7
sodium NEC 276.9
threonine 270.7
tryptophan 270.2
tyrosine 270.2
urea cycle 270.6
valine 270.3
motor 796.1
nervous functional 799.2
neuromuscular mechanism (eye) due to
syphilis 094.84
nutritional 269.9
nail 703.8
ocular motion 378.87
psychogenic 306.7
oculogyric 378.87
psychogenic 306.7

✓4ᵗʰ Fourth-digit Required   ✓5ᵗʰ Fifth-digit Required   ▶◀ Revised Text   ● New Line   ▲ Revised Code

Distortion — Disturbance

Disturbance — *see also* Disease — *continued*
oculomotor NEC 378.87
  psychogenic 306.7
olfactory nerve 781.1
optic nerve NEC 377.49
oral epithelium, including tongue 528.7
personality (pattern) (trait) (*see also* Disorder,
    personality) 301.9
  following organic brain damage 310.1
polyglandular 258.9
psychomotor 307.9
pupillary 379.49
reflex 796.1
rhythm, heart 427.9
  postoperative (immediate) 997.1
    long-term effect of cardiac surgery 429.4
  psychogenic 306.2
salivary secretion 527.7
sensation (cold) (heat) (localization) (tactile
    discrimination localization) (texture)
    (vibratory) NEC 782.0
  hysterical 300.11
  skin 782.0
  smell 781.1
  taste 781.1
sensory (*see also* Disturbance, sensation) 782.0
  innervation 782.0
situational (transient) (*see also* Reaction,
    adjustment) 309.9
  acute 308.3
sleep 780.50
  with apnea — *see* Apnea, sleep
  initiation or maintenance (*see also*
      Insomnia) 780.52
    nonorganic origin 307.41
  nonorganic origin 307.40
    specified type NEC 307.49
  specified NEC 780.59
    nonorganic origin 307.49
  wakefulness (*see also* Hypersomnia) 780.54
    nonorganic origin 307.43
sociopathic 301.7
speech NEC 784.5
  developmental 315.39
    associated with hyperkinesis 314.1
  secondary to organic lesion 784.5
stomach (functional) (*see also* Disturbance,
    gastric) 536.9
sympathetic (nerve) (*see also* Neuropathy,
    peripheral, autonomic) 337.9
temperature sense 782.0
  hysterical 300.11
tooth
  eruption 520.6
  formation 520.4
  structure, hereditary NEC 520.5
touch (*see also* Disturbance, sensation) 782.0
vascular 459.9
  arteriosclerotic — *see* Arteriosclerosis
vasomotor 443.9
vasospastic 443.9
vestibular labyrinth 386.9
vision, visual NEC 368.9
  psychophysical 368.16
  specified NEC 368.8
  subjective 368.10
voice 784.40
wakefulness (initiation or maintenance) (*see
    also* Hypersomnia) 780.54
  nonorganic origin 307.43

Disulfiduria, beta-mercaptolactate-cysteine
  270.0

Disuse atrophy, bone 733.7

Ditthomska syndrome 307.81

Diuresis 788.42

Divers'
  palsy or paralysis 993.3
  squeeze 993.3

Diverticula, diverticulosis, diverticulum (acute)
  (multiple) (perforated) (ruptured) 562.10
  with diverticulitis 562.11
  aorta (Kommerell's) 747.21
  appendix (noninflammatory) 543.9
  bladder (acquired) (sphincter) 596.3
    congenital 753.8
  broad ligament 620.8

Diverticula, diverticulosis, diverticulum —
  continued
  bronchus (congenital) 748.3
    acquired 494.0
      with acute exacerbation 494.1
  calyx, calyceal (kidney) 593.89
  cardia (stomach) 537.1
  cecum 562.10
    with
      diverticulitis 562.11
        with hemorrhage 562.13
      hemorrhage 562.12
    congenital 751.5
  colon (acquired) 562.10
    with
      diverticulitis 562.11
        with hemorrhage 562.13
      hemorrhage 562.12
    congenital 751.5
  duodenum 562.00
    with
      diverticulitis 562.01
        with hemorrhage 562.03
      hemorrhage 562.02
    congenital 751.5
  epiphrenic (esophagus) 530.6
  esophagus (congenital) 750.4
    acquired 530.6
    epiphrenic 530.6
    pulsion 530.6
    traction 530.6
    Zenker's 530.6
  Eustachian tube 381.89
  fallopian tube 620.8
  gallbladder (congenital) 751.69
  gastric 537.1
  heart (congenital) 746.89
  ileum 562.00
    with
      diverticulitis 562.01
        with hemorrhage 562.03
      hemorrhage 562.02
  intestine (large) 562.10
    with
      diverticulitis 562.11
        with hemorrhage 562.13
      hemorrhage 562.12
    congenital 751.5
    small 562.00
      with
        diverticulitis 562.01
          with hemorrhage 562.03
        hemorrhage 562.02
      congenital 751.5
  jejunum 562.00
    with
      diverticulitis 562.01
        with hemorrhage 562.03
      hemorrhage 562.02
  kidney (calyx) (pelvis) 593.89
    with calculus 592.0
  Kommerell's 747.21
  laryngeal ventricle (congenital) 748.3
  Meckel's (displaced) (hypertrophic) 751.0
  midthoracic 530.6
  organ or site, congenital NEC — *see* Distortion
  pericardium (congenital) (cyst) 746.89
    acquired (true) 423.8
  pharyngoesophageal (pulsion) 530.6
  pharynx (congenital) 750.27
  pulsion (esophagus) 530.6
  rectosigmoid 562.10
    with
      diverticulitis 562.11
        with hemorrhage 562.13
      hemorrhage 562.12
    congenital 751.5
  rectum 562.10
    with
      diverticulitis 562.11
        with hemorrhage 562.13
      hemorrhage 562.12
  renal (calyces) (pelvis) 593.89
    with calculus 592.0
  Rokitansky's 530.6
  seminal vesicle 608.0

Diverticula, diverticulosis, diverticulum —
  continued
  sigmoid 562.10
    with
      diverticulitis 562.11
        with hemorrhage 562.13
      hemorrhage 562.12
    congenital 751.5
  small intestine 562.00
    with
      diverticulitis 562.01
        with hemorrhage 562.03
      hemorrhage 562.02
  stomach (cardia) (juxtacardia) (juxtapyloric)
      (acquired) 537.1
    congenital 750.7
  subdiaphragmatic 530.6
  trachea (congenital) 748.3
    acquired 519.1
  traction (esophagus) 530.6
  ureter (acquired) 593.89
    congenital 753.4
  ureterovesical orifice 593.89
  urethra (acquired) 599.2
    congenital 753.8
  ventricle, left (congenital) 746.89
  vesical (urinary) 596.3
    congenital 753.8
  Zenker's (esophagus) 530.6

Diverticulitis (acute) (*see also* Diverticula) 562.11
  with hemorrhage 562.13
  bladder (urinary) 596.3
  cecum (perforated) 562.11
    with hemorrhage 562.13
  colon (perforated) 562.11
    with hemorrhage 562.13
  duodenum 562.01
    with hemorrhage 562.03
  esophagus 530.6
  ileum (perforated) 562.01
    with hemorrhage 562.03
  intestine (large) (perforated) 562.11
    with hemorrhage 562.13
    small 562.01
      with hemorrhage 562.03
  jejunum (perforated) 562.01
    with hemorrhage 562.03
  Meckel's (perforated) 751.0
  pharyngoesophageal 530.6
  rectosigmoid (perforated) 562.11
    with hemorrhage 562.13
  rectum 562.11
    with hemorrhage 562.13
  sigmoid (old) (perforated) 562.11
    with hemorrhage 562.13
  small intestine (perforated) 562.01
    with hemorrhage 562.03
  vesical (urinary) 596.3

Diverticulosis — *see* Diverticula

Division
  cervix uteri 622.8
    external os into two openings by frenum
      752.49
  external (cervical) into two openings by frenum
      752.49
  glans penis 752.69
  hymen 752.49
  labia minora (congenital) 752.49
  ligament (partial or complete) (current) — *see
      also* Sprain, by site
    with open wound — *see* Wound, open, by
        site
  muscle (partial or complete) (current) — *see
      also* Sprain, by site
    with open wound — *see* Wound, open, by
        site
  nerve — *see* Injury, nerve, by site
  penis glans 752.69
  spinal cord — *see* Injury, spinal, by site
  vein 459.9
    traumatic — *see* Injury, vascular, by site

Divorce V61.0

Dix-Hallpike neurolabyrinthitis 386.12

Dizziness 780.4
  hysterical 300.11
  psychogenic 306.9

Doan-Wiseman syndrome (primary splenic
neutropenia) 288.0
Dog bite — see Wound, open, by site
Döhle-Heller aortitis 093.1
Döhle body-panmyelopathic syndrome 288.2
Dolichocephaly, dolichocephalus 754.0
Dolichocolon 751.5
Dolichostenomelia 759.82
Donohue's syndrome (leprechaunism) 259.8
Donor
blood V59.01
other blood components V59.09
stem cells V59.02
whole blood V59.01
bone V59.2
marrow V59.3
cornea V59.5
heart V59.8
kidney V59.4
liver V59.6
lung V59.8
lymphocyte V59.8
organ V59.9
specified NEC V59.8
potential, examination of V70.8
skin V59.1
specified organ or tissue NEC V59.8
stem cells V59.02
tissue V59.9
specified type NEC V59.8
Donovanosis (granuloma venereum) 099.2
DOPS (diffuse obstructive pulmonary syndrome)
496
Double
albumin 273.8
aortic arch 747.21
auditory canal 744.29
auricle (heart) 746.82
bladder 753.8
external (cervical) os 752.49
kidney with double pelvis (renal) 753.3
larynx 748.3
meatus urinarius 753.8
organ or site NEC — see Accessory
orifice
heart valve NEC 746.89
pulmonary 746.09
outlet, right ventricle 745.11
pelvis (renal) with double ureter 753.4
penis 752.69
tongue 750.13
ureter (one or both sides) 753.4
with double pelvis (renal) 753.4
urethra 753.8
urinary meatus 753.8
uterus (any degree) 752.2
with doubling of cervix and vagina 752.2
in pregnancy or childbirth 654.0 ☑5ᵗʰ
affecting fetus or newborn 763.89
vagina 752.49
with doubling of cervix and uterus 752.2
vision 368.2
vocal cords 748.3
vulva 752.49
whammy (syndrome) 360.81
Douglas' pouch, cul-de-sac — see condition
Down's disease or syndrome (mongolism) 758.0
Down-growth, epithelial (anterior chamber)
364.61
Dracontiasis 125.7
Dracunculiasis 125.7
Drancunculosis 125.7
Drainage
abscess (spontaneous) — see Abscess
anomalous pulmonary veins to hepatic veins or
right atrium 747.41
stump (amputation) (surgical) 997.62
suprapubic, bladder 596.8
Dream state, hysterical 300.13
Drepanocytic anemia (see also Disease, sickle
cell) 282.60
Dresbach's syndrome (elliptocytosis) 282.1

Dreschlera (infection) 118
hawaiiensis 117.8
Dressler's syndrome (postmyocardial infarction)
411.0
Dribbling (post-void) 788.35
Drift, ulnar 736.09
Drinking (alcohol) — see also Alcoholism
excessive, to excess NEC (see also Abuse,
drugs, nondependent) 305.0 ☑5ᵗʰ
bouts, periodic 305.0 ☑5ᵗʰ
continual 303.9 ☑5ᵗʰ
episodic 305.0 ☑5ᵗʰ
habitual 303.9 ☑5ᵗʰ
periodic 305.0 ☑5ᵗʰ
Drip, postnasal (chronic) — see Sinusitis
Drivers' license examination V70.3
Droop
Cooper's 611.8
facial 781.99   ●
Drop
finger 736.29
foot 736.79
hematocrit (precipitous) 790.01
toe 735.8
wrist 736.05
Dropped
dead 798.1
heart beats 426.6
Dropsy, dropsical (see also Edema) 782.3
abdomen 789.5
amnion (see also Hydramnios) 657 ☑5ᵗʰ
brain — see Hydrocephalus
cardiac (see also Failure, heart) 428.0
cardiorenal (see also Hypertension, cardiorenal)
404.90
chest 511.9
fetus or newborn 778.0
due to isoimmunization 773.3
gangrenous (see also Gangrene) 785.4
heart (see also Failure, heart) 428.0
hepatic — see Cirrhosis, liver
infantile — see Hydrops, fetalis
kidney (see also Nephrosis) 581.9
liver — see Cirrhosis, liver
lung 514
malarial (see also Malaria) 084.9
neonatorum — see Hydrops, fetalis
nephritic 581.9
newborn — see Hydrops, fetalis
nutritional 269.9
ovary 620.8
pericardium (see also Pericarditis) 423.9
renal (see also Nephrosis) 581.9
uremic — see Uremia
Drowned, drowning 994.1
lung 518.5
Drowsiness 780.09
Drug — see also condition
addiction (see also listing under Dependence)
304.9 ☑5ᵗʰ
adverse effect NEC, correct substance properly
administered 995.2
dependence (see also listing under Dependence)
304.9 ☑5ᵗʰ
habit (see also listing under Dependence)
304.9 ☑5ᵗʰ
overdose — see Table of Drugs and Chemicals
poisoning — see Table of Drugs and Chemicals
therapy (maintenance) status NEC V58.1
anticoagulant V58.61
long-term (current) use V58.69
antibiotics V58.62
wrong substance given or taken in error — see
Table of Drugs and Chemicals
Drunkenness (see also Abuse, drugs,
nondependent) 305.0 ☑5ᵗʰ
acute in alcoholism (see also Alcoholism)
303.0 ☑5ᵗʰ
chronic (see also Alcoholism) 303.9 ☑5ᵗʰ
pathologic 291.4
simple (acute) 305.0 ☑5ᵗʰ
in alcoholism 303.0 ☑5ᵗʰ
sleep 307.47

Drusen
optic disc or papilla 377.21
retina (colloid) (hyaloid degeneration) 362.57
hereditary 362.77
Drusenfieber 075
Dry, dryness — see also condition
eye 375.15
syndrome 375.15
larynx 478.79
mouth 527.7
nose 478.1
skin syndrome 701.1
socket (teeth) 526.5
throat 478.29
DSAP (disseminated superficial actinic
porokeratosis) 692.75
Duane's retraction syndrome 378.71
Duane-Stilling-Türk syndrome (ocular retraction
syndrome) 378.71
Dubin-Johnson disease or syndrome 277.4
Dubini's disease (electric chorea) 049.8
Dubois' abscess or disease 090.5
Duchenne's
disease 094.0
locomotor ataxia 094.0
muscular dystrophy 359.1
pseudohypertrophy, muscles 359.1
paralysis 335.22
syndrome 335.22
Duchenne-Aran myelopathic, muscular atrophy
(nonprogressive) (progressive) 335.21
Duchenne-Griesinger disease 359.1
Ducrey's
bacillus 099.0
chancre 099.0
disease (chancroid) 099.0
Duct, ductus — see condition
Duengero 061
Duhring's disease (dermatitis herpetiformis)
694.0
Dukes (-Filatov) disease 057.8
Dullness
cardiac (decreased) (increased) 785.3
Dumb ague (see also Malaria) 084.6
Dumbness (see also Aphasia) 784.3
Dumdum fever 085.0
Dumping syndrome (postgastrectomy) 564.2
nonsurgical 536.8
Duodenitis (nonspecific) (peptic) 535.60
with hemorrhage 535.61
due to
Strongyloides stercoralis 127.2
Duodenocholangitis 575.8
Duodenum, duodenal — see condition
Duplay's disease, periarthritis, or syndrome
726.2
Duplex — see also Accessory
kidney 753.3
placenta — see Placenta, abnormal
uterus 752.2
Duplication — see also Accessory
anus 751.5
aortic arch 747.21
appendix 751.5
biliary duct (any) 751.69
bladder 753.8
cecum 751.5
and appendix 751.5
clitoris 752.49
cystic duct 751.69
digestive organs 751.8
duodenum 751.5
esophagus 750.4
fallopian tube 752.19
frontonasal process 756.0
gallbladder 751.69
ileum 751.5
intestine (large) (small) 751.5
jejunum 751.5
kidney 753.3
liver 751.69
nose 748.1

☑4ᵗʰ Fourth-digit Required   ☑5ᵗʰ Fifth-digit Required   ►◄ Revised Text   ● New Line   ▲ Revised Code

Duplication — *see also* Accessory — *continued*
  pancreas 751.7
  penis 752.69
  respiratory organs NEC 748.9
  salivary duct 750.22
  spinal cord (incomplete) 742.51
  stomach 750.7
  ureter 753.4
  vagina 752.49
  vas deferens 752.8
  vocal cords 748.3
Dupré's disease or syndrome (meningism) 781.6
Dupuytren's
  contraction 728.6
  disease (muscle contracture) 728.6
  fracture (closed) 824.4
    ankle (closed) 824.4
      open 824.5
    fibula (closed) 824.4
      open 824.5
    open 824.5
    radius (closed) 813.42
      open 813.52
  muscle contracture 728.6
Durand-Nicolas-Favre disease (climatic bubo) 099.1
Duroziez's disease (congenital mitral stenosis) 746.5
Dust
  conjunctivitis 372.05
  reticulation (occupational) 504
Dutton's
  disease (trypanosomiasis) 086.9
  relapsing fever (West African) 087.1
Dwarf, dwarfism 259.4
  with infantilism (hypophyseal) 253.3
  achondroplastic 756.4
  Amsterdam 759.89
  bird-headed 759.89
  congenital 259.4
  constitutional 259.4
  hypophyseal 253.3
  infantile 259.4
  Levi type 253.3
  Lorain-Levi (pituitary) 253.3
  Lorain type (pituitary) 253.3
  metatropic 756.4
  nephrotic-glycosuric, with hypophosphatemic rickets 270.0
  nutritional 263.2
  ovarian 758.6
  pancreatic 577.8
  pituitary 253.3
  polydystrophic 277.5
  primordial 253.3
  psychosocial 259.4
  renal 588.0
    with hypertension — *see* Hypertension, kidney
  Russell's (uterine dwarfism and craniofacial dysostosis) 759.89
Dyke-Young anemia or syndrome (acquired macrocytic hemolytic anemia) (secondary) (symptomatic) 283.9
Dynia abnormality (*see also* Defect, coagulation) 286.9
Dysacousis 388.40
Dysadrenocortism 255.9
  hyperfunction 255.3
  hypofunction 255.4
Dysarthria 784.5
Dysautonomia (*see also* Neuropathy, peripheral, autonomic) 337.9
  familial 742.8
Dysbarism 993.3
Dysbasia 719.7 ✓5ᵗʰ
  angiosclerotica intermittens 443.9
    due to atherosclerosis 440.21
  hysterical 300.11
  lordotica (progressiva) 333.6
  nonorganic origin 307.9
  psychogenic 307.9
Dysbetalipoproteinemia (familial) 272.2
Dyscalculia 315.1

Dyschezia (*see also* Constipation) 564.00
Dyschondroplasia (with hemangiomata) 756.4
  Voorhoeve's 756.4
Dyschondrosteosis 756.59
Dyschromia 709.00
Dyscollagenosis 710.9
Dyscoria 743.41
Dyscraniopyophalangy 759.89
Dyscrasia
  blood 289.9
    with antepartum hemorrhage 641.3 ✓5ᵗʰ
    fetus or newborn NEC 776.9
    hemorrhage, subungual 287.8
    puerperal, postpartum 666.3 ✓5ᵗʰ
  ovary 256.8
  plasma cell 273.9
  pluriglandular 258.9
  polyglandular 258.9
Dysdiadochokinesia 781.3
Dysectasia, vesical neck 596.8
Dysendocrinism 259.9
Dysentery, dysenteric (bilious) (catarrhal) (diarrhea) (epidemic) (gangrenous) (hemorrhagic) (infectious) (sporadic) (tropical) (ulcerative) 009.0
  abscess, liver (*see also* Abscess, amebic) 006.3
  amebic (*see also* Amebiasis) 006.9
    with abscess — *see* Abscess, amebic
    acute 006.0
    carrier (suspected) of V02.2
    chronic 006.1
  arthritis (*see also* Arthritis, due to, dysentery) 009.0 *[711.3]* ✓5ᵗʰ
    bacillary 004.9 *[711.3]* ✓5ᵗʰ
  asylum 004.9
  bacillary 004.9
    arthritis 004.9 *[711.3]* ✓5ᵗʰ
    Boyd 004.2
    Flexner 004.1
    Schmitz (-Stutzer) 004.0
    Shiga 004.0
    Shigella 004.9
      group A 004.0
      group B 004.1
      group C 004.2
      group D 004.3
      specified type NEC 004.8
    Sonne 004.3
    specified type NEC 004.8
  bacterium 004.9
  balantidial 007.0
  Balantidium coli 007.0
  Boyd's 004.2
  Chilomastix 007.8
  Chinese 004.9
  choleriform 001.1
  coccidial 007.2
  Dientamoeba fragilis 007.8
  due to specified organism NEC — *see* Enteritis, due to, by organism
  Embadomonas 007.8
  Endolimax nana — *see* Dysentery, amebic
  Entamoba, entamebic — *see* Dysentery, amebic
  Flexner's 004.1
  Flexner-Boyd 004.2
  giardial 007.1
  Giardia lamblia 007.1
  Hiss-Russell 004.1
  lamblia 007.1
  leishmanial 085.0
  malarial (*see also* Malaria) 084.6
  metazoal 127.9
  Monilia 112.89
  protozoal NEC 007.9
  Russell's 004.8
  salmonella 003.0
  schistosomal 120.1
  Schmitz (-Stutzer) 004.0
  Shiga 004.0
  Shigella NEC (*see also* Dysentery, bacillary) 004.9
    boydii 004.2
    dysenteriae 004.0
      Schmitz 004.0
      Shiga 004.0

Dysentery, dysenteric — *continued*
  Shigella NEC (*see also* Dysentery, bacillary) — *continued*
    flexneri 004.1
    Group A 004.0
    Group B 004.1
    Group C 004.2
    Group D 004.3
    Schmitz 004.0
    Shiga 004.0
    Sonnei 004.3
  Sonne 004.3
  strongyloidiasis 127.2
  trichomonal 007.3
  tuberculous (*see also* Tuberculosis) 014.8 ✓5ᵗʰ
  viral (*see also* Enteritis, viral) 008.8
Dysequilibrium 780.4
Dysesthesia 782.0
  hysterical 300.11
Dysfibrinogenemia (congenital) (*see also* Defect, coagulation) 286.3
Dysfunction
  adrenal (cortical) 255.9
    hyperfunction 255.3
    hypofunction 255.4
  associated with sleep stages or arousal from sleep 780.56
    nonorganic origin 307.47
  bladder NEC 596.59
  bleeding, uterus 626.8
  brain, minimal (*see also* Hyperkinesia) 314.9
  cerebral 348.3
  colon 564.9
    psychogenic 306.4
  colostomy or enterostomy 569.62
  cystic duct 575.8
  diastolic 429.9
    with heart failure — *see* Failure, heart
    due to
      cardiomyopathy — *see* Cardiomyopathy
      hypertension — *see* Hypertension, heart
  endocrine NEC 259.9
  endometrium 621.8
  enteric stoma 569.62
  enterostomy 569.62
  Eustachian tube 381.81
  gallbladder 575.8
  gastrointestinal 536.9
  gland, glandular NEC 259.9
  heart 427.9
    postoperative (immediate) 997.1
      long-term effect of cardiac surgery 429.4
  hemoglobin 288.8
  hepatic 573.9
  hepatocellular NEC 573.9
  hypophysis 253.9
    hyperfunction 253.1
    hypofunction 253.2
    posterior lobe 253.6
      hypofunction 253.5
  kidney (*see also* Disease, renal) 593.9
  labyrinthine 386.50
    specified NEC 386.58
  liver 573.9
    constitutional 277.4
  minimal brain (child) (*see also* Hyperkinesia) 314.9
  ovary, ovarian 256.9
    hyperfunction 256.1
      estrogen 256.0
    hypofunction 256.39
      postablative 256.2
    postablative 256.2
    specified NEC 256.8
  papillary muscle 429.81
    with myocardial infarction 410.8 ✓5ᵗʰ
  parathyroid 252.8
    hyperfunction 252.0
    hypofunction 252.1
  pineal gland 259.8
  pituitary (gland) 253.9
    hyperfunction 253.1
    hypofunction 253.2
    posterior 253.6
      hypofunction 253.5
  placental — *see* Placenta, insufficiency
  platelets (blood) 287.1

Dysfunction — continued
polyglandular 258.9
  specified NEC 258.8
psychosexual 302.70
  with
    dyspareunia (functional) (psychogenic)
      302.76
    frigidity 302.72
    impotence 302.72
    inhibition
      orgasm
        female 302.73
        male 302.74
      sexual
        desire 302.71
        excitement 302.72
    premature ejaculation 302.75
    sexual aversion 302.79
    specified disorder NEC 302.79
    vaginismus 306.51
pylorus 537.9
rectum 564.9
  psychogenic 306.4
segmental (see also Dysfunction, somatic)
  739.9
senile 797
sinoatrial node 427.81
somatic 739.9
  abdomen 739.9
  acromioclavicular 739.7
  cervical 739.1
  cervicothoracic 739.1
  costochondral 739.8
  costovertebral 739.8
  extremities
    lower 739.6
    upper 739.7
  head 739.0
  hip 739.5
  lumbar, lumbosacral 739.3
  occipitocervical 739.0
  pelvic 739.5
  pubic 739.5
  rib cage 739.8
  sacral 739.4
  sacrococcygeal 739.4
  sacroiliac 739.4
  specified site NEC 739.9
  sternochondral 739.8
  sternoclavicular 739.7
  temporomandibular 739.0
  thoracic, thoracolumbar 739.2
stomach 536.9
  psychogenic 306.4
suprarenal 255.9
  hyperfunction 255.3
  hypofunction 255.4
symbolic NEC 784.60
  specified type NEC 784.69
temporomandibular (joint) (joint-pain-
  syndrome) NEC 524.60
  specified NEC 524.69
testicular 257.9
  hyperfunction 257.0
  hypofunction 257.2
  specified type NEC 257.8
thymus 254.9
thyroid 246.9
  complicating pregnancy, childbirth or
    puerperium 648.1 ☑5ᵗʰ
  hyperfunction — see Hyperthyroidism
  hypofunction — see Hypothyroidism
uterus, complicating delivery 661.9 ☑5ᵗʰ
  affecting fetus or newborn 763.7
  hypertonic 661.4 ☑5ᵗʰ
  hypotonic 661.2 ☑5ᵗʰ
    primary 661.0 ☑5ᵗʰ
    secondary 661.1 ☑5ᵗʰ
velopharyngeal (acquired) 528.9
  congenital 750.29
ventricular 429.9
  with congestive heart failure (see also
    Failure, heart) 428.0
  due to
    cardiomyopathy — see Cardiomyopathy
    hypertension — see Hypertension, heart
vesicourethral NEC 596.59

Dysfunction — continued
vestibular 386.50
  specified type NEC 386.58
Dysgammaglobulinemia 279.06
Dysgenesis
gonadal (due to chromosomal anomaly) 758.6
  pure 752.7
kidney(s) 753.0
ovarian 758.6
renal 753.0
reticular 279.2
seminiferous tubules 758.6
tidal platelet 287.3
Dysgerminoma (M9060/3)
specified site — see Neoplasm, by site,
  malignant
unspecified site
  female 183.0
  male 186.9
Dysgeusia 781.1
Dysgraphia 781.3
Dyshidrosis 705.81
Dysidrosis 705.81
Dysinsulinism 251.8
Dyskaryotic cervical smear 795.09   ▲
Dyskeratosis (see also Keratosis) 701.1
bullosa hereditaria 757.39
cervix 622.1
congenital 757.39
follicularis 757.39
  vitamin A deficiency 264.8
gingiva 523.8
oral soft tissue NEC 528.7
tongue 528.7
uterus NEC 621.8
Dyskinesia 781.3
biliary 575.8
esophagus 530.5
hysterical 300.11
intestinal 564.89
nonorganic origin 307.9
orofacial 333.82
psychogenic 307.9
tardive (oral) 333.82
Dyslalia 784.5
developmental 315.39
Dyslexia 784.61
developmental 315.02
secondary to organic lesion 784.61
Dysmaturity (see also Immaturity) 765.1 ☑5ᵗʰ
lung 770.4
pulmonary 770.4
Dysmenorrhea (essential) (exfoliative) (functional)
  (intrinsic) (membranous) (primary)
  (secondary) 625.3
psychogenic 306.52
Dysmetabolic syndrome X 277.7
Dysmetria 781.3
Dysmorodystrophia mesodermalis congenita
  759.82
Dysnomia 784.3
Dysorexia 783.0
hysterical 300.11
Dysostosis
cleidocranial, cleidocranialis 755.59
craniofacial 756.0
Fairbank's (idiopathic familial generalized
  osteophytosis) 756.50
mandibularis 756.0
mandibulofacial, incomplete 756.0
multiplex 277.5
orodigitofacial 759.89
Dyspareunia (female) 625.0
male 608.89
psychogenic 302.76
Dyspepsia (allergic) (congenital) (fermentative)
  (flatulent) (functional) (gastric)
  (gastrointestinal) (neurogenic) (occupational)
  (reflex) 536.8
acid 536.8
atonic 536.3
  psychogenic 306.4

Dyspepsia — continued
diarrhea 787.91
  psychogenic 306.4
intestinal 564.89
  psychogenic 306.4
nervous 306.4
neurotic 306.4
psychogenic 306.4
Dysphagia 787.2
functional 300.11
hysterical 300.11
nervous 300.11
psychogenic 306.4
sideropenic 280.8
spastica 530.5
Dysphagocytosis, congenital 288.1
Dysphasia 784.5
Dysphonia 784.49
clericorum 784.49
functional 300.11
hysterical 300.11
psychogenic 306.1
spastica 478.79
Dyspigmentation — see also Pigmentation
eyelid (acquired) 374.52
Dyspituitarism 253.9
hyperfunction 253.1
hypofunction 253.2
posterior lobe 253.6
Dysplasia — see also Anomaly
artery
  fibromuscular NEC 447.8
    carotid 447.8
    renal 447.3
bladder 596.8
bone (fibrous) NEC 733.29
  diaphyseal, progressive 756.59
  jaw 526.89
  monostotic 733.29
  polyostotic 756.54
  solitary 733.29
brain 742.9
bronchopulmonary, fetus or newborn 770.7
cervix (uteri) 622.1
  cervical intraepithelial neoplasia I [CIN I]
    622.1
  cervical intraepithelial neoplasia II [CIN II]
    622.1
  cervical intraepithelial neoplasia III [CIN III]
    233.1
  CIN I 622.1
  CIN II 622.1
  CIN III 233.1
chondroectodermal 756.55
chondromatose 756.4
craniocarpotarsal 759.89
craniometaphyseal 756.89
dentinal 520.5
diaphyseal, progressive 756.59
ectodermal (anhidrotic) (Bason) (Clouston's)
  (congenital) (Feinmesser) (hereditary)
  (hidrotic) (Marshall) (Robinson's) 757.31
epiphysealis 756.9
  multiplex 756.56
  punctata 756.59
epiphysis 756.9
  multiple 756.56
epithelial
  epiglottis 478.79
  uterine cervix 622.1
erythroid NEC 289.8
eye (see also Microphthalmos) 743.10
familial metaphyseal 756.89
fibromuscular, artery NEC 447.8
  carotid 447.8
  renal 447.3
fibrous
  bone NEC 733.29
  diaphyseal, progressive 756.59
  jaw 526.89
  monostotic 733.29
  polyostotic 756.54
  solitary 733.29
high grade squamous intraepithelial   ●
  (HGSIL) 622.1   ●

Dysplasia — *see also* Anomaly — *continued*
- hip (congenital) 755.63
  - with dislocation (*see also* Dislocation, hip, congenital) 754.30
- hypohidrotic ectodermal 757.31
- joint 755.8
- kidney 753.15
- leg 755.69
- linguofacialis 759.89
- low grade squamous intraepithelial (LGSIL) 622.1 ●
- lung 748.5
- macular 743.55
- mammary (benign) (gland) 610.9
  - cystic 610.1
  - specified type NEC 610.8
- metaphyseal 756.9
  - familial 756.89
- monostotic fibrous 733.29
- muscle 756.89
- myeloid NEC 289.8
- nervous system (general) 742.9
- neuroectodermal 759.6
- oculoauriculovertebral 756.0
- oculodentodigital 759.89
- olfactogenital 253.4
- osteo-onycho-arthro (hereditary) 756.89
- periosteum 733.99
- polyostotic fibrous 756.54
- progressive diaphyseal 756.59
- prostate 602.3
  - intraepithelial neoplasia I [PIN I] 602.3
  - intraepithelial neoplasia II [PIN II] 602.3
  - intraepithelial neoplasia III [PIN III] 233.4
- renal 753.15
- renofacialis 753.0
- retinal NEC 743.56
- retrolental 362.21
- spinal cord 742.9
- thymic, with immunodeficiency 279.2
- vagina 623.0
- vocal cord 478.5
- vulva 624.8
  - intraepithelial neoplasia I [VIN I] 624.8
  - intraepithelial neoplasia II [VIN II] 624.8
  - intraepithelial neoplasia III [VIN III] 233.3
  - VIN I 624.8
  - VIN II 624.8
  - VIN III 233.3

Dyspnea (nocturnal) (paroxysmal) 786.09
- asthmatic (bronchial) (*see also* Asthma) 493.9 ✓5ᵗʰ
  - with bronchitis (*see also* Asthma) 493.9 ✓5ᵗʰ
    - chronic 493.2 ✓5ᵗʰ ▲
  - cardiac (*see also* Failure, ventricular, left) 428.1
- cardiac (*see also* Failure, ventricular, left) 428.1
- functional 300.11
- hyperventilation 786.01
- hysterical 300.11
- Monday morning 504
- newborn 770.89 ▲
- psychogenic 306.1
- uremic — *see* Uremia

Dyspraxia 781.3
- syndrome 315.4

Dysproteinemia 273.8
- transient with copper deficiency 281.4

Dysprothrombinemia (constitutional) (*see also* Defect, coagulation) 286.3

Dysreflexia, autonomic 337.3

Dysrhythmia
- cardiac 427.9
  - postoperative (immediate) 997.1
    - long-term effect of cardiac surgery 429.4
  - specified type NEC 427.89
- cerebral or cortical 348.3

Dyssecretosis, mucoserous 710.2

Dyssocial reaction, without manifest psychiatric disorder
- adolescent V71.02
- adult V71.01
- child V71.02

Dyssomnia NEC 780.56
- nonorganic origin 307.47

Dyssplenism 289.4

Dyssynergia
- biliary (*see also* Disease, biliary) 576.8
- cerebellaris myoclonica 334.2
- detrusor sphincter (bladder) 596.55
- ventricular 429.89

Dystasia, hereditary areflexic 334.3

Dysthymia 300.4

Dysthymic disorder 300.4

Dysthyroidism 246.9

Dystocia 660.9 ✓5ᵗʰ
- affecting fetus or newborn 763.1
- cervical 661.0 ✓5ᵗʰ
  - affecting fetus or newborn 763.7
- contraction ring 661.4 ✓5ᵗʰ
  - affecting fetus or newborn 763.7
- fetal 660.9 ✓5ᵗʰ
  - abnormal size 653.5 ✓5ᵗʰ
  - affecting fetus or newborn 763.1
  - deformity 653.7 ✓5ᵗʰ
- maternal 660.9 ✓5ᵗʰ
  - affecting fetus or newborn 763.1
- positional 660.0 ✓5ᵗʰ
  - affecting fetus or newborn 763.1
- shoulder (girdle) 660.4 ✓5ᵗʰ
  - affecting fetus or newborn 763.1
- uterine NEC 661.4 ✓5ᵗʰ
  - affecting fetus or newborn 763.7

Dystonia
- deformans progressiva 333.6
- due to drugs 333.7
- lenticularis 333.6
- musculorum deformans 333.6
- torsion (idiopathic) 333.6
  - fragments (of) 333.89
  - symptomatic 333.7

Dystonic
- movements 781.0

Dystopia kidney 753.3

Dystrophy, dystrophia 783.9
- adiposogenital 253.8
- asphyxiating thoracic 756.4
- Becker's type 359.1
- brevicollis 756.16
- Bruch's membrane 362.77
- cervical (sympathetic) NEC 337.0
- chondro-osseus with punctate epiphyseal dysplasia 756.59
- choroid (hereditary) 363.50
  - central (areolar) (partial) 363.53
    - total (gyrate) 363.54
  - circinate 363.53
  - circumpapillary (partial) 363.51
    - total 363.52
  - diffuse
    - partial 363.56
    - total 363.57
  - generalized
    - partial 363.56
    - total 363.57
  - gyrate
    - central 363.54
    - generalized 363.57
  - helicoid 363.52
  - peripapillary — *see* Dystrophy, choroid, circumpapillary
  - serpiginous 363.54
- cornea (hereditary) 371.50
  - anterior NEC 371.52
  - Cogan's 371.52
  - combined 371.57
  - crystalline 371.56
  - endothelial (Fuchs') 371.57
  - epithelial 371.50
    - juvenile 371.51
    - microscopic cystic 371.52
  - granular 371.53
  - lattice 371.54
  - macular 371.55
  - marginal (Terrien's) 371.48
  - Meesman's 371.51
  - microscopic cystic (epithelial) 371.52
  - nodular, Salzmann's 371.46
  - polymorphous 371.58
  - posterior NEC 371.58
  - ring-like 371.52
  - Salzmann's nodular 371.46

Dystrophy, dystrophia — *continued*
- cornea — *continued*
  - stromal NEC 371.56
- dermatochondrocorneal 371.50
- Duchenne's 359.1
- due to malnutrition 263.9
- Erb's 359.1
- familial
  - hyperplastic periosteal 756.59
  - osseous 277.5
- foveal 362.77
- Fuchs', cornea 371.57
- Gowers' muscular 359.1
- hair 704.2
- hereditary, progressive muscular 359.1
- hypogenital, with diabetic tendency 759.81
- Landouzy-Déjérine 359.1
- Leyden-Möbius 359.1
- mesodermalis congenita 759.82
- muscular 359.1
  - congenital (hereditary) 359.0
    - myotonic 359.2
  - distal 359.1
  - Duchenne's 359.1
  - Erb's 359.1
  - fascioscapulohumeral 359.1
  - Gowers' 359.1
  - hereditary (progressive) 359.1
  - Landouzy-Déjérine 359.1
  - limb-girdle 359.1
  - myotonic 359.2
  - progressive (hereditary) 359.1
    - Charcôt-Marie-Tooth 356.1
  - pseudohypertrophic (infantile) 359.1
- myocardium, myocardial (*see also* Degeneration, myocardial) 429.1
- myotonic 359.2
- myotonica 359.2
- nail 703.8
  - congenital 757.5
- neurovascular (traumatic) (*see also* Neuropathy, peripheral, autonomic) 337.9
- nutritional 263.9
- ocular 359.1
- oculocerebrorenal 270.8
- oculopharyngeal 359.1
- ovarian 620.8
- papillary (and pigmentary) 701.1
- pelvicrural atrophic 359.1
- pigmentary (*see also* Acanthosis) 701.2
- pituitary (gland) 253.8
- polyglandular 258.8
- posttraumatic sympathetic — *see* Dystrophy, sympathetic
- progressive ophthalmoplegic 359.1
- retina, retinal (hereditary) 362.70
  - albipunctate 362.74
  - Bruch's membrane 362.77
  - cone, progressive 362.75
  - hyaline 362.77
  - in
    - Bassen-Kornzweig syndrome 272.5 [362.72]
    - cerebroretinal lipidosis 330.1 [362.71]
    - Refsum's disease 356.3 [362.72]
    - systemic lipidosis 272.7 [362.71]
  - juvenile (Stargardt's) 362.75
  - pigmentary 362.74
  - pigment epithelium 362.76
  - progressive cone (-rod) 362.75
  - pseudoinflammatory foveal 362.77
  - rod, progressive 362.75
  - sensory 362.75
  - vitelliform 362.76
- Salzmann's nodular 371.46
- scapuloperoneal 359.1
- skin NEC 709.9
- sympathetic (posttraumatic) (reflex) 337.20
  - lower limb 337.22
  - specified NEC 337.29
  - upper limb 337.21
- tapetoretinal NEC 362.74
- thoracic asphyxiating 756.4
- unguium 703.8
  - congenital 757.5
- vitreoretinal (primary) 362.73
  - secondary 362.66
- vulva 624.0

✓4ᵗʰ Fourth-digit Required   ✓5ᵗʰ Fifth-digit Required   ►◄ Revised Text   ● New Line   ▲ Revised Code

Dysuria 788.1
  psychogenic 306.53

E

Eagle-Barrett syndrome 756.71
Eales' disease (syndrome) 362.18
Ear — *see also* condition
  ache 388.70
    otogenic 388.71
    referred 388.72
  lop 744.29
  piercing V50.3
  swimmers' acute 380.12
  tank 380.12
  tropical 111.8 *[380.15]*
  wax 380.4
Earache 388.70
  otogenic 388.71
  referred 388.72
Eaton-Lambert syndrome (*see also* Neoplasm, by
    site, malignant) 199.1 *[358.1]*
Eberth's disease (typhoid fever) 002.0
Ebstein's
  anomaly or syndrome (downward displacement,
    tricuspid valve into right ventricle) 746.2
  disease (diabetes) 250.4 ✓5ᵗʰ *[581.81]*
Eccentro-osteochondrodysplasia 277.5
Ecchondroma (M9210/0) — *see* Neoplasm, bone,
    benign
Ecchondrosis (M9210/1) 238.0
Ecchordosis physaliphora 756.0
Ecchymosis (multiple) 459.89
  conjunctiva 372.72
  eye (traumatic) 921.0
  eyelids (traumatic) 921.1
  newborn 772.6
  spontaneous 782.7
  traumatic — *see* Contusion
Echinococciasis — *see* Echinococcus
Echinococcosis — *see* Echinococcus
Echinococcus (infection) 122.9
  granulosus 122.4
    liver 122.0
    lung 122.1
    orbit 122.3 *[376.13]*
    specified site NEC 122.3
    thyroid 122.2
  liver NEC 122.8
    granulosus 122.0
    multilocularis 122.5
  lung NEC 122.9
    granulosus 122.1
    multilocularis 122.6
  multilocularis 122.7
    liver 122.5
    specified site NEC 122.6
  orbit 122.9 *[376.13]*
    granulosus 122.3 *[376.13]*
    multilocularis 122.6 *[376.13]*
  specified site NEC 122.9
    granulosus 122.3
    multilocularis 122.6 *[376.13]*
  thyroid NEC 122.9
    granulosus 122.2
    multilocularis 122.6
Echinorhynchiasis 127.7
Echinostomiasis 121.8
Echolalia 784.69
ECHO virus infection NEC 079.1
Eclampsia, eclamptic (coma) (convulsions)
    (delirium) 780.39
  female, child-bearing age NEC — *see*
      Eclampsia, pregnancy
  gravidarum — *see* Eclampsia, pregnancy
  male 780.39
  not associated with pregnancy or childbirth
      780.39
  pregnancy, childbirth, or puerperium 642.6 ✓5ᵗʰ
    with pre-existing hypertension 642.7 ✓5ᵗʰ
    affecting fetus or newborn 760.0
  uremic 586
Eclipse blindness (total) 363.31

Economic circumstance affecting care V60.9
  specified type NEC V60.8
Economo's disease (encephalitis lethargica) 049.8
Ectasia, ectasis
  aorta (*see also* Aneurysm, aorta) 441.9
    ruptured 441.5
  breast 610.4
  capillary 448.9
  cornea (marginal) (postinfectional) 371.71
  duct (mammary) 610.4
  kidney 593.89
  mammary duct (gland) 610.4
  papillary 448.9
  renal 593.89
  salivary gland (duct) 527.8
  scar, cornea 371.71
  sclera 379.11
Ecthyma 686.8
  contagiosum 051.2
  gangrenosum 686.09
  infectiosum 051.2
Ectocardia 746.87
Ectodermal dysplasia, congenital 757.31
Ectodermosis erosiva pluriorificialis 695.1
Ectopic, ectopia (congenital) 759.89
  abdominal viscera 751.8
    due to defect in anterior abdominal wall
        756.79
  ACTH syndrome 255.0
  adrenal gland 759.1
  anus 751.5
  auricular beats 427.61
  beats 427.60
  bladder 753.5
  bone and cartilage in lung 748.69
  brain 742.4
  breast tissue 757.6
  cardiac 746.87
  cerebral 742.4
  cordis 746.87
  endometrium 617.9
  gallbladder 751.69
  gastric mucosa 750.7
  gestation — *see* Pregnancy, ectopic
  heart 746.87
  hormone secretion NEC 259.3
  hyperparathyroidism 259.3
  kidney (crossed) (intrathoracic) (pelvis) 753.3
    in pregnancy or childbirth 654.4 ✓5ᵗʰ
      causing obstructed labor 660.2 ✓5ᵗʰ
  lens 743.37
  lentis 743.37
  mole — *see* Pregnancy, ectopic
  organ or site NEC — *see* Malposition,
      congenital
  ovary 752.0
  pancreas, pancreatic tissue 751.7
  pregnancy — *see* Pregnancy, ectopic
  pupil 364.75
  renal 753.3
  sebaceous glands of mouth 750.26
  secretion
    ACTH 255.0
    adrenal hormone 259.3
    adrenalin 259.3
    adrenocorticotropin 255.0
    antidiuretic hormone (ADH) 259.3
    epinephrine 259.3
    hormone NEC 259.3
    norepinephrine 259.3
    pituitary (posterior) 259.3
  spleen 759.0
  testis 752.51
  thyroid 759.2
  ureter 753.4
  ventricular beats 427.69
  vesicae 753.5
Ectrodactyly 755.4
  finger (*see also* Absence, finger, congenital)
      755.29
  toe (*see also* Absence, toe, congenital) 755.39
Ectromelia 755.4
  lower limb 755.30
  upper limb 755.20
Ectropion 374.10
  anus 569.49

Ectropion — *continued*
  cervix 622.0
    with mention of cervicitis 616.0
  cicatricial 374.14
  congenital 743.62
  eyelid 374.10
    cicatricial 374.14
    congenital 743.62
    mechanical 374.12
    paralytic 374.12
    senile 374.11
    spastic 374.13
  iris (pigment epithelium) 364.54
  lip (congenital) 750.26
    acquired 528.5
  mechanical 374.12
  paralytic 374.12
  rectum 569.49
  senile 374.11
  spastic 374.13
  urethra 599.84
  uvea 364.54
Eczema (acute) (allergic) (chronic) (erythematous)
    (fissum) (occupational) (rubrum) (squamous)
    692.9
  asteatotic 706.8
  atopic 691.8
  contact NEC 692.9
  dermatitis NEC 692.9
  due to specified cause — *see* Dermatitis, due to
  dyshidrotic 705.81
  external ear 380.22
  flexural 691.8
  gouty 274.89
  herpeticum 054.0
  hypertrophicum 701.8
  hypostatic — *see* Varicose, vein
  impetiginous 684
  infantile (acute) (chronic) (due to any
        substance) (intertriginous) (seborrheic)
        690.12
  intertriginous NEC 692.9
    infantile 690.12
  intrinsic 691.8
  lichenified NEC 692.9
  marginatum 110.3
  nummular 692.9
  pustular 686.8
  seborrheic 690.18
    infantile 690.12
  solare 692.72
  stasis (lower extremity) 454.1
    ulcerated 454.2
  vaccination, vaccinatum 999.0
  varicose (lower extremity) — *see* Varicose, vein
  verrucosum callosum 698.3
Eczematoid, exudative 691.8
Eddowes' syndrome (brittle bone and blue sclera)
    756.51
Edema, edematous 782.3
  with nephritis (*see also* Nephrosis) 581.9
  allergic 995.1
  angioneurotic (allergic) (any site) (with urticaria)
      995.1
    hereditary 277.6
  angiospastic 443.9
  Berlin's (traumatic) 921.3
  brain 348.5
    due to birth injury 767.8
    fetus or newborn 767.8
  cardiac (*see also* Failure, heart) 428.0
  cardiovascular (*see also* Failure, heart) 428.0
  cerebral — *see* Edema, brain
  cerebrospinal vessel — *see* Edema, brain
  cervix (acute) (uteri) 622.8
    puerperal, postpartum 674.8 ✓5ᵗʰ
  chronic hereditary 757.0
  circumscribed, acute 995.1
    hereditary 277.6
  complicating pregnancy (gestational) 646.1 ✓5ᵗʰ
    with hypertension — *see* Toxemia, of
      pregnancy
  conjunctiva 372.73
  connective tissue 782.3
  cornea 371.20
    due to contact lenses 371.24
    idiopathic 371.21

✓4ᵗʰ Fourth-digit Required   ✓5ᵗʰ Fifth-digit Required   ►◄ Revised Text   ● New Line   ▲ Revised Code

Edema, edematous — *continued*
cornea — *continued*
  secondary 371.22
 due to
  lymphatic obstruction — *see* Edema,
   lymphatic
  salt retention 276.0
 epiglottis — *see* Edema, glottis
 essential, acute 995.1
  hereditary 277.6
 extremities, lower — *see* Edema, legs
 eyelid NEC 374.82
 familial, hereditary (legs) 757.0
 famine 262
 fetus or newborn 778.5
 genital organs
  female 629.8
  male 608.86
 gestational 646.1 ✓5ᵗʰ
  with hypertension — *see* Toxemia, of
   pregnancy
 glottis, glottic, glottides (obstructive) (passive)
  478.6
  allergic 995.1
   hereditary 277.6
  due to external agent — *see* Condition,
   respiratory, acute, due to specified
   agent
 heart (*see also* Failure, heart) 428.0
  newborn 779.89   ▲
 heat 992.7
 hereditary (legs) 757.0
 inanition 262
 infectious 782.3
 intracranial 348.5
  due to injury at birth 767.8
 iris 364.8
 joint (*see also* Effusion, joint) 719.0 ✓5ᵗʰ
 larynx (*see also* Edema, glottis) 478.6
 legs 782.3
  due to venous obstruction 459.2
  hereditary 757.0
 localized 782.3
  due to venous obstruction 459.2
   lower extremity 459.2
 lower extremities — *see* Edema, legs
 lung 514
  acute 518.4
   with heart disease or failure (*see also*
    Failure, ventricular, left) 428.1
    congestive 428.0
   chemical (due to fumes or vapors) 506.1
   due to
    external agent(s) NEC 508.9
     specified NEC 508.8
    fumes and vapors (chemical)
     (inhalation) 506.1
    radiation 508.0
  chemical (acute) 506.1
   chronic 506.4
  chronic 514
   chemical (due to fumes or vapors) 506.4
   due to
    external agent(s) NEC 508.9
     specified NEC 508.8
    fumes or vapors (chemical) (inhalation)
     506.4
    radiation 508.1
  due to
   external agent 508.9
    specified NEC 508.8
   high altitude 993.2
   near drowning 994.1
  postoperative 518.4
  terminal 514
 lymphatic 457.1
  due to mastectomy operation 457.0
 macula 362.83
  cystoid 362.53
  diabetic 250.5 ✓5ᵗʰ [362.01]
 malignant (*see also* Gangrene, gas) 040.0
 Milroy's 757.0
 nasopharynx 478.25
 neonatorum 778.5
 nutritional (newborn) 262
  with dyspigmentation, skin and hair 260
 optic disc or nerve — *see* Papilledema

Edema, edematous — *continued*
 orbit 376.33
  circulatory 459.89
 palate (soft) (hard) 528.9
 pancrease 577.8
 penis 607.83
 periodic 995.1
  hereditary 277.6
 pharynx 478.25
 pitting 782.3
 pulmonary — *see* Edema, lung
 Quincke's 995.1
  hereditary 277.6
 renal (*see also* Nephrosis) 581.9
 retina (localized) (macular) (peripheral) 362.83
  cystoid 362.53
  diabetic 250.5 ✓5ᵗʰ [362.01]
 salt 276.0
 scrotum 608.86
 seminal vesicle 608.86
 spermatic cord 608.86
 spinal cord 336.1
 starvation 262
 stasis (*see also* Hypertension, venous)   ●
  459.30   ●
 subconjunctival 372.73
 subglottic (*see also* Edema, glottis) 478.6
 supraglottic (*see also* Edema, glottis) 478.6
 testis 608.86
 toxic NEC 782.3
 traumatic NEC 782.3
 tunica vaginalis 608.86
 vas deferens 608.86
 vocal cord — *see* Edema, glottis
 vulva (acute) 624.8

Edentia (complete) (partial) (*see also* Absence,
  tooth) 520.0
 acquired 525.10
  due to
   caries 525.13
   extraction 525.10
   periodontal disease 525.12
   specified NEC 525.19
   trauma 525.11
  causing malocclusion 524.3
 congenital (deficiency of tooth buds) 520.0

Edentulism 525.10

Edsall's disease 992.2

Educational handicap V62.3

Edwards' syndrome 758.2

Effect, adverse NEC
 abnormal gravitation (G) forces or states 994.9
 air pressure — *see* Effect, adverse, atmospheric
  pressure
 altitude (high) — *see* Effect, adverse, high
  altitude
 anesthetic
  in labor and delivery NEC 668.9 ✓5ᵗʰ
   affecting fetus or newborn 763.5
 antitoxin — *see* Complications, vaccination
 atmospheric pressure 993.9
  due to explosion 993.4
  high 993.3
  low — *see* Effect, adverse, high altitude
  specified effect NEC 993.8
 biological, correct substance properly
  administered (*see also* Effect, adverse,
  drug) 995.2
 blood (derivatives) (serum) (transfusion) — *see*
  Complications, transfusion
 chemical substance NEC 989.9
  specified — *see* Table of Drugs and
   Chemicals
 cobalt, radioactive (*see also* Effect, adverse,
  radioactive substance) 990
 cold (temperature) (weather) 991.9
  chilblains 991.5
  frostbite — *see* Frostbite
  specified effect NEC 991.8
 drugs and medicinals NEC 995.2
  correct substance properly administered
   995.2
  overdose or wrong substance given or taken
   977.9
   specified drug — *see* Table of Drugs and
    Chemicals

Effect, adverse NEC — *continued*
 electric current (shock) 994.8
  burn — *see* Burn, by site
 electricity (electrocution) (shock) 994.8
  burn — *see* Burn, by site
 exertion (excessive) 994.5
 exposure 994.9
  exhaustion 994.4
 external cause NEC 994.9
 fallout (radioactive) NEC 990
 fluoroscopy NEC 990
 foodstuffs
  allergic reaction (*see also* Allergy, food)
   693.1
   anaphylactic shock due to food NEC
    995.60
  noxious 988.9
   specified type NEC (*see also* Poisoning, by
    name of noxious foodstuff) 988.8
 gases, fumes, or vapors — *see* Table of Drugs
  and Chemicals
 glue (airplane) sniffing 304.6 ✓5ᵗʰ
 heat — *see* Heat
 high altitude NEC 993.2
  anoxia 993.2
  on
   ears 993.0
   sinuses 993.1
  polycythemia 289.0
 hot weather — *see* Heat
 hunger 994.2
 immersion, foot 991.4
 immunization — *see* Complications,
  vaccination
 immunological agents — *see* Complications,
  vaccination
 implantation (removable) of isotope or radium
  NEC 990
 infrared (radiation) (rays) NEC 990
  burn — *see* Burn, by site
  dermatitis or eczema 692.82
 infusion — *see* Complications, infusion
 ingestion or injection of isotope (therapeutic)
  NEC 990
 irradiation NEC (*see also* Effect, adverse,
  radiation) 990
 isotope (radioactive) NEC 990
 lack of care (child) (infant) (newborn) 995.52
  adult 995.84
 lightning 994.0
  burn — *see* Burn, by site
 Lirugin — *see* Complications, vaccination
 medicinal substance, correct, properly
  administered (*see also* Effect, adverse,
  drugs) 995.2
 mesothorium NEC 990
 motion 994.6
 noise, inner ear 388.10
 overheated places — *see* Heat
 polonium NEC 990
 psychosocial, of work environment V62.1
 radiation (diagnostic) (fallout) (infrared) (natural
  source) (therapeutic) (tracer) (ultraviolet)
  (x-ray) NEC 990
  with pulmonary manifestations
   acute 508.0
   chronic 508.1
  dermatitis or eczema 692.82
   due to sun NEC (*see also* Dermatitis, due
    to, sun) 692.70
  fibrosis of lungs 508.1
  maternal with suspected damage to fetus
   affecting management of pregnancy
   655.6 ✓5ᵗʰ
  pneumonitis 508.0
 radioactive substance NEC 990
  dermatitis or eczema 692.82
 radioactivity NEC 990
 radiotherapy NEC 990
  dermatitis or eczema 692.82
 radium NEC 990
 reduced temperature 991.9
  frostbite — *see* Frostbite
  immersion, foot (hand) 991.4
  specified effect NEC 991.8
 roentgenography NEC 990
 roentgenoscopy NEC 990

Edema — Effect

✓4ᵗʰ Fourth-digit Required   ✓5ᵗʰ Fifth-digit Required   ▶◀ Revised Text   ● New Line   ▲ Revised Code

Effect, adverse NEC — *continued*
  roentgen rays NEC 990
  serum (prophylactic) (therapeutic) NEC 999.5
  specified NEC 995.89
    external cause NEC 994.9
  strangulation 994.7
  submersion 994.1
  teletherapy NEC 990
  thirst 994.3
  transfusion — *see* Complications, transfusion
  ultraviolet (radiation) (rays) NEC 990
    burn — *see also* Burn, by site
      from sun (*see also* Sunburn) 692.71
    dermatitis or eczema 692.82
      due to sun NEC (*see also* Dermatitis, due
        to, sun) 692.70
  uranium NEC 990
  vaccine (any) — *see* Complications, vaccination
  weightlessness 994.9
  whole blood — *see also* Complications,
    transfusion
    overdose or wrong substance given (*see also*
      Table of Drugs and Chemicals) 964.7
  working environment V62.1
  x-rays NEC 990
    dermatitis or eczema 692.82
Effects, late — *see* Late, effect (of)
Effect, remote
  of cancer — *see* condition
Effluvium, telogen 704.02
Effort
  intolerance 306.2
  syndrome (aviators) (psychogenic) 306.2
Effusion
  amniotic fluid (*see also* Rupture, membranes,
    premature) 658.1 ☑5ᵗʰ
  brain (serous) 348.5
  bronchial (*see also* Bronchitis) 490
  cerebral 348.5
  cerebrospinal (*see also* Meningitis) 322.9
    vessel 348.5
  chest — *see* Effusion, pleura
  intracranial 348.5
  joint 719.00
    ankle 719.07
    elbow 719.02
    foot 719.07
    hand 719.04
    hip 719.05
    knee 719.06
    multiple sites 719.09
    pelvic region 719.05
    shoulder (region) 719.01
    specified site NEC 719.08
    wrist 719.03
  meninges (*see also* Meningitis) 322.9
  pericardium, pericardial (*see also* Pericarditis)
    423.9
    acute 420.90
  peritoneal (chronic) 568.82
  pleura, pleurisy, pleuritic, pleuropericardial
    511.9
    bacterial, nontuberculous 511.1
    fetus or newborn 511.9
    malignant 197.2
    nontuberculous 511.9
      bacterial 511.1
    pneumococcal 511.1
    staphylococcal 511.1
    streptococcal 511.1
    traumatic 862.29
      with open wound 862.39
    tuberculous (*see also* Tuberculosis, pleura)
      012.0 ☑5ᵗʰ
      primary progressive 010.1 ☑5ᵗʰ
  pulmonary — *see* Effusion, pleura
  spinal (*see also* Meningitis) 322.9
  thorax, thoracic — *see* Effusion, pleura
Eggshell nails 703.8
  congenital 757.5
Ego-dystonic
  homosexuality 302.0
  lesbianism 302.0
Egyptian splenomegaly 120.1
Ehlers-Danlos syndrome 756.83

Ehrlichiosis 082.40
  chaffeensis 082.41
  specified type NEC 082.49
Eichstedt's disease (pityriasis versicolor) 111.0
Eisenmenger's complex or syndrome
  (ventricular septal defect) 745.4
Ejaculation, semen
  painful 608.89
    psychogenic 306.59
  premature 302.75
  retrograde 608.87
Ekbom syndrome (restless legs) 333.99
Ekman's syndrome (brittle bones and blue sclera)
  756.51
Elastic skin 756.83
  acquired 701.8
Elastofibroma (M8820/0) — *see* Neoplasm,
  connective tissue, benign
Elastoidosis
  cutanea nodularis 701.8
  cutis cystica et comedonica 701.8
Elastoma 757.39
  juvenile 757.39
  Miescher's (elastosis perforans serpiginosa)
    701.1
Elastomyofibrosis 425.3
Elastosis 701.8
  atrophicans 701.8
  perforans serpiginosa 701.1
  reactive perforating 701.1
  senilis 701.8
  solar (actinic) 692.74
Elbow — *see* condition
Electric
  current, electricity, effects (concussion) (fatal)
    (nonfatal) (shock) 994.8
    burn — *see* Burn, by site
  feet (foot) syndrome 266.2
Electrocution 994.8
Electrolyte imbalance 276.9
  with
    abortion — *see* Abortion, by type with
      metabolic disorder
    ectopic pregnancy (*see also* categories
      633.0-633.9) 639.4
    hyperemesis gravidarum (before 22
      completed weeks gestation) 643.1 ☑5ᵗʰ
    molar pregnancy (*see also* categories 630-
      632) 639.4
  following
    abortion 639.4
    ectopic or molar pregnancy 639.4
Elephant man syndrome 237.71
Elephantiasis (nonfilarial) 457.1
  arabicum (*see also* Infestation, filarial) 125.9
  congenita hereditaria 757.0
  congenital (any site) 757.0
  due to
    Brugia (malayi) 125.1
    mastectomy operation 457.0
    Wuchereria (bancrofti) 125.0
      malayi 125.1
  eyelid 374.83
  filarial (*see also* Infestation, filarial) 125.9
  filariensis (*see also* Infestation, filarial) 125.9
  gingival 523.8
  glandular 457.1
  graecorum 030.9
  lymphangiectatic 457.1
  lymphatic vessel 457.1
    due to mastectomy operation 457.0
  neuromatosa 237.71
  postmastectomy 457.0
  scrotum 457.1
  streptococcal 457.1
  surgical 997.99
    postmastectomy 457.0
  telangiectodes 457.1
  vulva (nonfilarial) 624.8
Elevated — *see* Elevation
Elevation
  17-ketosteroids 791.9
  acid phosphatase 790.5
  alkaline phosphatase 790.5

Elevation — *continued*
  amylase 790.5
  antibody titers 795.79
  basal metabolic rate (BMR) 794.7
  blood pressure (*see also* Hypertension) 401.9
    reading (incidental) (isolated) (nonspecific),
      no diagnosis or hypertension 796.2
  body temperature (of unknown origin) (*see also*
    Pyrexia) 780.6
  conjugate, eye 378.81
  diaphragm, congenital 756.6
  immunoglobulin level 795.79
  indolacetic acid 791.9
  lactic acid dehydrogenase (LDH) level 790.4
  lipase 790.5
  prostate specific antigen (PSA) 790.93
  renin 790.99
    in hypertension (*see also* Hypertension,
      renovascular) 405.91
  Rh titer 999.7
  scapula, congenital 755.52
  sedimentation rate 790.1
  SGOT 790.4
  SGPT 790.4
  transaminase 790.4
  vanillylmandelic acid 791.9
  venous pressure 459.89
  VMA 791.9
Elliptocytosis (congenital) (hereditary) 282.1
  Hb-C (disease) 282.7
  hemoglobin disease 282.7
  sickle-cell (disease) 282.60
    trait 282.5
Ellis-van Creveld disease or syndrome
  (chondroectodermal dysplasia) 756.55
Ellison-Zollinger syndrome (gastric
  hypersecretion with pancreatic islet cell
  tumor) 251.5
Elongation, elongated (congenital) — *see also*
  Distortion
  bone 756.9
  cervix (uteri) 752.49
    acquired 622.6
    hypertrophic 622.6
  colon 751.5
  common bile duct 751.69
  cystic duct 751.69
  frenulum, penis 752.69
  labia minora, acquired 624.8
  ligamentum patellae 756.89
  petiolus (epiglottidis) 748.3
  styloid bone (process) 733.99
  tooth, teeth 520.2
  uvula 750.26
    acquired 528.9
Elschnig bodies or pearls 366.51
El Tor cholera 001.1
Emaciation (due to malnutrition) 261
Emancipation disorder 309.22
Embadomoniasis 007.8
Embarrassment heart, cardiac — *see* Disease,
  heart
Embedded tooth, teeth 520.6
  with abnormal position (same or adjacent
    tooth) 524.3
  root only 525.3
Embolic — *see* conditon
Embolism 444.9
  with
    abortion — *see* Abortion, by type, with
      embolism
    ectopic pregnancy (*see also* categories
      633.0-633.9) 639.6
    molar pregnancy (*see also* categories 630-
      632) 639.6
  air (any site) 958.0
    with
      abortion — *see* Abortion, by type, with
        embolism
      ectopic pregnancy (*see also* categories
        633.0-633.9) 639.6
      molar pregnancy (*see also* categories 630-
        632) 639.6

☑4ᵗʰ Fourth-digit Required   ☑5ᵗʰ Fifth-digit Required   ▶◀ Revised Text   ● New Line   ▲ Revised Code

Embolism — *continued*
air — *continued*
due to implanted device — *see*
Complications, due to (presence of)
any device, implant, or graft classified
to 996.0-996.5 NEC
following
abortion 639.6
ectopic or molar pregnancy 639.6
infusion, perfusion, or transfusion 999.1
in pregnancy, childbirth, or puerperium
673.0 ✓5ᵗʰ
traumatic 958.0
amniotic fluid (pulmonary) 673.1 ✓5ᵗʰ
with
abortion — *see* Abortion, by type, with
embolism
ectopic pregnancy (*see also* categories
633.0-633.9) 639.6
molar pregnancy (*see also* categories 630-
632) 639.6
following
abortion 639.6
ectopic or molar pregnancy 639.6
aorta, aortic 444.1
abdominal 444.0
bifurcation 444.0
saddle 444.0
thoracic 444.1
artery 444.9
auditory, internal 433.8 ✓5ᵗʰ
basilar (*see also* Occlusion, artery, basilar)
433.0 ✓5ᵗʰ
bladder 444.89
carotid (common) (internal) (*see also*
Occlusion, artery, carotid) 433.1 ✓5ᵗʰ
cerebellar (anterior inferior) (posterior
inferior) (superior) 433.8 ✓5ᵗʰ
cerebral (*see also* Embolism, brain)
434.1 ✓5ᵗʰ
choroidal (anterior) 433.8 ✓5ᵗʰ
communicating posterior 433.8 ✓5ᵗʰ
coronary (*see also* Infarct, myocardium)
410.9 ✓5ᵗʰ
without myocardial infarction 411.81
extremity 444.22
lower 444.22
upper 444.21
hypophyseal 433.8 ✓5ᵗʰ
mesenteric (with gangrene) 557.0
ophthalmic (*see also* Occlusion, retina)
362.30
peripheral 444.22
pontine 433.8 ✓5ᵗʰ
precerebral NEC — *see* Occlusion, artery,
precerebral
pulmonary — *see* Embolism, pulmonary
renal 593.81
retinal (*see also* Occlusion, retina) 362.30
specified site NEC 444.89
vertebral (*see also* Occlusion, artery,
vertebral) 433.2 ✓5ᵗʰ
auditory, internal 433.8 ✓5ᵗʰ
basilar (artery) (*see also* Occlusion, artery,
basilar) 433.0 ✓5ᵗʰ
birth, mother — *see* Embolism, obstetrical
blood-clot
with
abortion — *see* Abortion, by type, with
embolism
ectopic pregnancy (*see also* categories
633.0-633.9) 639.6
molar pregnancy (*see also* categories 630-
632) 639.6
following
abortion 639.6
ectopic or molar pregnancy 639.6
in pregnancy, childbirth, or puerperium
673.2 ✓5ᵗʰ
brain 434.1 ✓5ᵗʰ
with
abortion — *see* Abortion, by type, with
embolism
ectopic pregnancy (*see also* categories
633.0-633.9) 639.6
molar pregnancy (*see also* categories 630-
632) 639.6

Embolism — *continued*
brain — *continued*
following
abortion 639.6
ectopic or molar pregnancy 639.6
late effect — *see* Late effect(s) (of)
cerebrovascular disease
puerperal, postpartum, childbirth 674.0 ✓5ᵗʰ
capillary 448.9
cardiac (*see also* Infarct, myocardium)
410.9 ✓5ᵗʰ
carotid (artery) (common) (internal) (*see also*
Occlusion, artery, carotid) 433.1 ✓5ᵗʰ
cavernous sinus (venous) — *see* Embolism,
intracranial venous sinus
cerebral (*see also* Embolism, brain) 434.1 ✓5ᵗʰ ●
cholesterol — *see* Atheroembolism   ●
choroidal (anterior) (artery) 433.8 ✓5ᵗʰ
coronary (artery or vein) (systemic) (*see also*
Infarct, myocardium) 410.9 ✓5ᵗʰ
without myocardial infarction 411.81
due to (presence of) any device, implant, or
graft classifiable to 996.0-996.5 — *see*
Complications, due to (presence of) any
device, implant, or graft classified to
996.0-996.5 NEC
encephalomalacia (*see also* Embolism, brain)
434.1 ✓5ᵗʰ
extremities 444.22
lower 444.22
upper 444.21
eye 362.30
fat (cerebral) (pulmonary) (systemic) 958.1
with
abortion — *see* Abortion, by type, with
embolism
ectopic pregnancy (*see also* categories
633.0-633.9) 639.6
molar pregnancy (*see also* categories 630-
632) 639.6
complicating delivery or puerperium
673.8 ✓5ᵗʰ
following
abortion 639.6
ectopic or molar pregnancy 639.6
in pregnancy, childbirth, or the puerperium
673.8 ✓5ᵗʰ
femoral (artery) 444.22
vein 453.8
following
abortion 639.6
ectopic or molar pregnancy 639.6
infusion, perfusion, or transfusion
air 999.1
thrombus 999.2
heart (fatty) (*see also* Infarct, myocardium)
410.9 ✓5ᵗʰ
hepatic (vein) 453.0
iliac (artery) 444.81
iliofemoral 444.81
in pregnancy, childbirth, or puerperium
(pulmonary) — *see* Embolism, obstetrical
intestine (artery) (vein) (with gangrene) 557.0
intracranial (*see also* Embolism, brain)
434.1 ✓5ᵗʰ
venous sinus (any) 325
late effect — *see* category 326
nonpyogenic 437.6
in pregnancy or puerperium 671.5 ✓5ᵗʰ
kidney (artery) 593.81
lateral sinus (venous) — *see* Embolism,
intracranial venous sinus
longitudinal sinus (venous) — *see* Embolism,
intracranial venous sinus
lower extremity 444.22
lung (massive) — *see* Embolism, pulmonary
meninges (*see also* Embolism, brain) 434.1 ✓5ᵗʰ
mesenteric (artery) (with gangrene) 557.0
multiple NEC 444.9
obstetrical (pulmonary) 673.2 ✓5ᵗʰ
air 673.0 ✓5ᵗʰ
amniotic fluid (pulmonary) 673.1 ✓5ᵗʰ
blood-clot 673.2 ✓5ᵗʰ
cardiac 674.8 ✓5ᵗʰ
fat 673.8 ✓5ᵗʰ
heart 674.8 ✓5ᵗʰ
pyemic 673.3 ✓5ᵗʰ

Embolism — *continued*
obstetrical — *continued*
septic 673.3 ✓5ᵗʰ
specified NEC 674.8 ✓5ᵗʰ
ophthalmic (*see also* Occlusion, retina) 362.30
paradoxical NEC 444.9
penis 607.82
peripheral arteries NEC 444.22
lower 444.22
upper 444.21
pituitary 253.8
popliteal (artery) 444.22
portal (vein) 452
postoperative NEC 997.2
cerebral 997.02
mesenteric artery 997.71
other vessels 997.79
peripheral vascular 997.2
pulmonary 415.11
renal artery 997.72
precerebral artery (*see also* Occlusion, artery,
precerebral) 433.9 ✓5ᵗʰ
puerperal — *see* Embolism, obstetrical
pulmonary (artery) (vein) 415.1 ✓5ᵗʰ
with
abortion — *see* Abortion, by type, with
embolism
ectopic pregnancy (*see also* categories
633.0-633.9) 639.6
molar pregnancy (*see also* categories 630-
632) 639.6
following
abortion 639.6
ectopic or molar pregnancy 639.6
iatrogenic 415.11
in pregnancy, childbirth, or puerperium —
see Embolism, obstetrical
postoperative 415.11
pyemic (multiple) 038.9
with
abortion — *see* Abortion, by type, with
embolism
ectopic pregnancy (*see also* categories
633.0-633.9) 639.6
molar pregnancy (*see also* categories 630-
632) 639.6
Aerobacter aerogenes 038.49
enteric gram-negative bacilli 038.40
Enterobacter aerogenes 038.49
Escherichia coli 038.42
following
abortion 639.6
ectopic or molar pregnancy 639.6
Hemophilus influenzae 038.41
pneumococcal 038.2
Proteus vulgaris 038.49
Pseudomonas (aeruginosa) 038.43
puerperal, postparztum, childbirth (any
organism) 673.3 ✓5ᵗʰ
Serratia 038.44
specified organism NEC 038.8
staphylococcal 038.10
aureus 038.11
specified organism NEC 038.19
streptococcal 038.0
renal (artery) 593.81
vein 453.3
retina, retinal (*see also* Occlusion, retina)
362.30
saddle (aorta) 444.0
septicemic — *see* Embolism, pyemic
sinus — *see* Embolism, intracranial venous
sinus
soap
with
abortion — *see* Abortion, by type, with
embolism
ectopic pregnancy (*see also* categories
633.0-633.9) 639.6
molar pregnancy (*see also* categories 630-
632) 639.6
following
abortion 639.6
ectopic or molar pregnancy 639.6
spinal cord (nonpyogenic) 336.1
in pregnancy or puerperium 671.5 ✓5ᵗʰ

✓4ᵗʰ Fourth-digit Required   ✓5ᵗʰ Fifth-digit Required   ►◄ Revised Text   ● New Line   ▲ Revised Code

Embolism — *continued*
  spinal cord — *continued*
    pyogenic origin 324.1
      late effect — *see* category 326
  spleen, splenic (artery) 444.89
  thrombus (thromboembolism) following
    infusion, perfusion, or transfusion 999.2
  upper extremity 444.21
  vein 453.9
    with inflammation or phlebitis — *see*
      Thrombophlebitis
    cerebral (*see also* Embolism, brain)
      434.1 ✔5ᵗʰ
    coronary (*see also* Infarct, myocardium)
      410.9 ✔5ᵗʰ
      without myocardial infarction 411.81
    hepatic 453.0
    mesenteric (with gangrene) 557.0
    portal 452
    pulmonary — *see* Embolism, pulmonary
    renal 453.3
    specified NEC 453.8
      with inflammation or phlebitis — *see*
        Thrombophlebitis
  vena cava (inferior) (superior) 453.2
  vessels of brain (*see also* Embolism, brain)
    434.1 ✔5ᵗʰ

Embolization — *see* Embolism

Embolus — *see* Embolism

Embryoma (M9080/1) — *see also* Neoplasm, by
  site, uncertain behavior
  benign (M9080/0 — *see* Neoplasm, by site,
    benign
  kidney (M8960/3) 189.0
  liver (M8970/3) 155.0
  malignant (M9080/3) — *see also* Neoplasm, by
    site, malignant
    kidney (M8960/3) 189.0
    liver (M8970/3) 155.0
    testis (M9070/3) 186.9
      undescended 186.0
  testis (M9070/3) 186.9
    undescended 186.0

Embryonic
  circulation 747.9
  heart 747.9
  vas deferens 752.8

Embryopathia NEC 759.9

Embryotomy, fetal 763.89

Embryotoxon 743.43
  interfering with vision 743.42

Emesis — *see also* Vomiting
  gravidarum — *see* Hyperemesis, gravidarum

Emissions, nocturnal (semen) 608.89

Emotional
  crisis — *see* Crisis, emotional
  disorder (*see also* Disorder, mental) 300.9
  instability (excessive) 301.3
  overlay — *see* Reaction, adjustment
  upset 300.9

Emotionality, pathological 301.3

Emotogenic disease (*see also* Disorder,
  psychogenic) 306.9

Emphysema (atrophic) (centriacinar)
  (centrilobular) (chronic) (diffuse) (essential)
  (hypertrophic) (interlobular) (lung)
  (obstructive) (panlobular) (paracicatricial)
  (paracinar) (postural) (pulmonary) (senile)
  (subpleural) (traction) (unilateral)
  (unilobular) (vesicular) 492.8
  with
    bronchitis
      acute and chronic 491.21
      chronic 491.20
        with acute bronchitis or acute
          exacerbation 491.21
  bullous (giant) 492.0
  cellular tissue 958.7
    surgical 998.81
  compensatory 518.2
  congenital 770.2
  conjunctiva 372.89
  connective tissue 958.7
    surgical 998.81

Emphysema — *continued*
  due to fumes or vapors 506.4
  eye 376.89
  eyelid 374.85
    surgical 998.81
    traumatic 958.7
  fetus or newborn (interstitial) (mediastinal)
    (unilobular) 770.2
  heart 416.9
  interstitial 518.1
    congenital 770.2
    fetus or newborn 770.2
  laminated tissue 958.7
    surgical 998.81
  mediastinal 518.1
    fetus or newborn 770.2
  newborn (interstitial) (mediastinal) (unilobular)
    770.2
  obstructive diffuse with fibrosis 492.8
  orbit 376.89
  subcutaneous 958.7
    due to trauma 958.7
    nontraumatic 518.1
    surgical 998.81
  surgical 998.81
  thymus (gland) (congenital) 254.8
  traumatic 958.7
  tuberculous (*see also* Tuberculosis, pulmonary)
    011.9 ✔5ᵗʰ

Employment examination (certification) V70.5

Empty sella (turcica) syndrome 253.8

Empyema (chest) (diaphragmatic) (double)
  (encapsulated) (general) (interlobar) (lung)
  (medial) (necessitatis) (perforating chest wall)
  (pleura) (pneumococcal) (residual)
  (sacculated) (streptococcal)
  (supradiaphragmatic) 510.9
  with fistula 510.0
  accessory sinus (chronic) (*see also* Sinusitis)
    473.9
  acute 510.9
    with fistula 510.0
  antrum (chronic) (*see also* Sinusitis, maxillary)
    473.0
  brain (any part) (*see also* Abcess, brain) 324.0
  ethmoidal (sinus) (chronic) (*see also* Sinusitis,
    ethmoidal) 473.2
  extradural (*see also* Abscess, extradural) 324.9
  frontal (sinus) (chronic) (*see also* Sinusitis,
    frontal) 473.1
  gallbladder (*see also* Cholecystitis, acute) 575.0
  mastoid (process) (acute) (*see also* Mastoiditis,
    acute) 383.00
  maxilla, maxillary 526.4
    sinus (chronic) (*see also* Sinusitis, maxillary)
      473.0
  nasal sinus (chronic) (*see also* Sinusitis) 473.9
  sinus (accessory) (nasal) (*see also* Sinusitis)
    473.9
  sphenoidal (chronic) (sinus) (*see also* Sinusitis,
    sphenoidal) 473.3
  subarachnoid (*see also* Abscess, extradural)
    324.9
  subdural (*see also* Abscess, extradural) 324.9
  tuberculous (*see also* Tuberculosis, pleura)
    012.0 ✔5ᵗʰ
  ureter (*see also* Ureteritis) 593.89
  ventricular (*see also* Abscess, brain) 324.0

Enameloma 520.2

Encephalitis (bacterial) (chronic) (hemorrhagic)
  (idiopathic) (nonepidemic) (spurious)
  (subacute) 323.9
  acute — *see also* Encephalitis, viral
    disseminated (postinfectious) NEC
      136.9 *[323.6]*
      postimmunization or postvaccination
        323.5
    inclusional 049.8
    inclusion body 049.8
    necrotizing 049.8
  arboviral, arbovirus NEC 064
  arthropod-borne (*see also* Encephalitis, viral,
    arthropod-borne) 064
  Australian X 062.4
  Bwamba fever 066.3
  California (virus) 062.5
  Central European 063.2

Encephalitis — *continued*
  Czechoslovakian 063.2
  Dawson's (inclusion body) 046.2
  diffuse sclerosing 046.2
  due to
    actinomycosis 039.8 *[323.4]*
    cat-scratch disease 078.3 *[323.0]*
    infectious mononucleosis 075 *[323.0]*
    malaria (*see also* Malaria) 084.6 *[323.2]*
    Negishi virus 064
    ornithosis 073.7 *[323.0]*
    prophylactic inoculation against smallpox
      323.5
    rickettsiosis (*see also* Rickettsiosis)
      083.9 *[323.1]*
    rubella 056.01
    toxoplasmosis (acquired) 130.0
      congenital (active) 771.2 *[323.4]*
    typhus (fever) (*see also* Typhus)
      081.9 *[323.1]*
    vaccination (smallpox) 323.5
  Eastern equine 062.2
  endemic 049.8
  epidemic 049.8
  equine (acute) (infectious) (viral) 062.9
    Eastern 062.2
    Venezuelan 066.2
    Western 062.1
  Far Eastern 063.0
  following vaccination or other immunization
    procedure 323.5
  herpes 054.3
  Ilheus (virus) 062.8
  inclusion body 046.2
  infectious (acute) (virus) NEC 049.8
  influenzal 487.8 *[323.4]*
    lethargic 049.8
  Japanese (B type) 062.0
  La Crosse 062.5
  Langat 063.8
  late effect — *see* Late, effect, encephalitis
  lead 984.9 *[323.7]*
  lethargic (acute) (infectious) (influenzal) 049.8
  lethargica 049.8
  louping ill 063.1
  lupus 710.0 *[323.8]*
  lymphatica 049.0
  Mengo 049.8
  meningococcal 036.1
  mumps 072.2
  Murray Valley 062.4
  myoclonic 049.8
  Negishi virus 064
  otitic NEC 382.4 *[323.4]*
  parasitic NEC 123.9 *[323.4]*
  periaxialis (concentrica) (diffusa) 341.1
  postchickenpox 052.0
  postexanthematous NEC 057.9 *[323.6]*
  postimmunization 323.5
  postinfectious NEC 136.9 *[323.6]*
  postmeasles 055.0
  posttraumatic 323.8
  postvaccinal (smallpox) 323.5
  postvaricella 052.0
  postviral NEC 079.99 *[323.6]*
    postexanthematous 057.9 *[323.6]*
    specified NEC 057.8 *[323.6]*
  Powassan 063.8
  progressive subcortical (Binswanger's) 290.12
  Rio Bravo 049.8
  rubella 056.01
  Russian
    autumnal 062.0
    spring-summer type (taiga) 063.0
  saturnine 984.9 *[323.7]*
  Semliki Forest 062.8
  serous 048
  slow-acting virus NEC 046.8
  specified cause NEC 323.8
  St. Louis type 062.3
  subacute sclerosing 046.2
  subcorticalis chronica 290.12
  summer 062.0
  suppurative 324.0
  syphilitic 094.81
    congenital 090.41
  tick-borne 063.9
  torula, torular 117.5 *[323.4]*

✔4ᵗʰ Fourth-digit Required   ✔5ᵗʰ Fifth-digit Required   ►◄ Revised Text   ● New Line   ▲ Revised Code

Encephalitis — Endocarditis

Endocarditis — *continued*
  aortic — *continued*
    rheumatic — *continued*
      active or acute 391.1
        with chorea (acute) (rheumatic)
          (Sydenham's) 392.0
      specified cause, except rheumatic 424.1
      syphilitic 093.22
  arteriosclerotic or due to arteriosclerosis
    424.99
  atypical verrucous (Libman-Sacks)
    710.0 *[424.91]*
  bacterial (acute) (any valve) (chronic) (subacute)
    421.0
  blastomycotic 116.0 *[421.1]*
  candidal 112.81
  congenital 425.3
  constrictive 421.0
  Coxsackie 074.22
  due to
    blastomycosis 116.0 *[421.1]*
    candidiasis 112.81
    Coxsackie (virus) 074.22
    disseminated lupus erythematosus
      710.0 *[424.91]*
    histoplasmosis (*see also* Histoplasmosis)
      115.94
    hypertension (benign) 424.99
    moniliasis 112.81
    prosthetic cardiac valve 996.61
    Q fever 083.0 *[421.1]*
    serratia marcescens 421.0
    typhoid (fever) 002.0 *[421.1]*
  fetal 425.3
  gonococcal 098.84
  hypertensive 424.99
  infectious or infective (acute) (any valve)
    (chronic) (subacute) 421.0
  lenta (acute) (any valve) (chronic) (subacute)
    421.0
  Libman-Sacks 710.0 *[424.91]*
  Loeffler's (parietal fibroplastic) 421.0
  malignant (acute) (any valve) (chronic)
    (subacute) 421.0
  meningococcal 036.42
  mitral (chronic) (double) (fibroid) (heart)
    (inactive) (valve) (with chorea) 394.9
    with
      aortic (valve) disease 396.9
        active or acute 391.1
          with chorea (acute) (rheumatic)
            (Sydenham's) 392.0
      rheumatic fever (conditions classifiable to
        390)
        active — *see* Endocarditis, acute,
          rheumatic
        inactive or quiescent (with chorea)
          394.9
          with aortic valve disease 396.9
    active or acute 391.1
      with chorea (acute) (rheumatic)
        (Sydenham's) 392.0
      bacterial 421.0
    arteriosclerotic 424.0
    congenital 746.89
    hypertensive 424.0
    nonrheumatic 424.0
      acute or subacute 421.9
    syphilitic 093.21
  monilial 112.81
  mycotic (acute) (any valve) (chronic) (subacute)
    421.0
  pneumococcic (acute) (any valve) (chronic)
    (subacute) 421.0
  pulmonary (chronic) (heart) (valve) 424.3
    with
      rheumatic fever (conditions classifiable to
        390)
        active — *see* Endocarditis, acute,
          rheumatic
        inactive or quiescent (with chorea)
          397.1
    acute or subacute 421.9
      rheumatic 391.1
        with chorea (acute) (rheumatic)
          (Sydenham's) 392.0

Endocarditis — *continued*
  pulmonary — *continued*
    arteriosclerotic or due to arteriosclerosis
      424.3
    congenital 746.09
    hypertensive or due to hypertension (benign)
      424.3
    rheumatic (chronic) (inactive) (with chorea)
      397.1
      active or acute 391.1
        with chorea (acute) (rheumatic)
          (Sydenham's) 392.0
    syphilitic 093.24
  purulent (acute) (any valve) (chronic) (subacute)
    421.0
  rheumatic (chronic) (inactive) (with chorea)
    397.9
    active or acute (aortic) (mitral) (pulmonary)
      (tricuspid) 391.1
      with chorea (acute) (rheumatic)
        (Sydenham's) 392.0
  septic (acute) (any valve) (chronic) (subacute)
    421.0
  specified cause, except rheumatic 424.99
  streptococcal (acute) (any valve) (chronic)
    (subacute) 421.0
  subacute — *see* Endocarditis, acute
  suppurative (any valve) (acute) (chronic)
    (subacute) 421.0
  syphilitic NEC 093.20
  toxic (*see also* Endocarditis, acute) 421.9
  tricuspid (chronic) (heart) (inactive) (rheumatic)
    (valve) (with chorea) 397.0
    with
      rheumatic fever (conditions classifiable to
        390)
        active — *see* Endocarditis, acute,
          rheumatic
        inactive or quiescent (with chorea)
          397.0
    active or acute 391.1
      with chorea (acute) (rheumatic)
        (Sydenham's) 392.0
    arteriosclerotic 424.2
    congenital 746.89
    hypertensive 424.2
    nonrheumatic 424.2
      acute or subacute 421.9
    specified cause, except rheumatic 424.2
    syphilitic 093.23
  tuberculous (*see also* Tuberculosis)
    017.9 ☑5ᵗʰ *[424.91]*
  typhoid 002.0 *[421.1]*
  ulcerative (acute) (any valve) (chronic)
    (subacute) 421.0
  vegetative (acute) (any valve) (chronic)
    (subacute) 421.0
  verrucous (acute) (any valve) (chronic)
    (subacute) NEC 710.0 *[424.91]*
    nonbacterial 710.0 *[424.91]*
    nonrheumatic 710.0 *[424.91]*

Endocardium, endocardial — *see also* condition
  cushion defect 745.60
  specified type NEC 745.69

Endocervicitis (*see also* Cervicitis) 616.0
  due to
    intrauterine (contraceptive) device 996.65
  gonorrheal (acute) 098.15
    chronic or duration of 2 months or over
      098.35
  hyperplastic 616.0
  syphilitic 095.8
  trichomonal 131.09
  tuberculous (*see also* Tuberculosis) 016.7 ☑5ᵗʰ

Endocrine — *see* condition

Endocrinopathy, pluriglandular 258.9

Endodontitis 522.0

Endomastoiditis (*see also* Mastoiditis) 383.9

Endometrioma 617.9

Endometriosis 617.9
  appendix 617.5
  bladder 617.8
  bowel 617.5
  broad ligament 617.3
  cervix 617.0
  colon 617.5

Endometriosis — *continued*
  cul-de-sac (Douglas') 617.3
  exocervix 617.0
  fallopian tube 617.2
  female genital organ NEC 617.8
  gallbladder 617.8
  in scar of skin 617.6
  internal 617.0
  intestine 617.5
  lung 617.8
  myometrium 617.0
  ovary 617.1
  parametrium 617.3
  pelvic peritoneum 617.3
  peritoneal (pelvic) 617.3
  rectovaginal septum 617.4
  rectum 617.5
  round ligament 617.3
  skin 617.6
  specified site NEC 617.8
  stromal (M8931/1) 236.0
  umbilicus 617.8
  uterus 617.0
    internal 617.0
  vagina 617.4
  vulva 617.8

Endometritis (nonspecific) (purulent) (septic)
  (suppurative) 615.9
  with
    abortion — *see* Abortion, by type, with
      sepsis
    ectopic pregnancy (*see also* categories
      633.0-633.9) 639.0
    molar pregancy (*see also* categories 630-632)
      639.0
  acute 615.0
  blennorrhagic 098.16
    acute 098.16
    chronic or duration of 2 months or over
      098.36
  cervix, cervical (*see also* Cervicitis) 616.0
    hyperplastic 616.0
  chronic 615.1
  complicating pregnancy 646.6 ☑5ᵗʰ
    affecting fetus or newborn 760.8
  decidual 615.9
  following
    abortion 639.0
    ectopic or molar pregnancy 639.0
  gonorrheal (acute) 098.16
    chronic or duration of 2 months or over
      098.36
  hyperplastic 621.3
    cervix 616.0
  polypoid — *see* Endometritis, hyperplastic
  puerperal, postpartum, childbirth 670 ☑4ᵗʰ
  senile (atrophic) 615.9
  subacute 615.0
  tuberculous (*see also* Tuberculosis) 016.7 ☑5ᵗʰ

Endometrium — *see* condition

Endomyocardiopathy, South African 425.2

Endomyocarditis — *see* Endocarditis

Endomyofibrosis 425.0

Endomyometritis (*see also* Endometritis) 615.9

Endopericarditis — *see* Endocarditis

Endoperineuritis — *see* Disorder, nerve

Endophlebitis (*see also* Phlebitis) 451.9
  leg 451.2
    deep (vessels) 451.19
    superficial (vessels) 451.0
  portal (vein) 572.1
  retina 362.18
  specified site NEC 451.89
  syphilitic 093.89

Endophthalmia (*see also* Endophthalmitis)
  360.00
  gonorrheal 098.42

Endophthalmitis (globe) (infective) (metastatic)
  (purulent) (subacute) 360.00
  acute 360.01
  chronic 360.03
  parasitis 360.13
  phacoanaphylactic 360.19
  specified type NEC 360.19
  sympathetic 360.11

Endosalpingioma (M9111/1) 236.2

Endosteitis — see Osteomyelitis

Endothelioma, bone (M9260/3) — see Neoplasm, bone, malignant

Endotheliosis 287.8
   hemorrhagic infectional 287.8

Endotoxic shock 785.59

Endotrachelitis (see also Cervicitis) 616.0

Enema rash 692.89

Engel-von Recklinghausen disease or syndrome (osteitis fibrosa cystica) 252.0

Engelmann's disease (diaphyseal sclerosis) 756.9

English disease (see also Rickets) 268.0

Engman's disease (infectious eczematoid dermatitis) 690.8

Engorgement
   breast 611.79
      newborn 778.7
      puerperal, postpartum 676.2 ✓5ᵗʰ
   liver 573.9
   lung 514
   pulmonary 514
   retina, venous 362.37
   stomach 536.8
   venous, retina 362.37

Enlargement, enlarged — see also Hypertrophy
   abdomen 789.3 ✓5ᵗʰ
   adenoids 474.12
      and tonsils 474.10
   alveolar process or ridge 525.8
   apertures of diaphragm (congenital) 756.6
   blind spot, visual field 368.42
   gingival 523.8
   heart, cardiac (see also Hypertrophy, cardiac) 429.3
   lacrimal gland, chronic 375.03
   liver (see also Hypertrophy, liver) 789.1
   lymph gland or node 785.6
   orbit 376.46
   organ or site, congenital NEC — see Anomaly, specified type NEC
   parathyroid (gland) 252.0
   pituitary fossa 793.0
   prostate ▶(simple) (soft)◀ 600.0
   sella turcica 793.0
   spleen (see also Splenomegaly) 789.2
      congenital 759.0
   thymus (congenital) (gland) 254.0
   thyroid (gland) (see also Goiter) 240.9
   tongue 529.8
   tonsils 474.11
      and adenoids 474.10
   uterus 621.2

Enophthalmos 376.50
   due to
      atrophy of orbital tissue 376.51
      surgery 376.52
      trauma 376.52

Enostosis 526.89

Entamebiasis — see Amebiasis

Entamebic — see Amebiasis

Entanglement, umbilical cord(s) 663.3 ✓5ᵗʰ
   with compression 663.2 ✓5ᵗʰ
      affecting fetus or newborn 762.5
   around neck with compression 663.1 ✓5ᵗʰ
   twins in monoamniotic sac 663.2 ✓5ᵗʰ

Enteralgia 789.0 ✓5ᵗʰ

Enteric — see condition

Enteritis (acute) (catarrhal) (choleraic) (chronic) (congestive) (diarrheal) (exudative) (follicular) (hemorrhagic) (infantile) (lienteric) (noninfectious) (perforative) (phlegmonous) (presumed noninfectious) (pseudomembranous) 558.9
   adaptive 564.9
   aertrycke infection 003.0
   allergic 558.3
   amebic (see also Amebiasis) 006.9
      with abscess — see Abscess, amebic
      acute 006.0
         with abscess — see Abscess, amebic
         nondysenteric 006.2

Enteritis — continued
   amebic (see also Amebiasis) — continued
      chronic 006.1
         with abscess — see Abscess, amebic
         nondysenteric 006.2
      nondysenteric 006.2
   anaerobic (cocci) (gram-negative) (gram-positive) (mixed) NEC 008.46
   bacillary NEC 004.9
   bacterial NEC 008.5
      specified NEC 008.49
   Bacteroides (fragilis) (melaninogeniscus) (oralis) 008.46
   Butyrivibrio (fibriosolvens) 008.46
   Campylobacter 008.43
   Candida 112.85
   Chilomastix 007.8
   choleriformis 001.1
   chronic 558.9
      ulcerative (see also Colitis, ulcerative) 556.9
   cicatrizing (chronic) 555.0
   Clostridium
      botulinum 005.1
      difficile 008.45
      haemolyticum 008.46
      novyi 008.46
      perfringens (C) (F) 008.46
      specified type NEC 008.46
   coccidial 007.2
   dietetic 558.9
   due to
      achylia gastrica 536.8
      adenovirus 008.62
      Aerobacter aerogenes 008.2 ✓5ᵗʰ
      anaerobes — see Enteritis, anaerobic
      Arizona (bacillus) 008.1
      astrovirus 008.66
      Bacillus coli — see Enteritis, E. coli 008.0 ✓5ᵗʰ
      bacteria NEC 008.5
         specified NEC 008.49
      Bacteroides 008.46
      Butyrivibrio (fibriosolvens)
      Calcivirus 008.65
      Camplyobacter 008.43
      Clostridium — see Enteritis, Clostridium
      Cockle agent 008.64
      Coxsackie (virus) 008.67
      Ditchling agent 008.64
      ECHO virus 008.67
      Enterobacter aerogenes 008.2 ✓5ᵗʰ
      enterococci 008.49
      enterovirus NEC 008.67
      Escherichia coli — see Enteritis, E. coli 008.0 ✓5ᵗʰ
      Eubacterium 008.46
      Fusobacterium (nucleatum) 008.46
      gram-negative bacteria NEC 008.47
         anaerobic NEC 008.46
      Hawaii agent 008.63
      irritating foods 558.9
      Klebsiella aerogenes 008.47
      Marin County agent 008.66
      Montgomery County agent 008.63
      Norwalk-like agent 008.63
      Norwalk virus 008.63
      Otofuke agent 008.63
      Paracolobactrum arizonae 008.1
      paracolon bacillus NEC 008.47
         Arizona 008.1
      Paramatta agent 008.64
      Peptococcus 008.46
      Peptostreptococcus 008.46
      Proprionibacterium 008.46
      Proteus (bacillus) (mirabilis) (morganii) 008.3
      Pseudomonas aeruginosa 008.42
      Rotavirus 008.61
      Sapporo agent 008.63
      small round virus (SRV) NEC 008.64
         featureless NEC 008.63
         structured NEC 008.63
      Snow Mountain (SM) agent 008.63
      specified
         bacteria NEC 008.49
         organism, nonbacterial NEC 008.8
         virus (NEC) 008.69
      Staphylococcus 008.41

Enteritis — continued
   due to — continued
      Streptococcus 008.49
         anaerobic 008.46
      Taunton agent 008.63
      Torovirus 008.69
      Treponema 008.46
      Veillonella 008.46
      virus 008.8
         specified type NEC 008.69
      Wollan (W) agent 008.64
      Yersinia enterocolitica 008.44
   dysentery — see Dysentery
   E. coli 008.00
      enterohemorrhagic 008.04
      enteroinvasive 008.03
      enteropathogenic 008.01
      enterotoxigenic 008.02
      specified type NEC 008.09
   el tor 001.1
   embadomonial 007.8
   epidemic 009.0
   Eubacterium 008.46
   fermentative 558.9
   fulminant 557.0
   Fusobacterium (nucleatum) 008.46
   gangrenous (see also Enteritis, due to, by organism) 009.0
   giardial 007.1
   gram-negative bacteria NEC 008.47
      anaerobic NEC 008.46
   infectious NEC (see also Enteritis, due to, by organism) 009.0
      presumed 009.1
   influenzal 487.8
   ischemic 557.9
      acute 557.0
      chronic 557.1
      due to mesenteric artery insufficiency 557.1
   membranous 564.9
   mucous 564.9
   myxomembranous 564.9
   necrotic (see also Enteritis, due to, by organism) 009.0
   necroticans 005.2
   necrotizing of fetus or newborn 777.5
   neurogenic 564.9
   newborn 777.8
      necrotizing 777.5
   parasitic NEC 129
   paratyphoid (fever) (see also Fever, paratyphoid) 002.9
   Peptococcus 008.46
   Peptostreptococcus 008.46
   Proprionibacterium 008.46
   protozoal NEC 007.9
   radiation 558.1
   regional (of) 555.9
      intestine
         large (bowel, colon, or rectum) 555.1
            with small intestine 555.2
         small (duodenum, ileum, or jejunum) 555.0
            with large intestine 555.2
   Salmonella infection 003.0
   salmonellosis 003.0
   segmental (see also Enteritis, regional) 555.9
   septic (see also Enteritis, due to, by organism) 009.0
   Shigella 004.9
   simple 558.9
   spasmodic 564.9
   spastic 564.9
   staphylococcal 008.41
      due to food 005.0
   streptococcal 008.49
      anaerobic 008.46
   toxic 558.2
   Treponema (denticola) (macrodentium) 008.46
   trichomonal 007.3
   tuberculous (see also Tuberculosis) 014.8 ✓5ᵗʰ
   typhosa 002.0
   ulcerative (chronic) (see also Colitis, ulcerative) 556.9
   Veillonella 008.46
   viral 008.8
      adenovirus 008.62

Enteritis — *continued*
  viral — *continued*
    enterovirus 008.67
      specified virus NEC 008.69
    Yersinia enterocolitica 008.44
    zymotic 009.0
Enteroarticular syndrome 099.3
Enterobiasis 127.4
Enterobius vermicularis 127.4
Enterocele (*see also* Hernia) 553.9
  pelvis, pelvic (acquired) (congenital) 618.6
  vagina, vaginal (acquired) (congenital) 618.6
Enterocolitis — *see also* Enteritis
  fetus or newborn 777.8
    necrotizing 777.5
  fulminant 557.0
  granulomatous 555.2
  hemorrhagic (acute) 557.0
    chronic 557.1
  necrotizing (acute) (membranous) 557.0
  primary necrotizing 777.5
  pseudomembranous 008.45
  radiation 558.1
    newborn 777.5
  ulcerative 556.0
Enterocystoma 751.5
Enterogastritis — *see* Enteritis
Enterogenous cyanosis 289.7
Enterolith, enterolithiasis (impaction) 560.39
  with hernia — *see also* Hernia, by site, with obstruction
    gangrenous — *see* Hernia, by site, with gangrene
Enteropathy 569.9
  exudative (of Gordon) 579.8
  gluten 579.0
  hemorrhagic, terminal 557.0
  protein-losing 579.8
Enteroperitonitis (*see also* Peritonitis) 567.9
Enteroptosis 569.89
Enterorrhagia 578.9
Enterospasm 564.9
  psychogenic 306.4
Enterostenosis (*see also* Obstruction, intestine) 560.9
Enterostomy status V44.4
  with complication 569.60
Enthesopathy 726.39
  ankle and tarsus 726.70
  elbow region 726.30
    specified NEC 726.39
  hip 726.5
  knee 726.60
  peripheral NEC 726.8
  shoulder region 726.10
    adhesive 726.0
  spinal 720.1
  wrist and carpus 726.4
Entrance, air into vein — *see* Embolism, air
Entrapment, nerve — *see* Neuropathy, entrapment
Entropion (eyelid) 374.00
  cicatricial 374.04
  congenital 743.62
  late effect of trachoma (healed) 139.1
  mechanical 374.02
  paralytic 374.02
  senile 374.01
  spastic 374.03
Enucleation of eye (current) (traumatic) 871.3
Enuresis 788.30
  habit disturbance 307.6
  nocturnal 788.36
    psychogenic 307.6
  nonorganic origin 307.6
  psychogenic 307.6
Enzymopathy 277.9
Eosinopenia 288.0
Eosinophilia 288.3
  allergic 288.3
  hereditary 288.3
  idiopathic 288.3

Eosinophilia — *continued*
  infiltrative 518.3
  Loeffler's 518.3
  myalgia syndrome 710.5
  pulmonary (tropical) 518.3
  secondary 288.3
  tropical 518.3
Eosinophilic — *see also* condition
  fasciitis 728.89
  granuloma (bone) 277.8
  infiltration lung 518.3
Ependymitis (acute) (cerebral) (chronic) (granular) (*see also* Meningitis) 322.9
Ependymoblastoma (M9392/3)
  specified site — *see* Neoplasm, by site, malignant
  unspecified site 191.9
Ependymoma (epithelial) (malignant) (M9391/3)
  anaplastic type (M9392/3)
    specified site — *see* Neoplasm, by site, malignant
    unspecified site 191.9
  benign (M9391/0)
    specified site — *see* Neoplasm, by site, benign
    unspecified site 225.0
  myxopapillary (M9394/1) 237.5
  papillary (M9393/1) 237.5
  specified site — *see* Neoplasm, by site, malignant
  unspecified site 191.9
Ependymopathy 349.2
  spinal cord 349.2
Ephelides, ephelis 709.09
Ephemeral fever (*see also* Pyrexia) 780.6
Epiblepharon (congenital) 743.62
Epicanthus, epicanthic fold (congenital) (eyelid) 743.63
Epicondylitis (elbow) (lateral) 726.32
  medial 726.31
Epicystitis (*see also* Cystitis) 595.9
Epidemic — *see* condition
Epidermidalization, cervix — *see* condition
Epidermidization, cervix — *see* condition
Epidermis, epidermal — *see* condition
Epidermization, cervix — *see* condition
Epidermodysplasia verruciformis 078.19
Epidermoid
  cholesteatoma — *see* Cholesteatoma
  inclusion (*see also* Cyst, skin) 706.2
Epidermolysis
  acuta (combustiformis) (toxica) 695.1
  bullosa 757.39
  necroticans combustiformis 695.1
    due to drug
      correct substance properly administered 695.1
      overdose or wrong substance given or taken 977.9
        specified drug — *see* Table of Drugs and Chemicals
Epidermophytid — *see* Dermatophytosis
Epidermophytosis (infected) — *see* Dermatophytosis
Epidermosis, ear (middle) (*see also* Cholesteatoma) 385.30
Epididymis — *see* condition
Epididymitis (nonvenereal) 604.90
  with abscess 604.0
  acute 604.99
  blennorrhagic (acute) 098.0
    chronic or duration of 2 months or over 098.2
  caseous (*see also* Tuberculosis) 016.4 ✓5ᵗʰ
  chlamydial 099.54
  diphtheritic 032.89 [604.91]
  filarial 125.9 [604.91]
  gonococcal (acute) 098.0
    chronic or duration of 2 months or over 098.2
  recurrent 604.99
  residual 604.99
  syphilitic 095.8 [604.91]

Epididymitis — *continued*
  tuberculous (*see also* Tuberculosis) 016.4 ✓5ᵗʰ
Epididymo-orchitis (*see also* Epididymitis) 604.90
  with abscess 604.0
  chlamydial 099.54
  gonococcal (acute) 098.13
    chronic or duration of 2 months or over 098.33
Epidural — *see* condition
Epigastritis (*see also* Gastritis) 535.5 ✓5ᵗʰ
Epigastrium, epigastric — *see* condition
Epigastrocele (*see also* Hernia, epigastric) 553.29
Epiglottiditis (acute) 464.30
  with obstruction 464.31
  chronic 476.1
  viral 464.30
    with obstruction 464.31
Epiglottis — *see* condition
Epiglottitis (acute) 464.30
  with obstruction 464.31
  chronic 476.1
  viral 464.30
    with obstruction 464.31
Epignathus 759.4
Epilepsia
  partialis continua (*see also* Epilepsy) 345.7 ✓5ᵗʰ
  procursiva (*see also* Epilepsy) 345.8 ✓5ᵗʰ
Epilepsy, epileptic (idiopathic) 345.9 ✓5ᵗʰ

> *Note — use the following fifth-digit subclassification with categories 345.0, 345.1, 345.4–345.9:*
>
>   *0 without mention of intractable epilepsy*
>   *1 with intractable epilepsy*

  abdominal 345.5 ✓5ᵗʰ
  absence (attack) 345.0 ✓5ᵗʰ
  akinetic 345.0 ✓5ᵗʰ
    psychomotor 345.4 ✓5ᵗʰ
  automatism 345.4 ✓5ᵗʰ
  autonomic diencephalic 345.5 ✓5ᵗʰ
  brain 345.9 ✓5ᵗʰ
  Bravais-Jacksonian 345.5 ✓5ᵗʰ
  cerebral 345.9 ✓5ᵗʰ
  climacteric 345.9 ✓5ᵗʰ
  clonic 345.1 ✓5ᵗʰ
  clouded state 345.9 ✓5ᵗʰ
  coma 345.3
  communicating 345.4 ✓5ᵗʰ
  congenital 345.9 ✓5ᵗʰ
  convulsions 345.9 ✓5ᵗʰ
  cortical (focal) (motor) 345.5 ✓5ᵗʰ
  cursive (running) 345.8 ✓5ᵗʰ
  cysticercosis 123.1
  deterioration
    with behavioral disturbance 345.9 ✓5ᵗʰ [294.11]
    without behavioral disturbance 345.9 ✓5ᵗʰ [294.10]
  due to syphilis 094.89
  equivalent 345.5 ✓5ᵗʰ
  fit 345.9 ✓5ᵗʰ
  focal (motor) 345.5 ✓5ᵗʰ
  gelastic 345.8 ✓5ᵗʰ
  generalized 345.9 ✓5ᵗʰ
    convulsive 345.1 ✓5ᵗʰ
    flexion 345.1 ✓5ᵗʰ
    nonconvulsive 345.0 ✓5ᵗʰ
  grand mal (idiopathic) 345.1 ✓5ᵗʰ
  Jacksonian (motor) (sensory) 345.5 ✓5ᵗʰ
  Kojevnikof's, Kojevnikov's, Kojewnikoff's 345.7 ✓5ᵗʰ
  laryngeal 786.2
  limbic system 345.4 ✓5ᵗʰ
  major (motor) 345.1 ✓5ᵗʰ
  minor 345.0 ✓5ᵗʰ
  mixed (type) 345.9 ✓5ᵗʰ
  motor partial 345.5 ✓5ᵗʰ
  musicogenic 345.1 ✓5ᵗʰ
  myoclonus, myoclonic 345.1 ✓5ᵗʰ
    progressive (familial) 333.2
  nonconvulsive, generalized 345.0 ✓5ᵗʰ
  parasitic NEC 123.9

Enteritis — Epilepsy

Epilepsy — Eruption

Eruption — *continued*
teeth, tooth — *continued*
   natal 520.6
   neonatal 520.6
   obstructed 520.6
   partial 520.6
   persistent primary 520.6
   premature 520.6
   vesicular 709.8
Erysipelas (gangrenous) (infantile) (newborn) (phlegmonous) (suppurative) 035
  external ear 035 *[380.13]*
  puerperal, postpartum, childbirth 670 ✓5ᵗʰ
Erysipelatoid (Rosenbach's) 027.1
Erysipeloid (Rosenbach's) 027.1
Erythema, erythematous (generalized) 695.9
  ab igne — *see* Burn, by site, first degree
  annulare (centrifugum) (rheumaticum) 695.0
  arthriticum epidemicum 026.1
  brucellum (*see also* Brucellosis) 023.9
  bullosum 695.1
  caloricum — *see* Burn, by site, first degree
  chronicum migrans 088.81
    chronicum 088.81
  circinatum 695.1
  diaper 691.0
  due to
    chemical (contact) NEC 692.4
      internal 693.8
    drug (internal use) 693.0
      contact 692.3
  elevatum diutinum 695.89
  endemic 265.2
  epidemic, arthritic 026.1
  figuratum perstans 695.0
  gluteal 691.0
  gyratum (perstans) (repens) 695.1
  heat — *see* Burn, by site, first degree
  ichthyosiforme congenitum 757.1
  induratum (primary) (scrofulosorum) (*see also* Tuberculosis) 017.1 ✓5ᵗʰ
    nontuberculous 695.2
  infantum febrile 057.8
  infectional NEC 695.9
  infectiosum 057.0
  inflammation NEC 695.9
  intertrigo 695.89
  iris 695.1
  lupus (discoid) (localized) (*see also* Lupus erythematosus) 695.4
  marginatum 695.0
    rheumaticum — *see* Fever, rheumatic
  medicamentosum — *see* Dermatitis, due to, drug
  migrans 529.1
    chronicum 088.81
  multiforme 695.1
    bullosum 695.1
    conjunctiva 695.1
    exudativum (Hebra) 695.1
    pemphigoides 694.5
  napkin 691.0
  neonatorum 778.8
  nodosum 695.2
    tuberculous (*see also* Tuberculosis) 017.1 ✓5ᵗʰ
  nummular, nummulare 695.1
  palmar 695.0
  palmaris hereditarium 695.0
  pernio 991.5
  perstans solare 692.72
  rash, newborn 778.8
  scarlatiniform (exfoliative) (recurrent) 695.0
  simplex marginatum 057.8
  solare (*see also* Sunburn) 692.71
  streptogenes 696.5
  toxic, toxicum NEC 695.0
    newborn 778.8
  tuberculous (primary) (*see also* Tuberculosis) 017.0 ✓5ᵗʰ
  venenatum 695.0
Erythematosus — *see* condition
Erythematous — *see* condition
Erythermalgia (primary) 443.89
Erythralgia 443.89
Erythrasma 039.0

Erythredema 985.0
  polyneuritica 985.0
  polyneuropathy 985.0
Erythremia (acute) (M9841/3) 207.0 ✓5ᵗʰ
  chronic (M9842/3) 207.1 ✓5ᵗʰ
  secondary 289.0
Erythroblastopenia (acquired) 284.8
  congenital 284.0
Erythroblastophthisis 284.0
Erythroblastosis (fetalis) (newborn) 773.2
  due to
    ABO
      antibodies 773.1
      incompatibility, maternal/fetal 773.1
      isoimmunization 773.1
    Rh
      antibodies 773.0
      incompatibility, maternal/fetal 773.0
      isoimmunization 773.0
Erythrocyanosis (crurum) 443.89
Erythrocythemia — *see* Erythremia
Erythrocytopenia 285.9
Erythrocytosis (megalosplenic)
  familial 289.6
  oval, hereditary (*see also* Elliptocytosis) 282.1
  secondary 289.0
  stress 289.0
Erythroderma (*see also* Erythema) 695.9
  desquamativa (in infants) 695.89
  exfoliative 695.89
  ichthyosiform, congenital 757.1
  infantum 695.89
  maculopapular 696.2
  neonatorum 778.8
  psoriaticum 696.1
  secondary 695.9
Erythrogenesis imperfecta 284.0
Erythroleukemia (M9840/3) 207.0 ✓5ᵗʰ
Erythromelalgia 443.89
Erythromelia 701.8
Erythropenia 285.9
Erythrophagocytosis 289.9
Erythrophobia 300.23
Erythroplakia
  oral mucosa 528.7
  tongue 528.7
Erythroplasia (Queyrat) (M8080/2)
  specified site — *see* Neoplasm, skin, in situ
  unspecified site 233.5
Erythropoiesis, idiopathic ineffective 285.0
Escaped beats, heart 427.60
  postoperative 997.1
Esoenteritis — *see* Enteritis
Esophagalgia 530.89
Esophagectasis 530.89
  due to cardiospasm 530.0
Esophagismus 530.5
Esophagitis (alkaline) (chemical) (chronic) (infectional) (necrotic) (peptic) (postoperative) (regurgitant) 530.10
  acute 530.12
  candidal 112.84
  reflux 530.11
  specified NEC 530.19
  tuberculous (*see also* Tuberculosis) 017.8 ✓5ᵗʰ
  ulcerative 530.19
Esophagocele 530.6
Esophagodynia 530.89
Esophagomalacia 530.89
Esophagoptosis 530.89
Esophagospasm 530.5
Esophagostenosis 530.3
Esophagostomiasis 127.7
Esophagotracheal — *see* condition
Esophagus — *see* condition
Esophoria 378.41
  convergence, excess 378.84
  divergence, insufficiency 378.85
Esotropia (nonaccommodative) 378.00
  accommodative 378.35

Esotropia — *continued*
  alternating 378.05
    with
      A pattern 378.06
      specified noncomitancy NEC 378.08
      V pattern 378.07
      X pattern 378.08
      Y pattern 378.08
      intermittent 378.22
  intermittent 378.20
    alternating 378.22
    monocular 378.21
  monocular 378.01
    with
      A pattern 378.02
      specified noncomitancy NEC 378.04
      V pattern 378.03
      X pattern 378.04
      Y pattern 378.04
      intermittent 378.21
Espundia 085.5
Essential — *see* condition
Esterapenia 289.8
Esthesioneuroblastoma (M9522/3) 160.0
Esthesioneurocytoma (M9521/3) 160.0
Esthesioneuroepithelioma (M9523/3) 160.0
Esthiomene 099.1
Estivo-autumnal
  fever 084.0
  malaria 084.0
Estrangement V61.0
Estriasis 134.0
Ethanolaminuria 270.8
Ethanolism (*see also* Alcoholism) 303.9 ✓5ᵗʰ
Ether dependence, dependency (*see also* Dependence) 304.6 ✓5ᵗʰ
Etherism (*see also* Dependence) 304.6 ✓5ᵗʰ
Ethmoid, ethmoidal — *see* condition
Ethmoiditis (chronic) (nonpurulent) (purulent) (*see also* Sinusitis, ethmoidal) 473.2
  influenzal 487.1
  Woakes' 471.1
Ethylism (*see also* Alcoholism) 303.9 ✓5ᵗʰ
Eulenburg's disease (congenital paramyotonia) 359.2
Eunuchism 257.2
Eunuchoidism 257.2
  hypogonadotropic 257.2
European blastomycosis 117.5
Eustachian — *see* condition
Euthyroid sick syndrome 790.94
Euthyroidism 244.9
Evaluation
  fetal lung maturity 659.8
  for suspected condition (*see also* Observation) V71.9
    abuse V71.81
    exposure   ●
      anthrax V71.82   ●
      biologic agent NEC V71.83   ●
    neglect V71.81
    newborn — *see* Observation, suspected, condition, newborn
    specified condition NEC V71.89
  mental health V70.2
    requested by authority V70.1
  nursing care V63.8
  social service V63.8
Evan's syndrome (thrombocytopenic purpura) 287.3
Eventration
  colon into chest — *see* Hernia, diaphragm
  diaphragm (congenital) 756.6
Eversion
  bladder 596.8
  cervix (uteri) 622.0
    with mention of cervicitis 616.0
  foot NEC 736.79
    congenital 755.67
  lacrimal punctum 375.51
  punctum lacrimale (postinfectional) (senile) 375.51

Eruption — Eversion

Eversion — *continued*
ureter (meatus) 593.89
urethra (meatus) 599.84
uterus 618.1
complicating delivery 665.2 ✓5ᵗʰ
affecting fetus or newborn 763.89
puerperal, postpartum 674.8 ✓5ᵗʰ

Evisceration
birth injury 767.8
bowel (congenital) — *see* Hernia, ventral
congenital (*see also* Hernia, ventral) 553.29
operative wound 998.32   ▲
traumatic NEC 869.1
eye 871.3

Evulsion — *see* Avulsion

Ewing's
angioendothelioma (M9260/3) — *see* Neoplasm,
bone, malignant
sarcoma (M9260/3) — *see* Neoplasm, bone,
malignant
tumor (M9260/3) — *see* Neoplasm, bone,
malignant

Exaggerated lumbosacral angle (with impinging
spine) 756.12

Examination (general) (routine) (of) (for) V70.9
allergy V72.7
annual V70.0
cardiovascular preoperative V72.81
cervical Papanicolaou smear V76.2
as a part of routine gynecological
examination V72.3
child care (routine) V20.2
clinical research investigation (normal control
patient) (participant) V70.7
dental V72.2
developmental testing (child) (infant) V20.2
donor (potential) V70.8
ear V72.1
eye V72.0
following
accident (motor vehicle) V71.4
alleged rape or seduction (victim or culprit)
V71.5
inflicted injury (victim or culprit) NEC V71.6
rape or seduction, alleged (victim or culprit)
V71.5
treatment (for) V67.9
combined V67.6
fracture V67.4
involving high-risk medication NEC
V67.51
mental disorder V67.3
specified condition NEC V67.59
follow-up (routine) (following) V67.9
cancer chemotherapy V67.2
chemotherapy V67.2
disease NEC V67.59
high-risk medication NEC V67.51
injury NEC V67.59
population survey V70.6
postpartum V24.2
psychiatric V67.3
psychotherapy V67.3
radiotherapy V67.1
specified surgery NEC V67.09
surgery V67.00
vaginal pap smear V67.01
gynecological V72.3
for contraceptive maintenance V25.40
intrauterine device V25.42
pill V25.41
specified method NEC V25.49
health (of)
armed forces personnel V70.5
checkup V70.0
child, routine V20.2
defined subpopulation NEC V70.5
inhabitants of institutions V70.5
occupational V70.5
pre-employment screening V70.5
preschool children V70.5
for admission to school V70.3
prisoners V70.5
for entrance into prison V70.3
prostitutes V70.5
refugees V70.5

Examination — *continued*
health — *continued*
school children V70.5
students V70.5
hearing V72.1
infant V20.2
laboratory V72.6
lactating mother V24.1
medical (for) (of) V70.9
administrative purpose NEC V70.3
admission to
old age home V70.3
prison V70.3
school V70.3
adoption V70.3
armed forces personnel V70.5
at health care facility V70.0
camp V70.3
child, routine V20.2
clinical research investigation (control)
(normal comparison) (participant)
V70.7
defined subpopulation NEC V70.5
donor (potential) V70.8
driving license V70.3
general V70.9
routine V70.0
specified reason NEC V70.8
immigration V70.3
inhabitants of institutions V70.5
insurance certification V70.3
marriage V70.3
medicolegal reasons V70.4
naturalization V70.3
occupational V70.5
population survey V70.6
pre-employment V70.5
preschool children V70.5
for admission to school V70.3
prison V70.3
prisoners V70.5
for entrance into prison V70.3
prostitutes V70.5
refugees V70.5
school children V70.5
specified reason NEC V70.8
sport competition V70.3
students V70.5
medicolegal reason V70.4
pelvic (annual) (periodic) V72.3
periodic (annual) (routine) V70.0
postpartum
immediately after delivery V24.0
routine follow-up V24.2
pregnancy (unconfirmed) (possible) V72.4
prenatal V22.1
first pregnancy V22.0
high-risk pregnancy V23.9
specified problem NEC V23.8 ✓5ᵗʰ
preoperative V72.84
cardiovascular V72.81
respiratory V72.82
specified NEC V72.83
psychiatric V70.2
follow-up not needing further care V67.3
requested by authority V70.1
radiological NEC V72.5
respiratory preoperative V72.82
screening — *see* Screening
sensitization V72.7
skin V72.7
hypersensitivity V72.7
special V72.9
specified type or reason NEC V72.85
preoperative V72.83
specified NEC V72.83
teeth V72.2
victim or culprit following
alleged rape or seduction V71.5
inflicted injury NEC V71.6
vaginal Papanicolaou smear V76.47
following hysterectomy for malignant
condition V67.01
vision V72.0
well baby V20.2

Exanthem, exanthema (*see also* Rash) 782.1
Boston 048
epidemic, with meningitis 048
lichenoid psoriasiform 696.2
subitum 057.8
viral, virus NEC 057.9
specified type NEC 057.8

Excess, excessive, excessively
alcohol level in blood 790.3
carbohydrate tissue, localized 278.1
carotene (dietary) 278.3
cold 991.9
specified effect NEC 991.8
convergence 378.84
crying of infant (baby) 780.92   ●
development, breast 611.1
diaphoresis 780.8
divergence 378.85
drinking (alcohol) NEC (*see also* Abuse, drugs,
nondependent) 305.0 ✓5ᵗʰ
continual (*see also* Alcoholism) 303.9 ✓5ᵗʰ
habitual (*see also* Alcoholism) 303.9 ✓5ᵗʰ
eating 783.6
eyelid fold (congenital) 743.62
fat 278.00
in heart (*see also* Degeneration, myocardial)
429.1
tissue, localized 278.1
foreskin 605
gas 787.3
gastrin 251.5
glucagon 251.4
heat (*see also* Heat) 992.9
large
colon 564.7
congenital 751.3
fetus or infant 766.0
with obstructed labor 660.1 ✓5ᵗʰ
affecting management of pregnancy
656.6 ✓5ᵗʰ
causing disproportion 653.5 ✓5ᵗʰ
newborn (weight of 4500 grams or more)
766.0
organ or site, congenital NEC — *see*
Anomaly, specified type NEC
lid fold (congenital) 743.62
long
colon 751.5
organ or site, congenital NEC — *see*
Anomaly, specified type NEC
umbilical cord (entangled)
affecting fetus or newborn 762.5
in pregnancy or childbirth 663.3 ✓5ᵗʰ
with compression 663.2 ✓5ᵗʰ
menstruation 626.2
number of teeth 520.1
causing crowding 524.3
nutrients (dietary) NEC 783.6
potassium (K) 276.7
salivation (*see also* Ptyalism) 527.7
secretion — *see also* Hypersecretion
milk 676.6 ✓5ᵗʰ
sputum 786.4
sweat 780.8
short
organ or site, congenital NEC — *see*
Anomaly, specified type NEC
umbilical cord
affecting fetus or newborn 762.6
in pregnancy or childbirth 663.4 ✓5ᵗʰ
skin NEC 701.9
eyelid 743.62
acquired 374.30
sodium (Na) 276.0
sputum 786.4
sweating 780.8
tearing (ducts) (eye) (*see also* Epiphora) 375.20
thirst 783.5
due to deprivation of water 994.3
vitamin
A (dietary) 278.2
administered as drug (chronic) (prolonged
excessive intake) 278.2
reaction to sudden overdose 963.5

Excess, excessive, excessively — *continued*
vitamin — *continued*
D (dietary) 278.4
administered as drug (chronic) (prolonged excessive intake) 278.4
reaction to sudden overdose 963.5
weight 278.00
gain 783.1
of pregnancy 646.1 ✓5ᵗʰ
loss 783.21

Excitability, abnormal, under minor stress 309.29

Excitation
catatonic (*see also* Schizophrenia) 295.2 ✓5ᵗʰ
psychogenic 298.1
reactive (from emotional stress, psychological trauma) 298.1

Excitement
manic (*see also* Psychosis, affective) 296.0 ✓5ᵗʰ
recurrent episode 296.1 ✓5ᵗʰ
single episode 296.0 ✓5ᵗʰ
mental, reactive (from emotional stress, psychological trauma) 298.1
state, reactive (from emotional stress, psychological trauma) 298.1

Excluded pupils 364.76

Excoriation (traumatic) (*see also* Injury, superficial, by site) 919.8
neurotic 698.4

Excyclophoria 378.44

Excyclotropia 378.33

Exencephalus, exencephaly 742.0

Exercise
breathing V57.0
remedial NEC V57.1
therapeutic NEC V57.1

Exfoliation, teeth due to systemic causes 525.0

Exfoliative — *see also* condition dermatitis 695.89

Exhaustion, exhaustive (physical NEC) 780.79
battle (*see also* Reaction, stress, acute) 308.9
cardiac (*see also* Failure, heart) 428.9
delirium (*see also* Reaction, stress, acute) 308.9
due to
cold 991.8
excessive exertion 994.5
exposure 994.4
fetus or newborn 779.89 ▲
heart (*see also* Failure, heart) 428.9
heat 992.5
due to
salt depletion 992.4
water depletion 992.3
manic (*see also* Psychosis, affective) 296.0 ✓5ᵗʰ
recurrent episode 296.1 ✓5ᵗʰ
single episode 296.0 ✓5ᵗʰ
maternal, complicating delivery 669.8 ✓5ᵗʰ
affecting fetus or newborn 763.89
mental 300.5
myocardium, myocardial (*see also* Failure, heart) 428.9
nervous 300.5
old age 797
postinfectional NEC 780.79
psychogenic 300.5
psychosis (*see also* Reaction, stress, acute) 308.9
senile 797
dementia 290.0

Exhibitionism (sexual) 302.4

Exomphalos 756.79

Exophoria 378.42
convergence, insufficiency 378.83
divergence, excess 378.85

Exophthalmic
cachexia 242.0 ✓5ᵗʰ
goiter 242.0 ✓5ᵗʰ
ophthalmoplegia 242.0 ✓5ᵗʰ [376.22]

Exophthalmos 376.30
congenital 743.66
constant 376.31
endocrine NEC 259.9 [376.22]
hyperthyroidism 242.0 ✓5ᵗʰ [376.21]

Exophthalmos — *continued*
intermittent NEC 376.34
malignant 242.0 ✓5ᵗʰ [376.21]
pulsating 376.35
endocrine NEC 259.9 [376.22]
thyrotoxic 242.0 ✓5ᵗʰ [376.21]

Exostosis 726.91
cartilaginous (M9210/0) — *see* Neoplasm, bone, benign
congenital 756.4
ear canal, external 380.81
gonococcal 098.89
hip 726.5
intracranial 733.3
jaw (bone) 526.81
luxurians 728.11
multiple (cancellous) (congenital) (hereditary) 756.4
nasal bones 726.91
orbit, orbital 376.42
osteocartilaginous (M9210/0) — *see* Neoplasm, bone, benign
spine 721.8
with spondylosis — *see* Spondylosis
syphilitic 095.5
wrist 726.4

Exotropia 378.10
alternating 378.15
with
A pattern 378.16
specified noncomitancy NEC 378.18
V pattern 378.17
X pattern 378.18
Y pattern 378.18
intermittent 378.24
intermittent 378.20
alternating 378.24
monocular 378.23
monocular 378.11
with
A pattern 378.12
specified noncomitancy NEC 378.14
V pattern 378.13
X pattern 378.14
Y pattern 378.14
intermittent 378.23

Explanation of
investigation finding V65.4
medication V65.4

Exposure 994.9
cold 991.9
specified effect NEC 991.8
effects of 994.9
exhaustion due to 994.4
to
AIDS virus V01.7
anthrax V01.81 ●
asbestos V15.84
body fluids (hazardous) V15.85
cholera V01.0
communicable disease V01.9
specified type NEC V01.89 ▲
German measles V01.4
gonorrhea V01.6
hazardous body fluids V15.85
HIV V01.7
human immunodeficiency virus V01.7
lead V15.86
parasitic disease V01.89 ▲
poliomyelitis V01.2
potentially hazardous body fluids V15.85
rabies V01.5
rubella V01.4
smallpox V01.3
syphilis V01.6
tuberculosis V01.1
venereal disease V01.6
viral disease NEC V01.7

Exsanguination, fetal 772.0

Exstrophy
abdominal content 751.8
bladder (urinary) 753.5

Extensive — *see* condition

Extra — *see also* Accessory
rib 756.3
cervical 756.2

Extraction
with hook 763.89
breech NEC 669.6 ✓5ᵗʰ
affecting fetus or newborn 763.0
cataract postsurgical V45.61
manual NEC 669.8 ✓5ᵗʰ
affecting fetus or newborn 763.89

Extrasystole 427.60
atrial 427.61
postoperative 997.1
ventricular 427.69

Extrauterine gestation or pregnancy — *see* Pregnancy, ectopic

Extravasation
blood 459.0
lower extremity 459.0
chyle into mesentery 457.8
pelvicalyceal 593.4
pyelosinus 593.4
urine 788.8
from ureter 788.8

Extremity — *see* condition

Extrophy — *see* Exstrophy

Extroversion
bladder 753.5
uterus 618.1
complicating delivery 665.2 ✓5ᵗʰ
affecting fetus or newborn 763.89
postpartal (old) 618.1

Extrusion
breast implant (prosthetic) 996.54
device, implant, or graft — *see* Complications, mechanical
eye implant (ball) (globe) 996.59
intervertebral disc — *see* Displacement, intervertebral disc
lacrimal gland 375.43
mesh (reinforcing) 996.59
ocular lens implant 996.53
prosthetic device NEC — *see* Complications, mechanical
vitreous 379.26

Exudate, pleura — *see* Effusion, pleura

Exudates, retina 362.82

Exudative — *see* condition

Eye, eyeball, eyelid — *see* condition

Eyestrain 368.13

Eyeworm disease of Africa 125.2

Faber's anemia or syndrome (achlorhydric anemia) 280.9

Fabry's disease (angiokeratoma corporis diffusum) 272.7

Face, facial — *see* condition

Facet of cornea 371.44

Faciocephalalgia, autonomic (*see also* Neuropathy, peripheral, autonomic) 337.9

Facioscapulohumeral myopathy 359.1

Factitious disorder, illness — *see* Illness, factitious

Factor
deficiency — *see* Deficiency, factor
psychic, associated with diseases classified elsewhere 316
risk — *see* Problem

Fahr-Volhard disease (malignant nephrosclerosis) 403.00

Failure, failed
adenohypophyseal 253.2
attempted abortion (legal) (*see also* Abortion, failed) 638.9
bone marrow (anemia) 284.9
acquired (secondary) 284.8
congenital 284.0
idiopathic 284.9
cardiac (*see also* Failure, heart) 428.9
newborn 779.89 ▲
cardiorenal (chronic) 428.9
hypertensive (*see also* Hypertension, cardiorenal) 404.93

Failure — Failure

Failure, failed — *continued*
cardiorespiratory 799.1
specified during or due to a procedure 997.1
long-term effect of cardiac surgery 429.4
cardiovascular (chronic) 428.9
cerebrovascular 437.8
cervical dilatation in labor 661.0 ✓5ᵗʰ
affecting fetus or newborn 763.7
circulation, circulatory 799.8
fetus or newborn 779.89 ▲
peripheral 785.50
compensation — *see* Disease, heart
congestive (*see also* Failure, heart) 428.0
coronary (*see also* Insufficiency, coronary) 411.89
descent of head (at term) 652.5 ✓5ᵗʰ
affecting fetus or newborn 763.1
in labor 660.0 ✓5ᵗʰ
affecting fetus or newborn 763.1
device, implant, or graft — *see* Complications, mechanical
engagement of head NEC 652.5 ✓5ᵗʰ
in labor 660.0 ✓5ᵗʰ
extrarenal 788.9
fetal head to enter pelvic brim 652.5 ✓5ᵗʰ
affecting fetus or newborn 763.1
in labor 660.0 ✓5ᵗʰ
affecting fetus or newborn 763.1
forceps NEC 660.7 ✓5ᵗʰ
affecting fetus or newborn 763.1
fusion (joint) (spinal) 996.4
growth in childhood 783.43
heart (acute) (sudden) 428.9
with
abortion — *see* Abortion, by type, with specified complication NEC
acute pulmonary edema (*see also* Failure, ventricular, left) 428.1
with congestion ▶(*see also* Failure, heart)◀ 428.0
decompensation (*see also* Failure, heart) 428.0
dilation — *see* Disease, heart
ectopic pregnancy (*see also* categories 633.0-633.9) 639.8
molar pregnancy (*see also* categories 630-632) 639.8
arteriosclerotic 440.9
combined left-right sided 428.0
combined systolic and diastolic 428.40 ●
acute 428.41 ●
acute on chronic 428.43 ●
chronic 428.42 ●
compensated (*see also* Failure, heart) 428.0
complicating
abortion — *see* Abortion, by type, with specified complication NEC
delivery (cesarean) (instrumental) 669.4 ✓5ᵗʰ
ectopic pregnancy (*see also* categories 633.0-633.9) 639.8
molar pregnancy (*see also* categories 630-632) 639.8
obstetric anesthesia or sedation 668.1 ✓5ᵗʰ
surgery 997.1
congestive (compensated) (decompensated) ▶(*see also* Failure, heart)◀ 428.0
with rheumatic fever (conditions classifiable to 390)
active 391.8
inactive or quiescent (with chorea) 398.91
fetus or newborn 779.89 ▲
hypertensive (*see also* Hypertension, heart) 402.90
with renal disease (*see also* Hypertension, cardiorenal) 404.91
with renal failure 404.93
benign 402.11
malignant 402.01
rheumatic (chronic) (inactive) (with chorea) 398.91
active or acute 391.8
with chorea (Sydenham's) 392.0

Failure, failed — *continued*
heart — *continued*
decompensated (*see also* Failure, heart) 428.0
degenerative (*see also* Degeneration, myocardial) 429.1
diastolic 428.30 ●
acute 428.31 ●
acute on chronic 428.33 ●
chronic 428.32 ●
due to presence of (cardiac) prosthesis 429.4
fetus or newborn 779.89 ▲
following
abortion 639.8
cardiac surgery 429.4
ectopic or molar pregnancy 639.8
high output NEC 428.9
hypertensive (*see also* Hypertension, heart) 402.91
with renal disease (*see also* Hypertension, cardiorenal) 404.91
with renal failure 404.93
benign 402.11
malignant 402.01
left (ventricular) (*see also* Failure, ventricular, left) 428.1
with right-sided failure ▶(*see also* Failure, heart)◀ 428.0
low output (syndrome) NEC 428.9
organic — *see* Disease, heart
postoperative (immediate) 997.1
long term effect of cardiac surgery 429.4
rheumatic (chronic) (congestive) (inactive) 398.91
right (secondary to left heart failure, conditions classifiable to 428.1) (ventricular) (*see also* Failure, heart) 428.0
senile 797
specified during or due to a procedure 997.1
long-term effect of cardiac surgery 429.4
systolic 428.20 ●
acute 428.21 ●
acute on chronic 428.23 ●
chronic 428.22 ●
thyrotoxic (*see also* Thyrotoxicosis) 242.9 ✓5ᵗʰ [425.7]
valvular — *see* Endocarditis
hepatic 572.8
acute 570
due to a procedure 997.4
hepatorenal 572.4
hypertensive heart (*see also* Hypertension, heart) 402.91
benign 402.11
malignant 402.01
induction (of labor) 659.1 ✓5ᵗʰ
abortion (legal) (*see also* Abortion, failed) 638.9
affecting fetus or newborn 763.89
by oxytocic drugs 659.1 ✓5ᵗʰ
instrumental 659.0 ✓5ᵗʰ
mechanical 659.0 ✓5ᵗʰ
medical 659.1 ✓5ᵗʰ
surgical 659.0 ✓5ᵗʰ
initial alveolar expansion, newborn 770.4
involution, thymus (gland) 254.8
kidney — *see* Failure, renal
lactation 676.4 ✓5ᵗʰ
Leydig's cell, adult 257.2
liver 572.8
acute 570
medullary 799.8
mitral — *see* Endocarditis, mitral
myocardium, myocardial (*see also* Failure, heart) 428.9
chronic (*see also* Failure, heart) 428.0
congestive (*see also* Failure, heart) 428.0
ovarian (primary) 256.39
iatrogenic 256.2
postablative 256.2
postirradiation 256.2
postsurgical 256.2
ovulation 628.0
prerenal 788.9

Failure, failed — *continued*
renal 586
with
abortion — *see* Abortion, by type, with renal failure
ectopic pregnancy (*see also* categories 633.0-633.9) 639.3
edema (*see also* Nephrosis) 581.9
hypertension (*see also* Hypertension, kidney) 403.91
hypertensive heart disease (conditions classifiable to 402) 404.92
with heart failure 404.93
benign 404.12
with heart failure 404.13
malignant 404.02
with heart failure 404.03
molar pregnancy (*see also* categories 630-632) 639.3
tubular necrosis (acute) 584.5
acute 584.9
with lesion of
necrosis
cortical (renal) 584.6
medullary (renal) (papillary) 584.7
tubular 584.5
specified pathology NEC 584.8
chronic 585
hypertensive or with hypertension (*see also* Hypertension, kidney) 403.91
due to a procedure 997.5
following
abortion 639.3
crushing 958.5
ectopic or molar pregnancy 639.3
labor and delivery (acute) 669.3 ✓5ᵗʰ
hypertensive (*see also* Hypertension, kidney) 403.91
puerperal, postpartum 669.3 ✓5ᵗʰ
respiration, respiratory 518.81
acute 518.81
acute and chronic 518.84
center 348.8
newborn 770.84 ▲
chronic 518.83
due to trauma, surgery or shock 518.5
newborn 770.84 ▲
rotation
cecum 751.4
colon 751.4
intestine 751.4
kidney 753.3
segmentation — *see also* Fusion
fingers (*see also* Syndactylism, fingers) 755.11
toes (*see also* Syndactylism, toes) 755.13
seminiferous tubule, adult 257.2
senile (general) 797
with psychosis 290.20
testis, primary (seminal) 257.2
to progress 661.2 ✓5ᵗʰ
to thrive
adult 783.7
child 783.41
transplant 996.80
bone marrow 996.85
organ (immune or nonimmune cause) 996.80
bone marrow 996.85
heart 996.83
intestines 996.87
kidney 996.81
liver 996.82
lung 996.84
pancreas 996.86
specified NEC 996.89
skin 996.52
artificial 996.55
decellularized allodermis 996.55
temporary allograft or pigskin graft — *omit code*
trial of labor NEC 660.6 ✓5ᵗʰ
affecting fetus or newborn 763.1
urinary 586
vacuum extraction
abortion — *see* Abortion, failed
delivery NEC 660.7 ✓5ᵗʰ

✓4ᵗʰ Fourth-digit Required   ✓5ᵗʰ Fifth-digit Required   ▶◀ Revised Text   ● New Line   ▲ Revised Code

Failure, failed — *continued*
  vacuum extraction — *continued*
    delivery NEC — *continued*
      affecting fetus or newborn 763.1
    ventouse NEC 660.7 ✓5ᵗʰ
      affecting fetus or newborn 763.1
  ventricular (*see also* Failure, heart) 428.9
    left 428.1
      with rheumatic fever (conditions
        classifiable to 390)
        active 391.8
          with chorea 392.0
        inactive or quiescent (with chorea)
          398.91
      hypertensive (*see also* Hypertension,
        heart) 402.91
        benign 402.11
        malignant 402.01
      rheumatic (chronic) (inactive) (with
        chorea) 398.91
        active or acute 391.8
          with chorea 392.0
    right (*see also* Failure, heart) 428.0
  vital centers, fetus or newborn 779.8
  weight gain in childhood 783.41
Fainting (fit) (spell) 780.2
Falciform hymen 752.49
Fall, maternal, affecting fetus or newborn
  760.5
Fallen arches 734
Falling, any organ or part — *see* Prolapse
Fallopian
  insufflation
    fertility testing V26.21
    following sterilization reversal V26.22
  tube — *see* condition
Fallot's
  pentalogy 745.2
  tetrad or tetralogy 745.2
  triad or trilogy 746.09
Fallout, radioactive (adverse effect) NEC 990
False — *see also* condition
  bundle branch block 426.50
  bursa 727.89
  croup 478.75
  joint 733.82
  labor (pains) 644.1 ✓5ᵗʰ
  opening, urinary, male 752.69
  passage, urethra (prostatic) 599.4
  positive
    serological test for syphilis 795.6
    Wassermann reaction 795.6
  pregnancy 300.11
Family, familial — *see also* condition
  disruption V61.0
  planning advice V25.09
  problem V61.9
    specified circumstance NEC V61.8
Famine 994.2
  edema 262
Fanconi's anemia (congenital pancytopenia)
  284.0
Fanconi (-de Toni) (-Debré) syndrome
  (cystinosis) 270.0
Farber (-Uzman) syndrome or disease
  (disseminated lipogranulomatosis) 272.8
Farcin 024
Farcy 024
Farmers'
  lung 495.0
  skin 692.74
Farsightedness 367.0
Fascia — *see* condition
Fasciculation 781.0
Fasciculitis optica 377.32
Fasciitis 729.4
  eosinophilic 728.89
  necrotizing 728.86
  nodular 728.79
  perirenal 593.4
  plantar 728.71
  pseudosarcomatous 728.79

Fasciitis — *continued*
  traumatic (old) NEC 728.79
    current — *see* Sprain, by site
Fasciola hepatica infestation 121.3
Fascioliasis 121.3
Fasciolopsiasis (small intestine) 121.4
Fasciolopsis (small intestine) 121.4
Fast pulse 785.0
Fat
  embolism (cerebral) (pulmonary) (systemic)
    958.1
    with
      abortion — *see* Abortion, by type, with
        embolism
      ectopic pregnancy (*see also* categories
        633.0-633.9) 639.6
      molar pregnancy (*see also* categories 630-
        632) 639.6
    complicating delivery or puerperium
      673.8 ✓5ᵗʰ
    following
      abortion 639.6
      ectopic or molar pregnancy 639.6
    in pregnancy, childbirth, or the puerperium
      673.8 ✓5ᵗʰ
  excessive 278.00
    in heart (*see also* Degeneration, myocardial)
      429.1
  general 278.00
  hernia, herniation 729.30
    eyelid 374.34
    knee 729.31
    orbit 374.34
    retro-orbital 374.34
    retropatellar 729.31
    specified site NEC 729.39
  indigestion 579.8
  in stool 792.1
  localized (pad) 278.1
    heart (*see also* Degeneration, myocardial)
      429.1
    knee 729.31
    retropatellar 729.31
  necrosis — *see also* Fatty, degeneration breast
    (aseptic)
    (segmental) 611.3
    mesentery 567.8
    omentum 567.8
  pad 278.1
Fatal syncope 798.1
Fatigue 780.79
  auditory deafness (*see also* Deafness) 389.9
  chronic 780.7 ✓5ᵗʰ
  chronic, syndrome 780.71
  combat (*see also* Reaction, stress, acute) 308.9
  during pregnancy 646.8 ✓5ᵗʰ
  general 780.79
  psychogenic 300.5
  heat (transient) 992.6
  muscle 729.89
  myocardium (*see also* Failure, heart) 428.9
  nervous 300.5
  neurosis 300.5
  operational 300.89
  postural 729.89
  posture 729.89
  psychogenic (general) 300.5
  senile 797
  syndrome NEC 300.5
    chronic 780.71
  undue 780.79
  voice 784.49
Fatness 278.00
Fatty — *see also* condition
  apron 278.1
  degeneration (diffuse) (general) NEC 272.8
    localized — *see* Degeneration, by site, fatty
    placenta — *see* Placenta, abnormal
  heart (enlarged) (*see also* Degeneration,
    myocardial) 429.1
  infiltration (diffuse) (general) (*see also*
    Degeneration, by site, fatty) 272.8
    heart (enlarged) (*see also* Degeneration,
      myocardial) 429.1
  liver 571.8
    alcoholic 571.0

Fatty — *see also* condition — *continued*
  necrosis — *see* Degeneration, fatty
  phanerosis 272.8
Fauces — *see* condition
Fauchard's disease (periodontitis) 523.4
Faucitis 478.29
Faulty — *see also* condition
  position of teeth 524.3
Favism (anemia) 282.2
Favre-Racouchot disease (elastoidosis cutanea
  nodularis) 701.8
Favus 110.9
  beard 110.0
  capitis 110.0
  corporis 110.5
  eyelid 110.8
  foot 110.4
  hand 110.2
  scalp 110.0
  specified site NEC 110.8
Fear, fearfullness (complex) (reaction) 300.20
  child 313.0
  of
    animals 300.29
    closed spaces 300.29
    crowds 300.29
    eating in public 300.23
    heights 300.29
    open spaces 300.22
      with panic attacks 300.21
    public speaking 300.23
    streets 300.22
      with panic attacks 300.21
    travel 300.22
      with panic attacks 300.21
    washing in public 300.23
  transient 308.0
Feared complaint unfounded V65.5
Febricula (continued) (simple) (*see also* Pyrexia
  780.6
Febrile (*see also* Pyrexia) 780.6
  convulsion 780.31
  seizure 780.31
Febris (*see also* Fever) 780.6
  aestiva (*see also* Fever, hay) 477.9
  flava (*see also* Fever, yellow) 060.9
  melitensis 023.0
  pestis (*see also* Plague) 020.9
  puerperalis 672 ✓5ᵗʰ
  recurrens (*see also* Fever, relapsing) 087.9
    pediculo vestimenti 087.0
  rubra 034.1
  typhoidea 002.0
  typhosa 002.0
Fecal — *see* condition
Fecalith (impaction) 560.39
  with hernia — *see also* Hernia, by site, with
    obstruction
    gangrenous — *see* Hernia, by site, with
      gangrene
  appendix 543.9
  congenital 777.1
Fede's disease 529.0
Feeble-minded 317
Feeble rapid pulse due to shock following
  injury 958.4
Feeding
  faulty (elderly) (infant) 783.3
    newborn 779.3
  formula check V20.2
  improper (elderly) (infant) 783.3
    newborn 779.3
  problem (elderly) (infant) 783.3
    newborn 779.3
    nonorganic origin 307.59
Feer's disease 985.0
Feet — *see* condition
Feigned illness V65.2
Feil-Klippel syndrome (brevicollis) 756.16
Feinmesser's (hidrotic) **ectodermal dysplasia**
  757.31

Failure — Feinmesser's

Felix's disease (juvenile osteochondrosis, hip) 732.1

Felon (any digit) (with lymphangitis) 681.01
  herpetic 054.6

Felty's syndrome (rheumatoid arthritis with splenomegaly and leukopenia) 714.1

Feminism in boys 302.6

Feminization, testicular 257.8
  with pseudohermaphroditism, male 257.8

Femoral hernia — see Hernia, femoral

Femora vara 736.32

Femur, femoral — see condition

Fenestrata placenta — see Placenta, abnormal

Fenestration, fenestrated — see also Imperfect, closure
  aorta-pulmonary 745.0
  aorticopulmonary 745.0
  aortopulmonary 745.0
  cusps, heart valve NEC 746.89
    pulmonary 746.09
  hymen 752.49
  pulmonic cusps 746.09

Fenwick's disease 537.89

Fermentation (gastric) (gastrointestinal) (stomach) 536.8
  intestine 564.89
    psychogenic 306.4
  psychogenic 306.4

Fernell's disease (aortic aneurysm) 441.9

Fertile eunuch syndrome 257.2

Fertility, meaning multiparity — see Multiparity

Fetal alcohol syndrome 760.71

Fetalis uterus 752.3

Fetid
  breath 784.9
  sweat 705.89

Fetishism 302.81
  transvestic 302.3

Fetomaternal hemorrhage
  affecting management of pregnancy 656.0 ✓5ᵗʰ
  fetus or newborn 772.0

Fetus, fetal — see also condition
  papyraceous 779.89   ▲
  type lung tissue 770.4

Fever 780.6
  with chills 780.6
    in malarial regions (see also Malaria) 084.6
  abortus NEC 023.9
  Aden 061
  African tick-borne 087.1
  American
    mountain tick 066.1
    spotted 082.0
  and ague (see also Malaria) 084.6
  aphthous 078.4
  arbovirus hemorrhagic 065.9
  Assam 085.0
  Australian A or Q 083.0
  Bangkok hemorrhagic 065.4
  biliary, Charcôt's intermittent — see Choledocholithiasis
  bilious, hemoglobinuric 084.8
  blackwater 084.8
  blister 054.9
  Bonvale Dam 780.79
  boutonneuse 082.1
  brain 323.9
    late effect — see category 326
  breakbone 061
  Bullis 082.8
  Bunyamwera 066.3
  Burdwan 085.0
  Bwamba (encephalitis) 066.3
  Cameroon (see also Malaria) 084.6
  Canton 081.9
  catarrhal (acute) 460
    chronic 472.0
  cat-scratch 078.3
  cerebral 323.9
    late effect — see category 326
  cerebrospinal (meningococcal) (see also Meningitis, cerebrospinal) 036.0
  Chagres 084.0

Fever — continued
  Chandipura 066.8
  changuinola 066.0
  Charcôt's (biliary) (hepatic) (intermittent) see Choledocholithiasis
  Chikungunya (viral) 066.3
    hemorrhagic 065.4
  childbed 670 ✓4ᵗʰ
  Chitral 066.0
  Colombo (see also Fever, paratyphoid) 002.9
  Colorado tick (virus) 066.1
  congestive
    malarial (see also Malaria) 084.6
    remittent (see also Malaria) 084.6
  Congo virus 065.0
  continued 780.6
    malarial 084.0
  Corsican (see also Malaria) 084.6
  Crimean hemorrhagic 065.0
  Cyprus (see also Brucellosis) 023.9
  dandy 061
  deer fly (see also Tularemia) 021.9
  dehydration, newborn 778.4
  dengue (virus) 061
    hemorrhagic 065.4
  desert 114.0
  due to heat 992.0
  Dumdum 085.0
  enteric 002.0
  ephemeral (of unknown origin) (see also Pyrexia) 780.6
  epidemic, hemorrhagic of the Far East 065.0
  erysipelatous (see also Erysipelas) 035
  estivo-autumnal (malarial) 084.0
  etiocholanolone 277.3
  famine — see also Fever, relapsing
    meaning typhus — see Typhus
  Far Eastern hemorrhagic 065.0
  five day 083.1
  Fort Bragg 100.89
  gastroenteric 002.0
  gastromalarial (see also Malaria) 084.6
  Gibraltar (see also Brucellosis) 023.9
  glandular 075
  Guama (viral) 066.3
  Haverhill 026.1
  hay (allergic) (with rhinitis) 477.9
    with
      asthma (bronchial) (see also Asthma) 493.0 ✓5ᵗʰ
      due to
        dander 477.8
        dust 477.8
        fowl 477.8
        pollen, any plant or tree 477.0
        specified allergen other than pollen 477.8
  heat (effects) 992.0
  hematuric, bilious 084.8
  hemoglobinuric (malarial) 084.8
    bilious 084.8
  hemorrhagic (arthropod-borne) NEC 065.9
    with renal syndrome 078.6
    arenaviral 078.7
    Argentine 078.7
    Bangkok 065.4
    Bolivian 078.7
    Central Asian 065.0
    chikungunya 065.4
    Crimean 065.0
    dengue (virus) 065.4
    Ebola 065.8
    epidemic 078.6
      of Far East 065.0
    Far Eastern 065.0
    Junin virus 078.7
    Korean 078.6
    Kyasanur forest 065.2
    Machupo virus 078.7
    mite-borne NEC 065.8
    mosquito-borne 065.4
    Omsk 065.1
    Philippine 065.4
    Russian (Yaroslav) 078.6
    Singapore 065.4
    Southeast Asia 065.4
    Thailand 065.4
    tick-borne NEC 065.3

Fever — continued
  hepatic (see also Cholecystitis) 575.8
    intermittent (Charcôt's) — see Choledocholithiasis
  herpetic (see also Herpes) 054.9
  Hyalomma tick 065.0
  icterohemorrhagic 100.0
  inanition 780.6
    newborn 778.4
  infective NEC 136.9
  intermittent (bilious) (see also Malaria) 084.6
    hepatic (Charcôt) — see Choledocholithiasis
    of unknown origin (see also Pyrexia) 780.6
    pernicious 084.0
  iodide
    correct substance properly administered 780.6
    overdose or wrong substance given or taken 975.5
  Japanese river 081.2
  jungle yellow 060.0
  Junin virus, hemorrhagic 078.7
  Katayama 120.2
  Kedani 081.2
  Kenya 082.1
  Korean hemorrhagic 078.6
  Lassa 078.89
  Lone Star 082.8
  lung — see Pneumonia
  Machupo virus, hemorrhagic 078.7
  malaria, malarial (see also Malaria) 084.6
  Malta (see also Brucellosis) 023.9
  Marseilles 082.1
  marsh (see also Malaria) 084.6
  Mayaro (viral) 066.3
  Mediterranean (see also Brucellosis) 023.9
    familial 277.3
    tick 082.1
  meningeal — see Meningitis
  metal fumes NEC 985.8
  Meuse 083.1
  Mexican — see Typhus, Mexican
  Mianeh 087.1
  miasmatic (see also Malaria) 084.6
  miliary 078.2
  milk, female 672 ✓4ᵗʰ
  mill 504
  mite-borne hemorrhagic 065.8
  Monday 504
  mosquito-borne NEC 066.3
    hemorrhagic NEC 065.4
  mountain 066.1
    meaning
      Rocky Mountain spotted 082.0
      undulant fever (see also Brucellosis) 023.9
    tick (American) 066.1
  Mucambo (viral) 066.3
  mud 100.89
  Neapolitan (see also Brucellosis) 023.9
  neutropenic 288.0
  nine-mile 083.0
  nonexanthematous tick 066.1
  North Asian tick-borne typhus 082.2
  Omsk hemorrhagic 065.1
  O'nyong-nyong (viral) 066.3
  Oropouche (viral) 066.3
  Oroya 088.0
  paludal (see also Malaria) 084.6
  Panama 084.0
  pappataci 066.0
  paratyphoid 002.9
    A 002.1
    B (Schottmüller's) 002.2
    C (Hirschfeld) 002.3
  parrot 073.9
  periodic 277.3
  pernicious, acute 084.0
  persistent (of unknown origin) (see also Pyrexia) 780.6
  petechial 036.0
  pharyngoconjunctival 077.2
    adenoviral type 3 077.2
  Philippine hemorrhagic 065.4
  phlebotomus 066.0
  Piry 066.8
  Pixuna (viral) 066.3
  Plasmodium ovale 084.3

Felix's disease — Fever

Fever — *continued*
pleural (*see also* Pleurisy) 511.0
pneumonic — *see* Pneumonia
polymer fume 987.8
postoperative 998.89
   due to infection 998.59
pretibial 100.89
puerperal, postpartum 672 ☑4ᵗʰ
putrid — *see* Septicemia
pyemic — *see* Septicemia
Q 083.0
   with pneumonia 083.0 [484.8]
quadrilateral 083.0
quartan (malaria) 084.2
Queensland (coastal) 083.0
   seven-day 100.89
Quintan (A) 083.1
quotidian 084.0
rabbit (*see also* Tularemia) 021.9
rat-bite 026.9
   due to
      Spirillum minor or minus 026.0
      Spirochaeta morsus muris 026.0
      Streptobacillus moniliformis 026.1
recurrent — *see* Fever, relapsing
relapsing 087.9
   Carter's (Asiatic) 087.0
   Dutton's (West African) 087.1
   Koch's 087.9
   louse-borne (epidemic) 087.0
   Novy's (American) 087.1
   Obermeyer's (European) 087.0
   spirillum NEC 087.9
   tick-borne (endemic) 087.1
remittent (bilious) (congestive) (gastric) (*see also* Malaria) 084.6
rheumatic (active) (acute) (chronic) (subacute) 390
   with heart involvement 391.9
      carditis 391.9
      endocarditis (aortic) (mitral) (pulmonary) (tricuspid) 391.1
      multiple sites 391.8
      myocarditis 391.2
      pancarditis, acute 391.8
      pericarditis 391.0
      specified type NEC 391.8
      valvulitis 391.1
   inactive or quiescent with cardiac hypertrophy 398.99
      carditis 398.90
      endocarditis 397.9
         aortic (valve) 395.9
            with mitral (valve) disease 396.9
         mitral (valve) 394.9
            with aortic (valve) disease 396.9
         pulmonary (valve) 397.1
         tricuspid (valve) 397.0
      heart conditions (classifiable to 429.3, 429.6, 429.9) 398.99
      failure (congestive) (conditions classifiable to 428.0, 428.9) 398.91
      left ventricular failure (conditions classifiable to 428.1) 398.91
      myocardial degeneration (conditions classifiable to 429.1) 398.0
      myocarditis (conditions classifiable to 429.0) 398.0
      pancarditis 398.99
      pericarditis 393
Rift Valley (viral) 066.3
Rocky Mountain spotted 082.0
rose 477.0
Ross river (viral) 066.3
Russian hemorrhagic 078.6
sandfly 066.0
San Joaquin (valley) 114.0
São Paulo 082.0
scarlet 034.1
septic — *see* Septicemia
seven-day 061
   Japan 100.89
   Queensland 100.89
shin bone 083.1
Singapore hemorrhagic 065.4
solar 061

Fever — *continued*
sore 054.9
South African tick-bite 087.1
Southeast Asia hemorrhagic 065.4
spinal — *see* Meningitis
spirillary 026.0
splenic (*see also* Anthrax) 022.9
spotted (Rocky Mountain) 082.0
   American 082.0
   Brazilian 082.0
   Colombian 082.0
   meaning
      cerebrospinal meningitis 036.0
      typhus 082.9
spring 309.23
steroid
   correct substance properly administered 780.6
   overdose or wrong substance given or taken 962.0
streptobacillary 026.1
subtertian 084.0
Sumatran mite 081.2
sun 061
swamp 100.89
sweating 078.2
swine 003.8
sylvatic yellow 060.0
Tahyna 062.5
tertian — *see* Malaria, tertian
Thailand hemorrhagic 065.4
thermic 992.0
three day 066.0
   with Coxsackie exanthem 074.8
tick
   American mountain 066.1
   Colorado 066.1
   Kemerovo 066.1
   Mediterranean 082.1
   mountain 066.1
   nonexanthematous 066.1
   Quaranfil 066.1
tick-bite NEC 066.1
tick-borne NEC 066.1
   hemorrhagic NEC 065.3
transitory of newborn 778.4
trench 083.1
tsutsugamushi 081.2
typhogastric 002.0
typhoid (abortive) (ambulant) (any site) (hemorrhagic) (infection) (intermittent) (malignant) (rheumatic) 002.0
typhomalarial (*see also* Malaria) 084.6
typhus — *see* Typhus
undulant (*see also* Brucellosis) 023.9
unknown origin (*see also* Pyrexia) 780.6
uremic — *see* Uremia
uveoparotid 135
valley (Coccidioidomycosis) 114.0
Venezuelan equine 066.2
Volhynian 083.1
Wesselsbron (viral) 066.3
West
   African 084.8
   Nile (viral) 066.4 ▲
Whitmore's 025
Wolhynian 083.1
worm 128.9
Yaroslav hemorrhagic 078.6
yellow 060.9
   jungle 060.0
   sylvatic 060.0
   urban 060.1
   vaccination, prophylactic (against) V04.4
Zika (viral) 066.3

Fibrillation
atrial (established) (paroxysmal) 427.31
auricular (atrial) (established) 427.31
cardiac (ventricular) 427.41
coronary (*see also* Infarct, myocardium) 410.9 ☑5ᵗʰ
heart (ventricular) 427.41
muscular 728.9
postoperative 997.1
ventricular 427.41

Fibrin
ball or bodies, pleural (sac) 511.0
chamber, anterior (eye) (gelatinous exudate) 364.04
Fibrinogenolysis (hemorrhagic) — *see* Fibrinolysis
Fibrinogenopenia (congenital) (hereditary) (*see also* Defect, coagulation) 286.3
acquired 286.6
Fibrinolysis (acquired) (hemorrhagic) (pathologic) 286.6
with
   abortion — *see* Abortion, by type, with hemorrhage, delayed or excessive
   ectopic pregnancy (*see also* categories 633.0-633.9) 639.1
   molar pregnancy (*see also* categories 630-632) 639.1
antepartum or intrapartum 641.3 ☑5ᵗʰ
   affecting fetus or newborn 762.1
following
   abortion 639.1
   ectopic or molar pregnancy 639.1
newborn, transient 776.2
postpartum 666.3 ☑5ᵗʰ
Fibrinopenia (hereditary) (*see also* Defect, coagulation) 286.3
acquired 286.6
Fibrinopurulent — *see* condition
Fibrinous — *see* condition
Fibroadenoma (M9010/0)
cellular intracanalicular (M9020/0) 217
giant (intracanalicular) (M9020/0) 217
intracanalicular (M9011/0)
   cellular (M9020/0) 217
   giant (M9020/0) 217
   specified site — *see* Neoplasm, by site, benign
   unspecified site 217
juvenile (M9030/0) 217
pericanicular (M9012/0)
   specified site — *see* Neoplasm, by site, benign
   unspecified site 217
phyllodes (M9020/0) 217
prostate 600.2
specified site — *see* Neoplasm, by site, benign
unspecified site 217
Fibroadenosis, breast (chronic) (cystic) (diffuse) (periodic) (segmental) 610.2
Fibroangioma (M9160/0) — *see also* Neoplasm, by site, benign
juvenile (M9160/0)
   specified site — *see* Neoplasm, by site, benign
   unspecified site 210.7
Fibrocellulitis progressiva ossificans 728.11
Fibrochondrosarcoma (M9220/3) — *see* Neoplasm, cartilage, malignant
Fibrocystic
disease 277.00
   bone NEC 733.29
   breast 610.1
   jaw 526.2
   kidney (congenital) 753.19
   liver 751.62
   lung 518.89
      congenital 748.4
   pancreas 277.00
   kidney (congenital) 753.19
Fibrodysplasia ossificans multiplex (progressiva) 728.11
Fibroelastosis (cordis) (endocardial) (endomyocardial) 425.3
Fibroid (tumor) (M8890/0) — *see also* Neoplasm, connective tissue, benign
disease, lung (chronic) (*see also* Fibrosis, lung) 515
heart (disease) (*see also* Myocarditis) 429.0
induration, lung (chronic) (*see also* Fibrosis, lung) 515
in pregnancy or childbirth 654.1 ☑5ᵗʰ
   affecting fetus or newborn 763.89
   causing obstructed labor 660.2 ☑5ᵗʰ
      affecting fetus or newborn 763.1

Fever — Fibroid

Fibroid — *see also* Neoplasm, connective tissue, benign — *continued*
  liver — *see* Cirrhosis, liver
  lung (*see also* Fibrosis, lung) 515
  pneumonia (chronic) (*see also* Fibrosis, lung) 515
  uterus (M8890/0) (*see also* Leiomyoma, uterus) 218.9
Fibrolipoma (M8851/0) (*see also* Lipoma, by site) 214.9
Fibroliposarcoma (M8850/3) — *see* Neoplasm, connective tissue, malignant
Fibroma (M8810/0) — *see also* Neoplasm, connective tissue, benign
  ameloblastic (M9330/0) 213.1
    upper jaw (bone) 213.0
  bone (nonossifying) 733.99
    ossifying (M9262/0) — *see* Neoplasm, bone, benign
  cementifying (M9274/0) — *see* Neoplasm, bone, benign
  chondromyxoid (M9241/0) — *see* Neoplasm, bone, benign
  desmoplastic (M8823/1) — *see* Neoplasm, connective tissue, uncertain behavior
  facial (M8813/0) — *see* Neoplasm, connective tissue, benign
  invasive (M8821/1) — *see* Neoplasm, connective tissue, uncertain behavior
  molle (M8851/0) (*see also* Lipoma, by site) 214.9
  myxoid (M8811/0) — *see* Neoplasm, connective tissue, benign
  nasopharynx, nasopharyngeal (juvenile) (M9160/0) 210.7
  nonosteogenic (nonossifying) — *see* Dysplasia, fibrous
  odontogenic (M9321/0) 213.1
    upper jaw (bone) 213.0
  ossifying (M9262/0) — *see* Neoplasm, bone, benign
  periosteal (M8812/0) — *see* Neoplasm, bone, benign
  prostate 600.2
  soft (M8851/0) (*see also* Lipoma, by site) 214.9
Fibromatosis
  abdominal (M8822/1) — *see* Neoplasm, connective tissue, uncertain behavior
  aggressive (M8821/1) — *see* Neoplasm, connective tissue, uncertain behavior
  Dupuytren's 728.6
  gingival 523.8
  plantar fascia 728.71
  proliferative 728.79
  pseudosarcomatous (proliferative) (subcutaneous) 728.79
  subcutaneous pseudosarcomatous (proliferative) 728.79
Fibromyalgia 729.1
Fibromyoma (M8890/0) — *see also* Neoplasm, connective tissue, benign
  uterus (corpus) (*see also* Leiomyoma, uterus) 218.9
  in pregnancy or childbirth 654.1 ✓5ᵗʰ
    affecting fetus or newborn 763.89
    causing obstructed labor 660.2 ✓5ᵗʰ
      affecting fetus or newborn 763.1
Fibromyositis (*see also* Myositis) 729.1
  scapulohumeral 726.2
Fibromyxolipoma (M8852/0) (*see also* Lipoma, by site) 214.9
Fibromyxoma (M8811/0) — *see* Neoplasm, connective tissue, benign
Fibromyxosarcoma (M8811/3) — *see* Neoplasm, connective tissue, malignant
Fibro-odontoma, ameloblastic (M9290/0) 213.1
  upper jaw (bone) 213.0
Fibro-osteoma (M9262/0) — *see* Neoplasm, bone, benign
Fibroplasia, retrolental 362.21
Fibropurulent — *see* condition
Fibrosarcoma (M8810/3) — *see also* Neoplasm, connective tissue, malignant
  ameloblastic (M9330/3) 170.1
    upper jaw (bone) 170.0

Fibrosarcoma — *see also* Neoplasm, connective tissue, malignant — *continued*
  congenital (M8814/3) — *see* Neoplasm, connective tissue, malignant
  fascial (M8813/3) — *see* Neoplasm, connective tissue, malignant
  infantile (M8814/3) — *see* Neoplasm, connective tissue, malignant
  odontogenic (M9330/3) 170.1
    upper jaw (bone) 170.0
  periosteal (M8812/3) — *see* Neoplasm, bone, malignant
Fibrosclerosis
  breast 610.3
  corpora cavernosa (penis) 607.89
  familial multifocal NEC 710.8
  multifocal (idiopathic) NEC 710.8
  penis (corpora cavernosa) 607.89
Fibrosis, fibrotic
  adrenal (gland) 255.8
  alveolar (diffuse) 516.3
  amnion 658.8 ✓5ᵗʰ
  anal papillae 569.49
  anus 569.49
  appendix, appendiceal, noninflammatory 543.9
  arteriocapillary — *see* Arteriosclerosis
  bauxite (of lung) 503
  biliary 576.8
    due to Clonorchis sinensis 121.1
  bladder 596.8
    interstitial 595.1
    localized submucosal 595.1
    panmural 595.1
  bone, diffuse 756.59
  breast 610.3
  capillary — *see also* Arteriosclerosis
    lung (chronic) (*see also* Fibrosis, lung) 515
  cardiac (*see also* Myocarditis) 429.0
  cervix 622.8
  chorion 658.8 ✓5ᵗʰ
  corpus cavernosum 607.89
  cystic (of pancreas) 277.00
    with ●
      manifestations ●
        gastrointestinal 277.03 ●
        pulmonary 277.02 ●
        specified NEC 277.09 ●
      meconium ileus 277.01 ●
      pulmonary exacerbation 277.02 ●
  due to (presence of) any device, implant, or graft — *see* Complications, due to (presence of) any device, implant, or graft classified to 996.0-996.5 NEC
  ejaculatory duct 608.89
  endocardium (*see also* Endocarditis) 424.90
  endomyocardial (African) 425.0
  epididymis 608.89
  eye muscle 378.62
  graphite (of lung) 503
  heart (*see also* Myocarditis) 429.0
  hepatic — *see also* Cirrhosis, liver due to Clonorchis sinensis 121.1
  hepatolienal — *see* Cirrhosis, liver
  hepatosplenic — *see* Cirrhosis, liver
  infrapatellar fat pad 729.31
  interstitial pulmonary, newborn 770.7
  intrascrotal 608.89
  kidney (*see also* Sclerosis, renal) 587
  liver — *see* Cirrhosis, liver
  lung (atrophic) (capillary) (chronic) (confluent) (massive) (perialveolar) (peribronchial) 515
    with
      anthracosilicosis (occupational) 500
      anthracosis (occupational) 500
      asbestosis (occupational) 501
      bagassosis (occupational) 495.1
      bauxite 503
      berylliosis (occupational) 503
      byssinosis (occupational) 504
      calcicosis (occupational) 502
      chalicosis (occupational) 502
      dust reticulation (occupational) 504
      farmers' lung 495.0
      gannister disease (occupational) 502
      graphite 503
      pneumoconiosis (occupational) 505

Fibrosis, fibrotic — *continued*
  lung — *continued*
    with — *continued*
      pneumosiderosis (occupational) 503
      siderosis (occupational) 503
      silicosis (occupational) 502
      tuberculosis (*see also* Tuberculosis) 011.4 ✓5ᵗʰ
    diffuse (idiopathic) (interstitial) 516.3
    due to
      bauxite 503
      fumes or vapors (chemical) inhalation) 506.4
      graphite 503
    following radiation 508.1
    postinflammatory 515
    silicotic (massive) (occupational) 502
    tuberculous (*see also* Tuberculosis) 011.4 ✓5ᵗʰ
  lymphatic gland 289.3
  median bar 600.9
  mediastinum (idiopathic) 519.3
  meninges 349.2
  muscle NEC 728.2
    iatrogenic (from injection) 999.9
  myocardium, myocardial (*see also* Myocarditis) 429.0
  oral submucous 528.8
  ovary 620.8
  oviduct 620.8
  pancreas 577.8
    cystic 277.00 ●
      with ●
        manifestations ●
          gastrintestinal 277.03 ●
          pulmonary 277.02 ●
          specified NEC 277.09 ●
        meconium ileus 277.01 ●
        pulmonary exacerbation 277.02 ●
  penis 607.89
  periappendiceal 543.9
  periarticular (*see also* Ankylosis) 718.5 ✓5ᵗʰ
  pericardium 423.1
  perineum, in pregnancy or childbirth 654.8 ✓5ᵗʰ
    affecting fetus or newborn 763.89
    causing obstructed labor 660.2 ✓5ᵗʰ
      affecting fetus or newborn 763.1
  perineural NEC 355.9
    foot 355.6
  periureteral 593.89
  placenta — *see* Placenta, abnormal
  pleura 511.0
  popliteal fat pad 729.31
  preretinal 362.56
  prostate (chronic) 600.9
  pulmonary (chronic) (*see also* Fibrosis, lung) 515
    alveolar capillary block 516.3
    interstitial
      diffuse (idiopathic) 516.3
      newborn 770.7
  radiation — *see* Effect, adverse, radiation
  rectal sphincter 569.49
  retroperitoneal, idiopathic 593.4
  scrotum 608.89
  seminal vesicle 608.89
  senile 797
  skin NEC 709.2
  spermatic cord 608.89
  spleen 289.59
    bilharzial (*see also* Schistosomiasis) 120.9
  subepidermal nodular (M8832/0) — *see* Neoplasm, skin, benign
  submucous NEC 709.2
    oral 528.8
    tongue 528.8
  syncytium — *see* Placenta, abnormal
  testis 608.89
    chronic, due to syphilis 095.8
  thymus (gland) 254.8
  tunica vaginalis 608.89
  ureter 593.89
  urethra 599.84
  uterus (nonneoplastic) 621.8
    bilharzial (*see also* Schistosomiasis) 120.9
    neoplastic (*see also* Leiomyoma, uterus) 218.9

Fibroid — Fibrosis

Fibrosis — Findings

Findings, abnormal, without diagnosis —
continued
  radiologic — *continued*
    subcutaneous tissue 793.9
  red blood cell 790.09
    count 790.09
    morphology 790.09
    sickling 790.09
    volume 790.09
  saliva 792.4
  scan NEC 794.9
    bladder 794.9
    bone 794.9
    brain 794.09
    kidney 794.4
    liver 794.8
    lung 794.2
    pancreas 794.9
    placental 794.9
    spleen 794.9
    thyroid 794.5
  sedimentation rate, elevated 790.1
  semen 792.2
  serological (for)
    human immunodeficiency virus (HIV)
      inconclusive 795.71
      positive V08
    syphilis — *see* Findings, serology for syphilis
  serology for syphilis
    false positive 795.6
    positive 097.1
      false 795.6
      follow-up of latent syphilis — *see*
        Syphilis, latent
      only finding — *see* Syphilis, latent
  serum 790.99
    blood NEC 790.99
    enzymes NEC 790.5
    proteins 790.99
  SGOT 790.4
  SGPT 790.4
  sickling of red blood cells 790.09
  skin test, positive 795.79
    tuberculin (without active tuberculosis)
      795.5
  sodium 790.6
    deficiency 276.1
    excess 276.0
  spermatozoa 792.2
  spinal fluid 792.0
    culture, positive 792.0
  sputum culture, positive 795.39 ▲
    for acid-fast bacilli 795.39 ▲
  stool NEC 792.1
    bloody 578.1
      occult 792.1
    color 792.1
    culture, positive 792.1
    occult blood 792.1
  structure, body (echogram) (thermogram)
    (ultrasound) (x-ray) NEC 793.9
    abdomen 793.6
    breast 793.89
      abnormal mammogram 793.80
      mammographic microcalcification 793.81
    gastrointestinal tract 793.4
    genitourinary organs 793.5
    head 793.0
      echogram (ultrasound) 794.01
    intrathoracic organs NEC 793.2
    lung 793.1
    musculoskeletal 793.7
    placenta 793.9
    retroperitoneum 793.6
    skin 793.9
    subcutaneous tissue NEC 793.9
  synovial fluid 792.9
  thermogram — *see* Finding, abnormal,
    structure
  throat culture, positive 795.39 ▲
  thyroid (function) 794.5
    metabolism (rate) 794.5
    scan 794.5
    uptake 794.5
  total proteins 790.99
  toxicology (drugs) (heavy metals) 796.0
  transaminase (level) 790.4

Findings, abnormal, without diagnosis —
continued
  triglycerides 272.9
  tuberculin skin test (without active
    tuberculosis) 795.5
  ultrasound — *see also* Finding, abnormal,
    structure
    cardiogram 793.2
  uric acid, blood 790.6
  urine, urinary constituents 791.9
    acetone 791.6
    albumin 791.0
    bacteria 791.9
    bile 791.4
    blood 599.7
    casts or cells 791.7
    chyle 791.1
    culture, positive 791.9
    glucose 791.5
    hemoglobin 791.2
    ketone 791.6
    protein 791.0
    pus 791.9
    sugar 791.5
  vaginal fluid 792.9
  vanillylmandelic acid, elevated 791.9
  vectorcardiogram (VCG) 794.39
  ventriculogram (cerebral) 793.0
  VMA, elevated 791.9
  Wassermann reaction
    false positive 795.6
    positive 097.1
      follow-up of latent syphilis — *see*
        Syphilis, latent
      only finding — *see* Syphilis, latent
  white blood cell 288.9
    count 288.9
      elevated 288.8
      low 288.0
    differential 288.9
    morphology 288.9
  wound culture 795.39 ▲
  xerography 793.89
  zinc, blood 790.6

Finger — *see* condition

Fire, St. Anthony's (*see also* Erysipelas) 035

Fish
  hook stomach 537.89
  meal workers' lung 495.8

Fisher's syndrome 357.0

Fissure, fissured
  abdominal wall (congenital) 756.79
  anus, anal 565.0
    congenital 751.5
  buccal cavity 528.9
  clitoris (congenital) 752.49
  ear, lobule (congenital) 744.29
  epiglottis (congenital) 748.3
  larynx 478.79
    congenital 748.3
  lip 528.5
    congenital (*see also* Cleft, lip) 749.10
  nipple 611.2
    puerperal, postpartum 676.1 ✓5ᵗʰ
  palate (congenital) (*see also* Cleft, palate)
    749.00
  postanal 565.0
  rectum 565.0
  skin 709.8
    streptococcal 686.9
  spine (congenital) (*see also* Spina bifida)
    741.9 ✓5ᵗʰ
  sternum (congenital) 756.3
  tongue (acquired) 529.5
    congenital 750.13

Fistula (sinus) 686.9
  abdomen (wall) 569.81
    bladder 596.2
    intestine 569.81
    ureter 593.82
    uterus 619.2
  abdominorectal 569.81
  abdominosigmoidal 569.81
  abdominothoracic 510.0
  abdominouterine 619.2
    congenital 752.3

Fistula — *continued*
  abdominovesical 596.2
  accessory sinuses (*see also* Sinusitis) 473.9
  actinomycotic — *see* Actinomycosis
  alveolar
    antrum (*see also* Sinusitis, maxillary) 473.0
    process 522.7
  anorectal 565.1
  antrobuccal (*see also* Sinusitis, maxillary)
    473.0
  antrum (*see also* Sinusitis, maxillary) 473.0
  anus, anal (infectional) (recurrent) 565.1
    congenital 751.5
    tuberculous (*see also* Tuberculosis)
      014.8 ✓5ᵗʰ
  aortic sinus 747.29
  aortoduodenal 447.2
  appendix, appendicular 543.9
  arteriovenous (acquired) 447.0
    brain 437.3
      congenital 747.81
        ruptured (*see also* Hemorrhage,
          subarachnoid) 430
      ruptured (*see also* Hemorrhage,
        subarachnoid) 430
    cerebral 437.3
      congenital 747.81
    congenital (peripheral) 747.60
      brain — *see* Fistula, arteriovenous, brain,
        congenital
      coronary 746.85
      gastrointestinal 747.61
      lower limb 747.64
      pulmonary 747.3
      renal 747.62
      specified NEC 747.69
      upper limb 747.63
    coronary 414.19
      congenital 746.85
    heart 414.19
    pulmonary (vessels) 417.0
      congenital 747.3
    surgically created (for dialysis) V45.1
      complication NEC 996.73
        atherosclerosis — *see* Arteriosclerosis,
          extremities
        embolism 996.74
        infection or inflammation 996.62
        mechanical 996.1
        occlusion NEC 996.74
        thrombus 996.74
    traumatic — *see* Injury, blood vessel, by site
  artery 447.2
  aural 383.81
    congenital 744.49
  auricle 383.81
    congenital 744.49
  Bartholin's gland 619.8
  bile duct (*see also* Fistula, biliary) 576.4
  biliary (duct) (tract) 576.4
    congenital 751.69
  bladder (neck) (sphincter) 596.2
    into seminal vesicle 596.2
  bone 733.99
  brain 348.8
    arteriovenous — *see* Fistula, arteriovenous,
      brain
  branchial (cleft) 744.41
  branchiogenous 744.41
  breast 611.0
    puerperal, postpartum 675.1 ✓5ᵗʰ
  bronchial 510.0
  bronchocutaneous, bronchomediastinal,
    bronchopleural,
    bronchopleuromediastinal (infective)
    510.0
    tuberculous (*see also* Tuberculosis)
      011.3 ✓5ᵗʰ
  bronchoesophageal 530.89
    congenital 750.3
  buccal cavity (infective) 528.3
  canal, ear 380.89
  carotid-cavernous
    congenital 747.81
      with hemorrhage 430

Findings — Fistula

Fistula — *continued*
  carotid-cavernous — *continued*
    traumatic 900.82
      with hemorrhage (*see also* Hemorrhage,
        brain, traumatic) 853.0 ✓5ᵗʰ
      late effect 908.3
  cecosigmoidal 569.81
  cecum 569.81
  cerebrospinal (fluid) 349.81
  cervical, lateral (congenital) 744.41
  cervicoaural (congenital) 744.49
  cervicosigmoidal 619.1
  cervicovesical 619.0
  cervix 619.8
  chest (wall) 510.0
  cholecystocolic (*see also* Fistula, gallbladder)
    575.5
  cholecystocolonic (*see also* Fistula, gallbladder)
    575.5
  cholecystoduodenal (*see also* Fistula,
    gallbladder) 575.5
  cholecystoenteric (*see also* Fistula,
    gallbladder) 575.5
  cholecystogastric (*see also* Fistula, gallbladder)
    575.5
  cholecystointestinal (*see also* Fistula,
    gallbladder) 575.5
  choledochoduodenal 576.4
  cholocolic (*see also* Fistula, gallbladder) 575.5
  coccyx 685.1
    with abscess 685.0
  colon 569.81
  colostomy 569.69
  colovaginal (acquired) 619.1
  common duct (bile duct) 576.4
  congenital, NEC — *see* Anomaly, specified type
    NEC
  cornea, causing hypotony 360.32
  coronary, arteriovenous 414.19
    congenital 746.85
  costal region 510.0
  cul-de-sac, Douglas' 619.8
  cutaneous 686.9
  cystic duct (*see also* Fistula, gallbladder) 575.5
    congenital 751.69
  dental 522.7
  diaphragm 510.0
    bronchovisceral 510.0
    pleuroperitoneal 510.0
    pulmonoperitoneal 510.0
  duodenum 537.4
  ear (canal) (external) 380.89
  enterocolic 569.81
  enterocutaneous 569.81
  enteroenteric 569.81
  entero-uterine 619.1
    congenital 752.3
  enterovaginal 619.1
    congenital 752.49
  enterovesical 596.1
  epididymis 608.89
    tuberculous (*see also* Tuberculosis)
      016.4 ✓5ᵗʰ
  esophagobronchial 530.89
    congenital 750.3
  esophagocutaneous 530.89
  esophagopleurocutaneous 530.89
  esophagotracheal 530.84
    congenital 750.3
  esophagus 530.89
    congenital 750.4
  ethmoid (*see also* Sinusitis, ethmoidal) 473.2
  eyeball (cornea) (sclera) 360.32
  eyelid 373.11
  fallopian tube (external) 619.2
  fecal 569.81
    congenital 751.5
  from periapical lesion 522.7
  frontal sinus (*see also* Sinusitis, frontal) 473.1
  gallbladder 575.5
    with calculus, cholelithiasis, stones (*see also*
      Cholelithiasis) 574.2 ✓5ᵗʰ
    congenital 751.69
  gastric 537.4
  gastrocolic 537.4
    congenital 750.7
    tuberculous (*see also* Tuberculosis)
      014.8 ✓5ᵗʰ

Fistula — *continued*
  gastroenterocolic 537.4
  gastroesophageal 537.4
  gastrojejunal 537.4
  gastrojejunocolic 537.4
  genital
    organs
      female 619.9
        specified site NEC 619.8
      male 608.89
    tract-skin (female) 619.2
  hepatopleural 510.0
  hepatopulmonary 510.0
  horseshoe 565.1
  ileorectal 569.81
  ileosigmoidal 569.81
  ileostomy 569.69
  ileovesical 596.1
  ileum 569.81
  in ano 565.1
    tuberculous (*see also* Tuberculosis)
      014.8 ✓5ᵗʰ
  inner ear (*see also* Fistula, labyrinth) 386.40
  intestine 569.81
  intestinocolonic (abdominal) 569.81
  intestinoureteral 593.82
  intestinouterine 619.1
  intestinovaginal 619.1
    congenital 752.49
  intestinovesical 596.1
  involving female genital tract 619.9
    digestive-genital 619.1
    genital tract-skin 619.2
    specified site NEC 619.8
    urinary-genital 619.0
  ischiorectal (fossa) 566
  jejunostomy 569.69
  jejunum 569.81
  joint 719.89
    ankle 719.87
    elbow 719.82
    foot 719.87
    hand 719.84
    hip 719.85
    knee 719.86
    multiple sites 719.89
    pelvic region 719.85
    shoulder (region) 719.81
    specified site NEC 719.88
    tuberculous — *see* Tuberculosis, joint
    wrist 719.83
  kidney 593.89
  labium (majus) (minus) 619.8
  labyrinth, labyrinthine NEC 386.40
    combined sites 386.48
    multiple sites 386.48
    oval window 386.42
    round window 386.41
    semicircular canal 386.43
  lacrimal, lachrymal (duct) (gland) (sac) 375.61
  lacrimonasal duct 375.61
  laryngotracheal 748.3
  larynx 478.79
  lip 528.5
    congenital 750.25
  lumbar, tuberculous (*see also* Tuberculosis)
    015.0 ✓5ᵗʰ [730.8] ✓5ᵗʰ
  lung 510.0
  lymphatic (node) (vessel) 457.8
  mamillary 611.0
  mammary (gland) 611.0
    puerperal, postpartum 675.1 ✓5ᵗʰ
  mastoid (process) (region) 383.1
  maxillary (*see also* Sinusitis, maxillary) 473.0
  mediastinal 510.0
  mediastinobronchial 510.0
  mediastinocutaneous 510.0
  middle ear 385.89
  mouth 528.3
  nasal 478.1
    sinus (*see also* Sinusitis) 473.9
  nasopharynx 478.29
  nipple — *see* Fistula, breast
  nose 478.1
  oral (cutaneous) 528.3
    maxillary (*see also* Sinusitis, maxillary)
      473.0

Fistula — *continued*
  oral — *continued*
    nasal (with cleft palate) (*see also* Cleft,
      palate) 749.00
  orbit, orbital 376.10
  oro-antral (*see also* Sinusitis, maxillary) 473.0
  oval window (internal ear) 386.42
  oviduct (external) 619.2
  palate (hard) 526.89
    soft 528.9
  pancreatic 577.8
  pancreaticoduodenal 577.8
  parotid (gland) 527.4
    region 528.3
  pelvoabdominointestinal 569.81
  penis 607.89
  perianal 565.1
  pericardium (pleura) (sac) (*see also* Pericarditis)
    423.8
  pericecal 569.81
  perineal — *see* Fistula, perineum
  perineorectal 569.81
  perineosigmoidal 569.81
  perineo-urethroscrotal 608.89
  perineum, perineal (with urethral involvement)
    NEC 599.1
    tuberculous (*see also* Tuberculosis)
      017.9 ✓5ᵗʰ
    ureter 593.82
  perirectal 565.1
    tuberculous (*see also* Tuberculosis)
      014.8 ✓5ᵗʰ
  peritoneum (*see also* Peritonitis) 567.2
  periurethral 599.1
  pharyngo-esophageal 478.29
  pharynx 478.29
    branchial cleft (congenital) 744.41
  pilonidal (infected) (rectum) 685.1
    with abscess 685.0
  pleura, pleural, pleurocutaneous,
    pleuroperitoneal 510.0
    stomach 510.0
    tuberculous (*see also* Tuberculosis)
      012.0 ✓5ᵗʰ
  pleuropericardial 423.8
  postauricular 383.81
  postoperative, persistent 998.6
  preauricular (congenital) 744.46
  prostate 602.8
  pulmonary 510.0
    arteriovenous 417.0
      congenital 747.3
    tuberculous (*see also* Tuberculosis,
      pulmonary) 011.9 ✓5ᵗʰ
  pulmonoperitoneal 510.0
  rectolabial 619.1
  rectosigmoid (intercommunicating) 569.81
  rectoureteral 593.82
  rectourethral 599.1
    congenital 753.8
  rectouterine 619.1
    congenital 752.3
  rectovaginal 619.1
    congenital 752.49
    old, postpartal 619.1
    tuberculous (*see also* Tuberculosis)
      014.8 ✓5ᵗʰ
  rectovesical 596.1
    congenital 753.8
  rectovesicovaginal 619.1
  rectovulvar 619.1
    congenital 752.49
  rectum (to skin) 565.1
    tuberculous (*see also* Tuberculosis)
      014.8 ✓5ᵗʰ
  renal 593.89
  retroauricular 383.81
  round window (internal ear) 386.41
  salivary duct or gland 527.4
    congenital 750.24
  sclera 360.32
  scrotum (urinary) 608.89
    tuberculous (*see also* Tuberculosis)
      016.5 ✓5ᵗʰ
  semicircular canals (internal ear) 386.43
  sigmoid 569.81
    vesicoabdominal 596.1

Fistula — *continued*
  sigmoidovaginal 619.1
    congenital 752.49
  skin 686.9
    ureter 593.82
    vagina 619.2
  sphenoidal sinus (*see also* Sinusitis,
    sphenoidal) 473.3
  splenocolic 289.59
  stercoral 569.81
  stomach 537.4
  sublingual gland 527.4
    congenital 750.24
  submaxillary
    gland 527.4
      congenital 750.24
    region 528.3
  thoracic 510.0
    duct 457.8
  thoracicoabdominal 510.0
  thoracicogastric 510.0
  thoracicointestinal 510.0
  thoracoabdominal 510.0
  thoracogastric 510.0
  thorax 510.0
  thyroglossal duct 759.2
  thyroid 246.8
  trachea (congenital) (external) (internal) 748.3
  tracheoesophageal 530.84
    congenital 750.3
    following tracheostomy 519.09
  traumatic
    arteriovenous (*see also* Injury, blood vessel,
      by site) 904.9
      brain — *see* Injury, intracranial
  tuberculous — *see* Tuberculosis, by site
  typhoid 002.0
  umbilical 759.89
  umbilico-urinary 753.8
  urachal, urachus 753.7
  ureter (persistent) 593.82
  ureteroabdominal 593.82
  ureterocervical 593.82
  ureterorectal 593.82
  ureterosigmoido-abdominal 593.82
  ureterovaginal 619.0
  ureterovesical 596.2
  urethra 599.1
    congenital 753.8
    tuberculous (*see also* Tuberculosis)
      016.3 ✓5ᵗʰ
  urethroperineal 599.1
  urethroperineovesical 596.2
  urethrorectal 599.1
    congenital 753.8
  urethroscrotal 608.89
  urethrovaginal 619.0
  urethrovesical 596.2
  urethrovesicovaginal 619.0
  urinary (persistent) (recurrent) 599.1
  uteroabdominal (anterior wall) 619.2
    congenital 752.3
  uteroenteric 619.1
  uterofecal 619.1
  uterointestinal 619.1
    congenital 752.3
  uterorectal 619.1
    congenital 752.3
  uteroureteric 619.0
  uterovaginal 619.8
  uterovesical 619.0
    congenital 752.3
  uterus 619.8
  vagina (wall) 619.8
    postpartal, old 619.8
  vaginocutaneous (postpartal) 619.2
  vaginoileal (acquired) 619.1
  vaginoperineal 619.2
  vesical NEC 596.2
  vesicoabdominal 596.2
  vesicocervicovaginal 619.0
  vesicocolic 596.1
  vesicocutaneous 596.2
  vesicoenteric 596.1
  vesicointestinal 596.1
  vesicometrorectal 619.1
  vesicoperineal 596.2

Fistula — *continued*
  vesicorectal 596.1
    congenital 753.8
  vesicosigmoidal 596.1
  vesicosigmoidovaginal 619.1
  vesicoureteral 596.2
  vesicoureterovaginal 619.0
  vesicourethral 596.2
  vesicourethrorectal 596.1
  vesicouterine 619.0
    congenital 752.3
  vesicovaginal 619.0
  vulvorectal 619.1
    congenital 752.49
Fit 780.39
  apoplectic (*see also* Disease, cerebrovascular,
    acute) 436
    late effect — *see* Late effect(s) (of)
      cerebrovascular disease
  epileptic (*see also* Epilepsy) 345.9 ✓5ᵗʰ
  fainting 780.2
  hysterical 300.11
  newborn 779.0
Fitting (of)
  artificial
    arm (complete) (partial) V52.0
    breast V52.4
    eye(s) V52.2
    leg(s) (complete) (partial) V52.1
  brain neuropacemaker V53.02
  cardiac pacemaker V53.31
  carotid sinus pacemaker V53.39
  cerebral ventricle (communicating) shunt
    V53.01
  colostomy belt V53.5
  contact lenses V53.1
  cystostomy device V53.6
  defibrillator, automatic implantable cardiac
    V53.32
  dentures V52.3
  device NEC V53.9
    abdominal V53.5
    cardiac
      defibrillator, automatic implantable
        V53.32
      pacemaker V53.31
      specified NEC V53.39
    cerebral ventricle (communicating) shunt
      V53.01
    intrauterine contraceptive V25.1
    nervous system V53.09
    orthodontic V53.4
    orthoptic V53.1
    prosthetic V52.9
      breast V52.4
      dental V52.3
      eye V52.2
      specified type NEC V52.8
    special senses V53.09
    substitution
      auditory V53.09
      nervous system V53.09
      visual V53.09
    urinary V53.6
  diaphragm (contraceptive) V25.02
  glasses (reading) V53.1
  hearing aid V53.2
  ileostomy device V53.5
  intestinal appliance or device NEC V53.5
  intrauterine contraceptive device V25.1
  neuropacemaker (brain) (peripheral nerve)
    (spinal cord) V53.02
  orthodontic device V53.4
  orthopedic (device) V53.7
    brace V53.7
    cast V53.7
    corset V53.7
    shoes V53.7
  pacemaker (cardiac) V53.31
    brain V53.02
    carotid sinus V53.39
    peripheral nerve V53.02
    spinal cord V53.02
  prosthesis V52.9
    arm (complete) (partial) V52.0
    breast V52.4
    dental V52.3

Fitting — *continued*
  prosthesis — *continued*
    eye V52.2
    leg (complete) (partial) V52.1
    specified type NEC V52.8
  spectacles V53.1
  wheelchair V53.8
Fitz's syndrome (acute hemorrhagic pancreatitis)
  577.0
Fitz-Hugh and Curtis syndrome (gonococcal
  peritonitis) 098.86
Fixation
  joint — *see* Ankylosis
  larynx 478.79
  pupil 364.76
  stapes 385.22
    deafness (*see also* Deafness, conductive)
      389.04
  uterus (acquired) — *see* Malposition, uterus
  vocal cord 478.5
Flaccid — *see also* condition
  foot 736.79
  forearm 736.09
  palate, congenital 750.26
Flail
  chest 807.4
    newborn 767.3
  joint (paralytic) 718.80
    ankle 718.87
    elbow 718.82
    foot 718.87
    hand 718.84
    hip 718.85
    knee 718.86
    multiple sites 718.89
    pelvic region 718.85
    shoulder (region) 718.81
    specified site NEC 718.88
    wrist 718.83
Flajani (-Basedow) syndrome or disease
  (exophthalmic goiter) 242.0 ✓5ᵗʰ
Flap, liver 572.8
Flare, anterior chamber (aqueous) (eye) 364.04
Flashback phenomena (drug) (hallucinogenic)
  292.89
Flat
  chamber (anterior) (eye) 360.34
  chest, congenital 754.89
  electroencephalogram (EEG) 348.8
  foot (acquired) (fixed type) (painful) (postural)
    (spastic) 734
    congenital 754.61
      rocker bottom 754.61
      vertical talus 754.61
    rachitic 268.1
    rocker bottom (congenital) 754.61
    vertical talus, congenital 754.61
  organ or site, congenital NEC — *see* Anomaly,
    specified type NEC
  pelvis 738.6
    with disproportion (fetopelvic) 653.2 ✓5ᵗʰ
      affecting fetus or newborn 763.1
      causing obstructed labor 660.1 ✓5ᵗʰ
        affecting fetus or newborn 763.1
    congenital 755.69
Flatau-Schilder disease 341.1
Flattening
  head, femur 736.39
  hip 736.39
  lip (congenital) 744.89
  nose (congenital) 754.0
    acquired 738.0
Flatulence 787.3
Flatus 787.3
  vaginalis 629.8
Flax dressers' disease 504
Flea bite — *see* Injury, superficial, by site
Fleischer (-Kayser) ring (corneal pigmentation)
  275.1 *[371.14]*
Fleischner's disease 732.3
Fleshy mole 631
Flexibilitas cerea (*see also* Catalepsy) 300.11

Flexion
cervix (see also Malposition, uterus) 621.6
contracture, joint (see also Contraction, joint) 718.4 ✔5ᵗʰ
deformity, joint (see also Contraction, joint) 718.4 ✔5ᵗʰ
hip, congenital (see also Subluxation, congenital, hip) 754.32
uterus (see also Malposition, uterus) 621.6

Flexner's
bacillus 004.1
diarrhea (ulcerative) 004.1
dysentery 004.1

Flexner-Boyd dysentery 004.2

Flexure — see condition

Floater, vitreous 379.24

Floating
cartilage (joint) (see also Disorder, cartilage, articular) 718.0 ✔5ᵗʰ
knee 717.6
gallbladder (congenital) 751.69
kidney 593.0
congenital 753.3
liver (congenital) 751.69
rib 756.3
spleen 289.59

Flooding 626.2

Floor — see condition

Floppy
infant NEC 781.99
valve syndrome (mitral) 424.0

Flu — see also Influenza
gastric NEC 008.8

Fluctuating blood pressure 796.4

Fluid
abdomen 789.5
chest (see also Pleurisy, with effusion) 511.9
heart (see also Failure, heart) 428.0
joint (see also Effusion, joint) 719.0 ✔5ᵗʰ
loss (acute) 276.5
with
hypernatremia 276.0
hyponatremia 276.1
lung — see also Edema, lung encysted 511.8
peritoneal cavity 789.5
pleural cavity (see also Pleurisy, with effusion) 511.9
retention 276.6

Flukes NEC (see also Infestation, fluke) 121.9
blood NEC (see also Infestation, Schistosoma) 120.9
liver 121.3

Fluor (albus) (vaginalis) 623.5
trichomonal (Trichomonas vaginalis) 131.00

Fluorosis (dental) (chronic) 520.3

Flushing 782.62
menopausal 627.2

Flush syndrome 259.2

Flutter
atrial or auricular 427.32
heart (ventricular) 427.42
atrial 427.32
impure 427.32
postoperative 997.1
ventricular 427.42

Flux (bloody) (serosanguineous) 009.0

Focal — see condition

Fochier's abscess — see Abscess, by site

Focus, Assmann's (see also Tuberculosis) 011.0 ✔5ᵗʰ

Fogo selvagem 694.4

Foix-Alajouanine syndrome 336.1

Folds, anomalous — see also Anomaly, specified type NEC
Bowman's membrane 371.31
Descemet's membrane 371.32
epicanthic 743.63
heart 746.89
posterior segment of eye, congenital 743.54

Folie à deux 297.3

Follicle
cervix (nabothian) (ruptured) 616.0
graafian, ruptured, with hemorrhage 620.0

Follicle — continued
nabothian 616.0

Folliclis (primary) (see also Tuberculosis) 017.0 ✔5ᵗʰ

Follicular — see also condition
cyst (atretic) 620.0

Folliculitis 704.8
abscedens et suffodiens 704.8
decalvans 704.09
gonorrheal (acute) 098.0
chronic or duration of 2 months or more 098.2
keloid, keloidalis 706.1
pustular 704.8
ulerythematosa reticulata 701.8

Folliculosis, conjunctival 372.02

Følling's disease (phenylketonuria) 270.1

Follow-up (examination) (routine) (following) V67.9
cancer chemotherapy V67.2
chemotherapy V67.2
fracture V67.4
high-risk medication V67.51
injury NEC V67.59
postpartum
immediately after delivery V24.0
routine V24.2
psychiatric V67.3
psychotherapy V67.3
radiotherapy V67.1
specified condition NEC V67.59
specified surgery NEC V67.09
surgery V67.00
vaginal pap smear V67.01
treatment V67.9
combined NEC V67.6
fracture V67.4
involving high-risk medication NEC V67.51
mental disorder V67.3
specified NEC V67.59

Fong's syndrome (hereditary osteoonychodysplasia) 756.89

Food
allergy 693.1
anaphylactic shock — see Anaphylactic shock, due to, food
asphyxia (from aspiration or inhalation) (see also Asphyxia, food) 933.1
choked on (see also Asphyxia, food) 933.1
deprivation 994.2
specified kind of food NEC 269.8
intoxication (see also Poisoning, food) 005.9
lack of 994.2
poisoning (see also Poisoning, food) 005.9
refusal or rejection NEC 307.59
strangulation or suffocation (see also Asphyxia, food) 933.1
toxemia (see also Poisoning, food) 005.9

Foot — see also condition
and mouth disease 078.4
process disease 581.3

Foramen ovale (nonclosure) (patent) (persistent) 745.5

Forbes' (glycogen storage) **disease** 271.0

Forbes-Albright syndrome (nonpuerperal amenorrhea and lactation associated with pituitary tumor) 253.1

Forced birth or delivery NEC 669.8 ✔5ᵗʰ
affecting fetus or newborn NEC 763.89

Forceps
delivery NEC 669.6 ✔5ᵗʰ
affecting fetus or newborn 763.2

Fordyce's disease (ectopic sebaceous glands) (mouth) 750.26

Fordyce-Fox disease (apocrine miliaria) 705.82

Forearm — see condition

Foreign body

> Note — For foreign body with open wound or other injury, see Wound, open, or the type of injury specified.

accidentally left during a procedure 998.4

Foreign body — continued
anterior chamber (eye) 871.6
magnetic 871.5
retained or old 360.51
retained or old 360.61
ciliary body (eye) 871.6
magnetic 871.5
retained or old 360.52
retained or old 360.62
entering through orifice (current) (old)
accessory sinus 932
air passage (upper) 933.0
lower 934.8
alimentary canal 938
alveolar process 935.0
antrum (Highmore) 932
anus 937
appendix 936
asphyxia due to (see also Asphyxia, food) 933.1
auditory canal 931
auricle 931
bladder 939.0
bronchioles 934.8
bronchus (main) 934.1
buccal cavity 935.0
canthus (inner) 930.1
cecum 936
cervix (canal) uterine 939.1
coil, ileocecal 936
colon 936
conjunctiva 930.1
conjunctival sac 930.1
cornea 930.0
digestive organ or tract NEC 938
duodenum 936
ear (external) 931
esophagus 935.1
eye (external) 930.9
combined sites 930.8
intraocular — see Foreign body, by site
specified site NEC 930.8
eyeball 930.8
intraocular — see Foreign body, intraocular
eyelid 930.1
retained or old 374.86
frontal sinus 932
gastrointestinal tract 938
genitourinary tract 939.9
globe 930.8
penetrating 871.6
magnetic 871.5
retained or old 360.50
retained or old 360.60
gum 935.0
Highmore's antrum 932
hypopharynx 933.0
ileocecal coil 936
ileum 936
inspiration (of) 933.1
intestine (large) (small) 936
lacrimal apparatus, duct, gland, or sac 930.2
larynx 933.1
lung 934.8
maxillary sinus 932
mouth 935.0
nasal sinus 932
nasopharynx 933.0
nose (passage) 932
nostril 932
oral cavity 935.0
palate 935.0
penis 939.3
pharynx 933.0
pyriform sinus 933.0
rectosigmoid 937
junction 937
rectum 937
respiratory tract 934.9
specified part NEC 934.8
sclera 930.1
sinus 932
accessory 932
frontal 932
maxillary 932

Foreign body — *continued*
　entering through orifice — *continued*
　　sinus — *continued*
　　　nasal 932
　　　pyriform 933.0
　　small intestine 936
　　stomach (hairball) 935.2
　　suffocation by (*see also* Asphyxia, food)
　　　933.1
　　swallowed 938
　　　tongue 933.0
　　tear ducts or glands 930.2
　　throat 933.0
　　tongue 935.0
　　　swallowed 933.0
　　tonsil, tonsillar 933.0
　　　fossa 933.0
　　trachea 934.0
　　ureter 939.0
　　urethra 939.0
　　uterus (any part) 939.1
　　vagina 939.2
　　vulva 939.2
　　wind pipe 934.0
　granuloma (old) 728.82
　　bone 733.99
　　in operative wound (inadvertently left) 998.4
　　　due to surgical material intentionally left
　　　　— *see* Complications, due to
　　　　(presence of) any device, implant, or
　　　　graft classified to 996.0-996.5 NEC
　　muscle 728.82
　　skin 709.4
　　soft tissue 709.4
　　subcutaneous tissue 709.4
　in
　　bone (residual) 733.99
　　open wound — *see* Wound, open, by site
　　　complicated
　　soft tissue (residual) 729.6
　inadvertently left in operation wound (causing
　　adhesions, obstruction, or perforation)
　　998.4
　ingestion, ingested NEC 938
　inhalation or inspiration (*see also* Asphyxia,
　　food) 933.1
　internal organ, not entering through an orifice
　　— *see* Injury, internal, by site, with open
　　wound
　intraocular (nonmagnetic 871.6
　　combined sites 871.6
　　　magnetic 871.5
　　　　retained or old 360.59
　　　retained or old 360.69
　　magnetic 871.5
　　　retained or old 360.50
　　retained or old 360.60
　　specified site NEC 871.6
　　　magnetic 871.5
　　　　retained or old 360.59
　　　retained or old 360.69
　iris (nonmagnetic) 871.6
　　magnetic 871.5
　　　retained or old 360.52
　　retained or old 360.62
　lens (nonmagnetic) 871.6
　　magnetic 871.5
　　　retained or old 360.53
　　retained or old 360.63
　lid, eye 930.1
　ocular muscle 870.4
　　retained or old 376.6
　old or residual
　　bone 733.99
　　eyelid 374.86
　　middle ear 385.83
　　muscle 729.6
　　　ocular 376.6
　　retrobulbar 376.6
　　skin 729.6
　　　with granuloma 709.4
　　soft tissue 729.6
　　　with granuloma 709.4
　　subcutaneous tissue 729.6
　　　with granuloma 709.4
　operation wound, left accidentally 998.4

Foreign body — *continued*
　orbit 870.4
　　retained or old 376.6
　posterior wall, eye 871.6
　　magnetic 871.5
　　　retained or old 360.55
　　retained or old 360.65
　respiratory tree 934.9
　　specified site NEC 934.8
　retained (old) (nonmagnetic) (in)
　　anterior chamber (eye) 360.61
　　　magnetic 360.51
　　ciliary body 360.62
　　　magnetic 360.52
　　eyelid 374.86
　　globe 360.60
　　　magnetic 360.50
　　intraocular 360.60
　　　magnetic 360.50
　　　specified site NEC 360.69
　　　　magnetic 360.59
　　iris 360.62
　　　magnetic 360.52
　　lens 360.63
　　　magnetic 360.53
　　muscle 729.6
　　orbit 376.6
　　posterior wall of globe 360.65
　　　magnetic 360.55
　　retina 360.65
　　　magnetic 360.55
　　retrobulbar 376.6
　　soft tissue 729.6
　　vitreous 360.64
　　　magnetic 360.54
　　skin 729.6
　　　with granuloma 709.4
　　soft tissue 729.6
　　　with granuloma 709.4
　　subcutaneous tissue 729.6
　　　with granuloma 709.4
　retina 871.6
　　magnetic 871.5
　　　retained or old 360.55
　　retained or old 360.65
　superficial, without major open wound (*see
　　also* Injury, superficial, by site) 919.6
　swallowed NEC 938
　vitreous (humor) 871.6
　　magnetic 871.5
　　　retained or old 360.54
　　retained or old 360.64

Forking, aqueduct of Sylvius 742.3
　with spina bifida (*see also* Spina bifida)
　　741.0 ✓5ᵗʰ

Formation
　bone in scar tissue (skin) 709.3
　connective tissue in vitreous 379.25
　Elschnig pearls (postcataract extraction) 366.51
　hyaline in cornea 371.49
　sequestrum in bone (due to infection) (*see also*
　　Osteomyelitis) 730.1 ✓5ᵗʰ
　valve
　　colon, congenital 751.5
　　ureter (congenital) 753.29

Formication 782.0

Fort Bragg fever 100.89

Fossa — *see also* condition
　pyriform — *see* condition

Foster-Kennedy syndrome 377.04

Fothergill's
　disease, meaning scarlatina anginosa 034.1
　neuralgia (*see also* Neuralgia, trigeminal) 350.1

Foul breath 784.9

Found dead (cause unknown) 798.9

Foundling V20.0

Fournier's disease (idiopathic gangrene) 608.83

Fourth
　cranial nerve — *see* condition
　disease 057.8
　molar 520.1

Foville's syndrome 344.89

Fox's
　disease (apocrine miliaria) 705.82
　impetigo (contagiosa) 684
Fox-Fordyce disease (apocrine miliaria) 705.82
Fracture (abduction) (adduction) (avulsion)
　(compression) (crush) (dislocation) (oblique)
　(separation) (closed) 829.0

> *Note* — *For fracture of any of the following
> sites with fracture of other bones — see
> Fracture, multiple.*
> *"Closed" includes the following descriptions
> of fractures, with or without delayed healing,
> unless they are specified as open or
> compound:*
>
> | | |
> |---|---|
> | *comminuted* | *linear* |
> | *depressed* | *simple* |
> | *elevated* | *slipped epiphysis* |
> | *fissured* | *spiral* |
> | *greenstick* | *unspecified* |
> | *impacted* | |
>
> *"Open" includes the following descriptions of
> fractures, with or without delayed healing:*
>
> | | |
> |---|---|
> | *compound* | *puncture* |
> | *infected* | *with foreign body* |
> | *missile* | |
>
> *For late effect of fracture, see Late, effect,
> fracture, by site.*

　with
　　internal injuries in same region (conditions
　　　classifiable to 860-869) — *see also*
　　　Injury, internal, by site pelvic region —
　　　see Fracture, pelvis
　acetabulum (with visceral injury) (closed) 808.0
　　open 808.1
　acromion (process) (closed) 811.01
　　open 811.11
　alveolus (closed) 802.8
　　open 802.9
　ankle (malleolus) (closed) 824.8
　　bimalleolar (Dupuytren's) (Pott's) 824.4
　　　open 824.5
　　bone 825.21
　　　open 825.31
　　lateral malleolus only (fibular) 824.2
　　　open 824.3
　　medial malleolus only (tibial) 824.0
　　　open 824.1
　　open 824.9
　　pathologic 733.16
　　talus 825.21
　　　open 825.31
　　trimalleolar 824.6
　　　open 824.7
　antrum — *see* Fracture, skull, base
　arm (closed) 818.0
　　and leg(s) (any bones) 828.0
　　　open 828.1
　　both (any bones) (with rib(s)) (with sternum)
　　　819.0
　　　open 819.1
　　lower 813.80
　　　open 813.90
　　open 818.1
　　upper — *see* Fracture, humerus
　astragalus (closed) 825.21
　　open 825.31
　atlas — *see* Fracture, vertebra, cervical, first
　axis — *see* Fracture, vertebra, cervical, second
　back — *see* Fracture, vertebra, by site
　Barton's — *see* Fracture, radius, lower end
　basal (skull) — *see* Fracture, skull, base
　Bennett's (closed) 815.01
　　open 815.11
　bimalleolar (closed) 824.4
　　open 824.5
　bone (closed) NEC 829.0
　　birth injury NEC 767.3
　　open 829.1
　　pathologic NEC (*see also* Fracture,
　　　pathologic) 733.10
　　stress NEC (*see also* Fracture, stress)
　　　733.95
　boot top — *see* Fracture, fibula
　boxers' — *see* Fracture, metacarpal bone(s)
　breast bone — *see* Fracture, sternum

Fracture — *continued*
- bucket handle (semilunar cartilage) — *see* Tear, meniscus
- bursting — *see* Fracture, phalanx, hand, distal
- calcaneus (closed) 825.0
  - open 825.1
- capitate (bone) (closed) 814.07
  - open 814.17
- capitellum (humerus) (closed) 812.49
  - open 812.59
- carpal bone(s) (wrist NEC) (closed) 814.00
  - open 814.10
  - specified site NEC 814.09
    - open 814.19
- cartilage, knee (semilunar) — *see* Tear, meniscus
- cervical — *see* Fracture, vertebra, cervical
- chauffeur's — *see* Fracture, ulna, lower end
- chisel — *see* Fracture, radius, upper end
- clavicle (interligamentous part) (closed) 810.00
  - acromial end 810.03
    - open 810.13
  - due to birth trauma 767.2
  - open 810.10
  - shaft (middle third) 810.02
    - open 810.12
  - sternal end 810.01
    - open 810.11
- clayshovelers' — *see* Fracture, vertebra, cervical
- coccyx — *see also* Fracture, vertebra, coccyx
  - complicating delivery 665.6 ✔5ᵗʰ
- collar bone — *see* Fracture, clavicle
- Colles' (reversed) (closed) 813.41
  - open 813.51
- comminuted — *see* Fracture, by site
- compression — *see also* Fracture, by site
  - nontraumatic — *see* Fracture, pathologic
- congenital 756.9
- coracoid process (closed) 811.02
  - open 811.12
- coronoid process (ulna) (closed) 813.02
  - mandible (closed) 802.23
    - open 802.33
  - open 813.12
- costochondral junction — *see* Fracture, rib
- costosternal junction — *see* Fracture, rib
- cranium — *see* Fracture, skull, by site
- cricoid cartilage (closed) 807.5
  - open 807.6
- cuboid (ankle) (closed) 825.23
  - open 825.33
- cuneiform
  - foot (closed) 825.24
    - open 825.34
  - wrist (closed) 814.03
    - open 814.13
- due to
  - birth injury — *see* Birth injury, fracture
  - gunshot — *see* Fracture, by site, open
  - neoplasm — *see* Fracture, pathologic
  - osteoporosis — *see* Fracture, pathologic
- Dupuytren's (ankle) (fibula) (closed) 824.4
  - open 824.5
  - radius 813.42
    - open 813.52
- Duverney's — *see* Fracture, ilium
- elbow — *see also* Fracture, humerus, lower end
  - olecranon (process) (closed) 813.01
    - open 813.11
  - supracondylar (closed) 812.41
    - open 812.51
- ethmoid (bone) (sinus) — *see* Fracture, skull, base
- face bone(s) (closed) NEC 802.8
  - with
    - other bone(s) — *see* Fracture, multiple, skull
    - skull — *see also* Fracture, skull
      - involving other bones — *see* Fracture, multiple, skull
  - open 802.9
- fatigue — *see* Fracture, march
- femur, femoral (closed) 821.00
  - cervicotrochanteric 820.03
    - open 820.13
  - condyles, epicondyles 821.21
    - open 821.31

Fracture — *continued*
femur, femoral — *continued*
- distal end — *see* Fracture, femur, lower end
- epiphysis (separation)
  - capital 820.01
    - open 820.11
  - head 820.01
    - open 820.11
  - lower 821.22
    - open 821.32
  - trochanteric 820.01
    - open 820.11
  - upper 820.01
    - open 820.11
- head 820.09
  - open 820.19
- lower end or extremity (distal end) (closed) 821.20
  - condyles, epicondyles 821.21
    - open 821.31
  - epiphysis (separation) 821.22
    - open 821.32
  - multiple sites 821.29
    - open 821.39
  - open 821.30
  - specified site NEC 821.29
    - open 821.39
  - supracondylar 821.23
    - open 821.33
  - T-shaped 821.21
    - open 821.31
- neck (closed) 820.8
  - base (cervicotrochanteric) 820.03
    - open 820.13
  - extracapsular 820.20
    - open 820.30
  - intertrochanteric (section) 820.21
    - open 820.31
  - intracapsular 820.00
    - open 820.10
  - intratrochanteric 820.21
    - open 820.31
  - midcervical 820.02
    - open 820.12
  - open 820.9
  - pathologic 733.14
    - specified part NEC 733.15
  - specified site NEC 820.09
    - open 820.19
  - transcervical 820.02
    - open 820.12
  - transtrochanteric 820.20
    - open 820.30
- open 821.10
- pathologic 733.14
  - specified part NEC 733.15
- peritrochanteric (section) 820.20
  - open 820.30
- shaft (lower third) (middle third) (upper third) 821.01
  - open 821.11
- subcapital 820.09
  - open 820.19
- subtrochanteric (region) (section) 820.22
  - open 820.32
- supracondylar 821.23
  - open 821.33
- transepiphyseal 820.01
  - open 820.11
- trochanter (greater) (lesser) (*see also* Fracture, femur, neck, by site) 820.20
  - open 820.30
- T-shaped, into knee joint 821.21
  - open 821.31
- upper end 820.8
  - open 820.9
- fibula (closed) 823.81
  - with tibia 823.82
    - open 823.92
  - distal end 824.8
    - open 824.9
  - epiphysis
    - lower 824.8
      - open 824.9
    - upper — *see* Fracture, fibula, upper end

Fracture — *continued*
fibula — *continued*
- head — *see* Fracture, fibula, upper end
- involving ankle 824.2
  - open 824.3
- lower end or extremity 824.8
  - open 824.9
- malleolus (external) (lateral) 824.2
  - open 824.3
- open NEC 823.91
- pathologic 733.16
- proximal end — *see* Fracture, fibula, upper end
- shaft 823.21
  - with tibia 823.22
    - open 823.32
  - open 823.31
- stress 733.93
- torus 823.41 ●
  - with tibia 823.42 ●
- upper end or extremity (epiphysis) (head) (proximal end) (styloid) 823.01
  - with tibia 823.02
    - open 823.12
  - open 823.11
- finger(s), of one hand (closed) (*see also* Fracture, phalanx, hand) 816.00
  - with
    - metacarpal bone(s), of same hand 817.0
      - open 817.1
    - thumb of same hand 816.03
      - open 816.13
  - open 816.10
- foot, except toe(s) alone (closed) 825.20
  - open 825.30
- forearm (closed) NEC 813.80
  - lower end (distal end) (lower epiphysis) 813.40
    - open 813.50
  - open 813.90
  - shaft 813.20
    - open 813.30
  - upper end (proximal end) (upper epiphysis) 813.00
    - open 813.10
- fossa, anterior, middle, or posterior — *see* Fracture, skull, base
- frontal (bone) — *see also* Fracture, skull, vault
  - sinus — *see* Fracture, skull, base
- Galeazzi's — *see* Fracture, radius, lower end
- glenoid (cavity) (fossa) (scapula) (closed) 811.03
  - open 811.13
- Gosselin's — *see* Fracture, ankle
- greenstick — *see* Fracture, by site
- grenade-throwers' — *see* Fracture, humerus, shaft
- gutter — *see* Fracture, skull, vault
- hamate (closed) 814.08
  - open 814.18
- hand, one (closed) 815.00
  - carpals 814.00
    - open 814.10
    - specified site NEC 814.09
      - open 814.19
  - metacarpals 815.00
    - open 815.10
  - multiple, bones of one hand 817.0
    - open 817.1
  - open 815.10
  - phalanges (*see also* Fracture, phalanx, hand) 816.00
    - open 816.10
- healing
  - aftercare ▶(*see also* Aftercare, fracture)◀ V54.89 ▲
  - change of cast V54.89 ▲
  - complications — *see* condition
  - convalescence V66.4 ●
  - removal of
    - cast V54.89 ▲
    - fixation device
      - external V54.89 ▲
      - internal V54.0
- heel bone (closed) 825.0
  - open 825.1
- hip (closed) (*see also* Fracture, femur, neck) 820.8

Fracture — *continued*
  hip (*see also* Fracture, femur, neck) —
      continued
    open 820.9
    pathologic 733.14
  humerus (closed) 812.20
    anatomical neck 812.02
      open 812.12
    articular process (*see also* Fracture
        humerus, condyle(s)) 812.44
      open 812.54
    capitellum 812.49
      open 812.59
    condyle(s) 812.44
      lateral (external) 812.42
        open 812.52
      medial (internal epicondyle) 812.43
        open 812.53
      open 812.54
    distal end — *see* Fracture, humerus, lower
        end
    epiphysis
      lower (*see also* Fracture, humerus,
          condyle(s)) 812.44
        open 812.54
      upper 812.09
        open 812.19
    external condyle 812.42
      open 812.52
    great tuberosity 812.03
      open 812.13
    head 812.09
      open 812.19
    internal epicondyle 812.43
      open 812.53
    lesser tuberosity 812.09
      open 812.19
    lower end or extremity (distal end) (*see also*
        Fracture, humerus, by site) 812.40
      multiple sites NEC 812.49
        open 812.59
        open 812.50
      specified site NEC 812.49
        open 812.59
    neck 812.01
      open 812.11
    open 812.30
    pathologic 733.11
    proximal end — *see* Fracture, humerus,
        upper end
    shaft 812.21
      open 812.31
    supracondylar 812.41
      open 812.51
    surgical neck 812.01
      open 812.11
    trochlea 812.49
      open 812.59
    T-shaped 812.44
      open 812.54
    tuberosity — *see* Fracture, humerus, upper
        end
    upper end or extremity (proximal end) (*see
        also* Fracture, humerus, by site)
        812.00
      open 812.10
      specified site NEC 812.09
        open 812.19
  hyoid bone (closed) 807.5
    open 807.6
  hyperextension — *see* Fracture, radius, lower
      end
  ilium (with visceral injury) (closed) 808.41
    open 808.51
  impaction, impacted — *see* Fracture, by site
  incus — *see* Fracture, skull, base
  innominate bone (with visceral injury) (closed)
      808.49
    open 808.59
  instep, of one foot (closed) 825.20
    with toe(s) of same foot 827.0
      open 827.1
    open 825.30
  internal
    ear — *see* Fracture, skull, base
    semilunar cartilage, knee — *see* Tear,
        meniscus, medial

  intertrochanteric — *see* Fracture, femur, neck,
      intertrochanteric
  ischium (with visceral injury) (closed) 808.42
    open 808.52
  jaw (bone) (lower) (closed) (*see also* Fracture,
      mandible) 802.20
    angle 802.25
      open 802.35
    open 802.30
    upper — *see* Fracture, maxilla
  knee
    cap (closed) 822.0
      open 822.1
    cartilage (semilunar) — *see* Tear, meniscus
  labyrinth (osseous) — *see* Fracture, skull, base
  larynx (closed) 807.5
    open 807.6
  late effect — *see* Late, effects (of), fracture
  Le Fort's — *see* Fracture, maxilla
  leg (closed) 827.0
    with rib(s) or sternum 828.0
      open 828.1
    both (any bones) 828.0
      open 828.1
    lower — *see* Fracture, tibia
      open 827.1
    upper — *see* Fracture, femur
  limb
    lower (multiple) (closed) NEC 827.0
      open 827.1
    upper (multiple) (closed) NEC 818.0
      open 818.1
  long bones, due to birth trauma — *see* Birth
      injury, fracture
  lumbar — *see* Fracture, vertebra, lumbar
  lunate bone (closed) 814.02
    open 814.12
  malar bone (closed) 802.4
    open 802.5
  Malgaigne's (closed) 808.43
    open 808.53
  malleolus (closed) 824.8
    bimalleolar 824.4
      open 824.5
    lateral 824.2
      and medial — *see also* Fracture,
          malleolus, bimalleolar
        with lip of tibia — *see* Fracture,
            malleolus, trimalleolar
      open 824.3
    medial (closed) 824.0
      and lateral — *see also* Fracture,
          malleolus, bimalleolar
        with lip of tibia — *see* Fracture,
            malleolus, trimalleolar
      open 824.1
    open 824.9
    trimalleolar (closed) 824.6
      open 824.7
  malleus — *see* Fracture, skull, base
  malunion 733.81
  mandible (closed) 802.20
    angle 802.25
      open 802.35
    body 802.28
      alveolar border 802.27
        open 802.37
      open 802.38
      symphysis 802.26
        open 802.36
    condylar process 802.21
      open 802.31
    coronoid process 802.23
      open 802.33
    multiple sites 802.29
      open 802.39
    open 802.30
    ramus NEC 802.24
      open 802.34
    subcondylar 802.22
      open 802.32
  manubrium — *see* Fracture, sternum
  march 733.95
    fibula 733.94
    metatarsals 733.94
    tibia 733.94

  maxilla, maxillary (superior) (upper jaw)
      (closed) 802.4
    inferior — *see* Fracture, mandible
    open 802.5
  meniscus, knee — *see* Tear, meniscus
  metacarpus, metacarpal (bone(s)), of one hand
      (closed) 815.00
    with phalanx, phalanges, hand (finger(s))
        (thumb) of same hand 817.0
      open 817.1
    base 815.02
      first metacarpal 815.01
        open 815.11
      open 815.12
      thumb 815.01
        open 815.11
    multiple sites 815.09
      open 815.19
    neck 815.04
      open 815.14
    open 815.10
    shaft 815.03
      open 815.13
  metatarsus, metatarsal (bone(s)), of one foot
      (closed) 825.25
    with tarsal bone(s) 825.29
      open 825.39
    open 825.35
  Monteggia's (closed) 813.03
    open 813.13
  Moore's — *see* Fracture, radius, lower end
  multangular bone (closed)
    larger 814.05
      open 814.15
    smaller 814.06
      open 814.16
  multiple (closed) 829.0

Note — *Multiple fractures of sites classifiable to
the same three- or four-digit category are coded
to that category, except for sites classifiable to
810-818 or 820-827 in different limbs.*

*Multiple fractures of sites classifiable to different
fourth-digit subdivisions within the same three-
digit category should be dealt with according to
coding rules.*

*Multiple fractures of sites classifiable to different
three-digit categories (identifiable from the
listing under "Fracture"), and of sites
classifiable to 810-818 or 820-827 in different
limbs should be coded according to the following
list, which should be referred to in the following
priority order: skull or face bones, pelvis or
vertebral column, legs, arms.*

---

    arm (multiple bones in same arm except in
        hand alone) (sites classifiable to 810-
        817 with sites classifiable to a
        different three-digit category in 810-
        817 in same arm) (closed) 818.0
      open 818.1
    arms, both or arm(s) with rib(s) or sternum
        (sites classifiable to 810-818 with sites
        classifiable to same range of categories
        in other limb or to 807) (closed) 819.0
      open 819.1
    bones of trunk NEC (closed) 809.0
      open 809.1
    hand, metacarpal bone(s) with phalanx or
        phalanges of same hand (sites
        classifiable to 815 with sites
        classifiable to 816 in same hand)
        (closed) 817.0
      open 817.1
    leg (multiple bones in same leg) (sites
        classifiable to 820-826 with sites
        classifiable to a different three-digit
        category in that range in same leg)
        (closed) 827.0
      open 827.1
    legs, both or leg(s) with arm(s), rib(s), or
        sternum (sites classifiable to 820-827
        with sites classifiable to same range of
        categories in other leg or to 807 or
        810-819) (closed) 828.0
      open 828.1

▲
●
●
●

Fracture — *continued*
  Moore's — *see* Fracture, radius, lower end
  multangular bone — *continued*
    open 829.1
  pelvis with other bones except skull or face
    bones (sites classifiable to 808 with
    sites classifiable to 805-807 or 810-
    829) (closed) 809.0
    open 809.1
  skull, specified or unspecified bones, or face
    bone(s) with any other bone(s) (sites
    classifiable to 800-803 with sites
    classifiable to 805-829) (closed)
    804.0 ✓5ᵗʰ

> Note — Use the following fifth-digit
> subclassification with categories 800, 801,
> 803, and 804:
>
> 0   unspecified state of consciousness
> 1   with no loss of consciousness
> 2   with brief [less than one hour] loss
>   of consciousness
> 3   with moderate [1-24 hours] loss of
>   consciousness
> 4   with prolonged [more than 24 hours]
>   loss of consciousness and return to
>   pre-existing conscious level
> 5   with prolonged [more than 24 hours]
>   loss of consciousness, without
>   return to pre-existing conscious level
>
> Use fifth-digit 5 to designate when a
>   patient is unconscious and dies
>   before regaining consciousness,
>   regardless of the duration of the
>   loss of consciousness
> 6   with loss of consciousness of
>   unspecified duration
> 9   with concussion, unspecified

    with
      contusion, cerebral 804.1 ✓5ᵗʰ
      epidural hemorrhage 804.2 ✓5ᵗʰ
      extradural hemorrhage 804.2 ✓5ᵗʰ
      hemorrhage (intracranial) NEC
        804.3 ✓5ᵗʰ
      intracranial injury NEC 804.4 ✓5ᵗʰ
      laceration, cerebral 804.1 ✓5ᵗʰ
      subarachnoid hemorrhage 804.2 ✓5ᵗʰ
      subdural hemorrhage 804.2 ✓5ᵗʰ
    open 804.5 ✓5ᵗʰ
      with
        contusion, cerebral 804.6 ✓5ᵗʰ
        epidural hemorrhage 804.7 ✓5ᵗʰ
        extradural hemorrhage 804.7 ✓5ᵗʰ
        hemorrhage (intracranial) NEC
          804.8 ✓5ᵗʰ
        intracranial injury NEC 804.9 ✓5ᵗʰ
        laceration, cerebral 804.6 ✓5ᵗʰ
        subarachnoid hemorrhage
          804.7 ✓5ᵗʰ
        subdural hemorrhage 804.7 ✓5ᵗʰ
  vertebral column with other bones, except
    skull or face bones (sites classifiable to
    805 or 806 with sites classifiable to
    807-808 or 810-829) (closed) 809.0
    open 809.1
  nasal (bone(s)) (closed) 802.0
    open 802.1
    sinus — *see* Fracture, skull, base
  navicular
    carpal (wrist) (closed) 814.01
      open 814.11
    tarsal (ankle) (closed) 825.22
      open 825.32
  neck — *see* Fracture, vertebra, cervical
  neural arch — *see* Fracture, vertebra, by site
  nonunion 733.82
  nose, nasal, (bone) (septum) (closed) 802.0
    open 802.1
  occiput — *see* Fracture, skull, base
  odontoid process — *see* Fracture, vertebra,
    cervical
  olecranon (process) (ulna) (closed) 813.01
    open 813.11
    open 829.1

Fracture — *continued*
  orbit, orbital (bone) (region) (closed) 802.8
    floor (blow-out) 802.6
      open 802.7
    open 802.9
    roof — *see* Fracture, skull, base
    specified part NEC 802.8
      open 802.9
  os
    calcis (closed) 825.0
      open 825.1
    magnum (closed) 814.07
      open 814.17
    pubis (with visceral injury) (closed) 808.2
      open 808.3
    triquetrum (closed) 814.03
      open 814.13
  osseous
    auditory meatus — *see* Fracture, skull, base
    labyrinth — *see* Fracture, skull, base
      ossicles, auditory (incus) (malleus)
        (stapes) — *see* Fracture, skull, base
  osteoporotic — *see* Fracture, pathologic
  palate (closed) 802.8
    open 802.9
  paratrooper — *see* Fracture, tibia, lower end
  parietal bone — *see* Fracture, skull, vault
  parry — *see* Fracture, Monteggia's
  patella (closed) 822.0
    open 822.1
  pathologic (cause unknown) 733.10
    ankle 733.16
    femur (neck) 733.14
      specified NEC 733.15
    fibula 733.16
    hip 733.14
    humerus 733.11
    radius 733.12
    specified site NEC 733.19
    tibia 733.16
    ulna 733.12
    vertebrae (collapse) 733.13
    wrist 733.12
  pedicle (of vertebral arch) — *see* Fracture,
    vertebra, by site
  pelvis, pelvic (bone(s)) (with visceral injury)
    (closed) 808.8
    multiple (with disruption of pelvic circle)
      808.43
      open 808.53
    open 808.9
    rim (closed) 808.49
      open 808.59
  peritrochanteric (closed) 820.20
    open 820.30
  phalanx, phalanges, of one
    foot (closed) 826.0
      with bone(s) of same lower limb 827.0
        open 827.1
      open 826.1
    hand (closed) 816.00
      with metacarpal bone(s) of same hand
        817.0
        open 817.1
      distal 816.02
        open 816.12
      middle 816.01
        open 816.11
      multiple sites NEC 816.03
        open 816.13
      open 816.10
      proximal 816.01
        open 816.11
  pisiform (closed) 814.04
    open 814.14
  pond — *see* Fracture, skull, vault
  Pott's (closed) 824.4
    open 824.5
  prosthetic device, internal — *see*
    Complications, mechanical
  pubis (with visceral injury) (closed) 808.2
    open 808.3
  Quervain's (closed) 814.01
    open 814.11
  radius (alone) (closed) 813.81
    with ulna NEC 813.83
      open 813.93

Fracture — *continued*
  radius — *continued*
    distal end — *see* Fracture, radius, lower end
    epiphysis
      lower — *see* Fracture, radius, lower end
      upper — *see* Fracture, radius, upper end
    head — *see* Fracture, radius, upper end
    lower end or extremity (distal end) (lower
      epiphysis) 813.42
      with ulna (lower end) 813.44
        open 813.54
      torus 813.45   ●
      open 813.52
    neck — *see* Fracture, radius, upper end
    open NEC 813.91
    pathologic 733.12
    proximal end — *see* Fracture, radius, upper
      end
    shaft (closed) 813.21
      with ulna (shaft) 813.23
        open 813.33
      open 813.31
    upper end 813.07
      with ulna (upper end) 813.08
        open 813.18
      epiphysis 813.05
        open 813.15
      head 813.05
        open 813.15
      multiple sites 813.07
        open 813.17
      neck 813.06
        open 813.16
      open 813.17
      specified site NEC 813.07
        open 813.17
  ramus
    inferior or superior (with visceral injury)
      (closed) 808.2
      open 808.3
    ischium — *see* Fracture, ischium
    mandible 802.24
      open 802.34
  rib(s) (closed) 807.0

> Note — Use the following fifth-digit
> subclassification with categories 807.0-
> 807.1:
>
> 0   rib(s), unspecified
> 1   one rib
> 2   two ribs
> 3   three ribs
> 4   four ribs
> 5   five ribs
> 6   six ribs
> 7   seven ribs
> 8   eight or more ribs
> 9   multiple ribs, unspecified

    with flail chest (open) 807.4
    open 807.1 ✓5ᵗʰ
  root, tooth 873.63
    complicated 873.73
  sacrum — *see* Fracture, vertebra, sacrum
  scaphoid
    ankle (closed) 825.22
      open 825.32
    wrist (closed) 814.01
      open 814.11
  scapula (closed) 811.00
    acromial, acromion (process) 811.01
      open 811.11
    body 811.09
      open 811.19
    coracoid process 811.02
      open 811.12
    glenoid (cavity) (fossa) 811.03
      open 811.13
    neck 811.03
      open 811.13
      open 811.10
  semilunar
    bone, wrist (closed) 814.02
      open 814.12

Fracture — *Fracture* (vertical left margin)

Fracture — *continued*
  semilunar — *continued*
    cartilage (interior) (knee) — *see* Tear, meniscus
  sesamoid bone — *see* Fracture, by site
  Shepherd's (closed) 825.21
    open 825.31
  shoulder — *see also* Fracture, humerus, upper end
    blade — *see* Fracture, scapula
  silverfork — *see* Fracture, radius, lower end
  sinus (ethmoid) (frontal) (maxillary) (nasal) (sphenoidal) — *see* Fracture, skull, base
  Skillern's — *see* Fracture, radius, shaft
  skull (multiple NEC) (with face bones) (closed) 803.0 ✓5ᵗʰ

Note — *Use the following fifth digit subclassification with categories 800, 801, 803, and 804:*

  0   *unspecified state of consciousness*
  1   *with no loss of consciousness*
  2   *with brief [less than one hour] loss of consciousness*
  3   *with moderate [1-24 hours] loss of consciousness*
  4   *with prolonged [more than 24 hours] loss of consciousness and return to pre-existing conscious level*
  5   *with prolonged [more than 24 hours] loss of consciousness, without return to pre-existing conscious level*
  Use fifth-digit 5 to designate when a patient is unconscious and dies before regaining consciousness, regardles of the duration of loss of consciousness
  6   *with loss of consciousness of unspecified duration*
  9   *with concussion, unspecified*

---

    with
      contusion, cerebral 803.1 ✓5ᵗʰ
      epidural hemorrhage 803.2 ✓5ᵗʰ
      extradural hemorrhage 803.2 ✓5ᵗʰ
      hemorrhage (intracranial) NEC 803.3 ✓5ᵗʰ
      intracranial injury NEC 803.4 ✓5ᵗʰ
      laceration, cerebral 803.1 ✓5ᵗʰ
      other bones — *see* Fracture, multiple, skull
      subarachnoid hemorrhage 803.2 ✓5ᵗʰ
      subdural hemorrhage 803.2 ✓5ᵗʰ
    base (antrum) (ethmoid bone) (fossa) (internal ear) (nasal sinus) (occiput) (sphenoid) (temporal bone) (closed) 801.0 ✓5ᵗʰ
      with
        contusion, cerebral 801.1 ✓5ᵗʰ
        epidural hemorrhage 801.2 ✓5ᵗʰ
        extradural hemorrhage 801.2 ✓5ᵗʰ
        hemorrhage (intracranial) NEC 801.3 ✓5ᵗʰ
        intracranial injury NEC 801.4 ✓5ᵗʰ
        laceration, cerebral 801.1 ✓5ᵗʰ
        subarachnoid hemorrhage 801.2 ✓5ᵗʰ
        subdural hemorrhage 801.2 ✓5ᵗʰ
      open 801.5 ✓5ᵗʰ
        with
          contusion, cerebral 801.6 ✓5ᵗʰ
          epidural hemorrhage 801.7 ✓5ᵗʰ
          extradural hemorrhage 801.7 ✓5ᵗʰ
          hemorrhage (intracranial) NEC 801.8 ✓5ᵗʰ
          intracranial injury NEC 801.9 ✓5ᵗʰ
          laceration, cerebral 801.6 ✓5ᵗʰ
          subarachnoid hemorrhage 801.7 ✓5ᵗʰ
          subdural hemorrhage 801.7 ✓5ᵗʰ
    birth injury 767.3
    face bones — *see* Fracture, face bones
    open 803.5 ✓5ᵗʰ
      with
        contusion, cerebral 803.6 ✓5ᵗʰ
        epidural hemorrhage 803.7 ✓5ᵗʰ
        extradural hemorrhage 803.7 ✓5ᵗʰ

Fracture — *continued*
  skull — *continued*
    open — *continued*
      with — *continued*
        hemorrhage (intracranial) NEC 803.8 ✓5ᵗʰ
        intracranial injury NEC 803.9 ✓5ᵗʰ
        laceration, cerebral 803.6 ✓5ᵗʰ
        subarachnoid hemorrhage 803.7 ✓5ᵗʰ
        subdural hemorrhage 803.7 ✓5ᵗʰ
    vault (frontal bone) (parietal bone) (vertex) (closed) 800.0 ✓5ᵗʰ
      with
        contusion, cerebral 800.1 ✓5ᵗʰ
        epidural hemorrhage 800.2 ✓5ᵗʰ
        extradural hemorrhage 800.2 ✓5ᵗʰ
        hemorrhage (intracranial) NEC 800.3 ✓5ᵗʰ
        intracranial injury NEC 800.4 ✓5ᵗʰ
        laceration, cerebral 800.1 ✓5ᵗʰ
        subarachnoid hemorrhage 800.2 ✓5ᵗʰ
        subdural hemorrhage 800.2 ✓5ᵗʰ
      open 800.5 ✓5ᵗʰ
        with
          contusion, cerebral 800.6 ✓5ᵗʰ
          epidural hemorrhage 800.7 ✓5ᵗʰ
          extradural hemorrhage 800.7 ✓5ᵗʰ
          hemorrhage (intracranial) NEC 800.8 ✓5ᵗʰ
          intracranial injury NEC 800.9 ✓5ᵗʰ
          laceration, cerebral 800.6 ✓5ᵗʰ
          subarachnoid hemorrhage 800.7 ✓5ᵗʰ
          subdural hemorrhage 800.7 ✓5ᵗʰ
  Smith's 813.41
    open 813.51
  sphenoid (bone) (sinus) — *see* Fracture, skull, base
  spine — *see also* Fracture, vertebra, by site due to birth trauma 767.4
  spinous process — *see* Fracture, vertebra, by site
  spontaneous — *see* Fracture, pathologic
  sprinters' — *see* Fracture, ilium
  stapes — *see* Fracture, skull, base
  stave — *see also* Fracture, metacarpus, metacarpal bone(s)
    spine — *see* Fracture, tibia, upper end
  sternum (closed) 807.2
    with flail chest (open) 807.4
    open 807.3
  Stieda's — *see* Fracture, femur, lower end
  stress 733.95
    fibula 733.93
    metatarsals 733.94
    specified site NEC 733.95
    tibia 733.93
  styloid process
    metacarpal (closed) 815.02
      open 815.12
    radius — *see* Fracture, radius, lower end
    temporal bone — *see* Fracture, skull, base
    ulna — *see* Fracture, ulna, lower end
  supracondylar, elbow 812.41
    open 812.51
  symphysis pubis (with visceral injury) (closed) 808.2
    open 808.3
  talus (ankle bone) (closed) 825.21
    open 825.31
  tarsus, tarsal bone(s) (with metatarsus) of one foot (closed) NEC 825.29
    open 825.39
  temporal bone (styloid) — *see* Fracture, skull, base
  tendon — *see* Sprain, by site
  thigh — *see* Fracture, femur, shaft
  thumb (and finger(s)) of one hand (closed) (*see also* Fracture, phalanx, hand) 816.00
    with metacarpal bone(s) of same hand 817.0
    open 817.1
    metacarpal(s) — *see* Fracture, metacarpus
    open 816.10
  thyroid cartilage (closed) 807.5
    open 807.6

Fracture — *continued*
  tibia (closed) 823.80
    with fibula 823.82
      open 823.92
    condyles — *see* Fracture, tibia, upper end
    distal end 824.8
      open 824.9
    epiphysis
      lower 824.8
        open 824.9
      upper — *see* Fracture, tibia, upper end
    head (involving knee joint) — *see* Fracture, tibia, upper end
    intercondyloid eminence — *see* Fracture, tibia, upper end
    involving ankle 824.0
      open 824.9
    malleolus (internal) (medial) 824.0
      open 824.1
    open NEC 823.90
    pathologic 733.16
    proximal end — *see* Fracture, tibia, upper end
    shaft 823.20
      with fibula 823.22
        open 823.32
      open 823.30
    spine — *see* Fracture, tibia, upper end
    stress 733.93
    torus 823.40   ●
      with tibia 823.42
    tuberosity — *see* Fracture, tibia, upper end
    upper end or extremity (condyle) (epiphysis) (head) (spine) (proximal end) (tuberosity) 823.00
      with fibula 823.02
        open 823.12
      open 823.10
  toe(s), of one foot (closed) 826.0
    with bone(s) of same lower limb 827.0
      open 827.1
    open 826.1
  tooth (root) 873.63
    complicated 873.73   ●
  torus   ●
    fibula 823.41   ●
      with tibia 823.42   ●
    radius 813.45   ●
    tibia 823.40   ●
      with fibula 823.42   ●
  trachea (closed) 807.5
    open 807.6
  transverse process — *see* Fracture, vertebra, by site
  trapezium (closed) 814.05
    open 814.15
  trapezoid bone (closed) 814.06
    open 814.16
  trimalleolar (closed) 824.6
    open 824.7
  triquetral (bone) (closed) 814.03
    open 814.13
  trochanter (greater) (lesser) (closed) (*see also* Fracture, femur, neck, by site) 820.20
    open 820.30
  trunk (bones) (closed) 809.0
    open 809.1
  tuberosity (external) — *see* Fracture, by site
  ulna (alone) (closed) 813.82
    with radius NEC 813.83
      open 813.93
    coronoid process (closed) 813.02
      open 813.12
    distal end — *see* Fracture, ulna, lower end
    epiphysis
      lower — *see* Fracture, ulna, lower end
      upper — *see* Fracture, ulna, upper end
    head — *see* Fracture, ulna, lower end
    lower end (distal end) (head) (lower epiphysis) (styloid process) 813.43
      with radius (lower end) 813.44
        open 813.54
      open 813.53
    olecranon process (closed) 813.01
      open 813.11
    open NEC 813.92

Fracture — *continued*
  ulna — *continued*
    pathologic 733.12
    proximal end — *see* Fracture, ulna, upper
      end
    shaft 813.22
      with radius (shaft) 813.23
        open 813.33
      open 813.32
    styloid process — *see* Fracture, ulna, lower
      end
    transverse — *see* Fracture, ulna, by site
    upper end (epiphysis) 813.04
      with radius (upper end) 813.08
        open 813.18
      multiple sites 813.04
        open 813.14
      open 813.14
      specified site NEC 813.04
        open 813.14
  unciform (closed) 814.08
    open 814.18
  vertebra, vertebral (back) (body) (column)
    (neural arch) (pedicle) (spine) (spinous
    process) (transverse process) (closed)
    805.8
    with
      hematomyelia — *see* Fracture, vertebra,
        by site, with spinal cord injury
      injury to
        cauda equina — *see* Fracture,
          vertebra, sacrum, with spinal
          cord injury
        nerve — *see* Fracture, vertebra, by
          site, with spinal cord injury
      paralysis — *see* Fracture, vertebra, by
        site, with spinal cord injury
      paraplegia — *see* Fracture, vertebra, by
        site, with spinal cord injury
      quadriplegia — *see* Fracture, vertebra, by
        site, with spinal cord injury
      spinal concussion — *see* Fracture,
        vertebra, by site, with spinal cord
        injury
      spinal cord injury (closed) NEC 806.8

> Note — Use the following fifth-digit subclassification with categories 806.0-806.3:
>
> C_1-C_4 or unspecified level and D_1-D_6 (T_1-T_6) or unspecified level with
>
> 0   unspecified spinal cord injury
> 1   complete lesion of cord
> 2   anterior cord syndrome
> 3   central cord syndrome
> 4   specified injury NEC
>
> C_5-C_7 level and D_7-D_{12} level with:
>
> 5   unspecified spinal cord injury
> 6   complete lesion of cord
> 7   anterior cord syndrome
> 8   central cord syndrome
> 9   specified injury NEC

        cervical 806.0 ✓5ᵗʰ
          open 806.1 ✓5ᵗʰ
        dorsal, dorsolumbar 806.2 ✓5ᵗʰ
          open 806.3 ✓5ᵗʰ
        open 806.9
        thoracic, thoracolumbar 806.2 ✓5ᵗʰ
          open 806.3 ✓5ᵗʰ
      atlanto-axial — *see* Fracture, vertebra,
        cervical
      cervical (hangman) (teardrop) (closed) 805.00
        with spinal cord injury — *see* Fracture,
          vertebra, with spinal cord injury,
          cervical
        first (atlas) 805.01
          open 805.11
        second (axis) 805.02
          open 805.12
        third 805.03
          open 805.13
        fourth 805.04
          open 805.14

Fracture — *continued*
  vertebra, vertebral — *continued*
    cervical — *continued*
      fifth 805.05
        open 805.15
      sixth 805.06
        open 805.16
      seventh 805.07
        open 805.17
      multiple sites 805.08
        open 805.18
      open 805.10
    coccyx (closed) 805.6
      with spinal cord injury (closed) 806.60
        cauda equina injury 806.62
          complete lesion 806.61
            open 806.71
          open 806.72
        open 806.70
        specified type NEC 806.69
          open 806.79
      open 805.7
    collapsed 733.13
    compression, not due to trauma 733.13
    dorsal (closed) 805.2
      with spinal cord injury — *see* Fracture,
        vertebra, with spinal cord injury,
        dorsal
      open 805.3
    dorsolumbar (closed) 805.2
      with spinal cord injury — *see* Fracture,
        vertebra, with spinal cord injury,
        dorsal
      open 805.3
    due to osteoporosis 733.13
    fetus or newborn 767.4
    lumbar (closed) 805.4
      with spinal cord injury (closed) 806.4
        open 806.5
      open 805.5
    nontraumatic 733.13
    open NEC 805.9
    pathologic (any site) 733.13
    sacrum (closed) 805.6
      with spinal cord injury 806.60
        cauda equina injury 806.62
          complete lesion 806.61
            open 806.71
          open 806.72
        open 806.70
        specified type NEC 806.69
          open 806.79
      open 805.7
    site unspecified (closed) 805.8
      with spinal cord injury (closed) 806.8
        open 806.9
      open 805.9
    stress (any site) 733.95
    thoracic (closed) 805.2
      with spinal cord injury — *see* Fracture,
        vertebra, with spinal cord injury,
        thoracic
      open 805.3
  vertex — *see* Fracture, skull, vault
  vomer (bone) 802.0
    open 802.1
  Wagstaffe's — *see* Fracture, ankle
  wrist (closed) 814.00
    open 814.10
    pathologic 733.12
  xiphoid (process) — *see* Fracture, sternum
  zygoma (zygomatic arch) (closed) 802.4
    open 802.5
Fragile X syndrome 759.83
Fragilitas
  crinium 704.2
  hair 704.2
  ossium 756.51
    with blue sclera 756.51
  unguium 703.8
    congenital 757.5
Fragility
  bone 756.51
    with deafness and blue sclera 756.51
  capillary (hereditary) 287.8

Fragility — *continued*
  hair 704.2
  nails 703.8
Fragmentation — *see* Fracture, by site
Frambesia, frambesial (tropica) (*see also* Yaws)
  102.9
  initial lesion or ulcer 102.0
  primary 102.0
Frambeside
  gummatous 102.4
  of early yaws 102.2
Frambesioma 102.1
Franceschetti's syndrome (mandibulofacial
  dysotosis) 756.0
Francis' disease (*see also* Tularemia) 021.9
Frank's essential thrombocytopenia (*see also*
  Purpura, thrombocytopenic) 287.3
Franklin's disease (heavy chain) 273.2
Fraser's syndrome 759.89
Freckle 709.09
  malignant melanoma in (M8742/3) — *see*
    Melanoma
  melanotic (of Hutchinson) (M8742/2) — *see*
    Neoplasm, skin, in situ
Freeman-Sheldon syndrome 759.89
Freezing 991.9
  specified effect NEC 991.8
Frei's disease (climatic bubo) 099.1
Freiberg's
  disease (osteochondrosis, second metatarsal)
    732.5
  infraction of metatarsal head 732.5
  osteochondrosis 732.5
Fremitus, friction, cardiac 785.3
Frenulum linguae 750.0
Frenum
  external os 752.49
  tongue 750.0
Frequency (urinary) NEC 788.41
  micturition 788.41
  nocturnal 788.43
  psychogenic 306.53
Frey's syndrome (auriculotemporal syndrome)
  350.8
Friction
  burn (*see also* Injury, superficial, by site) 919.0
  fremitus, cardiac 785.3
  precordial 785.3
  sounds, chest 786.7
Friderichsen-Waterhouse syndrome or disease
  036.3
Friedländer's
  B (bacillus) NEC (*see also* condition) 041.3
    sepsis or septicemia 038.49
  disease (endarteritis obliterans) — *see*
    Arteriosclerosis
Friedreich's
  ataxia 334.0
  combined systemic disease 334.0
  disease 333.2
    combined systemic 334.0
  myoclonia 333.2
  sclerosis (spinal cord) 334.0
Friedrich-Erb-Arnold syndrome
  (acropachyderma) 757.39
Frigidity 302.72
  psychic or psychogenic 302.72
Fröhlich's disease or syndrome (adiposogenital
  dystrophy) 253.8
Froin's syndrome 336.8
Frommel's disease 676.6 ✓5ᵗʰ
Frommel-Chiari syndrome 676.6 ✓5ᵗʰ
Frontal — *see also* condition
  lobe syndrome 310.0
Frostbite 991.3
  face 991.0
  foot 991.2
  hand 991.1
  specified site NEC 991.3
Frotteurism 302.89

Frozen 991.9
  pelvis 620.8
  shoulder 726.0
Fructosemia 271.2
Fructosuria (benign) (essential) 271.2
Fuchs'
  black spot (myopic) 360.21
  corneal dystrophy (endothelial) 371.57
  heterochromic cyclitis 364.21
Fucosidosis 271.8
Fugue 780.99 ▲
  hysterical (dissociative) 300.13
  reaction to exceptional stress (transient) 308.1
Fuller Albright's syndrome (osteitis fibrosa disseminata) 756.59
Fuller's earth disease 502
Fulminant, fulminating — see condition
Functional — see condition
Fundus — see also condition
  flavimaculatus 362.76
Fungemia 117.9
Fungus, fungous
  cerebral 348.8
  disease NEC 117.9
  infection — see Infection, fungus
  testis (see also Tuberculosis) 016.5 ✓5ᵗʰ [608.81]
Funiculitis (acute) 608.4
  chronic 608.4
  endemic 608.4
  gonococcal (acute) 098.14
    chronic or duration of 2 months or over 098.34
  tuberculous (see also Tuberculosis) 016.5 ✓5ᵗʰ
Funnel
  breast (acquired) 738.3
    congenital 754.81
    late effect of rickets 268.1
  chest (acquired) 738.3
    congenital 754.81
    late effect of rickets 268.1
  pelvis (acquired) 738.6
    with disproportion (fetopelvic) 653.3 ✓5ᵗʰ
      affecting fetus or newborn 763.1
      causing obstructed labor 660.1 ✓5ᵗʰ
        affecting fetus or newborn 763.1
    congenital 755.69
    tuberculous (see also Tuberculosis) 016.9 ✓5ᵗʰ
F.U.O. (see also Pyrexia) 780.6
Furfur 690.18
  microsporon 111.0
Furor, paroxysmal (idiopathic) (see also Epilepsy) 345.8 ✓5ᵗʰ
Furriers' lung 495.8
Furrowed tongue 529.5
  congenital 750.13
Furrowing nail(s) (transverse) 703.8
  congenital 757.5
Furuncle 680.9
  abdominal wall 680.2
  ankle 680.6
  anus 680.5
  arm (any part, above wrist) 680.3
  auditory canal, external 680.0
  axilla 680.3
  back (any part) 680.2
  breast 680.2
  buttock 680.5
  chest wall 680.2
  corpus cavernosum 607.2
  ear (any part) 680.0
  eyelid 373.13
  face (any part, except eye) 680.0
  finger (any) 680.4
  flank 680.2
  foot (any part) 680.7
  forearm 680.3
  gluteal (region) 680.5
  groin 680.2
  hand (any part) 680.4
  head (any part, except face) 680.8
  heel 680.7

Furuncle — continued
  hip 680.6
  kidney (see also Abscess, kidney) 590.2
  knee 680.6
  labium (majus) (minus) 616.4
  lacrimal
    gland (see also Dacryoadenitis) 375.00
    passages (duct) (sac) (see also Dacryocystitis) 375.30
  leg, any part except foot 680.6
  malignant 022.0
  multiple sites 680.9
  neck 680.1
  nose (external) (septum) 680.0
  orbit 376.01
  partes posteriores 680.5
  pectoral region 680.2
  penis 607.2
  perineum 680.2
  pinna 680.0
  scalp (any part) 680.8
  scrotum 608.4
  seminal vesicle 608.0
  shoulder 680.3
  skin NEC 680.9
  specified site NEC 680.8
  spermatic cord 608.4
  temple (region) 680.0
  testis 604.90
  thigh 680.6
  thumb 680.4
  toe (any) 680.7
  trunk 680.2
  tunica vaginalis 608.4
  umbilicus 680.2
  upper arm 680.3
  vas deferens 608.4
  vulva 616.4
  wrist 680.4
Furunculosis (see also Furuncle) 680.9
  external auditory meatus 680.0 [380.13]
Fusarium (infection) 118
Fusion, fused (congenital)
  anal (with urogenital canal) 751.5
  aorta and pulmonary artery 745.0
  astragaloscaphoid 755.67
  atria 745.5
  atrium and ventricle 745.69
  auditory canal 744.02
  auricles, heart 745.5
  binocular, with defective stereopsis 368.33
  bone 756.9
  cervical spine — see Fusion, spine
  choanal 748.0
  commissure, mitral valve 746.5
  cranial sutures, premature 756.0
  cusps, heart valve NEC 746.89
    mitral 746.5
    tricuspid 746.89
  ear ossicles 744.04
  fingers (see also Syndactylism, fingers) 755.11
  hymen 752.42
  hymeno-urethral 599.89
    causing obstructed labor 660.1 ✓5ᵗʰ
      affecting fetus or newborn 763.1
  joint (acquired) — see also Ankylosis
    congenital 755.8
  kidneys (incomplete) 753.3
  labium (majus) (minus) 752.49
  larynx and trachea 748.3
  limb 755.8
    lower 755.69
    upper 755.59
  lobe, lung 748.5
  lumbosacral (acquired) 724.6
    congenital 756.15
    surgical V45.4
  nares (anterior) (posterior) 748.0
  nose, nasal 748.0
  nostril(s) 748.0
  organ or site NEC — see Anomaly, specified type NEC
  ossicles 756.9
    auditory 744.04
  pulmonary valve segment 746.02

Fusion, fused — continued
  pulmonic cusps 746.02
  ribs 756.3
  sacroiliac (acquired) (joint) 724.6
    congenital 755.69
    surgical V45.4
  skull, imperfect 756.0
  spine (acquired) 724.9
    arthrodesis status V45.4
    congenital (vertebra) 756.15
    postoperative status V45.4
  sublingual duct with submaxillary duct at opening in mouth 750.26
  talonavicular (bar) 755.67
  teeth, tooth 520.2
  testes 752.8
  toes (see also Syndactylism, toes) 755.13
  trachea and esophagus 750.3
  twins 759.4
  urethral-hymenal 599.89
  vagina 752.49
  valve cusps — see Fusion, cusps, heart valve
  ventricles, heart 745.4
  vertebra (arch) — see Fusion, spine
  vulva 752.49
Fusospirillosis (mouth) (tongue) (tonsil) 101
Fussy infant (baby) 780.91 ●

G

Gafsa boil 085.1

Gain, weight (abnormal) (excessive) (*see also*
Weight, gain) 783.1

Gaisböck's disease or syndrome
(polycythemia hypertonica) 289.0

Gait
abnormality 781.2
  hysterical 300.11
ataxic 781.2
  hysterical 300.11
disturbance 781.2
  hysterical 300.11
paralytic 781.2
scissor 781.2
spastic 781.2
staggering 781.2
  hysterical 300.11

Galactocele (breast) (infected) 611.5
puerperal, postpartum 676.8 ✓5ᵗʰ

Galactophoritis 611.0
puerperal, postpartum 675.2 ✓5ᵗʰ

Galactorrhea 676.6 ✓5ᵗʰ
not associated with childbirth 611.6

Galactosemia (classic) (congenital) 271.1

Galactosuria 271.1

Galacturia 791.1
bilharziasis 120.0

Galen's vein — *see* condition

Gallbladder — *see also* condition
acute (*see also* Disease, gallbladder) 575.0

Gall duct — *see* condition

Gallop rhythm 427.89

Gallstone (cholemic) (colic) (impacted) — *see also*
Cholelithiasis
causing intestinal obstruction 560.31

Gambling, pathological 312.31

Gammaloidosis 277.3

Gammopathy 273.9
macroglobulinemia 273.3
monoclonal (benign) (essential) (idiopathic)
  (with lymphoplasmacytic dyscrasia) 273.1

Gamna's disease (siderotic splenomegaly) 289.51

Gampsodactylia (congenital) 754.71

Gamstorp's disease (adynamia episodica
hereditaria) 359.3

Gandy-Nanta disease (siderotic splenomegaly)
289.51

**Gang activity, without manifest psychiatric
disorder** V71.09
adolescent V71.02
adult V71.01
child V71.02

Gangliocytoma (M9490/0) — *see* Neoplasm,
connective tissue, benign

Ganglioglioma (M9505/1) — *see* Neoplasm, by
site, uncertain behavior

Ganglion 727.43
joint 727.41
of yaws (early) (late) 102.6
periosteal (*see also* Periostitis) 730.3 ✓5ᵗʰ
tendon sheath (compound) (diffuse) 727.42
tuberculous (*see also* Tuberculosis) 015.9 ✓5ᵗʰ

Ganglioneuroblastoma (M9490/3) — *see*
Neoplasm, connective tissue, malignant

Ganglioneuroma (M9490/0) — *see also*
Neoplasm, connective tissue, benign
malignant (M9490/3) — *see* Neoplasm,
connective tissue, malignant

Ganglioneuromatosis (M9491/0) — *see*
Neoplasm, connective tissue, benign

Ganglionitis
fifth nerve (*see also* Neuralgia, trigeminal)
  350.1
gasserian 350.1
geniculate 351.1
  herpetic 053.11
  newborn 767.5
herpes zoster 053.11
herpetic geniculate (Hunt's syndrome) 053.11

Gangliosidosis 330.1

Gangosa 102.5

Gangrene, gangrenous (anemia) (artery) (cellulitis)
(dermatitis) (dry) (infective) (moist)
(pemphigus) (septic) (skin) (stasis) (ulcer)
785.4
with
  arteriosclerosis (native artery) 440.24
    bypass graft 440.30
      autologous vein 440.31
      nonautologous biological 440.32
  diabetes (mellitus) 250.7 ✓5ᵗʰ [785.4]
abdomen (wall) 785.4
  arteriosclerosis 440.29 [785.4]
adenitis 683
alveolar 526.5
angina 462
  diphtheritic 032.0
anus 569.49
appendices epiploicae — *see* Gangrene,
  mesentery
appendix — *see* Appendicitis, acute
arteriosclerotic — *see* Arteriosclerosis, with,
  gangrene
auricle 785.4
Bacillus welchii (*see also* Gangrene, gas) 040.0
bile duct (*see also* Cholangitis) 576.8
bladder 595.89
bowel — *see* Gangrene, intestine
cecum — *see* Gangrene, intestine
Clostridium perfringens or welchii (*see also*
  Gangrene, gas) 040.0
colon — *see* Gangrene, intestine
connective tissue 785.4
cornea 371.40
corpora cavernosa (infective) 607.2
  noninfective 607.89
cutaneous, spreading 785.4
decubital 707.0 [785.4]
diabetic (any site) 250.7 ✓5ᵗʰ [785.4]
dropsical 785.4
emphysematous (*see also* Gangrene, gas) 040.0
epidemic (ergotized grain) 988.2
epididymis (infectional) (*see also* Epididymitis)
  604.99
erysipelas (*see also* Erysipelas) 035
extremity (lower) (upper) 785.4
gallbladder or duct (*see also* Cholecystitis,
  acute) 575.0
gas (bacillus) 040.0
  with
    abortion — *see* Abortion, by type, with
      sepsis
    ectopic pregnancy (*see also* categories
      633.0-633.9) 639.0
    molar pregnancy (*see also* categories 630-
      632) 639.0
  following
    abortion 639.0
    ectopic or molar pregnancy 639.0
  puerperal, postpartum, childbirth 670 ✓4ᵗʰ
glossitis 529.0
gum 523.8
hernia — *see* Hernia, by site, with gangrene
hospital noma 528.1
intestine, intestinal (acute) (hemorrhagic)
  (massive) 557.0
  with
    hernia — *see* Hernia, by site, with
      gangrene
    mesenteric embolism or infarction 557.0
    obstruction (*see also* Obstruction,
      intestine) 560.9
laryngitis 464.00
  with obstruction 464.01
liver 573.8
lung 513.0
  spirochetal 104.8
lymphangitis 457.2
Meleney's (cutaneous) 686.09
mesentery 557.0
  with
    embolism or infarction 557.0
    intestinal obstruction (*see also*
      Obstruction, intestine) 560.9
mouth 528.1
noma 528.1
orchitis 604.90

Gangrene, gangrenous — *continued*
ovary (*see also* Salpingo-oophoritis) 614.2
pancreas 577.0
penis (infectional) 607.2
  noninfective 607.89
perineum 785.4
pharynx 462
septic 034.0
pneumonia 513.0
Pott's 440.24
presenile 443.1
pulmonary 513.0
pulp, tooth 522.1
quinsy 475
Raynaud's (symmetric gangrene) 443.0 [785.4]
rectum 569.49
retropharyngeal 478.24
rupture — *see* Hernia, by site, with gangrene
scrotum 608.4
  noninfective 608.83
senile 440.24
sore throat 462
spermatic cord 608.4
  noninfective 608.89
spine 785.4
spirochetal NEC 104.8
spreading cutaneous 785.4
stomach 537.89
stomatitis 528.1
symmetrical 443.0 [785.4]
testis (infectional) (*see also* Orchitis) 604.99
  noninfective 608.89
throat 462
  diphtheritic 032.0
thyroid (gland) 246.8
tonsillitis (acute) 463
tooth (pulp) 522.1
tuberculous NEC (*see also* Tuberculosis)
  011.9 ✓5ᵗʰ
tunica vaginalis 608.4
  noninfective 608.89
umbilicus 785.4
uterus (*see also* Endometritis) 615.9
uvulitis 528.3
vas deferens 608.4
  noninfective 608.89
vulva (*see also* Vulvitis) 616.10

Gannister disease (occupational) 502
with tuberculosis — *see* Tuberculosis,
  pulmonary

Ganser's syndrome, hysterical 300.16

Gardner-Diamond syndrome (autoerythrocyte
sensitization) 287.2

Gargoylism 277.5

Garré's
disease (*see also* Osteomyelitis) 730.1 ✓5ᵗʰ
osteitis (sclerosing) (*see also* Osteomyelitis)
  730.1 ✓5ᵗʰ
osteomyelitis (*see also* Osteomyelitis) 730.1 ✓5ᵗʰ

Garrod's pads, knuckle 728.79

Gartner's duct
cyst 752.11
persistent 752.11

Gas
asphyxia, asphyxiation, inhalation, poisoning,
  suffocation NEC 987.9
  specified gas — *see* Table of Drugs and
    Chemicals
bacillus gangrene or infection — *see* Gas,
  gangrene
cyst, mesentery 568.89
excessive 787.3
gangrene 040.0
  with
    abortion — *see* Abortion, by type, with
      sepsis
    ectopic pregnancy (*see also* categories
      633.0-633.9) 639.0
    molar pregnancy (*see also* categories 630-
      632) 639.0
  following
    abortion 639.0
    ectopic or molar pregnancy 639.0
  puerperal, postpartum, childbirth 670 ✓4ᵗʰ
on stomach 787.3
pains 787.3

Gastradenitis 535.0 E
Gastralgia 536.8
  psychogenic 307.89
Gastrectasis, gastrectasia 536.1
  psychogenic 306.4
Gastric — *see* condition
Gastrinoma (M8153/1)
  malignant (M8153/3)
    pancreas 157.4
    specified site NEC — *see* Neoplasm, by site,
      malignant
    unspecified site 157.4
  specified site — *see* Neoplasm, by site,
    uncertain behavior
  unspecified site 235.5
Gastritis 535.5 ✓5ᵗʰ

> *Note* — Use the following fifth-digit
> subclassification for category 535:
>
>   0   *without mention of hemorrhage*
>   1   *with hemorrhage*

  acute 535.0 ✓5ᵗʰ
  alcoholic 535.3 ✓5ᵗʰ
  allergic 535.4 ✓5ᵗʰ
  antral 535.4 ✓5ᵗʰ
  atrophic 535.1 ✓5ᵗʰ
  atrophic-hyperplastic 535.1 ✓5ᵗʰ
  bile-induced 535.4 ✓5ᵗʰ
  catarrhal 535.0 ✓5ᵗʰ
  chronic (atrophic) 535.1 ✓5ᵗʰ
  cirrhotic 535.4 ✓5ᵗʰ
  corrosive (acute) 535.4 ✓5ᵗʰ
  dietetic 535.4 ✓5ᵗʰ
  due to diet deficiency 269.9 [535.4]
  eosinophilic 535.4 ✓5ᵗʰ
  erosive 535.4 ✓5ᵗʰ
  follicular 535.4 ✓5ᵗʰ
    chronic 535.1 ✓5ᵗʰ
  giant hypertrophic 535.2 ✓5ᵗʰ
  glandular 535.4 ✓5ᵗʰ
    chronic 535.1 ✓5ᵗʰ
  hypertrophic (mucosa) 535.2 ✓5ᵗʰ
    chronic giant 211.1
  irritant 535.4 ✓5ᵗʰ
  nervous 306.4
  phlegmonous 535.0 ✓5ᵗʰ
  psychogenic 306.4
  sclerotic 535.4 ✓5ᵗʰ
  spastic 536.8
  subacute 535.0 ✓5ᵗʰ
  superficial 535.4 ✓5ᵗʰ
  suppurative 535.0 ✓5ᵗʰ
  toxic 535.4 ✓5ᵗʰ
  tuberculous (*see also* Tuberculosis) 017.9 ✓5ᵗʰ
Gastrocarcinoma (M8010/3) 151.9
Gastrocolic — *see* condition
Gastrocolitis — *see* Enteritis
Gastrodisciasis 121.8
Gastroduodenitis (*see also* Gastritis) 535.5 ✓5ᵗʰ
  catarrhal 535.0 ✓5ᵗʰ
  infectional 535.0 ✓5ᵗʰ
  virus, viral 008.8
    specified type NEC 008.69
Gastrodynia 536.8
Gastroenteritis (acute) (catarrhal) (congestive)
  (hemorrhagic) (noninfectious) (*see also*
  Enteritis) 558.9
  aertrycke infection 003.0
  allergic 558.3
  chronic 558.9
    ulcerative (*see also* Colitis, ulcerative) 556.9
  dietetic 558.9
  due to
    food poisoning (*see also* Poisoning, food)
      005.9
    radiation 558.1
  epidemic 009.0
  functional 558.9
  infectious (*see also* Enteritis, due to, by
    organism) 009.0
    presumed 009.1
  salmonella 003.0
  septic (*see also* Enteritis, due to, by organism)
    009.0

Gastroenteritis — *continued*
  toxic 558.2
  tuberculous (*see also* Tuberculosis) 014.8 ✓5ᵗʰ
  ulcerative (*see also* Colitis, ulcerative) 556.9
  viral NEC 008.8
    specified type NEC 008.69
  zymotic 009.0
Gastroenterocolitis — *see* Enteritis
Gastroenteropathy, protein-losing 579.8
Gastroenteroptosis 569.89
Gastroesophageal laceration-hemorrhage
  syndrome 530.7
Gastroesophagitis 530.19
Gastrohepatitis (*see also* Gastritis) 535.5 ✓5ᵗʰ
Gastrointestinal — *see* condition
Gastrojejunal — *see* condition
Gastrojejunitis (*see also* Gastritis) 535.5 ✓5ᵗʰ
Gastrojejunocolic — *see* condition
Gastroliths 537.89
Gastromalacia 537.89
Gastroparalysis 536.8
  diabetic 250.6 ✓5ᵗʰ [536.3]
Gastroparesis 536.3
  diabetic 250.6 ✓5ᵗʰ [536.3]
Gastropathy, exudative 579.8
Gastroptosis 537.5
Gastrorrhagia 578.0
Gastorrhea 536.8
  psychogenic 306.4
Gastroschisis (congenital) 756.79
  acquired 569.89
Gastrospasm (neurogenic) (reflex) 536.8
  neurotic 306.4
  psychogenic 306.4
Gastrostaxis 578.0
Gastrostenosis 537.89
Gastrostomy
  attention to V55.1
  complication 536.40
    specified type 536.49
  infection 536.41
  malfunctioning 536.42
  status V44.1
Gastrosuccorrhea (continous) (intermittent) 536.8
  neurotic 306.4
  psychogenic 306.4
Gaucher's
  disease (adult) (cerebroside lipidosis) (infantile)
    272.7
  hepatomegaly 272.7
  splenomegaly (cerebroside lipidosis) 272.7
Gayet's disease (superior hemorrhagic
  polioencephalitis) 265.1
Gayet-Wernicke's syndrome (superior
  hemorrhagic polioencephalitis) 265.1
Gee (-Herter) (-Heubner) (-Thaysen) disease or
  syndrome (nontropical sprue) 579.0
Gélineau's syndrome 347
Gemination, teeth 520.2
Gemistocytoma (M9411/3)
  specified site — *see* Neoplasm, by site,
    malignant
  unspecified site 191.9
General, generalized — *see* condtion
Genital — *see* condition
Genito-anorectal syndrome 099.1
Genitourinary system — *see* condition
Genu
  congenital 755.64
  extrorsum (acquired) 736.42
    congenital 755.64
    late effects of rickets 268.1
  introrsum (acquired) 736.41
    congenital 755.64
    late effects of rickets 268.1
  rachitic (old) 268.1
  recurvatum (acquired) 736.5
    congenital 754.40
      with dislocation of knee 754.41
    late effects or rickets 268.1

Genu — *continued*
  valgum (acquired) (knock-knee) 736.41
    congenital 755.64
    late effects of rickets 268.1
  varum (acquired) (bowleg) 736.42
    congenital 755.64
    late effect of rickets 268.1
Geographic tongue 529.1
Geophagia 307.52
Geotrichosis 117.9
  intestine 117.9
  lung 117.9
  mouth 117.9
Gephyrophobia 300.29
Gerbode defect 745.4
Gerhardt's
  disease (erythromelalgia) 443.89
  syndrome (vocal cord paralysis) 478.30
Gerlier's disease (epidemic vertigo) 078.81
German measles 056.9
  exposure to V01.4
Germinoblastoma (diffuse) (M9614/3) 202.8 ✓5ᵗʰ
  follicular (M9692/3) 202.0 ✓5ᵗʰ
Germinoma (M9064/3) — *see* Neoplasm, by site,
  malignant
Gerontoxon 371.41
Gerstmann's syndrome (finger agnosia) 784.69
Gestation (period) — *see also* Pregnancy
  ectopic NEC (*see also* Pregnancy, ectopic)
    633.90 ▲
    with intrauterine pregnancy 633.91 ●
Gestational proteinuria 646.2 ✓5ᵗʰ
  with hypertension — *see* Toxemia, of pregnancy
Ghon tubercle primary infection (*see also*
  Tuberculosis) 010.0 ✓5ᵗʰ
Ghost
  teeth 520.4
  vessels, cornea 370.64
Ghoul hand 102.3
Giant
  cell
    epulis 523.8
    peripheral (gingiva) 523.8
    tumor, tendon sheath 727.02
  colon (congenital) 751.3
  esophagus (congenital) 750.4
  kidney 753.3
  urticaria 995.1
    hereditary 277.6
Giardia lamblia infestation 007.1
Giardiasis 007.1
Gibert's disease (pityriasis rosea) 696.3
Gibraltar fever — *see* Brucellosis
Giddiness 780.4
  hysterical 300.11
  psychogenic 306.9
Gierke's disease (glycogenosis I) 271.0
Gigantism (cerebral) (hypophyseal) (pituitary)
  253.0
Gilbert's disease or cholemia (familial
  nonhemolytic jaundice) 277.4
Gilchrist's disease (North American
  blastomycosis) 116.0
Gilford (-Hutchinson) disease or syndrome
  (progeria) 259.8
Gilles de la Tourette's disease (motor-verbal tic)
  307.23
Gillespie's syndrome (dysplasia
  oculodentodigitalis) 759.89
Gingivitis 523.1
  acute 523.0
    necrotizing 101
  catarrhal 523.0
  chronic 523.1
  desquamative 523.1
  expulsiva 523.4
  hyperplastic 523.1
  marginal, simple 523.1
  necrotizing, acute 101
  pellagrous 265.2
  ulcerative 523.1
    acute necrotizing 101

Gastradenitis — Gingivitis

✓4ᵗʰ Fourth-digit Required   ✓5ᵗʰ Fifth-digit Required   ▶◀ Revised Text   ● New Line   ▲ Revised Code

Gingivitis — *continued*
Vincent's 101
Gingivoglossitis 529.0
Gingivopericementitis 523.4
Gingivosis 523.1
Gingivostomatitis 523.1
herpetic 054.2
Giovannini's disease 117.9
Gland, glandular — *see* condition
Glanders 024
**Glanzmann (-Naegeli) disease or
thrombasthenia** 287.1
Glassblowers' disease 527.1
Glaucoma (capsular) (inflammatory)
(noninflammatory) (primary) 365.9
with increased episcleral venous pressure
365.82
absolute 360.42
acute 365.22
narrow angle 365.22
secondary 365.60
angle closure 365.20
acute 365.22
chronic 365.23
intermittent 365.21
interval 365.21
residual stage 365.24
subacute 365.21
borderline 365.00
chronic 365.11
noncongestive 365.11
open angle 365.11
simple 365.11
closed angle — *see* Glaucoma, angle closure
congenital 743.20
associated with other eye anomalies 743.22
simple 743.21
congestive — *see* Glaucoma, narrow angle
corticosteroid-induced (glaucomatous stage)
365.31
residual stage 365.32
hemorrhagic 365.60
hypersecretion 365.81
in or with
aniridia 743.45 *[365.42]*
Axenfeld's anomaly 743.44 *[365.41]*
concussion of globe 921.3 *[365.65]*
congenital syndromes NEC 759.89 *[365.44]*
dislocation of lens
anterior 379.33 *[365.59]*
posterior 379.34 *[365.59]*
disorder of lens NEC 365.59
epithelial down-growth 364.61 *[365.64]*
glaucomatocyclitic crisis 364.22 *[365.62]*
hypermature cataract 366.18 *[365.51]*
hyphema 364.41 *[365.63]*
inflammation, ocular 365.62
iridocyclitis 364.3 *[365.62]*
iris
anomalies NEC 743.46 *[365.42]*
atrophy, essential 364.51 *[365.42]*
bombé 364.74 *[365.61]*
rubeosis 364.42 *[365.63]*
microcornea 743.41 *[365.43]*
neurofibromatosis 237.71 *[365.44]*
ocular
cysts NEC 365.64
disorders NEC 365.60
trauma 365.65
tumors NEC 365.64
postdislocation of lens
anterior 379.33 *[365.59]*
posterior 379.34 *[365.59]*
pseudoexfoliation of capsule 366.11 *[365.52]*
pupillary block or seclusion 364.74 *[365.61]*
recession of chamber angle 364.77 *[365.65]*
retinal vein occlusion 362.35 *[365.63]*
Rieger's anomaly or syndrome 743.44
[365.41]
rubeosis of iris 364.42 *[365.63]*
seclusion of pupil 364.74 *[365.61]*
spherophakia 743.36 *[365.59]*
Sturge-Weber (-Dimitri) syndrome
759.6 *[365.44]*
systemic syndrome NEC 365.44

Glaucoma — *continued*
in or with — *continued*
tumor of globe 365.64
vascular disorders NEC 365.63
infantile 365.14
congenital 743.20
associated with other eye anomalies
743.22
simple 743.21
juvenile 365.14
low tension 365.12
malignant 365.83   ▲
narrow angle (primary) 365.20
acute 365.22
chronic 365.23
intermittent 365.21
interval 365.21
residual stage 365.24
subacute 365.21
newborn 743.20
associated with other eye anomalies 743.22
simple 743.21
noncongestive (chronic) 365.11
nonobstructive (chronic) 365.11
obstructive 365.60
due to lens changes 365.59
open angle 365.10
with
borderline intraocular pressure 365.01
cupping of optic discs 365.01
primary 365.11
residual stage 365.15
phacolytic 365.51
with hypermature cataract 366.18 *[365.51]*
pigmentary 365.13
postinfectious 365.60
pseudoexfoliation 365.52
with pseudoexfoliation of capsule
366.11 *[365.52]*
secondary NEC 365.60
simple (chronic) 365.11
simplex 365.11
steroid responders 365.03
suspect 365.00
syphilitic 095.8
traumatic NEC 365.65
newborn 767.8
tuberculous (*see also* Tuberculosis)
017.3 ✓5ᵗʰ *[365.62]*
wide angle (*see also* Glaucoma, open angle)
365.10
Glaucomatous flecks (subcapsular) 366.31
Glazed tongue 529.4
Gleet 098.2
Glénard's disease or syndrome (enteroptosis)
569.89
Glinski-Simmonds syndrome (pituitary cachexia)
253.2
Glioblastoma (multiforme) (M9440/3)
with sarcomatous component (M9442/3)
specified site — *see* Neoplasm, by site,
malignant
unspecified site 191.9
giant cell (M9441/3)
specified site — *see* Neoplasm, by site,
malignant
unspecified site 191.9
specified site — *see* Neoplasm, by site,
malignant
unspecified site 191.9
Glioma (malignant) (M9380/3)
astrocytic (M9400/3)
specified site — *see* Neoplasm, by site,
malignant
unspecified site 191.9
mixed (M9382/3)
specified site — *see* Neoplasm, by site,
malignant
unspecified site 191.9
nose 748.1
specified site NEC — *see* Neoplasm, by site,
malignant
subependymal (M9383/1) 237.5
unspecified site 191.9
Gliomatosis cerebri (M9381/3) 191.0

Glioneuroma (M9505/1) — *see* Neoplasm, by site,
uncertain behavior
Gliosarcoma (M9380/3)
specified site — *see* Neoplasm, by site,
malignant
unspecified site 191.9
Gliosis (cerebral) 349.89
spinal 336.0
Glisson's
cirrhosis — *see* Cirrhosis, portal
disease (*see also* Rickets) 268.0
Glissonitis 573.3
Globinuria 791.2
Globus 306.4
hystericus 300.11
Glomangioma (M8712/0) (*see also* Hemangioma)
228.00
Glomangiosarcoma (M8710/3) — *see* Neoplasm,
connective tissue, malignant
Glomerular nephritis (*see also* Nephritis) 583.9
Glomerulitis (*see also* Nephritis) 583.9
Glomerulonephritis (*see also* Nephritis) 583.9
with
edema (*see also* Nephrosis) 581.9
lesion of
exudative nephritis 583.89
interstitial nephritis (diffuse) (focal)
583.89
necrotizing glomerulitis 583.4
acute 580.4
chronic 582.4
renal necrosis 583.9
cortical 583.6
medullary 583.7
specified pathology NEC 583.89
acute 580.89
chronic 582.89
necrosis, renal 583.9
cortical 583.6
medullary (papillary) 583.7
specified pathology or lesion NEC 583.89
acute 580.9
with
exudative nephritis 580.89
interstitial nephritis (diffuse) (focal)
580.89
necrotizing glomerulitis 580.4
extracapillary with epithelial crescents 580.4
poststreptococcal 580.0
proliferative (diffuse) 580.0
rapidly progressive 580.4
specified pathology NEC 580.89
arteriolar (*see also* Hypertension, kidney)
403.90
arteriosclerotic (*see also* Hypertension, kidney)
403.90
ascending (*see also* Pyelitis) 590.80
basement membrane NEC 583.89
with
pulmonary hemorrhage (Goodpasture's
syndrome) 446.21 *[583.81]*
chronic 582.9
with
exudative nephritis 582.89
interstitial nephritis (diffuse) (focal)
582.89
necrotizing glomerulitis 582.4
specified pathology or lesion NEC 582.89
endothelial 582.2
extracapillary with epithelial crescents 582.4
hypocomplementemic persistent 582.2
lobular 582.2
membranoproliferative 582.2
membranous 582.1
and proliferative (mixed) 582.2
sclerosing 582.1
mesangiocapillary 582.2
mixed membranous and proliferative 582.2
proliferative (diffuse) 582.0
rapidly progressive 582.4
sclerosing 582.1
cirrhotic — *see* Sclerosis, renal
desquamative — *see* Nephrosis

Glomerulonephritis — Goldscheider's disease

Glomerulonephritis (*see also* Nephritis) — *continued*
  due to or associated with
    amyloidosis 277.3 *[583.81]*
      with nephrotic syndrome 277.3 *[581.81]*
      chronic 277.3 *[582.81]*
    diabetes mellitus 250.4 ✓5ᵗʰ *[583.81]*
      with nephrotic syndrome
        250.4 ✓5ᵗʰ *[581.81]*
    diphtheria 032.89 *[580.81]*
    gonococcal infection (acute) 098.19 *[583.81]*
      chronic or duration of 2 months or over 098.39 *[583.81]*
    infectious hepatitis 070.9 *[580.81]*
    malaria (with nephrotic syndrome) 084.9 *[581.81]*
    mumps 072.79 *[580.81]*
    polyarteritis (nodosa) (with nephrotic syndrome) 446.0 *[581.81]*
    specified pathology NEC 583.89
      acute 580.89
      chronic 582.89
    streptotrichosis 039.8 *[583.81]*
    subacute bacterial endocarditis 421.0 *[580.81]*
    syphilis (late) 095.4
      congenital 090.5 *[583.81]*
      early 091.69 *[583.81]*
    systemic lupus erythematosus 710.0 *[583.81]*
      with nephrotic syndrome 710.0 *[581.81]*
      chronic 710.0 *[582.81]*
    tuberculosis (*see also* Tuberculosis) 016.0 ✓5ᵗʰ *[583.81]*
    typhoid fever 002.0 *[580.81]*
  extracapillary with epithelial crescents 583.4
    acute 580.4
    chronic 582.4
  exudative 583.89
    acute 580.89
    chronic 582.89
  focal (*see also* Nephritis) 583.9
    embolic 580.4
  granular 582.89
  granulomatous 582.89
  hydremic (*see also* Nephrosis) 581.9
  hypocomplementemic persistent 583.2
    with nephrotic syndrome 581.2
    chronic 582.2
  immune complex NEC 583.89
  infective (*see also* Pyelitis) 590.80
  interstitial (diffuse) (focal) 583.89
    with nephrotic syndrome 581.89
    acute 580.89
    chronic 582.89
  latent or quiescent 582.9
  lobular 583.2
    with nephrotic syndrome 581.2
    chronic 582.2
  membranoproliferative 583.2
    with nephrotic syndrome 581.2
    chronic 582.2
  membranous 583.1
    with nephrotic syndrome 581.1
    and proliferative (mixed) 583.2
      with nephrotic syndrome 581.2
      chronic 582.2
    chronic 582.1
    sclerosing 582.1
      with nephrotic syndrome 581.1
  mesangiocapillary 583.2
    with nephrotic syndrome 581.2
    chronic 582.2
  minimal change 581.3
  mixed membranous and proliferative 583.2
    with nephrotic syndrome 581.2
    chronic 582.2
  necrotizing 583.4
    acute 580.4
    chronic 582.4
  nephrotic (*see also* Nephrosis) 581.9
  old — *see* Glomerulonephritis, chronic
  parenchymatous 581.89
  poststreptococcal 580.0
  proliferative (diffuse) 583.0
    with nephrotic syndrome 581.0
    acute 580.0
    chronic 582.0

Glomerulonephritis (*see also* Nephritis) — *continued*
  purulent (*see also* Pyelitis) 590.80
  quiescent — *see* Nephritis, chronic
  rapidly progressive 583.4
    acute 580.4
    chronic 582.4
  sclerosing membranous (chronic) 582.1
    with nephrotic syndrome 581.1
  septic (*see also* Pyelitis) 590.80
  specified pathology or lesion NEC 583.89
    with nephrotic syndrome 581.89
    acute 580.89
    chronic 582.89
  suppurative (acute) (disseminated) (*see also* Pyelitis) 590.80
  toxic — *see* Nephritis, acute
  tubal, tubular — *see* Nephrosis, tubular
  type II (Ellis) — *see* Nephrosis
  vascular — *see* Hypertension, kidney
Glomerulosclerosis (*see also* Sclerosis, renal) 587
  focal 582.1
    with nephrotic syndrome 581.1
  intercapillary (nodular) (with diabetes) 250.4 ✓5ᵗʰ *[581.81]*
Glossagra 529.6
Glossalgia 529.6
Glossitis 529.0
  areata exfoliativa 529.1
  atrophic 529.4
  benign migratory 529.1
  gangrenous 529.0
  Hunter's 529.4
  median rhomboid 529.2
  Moeller's 529.4
  pellagrous 265.2
Glossocele 529.8
Glossodynia 529.6
  exfoliativa 529.4
Glossoncus 529.8
Glossophytia 529.3
Glossoplegia 529.8
Glossoptosis 529.8
Glossopyrosis 529.6
Glossotrichia 529.3
Glossy skin 710.9
Glottis — *see* condition
Glottitis — *see* Glossitis
Glucagonoma (M8152/0)
  malignant (M8152/3)
    pancreas 157.4
    specified site NEC — *see* Neoplasm, by site, malignant
    unspecified site 157.4
  pancreas 211.7
  specified site NEC — *see* Neoplasm, by site, benign
  unspecified site 211.7
Glucoglycinuria 270.7
Glue ear syndrome 381.20
Glue sniffing (airplane glue) (*see also* Dependence) 304.6 ✓5ᵗʰ
Glycinemia (with methylmalonic acidemia) 270.7
Glycinuria (renal) (with ketosis) 270.0
Glycogen
  infiltration (*see also* Disease, glycogen storage) 271.0
  storage disease (*see also* Disease, glycogen storage) 271.0
Glycogenosis (*see also* Disease, glycogen storage) 271.0
  cardiac 271.0 *[425.7]*
  Cori, types I-VII 271.0
  diabetic, secondary 250.8 ✓5ᵗʰ *[259.8]*
  diffuse (with hepatic cirrhosis) 271.0
  generalized 271.0
  glucose-6-phosphatase deficiency 271.0
  hepatophosphorylase deficiency 271.0
  hepatorenal 271.0
  myophosphorylase deficiency 271.0
Glycopenia 251.2
Glycoprolinuria 270.8

Glycosuria 791.5
  renal 271.4
Gnathostoma (spinigerum) (infection) (infestation) 128.1
  wandering swellings from 128.1
Gnathostomiasis 128.1
Goiter (adolescent) (colloid) (diffuse) (dipping) (due to iodine deficiency) (endemic) (euthyroid) (heart) (hyperplastic) (internal) (intrathoracic) (juvenile) (mixed type) (nonendemic) (parenchymatous) (plunging) (sporadic) (subclavicular) (substernal) 240.9
  with
    hyperthyroidism (recurrent) (*see also* Goiter, toxic) 242.0 ✓5ᵗʰ
    thyrotoxicosis (*see also* Goiter, toxic) 242.0 ✓5ᵗʰ
  adenomatous (*see also* Goiter, nodular) 241.9
  cancerous (M8000/3) 193
  complicating pregnancy, childbirth, or puerperium 648.1 ✓5ᵗʰ
  congenital 246.1
  cystic (*see also* Goiter, nodular) 241.9
  due to enzyme defect in synthesis of thyroid hormone (butane-insoluble iodine) (coupling) (deiodinase) (iodide trapping or organificaiton) (iodotyrosine dehalogenase) (peroxidase) 246.1
  dyshormonogenic 246.1
  exophthalmic (*see also* Goiter, toxic) 242.0 ✓5ᵗʰ
  familial (with deaf-mutism) 243
  fibrous 245.3
  lingual 759.2
  lymphadenoid 245.2
  malignant (M8000/3) 193
  multinodular (nontoxic) 241.1
    toxic or with hyperthyroidism (*see also* Goiter, toxic) 242.2 ✓5ᵗʰ
  nodular (nontoxic) 241.9
    with
      hyperthyroidism (*see also* Goiter, toxic) 242.3 ✓5ᵗʰ
      thyrotoxicosis (*see also* Goiter, toxic) 242.3 ✓5ᵗʰ
    endemic 241.9
    exophthalmic (diffuse) (*see also* Goiter, toxic) 242.0 ✓5ᵗʰ
    multinodular (nontoxic) 241.1
    sporadic 241.9
    toxic (*see also* Goiter, toxic) 242.3 ✓5ᵗʰ
    uninodular (nontoxic) 241.0
  nontoxic (nodular) 241.9
    multinodular 241.1
    uninodular 241.0
  pulsating (*see also* Goiter, toxic) 242.0 ✓5ᵗʰ
  simple 240.0
  toxic 242.0 ✓5ᵗʰ

Note — Use the following fifth-digit subclassification with category 242:

  0   without mention of thyrotoxic crisis or storm

  1   with mention of thyrotoxic crisis or storm

    adenomatous 242.3 ✓5ᵗʰ
      multinodular 242.2 ✓5ᵗʰ
      uninodular 242.1 ✓5ᵗʰ
    multinodular 242.2 ✓5ᵗʰ
    nodular 242.3 ✓5ᵗʰ
      multinodular 242.2 ✓5ᵗʰ
      uninodular 242.1 ✓5ᵗʰ
    uninodular 242.1 ✓5ᵗʰ
  uninodular (nontoxic) 241.0
    toxic or with hyperthyroidism (*see also* Goiter, toxic) 242.1 ✓5ᵗʰ
Goldberg (-Maxwell) (-Morris) syndrome (testicular feminization) 257.8
Goldblatt's
  hypertension 440.1
  kidney 440.1
Goldenhar's syndrome (oculoauriculovertebral dysplasia) 756.0
Goldflam-Erb disease or syndrome 358.0
Goldscheider's disease (epidermolysis bullosa) 757.39

Goldstein's disease (familial hemorrhagic telangiectasia) 448.0

Golfer's elbow 726.32

Goltz-Gorlin syndrome (dermal hypoplasia) 757.39

Gonadoblastoma (M9073/1)
  specified site — *see* Neoplasm, by site, uncertain behavior
  unspecified site
    female 236.2
    male 236.4

Gonecystitis (*see also* Vesiculitis) 608.0

Gongylonemiasis 125.6
  mouth 125.6

Goniosynechiae 364.73

Gonococcemia 098.89

Gonococcus, gonococcal (disease) (infection) (*see also* condition) 098.0
  anus 098.7
  bursa 098.52
  chronic NEC 098.2
  complicating pregnancy, childbirth, or puerperium 647.1 ✔5ᵗʰ
    affecting fetus or newborn 760.2
  conjunctiva, conjunctivitis (neonatorum) 098.40
  dermatosis 098.89
  endocardium 098.84
  epididymo-orchitis 098.13
    chronic or duration of 2 months or over 098.33
  eye (newborn) 098.40
  fallopian tube (chronic) 098.37
    acute 098.17
  genitourinary (acute) (organ) (system) (tract) (*see also* Gonnorrhea) 098.0
    lower 098.0
      chronic 098.2
    upper 098.10
      chronic 098.30
  heart NEC 098.85
  joint 098.50
  keratoderma 098.81
  keratosis (blennorrhagica) 098.81
  lymphatic (gland) (node) 098.89
  meninges 098.82
  orchitis (acute) 098.13
    chronic or duration of 2 months or over 098.33
  pelvis (acute) 098.19
    chronic or duration of 2 months or over 098.39
  pericarditis 098.83
  peritonitis 098.86
  pharyngitis 098.6
  pharynx 098.6
  proctitis 098.7
  pyosalpinx (chronic) 098.37
    acute 098.17
  rectum 098.7
  septicemia 098.89
  skin 098.89
  specified site NEC 098.89
  synovitis 098.51
  tendon sheath 098.51
  throat 098.6
  urethra (acute) 098.0
    chronic or duration of 2 months or over 098.2
  vulva (acute) 098.0
    chronic or duration of 2 months or over 098.2

Gonocytoma (M9073/1)
  specified site — *see* Neoplasm, by site, uncertain behavior
  unspecified site
    female 236.2
    male 236.4

Gonorrhea 098.0
  acute 098.0
  Bartholin's gland (acute) 098.0
    chronic or duration of 2 months or over 098.2
  bladder (acute) 098.11
    chronic or duration of 2 months or over 098.31

Gonorrhea — *continued*
  carrier (suspected of) V02.7
  cervix (acute) 098.15
    chronic or duration of 2 months or over 098.35
  chronic 098.2
  complicating pregnancy, childbirth, or puerperium 647.1 ✔5ᵗʰ
    affecting fetus or newborn 760.2
  conjunctiva, conjunctivitis (neonatorum) 098.40
  contact V01.6
  Cowper's gland (acute) 098.0
    chronic or duration of 2 months or over 098.2
  duration of two months or over 098.2
  exposure to V01.6
  fallopian tube (chronic) 098.37
    acute 098.17
  genitourinary (acute) (organ) (system) (tract) 098.0
    chronic 098.2
    duration of two months or over 098.2
  kidney (acute) 098.19
    chronic or duration of 2 months or over 098.39
  ovary (acute) 098.19
    chronic or duration of 2 months or over 098.39
  pelvis (acute) 098.19
    chronic or duration of 2 months or over 098.39
  penis (acute) 098.0
    chronic or duration of 2 months or over 098.2
  prostate (acute) 098.12
    chronic or duration of 2 months or over 098.32
  seminal vesicle (acute) 098.14
    chronic or duration of 2 months or over 098.34
  specified site NEC — *see* Gonococcus
  spermatic cord (acute) 098.14
    chronic or duration of 2 months or over 098.34
  urethra (acute) 098.0
    chronic or duration of 2 months or over 098.2
  vagina (acute) 098.0
    chronic or duration of 2 months or over 098.2
  vas deferens (acute) 098.14
    chronic or duration of 2 months or over 098.34
  vulva (acute) 098.0
    chronic or duration of 2 months or over 098.2

Goodpasture's syndrome (pneumorenal) 446.21

Gopalan's syndrome (burning feet) 266.2

Gordon's disease (exudative enteropathy) 579.8

Gorlin-Chaudhry-Moss syndrome 759.89

Gougerot's syndrome (trisymptomatic) 709.1

Gougerot-Blum syndrome (pigmented purpuric lichenoid dermatitis) 709.1

Gougerot-Carteaud disease or syndrome (confluent reticulate papillomatosis) 701.8

Gougerot-Hailey-Hailey disease (benign familial chronic pemphigus) 757.39

Gougerot (-Houwer) - Sjögren syndrome (keratoconjunctivitis sicca) 710.2

Gouley's syndrome (constrictive pericarditis) 423.2

Goundou 102.6

Gout, gouty 274.9
  with specified manifestations NEC 274.89
  arthritis (acute) 274.0
  arthropathy 274.0
  degeneration, heart 274.82
  diathesis 274.9
  eczema 274.89
  episcleritis 274.89 [379.09]
  external ear (tophus) 274.81
  glomerulonephritis 274.10
  iritis 274.89 [364.11]
  joint 274.0

Gout, gouty — *continued*
  kidney 274.10
  lead 984.9
    specified type of lead — *see* Table of Drugs and Chemicals
  nephritis 274.10
  neuritis 274.89 [357.4]
  phlebitis 274.89 [451.9]
  rheumatic 714.0
  saturnine 984.9
    specified type of lead — *see* Table of Drugs and Chemicals
  spondylitis 274.0
  synovitis 274.0
  syphilitic 095.8
  tophi 274.0
    ear 274.81
    heart 274.82
    specified site NEC 274.82

Gowers'
  muscular dystrophy 359.1
  syndrome (vasovagal attack) 780.2

Gowers-Paton-Kennedy syndrome 377.04

Gradenigo's syndrome 383.02

Graft-versus-host disease (bone marrow) 996.85
  due to organ transplant NEC — *see* Complications, transplant, organ

Graham Steell's murmur (pulmonic regurgitation) (*see also* Endocarditis, pulmonary) 424.3

Grain-handlers' disease or lung 495.8

Grain mite (itch) 133.8

Grand
  mal (idiopathic) (*see also* Epilepsy) 345.1 ✔5ᵗʰ
    hysteria of Charcôt 300.11
    nonrecurrent or isolated 780.39
  multipara
    affecting management of labor and delivery 659.4 ✔5ᵗʰ
    status only (not pregnant) V61.5

Granite workers' lung 502

Granular — *see also* condition
  inflammation, pharynx 472.1
  kidney (contracting) (*see also* Sclerosis, renal) 587
  liver — *see* Cirrhosis, liver
  nephritis — *see* Nephritis

Granulation tissue, abnormal — *see also* Granuloma
  abnormal or excessive 701.5
  postmastoidectomy cavity 383.33
  postoperative 701.5
  skin 701.5

Granulocytopenia, granulocytopenic (primary) 288.0
  malignant 288.0

Granuloma NEC 686.1
  abdomen (wall) 568.89
    skin (pyogenicum) 686.1
      from residual foreign body 709.4
  annulare 695.89
  anus 569.49
  apical 522.6
  appendix 543.9
  aural 380.23
  beryllium (skin) 709.4
    lung 503
  bone (*see also* Osteomyelitis) 730.1 ✔5ᵗʰ
    eosinophilic 277.8
    from residual foreign body 733.99
  canaliculus lacrimalis 375.81
  cerebral 348.8
  cholesterin, middle ear 385.82
  coccidioidal (progressive) 114.3
    lung 114.4
    meninges 114.2
    primary (lung) 114.0
  colon 569.89
  conjunctiva 372.61
  dental 522.6
  ear, middle (cholesterin) 385.82
    with otitis media — *see* Otitis media
  eosinophilic 277.8
    bone 277.8
    lung 277.8

✔4ᵗʰ Fourth-digit Required   ✔5ᵗʰ Fifth-digit Required   ▶◀ Revised Text   ● New Line   ▲ Revised Code

Granuloma NEC — *continued*
  eosinophilic — *continued*
    oral mucosa 528.9
  exuberant 701.5
  eyelid 374.89
  facial
    lethal midline 446.3
    malignant 446.3
  faciale 701.8
  fissuratum (gum) 523.8
  foot NEC 686.1
  foreign body (in soft tissue) NEC 728.82
    bone 733.99
    in operative wound 998.4
    muscle 728.82
    skin 709.4
    subcutaneous tissue 709.4
  fungoides 202.1 ✓5ᵗʰ
  gangraenescens 446.3
  giant cell (central) (jaw) (reparative) 526.3
    gingiva 523.8
    peripheral (gingiva) 523.8
  gland (lymph) 289.3
  Hodgkin's (M9661/3) 201.1 ✓5ᵗʰ
  ileum 569.89
  infectious NEC 136.9
  inguinale (Donovan) 099.2
    venereal 099.2
  intestine 569.89
  iridocyclitis 364.10
  jaw (bone) 526.3
    reparative giant cell 526.3
  kidney (*see also* Infection, kidney) 590.9
  lacrimal sac 375.81
  larynx 478.79
  lethal midline 446.3
  lipid 277.8
  lipoid 277.8
  liver 572.8
  lung (infectious) (*see also* Fibrosis, lung) 515
    coccidioidal 114.4
    eosinophilic 277.8
  lymph gland 289.3
  Majocchi's 110.6
  malignant, face 446.3
  mandible 526.3
  mediastinum 519.3
  midline 446.3
  monilial 112.3
  muscle 728.82
    from residual foreign body 728.82
  nasal sinus (*see also* Sinusitis) 473.9
  operation wound 998.59
    foreign body 998.4
    stitch (external) 998.89
      internal organ 996.7 ✓5ᵗʰ
      internal wound 998.89
    talc 998.7
  oral mucosa, eosinophilic or pyogenic 528.9
  orbit, orbital 376.11
  paracoccidiodal 116.1
  penis, venereal 099.2
  periapical 522.6
  peritoneum 568.89
    due to ova of helminths NEC (*see also* Helminthiasis) 128.9
  postmastoidectomy cavity 383.33
  postoperative — *see* Granuloma, operation wound
  prostate 601.8
  pudendi (ulcerating) 099.2
  pudendorum (ulcerative) 099.2
  pulp, internal (tooth) 521.4
  pyogenic, pyogenicum (skin) 686.1
    maxillary alveolar ridge 522.6
    oral mucosa 528.9
  rectum 569.49
  reticulohistiocytic 277.8
  rubrum nasi 705.89
  sarcoid 135
  Schistosoma 120.9
  septic (skin) 686.1
  silica (skin) 709.4
  sinus (accessory) (infectional) (nasal) (*see also* Sinusitis) 473.9
  skin (pyogenicum) 686.1
    from foreign body or material 709.4
  sperm 608.89

Granuloma NEC — *continued*
  spine
    syphilitic (epidural) 094.89
    tuberculous (*see also* Tuberculosis)
      015.0 ✓5ᵗʰ *[730.88]*
  stitch (postoperative) 998.89
    internal wound 998.89
  suppurative (skin) 686.1
  suture (postoperative) 998.89
    internal wound 998.89
  swimming pool 031.1
  talc 728.82
    in operation wound 998.7
  telangiectaticum (skin) 686.1
  trichophyticum 110.6
  tropicum 102.4
  umbilicus 686.1
    newborn 771.4
  urethra 599.84
  uveitis 364.10
  vagina 099.2
  venereum 099.2
  vocal cords 478.5
  Wegener's (necrotizing respiratory granulomatosis) 446.4
Granulomatosis NEC 686.1
  disciformis chronica et progressiva 709.3
  infantiseptica 771.2
  lipoid 277.8
  lipohagic, intestinal 040.2
  miliary 027.0
  necrotizing, respiratory 446.4
  progressive, septic 288.1
  Wegener's (necrotizing respiratory) 446.4
Granulomatous tissue — *see* Granuloma
Granulosis rubra nasi 705.89
Graphite fibrosis (of lung) 503
Graphospasm 300.89
  organic 333.84
Grating scapula 733.99
Gravel (urinary) (*see also* Calculus) 592.9
Graves' disease (exophthalmic goiter) (*see also* Goiter, toxic) 242.0 ✓5ᵗʰ
Gravis — *see* condition
Grawitz's tumor (hypernephroma) (M8312/3) 189.0
Grayness, hair (premature) 704.3
  congenital 757.4
Gray or grey syndrome (chloramphenicol) (newborn) 779.4
Greenfield's disease 330.0
Green sickness 280.9
Greenstick fracture — *see* Fracture, by site
Greig's syndrome (hypertelorism) 756.0
Griesinger's disease (*see also* Ancylostomiasis) 126.9
Grinders'
  asthma 502
  lung 502
  phthisis (*see also* Tuberculosis) 011.4 ✓5ᵗʰ
Grinding, teeth 306.8
Grip
  Dabney's 074.1
  devil's 074.1
Grippe, grippal — *see also* Influenza
  Balkan 083.0
  intestinal 487.8
  summer 074.8
Grippy cold 487.1
Grisel's disease 723.5
Groin — *see* condition
Grooved
  nails (transverse) 703.8
  tongue 529.5
    congenital 750.13
Ground itch 126.9
Growing pains, children 781.99
Growth (fungoid) (neoplastic) (new) (M8000/1) — *see also* Neoplasm, by site, unspecified nature
  adenoid (vegetative) 474.12

Growth — *see also* Neoplasm, by site, unspecified nature — *continued*
  benign (M8000/0) — *see* Neoplasm, by site, benign
  fetal, poor 764.9 ✓5ᵗʰ
    affecting management of pregnancy 656.5 ✓5ᵗʰ
  malignant (M8000/3) — *see* Neoplasm, by site, malignant
  rapid, childhood V21.0
  secondary (M8000/6) — *see* Neoplasm, by site, malignant, secondary
Gruber's hernia — *see* Hernia, Gruber's
Gruby's disease (tinea tonsurans) 110.0
G-trisomy 758.0
Guama fever 066.3
Gubler (-Millard) paralysis or syndrome 344.89
Guérin-Stern syndrome (arthorgryposis multiplex congenita) 754.89
Guertin's disease (electric chorea) 049.8
Guillain-Barré disease or syndrome 357.0
Guinea worms (infection) (infestation) 125.7
Guinon's disease (motor-verbal tic) 307.23
Gull's disease (thyroid atrophy with myxedema) 244.8
Gull and Sutton's disease — *see* Hypertension, kidney
Gum — *see* condition
Gumboil 522.7
Gumma (syphilitic) 095.9
  artery 093.89
    cerebral or spinal 094.89
  bone 095.5
    of yaws (late) 102.6
  brain 094.89
  cauda equina 094.89
  central nervous system NEC 094.9
  ciliary body 095.8 *[364.11]*
  congenital 090.5
    testis 090.5
  eyelid 095.8 *[373.5]*
  heart 093.89
  intracranial 094.89
  iris 095.8 *[364.11]*
  kidney 095.4
  larynx 095.8
  leptomeninges 094.2
  liver 095.3
  meninges 094.2
  myocardium 093.82
  nasopharynx 095.8
  neurosyphilitic 094.9
  nose 095.8
  orbit 095.8
  palate (soft) 095.8
  penis 095.8
  pericardium 093.81
  pharynx 095.8
  pituitary 095.8
  scrofulous (see also Tuberculosis) 017.0 ✓5ᵗʰ
  skin 095.8
  specified site NEC 095.8
  spinal cord 094.89
  tongue 095.8
  tonsil 095.8
  trachea 095.8
  tuberculous (*see also* Tuberculosis) 017.0 ✓5ᵗʰ
  ulcerative due to yaws 102.4
  ureter 095.8
  yaws 102.4
    bone 102.6
Gunn's syndrome (jaw-winking syndrome) 742.8
Gunshot wound — *see also* Wound, open, by site
  fracture — *see* Fracture, by site, open
  internal organs (abdomen, chest, or pelvis) — *see* Injury, internal, by site, with open wound
  intracranial — *see* Laceration, brain, with open intracranial wound
Günther's disease or syndrome (congenital erythropoietic porphyria) 277.1
Gustatory hallucination 780.1
Gynandrism 752.7

Granuloma — Gynandrism

Gynanadroblastoma (M8632/1)
  specified site — *see* Neoplasm, by site,
    uncertain behavior
  unspecified site
    female 236.2
    male 236.4
Gynandromorphism 752.7
Gynatresia (congenital) 752.49
Gynecoid pelvis, male 738.6
Gynecological examination V72.3
  for contraceptive maintenance V25.40
Gynecomastia 611.1
Gynephobia 300.29
Gyrate scalp 757.39

H

Haas' disease (osteochondrosis head of humerus)
  732.3
Habermann's disease (acute parapsoriasis
  varioliformis) 696.2
Habit, habituation
  chorea 307.22
  disturbance, child 307.9
  drug (*see also* Dependence) 304.9 ✓5ᵗʰ
  laxative (*see also* Abuse, drugs, nondependent)
    305.9 ✓5ᵗʰ
  spasm 307.20
    chronic 307.22
    transient of childhood 307.21
  tic 307.20
    chronic 307.22
    transient of childhood 307.21
  use of
    nonprescribed drugs (*see also* Abuse, drugs,
      nondependent) 305.9 ✓5ᵗʰ
    patent medicines (*see also* Abuse, drugs,
      nondependent) 305.9 ✓5ᵗʰ
  vomiting 536.2
Hadfield-Clarke syndrome (pancreatic
  infantilism) 577.8
Haff disease 985.1
Hageman factor defect, deficiency, or disease
  (*see also* Defect, coagulation) 286.3
Haglund's disease (osteochondrosis os tibiale
  externum) 732.5
Haglund-Läwen-Fründ syndrome 717.89
Hagner's disease (hypertrophic pulmonary
  osteoarthropathy) 731.2
Hag teeth, tooth 524.3
Hailey-Hailey disease (benign familial chronic
  pemphigus) 757.39
Hair — *see also* condition
  plucking 307.9
Hairball in stomach 935.2
Hairy black tongue 529.3
Half vertebra 756.14
Halitosis 784.9
Hallermann-Streiff syndrome 756.0
Hallervorden-Spatz disease or syndrome 333.0
Hallopeau's
  acrodermatitis (continua) 696.1
  disease (lichen sclerosis et atrophicus) 701.0
Hallucination (auditory) (gustatory) (olfactory)
  (tactile) 780.1
  alcoholic 291.3
  drug-induced 292.12
  visual 368.16
Hallucinosis 298.9
  alcoholic (acute) 291.3
  drug-induced 292.12
Hallus — *see* Hallux
Hallux 735.9
  malleus (acquired) 735.3
  rigidus (acquired) 735.2
    congenital 755.66
    late effects of rickets 268.1
  valgus (acquired) 735.0
    congenital 755.66
  varus (acquired) 735.1
    congenital 755.66

Halo, visual 368.15
Hamartoblastoma 759.6
Hamartoma 759.6
  epithelial (gingival), odontogenic, central, or
    peripheral (M9321/0) 213.1
    upper jaw (bone) 213.0
  vascular 757.32
Hamartosis, hamartoses NEC 759.6
Hamman's disease or syndrome (spontaneous
  mediastinal emphysema) 518.1
Hamman-Rich syndrome (diffuse interstitial
  pulmonary fibrosis) 516.3
Hammer toe (acquired) 735.4
  congenital 755.66
  late effects of rickets 268.1
Hand — *see* condition
Hand-Schüller-Christian disease or syndrome
  (chronic histiocytosis x) 277.8
Hand-foot syndrome 282.61
Hanging (asphyxia) (strangulation) (suffocation)
  994.7
Hangnail (finger) (with lymphangitis) 681.02
Hangover (alcohol) (*see also* Abuse, drugs,
  nondependent) 305.0 ✓5ᵗʰ
Hanot's cirrhosis or disease — *see* Cirrhosis,
  biliary
Hanot-Chauffard (-Troisier) syndrome (bronze
  diabetes) 275.0
Hansen's disease (leprosy) 030.9
  benign form 030.1
  malignant form 030.0
Harada's disease or syndrome 363.22
Hard chancre 091.0
Hard firm prostate 600.1
Hardening
  artery — *see* Arteriosclerosis
  brain 348.8
  liver 571.8
Hare's syndrome (M8010/3) (carcinoma,
  pulmonary apex) 162.3
Harelip (*see also* Cleft, lip) 749.10
Harkavy's syndrome 446.0
Harlequin (fetus) 757.1
  color change syndrome 779.89 ▲
Harley's disease (intermittent hemoglobinuria)
  283.2
Harris'
  lines 733.91
  syndrome (organic hyperinsulinism) 251.1
Hart's disease or syndrome (pellagra-cerebellar
  ataxia-renal aminoaciduria) 270.0
Hartmann's pouch (abnormal sacculation of
  gallbladder neck) 575.8
  of intestine V44.3
    attention to V55.3
Hartnup disease (pellagra-cerebellar ataxia-renal
  aminoaciduria) 270.0
Harvester lung 495.0
Hashimoto's disease or struma (struma
  lymphomatosa) 245.2
Hassell-Henle bodies (corneal warts) 371.41
Haut mal (*see also* Epilepsy) 345.1 ✓5ᵗʰ
Haverhill fever 026.1
Hawaiian wood rose dependence 304.5 ✓5ᵗʰ
Hawkins' keloid 701.4
Hay
  asthma (*see also* Asthma) 493.0 ✓5ᵗʰ
  fever (allergic) (with rhinitis) 477.9
    with asthma (bronchial) (*see also* Asthma)
      493.0 ✓5ᵗʰ
    allergic, due to grass, pollen, ragweed, or
      tree 477.0
    conjunctivitis 372.05
    due to
      dander 477.8
      dust 477.8
      fowl 477.8
      pollen 477.8
      specified allergen other than pollen 477.8

Hayem-Faber syndrome (achlorhydric anemia)
  280.9
Hayem-Widal syndrome (acquired hemolytic
  jaundice) 283.9
Haygarth's nodosities 715.04
Hazard-Crile tumor (M8350/3) 193
Hb (abnormal)
  disease — *see* Disease, hemoglobin
  trait — *see* Trait
H disease 270.0
Head — *see also* condition
  banging 307.3
Headache 784.0
  allergic 346.2 ✓5ᵗʰ
  cluster 346.2 ✓5ᵗʰ
  due to
    loss, spinal fluid 349.0
    lumbar puncture 349.0
    saddle block 349.0
  emotional 307.81
  histamine 346.2 ✓5ᵗʰ
  lumbar puncture 349.0
  menopausal 627.2
  migraine 346.9 ✓5ᵗʰ
  nonorganic origin 307.81
  postspinal 349.0
  psychogenic 307.81
  psychophysiologic 307.81
  sick 346.1 ✓5ᵗʰ
  spinal 349.0
    complicating labor and
      delivery 668.8 ✓5ᵗʰ   ●
    postpartum 668.8 ✓5ᵗʰ   ●
  spinal fluid loss 349.0
  tension 307.81
  vascular 784.0
    migraine type 346.9 ✓5ᵗʰ
  vasomotor 346.9 ✓5ᵗʰ
Health
  advice V65.4
  audit V70.0
  checkup V70.0
  education V65.4
  hazard (*see also* History of) V15.9
    specified cause NEC V15.89
  instruction V65.4
  services provided because (of)
    boarding school residence V60.6
    holiday relief for person providing home care
      V60.5
    inadequate
      housing V60.1
      resources V60.2
    lack of housing V60.0
    no care available in home V60.4
    person living alone V60.3
    poverty V60.3
    residence in institution V60.6
    specified cause NEC V60.8
    vacation relief for person providing home
      care V60.5
Healthy
  donor (*see also* Donor) V59.9
  infant or child
    accompanying sick mother V65.0
    receiving care V20.1
  person
    accompanying sick relative V65.0
    admitted for sterilization V25.2
    receiving prophylactic inoculation or
      vaccination (*see also* Vaccination,
      prophylactic) V05.9
Hearing examination V72.1
Heart — *see* condition
Heartburn 787.1
  psychogenic 306.4
Heat (effects) 992.9
  apoplexy 992.0
  burn — *see also* Burn, by site
    from sun (*see also* Sunburn) 692.71
  collapse 992.1
  cramps 992.2
  dermatitis or eczema 692.89
  edema 992.7
  erythema — *see* Burn, by site

Gynanadroblastoma — Heat

Heat — *continued*
excessive 992.9
specified effect NEC 992.8
exhaustion 992.5
anhydrotic 992.3
due to
salt (and water) depletion 992.4
water depletion 992.3
fatigue (transient) 992.6
fever 992.0
hyperpyrexia 992.0
prickly 705.1
prostration — *see* Heat, exhaustion
pyrexia 992.0
rash 705.1
specified effect NEC 992.8
stroke 992.0
sunburn (*see also* Sunburn) 692.71
syncope 992.1
Heavy-chain disease 273.2
Heavy-for-dates (fetus or infant) 766.1
4500 grams or more 766.0
exceptionally 766.0
Hebephrenia, hebephrenic (acute) (*see also* Schizophrenia) 295.1 ✔5ᵗʰ
dementia (praecox) (*see also* Schizophrenia) 295.1 ✔5ᵗʰ
schizophrenia (*see also* Schizophrenia) 295.1 ✔5ᵗʰ
Heberden's
disease or nodes 715.04
syndrome (angina pectoris) 413.9
Hebra's disease
dermatitis exfoliativa 695.89
erythema multiforme exudativum 695.1
pityriasis 695.89
maculata et circinata 696.3
rubra 695.89
pilaris 696.4
prurigo 698.2
Hebra, nose 040.1
Hedinger's syndrome (malignant carcinoid) 259.2
Heel — *see* condition
Heerfordt's disease or syndrome (uveoparotitis) 135
Hegglin's anomaly or syndrome 288.2
Heidenhain's disease 290.10
with dementia 290.10
Heilmeyer-Schöner disease (M9842/3) 207.1 ✔5ᵗʰ
Heine-Medin disease (*see also* Poliomyelitis) 045.9 ✔5ᵗʰ
Heinz-body anemia, congenital 282.7
Heller's disease or syndrome (infantile psychosis) (*see also* Psychosis, childhood) 299.1 ✔5ᵗʰ
H.E.L.L.P 642.5 ✔5ᵗʰ
Helminthiasis (*see also* Infestation, by specific parasite) 128.9
Ancylostoma (*see also* Ancylostoma) 126.9
intestinal 127.9
mixed types (types classifiable to more than one of the titles 120.0-127.7) 127.8
specified type 127.7
mixed types (intestinal) (types classifiable to more than one of the titles 120.0-127.7) 127.8
Necator americanus 126.1
specified type NEC 128.8
Trichinella 124
Heloma 700
Hemangioblastoma (M9161/1) — *see also* Neoplasm, connective tissue, uncertain behavior
malignant (M9161/3) — *see* Neoplasm, connective tissue, malignant
Hemangioblastomatosis, cerebelloretinal 759.6
Hemangioendothelioma (M9130/1) — *see also* Neoplasm, by site, uncertain behavior
benign (M9130/0) 228.00
bone (diffuse) (M9130/3) — *see* Neoplasm, bone, malignant
malignant (M9130/3) — *see* Neoplasm, connective tissue, malignant

Hemangioendothelioma — *see also* Neoplasm, by site, uncertain behavior — *continued*
nervous system (M9130/0) 228.09
Hemangioendotheliosarcoma (M9130/3) — *see* Neoplasm, connective tissue, malignant
Hemangiofibroma (M9160/0) — *see* Neoplasm, by site, benign
Hemangiolipoma (M8861/0) — *see* Lipoma
Hemangioma (M9120/0) 228.00
arteriovenous (M9123/0) — *see* Hemangioma, by site
brain 228.02
capillary (M9131/0) — *see* Hemangioma, by site
cavernous (M9121/0) — *see* Hemangioma, by site
central nervous system NEC 228.09
choroid 228.09
heart 228.09
infantile (M9131/0) — *see* Hemangioma, by site
intra-abdominal structures 228.04
intracranial structures 228.02
intramuscular (M9132/0) — *see* Hemangioma, by site
iris 228.09
juvenile (M9131/0) — *see* Hemangioma, by site
malignant (M9120/3) — *see* Neoplasm, connective tissue, malignant
meninges 228.09
brain 228.02
spinal cord 228.09
peritoneum 228.04
placenta — *see* Placenta, abnormal
plexiform (M9131/0) — *see* Hemangioma, by site
racemose (M9123/0) — *see* Hemangioma, by site
retina 228.03
retroperitoneal tissue 228.04
sclerosing (M8832/0) — *see* Neoplasm, skin, benign
simplex (M9131/0) — *see* Hemangioma, by site
skin and subcutaneous tissue 228.01
specified site NEC 228.09
spinal cord 228.09
venous (M9122/0) — *see* Hemangioma, by site
verrucous keratotic (M9142/0) — *see* Hemangioma, by site
Hemangiomatosis (systemic) 757.32
involving single site — *see* Hemangioma
Hemangiopericytoma (M9l50/1) — *see also* Neoplasm, connective tissue, uncertain behavior
benign (M9150/0) — *see* Neoplasm, connective tissue, benign
malignant (M9150/3) — *see* Neoplasm, connective tissue, malignant
Hemangiosarcoma (M9120/3) — *see* Neoplasm, connective tissue, malignant
Hemarthrosis (nontraumatic) 719.10
ankle 719.17
elbow 719.12
foot 719.17
hand 719.14
hip 719.15
knee 719.16
multiple sites 719.19
pelvic region 719.15
shoulder (region) 719.11
specified site NEC 719.18
traumatic — *see* Sprain, by site
wrist 719.13
Hematemesis 578.0
with ulcer — *see* Ulcer, by site, with hemorrhage
due to S. japonicum 120.2
Goldstein's (familial hemorrhagic telangiectasia) 448.0
newborn 772.4
due to swallowed maternal blood 777.3
Hematidrosis 705.89
Hematinuria (*see also* Hemoglobinuria) 791.2
malarial 084.8
paroxysmal 283.2
Hematite miners' lung 503

Hematobilia 576.8
Hematocele (congenital) (diffuse) (idiopathic) 608.83
broad ligament 620.7
canal of Nuck 629.0
cord male 608.83
fallopian tube 620.8
female NEC 629.0
ischiorectal 569.89
male NEC 608.83
ovary 629.0
pelvis, pelvic
female 629.0
with ectopic pregnancy (*see also* Pregnancy, ectopic) 633.90 ▲
with intrauterine pregnancy 633.91 ●
male 608.83
periuterine 629.0
retrouterine 629.0
scrotum 608.83
spermatic cord (diffuse) 608.83
testis 608.84
traumatic — *see* Injury, internal, pelvis
tunica vaginalis 608.83
uterine ligament 629.0
uterus 621.4
vagina 623.6
vulva 624.5
Hematocephalus 742.4
Hematochezia (*see also* Melena) 578.1
Hematochyluria (*see also* Infestation, filarial) 125.9
Hematocolpos 626.8
Hematocornea 371.12
Hematogenous — *see* condition
Hematoma (skin surface intact) (traumatic) — *see also* Contusion

> *Note* — *Hematomas are coded according to origin and the nature and site of the hematoma or the accompanying injury. Hematomas of unspecified origin are coded as injuries of the sites involved, except:*
>
> (a) *hematomas of genital organs which are coded as diseases of the organ involved unless they complicate pregnancy or delivery*
>
> (b) *hematomas of the eye which are coded as diseases of the eye.*
>
> *For late effect of hematoma classifiable to 920-924 see Late, effect, contusion*

with
crush injury — *see* Crush
fracture — *see* Fracture, by site
injury of internal organs — *see also* Injury, internal, by site
kidney — *see* Hematoma, kidney traumatic
liver — *see* Hematoma, liver, traumatic
spleen — *see* Hematoma, spleen
nerve injury — *see* Injury, nerve
open wound — *see* Wound, open, by site
skin surface intact — *see* Contusion
abdomen (wall) — *see* Contusion, abdomen
amnion 658.8 ✔5ᵗʰ
aorta, dissecting 441.00
abdominal 441.02
thoracic 441.01
thoracoabdominal 441.03
arterial (complicating trauma) 904.9
specified site — *see* Injury, blood vessel, by site
auricle (ear) 380.31
birth injury 767.8
skull 767.1

Hematoma — *see also* Contusion — *continued*
 brain (traumatic) 853.0 ☑5ᵗʰ

> *Note* — *Use the following fifth-digit subclassification with categories 851-854:*
>
> *0 unspecified state of consciousness*
> *1 with no loss of consciousness*
> *2 with brief [less than one hour] loss of consciousness*
> *3 with moderate [1-24 hours] loss of consciousness*
> *4 with prolonged [more than 24 hours] loss of consciousness and return to pre-existing conscious level*
> *5 with prolonged [more than 24 hours] loss of consciousness, without return to pre-existing conscious level*
> *Use fifth-digit 5 to designate when a patient is unconscious and dies before regaining consciousness, regardless of the duration of the loss of consciousness*
> *6 with loss of consciousness of unspecified duration*
> *9 with concussion, unspecified*

 with
  cerebral
   contusion — *see* Contusion, brain
   laceration — *see* Laceration, brain
   open intracranial wound 853.1 ☑5ᵗʰ
   skull fracture — *see* Fracture, skull, by site
  extradural or epidural 852.4 ☑5ᵗʰ
   with open intracranial wound 852.5 ☑5ᵗʰ
   fetus or newborn 767.0
   nontraumatic 432.0
  fetus or newborn NEC 767.0
  nontraumatic (*see also* Hemorrhage, brain) 431
   epidural or extradural 432.0
   newborn NEC 772.8
   subarachnoid, arachnoid, or meningeal (*see also* Hemorrhage, subarachnoid) 430
   subdural (*see also* Hemorrhage, subdural) 432.1
  subarachnoid, arachnoid, or meningeal 852.0 ☑5ᵗʰ
   with open intracranial wound 852.1 ☑5ᵗʰ
   fetus or newborn 772.2
   nontraumatic (*see also* Hemorrhage, subarachnoid) 430
  subdural 852.2 ☑5ᵗʰ
   with open intracranial wound 852.3 ☑5ᵗʰ
   fetus or newborn (localized) 767.0
   nontraumatic (*see also* Hemorrhage, subdural) 432.1
 breast (nontraumatic) 611.8
 broad ligament (nontraumatic) 620.7
  complicating delivery 665.7 ☑5ᵗʰ
  traumatic — *see* Injury, internal, broad ligament
 calcified NEC 959.9
 capitis 920
  due to birth injury 767.1
  newborn 767.1
 cerebral — *see* Hematoma, brain
 cesarean section wound 674.3 ☑5ᵗʰ
 chorion — *see* Placenta, abnormal
 complicating delivery (perineum) (vulva) 664.5 ☑5ᵗʰ
  pelvic 665.7 ☑5ᵗʰ
  vagina 665.7 ☑5ᵗʰ
 corpus
  cavernosum (nontraumatic) 607.82
  luteum (nontraumatic) (ruptured) 620.1
 dura (mater) — *see* Hematoma, brain, subdural
 epididymis (nontraumatic) 608.83
 epidural (traumatic) — *see also* Hematoma, brain, extradural
  spinal — *see* Injury, spinal, by site
 episiotomy 674.3 ☑5ᵗʰ
 external ear 380.31

Hematoma — *see also* Contusion — *continued*
 extradural — *see also* Hematoma, brain, extradural
  fetus or newborn 767.0
  nontraumatic 432.0
   fetus or newborn 767.0
 fallopian tube 620.8
 genital organ (nontraumatic)
  female NEC 629.8
  male NEC 608.83
  traumatic (external site) 922.4
   internal — *see* Injury, internal, genital organ
 graafian follicle (ruptured) 620.0
 internal organs (abdomen, chest, or pelvis) — *see also* Injury, internal, by site
  kidney — *see* Hematoma, kidney, traumatic
  liver — *see* Hematoma, liver, traumatic
  spleen — *see* Hematoma, brain
 intracrainal — *see* Hematoma, brain
 kidney, cystic 593.81
  traumatic 866.01
   with open wound into cavity 866.11
 labia (nontraumatic) 624.5
 lingual (and other parts of neck, scalp, or face, except eye) 920
 liver (subcapsular) 573.8
  birth injury 767.8
  fetus or newborn 767.8
  traumatic NEC 864.01
   with
    laceration — *see* Laceration, liver
    open wound into cavity 864.11
 mediastinum — *see* Injury, internal, mediastinum
 meninges, meningeal (brain) — *see also* Hematoma, brain, subarachnoid
  spinal — *see* Injury, spinal, by site
 mesosalpinx (nontraumatic) 620.8
  traumatic — *see* Injury, internal, pelvis
 muscle (traumatic — *see* Contusion, by site
 nasal (septum) (and other part(s) of neck, scalp, or face, except eye) 920
 obstetrical surgical wound 674.3 ☑5ᵗʰ
 orbit, orbital (nontraumatic) 376.32
  traumatic 921.2
 ovary (corpus luteum) (nontraumatic) 620.1
  traumatic — *see* Injury, internal, ovary
 pelvis (female) (nontraumatic) 629.8
  complicating delivery 665.7 ☑5ᵗʰ
  male 608.83
  traumatic — *see also* Injury, internal, pelvis
   specified organ NEC (*see also* Injury, internal, pelvis) 867.6
 penis (nontraumatic) 607.82
 pericranial (and neck, or face any part, except eye) 920
  due to injury at birth 767.1
 perineal wound (obstetrical) 674.3 ☑5ᵗʰ
  complicating delivery 664.5 ☑5ᵗʰ
 perirenal, cystic 593.81
 pinna 380.31
 placenta — *see* Placenta, abnormal
 postoperative 998.12
 retroperitoneal (nontraumatic) 568.81
  traumatic — *see* Injury, internal, retroperitoneum
 retropubic, male 568.81
 scalp (and neck, or face any part, except eye) 920
  fetus or newborn 767.1
 scrotum (nontraumatic) 608.83
  traumatic 922.4
 seminal vesicle (nontraumatic) 608.83
  traumatic — *see* Injury, internal, seminal, vesicle
 spermatic cord — *see also* Injury, internal, spermatic cord
  nontraumatic 608.83
 spinal (cord) (meninges) — *see also* Injury, spinal, by site
  fetus or newborn 767.4
  nontraumatic 336.1
 spleen 865.01
  with
   laceration — *see* Laceration, spleen
   open wound into cavity 865.11

Hematoma — *see also* Contusion — *continued*
 sternocleidomastoid, birth injury 767.8
 sternomastoid, birth injury 767.8
 subarachnoid — *see also* Hematoma, brain, subarachnoid
  fetus or newborn 772.2
  nontraumatic (*see also* Hemorrhage, subarachnoid) 430
  newborn 772.2
 subdural — *see also* Hematoma, brain, subdural
  fetus or newborn (localized) 767.0
  nontraumatic (*see also* Hemorrhage, subdural) 432.1
 subperiosteal (syndrome) 267
  traumatic — *see* Hematoma, by site
 superficial, fetus or newborn 772.6
 syncytium — *see* Placenta, abnormal
 testis (nontraumatic) 608.83
  birth injury 767.8
  traumatic 922.4
 tunica vaginalis (nontraumatic) 608.83
 umbilical cord 663.6 ☑5ᵗʰ
  affecting fetus or newborn 762.6
 uterine ligament (nontraumatic) 620.7
  traumatic — *see* Injury, internal, pelvis
 uterus 621.4
  traumatic — *see* Injury, internal, pelvis
 vagina (nontraumatic) (ruptured) 623.6
  complicating delivery 665.7 ☑5ᵗʰ
  traumatic 922.4
 vas deferens (nontraumatic) 608.83
  traumatic — *see* Injury, internal, vas deferens
 vitreous 379.23
 vocal cord 920
 vulva (nontraumatic) 624.5
  complicating delivery 664.5 ☑5ᵗʰ
  fetus or newborn 767.8
  traumatic 922.4

Hematometra 621.4
Hematomyelia 336.1
 with fracture of vertebra (*see also* Fracture, vertebra, by site, with spinal cord injury) 806.8
 fetus or newborn 767.4
Hematomyelitis 323.9
 late effect — *see* category 326
Hematoperitoneum (*see also* Hemoperitoneum) 568.81
Hematopneumothorax (*see also* Hemothorax) 511.8
Hematoporphyria (acquired) (congenital) 277.1
Hematoporphyrinuria (acquired) (congenital) 277.1
Hematorachis, hematorrhachis 336.1
 fetus or newborn 767.4
Hematosalpinx 620.8
 with
  ectopic pregnancy (*see also* categories 633.0-633.9) 639.2
  molar pregnancy (*see also* categories 630-632) 639.2
 infectional (*see also* Salpingo-oophoritis) 614.2
Hematospermia 608.82
Hematothorax (*see also* Hemothorax) 511.8
Hematotympanum 381.03
Hematuria (benign) (essential) (idiopathic) 599.7
 due to S. hematobium 120.0
 endemic 120.0
 intermittent 599.7
 malarial 084.8
 paroxysmal 599.7
 sulfonamide
  correct substance properly administered 599.7
  overdose or wrong substance given or taken 961.0
 tropical (bilharziasis) 120.0
 tuberculous (*see also* Tuberculosis) 016.9 ☑5ᵗʰ
Hematuric bilious fever 084.8
Hemeralopia 368.10 ▲

Hemiabiotrophy 799.8

Hemi-akinesia 781.8

Hemianalgesia (see also Disturbance, sensation) 782.0

Hemianencephaly 740.0

Hemianesthesia (see also Disturbance, sensation) 782.0

Hemianopia, hemianopsia (altitudinal) (homonymous) 368.46
  binasal 368.47
  bitemporal 368.47
  heteronymous 368.47
  syphilitic 095.8

Hemiasomatognosia 307.9

Hemiathetosis 781.0

Hemiatrophy 799.8
  cerebellar 334.8
  face 349.89
    progressive 349.89
  fascia 728.9
  leg 728.2
  tongue 529.8

Hemiballism(us) 333.5

Hemiblock (cardiac) (heart) (left) 426.2

Hemicardia 746.89

Hemicephalus, hemicephaly 740.0

Hemichorea 333.5

Hemicrania 346.9 ✓5ᵗʰ
  congenital malformation 740.0

Hemidystrophy — see Hemiatrophy

Hemiectromelia 755.4

Hemihypalgesia (see also Disturbance, sensation) 782.0

Hemihypertrophy (congenital) 759.89
  cranial 756.0

Hemihypesthesia (see also Disturbance, sensation) 782.0

Hemi-inattention 781.8

Hemimelia 755.4
  lower limb 755.30
    paraxial (complete) (incomplete) (intercalary) (terminal) 755.32
      fibula 755.37
      tibia 755.36
    transverse (complete) (partial) 755.31
  upper limb 755.20
    paraxial (complete) (incomplete) (intercalary) (terminal) 755.22
      radial 755.26
      ulnar 755.27
    transverse (complete) (partial) 755.21

Hemiparalysis (see also Hemiplegia) 342.9 ✓5ᵗʰ

Hemiparesis (see also Hemiplegia) 342.9 ✓5ᵗʰ

Hemiparesthesia (see also Disturbance, sensation) 782.0

Hemiplegia 342.9 ✓5ᵗʰ
  acute (see also Disease, cerebrovascular, acute) 436
  alternans facialis 344.89
  apoplectic (see also Disease, cerebrovascular, acute) 436
    late effect or residual
      affecting
        dominant side 438.21
        nondominant side 438.22
        unspecified side 438.20
  arteriosclerotic 437.0
    late effect or residual
      affecting
        dominant side 438.21
        nondominant side 438.22
        unspecified side 438.20
  ascending (spinal) NEC 344.89
  attack (see also Disease, cerebrovascular, acute) 436
  brain, cerebral (current episode) 437.8
    congenital 343.1
  cerebral — see Hemiplegia, brain
  congenital (cerebral) (spastic) (spinal) 343.1
  conversion neurosis (hysterical) 300.11

Hemiplegia — continued
  cortical — see Hemiplegia, brain
  due to
    arteriosclerosis 437.0
      late effect or residual
        affecting
          dominant side 438.21
          nondominant side 438.22
          unspecified side 438.20
    cerebrovascular lesion (see also Disease, cerebrovascular, acute) 436
      late effect
        affecting
          dominant side 438.21
          nondominant side 438.22
          unspecified side 438.20
  embolic (current) (see also Embolism, brain) 434.1 ✓5ᵗʰ
    late effect
      affecting
        dominant side 438.21
        nondominant side 438.22
        unspecified side 438.20
  flaccid 342.0
  hypertensive (current episode) 437.8
  infantile (postnatal) 343.4
  late effect
    birth injury, intracranial or spinal 343.4
    cerebrovascular lesion — see Late effect(s) (of) cerebrovascular disease
    viral encephalitis 139.0
  middle alternating NEC 344.89
  newborn NEC 767.0
  seizure (current episode) (see also Disease, cerebrovascular, acute) 436
  spastic 342.1
    congenital or infantile 343.1
  specified NEC 342.8
  thrombotic (current) (see also Thrombosis, brain) 434.0 ✓5ᵗʰ
    late effect — see Late effect(s) (of) cerebrovascular disease

Hemisection, spinal cord — see Fracture, vertebra, by site, with spinal cord injury

Hemispasm 781.0
  facial 781.0

Hemispatial neglect 781.8

Hemisporosis 117.9

Hemitremor 781.0

Hemivertebra 756.14

Hemobilia 576.8

Hemocholecyst 575.8

Hemochromatosis (acquired) (diabetic) (hereditary) (liver) (myocardium) (primary idiopathic) (secondary) 275.0
  with refractory anemia 285.0

Hemodialysis V56.0

Hemoglobin — see also condition
  abnormal (disease) — see Disease, hemoglobin
  AS genotype 282.5
  fetal, hereditary persistence 282.7
  high-oxygen-affinity 289.0
  low NEC 285.9
  S (Hb-S), heterozygous 282.5

Hemoglobinemia 283.2
  due to blood transfusion NEC 999.8
    bone marrow 996.85
  paroxysmal 283.2

Hemoglobinopathy (mixed) (see also Disease, hemoglobin) 282.7
  with thalassemia 282.4
  sickle-cell 282.60
    with thalassemia 282.4

Hemoglobinuria, hemoglobinuric 791.2
  with anemia, hemolytic, acquired (chronic) NEC 283.2
  cold (agglutinin) (paroxysmal) (with Raynaud's syndrome) 283.2
  due to
    exertion 283.2
    hemolysis (from external causes) NEC 283.2
  exercise 283.2
  fever (malaria) 084.8
  infantile 791.2

Hemoglobinuria, hemoglobinuric — continued
  intermittent 283.2
  malarial 084.8
  march 283.2
  nocturnal (paroxysmal) 283.2
  paroxysmal (cold) (nocturnal) 283.2

Hemolymphangioma (M9175/0) 228.1

Hemolysis
  fetal — see Jaundice, fetus or newborn
  intravascular (disseminated) NEC 286.6
    with
      abortion — see Abortion, by type, with hemorrhage, delayed or excessive
      ectopic pregnancy (see also categories 633.0-633.9) 639.1
      hemorrhage of pregnancy 641.3 ✓5ᵗʰ
        affecting fetus or newborn 762.1
      molar pregnancy (see also categories 630-632) 639.1
    acute 283.2
    following
      abortion 639.1
      ectopic or molar pregnancy 639.1
  neonatal — see Jaundice, fetus or newborn
  transfusion NEC 999.8
    bone marrow 996.85

Hemolytic — see also condition
  anemia — see Anemia, hemolytic
  uremic syndrome 283.11

Hemometra 621.4

Hemopericardium (with effusion) 423.0
  newborn 772.8
  traumatic (see also Hemothorax, traumatic) 860.2
    with open wound into thorax 860.3

Hemoperitoneum 568.81
  infectional (see also Peritonitis) 567.2
  traumatic — see Injury, internal, peritoneum

Hemophilia (familial) (hereditary) 286.0
  A 286.0
    carrier (asymptomatic) V83.01
      symptomatic V83.02
  acquired 286.5   ●
  B (Leyden) 286.1
  C 286.2
  calcipriva (see also Fibrinolysis) 286.7
  classical 286.0
  nonfamilial 286.7
  vascular 286.4

Hemophilus influenzae NEC 041.5
  arachnoiditis (basic) (brain) (spinal) 320.0
    late effect — see category 326
  bronchopneumonia 482.2
  cerebral ventriculitis 320.0
    late effect — see category 326
  cerebrospinal inflammation 320.0
    late effect — see category 326
  infection NEC 041.5
  leptomeningitis 320.0
    late effect — see category 326
  meningitis (cerebral) (cerebrospinal) (spinal) 320.0
    late effect — see category 326
  meningomyelitis 320.0
    late effect — see category 326
  pachymeningitis (adhesive) (fibrous) (hemorrhagic) (hypertrophic) (spinal) 320.0
    late effect — see category 326
  pneumonia (broncho-) 482.2

Hemophthalmos 360.43

Hemopneumothorax (see also Hemothorax) 511.8
  traumatic 860.4
    with open wound into thorax 860.5

Hemoptysis 786.3
  due to Paragonimus (westermani) 121.2
  newborn 770.3
  tuberculous (see also Tuberculosis, pulmonary) 011.9 ✓5ᵗʰ

Hemorrhage, hemorrhagic (nontraumatic) 459.0
  abdomen 459.0
  accidental (antepartum) 641.2 ✓5ᵗʰ
    affecting fetus or newborn 762.1
  adenoid 474.8

Hemorrhage, hemorrhagic — *continued*
adrenal (capsule) (gland) (medulla) 255.4
  newborn 772.5
after labor — *see* Hemorrhage, postpartum
alveolar
  lung, newborn 770.3
  process 525.8
alveolus 525.8
amputation stump (surgical) 998.11
  secondary, delayed 997.69
anemia (chronic) 280.0
  acute 285.1
antepartum — *see* Hemorrhage, pregnancy
anus (sphincter) 569.3
apoplexy (stroke) 432.9
arachnoid — *see* Hemorrhage, subarachnoid
artery NEC 459.0
  brain (*see also* Hemorrhage, brain) 431
  middle meningeal — *see* Hemorrhage,
    subarachnoid
basilar (ganglion) (*see also* Hemorrhage, brain)
  431
bladder 596.8
blood dyscrasia 289.9
bowel 578.9
  newborn 772.4
brain (miliary) (nontraumatic) 431
  with
    birth injury 767.0
  arachnoid — *see* Hemorrhage, subarachnoid
  due to
    birth injury 767.0
    rupture of aneurysm (congenital) (*see*
      also Hemorrhage, subarachnoid)
      430
      mycotic 431
    syphilis 094.89
  epidural or extradural — *see* Hemorrhage,
    extradural
  fetus or newborn (anoxic) (hypoxic) (due to
    birth trauma) (nontraumatic) 767.0
    intraventricular 772.10
      grade I 772.11
      grade II 772.12
      grade III 772.13
      grade IV 772.14
  iatrogenic 997.02
  postoperative 997.02
  puerperal, postpartum, childbirth 674.0 ✓5ᵗʰ
  stem 431
  subarachnoid, arachnoid, or meningeal —
    see Hemorrhage, subarachnoid
  subdural — *see* Hemorrhage, subdural
  traumatic NEC 853.0 ✓5ᵗʰ

Note — *Use the following fifth-digit*
subclassification with categories 851-854:

0 *unspecified state of consciousness*

1 *with no loss of consciousness*

2 *with brief [less than one hour] loss of*
   consciousness

3 *with moderate [1-24 hours] loss of*
   consciousness

4 *with prolonged [more than 24 hours]*
   loss of consciousness and return to
   pre-existing conscious level

5 *with prolonged [more than 24 hours]*
   loss of consciousness, without return
   to pre-existing conscious level

Use fifth-digit 5 to designate when a patient
is unconscious and dies before
regaining consciousness, regardless
of the duration of the loss of
consciousness

6 *with loss of consciousness of*
   unspecified duration

9 *with concussion, unspecified*

---

    with
      cerebral
        contusion — *see* Contusion, brain
        laceration — *see* Laceration, brain
      open intracranial wound 853.1 ✓5ᵗʰ
      skull fracture — *see* Fracture, skull,
        by site

Hemorrhage, hemorrhagic — *continued*
brain — *continued*
  traumatic NEC — *continued*
    extradural or epidural 852.4 ✓5ᵗʰ
      with open intracranial wound
        852.5 ✓5ᵗʰ
    subarachnoid 852.0 ✓5ᵗʰ
      with open intracranial wound
        852.1 ✓5ᵗʰ
    subdural 852.2 ✓5ᵗʰ
      with open intracranial wound
        852.3 ✓5ᵗʰ
breast 611.79
bronchial tube — *see* Hemorrhage, lung
bronchopulmonary — *see* Hemorrhage, lung
bronchus (cause unknown) (*see also*
  Hemorrhage, lung) 786.3
bulbar (*see also* Hemorrhage, brain) 431
bursa 727.89
capillary 448.9
  primary 287.8
capsular — *see* Hemorrhage, brain
cardiovascular 429.89
cecum 578.9
cephalic (*see also* Hemorrhage, brain) 431
cerebellar (*see also* Hemorrhage, brain) 431
cerebellum (*see also* Hemorrhage, brain) 431
cerebral (*see also* Hemorrhage, brain) 431
  fetus or newborn (anoxic) (traumatic) 767.0
cerebromeningeal (*see also* Hemorrhage, brain)
  431
cerebrospinal (*see also* Hemorrhage, brain) 431
cerebrum (*see also* Hemorrhage, brain) 431
cervix (stump) (uteri) 622.8
cesarean section wound 674.3 ✓5ᵗʰ
chamber, anterior (eye) 364.41
childbirth — *see* Hemorrhage, complicating,
  delivery
choroid 363.61
  expulsive 363.62
ciliary body 364.41
cochlea 386.8
colon — *see* Hemorrhage, intestine
complicating
  delivery 641.9 ✓5ᵗʰ
    affecting fetus or newborn 762.1
    associated with
      afibrinogenemia 641.3 ✓5ᵗʰ
        affecting fetus or newborn 763.89
      coagulation defect 641.3 ✓5ᵗʰ
        affecting fetus or newborn 763.89
      hyperfibrinolysis 641.3 ✓5ᵗʰ
        affecting fetus or newborn 763.89
      hypofibrinogenemia 641.3 ✓5ᵗʰ
        affecting fetus or newborn 763.89
    due to
      low-lying placenta 641.1 ✓5ᵗʰ
        affecting fetus or newborn 762.0
      placenta previa 641.1 ✓5ᵗʰ
        affecting fetus or newborn 762.0
      premature separation of placenta
        641.2 ✓5ᵗʰ
        affecting fetus or newborn 762.1
      retained
        placenta 666.0 ✓5ᵗʰ
        secundines 666.2 ✓5ᵗʰ
      trauma 641.8 ✓5ᵗʰ
        affecting fetus or newborn 763.89
      uterine leiomyoma 641.8 ✓5ᵗʰ
        affecting fetus or newborn 763.89
  surgical procedure 998.11
concealed NEC 459.0
congenital 772.9
conjunctiva 372.72
  newborn 772.8
cord, newborn 772.0
  slipped ligature 772.3
  stump 772.3
corpus luteum (ruptured) 620.1
cortical (*see also* Hemorrhage, brain) 431
cranial 432.9
cutaneous 782.7
  newborn 772.6
cyst, pancreas 577.2
cystitis — *see* Cystitis

Hemorrhage, hemorrhagic — *continued*
delayed
  with
    abortion — *see* Abortion, by type, with
      hemorrhage, delayed or excessive
    ectopic pregnancy (*see also* categories
      633.0-633.9) 639.1
    molar pregnancy (*see also* categories 630-
      632) 639.1
  following
    abortion 639.1
    ectopic or molar pregnancy 639.1
  postpartum 666.2 ✓5ᵗʰ
diathesis (familial) 287.9
  newborn 776.0
disease 287.9
  newborn 776.0
  specified type NEC 287.8
disorder 287.9
  due to circulating anticoagulants 286.5
  specified type NEC 287.8
due to
  any device, implant or graft (presence of)
    classifiable to 996.0-996.5 — *see*
      Complications, due to (presence of)
      any device, implant, or graft classified
      to 996.0-996.5 NEC
  circulating anticoagulant 286.5
duodenum, duodenal 537.89
  ulcer — *see* Ulcer, duodenum, with
    hemorrhage
dura mater — *see* Hemorrhage, subdural
endotracheal — *see* Hemorrhage, lung
epidural — *see* Hemorrhage, extradural
episiotomy 674.3 ✓5ᵗʰ
esophagus 530.82
  varix (*see also* Varix, esophagus, bleeding)
    456.0
excessive
  with
    abortion — *see* Abortion, by type, with
      hemorrhage, delayed or excessive
    ectopic pregnancy (*see also* categories
      633.0-633.9) 639.1
    molar pregnancy (*see also* categories 630-
      632) 639.1
  following
    abortion 639.1
    ectopic or molar pregnancy 639.1
external 459.0
extradural (traumatic) — *see also* Hemorrhage,
  brain, traumatic, extradural
  birth injury 767.0
  fetus or newborn (anoxic) (traumatic) 767.0
  nontraumatic 432.0
eye 360.43
  chamber (anterior) (aqueous) 364.41
  fundus 362.81
eyelid 374.81
fallopian tube 620.8
fetomaternal 772.0
  affecting management of pregnancy or
    puerperium 656.0 ✓5ᵗʰ
fetus, fetal 772.0
  from
    cut end of co-twin's cord 772.0
    placenta 772.0
    ruptured cord 772.0
    vasa previa 772.0
  into
    co-twin 772.0
    mother's circulation 772.0
      affecting management of pregnancy or
        puerperium 656.0 ✓5ᵗʰ
fever (*see also* Fever, hemorrhagic) 065.9
  with renal syndrome 078.6
  arthropod-borne NEC 065.9
  Bangkok 065.4
  Crimean 065.0
  dengue virus 065.4
  epidemic 078.6
  Junin virus 078.7
  Korean 078.6
  Machupo virus 078.7
  mite-borne 065.8
  mosquito-borne 065.4
  Philippine 065.4

Hemorrhage — Hemorrhage

Hemorrhage, hemorrhagic — *continued*
  fever (*see also* Fever, hemorrhagic) — *continued*
    Russian (Yaroslav) 078.6
    Singapore 065.4
    southeast Asia 065.4
    Thailand 065.4
    tick-borne NEC 065.3
  fibrinogenolysis (*see also* Fibrinolysis) 286.6
  fibrinolytic (acquired) (*see also* Fibrinolysis) 286.6
  fontanel 767.1
  from tracheostomy stoma 519.09
  fundus, eye 362.81
  funis
    affecting fetus or newborn 772.0
    complicating delivery 663.8 ☑5ᵗʰ
  gastric (*see also* Hemorrhage, stomach) 578.9
  gastroenteric 578.9
    newborn 772.4
  gastrointestinal (tract) 578.9
    newborn 772.4
  genitourinary (tract) NEC 599.89
  gingiva 523.8
  globe 360.43
  gravidarum — *see* Hemorrhage, pregnancy
  gum 523.8
  heart 429.89
  hypopharyngeal (throat) 784.8
  intermenstrual 626.6
    irregular 626.6
    regular 626.5
  internal (organs) 459.0
    capsule (*see also* Hemorrhage, brain) 431
    ear 386.8
    newborn 772.8
  intestine 578.9
    congenital 772.4
    newborn 772.4
  into
    bladder wall 596.7
    bursa 727.89
    corpus luysii (*see also* Hemorrhage, brain) 431
  intra-abdominal 459.0
    during or following surgery 998.11
  intra-alveolar, newborn (lung) 770.3
  intracerebral (*see also* Hemorrhage, brain) 431
  intracranial NEC 432.9
    puerperal, postpartum, childbirth 674.0 ☑5ᵗʰ
    traumatic — *see* Hemorrhage, brain, traumatic
  intramedullary NEC 336.1
  intraocular 360.43
  intraoperative 998.11
  intrapartum — *see* Hemorrhage, complicating, delivery
  intrapelvic
    female 629.8
    male 459.0
  intraperitoneal 459.0
  intrapontine (*see also* Hemorrhage, brain) 431
  intrauterine 621.4
    complicating delivery — *see* Hemorrhage, complicating, delivery
    in pregnancy or childbirth — *see* Hemorrhage, pregnancy
    postpartum (*see also* Hemorrhage, postpartum) 666.1 ☑5ᵗʰ
  intraventricular (*see also* Hemorrhage, brain) 431
    fetus or newborn (anoxic) (traumatic) 772.10
      grade I 772.11
      grade II 772.12
      grade III 772.13
      grade IV 772.14
  intravesical 596.7
  iris (postinfectional) (postinflammatory) (toxic) 364.41
  joint (nontraumatic) 719.10
    ankle 719.17
    elbow 719.12
    foot 719.17
    forearm 719.13
    hand 719.14
    hip 719.15
    knee 719.16
    lower leg 719.16
    multiple sites 719.19

Hemorrhage, hemorrhagic — *continued*
  joint — *continued*
    pelvic region 719.15
    shoulder (region) 719.11
    specified site NEC 719.18
    thigh 719.15
    upper arm 719.12
    wrist 719.13
  kidney 593.81
  knee (joint) 719.16
  labyrinth 386.8
  leg NEC 459.0
  lenticular striate artery (*see also* Hemorrhage, brain) 431
  ligature, vessel 998.11
  liver 573.8
  lower extremity NEC 459.0
  lung 786.3
    newborn 770.3
    tuberculous (*see also* Tuberculosis, pulmonary) 011.9 ☑5ᵗʰ
  malaria 084.8
  marginal sinus 641.2 ☑5ᵗʰ
  massive subaponeurotic, birth injury 767.1
  maternal, affecting fetus or newborn 762.1
  mediastinum 786.3
  medulla (*see also* Hemorrhage, brain) 431
  membrane (brain) (*see also* Hemorrhage, subarachnoid) 430
    spinal cord — *see* Hemorrhage, spinal cord
  meninges, meningeal (brain) (middle) (*see also* Hemorrhage, subarachnoid) 430
    spinal cord — *see* Hemorrhage, spinal cord
  mesentery 568.81
  metritis 626.8
  midbrain (*see also* Hemorrhage, brain) 431
  mole 631
  mouth 528.9
  mucous membrane NEC 459.0
    newborn 728.8 ☑5ᵗʰ
  muscle 728.89
  nail (subungual) 703.8
  nasal turbinate 784.7
    newborn 772.8
  nasopharynx 478.29
  navel, newborn 772.3
  newborn 772.9
    adrenal 772.5
    alveolar (lung) 770.3
    brain (anoxic) (hypoxic) (due to birth trauma) 767.0
    cerebral (anoxic) (hypoxic) (due to birth trauma) 767.0
    conjunctiva 772.8
    cutaneous 772.6
    diathesis 776.0
    due to vitamin K deficiency 776.0
    gastrointestinal 772.4
    internal (organs) 772.8
    intestines 772.4
    intra-alveolar (lung) 770.3
    intracranial (from any perinatal cause) 767.0
    intraventricular (from any perinatal cause) 772.10
      grade I 772.11
      grade II 772.12
      grade III 772.13
      grade IV 772.14
    lung 770.3
    pulmonary (massive) 770.3
    spinal cord, traumatic 767.4
    stomach 772.4
    subaponeurotic (massive) 767.1
    subarachnoid (from any perinatal cause) 772.2
    subconjunctival 772.8
    umbilicus 772.0
      slipped ligature 772.3
      vasa previa 772.0
  nipple 611.79
  nose 784.7
    newborn 772.8
  obstetrical surgical wound 674.3 ☑5ᵗʰ
  omentum 568.89
    newborn 772.4
  optic nerve (sheath) 377.42
  orbit 376.32
  ovary 620.1

Hemorrhage, hemorrhagic — *continued*
  oviduct 620.8
  pancreas 577.8
  parathyroid (gland) (spontaneous) 252.8
  parturition — *see* Hemorrhage, complicating, delivery
  penis 607.82
  pericardium, paricarditis 423.0
  perineal wound (obstetrical) 674.3 ☑5ᵗʰ
  peritoneum, peritoneal 459.0
  peritonsillar tissue 474.8
    after operation on tonsils 998.11
    due to infection 475
  petechial 782.7
  pituitary (gland) 253.8
  placenta NEC 641.9 ☑5ᵗʰ
    affecting fetus or newborn 762.1
    from surgical or instrumental damage 641.8 ☑5ᵗʰ
      affecting fetus or newborn 762.1
    previa 641.8 ☑5ᵗʰ
      affecting fetus or newborn 762.0
  pleura — *see* Hemorrhage, lung
  polioencephalitis, superior 265.1
  polymyositis — *see* Polymyositis
  pons (*see also* Hemorrhage, brain) 431
  pontine (*see also* Hemorrhage, brain) 431
  popliteal 459.0
  postcoital 626.7
  postextraction (dental) 998.11
  postmenopausal 627.1
  postnasal 784.7
  postoperative 998.11
  postpartum (atonic) (following delivery of placenta) 666. ☑5ᵗʰ
    delayed or secondary (after 24 hours) 666.2 ☑5ᵗʰ
    retained placenta 666.0 ☑5ᵗʰ
    third stage 666.0 ☑5ᵗʰ
  pregnancy (concealed) 641.9 ☑5ᵗʰ
    accidental 641.2 ☑5ᵗʰ
      affecting fetus or newborn 762.1
    affecting fetus or newborn 762.1
    before 22 completed weeks gestation 640.9 ☑5ᵗʰ
      affecting fetus or newborn 762.1
    due to
      abruptio placenta 641.2 ☑5ᵗʰ
        affecting fetus or newborn 762.1
      afibrinogenemia or other coagulation defect (conditions classifiable to 286.0-286.9) 641.3 ☑5ᵗʰ
        affecting fetus or newborn 762.1
      coagulation defect 641.3 ☑5ᵗʰ
        affecting fetus or newborn 762.1
      hyperfibrinolysis 641.3 ☑5ᵗʰ
        affecting fetus or newborn 762.1
      hypofibrinogenemia 641.3 ☑5ᵗʰ
        affecting fetus or newborn 762.1
      leiomyoma, uterus 641.8 ☑5ᵗʰ
        affecting fetus or newborn 762.1
      low-lying placenta 641.1 ☑5ᵗʰ
        affecting fetus or newborn 762.1
      marginal sinus (rupture) 641.2 ☑5ᵗʰ
        affecting fetus or newborn 762.1
      placenta previa 641.1 ☑5ᵗʰ
        affecting fetus or newborn 762.0
      premature separation of placenta (normally implanted) 641.2 ☑5ᵗʰ
        affecting fetus or newborn 762.1
      threatend abortion 640.0 ☑5ᵗʰ
        affecting fetus or newborn 762.1
      trauma 641.8 ☑5ᵗʰ
        affecting fetus or newborn 762.1
    early (before 22 completed weeks gestation) 640.9 ☑5ᵗʰ
      affecting fetus or newborn 762.1
    previous, affecting management of pregnancy or childbirth V23.49 ▲
    unavoidable — *see* Hemorrhage, pregnancy, due to placenta previa
  prepartum (mother) — *see* Hemorrhage, pregnancy
  preretinal, cause unspecified 362.81
  prostate 602.1
  puerperal (*see also* Hemorrhage, postpartum) 666.1 ☑5ᵗʰ

Hemorrhage, hemorrhagic — *continued*
pulmonary — *see also* Hemorrhage, lung
  newborn (massive) 770.3
  renal syndrome 446.21
purpura (primary) (*see also* Purpura,
  thrombocytopenic) 287.3
rectum (sphincter) 569.3
recurring, following initial hemorrhage at time
  of injury 958.2
renal 593.81
  pulmonary syndrome 446.21
respiratory tract (*see also* Hemorrhage, lung)
  786.3
retina, retinal (deep) (superficial) (vessels)
  362.81
  diabetic 250.5 ✓5ᵗʰ *[362.01]*
  due to birth injury 772.8
retrobulbar 376.89
retroperitoneal 459.0
retroplacental (*see also* Placenta, separation)
  641.2 ✓5ᵗʰ
scalp 459.0
  due to injury at birth 767.1
scrotum 608.83
secondary (nontraumatic) 459.0
  following initial hemorrhage at time of injury
    958.2
seminal vesicle 608.83
skin 782.7
  newborn 772.6
spermatic cord 608.83
spinal (cord) 336.1
  aneurysm (ruptured) 336.1
    syphilitic 094.89
  due to birth injury 767.4
  fetus or newborn 767.4
spleen 289.59
spontaneous NEC 459.0
  petechial 782.7
stomach 578.9
  newborn 772.4
  ulcer — *see* Ulcer, stomach, with
    hemorrhage
subaponeurotic, newborn 767.1
  massive (birth injury) 767.1
subarachnoid (nontraumatic) 430
  fetus or newborn (anoxic) (traumatic) 772.2
  puerperal, postpartum, childbirth 674.0 ✓5ᵗʰ
  traumatic — *see* Hemorrhage, brain,
    traumatic, subarachnoid
subconjunctival 372.72
  due to birth injury 772.8
  newborn 772.8
subcortical (*see also* Hemorrhage, brain) 431
subcutaneous 782.7
subdiaphragmatic 459.0
subdural (nontraumatic) 432.1
  due to birth injury 767.0
  fetus or newborn (anoxic) (hypoxic) (due to
    birth trauma) 767.0
  puerperal, postpartum, childbirth 674.0 ✓5ᵗʰ
  spinal 336.1
  traumatic — *see* Hemorrhage, brain,
    traumatic, subdural
subhyaloid 362.81
subperiosteal 733.99
subretinal 362.81
subtentorial (*see also* Hemorrhage, subdural
  432.1
subungual 703.8
  due to blood dyscrasia 287.8
suprarenal (capsule) (gland) 255.4
  fetus or newborn 772.5
tentorium (traumatic) — *see also* Hemorrhage,
  brain, traumatic
  fetus or newborn 767.0
  nontraumatic — *see* Hemorrhage, subdural
testis 608.83
thigh 459.0
third stage 666.0 ✓5ᵗʰ
thorax — *see* Hemorrhage, lung
throat 784.8
thrombocythemia 238.7
thymus (gland) 254.8
thyroid (gland) 246.3
  cyst 246.3
tongue 529.8

Hemorrhage, hemorrhagic — *continued*
tonsil 474.8
  postoperative 998.11
tooth socket (postextraction) 998.11
trachea — *see* Hemorrhage, lung
traumatic — *see also* nature of injury
  brain — *see* Hemorrhage, brain, traumatic
  recurring or secondary (following initial
    hemorrhage at time of injury) 958.2
tuberculous NEC (*see also* Tuberculosis,
  pulmonary) 011.9 ✓5ᵗʰ
tunica vaginalis 608.83
ulcer — *see* Ulcer, by site, with hemorrhage
umbilicus, umbilical cord 772.0
  after birth, newborn 772.3
  complicating delivery 663.8 ✓5ᵗʰ
    affecting fetus or newborn 772.0
  slipped ligature 772.3
  stump 772.3
unavoidable (due to placenta previa) 641.1 ✓5ᵗʰ
  affecting fetus or newborn 762.0
upper extremity 459.0
urethra (idiopathic) 599.84
uterus, uterine (abnormal) 626.9
  climacteric 627.0
  complicating delivery — *see* Hemorrhage,
    complicating delivery
  due to
    intrauterine contraceptive device 996.76
      perforating uterus 996.32
  functional or dysfunctional 626.8
  in pregnancy — *see* Hemorrhage, pregnancy
  intermenstrual 626.6
    irregular 626.6
    regular 626.5
  postmenopausal 627.1
  postpartum (*see also* Hemorrhage,
    postpartum) 666.1 ✓5ᵗʰ
  prepubertal 626.8
  pubertal 626.3
  puerperal (immediate) 666.1 ✓5ᵗʰ
vagina 623.8
vasa previa 663.5 ✓5ᵗʰ
  affecting fetus or newborn 772.0
vas deferens 608.83
ventricular (*see also* Hemorrhage, brain) 431
vesical 596.8
viscera 459.0
  newborn 772.8
vitreous (humor) (intraocular) 379.23
vocal cord 478.5
vulva 624.8

Hemorrhoids (anus) (rectum) (without
  complication) 455.6
bleeding, prolapsed, strangulated, or ulcerated
  NEC 455.8
  external 455.5
  internal 455.2
complicated NEC 455.8
complicating pregnancy and puerperium
  671.8 ✓5ᵗʰ
external 455.3
  with complication NEC 455.5
  bleeding, prolapsed, strangulated, or
    ulcerated 455.5
  thrombosed 455.4
internal 455.0
  with complication NEC 455.2
  bleeding, prolapsed, strangulated, or
    ulcerated 455.2
  thrombosed 455.1
residual skin tag 455.9
sentinel pile 455.9
thrombosed NEC 455.7
  external 455.4
  internal 455.1

Hemosalpinx 620.8

Hemosiderosis 275.0
dietary 275.0
pulmonary (idiopathic) 275.0 *[516.1]*
transfusion NEC 999.8
  bone marrow 996.85

Hemospermia 608.82

Hemothorax 511.8
bacterial, nontuberculous 511.1
newborn 772.8

Hemothorax — *continued*
nontuberculous 511.8
  bacterial 511.1
pneumococcal 511.1
postoperative 998.11
staphylococcal 511.1
streptococcal 511.1
traumatic 860.2
  with
    open wound into thorax 860.3
    pneumothorax 860.4
      with open wound into thorax 860.5
tuberculous (*see also* Tuberculosis, pleura)
  012.0 ✓5ᵗʰ

Hemotympanum 385.89

Hench-Rosenberg syndrome (palindromic
  arthritis) (*see also* Rheumatism,
  palindromic) 719.3 ✓5ᵗʰ

Henle's warts 371.41

Henoch (-Schönlein)
disease or syndrome (allergic purpura) 287.0
purpura (allergic) 287.0

Henpue, henpuye 102.6

Heparitinuria 277.5

Hepar lobatum 095.3

Hepatalgia 573.8

Hepatic — *see also* conditon
flexure syndrome 569.89

Hepatitis 573.3
acute (*see also* Necrosis, liver) 570
  alcoholic 571.1
  infective 070.1
    with hepatic coma 070.0
alcoholic 571.1
amebic — *see* Abscess, liver, amebic
anicteric (acute) — *see* Hepatitis, viral
antigen-associated (HAA) — *see* Hepatitis, viral,
  type B
Australian antigen (positive) — *see* Hepatitis,
  viral, type B
catarrhal (acute) 070.1
  with hepatic coma 070.0
  chronic 571.40
  newborn 070.1
    with hepatic coma 070.0
chemical 573.3
cholangiolitic 573.8
cholestatic 573.8
chronic 571.40
  active 571.49
    viral — *see* Hepatitis, viral
  aggressive 571.49
  persistent 571.41
  viral — *see* Hepatitis, viral
cytomegalic inclusion virus 078.5 *[573.1]*
diffuse 573.3
"dirty needle" — *see* Hepatitis, viral
  with hepatic coma 070.2 ✓5ᵗʰ
drug-induced 573.3
due to
  Coxsackie 074.8 *[573.1]*
  cytomegalic inclusion virus 078.5 *[573.1]*
  infectious mononucleosis 075 *[573.1]*
  malaria 084.9 *[573.2]*
  mumps 072.71
  secondary syphilis 091.62
  toxoplasmosis (acquired) 130.5
    congenital (active) 771.2
epidemic — *see* Hepatitis, viral, type A
fetus or newborn 774.4
fibrous (chronic) 571.49
  acute 570
from injection, inoculation, or transfusion
  (blood) (other substance) (plasma) serum)
  (onset within 8 months after
  administration) — *see* Hepatitis, viral
fulminant (viral) (*see also* Hepatitis, viral) 070.9
  with hepatic coma 070.6
  type A 070.1
    with hepatic coma 070.0
  type B — *see* Hepatitis, viral, type B
giant cell (neonatal) 774.4
hemorrhagic 573.8
homologous serum — *see* Hepatitis, viral
hypertrophic (chronic) 571.49
  acute 570

Hepatitis — *continued*
  infectious, infective (acute) (chronic) (subacute)
      070.1
    with hepatic coma 070.0
  inoculation — *see* Hepatitis, viral
  interstitial (chronic) 571.49
    acute 570
  lupoid 571.49
  malarial 084.9 *[573.2]*
  malignant (*see also* Necrosis, liver) 570
  neonatal (toxic) 774.4
  newborn 774.4
  parenchymatous (acute) (*see also* Necrosis,
      liver) 570
  peliosis 573.3
  persistent, chronic 571.41
  plasma cell 571.49
  postimmunization — *see* Hepatitis, viral
  postnecrotic 571.49
  posttransfusion — *see* Hepatitis, viral
  recurrent 571.49
  septic 573.3
  serum — *see* Hepatitis, viral
    carrier (suspected of) V02.61
  subacute (*see also* Necrosis, liver) 570
  suppurative (diffuse) 572.0
  syphilitic (late) 095.3
    congenital (early) 090.0 *[573.2]*
      late 090.5 *[573.2]*
    secondary 091.62
  toxic (noninfectious) 573.3
    fetus or newborn 774.4
  tuberculous (*see also* Tuberculosis) 017.9 ✓5ᵗʰ
  viral (acute) (anicteric) (cholangiolitic)
      (cholestatic) (chronic) (subacute) 070.9
    with hepatic coma 070.6
    AU-SH type virus — *see* Hepatitis, viral, type
        B
    Australian antigen — *see* Hepatitis, viral,
        type B
    B-antigen — *see* Hepatitis, viral, type B
    Coxsackie 074.8 *[573.1]*
    cytomegalic inclusion 078.5 *[573.1]*
    IH (virus) — *see* Hepatitis, viral, type A
    infectious hepatitis, viral, type A
    serum hepatitis virus — *see* Hepatitis, viral,
        type B
    SH — *see* Hepatitis, viral, type B
    specified type NEC 070.59
      with hepatic coma 070.49
    type A 070.1
      with hepatic coma 070.0
    type B (acute) 070.30
      with
        hepatic coma 070.20
          with hepatitis delta 070.21
        hepatitis delta 070.31
          with hepatic coma 070.21
      carrier status V02.61
      chronic 070.32
        with
          hepatic coma 070.22
            with hepatitis delta 070.23
          hepatitis delta 070.33
            with hepatic coma 070.23
    type C (acute) 070.51
      with hepatic coma 070.41
      carrier status V02.62
      chronic 070.54
        with hepatic coma 070.44
    type delta (with hepatitis B carrier state)
        070.52
      with
        active hepatitis B disease — *see*
            Hepatitis, viral, type B
        hepatic coma 070.42
    type E 070.53
      with hepatic coma 070.43
    vaccination and inoculation (prophylactic)
        V05.3
  Waldenstrom's (lupoid hepatitis) 571.49
Hepatization, lung (acute) — *see also*
    Pneumonia, lobar
  chronic (*see also* Fibrosis, lung) 515
Hepatoblastoma (M8970/3) 155.0
Hepatocarcinoma (M8170/3) 155.0
Hepatocholangiocarcinoma (M8180/3) 155.0

Hepatocholangioma, benign (M8180/0) 211.5
Hepatocholangitis 573.8
Hepatocystitis (*see also* Cholecystitis) 575.10
Hepatodystrophy 570
Hepatolenticular degeneration 275.1
Hepatolithiasis — *see* Choledocholithiasis
Hepatoma (malignant) (M8170/3) 155.0
  benign (M8170/0) 211.5
  congenital (M8970/3) 155.0
  embryonal (M8970/3) 155.0
Hepatomegalia glycogenica diffusa 271.0
Hepatomegaly (*see also* Hypertrophy, liver) 789.1
  congenital 751.69
    syphilitic 090.0
  due to Clonorchis sinensis 121.1
  Gaucher's 272.7
  syphilitic (congenital) 090.0
Hepatoptosis 573.8
Hepatorrhexis 573.8
Hepatosis, toxic 573.8
Hepatosplenomegaly 571.8
  due to S. japonicum 120.2
  hyperlipemic (Burger-Grutz type) 272.3
Herald patch 696.3
Hereditary — *see* condition
Heredodegeneration 330.9
  macular 362.70
Heredopathia atactica polyneuritiformis 356.3
Heredosyphilis (*see also* Syphilis, congenital)
    090.9 ✓5ᵗʰ
Hermaphroditism (true) 752.7
  with specified chromosomal anomaly — *see*
      Anomaly, chromosomes, sex
Hernia, hernial (acquired) (recurrent) 553.9
  with
    gangrene (obstructed) NEC 551.9
    obstruction NEC 552.9
      and gangrene 551.9
  abdomen (wall) — *see* Hernia, ventral
  abdominal, specified site NEC 553.8
    with
      gangrene (obstructed) 551.8
      obstruction 552.8
        and gangrene 551.8
  appendix 553.8
    with
      gangrene (obstructed) 551.8
      obstruction 552.8
        and gangrene 551.8
  bilateral (inguinal) — *see* Hernia, inguinal
  bladder (sphincter)
    congenital (female) (male) 756.71
    female 618.0
    male 596.8
  brain 348.4
    congenital 742.0
  broad ligament 553.8
  cartilage, vertebral — *see* Displacement,
      intervertebral disc
  cerebral 348.4
    congenital 742.0
    endaural 742.0
  ciliary body 364.8
    traumatic 871.1
  colic 553.9
    with
      gangrene (obstructed) 551.9
      obstruction 552.9
        and gangrene 551.9
  colon 553.9
    with
      gangrene (obstructed) 551.9
      obstruction 552.9
        and gangrene 551.9
  colostomy (stoma) 569.69
  Cooper's (retroperitoneal) 553.8
    with
      gangrene (obstructed) 551.8
      obstruction 552.8
        and gangrene 551.8
  crural — *see* Hernia, femoral

Hernia, hernial — *continued*
  diaphragm, diaphragmatic 553.3
    with
      gangrene (obstructed) 551.3
      obstruction 552.3
        and gangrene 551.3
    congenital 756.6
    due to gross defect of diaphragm 756.6
    traumatic 862.0
      with open wound into cavity 862.1
  direct (inguinal) — *see* Hernia, inguinal
  disc, intervetebral — *see* Displacement,
      intervetebral disc
  diverticulum, intestine 553.9
    with
      gangrene (obstructed) 551.9
      obstruction 552.9
        and gangrene 551.9
  double (inguinal) — *see* Hernia, inguinal
  duodenojejunal 553.8
    with
      gangrene (obstructed) 551.8
      obstruction 552.8
        and gangrene 551.8
  en glissade — *see* Hernia, inguinal
  enterostomy (stoma) 569.69
  epigastric 553.29
    with
      gangrene (obstruction) 551.29
      obstruction 552.29
        and gangrene 551.29
    recurrent 553.21
      with
        gangrene (obstructed) 551.21
        obstruction 552.21
          and gangrene 551.21
  esophageal hiatus (sliding) 553.3
    with
      gangrene (obstructed) 551.3
      obstruction 552.3
        and gangrene 551.3
    congenital 750.6
  external (inguinal) — *see* Hernia, inguinal
  fallopian tube 620.4
  fascia 728.89
  fat 729.30
    eyelid 374.34
    orbital 374.34
    pad 729.30
      eye, eyelid 374.34
      knee 729.31
      orbit 374.34
      popliteal (space) 729.31
      specified site NEC 729.39
  femoral (unilateral) 553.00
    with
      gangrene (obstructed) 551.00
      obstruction 552.00
        with gangrene 551.0 ✓5ᵗʰ
    bilateral 553.02
      gangrenous (obstructed) 551.02
      obstructed 552.02
        with gangrene 551.02
      recurrent 553.03
        gangrenous (obstructed) 551.03
        obstructed 552.03
          with gangrene 551.03
    recurrent (unilateral) 553.01
      bilateral 553.03
        gangrenous (obstructed) 551.03
        obstructed 552.03
          with gangrene 551.03
      gangrenous (obstructed) 551.01
      obstructed 552.01
        with gangrene
  foramen
    Bochdalek 553.3
      with
        gangrene (obstructed) 551.3
        obstruction 552.3
          and gangrene 551.3
      congenital 756.6
    magnum 348.4
    Morgagni, Morgagnian 553.3
      with
        gangrene 551.3

Hernia, hernial — *continued*
  foramen — *continued*
    Morgagni, Morgagnian — *continued*
      with — *continued*
        obstruction 552.3
          and gangrene 551.3
      congenital 756.6
  funicular (umbilical) 553.1
    with
      gangrene (obstructed) 551.1
      obstruction 552.1
        and gangrene 551.1
    spermatic cord — *see* Hernia, inguinal
  gangrenous — *see* Hernia, by site, with
    gangrene
  gastrointestinal tract 553.9
    with
      gangrene (obstructed) 551.9
      obstruction 552.9
        and gangrene 551.9
  gluteal — *see* Hernia, femoral
  Gruber's (internal mesogastric) 553.8
    with
      gangrene (obstructed) 551.8
      obstruction 552.8
        and gangrene 551.8
  Hesselbach's 553.8
    with
      gangrene (obstructed) 551.8
      obstruction 552.8
        and gangrene 551.8
  hiatal (esophageal) (sliding) 553.3
    with
      gangrene (obstructed) 551.3
      obstruction 552.3
        and gangrene 551.3
    congenital 750.6
  incarcerated (*see also* Hernia, by site, with
    obstruction) 552.9
    gangrenous (*see also* Hernia, by site, with
      gangrene) 551.9
  incisional 553.21
    with
      gangrene (obstructed) 551.21
      obstruction 552.21
        and gangrene 551.21
    lumbar — *see* Hernia, lumbar
    recurrent 553.21
      with
        gangrene (obstructed) 551.21
        obstruction 552.21
          and gangrene 551.21
  indirect (inguinal) — *see* Hernia, inguinal
  infantile — *see* Hernia, inguinal
  infrapatellar fat pad 729.31
  inguinal (direct) (double) (encysted) (external)
    (funicular) (indirect) (infantile) (internal)
    (interstitial) (oblique) (scrotal) (sliding)
    550.9 ✓5ᵗʰ

Note — *Use the following fifth-digit*
subclassification with category 550:

  0   *unilateral or unspecified (not*
      specified as recurrent)

  1   *unilateral or unspecified, recurrent*

  2   *bilateral (not specified as recurrent)*

  3   *bilateral, recurrent*

---

    with
      gangrene (obstructed) 550.0 ✓5ᵗʰ
      obstruction 550.1 ✓5ᵗʰ
        and gangrene 550.0 ✓5ᵗʰ
  internal 553.8
    with
      gangrene (obstructed) 551.8
      obstruction 552.8
        and gangrene 551.8
    inguinal — *see* Hernia, inguinal
  interstitial 553.9
    with
      gangrene (obstructed) 551.9
      obstruction 552.9
        and gangrene 551.9
    inguinal — *see* Hernia, inguinal
  intervertebral cartilage or disc — *see*
    Displacement, intervertebral disc

Hernia, hernial — *continued*
  intestine, intestinal 553.9
    with
      gangrene (obstructed) 551.9
      obstruction 552.9
        and gangrene 551.9
  intra-abdominal 553.9
    with
      gangrene (obstructed) 551.9
      obstruction 552.9
        and gangrene 551.9
  intraparietal 553.9
    with
      gangrene (obstructed) 551.9
      obstruction 552.9
        and gangrene 551.9
  iris 364.8
    traumatic 871.1
  irreducible (*see also* Hernia, by site, with
    obstruction) 552.9
    gangrenous (with obstruction) (*see also*
      Hernia, by site, with gangrene) 551.9
  ischiatic 553.8
    with
      gangrene (obstructed) 551.8
      obstruction 552.8
        and gangrene 551.8
  ischiorectal 553.8
    with
      gangrene (obstructed) 551.8
      obstruction 552.8
        and gangrene 551.8
  lens 379.32
    traumatic 871.1
  linea
    alba — *see* Hernia, epigastric
    semilunaris — *see* Hernia, spigelian
  Littre's (diverticular) 553.9
    with
      gangrene (obstructed) 551.9
      obstruction 552.9
        and gangrene 551.9
  lumbar 553.8
    with
      gangrene (obstructed) 551.8
      obstruction 552.8
        and gangrene 551.8
    intervertebral disc 722.10
  lung (subcutaneous) 518.89
    congenital 748.69
  mediastinum 519.3
  mesenteric (internal) 553.8
    with
      gangrene (obstructed) 551.8
      obstruction 552.8
        and gangrene 551.8
  mesocolon 553.8
    with
      gangrene (obstructed) 551.8
      obstruction 552.8
        and gangrene 551.8
  muscle (sheath) 728.89
  nucleus pulposus — *see* Displacement,
    intervertebral disc
  oblique (inguinal) — *see* Hernia, inguinal
  obstructive (*see also* Hernia, by site, with
    obstruction) 552.9
    gangrenous (with obstruction) (*see also*
      Hernia, by site, with gangrene) 551.9
  obturator 553.8
    with
      gangrene (obstructed) 551.8
      obstruction 552.8
        and gangrene 551.8
  omental 553.8
    with
      gangrene (obstructed) 551.8
      obstruction 552.8
        and gangrene 551.8
  orbital fat (pad) 374.34
  ovary 620.4
  oviduct 620.4
  paracolostomy (stoma) 569.69
  paraduodenal 553.8
    with
      gangrene (obstructed) 551.8
      obstruction 552.8
        and gangrene 551.8

Hernia, hernial — *continued*
  paraesophageal 553.3
    with
      gangrene (obstructed) 551.3
      obstruction 552.3
        and gangrene 551.3
    congenital 750.6
  parahiatal 553.3
    with
      gangrene (obstructed) 551.3
      obstruction 552.3
        and gangrene 551.3
  paraumbilical 553.1
    with
      gangrene (obstructed) 551.1
      obstruction 552.1
        and gangrene 551.1
  parietal 553.9
    with
      gangrene (obstructed) 551.9
      obstruction 552.9
        and gangrene 551.9
  perineal 553.8
    with
      gangrene (obstructed) 551.8
      obstruction 552.8
        and gangrene 551.8
  peritoneal sac, lesser 553.8
    with
      gangrene (obstructed) 551.8
      obstruction 552.8
        and gangrene 551.8
  popliteal fat pad 729.31
  postoperative 553.21
    with
      gangrene (obstructed) 551.21
      obstruction 552.21
        and gangrene 551.21
  pregnant uterus 654.4 ✓5ᵗʰ
  prevesical 596.8
  properitoneal 553.8
    with
      gangrene (obstructed) 551.8
      obstruction 552.8
        and gangrene 551.8
  pudendal 553.8
    with
      gangrene (obstructed) 551.8
      obstruction 552.8
        and gangrene 551.8
  rectovaginal 618.6
  retroperitoneal 553.8
    with
      gangrene (obstructed) 551.8
      obstruction 552.8
        and gangrene 551.8
  Richter's (parietal) 553.9
    with
      gangrene (obstructed) 551.9
      obstruction 552.9
        and gangrene 551.9
  Rieux's, Riex's (retrocecal) 553.8
    with
      gangrene (obstructed) 551.8
      obstruction 552.8
        and gangrene 551.8
  sciatic 553.8
    with
      gangrene (obstructed) 551.8
      obstruction 552.8
        and gangrene 551.8
  scrotum, scrotal — *see* Hernia, inguinal
  sliding (inguinal) — *see also* Hernia, inguinal
    hiatus — *see* Hernia, hiatal
  spigelian 553.29
    with
      gangrene (obstructed) 551.29
      obstruction 552.29
        and gangrene 551.29
  spinal (*see also* Spina bifida) 741.9 ✓5ᵗʰ
    with hydrocephalus 741.0 ✓5ᵗʰ
  strangulated (*see also* Hernia, by site, with
    obstruction) 552.9
    gangrenous (with obstruction) (*see also*
      Hernia, by site, with gangrene) 551.9
  supraumbilicus (linea alba) — *see* Hernia,
    epigastric

✓4ᵗʰ Fourth-digit Required   ✓5ᵗʰ Fifth-digit Required   ▶◀ Revised Text   ● New Line   ▲ Revised Code

Hernia, hernial — *continued*
tendon 727.9
testis (nontraumatic) 550.9
meaning
scrotal hernia 550.9
symptomatic late syphilis 095.8
Treitz's (fossa) 553.8
with
gangrene (obstructed) 551.8
obstruction 552.8
and gangrene 551.8
tunica
albuginea 608.89
vaginalis 752.8
umbilicus, umbilical 553.1
with
gangrene (obstructed) 551.1
obstruction 552.1
and gangrene 551.1
ureter 593.89
with obstruction 593.4
uterus 621.8
pregnant 654.4 ✓5ᵗʰ
vaginal (posterior) 618.6
Velpeau's (femoral) (*see also* Hernia, femoral) 553.00
ventral 553.20
with
gangrene (obstructed) 551.20
obstruction 552.20
and gangrene 551.20
recurrent 553.21
with
gangrene (obstructed) 551.21
obstruction 552.21
and gangrene 551.21
vesical
congenital (female) (male) 756.71
female 618.0
male 596.8
vitreous (into anterior chamber) 379.21
traumatic 871.1
Herniation — *see also* Hernia
brain (stem) 348.4
cerebral 348.4
gastric mucosa (into duodenal bulb) 537.89
mediastinum 519.3
nucleus pulposus — *see* Displacement, intervertebral disc
Herpangina 074.0
Herpes, herpetic 054.9
auricularis (zoster) 053.71
simplex 054.73
blepharitis (zoster) 053.20
simplex 054.41
circinate 110.5
circinatus 110.5
bullous 694.5
conjunctiva (simplex) 054.43
zoster 053.21
cornea (simplex) 054.43
disciform (simplex) 054.43
zoster 053.21
encephalitis 054.3
eye (zoster) 053.29
simplex 054.40
eyelid (zoster) 053.20
simplex 054.41
febrilis 054.9
fever 054.9
geniculate ganglionitis 053.11
genital, genitalis 054.10
specified site NEC 054.19
gestationis 646.8 ✓5ᵗʰ
gingivostomatitis 054.2
iridocyclitis (simplex) 054.44
zoster 053.22
iris (any site) 695.1
iritis (simplex) 054.44
keratitis (simplex) 054.43
dendritic 054.42
disciform 054.43
interstitial 054.43
zoster 053.21
keratoconjunctivitis (simplex) 054.43
zoster 053.21

Herpes, herpetic — *continued*
labialis 054.9
meningococcal 036.89
lip 054.9
meningitis (simplex) 054.72
zoster 053.0
ophthalmicus (zoster) 053.20
simplex 054.40
otitis externa (zoster) 053.71
simplex 054.73
penis 054.13
perianal 054.10
pharyngitis 054.79
progenitalis 054.10
scrotum 054.19
septicemia 054.4 ✓5ᵗʰ
simplex 054.9
complicated 054.8
ophthalmic 054.40
specified NEC 054.49
specified NEC 054.79
congenital 771.2
external ear 054.73
keratitis 054.43
dendritic 054.42
meningitis 054.72
neuritis 054.79
specified complication NEC 054.79
ophthalmic 054.49
visceral 054.71
stomatitis 054.2
tonsurans 110.0
maculosus (of Hebra) 696.3
visceral 054.71
vulva 054.12
vulvovaginitis 054.11
whitlow 054.6
zoster 053.9
auricularis 053.71
complicated 053.8
specified NEC 053.79
conjunctiva 053.21
cornea 053.21
ear 053.71
eye 053.29
geniculate 053.11
keratitis 053.21
interstitial 053.21
neuritis 053.10
ophthalmicus(a) 053.20
oticus 053.71
otitis externa 053.71
specified complication NEC 053.79
specified site NEC 053.9
zosteriform, intermediate type 053.9
Herrick's
anemia (hemoglobin S disease) 282.61
syndrome (hemoglobin S disease) 282.61
Hers' disease (glycogenosis VI) 271.0
Herter's infantilism (nontropical sprue) 579.0
Herter (-Gee) disease or syndrome (nontropical sprue) 579.0
Herxheimer's disease (diffuse idiopathic cutaneous atrophy) 701.8
Herxheimer's reaction 995.0
Hesselbach's hernia — *see* Hernia, Hesselbach's
Heterochromia (congenital) 743.46
acquired 364.53
cataract 366.33
cyclitis 364.21
hair 704.3
iritis 364.21
retained metallic foreign body 360.62
magnetic 360.52
uveitis 364.21
Heterophoria 378.40
alternating 378.45
vertical 378.43
Heterophyes, small intestine 121.6
Heterophyiasis 121.6
Heteropsia 368.8
Heterotopia, heterotopic — *see also* Malposition, congenital
cerebralis 742.4
pancreas, pancreatic 751.7

Heterotopia, heterotopic — *see also* Malposition, congenital — *continued*
spinalis 742.59
Heterotropia 378.30
intermittent 378.20
vertical 378.31
vertical (constant) (intermittent) 378.31
Heubner's disease 094.89
Heubner-Herter disease or syndrome (nontropical sprue) 579.0
Hexadactylism 755.0 ✓5ᵗʰ
Heyd's syndrome (hepatorenal) 572.4
HGSIL (high grade squamous intraepithelial ● dysplasia) 622.1 ●
Hibernoma (M8880/0) — *see* Lipoma
Hiccough 786.8
epidemic 078.89
psychogenic 306.1
Hiccup (*see also* Hiccough) 786.8
Hicks (-Braxton) contractures 644.1 ✓5ᵗʰ
Hidden penis 752.65
Hidradenitis (axillaris) (suppurative) 705.83
Hidradenoma (nodular) (M8400/0) — *see also* Neoplasm, skin, benign
clear cell (M8402/0) — *see* Neoplasm, skin, benign
papillary (M8405/0) — *see* Neoplasm, skin, benign
Hidrocystoma (M8404/0) — *see* Neoplasm, skin, benign
High
A₂ anemia 282.4
altitude effects 993.2
anoxia 993.2
on
ears 993.0
sinuses 993.1
polycythemia 289.0
arch
foot 755.67
palate 750.26
artery (arterial) tension (*see also* Hypertension) 401.9
without diagnosis of hypertension 796.2
basal metabolic rate (BMR) 794.7
blood pressure (*see also* Hypertension) 401.9
incidental reading (isolated) (nonspecific), no diagnosis of hypertension 796.2
compliance bladder 596.4
diaphragm (congenital) 756.6
frequency deafness (congenital) (regional) 389.8
head at term 652.5 ✓5ᵗʰ
affecting fetus or newborn 763.1
output failure (cardiac) (*see also* Failure, heart) 428.9
oxygen-affinity hemoglobin 289.0
palate 750.26
risk
behavior — *see* Problem
family situation V61.9
specified circumstance NEC V61.8
individual NEC V62.89
infant NEC V20.1
patient taking drugs (prescribed) V67.51
nonprescribed (*see also* Abuse, drugs, nondependent) 305.9 ✓5ᵗʰ
pregnancy V23.9
inadequate prenatal care V23.7
specified problem NEC V23.8 ✓5ᵗʰ
temperature (of unknown origin) (*see also* Pyrexia) 780.6
thoracic rib 756.3
Hildenbrand's disease (typhus) 081.9
Hilger's syndrome 337.0
Hill diarrhea 579.1
Hilliard's lupus (*see also* Tuberculosis) 017.0 ✓5ᵗʰ
Hilum — *see* condition
Hip — *see* condition
Hippel's disease (retinocerebral angiomatosis) 759.6
Hippus 379.49
Hirschfeld's disease (acute diabetes mellitus) (*see also* Diabetes) 250.0 ✓5ᵗʰ

✓4ᵗʰ Fourth-digit Required   ✓5ᵗʰ Fifth-digit Required   ►◄ Revised Text   ● New Line   ▲ Revised Code

Hirschsprung's disease or megacolon (congenital) 751.3

Hirsuties (*see also* Hypertrichosis) 704.1

Hirsutism (*see also* Hypertrichosis) 704.1

Hirudiniasis (external) (internal) 134.2

His-Werner disease (trench fever) 083.1

Hiss-Russell dysentery 004.1

Histamine cephalgia 346.2 ✓5ᵗʰ

Histidinemia 270.5

Histidinuria 270.5

Histiocytoma (M8832/0) — *see also* Neoplasm, skin, benign
  fibrous (M8830/0) — *see also* Neoplasm, skin, benign
    atypical (M8830/1) — *see* Neoplasm, connective tissue, uncertain behavior
    malignant (M8830/3) — *see* Neoplasm, connective tissue, malignant

Histiocytosis (acute) (chronic) (subacute) 277.8
  acute differentiated progressive (M9722/3) 202.5 ✓5ᵗʰ
  cholesterol 277.8
  essential 277.8
  lipid, lipoid (essential) 272.7
  lipochrome (familial) 288.1
  malignant (M9720/3) 202.3 ✓5ᵗʰ
  X (chronic) 277.8
    acute (progressive) (M9722/3) 202.5 ✓5ᵗʰ

Histoplasmosis 115.90
  with
    endocarditis 115.94
    meningitis 115.91
    pericarditis 115.93
    pneumonia 115.95
    retinitis 115.92
    specified manifestation NEC 115.99
  African (due to Histoplasma duboisii) 115.10
    with
      endocarditis 115.14
      meningitis 115.11
      pericarditis 115.13
      pneumonia 115.15
      retinitis 115.12
      specified manifestation NEC 115.19
  American (due to Histoplasma capsulatum) 115.00
    with
      endocarditis 115.04
      meningitis 115.01
      pericarditis 115.03
      pneumonia 115.05
      retinitis 115.02
      specified manifestation NEC 115.09
  Darling's — *see* Histoplasmosis, American
  large cell (*see also* Histoplasmosis, African) 115.10
  lung 115.05
  small form (*see also* Histoplasmosis, American) 115.00

History (personal) of
  abuse
    emotional V15.42
    neglect V15.42
    physical V15.41
    sexual V15.41
  affective psychosis V11.1
  alcoholism V11.3
    specified as drinking problem (*see also* Abuse, drugs, nondependent) 305.0 ✓5ᵗʰ
  allergy to
    analgesic agent NEC V14.6
    anesthetic NEC V14.4
    antibiotic agent NEC V14.1
      penicillin V14.0
    anti-infective agent NEC V14.3
    diathesis V15.09
    drug V14.9
      specified type NEC V14.8
    eggs V15.03
    food additives V15.05
    insect bite V15.06
    latex V15.07
    medicinal agents V14.9
      specified type NEC V14.8

History (personal) of — *continued*
  allergy to — *continued*
    milk products V15.02
    narcotic agent NEC V14.5
    nuts V15.05
      peanuts V15.01
    penicillin V14.0
    radiographic dye V15.08
    seafood V15.04
    serum V14.7
    specified food NEC V15.05
    specified nonmedicinal agents NEC V15.09
    spider bite V15.06
    sulfa V14.2
    sulfonamides V14.2
    therapeutic agent NEC V15.09
    vaccine V14.7
  anemia V12.3
  arthritis V13.4
  benign neoplasm of brain V12.41
  blood disease V12.3
  calculi, urinary V13.01
  cardiovascular disease V12.50
    myocardial infarction 412
  child abuse V15.41
  cigarette smoking V15.82
  circulatory system disease V12.50
    myocardial infarction 412
  congenital malformation V13.69
  contraception V15.7
  diathesis, allergic V15.09
  digestive system disease V12.70
    peptic ulcer V12.71
    polyps, colonic V12.72
    specified NEC V12.79
  disease (of) V13.9
    blood V12.3
    blood-forming organs V12.3
    cardiovascular system V12.50
    circulatory system V12.50
    digestive system V12.70
      peptic ulcer V12.71
      polyps, colonic V12.72
      specified NEC V12.79
    infectious V12.00
      malaria V12.03
      poliomyelitis V12.02
      specified NEC V12.09
      tuberculosis V12.01
    parasitic V12.00
      specified NEC V12.09
    respiratory system V12.6
    skin V13.3
    specified site NEC V13.8
    subcutaneous tissue V13.3
    trophoblastic V13.1
      affecting management of pregnant V23.1
  disorder (of) V13.9
    endocrine V12.2
    genital system V13.29 ▲
    hematological V12.3
    immunity V12.2
    mental V11.9
      affective type V11.1
      manic-depressive V11.1
      neurosis V11.2
      schizophrenia V11.0
      specified type NEC V11.8
    metabolic V12.2
    musculoskeletal NEC V13.5
    nervous system V12.40
      specified type NEC V12.49
    obstetric V13.29 ▲
      affecting management of current pregnancy V23.49 ▲
        pre-term labor V23.41 ●
      pre-term labor V13.21 ●
    sense organs V12.40
      specified type NEC V12.49
    specified site NEC V13.8
    urinary system V13.00
      calculi V13.01
      specified NEC V13.09
  drug use
    nonprescribed (*see also* Abuse, drugs, nondependent) 305.9 ✓5ᵗʰ

History (personal) of — *continued*
  drug use — *continued*
    patent (*see also* Abuse, drugs, nondependent) 305.9 ✓5ᵗʰ
  effect NEC of external cause V15.89
  embolism (pulmonary) V12.51
  emotional abuse V15.42
  endocrine disorder V12.2
  family
    allergy V19.6
    anemia V18.2
    arteriosclerosis V17.4
    arthritis V17.7
    asthma V17.5
    blindness V19.0
    blood disorder NEC V18.3
    cardiovascular disease V17.4
    cerebrovascular disease V17.1
    chronic respiratory condition NEC V17.6
    congenital anomalies V19.5
    consanguinity V19.7
    coronary artery disease V17.3
    cystic fibrosis V18.1
    deafness V19.2
    diabetes mellitus V18.0
    digestive disorders V18.5
    disease or disorder (of)
      allergic V19.6
      blood NEC V18.3
      cardiovascular NEC V17.4
      cerebrovascular V17.1
      coronary artery V17.3
      digestive V18.5
      ear NEC V19.3
      endocrine V18.1
      eye NEC V19.1
      genitourinary NEC V18.7
      hypertensive V17.4
      infectious V18.8
      ischemic heart V17.3
      kidney V18.69
        polycystic V18.61
      mental V17.0
      metabolic V18.1
      musculoskeletal NEC V17.8
      neurological NEC V17.2
      parasitic V18.8
      psychiatric condition V17.0
      skin condition V19.4
    ear disorder NEC V19.3
    endocrine disease V18.1
    epilepsy V17.2
    eye disorder NEC V19.1
    genitourinary disease NEC V18.7
    glomerulonephritis V18.69
    gout V18.1
    hay fever V17.6
    hearing loss V19.2
    hematopoietic neoplasia V16.7
    Hodgkin's disease V16.7
    Huntington's chorea V17.2
    hydrocephalus V19.5
    hypertension V17.4
    hypospadias V13.61
    infectious disease V18.8
    ischemia heart disease V17.3
    kidney disease V18.69
      polycystic V18.61
    leukemia V16.6
    lymphatic malignant neoplasia NEC V16.7
    malignant neoplasm (of) NEC V16.9
      anorectal V16.0
      anus V16.0
      appendix V16.0
      bladder V16.59
      bone V16.8
      brain V16.8
      breast V16.3
        male V16.8
      bronchus V16.1
      cecum V16.0
      cervix V16.49
      colon V16.0
      duodenum V16.0
      esophagus V16.0
      eye V16.8
      gallbladder V16.0

✓4ᵗʰ Fourth-digit Required   ✓5ᵗʰ Fifth-digit Required   ▶◀ Revised Text   ● New Line   ▲ Revised Code

History (personal) of — *continued*
  family — *continued*
    malignant neoplasm (of) NEC — *continued*
      gastrointestinal tract V16.0
      genital organs V16.40
      hemopoietic NEC V16.7
      ileum V16.0
      ilium V16.8
      intestine V16.0
      intrathoracic organs NEC V16.2
      kidney V16.51
      larynx V16.2
      liver V16.0
      lung V16.1
      lymphatic NEC V16.7
      ovary V16.41
      oviduct V16.41
      pancreas V16.0
      penis V16.49
      prostate V16.42
      rectum V16.0
      respiratory organs NEC V16.2
      skin V16.8
      specified site NEC V16.8
      stomach V16.0
      testis V16.43
      trachea V16.1
      ureter V16.59
      urethra V16.59
      urinary organs V16.59
      uterus V16.49
      vagina V16.49
      vulva V16.49
    mental retardation V18.4
    metabolic disease NEC V18.1
    mongolism V19.5
    multiple myeloma V16.7
    musculoskeletal disease NEC V17.8
    nephritis V18.69
    nephrosis V18.69
    parasitic disease V18.8
    polycystic kidney disease V18.61
    psychiatric disorder V17.0
    psychosis V17.0
    retardation, mental V18.4
    retinitis pigmentosa V19.1
    schizophrenia V17.0
    skin conditions V19.4
    specified condition NEC V19.8
    stroke (cerebrovascular) V17.1
    visual loss V19.0
  genital system disorder V13.29   ▲
    pre-term labor V13.21   ●
  health hazard V15.9
    specified cause NEC V15.89
  Hodgkin's disease V10.72
  immunity disorder V12.2
  infectious disease V12.00
    malaria V12.03
    poliomyelitis V12.02
    specified NEC V12.09
    tuberculosis V12.01
  injury NEC V15.5
  insufficient prenatal care V23.7
  irradiation V15.3
  leukemia V10.60
    lymphoid V10.61
    monocytic V10.63
    myeloid V10.62
    specified type NEC V10.69
  little or no prenatal care V23.7
  low birth weight (*see also* Status, low birth
    weight) V21.30
  lymphosarcoma V10.71
  malaria V12.03
  malignant neoplasm (of) V10.9
    accessory sinus V10.22
    adrenal V10.88
    anus V10.06
    bile duct V10.09
    bladder V10.51
    bone V10.81
    brain V10.85
    breast V10.3
    bronchus V10.11
    cervix uteri V10.41
    colon V10.05

History (personal) of — *continued*
  malignant neoplasm (of) — *continued*
    connective tissue NEC V10.89
    corpus uteri V10.42
    digestive system V10.00
      specified part NEC V10.09
    duodenum V10.09
    endocrine gland NEC V10.88
    epididymis V10.48
    esophagus V10.03
    eye V10.84
    fallopian tube V10.44
    female genital organ V10.40
      specified site NEC V10.44
    gallbladder V10.09
    gastrointestinal tract V10.00
    gum V10.02
    hematopoietic NEC V10.79
    hypopharynx V10.02
    ileum V10.09
    intrathoracic organs NEC V10.20
    jejunum V10.09
    kidney V10.52
    large intestine V10.05
    larynx V10.21
    lip V10.02
    liver V10.07
    lung V10.11
    lymphatic NEC V10.79
    lymph glands or nodes NEC V10.79
    male genital organ V10.45
      specified site NEC V10.49
    mediastinum V10.29
    melanoma (of skin) V10.82
    middle ear V10.22
    mouth V10.02
      specified part NEC V10.02
    nasal cavities V10.22
    nasopharynx V10.02
    nervous system NEC V10.86
    nose V10.22
    oropharynx V10.02
    ovary V10.43
    pancreas V10.09
    parathyroid V10.88
    penis V10.49
    pharynx V10.02
    pineal V10.88
    pituitary V10.88
    placenta V10.44
    pleura V10.29
    prostate V10.46
    rectosigmoid junction V10.06
    rectum V10.06
    renal pelvis V10.53
    respiratory organs NEC V10.20
    salivary gland V10.02
    skin V10.83
      melanoma V10.82
    small intestine NEC V10.09
    soft tissue NEC V10.89
    specified site NEC V10.89
    stomach V10.04
    testis V10.47
    thymus V10.29
    thyroid V10.87
    tongue V10.01
    trachea V10.12
    ureter V10.59
    urethra V10.59
    urinary organ V10.50
    uterine adnexa V10.44
    uterus V10.42
    vagina V10.44
    vulva V10.44
  manic-depressive psychosis V11.1
  mental disorder V11.9
    affective type V11.1
    manic-depressive V11.1
    neurosis V11.2
    schizophrenia V11.0
    specified type NEC V11.8
  metabolic disorder V12.2
  musculoskeletal disorder NEC V13.5
  myocardial infarction 412
  neglect (emotional) V15.42
  nervous system disorder V12.40
    specified type NEC V12.49

History (personal) of — *continued*
  neurosis V11.2
  noncompliance with medical treatment V15.81
  nutritional deficiency V12.1
  obstetric disorder V13.29   ●
    affecting management of current
      pregnancy V23.49   ▲
      pre-term labor V23.41   ●
    pre-term labor V13.21   ●
  parasitic disease V12.00
    specified NEC V12.09
  perinatal problems V13.7
    low birth weight (*see also* Status, low birth
      weight) V21.30
  physical abuse V15.41
  poisoning V15.6
  poliomyelitis V12.02
  polyps, colonic V12.72
  poor obstetric V13.29   ▲
    affecting management of current   ●
      pregnancy V23.49   ●
      pre-term labor V23.41   ●
      pre-term labor V13.21   ●
  psychiatric disorder V11.9
    affective type V11.1
    manic-depressive V11.1
    neurosis V11.2
    schizophrenia V11.0
    specified type NEC V11.8
  psychological trauma V15.49
    emotional abuse V15.42
    neglect V15.42
    physical abuse V15.41
    rape V15.41
  psychoneurosis V11.2
  radiation therapy V15.3
  rape V15.41
  respiratory system disease V12.6
  reticulosarcoma V10.71
  schizophrenia V11.0
  skin disease V13.3
  smoking (tobacco) V15.82
  subcutaneous tissue disease V13.3
  surgery (major) to
    great vessels V15.1
    heart V15.1
    major organs NEC V15.2
  thrombophlebitis V12.52
  thrombosis V12.51
  tobacco use V15.82
  trophoblastic disease V13.1
    affecting management of pregnancy V23.1
  tuberculosis V12.01
  ulcer, peptic V12.71
  urinary system disorder V13.00
    calculi V13.01
    specified NEC V13.09

HIV infection (disease) (illness) — *see* Human immunodeficiency virus (disease) (illness) (infection)

Hives (bold) (*see also* Urticaria) 708.9

Hoarseness 784.49

Hobnail liver — *see* Cirrhosis, portal

Hobo, hoboism V60.0

Hodgkins
  disease (M9650/3) 201.9 ✓5ᵗʰ
    lymphocytic
      depletion (M9653/3) 201.7 ✓5ᵗʰ
        diffuse fibrosis (M9654/3) 201.7 ✓5ᵗʰ
        reticular type (M9655/3) 201.7 ✓5ᵗʰ
      predominance (M9651/3) 201.4 ✓5ᵗʰ
    lymphocytic-histiocytic predominance
      (M9651/3) 201.4 ✓5ᵗʰ
    mixed cellularity (M9652/3) 201.6 ✓5ᵗʰ
    nodular sclerosis (M9656/3) 201.5 ✓5ᵗʰ
      cellular phase (M9657/3) 201.5 ✓5ᵗʰ
  granuloma (M9661/3) 201.1 ✓5ᵗʰ
  lymphogranulomatosis (M9650/3) 201.9 ✓5ᵗʰ
  lymphoma (M9650/3) 201.9 ✓5ᵗʰ
  lymphosarcoma (M9650/3) 201.9 ✓5ᵗʰ
  paragranuloma (M9660/3) 201.0 ✓5ᵗʰ
  sarcoma (M9662/3) 201.2 ✓5ᵗʰ

Hodgson's disease (aneurysmal dilatation of
  aorta) 441.9
  ruptured 441.5

Hodi-potsy 111.0

✓4ᵗʰ Fourth-digit Required   ✓5ᵗʰ Fifth-digit Required   ▶◀ Revised Text   ● New Line   ▲ Revised Code

Hoffa (-Kastert) disease or syndrome (liposynovitis prepatellaris) 272.8

Hoffman's syndrome 244.9 [359.5]

Hoffmann-Bouveret syndrome (paroxysmal tachycardia) 427.2

Hole
macula 362.54
optic disc, crater-like 377.22
retina (macula) 362.54
round 361.31
with detachment 361.01

Holla disease (see also Spherocytosis) 282.0

Holländer-Simons syndrome (progressive lipodystrophy) 272.6

Hollow foot (congenital) 754.71
acquired 736.73

Holmes' syndrome (visual disorientation) 368.16

Holoprosencephaly 742.2
due to
trisomy 13 758.1
trisomy 18 758.2

Holthouse's hernia — see Hernia, inguinal

Homesickness 309.89

Homocystinemia 270.4

Homocystinuria 270.4

Homologous serum jaundice (prophylactic) (therapeutic) — see Hepatitis, viral

Homosexuality — omit code
ego-dystonic 302.0
pedophilic 302.2
problems with 302.0

Homozygous Hb-S disease 282.61

Honeycomb lung 518.89
congenital 748.4

Hong Kong ear 117.3

HOOD (hereditary osteo-onychodysplasia) 756.89

Hooded
clitoris 752.49
penis 752.69

Hookworm (anemia) (disease) (infestation) — see Ancylostomiasis

Hoppe-Goldflam syndrome 358.0

Hordeolum (external) (eyelid) 373.11
internal 373.12

Horn
cutaneous 702.8
cheek 702.8
eyelid 702.8
penis 702.8
iliac 756.89
nail 703.8
congenital 757.5
papillary 700

Horner's
syndrome (see also Neuropathy, peripheral, autonomic) 337.9
traumatic 954.0
teeth 520.4

Horseshoe kidney (congenital) 753.3

Horton's
disease (temporal arteritis) 446.5
headache or neuralgia 346.2 ✔5ᵗʰ

Hospice care V66.7

Hospitalism (in children) NEC 309.83

Hourglass contraction, contracture
bladder 596.8
gallbladder 575.2
congenital 751.69
stomach 536.8
congenital 750.7
psychogenic 306.4
uterus 661.4 ✔5ᵗʰ
affecting fetus or newborn 763.7

Household circumstance affecting care V60.9
specified type NEC V60.8

Housemaid's knee 727.2

Housing circumstance affecting care V60.9
specified type NEC V60.8

Huchard's disease (continued arterial hypertension) 401.9

Hudson-Stähli lines 371.11

Huguier's disease (uterine fibroma) 218.9

Hum, venous — omit code

Human bite (open wound) — see also Wound, open, by site
intact skin surface — see Contusion

Human immunodeficiency virus (disease) (illness) 042
infection V08
with symptoms, symptomatic 042

Human immunodeficiency virus-2 infection 079.53

Human immunovirus (disease) (illness) (infection) — see Human immunodeficiency virus (disease) (illness) (infection)

Human papillomavirus 079.4

Human T-cell lymphotrophic virus-I infection 079.51

Human T-cell lymphotrophic virus-II infection 079.52

Human T-cell lymphotrophic virus-III (disease) (illness) (infection) — see Human immunodeficiency virus (disease) (illness) (infection)

HTLV-I infection 079.51

HTLV-II infection 079.52

HTLV-III (disease) (illness) (infection) — see Human immunodeficiency virus (disease) (illness) (infection)

HTLV-III/LAV (disease) (illness) (infection) — see Human immunodeficiency virus (disease) (illness) (infection)

Humpback (acquired) 737.9
congenital 756.19

Hunchback (acquired) 737.9
congenital 756.19

Hunger 994.2
air, psychogenic 306.1
disease 251.1

Hunner's ulcer (see also Cystitis) 595.1

Hunt's
neuralgia 053.11
syndrome (herpetic geniculate ganglionitis) 053.11
dyssynergia cerebellaris myoclonica 334.2

Hunter's glossitis 529.4

Hunter (-Hurler) syndrome (mucopolysaccharidosis II) 277.5

Hunterian chancre 091.0

Huntington's
chorea 333.4
disease 333.4

Huppert's disease (multiple myeloma) (M9730/3) 203.0 ✔5ᵗʰ

Hurier (-Hunter) disease or syndrome (mucopolysaccharidosis II) 277.5

Hürthle cell
adenocarcinoma (M8290/3) 193
adenoma (M8290/0) 226
carcinoma (M8290/3) 193
tumor (M8290/0) 226

Hutchinson's
disease meaning
angioma serpiginosum 709.1
cheiropompholyx 705.81
prurigo estivalis 692.72
summer eruption, or summer prurigo 692.72
incisors 090.5
melanotic freckle (M8742/2) — see also Neoplasm, skin, in situ
malignant melanoma in (M8742/3) — see Melanoma
teeth or incisors (congenital syphilis) 090.5

Hutchinson-Boeck disease or syndrome (sarcoidosis) 135

Hutchinson-Gilford disease or syndrome (progeria) 259.8

Hyaline
degeneration (diffuse) (generalized) 728.9
localized — see Degeneration, by site

Hyaline — continued
membrane (disease) (lung) (newborn) 769

Hyalinosis cutis et mucosae 272.8

Hyalin plaque, sclera, senile 379.16

Hyalitis (asteroid) 379.22
syphilitic 095.8

Hydatid
cyst or tumor — see also Echinococcus
fallopian tube 752.11
mole — see Hydatidiform mole
Morgagni (congenital) 752.8
fallopian tube 752.11

Hydatidiform mole (benign) (complicating pregnancy) (delivered) (undelivered) 630
invasive (M9100/1) 236.1
malignant (M9100/1) 236.1
previous, affecting management of pregnancy V23.1

Hydatidosis — see Echinococcus

Hyde's disease (prurigo nodularis) 698.3

Hydradenitis 705.83

Hydradenoma (M8400/0) — see Hidradenoma

Hydralazine lupus or syndrome
correct substance properly administered 695.4
overdose or wrong substance given or taken 972.6

Hydramnios 657 ✔4ᵗʰ
affecting fetus or newborn 761.3

Hydrancephaly 742.3
with spina bifida (see also Spina bifida) 741.0 ✔5ᵗʰ

Hydranencephaly 742.3
with spina bifida (see also Spina bifida) 741.0 ✔5ᵗʰ

Hydrargyrism NEC 985.0

Hydrarthrosis (see also Effusion, joint) 719.0 ✔5ᵗʰ
gonococcal 098.50
intermittent (see also Rheumatism, palindromic) 719.3 ✔5ᵗʰ
of yaws (early) (late) 102.6
syphilitic 095.8
congenital 090.5

Hydremia 285.9

Hydrencephalocele (congenital) 742.0

Hydrencephalomeningocele (congenital) 742.0

Hydroa 694.0
aestivale 692.72
gestationis 646.8 ✔5ᵗʰ
herpetiformis 694.0
pruriginosa 694.0
vacciniforme 692.72

Hydroadenitis 705.83

Hydrocalycosis (see also Hydronephrosis) 591
congenital 753.29

Hydrocalyx (see also Hydronephrosis) 591

Hydrocele (calcified) (chylous) (idiopathic) (infantile) (inguinal canal) (recurrent) (senile) (spermatic cord) (testis) (tunica vaginalis) 603.9
canal of Nuck (female) 629.1
male 603.9
congenital 778.6
encysted 603.0
congenital 778.6
female NEC 629.8
infected 603.1
round ligament 629.8
specified type NEC 603.8
congenital 778.6
spinalis (see also Spina bifida) 741.9 ✔5ᵗʰ
vulva 624.8

Hydrocephalic fetus
affecting management or pregnancy 655.0 ✔5ᵗʰ
causing disproportion 653.6 ✔5ᵗʰ
with obstructed labor 660.1 ✔5ᵗʰ
affecting fetus or newborn 763.1

Hydrocephalus (acquired) (external) (internal) (malignant) (noncommunicating) (obstructive) (recurrent) 331.4
aqueduct of Sylvius structure 742.3
with spina bifida (see also Spina bifida) 741.0 ✔5ᵗʰ

Hydrocephalus — *continued*
  chronic 742.3
    with spina bifida (*see also* Spina bifida)
      741.0 ✔5ᵗʰ
  communicating 331.3
  congenital (external) (internal) 742.3
    with spina bifida (*see also* Spina bifida)
      741.0 ✔5ᵗʰ
  due to
    structure of aqueduct of Sylvius 742.3
      with spina bifida (*see also* Spina bifida)
        741.0 ✔5ᵗʰ
    toxoplasmosis (congenital) 771.2
  fetal affecting management of pregnancy
    655.0 ✔5ᵗʰ
  foramen Magendie block (acquired) 331.3
    congenital 742.3
      with spina bifida (*see also* Spina bifida)
        741.0 ✔5ᵗʰ
  newborn 742.3
    with spina bifida (*see also* Spina bifida)
      741.0 ✔5ᵗʰ
  otitic 331.4
  syphilitic, congenital 090.49
  tuberculous (*see also* Tuberculosis) 013.8 ✔5ᵗʰ
Hydrocolpos (congenital) 623.8
Hydrocystoma (M8404/0) — *see* Neoplasm, skin,
  benign
Hydroencephalocele (congenital) 742.0
Hydroencephalomeningocele (congenital) 742.0
Hydrohematopneumothorax (*see also*
  Hemothorax) 511.8
Hydromeningitis — *see* Meningitis
Hydromeningocele (spinal) (*see also* Spina bifida)
  741.9 ✔5ᵗʰ
  cranial 742.0
Hydrometra 621.8
Hydrometrocolpos 623.8
Hydromicrocephaly 742.1
Hydromphalus (congenital) (since birth) 757.39
Hydromyelia 742.53
Hydromyelocele (*see also* Spina bifida) 741.9 ✔5ᵗʰ
Hydronephrosis 591
  atrophic 591
  congenital 753.29
  due to S. hematobium 120.0
  early 591
  functionless (infected) 591
  infected 591
  intermittent 591
  primary 591
  secondary 591
  tuberculous (*see also* Tuberculosis) 016.0 ✔5ᵗʰ
Hydropericarditis (*see also* Pericarditis) 423.9
Hydropericardium (*see also* Pericarditis) 423.9
Hydroperitoneum 789.5
Hydrophobia 071
Hydrophthalmos (*see also* Buphthalmia) 743.20
Hydropneumohemothorax (*see also* Hemothorax)
  511.8
Hydropneumopericarditis (*see also* Pericarditis)
  423.9
Hydropneumopericardium (*see also* Pericarditis)
  423.9
Hydropneumothorax 511.8
  nontuberculous 511.8
    bacterial 511.1
  pneumococcal 511.1
  staphylococcal 511.1
  streptococcal 511.1
  traumatic 860.0
    with open wound into thorax 860.1
  tuberculous (*see also* Tuberculosis, pleura)
    012.0 ✔5ᵗʰ
Hydrops 782.3
  abdominis 789.5
  amnii (complicating pregnancy) (*see also*
    Hydramnios) 657 ✔4ᵗʰ
  articulorum intermittens (*see also*
    Rheumatism, palindromic) 719.3 ✔5ᵗʰ
  cardiac (*see also* Failure, heart) 428.0
  congenital — *see* Hydrops, fetalis

Hydrops — *continued*
  endolymphatic (*see also* Disease, Ménière's)
    386.00
  fetal(is) or newborn 778.0
    due to isoimmunization 773.3
    not due to isoimmunization 778.0
  gallbladder 575.3
  idiopathic (fetus or newborn) 778.0
  joint (*see also* Effusion, joint) 719.0 ✔5ᵗʰ
  labyrinth (*see also* Disease, Ménière's) 386.00
  meningeal NEC 331.4
  nutritional 262
  pericardium — *see* Pericarditis
  pleura (*see also* Hydrothorax) 511.8
  renal (*see also* Nephrosis) 581.9
  spermatic cord (*see also* Hydrocele) 603.9
Hydropyonephrosis (*see also* Pyelitis) 590.80
  chronic 590.00
Hydrorachis 742.53
Hydrorrhea (nasal) 478.1
  gravidarum 658.1 ✔5ᵗʰ
  pregnancy 658.1 ✔5ᵗʰ
Hydrosadenitis 705.83
Hydrosalpinx (fallopian tube) (follicularis) 614.1
Hydrothorax (double) (pleural) 511.8
  chylous (nonfilarial) 457.8
    filaria (*see also* Infestation, filarial) 125.9
  nontuberculous 511.8
    bacterial 511.1
  pneumococcal 511.1
  staphylococcal 511.1
  streptococcal 511.1
  traumatic 862.29
    with open wound into thorax 862.39
  tuberculous (*see also* Tuberculosis, pleura)
    012.0 ✔5ᵗʰ
Hydroureter 593.5
  congenital 753.22
Hydroureteronephrosis (*see also* Hydronephrosis)
  591
Hydrourethra 599.84
Hydroxykynureninuria 270.2
Hydroxyprolinemia 270.8
Hydroxyprolinuria 270.8
Hygroma (congenital) (cystic) (M9173/0) 228.1
  prepatellar 727.3
  subdural — *see* Hematoma, subdural
Hymen — *see* condition
Hymenolepiasis (diminuta) (infection) (infestation)
  (nana) 123.6
Hymenolepis (diminuta) (infection) (infestation)
  (nana) 123.6
Hypalgesia (*see also* Disturbance, sensation)
  782.0
Hyperabduction syndrome 447.8
Hyperacidity, gastric 536.8
  psychogenic 306.4
Hyperactive, hyperactivity
  basal cell, uterine cervix 622.1
  bladder 596.51
  bowel (syndrome) 564.9
    sounds 787.5
  cervix epithelial (basal) 622.1
  child 314.01
  colon 564.9
  gastrointestinal 536.8
    psychogenic 306.4
  intestine 564.9
  labyrinth (unilateral) 386.51
    with loss of labyrinthine reactivity 386.58
    bilateral 386.52
  nasal mucous membrane 478.1
  stomach 536.8
  thyroid (gland) (*see also* Thyrotoxicosis)
    242.9 ✔5ᵗʰ
Hyperacusis 388.42
Hyperadrenalism (cortical) 255.3
  medullary 255.6
Hyperadrenocorticism 255.3
  congenital 255.2
  iatrogenic
    correct substance properly administered
      255.3

Hyperadrenocorticism — *continued*
  iatrogenic — *continued*
    overdose or wrong substance given or taken
      962.0
Hyperaffectivity 301.11
Hyperaldosteronism (atypical) (hyperplastic)
  (normoaldosteronal) (normotensive)
  (primary) (secondary) 255.1
Hyperalgesia (*see also* Disturbance, sensation)
  782.0
Hyperalimentation 783.6
  carotene 278.3
  specified NEC 278.8
  vitamin A 278.2
  vitamin D 278.4
Hyperaminoaciduria 270.9
  arginine 270.6
  citrulline 270.6
  cystine 270.0
  glycine 270.0
  lysine 270.7
  ornithine 270.6
  renal (types I, II, III) 270.0
Hyperammonemia (congenital) 270.6
Hyperamnesia 780.99   ▲
Hyperamylasemia 790.5
Hyperaphia 782.0
Hyperazotemia 791.9
Hyperbetalipoproteinemia (acquired) (essential)
  (familial) (hereditary) (primary) (secondary)
  272.0
  with prebetalipoproteinemia 272.2
Hyperbilirubinemia 782.4
  congenital 277.4
  constitutional 277.4
  neonatal (transient) (*see also* Jaundice, fetus or
    newborn) 774.6
  of prematurity 774.2
Hyperbilirubinemica encephalopathia, newborn
  774.7
  due to isoimmunization 773.4
Hypercalcemia, hypercalcemic (idiopathic)
  275.42
  nephropathy 588.8
Hypercalcinuria 275.40
Hypercapnia 786.09
  with mixed acid-base disorder 276.4
  fetal, affecting newborn 770.89   ▲
Hypercarotinemia 278.3
Hypercementosis 521.5
Hyperchloremia 276.9
Hyperchlorhydria 536.8
  neurotic 306.4
  psychogenic 306.4
Hypercholesterinemia — *see*
  Hypercholesterolemia
Hypercholesterolemia 272.0
  with hyperglyceridemia, endogenous 272.2
  essential 272.0
  familial 272.0
  hereditary 272.0
  primary 272.0
  pure 272.0
Hypercholesterolosis 272.0
Hyperchylia gastrica 536.8
  psychogenic 306.4
Hyperchylomicronemia (familial) (with
  hyperbetalipoproteinemia) 272.3
Hypercoagulation syndrome 289.8
Hypercorticosteronism
  correct substance properly administered 255.3
  overdose or wrong substance given or taken
    962.0
Hypercortisonism
  correct substance properly administered 255.3
  overdose or wrong substance given or taken
    962.0
Hyperdynamic beta-adrenergic state or
  syndrome (circulatory) 429.82
Hyperelectrolytemia 276.9

✔4ᵗʰ Fourth-digit Required   ✔5ᵗʰ Fifth-digit Required   ►◄ Revised Text   ● New Line   ▲ Revised Code

Hyperemesis 536.2
  arising during pregnancy — *see* Hyperemesis,
    gravidarum
  gravidarum (mild) (before 22 completed weeks
    gestation) 643.0 ✓5ᵗʰ
    with
      carbohydrate depletion 643.1 ✓5ᵗʰ
      dehydration 643.1 ✓5ᵗʰ
      electrolyte imbalance 643.1 ✓5ᵗʰ
      metabolic disturbance 643.1 ✓5ᵗʰ
    affecting fetus or newborn 761.8
    severe (with metabolic disturbance)
      643.1 ✓5ᵗʰ
  psychogenic 306.4
Hyperemia (acute) 780.99   ▲
  anal mucosa 569.49
  bladder 596.7
  cerebral 437.8
  conjunctiva 372.71
  ear, internal, acute 386.30
  enteric 564.89
  eye 372.71
  eyelid (active) (passive) 374.82
  intestine 564.89
  iris 364.41
  kidney 593.81
  labyrinth 386.30
  liver (active) (passive) 573.8
  lung 514
  ovary 620.8
  passive 780.99   ▲
  pulmonary 514
  renal 593.81
  retina 362.89
  spleen 289.59
  stomach 537.89
Hyperesthesia (body surface) (*see also*
  Disturbance, sensation) 782.0
  larynx (reflex) 478.79
    hysterical 300.11
  pharynx (reflex) 478.29
Hyperestrinism 256.0
Hyperestrogenism 256.0
Hyperestrogenosis 256.0
Hyperextension, joint 718.80
  ankle 718.87
  elbow 718.82
  foot 718.87
  hand 718.84
  hip 718.85
  knee 718.86
  multiple sites 718.89
  pelvic region 718.85
  shoulder (region) 718.81
  specified site NEC 718.88
  wrist 718.83
Hyperfibrinolysis — *see* Fibrinolysis
Hyperfolliculinism 256.0
Hyperfructosemia 271.2
Hyperfunction
  adrenal (cortex) 255.3
    androgenic, acquired benign 255.3
    medulla 255.6
    virilism 255.2
  corticoadrenal NEC 255.3
  labyrinth — *see* Hyperactive, labyrinth
  medulloadrenal 255.6
  ovary 256.1
    estrogen 256.0
  pancreas 577.8
  parathyroid (gland) 252.0
  pituitary (anterior) (gland) (lobe) 253.1
  testicular 257.0
Hypergammaglobulinemia 289.8
  monoclonal, benign (BMH) 273.1
  polyclonal 273.0
  Waldenström's 273.0
Hyperglobulinemia 273.8
Hyperglycemia 790.6
  maternal
    affecting fetus or newborn 775.0
      manifest diabetes in infant 775.1
  postpancreatectomy (complete) (partial) 251.3

Hyperglyceridemia 272.1
  endogenous 272.1
  essential 272.1
  familial 272.1
  hereditary 272.1
  mixed 272.3
  pure 272.1
Hyperglycinemia 270.7
Hypergonadism
  ovarian 256.1
  testicular (infantile) (primary) 257.0
Hyperheparinemia (*see also* Circulating
  anticoagulants) 286.5
Hyperhidrosis, hyperidrosis 780.8
  psychogenic 306.3
Hyperhistidinemia 270.5
Hyperinsulinism (ectopic) (functional) (organic)
  NEC 251.1
  iatrogenic 251.0
  reactive 251.2
  spontaneous 251.2
  therapeutic misadventure (from administration
    of insulin) 962.3
Hyperiodemia 276.9
Hyperirritability (cerebral), in newborn 779.1
Hyperkalemia 276.7
Hyperkeratosis (*see also* Keratosis) 701.1
  cervix 622.1
  congenital 757.39
  cornea 371.89
  due to yaws (early) (late) (palmar or plantar)
    102.3
  eccentrica 757.39
  figurata centrifuga atrophica 757.39
  follicularis 757.39
    in cutem penetrans 701.1
  limbic (comea) 371.89
  palmoplantaris climacterica 701.1
  pinta (carate) 103.1
  senile (with pruritus) 702.0
  tongue 528.7
  universalis congenita 757.1
  vagina 623.1
  vocal cord 478.5
  vulva 624.0
Hyperkinesia, hyperkinetic (disease) (reaction)
  (syndrome) 314.9
  with
    attention deficit — *see* Disorder, attention
      deficit
    conduct disorder 314.2
    developmental delay 314.1
    simple disturbance of activity and attention
      314.01
    specified manifestation NEC 314.8
  heart (disease) 429.82
  of childhood or adolescence NEC 314.9
Hyperlacrimation (*see also* Epiphora) 375.20
Hyperlipemia (*see also* Hyperlipidemia) 272.4
Hyperlipidemia 272.4
  carbohydrate-induced 272.1
  combined 272.4
  endogenous 272.1
  exogenous 272.3
  fat-induced 272.3
  group
    A 272.0
    B 272.1
    C 272.2
    D 272.3
  mixed 272.2
  specified type NEC 272.4
Hyperlipidosis 272.7
  hereditary 272.7
Hyperlipoproteinemia (acquired) (essential)
  (familial) (hereditary) (primary) (secondary)
  272.4
  Fredrickson type
    I 272.3
    IIa 272.0
    IIb 272.2
    III 272.2
    IV 272.1
    V 272.3

Hyperlipoproteinemia — *continued*
  low-density-lipoid-type (LDL) 272.0
  very-low-density-lipoid-type (VLDL) 272.1
Hyperlucent lung, unilateral 492.8
Hyperluteinization 256.1
Hyperlysinemia 270.7
Hypermagnesemia 275.2
  neonatal 775.5
Hypermaturity (fetus or newborn) 766.2
Hypermenorrhea 626.2
Hypermetabolism 794.7
Hypermethioninemia 270.4
Hypermetropia (congenital) 367.0
Hypermobility
  cecum 564.9
  coccyx 724.71
  colon 564.9
    psychogenic 306.4
  ileum 564.89
  joint (acquired) 718.80
    ankle 718.87
    elbow 718.82
    foot 718.87
    hand 718.84
    hip 718.85
    knee 718.86
    multiple sites 718.89
    pelvic region 718.85
    shoulder (region) 718.81
    specified site NEC 718.88
    wrist 718.83
  kidney, congenital 753.3
  meniscus (knee) 717.5
  scapula 718.81
  stomach 536.8
    psychogenic 306.4
  syndrome 728.5
  testis, congenital 752.52
  urethral 599.81
Hypermotility
  gastrointestinal 536.8
  intestine 564.9
    psychogenic 306.4
  stomach 536.8
Hypernasality 784.49
Hypernatremia 276.0
  with water depletion 276.0
Hypernephroma (M8312/3) 189.0
Hyperopia 367.0
Hyperorexia 783.6
Hyperornithinemia 270.6
Hyperosmia (*see also* Disturbance, sensation)
  781.1
Hyperosmolality 276.0
Hyperosteogenesis 733.99
Hyperostosis 733.99
  calvarial 733.3
  cortical 733.3
    infantile 756.59
  frontal, internal of skull 733.3
  interna frontalis 733.3
  monomelic 733.99
  skull 733.3
    congenital 756.0
  vertebral 721.8
    with spondylosis — *see* Spondylosis
    ankylosing 721.6
Hyperovarianism 256.1
Hyperovarism, hyperovaria 256.1
Hyperoxaluria (primary) 271.8
Hyperoxia 987.8
Hyperparathyroidism 252.0
  ectopic 259.3
  secondary, of renal origin 588.8
Hyperpathia (*see also* Disturbance, sensation)
  782.0
  psychogenic 307.80
Hyperperistalsis 787.4
  psychogenic 306.4
Hyperpermeability, capillary 448.9
Hyperphagia 783.6

✓4ᵗʰ Fourth-digit Required   ✓5ᵗʰ Fifth-digit Required   ▶◀ Revised Text   ● New Line   ▲ Revised Code

Hyperphenylalaninemia 270.1

Hyperphoria 378.40
   alternating 378.45

Hyperphosphatemia 275.3

Hyperpiesia (*see also* Hypertension) 401.9

Hyperpiesis (*see also* Hypertension) 401.9

Hyperpigmentation — *see* Pigmentation

Hyperpinealism 259.8

Hyperpipecolatemia 270.7

Hyperpituitarism 253.1

Hyperplasia, hyperplastic
   adenoids (lymphoid tissue) 474.12
      and tonsils 474.10
   adrenal (capsule) (cortex) (gland) 255.8
      with
         sexual precocity (male) 255.2
         virilism, adrenal 255.2
         virilization (female) 255.2
      congenital 255.2
      due to excess ACTH (ectopic) (pituitary)
         255.0
      medulla 255.8
   alpha cells (pancreatic)
      with
         gastrin excess 251.5
         glucagon excess 251.4
   appendix (lymphoid) 543.0
   artery, fibromuscular NEC 447.8
      carotid 447.8
      renal 447.3
   bone 733.99
      marrow 289.9
   breast (*see also* Hypertrophy, breast) 611.1
   carotid artery 447.8
   cementation, cementum (teeth) (tooth) 521.5
   cervical gland 785.6
   cervix (uteri) 622.1
      basal cell 622.1
      congenital 752.49
      endometrium 622.1
      polypoid 622.1
   chin 524.05
   clitoris, congenital 752.49
   dentin 521.5
   endocervicitis 616.0
   endometrium, endometrial (adenomatous)
         (atypical) (cystic) (glandular) (polypoid)
         (uterus) 621.3
      cervix 622.1
   epithelial 709.8
      focal, oral, including tongue 528.7
      mouth (focal) 528.7
      nipple 611.8
      skin 709.8
      tongue (focal) 528.7
      vaginal wall 623.0
   erythroid 289.9
   fascialis ossificans (progressiva) 728.11
   fibromuscular, artery NEC 447.8
      carotid 447.8
      renal 447.3
   genital
      female 629.8
      male 608.89
   gingiva 523.8
   glandularis
      cystica uteri 621.3
      endometrium (uterus) 621.3
      interstitialis uteri 621.3
   granulocytic 288.8
   gum 523.8
   hymen, congenital 752.49
   islands of Langerhans 251.1
   islet cell (pancreatic) 251.9
      alpha cells
         with excess
            gastrin 251.5
            glucagon 251.4
      beta cells 251.1
   juxtaglomerular (complex) (kidney) 593.89
   kidney (congenital) 753.3
   liver (congenital) 751.69
   lymph node (gland) 785.6
   lymphoid (diffuse) (nodular) 785.6
      appendix 543.0

Hyperplasia, hyperplastic — *continued*
   lymphoid — *continued*
      intestine 569.89
   mandibular 524.02
      alveolar 524.72
      unilateral condylar 526.89
   Marchand multiple nodular (liver) — *see*
      Cirrhosis, postnecrotic
   maxillary 524.01
      alveolar 524.71
   medulla, adrenal 255.8
   myometrium, myometrial 621.2
   nose (lymphoid) (polypoid) 478.1
   oral soft tissue (inflammatory) (irritative)
         (mucosa) NEC 528.9
      gingiva 523.8
      tongue 529.8
   organ or site, congenital NEC — *see* Anomaly,
      specified type NEC
   ovary 620.8
   palate, papillary 528.9
   pancreatic islet cells 251.9
      alpha
         with excess
            gastrin 251.5
            glucagon 251.4
      beta 251.1
   parathyroid (gland) 252.0
   persistent, vitreous (primary) 743.51
   pharynx (lymphoid) 478.29
   prostate 600.9   ▲
      adenofibromatous 600.2
      nodular 600.1
   renal artery (fibromuscular) 447.3
   reticuloendothelial (cell) 289.9
   salivary gland (any) 527.1
   Schimmelbusch's 610.1
   suprarenal (capsule) (gland) 255.8
   thymus (gland) (persistent) 254.0
   thyroid (*see also* Goiter) 240.9
      primary 242.0 ✓5ᵗʰ
      secondary 242.2 ✓5ᵗʰ
   tonsil (lymphoid tissue) 474.11
      and adenoids 474.10
   urethrovaginal 599.89
   uterus, uterine (myometrium) 621.2
      endometrium 621.3
   vitreous (humor), primary persistent 743.51
   vulva 624.3
   zygoma 738.11

Hyperpnea (*see also* Hyperventilation) 786.01

Hyperpotassemia 276.7

Hyperprebetalipoproteinemia 272.1
   with chylomicronemia 272.3
   familial 272.1

Hyperprolactinemia 253.1

Hyperprolinemia 270.8

Hyperproteinemia 273.8

Hyperprothrombinemia 289.8

Hyperpselaphesia 782.0

Hyperpyrexia 780.6
   heat (effects of) 992.0
   malarial (*see also* Malaria) 084.6
   malignant, due to anesthetic 995.86
   rheumatic — *see* Fever, rheumatic
   unknown origin (*see also* Pyrexia) 780.6

Hyperreactor, vascular 780.2

Hyperreflexia 796.1
   bladder, autonomic 596.54
      with cauda equina 344.61
   detrusor 344.61

Hypersalivation (*see also* Ptyalism) 527.7

Hypersarcosinemia 270.8

Hypersecretion
   ACTH 255.3
   androgens (ovarian) 256.1
   calcitonin 246.0
   corticoadrenal 255.3
   cortisol 255.0
   estrogen 256.0
   gastric 536.8
      psychogenic 306.4
   gastrin 251.5
   glucagon 251.4

Hypersecretion — *continued*
   hormone
      ACTH 255.3
      anterior pituitary 253.1
      growth NEC 253.0
      ovarian androgen 256.1
      testicular 257.0
      thyroid stimulating 242.8 ✓5ᵗʰ
   insulin — *see* Hyperinsulinism
   lacrimal glands (*see also* Epiphora) 375.20
   medulloadrenal 255.6
   milk 676.6 ✓5ᵗʰ
   ovarian androgens 256.1
   pituitary (anterior) 253.1
   salivary gland (any) 527.7
   testicular hormones 257.0
   thyrocalcitonin 246.0
   upper respiratory 478.9

Hypersegmentation, hereditary 288.2
   eosinophils 288.2
   neutrophil nuclei 288.2

**Hypersensitive, hypersensitiveness,
   hypersensitivity** — *see also* Allergy
   angiitis 446.20
      specified NEC 446.29
   carotid sinus 337.0
   colon 564.9
      psychogenic 306.4
   DNA (deoxyribonucleic acid) NEC 287.2
   drug (*see also* Allergy, drug) 995.2
   esophagus 530.89
   insect bites — *see* Injury, superficial, by site
   labyrinth 386.58
   pain (*see also* Disturbance, sensation) 782.0
   pneumonitis NEC 495.9
   reaction (*see also* Allergy) 995.3
      upper respiratory tract NEC 478.8
   stomach (allergic) (nonallergic) 536.8
      psychogenic 306.4

Hypersomatotropism (classic) 253.0

Hypersomnia 780.54
   with sleep apnea 780.53
   nonorganic origin 307.43
      persistent (primary) 307.44
      transient 307.43

Hypersplenia 289.4

Hypersplenism 289.4

Hypersteatosis 706.3

Hyperstimulation, ovarian 256.1

Hypersuprarenalism 255.3

Hypersusceptibility — *see* Allergy

Hyper-TBG-nemia 246.8

Hypertelorism 756.0
   orbit, orbital 376.41

	Malignant	Benign	Unspecified
Hypertension, hypertensive (arterial) (arteriolar) (crisis) (degeneration) (disease) (essential) (fluctuating) (idiopathic) (intermittent) (labile) (low renin) (orthostatic) (paroxysmal) (primary) (systemic) (uncontrolled) (vascular)	401.0	401.1	401.9
with			
heart involvement (conditions classifiable to 425.8, 428, 429.0-429.3, 429.8, 429.9 due to hypertension) (*see also* Hypertension, heart)	402.00	402.10	402.90
with kidney involvement — *see* Hypertension, cardiorenal			
renal involvement (only conditions classifiable to 585, 586, 587) (excludes conditions classifiable to 584) (*see also* Hypertension, kidney)	403.00	403.10	403.90
renal sclerosis or failure	403.00	403.10	403.90
with heart involvement — *see* Hypertension, cardiorenal			
failure (and sclerosis) (*see also* Hypertension, kidney)	403.01	403.11	403.91
sclerosis without failure (*see also* Hypertension, kidney)	403.00	403.10	403.90
accelerated — (*see also* Hypertension, by type, malignant)	401.0	—	—
antepartum — *see* Hypertension, complicating pregnancy, childbirth, or the puerperium			
cardiorenal (disease)	404.00	404.10	404.90
with			
heart failure	404.01	404.11	404.91
and renal failure	404.03	404.13	404.93
renal failure	404.02	404.12	404.92
and heart failure	404.03	404.13	404.93
cardiovascular disease (arteriosclerotic) (sclerotic)	402.00	402.10	402.90
with			
heart failure	402.01	402.11	402.91
renal involvement (conditions classifiable to 403) (*see also* Hypertension, cardiorenal)	404.00	404.10	404.90
cardiovascular renal (disease) (sclerosis) (*see also* Hypertension, cardiorenal)	404.00	404.10	404.90
cerebrovascular disease NEC	437.2	437.2	437.2
complicating pregnancy, childbirth, or the puerperium	642.2 ✓5ᵗʰ	642.0	642.9 ✓5ᵗʰ
with			
albuminuria (and edema) (mild)	—	—	642.4 ✓5ᵗʰ
severe	—	—	642.5 ✓5ᵗʰ
edema (mild)	—	—	642.4 ✓5ᵗʰ
severe	—	—	642.5 ✓5ᵗʰ
heart disease	642.2 ✓5ᵗʰ	642.2 ✓5ᵗʰ	642.2 ✓5ᵗʰ
and renal disease	642.2 ✓5ᵗʰ	642.2 ✓5ᵗʰ	642.2 ✓5ᵗʰ
renal disease	642.2 ✓5ᵗʰ	642.2 ✓5ᵗʰ	642.2 ✓5ᵗʰ
and heart disease	642.2 ✓5ᵗʰ	642.2 ✓5ᵗʰ	642.2 ✓5ᵗʰ
chronic	642.2 ✓5ᵗʰ	642.0 ✓5ᵗʰ	642.0 ✓5ᵗʰ
with pre-eclampsia or eclampsia	642.7 ✓5ᵗʰ	642.7 ✓5ᵗʰ	642.7 ✓5ᵗʰ
fetus or newborn	760.0	760.0	760.0
essential	—	642.0	642.0 ✓5ᵗʰ
with pre-eclampsia or eclampsia	—	642.7 ✓5ᵗʰ	642.7 ✓5ᵗʰ
fetus or newborn	760.0	760.0	760.0
fetus or newborn	760.0	760.0	760.0
gestational	—	—	642.3 ✓5ᵗʰ
pre-existing	642.2 ✓5ᵗʰ	642.0	642.0 ✓5ᵗʰ
with pre-eclampsia or eclampsia	642.7 ✓5ᵗʰ	642.7 ✓5ᵗʰ	642.7 ✓5ᵗʰ
fetus or newborn	760.0	760.0	760.0
secondary to renal disease	642.1 ✓5ᵗʰ	642.1 ✓5ᵗʰ	642.1 ✓5ᵗʰ
with pre-eclampsia or eclampsia	642.7 ✓5ᵗʰ	642.7 ✓5ᵗʰ	642.7 ✓5ᵗʰ
fetus or newborn	760.0	760.0	760.0
transient	—	—	642.3 ✓5ᵗʰ
due to			
aldosteronism, primary	405.09	405.19	405.99
brain tumor	405.09	405.19	405.99
bulbar poliomyelitis	405.09	405.19	405.99
calculus			
kidney	405.09	405.19	405.99
ureter	405.09	405.19	405.99
coarctation, aorta	405.09	405.19	405.99
Cushing's disease	405.09	405.19	405.99
glomerulosclerosis (*see also* Hypertension, kidney)	403.00	403.10	403.90
periarteritis nodosa	405.09	405.19	405.99
pheochromocytoma	405.09	405.19	405.99
polycystic kidney(s)	405.09	405.19	405.99

✓4ᵗʰ Fourth-digit Required   ✓5ᵗʰ Fifth-digit Required   ►◄ Revised Text   ● New Line   ▲ Revised Code

Hypertension — Hypertension

	Malignant	Benign	Unspecified
Hypertension, hypertensive — *continued*			
due to — *continued*			
polycythemia	405.09	405.19	405.99
porphyria	405.09	405.19	405.99
pyelonephritis	405.09	405.19	405.99
renal (artery)			
aneurysm	405.01	405.11	405.91
anomaly	405.01	405.11	405.91
embolism	405.01	405.11	405.91
fibromuscular hyperplasia	405.01	405.11	405.91
occlusion	405.01	405.11	405.91
stenosis	405.01	405.11	405.91
thrombosis	405.01	405.11	405.91
encephalopathy	437.2	437.2	437.2
gestational (transient) NEC	—	—	642.3 ✓5ᵗʰ
Goldblatt's	440.1	440.1	440.1
heart (disease) (conditions classifiable to 425.8, 428, 429.0-429.3, 429.8, 429.9 due to hypertension)	402.00	402.10	402.90
with heart failure	402.01	402.11	402.91
hypertensive kidney disease (conditions classifiable to 403) (*see also* Hypertension, cardiorenal)	404.00	404.10	404.90
renal sclerosis (*see also* Hypertension, cardiorenal)	404.00	404.10	404.90
intracranial, benign	—	348.2	—
intraocular	—	—	365.04
kidney	403.00	403.10	403.90
with			
heart involvement (conditions classifiable to 425.8, 428, 429.0-429.3, 429.8, 429.9 due to hypertension) (*see also* Hypertension, cardiorenal)	404.00	404.10	404.90
hypertensive heart (disease) (conditions classifiable to 402) (*see also* Hypertension, cardiorenal)	404.00	404.10	404.90
lesser circulation	—	—	416.0
necrotizing	401.0	—	—
ocular	—	—	365.04
portal (due to chronic liver disease)	—	—	572.3
postoperative	—	—	997.91
psychogenic	—	—	306.2
puerperal, postpartum — *see* Hypertension, complicating pregnancy, childbirth, or the puerperium			
pulmonary (artery)	—	—	416.8
with cor pulmonale (chronic)	—	—	416.8
acute	—	—	415.0
idiopathic	—	—	416.0
primary	—	—	416.0
of newborn	—	—	747.83 ●
secondary	—	—	416.8
renal (disease) (*see also* Hypertension, kidney)	403.00	403.10	403.90
renovascular NEC	405.01	405.11	405.91
secondary NEC	405.09	405.19	405.99
due to			
aldosteronism, primary	405.09	405.19	405.99
brain tumor	405.09	405.19	405.99
bulbar poliomyelitis	405.09	405.19	405.99
calculus			
kidney	405.09	405.19	405.99
ureter	405.09	405.19	405.99
coarctation, aorta	405.09	405.19	405.99
Cushing's disease	405.09	405.19	405.99
glomerulosclerosis (*see also* Hypertension, kidney)	403.00	403.10	403.90
periarteritis nodosa	405.09	405.19	405.99
pheochromocytoma	405.09	405.19	405.99
polycystic kidney(s)	405.09	405.19	405.99
polycythemia	405.09	405.19	405.99
porphyria	405.09	405.19	405.99
pyelonephritis	405.09	405.19	405.99
renal (artery)			
aneurysm	405.01	405.11	405.91
anomaly	405.01	405.11	405.91
embolism	405.01	405.11	405.91
fibromuscular hyperplasia	405.01	405.11	405.91
occlusion	405.01	405.11	405.91
stenosis	405.01	405.11	405.91
thrombosis	405.01	405.11	405.91
transient	—	—	796.2
of pregnancy	—	—	642.3 ✓5ᵗʰ

	Malignant	Benign	Unspecified
Hypertension, hypertensive — *continued*			
venous, chronic (asymptomatic) (idiopathic)	—	—	459.30 ●
			●
due to			●
deep vein thrombosis (see also Syndrome, postphlebetic)	—	—	459.10 ●
			●
with			●
complication, NEC	—	—	459.39 ●
inflammation	—	—	459.32 ●
with ulcer	—	—	459.33 ●
ulcer	—	—	459.31 ●
with inflammation	—	—	459.33 ●

Hyperthecosis, ovary 256.8

Hyperthermia (of unknown origin) (*see also* Pyrexia) 780.6
   malignant (due to anesthesia) 995.86
   newborn 778.4

Hyperthymergasia (*see also* Psychosis, affective) 296.0 ✓5th
   reactive (from emotional stress, psychological trauma) 298.1
   recurrent episode 296.1 ✓5th
   single episode 296.0 ✓5th

Hyperthymism 254.8

Hyperthyroid (recurrent) — *see* Hyperthyroidism

Hyperthyroidism (latent) (preadult) (recurrent) (without goiter) 242.9 ✓5th

> Note — Use the following fifth-digit subclassification with category 242:
>
> 0   without mention of thyrotoxic crisis or storm
>
> 1   with mention of thyrotoxic crisis or storm

   with
      goiter (diffuse) 242.0 ✓5th
         adenomatous 242.3 ✓5th
            multinodular 242.2 ✓5th
            uninodular 242.1 ✓5th
         nodular 242.3 ✓5th
            multinodular 242.2 ✓5th
            uninodular 242.1 ✓5th
      thyroid nodule 242.1 ✓5th
   complicating pregnancy, childbirth, or puerperium 648.1 ✓5th
   neonatal (transient) 775.3

Hypertonia — *see* Hypertonicity

Hypertonicity
   bladder 596.51
   fetus or newborn 779.89 ▲
   gastrointestinal (tract) 536.8
   infancy 779.89 ▲
      due to electrolyte imbalance 779.89 ▲
   muscle 728.85
   stomach 536.8
      psychogenic 306.4
   uterus, uterine (contractions) 661.4 ✓5th
      affecting fetus or newborn 763.7

Hypertony — *see* Hypertonicity

Hypertransaminemia 790.4

Hypertrichosis 704.1
   congenital 757.4
   eyelid 374.54
   lanuginosa 757.4
      acquired 704.1

Hypertriglyceridemia, essential 272.1

Hypertrophy, hypertrophic
   adenoids (infectional) 474.12
      and tonsils (faucial) (infective) (lingual) (lymphoid) 474.10
   adrenal 255.8
   alveolar process or ridge 525.8
   anal papillae 569.49
   apocrine gland 705.82
   artery NEC 447.8
      carotid 447.8
      congenital (peripheral) NEC 747.60
         gastrointestinal 747.61
         lower limb 747.64
         renal 747.62
         specified NEC 747.69
         spinal 747.82
         upper limb 747.63
   arthritis (chronic) (*see also* Osteoarthrosis) 715.9 ✓5th
      spine (*see also* Spondylosis) 721.90
   arytenoid 478.79
   asymmetrical (heart) 429.9
   auricular — *see* Hypertrophy, cardiac
   Bartholin's gland 624.8
   bile duct 576.8
   bladder (sphincter) (trigone) 596.8
   blind spot, visual field 368.42
   bone 733.99

Hypertrophy, hypertrophic — *continued*
brain 348.8
breast 611.1
  cystic 610.1
  fetus or newborn 778.7
  fibrocystic 610.1
  massive pubertal 611.1
  puerperal, postpartum 676.3 ✓5th
  senile (parenchymatous) 611.1
cardiac (chronic) (idiopathic) 429.3
  with
    rheumatic fever (conditions classifiable to
      390)
      active 391.8
        with chorea 392.0
      inactive or quiescent (with chorea)
        398.99
  congenital NEC 746.89
  fatty (*see also* Degeneration, myocardial)
    429.1
  hypertensive (*see also* Hypertension, heart)
    402.90
  rheumatic (with chorea) 398.99
    active or acute 391.8
      with chorea 392.0
  valve (*see also* Endocarditis) 424.90
    congenital NEC 746.89
cartilage 733.99
cecum 569.89
cervix (uteri) 622.6
  congenital 752.49
  elongation 622.6
clitoris (cirrhotic) 624.2
  congenital 752.49
colon 569.89
  congenital 751.3
conjunctiva, lymphoid 372.73
cornea 371.89
corpora cavernosa 607.89
duodenum 537.89
endometrium (uterus) 621.3
  cervix 622.6
epididymis 608.89
esophageal hiatus (congenital) 756.6
  with hernia — *see* Hernia, diaphragm
eyelid 374.30
falx, skull 733.99
fat pad 729.30
  infrapatellar 729.31
  knee 729.31
  orbital 374.34
  popliteal 729.31
  prepatellar 729.31
  retropatellar 729.31
  specified site NEC 729.39
foot (congenital) 755.67
frenum, frenulum (tongue) 529.8
  linguae 529.8
  lip 528.5
gallbladder or cystic duct 575.8
gastric mucosa 535.2 ✓5th
gingiva 523.8
gland, glandular (general) NEC 785.6
gum (mucous membrane) 523.8
heart (idiopathic) — *see also* Hypertrophy,
    cardiac
  valve — *see also* Endocarditis
    congenital NEC 746.89
hemifacial 754.0
hepatic — *see* Hypertrophy, liver
hiatus (esophageal) 756.6
hilus gland 785.6
hymen, congenital 752.49
ileum 569.89
infrapatellar fat pad 729.31
intestine 569.89
jejunum 569.89
kidney (compensatory) 593.1
  congenital 753.3
labial frenulum 528.5
labium (majus) (minus) 624.3
lacrimal gland, chronic 375.03
ligament 728.9
  spinal 724.8
linguae frenulum 529.8
lingual tonsil (infectional) 474.11

Hypertrophy, hypertrophic — *continued*
lip (frenum) 528.5
  congenital 744.81
liver 789.1
  acute 573.8
  cirrhotic — *see* Cirrhosis, liver
  congenital 751.69
  fatty — *see* Fatty, liver
lymph gland 785.6
  tuberculous — *see* Tuberculosis, lymph
    gland
mammary gland — *see* Hypertrophy, breast
maxillary frenuium 528.5
Meckel's diverticulum (congenital) 751.0
medial meniscus, acquired 717.3
median bar 600.9
mediastinum 519.3
meibomian gland 373.2
meniscus, knee, congenital 755.64
metatarsal head 733.99
metatarsus 733.99
mouth 528.9
mucous membrane
  alveolar process 523.8
  nose 478.1
  turbinate (nasal) 478.0
muscle 728.9
muscular coat, artery NEC 447.8
  carotid 447.8
  renal 447.3
myocardium (*see also* Hypertrophy, cardiac)
    429.3
  idiopathic 425.4
myometrium 621.2
nail 703.8
  congenital 757.5
nasal 478.1
  alae 478.1
  bone 738.0
  cartilage 478.1
  mucous membrane (septum) 478.1
  sinus (*see also* Sinusitis) 473.9
  turbinate 478.0
nasopharynx, lymphoid (infectional) (tissue)
    (wall) 478.29
neck, uterus 622.6
nipple 611.1
normal aperture diaphragm (congenital) 756.6
nose (*see also* Hypertrophy, nasal) 478.1
orbit 376.46
organ or site, congenital NEC — *see* Anomaly,
    specified type NEC
osteoarthropathy (pulmonary) 731.2
ovary 620.8
palate (hard) 526.89
  soft 528.9
pancreas (congenital) 751.7
papillae
  anal 569.49
  tongue 529.3
parathyroid (gland) 252.0
parotid gland 527.1
penis 607.89
phallus 607.89
  female (clitoris) 624.2
pharyngeal tonsil 474.12
pharyngitis 472.1
pharynx 478.29
  lymphoid (infectional) (tissue) (wall) 478.29
pituitary (fossa) (gland) 253.8
popliteal fat pad 729.31
preauricular (lymph) gland (Hampstead) 785.6
prepuce (congenital) 605
  female 624.2
prostate (asymptomatic) (early) (recurrent)
    600.9
  adenofibromatous 600.2
  benign 600.0
  congenital 752.8
pseudoedematous hypodermal 757.0
pseudomuscular 359.1
pylorus (muscle) (sphincter) 537.0
  congenital 750.5
  infantile 750.5
rectal sphincter 569.49
rectum 569.49
renal 593.1
rhinitis (turbinate) 472.0

Hypertrophy, hypertrophic — *continued*
salivary duct or gland 527.1
  congenital 750.26
scaphoid (tarsal) 733.99
scar 701.4
scrotum 608.89
sella turcica 253.8
seminal vesicle 608.89
sigmoid 569.89
skin condition NEC 701.9
spermatic cord 608.89
spinal ligament 728.9
spleen — *see* Splenomegaly
spondylitis (spine) (*see also* Spondylosis)
    721.90
stomach 537.89
subaortic stenosis (idiopathic) 425.1
sublingual gland 527.1
  congenital 750.26
submaxillary gland 527.1
suprarenal (gland) 255.8
tendon 727.9
testis 608.89
  congenital 752.8
thymic, thymus (congenital) (gland) 254.0
thyroid (gland) (*see also* Goiter) 240.9
  primary 242.0 ✓5th
  secondary 242.2 ✓5th
toe (congenital) 755.65
  acquired 735.8
tongue 529.8
  congenital 750.15
  frenum 529.8
  papillae (foliate) 529.3
tonsil (faucial) (infective) (lingual) (lymphoid)
    474.11
  with
    adenoiditis 474.01
    tonsillitis 474.00
      and adenoiditis 474.02
  and adenoids 474.10
tunica vaginalis 608.89
turbinate (mucous membrane) 478.0
ureter 593.89
urethra 599.84
uterus 621.2
  puerperal, postpartum 674.8 ✓5th
uvula 528.9
vagina 623.8
vas deferens 608.89
vein 459.89
ventricle, ventricular (heart) (left) (right) — *see
    also* Hypertrophy, cardiac
  congenital 746.89
  due to hypertension (left) (right) (*see also*
      Hypertension, heart) 402.90
    benign 402.10
    malignant 402.00
  right with ventricular septal defect,
      pulmonary stenosis or atresia, and
      dextraposition of aorta 745.2
verumontanum 599.89
vesical 596.8
vocal cord 478.5
vulva 624.3
  stasis (nonfilarial) 624.3
Hypertropia (intermittent) (periodic) 378.31
Hypertyrosinemia 270.2
Hyperuricemia 790.6
Hypervalinemia 270.3
Hyperventilation (tetany) 786.01
  hysterical 300.11
  psychogenic 306.1
  syndrome 306.1
Hyperviscidosis 277.00
Hyperviscosity (of serum) (syndrome) NEC 273.3
  polycythemic 289.0
  sclerocythemic 282.8
Hypervitaminosis (dietary) NEC 278.8
  A (dietary) 278.2
  D (dietary) 278.4
  from excessive administration or use of vitamin
      preparations (chronic) 278.8
    reaction to sudden overdose 963.5

Hypertrophy — Hypervitaminosis

Hypervitaminosis (dietary) NEC
　from excessive administration or use of vitamin
　　preparations — *continued*
　　vitamin A 278.2
　　　reaction to sudden overdose 963.5
　　vitamin D 278.4
　　　reaction to sudden overdose 963.5
　　vitamin K
　　　correct substance properly administered
　　　　278.8
　　　overdose or wrong substance given or
　　　　taken 964.3
Hypervolemia 276.6
Hypesthesia (*see also* Disturbance, sensation)
　782.0
　cornea 371.81
Hyphema (anterior chamber) (ciliary body) (iris)
　364.41
　traumatic 921.3
Hyphemia — *see* Hyphema
Hypoacidity, gastric 536.8
　psychogenic 306.4
Hypoactive labyrinth (function) — *see*
　Hypofunction, labyrinth
Hypoadrenalism 255.4
　tuberculous (*see also* Tuberculosis) 017.6 ✓5ᵗʰ
Hypoadrenocorticism 255.4
　pituitary 253.4
Hypoalbuminemia 273.8
Hypoalphalipoproteinemia 272.5
Hypobarism 993.2
Hypobaropathy 993.2
Hypobetalipoproteinemia (familial) 272.5
Hypocalcemia 275.41
　cow's milk 775.4
　dietary 269.3
　neonatal 775.4
　phosphate-loading 775.4
Hypocalcification, teeth 520.4
Hypochloremia 276.9
Hypochlorhydria 536.8
　neurotic 306.4
　psychogenic 306.4
Hypocholesteremia 272.5
Hypochondria (reaction) 300.7
Hypochondriac 300.7
Hyponchondriasis 300.7
Hypochromasia blood cells 280.9
Hypochromic anemia 280.9
　due to blood loss (chronic) 280.0
　　acute 285.1
　microcytic 280.9
Hypocoagulability (*see also* Defect, coagulation)
　286.9
Hypocomplementemia 279.8
Hypocythemia (progressive) 284.9
Hypodontia (*see also* Anodontia) 520.0
Hypoeosinophilia 288.8
Hypoesthesia (*see also* Disturbance, sensation)
　782.0
　cornea 371.81
　tactile 782.0
Hypoestrinism 256.39
Hypoestrogenism 256.39
Hypoferremia 280.9
　due to blood loss (chronic) 280.0
Hypofertility
　female 628.9
　male 606.1
Hypofibrinogenemia 286.3
　acquired 286.6
　congenital 286.3
Hypofunction
　adrenal (gland) 255.4
　　cortex 255.4
　　medulla 255.5
　　specified NEC 255.5
　cerebral 331.9
　corticoadrenal NEC 255.4
　intestinal 564.89

Hypofunction — *continued*
　labyrinth (unilateral) 386.53
　　with loss of labyrinthine reactivity 386.55
　　bilateral 386.54
　　　with loss of labyrinthine reactivity 386.56
　Leydig cell 257.2
　ovary 256.39
　　postablative 256.2
　pituitary (anterior) (gland) (lobe) 253.2
　　posterior 253.5
　testicular 257.2
　　iatrogenic 257.1
　　postablative 257.1
　　postirradiation 257.1
　　postsurgical 257.1
Hypogammaglobulinemia 279.00
　acquired primary 279.06
　non-sex-linked, congenital 279.06
　sporadic 279.06
　transient of infancy 279.09
Hypogenitalism (congenital) (female) (male) 752.8
　penis 752.69
Hypoglycemia (spontaneous) 251.2
　coma 251.0
　　diabetic 250.3 ✓5ᵗʰ
　　diabetic 250.8 ✓5ᵗʰ
　due to insulin 251.0
　　therapeutic misadventure 962.3
　familial (idiopathic) 251.2
　following gastrointestinal surgery 579.3
　infantile (idiopathic) 251.2
　in infant of diabetic mother 775.0
　leucine-induced 270.3
　neonatal 775.6
　reactive 251.2
　specified NEC 251.1
Hypoglycemic shock 251.0
　diabetic 250.8 ✓5ᵗʰ
　due to insulin 251.0
　functional (syndrome) 251.1
Hypogonadism
　female 256.39
　gonadotrophic (isolated) 253.4
　hypogonadotropic (isolated) (with anosmia)
　　253.4
　isolated 253.4
　male 257.2
　ovarian (primary) 256.39
　pituitary (secondary) 253.4
　testicular (primary) (secondary) 257.2
Hypohidrosis 705.0
Hypohidrotic ectodermal dysplasia 757.31
Hypoidrosis 705.0
Hypoinsulinemia, postsurgical 251.3
　postpancreatectomy (complete) (partial) 251.3
Hypokalemia 276.8
Hypokinesia 780.99　　　　　　　　　　　　▲
Hypoleukia splenica 289.4
Hypoleukocytosis 288.8
Hypolipidemia 272.5
Hypolipoproteinemia 272.5
Hypomagnesemia 275.2
　neonatal 775.4
Hypomania, hypomanic reaction (*see also*
　Psychosis, affective) 296.0 ✓5ᵗʰ
　recurrent episode 296.1 ✓5ᵗʰ
　single episode 296.0 ✓5ᵗʰ
Hypomastia (congenital) 757.6
Hypomenorrhea 626.1
Hypometabolism 783.9
Hypomotility
　gastrointestinal tract 536.8
　　psychogenic 306.4
　intestine 564.89
　　psychogenic 306.4
　stomach 536.8
　　psychogenic 306.4
Hyponasality 784.49
Hyponatremia 276.1
Hypo-ovarianism 256.39
Hypo-ovarism 256.39

Hypoparathyroidism (idiopathic) (surgically
　induced) 252.1
　neonatal 775.4
Hypopharyngitis 462
Hypophoria 378.40
Hypophosphatasia 275.3
Hypophosphatemia (acquired) (congenital)
　(familial) 275.3
　renal 275.3
Hypophyseal, hypophysis — *see also* condition
　dwarfism 253.3
　gigantism 253.0
　syndrome 253.8
Hypophyseothalamic syndrome 253.8
Hypopiesis — *see* Hypotension
Hypopigmentation 709.00
　eyelid 374.53
Hypopinealism 259.8
Hypopituitarism (juvenile) (syndrome) 253.2
　due to
　　hormone therapy 253.7
　　hypophysectomy 253.7
　　radiotherapy 253.7
　postablative 253.7
　postpartum hemorrhage 253.2
Hypoplasia, hypoplasis 759.89
　adrenal (gland) 759.1
　alimentary tract 751.8
　　lower 751.2
　　upper 750.8
　anus, anal (canal) 751.2
　aorta 747.22
　aortic
　　arch (tubular) 747.10
　　orifice or valve with hypoplasia of ascending
　　　aorta and defective development of left
　　　ventricle (with mitral valve atresia)
　　　746.7
　appendix 751.2
　areola 757.6
　arm (*see also* Absence, arm, congenital) 755.20
　artery (congenital) (peripheral) NEC 747.60
　　brain 747.81
　　cerebral 747.81
　　coronary 746.85
　　gastrointestinal 747.61
　　lower limb 747.64
　　pulmonary 747.3
　　renal 747.62
　　retinal 743.58
　　specified NEC 747.69
　　spinal 747.82
　　umbilical 747.5
　　upper limb 747.63
　auditory canal 744.29
　　causing impairment of hearing 744.02
　biliary duct (common) or passage 751.61
　bladder 753.8
　bone NEC 756.9
　　face 756.0
　　malar 756.0
　　mandible 524.04
　　　alveolar 524.74
　　marrow 284.9
　　　acquired (secondary) 284.8
　　　congenital 284.0
　　　idiopathic 284.9
　　maxilla 524.03
　　　alveolar 524.73
　　skull (*see also* Hypoplasia, skull) 756.0
　brain 742.1
　　gyri 742.2
　　specified part 742.2
　breast (areola) 757.6
　bronchus (tree) 748.3
　cardiac 746.89
　　valve — *see* Hypoplasia, heart, valve
　　vein 746.89
　carpus (*see also* Absence, carpal, congenital)
　　755.28
　cartilaginous 756.9
　cecum 751.2
　cementum 520.4
　　hereditary 520.5
　cephalic 742.1

Hypoplasia, hypoplasis — *continued*
cerebellum 742.2
cervix (uteri) 752.49
chin 524.06
clavicle 755.51
coccyx 756.19
colon 751.2
corpus callosum 742.2
cricoid cartilage 748.3
dermal, focal (Goltz) 757.39
digestive organ(s) or tract NEC 751.8
  lower 751.2
  upper 750.8
ear 744.29
  auricle 744.23
  lobe 744.29
  middle, except ossicles 744.03
    ossicles 744.04
  ossicles 744.04
enamel of teeth (neonatal) (postnatal) (prenatal) 520.4
  hereditary 520.5
endocrine (gland) NEC 759.2
endometrium 621.8
epididymis 752.8
epiglottis 748.3
erythroid, congenital 284.0
erythropoietic, chronic acquired 284.8
esophagus 750.3
Eustachian tube 744.24
eye (*see also* Microphthalmos) 743.10
  lid 743.62
face 744.89
  bone(s) 756.0
fallopian tube 752.19
femur (*see also* Absence, femur, congenital) 755.34
fibula (*see also* Absence, fibula, congenital) 755.37
finger (*see also* Absence, finger, congenital) 755.29
focal dermal 757.39
foot 755.31
gallbladder 751.69
genitalia, genital organ(s)
  female 752.8
    external 752.49
    internal NEC 752.8
  in adiposogenital dystrophy 253.8
  male 752.8
    penis 752.69
glottis 748.3
hair 757.4
hand 755.21
heart 746.89
  left (complex) (syndrome) 746.7
  valve NEC 746.89
    pulmonary 746.01
humerus (*see also* Absence, humerus, congenital) 755.24
hymen 752.49
intestine (small) 751.1
  large 751.2
iris 743.46
jaw 524.09
kidney(s) 753.0
labium (majus) (minus) 752.49
labyrinth, membranous 744.05
lacrimal duct (apparatus) 743.65
larynx 748.3
leg (*see also* Absence, limb, congenital, lower) 755.30
limb 755.4
  lower (*see also* Absence, limb, congenital, lower) 755.30
  upper (*see also* Absence, limb, congenital, upper) 755.20
liver 751.69
lung (lobe) 748.5
mammary (areolar) 757.6
mandibular 524.04
  alveolar 524.74
  unilateral condylar 526.89
maxillary 524.03
  alveolar 524.73
medullary 284.9
megakaryocytic 287.3

Hypoplasia, hypoplasis — *continued*
metacarpus (*see also* Absence, metacarpal, congenital) 755.28
metatarsus (*see also* Absence, metatarsal, congenital) 755.38
muscle 756.89
  eye 743.69
myocardium (congenital) (Uhl's anomaly) 746.84
nail(s) 757.5
nasolacrimal duct 743.65
nervous system NEC 742.8
neural 742.8
nose, nasal 748.1
ophthalmic (*see also* Microphthalmos) 743.10
organ
  of Corti 744.05
  or site NEC — *see* Anomaly, by site
osseous meatus (ear) 744.03
ovary 752.0
oviduct 752.19
pancreas 751.7
parathyroid (gland) 759.2
parotid gland 750.26
patella 755.64
pelvis, pelvic girdle 755.69
penis 752.69
peripheral vascular system (congenital) NEC 747.60
  gastrointestinal 747.61
  lower limb 747.64
  renal 747.62
  specified NEC 747.69
  spinal 747.82
  upper limb 747.63
pituitary (gland) 759.2
pulmonary 748.5
  arteriovenous 747.3
  artery 747.3
  valve 746.01
punctum lacrimale 743.65
radioulnar (*see also* Absence, radius, congenital, with ulna) 755.25
radius (*see also* Absence, radius, congenital) 755.26
rectum 751.2
respiratory system NEC 748.9
rib 756.3
sacrum 756.19
scapula 755.59
shoulder girdle 755.59
skin 757.39
skull (bone) 756.0
  with
    anencephalus 740.0
    encephalocele 742.0
    hydrocephalus 742.3
      with spina bifida (*see also* Spina bifida) 741.0 ✓5ᵗʰ
    microcephalus 742.1
spinal (cord) (ventral horn cell) 742.59
  vessel 747.82
spine 756.19
spleen 759.0
sternum 756.3
tarsus (*see also* Absence, tarsal, congenital) 755.38
testis, testicle 752.8
thymus (gland) 279.11
thyroid (gland) 243
  cartilage 748.3
tibiofibular (*see also* Absence, tibia, congenital, with fibula) 755.35
toe (*see also* Absence, toe, congenital) 755.39
tongue 750.16
trachea (cartilage) (rings) 748.3
Turner's (tooth) 520.4
ulna (*see also* Absence, ulna, congenital) 755.27
umbilical artery 747.5
ureter 753.29
uterus 752.3
vagina 752.49
vascular (peripheral) NEC (*see also* Hypoplasia, peripheral vascular system) 747.60
  brain 747.81

Hypoplasia, hypoplasis — *continued*
vein(s) (peripheral) NEC (*see also* Hypoplasia, peripheral vascular system) 747.60
  brain 747.81
  cardiac 746.89
  great 747.49
  portal 747.49
  pulmonary 747.49
  vena cava (inferior) (superior) 747.49
  vertebra 756.19
  vulva 752.49
  zonule (ciliary) 743.39
  zygoma 738.12

Hypopotassemia 276.8

Hypoproaccelerinemia (*see also* Defect, coagulation) 286.3

Hypoproconvertinemia (congenital) (*see also* Defect, coagulation) 286.3

Hypoproteinemia (essential) (hypermetabolic) (idiopathic) 273.8

Hypoproteinosis 260

Hypoprothrombinemia (congenital) (hereditary) (idiopathic) (*see also* Defect, coagulation) 286.3
  acquired 286.7
  newborn 776.3

Hypopselaphesia 782.0

Hypopyon (anterior chamber) (eye) 364.05
  iritis 364.05
  ulcer (cornea) 370.04

Hypopyrexia 780.99   ▲

Hyporeflex 796.1

Hyporeninemia, extreme 790.99
  in primary aldosteronism 255.1

Hyporesponsive episode 780.09

Hyposecretion
  ACTH 253.4
  ovary 256.39
    postblative 256.2
  salivary gland (any) 527.7

Hyposegmentation of neutrophils, hereditary 288.2

Hyposiderinemia 280.9

Hyposmolality 276.1
  syndrome 276.1

Hyposomatotropism 253.3

Hyposomnia (*see also* Insomnia) 780.52

Hypospadias (male) 752.61
  female 753.8

Hypospermatogenesis 606.1

Hyposphagma 372.72

Hyposplenism 289.59

Hypostasis, pulmonary 514

Hypostatic — *see* condition

Hyposthenuria 593.89

Hyposuprarenalism 255.4

Hypo-TBG-nemia 246.8

Hypotension (arterial) (constitutional) 458.9
  chronic 458.1
  iatrogenic 458.2
  maternal, syndrome (following labor and delivery) 669.2 ✓5ᵗʰ
  orthostatic (chronic) 458.0
    dysautonomic-dyskinetic syndrome 333.0
  permanent idiopathic 458.1
  postoperative 458.2
  postural 458.0
  specified type NEC 458.8
  transient 796.3

Hypothermia (accidental) 991.6
  anesthetic 995.89
  newborn NEC 778.3
  not associated with low environmental temperature 780.99   ▲

Hypothymergasia (*see also* Psychosis, affective) 296.2 ✓5ᵗʰ
  recurrent episode 296.3 ✓5ᵗʰ
  single episode 296.2 ✓5ᵗʰ

Hypothyroidism (acquired) 244.9
  complicating pregnancy, childbirth, or puerperium 648.1 ✓5ᵗʰ
  congenital 243

Hypothyroidism — continued
 due to
  ablation 244.1
   radioactive iodine 244.1
   surgical 244.0
  iodine (administration) (ingestion) 244.2
   radioactive 244.1
  irradiation therapy 244.1
  p-aminosalicylic acid (PAS) 244.3
  phenylbutazone 244.3
  resorcinol 244.3
  specified cause NEC 244.8
  surgery 244.0
 goitrous (sporadic) 246.1
 iatrogenic NEC 244.3
 iodine 244.2
 pituitary 244.8
 postablative NEC 244.1
 postsurgical 244.0
 primary 244.9
 secondary NEC 244.8
 specified cause NEC 244.8
 sporadic goitrous 246.1
Hypotonia, hypotonicity, hypotony 781.3
 benign congenital 358.8
 bladder 596.4
 congenital 779.89   ▲
  benign 358.8
 eye 360.30
  due to
   fistula 360.32
   ocular disorder NEC 360.33
  following loss of aqueous or vitreous 360.33
  primary 360.31
 infantile muscular (benign) 359.0
 muscle 728.9
 uterus, uterine (contractions) — see Inertia,
  uterus
Hypotrichosis 704.09
 congenital 757.4
 lid (congenital) 757.4
  acquired 374.55
 postinfectional NEC 704.09
Hypotropia 378.32
Hypoventilation 786.09
Hypovitaminosis (see also Deficiency, vitamin)
 269.2
Hypovolemia 276.5
 surgical shock 998.0
 traumatic (shock) 958.4
Hypoxemia (see also Anoxia) 799.0
Hypoxia (see also Anoxia) 799.0
 cerebral 348.1
  during or resulting from a procedure 997.01
  newborn 768.9
   mild or moderate 768.6
   severe 768.5
 fetal, affecting newborn 768.9   ▲
 intrauterine — see Distress, fetal
 myocardial (see also Insufficiency, coronary)
  411.89
  arteriosclerotic — see Arteriosclerosis,
   coronary
 newborn 768.9   ▲
Hypsarrhythmia (see also Epilepsy) 345.6 ✓5ᵗʰ
Hysteralgia, pregnant uterus 646.8 ✓5ᵗʰ
Hysteria, hysterical 300.10
 anxiety 300.20
 Charcôt's gland 300.11
 conversion (any manifestation) 300.11
 dissociative type NEC 300.15
 psychosis, acute 298.1
Hysteroepilepsy 300.11
Hysterotomy, affecting fetus or newborn
 763.89

I

Iatrogenic syndrome of excess cortisol 255.0
Iceland disease (epidemic neuromyasthenia)
 049.8
Ichthyosis (congenita) 757.1
 acquired 701.1
 fetalis gravior 757.1

Ichthyosis — continued
 follicularis 757.1
 hystrix 757.39
 lamellar 757.1
 lingual 528.6
 palmaris and plantaris 757.39
 simplex 757.1
 vera 757.1
 vulgaris 757.1
Ichthyotoxism 988.0
 bacterial (see also Poisoning, food) 005.9
Icteroanemia, hemolytic (acquired) 283.9
 congenital (see also Spherocytosis) 282.0
Icterus (see also Jaundice) 782.4
 catarrhal — see Icterus, infectious
 conjunctiva 782.4
  newborn 774.6
 epidemic — see Icterus, infectious
 febrilis — see Icterus, infectious
 fetus or newborn — see Jaundice, fetus or
  newborn
 gravis (see also Necrosis, liver) 570
  complicating pregnancy 646.7 ✓5ᵗʰ
   affecting fetus or newborn 760.8
  fetus or newborn NEC 773.0
  obstetrical 646.7 ✓5ᵗʰ
   affecting fetus or newborn 760.8
 hematogenous (acquired) 283.9
 hemolytic (acquired) 283.9
  congenital (see also Spherocytosis) 282.0
 hemorrhagic (acute) 100.0
  leptospiral 100.0
  newborn 776.0
  spirochetal 100.0
 infectious 070.1
  with hepatic coma 070.0
  leptospiral 100.0
  spirochetal 100.0
 intermittens juvenilis 277.4
 malignant (see also Necrosis, liver) 570
 neonatorum (see also Jaundice, fetus or
  newborn) 774.6
 pernicious (see also Necrosis, liver) 570
 spirochetal 100.0
Ictus solaris, solis 992.0
Identity disorder 313.82
 dissociative 300.14
 gender role (child) 302.6
  adult 302.85
 psychosexual (child) 302.6
  adult 302.85
Idioglossia 307.9
Idiopathic — see condition
Idiosyncrasy (see also Allergy) 995.3
 drug, medicinal substance, and biological —
  see Allergy, drug
Idiot, idiocy (congenital) 318.2
 amaurotic (Bielschowsky) (-Jansky) (family)
  (infantile (late)) (juvenile (late)) (Vogt-
  Spielmeyer) 330.1
 microcephalic 742.1
 Mongolian 758.0
 oxycephalic 756.0
Id reaction (due to bacteria) 692.89
IgE asthma 493.0 ✓5ᵗʰ
Ileitis (chronic) (see also Enteritis) 558.9
 infectious 009.0
 noninfectious 558.9
 regional (ulcerative) 555.0
  with large intestine 555.2
 segmental 555.0
  with large intestine 555.2
 terminal (ulcerative) 555.0
  with large intestine 555.2
Ileocolitis (see also Enteritis) 558.9
 infectious 009.0
 regional 555.2
 ulcerative 556.1
Ileostomy status V44.2
 with complication 569.60
Ileotyphus 002.0
Ileum — see condition

Ileus (adynamic) (bowel) (colon) (inhibitory)
 (intestine) (neurogenic) (paralytic) 560.1
 arteriomesenteric duodenal 537.2
 due to gallstone (in intestine) 560.31
 duodenal, chronic 537.2
 following gastrointestinal surgery 997.4
 gallstone 560.31
 mechanical (see also Obstruction, intestine)
  560.9
 meconium 777.1
  due to cystic fibrosis 277.01
 myxedema 564.89
 postoperative 997.4
 transitory, newborn 777.4
Iliac — see condition
Iliotibial band friction syndrome 728.89
Ill, louping 063.1
Illegitimacy V61.6
Illness — see also Disease
 factitious 300.19
  with
   combined physical and psychological
    symptoms 300.19
   physical symptoms 300.19
   psychological symptoms 300.16
  chronic (with physical symptoms) 301.51
 heart — see Disease, heart
 manic-depressive (see also Psychosis, affective)
  296.80
 mental (see also Disorder, mental) 300.9
Imbalance 781.2
 autonomic (see also Neuropathy, peripheral,
  autonomic) 337.9
 electrolyte 276.9
  with
   abortion — see Abortion, by type, with
    metabolic disorder
   ectopic pregnancy (see also categories
    633.0-633.9) 639.4
   hyperemesis gravidarum (before 22
    completed weeks gestation)
    643.1 ✓5ᵗʰ
   molar pregnancy (see also categories 630-
    632) 639.4
  following
   abortion 639.4
   ectopic or molar pregnancy 639.4
  neonatal, transitory NEC 775.5
 endocrine 259.9
 eye muscle NEC 378.9
  heterophoria — see Heterophoria
 glomerulotubular NEC 593.89
 hormone 259.9
 hysterical (see also Hysteria) 300.10
 labyrinth NEC 386.50
 posture 729.9
 sympathetic (see also Neuropathy, peripheral,
  autonomic) 337.9
Imbecile, imbecility 318.0
 moral 301.7
 old age 290.9
 senile 290.9
 specified IQ — see IQ
 unspecified IQ 318.0
Imbedding, intrauterine device 996.32
Imbibition, cholesterol (gallbladder) 575.6
Imerslund (-Gräsbeck) syndrome (anemia due to
 familial selective vitamin B₁₂ malabsorption)
 281.1
Iminoacidopathy 270.8
Iminoglycinuria, familial 270.8
Immature — see also Immaturity
 personality 301.89
Immaturity 765.1 ✓5ᵗʰ
 extreme 765.0 ✓5ᵗʰ
 fetus or infant light-for-dates — see Light-for-
  dates
 lung, fetus or newborn 770.4
 organ or site NEC — see Hypoplasia
 pulmonary, fetus or newborn 770.4
 reaction 301.89
 sexual (female) (male) 259.0

Immersion 994.1
  foot 991.4
  hand 991.4
Immobile, immobility
  intestine 564.89
  joint — see Ankylosis
  syndrome (paraplegic) 728.3
Immunization
  ABO
    affecting management of pregnancy 656.2 ✓5ᵗʰ
      fetus or newborn 773.1
    complication — see Complications, vaccination
  Rh factor
    affecting management of pregnancy 656.1 ✓5ᵗʰ
      fetus or newborn 773.0
      from transfusion 999.7
Immunodeficiency 279.3
  with
    adenosine-deaminase deficiency 279.2
    defect, predominant
      B-cell 279.00
      T-cell 279.10
    hyperimmunoglobulinemia 279.2
    lymphopenia, hereditary 279.2
    thrombocytopenia and eczema 279.12
    thymic
      aplasia 279.2
      dysplasia 279.2
  autosomal recessive, Swiss-type 279.2
  common variable 279.06
  severe combined (SCID) 279.2
  to Rh factor
    affecting management of pregnancy 656.1 ✓5ᵗʰ
      fetus or newborn 773.0
  X-linked, with increased IgM 279.05
Immunotherapy, prophylactic V07.2
Impaction, impacted
  bowel, colon, rectum 560.30
    with hernia — see also Hernia, by site, with obstruction
      gangrenous — see Hernia, by site, with gangrene
    by
      calculus 560.39
      gallstone 560.31
    fecal 560.39
    specified type NEC 560.39
  calculus — see Calculus
  cerumen (ear) (external) 380.4
  cuspid 520.6
    with abnormal position (same or adjacent tooth) 524.3
  dental 520.6
    with abnormal position (same or adjacent tooth) 524.3
  fecal, feces 560.39
    with hernia — see also Hernia, by site, with obstruction
      gangrenous — see Hernia, by site, with gangrene
  fracture — see Fracture, by site
  gallbladder — see Cholelithiasis
  gallstone(s) — see Cholelithiasis
    in intestine (any part) 560.31
  intestine(s) 560.30
    with hernia — see also Hernia, by site, with obstruction
      grangrenous — see Hernia, by site, with gangrene
    by
      calculus 560.39
      gallstone 560.31
    fecal 560.39
    specified type NEC 560.39
  intrauterine device (IUD) 996.32
  molar 520.6
    with abnormal position (same or adjacent tooth) 524.3
  shoulder 660.4 ✓5ᵗʰ
    affecting fetus or newborn 763.1
  tooth, teeth 520.6
    with abnormal position (same or adjacent tooth) 524.3

Impaction, impacted — continued
  turbinate 733.99
Impaired, impairment (function)
  arm V49.1
    movement, involving
      musculoskeletal system V49.1
      nervous system V49.2
  auditory discrimination 388.43
  back V48.3
  body (entire) V49.89
  hearing (see also Deafness) 389.9
  heart — see Disease, heart
  kidney (see also Disease, renal) 593.9
    disorder resulting from 588.9
      specified NEC 588.8
  leg V49.1
    movement, involving
      musculoskeletal system V49.1
      nervous system V49.2
  limb V49.1
    movement, involving
      musculoskeletal system V49.1
      nervous system V49.2
  liver 573.8
  mastication 524.9
  mobility
    ear ossicles NEC 385.22
    incostapedial joint 385.22
    malleus 385.21
  myocardium, myocardial (see also Insufficiency, myocardial) 428.0
  neuromusculoskeletal NEC V49.89
    back V48.3
    head V48.2
    limb V49.2
    neck V48.3
    spine V48.3
    trunk V48.3
  rectal sphincter 787.99
  renal (see also Disease, renal) 593.9
    disorder resulting from 588.9
      specified NEC 588.8
  spine V48.3
  vision NEC 369.9
    both eyes NEC 369.3
    moderate 369.74
      both eyes 369.25
        with impairment of lesser eye (specified as)
          blind, not further specified 369.15
          low vision, not further specified 369.23
          near-total 369.17
          profound 369.18
          severe 369.24
          total 369.16
      one eye 369.74
        with vision of other eye (specified as)
          near-normal 369.75
          normal 369.76
    near-total 369.64
      both eyes 369.04
        with impairment of lesser eye (specified as)
          blind, not further specified 369.02
          total 369.03
      one eye 369.64
        with vision of other eye (specified as)
          near normal 369.65
          normal 369.66
    one eye 369.60
      with low vision of other eye 369.10
    profound 369.67
      both eyes 369.08
        with impairment of lesser eye (specified as)
          blind, not further specified 369.05
          near-total 369.07
          total 369.06
      one eye 369.67
        with vision of other eye (specified as)
          near-normal 369.68
          normal 369.69

Impaired, impairment — continued
  vision NEC — continued
    severe 369.71
      both eyes 369.22
        with impairment of lesser eye (specified as)
          blind, not further specified 369.11
          low vision, not further specified 369.21
          near-total 369.13
          profound 369.14
          total 369.12
      one eye 369.71
        with vision of other eye (specified as)
          near-normal 369.72
          normal 369.73
    total
      both eyes 369.01
      one eye 369.61
        with vision of other eye (specified as)
          near-normal 369.62
          normal 369.63
Impaludism — see Malaria
Impediment, speech NEC 784.5
  psychogenic 307.9
  secondary to organic lesion 784.5
Impending
  cerebrovascular accident or attack 435.9
  coronary syndrome 411.1
  delirium tremens 291.0
  myocardial infarction 411.1
Imperception, auditory (acquired) (congenital) 389.9
Imperfect
  aeration, lung (newborn) 770.5
  closure (congenital)
    alimentary tract NEC 751.8
      lower 751.5
      upper 750.8
    atrioventricular ostium 745.69
    atrium (secundum) 745.5
      primum 745.61
    branchial cleft or sinus 744.41
    choroid 743.59
    cricoid cartilage 748.3
    cusps, heart valve NEC 746.89
      pulmonary 746.09
    ductus
      arteriosus 747.0
      Botalli 747.0
    ear drum 744.29
      causing impairment of hearing 744.03
    endocardial cushion 745.60
    epiglottis 748.3
    esophagus with communication to bronchus or trachea 750.3
    Eustachian valve 746.89
    eyelid 743.62
    face, facial (see also Cleft, lip) 749.10
    foramen
      Botalli 745.5
      ovale 745.5
    genitalia, genital organ(s) or system
      female 752.8
        external 752.49
        internal NEC 752.8
        uterus 752.3
      male 752.8
        penis 752.69
    glottis 748.3
    heart valve (cusps) NEC 746.89
    interatrial ostium or septum 745.5
    interauricular ostium or septum 745.5
    interventricular ostium or septum 745.4
    iris 743.46
    kidney 753.3
    larynx 748.3
    lens 743.36
    lip (see also Cleft, lip) 749.10
    nasal septum or sinus 748.1
    nose 748.1
    omphalomesenteric duct 751.0
    optic nerve entry 743.57
    organ or site NEC — see Anomaly, specified type, by site

Immersion — Imperfect

Imperfect — continued
closure — continued
ostium
interatrial 745.5
interauricular 745.5
interventricular 745.4
palate (see also Cleft, palate) 749.00
preauricular sinus 744.46
retina 743.56
roof of orbit 742.0
sclera 743.47
septum
aortic 745.0
aorticopulmonary 745.0
atrial (secundum) 745.5
primum 745.61
between aorta and pulmonary artery
745.0
heart 745.9
interatrial (secundum) 745.5
primum 745.61
interauricular (secundum) 745.5
primum 745.61
interventricular 745.4
with pulmonary stenosis or atresia,
dextraposition of aorta, and
hypertrophy of right ventricle
745.2
in tetralogy of Fallot 745.2
nasal 748.1
ventricular 745.4
with pulmonary stenosis or atresia,
dextraposition of aorta, and
hypertrophy of right ventricle
745.2
in tetralogy of Fallot 745.2
skull 756.0
with
anencephalus 740.0
encephalocele 742.0
hydrocephalus 742.3
with spina bifida (see also Spina
bifida) 741.0 ✔5ᵗʰ
microcephalus 742.1
spine (with meningocele) (see also Spina
bifida) 741.90
thyroid cartilage 748.3
trachea 748.3
tympanic membrane 744.29
causing impairment of hearing 744.03
uterus (with communication to bladder,
intestine, or rectum) 752.3
uvula 749.02
with cleft lip (see also Cleft, palate, with
cleft lip) 749.20
vitelline duct 751.0
development — see Anomaly, by site
erection 607.84
fusion — see Imperfect, closure
inflation lung (newborn) 770.5
intestinal canal 751.5
poise 729.9
rotation — see Malrotation
septum, ventricular 745.4
Imperfectly descended testis 752.51
Imperforate (congenital) — see also Atresia
anus 751.2
bile duct 751.61
cervix (uteri) 752.49
esophagus 750.3
hymen 752.42
intestine (small) 751.1
large 751.2
jejunum 751.1
pharynx 750.29
rectum 751.2
salivary duct 750.23
urethra 753.6
urinary meatus 753.6
vagina 752.49
Impervious (congenital) — see also Atresia
anus 751.2
bile duct 751.61
esophagus 750.3
intestine (small) 751.1
large 751.5
rectum 751.2
urethra 753.6

Impetiginization of other dermatoses 684
Impetigo (any organism) (any site) (bullous)
(circinate) (contagiosa) (neonatorum)
(simplex) 684
Bockhart's (superficial folliculitis) 704.8
external ear 684 [380.13]
eyelid 684 [373.5]
Fox's (contagiosa) 684
furfuracea 696.5
herpetiformis 694.3
nonobstetrical 694.3
staphylococcal infection 684
ulcerative 686.8
vulgaris 684
Impingement, soft tissue between teeth 524.2
Implant, endometrial 617.9
Implantation
anomalous — see also Anomaly, specified type,
by site
ureter 753.4
cyst
external area or site (skin) NEC 709.8
iris 364.61
vagina 623.8
vulva 624.8
dermoid (cyst)
external area or site (skin) NEC 709.8
iris 364.61
vagina 623.8
vulva 624.8
placenta, low or marginal — see Placenta
previa
Impotence (sexual) (psychogenic) 302.72
organic origin NEC 607.84
Impoverished blood 285.9
Impression, basilar 756.0
Imprisonment V62.5
Improper
development, infant 764.9 ✔5ᵗʰ
Improperly tied umbilical cord (causing
hemorrhage) 772.3
Impulses, obsessional 300.3
Impulsive neurosis 300.3
Inaction, kidney (see also Disease, renal) 593.9
Inactive — see condition
Inadequate, inadequacy
biologic 301.6
cardiac and renal — see Hypertension,
cardiorenal
constitutional 301.6
development
child 783.40
fetus 764.9 ✔5ᵗʰ
affecting management of pregnancy
656.5 ✔5ᵗʰ
genitalia
after puberty NEC 259.0
congenital — see Hypoplasia, genitalia
lungs 748.5
organ or site NEC — see Hypoplasia, by site
dietary 269.9
education V62.3
environment
economic problem V60.2
household condition NEC V60.1
poverty V60.2
unemployment V62.0
functional 301.6
household care, due to
family member
handicapped or ill V60.4
temporarily away from home V60.4
on vacation V60.5
technical defects in home V60.1
temporary absence from home of person
rendering care V60.4
housing (heating) (space) V60.1
material resources V60.2
mental (see also Retardation, mental) 319
nervous system 799.2
personality 301.6
prenatal care in current pregnancy V23.7
pulmonary
function 786.09
newborn 770.89   ▲
ventilation, newborn 770.89   ▲

Inadequate, inadequacy — continued
respiration 786.09
newborn 770.89   ▲
social 301.6
Inanition 263.9
with edema 262
due to
deprivation of food 994.2
malnutrition 263.9
fever 780.6
Inappropriate secretion
ACTH 255.0
antidiuretic hormone (ADH) (excessive) 253.6
deficiency 253.5
ectopic hormone NEC 259.3
pituitary (posterior) 253.6
Inattention after or at birth 995.52
Inborn errors of metabolism — see Disorder,
metabolism
Incarceration, incarcerated
bubonocele — see also Hernia, inguinal, with
obstruction
gangrenous — see Hernia, inguinal, with
gangrene
colon (by hernia) — see also Hernia, by site
with obstruction
gangrenous — see Hernia, by site, with
gangrene
enterocele 552.9
gangrenous 551.9
epigastrocele 552.29
gangrenous 551.29
epiplocele 552.9
gangrenous 551.9
exomphalos 552.1
gangrenous 551.1
fallopian tube 620.8
hernia — see also Hernia, by site, with
obstruction
gangrenous — see Hernia, by site, with
gangrene
iris, in wound 871.1
lens, in wound 871.1
merocele (see also Hernia, femoral, with
obstruction) 552.00
omentum (by hernia) — see also Hernia, by
site, with obstruction
gangrenous — see Hernia, by site, with
gangrene
omphalocele 756.79
rupture (meaning hernia) (see also Hernia, by
site, with obstruction) 552.9
gangrenous (see also Hernia, by site, with
gangrene) 551.9
sarcoepiplocele 552.9
gangrenous 551.9
sarcoepiplomphalocele 552.1
with gangrene 551.1
uterus 621.8
gravid 654.3 ✔5ᵗʰ
causing obstructed labor 660.2 ✔5ᵗʰ
affecting fetus or newborn 763.1
Incident, cerebrovascular (see also Disease,
cerebrovascular, acute) 436
Incineration (entire body) (from fire,
conflagration, electricity, or lightning) — see
Burn, multiple, specified sites
Incised wound
external — see Wound, open, by site
internal organs (abdomen, chest, or pelvis) —
see Injury, internal, by site, with open
wound
Incision, incisional
hernia — see Hernia, incisional
surgical, complication — see Complications,
surgical procedures
traumatic
external — see Wound, open, by site
internal organs (abdomen, chest, or pelvis)
— see Injury, internal, by site, with
open wound
Inclusion
azurophilic leukocytic 288.2
blennorrhea (neonatal) (newborn) 771.6
cyst — see Cyst, skin
gallbladder in liver (congenital) 751.69

Incompatibility
  ABO
    affecting management of pregnancy 656.2 ✓5ᵗʰ
    fetus or newborn 773.1
    infusion or transfusion reaction 999.6
  blood (group) (Duffy) (E) (K(ell)) (Kidd) (Lewis) (M) (N) (P) (S) NEC
    affecting management of pregnancy 656.2 ✓5ᵗʰ
    fetus or newborn 773.2
    infusion or transfusion reaction 999.6
  marital V61.10
    involving divorce or estrangement V61.0
  Rh (blood group) (factor)
    affecting management of pregnancy 656.1 ✓5ᵗʰ
    fetus or newborn 773.0
    infusion or transfusion reaction 999.7
  Rhesus — see Incompatibility, Rh
Incompetency, incompetence, incompetent
  annular
    aortic (valve) (see also Insufficiency, aortic) 424.1
    mitral (valve) — (see also Insufficiency, mitral) 424.0
    pulmonary valve (heart) (see also Endocarditis, pulmonary) 424.3
  aortic (valve) (see also Insufficiency, aortic) 424.1
    syphilitic 093.22
  cardiac (orifice) 530.0
    valve — see Endocarditis
  cervix, cervical (os) 622.5
    in pregnancy 654.5 ✓5ᵗʰ
      affecting fetus or newborn 761.0
  esophagogastric (junction) (sphincter) 530.0
  heart valve, congenital 746.89
  mitral (valve) — see Insufficiency, mitral
  papillary muscle (heart) 429.81
  pelvic fundus 618.8
  pulmonary valve (heart) (see also Endocarditis, pulmonary) 424.3
    congenital 746.09
  tricuspid (annular) (rheumatic) (valve) (see also Endocarditis, tricuspid) 397.0
  valvular — see Endocarditis
  vein, venous (saphenous) (varicose) (see also Varicose, vein) 454.9
  velopharyngeal (closure)
    acquired 528.9
    congenital 750.29
Incomplete — see also condition
  bladder emptying 788.21
  expansion lungs (newborn) 770.5
  gestation (liveborn) — see Immaturity
  rotation — see Malrotation
Incontinence 788.30
  without sensory awareness 788.34
  anal sphincter 787.6
  continuous leakage 788.37
  feces 787.6
    due to hysteria 300.11
    nonorganic origin 307.7
  hysterical 300.11
  mixed (male) (female) (urge and stress) 788.33
  overflow 788.39
  paradoxical 788.39
  rectal 787.6
  specified NEC 788.39
  stress (female) 625.6
    male NEC 788.32
  urethral sphincter 599.84
  urge 788.31
    and stress (male) (female) 788.33
  urine 788.30
    active 788.30
    male 788.30
      stress 788.32
        and urge 788.33
      neurogenic 788.39
    nonorganic origin 307.6
    stress (female) 625.6
      male NEC 788.32
    urge 788.31
      and stress 788.33
Incontinentia pigmenti 757.33

Incoordinate
  uterus (action) (contractions) 661.4 ✓5ᵗʰ
    affecting fetus or newborn 763.7
Incoordination
  esophageal-pharyngeal (newborn) 787.2
  muscular 781.3
  papillary muscle 429.81
Increase, increased
  abnormal, in development 783.9
  androgens (ovarian) 256.1
  anticoagulants (antithrombin) (anti-VIIIa) (anti-IXa) (anti-Xa) (anti-XIa) 286.5
    postpartum 666.3 ✓5ᵗʰ
  cold sense (see also Disturbance, sensation) 782.0
  estrogen 256.0
  function
    adrenal (cortex) 255.3
      medulla 255.6
    pituitary (anterior) (gland) (lobe) 253.1
      posterior 253.6
  heat sense (see also Disturbance, sensation) 782.0
  intracranial pressure 781.99
    injury at birth 767.8
  light reflex of retina 362.13
  permeability, capillary 448.9
  pressure
    intracranial 781.99
      injury at birth 767.8
    intraocular 365.00
  pulsations 785.9
  pulse pressure 785.9
  sphericity, lens 743.36
  splenic activity 289.4
  venous pressure 459.89
    portal 572.3
Incrustation, cornea, lead or zinc 930.0
Incyclophoria 378.44
Incyclotropia 378.33
Indeterminate sex 752.7
India rubber skin 756.83
Indicanuria 270.2
Indigestion (bilious) (functional) 536.8
  acid 536.8
  catarrhal 536.8
  due to decomposed food NEC 005.9
  fat 579.8
  nervous 306.4
  psychogenic 306.4
Indirect — see condition
Indolent bubo NEC 099.8
Induced
  abortion — see Abortion, induced
  birth, affecting fetus or newborn 763.89
  delivery — see Delivery
  labor — see Delivery
Induration, indurated
  brain 348.8
  breast (fibrous) 611.79
    puerperal, postpartum 676.3 ✓5ᵗʰ
  broad ligament 620.8
  chancre 091.0
    anus 091.1
    congenital 090.0
    extragenital NEC 091.2
  corpora cavernosa (penis) (plastic) 607.89
  liver (chronic) 573.8
    acute 573.8
  lung (black) (brown) (chronic) (fibroid) (see also Fibrosis, lung) 515
    essential brown 275.0 [516.1]
  penile 607.89
  phlebitic — see Phlebitis
  skin 782.8
  stomach 537.89
Induratio penis plastica 607.89
Industrial — see condition
Inebriety (see also Abuse, drugs, nondependent) 305.0 ✓5ᵗʰ
Inefficiency
  kidney (see also Disease, renal) 593.9
  thyroid (acquired) (gland) 244.9
Inelasticity, skin 782.8

Inequality, leg (acquired) (length) 736.81
  congenital 755.30
Inertia
  bladder 596.4
    neurogenic 596.54
      with cauda equina syndrome 344.61
  stomach 536.8
    psychogenic 306.4
  uterus, uterine 661.2 ✓5ᵗʰ
    affecting fetus or newborn 763.7
    primary 661.0 ✓5ᵗʰ
    secondary 661.1 ✓5ᵗʰ
  vesical 596.4
    neurogenic 596.54
      with cauda equina 344.61
Infant — see also condition
  • excessive crying of 780.92
  • fussy (baby) 780.91
  held for adoption V68.89
  newborn — see Newborn
  syndrome of diabetic mother 775.0
"Infant Hercules" syndrome 255.2
Infantile — see also condition
  genitalia, genitals 259.0
    in pregnancy or childbirth NEC 654.4 ✓5ᵗʰ
      affecting fetus or newborn 763.89
      causing obstructed labor 660.2 ✓5ᵗʰ
        affecting fetus or newborn 763.1
  heart 746.9
  kidney 753.3
  lack of care 995.52
  macula degeneration 362.75
  melanodontia 521.05
  os, uterus (see also Infantile, genitalia) 259.0
  pelvis 738.6
    with disproportion (fetopelvic) 653.1 ✓5ᵗʰ
      affecting fetus or newborn 763.1
      causing obstructed labor 660.1 ✓5ᵗʰ
        affecting fetus or newborn 763.1
  penis 259.0
  testis 257.2
  uterus (see also Infantile, genitalia) 259.0
  vulva 752.49
Infantilism 259.9
  with dwarfism (hypophyseal) 253.3
  Brissaud's (infantile myxedema) 244.9
  celiac 579.0
  Herter's (nontropical sprue) 579.0
  hypophyseal 253.3
  hypothalamic (with obesity) 253.8
  idiopathic 259.9
  intestinal 579.0
  pancreatic 577.8
  pituitary 253.3
  renal 588.0
  sexual (with obesity) 259.0
Infants, healthy liveborn — see Newborn
Infarct, infarction
  adrenal (capsule) (gland) 255.4
  amnion 658.8 ✓5ᵗʰ
  anterior (with contiguous portion of intraventricular septum) NEC (see also Infarct, myocardium) 410.1 ✓5ᵗʰ
  appendices epiploicae 557.0
  bowel 557.0
  brain (stem) 434.91
    embolic (see also Embolism, brain) 434.11
    healed or old without residuals V12.59
    iatrogenic 997.02
    postoperative 997.02
    puerperal, postpartum, childbirth 674.0 ✓5ᵗʰ
    thrombotic (see also Thrombosis, brain) 434.01
  breast 611.8
  Brewer's (kidney) 593.81
  cardiac (see also Infarct, myocardium) 410.9 ✓5ᵗʰ
  cerebellar (see also Infarct, brain) 434.91
    embolic (see also Embolism, brain) 434.11
  cerebral (see also Infarct, brain) 434.91
    embolic (see also Embolism, brain) 434.11
  chorion 658.8 ✓5ᵗʰ
  colon (acute) (agnogenic) (embolic) (hemorrhagic) (nonocclusive) (nonthrombotic) (occlusive) (segmental) (thrombotic) (with gangrene) 557.0

Infarct, infarction — *continued*
  coronary artery (*see also* Infarct, myocardium)
    410.9 ✓5th
  embolic (*see also* Embolism) 444.9
  fallopian tube 620.8
  gallbladder 575.8
  heart (*see also* Infarct, myocardium) 410.9 ✓5th
  hepatic 573.4
  hypophysis (anterior lobe) 253.8
  impending (myocardium) 411.1
  intestine (acute) (agnogenic) (embolic)
    (hemorrhagic) (nonocclusive)
    (nonthrombotic) (occlusive) (thrombotic)
    (with gangrene) 557.0
  kidney 593.81
  liver 573.4
  lung (embolic) (thrombotic) 415.1 ✓5th
    with
      abortion — *see* Abortion, by type, with
        embolism
      ectopic pregnancy (*see also* categories
        633.0-633.9) 639.6
      molar pregnancy (*see also* categories 630-
        632) 639.6
    following
      abortion 639.6
      ectopic or molar pregnancy 639.6
    iatrogenic 415.11
    in pregnancy, childbirth, or puerperium —
      see Embolism, obstetrical
    postoperative 415.11
  lymph node or vessel 457.8
  medullary (brain) — *see* Infarct, brain
  meibomian gland (eyelid) 374.85
  mesentary, mesenteric (embolic) (thrombotic)
    (with gangrene) 557.0
  midbrain — *see* Infarct, brain
  myocardium, myocardial (acute or with a
    stated duration of 8 weeks or less) (with
    hypertension) 410.9 ✓5th

> Note — Use the following fifth-digit
> subclassification with category 410:
>
> 0   episode unspecified
>
> 1   initial episode
>
> 2   subsequent episode without
>   recurrence

    with symptoms after 8 weeks from date of
      infarction 414.8
    anterior (wall) (with contiguous portion of
      intraventricular septum)
      NEC 410.1 ✓5th
    anteroapical (with contiguous portion of
      intraventricular septum) 410.1 ✓5th
    anterolateral (wall) 410.0 ✓5th
    anteroseptal (with contiguous portion of
      intraventricular septum) 410.1 ✓5th
    apical-lateral 410.5 ✓5th
    atrial 410.8 ✓5th
    basal-lateral 410.5 ✓5th
    chronic (with symptoms after 8 weeks from
      date of infarction) 414.8
    diagnosed on ECG, but presenting no
      symptoms 412
    diaphragmatic wall (with contiguous portion
      of intraventricular septum) 410.4 ✓5th
    healed or old, currently presenting no
      symptoms 412
    high lateral 410.5 ✓5th
    impending 411.1
    inferior (wall) (with contiguous portion of
      intraventricular septum) 410.4 ✓5th
    inferolateral (wall) 410.2 ✓5th
    inferoposterior wall 410.3 ✓5th
    lateral wall 410.5 ✓5th
    nontransmural 410.7 ✓5th
    papillary muscle 410.8 ✓5th
    past (diagnosed on ECG or other special
      investigation, but currently presenting
      no symptoms) 412
      with symptoms NEC 414.8
    posterior (strictly) (true) (wall) 410.6 ✓5th
    posterobasal 410.6 ✓5th
    posteroinferior 410.3 ✓5th
    posterolateral 410.5 ✓5th

Infarct, infarction — *continued*
  myocardium, myocardial — *continued*
    previous, currently presenting no symptoms
      412
    septal 410.8 ✓5th
    specified site NEC 410.8 ✓5th
    subendocardial 410.7 ✓5th
    syphilitic 093.82
  nontransmural 410.7 ✓5th
  omentum 557.0
  ovary 620.8
  pancreas 577.8
  papillary muscle (*see also* Infarct, myocardium)
    410.8 ✓5th
  parathyroid gland 252.8
  pituitary (gland) 253.8
  placenta (complicating pregnancy) 656.7 ✓5th
    affecting fetus or newborn 762.2
  pontine — *see* Infarct, brain
  posterior NEC (*see also* Infarct, myocardium)
    410.6 ✓5th
  prostate 602.8
  pulmonary (artery) (hemorrhagic) (vein)
    415.1 ✓5th
    with
      abortion — *see* Abortion, by type, with
        embolism
      ectopic pregnancy (*see also* categories
        633.0-633.9) 639.6
      molar pregnancy (*see also* categories 630-
        632) 639.6
    following
      abortion 639.6
      ectopic or molar pregnancy 639.6
    iatrogenic 415.11
    in pregnancy, childbirth, or puerperium —
      see Embolism, obstetrical
    postoperative 415.11
  renal 593.81
    embolic or thrombotic 593.81
  retina, retinal 362.84
    with occlusion — *see* Occlusion, retina
  spinal (acute) (cord) (embolic) (nonembolic)
    336.1
  spleen 289.59
    embolic or thrombotic 444.89
  subchorionic — *see* Infarct, placenta
  subendocardial (*see also* Infarct, myocardium)
    410.7 ✓5th
  suprarenal (capsule) (gland) 255.4
  syncytium — *see* Infarct, placenta
  testis 608.83
  thrombotic (*see also* Thrombosis) 453.9
    artery, arterial — *see* Embolism
  thyroid (gland) 246.3
  ventricle (heart) (*see also* Infarct, myocardium)
    410.9 ✓5th

Infecting — *see* condition
Infection, infected, infective (opportunistic)
  136.9
  with lymphangitis — *see* Lymphangitis
  abortion — *see* Abortion, by type, with sepsis
  abscess (skin) — *see* Abscess, by site
  Absidia 117.7
  Acanthocheilonema (perstans) 125.4
    streptocerca 125.6
  accessory sinus (chronic) (*see also* Sinusitis)
    473.9
  Achorion — *see* Dermatophytosis
  Acremonium falciforme 117.4
  acromioclavicular (joint) 711.91
  actinobacillus
    lignieresii 027.8
    mallei 024
    muris 026.1
  actinomadura — *see* Actinomycosis
  Actinomyces (israelii) — *see also* Actinomycosis
    muris-ratti 026.1
  Actinomycetales (actinomadura) (Actinomyces)
    (Nocardia) (Streptomyces) — *see*
    Actinomycosis
  actinomycotic NEC (*see also* Actinomycosis)
    039.9
  adenoid (chronic) 474.01
    acute 463
    and tonsil (chronic) 474.02
      acute or subacute 463

Infection, infected, infective — *continued*
  adenovirus NEC 079.0
    in diseases classified elsewhere — *see*
      category 079 ✓4th
    unspecified nature or site 079.0
  Aerobacter aerogenes NEC 041.85
    enteritis 008.2
  aerogenes capsulatus (*see also* Gangrene, gas)
    040.0
  aertrycke (*see also* Infection, Salmonella) 003.9
  ajellomyces dermatitidis 116.0
  alimentary canal NEC (*see also* Enteritis, due
    to, by organism) 009.0
  Allescheria boydii 117.6
  Alternaria 118
  alveolus, alveolar (process) (pulpal origin) 522.4
  ameba, amebic (histolytica) (*see also* Amebiasis)
    006.9
    acute 006.0
    chronic 006.1
    free-living 136.2
    hartmanni 007.8
    specified
      site NEC 006.8
      type NEC 007.8
  amniotic fluid or cavity 658.4 ✓5th
    affecting fetus or newborn 762.7
  anaerobes (cocci) (gram-negative) (gram-
    positive) (mixed) NEC 041.84
  anal canal 569.49
  Ancylostoma braziliense 126.2
  Angiostrongylus cantonensis 128.8
  anisakiasis 127.1
  Anisakis larva 127.1
  anthrax (*see also* Anthrax) 022.9
  antrum (chronic) (*see also* Sinusitis, maxillary)
    473.0
  anus (papillae) (sphincter) 569.49
  arbor virus NEC 066.9
  arbovirus NEC 066.9
  argentophil-rod 027.0
  Ascaris lumbricoides 127.0
  ascomycetes 117.4
  Aspergillus (flavus) (fumigatus) (terreus) 117.3
  atypical
    acid-fast (bacilli) (*see also* Mycobacterium,
      atypical) 031.9
    mycobacteria (*see also* Mycobacterium,
      atypical) 031.9
  auditory meatus (circumscribed) (diffuse)
    (external) (*see also* Otitis, externa) 380.10
  auricle (ear) (*see also* Otitis, externa) 380.10
  axillary gland 683
  Babesiasis 088.82
  Babesiosis 088.82
  Bacillus NEC 041.89
    abortus 023.1
    anthracis (*see also* Anthrax) 022.9
    cereus (food poisoning) 005.89
    coli — *see* Infection, Escherichia coli
    coliform NEC 041.85
    Ducrey's (any location) 099.0
    Flexner's 004.1
    fragilis NEC 041.82
    Friedländer's NEC 041.3
    fusiformis 101
    gas (gangrene) (*see also* Gangrene, gas)
      040.0
    mallei 024
    melitensis 023.0
    paratyphoid, paratyphosus 002.9
      A 002.1
      B 002.2
      C 002.3
    Schmorl's 040.3
    Shiga 004.0
    suipestifer (*see also* Infection, Salmonella)
      003.9
    swimming pool 031.1
    typhosa 002.0
    welchii (*see also* Gangrene, gas) 040.0
    Whitmore's 025
  bacterial NEC 041.9
    specified NEC 041.89
      anaerobic NEC 041.84
      gram-negative NEC 041.85
        anaerobic NEC 041.84

✓4th Fourth-digit Required   ✓5th Fifth-digit Required   ▶◀ Revised Text   ● New Line   ▲ Revised Code

Infection, infected, infective — *continued*
Bacterium
   paratyphosum 002.9
     A 002.1
     B 002.2
     C 002.3
   typhosum 002.0
Bacteroides (fragilis) (melaninogenicus) (oralis)
   NEC 041.84
balantidium coli 007.0
Bartholin's gland 616.8
Basidiobolus 117.7
Bedsonia 079.98
   specified NEC 079.88
bile duct 576.1
bladder (*see also* Cystitis) 595.9
Blastomyces, blastomycotic 116.0
   brasiliensis 116.1
   dermatitidis 116.0
   European 117.5
   Loboi 116.2
   North American 116.0
   South American 116.1
blood stream — *see* Septicemia
bone 730.9 ✓5ᵗʰ
   specified — *see* Osteomyelitis
Bordetella 033.9
   bronchiseptica 033.8
   parapertussis 033.1
   pertussis 033.0
Borrelia
   bergdorfi 088.81
   vincentii (mouth) (pharynx) (tonsil) 101
brain (*see also* Encephalitis) 323.9
   late effect — *see* category 326
   membranes — (*see also* Meningitis) 322.9
   septic 324.0
     late effect — *see* category 326
     meninges (*see also* Meningitis) 320.9
branchial cyst 744.42
breast 611.0
   puerperal, postpartum 675.2 ✓5ᵗʰ
     with nipple 675.9 ✓5ᵗʰ
       specified type NEC 675.8 ✓5ᵗʰ
     nonpurulent 675.2 ✓5ᵗʰ
     purulent 675.1 ✓5ᵗʰ
bronchus (*see also* Bronchitis) 490
   fungus NEC 117.9
Brucella 023.9
   abortus 023.1
   canis 023.3
   melitensis 023.0
   mixed 023.8
   suis 023.2
Brugia (Wuchereria) malayi 125.1
bursa — *see* Bursitis
buttocks (skin) 686.9
Candida (albicans) (tropicalis) (*see also*
   Candidiasis) 112.9
   congenital 771.7
Candiru 136.8
Capillaria
   hepatica 128.8
   philippinensis 127.5
cartilage 733.99
cat liver fluke 121.0
cellulitis — *see* Cellulitis, by site
Cephalosporum falciforme 117.4
Cercomonas hominis (intestinal) 007.3
cerebrospinal (*see also* Meningitis) 322.9
   late effect — *see* category 326
cervical gland 683
cervix (*see also* Cervicitis) 616.0
cesarean section wound 674.3 ✓5ᵗʰ
Chilomastix (intestinal) 007.8
Chlamydia 079.98
   specified NEC 079.88
cholera (*see also* Cholera) 001.9
chorionic plate 658.8 ✓5ᵗʰ
Cladosporium
   bantianum 117.8
   carrionii 117.2
   mansoni 111.1
   trichoides 117.8
   wernecki 111.1
Clonorchis (sinensis) (liver) 121.1

Infection, infected, infective — *continued*
Clostridium (haemolyticum) (novyi) NEC 041.84
   botulinum 005.1
     congenital 771.89 ▲
   histolyticum (*see also* Gangrene, gas) 040.0
   oedematiens (*see also* Gangrene, gas) 040.0
   perfringens 041.83
     due to food 005.2
   septicum (*see also* Gangrene, gas) 040.0
   sordellii (*see also* Gangrene, gas) 040.0
   welchii (*see also* Gangrene, gas) 040.0
     due to food 005.2
Coccidioides (immitis) (*see also*
   Coccidioidomycosis) 114.9
coccus NEC 041.89
colon (*see also* Enteritis, due to, by organism)
   009.0
   bacillus — *see* Infection, Escherichia coli
colostomy or enterostomy 569.61
common duct 576.1
complicating pregnancy, childbirth, or
   puerperium NEC 647.9 ✓5ᵗʰ
   affecting fetus or newborn 760.2
Condiobolus 117.7
congenital NEC 771.89 ▲
   Candida albicans 771.7
   chronic 771.2
   clostridial 771.89 ▲
   cytomegalovirus 771.1
   Escherichia coli 771.89 ▲
   hepatitis, viral 771.2
   herpes simplex 771.2
   listeriosis 771.2
   malaria 771.2
   poliomyelitis 771.2
   rubella 771.0
   Salmonella 771.89 ▲
   streptococcal 771.89 ▲
   toxoplasmosis 771.2
   tuberculosis 771.2
   urinary (tract) 771.82 ▲
   vaccinia 771.2
corpus luteum (*see also* Salpingo-oophoritis)
   614.2
Corynebacterium diphtheriae — *see* Diphtheria
Coxsackie (*see also* Coxsackie) 079.2
   endocardium 074.22
   heart NEC 074.20
   in diseases classified elsewhere — *see*
     category 079 ✓5ᵗʰ
   meninges 047.0
   myocardium 074.23
   pericardium 074.21
   pharynx 074.0
   specified disease NEC 074.8
   unspecified nature or site 079.2
Cryptococcus neoformans 117.5
Cryptosporidia 007.4
Cunninghamella 117.7
cyst — *see* Cyst
Cysticercus cellulosae 123.1
cytomegalovirus 078.5
   congenital 771.1
dental (pulpal origin) 522.4
deuteromycetes 117.4
Dicrocoelium dendriticum 121.8
Dipetalonema (perstans) 125.4
   streptocerca 125.6
diphtherial — *see* Diphtheria
Diphyllobothrium (adult) (latum) (pacificum)
   123.4
   larval 123.5
Diplogonoporus (grandis) 123.8
Dipylidium (caninum) 123.8
Dirofilaria 125.6
dog tapeworm 123.8
Dracunculus medinensis 125.7
Dreschlera 118
   hawaiiensis 117.8
Ducrey's bacillus (any site) 099.0
due to or resulting from
   device, implant, or graft (any) (presence of)
     — *see* Complications, infection and
     inflammation, due to (presence of) any
     device, implant, or graft classified to
     996.0-996.5 NEC

Infection, infected, infective — *continued*
due to or resulting from — *continued*
   injection, inoculation, infusion, transfusion,
     or vaccination (prophylactic)
     (therapeutic) 999.3
   injury NEC — *see* Wound, open, by site,
     complicated
   surgery 998.59
duodenum 535.6 ✓5ᵗʰ
ear — *see also* Otitis
   external (*see also* Otitis, externa) 380.10
   inner (*see also* Labyrinthitis) 386.30
   middle — *see* Otitis, media
Eaton's agent NEC 041.81
Eberthella typhosa 002.0
Ebola 065.8
echinococcosis 122.9
Echinococcus (*see also* Echinococcus) 122.9
Echinostoma 121.8
ECHO virus 079.1
   in diseases classified elsewhere — *see*
     category 079 ✓4ᵗʰ
   unspecified nature or site 079.1
Ehrlichiosis 082.40
   chaffeensis 082.41
   specified type NEC 082.49
Endamoeba — *see* Infection, ameba
endocardium (*see also* Endocarditis) 421.0
endocervix (*see also* Cervicitis) 616.0
Entamoeba — *see* Infection, ameba
enteric (*see also* Enteritis, due to, by organism)
   009.0
Enterobacter aerogenes NEC 041.85
Enterobius vermicularis 127.4
enterococcus NEC 041.04
enterovirus NEC 079.89
   central nervous system NEC 048
   enteritis 008.67
   meningitis 047.9
Entomophthora 117.7
Epidermophyton — *see* Dermatophytosis
epidermophytosis — *see* Dermatophytosis
episiotomy 674.3 ✓5ᵗʰ
Epstein-Barr virus 075
   chronic 780.79 *[139.8]*
erysipeloid 027.1
Erysipelothrix (insidiosa) (rhusiopathiae) 027.1
erythema infectiosum 057.0
Escherichia coli NEC 041.4
   congenital 771.89 ▲
   enteritis — *see* Enteritis, E. coli
   generalized 038.42
   intestinal — *see* Enteritis, E. coli
ethmoidal (chronic) (sinus) (*see also* Sinusitis,
   ethmoidal) 473.2
Eubacterium 041.84
Eustachian tube (ear) 381.50
   acute 381.51
   chronic 381.52
exanthema subitum 057.8
external auditory canal (meatus) (*see also*
   Otitis, externa) 380.10
eye NEC 360.00
eyelid 373.9
   specified NEC 373.8
fallopian tube (*see also* Salpingo-oophoritis)
   614.2
fascia 728.89
Fasciola
   gigantica 121.3
   hepatica 121.3
Fasciolopsis (buski) 121.4
fetus (intra-amniotic) — *see* Infection,
   congenital
filarial — *see* Infestation, filarial
finger (skin) 686.9
   abscess (with lymphangitis) 681.00
     pulp 681.01
   cellulitis (with lymphangitis) 681.00
   distal closed space (with lymphangitis)
     681.00
   nail 681.02
     fungus 110.1
fish tapeworm 123.4
   larval 123.5
flagellate, intestinal 007.9
fluke — *see* Infestation, fluke

Infection, infected, infective — *continued*
focal
  teeth (pulpal origin) 522.4
  tonsils 474.00
    and adenoids 474.02
Fonsecaea
  compactum 117.2
  pedrosoi 117.2
food (*see also* Poisoning, food) 005.9
foot (skin) 686.9
  fungus 110.4
Francisella tularensis (*see also* Tularemia)
  021.9
frontal sinus (chronic) (*see also* Sinusitis,
  frontal) 473.1
fungus NEC 117.9
  beard 110.0
  body 110.5
  dermatiacious NEC 117.8
  foot 110.4
  groin 110.3
  hand 110.2
  nail 110.1
  pathogenic to compromised host only 118
  perianal (area) 110.3
  scalp 110.0
  scrotum 110.8
  skin 111.9
    foot 110.4
    hand 110.2
  toenails 110.1
  trachea 117.9
Fusarium 118
Fusobacterium 041.84
gallbladder (*see also* Cholecystitis, acute) 575.0
Gardnerella vaginalis 041.89 ●
gas bacillus (*see also* Gas, gangrene) 040.0
gastric (*see also* Gastritis) 535.5 ✓5ᵗʰ
Gastrodiscoides hominis 121.8
gastroenteric (*see also* Enteritis, due to, by
  organism) 009.0
gastrointestinal (*see also* Enteritis, due to, by
  organism) 009.0
gastrostomy 536.41
generalized NEC (*see also* Septicemia) 038.9
genital organ or tract NEC
  female 614.9
    with
      abortion — *see* Abortion, by type, with
        sepsis
      ectopic pregnancy (*see also* categories
        633.0-633.9) 639.0
      molar pregnancy (*see also* categories
        630-632) 639.0
    complicating pregnancy 646.6 ✓5ᵗʰ
      affecting fetus or newborn 760.8
    following
      abortion 639.0
      ectopic or molar pregnancy 639.0
    puerperal, postpartum, childbirth
      670 ✓4ᵗʰ
      minor or localized 646.6 ✓5ᵗʰ
        affecting fetus or newborn 760.8
  male 608.4
genitourinary tract NEC 599.0
Ghon tubercle, primary (*see also* Tuberculosis)
  010.0 ✓5ᵗʰ
Giardia lamblia 007.1
gingival (chronic) 523.1
  acute 523.0
  Vincent's 101
glanders 024
Glenosporopsis amazonica 116.2
Gnathostoma spinigerum 128.1
Gongylonema 125.6
gonococcal NEC (*see also* Gonococcus) 098.0
gram-negative bacilli NEC 041.85
  anaerobic 041.84
guinea worm 125.7
gum (*see also* Infection, gingival) 523.1
Hantavirus 079.81
heart 429.89
Helicobacter pylori (H. pylori) 041.86
helminths NEC 128.9
  intestinal 127.9
    mixed (types classifiable to more than one
      category in 120.0-127.7) 127.8

Infection, infected, infective — *continued*
helminths NEC — *continued*
  intestinal — *continued*
    specified type NEC 127.7
  specified type NEC 128.8
Hemophilus influenzae NEC 041.5
  generalized 038.41
herpes (simplex) (*see also* Herpes, simplex)
  054.9
  congenital 771.2
  zoster (*see also* Herpes, zoster) 053.9
    eye NEC 053.29
Heterophyes heterophyes 121.6
Histoplasma (*see also* Histoplasmosis) 115.90
  capsulatum (*see also* Histoplasmosis,
    American) 115.00
  duboisii (*see also* Histoplasmosis, African)
    115.10
HIV V08
  with symptoms, symptomatic 042
hookworm (*see also* Ancylostomiasis) 126.9
human immunodeficiency virus V08
  with symptoms, symptomatic 042
human papillomavirus 079.4
hydrocele 603.1
hydronephrosis 591
Hymenolepis 123.6
hypopharynx 478.29
inguinal glands 683
  due to soft chancre 099.0
intestine, intestinal (*see also* Enteritis, due to,
  by organism) 009.0
intrauterine (*see also* Endometritis) 615.9
  complicating delivery 646.6 ✓5ᵗʰ
isospora belli or hominis 007.2
Japanese B encephalitis 062.0
jaw (bone) (acute) (chronic) (lower) (subacute)
  (upper) 526.4
joint — *see* Arthritis, infectious or infective
kidney (cortex) (hematogenous) 590.9
  with
    abortion — *see* Abortion, by type, with
      urinary tract infection
    calculus 592.0
    ectopic pregnancy (*see also* categories
      633.0-633.9) 639.8
    molar pregnancy (*see also* categories 630-
      632) 639.8
  complicating pregnancy or puerperium
    646.6 ✓5ᵗʰ
    affecting fetus or newborn 760.1
  following
    abortion 639.8
    ectopic or molar pregnancy 639.8
  pelvis and ureter 590.3
Klebsiella pneumoniae NEC 041.3
knee (skin) NEC 686.9
  joint — *see* Arthritis, infectious
Koch's (*see also* Tuberculosis, pulmonary)
  011.9 ✓5ᵗʰ
labia (majora) (minora) (*see also* Vulvitis)
  616.10
lacrimal
  gland (*see also* Dacryoadenitis) 375.00
  passages (duct) (sac) (*see also*
    Dacryocystitis) 375.30
larynx NEC 478.79
leg (skin) NEC 686.9
Leishmania (*see also* Leishmaniasis) 085.9
  braziliensis 085.5
  donovani 085.0
  Ethiopica 085.3
  furunculosa 085.1
  infantum 085.0
  mexicana 085.4
  tropica (minor) 085.1
    major 085.2
Leptosphaeria senegalensis 117.4
leptospira (*see also* Leptospirosis) 100.9
  Australis 100.89
  Bataviae 100.89
  pyrogenes 100.89
  specified type NEC 100.89
leptospirochetal NEC (*see also* Leptospirosis)
  100.9
Leptothrix — *see* Actinomycosis

Infection, infected, infective — *continued*
Listeria monocytogenes (listeriosis) 027.0
  congenital 771.2
liver fluke — *see* Infestation, fluke, liver
Loa loa 125.2
  eyelid 125.2 [373.6]
Loboa loboi 116.2
local, skin (staphylococcal) (streptococcal)
  NEC 686.9
  abscess — *see* Abscess, by site
  cellulitis — *see* Cellulitis, by site
  ulcer (*see also* Ulcer, skin) 707.9
Loefflerella
  mallei 024
  whitmori 025
lung 518.89
  atypical Mycobacterium 031.0
    tuberculous (*see also* Tuberculosis,
      pulmonary) 011.9 ✓5ᵗʰ
  basilar 518.89
  chronic 518.89
  fungus NEC 117.9
  spirochetal 104.8
  virus — *see* Pneumonia, virus
lymph gland (axillary) (cervical) (inguinal) 683
  mesenteric 289.2
lymphoid tissue, base of tongue or posterior
  pharynx, NEC 474.00
madurella
  grisea 117.4
  mycetomii 117.4
major
  with
    abortion — *see* Abortion, by type, with
      sepsis
    ectopic pregnancy (*see also* categories
      633.0-633.9) 639.0
    molar pregnancy (*see also* categories 630-
      632) 639.0
  following
    abortion 639.0
    ectopic or molar pregnancy 639.0
  puerperal, postpartum, childbirth 670 ✓4ᵗʰ
Malassezia furfur 111.0
Malleomyces
  mallei 024
  pseudomallei 025
mammary gland 611.0
  puerperal, postpartum 675.2 ✓5ᵗʰ
Mansonella (ozzardi) 125.5
mastoid (suppurative) — *see* Mastoiditis
maxilla, maxillary 526.4
  sinus (chronic) (*see also* Sinusitis, maxillary)
    473.0
mediastinum 519.2
medina 125.7
meibomian
  cyst 373.12
  gland 373.12
melioidosis 025
meninges (*see also* Meningitis) 320.9
meningococcal (*see also* condition) 036.9
  brain 036.1
  cerebrospinal 036.0
  endocardium 036.42
  generalized 036.2
  meninges 036.0
  meningococcemia 036.2
  specified site NEC 036.89
mesenteric lymph nodes or glands NEC 289.2
Metagonimus 121.5
metatarsophalangeal 711.97
microorganism resistant to drugs — *see*
  Resistance (to), drugs by microorganisms
Microsporidia 136.8
microsporum, microsporic — *see*
  Dermatophytosis
Mima polymorpha NEC 041.85
mixed flora NEC 041.89
Monilia (*see also* Candidiasis) 112.9
  neonatal 771.7
Monosporium apiospermum 117.6
mouth (focus) NEC 528.9
  parasitic 112.0
Mucor 117.7
muscle NEC 728.89

✓4ᵗʰ Fourth-digit Required   ✓5ᵗʰ Fifth-digit Required   ▶◀ Revised Text   ● New Line   ▲ Revised Code

Infection, infected, infective — *continued*
mycelium NEC 117.9
mycetoma
actinomycotic NEC (*see also* Actinomycosis)
039.9
mycotic NEC 117.4
Mycobacterium, mycobacterial (*see also*
Mycobacterium) 031.9
mycoplasma NEC 041.81
mycotic NEC 117.9
pathogenic to compromised host only 118
skin NEC 111.9
systemic 117.9
myocardium NEC 422.90
nail (chronic) (with lymphangitis) 681.9
finger 681.02
fungus 110.1
ingrowing 703.0
toe 681.11
fungus 110.1
nasal sinus (chronic) (*see also* Sinusitis) 473.9
nasopharynx (chronic) 478.29
acute 460
navel 686.9
newborn 771.4
Neisserian — *see* Gonococcus
Neotestudina rosatii 117.4
newborn, generalized 771.89   ▲
nipple 611.0
puerperal, postpartum 675.0 ☑5ᵗʰ
with breast 675.9 ☑5ᵗʰ
specified type NEC 675.8 ☑5ᵗʰ
Nocardia — *see* Actinomycosis
nose 478.1
nostril 478.1
obstetrical surgical wound 674.3 ☑5ᵗʰ
Oesophagostomum (apiostomum) 127.7
Oestrus ovis 134.0
Oidium albicans (*see also* Candidiasis) 112.9
Onchocerca (volvulus) 125.3
eye 125.3 [360.13]
eyelid 125.3 [373.6]
operation wound 998.59
Opisthorchis (felineus) (tenuicollis) (viverrini)
121.0
orbit 376.00
chronic 376.10
ovary (*see also* Salpingo-oophoritis) 614.2
Oxyuris vermicularis 127.4
pancreas 577.0
Paracoccidioides brasiliensis 116.1
Paragonimus (westermani) 121.2
parainfluenza virus 079.89
parameningococcus NEC 036.9
with meningitis 036.0
parasitic NEC 136.9
paratyphoid 002.9
Type A 002.1
Type B 002.2
Type C 002.3
paraurethral ducts 597.89
parotid gland 527.2
Pasteurella NEC 027.2
multocida (cat-bite) (dog-bite) 027.2
pestis (*see also* Plague) 020.9
pseudotuberculosis 027.2
septica (cat-bite) (dog-bite) 027.2
tularensis (*see also* Tularemia) 021.9
pelvic, female (*see also* Disease, pelvis,
inflammatory) 614.9
penis (glans) (retention) NEC 607.2
herpetic 054.13
Peptococcus 041.84
Peptostreptococcus 041.84
periapical (pulpal origin) 522.4
peridental 523.3
perineal wound (obstetrical) 674.3 ☑5ᵗʰ
periodontal 523.3
periorbital 376.00
chronic 376.10
perirectal 569.49
perirenal (*see also* Infection, kidney) 590.9
peritoneal (*see also* Peritonitis) 567.9
periureteral 593.89
periurethral 597.89
Petriellidium boydii 117.6

Infection, infected, infective — *continued*
pharynx 478.29
Coxsackievirus 074.0
phlegmonous 462
posterior, lymphoid 474.00
Phialophora
gougerotii 117.8
jeanselmei 117.8
verrucosa 117.2
Piedraia hortai 111.3
pinna, acute 380.11
pinta 103.9
intermediate 103.1
late 103.2
mixed 103.3
primary 103.0
pinworm 127.4
pityrosporum furfur 111.0
pleuropneumonia-like organisms NEC (PPLO)
041.81
pneumococcal NEC 041.2
generalized (purulent) 038.2
Pneumococcus NEC 041.2
postoperative wound 998.59
posttraumatic NEC 958.3
postvaccinal 999.3
prepuce NEC 607.1
Proprionibacterium 041.84
prostate (capsule) (*see also* Prostatitis) 601.9
Proteus (mirabilis) (morganii) (vulgaris)
NEC 041.6
enteritis 008.3
protozoal NEC 136.8
intestinal NEC 007.9
Pseudomonas NEC 041.7
mallei 024
pneumonia 482.1
pseudomallei 025
psittacosis 073.9
puerperal, postpartum (major) 670 ☑4ᵗʰ
minor 646.6 ☑5ᵗʰ
pulmonary — *see* Infection, lung
purulent — *see* Abscess
putrid, generalized — *see* Septicemia
pyemic — *see* Septicemia
Pyrenochaeta romeroi 117.4
Q fever 083.0
rabies 071
rectum (sphincter) 569.49
renal (*see also* Infection, kidney) 590.9
pelvis and ureter 590.3
resistant to drugs — *see* Resistance (to), drugs
by microorganisms
respiratory 519.8
chronic 519.8
influenzal (acute) (upper) 487.1
lung 518.89
rhinovirus 460
syncytial virus 079.6
upper (acute) (infectious) NEC 465.9
with flu, grippe, or influenza 487.1
influenzal 487.1
multiple sites NEC 465.8
streptococcal 034.0
viral NEC 465.9
respiratory syncytial virus (RSV) 079.6
resulting from presence of shunt or other
internal prosthetic device — *see*
Complications, infection and
inflammation, due to (presence of) any
device, implant, or graft classified to
996.0-996.5 NEC
retrovirus 079.50
human immunodeficiency virus type 2 [HIV
2] 079.53
human T-cell lymphotrophic virus type I
[HTLV-I] 079.51
human T-cell lymphotrophic virus type II
[HTLV-II] 079.52
specified NEC 079.59
Rhinocladium 117.1
Rhinosporidium (seeberi) 117.0
rhinovirus
in diseases classified elsewhere — *see*
category 079 ☑4ᵗʰ
unspecified nature or site 079.3
Rhizopus 117.7
rickettsial 083.9

Infection, infected, infective — *continued*
rickettsialpox 083.2
rubella (*see also* Rubella) 056.9
congenital 771.0
Saccharomyces (*see also* Candidiasis) 112.9
Saksenaea 117.7
salivary duct or gland (any) 527.2
Salmonella (aertrycke) (callinarum)
(choleraesuis) (enteritidis) (suipestifer)
(typhimurium) 003.9
with
arthritis 003.23
gastroenteritis 003.0
localized infection 003.20
specified type NEC 003.29
meningitis 003.21
osteomyelitis 003.24
pneumonia 003.22
septicemia 003.1
specified manifestation NEC 003.8
congenital 771.89   ▲
due to food (poisoning) (any serotype) (*see
also* Poisoning, food, due to,
Salmonella)
hirschfeldii 002.3
localized 003.20
specified type NEC 003.29
paratyphi 002.9
A 002.1
B 002.2
C 002.3
schottmuelleri 002.2
specified type NEC 003.8
typhi 002.0
typhosa 002.0
saprophytic 136.8
Sarcocystis, lindemanni 136.5
scabies 133.0
Schistosoma — *see* Infestation, Schistosoma
Schmorl's bacillus 040.3
scratch or other superficial injury — *see* Injury,
superficial, by site
scrotum (acute) NEC 608.4
secondary, burn or open wound (dislocation)
(fracture) 958.3
seminal vesicle (*see also* Vesiculitis) 608.0
septic
generalized — *see* Septicemia
localized, skin (*see also* Abscess) 682.9
septicemic — *see* Septicemia
seroma 998.51
Serratia (marcescens) 041.85
generalized 038.44
sheep liver fluke 121.3
Shigella 004.9
boydii 004.2
dysenteriae 004.0
flexneri 004.1
group
A 004.0
B 004.1
C 004.2
D 004.3
Schmitz (-Stutzer) 004.0
schmitzii 004.0
shiga 004.0
sonnei 004.3
specified type NEC 004.8
Sin Nombre virus 079.81
sinus (*see also* Sinusitis) 473.9
pilonidal 685.1
with abscess 685.0
skin NEC 686.9
Skene's duct or gland (*see also* Urethritis)
597.89
skin (local) (staphylococcal) (streptococcal)
NEC 686.9
abscess — *see* Abscess, by site
cellulitis — *see* Cellulitis, by site
due to fungus 111.9
specified type NEC 111.8
mycotic 111.9
specified type NEC 111.8
ulcer (*see also* Ulcer, skin) 707.9
slow virus 046.9
specified condition NEC 046.8
Sparganum (mansoni) (proliferum) 123.5

Infection, infected, infective — *continued*
   spermatic cord NEC 608.4
   sphenoidal (chronic) (sinus) (*see also* Sinusitis,
      sphenoidal 473.3)
   Spherophorus necrophorus 040.3
   spinal cord NEC (*see also* Encephalitis) 323.9
      abscess 324.1
         late effect — *see* category 326
      late effect — *see* category 326
      meninges — *see* Meningitis
      streptococcal 320.2
   Spirillum
      minus or minor 026.0
      morsus muris 026.0
      obermeieri 087.0
   spirochetal NEC 104.9
      lung 104.8
      specified nature or site NEC 104.8
   spleen 289.59
   Sporothrix schenckii 117.1
   Sporotrichum (schenckii) 117.1
   Sporozoa 136.8
   staphylococcal NEC 041.10
      aureus 041.11
      food poisoning 005.0
      generalized (purulent) 038.10
         aureus 038.11
         specified organism NEC 038.19
      pneumonia 482.40
         aureus 482.41
         specified type NEC 482.49
      septicemia 038.10
         aureus 038.11
         specified organism NEC 038.19
      specified NEC 041.19
   steatoma 706.2
   Stellantchasmus falcatus 121.6
   Streptobacillus moniliformis 026.1
   streptococcal NEC 041.00
      congenital 771.89   ▲
      generalized (purulent) 038.0
      Group
         A 041.01
         B 041.02
         C 041.03
         D [enterococcus] 041.04
         G 041.05
      pneumonia — *see* Pneumonia, streptococcal
         482.3 ☑5ᵗʰ
      septicemia 038.0
      sore throat 034.0
      specified NEC 041.09
   Streptomyces — *see* Actinomycosis
   streptotrichosis — *see* Actinomycosis
   Strongyloides (stercoralis) 127.2
   stump (amputation) (posttraumatic) (surgical)
      997.62
         traumatic — *see* Amputation, traumatic, by
            site, complicated
   subcutaneous tissue, local NEC 686.9
   submaxillary region 528.9
   suipestifer (*see also* Infection, Salmonella)
      003.9
   swimming pool bacillus 031.1
   syphilitic — *see* Syphilis
   systemic — *see* Septicemia
   Taenia — *see* Infestation, Taenia
   Taeniarhynchus saginatus 123.2
   tapeworm — *see* Infestation, tapeworm
   tendon (sheath) 727.89
   Ternidens diminutus 127.7
   testis (*see also* Orchitis) 604.90
   thigh (skin) 686.9
   threadworm 127.4
   throat 478.29
      pneumococcal 462
      staphylococcal 462
      streptococcal 034.0
      viral NEC (*see also* Pharyngitis) 462
   thumb (skin) 686.9
      abscess (with lymphangitis) 681.00
         pulp 681.01
      cellulitis (with lymphangitis) 681.00
      nail 681.02
   thyroglossal duct 529.8
   toe (skin) 686.9
      abscess (with lymphangitis) 681.10

Infection, infected, infective — *continued*
   toe — *continued*
      cellulitis (with lymphangitis) 681.10
      nail 681.11
         fungus 110.1
   tongue NEC 529.0
      parasitic 112.0
   tonsil (faucial) (lingual) (pharyngeal) 474.00
      acute or subacute 463
      and adenoid 474.02
      tag 474.00
   tooth, teeth 522.4
      periapical (pulpal origin) 522.4
      peridental 523.3
      periodontal 523.3
      pulp 522.0
      socket 526.5
   Torula histolytica 117.5
   Toxocara (cani) (cati) (felis) 128.0
   Toxoplasma gondii (*see also* Toxoplasmosis)
      130.9
   trachea, chronic 491.8
      fungus 117.9
   traumatic NEC 958.3
   trematode NEC 121.9
   trench fever 083.1
   Treponema
      denticola 041.84
      macrodenticum 041.84
      pallidum (*see also* Syphilis) 097.9
   Trichinella (spiralis) 124
   Trichomonas 131.9
      bladder 131.09
      cervix 131.09
      hominis 007.3
      intestine 007.3
      prostate 131.03
      specified site NEC 131.8
      urethra 131.02
      urogenitalis 131.00
      vagina 131.01
      vulva 131.01
   Trichophyton, trichophytid — *see*
      Dermatophytosis
   Trichosporon (beigelii) cutaneum 111.2
   Trichostrongylus 127.6
   Trichuris (trichiuria) 127.3
   Trombicula (irritans) 133.8
   Trypanosoma (*see also* Trypanosomiasis) 086.9
      cruzi 086.2
   tubal (*see also* Salpingo-oophoritis) 614.2
   tuberculous NEC (*see also* Tuberculosis)
      011.9 ☑5ᵗʰ
   tubo-ovarian (*see also* Salpingo-oophoritis)
      614.2
   tunica vaginalis 608.4
   tympanic membrane — *see* Myringitis
   typhoid (abortive) (ambulant) (bacillus) 002.0
   typhus 081.9
      flea-borne (endemic) 081.0
      louse-borne (epidemic) 080
      mite-borne 081.2
      recrudescent 081.1
      tick-borne 082.9
         African 082.1
         North Asian 082.2
   umbilicus (septic) 686.9
      newborn NEC 771.4
   ureter 593.89
   urethra (*see also* Urethritis) 597.80
   urinary (tract) NEC 599.0
      with
         abortion — *see* Abortion, by type, with
            urinary tract infection
         ectopic pregnancy (*see also* categories
            633.0-633.9) 639.8
         molar pregnancy (*see also* categories 630-
            632) 639.8
      candidal 112.2
      complicating pregnancy, childbirth, or
         puerperium 646.6 ☑5ᵗʰ
         affecting fetus or newborn 760.1
      asymptomatic 646.5 ☑5ᵗʰ
         affecting fetus or newborn 760.1
      diplococcal (acute) 098.0
         chronic 098.2

Infection, infected, infective — *continued*
   urinary (tract) NEC — *continued*
      due to Trichomonas (vaginalis) 131.00
      following
         abortion 639.8
         ectopic or molar pregnancy 639.8
      gonococcal (acute) 098.0
         chronic or duration of 2 months or
            over 098.2
      newborn 771.82   ▲
      trichomonal 131.00
      tuberculous (*see also* Tuberculosis)
         016.3 ☑5ᵗʰ
   uterus, uterine (*see also* Endometritis) 615.9
   utriculus masculinus NEC 597.89
   vaccination 999.3
   vagina (granulation tissue) (wall) (*see also*
      Vaginitis) 616.10
   varicella 052.9
   varicose veins — *see* Varicose, veins
   variola 050.9
      major 050.0
      minor 050.1
   vas deferens NEC 608.4
   Veillonella 041.84
   verumontanum 597.89
   vesical (*see also* Cystitis) 595.9
   Vibrio
      cholerae 001.0
         El Tor 001.1
      parahaemolyticus (food poisoning) 005.4
      vulnificus 041.85
   Vincent's (gums) (mouth) (tonsil) 101
   virus, viral 079.99
      adenovirus
         in diseases classified elsewhere — *see*
            category 079 ☑4ᵗʰ
         unspecified nature or site 079.0
      central nervous system NEC 049.9
         enterovirus 048
            meningitis 047.9
               specified type NEC 047.8
         slow virus 046.9
            specified condition NEC 046.8
      chest 519.8
      conjunctivitis 077.99
         specified type NEC 077.8
      Coxsackie (*see also* Infection, Coxsackie)
         079.2
      Ebola 065.8
      ECHO
         in diseases classified elsewhere — *see*
            category 079 ☑4ᵗʰ
         unspecified nature or site 079.1
      encephalitis 049.9
         arthropod-borne NEC 064
            tick-borne 063.9
               specified type NEC 063.8
      enteritis NEC (*see also* Enteritis, viral) 008.8
      exanthem NEC 057.9
      Hantavirus 079.81
      human papilloma 079.4
      in diseases classified elsewhere — *see*
         category 079 ☑4ᵗʰ
      intestine (*see also* Enteritis, viral) 008.8
      lung — *see* Pneumonia, viral
      respiratory syncytial (RSV) 079.6
      retrovirus 079.50
      rhinovirus
         in diseases classified elsewhere — *see*
            category 079 ☑4ᵗʰ
         unspecified nature or site 079.3
      salivary gland disease 078.5
      slow 046.9
         specified condition NEC 046.8
      specified type NEC 079.89
         in diseases classified elsewhere — *see*
            category 079 ☑4ᵗʰ
      unspecified nature or site 079.99
      warts NEC 078.10
   vulva (*see also* Vulvitis) 616.10
   whipworm 127.3
   Whitmore's bacillus 025
   wound (local) (posttraumatic) NEC 958.3
      with
         dislocation — *see* Dislocation, by site,
            open

☑4ᵗʰ Fourth-digit Required   ☑5ᵗʰ Fifth-digit Required   ►◄ Revised Text   ● New Line   ▲ Revised Code

Infection, infected, infective — *continued*
  wound` — *continued*
    with — *continued*
      fracture — *see* Fracture, by site, open
      open wound — *see* Wound, open, by site, complicated
      postoperative 998.59
      surgical 998.59
    Wuchereria 125.0
      bancrofti 125.0
      malayi 125.1
  yaws — *see* Yaws
  yeast (*see also* Candidiasis) 112.9
  yellow fever (*see also* Fever, yellow) 060.9
  Yersinia pestis (*see also* Plague) 020.9
  Zeis' gland 373.12
  zoonotic bacterial NEC 027.9
  Zopfia senegalensis 117.4
Infective, infectious — *see* condition
Inferiority complex 301.9
  constitutional psychopathic 301.9
Infertility
  female 628.9
    associated with
      adhesions, peritubal 614.6 *[628.2]*
      anomaly
        cervical mucus 628.4
        congenital
          cervix 628.4
          fallopian tube 628.2
          uterus 628.3
          vagina 628.4
      anovulation 628.0
      dysmucorrhea 628.4
      endometritis, tuberculous (*see also* Tuberculosis) 016.7 ✓5th *[628.3]*
      Stein-Leventhal syndrome 256.4 *[628.0]*
    due to
      adiposogenital dystrophy 253.8 *[628.1]*
      anterior pituitary disorder NEC 253.4 *[628.1]*
        hyperfunction 253.1 *[628.1]*
      cervical anomaly 628.4
      fallopian tube anomaly 628.2
      ovarian failure 256.39 *[628.0]*
      Stein-Leventhal syndrome 256.4 *[628.0]*
      uterine anomaly 628.3
      vaginal anomaly 628.4
    nonimplantation 628.3
    origin
      cervical 628.4
      pituitary-hypothalamus NEC 253.8 *[628.1]*
        anterior pituitary NEC 253.4 *[628.1]*
          hyperfunction NEC 253.1 *[628.1]*
        dwarfism 253.3 *[628.1]*
        panhypopituitarism 253.2 *[628.1]*
      specified NEC 628.8
      tubal (block) (occlusion) (stenosis) 628.2
        adhesions 614.6 *[628.2]*
      uterine 628.3
      vaginal 628.4
    previous, requiring supervision of pregnancy V23.0
  male 606.9
    absolute 606.0
    due to
      azoospermia 606.0
      drug therapy 606.8
      extratesticular cause NEC 606.8
      germinal cell
        aplasia 606.0
        desquamation 606.1
      hypospermatogenesis 606.1
      infection 606.8
      obstruction, afferent ducts 606.8
      oligospermia 606.1
      radiation 606.8
      spermatogenic arrest (complete) 606.0
        incomplete 606.1
      systemic disease 606.8
Infestation 134.9
  Acanthocheilonema (perstans) 125.4
    streptocerca 125.6
  Acariasis 133.9
    demodex folliculorum 133.8

Infestation — *continued*
  Acariasis — *continued*
    Sarcoptes scabiei 133.0
    trombiculae 133.8
  Agamofilaria streptocerca 125.6
  Ancylostoma, Ankylostoma 126.9
    americanum 126.1
    braziliense 126.2
    canium 126.8
    ceylanicum 126.3
    duodenale 126.0
    new world 126.1
    old world 126.0
  Angiostrongylus cantonensis 128.8
  anisakiasis 127.1
  Anisakis larva 127.1
  arthropod NEC 134.1
  Ascaris lumbricoides 127.0
  Bacillus fusiformis 101
  Balantidium coli 007.0
  beef tapeworm 123.2
  Bothriocephalus (latus) 123.4
    larval 123.5
  broad tapeworm 123.4
    larval 123.5
  Brugia malayi 125.1
  Candiru 136.8
  Capillaria
    hepatica 128.8
    philippinensis 127.5
  cat liver fluke 121.0
  Cercomonas hominis (intestinal) 007.3
  cestodes 123.9
    specified type NEC 123.8
  chigger 133.8
  chigoe 134.1
  Chilomastix 007.8
  Clonorchis (sinensis) (liver) 121.1
  coccidia 007.2
  complicating pregnancy, childbirth, or puerperium 647.9 ✓5th
    affecting fetus or newborn 760.8
  Cysticercus cellulosae 123.1
  Demodex folliculorum 133.8
  Dermatobia (hominis) 134.0
  Dibothriocephalus (latus) 123.4
    larval 123.5
  Dicrocoelium dendriticum 121.8
  Diphyllobothrium (adult) (intestinal) (latum) (pacificum) 123.4
    larval 123.5
  Diplogonoporus (grandis) 123.8
  Dipylidium (caninum) 123.8
  Distoma hepaticum 121.3
  dog tapeworm 123.8
  Dracunculus medinensis 125.7
  dragon worm 125.7
  dwarf tapeworm 123.6
  Echinococcus (*see also* Echinococcus) 122.9
  Echinostoma ilocanum 121.8
  Embadomonas 007.8
  Endamoeba (histolytica) — *see* Infection, ameba
  Entamoeba (histolytica) — *see* Infection, ameba
  Enterobius vermicularis 127.4
  Epidermophyton — *see* Dermatophytosis
  eyeworm 125.2
  Fasciola
    gigantica 121.3
    hepatica 121.3
  Fasciolopsis (buski) (small intestine) 121.4
    filarial 125.9
      due to
        Acanthocheilonema (perstans) 125.4
          streptocerca 125.6
        Brugia (Wuchereria) malayi 125.1
        Dracunculus medinensis 125.7
        guinea worms 125.7
        Mansonella (ozzardi) 125.5
        Onchocerca volvulus 125.3
          eye 125.3 *[360.13]*
          eyelid 125.3 *[373.6]*
        Wuchereria (bancrofti) 125.0
          malayi 125.1
      specified type NEC 125.6
  fish tapeworm 123.4
    larval 123.5

Infestation — *continued*
  Fasciolopsis — *continued*
    fluke 121.9
    blood NEC (*see also* Schistosomiasis) 120.9
    cat liver 121.0
    intestinal (giant) 121.4
    liver (sheep) 121.3
      cat 121.0
      Chinese 121.1
      clonorchiasis 121.1
      fascioliasis 121.3
      Oriental 121.1
    lung (oriental) 121.2
    sheep liver 121.3
  fly larva 134.0
  Gasterophilus (intestinalis) 134.0
  Gastrodiscoides hominis 121.8
  Giardia lamblia 007.1
  Gnathostoma (spinigerum) 128.1
  Gongylonema 125.6
  guinea worm 125.7
  helminth NEC 128.9
    intestinal 127.9
      mixed (types classifiable to more than one category in 120.0-127.7) 127.8
      specified type NEC 127.7
    specified type NEC 128.8
  Heterophyes heterophyes (small intestine) 121.6
  hookworm (*see also* Infestation, ancylostoma) 126.9
  Hymenolepis (diminuta) (nana) 123.6
  intestinal NEC 129
  leeches (aquatic) (land) 134.2
  Leishmania — *see* Leishmaniasis
  lice (*see also* Infestation, pediculus) 132.9
  Linguatulidae, linguatula (pentastoma) (serrata) 134.1
  Loa loa 125.2
    eyelid 125.2 *[373.6]*
  louse (*see also* Infestation, pediculus) 132.9
    body 132.1
    head 132.0
    pubic 132.2
  maggots 134.0
  Mansonella (ozzardi) 125.5
  medina 125.7
  Metagonimus yokogawai (small intestine) 121.5
  Microfilaria streptocerca 125.3
    eye 125.3 *[360.13]*
    eyelid 125.3 *[373.6]*
  Microsporon furfur 111.0
  microsporum — *see* Dermatophytosis
  mites 133.9
    scabic 133.0
    specified type NEC 133.8
  Monilia (albicans) (*see also* Candidiasis) 112.9
    vagina 112.1
    vulva 112.1
  mouth 112.0
  Necator americanus 126.1
  nematode (intestinal) 127.9
    Ancylostoma (*see also* Ancylostoma) 126.9
    Ascaris lumbricoides 127.0
    conjunctiva NEC 128.9
    Dioctophyma 128.8
    Enterobius vermicularis 127.4
    Gnathostoma spinigerum 128.1
    Oesophagostomum (apiostomum) 127.7
    Physaloptera 127.4
    specified type NEC 127.7
    Strongyloides stercoralis 127.2
    Ternidens diminutus 127.7
    Trichinella spiralis 124
    Trichostrongylus 127.6
    Trichuris (trichiuria) 127.3
  Oesophagostomum (apiostomum) 127.7
  Oestrus ovis 134.0
  Onchocerca (volvulus) 125.3
    eye 125.3 *[360.13]*
    eyelid 125.3 *[373.6]*
  Opisthorchis (felineus) (tenuicollis) (viverrini) 121.0
  Oxyuris vermicularis 127.4
  Paragonimus (westermani) 121.2
  parasite, parasitic NEC 136.9
    eyelid 134.9 *[373.6]*

Infestation — *continued*
parasite, parasitic NEC — *continued*
intestinal 129
mouth 112.0
orbit 376.13
skin 134.9
tongue 112.0
pediculus 132.9
capitis (humanus) (any site) 132.0
corporis (humanus) (any site) 132.1
eyelid 132.0 *[373.6]*
mixed (classifiable to more than one category in 132.0-132.2) 132.3
pubis (any site) 132.2
phthirus (pubis) (any site) 132.2
with any infestation classifiable to 132.0, 132.1 and 132.3
pinworm 127.4
pork tapeworm (adult) 123.0
protozoal NEC 136.8
pubic louse 132.2
rat tapeworm 123.6
red bug 133.8
roundworm (large) NEC 127.0
sand flea 134.1
saprophytic NEC 136.8
Sarcoptes scabiei 133.0
scabies 133.0
Schistosoma 120.9
bovis 120.8
cercariae 120.3
hematobium 120.0
intercalatum 120.8
japonicum 120.2
mansoni 120.1
mattheii 120.8
specified
site — *see* Schistosomiasis
type NEC 120.8
spindale 120.8
screw worms 134.0
skin NEC 134.9
Sparganum (mansoni) (proliferum) 123.5
larval 123.5
specified type NEC 134.8
Spirometra larvae 123.5
Sporozoa NEC 136.8
Stellantchasmus falcatus 121.6
Strongyloides 127.2
Strongylus (gibsoni) 127.7
Taenia 123.3
diminuta 123.6
Echinococcus (*see also* Echinococcus) 122.9
mediocanellata 123.2
nana 123.6
saginata (mediocanellata) 123.2
solium (intestinal form) 123.0
larval form 123.1
Taeniarhynchus saginatus 123.2
tapeworm 123.9
beef 123.2
broad 123.4
larval 123.5
dog 123.8
dwarf 123.6
fish 123.4
larval 123.5
pork 123.0
rat 123.6
Ternidens diminutus 127.7
Tetranychus molestissimus 133.8
threadworm 127.4
tongue 112.0
Toxocara (cani) (cati) (felis) 128.0
trematode(s) NEC 121.9
Trichina spiralis 124
Trichinella spiralis 124
Trichocephalus 127.3
Trichomonas 131.9
bladder 131.09
cervix 131.09
intestine 007.3
prostate 131.03
specified site NEC 131.8
urethra (female) (male) 131.02
urogenital 131.00

Infestation — *continued*
Trichomonas — *continued*
vagina 131.01
vulva 131.01
Trichophyton — *see* Dermatophytosis
Trichostrongylus instabilis 127.6
Trichuris (trichiuria) 127.3
Trombicula (irritans) 133.8
Trypanosoma — *see* Trypanosomiasis
Tunga penetrans 134.1
Uncinaria americana 126.1
whipworm 127.3
worms NEC 128.9
intestinal 127.9
Wuchereria 125.0
bancrofti 125.0
malayi 125.1

Infiltrate, infiltration
with an iron compound 275.0
amyloid (any site) (generalized) 277.3
calcareous (muscle) NEC 275.49
localized — *see* Degeneration, by site
calcium salt (muscle) 275.49
corneal (*see also* Edema, cornea) 371.20
eyelid 373.9
fatty (diffuse) (generalized) 272.8
localized — *see* Degeneration, by site, fatty
glycogen, glycogenic (*see also* Disease, glycogen storage) 271.0
heart, cardiac
fatty (*see also* Degeneration, myocardial) 429.1
glycogenic 271.0 *[425.7]*
inflammatory in vitreous 379.29
kidney (*see also* Disease, renal) 593.9
leukemic (M9800/3) — *see* Leukemia
liver 573.8
fatty — *see* Fatty, liver
glycogen (*see also* Disease, glycogen storage) 271.0
lung (*see also* Infiltrate, pulmonary) 518.3
eosinophilic 518.3
x-ray finding only 793.1
lymphatic (*see also* Leukemia, lymphatic) 204.9 ✓5ᵗʰ
gland, pigmentary 289.3
muscle, fatty 728.9
myelogenous (*see also* Leukemia, myeloid) 205.9 ✓5ᵗʰ
myocardium, myocardial
fatty (*see also* Degeneration, myocardial) 429.1
glycogenic 271.0 *[425.7]*
pulmonary 518.3
with
eosinophilia 518.3
pneumonia — *see* Pneumonia, by type
x-ray finding only 793.1
Ranke's primary (*see also* Tuberculosis) 010.0 ✓5ᵗʰ
skin, lymphocytic (benign) 709.8
thymus (gland) (fatty) 254.8
urine 788.8
vitreous humor 379.29

Infirmity 799.8
senile 797

Inflammation, inflamed, inflammatory (with exudation)
abducens (nerve) 378.54
accessory sinus (chronic) (*see also* Sinusitis) 473.9
adrenal (gland) 255.8
alimentary canal — *see* Enteritis
alveoli (teeth) 526.5
scorbutic 267
amnion — *see* Amnionitis
anal canal 569.49
antrum (chronic) (*see also* Sinusitis, maxillary) 473.0
anus 569.49
appendix (*see also* Appendicitis) 541
arachnoid — *see* Meningitis
areola 611.0
puerperal, postpartum 675.0 ✓5ᵗʰ
areolar tissue NEC 686.9
artery — *see* Arteritis

Inflammation, inflamed, inflammatory — *continued*
auditory meatus (external) (*see also* Otitis, externa) 380.10
Bartholin's gland 616.8
bile duct or passage 576.1
bladder (*see also* Cystitis) 595.9
bone — *see* Osteomyelitis
bowel (*see also* Enteritis) 558.9
brain (*see also* Encephalitis) 323.9
late effect — *see* category 326
membrane — *see* Meningitis
breast 611.0
puerperal, postpartum 675.2 ✓5ᵗʰ
broad ligament (*see also* Disease, pelvis, inflammatory) 614.4
acute 614.3
bronchus — *see* Bronchitis
bursa — *see* Bursitis
capsule
liver 573.3
spleen 289.59
catarrhal (*see also* Catarrh) 460
vagina 616.10
cecum (*see also* Appendicitis) 541
cerebral (*see also* Encephalitis) 323.9
late effect — *see* category 326
membrane — *see* Meningitis
cerebrospinal (*see also* Meningitis) 322.9
late effect — *see* category 326
meningococcal 036.0
tuberculous (*see also* Tuberculosis) 013.6 ✓5ᵗʰ
cervix (uteri) (*see also* Cervicitis) 616.0
chest 519.9
choroid NEC (*see also* Choroiditis) 363.20
cicatrix (tissue) — *see* Cicatrix
colon (*see also* Enteritis) 558.9
granulomatous 555.1
newborn 558.9
connective tissue (diffuse) NEC 728.9
cornea (*see also* Keratitis) 370.9
with ulcer (*see also* Ulcer, cornea) 370.00
corpora cavernosa (penis) 607.2
cranial nerve — *see* Disorder, nerve, cranial
diarrhea — *see* Diarrhea
disc (intervertebral) (space) 722.90
cervical, cervicothoracic 722.91
lumbar, lumbosacral 722.93
thoracic, thoracolumbar 722.92
Douglas' cul-de-sac or pouch (chronic) (*see also* Disease, pelvis, inflammatory) 614.4
acute 614.3
due to (presence of) any device, implant, or graft classifiable to 996.0-996.5 — *see* Complications, infection and inflammation, due to (presence of) any device, implant, or graft classified to 996.0-996.5 NEC
duodenum 535.6 ✓5ᵗʰ
dura mater — *see* Meningitis
ear — *see also* Otitis
external (*see also* Otitis, externa) 380.10
inner (*see also* Labyrinthitis) 386.30
middle — *see* Otitis media
esophagus 530.10
ethmoidal (chronic) (sinus) (*see also* Sinusitis, ethmoidal) 473.2
Eustachian tube (catarrhal) 381.50
acute 381.51
chronic 381.52
extrarectal 569.49
eye 379.99
eyelid 373.9
specified NEC 373.8
fallopian tube (*see also* Salpingo-oophoritis) 614.2
fascia 728.9
fetal membranes (acute) 658.4 ✓5ᵗʰ
affecting fetus or newborn 762.7
follicular, pharynx 472.1
frontal (chronic) (sinus) (*see also* Sinusitis, frontal) 473.1
gallbladder (*see also* Cholecystitis, acute) 575.0
gall duct (*see also* Cholecystitis) 575.10
gastrointestinal (*see also* Enteritis) 558.9

Inflammation — Inhalation

Inflammation, inflamed, inflammatory —
  continued
  genital organ (diffuse) (internal)
    female 614.9
      with
        abortion — *see* Abortion, by type, with
          sepsis
        ectopic pregnancy (*see also* categories
          633.0-633.9) 639.0
        molar pregnancy (*see also* categories
          630-632) 639.0
        complicating pregnancy, childbirth, or
          puerperium 646.6 ☑5ᵗʰ
        affecting fetus or newborn 760.8
      following
        abortion 639.0
        ectopic or molar pregnancy 639.0
    male 608.4
  gland (lymph) (*see also* Lymphadenitis) 289.3
  glottis (*see also* Laryngitis) 464.00
    with obstruction 464.01
  granular, pharynx 472.1
  gum 523.1
  heart (*see also* Carditis) 429.89
  hepatic duct 576.8
  hernial sac — *see* Hernia, by site
  ileum (*see also* Enteritis) 558.9
    terminal or regional 555.0
      with large intestine 555.2
  intervertebral disc 722.90
    cervical, cervicothoracic 722.91
    lumbar, lumbosacral 722.93
    thoracic, thoracolumbar 722.92
  intestine (*see also* Enteritis) 558.9
  jaw (acute) (bone) (chronic) (lower) (suppurative)
    (upper) 526.4
  jejunum — *see* Enteritis
  joint NEC (*see also* Arthritis) 716.9 ☑5ᵗʰ
    sacroiliac 720.2
  kidney (*see also* Nephritis) 583.9
  knee (joint) 716.66
    tuberculous (active) (*see also* Tuberculosis)
      015.2 ☑5ᵗʰ
  labium (majus) (minus) (*see also* Vulvitis)
    616.10
  lacrimal
    gland (*see also* Dacryoadenitis) 375.00
    passages (duct) (sac) (*see also*
      Dacryocystitis) 375.30
  larynx (*see also* Laryngitis) 464.00
    with obstruction 464.01
    diphtheritic 032.3
  leg NEC 686.9
  lip 528.5
  liver (capsule) (*see also* Hepatitis) 573.3
    acute 570
    chronic 571.40
    suppurative 572.0
  lung (acute) (*see also* Pneumonia) 486
    chronic (interstitial) 518.89
  lymphatic vessel (*see also* Lymphangitis) 457.2
  lymph node or gland (*see also* Lymphadenitis)
    289.3
  mammary gland 611.0
    puerperal, postpartum 675.2 ☑5ᵗʰ
  maxilla, maxillary 526.4
    sinus (chronic) (*see also* Sinusitis, maxillary)
      473.0
  membranes of brain or spinal cord — *see*
    Meningitis
  meninges — *see* Meningitis
  mouth 528.0
  muscle 728.9
  myocardium (*see also* Myocarditis) 429.0
  nasal sinus (chronic) (*see also* Sinusitis) 473.9
  nasopharynx — *see* Nasopharyngitis
  navel 686.9
    newborn NEC 771.4
  nerve NEC 729.2
  nipple 611.0
    puerperal, postpartum 675.0 ☑5ᵗʰ
  nose 478.1
    suppurative 472.0
  oculomotor nerve 378.51
  optic nerve 377.30
  orbit (chronic) 376.10
    acute 376.00

Inflammation, inflamed, inflammatory —
  continued
  orbit — *continued*
    chronic 376.10
  ovary (*see also* Salpingo-oophoritis) 614.2
  oviduct (*see also* Salpingo-oophoritis) 614.2
  pancreas — *see* Pancreatitis
  parametrium (chronic) (*see also* Disease, pelvis,
    inflammatory) 614.4
    acute 614.3
  parotid region 686.9
    gland 527.2
  pelvis, female (*see also* Disease, pelvis,
    inflammatory) 614.9
  penis (corpora cavernosa) 607.2
  perianal 569.49
  pericardium (*see also* Pericarditis) 423.9
  perineum (female) (male) 686.9
  perirectal 569.49
  peritoneum (*see also* Peritonitis) 567.9
  periuterine (*see also* Disease, pelvis,
    inflammatory) 614.9
  perivesical (*see also* Cystitis) 595.9
  petrous bone (*see also* Petrositis) 383.20
  pharynx (*see also* Pharyngitis) 462
    follicular 472.1
    granular 472.1
  pia mater — *see* Meningitis
  pleura — *see* Pleurisy
  postmastoidectomy cavity 383.30
    chronic 383.33
  prostate (*see also* Prostatitis) 601.9
  rectosigmoid — *see* Rectosigmoiditis
  rectum (*see also* Proctitis) 569.49
  respiratory, upper (*see also* Infection,
    respiratory, upper) 465.9
    chronic, due to external agent — *see*
      Condition, respiratory, chronic, due to,
      external agent
    due to
      fumes or vapors (chemical) (inhalation)
        506.2
      radiation 508.1
  retina (*see also* Retinitis) 363.20
  retrocecal (*see also* Appendicitis) 541
  retroperitoneal (*see also* Peritonitis) 567.9
  salivary duct or gland (any) (suppurative) 527.2
  scorbutic, alveoli, teeth 267
  scrotum 608.4
  sigmoid — *see* Enteritis
  sinus (*see also* Sinusitis) 473.9
  Skene's duct or gland (*see also* Urethritis)
    597.89
  skin 686.9
  spermatic cord 608.4
  sphenoidal (sinus) (*see also* Sinusitis,
    sphenoidal) 473.3
  spinal
    cord (*see also* Encephalitis) 323.9
      late effect — *see* category 326
    membrane — *see* Meningitis
    nerve — *see* Disorder, nerve
  spine (*see also* Spondylitis) 720.9
  spleen (capsule) 289.59
  stomach — *see* Gastritis
  stricture, rectum 569.49
  subcutaneous tissue NEC 686.9
  suprarenal (gland) 255.8
  synovial (fringe) (membrane) — *see* Bursitis
  tendon (sheath) NEC 726.90
  testis (*see also* Orchitis) 604.90
  thigh 686.9
  throat (*see also* Sore throat) 462
  thymus (gland) 254.8
  thyroid (gland) (*see also* Thyroiditis) 245.9
  tongue 529.0
  tonsil — *see* Tonsillitis
  trachea — *see* Tracheitis
  trochlear nerve 378.53
  tubal (*see also* Salpingo-oophoritis) 614.2
  tuberculous NEC (*see also* Tuberculosis)
    011.9 ☑5ᵗʰ
  tubo-ovarian (*see also* Salpingo-oophoritis)
    614.2
  tunica vaginalis 608.4
  tympanic membrane — *see* Myringitis
  umbilicus, umbilical 686.9
    newborn NEC 771.4

Inflammation, inflamed, inflammatory —
  continued
  uterine ligament (*see also* Disease, pelvis,
    inflammatory) 614.4
    acute 614.3
  uterus (catarrhal) (*see also* Endometritis) 615.9
  uveal tract (anterior) (*see also* Iridocyclitis)
    364.3
    posterior — *see* Chorioretinitis
    sympathetic 360.11
  vagina (*see also* Vaginitis) 616.10
  vas deferens 608.4
  vein (*see also* Phlebitis) 451.9
    thrombotic 451.9
      cerebral (*see also* Thrombosis, brain)
        434.0 ☑5ᵗʰ
      leg 451.2
        deep (vessels) NEC 451.19
        superficial (vessels) 451.0
      lower extremity 451.2
        deep (vessels) NEC 451.19
        superficial (vessels) 451.0
  vocal cord 478.5
  vulva (*see also* Vulvitis) 616.10
Inflation, lung imperfect (newborn) 770.5
Influenza, influenzal 487.1
  with
    bronchitis 487.1
    bronchopneumonia 487.0
    cold (any type) 487.1
    digestive manifestations 487.8
    hemoptysis 487.1
    involvement of
      gastrointestinal tract 487.8
      nervous system 487.8
    laryngitis 487.1
    manifestations NEC 487.8
      respiratory 487.1
        pneumonia 487.0
    pharyngitis 487.1
    pneumonia (any form classifiable to 480-
      483, 485-486) 487.0
    respiratory manifestations NEC 487.1
    sinusitis 487.1
    sore throat 487.1
    tonsillitis 487.1
    tracheitis 487.1
    upper respiratory infection (acute) 487.1
  abdominal 487.8
  Asian 487.1
  bronchial 487.1
  bronchopneumonia 487.0
  catarrhal 487.1
  epidemic 487.1
  gastric 487.8
  intestinal 487.8
  laryngitis 487.1
  maternal affecting fetus or newborn 760.2
    manifest influenza in infant 771.2
  pharyngitis 487.1
  pneumonia (any form) 487.0
  respiratory (upper) 487.1
  stomach 487.8
  vaccination, prophylactic (against) V04.8
Influenza-like disease 487.1
Infraction, Freiberg's (metatarsal head) 732.5
**Infusion complication, misadventure, or
  reaction** — *see* Complication, infusion
Ingestion
  chemical — *see* Table of Drugs and Chemicals
  drug or medicinal substance
    overdose or wrong substance given or taken
      977.9
      specified drug — *see* Table of Drugs and
        Chemicals
  foreign body NEC (*see also* Foreign body) 938
Ingrowing
  hair 704.8
  nail (finger) (toe) (infected) 703.0
Inguinal — *see also* condition
  testis 752.51
Inhalation
  carbon monoxide 986
  flame
    mouth 947.0

Inhalation — *continued*
  flame — *continued*
    lung 947.1
  food or foreign body (*see also* Asphyxia, food or
      foreign body) 933.1
  gas, fumes, or vapor (noxious) 987.9
    specified agent — *see* Table of Drugs and
      Chemicals
  liquid or vomitus (*see also* Asphyxia, food or
      foreign body) 933.1
    lower respiratory tract NEC 934.9
  meconium (fetus or newborn) 770.1
  mucus (*see also* Asphyxia, mucus) 933.1
  oil (causing suffocation) (*see also* Asphyxia,
      food or foreign body) 933.1
  pneumonia — *see* Pneumonia, aspiration
  smoke 987.9
  steam 987.9
  stomach contents or secretions (*see also*
      Asphyxia, food or foreign body) 933.1
    in labor and delivery 668.0 ✓5ᵗʰ
Inhibition, inhibited
  academic as adjustment reaction 309.23
  orgasm
    female 302.73
    male 302.74
  sexual
    desire 302.71
    excitement 302.72
  work as adjustment reaction 309.23
Inhibitor, systemic lupus erythematosus
    (presence of) 286.5
Iniencephalus, iniencephaly 740.2
Injected eye 372.74
Injury 959.9

> Note — For abrasion, insect bite
> (nonvenomous), blister, or scratch, see Injury,
> superficial.
>
> For laceration, traumatic rupture, tear, or
> penetrating wound of internal organs, such
> as heart, lung, liver, kidney, pelvic organs,
> whether or not accompanied by open wound
> in the same region, see Injury, internal.
>
> For nerve injury, see Injury, nerve.
>
> For late effect of injuries classifiable to 850-
> 854, 860-869, 900-919, 950-959, see Late,
> effect, injury, by type.

  abdomen, abdominal (viscera) — *see also*
      Injury, internal, abdomen
    muscle or wall 959.1
  acoustic, resulting in deafness 951.5
  adenoid 959.09
  adrenal (gland) — *see* Injury, internal, adrenal
  alveolar (process) 959.09
  ankle (and foot) (and knee) (and leg, except
      thigh) 959.7
  anterior chamber, eye 921.3
  anus 959.1
  aorta (thoracic) 901.0
    abdominal 902.0
  appendix — *see* Injury, internal, appendix
  arm, upper (and shoulder) 959.2
  artery (complicating trauma) (*see also* Injury,
      blood vessel, by site) 904.9
    cerebral or meningeal (*see also* Hemorrhage,
      brain, traumatic, subarachnoid)
      852.0 ✓5ᵗʰ
  auditory canal (external) (meatus) 959.09
  auricle, auris, ear 959.09
  axilla 959.2
  back 959.1
  bile duct — *see* Injury, internal, bile duct
  birth — *see also* Birth, injury
    canal NEC, complicating delivery 665.9 ✓5ᵗʰ
  bladder (sphincter) — *see* Injury, internal,
      bladder
  blast (air) (hydraulic) (immersion) (underwater)
      NEC 869.0
    with open wound into cavity NEC 869.1
    abdomen or thorax — *see* Injury, internal,
      by site
    brain — *see* Concussion, brain

Injury — *continued*
  blast — *continued*
    ear (acoustic nerve trauma) 951.5
      with perforation of tympanic membrane
        — *see* Wound, open, ear, drum
  blood vessel NEC 904.9
    abdomen 902.9
      multiple 902.87
      specified NEC 902.89
    aorta (thoracic) 901.0
      abdominal 902.0
    arm NEC 903.9
    axillary 903.00
      artery 903.01
      vein 903.02
    azygos vein 901.89
    basilic vein 903.1
    brachial (artery) (vein) 903.1
    bronchial 901.89
    carotid artery 900.00
      common 900.01
      external 900.02
      internal 900.03
    celiac artery 902.20
      specified branch NEC 902.24
    cephalic vein (arm) 903.1
    colica dextra 902.26
    cystic
      artery 902.24
      vein 902.39
    deep plantar 904.6
    digital (artery) (vein) 903.5
    due to accidental puncture or laceration
        during procedure 998.2
    extremity
      lower 904.8
        multiple 904.7
        specified NEC 904.7
      upper 903.9
        multiple 903.8
        specified NEC 903.8
    femoral
      artery (superficial) 904.1
        above profunda origin 904.0
        common 904.0
      vein 904.2
    gastric
      artery 902.21
      vein 902.39
    head 900.9
      intracranial — *see* Injury, intracranial
      multiple 900.82
      specified NEC 900.89
    hemiazygos vein 901.89
    hepatic
      artery 902.22
      vein 902.11
    hypogastric 902.59
      artery 902.51
      vein 902.52
    ileocolic
      artery 902.26
      vein 902.31
    iliac 902.50
      artery 902.53
      specified branch NEC 902.59
      vein 902.54
    innominate
      artery 901.1
      vein 901.3
    intercostal (artery) (vein) 901.81
    jugular vein (external) 900.81
      internal 900.1
    leg NEC 904.8
    mammary (artery) (vein) 901.82
    mesenteric
      artery 902.20
        inferior 902.27
        specified branch NEC 902.29
        superior (trunk) 902.25
          branches, primary 902.26
      vein 902.39
        inferior 902.32
        superior (and primary subdivisions)
          902.31

Injury — *continued*
  blood vessel NEC — *continued*
    neck 900.9
      multiple 900.82
      specified NEC 900.89
    ovarian 902.89
      artery 902.81
      vein 902.82
    palmar artery 903.4
    pelvis 902.9
      multiple 902.87
      specified NEC 902.89
    plantar (deep) (artery) (vein) 904.6
    popliteal 904.40
      artery 904.41
      vein 904.42
    portal 902.33
    pulmonary 901.40
      artery 901.41
      vein 901.42
    radial (artery) (vein) 903.2
    renal 902.40
      artery 902.41
      specified NEC 902.49
      vein 902.42
    saphenous
      artery 904.7
      vein (greater) (lesser) 904.3
    splenic
      artery 902.23
      vein 902.34
    subclavian
      artery 901.1
      vein 901.3
    suprarenal 902.49
    thoracic 901.9
      multiple 901.83
      specified NEC 901.89
    tibial 904.50
      artery 904.50
        anterior 904.51
        posterior 904.53
      vein 904.50
        anterior 904.52
        posterior 904.54
    ulnar (artery) (vein) 903.3
    uterine 902.59
      artery 902.55
      vein 902.56
    vena cava
      inferior 902.10
        specified branches NEC 902.19
      superior 901.2
  brachial plexus 953.4
    newborn 767.6
  brain NEC (*see also* Injury, intracranial)
      854.0 ✓5ᵗʰ
  breast 959.1
  broad ligament — *see* Injury, internal, broad
      ligament
  bronchus, bronchi — *see* Injury, internal,
      bronchus
  brow 959.09
  buttock 959.1
  canthus, eye 921.1
  cathode ray 990
  cauda equina 952.4
    with fracture, vertebra — *see* Fracture,
      vertebra, sacrum
  cavernous sinus (*see also* Injury, intracranial)
      854.0 ✓5ᵗʰ
  cecum — *see* Injury, internal, cecum
  celiac ganglion or plexus 954.1
  cerebellum (*see also* Injury, intracranial)
      854.0 ✓5ᵗʰ
  cervix (uteri) — *see* Injury, internal, cervix
  cheek 959.09
  chest — *see also* Injury, internal, chest
      wall 959.1
  childbirth — *see also* Birth, injury
    maternal NEC 665.9 ✓5ᵗʰ
  chin 959.09
  choroid (eye) 921.3
  clitoris 959.1
  coccyx 959.1
    complicating delivery 665.6 ✓5ᵗʰ
  colon — *see* Injury, internal, colon

Injury — *continued*
  common duct — *see* Injury, internal, common
    duct
  conjunctiva 921.1
    superficial 918.2
  cord
    spermatic — *see* Injury, internal, spermatic
      cord
    spinal — *see* Injury, spinal, by site
  cornea 921.3
    abrasion 918.1
    due to contact lens 371.82
    penetrating — *see* Injury, eyeball,
      penetrating
    superficial 918.1
    due to contact lens 371.82
  cortex (cerebral) (*see also* Injury, intracranial)
    854.0 ✓5ᵗʰ
    visual 950.3
  costal region 959.1
  costochondral 959.1
  cranial
    bones — *see* Fracture, skull, by site
    cavity (*see also* Injury, intracranial)
      854.0 ✓5ᵗʰ
    nerve — *see* Injury, nerve, cranial
  crushing — *see* Crush
  cutaneous sensory nerve
    lower limb 956.4
    upper limb 955.5 ✓5ᵗʰ
  delivery — *see also* Birth, injury
    maternal NEC 665.9 ✓5ᵗʰ
  Descemet's membrane — *see* Injury, eyeball,
    penetrating
  diaphragm — *see* Injury, internal, diaphragm
  duodenum — *see* Injury, internal, duodenum
  ear (auricle) (canal) (drum) (external) 959.09
  elbow (and forearm) (and wrist) 959.3
  epididymis 959.1
  epigastric region 959.1
  epiglottis 959.09
  epiphyseal, current — *see* Fracture, by site
  esophagus — *see* Injury, internal, esophagus
  Eustachian tube 959.09
  extremity (lower) (upper) NEC 959.8
  eye 921.9
    penetrating eyeball — *see* Injury, eyeball,
      penetrating
    superficial 918.9
  eyeball 921.3
    penetrating 871.7
      with
        partial loss (of intraocular tissue)
          871.2
        prolapse or exposure (of intraocular
          tissue) 871.1
        without prolapse 871.0
      foreign body (nonmagnetic) 871.6
        magnetic 871.5
    superficial 918.9
  eyebrow 959.09
  eyelid(s) 921.1
    laceration — *see* Laceration, eyelid
    superficial 918.0
  face (and neck) 959.09
  fallopian tube — *see* Injury, internal, fallopian
    tube
  finger(s) (nail) 959.5
  flank 959.1
  foot (and ankle) (and knee) (and leg except
    thigh) 959.7
  forceps NEC 767.9
    scalp 767.1
  forearm (and elbow) (and wrist) 959.3
  forehead 959.09
  gallbladder — *see* Injury, internal, gallbladder
  gasserian ganglion 951.2
  gastrointestinal tract — *see* Injury, internal,
    gastrointestinal tract
  genital organ(s)
    with
      abortion — *see* Abortion, by type, with,
        damage to pelvic organs
      ectopic pregnancy (*see also* categories
        633.0-633.9) 639.2
      molar pregnancy (*see also* categories 630-
        632) 639.2

Injury — *continued*
  genital organ(s) — *continued*
    external 959.1
    following
      abortion 639.2
      ectopic or molar pregnancy 639.2
    internal — *see* Injury, internal, genital
      organs
    obstetrical trauma NEC 665. ✓5ᵗʰ
      affecting fetus or newborn 763.89
  gland
    lacrimal 921.1
      laceration 870.8
    parathyroid 959.09
    salivary 959.09
    thyroid 959.09
  globe (eye) (*see also* Injury, eyeball) 921.3
  grease gun — *see* Wound, open, by site,
    complicated
  groin 959.1
  gum 959.09
  hand(s) (except fingers) 959.4
  head NEC 959.01
    with
      loss of consciousness 850.5   ●
      skull fracture — *see* Fracture, skull, by
        site
  heart — *see* Injury, internal, heart
  heel 959.7
  hip (and thigh) 959.6
  hymen 959.1
  hyperextension (cervical) (vertebra) 847.0
  ileum — *see* Injury, internal, ileum
  iliac region 959.1
  infrared rays NEC 990
  instrumental (during surgery) 998.2
    birth injury — *see* Birth, injury
    nonsurgical (*see also* Injury, by site) 959.9
    obstetrical 665.9 ✓5ᵗʰ
      affecting fetus or newborn 763.89
      bladder 665.5 ✓5ᵗʰ
      cervix 665.3 ✓5ᵗʰ
      high vaginal 665.4 ✓5ᵗʰ
      perineal NEC 664.9 ✓5ᵗʰ
      urethra 665.5 ✓5ᵗʰ
      uterus 665.5 ✓5ᵗʰ
  internal 869.0

> *Note* — *For injury of internal organ(s) by*
> *foreign body entering through a natural*
> *orifice (e.g., inhaled, ingested, or swallowed)*
> *— see Foreign body, entering through orifice.*
>
> *For internal injury of any of the following*
> *sites with internal injury of any other of the*
> *sites — see Injury, internal, multiple.*

    with
      fracture
        open wound into cavity 869.1
        pelvis — *see* Fracture, pelvis
        specified site, except pelvis — *see*
          Injury, internal, by site
    abdomen, abdominal (viscera) NEC 868.00
      with
        fracture, pelvis — *see* Fracture, pelvis
        open wound into cavity 868.10
      specified site NEC 868.09
        with open wound into cavity 868.19
    adrenal (gland) 868.01
      with open wound into cavity 868.11
    aorta (thoracic) 901.0
      abdominal 902.0
    appendix 863.85
      with open wound into cavity 863.95
    bile duct 868.02
      with open wound into cavity 868.12
    bladder (sphincter) 867.0
      with
        abortion — *see* Abortion, by type, with
          damage to pelvic organs
        ectopic pregnancy (*see also* categories
          633.0-633.9) 639.2
        molar pregnancy (*see also* categories
          630-632) 639.2
        open wound into cavity 867.1

Injury — *continued*
  internal — *continued*
    bladder — *continued*
      following
        abortion 639.2
        ectopic or molar pregnancy 639.2
      obstetrical trauma 665.5 ✓5ᵗʰ
        affecting fetus or newborn 763.89
    blood vessel — *see* Injury, blood vessel, by
      site
    broad ligament 867.6
      with open wound into cavity 867.7
    bronchus, bronchi 862.21
      with open wound into cavity 862.31
    cecum 863.89
      with open wound into cavity 863.99
    cervix (uteri) 867.4
      with
        abortion — *see* Abortion, by type, with
          damage to pelvic organs
        ectopic pregnancy (*see also* categories
          633.0-633.9) 639.2
        molar pregnancy (*see also* categories
          630-632) 639.2
        open wound into cavity 867.5
      following
        abortion 639.2
        ectopic or molar pregnancy 639.2
      obstetrical trauma 665.3 ✓5ᵗʰ
        affecting fetus or newborn 763.89
    chest (*see also* Injury, internal, intrathoracic
      organs) 862.8
      with open wound into cavity 862.9
    colon 863.40
      with
        open wound into cavity 863.50
        rectum 863.46
          with open wound into cavity 863.56
      ascending (right) 863.41
        with open wound into cavity 863.51
      descending (left) 863.43
        with open wound into cavity 863.53
      multiple sites 863.46
        with open wound into cavity 863.56
      sigmoid 863.44
        with open wound into cavity 863.54
      specified site NEC 863.49
        with open wound into cavity 863.59
      transverse 863.42
        with open wound into cavity 863.52
    common duct 868.02
      with open wound into cavity 868.12
    complicating delivery 665.9 ✓5ᵗʰ
      affecting fetus or newborn 763.89
    diaphragm 862.0
      with open wound into cavity 862.1
    duodenum 863.21
      with open wound into cavity 863.31
    esophagus (intrathoracic) 862.22
      with open wound into cavity 862.32
      cervical region 874.4
        complicated 874.5
    fallopian tube 867.6
      with open wound into cavity 867.7
    gallbladder 868.02
      with open wound into cavity 868.12
    gastrointestinal tract NEC 863.80
      with open wound into cavity 863.90
    genital organ NEC 867.6
      with open wound into cavity 867.7
    heart 861.00
      with open wound into thorax 861.10
    ileum 863.29
      with open wound into cavity 863.39
    intestine NEC 863.89
      with open wound into cavity 863.99
      large NEC 863.40
        with open wound into cavity 863.50
      small NEC 863.20
        with open wound into cavity 863.30
    intra-abdominal (organ) 868.00
      with open wound into cavity 868.10
      multiple sites 868.09
        with open wound into cavity 868.19
      specified site NEC 868.09
        with open wound into cavity 868.19

✓4ᵗʰ Fourth-digit Required   ✓5ᵗʰ Fifth-digit Required   ►◄ Revised Text   ● New Line   ▲ Revised Code

Injury — *continued*
  internal — *continued*
    intrathoracic organs (multiple) 862.8
      with open wound into cavity 862.9
      diaphragm (only) — *see* Injury, internal, diaphragm
      heart (only) — *see* Injury, internal, heart
      lung (only) — *see* Injury, internal, lung
      specified site NEC 862.29
        with open wound into cavity 862.39
    intrauterine (*see also* Injury, internal, uterus) 867.4
      with open wound into cavity 867.5
    jejunum 863.29
      with open wound into cavity 863.39
    kidney (subcapsular) 866.00
      with
        disruption of parenchyma (complete) 866.03
          with open wound into cavity 866.13
        hematoma (without rupture of capsule) 866.01
          with open wound into cavity 866.11
        laceration 866.02
          with open wound into cavity 866.12
        open wound into cavity 866.10
    liver 864.00
      with
        contusion 864.01
          with open wound into cavity 864.11
        hematoma 864.01
          with open wound into cavity 864.11
        laceration 864.05
          with open wound into cavity 864.15
          major (disruption of hepatic parenchyma) 864.04
            with open wound into cavity 864.14
          minor (capsule only) 864.02
            with open wound into cavity 864.12
          moderate (involving parenchyma) 864.03
            with open wound into cavity 864.13
          multiple 864.04
          stellate 864.04
            with open wound into cavity 864.14
        open wound into cavity 864.10
    lung 861.20
      with open wound into thorax 861.30
      hemopneumothorax — *see* Hemopneumothorax, traumatic
      hemothorax — *see* Hemothorax, traumatic
      pneumohemothorax — *see* Pneumohemothorax, traumatic
      pneumothorax — *see* Pneumothorax, traumatic
    mediastinum 862.29
      with open wound into cavity 862.39
    mesentery 863.89
      with open wound into cavity 863.99
    mesosalpinx 867.6
      with open wound into cavity 867.7
    multiple 869.0

> Note — Multiple internal injuries of sites classifiable to the same three- or four-digit category should be classified to that category.
>
> Multiple injuries classifiable to different fourth-digit subdivisions of 861 (heart and lung injuries) should be dealt with according to coding rules.

    internal
      with open wound into cavity 869.1
      intra-abdominal organ (sites classifiable to 863-868)
        with
          intrathoracic organ(s) (sites classifiable to 861-862) 869.0
            with open wound into cavity 869.1

Injury — *continued*
  internal — *continued*
    multiple — *continued*
      intra-abdominal organ — *continued*
        with — *continued*
          other intra-abdominal organ(s) (sites classifiable to 863-868, except where classifiable to the same three-digit category) 868.09
            with open wound into cavity 868.19
      intrathoracic organ (sites classifiable to 861-862)
        with
          intra-abdominal organ(s) (sites classifiable to 863-868) 869.0
            with open wound into cavity 869.1
          other intrathoracic organ(s) (sites classifiable to 861-862, except where classifiable to the same three-digit category) 862.8
            with open wound into cavity 862.9
    myocardium — *see* Injury, internal, heart
    ovary 867.6
      with open wound into cavity 867.7
    pancreas (multiple sites) 863.84
      with open wound into cavity 863.94
      body 863.82
        with open wound into cavity 863.92
      head 863.81
        with open wound into cavity 863.91
      tail 863.83
        with open wound into cavity 863.93
    pelvis, pelvic (organs) (viscera) 867.8
      with
        fracture, pelvis — *see* Fracture, pelvis
        open wound into cavity 867.9
      specified site NEC 867.6
        with open wound into cavity 867.7
    peritoneum 868.03
      with open wound into cavity 868.13
    pleura 862.29
      with open wound into cavity 862.39
    prostate 867.6
      with open wound into cavity 867.7
    rectum 863.45
      with
        colon 863.46
          with open wound into cavity 863.56
        open wound into cavity 863.55
    retroperitoneum 868.04
      with open wound into cavity 868.14
    round ligament 867.6
      with open wound into cavity 867.7
    seminal vesicle 867.6
      with open wound into cavity 867.7
    spermatic cord 867.6
      with open wound into cavity 867.7
      scrotal — *see* Wound, open, spermatic cord
    spleen 865.00
      with
        disruption of parenchyma (massive) 865.04
          with open wound into cavity 865.14
        hematoma (without rupture of capsule) 865.01
          with open wound into cavity 865.11
        open wound into cavity 865.10
        tear, capsular 865.02
          with open wound into cavity 865.12
          extending into parenchyma 865.03
            with open wound into cavity 865.13
    stomach 863.0
      with open wound into cavity 863.1
    suprarenal gland (multiple) 868.01
      with open wound into cavity 868.11
    thorax, thoracic (cavity) (organs) (multiple) (*see also* Injury, internal, intrathoracic organs) 862.8
      with open wound into cavity 862.9
    thymus (gland) 862.29
      with open wound into cavity 862.39

Injury — *continued*
  internal — *continued*
    trachea (intrathoracic) 862.29
      with open wound into cavity 862.39
      cervical region (*see also* Wound, open, trachea) 874.02
    ureter 867.2
      with open wound into cavity 867.3
    urethra (sphincter) 867.0
      with
        abortion — *see* Abortion, by type, with damage to pelvic organs
        ectopic pregnancy (*see also* categories 633.0-633.9) 639.2
        molar pregnancy (*see also* categories 630-632) 639.2
        open wound into cavity 867.1
      following
        abortion 639.2
        ectopic or molar pregnancy 639.2
      obstetrical trauma 665.5 ✓5ᵗʰ
        affecting fetus or newborn 763.89
    uterus 867.4
      with
        abortion — *see* Abortion, by type, with damage to pelvic organs
        ectopic pregnancy (*see also* categories 633.0-633.9) 639.2
        molar pregnancy (*see also* categories 630-632) 639.2
        open wound into cavity 867.5
      following
        abortion 639.2
        ectopic or molar pregnancy 639.2
      obstetrical trauma NEC 665.5 ✓5ᵗʰ
        affecting fetus or newborn 763.89
    vas deferens 867.6
      with open wound into cavity 867.7
    vesical (sphincter) 867.0
      with open wound into cavity 867.1
    viscera (abdominal) (*see also* Injury, internal, multiple) 868.00
      with
        fracture, pelvis — *see* Fracture, pelvis
        open wound into cavity 868.10
      thoracic NEC (*see also* Injury, internal, intrathoracic organs) 862.8
        with open wound into cavity 862.9
  interscapular region 959.1
  intervertebral disc 959.1
  intestine — *see* Injury, internal, intestine
  intra-abdominal (organs) NEC — *see* Injury, internal, intra-abdominal
  intracranial 854.0 ✓5ᵗʰ

> Note — Use the following fifth-digit subclassification with categories 851-854:
>
> 0 unspecified state of consciousness
>
> 1 with no loss of consciousness
>
> 2 with brief [less than one hour] loss of consciousness
>
> 3 with moderate [1-24 hours] loss of consciousness
>
> 4 with prolonged [more than 24 hours] loss of consciousness and return to pre-existing conscious level
>
> 5 with prolonged [more than 24 hours] loss of consciousness, without return to pre-existing conscious level
>
> Use fifth-digit 5 to designate when a patient is unconscious and dies before regaining consciousness, regardless of the duration of the loss of consciousness
>
> 6 with loss of consciousness of unspecified duration
>
> 9 with concussion, unspecified

    with
      open intracranial wound 854.1 ✓5ᵗʰ
      skull fracture — *see* Fracture, skull, by site
    contusion 851.8 ✓5ᵗʰ
      with open intracranial wound 851.9 ✓5ᵗʰ

Injury — *continued*
  intracranial — *continued*
    contusion — *continued*
      brain stem 851.4 ✓5ᵗʰ
        with open intracranial wound
          851.5 ✓5ᵗʰ
      cerebellum 851.4 ✓5ᵗʰ
        with open intracranial wound
          851.5 ✓5ᵗʰ
      cortex (cerebral) 851.0 ✓5ᵗʰ
        with open intracranial wound
          851.2 ✓5ᵗʰ
    hematoma — *see* Injury, intracranial,
      hemorrhage
    hemorrhage 853.0 ✓5ᵗʰ
      with
        laceration — *see* Injury, intracranial,
          laceration
        open intracranial wound 853.1 ✓5ᵗʰ
      extradural 852.4 ✓5ᵗʰ
        with open intracranial wound
          852.5 ✓5ᵗʰ
      subarachnoid 852.0 ✓5ᵗʰ
        with open intracranial wound
          852.1 ✓5ᵗʰ
      subdural 852.2 ✓5ᵗʰ
        with open intracranial wound
          852.3 ✓5ᵗʰ
    laceration 851.8 ✓5ᵗʰ
      with open intracranial wound 851.9 ✓5ᵗʰ
      brain stem 851.6 ✓5ᵗʰ
        with open intracranial wound
          851.7 ✓5ᵗʰ
      cerebellum 851.6 ✓5ᵗʰ
        with open intracranial wound
          851.7 ✓5ᵗʰ
      cortex (cerebral) 851.2 ✓5ᵗʰ
        with open intracranial wound
          851.3 ✓5ᵗʰ
  intraocular — *see* Injury, eyeball, penetrating
  intrathoracic organs (multiple) — *see* Injury,
    internal, intrathoracic organs
  intrauterine — *see* Injury, internal, intrauterine
  iris 921.3
    penetrating — *see* Injury, eyeball,
      penetrating
  jaw 959.09
  jejunum — *see* Injury, internal, jejunum
  joint NEC 959.9
    old or residual 718.80
      ankle 718.87
      elbow 718.82
      foot 718.87
      hand 718.84
      hip 718.85
      knee 718.86
      multiple sites 718.89
      pelvic region 718.85
      shoulder (region) 718.81
      specified site NEC 718.88
      wrist 718.83
  kidney — *see* Injury, internal, kidney
  knee (and ankle) (and foot) (and leg, except
    thigh) 959.7
  labium (majus) (minus) 959.1
  labyrinth, ear 959.09
  lacrimal apparatus, gland, or sac 921.1
    laceration 870.8
  larynx 959.09
  late effect — *see* Late, effects (of), injury
  leg except thigh (and ankle) (and foot) (and
    knee) 959.7
    upper or thigh 959.6
  lens, eye 921.3
    penetrating — *see* Injury, eyeball,
      penetrating
  lid, eye — *see* Injury, eyelid
  lip 959.09
  liver — *see* Injury, internal, liver
  lobe, parietal — *see* Injury, intracranial
  lumbar (region) 959.1
    plexus 953.5
  lumbosacral (region) 959.1
    plexus 953.5
  lung — *see* Injury, internal, lung
  malar region 959.09
  mastoid region 959.09

Injury — *continued*
  maternal, during pregnancy, affecting fetus or
    newborn 760.5
  maxilla 959.09
  mediastinum — *see* Injury, internal,
    mediastinum
  membrane
    brain (*see also* Injury, intracranial)
      854.0 ✓5ᵗʰ
    tympanic 959.09
  meningeal artery — *see* Hemorrhage, brain,
    traumatic, subarachnoid
  meninges (cerebral) — *see* Injury, intracranial
  mesenteric
    artery — *see* Injury, blood vessel,
      mesenteric, artery
    plexus, inferior 954.1
    vein — *see* Injury, blood vessel, mesenteric,
      vein
  mesentery — *see* Injury, internal, mesentery
  mesosalpinx — *see* Injury, internal,
    mesosalpinx
  middle ear 959.09
  midthoracic region 959.1
  mouth 959.09
  multiple (sites not classifiable to the same four-
    digit category in 959.0-959.7) 959.8
    internal 869.0
      with open wound into cavity 869.1
  musculocutaneous nerve 955.4
  nail
    finger 959.5
    toe 959.7
  nasal (septum) (sinus) 959.09
  nasopharynx 959.09
  neck (and face) 959.09
  nerve 957.9
    abducens 951.3
    abducent 951.3
    accessory 951.6
    acoustic 951.5
    ankle and foot 956.9
    anterior crural, femoral 956.1
    arm (*see also* Injury, nerve, upper limb)
      955.9
    auditory 951.5
    axillary 955.0
    brachial plexus 953.4
    cervical sympathetic 954.0
    cranial 951.9
      first or olfactory 951.8
      second or optic 950.0
      third or oculomotor 951.0
      fourth or trochlear 951.1
      fifth or trigeminal 951.2
      sixth or abducens 951.3
      seventh or facial 951.4
      eighth, acoustic, or auditory 951.5
      ninth or glossopharyngeal 951.8
      tenth, pneumogastric, or vagus 951.8
      eleventh or accessory 951.6
      twelfth or hypoglossal 951.7
      newborn 767.7
    cutaneous sensory
      lower limb 956.4
      upper limb 955.5 ✓5ᵗʰ
    digital (finger) 955.6
      toe 956.5
    facial 951.4
      newborn 767.5
    femoral 956.1
    finger 955.9
    foot and ankle 956.9
    forearm 955.9
    glossopharyngeal 951.8
    hand and wrist 955.9
    head and neck, superficial 957.0
    hypoglossal 951.7
    involving several parts of body 957.8
    leg (*see also* Injury, nerve, lower limb) 956.9
    lower limb 956.9
      multiple 956.8
      specified site NEC 956.5
    lumbar plexus 953.5
    lumbosacral plexus 953.5
    median 955.1
      forearm 955.1

Injury — *continued*
  nerve — *continued*
    median — *continued*
      wrist and hand 955.1
    multiple (in several parts of body) (sites not
      classifiable to the same three-digit
      category) 957.8
    musculocutaneous 955.4
    musculospiral 955.3
      upper arm 955.3
    oculomotor 951.0
    olfactory 951.8
    optic 950.0
    pelvic girdle 956.9
      multiple sites 956.8
      specified site NEC 956.5
    peripheral 957.9
      multiple (in several regions) (sites not
        classifiable to the same three-digit
        category) 957.8
      specified site NEC 957.1
    peroneal 956.3
      ankle and foot 956.3
      lower leg 956.3
    plantar 956.5
    plexus 957.9
      celiac 954.1
      mesenteric, inferior 954.1
      spinal 953.9
        brachial 953.4
        lumbosacral 953.5
        multiple sites 953.8
      sympathetic NEC 954.1
    pneumogastric 951.8
    radial 955.3
      wrist and hand 955.3
    sacral plexus 953.5
    sciatic 956.0
      thigh 956.0
    shoulder girdle 955.9
      multiple 955.8
      specified site NEC 955.7
    specified site NEC 957.1
    spinal 953.9
      plexus — *see* Injury, nerve, plexus, spinal
      root 953.9
        cervical 953.0
        dorsal 953.1
        lumbar 953.2
        multiple sites 953.8
        sacral 953.3
    splanchnic 954.1
    sympathetic NEC 954.1
      cervical 954.0
    thigh 956.9
    tibial 956.5
      ankle and foot 956.2
      lower leg 956.5
      posterior 956.2
    toe 956.9
    trigeminal 951.2
    trochlear 951.1
    trunk, excluding shoulder and pelvic girdles
      954.9
      specified site NEC 954.8
      sympathetic NEC 954.1
    ulnar 955.2
      forearm 955.2
      wrist (and hand) 955.2
    upper limb 955.9
      multiple 955.8
      specified site NEC 955.7
    vagus 951.8
    wrist and hand 955.9
  nervous system, diffuse 957.8
  nose (septum) 959.09
  obstetrical NEC 665.9 ✓5ᵗʰ
    affecting fetus or newborn 763.89
  occipital (region) (scalp) 959.09
    lobe (*see also* Injury, intracranial) 854.0 ✓5ᵗʰ
  optic 950.9
    chiasm 950.1
    cortex 950.3
    nerve 950.0
    pathways 950.2

Injury — *continued*
orbit, orbital (region) 921.2
  penetrating 870.3
    with foreign body 870.4
ovary — *see* Injury, internal, ovary
paint-gun — *see* Wound, open, by site, complicated
palate (soft) 959.09
pancreas — *see* Injury, internal, pancreas
parathyroid (gland) 959.09
parietal (region) (scalp) 959.09
  lobe — *see* Injury, intracranial
pelvic
  floor 959.1
    complicating delivery 664.1 ✔5th
      affecting fetus or newborn 763.89
  joint or ligament, complicating delivery 665.6 ✔5th
    affecting fetus or newborn 763.89
  organs — *see also* Injury, internal, pelvis
    with
      abortion — *see* Abortion, by type, with damage to pelvic organs
      ectopic pregnancy (*see also* categories 633.0-633.9) 639.2
      molar pregnancy (*see also* categories 633.0-633.9) 639.2
    following
      abortion 639.2
      ectopic or molar pregnancy 639.2
    obstetrical trauma 665.5 ✔5th
      affecting fetus or newborn 763.89
pelvis 959.1
penis 959.1
perineum 959.1
peritoneum — *see* Injury, internal, peritoneum
periurethral tissue
  with
    abortion — *see* Abortion, by type, with damage to pelvic organs
    ectopic pregnancy (*see also* categories 633.0-633.9) 639.2
    molar pregnancy (*see also* categories 630-632) 639.2
    complicating delivery 665.5 ✔5th
      affecting fetus or newborn 763.89
  following
    abortion 639.2
    ectopic or molar pregnancy 639.2
phalanges
  foot 959.7
  hand 959.5
pharynx 959.09
pleura — *see* Injury, internal, pleura
popliteal space 959.7
prepuce 959.1
prostate — *see* Injury, internal, prostate
pubic region 959.1
pudenda 959.1
radiation NEC 990
radioactive substance or radium NEC 990
rectovaginal septum 959.1
rectum — *see* Injury, internal, rectum
retina 921.3
  penetrating — *see* Injury, eyeball, penetrating
retroperitoneal — *see* Injury, internal, retroperitoneum
roentgen rays NEC 990
round ligament — *see* Injury, internal, round ligament
sacral (region) 959.1
  plexus 953.5
sacroiliac ligament NEC 959.1
sacrum 959.1
salivary ducts or glands 959.09
scalp 959.09
  due to birth trauma 767.1
  fetus or newborn 767.1
scapular region 959.2
sclera 921.3
  penetrating — *see* Injury, eyeball, penetrating
  superficial 918.2
scrotum 959.1
seminal vesicle — *see* Injury, internal, seminal vesicle
shoulder (and upper arm) 959.2

Injury — *continued*
sinus
  cavernous (*see also* Injury, intracranial) 854.0 ✔5th
  nasal 959.09
skeleton NEC, birth injury 767.3
skin NEC 959.9
skull — *see* Fracture, skull, by site
soft tissue (of external sites) (severe) — *see* Wound, open, by site
specified site NEC 959.8
spermatic cord — *see* Injury, internal, spermatic cord
spinal (cord) 952.9
  with fracture, vertebra — *see* Fracture, vertebra, by site, with spinal cord injury
  cervical (C$_1$-C$_4$) 952.00
    with
      anterior cord syndrome 952.02
      central cord syndrome 952.03
      complete lesion of cord 952.01
      incomplete lesion NEC 952.04
      posterior cord syndrome 952.04
    C$_5$-C$_7$ level 952.05
      with
        anterior cord syndrome 952.07
        central cord syndrome 952.08
        complete lesion of cord 952.06
        incomplete lesion NEC 952.09
        posterior cord syndrome 952.09
      specified type NEC 952.09
    specified type NEC 952.04
  dorsal (D$_1$-D$_6$) (T$_1$-T$_6$) (thoracic) 952.10
    with
      anterior cord syndrome 952.12
      central cord syndrome 952.13
      complete lesion of cord 952.11
      incomplete lesion NEC 952.14
      posterior cord syndrome 952.14
    D$_7$-D$_{12}$ level (T$_7$-T$_{12}$) 952.15
      with
        anterior cord syndrome 952.17
        central cord syndrome 952.18
        complete lesion of cord 952.16
        incomplete lesion NEC 952.19
        posterior cord syndrome 952.19
      specified type NEC 952.19
    specified type NEC 952.14
  lumbar 952.2
  multiple sites 952.8
  nerve (root) NEC — *see* Injury, nerve, spinal, root
  plexus 953.9
    brachial 953.4
    lumbosacral 953.5
    multiple sites 953.8
  sacral 952.3
  thoracic (*see also* Injury, spinal, dorsal) 952.10
spleen — *see* Injury, internal, spleen
stellate ganglion 954.1
sternal region 959.1
stomach — *see* Injury, internal, stomach
subconjunctival 92l.l
subcutaneous 959.9
subdural — *see* Injury, intracranial
submaxillary region 959.09
submental region 959.09
subungual
  fingers 959.5
  toes 959.7
superficial 919 ✔4th

Injury — *continued*
superficial — *continued*

> Note — Use the following fourth-digit subdivisions with categories 910-919:
>
> 0   Abrasion or friction burn without mention of infection
> 1   Abrasion or friction burn, infected
> 2   Blister without mention of infection
> 3   Blister, infected
> 4   Insect bite, nonvenomous, without mention of infection
> 5   Insect bite, nonvenomous, infected
> 6   Superficial foreign body (splinter) without major open wound and without mention of infection
> 7   Superficial foreign body (splinter) without major open wound, infected
> 8   Other and unspecified superficial injury without mention of infection
> 9   Other and unspecified superficial injury, infected
>
> For late effects of superficial injury, see category 906.2.

abdomen, abdominal (muscle) (wall) (and other part(s) of trunk) 911 ✔4th
ankle (and hip, knee, leg, or thigh) 916 ✔4th
anus (and other part(s) of trunk) 911 ✔4th
arm 913 ✔4th
  upper (and shoulder) 912 ✔4th
auditory canal (external) (meatus) (and other part(s) of face, neck, or scalp, except eye) 910 ✔4th
axilla (and upper arm) 912 ✔4th
back (and other part(s) of trunk) 911 ✔4th
breast (and other part(s) of trunk) 911 ✔4th
brow (and other part(s) of face, neck, or scalp, except eye) 910 ✔4th
buttock (and other part(s) of trunk) 911 ✔4th
canthus, eye 918.0
cheek(s) (and other part(s) of face, neck, or scalp, except eye) 910 ✔4th
chest wall (and other part(s) of trunk) 911 ✔4th
chin (and other part(s) of face, neck, or scalp, except eye) 910 ✔4th
clitoris (and other part(s) of trunk) 911 ✔4th
conjunctiva 918.2
cornea 918.1
  due to contact lens 371.82
costal region (and other part(s) of trunk) 911 ✔4th
ear(s) (auricle) (canal) (drum) (external) (and other part(s) of face, neck, or scalp, except eye) 910 ✔4th
elbow (and forearm) (and wrist) 913 ✔4th
epididymis (and other part(s) of trunk) 911 ✔4th
epigastric region (and other part(s) of trunk) 911 ✔4th
epiglottis (and other part(s) of face, neck, or scalp, except eye) 910 ✔4th
eye(s) (and adnexa) NEC 918.9
eyelid(s) (and periocular area) 918.0
face (any part(s), except eye) (and neck or scalp) 910 ✔4th
finger(s) (nail) (any) 915 ✔4th
flank (and other part(s) of trunk) 911 ✔4th
foot (phalanges) (and toe(s)) 917 ✔4th
forearm (and elbow) (and wrist) 913 ✔4th
forehead (and other part(s) of face, neck, or scalp, except eye) 910 ✔4th
globe (eye) 918.9
groin (and other part(s) of trunk) 911 ✔4th
gum(s) (and other part(s) of face, neck, or scalp, except eye) 910 ✔4th
hand(s) (except fingers alone) 914 ✔4th
head (and other part(s) of face, neck, or scalp, except eye) 910 ✔4th
heel (and foot or toe) 917 ✔4th
hip (and ankle, knee, leg, or thigh) 916 ✔4th
iliac region (and other part(s) of trunk) 911 ✔4th

Injury — continued
superficial — continued
interscapular region (and other part(s) of trunk) 911 ✓4ᵗʰ

iris 918.9

knee (and ankle, hip, leg, or thigh) 916 ✓4ᵗʰ

labium (majus) (minus) (and other part(s) of trunk) 911 ✓4ᵗʰ

lacrimal (apparatus) (gland) (sac) 918.0

leg (lower) (upper) (and ankle, hip, knee, or thigh) 916 ✓4ᵗʰ

lip(s) (and other part(s) of face, neck, or scalp, except eye) 910 ✓4ᵗʰ

lower extremity (except foot) 916 ✓4ᵗʰ

lumbar region (and other part(s) of trunk) 911 ✓4ᵗʰ

malar region (and other part(s) of face, neck, or scalp, except eye) 910 ✓4ᵗʰ

mastoid region (and other part(s) of face, neck, or scalp, except eye) 910 ✓4ᵗʰ

midthoracic region (and other part(s) of trunk) 911 ✓4ᵗʰ

mouth (and other part(s) of face, neck, or scalp, except eye) 910 ✓4ᵗʰ

multiple sites (not classifiable to the same three-digit category) 919 ✓4ᵗʰ

nasal (septum) (and other part(s) of face, neck, or scalp, except eye) 910 ✓4ᵗʰ

neck (and face or scalp, any part(s), except eye) 910 ✓4ᵗʰ

nose (septum) (and other part(s) of face, neck, or scalp, except eye) 910 ✓4ᵗʰ

occipital region (and other part(s) of face, neck, or scalp, except eye) 910 ✓4ᵗʰ

orbital region 918.0

palate (soft) (and other part(s) of face, neck, or scalp, except eye) 910 ✓4ᵗʰ

parietal region (and other part(s) of face, neck, or scalp, except eye) 910 ✓4ᵗʰ

penis (and other part(s) of trunk) 911 ✓4ᵗʰ

perineum (and other part(s) of trunk) 911 ✓4ᵗʰ

periocular area 918.0

pharynx (and other part(s) of face, neck, or scalp, except eye) 910 ✓4ᵗʰ

popliteal space (and ankle, hip, leg, or thigh) 916 ✓4ᵗʰ

prepuce (and other part(s) of trunk) 911 ✓4ᵗʰ

pubic region (and other part(s) of trunk) 911 ✓4ᵗʰ

pudenda (and other part(s) of trunk) 911 ✓4ᵗʰ

sacral region (and other part(s) of trunk) 911 ✓4ᵗʰ

salivary (ducts) (glands) (and other part(s) of face, neck, or scalp, except eye) 910 ✓4ᵗʰ

scalp (and other part(s) of face or neck, except eye) 910 ✓4ᵗʰ

scapular region (and upper arm) 912 ✓4ᵗʰ

sclera 918.2

scrotum (and other part(s) of trunk) 911 ✓4ᵗʰ

shoulder (and upper arm) 912 ✓4ᵗʰ

skin NEC 919 ✓4ᵗʰ

specified site(s) NEC 919 ✓4ᵗʰ

sternal region (and other part(s) of trunk) 911 ✓4ᵗʰ

subconjunctival 918.2

subcutaneous NEC 919 ✓4ᵗʰ

submaxillary region (and other part(s) of face, neck, or scalp, except eye) 910 ✓4ᵗʰ

submental region (and other part(s) of face, neck, or scalp, except eye) 910 ✓4ᵗʰ

supraclavicular fossa (and other part(s) of face, neck or scalp, except eye) 910 ✓4ᵗʰ

supraorbital 918.0

temple (and other part(s) of face, neck, or scalp, except eye) 910 ✓4ᵗʰ

temporal region (and other part(s) of face, neck, or scalp, except eye) 910 ✓4ᵗʰ

testis (and other part(s) of trunk) 911 ✓4ᵗʰ

thigh (and ankle, hip, knee, or leg) 916 ✓4ᵗʰ

thorax, thoracic (external) (and other part(s) of trunk) 911 ✓4ᵗʰ

throat (and other part(s) of face, neck, or scalp, except eye) 910 ✓4ᵗʰ

thumb(s) (nail) 915 ✓4ᵗʰ

Injury — continued
superficial — continued
toe(s) (nail) (subungual) (and foot) 917 ✓4ᵗʰ

tongue (and other part(s) of face, neck, or scalp, except eye) 910 ✓4ᵗʰ

tooth, teeth 521.2

trunk (any part(s)) 911 ✓4ᵗʰ

tunica vaginalis (and other part(s) of trunk) 911 ✓4ᵗʰ

tympanum, tympanic membrane (and other part(s) of face, neck, or scalp, except eye) 910 ✓4ᵗʰ

upper extremity NEC 913 ✓4ᵗʰ

uvula (and other part(s) of face, neck, or scalp, except eye) 910 ✓4ᵗʰ

vagina (and other part(s) of trunk) 911 ✓4ᵗʰ

vulva (and other part(s) of trunk) 911 ✓4ᵗʰ

wrist (and elbow) (and forearm) 913 ✓4ᵗʰ

supraclavicular fossa 959.1

supraorbital 959.09

surgical complication (external or internal site) 998.2

symphysis pubis 959.1

complicating delivery 665.6 ✓5ᵗʰ

affecting fetus or newborn 763.89

temple 959.09

temporal region 959.09

testis 959.1

thigh (and hip) 959.6

thorax, thoracic (external) 959.1

cavity — see Injury, internal, thorax

internal — see Injury, internal, intrathoracic organs

throat 959.09

thumb(s) (nail) 959.5

thymus — see Injury, internal, thymus

thyroid (gland) 959.09

toe (nail) (any) 959.7

tongue 959.09

tonsil 959.09

tooth NEC 873.63

complicated 873.73

trachea — see Injury, internal, trachea

trunk 959.1

tunica vaginalis 959.1

tympanum, tympanic membrane 959.09

ultraviolet rays NEC 990

ureter — see Injury, internal, ureter

urethra (sphincter) — see Injury, internal, urethra

uterus — see Injury, internal, uterus

uvula 959.09

vagina 959.1

vascular — see Injury, blood vessel

vas deferens — see Injury, internal, vas deferens

vein (see also Injury, blood vessel, by site) 904.9

vena cava

inferior 902.10

superior 901.2

vesical (sphincter) — see Injury, internal, vesical

viscera (abdominal) — see also Injury, internal, viscera

with fracture, pelvis — see Fracture, pelvis

visual 950.9

cortex 950.3

vitreous (humor) 871.2

vulva 959.1

whiplash (cervical spine) 847.0

wringer — see Crush, by site

wrist (and elbow) (and forearm) 959.3

x-ray NEC 990

Inoculation — see also Vaccination

complication or reaction — see Complication, vaccination

Insanity, insane (see also Psychosis) 298.9

adolescent (see also Schizophrenia) 295.9 ✓5ᵗʰ

alternating (see also Psychosis, affective, circular) 296.7

confusional 298.9

acute 293.0

subacute 293.1

delusional 298.9

Insanity, insane (see also Psychosis) — continued
paralysis, general 094.1

progressive 094.1

paresis, general 094.1

senile 290.20

Insect
bite — see Injury, superficial, by site

venomous, poisoning by 989.5

Insemination, artificial V26.1

Insertion
cord (umbilical) lateral or velamentous 663.8 ✓5ᵗʰ

affecting fetus or newborn 762.6

intrauterine contraceptive device V25.1

placenta, vicious — see Placenta, previa

subdermal implantable contraceptive V25.5

velamentous, umbilical cord 663.8 ✓5ᵗʰ

affecting fetus or newborn 762.6

Insolation 992.0
meaning sunstroke 992.0

Insomnia 780.52
with sleep apnea 780.51

nonorganic origin 307.41

persistent (primary) 307.42

transient 307.41

subjective complaint 307.49

Inspiration
food or foreign body (see also Asphyxia, food or foreign body) 933.1

mucus (see also Asphyxia, mucus) 933.1

Inspissated bile syndrome, newborn 774.4

Instability
detrusor 596.59

emotional (excessive) 301.3

joint (posttraumatic) 718.80

ankle 718.87

elbow 718.82

foot 718.87

hand 718.84

hip 718.85

knee 718.86

lumbosacral 724.6

multiple sites 718.89

pelvic region 718.85

sacroiliac 724.6

shoulder (region) 718.81

specified site NEC 718.88

wrist 718.83

lumbosacral 724.6

nervous 301.89

personality (emotional) 301.59

thyroid, paroxysmal 242.9 ✓5ᵗʰ

urethral 599.83

vasomotor 780.2

Insufficiency, insufficient
accommodation 367.4

adrenal (gland) (acute) (chronic) 255.4

medulla 255.5

primary 255.4

specified NEC 255.5

adrenocortical 255.4

anus 569.49

aortic (valve) 424.1

with

mitral (valve) disease 396.1

insufficiency, incompetence, or regurgitation 396.3

stenosis or obstruction 396.1

stenosis or obstruction 424.1

with mitral (valve) disease 396.8

congenital 746.4

rheumatic 395.1

with

mitral (valve) disease 396.1

insufficiency, incompetence, or regurgitation 396.3

stenosis or obstruction 396.1

stenosis or obstruction 395.2

with mitral (valve) disease 396.8

specified cause NEC 424.1

syphilitic 093.22

arterial 447.1

basilar artery 435.0

carotid artery 435.8

cerebral 437.1

coronary (acute or subacute) 411.89

Injury — Insufficiency

Insufficiency, insufficient — *continued*
arterial — *continued*
   mesenteric 557.1
   peripheral 443.9
   precerebral 435.9
   vertebral artery 435.1
   vertebrobasilar 435.3
arteriovenous 459.9
basilar artery 435.0
biliary 575.8
cardiac (*see also* Insufficiency, myocardial)
   428.0
   complicating surgery 997.1
   due to presence of (cardiac) prosthesis 429.4
   postoperative 997.1
     long-term effect of cardiac surgery 429.4
   specified during or due to a procedure 997.1
     long-term effect of cardiac surgery 429.4
cardiorenal (*see also* Hypertension, cardiorenal)
   404.90
cardiovascular (*see also* Disease,
   cardiovascular) 429.2
   renal (*see also* Hypertension, cardiorenal)
     404.90
carotid artery 435.8
cerebral (vascular) 437.9
cerebrovascular 437.9
   with transient focal neurological signs and
     symptoms 435.9
   acute 437.1
     with transient focal neurological signs
      and symptoms 435.9
circulatory NEC 459.9
   fetus or newborn 779.89 ▲
convergence 378.83
coronary (acute or subacute) 411.89
   chronic or with a stated duration of over 8
     weeks 414.8
corticoadrenal 255.4
dietary 269.9
divergence 378.85
food 994.2
gastroesophageal 530.89
gonadal
   ovary 256.39
   testis 257.2
gonadotropic hormone secretion 253.4
heart — *see also* Insufficiency, myocardial
   fetus or newborn 779.89 ▲
   valve (*see also* Endocarditis) 424.90
     congenital NEC 746.89
hepatic 573.8
idiopathic autonomic 333.0
kidney ▶(acute) (chronic)◀ 593.9
labyrinth, labyrinthine (function) 386.53
   bilateral 386.54
   unilateral 386.53
lacrimal 375.15
liver 573.8
lung (acute) (*see also* Insufficiency, pulmonary)
   518.82
   following trauma, surgery, or shock 518.5
   newborn 770.89 ▲
mental (congenital) (*see also* Retardation,
   mental) 319
mesenteric 557.1
mitral (valve) 424.0
   with
     aortic (valve) disease 396.3
       insufficiency, incompetence, or
         regurgitation 396.3
       stenosis or obstruction 396.2
     obstruction or stenosis 394.2
       with aortic valve disease 396.8
   congenital 746.6
   rheumatic 394.1
     with
       aortic (valve) disease 396.3
         insufficiency, incompetence, or
           regurgitation 396.3
         stenosis or obstruction 396.2
       obstruction or stenosis 394.2
         with aortic valve disease 396.8
     active or acute 391.1
       with chorea, rheumatic (Sydenham's)
         392.0
   specified cause, except rheumatic 424.0

Insufficiency, insufficient — *continued*
muscle
   heart — *see* Insufficiency, myocardial
   ocular (*see also* Strabismus) 378.9
myocardial, myocardium (with arteriosclerosis)
   428.0
   with rheumatic fever (conditions classifiable
     to 390)
     active, acute, or subacute 391.2
       with chorea 392.0
     inactive or quiescent (with chorea) 398.0
   congenital 746.89
   due to presence of (cardiac)
     prosthesis 429.4
   fetus or newborn 779.89 ▲
   following cardiac surgery 429.4
   hypertensive (*see also* Hypertension, heart)
     402.91
     benign 402.11
     malignant 402.01
   postoperative 997.1
     long-term effect of cardiac surgery 429.4
   rheumatic 398.0
     active, acute, or subacute 391.2
       with chorea (Sydenham's) 392.0
   syphilitic 093.82
nourishment 994.2
organic 799.8
ovary 256.39
   postablative 256.2
pancreatic 577.8
parathyroid (gland) 252.1
peripheral vascular (arterial) 443.9
pituitary (anterior) 253.2
   posterior 253.5
placental — *see* Placenta, insufficiency
platelets 287.5
prenatal care in current pregnancy V23.7
progressive pluriglandular 258.9
pseudocholinesterase 289.8
pulmonary (acute) 518.82
   following
     shock 518.5
     surgery 518.5
     trauma 518.5
   newborn 770.89 ▲
   valve (*see also* Endocarditis, pulmonary)
     424.3
     congenital 746.09
pyloric 537.0
renal ▶(acute) (chronic)◀ 593.9
   due to a procedure 997.5
respiratory 786.09
   acute 518.82
     following shock, surgery,
       or trauma 518.5
     newborn 770.89 ▲
rotation — *see* Malrotation
suprarenal 255.4
   medulla 255.5
tarso-orbital fascia, congenital 743.66
tear film 375.15
testis 257.2
thyroid (gland) (acquired) — *see also*
   Hypothyroidism
   congenital 243
tricuspid (*see also* Endocarditis, tricuspid)
   397.0
   congenital 746.89
   syphilitic 093.23
urethral sphincter 599.84
valve, valvular (heart) (*see also* Endocarditis)
   424.90
vascular 459.9
   intestine NEC 557.9
   mesenteric 557.1
   peripheral 443.9
   renal (*see also* Hypertension, kidney) 403.90
velopharyngeal
   acquired 528.9
   congenital 750.29
venous (peripheral) 459.81
ventricular — *see* Insufficiency, myocardial
vertebral artery 435.1
vertebrobasilar artery 435.3
weight gain during pregnancy 646.8 ✓5ᵗʰ
zinc 269.3

Insufflation
fallopian
   fertility testing V26.21
   following sterilization reversal V26.22
meconium 770.1
Insular — *see* condition
Insulinoma (M8151/0)
malignant (M8151/3)
   pancreas 157.4
   specified site — *see* Neoplasm, by site,
     malignant
   unspecified site 157.4
pancreas 211.7
specified site — *see* Neoplasm, by site, benign
unspecified site 211.7
Insuloma — *see* Insulinoma
Insult
brain 437.9
   acute 436
cerebral 437.9
   acute 436
cerebrovascular 437.9
   acute 436
vascular NEC 437.9
   acute 436
Insurance examination (certification) V70.3
Intemperance (*see also* Alcoholism) 303.9 ✓5ᵗʰ
Interception of pregnancy (menstrual extraction)
   V25.3
Intermenstrual
bleeding 626.6
   irregular 626.6
   regular 626.5
hemorrhage 626.6
   irregular 626.6
   regular 626.5
pain(s) 625.2
Intermittent — *see* condition
Internal — *see* condition
Interproximal wear 521.1
Interruption
aortic arch 747.11
bundle of His 426.50
fallopian tube (for sterilization) V25.2
phase-shift, sleep cycle 307.45
repeated REM-sleep 307.48
sleep
   due to perceived environmental disturbances
     307.48
   phase-shift, of 24-hour sleep-wake cycle
     307.45
   repeated REM-sleep type 307.48
vas deferens (for sterilization) V25.2
Intersexuality 752.7
Interstitial — *see* condition
Intertrigo 695.89
labialis 528.5
Intervertebral disc — *see* condition
Intestine, intestinal — *see also* condition
flu 487.8
Intolerance
carbohydrate NEC 579.8
cardiovascular exercise, with pain (at rest)
   (with less than ordinary activity) (with
   ordinary activity) V47.2
cold 780.99 ▲
dissacharide (hereditary) 271.3
drug
   correct substance properly administered
     995.2
   wrong substance given or taken in error
     977.9
     specified drug — *see* Table of Drugs and
       Chemicals
effort 306.2
fat NEC 579.8
foods NEC 579.8
fructose (hereditary) 271.2
glucose (-galactose) (congenital) 271.3
gluten 579.0
lactose (hereditary) (infantile) 271.3
lysine (congenital) 270.7
milk NEC 579.8
protein (familial) 270.7
starch NEC 579.8

Intolerance — *continued*
  sucrose (-isomaltose) (congenital) 271.3
Intoxicated NEC (*see also* Alcoholism) 305.0 ☑5ᵗʰ
Intoxication
  acid 276.2
  acute
    alcoholic 305.0 ☑5ᵗʰ
      with alcoholism 303.0 ☑5ᵗʰ
      hangover effects 305.0 ☑5ᵗʰ
    caffeine 305.9 ☑5ᵗʰ
    hallucinogenic (*see also* Abuse, drugs,
      nondependent) 305.3 ☑5ᵗʰ
  alcohol (acute) 305.0 ☑5ᵗʰ
    with alcoholism 303.0 ☑5ᵗʰ
    hangover effects 305.0 ☑5ᵗʰ
    idiosyncratic 291.4
    pathological 291.4
  alimentary canal 558.2
  ammonia (hepatic) 572.2
  chemical — *see also* Table of Drugs and
    Chemicals
    via placenta or breast milk 760.70
      alcohol 760.71
      anti-infective agents 760.74
      cocaine 760.75
      "crack" 760.75
      hallucinogenic agents NEC 760.73
      medicinal agents NEC 760.79
  chemical — *see also* Table of Drugs and
    Chemicals — *continued*
    via placenta or breast milk — *continued*
      narcotics 760.72
      obstetric anesthetic or analgesic drug
        763.5
      specified agent NEC 760.79
      suspected, affecting management of
        pregnancy 655.5 ☑5ᵗʰ
  cocaine, through placenta or breast milk
    760.75
  delirium
    alcohol 291.0
    drug 292.81
  drug
    with delirium 292.81
    correct substance properly administered (*see
      also* Allergy, drug) 995.2
    newborn 779.4
    obstetric anesthetic or sedation 668.9 ☑5ᵗʰ
      affecting fetus or newborn 763.5
    overdose or wrong substance given or taken
      — *see* Table of Drugs and Chemicals
    pathologic 292.2
    specific to newborn 779.4
    via placenta or breast milk 760.70
      alcohol 760.71
      anti-infective agents 760.74
      cocaine 760.75
      "crack" 760.75
      hallucinogenic agents 760.73
      medicinal agents NEC 760.79
      narcotics 760.72
      obstetric anesthetic or analgesic drug
        763.5
      specified agent NEC 760.79
      suspected, affecting management of
        pregnancy 655.5 ☑5ᵗʰ
  enteric — *see* Intoxication, intestinal
  fetus or newborn, via placenta or breast milk
    760.70
    alcohol 760.71
    anti-infective agents 760.74
    cocaine 760.75
    "crack" 760.75
    hallucinogenic agents 760.73
    medicinal agents NEC 760.79
    narcotics 760.72
    obstetric anesthetic or analgesic drug 763.5
    specified agent NEC 760.79
    suspected, affecting management of
      pregnancy 655.5 ☑5ᵗʰ
  food — *see* Poisoning, food
  gastrointestinal 558.2
  hallucinogenic (acute) 305.3 ☑5ᵗʰ
  hepatocerebral 572.2
  idiosyncratic alcohol 291.4
  intestinal 569.89
    due to putrefaction of food 005.9

Intoxication — *continued*
  methyl alcohol (*see also* Alcoholism) 305.0 ☑5ᵗʰ
    with alcoholism 303.0 ☑5ᵗʰ
  pathologic 291.4
    drug 292.2
  potassium (K) 276.7
  septic
    with
      abortion — *see* Abortion, by type, with
        sepsis
      ectopic pregnancy (*see also* categories
        633.0-633.9) 639.0
      molar pregnancy (*see also* categories 630-
        632) 639.0
    during labor 659.3 ☑5ᵗʰ
    following
      abortion 639.0
      ectopic or molar pregnancy 639.0
    generalized — *see* Septicemia
    puerperal, postpartum, childbirth 670 ☑4ᵗʰ
  serum (prophylactic) (therapeutic) 999.5
  uremic — *see* Uremia
  water 276.6
Intracranial — *see* condition
Intrahepatic gallbladder 751.69
Intraligamentous — *see also* condition
  pregnancy — *see* Pregnancy, cornual
Intraocular — *see also* condition
  sepsis 360.00
Intrathoracic — *see also* condition
  kidney 753.3
  stomach — *see* Hernia, diaphragm
Intrauterine contraceptive device
  checking V25.42
  insertion V25.1
  in situ V45.51
  management V25.42
  prescription V25.02
    repeat V25.42
  reinsertion V25.42
  removal V25.42
Intraventricular — *see* condition
Intrinsic deformity — *see* Deformity
Intrusion, repetitive, of sleep (due to
  environmental disturbances) (with atypical
  polysomnographic features) 307.48
Intumescent, lens (eye) NEC 366.9
  senile 366.12
Intussusception (colon) (enteric) (intestine)
  (rectum) 560.0
  appendix 543.9
  congenital 751.5
  fallopian tube 620.8
  ileocecal 560.0
  ileocolic 560.0
  ureter (with obstruction) 593.4
Invagination
  basilar 756.0
  colon or intestine 560.0
Invalid (since birth) 799.8
Invalidism (chronic) 799.8
Inversion
  albumin-globulin (A-G) ratio 273.8
  bladder 596.8
  cecum (*see also* Intussusception) 560.0
  cervix 622.8
  nipple 611.79
    congenital 757.6
    puerperal, postpartum 676.3 ☑5ᵗʰ
  optic papilla 743.57
  organ or site, congenital NEC — *see* Anomaly,
    specified type NEC
  sleep rhythm 780.55
    nonorganic origin 307.45
  testis (congenital) 752.51
  uterus (postinfectional) (postpartal, old) 621.7
    chronic 621.7
    complicating delivery 665.2 ☑5ᵗʰ
      affecting fetus or newborn 763.89
  vagina — *see* Prolapse, vagina
Investigation
  allergens V72.7
  clinical research (control) (normal comparison)
    (participant) V70.7

Inviability — *see* Immaturity
Involuntary movement, abnormal 781.0
Involution, involutional — *see also* condition
  breast, cystic or fibrocystic 610.1
  depression (*see also* Psychosis, affective)
    296.2 ☑5ᵗʰ
    recurrent episode 296.3 ☑5ᵗʰ
    single episode 296.2 ☑5ᵗʰ
  melancholia (*see also* Psychosis, affective)
    296.2 ☑5ᵗʰ
    recurrent episode 296.3 ☑5ᵗʰ
    single episode 296.2 ☑5ᵗʰ
  ovary, senile 620.3
  paranoid state (reaction) 297.2
  paraphrenia (climacteric) (menopause) 297.2
  psychosis 298.8
  thymus failure 254.8
IQ
  under 20 318.2
  20-34 318.1
  35-49 318.0
  50-70 317
IRDS 769
Irideremia 743.45
Iridis rubeosis 364.42
  diabetic 250.5 ☑5ᵗʰ [364.42]
Iridochoroiditis (panuveitis) 360.12
Iridocyclitis NEC 364.3
  acute 364.00
    primary 364.01
    recurrent 364.02
  chronic 364.10
    in
      lepromatous leprosy 030.0 [364.11]
      sarcoidosis 135 [364.11]
      tuberculosis (*see also* Tuberculosis)
        017.3 ☑5ᵗʰ [364.11]
  due to allergy 364.04
  endogenous 364.01
  gonococcal 098.41
  granulomatous 364.10
  herpetic (simplex) 054.44
    zoster 053.22
  hypopyon 364.05
  lens induced 364.23
  nongranulomatous 364.00
  primary 364.01
  recurrent 364.02
  rheumatic 364.10
  secondary 364.04
    infectious 364.03
    noninfectious 364.04
  subacute 364.00
    primary 364.01
    recurrent 364.02
  sympathetic 360.11
  syphilitic (secondary) 091.52
  tuberculous (chronic) (*see also* Tuberculosis)
    017.3 ☑5ᵗʰ [364.11]
Iridocyclochoroiditis (panuveitis) 360.12
Iridodialysis 364.76
Iridodonesis 364.8
Iridoplegia (complete) (partial) (reflex) 379.49
Iridoschisis 364.52
Iris — *see* condition
Iritis 364.3
  acute 364.00
    primary 364.01
    recurrent 364.02
  chronic 364.10
    in
      sarcoidosis 135 [364.11]
      tuberculosis (*see also* Tuberculosis)
        017.3 ☑5ᵗʰ [364.11]
  diabetic 250.5 ☑5ᵗʰ [364.42]
  due to
    allergy 364.04
    herpes simplex 054.44
    leprosy 030.0 [364.11]
  endogenous 364.01
  gonococcal 098.41
  gouty 274.89 [364.11]
  granulomatous 364.10
  hypopyon 364.05
  lens induced 364.23

Iritis — *continued*
- nongranulomatous 364.00
- papulosa 095.8 *[364.11]*
- primary 364.01
- recurrent 364.02
- rheumatic 364.10
- secondary 364.04
  - infectious 364.03
  - noninfectious 364.04
- subacute 364.00
  - primary 364.01
  - recurrent 364.02
- sympathetic 360.11
- syphilitic (secondary) 091.52
  - congenital 090.0 *[364.11]*
  - late 095.8 *[364.11]*
- tuberculous (*see also* Tuberculosis) 017.3 ✓5ᵗʰ *[364.11]*
- uratic 274.89 *[364.11]*

Iron
- deficiency anemia 280.9
- metabolism disease 275.0
- storage disease 275.0

Iron-miners' lung 503

Irradiated enamel (tooth, teeth) 521.8

Irradiation
- burn — *see* Burn, by site
- effects, adverse 990

Irreducible, irreducibility — *see* condition

Irregular, irregularity
- action, heart 427.9
- alveolar process 525.8
- bleeding NEC 626.4
- breathing 786.09
- colon 569.89
- contour of cornea 743.41
  - acquired 371.70
- dentin in pulp 522.3
- eye movements NEC 379.59
- menstruation (cause unknown) 626.4
- periods 626.4
- prostate 602.9
- pupil 364.75
- respiratory 786.09
- septum (nasal) 470
- shape, organ or site, congenital NEC — *see* Distortion
- sleep-wake rhythm (non-24-hour) 780.55
  - nonorganic origin 307.45
- vertebra 733.99

Irritability (nervous) 799.2
- bladder 596.8
  - neurogenic 596.54
    - with cauda equina syndrome 344.61
- bowel (syndrome) 564.1
- bronchial (*see also* Bronchitis) 490
- cerebral, newborn 779.1
- colon 564.1
  - psychogenic 306.4
- duodenum 564.89
- heart (psychogenic) 306.2
- ileum 564.89
- jejunum 564.89
- myocardium 306.2
- rectum 564.89
- stomach 536.9
  - psychogenic 306.4
- sympathetic (nervous system) (*see also* Neuropathy, peripheral, autonomic) 337.9
- urethra 599.84
- ventricular (heart) (psychogenic) 306.2

Irritable — *see* Irritability

Irritation
- anus 569.49
- axillary nerve 353.0
- bladder 596.8
- brachial plexus 353.0
- brain (traumatic) (*see also* Injury, intracranial) 854.0 ✓5ᵗʰ
  - nontraumatic — *see* Encephalitis
- bronchial (*see also* Bronchitis) 490
- cerebral (traumatic) (*see also* Injury, intracranial) 854.0 ✓5ᵗʰ
  - nontraumatic — *see* Encephalitis
- cervical plexus 353.2
- cervix (*see also* Cervicitis) 616.0

Irritation — *continued*
- choroid, sympathetic 360.11
- cranial nerve — *see* Disorder, nerve, cranial
- digestive tract 536.9
  - psychogenic 306.4
- gastric 536.9
  - psychogenic 306.4
- gastrointestinal (tract) 536.9
  - functional 536.9
  - psychogenic 306.4
- globe, sympathetic 360.11
- intestinal (bowel) 564.9
- labyrinth 386.50
- lumbosacral plexus 353.1
- meninges (traumatic) (*see also* Injury, intracranial) 854.0 ✓5ᵗʰ
  - nontraumatic — *see* Meningitis
- myocardium 306.2
- nerve — *see* Disorder, nerve
- nervous 799.2
- nose 478.1
- penis 607.89
- perineum 709.9
- peripheral
  - autonomic nervous system (*see also* Neuropathy, peripheral, autonomic) 337.9
  - nerve — *see* Disorder, nerve
- peritoneum (*see also* Peritonitis) 567.9
- pharynx 478.29
- plantar nerve 355.6
- spinal (cord) (traumatic) — *see also* Injury, spinal, by site
  - nerve — *see also* Disorder, nerve
    - root NEC 724.9
  - traumatic — *see* Injury, nerve, spinal
  - nontraumatic — *see* Myelitis
- stomach 536.9
  - psychogenic 306.4
- sympathetic nerve NEC (*see also* Neuropathy, peripheral, autonomic) 337.9
- ulnar nerve 354.2
- vagina 623.9

Isambert's disease 012.3 ✓5ᵗʰ

Ischemia, ischemic 459.9
- basilar artery (with transient neurologic deficit) 435.0
- bone NEC 733.40
- bowel (transient) 557.9
  - acute 557.0
  - chronic 557.1
  - due to mesenteric artery insufficiency 557.1
- brain — *see also* Ischemia, cerebral
  - recurrent focal 435.9
- cardiac (*see also* Ischemia, heart) 414.9
- cardiomyopathy 414.8
- carotid artery (with transient neurologic deficit) 435.8
- cerebral (chronic) (generalized) 437.1
  - arteriosclerotic 437.0
  - intermittent (with transient neurologic deficit) 435.9
  - puerperal, postpartum, childbirth 674.0 ✓5ᵗʰ
  - recurrent focal (with transient neurologic deficit) 435.9
  - transient (with transient neurologic deficit) 435.9
- colon 557.9
  - acute 557.0
  - chronic 557.1
  - due to mesenteric artery insufficiency 557.1
- coronary (chronic) (*see also* Ischemia, heart) 414.9
- heart (chronic or with a stated duration of over 8 weeks) 414.9
  - acute or with a stated duration of 8 weeks or less (*see also* Infarct, myocardium) 410.9 ✓5ᵗʰ
    - without myocardial infarction 411.89
      - with coronary (artery) occlusion 411.81
  - subacute 411.89
- intestine (transient) 557.9
  - acute 557.0
  - chronic 557.1
  - due to mesenteric artery insufficiency 557.1
- kidney 593.81

Ischemia, ischemic — *continued*
- labyrinth 386.50
- muscles, leg 728.89
- myocardium, myocardial (chronic or with a stated duration of over 8 weeks) 414.8
  - acute (*see also* Infarct, myocardium) 410.9 ✓5ᵗʰ
    - without myocardial infarction 411.89
      - with coronary (artery) occlusion 411.81
- renal 593.81
- retina, retinal 362.84
- small bowel 557.9
  - acute 557.0
  - chronic 557.1
  - due to mesenteric artery insufficiency 557.1
- spinal cord 336.1
- subendocardial (*see also* Insufficiency, coronary) 411.89
- vertebral artery (with transient neurologic deficit) 435.1

Ischialgia (*see also* Sciatica) 724.3

Ischiopagus 759.4

Ischium, ischial — *see* condition

Ischomenia 626.8

Ischuria 788.5

Iselin's disease or osteochondrosis 732.5

Islands of
- parotid tissue in
  - lymph nodes 750.26
  - neck structures 750.26
- submaxillary glands in
  - fascia 750.26
  - lymph nodes 750.26
  - neck muscles 750.26

Islet cell tumor, pancreas (M8150/0) 211.7

Isoimmunization NEC (*see also* Incompatibility) 656.2 ✓5ᵗʰ
- fetus or newborn 773.2
  - ABO blood groups 773.1
  - Rhesus (Rh) factor 773.0

Isolation V07.0
- social V62.4

Isosporosis 007.2

Issue
- medical certificate NEC V68.0
  - cause of death V68.0
  - fitness V68.0
  - incapacity V68.0
- repeat prescription NEC V68.1
  - appliance V68.1
  - contraceptive V25.40
    - device NEC V25.49
      - intrauterine V25.42
      - specified type NEC V25.49
    - pill V25.41
  - glasses V68.1
  - medicinal substance V68.1

Itch (*see also* Pruritus) 698.9
- bakers' 692.89
- barbers' 110.0
- bricklayers' 692.89
- cheese 133.8
- clam diggers' 120.3
- coolie 126.9
- copra 133.8
- Cuban 050.1
- dew 126.9
- dhobie 110.3
- eye 379.99
- filarial (*see also* Infestation, filarial) 125.9
- grain 133.8
- grocers' 133.8
- ground 126.9
- harvest 133.8
- jock 110.3
- Malabar 110.9
  - beard 110.0
  - foot 110.4
  - scalp 110.0
- meaning scabies 133.0
- Norwegian 133.0
- perianal 698.0
- poultrymen's 133.8

Itch (*see also* Pruritus) — *continued*
   sarcoptic 133.0
   scrub 134.1
   seven year V61.10
      meaning scabies 133.0
   straw 133.8
   swimmers' 120.3
   washerwoman's 692.4
   water 120.3
   winter 698.8
Itsenko-Cushing syndrome (pituitary
   basophilism) 255.0
Ivemark's syndrome (asplenia with congenital
   heart disease) 759.0
Ivory bones 756.52
Ixodes 134.8
Ixodiasis 134.8

J

Jaccoud's nodular fibrositis, chronic (Jaccoud's syndrome) 714.4

Jackson's
   membrane 751.4
   paralysis or syndrome 344.89
   veil 751.4

Jacksonian
   epilepsy (see also Epilepsy) 345.5 ✓5ᵗʰ
   seizures (focal) (see also Epilepsy) 345.5 ✓5ᵗʰ

Jacob's ulcer (M8090/3) — see Neoplasm, skin, malignant, by site

Jacquet's dermatitis (diaper dermatitis) 691.0

Jadassohn's
   blue nevus (M8780/0) — see Neoplasm, skin, benign
   disease (maculopapular erythroderma) 696.2
   intraepidermal epithelioma (M8096/0) — see Neoplasm, skin, benign

Jadassohn-Lewandowski syndrome (pachyonychia congenita) 757.5

Jadassohn-Pellizari's disease (anetoderma) 701.3

Jadassohn-Tièche nevus (M8780/0) — see Neoplasm, skin, benign

Jaffe-Lichtenstein (-Uehlinger) syndrome 252.0

Jahnke's syndrome (encephalocutaneous angiomatosis) 759.6

Jakob-Creutzfeldt disease or syndrome 046.1
   with dementia
      with behavioral disturbance 046.1 [294.11]
      without behavioral disturbance 046.1 [294.10]

Jaksch (-Luzet) disease or syndrome (pseudoleukemia infantum) 285.8

Jamaican
   neuropathy 349.82
   paraplegic tropical ataxic-spastic syndrome 349.82

Janet's disease (psychasthenia) 300.89

Janiceps 759.4

Jansky-Bielschowsky amaurotic familial idiocy 330.1

Japanese
   B type encephalitis 062.0
   river fever 081.2
   seven-day fever 100.89

Jaundice (yellow) 782.4
   acholuric (familial) (splenomegalic) (see also Spherocytosis) 282.0
      acquired 283.9
   breast milk 774.39
   catarrhal (acute) 070.1
      with hepatic coma 070.0
      chronic 571.9
      epidemic — see Jaundice, epidemic
   cholestatic (benign) 782.4
   chronic idiopathic 277.4
   epidemic (catarrhal) 070.1
      with hepatic coma 070.0
      leptospiral 100.0
      spirochetal 100.0
   febrile (acute) 070.1
      with hepatic coma 070.0
      leptospiral 100.0
      spirochetal 100.0
   fetus or newborn 774.6
      due to or associated with
         ABO
            antibodies 773.1
            incompatibility, maternal/fetal 773.1
            isoimmunization 773.1
         absence or deficiency of enzyme system for bilirubin conjugation (congenital) 774.39
         blood group incompatibility NEC 773.2
         breast milk inhibitors to conjugation 774.39
            associated with preterm delivery 774.2
         bruising 774.1
         Crigler-Najjar syndrome 277.4 [774.31]
         delayed conjugation 774.30
            associated with preterm delivery 774.2
            development 774.39

Jaundice — continued
   fetus or newborn — continued
      due to or associated with — continued
         drugs or toxins transmitted from mother 774.1
         G-6-PD deficiency 282.2 [774.0]
         galactosemia 271.1 [774.5]
         Gilbert's syndrome 277.4 [774.31]
         hepatocellular damage 774.4
         hereditary hemolytic anemia (see also Anemia, hemolytic) 282.9 [774.0]
         hypothyroidism, congenital 243 [774.31]
         incompatibility, maternal/fetal NEC 773.2
         infection 774.1
         inspissated bile syndrome 774.4
         isoimmunization NEC 773.2
         mucoviscidosis 277.01 [774.5]
         obliteration of bile duct, congenital 751.61 [774.5]
         polycythemia 774.1
         preterm delivery 774.2
         red cell defect 282.9 [774.0]
         Rh
            antibodies 773.0
            incompatibility, maternal/fetal 773.0
            isoimmunization 773.0
         spherocytosis (congenital) 282.0 [774.0]
         swallowed maternal blood 774.1
      physiological NEC 774.6
   from injection, inoculation, infusion, or transfusion (blood) (plasma) (serum) (other substance) (onset within 8 months after administration) — see Hepatitis, viral
   Gilbert's (familial nonhemolytic) 277.4
   hematogenous 283.9
   hemolytic (acquired) 283.9
      congenital (see also Spherocytosis) 282.0
   hemorrhagic (acute) 100.0
      leptospiral 100.0
      newborn 776.0
   hemorrhagic
      spirochetal 100.0
   hepatocellular 573.8
   homologous (serum) — see Hepatitis, viral
   idiopathic, chronic 277.4
   infectious (acute) (subacute) 070.1
      with hepatic coma 070.0
      leptospiral 100.0
      spirochetal 100.0
   leptospiral 100.0
   malignant (see also Necrosis, liver) 570
   newborn (physiological) (see also Jaundice, fetus or newborn) 774.6
   nonhemolytic, congenital familial (Gilbert's) 277.4
   nuclear, newborn (see also Kernicterus of newborn) 774.7
   obstructive NEC (see also Obstruction, biliary) 576.8
   postimmunization — see Hepatitis, viral
   posttransfusion — see Hepatitis, viral
   regurgitation (see also Obstruction, biliary) 576.8
   serum (homologous) (prophylactic) (therapeutic) — see Hepatitis, viral
   spirochetal (hemorrhagic) 100.0
   symptomatic 782.4
      newborn 774.6

Jaw — see condition

Jaw-blinking 374.43
   congenital 742.8

Jaw-winking phenomenon or syndrome 742.8

Jealousy
   alcoholic 291.5
   childhood 313.3
   sibling 313.3

Jejunitis (see also Enteritis) 558.9

Jejunostomy status V44.4

Jejunum, jejunal — see condition

Jensen's disease 363.05

Jericho boil 085.1

Jerks, myoclonic 333.2

Jeune's disease or syndrome (asphyxiating thoracic dystrophy) 756.4

Jigger disease 134.1

Job's syndrome (chronic granulomatous disease) 288.1

Jod-Basedow phenomenon 242.8 ✓5ᵗʰ

Johnson-Stevens disease (erythema multiforme exudativum) 695.1

Joint — see also condition
   Charcôt's 094.0 [713.5]
   false 733.82
   flail — see Flail, joint
   mice — see Loose, body, joint, by site
   sinus to bone 730.9 ✓5ᵗʰ
   von Gies' 095.8

Jordan's anomaly or syndrome 288.2

Josephs-Diamond-Blackfan anemia (congenital hypoplastic) 284.0

Joubert syndrome 759.89

Jumpers' knee 727.2

Jungle yellow fever 060.0

Jüngling's disease (sarcoidosis) 135

Junin virus hemorrhagic fever 078.7

Juvenile — see also condition
   delinquent 312.9
      group (see also Disturbance, conduct) 312.2 ✓5ᵗʰ
      neurotic 312.4

K

Kahler (-Bozzolo) disease (multiple myeloma) (M9730/3) 203.0 ✓5ᵗʰ

Kakergasia 300.9

Kakke 265.0

Kala-azar (Indian) (infantile) (Mediterranean) (Sudanese) 085.0

Kalischer's syndrome (encephalocutaneous angiomatosis) 759.6

Kallmann's syndrome (hypogonadotropic hypogonadism with anosmia) 253.4

Kanner's syndrome (autism) (see also Psychosis, childhood) 299.0 ✓5ᵗʰ

Kaolinosis 502

Kaposi's
   disease 757.33
      lichen ruber 696.4
         acuminatus 696.4
         moniliformis 697.8
      xeroderma pigmentosum 757.33
   sarcoma (M9140/3) 176.9
      adipose tissue 176.1
      aponeurosis 176.1
      artery 176.1
      blood vessel 176.1
      bursa 176.1
      connective tissue 176.1
      external genitalia 176.8
      fascia 176.1
      fatty tissue 176.1
      fibrous tissue 176.1
      gastrointestinal tract NEC 176.3
      ligament 176.1
      lung 176.4
      lymph
         gland(s) 176.5
         node(s) 176.5
      lymphatic(s) NEC 176.1
      muscle (skeletal) 176.1
      oral cavity NEC 176.8
      palate 176.2
      scrotum 176.8
      skin 176.0
      soft tissue 176.1
      specified site NEC 176.8
      subcutaneous tissue 176.1
      synovia 176.1
      tendon (sheath) 176.1
      vein 176.1
      vessel 176.1
      viscera NEC 176.9
      vulva 176.8

Kaposi's — continued
varicelliform eruption 054.0
vaccinia 999.0
Kartagener's syndrome or triad (sinusitis, bronchiectasis, situs inversus) 759.3
Kasabach-Merritt syndrome (capillary hemangioma associated with thrombocytopenic purpura) 287.3
Kaschin-Beck disease (endemic polyarthritis) — see Disease, Kaschin-Beck
Kast's syndrome (dyschondroplasia with hemangiomas) 756.4
Katatonia (see also Schizophrenia) 295.2 ☑5ᵗʰ
Katayama disease or fever 120.2
Kathisophobia 781.0
Kawasaki disease 446.1
Kayser-Fleischer ring (cornea) (pseudosclerosis) 275.1 [371.14]
Kaznelson's syndrome (congenital hypoplastic anemia) 284.0
Kedani fever 081.2
Kelis 701.4
Kelly (-Patterson) syndrome (sideropenic dysphagia) 280.8
Keloid, cheloid 701.4
Addison's (morphea) 701.0
cornea 371.00
Hawkins' 701.4
scar 701.4
Keloma 701.4
Kenya fever 082.1
Keratectasia 371.71
congenital 743.41
Keratitis (nodular) (nonulcerative) (simple) (zonular) NEC 370.9
with ulceration (see also Ulcer, cornea) 370.00
actinic 370.24
arborescens 054.42
areolar 370.22
bullosa 370.8
deep — see Keratitis, interstitial
dendritic(a) 054.42
desiccation 370.34
diffuse interstitial 370.52
disciform(is) 054.43
varicella 052.7 [370.44]
epithelialis vernalis 372.13 [370.32]
exposure 370.34
filamentary 370.23
gonococcal (congenital) (prenatal) 098.43
herpes, herpetic (simplex) NEC 054.43
zoster 053.21
hypopyon 370.04
in
chickenpox 052.7 [370.44]
exanthema (see also Exanthem) 057.9 [370.44]
paravaccinia (see also Paravaccinia) 051.9 [370.44]
smallpox (see also Smallpox) 050.9 [370.44]
vernal conjunctivitis 372.13 [370.32]
interstitial (nonsyphilitic) 370.50
with ulcer (see also Ulcer, cornea) 370.00
diffuse 370.52
herpes, herpetic (simplex) 054.43
zoster 053.21
syphilitic (congenital) (hereditary) 090.3
tuberculous (see also Tuberculosis) 017.3 ☑5ᵗʰ [370.59]
lagophthalmic 370.34
macular 370.22
neuroparalytic 370.35
neurotrophic 370.35
nummular 370.22
oyster-shuckers' 370.8
parenchymatous — see Keratitis, interstitial
petrificans 370.8
phlyctenular 370.31
postmeasles 055.71
punctata, punctate 370.21
leprosa 030.0 [370.21]
profunda 090.3
superficial (Thygeson's) 370.21
purulent 370.8

Keratitis — continued
pustuliformis profunda 090.3
rosacea 695.3 [370.49]
sclerosing 370.54
specified type NEC 370.8
stellate 370.22
striate 370.22
superficial 370.20
with conjunctivitis (see also Keratoconjunctivitis) 370.40
punctate (Thygeson's) 370.21
suppurative 370.8
syphilitic (congenital) (prenatal) 090.3
trachomatous 076.1
late effect 139.1
tuberculous (phlyctenular) (see also Tuberculosis) 017.3 ☑5ᵗʰ [370.31]
ulcerated (see also Ulcer, cornea) 370.00
vesicular 370.8
welders' 370.24
xerotic (see also Keratomalacia) 371.45
vitamin A deficiency 264.4
Keratoacanthoma 238.2
Keratocele 371.72
Keratoconjunctivitis (see also Keratitis) 370.40
adenovirus type 8 077.1
epidemic 077.1
exposure 370.34
gonococcal 098.43
herpetic (simplex) 054.43
zoster 053.21
in
chickenpox 052.7 [370.44]
exanthema (see also Exanthem) 057.9 [370.44]
paravaccinia (see also Paravaccinia) 051.9 [370.44]
smallpox (see also Smallpox) 050.9 [370.44]
infectious 077.1
neurotrophic 370.35
phlyctenular 370.31
postmeasles 055.71
shipyard 077.1
sicca (Sjögren's syndrome) 710.2
not in Sjögren's syndrome 370.33
specified type NEC 370.49
tuberculous (phlyctenular) (see also Tuberculosis) 017.3 ☑5ᵗʰ [370.31]
Keratoconus 371.60
acute hydrops 371.62
congenital 743.41
stable 371.61
Keratocyst (dental) 526.0
Keratoderma, keratodermia (congenital) (palmaris et plantaris) (symmetrical) 757.39
acquired 701.1
blennorrhagica 701.1
gonococcal 098.81
climacterium 701.1
eccentrica 757.39
gonorrheal 098.81
punctata 701.1
tylodes, progressive 701.1
Keratodermatocele 371.72
Keratoglobus 371.70
congenital 743.41
associated with buphthalmos 743.22
Keratohemia 371.12
Keratoiritis (see also Iridocyclitis) 364.3
syphilitic 090.3
tuberculous (see also Tuberculosis) 017.3 ☑5ᵗʰ [364.11]
Keratolysis exfoliativa (congenital) 757.39
acquired 695.89
neonatorum 757.39
Keratoma 701.1
congenital 757.39
malignum congenitale 757.1
palmaris et plantaris hereditarium 757.39
senile 702.0
Keratomalacia 371.45
vitamin A deficiency 264.4
Keratomegaly 743.41
Keratomycosis 111.1
nigricans (palmaris) 111.1

Keratopathy 371.40
band (see also Keratitis) 371.43
bullous (see also Keratitis) 371.23
degenerative (see also Degeneration, cornea) 371.40
hereditary (see also Dystrophy, cornea) 371.50
discrete colliquative 371.49
Keratoscleritis, tuberculous (see also Tuberculosis) 017.3 ☑5ᵗʰ [370.31]
Keratosis 701.1
actinic 702.0
arsenical 692.4
blennorrhagica 701.1
gonococcal 098.81
congenital (any type) 757.39
ear (middle) (see also Cholesteatoma) 385.30
female genital (external) 629.8
follicular, vitamin A deficiency 264.8
follicularis 757.39
acquired 701.1
congenital (acneiformis) (Siemens') 757.39
spinulosa (decalvans) 757.39
vitamin A deficiency 264.8
gonococcal 098.81
larynx, laryngeal 478.79
male genital (external) 608.89
middle ear (see also Cholesteatoma) 385.30
nigricans 701.2
congenital 757.39
obturans 380.21
palmaris et plantaris (symmetrical) 757.39
penile 607.89
pharyngeus 478.29
pilaris 757.39
acquired 701.1
punctata (palmaris et plantaris) 701.1
scrotal 608.89
seborrheic 702.19
inflamed 702.11
senilis 702.0
solar 702.0
suprafollicularis 757.39
tonsillaris 478.29
vagina 623.1
vegetans 757.39
vitamin A deficiency 264.8
Kerato-uveitis (see also Iridocyclitis) 364.3
Keraunoparalysis 994.0
Kerion (celsi) 110.0
Kernicterus of newborn (not due to isoimmunization) 774.7
due to isoimmunization (conditions classifiable to 773.0-773.2) 773.4
Ketoacidosis 276.2
diabetic 250.1 ☑5ᵗʰ
Ketonuria 791.6
branched-chain, intermittent 270.3
Ketosis 276.2
diabetic 250.1 ☑5ᵗʰ
Kidney — see condition
Kienböck's
disease 732.3
adult 732.8
osteochondrosis 732.3
Kimmelstiel (-Wilson) disease or syndrome (intercapillary glomerulosclerosis) 250.4 ☑5ᵗʰ [581.81]
Kink, kinking
appendix 543.9
artery 447.1
cystic duct, congenital 751.61
hair (acquired) 704.2
ileum or intestine (see also Obstruction, intestine) 560.9
Lane's (see also Obstruction, intestine) 560.9
organ or site, congenital NEC — see Anomaly, specified type NEC, by site
ureter (pelvic junction) 593.3
congenital 753.20
vein(s) 459.2
caval 459.2
peripheral 459.2
Kinnier Wilson's disease (hepatolenticular degeneration) 275.1

☑4ᵗʰ Fourth-digit Required   ☑5ᵗʰ Fifth-digit Required   ▶◀ Revised Text   ● New Line   ▲ Revised Code

Kissing
  osteophytes 721.5
  spine 721.5
  vertebra 721.5
Klauder's syndrome (erythema multiforme, exudativum) 695.1
Klebs' disease (see also Nephritis) 583.9
Klein-Waardenburg syndrome (ptosisepicanthus) 270.2
Kleine-Levin syndrome 349.89
Kleptomania 312.32
Klinefelter's syndrome 758.7
Klinger's disease 446.4
Klippel's disease 723.8
Klippel-Feil disease or syndrome (brevicollis) 756.16
Klippel-Trenaunay syndrome 759.89
Klumpke (-Déjérine) palsy, paralysis (birth) (newborn) 767.6
Klüver-Bucy (-Terzian) syndrome 310.0
Knee — see condition
Knifegrinders' rot (see also Tuberculosis) 011.4 ✓5ᵗʰ
Knock-knee (acquired) 736.41
  congenital 755.64
Knot
  intestinal, syndrome (volvulus) 560.2
  umbilical cord (true) 663.2 ✓5ᵗʰ
    affecting fetus or newborn 762.5
Knots, surfer 919.8
  infected 919.9
Knotting (of)
  hair 704.2
  intestine 560.2
Knuckle pads (Garrod's) 728.79
Köbner's disease (epidermolysis bullosa) 757.39
Koch's
  infection (see also Tuberculosis, pulmonary) 011.9 ✓5ᵗʰ
  relapsing fever 087.9
Koch-Weeks conjunctivitis 372.03
Koenig-Wichman disease (pemphigus) 694.4
Köhler's disease (osteochondrosis) 732.5
  first (osteochondrosis juvenilis) 732.5
  second (Freiburg's infarction, metatarsal head) 732.5
  patellar 732.4
  tarsal navicular (bone) (osteoarthrosis juvenilis) 732.5
Köhler-Mouchet disease (osteoarthrosis juvenilis) 732.5
Köhler-Pellegrini-Stieda disease or syndrome (calcification, knee joint) 726.62
Koilonychia 703.8
  congenital 757.5
Kojevnikov's, Kojewnikoff's epilepsy (see also Epilepsy) 345.7 ✓5ᵗʰ
König's
  disease (osteochondritis dissecans) 732.7
  syndrome 564.89
Koniophthisis (see also Tuberculosis) 011.4 ✓5ᵗʰ
Koplik's spots 055.9
Kopp's asthma 254.8
Korean hemorrhagic fever 078.6
Korsakoff (-Wernicke) disease, psychosis, or syndrome (nonalcoholic) 294.0
  alcoholic 291.1
Korsakov's disease — see Korsakoff's disease
Korsakow's disease — see Korsakoff's disease
Kostmann's disease or syndrome (infantile genetic agranulocytosis) 288.0
Krabbe's
  disease (leukodystrophy) 330.0
  syndrome
    congenital muscle hypoplasia 756.89
    cutaneocerebral angioma 759.6
Kraepelin-Morel disease (see also Schizophrenia) 295.9 ✓5ᵗʰ
Kraft-Weber-Dimitri disease 759.6

Kraurosis
  ani 569.49
  penis 607.0
  vagina 623.8
  vulva 624.0
Kreotoxism 005.9
Krukenberg's
  spindle 371.13
  tumor (M8490/6) 198.6
Kufs' disease 330.1
Kugelberg-Welander disease 335.11
Kuhnt-Junius degeneration or disease 362.52
Kulchitsky's cell carcinoma (carcinoid tumor of intestine) 259.2
Kümmell's disease or spondylitis 721.7
Kundrat's disease (lymphosarcoma) 200.1 ✓5ᵗʰ
Kunekune — see Dermatophytosis
Kunkel syndrome (lupoid hepatitis) 571.49
Kupffer cell sarcoma (M9124/3) 155.0
Kuru 046.0
Kussmaul's
  coma (diabetic) 250.3 ✓5ᵗʰ
  disease (polyarteritis nodosa) 446.0
  respiration (air hunger) 786.09
Kwashiorkor (marasmus type) 260
Kyasanur Forest disease 065.2
Kyphoscoliosis, kyphoscoliotic (acquired) (see also Scoliosis) 737.30
  congenital 756.19
  due to radiation 737.33
  heart (disease) 416.1
  idiopathic 737.30
    infantile
      progressive 737.32
      resolving 737.31
  late effect of rickets 268.1 [737.43]
  specified NEC 737.39
  thoracogenic 737.34
  tuberculous (see also Tuberculosis) 015.0 ✓5ᵗʰ [737.43]
Kyphosis, kyphotic (acquired) (postural) 737.10
  adolescent postural 737.0
  congenital 756.19
  dorsalis juvenilis 732.0
  due to or associated with
    Charcôt-Marie-Tooth disease 356.1 [737.41]
    mucopolysaccharidosis 277.5 [737.41]
    neurofibromatosis 237.71 [737.41]
    osteitis
      deformans 731.0 [737.41]
      fibrosa cystica 252.0 [737.41]
    osteoporosis (see also Osteoporosis) 733.0 ✓5ᵗʰ [737.41]
    poliomyelitis (see also Poliomyelitis) 138 [737.41]
    radiation 737.11
    tuberculosis (see also Tuberculosis) 015.0 ✓5ᵗʰ [737.41]
  Kümmell's 721.7
  late effect of rickets 268.1 [737.41]
  Morquio-Brailsford type (spinal) 277.5 [737.41]
  pelvis 738.6
  postlaminectomy 737.12
  specified cause NEC 737.19
  syphilitic, congenital 090.5 [737.41]
  tuberculous (see also Tuberculosis) 015.0 ✓5ᵗʰ [737.41]
Kyrle's disease (hyperkeratosis follicularis in cutem penetrans) 701.1

L

Labia, labium — see condition
Labiated hymen 752.49
Labile
  blood pressure 796.2
  emotions, emotionality 301.3
  vasomotor system 443.9
Labioglossal paralysis 335.22
Labium leporinum (see also Cleft, lip) 749.10
Labor (see also Delivery)
  with complications — see Delivery, complicated

Labor (see also Delivery) — continued
  abnormal NEC 661.9 ✓5ᵗʰ
    affecting fetus or newborn 763.7
  arrested active phase 661.1 ✓5ᵗʰ
    affecting fetus or newborn 763.7
  desultory 661.2 ✓5ᵗʰ
    affecting fetus or newborn 763.7
  dyscoordinate 661.4 ✓5ᵗʰ
    affecting fetus or newborn 763.7
  early onset (22-36 weeks gestation) 644.2 ✓5ᵗʰ
  failed
    induction 659.1 ✓5ᵗʰ
      mechanical 659.0 ✓5ᵗʰ
      medical 659.1 ✓5ᵗʰ
      surgical 659.0 ✓5ᵗʰ
    trial (vaginal delivery) 660.6 ✓5ᵗʰ
  false 644.1 ✓5ᵗʰ
  forced or induced, affecting fetus or newborn 763.89
  hypertonic 661.4 ✓5ᵗʰ
    affecting fetus or newborn 763.7
  hypotonic 661.2 ✓5ᵗʰ
    affecting fetus or newborn 763.7
    primary 661.0 ✓5ᵗʰ
      affecting fetus or newborn 763.7
    secondary 661.1 ✓5ᵗʰ
      affecting fetus or newborn 763.7
  incoordinate 661.4 ✓5ᵗʰ
    affecting fetus or newborn 763.7
  irregular 661.2 ✓5ᵗʰ
    affecting fetus or newborn 763.7
  long — see Labor, prolonged
  missed (at or near term) 656.4 ✓5ᵗʰ
  obstructed NEC 660.9 ✓5ᵗʰ
    affecting fetus or newborn 763.1
    specified cause NEC 660.8 ✓5ᵗʰ
      affecting fetus or newborn 763.1
  pains, spurious 644.1 ✓5ᵗʰ
  precipitate 661.3 ✓5ᵗʰ
    affecting fetus or newborn 763.6
  premature 644.2 ✓5ᵗʰ
    threatened 644.0 ✓5ᵗʰ
  prolonged or protracted 662.1 ✓5ᵗʰ
    affecting fetus or newborn 763.89
    first stage 662.0 ✓5ᵗʰ
      affecting fetus or newborn 763.89
    second stage 662.2 ✓5ᵗʰ
      affecting fetus or newborn 763.89
  threatened NEC 644.1 ✓5ᵗʰ
  undelivered 644.1 ✓5ᵗʰ
Labored breathing (see also Hyperventilation) 786.09
Labyrinthitis (inner ear) (destructive) (latent) 386.30
  circumscribed 386.32
  diffuse 386.31
  focal 386.32
  purulent 386.33
  serous 386.31
  suppurative 386.33
  syphilitic 095.8
  toxic 386.34
  viral 386.35
Laceration — see also Wound, open, by site
  accidental, complicating surgery 998.2
  Achilles tendon 845.09
    with open wound 892.2
  anus (sphincter) 863.89
    with
      abortion — see Abortion, by type, with damage to pelvic organs
      ectopic pregnancy (see also categories 633.0-633.9) 639.2
      molar pregnancy (see also categories 630-632) 639.2
    complicating delivery 664.2 ✓5ᵗʰ
      with laceration of anal or rectal mucosa 664.3 ✓5ᵗʰ
    following
      abortion 639.2
      ectopic or molar pregnancy 639.2
    nontraumatic, nonpuerperal 565.0
  bladder (urinary)
    with
      abortion — see Abortion, by type, with damage to pelvic organs

Laceration — *see also* Wound, open, by site —
  continued
  bladder (urinary) — *continued*
    with — *continued*
      ectopic pregancy (*see also* categories
        633.0-633.9) 639.2
      molar pregnancy (*see also* categories 630-
        632) 639.2
    following
      abortion 639.2
      ectopic or molar pregnancy 639.2
    obstetrical trauma 665.5 ✓5ᵗʰ
  blood vessel — *see* Injury, blood vessel, by site
  bowel
    with
      abortion — *see* Abortion, by type, with
        damage to pelvic organs
      ectopic pregnancy (*see also* categories
        633.0-633.9) 639.2
      molar pregnancy (*see also* categories 630-
        632) 639.2
    following
      abortion 639.2
      ectopic or molar pregnancy 639.2
    obstetrical trauma 665.5 ✓5ᵗʰ
  brain (with hemorrhage) (cerebral) (membrane)
    851.8 ✓5ᵗʰ
  brain (cerebral) (membrane) 851.8 ✓5ᵗʰ

Note — *Use the following fifth-digit*
subclassification with categories 851–854:

0 *unspecified state of consciousness*
1 *with no loss of consciousness*
2 *with brief [less than one hour] loss*
   of consciousness
3 *with moderate [1-24 hours] loss of*
   consciousness
4 *with prolonged [more than 24 hours]*
   loss of consciousness and return to
   pre-existing conscious level
5 *with prolonged [more than 24 hours]*
   loss of consciousness, without
   return to pre-existing conscious level
Use fifth-digit 5 to designate when a
patient is unconscious and dies
before regaining consciousness,
regardless of the duration of the
loss of consciousness
6 *with loss of consciousness of*
   unspecified duration
9 *with concussion, unspecified*

---

    with
      open intracranial wound 851.9 ✓5ᵗʰ
      skull fracture — *see* Fracture, skull, by
        site
    cerebellum 851.6 ✓5ᵗʰ
      with open intracranial wound 851.7 ✓5ᵗʰ
    cortex 851.2 ✓5ᵗʰ
      with open intracranial wound 851.3 ✓5ᵗʰ
    during birth 767.0
    stem 851.6 ✓5ᵗʰ
      with open intracranial wound 851.7 ✓5ᵗʰ
  broad ligament
    with
      abortion — *see* Abortion, by type, with
        damage to pelvic organs
      ectopic pregnancy (*see also* categories
        633.0-633.9) 639.2
      molar pregnancy (*see also* categories 630-
        632) 639.2
    following
      abortion 639.2
      ectopic or molar pregnancy 639.2
    nontraumatic 620.6
    obstetrical trauma 665.6 ✓5ᵗʰ
    syndrome (nontraumatic) 620.6
  capsule, joint — *see* Sprain, by site
  cardiac — *see* Laceration, heart
  causing eversion of cervix uteri (old) 622.0
  central, complicating delivery 664.4 ✓5ᵗʰ
  cerebellum — *see* Laceration, brain, cerebellum
  cerebral — *see also* Laceration, brain during
    birth 767.0

Laceration — *see also* Wound, open, by site —
  continued
  cervix (uteri)
    with
      abortion — *see* Abortion, by type, with
        damage to pelvic organs
      ectopic pregnancy (*see also* categories
        633.0-633.9) 639.2
      molar pregnancy (*see also* categories 630-
        632) 639.2
    following
      abortion 639.2
      ectopic or molar pregnancy 639.2
    nonpuerperal, nontraumatic 622.3
    obstetrical trauma (current) 665.3 ✓5ᵗʰ
    old (postpartal) 622.3
    traumatic — *see* Injury, internal, cervix
  chordae heart 429.5
  complicated 879.9
  cornea — *see* Laceration, eyeball
    superficial 918.1
  cortex (cerebral) — *see* Laceration, brain,
    cortex
  esophagus 530.89
  eye(s) — *see* Laceration, ocular
  eyeball NEC 871.4
    with prolapse or exposure of intraocular
      tissue 871.1
    penetrating — *see* Penetrating wound,
      eyeball
    specified as without prolapse of intraocular
      tissue 871.0
  eyelid NEC 870.8
    full thickness 870.1
      involving lacrimal passages 870.2
    skin (and periocular area) 870.0
      penetrating — *see* Penetrating wound,
        orbit
  fourchette
    with
      abortion — *see* Abortion, by type, with
        damage to pelvic organs
      ectopic pregnancy (*see also* categories
        633.0-633.9) 639.2
      molar pregnancy (*see also* categories 630-
        632) 639.2
    complicating delivery 664.0 ✓5ᵗʰ
    following
      abortion 639.2
      ectopic or molar pregnancy 639.2
  heart (without penetration of heart chambers)
    861.02
    with
      open wound into thorax 861.12
      penetration of heart chambers 861.03
        with open wound into thorax 861.13
  hernial sac — *see* Hernia, by site
  internal organ (abdomen) (chest) (pelvis)
    NEC — *see* Injury, internal, by site
  kidney (parenchyma) 866.02
    with
      complete disruption of parenchyma
        (rupture) 866.03
        with open wound into cavity 866.13
      open wound into cavity 866.12
  labia
    complicating delivery 664.0 ✓5ᵗʰ
  ligament — *see also* Sprain, by site
    with open wound — *see* Wound, open, by
      site
  liver 864.05
    with open wound into cavity 864.15
    major (disruption of hepatic parenchyma)
      864.04
      with open wound into cavity 864.14
    minor (capsule only) 864.02
      with open wound into cavity 864.12
    moderate (involving parenchyma without
      major disruption) 864.03
      with open wound into cavity 864.13
    multiple 864.04
      with open wound into cavity 864.14
    stellate 864.04
      with open wound into cavity 864.14
  lung 861.22
    with open wound into thorax 861.32
  meninges — *see* Laceration, brain

Laceration — *see also* Wound, open, by site —
  continued
  meniscus (knee) (*see also* Tear, meniscus)
    836.2
    old 717.5
    site other than knee — *see also* Sprain, by
      site
      old NEC (*see also* Disorder, cartilage,
        articular) 718.0 ✓5ᵗʰ
  muscle — *see also* Sprain, by site
    with open wound — *see* Wound, open, by
      site
  myocardium — *see* Laceration, heart
  nerve — *see* Injury, nerve, by site
  ocular NEC (*see also* Laceration, eyeball) 871.4
    adnexa NEC 870.8
      penetrating 870.3
        with foreign body 870.4
  orbit (eye) 870.8
    penetrating 870.3
      with foreign body 870.4
  pelvic
    floor (muscles)
      with
        abortion — *see* Abortion, by type, with
          damage to pelvic organs
        ectopic pregnancy (*see also* categories
          633.0-633.9) 639.2
        molar pregnancy (*see also* categories
          630-632) 639.2
      complicating delivery 664.1 ✓5ᵗʰ
      following
        abortion 639.2
        ectopic or molar pregnancy 639.2
      nonpuerperal 618.7
      old (postpartal) 618.7
    organ NEC
      with
        abortion — *see* Abortion, by type, with
          damage to pelvic organs
        ectopic pregnancy (*see also* categories
          633.0-633.9) 639.2
        molar pregnancy (*see also* categories
          630-632) 639.2
      complicating delivery 665.5 ✓5ᵗʰ
        affecting fetus or newborn 763.89
      following
        abortion 639.2
        ectopic or molar pregnancy 639.2
      obstetrical trauma 665.5 ✓5ᵗʰ
  perineum, perineal (old) (postpartal) 618.7
    with
      abortion — *see* Abortion, by type, with
        damage to pelvic floor
      ectopic pregnancy (*see also* categories
        633.0-633.9) 639.2
      molar pregnancy (*see also* categories 630-
        632) 639.2
    complicating delivery 664.4 ✓5ᵗʰ
      first degree 664.0 ✓5ᵗʰ
      second degree 664.1 ✓5ᵗʰ
      third degree 664.2 ✓5ᵗʰ
      fourth degree 664.3 ✓5ᵗʰ
      central 664.4 ✓5ᵗʰ
      involving
        anal sphincter 664.2 ✓5ᵗʰ
        fourchette 664.0 ✓5ᵗʰ
        hymen 664.0 ✓5ᵗʰ
        labia 664.0 ✓5ᵗʰ
        pelvic floor 664.1 ✓5ᵗʰ
        perineal muscles 664.1 ✓5ᵗʰ
        rectovaginal septum 664.2 ✓5ᵗʰ
          with anal mucosa 664.3 ✓5ᵗʰ
        skin 664.0 ✓5ᵗʰ
        sphincter (anal) 664.2 ✓5ᵗʰ
          with anal mucosa 664.3 ✓5ᵗʰ
        vagina 664.0 ✓5ᵗʰ
        vaginal muscles 664.1 ✓5ᵗʰ
        vulva 664.0 ✓5ᵗʰ
      secondary 674.2 ✓5ᵗʰ
    following
      abortion 639.2
      ectopic or molar pregnancy 639.2
  male 879.6
    complicated 879.7
  muscles, complicating delivery 664.1 ✓5ᵗʰ

Laceration — see also Wound, open, by site — continued
  perineum, perineal — continued
    nonpuerperal, current injury 879.6
      complicated 879.7
    secondary (postpartal) 674.2 ☑5ᵗʰ
  peritoneum
    with
      abortion — see Abortion, by type, with damage to pelvic organs
      ectopic pregnancy (see also categories 633.0-633.9) 639.2
      molar pregnancy (see also categories 630-632) 639.2
    following
      abortion 639.2
      ectopic or molar pregnancy 639.2
    obstetrical trauma 665.5 ☑5ᵗʰ
  periurethral tissue
    with
      abortion — see Abortion, by type, with damage to pelvic organs
      ectopic pregnancy (see also categories 633.0-633.9) 639.2
      molar pregnancy (see also categories 630-632) 639.2
    following
      abortion 639.2
      ectopic or molar pregnancy 639.2
    obstetrical trauma 665.5 ☑5ᵗʰ
  rectovaginal (septum)
    with
      abortion — see Abortion, by type, with damage to pelvic organs
      ectopic pregnancy (see also categories 633.0-633.9) 639.2
      molar pregnancy (see also categories 630-632) 639.2
    complicating delivery 665.4 ☑5ᵗʰ
      with perineum 664.2 ☑5ᵗʰ
        involving anal or rectal mucosa 664.3 ☑5ᵗʰ
    following
      abortion 639.2
      ectopic or molar pregnancy 639.2
    nonpuerperal 623.4
    old (postpartal) 623.4
  spinal cord (meninges) — see also Injury, spinal, by site
    due to injury at birth 767.4
    fetus or newborn 767.4
  spleen 865.09
    with
      disruption of parenchyma (massive) 865.04
        with open wound into cavity 865.14
      open wound into cavity 865.19
    capsule (without disruption of parenchyma) 865.02
      with open wound into cavity 865.12
    parenchyma 865.03
      with open wound into cavity 865.13
      massive disruption (rupture) 865.04
        with open wound into cavity 865.14
  tendon 848.9
    with open wound — see Wound, open, by site
    Achilles 845.09
      with open wound 892.2
    lower limb NEC 844.9
      with open wound NEC 894.2
    upper limb NEC 840.9
      with open wound NEC 884.2
  tentorium cerebelli — see Laceration, brain, cerebellum
  tongue 873.64
    complicated 873.74
  urethra
    with
      abortion — see Abortion, by type, with damage to pelvic organs
      ectopic pregnancy (see also categories 633.0-633.9) 639.2
      molar pregnancy (see also categories 630-632) 639.2

Laceration — see also Wound, open, by site — continued
  urethra — continued
    following
      abortion 639.2
      ectopic or molar pregnancy 639.2
    nonpuerperal, nontraumatic 599.84
    obstetrical trauma 665.5 ☑5ᵗʰ
  uterus
    with
      abortion — see Abortion, by type, with damage to pelvic organs
      ectopic pregnancy (see also categories 633.0-633.9) 639.2
      molar pregnancy (see also categories 630-632) 639.2
    following
      abortion 639.2
      ectopic or molar pregnancy 639.2
    nonpuerperal, nontraumatic 621.8
    obstetrical trauma NEC 665.8 ☑5ᵗʰ ▲
    old (postpartal) 621.8
  vagina
    with
      abortion — see Abortion, by type, with damage to pelvic organs
      ectopic pregnancy (see also categories 633.0-633.9) 639.2
      molar pregnancy (see also categories 630-632) 639.2
    perineal involvement, complicating delivery 664.0 ☑5ᵗʰ
    complicating delivery 665.4 ☑5ᵗʰ
      first degree 664.0 ☑5ᵗʰ
      second degree 664.1 ☑5ᵗʰ
      third degree 664.2 ☑5ᵗʰ
      fourth degree 664.3 ☑5ᵗʰ
      high 665.4 ☑5ᵗʰ
      muscles 664.1 ☑5ᵗʰ
      sulcus 665.4 ☑5ᵗʰ
      wall 665.4 ☑5ᵗʰ
    following
      abortion 639.2
      ectopic or molar pregnancy 639.2
    nonpuerperal, nontraumatic 623.4
    old (postpartal) 623.4
  valve, heart — see Endocarditis
  vulva
    with
      abortion — see Abortion, by type, with damage to pelvic organs,
      ectopic pregnancy (see also categories 633.0-633.9) 639.2
      molar pregnancy (see also categories 630-632) 639.2
    complicating delivery 664.0 ☑5ᵗʰ
    following
      abortion 639.2
      ectopic or molar pregnancy 639.2
    nonpuerperal, nontraumatic 624.4
    old (postpartal) 624.4
Lachrymal — see condition
Lachrymonasal duct — see condition
Lack of
  appetite (see also Anorexia) 783.0
  care
    in home V60.4
    of adult 995.84
    of infant (at or after birth) 995.52
  coordination 781.3
  development — see also Hypoplasia
    physiological in childhood 783.40
  education V62.3
  energy 780.79
  financial resources V60.2
  food 994.2
    in environment V60.8
  growth in childhood 783.43
  heating V60.1
  housing (permanent) (temporary) V60.0
    adequate V60.1
  material resources V60.2
  medical attention 799.8
  memory (see also Amnesia) 780.99 ▲
    mild, following organic brain damage 310.1
  ovulation 628.0

Lack of — continued
  person able to render necessary care V60.4
  physical exercise V69.0
  physiologic development in childhood 783.40
  prenatal care in current pregnancy V23.7
  shelter V60.0
  water 994.3
Lacrimal — see condition
Lacrimation, abnormal (see also Epiphora) 375.20
Lacrimonasal duct — see condition
Lactation, lactating (breast) (puerperal) (postpartum)
  defective 676.4 ☑5ᵗʰ
  disorder 676.9 ☑5ᵗʰ
    specified type NEC 676.8 ☑5ᵗʰ
  excessive 676.6 ☑5ᵗʰ
  failed 676.4 ☑5ᵗʰ
  mastitis NEC 675.2 ☑5ᵗʰ
  mother (care and/or examination) V24.1
  nonpuerperal 611.6
  suppressed 676.5 ☑5ᵗʰ
Lacticemia 271.3
  excessive 276.2
Lactosuria 271.3
Lacunar skull 756.0
Laennec's cirrhosis (alcoholic) 571.2
  nonalcoholic 571.5
Lafora's disease 333.2
Lag, lid (nervous) 374.41
Lagleyze-von Hippel disease (retinocerebral angiomatosis) 759.6
Lagophthalmos (eyelid) (nervous) 374.20
  cicatricial 374.23
  keratitis (see also Keratitis) 370.34
  mechanical 374.22
  paralytic 374.21
La grippe — see Influenza
Lahore sore 085.1
Lakes, venous (cerebral) 437.8
Laki-Lorand factor deficiency (see also Defect, coagulation) 286.3
Lalling 307.9
Lambliasis 007.1
Lame back 724.5
Lancereaux's diabetes (diabetes mellitus with marked emaciation) 250.8 ☑5ᵗʰ [261]
Landouzy-Déjérine dystrophy (fascioscapulohumeral atrophy) 359.1
Landry's disease or paralysis 357.0
Landry-Guillain-Barré syndrome 357.0
Lane's
  band 751.4
  disease 569.89
  kink (see also Obstruction, intestine) 560.9
Langdon Down's syndrome (mongolism) 758.0
Language abolition 784.69
Lanugo (persistent) 757.4
Laparoscopic surgical procedure converted to open procedure V64.4
Lardaceous
  degeneration (any site) 277.3
  disease 277.3
  kidney 277.3 [583.81]
  liver 277.3
Large
  baby (regardless of gestational age) 766.1
    exceptionally (weight of 4500 grams or more) 766.1
    of diabetic mother 775.0
  ear 744.22
  fetus — see also Oversize, fetus
    causing disproportion 653.5 ☑5ᵗʰ
      with obstructed labor 660.1 ☑5ᵗʰ
  for dates
    fetus or newborn (regardless of gestational age) 766.1
      affecting management of pregnancy 656.6 ☑5ᵗʰ
    exceptionally (weight of 4500 grams or more) 766.0

Large — *continued*
  physiological cup 743.57
  waxy liver 277.3
  white kidney — *see* Nephrosis

Larsen's syndrome (flattened facies and multiple congenital dislocations) 755.8

Larsen-Johansson disease (juvenile osteopathia patellae) 732.4

Larva migrans
  cutaneous NEC 126.9
    ancylostoma 126.9
  of Diptera in vitreous 128.0
  visceral NEC 128.0

Laryngeal — *see also* condition syncope 786.2

Laryngismus (acute) (infectious) (stridulous) 478.75
  congenital 748.3
  diphtheritic 032.3

Laryngitis (acute) (edematous) (fibrinous) (gangrenous) (infective) (infiltrative) (malignant) (membranous) (phlegmonous) (pneumococcal) (pseudomembranous) (septic) (subglottic) (suppurative) (ulcerative) (viral) 464.00
  with
    influenza, flu, or grippe 487.1
    obstruction 464.01
    tracheitis (*see also* Laryngotracheitis) 464.20
      with obstruction 464.21
      acute 464.20
        with obstruction 464.21
      chronic 476.1
  atrophic 476.0
  Borrelia vincentii 101
  catarrhal 476.0
  chronic 476.0
    with tracheitis (chronic) 476.1
    due to external agent — *see* Condition, respiratory, chronic, due to
  diphtheritic (membranous) 032.3
  due to external agent — *see* Inflammation, respiratory, upper, due to
  H. influenzae 464.00
    with obstruction 464.01
  Hemophilus influenzae 464.00
    wtih obstruction 464.01
  hypertrophic 476.0
  influenzal 487.1
  pachydermic 478.79
  sicca 476.0
  spasmodic 478.75
    acute 464.00
      with obstruction 464.01
  streptococcal 034.0
  stridulous 478.75
  syphilitic 095.8
    congenital 090.5
  tuberculous (*see also* Tuberculosis, larynx) 012.3 ✓5ᵗʰ
  Vincent's 101

Laryngocele (congenital) (ventricular) 748.3

Laryngofissure 478.79
  congenital 748.3

Laryngomalacia (congenital) 748.3

Laryngopharyngitis (acute) 465.0
  chronic 478.9
    due to external agent — *see* Condition, respiratory, chronic, due to
  due to external agent — *see* Inflammation, respiratory, upper, due to
  septic 034.0

Laryngoplegia (*see also* Paralysis, vocal cord) 478.30

Laryngoptosis 478.79

Laryngospasm 478.75
  due to external agent — *see* Condition, respiratory, acute, due to

Laryngostenosis 478.74
  congenital 748.3

Laryngotracheitis (acute) (infectional) (viral) (*see also* Laryngitis) 464.20
  with obstruction 464.21
  atrophic 476.1
  Borrelia vincenti 101

Laryngotracheitis (*see also* Laryngitis) — *continued*
  catarrhal 476.1
  chronic 476.1
    due to external agent — *see* Condition, respiratory, chronic, due to
  diphtheritic (membranous) 032.3
  due to external agent — *see* Inflammation, respiratory, upper, due to
  H. influenzae 464.20
    with obstruction 464.21
  hypertrophic 476.1
  influenzal 487.1
  pachydermic 478.75
  sicca 476.1
  spasmodic 478.75
    acute 464.20
      with obstruction 464.21
  streptococcal 034.0
  stridulous 478.75
  syphilitic 095.8
    congenital 090.5
  tuberculous (*see also* Tuberculosis, larynx) 012.3 ✓5ᵗʰ
  Vincent's 101

Laryngotracheobronchitis (*see also* Bronchitis) 490
  acute 466.0
  chronic 491.8
  viral 466.0

Laryngotracheobronchopneumonitis — *see* Pneumonia, broncho-

Larynx, laryngeal — *see* condition

Lasègue's disease (persecution mania) 297.9

Lassa fever 078.89

Lassitude (*see also* Weakness) 780.79

Late — *see also* condition
  effect(s) (of) — *see also* condition
    abscess
      intracranial or intraspinal (conditions classifiable to 324) — *see* category 326
    adverse effect of drug, medicinal or biological substance 909.5
    amputation
      postoperative (late) 997.60
      traumatic (injury classifiable to 885-887 and 895-897) 905.9
    burn (injury classifiable to 948-949) 906.9
      extremities NEC (injury classifiable to 943 or 945) 906.7
      hand or wrist (injury classifiable to 944) 906.6
      eye (injury classifiable to 940) 906.5
      face, head, and neck (injury classifiable to 941) 906.5
      specified site NEC (injury classifiable to 942 and 946-947) 906.8
    cerebrovascular disease (conditions classifiable to 430-437) 438.9
      with
        alterations of sensations 438.6 ●
        aphasia 438.11
        apraxia 438.81
        ataxia 438.84 ●
        cognitive deficits 438.0
        disturbances of vision 438.7 ●
        dysphagia 438.82
        dysphasia 438.12
        facial droop 438.83 ●
        facial weakness 438.83 ●
        hemiplegia/hemiparesis
          affecting
            dominant side 438.21
            nondominant side 438.22
            unspecified side 438.20
        monoplegia of lower limb
          affecting
            dominant side 438.41
            nondominant side 438.42
            unspecified side 438.40
        monoplegia of upper limb
          affecting
            dominant side 438.31

Late — *see also* condition — *continued*
  effect(s) (of) — *see also* condition — *continued*
    cerebrovascular disease — *continued*
      with — *continued*
        monoplegia of upper limb — *continued*
          affecting — *continued*
            nondominant side 438.32
            unspecified side 438.30
        paralytic syndrome NEC
          affecting
            bilateral 438.53
            dominant side 438.51
            nondominant side 438.52
            unspecified side 438.50
        speech and language deficit 438.10
        vertigo 438.85 ●
      specified type NEC 438.89
    childbirth complication(s) 677
    complication(s) of
      childbirth 677
      delivery 677
      pregnancy 677
      puerperium 677
      surgical and medical care (conditions classifiable to 996-999) 909.3
    complication(s) of — *continued*
      trauma (conditions classifiable to 958) 908.6
    contusion (injury classifiable to 920-924) 906.3
    crushing (injury classifiable to 925-929) 906.4
    delivery complication(s) 677
    dislocation (injury classifiable to 830-839) 905.6
    encephalitis or encephalomyelitis (conditions classifiable to 323) — *see* category 326
      in infectious diseases 139.8
      viral (conditions classifiable to 049.8, 049.9, 062-064) 139.0
    external cause NEC (conditions classifiable to 995) 909.9
      certain conditions classifiable to categories 991-994 909.4
    foreign body in orifice (injury classifiable to 930-939) 908.5
    fracture (multiple) (injury classifiable to 828-829) 905.5
      extremity
        lower (injury classifiable to 821-827) 905.4
          neck of femur (injury classifiable to 820) 905.3
        upper (injury classifiable to 810-819) 905.2
      face and skull (injury classifiable to 800-804) 905.0
      skull and face (injury classifiable to 800-804) 905.0
      spine and trunk (injury classifiable to 805 and 807-809) 905.1
        with spinal cord lesion (injury classifiable to 806) 907.2
    infection
      pyogenic, intracranial — *see* category 326
    infectious diseases (conditions classifiable to 001-136) NEC 139.8
    injury (injury classifiable to 959) 908.9
      blood vessel 908.3
        abdomen and pelvis (injury classifiable to 902) 908.4
        extremity (injury classifiable to 903-904) 908.3
        head and neck (injury classifiable to 900) 908.3
        intracranial (injury classifiable to 850-854) 907.0
          with skull fracture 905.0
        thorax (injury classifiable to 901) 908.4
      internal organ NEC (injury classifiable to 867 and 869) 908.2
        abdomen (injury classifiable to 863-866 and 868) 908.1
        thorax (injury classifiable to 860-862) 908.0

Late — *see also* condition — *continued*
  effect(s) (of) — *see also* condition — *continued*
    injury — *continued*
      intracranial (injury classifiable to 850-854) 907.0
        with skull fracture (injury classifiable to 800-801 and 803-804) 905.0
      nerve NEC (injury classifiable to 957) 907.9
        cranial (injury classifiable to 950-951) 907.1
        peripheral NEC (injury classifiable to 957) 907.9
          lower limb and pelvic girdle (injury classifiable to 956) 907.5
          upper limb and shoulder girdle (injury classifiable to 955) 907.4
        roots and plexus(es), spinal (injury classifiable to 953) 907.3
        trunk (injury classifiable to 954) 907.3
      spinal
        cord (injury classifiable to 806 and 952) 907.2
        nerve root(s) and plexus(es) (injury classifiable to 953) 907.3
      superficial (injury classifiable to 910-919) 906.2
      tendon (tendon injury classifiable to 840-848, 880-884 with .2, and 890-894 with .2) 905.8
    meningitis
      bacterial (conditions classifiable to 320) — *see* category 326
      unspecified cause (conditions classifiable to 322) — *see* category 326
    myelitis (*see also* Late, effect(s) (of), encephalitis) — *see* category 326
    parasitic diseases (conditions classifiable to 001-136 NEC) 139.8
    phlebitis or thrombophlebitis of intracranial venous sinuses (conditions classifiable to 325) — *see* category 326
    poisoning due to drug, medicinal or biological substance (conditions classifiable to 960-979) 909.0
    poliomyelitis, acute (conditions classifiable to 045) 138
    pregnancy complication(s) 677
    puerperal complication(s) 677
    radiation (conditions classifiable to 990) 909.2
    rickets 268.1
    sprain and strain without mention of tendon injury (injury classifiable to 840-848, except tendon injury) 905.7
      tendon involvement 905.8
    toxic effect of
      drug, medicinal or biological substance (conditions classifiable to 960-979) 909.0
      nonmedical substance (conditions classifiable to 980-989) 909.1
    trachoma (conditions classifiable to 076) 139.1
    tuberculosis 137.0
      bones and joints (conditions classifiable to 015) 137.3
      central nervous system (conditions classifiable to 013) 137.1
      genitourinary (conditions classifiable to 016) 137.2
      pulmonary (conditions classifiable to 010-012) 137.0
      specified organs NEC (conditions classifiable to 014, 017-018) 137.4
    viral encephalitis (conditions classifiable to 049.8, 049.9, 062-064) 139.0
    wound, open
      extremity (injury classifiable to 880-884 and 890-894, except .2) 906.1
        tendon (injury classifiable to 880-884 with .2 and 890-894 with.2) 905.8
      head, neck, and trunk (injury classifiable to 870-879) 906.0

Latent — *see* condition
Lateral — *see* condition
Laterocession — *see* Lateroversion
Lateroflexion — *see* Lateroversion
Lateroversion
  cervix — *see* Lateroversion, uterus
  uterus, uterine (cervix) (postinfectional) (postpartal, old) 621.6
    congenital 752.3
    in pregnancy or childbirth 654.4 ☑5ᵗʰ
      affecting fetus or newborn 763.89
Lathyrism 988.2
Launois' syndrome (pituitary gigantism) 253.0
Launois-Bensaude's lipomatosis 272.8
Launois-Cléret syndrome (adiposogenital dystrophy) 253.8
Laurence-Moon-Biedl syndrome (obesity, polydactyly, and mental retardation) 759.89
LAV (disease) (illness) (infection) — *see* Human immunodeficiency virus (disease) (illness) (infection)
LAV/HTLV-III (disease) (illness) (infection) — *see* Human immunodeficiency virus (disease) (illness) (infection)
Lawford's syndrome (encephalocutaneous angiomatosis) 759.6
Lax, laxity — *see also* Relaxation
  ligament 728.4
  skin (acquired) 701.8
    congenital 756.83
Laxative habit (*see also* Abuse, drugs, nondependent) 305.9 ☑5ᵗʰ
Lazy leukocyte syndrome 288.0
Lead — *see also* condition
  exposure to V15.86
  incrustation of cornea 371.15
  poisoning 984.9
    specified type of lead — *see* Table of Drugs and Chemicals
Lead miners' lung 503
Leakage
  amniotic fluid 658.1 ☑5ᵗʰ
    with delayed delivery 658.2 ☑5ᵗʰ
    affecting fetus or newborn 761.1
  bile from drainage tube (T tube) 997.4
  blood (microscopic), fetal, into maternal circulation 656.0 ☑5ᵗʰ
    affecting management of pregnancy or puerperium 656.0 ☑5ᵗʰ
  device, implant, or graft — *see* Complications, mechanical
  spinal fluid at lumbar puncture site 997.09
  urine, continuous 788.37
Leaky heart — *see* Endocarditis
Learning defect, specific NEC (strephosymbolia) 315.2
Leather bottle stomach (M8142/3) 151.9
Leber's
  congenital amaurosis 362.76
  optic atrophy (hereditary) 377.16
Lederer's anemia or disease (acquired infectious hemolytic anemia) 283.19
Lederer-Brill syndrome (acquired infectious hemolytic anemia) 283.19
Leeches (aquatic) (land) 134.2
Left-sided neglect 781.8
Leg — *see* condition
Legal investigation V62.5
Legg (-Calvé) -Perthes disease or syndrome (osteochondrosis, femoral capital) 732.1
Legionnaires' disease 482.84
Leigh's disease 330.8
Leiner's disease (exfoliative dermatitis) 695.89
Leiofibromyoma (M8890/0) — *see also* Leiomyoma
  uterus (cervix) (corpus) (*see also* Leiomyoma, uterus) 218.9
Leiomyoblastoma (M8891/1) — *see* Neoplasm, connective tissue, uncertain behavior

Leiomyofibroma (M8890/0) — *see also* Neoplasm, connective tissue, benign
  uterus (cervix) (corpus) (*see also* Leiomyoma, uterus) 218.9
Leiomyoma (M8890/0) — *see also* Neoplasm, connective tissue, benign
  bizarre (M8893/0) — *see* Neoplasm, connective tissue, benign
  cellular (M8892/1) — *see* Neoplasm, connective tissue, uncertain behavior
  epithelioid (M8891/1) — *see* Neoplasm, connective tissue, uncertain behavior
  prostate (polypoid) 600.2
  uterus (cervix) (corpus) 218.9
    interstitial 218.1
    intramural 218.1
    submucous 218.0
    subperitoneal 218.2
    subserous 218.2
  vascular (M8894/0) — *see* Neoplasm, connective tissue, benign
Leiomyomatosis (intravascular) (M8890/1) — *see* Neoplasm, connective tissue, uncertain behavior
Leiomyosarcoma (M8890/3) — *see also* Neoplasm, connective tissue, malignant
  epithelioid (M8891/3) — *see* Neoplasm, connective tissue, malignant
Leishmaniasis 085.9
  American 085.5
    cutaneous 085.4
    mucocutaneous 085.5
  Asian desert 085.2
  Brazilian 085.5
  cutaneous 085.9
    acute necrotizing 085.2
    American 085.4
    Asian desert 085.2
    diffuse 085.3
    dry form 085.1
    Ethiopian 085.3
    eyelid 085.5 *[373.6]*
    late 085.1
    lepromatous 085.3
    recurrent 085.1
    rural 085.2
    ulcerating 085.1
    urban 085.1
    wet form 085.2
    zoonotic form 085.2
  dermal — *see also* Leishmaniasis, cutaneous
    post kala-azar 085.0
  eyelid 085.5 *[373.6]*
  infantile 085.0
  Mediterranean 085.0
  mucocutaneous (American) 085.5
  naso-oral 085.5
  nasopharyngeal 085.5
  Old World 085.1
  tegumentaria diffusa 085.4
  vaccination, prophylactic (against) V05.2
  visceral (Indian) 085.0
Leishmanoid, dermal — *see also* Leishmaniasis, cutaneous
  post kala-azar 085.0
Leloir's disease 695.4
Lenegre's disease 426.0
Lengthening, leg 736.81
Lennox's syndrome (*see also* Epilepsy) 345.0 ☑5ᵗʰ
Lens — *see* condition
Lenticonus (anterior) (posterior) (congenital) 743.36
Lenticular degeneration, progressive 275.1
Lentiglobus (posterior) (congenital) 743.36
Lentigo (congenital) 709.09
  juvenile 709.09
  Maligna (M8742/2) — *see also* Neoplasm, skin, in situ
    melanoma (M8742/3) — *see* Melanoma
  senile 709.09
Leonine leprosy 030.0
Leontiasis
  ossium 733.3
  syphilitic 095.8
    congenital 090.5

Léopold-Lévi's syndrome (paroxysmal thyroid instability) 242.9 ☑5ᵗʰ

Lepore hemoglobin syndrome 282.4

Lepothrix 039.0

Lepra 030.9
Willan's 696.1

Leprechaunism 259.8

Lepromatous leprosy 030.0

Leprosy 030.9
anesthetic 030.1
beriberi 030.1
borderline (group B) (infiltrated) (neuritic) 030.3
cornea (see also Leprosy, by type) 030.9 [371.89]
dimorphous (group B) (infiltrated) (lepromatous) (neuritic) (tuberculoid) 030.3
eyelid 030.0 [373.4]
indeterminate (group I) (macular) (neuritic) (uncharacteristic) 030.2
leonine 030.0
lepromatous (diffuse) (infiltrated) (macular) (neuritic) (nodular) (type L) 030.0
macular (early) (neuritic) (simple) 030.2
maculoanesthetic 030.1
mixed 030.0
neuro 030.1
nodular 030.0
primary neuritic 030.3
specified type or group NEC 030.8
tubercular 030.1
tuberculoid (macular) (maculoanesthetic) (major) (minor) (neuritic) (type T) 030.1

Leptocytosis, hereditary 282.4

Leptomeningitis (chronic) (circumscribed) (hemorrhagic) (nonsuppurative) (see also Meningitis) 322.9
aseptic 047.9
adenovirus 049.1
Coxsackie virus 047.0
ECHO virus 047.1
enterovirus 047.9
lymphocytic choriomeningitis 049.0
epidemic 036.0
late effect — see category 326
meningococcal 036.0
pneumococcal 320.1
syphilitic 094.2
tuberculous (see also Tuberculosis, meninges) 013.0 ☑5ᵗʰ

Leptomeningopathy (see also Meningitis) 322.9

Leptospiral — see condition

Leptospirochetal — see condition

Leptospirosis 100.9
autumnalis 100.89
canicula 100.89
grippotyphosa 100.89
hebdomidis 100.89
icterohemorrhagica 100.0
nanukayami 100.89
pomona 100.89
Weil's disease 100.0

Leptothricosis — see Actinomycosis

Leptothrix infestation — see Actinomycosis

Leptotricosis — see Actinomycosis

Leptus dermatitis 133.8

Léris pleonosteosis 756.89

Léri-Weill syndrome 756.59

Leriche's syndrome (aortic bifurcation occlusion) 444.0

Lermoyez's syndrome (see also Disease, Ménière's) 386.00

Lesbianism — omit code
ego-dystonic 302.0
problems with 302.0

Lesch-Nyhan syndrome (hypoxanthineguanine-phosphoribosyltransferase deficiency) 277.2

Lesion
abducens nerve 378.54
alveolar process 525.8
anorectal 569.49
aortic (valve) — see Endocarditis, aortic
auditory nerve 388.5
basal ganglion 333.90

Lesion — continued
bile duct (see also Disease, biliary) 576.8
bladder 596.9
bone 733.90
brachial plexus 353.0
brain 348.8
congenital 742.9
vascular (see also Lesion, cerebrovascular) 437.9
degenerative 437.1
healed or old without residuals V12.59
hypertensive 437.2
late effect — see Late effect(s) (of) cerebrovascular disease
buccal 528.9
calcified — see Calcification
canthus 373.9
carate — see Pinta, lesions
cardia 537.89
cardiac — see also Disease, heart
congenital 746.9
valvular — see Endocarditis
cauda equina 344.60
with neurogenic bladder 344.61
cecum 569.89
cerebral — see Lesion, brain
cerebrovascular (see also Disease, cerebrovascular NEC) 437.9
degenerative 437.1
healed or old without residuals V12.59
hypertensive 437.2
specified type NEC 437.8
cervical root (nerve) NEC 353.2
chiasmal 377.54
associated with
inflammatory disorders 377.54
neoplasm NEC 377.52
pituitary 377.51
pituitary disorders 377.51
vascular disorders 377.53
chorda tympani 351.8
coin, lung 793.1
colon 569.89
congenital — see Anomaly
conjunctiva 372.9
coronary artery (see also Ischemia, heart) 414.9
cranial nerve 352.9
first 352.0
second 377.49
third
partial 378.51
total 378.52
fourth 378.53
fifth 350.9
sixth 378.54
seventh 351.9
eighth 388.5
ninth 352.2
tenth 352.3
eleventh 352.4
twelfth 352.5
cystic — see Cyst
degenerative — see Degeneration
dermal (skin) 709.9
Dieulafoy (hemorrhagic) ●
of ●
duodenum 537.84 ●
intestine 569.86 ●
stomach 537.84 ●
duodenum 537.89
with obstruction 537.3
eyelid 373.9
gasserian ganglion 350.8
gastric 537.89
gastroduodenal 537.89
gastrointestinal 569.89
glossopharyngeal nerve 352.2
heart (organic) — see also Disease, heart
vascular — see Disease, cardiovascular
helix (ear) 709.9
hyperchromic, due to pinta (carate) 103.1
hyperkeratotic (see also Hyperkeratosis) 701.1
hypoglossal nerve 352.5
hypopharynx 478.29
hypothalamic 253.9
ileocecal coil 569.89
ileum 569.89

Lesion — continued
iliohypogastric nerve 355.79
ilioinguinal nerve 355.79
in continuity — see Injury, nerve, by site
inflammatory — see Inflammation
intestine 569.89
intracerebral — see Lesion, brain
intrachiasmal (optic) (see also Lesion, chiasmal) 377.54
intracranial, space-occupying NEC 784.2
joint 719.90
ankle 719.97
elbow 719.92
foot 719.97
hand 719.94
hip 719.95
knee 719.96
multiple sites 719.99
pelvic region 719.95
sacroiliac (old) 724.6
shoulder (region) 719.91
specified site NEC 719.98
wrist 719.93
keratotic (see also Keratosis) 701.1
kidney (see also Disease, renal) 593.9
laryngeal nerve (recurrent) 352.3
leonine 030.0
lip 528.5
liver 573.8
lumbosacral
plexus 353.1
root (nerve) NEC 353.4
lung 518.89
coin 793.1
maxillary sinus 473.0
mitral — see Endocarditis, mitral
motor cortex 348.8
nerve (see also Disorder, nerve) 355.9
nervous system 349.9
congenital 742.9
nonallopathic NEC 739.9
in region (of)
abdomen 739.9
acromioclavicular 739.7
cervical, cervicothoracic 739.1
costochondral 739.8
costovertebral 739.8
extremity
lower 739.6
upper 739.7
head 739.0
hip 739.5
lower extremity 739.6
lumbar, lumbosacral 739.3
occipitocervical 739.0
pelvic 739.5
pubic 739.5
rib cage 739.8
sacral, sacrococcygeal, sacroiliac 739.4
sternochondral 739.8
sternoclavicular 739.7
thoracic, thoracolumbar 739.2
upper extremity 739.7
nose (internal) 478.1
obstructive — see Obstruction
obturator nerve 355.79
occlusive
artery — see Embolism, artery
organ or site NEC — see Disease, by site
osteolytic 733.90
paramacular, of retina 363.32
peptic 537.89
periodontal, due to traumatic occlusion 523.8
perirectal 569.49
peritoneum (granulomatous) 568.89
pigmented (skin) 709.00
pinta — see Pinta, lesions
polypoid — see Polyp
prechiasmal (optic) (see also Lesion, chiasmal) 377.54
primary — see also Syphilis, primary
carate 103.0
pinta 103.0
yaws 102.0
pulmonary 518.89
valve (see also Endocarditis, pulmonary) 424.3

☑4ᵗʰ Fourth-digit Required   ☑5ᵗʰ Fifth-digit Required   ▶◀ Revised Text   ● New Line   ▲ Revised Code

Lesion — *continued*
pylorus 537.89
radiation NEC 990
radium NEC 990
rectosigmoid 569.89
retina, retinal — *see also* Retinopathy
  vascular 362.17
retroperitoneal 568.89
romanus 720.1
sacroiliac (joint) 724.6
salivary gland 527.8
  benign lymphoepithelial 527.8
saphenous nerve 355.79
secondary — *see* Syphilis, secondary
sigmoid 569.89
sinus (accessory) (nasal) (*see also* Sinusitis)
  473.9
skin 709.9
  suppurative 686.00
SLAP (superior glenoid labrum) 840.7
space-occupying, intracranial NEC 784.2
spinal cord 336.9
  congenital 742.9
  traumatic (complete) (incomplete)
    (transverse) — *see also* Injury, spinal,
    by site
    with
      broken
        back — *see* Fracture, vertebra, by
          site, with spinal cord injury
        neck — *see* Fracture, vertebra,
          cervical, with spinal cord
          injury
      fracture, vertebra — *see* Fracture,
        vertebra, by site, with spinal
        cord injury
spleen 289.50
stomach 537.89
superior glenoid labrum (SLAP) 840.7
syphilitic — *see* Syphilis
tertiary — *see* Syphilis, tertiary
thoracic root (nerve) 353.3
tonsillar fossa 474.9
tooth, teeth 525.8
  white spot 521.01
traumatic NEC (*see also* nature and site of
  injury) 959.9
tricuspid (valve) — *see* Endocarditis, tricuspid
trigeminal nerve 350.9
ulcerated or ulcerative — *see* Ulcer
uterus NEC 621.9
vagina 623.8
vagus nerve 352.3
valvular — *see* Endocarditis
vascular 459.9
  affecting central nervous system (*see also*
    Lesion, cerebrovascular) 437.9
  following trauma (*see also* Injury, blood
    vessel, by site) 904.9
  retina 362.17
  traumatic — *see* Injury, blood vessel, by site
  umbilical cord 663.6 ✓5ᵗʰ
    affecting fetus or newborn 762.6
visual
  cortex NEC (*see also* Disorder, visual, cortex)
    377.73
  pathway NEC (*see also* Disorder, visual,
    pathway) 377.63
warty — *see* Verruca
white spot, on teeth 521.01
x-ray NEC 990
Lethargic — *see* condition
Lethargy 780.79
Letterer-Siwe disease (acute histiocytosis X)
  (M9722/3) 202.5 ✓5ᵗʰ
Leucinosis 270.3
Leucocoria 360.44
Leucosarcoma (M9850/3) 207.8 ✓5ᵗʰ
Leukasmus 270.2

Leukemia, leukemic (congenital) (M9800/3)
  208.9 ✓5ᵗʰ

> *Note* — Use the following fifth-digit
> subclassification for categories 203–208:
>
>   0   without mention of remission
>   1   with remission

  acute NEC (M9801/3) 208.0 ✓5ᵗʰ
  aleukemic NEC (M9804/3) 208.8 ✓5ᵗʰ
    granulocytic (M9864/3) 205.8 ✓5ᵗʰ
  basophilic (M9870/3) 205.1 ✓5ᵗʰ
  blast (cell) (M9801/3) 208.0 ✓5ᵗʰ
  blastic (M9801/3) 208.0 ✓5ᵗʰ
    granulocytic (M9861/3) 205.0 ✓5ᵗʰ
  chronic NEC (M9803/3) 208.1 ✓5ᵗʰ
  compound (M9810/3) 207.8 ✓5ᵗʰ
  eosinophilic (M9880/3) 205.1 ✓5ᵗʰ
  giant cell (M9910/3) 207.2 ✓5ᵗʰ
  granulocytic (M9860/3) 205.9 ✓5ᵗʰ
    acute (M9861/3) 205.0 ✓5ᵗʰ
    aleukemic (M9864/3) 205.8 ✓5ᵗʰ
    blastic (M9861/3) 205.0 ✓5ᵗʰ
    chronic (M9863/3) 205.1 ✓5ᵗʰ
    subacute (M9862/3) 205.2 ✓5ᵗʰ
    subleukemic (M9864/3) 205.8 ✓5ᵗʰ
  hairy cell (M9940/3) 202.4 ✓5ᵗʰ
  hemoblastic (M9801/3) 208.0 ✓5ᵗʰ
  histiocytic (M9890/3) 206.9 ✓5ᵗʰ
  lymphatic (M9820/3) 204.9 ✓5ᵗʰ
    acute (M9821/3) 204.0 ✓5ᵗʰ
    aleukemic (M9824/3) 204.8 ✓5ᵗʰ
    chronic (M9823/3) 204.1 ✓5ᵗʰ
    subacute (M9822/3) 204.2 ✓5ᵗʰ
    subleukemic (M9824/3) 204.8 ✓5ᵗʰ
  lymphoblastic (M9821/3) 204.0 ✓5ᵗʰ
  lymphocytic (M9820/3) 204.9 ✓5ᵗʰ
    acute (M9821/3) 204.0 ✓5ᵗʰ
    aleukemic (M9824/3) 204.8 ✓5ᵗʰ
    chronic (M9823/3) 204.1 ✓5ᵗʰ
    subacute (M9822/3) 204.2 ✓5ᵗʰ
    subleukemic (M9824/3) 204.8 ✓5ᵗʰ
  lymphogenous (M9820/3) — *see* Leukemia,
    lymphoid
  lymphoid (M9820/3) 204.9 ✓5ᵗʰ
    acute (M9821/3) 204.0 ✓5ᵗʰ
    aleukemic (M9824/3) 204.8 ✓5ᵗʰ
    blastic (M9821/3) 204.0 ✓5ᵗʰ
    chronic (M9823/3) 204.1 ✓5ᵗʰ
    subacute (M9822/3) 204.2 ✓5ᵗʰ
    subleukemic (M9824/3) 204.8 ✓5ᵗʰ
  lymphosarcoma cell (M9850/3) 207.8 ✓5ᵗʰ
  mast cell (M9900/3) 207.8 ✓5ᵗʰ
  megakaryocytic (M9910/3) 207.2 ✓5ᵗʰ
  megakaryocytoid (M9910/3) 207.2 ✓5ᵗʰ
  mixed (cell) (M9810/3) 207.8 ✓5ᵗʰ
  monoblastic (M9891/3) 206.0 ✓5ᵗʰ
  monocytic (Schilling-type) (M9890/3) 206.9 ✓5ᵗʰ
    acute (M9891/3) 206.0 ✓5ᵗʰ
    aleukemic (M9894/3) 206.8 ✓5ᵗʰ
    chronic (M9893/3) 206.1 ✓5ᵗʰ
    Naegeli-type (M9863/3) 205.1 ✓5ᵗʰ
    subacute (M9892/3) 206.2 ✓5ᵗʰ
    subleukemic (M9894/3) 206.8 ✓5ᵗʰ
  monocytoid (M9890/3) 206.9 ✓5ᵗʰ
    acute (M9891/3) 206.0 ✓5ᵗʰ
    aleukemic (M9894/3) 206.8 ✓5ᵗʰ
    chronic (M9893/3) 206.1 ✓5ᵗʰ
    myelogenous (M9863/3) 205.1 ✓5ᵗʰ
    subacute (M9892/3) 206.2 ✓5ᵗʰ
    subleukemic (M9894/3) 206.8 ✓5ᵗʰ
  monomyelocytic (M9860/3) — *see* Leukemia,
    myelomonocytic
  myeloblastic (M9861/3) 205.0 ✓5ᵗʰ
  myelocytic (M9863/3) 205.1 ✓5ᵗʰ
    acute (M9861/3) 205.0 ✓5ᵗʰ
  myelogenous (M9860/3) 205.9 ✓5ᵗʰ
    acute (M9861/3) 205.0 ✓5ᵗʰ
    aleukemic (M9864/3) 205.8 ✓5ᵗʰ
    chronic (M9863/3) 205.1 ✓5ᵗʰ
    monocytoid (M9863/3) 205.1 ✓5ᵗʰ
    subacute (M9862/3) 205.2 ✓5ᵗʰ
    subleukemic (M9864) 205.8 ✓5ᵗʰ
  myeloid (M9860/3) 205.9 ✓5ᵗʰ
    acute (M9861/3) 205.0 ✓5ᵗʰ
    aleukemic (M9864/3) 205.8 ✓5ᵗʰ
    chronic (M9863/3) 205.1 ✓5ᵗʰ

Leukemia, leukemic — *continued*
  myeloid — *continued*
    subacute (M9862/3) 205.2 ✓5ᵗʰ
    subleukemic (M9864/3) 205.8 ✓5ᵗʰ
  myelomonocytic (M9860/3) 205.9 ✓5ᵗʰ
    acute (M9861/3) 205.0 ✓5ᵗʰ
    chronic (M9863/3) 205.1 ✓5ᵗʰ
  Naegeli-type monocytic (M9863/3) 205.1 ✓5ᵗʰ
  neutrophilic (M9865/3) 205.1 ✓5ᵗʰ
  plasma cell (M9830/3) 203.1 ✓5ᵗʰ
  plasmacytic (M9830/3) 203.1 ✓5ᵗʰ
  prolymphocytic (M9825/3) — *see* Leukemia,
    lymphoid
  promyelocytic, acute (M9866/3) 205.0 ✓5ᵗʰ
  Schilling-type monocytic (M9890/3) — *see*
    Leukemia, monocytic
  stem cell (M9801/3) 208.0 ✓5ᵗʰ
  subacute NEC (M9802/3) 208.2 ✓5ᵗʰ
  subleukemic NEC (M9804/3) 208.8 ✓5ᵗʰ
  thrombocytic (M9910/3) 207.2 ✓5ᵗʰ
  undifferentiated (M9801/3) 208.0 ✓5ᵗʰ
Leukemoid reaction (lymphocytic) (monocytic)
  (myelocytic) 288.8
Leukoclastic vasculitis 446.29
Leukocoria 360.44
Leukocythemia — *see* Leukemia
Leukocytosis 288.8
  basophilic 288.8
  eosinophilic 288.3
  lymphocytic 288.8
  monocytic 288.8
  neutrophilic 288.8
Leukoderma 709.09
  syphilitic 091.3
    late 095.8
Leukodermia (*see also* Leukoderma) 709.09
Leukodystrophy (cerebral) (globoid cell)
  (metachromatic) (progressive) (sudanophilic)
  330.0
Leukoedema, mouth or tongue 528.7
Leukoencephalitis
  acute hemorrhagic (postinfectious) NEC
    136.9 *[323.6]*
    postimmunization or postvaccinal 323.5
  subacute sclerosing 046.2
    van Bogaert's 046.2
  van Bogaert's (sclerosing) 046.2
Leukoencephalopathy (*see also* Encephalitis)
  323.9
  acute necrotizing hemorrhagic (postinfectious)
    136.9 *[323.6]*
    postimmunization or postvaccinal 323.5
  metachromatic 330.0
  multifocal (progressive) 046.3
  progressive multifocal 046.3
Leukoerythroblastosis 289.0
Leukoerythrosis 289.0
Leukokeratosis (*see also* Leukoplakia) 702.8
  mouth 528.6
  nicotina palati 528.7
  tongue 528.6
Leukokoria 360.44
Leukokraurosis vulva, vulvae 624.0
Leukolymphosarcoma (M9850/3) 207.8 ✓5ᵗʰ
Leukoma (cornea) (interfering with central vision)
  371.03
  adherent 371.04
Leukomalacia, periventricular 779.7
Leukomelanopathy, hereditary 288.2
Leukonychia (punctata) (striata) 703.8
  congenital 757.5
Leukopathia
  unguium 703.8
    congenital 757.5
Leukopenia 288.0
  cyclic 288.0
  familial 288.0
  malignant 288.0
  periodic 288.0
  transitory neonatal 776.7
Leukopenic — *see* condition
Leukoplakia 702.8
  anus 569.49

Leukoplakia — Lipomatosis *(side tab)*

Leukoplakia — *continued*
 bladder (postinfectional) 596.8
 buccal 528.6
 cervix (uteri) 622.2
 esophagus 530.83
 gingiva 528.6
 kidney (pelvis) 593.89
 larynx 478.79
 lip 528.6
 mouth 528.6
 oral soft tissue (including tongue) (mucosa)
   528.6
 palate 528.6
 pelvis (kidney) 593.89
 penis (infectional) 607.0
 rectum 569.49
 syphilitic 095.8
 tongue 528.6
 tonsil 478.29
 ureter (postinfectional) 593.89
 urethra (postinfectional) 599.84
 uterus 621.8
 vagina 623.1
 vesical 596.8
 vocal cords 478.5
 vulva 624.0
Leukopolioencephalopathy 330.0
Leukorrhea (vagina) 623.5
 due to trichomonas (vaginalis) 131.00
 trichomonal (Trichomonas vaginalis) 131.00
Leukosarcoma (M9850/3) 207.8 ☑5ᵗʰ
Leukosis (M9800/3) — *see* Leukemia
Lev's disease or syndrome (acquired complete
   heart block) 426.0
Levi's syndrome (pituitary dwarfism) 253.3
Levocardia (isolated) 746.87
 with situs inversus 759.3
Levulosuria 271.2
Lewandowski's disease (primary) (*see also*
   Tuberculosis) 017.0 ☑5ᵗʰ
Lewandowski-Lutz disease (epidermodysplasia
   verruciformis) 078.19
Leyden's disease (periodic vomiting) 536.2
Leyden-Möbius dystrophy 359.1
Leydig cell
 carcinoma (M8650/3)
  specified site — *see* Neoplasm, by site,
    malignant
  unspecified site
    female 183.0
    male 186.9
 tumor (M8650/1)
  benign (M8650/0)
    specified site — *see* Neoplasm, by site,
      benign
    unspecified site
      female 220
      male 222.0
  malignant (M8650/3)
    specified site — *see* Neoplasm, by site,
      malignant
    unspecified site
      female 183.0
      male 186.9
  specified site — *see* Neoplasm, by site,
    uncertain behavior
  unspecified site
    female 236.2
    male 236.4
Leydig-Sertoli cell tumor (M8631/0)
 specified site — *see* Neoplasm, by site, benign
 unspecified site
  female 220
  male 222.0
LGSIL (low grade squamous intraepithelial ●
   dysplasia) 622.1 ●
Liar, pathologic 301.7
Libman-Sacks disease or syndrome
   710.0 *[424.91]*
Lice (infestation) 132.9
 body (pediculus corporis) 132.1
 crab 132.2
 head (pediculus capitis) 132.0

Lice — *continued*
 mixed (classifiable to more than one of the
   categories 132.0-132.2) 132.3
 pubic (pediculus pubis) 132.2
Lichen 697.9
 albus 701.0
 annularis 695.89
 atrophicus 701.0
 corneus obtusus 698.3
 myxedematous 701.8
 nitidus 697.1
 pilaris 757.39
  acquired 701.1
 planopilaris 697.0
 planus (acute) (chronicus) (hypertrophic)
   (verrucous) 697.0
  morphoeicus 701.0
  sclerosus (et atrophicus) 701.0
 ruber 696.4
  acuminatus 696.4
  moniliformis 697.8
  obtusus corneus 698.3
  of Wilson 697.0
  planus 697.0
 sclerosus (et atrophicus) 701.0
 scrofulosus (primary) (*see also* Tuberculosis)
   017.0 ☑5ᵗʰ
 simplex (Vidal's) 698.3
  chronicus 698.3
  circumscriptus 698.3
 spinulosus 757.39
  mycotic 117.9
 striata 697.8
 urticatus 698.2
Lichenification 698.3
 nodular 698.3
Lichenoides tuberculosis (primary) (*see also*
   Tuberculosis) 017.0 ☑5ᵗʰ
Lichtheim's disease or syndrome (subacute
   combined sclerosis with pernicious anemia)
   281.0 *[336.2]*
Lien migrans 289.59
Lientery (*see also* Diarrhea) 787.91
 infectious 009.2
Life circumstance problem NEC V62.89
Li-Fraumeni cancer syndrome 758.3
Ligament — *see* condition
Light-for-dates (infant) 764.0 ☑5ᵗʰ
 with signs of fetal malnutrition 764.1 ☑5ᵗʰ
 affecting management of pregnancy 656.5 ☑5ᵗʰ
Light-headedness 780.4
Lightning (effects) (shock) (stroke) (struck by)
   994.0
 burn — *see* Burn, by site
 foot 266.2
Lightwood's disease or syndrome (renal tubular
   acidosis) 588.8
Lignac's disease (cystinosis) 270.0
Lignac (-de Toni) (-Fanconi) (-Debré) syndrome
   (cystinosis) 270.0
Lignac (-Fanconi) syndrome (cystinosis) 270.0
Ligneous thyroiditis 245.3
Likoff's syndrome (angina in menopausal
   women) 413.9
Limb — *see* condition
Limitation of joint motion (*see also* Stiffness,
   joint) 719.5 ☑5ᵗʰ
 sacroiliac 724.6
Limit dextrinosis 271.0
Limited
 cardiac reserve — *see* Disease, heart
 duction, eye NEC 378.63
Lindau's disease (retinocerebral angiomatosis)
   759.6
Lindau (-von Hippel) disease (angiomatosis
   retinocerebellosa) 759.6
Linea corneae senilis 371.41
Lines
 Beau's (transverse furrows on fingernails)
   703.8
 Harris' 733.91
 Hudson-Stähli 371.11
 Stähli's 371.11

Lingua
 geographical 529.1
 nigra (villosa) 529.3
 plicata 529.5
  congenital 750.13
 tylosis 528.6
Lingual (tongue) — *see also* condition
 thyroid 759.2
Linitis (gastric) 535.4 ☑5ᵗʰ
 plastica (M8142/3) 151.9
Lioderma essentialis (cum melanosis et
   telangiectasia) 757.33
Lip — *see also* condition
 biting 528.9
Lipalgia 272.8
Lipedema — *see* Edema
Lipemia (*see also* Hyperlipidemia) 272.4
 retina, retinalis 272.3
Lipidosis 272.7
 cephalin 272.7
 cerebral (infantile) (juvenile) (late) 330.1
 cerebroretinal 330.1 *[362.71]*
 cerebroside 272.7
 cerebrospinal 272.7
 chemically-induced 272.7
 cholesterol 272.7
 diabetic 250.8 ☑5ᵗʰ *[272.7]*
 dystopic (hereditary) 272.7
 glycolipid 272.7
 hepatosplenomegalic 272.3
 hereditary, dystopic 272.7
 sulfatide 330.0
Lipoadenoma (M8324/0) — *see* Neoplasm, by
   site, benign
Lipoblastoma (M8881/0) — *see* Lipoma, by site
Lipoblastomatosis (M8881/0) — *see* Lipoma, by
   site
Lipochondrodystrophy 277.5
Lipochrome histiocytosis (familial) 288.1
Lipodystrophia progressiva 272.6
Lipodystrophy (progressive) 272.6
 insulin 272.6
 intestinal 040.2
Lipofibroma (M8851/0) — *see* Lipoma, by site
Lipoglycoproteinosis 272.8
Lipogranuloma, sclerosing 709.8
Lipogranulomatosis (disseminated) 272.8
 kidney 272.8
Lipoid — *see also* condition
 histiocytosis 272.7
  essential 272.7
 nephrosis (*see also* Nephrosis) 581.3
 proteinosis of Urbach 272.8
Lipoidemia (*see also* Hyperlipidemia) 272.4
Lipoidosis (*see also* Lipidosis) 272.7
Lipoma (M8850/0) 214.9
 breast (skin) 214.1
 face 214.0
 fetal (M8881/0) — *see also* Lipoma, by site
  fat cell (M8880/0) — *see* Lipoma, by site
 infiltrating (M8856/0) — *see* Lipoma, by site
 intra-abdominal 214.3
 intramuscular (M8856/0) — *see* Lipoma, by
   site
 intrathoracic 214.2
 kidney 214.3
 mediastinum 214.2
 muscle 214.8
 peritoneum 214.3
 retroperitoneum 214.3
 skin 214.1
  face 214.0
 spermatic cord 214.4
 spindle cell (M8857/0) — *see* Lipoma, by site
 stomach 214.3
 subcutaneous tissue 214.1
  face 214.0
 thymus 214.2
 thyroid gland 214.2
Lipomatosis (dolorosa) 272.8
 epidural 214.8
 fetal (M8881/0) — *see* Lipoma, by site

Lipomatosis — *continued*
  Launois-Bensaude's 272.8
Lipomyohemangioma (M8860/0)
  specified site — *see* Neoplasm, connective
    tissue, benign
  unspecified site 223.0
Lipomyoma (M8860/0)
  specified site — *see* Neoplasm, connective
    tissue, benign
  unspecified site 223.0
Lipomyxoma (M8852/0) — *see* Lipoma, by site
Lipomyxosarcoma (M8852/3) — *see* Neoplasm,
  connective tissue, malignant
Lipophagocytosis 289.8
Lipoproteinemia (alpha) 272.4
  broad-beta 272.2
  floating-beta 272.2
  hyper-pre-beta 272.1
Lipoproteinosis (Rössle-Urbach-Wiethe) 272.8
Liposarcoma (M8850/3) — *see also* Neoplasm,
  connective tissue, malignant
  differentiated type (M8851/3) — *see* Neoplasm,
    connective tissue, malignant
  embryonal (M8852/3) — *see* Neoplasm,
    connective tissue, malignant
  mixed type (M8855/3) — *see* Neoplasm,
    connective tissue, malignant
  myxoid (M8852/3) — *see* Neoplasm, connective
    tissue, malignant
  pleomorphic (M8854/3) — *see* Neoplasm,
    connective tissue, malignant
  round cell (M8853/3) — *see* Neoplasm,
    connective tissue, malignant
  well differentiated type (M8851/3) — *see*
    Neoplasm, connective tissue, malignant
Lipsynovitis prepatellaris 272.8
Lipping
  cervix 622.0
  spine (*see also* Spondylosis) 721.90
  vertebra (*see also* Spondylosis) 721.90
Lip pits (mucus), congenital 750.25
Lipschütz disease or ulcer 616.50
Lipuria 791.1
  bilharziasis 120.0
Liquefaction, vitreous humor 379.21
Lisping 307.9
Lissauer's paralysis 094.1
Lissencephalia, lissencephaly 742.2
Listerellose 027.0
Listeriose 027.0
Listeriosis 027.0
  congenital 771.2
  fetal 771.2
  suspected fetal damage affecting management
    of pregnancy 655.4 ✓5ᵗʰ
Listlessness 780.79
Lithemia 790.6
Lithiasis — *see also* Calculus
  hepatic (duct) — *see* Choledocholithiasis
  urinary 592.9
Lithopedion 779.9
  affecting management of pregnancy 656.8 ✓5ᵗʰ
Lithosis (occupational) 502
  with tuberculosis — *see* Tuberculosis,
    pulmonary
Lithuria 791.9
Litigation V62.5
Little
  league elbow 718.82
  stroke syndrome 435.9
Little's disease — *see* Palsy, cerebral
Littre's
  gland — *see* condition
  hernia — *see* Hernia, Littre's
Littritis (*see also* Urethritis) 597.89
Livedo 782.61
  annularis 782.61
  racemose 782.61
  reticularis 782.61
Live flesh 781.0

Liver — *see also* condition
  donor V59.6
Livida, asphyxia
  newborn 768.6
Living
  alone V60.3
  with handicapped person V60.4
Lloyd's syndrome 258.1
Loa loa 125.2
Loasis 125.2
Lobe, lobar — *see* condition
Lobo's disease or blastomycosis 116.2
Lobomycosis 116.2
Lobotomy syndrome 310.0
Lobstein's disease (brittle bones and blue sclera)
  756.51
Lobster-claw hand 755.58
Lobulation (congenital) — *see also* Anomaly,
    specified type NEC, by site
  kidney, fetal 753.3
  liver, abnormal 751.69
  spleen 759.0
Lobule, lobular — *see* condition
Local, localized — *see* condition
Locked bowel or intestine (*see also* Obstruction,
  intestine) 560.9
Locked-in state 344.81
Locked twins 660.5 ✓5ᵗʰ
  affecting fetus or newborn 763.1
Locking
  joint (*see also* Derangement, joint) 718.90
  knee 717.9
Lockjaw (*see also* Tetanus) 037
Locomotor ataxia (progressive) 094.0
Löffler's
  endocarditis 421.0
  eosinophilia or syndrome 518.3
  pneumonia 518.3
  syndrome (eosinophilic pneumonitis) 518.3
Löfgren's syndrome (sarcoidosis) 135
Loiasis 125.2
  eyelid 125.2 *[373.6]*
Loneliness V62.89
Lone star fever 082.8
Long labor 662.1 ✓5ᵗʰ
  affecting fetus or newborn 763.89
  first stage 662.0 ✓5ᵗʰ
  second stage 662.2 ✓5ᵗʰ
Longitudinal stripes or grooves, nails 703.8
  congenital 757.5
Long-term (current) drug use V58.69
  antibiotics V58.62
  anticoagulants V58.61
Loop
  intestine (*see also* Volvulus) 560.2
  intrascleral nerve 379.29
  vascular on papilla (optic) 743.57
Loose — *see also* condition
  body
    in tendon sheath 727.82
    joint 718.10
      ankle 718.17
      elbow 718.12
      foot 718.17
      hand 718.14
      hip 718.15
      knee 717.6
      multiple sites 718.19
      pelvic region 718.15
      prosthetic implant — *see* Complications,
        mechanical
      shoulder (region) 718.11
      specified site NEC 718.18
      wrist 718.13
    cartilage (joint) (*see also* Loose, body, joint)
      718.1 ✓5ᵗʰ
      knee 717.6
    facet (vertebral) 724.9
    prosthetic implant — *see* Complications,
      mechanical

Loose — *see also* condition — *continued*
  sesamoid, joint (*see also* Loose, body, joint)
    718.1 ✓5ᵗʰ
  tooth, teeth 525.8
Loosening epiphysis 732.9
Looser (-Debray) -Milkman syndrome
  (osteomalacia with pseudofractures) 268.2
Lop ear (deformity) 744.29
Lorain's disease or syndrome (pituitary
  dwarfism) 253.3
Lorain-Levi syndrome (pituitary dwarfism) 253.3
Lordosis (acquired) (postural) 737.20
  congenital 754.2
  due to or associated with
    Charcôt-Marie-Tooth disease 356.1 *[737.42]*
    mucopolysaccharidosis 277.5 *[737.42]*
    neurofibromatosis 237.71 *[737.42]*
    osteitis
      deformans 731.0 *[737.42]*
      fibrosa cystica 252.0 *[737.42]*
    osteoporosis (*see also* Osteoporosis)
      733.00 *[737.42]*
    poliomyelitis (*see also* Poliomyelitis)
      138 *[737.42]*
    tuberculosis (*see also* Tuberculosis)
      015.0 ✓5ᵗʰ *[737.42]*
  late effect of rickets 268.1 *[737.42]*
  postlaminectomy 737.21
  postsurgical NEC 737.22
  rachitic 268.1 *[737.42]*
  specified NEC 737.29
  tuberculous (*see also* Tuberculosis)
    015.0 ✓5ᵗʰ *[737.42]*
Loss
  appetite 783.0
    hysterical 300.11
    nonorganic origin 307.59
    psychogenic 307.59
  blood — *see* Hemorrhage
  central vision 368.41
  consciousness 780.09
    transient 780.2
  control, sphincter, rectum 787.6
    nonorganic origin 307.7
  ear ossicle, partial 385.24
  elasticity, skin 782.8
  extremity or member, traumatic, current — *see*
    Amputation, traumatic
  fluid (acute) 276.5
    with
      hypernatremia 276.0
      hyponatremia 276.1
    fetus or newborn 775.5
  hair 704.00
  hearing — *see also* Deafness
    central 389.14
    conductive (air) 389.00
      with sensorineural hearing loss 389.2
      combined types 389.08
      external ear 389.01
      inner ear 389.04
      middle ear 389.03
      multiple types 389.08
      tympanic membrane 389.02
    mixed type 389.2
    nerve 389.12
    neural 389.12
    noise-induced 388.12
    perceptive NEC (*see also* Loss, hearing,
      sensorineural) 389.10
    sensorineural 389.10
      with conductive hearing loss 389.2
      central 389.14
      combined types 389.18
      multiple types 389.18
      neural 389.12
      sensory 389.11
    sensory 389.11
    specified type NEC 389.8
    sudden NEC 388.2
  height 781.91
  labyrinthine reactivity (unilateral) 386.55
    bilateral 386.56
  memory (*see also* Amnesia) 780.99 ▲
    mild, following organic brain damage 310.1

Loss — continued
mind (*see also* Psychosis) 298.9
organ or part — *see* Absence, by site, acquired
sensation 782.0
sense of
smell (*see also* Disturbance, sensation) 781.1
taste (*see also* Disturbance, sensation) 781.1
touch (*see also* Disturbance, sensation) 781.1
sight (acquired) (complete) (congenital) *see* Blindness
spinal fluid
headache 349.0
substance of
bone (*see also* Osteoporosis) 733.00
cartilage 733.99
ear 380.32
vitreous (humor) 379.26
tooth, teeth
acquired 525.10
due to
caries 525.13
extraction 525.10
periodontal disease 525.12
specified NEC 525.19
trauma 525.11
vision, visual (*see also* Blindness) 369.9
both eyes (*see also* Blindness, both eyes) 369.3
complete (*see also* Blindness, both eyes) 369.00
one eye 369.8
sudden 368.11
transient 368.12
vitreous 379.26
voice (*see also* Aphonia) 784.41
weight (cause unknown) 783.21
Lou Gehrig's disease 335.20
Louis-Bar syndrome (ataxia-telangiectasia) 334.8
Louping ill 063.1
Lousiness — *see* Lice
Low
back syndrome 724.2
basal metabolic rate (BMR) 794.7
birthweight 765.1 ✔5ᵗʰ
extreme (less than 1000 grams) 765.0 ✔5ᵗʰ
for gestational age 764.0 ✔5ᵗʰ
status (*see also* Status, low birth weight) V21.30
bladder compliance 596.52
blood pressure (*see also* Hypotension) 458.9
reading (incidental) (isolated) (nonspecific) 796.3
cardiac reserve — *see* Disease, heart
compliance bladder 596.52
frequency deafness — *see* Disorder, hearing
function — *see also* Hypofunction
kidney (*see also* Disease, renal) 593.9
liver 573.9
hemoglobin 285.9
implantation, placenta — *see* Placenta, previa
insertion, placenta — *see* placenta, previa
lying
kidney 593.0
organ or site, congenital — *see* Malposition, congenital
placenta — *see* Placenta, previa
output syndrome (cardiac) (*see also* Failure, heart) 428.9
platelets (blood) (*see also* Thrombocytopenia) 287.5
reserve, kidney (*see also* Disease, renal) 593.9
salt syndrome 593.9
tension glaucoma 365.12
vision 369.9
both eyes 369.20
one eye 369.70
Lowe (-Terrey-MacLachlan) syndrome (oculocerebrorenal dystrophy) 270.8
Lower extremity — *see* condition
Lown (-Ganong) -Levine syndrome (short P-R interval, normal QRS complex, and paroxysmal supraventricular tachycardia) 426.81

LSD reaction (*see also* Abuse, drugs, nondependent) 305.3 ✔5ᵗʰ
L-shaped kidney 753.3
Lucas-Championnière disease (fibrinous bronchitis) 466.0
Lucey-Driscoll syndrome (jaundice due to delayed conjugation) 774.30
Ludwig's
angina 528.3
disease (submaxillary cellulitis) 528.3
Lues (venerea), luetic — *see* Syphilis
Luetscher's syndrome (dehydration) 276.5
Lumbago 724.2
due to displacement, intervertebral disc 722.10
Lumbalgia 724.2
due to displacement, intervertebral disc 722.10
Lumbar — *see* condition
Lumbarization, vertebra 756.15
Lumbermen's itch 133.8
Lump — *see also* Mass
abdominal 789.3 ✔5ᵗʰ
breast 611.72
chest 786.6
epigastric 789.3 ✔5ᵗʰ
head 784.2
kidney 753.3
liver 789.1
lung 786.6
mediastinal 786.6
neck 784.2
nose or sinus 784.2
pelvic 789.3 ✔5ᵗʰ
skin 782.2
substernal 786.6
throat 784.2
umbilicus 789.3 ✔5ᵗʰ
Lunacy (*see also* Psychosis) 298.9
Lunatomalacia 732.3
Lung — *see also* condition
donor V59.8
drug addict's 417.8
mainliners' 417.8
vanishing 492.0
Lupoid (miliary) **of Boeck** 135
Lupus 710.0
Cazenave's (erythematosus) 695.4
discoid (local) 695.4
disseminated 710.0
erythematosus (discoid) (local) 695.4
disseminated 710.0
eyelid 373.34
systemic 710.0
with
encephalitis 710.0 [323.8]
lung involvement 710.0 [517.8]
inhibitor (presence of) 286.5
exedens 017.0 ✔5ᵗʰ
eyelid (*see also* Tuberculosis) 017.0 ✔5ᵗʰ [373.4]
Hilliard's 017.0 ✔5ᵗʰ
hydralazine
correct substance properly administered 695.4
overdose or wrong substance given or taken 972.6
miliaris disseminatus faciei 017.0 ✔5ᵗʰ
nephritis 710.0 [583.81]
acute 710.0 [580.81]
chronic 710.0 [582.81]
nontuberculous, not disseminated 695.4
pernio (Besnier) 135
tuberculous (*see also* Tuberculosis) 017.0 ✔5ᵗʰ
eyelid (*see also* Tuberculosis) 017.0 ✔5ᵗʰ [373.4]
vulgaris 017.0 ✔5ᵗʰ
Luschka's joint disease 721.90
Luteinoma (M8610/0) 220
Lutembacher's disease or syndrome (atrial septal defect with mitral stenosis) 745.5
Luteoma (M8610/0) 220
Lutz-Miescher disease (elastosis perforans serpiginosa) 701.1
Lutz-Splendore-de Almeida disease (Brazilian blastomycosis) 116.1

Luxatio
bulbi due to birth injury 767.8
coxae congenita (*see also* Dislocation, hip, congenital) 754.30
erecta — *see* Dislocation, shoulder
imperfecta — *see* Sprain, by site
perinealis — *see* Dislocation, hip
Luxation — *see also* Dislocation, by site
eyeball 360.81
due to birth injury 767.8
lateral 376.36
genital organs (external) NEC — *see* Wound, open, genital organs
globe (eye) 360.81
lateral 376.36
lacrimal gland (postinfectional) 375.16
lens (old) (partial) 379.32
congenital 743.37
syphilitic 090.49 [379.32]
Marfan's disease 090.49
spontaneous 379.32
penis — *see* Wound, open, penis
scrotum — *see* Wound, open, scrotum
testis — *see* Wound, open, testis
L-xyloketosuria 271.8
Lycanthropy (*see also* Psychosis) 298.9
Lyell's disease or syndrome (toxic epidermal necrolysis) 695.1
due to drug
correct substance properly administered 695.1
overdose or wrong substance given or taken 977.9
specified drug — *see* Table of Drugs and Chemicals
Lyme disease 088.81
Lymph
gland or node — *see* condition
scrotum (*see also* Infestation, filarial) 125.9
Lymphadenitis 289.3
with
abortion — *see* Abortion, by type, with sepsis
ectopic pregnancy (*see also* categories 633.0-633.9) 639.0
molar pregnancy (*see also* categories 630-632) 639.0
acute 683
mesenteric 289.2
any site, except mesenteric 289.3
acute 683
chronic 289.1
mesenteric (acute) (chronic) (nonspecific) (subacute) 289.2
subacute 289.1
mesenteric 289.2
breast, puerperal, postpartum 675.2 ✔5ᵗʰ
chancroidal (congenital) 099.0
chronic 289.1
mesenteric 289.2
dermatopathic 695.89
due to
anthracosis (occupational) 500
Brugia (Wuchereria) malayi 125.1
diphtheria (toxin) 032.89
lymphogranuloma venereum 099.1
Wuchereria bancrofti 125.0
following
abortion 639.0
ectopic or molar pregnancy 639.0
generalized 289.3
gonorrheal 098.89
granulomatous 289.1
infectional 683
mesenteric (acute) (chronic) (nonspecific) (subacute) 289.2
due to Bacillus typhi 002.0
tuberculous (*see also* Tuberculosis) 014.8 ✔5ᵗʰ
mycobacterial 031.8
purulent 683
pyogenic 683
regional 078.3
septic 683
streptococcal 683
subacute, unspecified site 289.1

✔4ᵗʰ Fourth-digit Required ✔5ᵗʰ Fifth-digit Required ▶◀ Revised Text ● New Line ▲ Revised Code

Loss — Lymphadenitis

Lymphadenitis — *continued*
  suppurative 683
  syphilitic (early) (secondary) 091.4
    late 095.8
  tuberculous — *see* Tuberculosis, lymph gland
  venereal 099.1
Lymphadenoid goiter 245.2
Lymphadenopathy (general) 785.6
  due to toxoplasmosis (acquired) 130.7
    congenital (active) 771.2
Lymphadenopathy-associated virus (disease)
  (illness) (infection) — *see* Human
  immunodeficiency virus (disease) (illness)
  (infection)
Lymphadenosis 785.6
  acute 075
Lymphangiectasis 457.1
  conjunctiva 372.89
  postinfectional 457.1
  scrotum 457.1
Lymphangiectatic elephantiasis, nonfilarial
  457.1
Lymphangioendothelioma (M9170/0) 228.1
  malignant (M9170/3) — *see* Neoplasm,
    connective tissue, malignant
Lymphangioma (M9170/0) 228.1
  capillary (M9171/0) 228.1
  cavernous (M9172/0) 228.1
  cystic (M9173/0) 228.1
  malignant (M9170/3) — *see* Neoplasm,
    connective tissue, malignant
Lymphangiomyoma (M9174/0) 228.1
Lymphangiomyomatosis (M9174/1) — *see*
  Neoplasm, connective tissue, uncertain
  behavior
Lymphangiosarcoma (M9170/3) — *see*
  Neoplasm, connective tissue, malignant
Lymphangitis 457.2
  with
    abortion — *see* Abortion, by type, with
      sepsis
    abscess — *see* Abscess, by site
    cellulitis — *see* Abscess, by site
    ectopic pregnancy (*see also* categories
      633.0-633.9) 639.0
    molar pregnancy (*see also* categories 630-
      632) 639.0
  acute (with abscess or cellulitis) 682.9
    specified site — *see* Abscess, by site
  breast, puerperal, postpartum 675.2 ☑5ᵗʰ
  chancroidal 099.0
  chronic (any site) 457.2
  due to
    Brugia (Wuchereria) malayi 125.1
    Wuchereria bancrofti 125.0
  following
    abortion 639.0
    ectopic or molar pregnancy 639.0
  gangrenous 457.2
  penis
    acute 607.2
    gonococcal (acute) 098.0
      chronic or duration of 2 months or more
        098.2
  puerperal, postpartum, childbirth 670 ☑4ᵗʰ
  strumous, tuberculous (*see also* Tuberculosis)
    017.2 ☑5ᵗʰ
  subacute (any site) 457.2
  tuberculous — *see* Tuberculosis, lymph gland
Lymphatic (vessel) — *see* condition
Lymphatism 254.8
  scrofulous (*see also* Tuberculosis) 017.2 ☑5ᵗʰ
Lymphectasia 457.1
Lymphedema (*see also* Elephantiasis) 457.1
  acquired (chronic) 457.1
  chronic hereditary 757.0
  congenital 757.0
  idiopathic hereditary 757.0
  praecox 457.1
  secondary 457.1
  surgical NEC 997.99
    postmastectomy (syndrome) 457.0
Lymph-hemangioma (M9120/0) — *see*
  Hemangioma, by site

Lymphoblastic — *see* condition
Lymphoblastoma (diffuse) (M9630/3) 200.1 ☑5ᵗʰ
  giant follicular (M9690/3) 202.0 ☑5ᵗʰ
  macrofollicular (M9690/3) 202.0 ☑5ᵗʰ
Lymphoblastosis, acute benign 075
Lymphocele 457.8
Lymphocythemia 288.8
Lymphocytic — *see also* condition
  chorioencephalitis (acute) (serous) 049.0
  choriomeningitis (acute) (serous) 049.0
Lymphocytoma (diffuse) (malignant) (M9620/3)
  200.1 ☑5ᵗʰ
Lymphocytomatosis (M9620/3) 200.1 ☑5ᵗʰ
Lymphocytopenia 288.8
Lymphocytosis (symptomatic) 288.8
  infectious (acute) 078.89
Lymphoepithelioma (M8082/3) — *see* Neoplasm,
  by site, malignant
Lymphogranuloma (malignant) (M9650/3)
  201.9 ☑5ᵗʰ
  inguinale 099.1
  venereal (any site) 099.1
    with stricture of rectum 099.1
  venereum 099.1
Lymphogranulomatosis (malignant) (M9650/3)
  201.9 ☑5ᵗʰ
  benign (Boeck's sarcoid) (Schaumann's) 135
  Hodgkin's (M9650/3) 201.9 ☑5ᵗʰ
Lymphoid — *see* condition
Lympholeukoblastoma (M9850/3) 207.8 ☑5ᵗʰ
Lympholeukosarcoma (M9850/3) 207.8 ☑5ᵗʰ
Lymphoma (malignant) (M9590/3) 202.8 ☑5ᵗʰ

> *Note* — *Use the following fifth-digit*
> *subclassification with categories 200–202:*
>
>   0   *unspecified site*
>   1   *lymph nodes of head, face, and*
>   *neck*
>   2   *intrathoracic lymph nodes*
>   3   *intra-abdominal lymph nodes*
>   4   *lymph nodes of axilla and upper*
>   *limb*
>   5   *lymph nodes of inguinal region and*
>   *lower limb*
>   6   *intrapelvic lymph nodes*
>   7   *spleen*
>   8   *lymph nodes of multiple sites*

  benign (M9590/0) — *see* Neoplasm, by site,
    benign
  Burkitt's type (lymphoblastic) (undifferentiated)
    (M9750/3) 200.2 ☑5ᵗʰ
  Castleman's (mediastinal lymph node
    hyperplasia) 785.6
  centroblastic-centrocytic
    diffuse (M9614/3) 202.8 ☑5ᵗʰ
    follicular (M9692/3) 202.0 ☑5ᵗʰ
  centroblastic type (diffuse) (M9632/3)
    202.8 ☑5ᵗʰ
    follicular (M9697/3) 202.0 ☑5ᵗʰ
  centrocytic (M9622/3) 202.8 ☑5ᵗʰ
  compound (M9613/3) 200.8 ☑5ᵗʰ
  convoluted cell type (lymphoblastic) (M9602/3)
    202.8 ☑5ᵗʰ
  diffuse NEC (M9590/3) 202.8 ☑5ᵗʰ
  follicular (giant) (M9690/3) 202.0 ☑5ᵗʰ
    center cell (diffuse) (M9615/3) 202.8 ☑5ᵗʰ
    cleaved (diffuse) (M9623/3) 202.8 ☑5ᵗʰ
      follicular (M9695/3) 202.0 ☑5ᵗʰ
    non-cleaved (diffuse) (M9633/3)
      202.8 ☑5ᵗʰ
      follicular (M9698/3) 202.0 ☑5ᵗʰ
  centroblastic-centrocytic (M9692/3)
    202.0 ☑5ᵗʰ
  centroblastic type (diffuse) (M9697/3) 202.0 ☑5ᵗʰ
  lymphocytic
    intermediate differentiation (M9694/3)
      202.0 ☑5ᵗʰ
    poorly differentiated (M9696/3) 202.0 ☑5ᵗʰ
    mixed (cell type) (lymphocytic-histiocytic)
      (small cell and large cell) (M9691/3)
      202.0 ☑5ᵗʰ

Lymphoma — *continued*
  germinocytic (M9622/3) 202.8 ☑5ᵗʰ
  giant, follicular or follicle (M9690/3) 202.0 ☑5ᵗʰ
  histiocytic (diffuse) (M9640/3) 200.0 ☑5ᵗʰ
    nodular (M9642/3) 200.0 ☑5ᵗʰ
    pleomorphic cell type (M9641/3) 200.0 ☑5ᵗʰ
  Hodgkin's (M9650/3) (*see also* Disease,
    Hodgkin's) 201.9 ☑5ᵗʰ
  immunoblastic (type) (M9612/3) 200.8 ☑5ᵗʰ
  large cell (M9640/3) 200.0 ☑5ᵗʰ
    nodular (M9642/3) 200.0 ☑5ᵗʰ
    pleomorphic cell type (M9641/3) 200.0 ☑5ᵗʰ
  lymphoblastic (diffuse) (M9630/3) 200.1 ☑5ᵗʰ
    Burkitt's type (M9750/3) 200.2 ☑5ᵗʰ
    convoluted cell type (M9602/3) 202.8 ☑5ᵗʰ
  lymphocytic (cell type) (diffuse) (M9620/3)
    200.1 ☑5ᵗʰ
    with plasmacytoid differentiation, diffuse
      (M9611/3) 200.8 ☑5ᵗʰ
    intermediate differentiation (diffuse)
      (M9621/3) 200.1 ☑5ᵗʰ
      follicular (M9694/3) 202.0 ☑5ᵗʰ
      nodular (M9694/3) 202.0 ☑5ᵗʰ
    nodular (M9690/3) 202.0 ☑5ᵗʰ
    poorly differentiated (diffuse) (M9630/3)
      200.1 ☑5ᵗʰ
      follicular (M9696/3) 202.0 ☑5ᵗʰ
      nodular (M9696/3) 202.0 ☑5ᵗʰ
    well differentiated (diffuse) (M9620/3)
      200.1 ☑5ᵗʰ
      follicular (M9693/3) 202.0 ☑5ᵗʰ
      nodular (M9693/3) 202.0 ☑5ᵗʰ
  lymphocytic-histiocytic, mixed (diffuse)
    (M9613/3) 200.8 ☑5ᵗʰ
    follicular (M9691/3) 202.0 ☑5ᵗʰ
    nodular (M9691/3) 202.0 ☑5ᵗʰ
  lymphoplasmacytoid type (M9611/3) 200.8 ☑5ᵗʰ
  lymphosarcoma type (M9610/3) 200.1 ☑5ᵗʰ
  macrofollicular (M9690/3) 202.0 ☑5ᵗʰ
  mixed cell type (diffuse) (M9613/3) 200.8 ☑5ᵗʰ
    follicular (M9691/3) 202.0 ☑5ᵗʰ
    nodular (M9691/3) 202.0 ☑5ᵗʰ
  nodular (M9690/3) 202.0 ☑5ᵗʰ
    histiocytic (M9642/3) 200.0 ☑5ᵗʰ
    lymphocytic (M9690/3) 202.0 ☑5ᵗʰ
      intermediate differentiation (M9694/3)
        202.0 ☑5ᵗʰ
      poorly differentiated (M9696/3) 202.0 ☑5ᵗʰ
    mixed (cell type) (lymphocytic-histiocytic)
      (small cell and large cell) (M9691/3)
      202.0 ☑5ᵗʰ
  non-Hodgkin's type NEC (M9591/3) 202.8 ☑5ᵗʰ
  reticulum cell (type) (M9640/3) 200.0 ☑5ᵗʰ
  small cell and large cell, mixed (diffuse)
    (M9613/3) 200.8 ☑5ᵗʰ
    follicular (M9691/3) 202.0 ☑5ᵗʰ
    nodular (9691/3) 202.0 ☑5ᵗʰ
  stem cell (type) (M9601/3) 202.8 ☑5ᵗʰ
  T-cell 202.1 ☑5ᵗʰ
  undifferentiated (cell type) (non-Burkitt's)
    (M9600/3) 202.8 ☑5ᵗʰ
    Burkitt's type (M9750/3) 200.2 ☑5ᵗʰ
Lymphomatosis (M9590/3) — *see also*
  Lymphoma
  granulomatous 099.1
Lymphopathia
  venereum 099.1
  veneris 099.1
Lymphopenia 288.8
  familial 279.2
Lymphoreticulosis, benign (of inoculation) 078.3
Lymphorrhea 457.8
Lymphosarcoma (M9610/3) 200.1 ☑5ᵗʰ
  diffuse (M9610/3) 200.1 ☑5ᵗʰ
    with plasmacytoid differentiation (M9611/3)
      200.8 ☑5ᵗʰ
    lymphoplasmacytic (M9611/3) 200.8 ☑5ᵗʰ
  follicular (giant) (M9690/3) 202.0 ☑5ᵗʰ
    lymphoblastic (M9696/3) 202.0 ☑5ᵗʰ
    lymphocytic, intermediate differentiation
      (M9694/3) 202.0 ☑5ᵗʰ
    mixed cell type (M9691/3) 202.0 ☑5ᵗʰ
  giant follicular (M9690/3) 202.0 ☑5ᵗʰ
  Hodgkin's (M9650/3) 201.9 ☑5ᵗʰ
  immunoblastic (M9612/3) 200.8 ☑5ᵗʰ

☑4ᵗʰ Fourth-digit Required   ☑5ᵗʰ Fifth-digit Required   ►◄ Revised Text   ● New Line   ▲ Revised Code

Lymphosarcoma — *continued*
  lymphoblastic (diffuse) (M9630/3) 200.1 ✓5ᵗʰ
    follicular (M9696/3) 202.0 ✓5ᵗʰ
    nodular (M9696/3) 202.0 ✓5ᵗʰ
  lymphocytic (diffuse) (M9620/3) 200.1 ✓5ᵗʰ
    intermediate differentiation (diffuse)
        (M9621/3) 200.1 ✓5ᵗʰ
      follicular (M9694/3) 202.0 ✓5ᵗʰ
      nodular (M9694/3) 202.0 ✓5ᵗʰ
  mixed cell type (diffuse) (M9613/3) 200.8 ✓5ᵗʰ
    follicular (M9691/3) 202.0 ✓5ᵗʰ
    nodular (M9691/3) 202.0 ✓5ᵗʰ
  nodular (M9690/3) 202.0 ✓5ᵗʰ
    lymphoblastic (M9696/3) 202.0 ✓5ᵗʰ
    lymphocytic, intermediate differentiation
        (M9694/3) 202.0 ✓5ᵗʰ
    mixed cell type (M9691/3) 202.0 ✓5ᵗʰ
  prolymphocytic (M9631/3) 200.1 ✓5ᵗʰ
  reticulum cell (M9640/3) 200.0 ✓5ᵗʰ
Lymphostasis 457.8
Lypemania (*see also* Melancholia) 296.2 ✓5ᵗʰ
Lyssa 071

M

Macacus ear 744.29
Maceration
  fetus (cause not stated) 779.9
  wet feet, tropical (syndrome) 991.4
Machado-Joseph disease 334.8
Machupo virus hemorrhagic fever 078.7
Macleod's syndrome (abnormal transradiancy,
    one lung) 492.8
Macrocephalia, macrocephaly 756.0
Macrocheilia (congenital) 744.81
Macrochilia (congenital) 744.81
Macrocolon (congenital) 751.3
Macrocornea 743.41
  associated with buphthalmos 743.22
Macrocytic — *see* condition
Macrocytosis 289.8
Macrodactylia, macrodactylism (fingers)
    (thumbs) 755.57
  toes 755.65
Macrodontia 520.2
Macroencephaly 742.4
Macrogenia 524.05
Macrogenitosomia (female) (male) (praecox) 255.2
Macrogingivae 523.8
Macroglobulinemia (essential) (idiopathic)
    (monoclonal) (primary) (syndrome)
    (Waldenström's) 273.3
Macroglossia (congenital) 750.15
  acquired 529.8
Macrognathia, macrognathism (congenital)
    524.00
  mandibular 524.02
    alveolar 524.72
  maxillary 524.01
    alveolar 524.71
Macrogyria (congenital) 742.4
Macrohydrocephalus (*see also* Hydrocephalus)
    331.4
Macromastia (*see also* Hypertrophy, breast) 611.1
Macropsia 368.14
Macrosigmoid 564.7
  congenital 751.3
Macrospondylitis, acromegalic 253.0
Macrostomia (congenital) 744.83
Macrotia (external ear) (congenital) 744.22
Macula
  cornea, corneal
    congenital 743.43
      interfering with vision 743.42
    interfering with central vision 371.03
    not interfering with central vision 371.02
  degeneration (*see also* Degeneration, macula)
    362.50
    hereditary (*see also* Dystrophy, retina)
      362.70

Macula — *continued*
  edema, cystoid 362.53
Maculae ceruleae 132.1
Macules and papules 709.8
Maculopathy, toxic 362.55
Madarosis 374.55
Madelung's
  deformity (radius) 755.54
  disease (lipomatosis) 272.8
  lipomatosis 272.8
Madness (*see also* Psychosis) 298.9
  myxedema (acute) 293.0
    subacute 293.1
Madura
  disease (actinomycotic) 039.9
    mycotic 117.4
  foot (actinomycotic) 039.4
    mycotic 117.4
Maduromycosis (actinomycotic) 039.9
  mycotic 117.4
Maffucci's syndrome (dyschondroplasia with
    hemangiomas) 756.4
Magenblase syndrome 306.4
Main en griffe (acquired) 736.06
  congenital 755.59
Maintenance
  chemotherapy regimen or treatment V58.1
  dialysis regimen or treatment
    extracorporeal (renal) V56.0
    peritoneal V56.8
    renal V56.0
  drug therapy or regimen V58.1
  external fixation NEC V54.89   ▲
  radiotherapy V58.0
  traction NEC V54.89   ▲
Majocchi's
  disease (purpura annularis telangiectodes)
    709.1
  granuloma 110.6
Major — *see* condition
Mal
  cerebral (idiopathic) (*see also* Epilepsy)
    345.9 ✓5ᵗʰ
  comital (*see also* Epilepsy) 345.9 ✓5ᵗʰ
  de los pintos (*see also* Pinta) 103.9
  de Meleda 757.39
  de mer 994.6
  lie — *see* Presentation, fetal
  perforant (*see also* Ulcer, lower extremity)
    707.15
Malabar itch 110.9
  beard 110.0
  foot 110.4
  scalp 110.0
Malabsorption 579.9
  calcium 579.8
  carbohydrate 579.8
  disaccharide 271.3
  drug-induced 579.8
  due to bacterial overgrowth 579.8
  fat 579.8
  folate, congenital 281.2
  galactose 271.1
  glucose-galactose (congenital) 271.3
  intestinal 579.9
  isomaltose 271.3
  lactose (hereditary) 271.3
  methionine 270.4
  monosaccharide 271.8
  postgastrectomy 579.3
  postsurgical 579.3
  protein 579.8
  sucrose (-isomaltose) (congenital) 271.3
  syndrome 579.9
    postgastrectomy 579.3
    postsurgical 579.3
Malacia, bone 268.2
  juvenile (*see also* Rickets) 268.0
  Kienböck's (juvenile) (lunate) (wrist) 732.3
    adult 732.8
Malacoplakia
  bladder 596.8
  colon 569.89
  pelvis (kidney) 593.89

Malacoplakia — *continued*
  ureter 593.89
  urethra 599.84
Malacosteon 268.2
  juvenile (*see also* Rickets) 268.0
Maladaptation — *see* Maladjustment
Maladie de Roger 745.4
Maladjustment
  conjugal V61.10
    involving divorce or estrangement V61.0
  educational V62.3
  family V61.9
    specified circumstance NEC V61.8
  marital V61.10
    involving divorce or estrangement V61.0
  occupational V62.2
  simple, adult (*see also* Reaction, adjustment)
    309.9
  situational acute (*see also* Reaction,
    adjustment) 309.9
  social V62.4
Malaise 780.79
Malakoplakia — *see* Malacoplakia
Malaria, malarial (fever) 084.6
  algid 084.9
  any type, with
    algid malaria 084.9
    blackwater fever 084.8
    fever
      blackwater 084.8
      hemoglobinuric (bilious) 084.8
    hemoglobinuria, malarial 084.8
    hepatitis 084.9 *[573.2]*
    nephrosis 084.9 *[581.81]*
    pernicious complication NEC 084.9
      cardiac 084.9
      cerebral 084.9
  cardiac 084.9
  carrier (suspected) of V02.9
  cerebral 084.9
  complicating pregnancy, childbirth, or
    puerperium 647.4 ✓5ᵗʰ
  congenital 771.2
  congestion, congestive 084.6
    brain 084.9
  continued 084.0
  estivo-autumnal 084.0
  falciparum (malignant tertian) 084.0
  hematinuria 084.8
  hematuria 084.8
  hemoglobinuria 084.8
  hemorrhagic 084.6
  induced (therapeutically) 084.7
    accidental — *see* Malaria, by type
  liver 084.9 *[573.2]*
  malariae (quartan) 084.2
  malignant (tertian) 084.0
  mixed infections 084.5
  monkey 084.4
  ovale 084.3
  pernicious, acute 084.0
  Plasmodium, P.
    falciparum 084.0
    malariae 084.2
    ovale 084.3
    vivax 084.1
  quartan 084.2
  quotidian 084.0
  recurrent 084.6
    induced (therapeutically) 084.7
      accidental — *see* Malaria, by type
  remittent 084.6
  specified types NEC 084.4
  spleen 084.6
  subtertian 084.0
  tertian (benign) 084.1
    malignant 084.0
  tropical 084.0
  typhoid 084.6
  vivax (benign tertian) 084.1
Malassez's disease (testicular cyst) 608.89
Malassimilation 579.9
Maldescent, testis 752.51

Maldevelopment — *see also* Anomaly, by site
   brain 742.9
   colon 751.5
   hip (joint) 755.63
      congenital dislocation (*see also* Dislocation,
         hip, congenital) 754.30
   mastoid process 756.0
   middle ear, except ossicles 744.03
      ossicles 744.04
   newborn (not malformation) 764.9 ☑5ᵗʰ
   ossicles, ear 744.04
   spine 756.10
   toe 755.66
Male type pelvis 755.69
   with disproportion (fetopelvic) 653.2 ☑5ᵗʰ
      affecting fetus or newborn 763.1
      causing obstructed labor 660.1 ☑5ᵗʰ
         affecting fetus or newborn 763.1
Malformation (congenital) — *see also* Anomaly
   bone 756.9
   bursa 756.9
   circulatory system NEC 747.9
      specified type NEC 747.89
   Chiari
      type I 348.4
      type II (*see also* Spina bifida) 741.0 ☑5ᵗʰ
      type III 742.0
      type IV 742.2
   cochlea 744.05
   digestive system NEC 751.9
      lower 751.5
      specified type NEC 751.8
      upper 750.9
   eye 743.9
   gum 750.9
   heart NEC 746.9
      specified type NEC 746.89
      valve 746.9
   internal ear 744.05
   joint NEC 755.9
      specified type NEC 755.8
   Mondini's (congenital) (malformation, cochlea)
      744.05
   muscle 756.9
   nervous system (central) 742.9
   pelvic organs or tissues
      in pregnancy or childbirth 654.9 ☑5ᵗʰ
         affecting fetus or newborn 763.89
         causing obstructed labor 660.2 ☑5ᵗʰ
            affecting fetus or newborn 763.1
   placenta (*see also* Placenta, abnormal)
      656.7 ☑5ᵗʰ
   respiratory organs 748.9
      specified type NEC 748.8
   Rieger's 743.44
   sense organs NEC 742.9
      specified type NEC 742.8
   skin 757.9
      specified type NEC 757.8
   spinal cord 742.9
   teeth, tooth NEC 520.9
   tendon 756.9
   throat 750.9
   umbilical cord (complicating delivery) 663.9 ☑5ᵗʰ
      affecting fetus or newborn 762.6
   umbilicus 759.9
   urinary system NEC 753.9
      specified type NEC 753.8
Malfunction — *see also* Dysfunction
   arterial graft 996.1
   cardiac pacemaker 996.01
   catheter device — *see* Complications,
      mechanical, catheter
   colostomy 569.62
   cystostomy 997.5
   device, implant, or graft NEC — *see*
      Complications, mechanical
   enteric stoma 569.62
   enterostomy 569.62
   gastroenteric 536.8
   gastrostomy 536.42
   nephrostomy 997.5
   pacemaker — *see* Complications, mechanical,
      pacemaker
   prosthetic device, internal — *see*
      Complications, mechanical
   tracheostomy 519.02

Malfunction — *see also* Dysfunction — *continued*
   vascular graft or shunt 996.1
Malgaigne's fracture (closed) 808.43
   open 808.53
Malherbe's
   calcifying epithelioma (M8110/0) — *see*
      Neoplasm, skin, benign
   tumor (M8110/0) — *see* Neoplasm, skin,
      benign
Malibu disease 919.8
   infected 919.9
Malignancy (M8000/3) — *see* Neoplasm, by site,
   malignant
Malignant — *see* condition
Malingerer, malingering V65.2
Mallet, finger (acquired) 736.1
   congenital 755.59
   late effect of rickets 268.1
Malleus 024
Mallory's bodies 034.1
Mallory-Weiss syndrome 530.7
Malnutrition (calorie) 263.9
   complicating pregnancy 648.9 ☑5ᵗʰ
   degree
      first 263.1
      second 263.0
      third 262
      mild 263.1
      moderate 263.0
      severe 261
         protein-calorie 262
   fetus 764.2 ☑5ᵗʰ
      "light-for-dates" 764.1 ☑5ᵗʰ
   following gastrointestinal surgery 579.3
   intrauterine or fetal 764.2 ☑5ᵗʰ
      fetus or infant "light-for-dates" 764.1 ☑5ᵗʰ
   lack of care, or neglect (child) (infant) 995.52
      adult 995.84
   malignant 260
   mild 263.1
   moderate 263.0
   protein 260
   protein-calorie 263.9
      severe 262
      specified type NEC 263.8
   severe 261
      protein-calorie NEC 262
Malocclusion (teeth) 524.4
   due to
      abnormal swallowing 524.5
      accessory teeth (causing crowding) 524.3
      dentofacial abnormality NEC 524.8
      impacted teeth (causing crowding) 524.3
      missing teeth 524.3
      mouth breathing 524.5
      supernumerary teeth (causing crowding)
         524.3
      thumb sucking 524.5
      tongue, lip, or finger habits 524.5
   temporomandibular (joint) 524.69
Malposition
   cardiac apex (congenital) 746.87
   cervix — *see* Malposition, uterus
   congenital
      adrenal (gland) 759.1
      alimentary tract 751.8
         lower 751.5
         upper 750.8
      aorta 747.21
      appendix 751.5
      arterial trunk 747.29
      artery (peripheral) NEC (*see also*
         Malposition, congenital, peripheral
         vascular system) 747.60
         coronary 746.85
         pulmonary 747.3
      auditory canal 744.29
         causing impairment of hearing 744.02
      auricle (ear) 744.29
         causing impairment of hearing 744.02
         cervical 744.43
      biliary duct or passage 751.69
      bladder (mucosa) 753.8
         exteriorized or extroverted 753.5
      brachial plexus 742.8

Malposition — *continued*
   congenital — *continued*
      brain tissue 742.4
      breast 757.6
      bronchus 748.3
      cardiac apex 746.87
      cecum 751.5
      clavicle 755.51
      colon 751.5
      digestive organ or tract NEC 751.8
         lower 751.5
         upper 750.8
      ear (auricle) (external) 744.29
         ossicles 744.04
      endocrine (gland) NEC 759.2
      epiglottis 748.3
      Eustachian tube 744.24
      eye 743.8
      facial features 744.89
      fallopian tube 752.19
      finger(s) 755.59
         supernumerary 755.01
      foot 755.67
      gallbladder 751.69
      gastrointestinal tract 751.8
      genitalia, genital organ(s) or tract
         female 752.8
            external 752.49
            internal NEC 752.8
         male 752.8
            penis 752.69
      glottis 748.3
      hand 755.59
      heart 746.87
         dextrocardia 746.87
            with complete transposition of viscera
               759.3
      hepatic duct 751.69
      hip (joint) (*see also* Dislocation, hip,
         congenital) 754.30
      intestine (large) (small) 751.5
         with anomalous adhesions, fixation, or
            malrotation 751.4
      joint NEC 755.8
      kidney 753.3
      larynx 748.3
      limb 755.8
         lower 755.69
         upper 755.59
      liver 751.69
      lung (lobe) 748.69
      nail(s) 757.5
      nerve 742.8
      nervous system NEC 742.8
      nose, nasal (septum) 748.1
      organ or site NEC — *see* Anomaly, specified
         type NEC, by site
      ovary 752.0
      pancreas 751.7
      parathyroid (gland) 759.2
      patella 755.64
      peripheral vascular system 747.60
         gastrointestinal 747.61
         lower limb 747.64
         renal 747.62
         specified NEC 747.69
         spinal 747.82
         upper limb 747.63
      pituitary (gland) 759.2
      respiratory organ or system NEC 748.9
      rib (cage) 756.3
         supernumerary in cervical region 756.2
      scapula 755.59
      shoulder 755.59
      spinal cord 742.59
      spine 756.19
      spleen 759.0
      sternum 756.3
      stomach 750.7
      symphysis pubis 755.69
      testis (undescended) 752.51
      thymus (gland) 759.2
      thyroid (gland) (tissue) 759.2
         cartilage 748.3
      toe(s) 755.66
         supernumerary 755.02
      tongue 750.19

Malposition — *continued*
  congenital — *continued*
    trachea 748.3
    uterus 752.3
    vein(s) (peripheral) NEC (*see also*
      Malposition, congenital, peripheral
      vascular system) 747.60
      great 747.49
      portal 747.49
      pulmonary 747.49
      vena cava (inferior) (superior) 747.49
  device, implant, or graft — *see* Complications,
    mechanical
  fetus NEC — (*see also* Presentation, fetal)
    652.9 ✓5ᵗʰ
    with successful version 652.1 ✓5ᵗʰ
    affecting fetus or newborn 763.1
    before labor, affecting fetus or newborn
      761.7
    causing obstructed labor 660.0 ✓5ᵗʰ
    in multiple gestation (one fetus or more)
      652.6 ✓5ᵗʰ
      with locking 660.5 ✓5ᵗʰ
      causing obstructed labor 660.0 ✓5ᵗʰ
  gallbladder — (*see also* Disease, gallbladder)
    575.8
  gastrointestinal tract 569.89
    congenital 751.8
  heart (*see also* Malposition, congenital, heart)
    746.87
  intestine 569.89
    congenital 751.5
  pelvic organs or tissues
    in pregnancy or childbirth 654.4 ✓5ᵗʰ
      affecting fetus or newborn 763.89
      causing obstructed labor 660.2 ✓5ᵗʰ
        affecting fetus or newborn 763.1
  placenta — *see* Placenta, previa
  stomach 537.89
    congenital 750.7
  tooth, teeth (with impaction) 524.3
  uterus or cervix (acquired) (acute) (adherent)
    (any degree) (asymptomatic)
    (postinfectional) (postpartal, old) 621.6
    anteflexion or anteversion (*see also*
      Anteversion, uterus) 621.6
    congenital 752.3
    flexion 621.6
      lateral (*see also* Lateroversion, uterus)
        621.6
    in pregnancy or childbirth 654.4 ✓5ᵗʰ
      affecting fetus or newborn 763.89
      causing obstructed labor 660.2 ✓5ᵗʰ
        affecting fetus or newborn 763.1
    inversion 621.6
    lateral (flexion) (version) (*see also*
      Lateroversion, uterus) 621.6
    lateroflexion (*see also* Lateroversion, uterus)
      621.6
    lateroversion (*see also* Lateroversion, uterus)
      621.6
    retroflexion or retroversion (*see also*
      Retroversion, uterus) 621.6
Malposture 729.9
Malpresentation, fetus — (*see also* Presentation,
  fetal) 652.9 ✓5ᵗʰ
Malrotation
  cecum 751.4
  colon 751.4
  intestine 751.4
  kidney 753.3
Malta fever (*see also* Brucellosis) 023.9
Maltosuria 271.3
Maltreatment (of)
  adult 995.80
    emotional 995.82
    multiple forms 995.85
    neglect (nutritional) 995.84
    physical 995.81
    psychological 995.82
    sexual 995.83
  child 995.50
    emotional 995.51
    multiple forms 995.59
    neglect (nutritional) 995.52

Maltreatment — *continued*
  child — *continued*
    physical 995.54
      shaken infant syndrome 995.55
    psychological 995.51
    sexual 995.53
  spouse 995.80 — (*see also* Maltreatment,
    adult)
Malt workers' lung 495.4
Malum coxae senilis 715.25
Malunion, fracture 733.81
Mammillitis (*see also* Mastitis) 611.0
  puerperal, postpartum 675.2 ✓5ᵗʰ
Mammitis (*see also* Mastitis) 611.0
  puerperal, postpartum 675.2 ✓5ᵗʰ
Mammographic microcalcification 793.81
Mammoplasia 611.1
Management
  contraceptive V25.9
    specified type NEC V25.8
  procreative V26.9
    specified type NEC V26.8
Mangled NEC (*see also* nature and site of injury)
  959.9
Mania (monopolar) — (*see also* Psychosis,
  affective) 296.0 ✓5ᵗʰ
  alcoholic (acute) (chronic) 291.9
  Bell's — *see* Mania, chronic
  chronic 296.0 ✓5ᵗʰ
    recurrent episode 296.1 ✓5ᵗʰ
    single episode 296.0 ✓5ᵗʰ
  compulsive 300.3
  delirious (acute) 296.0 ✓5ᵗʰ
    recurrent episode 296.1 ✓5ᵗʰ
    single episode 296.0 ✓5ᵗʰ
  epileptic (*see also* Epilepsy) 345.4 ✓5ᵗʰ
  hysterical 300.10
  inhibited 296.89
  puerperal (after delivery) 296.0 ✓5ᵗʰ
    recurrent episode 296.1 ✓5ᵗʰ
    single episode 296.0 ✓5ᵗʰ
  recurrent episode 296.1 ✓5ᵗʰ
  senile 290.8
  single episode 296.0 ✓5ᵗʰ
  stupor 296.89
  stuporous 296.89
  unproductive 296.89
Manic-depressive insanity, psychosis, reaction,
  or syndrome (*see also* Psychosis, affective)
  296.80
  circular (alternating) 296.7
    currently
      depressed 296.5 ✓5ᵗʰ
      episode unspecified 296.7
      hypomanic, previously depressed
        296.4 ✓5ᵗʰ
      manic 296.4 ✓5ᵗʰ
      mixed 296.6 ✓5ᵗʰ
  depressed (type), depressive 296.2 ✓5ᵗʰ
    atypical 296.82
    recurrent episode 296.3 ✓5ᵗʰ
    single episode 296.2 ✓5ᵗʰ
  hypomanic 296.0 ✓5ᵗʰ
    recurrent episode 296.1 ✓5ᵗʰ
    single episode 296.0 ✓5ᵗʰ
  manic 296.0 ✓5ᵗʰ
    atypical 296.81
    recurrent episode 296.1 ✓5ᵗʰ
    single episode 296.0 ✓5ᵗʰ
  mixed NEC 296.89
  perplexed 296.89
  stuporous 296.89
Manifestations, rheumatoid
  lungs 714.81
  pannus — *see* Arthritis, rheumatoid
  subcutaneous nodules — *see* Arthritis,
    rheumatoid
Mankowsky's syndrome (familial dysplastic
  osteopathy) 731.2
Mannoheptulosuria 271.8
Mannosidosis 271.8
Manson's
  disease (schistosomiasis) 120.1
  pyosis (pemphigus contagiosus) 684
  schistosomiasis 120.1

Mansonellosis 125.5
Manual — *see* condition
Maple bark disease 495.6
Maple bark-strippers' lung 495.6
Maple syrup (urine) disease or syndrome 270.3
Marable's syndrome (celiac artery compression)
  447.4
Marasmus 261
  brain 331.9
  due to malnutrition 261
  intestinal 569.89
  nutritional 261
  senile 797
  tuberculous NEC (*see also* Tuberculosis)
    011.9 ✓5ᵗʰ
Marble
  bones 756.52
  skin 782.61
Marburg disease (virus) 078.89
March
  foot 733.94   ▲
  hemoglobinuria 283.2
Marchand multiple nodular hyperplasia (liver)
  571.5
Marchesani (-Weill) syndrome (brachymorphism
  and ectopia lentis) 759.89
Marchiafava (-Bignami) disease or syndrome
  341.8
Marchiafava-Micheli syndrome (paroxysmal
  nocturnal hemoglobinuria) 283.2
Marcus Gunn's syndrome (jaw-winking
  syndrome) 742.8
Marfan's
  congenital syphilis 090.49
  disease 090.49
  syndrome (arachnodactyly) 759.82
    meaning congenital syphilis 090.49
      with luxation of lens 090.49 [379.32]
Marginal
  implantation, placenta — *see* Placenta, previa
  placenta — *see* Placenta, previa
  sinus (hemorrhage) (rupture) 641.2 ✓5ᵗʰ
    affecting fetus or newborn 762.1
Marie's
  cerebellar ataxia 334.2
  syndrome (acromegaly) 253.0
Marie-Bamberger disease or syndrome
  (hypertrophic) (pulmonary) (secondary)
  731.2
  idiopathic (acropachyderma) 757.39
  primary (acropachyderma) 757.39
Marie-Charcôt-Tooth neuropathic atrophy,
  muscle 356.1
Marie-Strümpell arthritis or disease (ankylosing
  spondylitis) 720.0
Marihuana, marijuana
  abuse (*see also* Abuse, drugs, nondependent)
    305.2 ✓5ᵗʰ
  dependence (*see also* Dependence) 304.3 ✓5ᵗʰ
Marion's disease (bladder neck obstruction)
  596.0
Marital conflict V61.10
Mark
  port wine 757.32
  raspberry 757.32
  strawberry 757.32
  stretch 701.3
  tattoo 709.09
Maroteaux-Lamy syndrome
  (mucopolysaccharidosis VI) 277.5
Marriage license examination V70.3
Marrow (bone)
  arrest 284.9
  megakaryocytic 287.3
  poor function 289.9
Marseilles fever 082.1
Marsh's disease (exophthalmic goiter) 242.0 ✓5ᵗʰ
Marshall's (hidrotic) **ectodermal dysplasia**
  757.31
Marsh fever (*see also* Malaria) 084.6
Martin's disease 715.27

(side tab) Malposition—Martin's disease

Martin-Albright syndrome
(pseudohypoparathyroidism) 275.49
Martorell-Fabre syndrome (pulseless disease) 446.7
Masculinization, female, with adrenal hyperplasia 255.2
Masculinovoblastoma (M8670/0) 220
Masochism 302.83
Masons' lung 502
Mass
abdominal 789.3 ✓5ᵗʰ
anus 787.99
bone 733.90
breast 611.72
cheek 784.2
chest 786.6
cystic — see Cyst
ear 388.8
epigastric 789.3 ✓5ᵗʰ
eye 379.92
female genital organ 625.8
gum 784.2
head 784.2
intracranial 784.2
joint 719.60
ankle 719.67
elbow 719.62
foot 719.67
hand 719.64
hip 719.65
knee 719.66
multiple sites 719.69
pelvic region 719.65
shoulder (region) 719.61
specified site NEC 719.68
wrist 719.63
kidney (see also Disease, kidney) 593.9
lung 786.6
lymph node 785.6
malignant (M8000/3) — see Neoplasm, by site, malignant
mediastinal 786.6
mouth 784.2
muscle (limb) 729.89
neck 784.2
nose or sinus 784.2
palate 784.2
pelvis, pelvic 789.3 ✓5ᵗʰ
penis 607.89
perineum 625.8
rectum 787.99
scrotum 608.89
skin 782.2
specified organ NEC — see Disease of specified organ or site
splenic 789.2
substernal 786.6
thyroid (see also Goiter) 240.9
superficial (localized) 782.2
testes 608.89
throat 784.2
tongue 784.2
umbilicus 789.3 ✓5ᵗʰ
uterus 625.8
vagina 625.8
vulva 625.8
Massive — see condition
Mastalgia 611.71
psychogenic 307.89
Mast cell
disease 757.33
systemic (M9741/3) 202.6 ✓5ᵗʰ
leukemia (M9900/3) 207.8 ✓5ᵗʰ
sarcoma (M9742/3) 202.6 ✓5ᵗʰ
tumor (M9740/1) 238.5
malignant (M9740/3) 202.6 ✓5ᵗʰ
Masters-Allen syndrome 620.6
Mastitis (acute) (adolescent) (diffuse) (interstitial) (lobular) (nonpuerperal) (nonsuppurative) (parenchymatous) (phlegmonous) (simple) (subacute) (suppurative) 611.0
chronic (cystic) (fibrocystic) 610.1
cystic 610.1
Schimmelbusch's type 610.1
fibrocystic 610.1

Mastitis — continued
infective 611.0
lactational 675.2 ✓5ᵗʰ
lymphangitis 611.0
neonatal (noninfective) 778.7
infective 771.5
periductal 610.4
plasma cell 610.4
puerperal, postpartum, (interstitial) (nonpurulent) (parenchymatous) 675.2 ✓5ᵗʰ
purulent 675.1 ✓5ᵗʰ
stagnation 676.2 ✓5ᵗʰ
puerperalis 675.2 ✓5ᵗʰ
retromammary 611.0
puerperal, postpartum 675.1 ✓5ᵗʰ
submammary 611.0
puerperal, postpartum 675.1 ✓5ᵗʰ
Mastocytoma (M9740/1) 238.5
malignant (M9740/3) 202.6 ✓5ᵗʰ
Mastocytosis 757.33
malignant (M9741/3) 202.6 ✓5ᵗʰ
systemic (M9741/3) 202.6 ✓5ᵗʰ
Mastodynia 611.71
psychogenic 307.89
Mastoid — see condition
Mastoidalgia (see also Otalgia) 388.70
Mastoiditis (coalescent) (hemorrhagic) (pneumococcal) (streptococcal) (suppurative) 383.9
acute or subacute 383.00
with
Gradenigo's syndrome 383.02
petrositis 383.02
specified complication NEC 383.02
subperiosteal abscess 383.01
chronic (necrotic) (recurrent) 383.1
tuberculous (see also Tuberculosis) 015.6 ✓5ᵗʰ
Mastopathy, mastopathia 611.9
chronica cystica 610.1
diffuse cystic 610.1
estrogenic 611.8
ovarian origin 611.8
Mastoplasia 611.1
Masturbation 307.9
Maternal condition, affecting fetus or newborn
acute yellow atrophy of liver 760.8
albuminuria 760.1
anesthesia or analgesia 763.5
blood loss 762.1
chorioamnionitis 762.7
circulatory disease, chronic (conditions classifiable to 390-459, 745-747) 760.3
congenital heart disease (conditions classifiable to 745-746) 760.3
cortical necrosis of kidney 760.1
death 761.6
diabetes mellitus 775.0
manifest diabetes in the infant 775.1
disease NEC 760.9
circulatory system, chronic (conditions classifiable to 390-459, 745-747) 760.3
genitourinary system (conditions classifiable to 580-599) 760.1
respiratory (conditions classifiable to 490-519, 748) 760.3
eclampsia 760.0
hemorrhage NEC 762.1
hepatitis acute, malignant, or subacute 760.8
hyperemesis (gravidarum) 761.8
hypertension (arising during pregnancy) (conditions classifiable to 642) 760.0
infection
disease classifiable to 001-136 760.2
genital tract NEC 760.8
urinary tract 760.1
influenza 760.2
manifest influenza in the infant 771.2
injury (conditions classifiable to 800-996) 760.5
malaria 760.2
manifest malaria in infant or fetus 771.2
malnutrition 760.4
necrosis of liver 760.8
nephritis (conditions classifiable to 580-583) 760.1

Maternal condition, affecting fetus or newborn
— continued
nephrosis (conditions classifiable to 581) 760.1
noxious substance transmitted via breast milk or placenta 760.70
alcohol 760.71
anti-infective agents 760.74
cocaine 760.75
"crack" 760.75
diethylstilbestrol [DES] 760.76
hallucinogenic agents 760.73
medicinal agents NEC 760.79
narcotics 760.72
obstetric anesthetic or analgesic drug 760.72
specified agent NEC 760.79
nutritional disorder (conditions classifiable to 260-269) 760.4
operation unrelated to current delivery 760.6
preeclampsia 760.0
pyelitis or pyelonephritis, arising during pregnancy (conditions classifiable to 590) 760.1
renal disease or failure 760.1
respiratory disease, chronic (conditions classifiable to 490-519, 748) 760.3
rheumatic heart disease (chronic) (conditions classifiable to 393-398) 760.3
rubella (conditions classifiable to 056) 760.2
manifest rubella in the infant or fetus 771.0
surgery unrelated to current delivery 760.6
to uterus or pelvic organs 763.89
syphilis (conditions classifiable to 090-097) 760.2
manifest syphilis in the infant or fetus 090.0
thrombophlebitis 760.3
toxemia (of pregnancy) 760.0
preeclamptic 760.0
toxoplasmosis (conditions classifiable to 130) 760.2
manifest toxoplasmosis in the infant or fetus 771.2
transmission of chemical substance through the placenta 760.70
alcohol 760.71
anti-infective 760.74
cocaine 760.75
"crack" 760.75
diethylstilbestrol [DES] 760.76
hallucinogenic agents 760.73
narcotics 760.72
specified substance NEC 760.79
uremia 760.1
urinary tract conditions (conditions classifiable to 580-599) 760.1
vomiting (pernicious) (persistent) (vicious) 761.8
Maternity — see Delivery
Matheiu's disease (leptospiral jaundice) 100.0
Mauclaire's disease or osteochondrosis 732.3
Maxcy's disease 081.0
Maxilla, maxillary — see condition
May (-Hegglin) anomaly or syndrome 288.2
Mayaro fever 066.3
Mazoplasia 610.8
MBD (minimal brain dysfunction), child (see also Hyperkinesia) 314.9
McArdle (-Schmid-Pearson) disease or syndrome (glycogenosis V) 271.0
McCune-Albright syndrome (osteitis fibrosa disseminata) 756.59
MCLS (mucocutaneous lymph node syndrome) 446.1
McQuarrie's syndrome (idiopathic familial hypoglycemia) 251.2
Measles (black) (hemorrhagic) (suppressed) 055.9
with
encephalitis 055.0
keratitis 055.71
keratoconjunctivitis 055.71
otitis media 055.2
pneumonia 055.1
complication 055.8
specified type NEC 055.79
encephalitis 055.0

✓4ᵗʰ Fourth-digit Required   ✓5ᵗʰ Fifth-digit Required   ▶◀ Revised Text   ● New Line   ▲ Revised Code

Measles — continued
French 056.9
German 056.9
keratitis 055.71
keratoconjunctivitis 055.71
liberty 056.9
otitis media 055.2
pneumonia 055.1
specified complications NEC 055.79
vaccination, prophylactic (against) V04.2
Meatitis, urethral (see also Urethritis) 597.89
Meat poisoning — see Poisoning, food
Meatus, meatal — see condition
Meat-wrappers' asthma 506.9
Meckel's
diverticulitis 751.0
diverticulum (displaced) (hypertrophic) 751.0
Meconium
aspiration 770.1
delayed passage in newborn 777.1
ileus 777.1
due to cystic fibrosis 277.01
in liquor 792.3
noted during delivery 656.8 ✓5ᵗʰ
insufflation 770.1
obstruction
fetus or newborn 777.1
in mucoviscidosis 277.01
passage of 792.3
noted during delivery — omit code
peritonitis 777.6
plug syndrome (newborn) NEC 777.1
Median — see also condition
arcuate ligament syndrome 447.4
bar (prostate) 600.9
vesical orifice 600.9
rhomboid glossitis 529.2
Mediastinal shift 793.2
Mediastinitis (acute) (chronic) 519.2
actinomycotic 039.8
syphilitic 095.8
tuberculous (see also Tuberculosis) 012.8 ✓5ᵗʰ
Mediastinopericarditis (see also Pericarditis)
423.9
acute 420.90
chronic 423.8
rheumatic 393
rheumatic, chronic 393
Mediastinum, mediastinal — see condition
Medical services provided for — see Health,
services provided because (of)
Medicine poisoning (by overdose) (wrong
substance given or taken in error) 977.9
specified drug or substance — see Table of
Drugs and Chemicals
Medin's disease (poliomyelitis) 045.9 ✓5ᵗʰ
Mediterranean
anemia (with other hemoglobinopathy) 282.4
disease or syndrome (hemipathic) 282.4
fever (see also Brucellosis) 023.9
familial 277.3
kala-azar 085.0
leishmaniasis 085.0
tick fever 082.1
Medulla — see condition
Medullary
cystic kidney 753.16
sponge kidney 753.17
Medullated fibers
optic (nerve) 743.57
retina 362.85
Medulloblastoma (M9470/3)
desmoplastic (M9471/3) 191.6
specified site — see Neoplasm, by site,
malignant
unspecified site 191.6
Medulloepithelioma (M9501/3) — see also
Neoplasm, by site, malignant
teratoid (M9502/3) — see Neoplasm, by site,
malignant
Medullomyoblastoma (M9472/3)
specified site — see Neoplasm, by site,
malignant

Medullomyoblastoma — continued
unspecified site 191.6
Meekeren-Ehlers-Danlos syndrome 756.83
Megacaryocytic — see condition
Megacolon (acquired) (functional) (not
Hirschsprung's disease) 564.7
aganglionic 751.3
congenital, congenitum 751.3
Hirschsprung's (disease) 751.3
psychogenic 306.4
toxic (see also Colitis, ulcerative) 556.9
Megaduodenum 537.3
Megaesophagus (functional) 530.0
congenital 750.4
Megakaryocytic — see condition
Megalencephaly 742.4
Megalerythema (epidermicum) (infectiosum)
057.0
Megalia, cutis et ossium 757.39
Megaloappendix 751.5
Megalocephalus, megalocephaly NEC 756.0
Megalocornea 743.41
associated with buphthalmos 743.22
Megalocytic anemia 281.9
Megalodactylia (fingers) (thumbs) 755.57
toes 755.65
Megaloduodenum 751.5
Megaloesophagus (functional) 530.0
congenital 750.4
Megalogastria (congenital) 750.7
Megalomania 307.9
Megalophthalmos 743.8
Megalopsia 368.14
Megalosplenia (see also Splenomegaly) 789.2
Megaloureter 593.89
congenital 753.22
Megarectum 569.49
Megasigmoid 564.7
congenital 751.3
Megaureter 593.89
congenital 753.22
Megrim 346.9 ✓5ᵗʰ
Meibomian
cyst 373.2
infected 373.12
gland — see condition
infarct (eyelid) 374.85
stye 373.11
Meibomitis 373.12
Meige
-Milroy disease (chronic hereditary edema)
757.0
syndrome (blepharospasm-oromandibular
dystonia) 333.82
Melalgia, nutritional 266.2
Melancholia (see also Psychosis, affective) 296.90
climacteric 296.2 ✓5ᵗʰ
recurrent episode 296.3 ✓5ᵗʰ
single episode 296.2 ✓5ᵗʰ
hypochondriac 300.7
intermittent 296.2 ✓5ᵗʰ
recurrent episode 296.3 ✓5ᵗʰ
single episode 296.2 ✓5ᵗʰ
involutional 296.2 ✓5ᵗʰ
recurrent episode 296.3 ✓5ᵗʰ
single episode 296.2 ✓5ᵗʰ
menopausal 296.2 ✓5ᵗʰ
recurrent episode 296.3 ✓5ᵗʰ
single episode 296.2 ✓5ᵗʰ
puerperal 296.2 ✓5ᵗʰ
reactive (from emotional stress, psychological
trauma) 298.0
recurrent 296.3 ✓5ᵗʰ
senile 290.21
stuporous 296.2 ✓5ᵗʰ
recurrent episode 296.3 ✓5ᵗʰ
single episode 296.2 ✓5ᵗʰ
Melanemia 275.0
Melanoameloblastoma (M9363/0) — see
Neoplasm, bone, benign
Melanoblastoma (M8720/3) — see Melanoma

Melanoblastosis
Block-Sulzberger 757.33
cutis linearis sive systematisata 757.33
Melanocarcinoma (M8720/3) — see Melanoma
Melanocytoma, eyeball (M8726/0) 224.0
Melanoderma, melanodermia 709.09
Addison's (primary adrenal insufficiency) 255.4
Melanodontia, infantile 521.05
Melanodontoclasia 521.05
Melanoepithelioma (M8720/3) — see Melanoma
Melanoma (malignant) (M8720/3) 172.9

Note — Except where otherwise indicated,
the morphological varieties of melanoma in
the list below should be coded by site as for
"Melanoma (malignant)". Internal sites
should be coded to malignant neoplasm of
those sites.

abdominal wall 172.5
ala nasi 172.3
amelanotic (M8730/3) — see Melanoma, by site
ankle 172.7
anus, anal 154.3
canal 154.2
arm 172.6
auditory canal (external) 172.2
auricle (ear) 172.2
auricular canal (external) 172.2
axilla 172.5
axillary fold 172.5
back 172.5
balloon cell (M8722/3) — see Melanoma, by
site
benign (M8720/0) — see Neoplasm, skin,
benign
breast (female) (male) 172.5
brow 172.3
buttock 172.5
canthus (eye) 172.1
cheek (external) 172.3
chest wall 172.5
chin 172.3
choroid 190.6
conjunctiva 190.3
ear (external) 172.2
epithelioid cell (M8771/3) — see also
Melanoma, by site
and spindle cell, mixed (M8775/3) — see
Melanoma, by site
external meatus (ear) 172.2
eye 190.9
eyebrow 172.3
eyelid (lower) (upper) 172.1
face NEC 172.3
female genital organ (external) NEC 184.4
finger 172.6
flank 172.5
foot 172.7
forearm 172.6
forehead 172.3
foreskin 187.1
gluteal region 172.5
groin 172.5
hand 172.6
heel 172.7
helix 172.2
hip 172.7
in
giant pigmented nevus (M8761/3) — see
Melanoma, by site
Hutchinson's melanotic freckle (M8742/3) —
see Melanoma, by site
junctional nevus (M8740/3) — see
Melanoma, by site
precancerous melanosis (M8741/3) — see
Melanoma, by site
interscapular region 172.5
iris 190.0
jaw 172.3
juvenile (M8770/0) — see Neoplasm, skin,
benign
knee 172.7
labium
majus 184.1
minus 184.2

Melanoma — *continued*
lacrimal gland 190.2
leg 172.7
lip (lower) (upper) 172.0
liver 197.7
lower limb NEC 172.7
male genital organ (external) NEC 187.9
meatus, acoustic (external) 172.2
meibomian gland 172.1
metastatic
of or from specified site — *see* Melanoma, by site
site not of skin — *see* Neoplasm, by site, malignant, secondary
to specified site — *see* Neoplasm, by site, malignant, secondary
unspecified site 172.9
nail 172.9
finger 172.6
toe 172.7
neck 172.4
nodular (M8721/3) — *see* Melanoma, by site
nose, external 172.3
orbit 190.1
penis 187.4
perianal skin 172.5
perineum 172.5
pinna 172.2
popliteal (fossa) (space) 172.7
prepuce 187.1
pubes 172.5
pudendum 184.4
retina 190.5
scalp 172.4
scrotum 187.7
septum nasal (skin) 172.3
shoulder 172.6
skin NEC 172.8
spindle cell (M8772/3) — *see also* Melanoma, by site
type A (M8773/3) 190.0
type B (M8774/3) 190.0
submammary fold 172.5
superficial spreading (M8743/3) — *see* Melanoma, by site
temple 172.3
thigh 172.7
toe 172.7
trunk NEC 172.5
umbilicus 172.5
upper limb NEC 172.6
vagina vault 184.0
vulva 184.4
Melanoplakia 528.9
Melanosarcoma (M8720/3) — *see also* Melanoma
epithelioid cell (M8771/3) — *see* Melanoma
Melanosis 709.09
addisonian (primary adrenal insufficiency) 255.4
tuberculous (*see also* Tuberculosis) 017.6 ✓5ᵗʰ
adrenal 255.4
colon 569.89
conjunctiva 372.55
congenital 743.49
corii degenerativa 757.33
cornea (presenile) (senile) 371.12
congenital 743.43
interfering with vision 743.42
prenatal 743.43
interfering with vision 743.42
eye 372.55
congenital 743.49
jute spinners' 709.09
lenticularis progressiva 757.33
liver 573.8
precancerous (M8741/2) — *see also* Neoplasm, skin, in situ
malignant melanoma in (M8741/3) — *see* Melanoma
Riehl's 709.09
sclera 379.19
congenital 743.47
suprarenal 255.4
tar 709.09
toxic 709.09
Melanuria 791.9

MELAS 758.89
Melasma 709.09
adrenal (gland) 255.4
suprarenal (gland) 255.4
Melena 578.1
due to
swallowed maternal blood 777.3
ulcer — *see* Ulcer, by site, with hemorrhage
newborn 772.4
due to swallowed maternal blood 777.3
Meleney's
gangrene (cutaneous) 686.09
ulcer (chronic undermining) 686.09
Melioidosis 025
Melitensis, febris 023.0
Melitococcosis 023.0
Melkersson (-Rosenthal) syndrome 351.8
Mellitus, diabetes — *see* Diabetes
Melorheostosis (bone) (leri) 733.99
Meloschisis 744.83
Melotia 744.29
Membrana
capsularis lentis posterior 743.39
epipapillaris 743.57
Membranacea placenta — *see* Placenta, abnormal
Membranaceous uterus 621.8
Membrane, membranous — *see also* condition
folds, congenital — *see* Web
Jackson's 751.4
over face (causing asphyxia), fetus or newborn 768.9
premature rupture — *see* Rupture, membranes, premature
pupillary 364.74
persistent 743.46
retained (complicating delivery) (with hemorrhage) 666.2 ✓5ᵗʰ
without hemorrhage 667.1 ✓5ᵗʰ
secondary (eye) 366.50
unruptured (causing asphyxia) 768.9
vitreous humor 379.25
Membranitis, fetal 658.4 ✓5ᵗʰ
affecting fetus or newborn 762.7
Memory disturbance, loss or lack (*see also* Amnesia) 780.99 ▲
mild, following organic brain damage 310.1
Menadione (vitamin K) deficiency 269.0
Menarche, precocious 259.1
Mendacity, pathologic 301.7
Mende's syndrome (ptosis-epicanthus) 270.2
Mendelson's syndrome (resulting from a procedure) 997.3
obstetric 668.0 ✓5ᵗʰ
Ménétrier's disease or syndrome (hypertrophic gastritis) 535.2 ✓5ᵗʰ
Ménière's disease, syndrome, or vertigo 386.00
cochlear 386.02
cochleovestibular 386.01
inactive 386.04
in remission 386.04
vestibular 386.03
Meninges, meningeal — *see* condition
Meningioma (M9530/0) — *see also* Neoplasm, meninges, benign
angioblastic (M9535/0) — *see* Neoplasm, meninges, benign
angiomatous (M9534/0) — *see* Neoplasm, meninges, benign
endotheliomatous (M9531/0) — *see* Neoplasm, meninges, benign
fibroblastic (M9532/0) — *see* Neoplasm, meninges, benign
fibrous (M9532/0) — *see* Neoplasm, meninges, benign
hemangioblastic (M9535/0) — *see* Neoplasm, meninges, benign
hemangiopericytic (M9536/0) — *see* Neoplasm, meninges, benign
malignant (M9530/3) — *see* Neoplasm, meninges, malignant
meningiothelial (M9531/0) — *see* Neoplasm, meninges, benign

Meningioma — *see also* Neoplasm, meninges, benign — *continued*
meningotheliomatous (M9531/0) — *see* Neoplasm, meninges, benign
mixed (M9537/0) — *see* Neoplasm, meninges, benign
multiple (M9530/1) 237.6
papillary (M9538/1) 237.6
psammomatous (M9533/0) — *see* Neoplasm, meninges, benign
syncytial (M9531/0) — *see* Neoplasm, meninges, benign
transitional (M9537/0) — *see* Neoplasm, meninges, benign
Meningiomatosis (diffuse) (M9530/1) 237.6
Meningism (*see also* Meningismus) 781.6
Meningismus (infectional) (pneumococcal) 781.6
due to serum or vaccine 997.09 *[321.8]*
influenzal NEC 487.8
Meningitis (basal) (basic) (basilar) (brain) (cerebral) (cervical) (congestive) (diffuse) (hemorrhagic) (infantile) (membranous) (metastatic) (nonspecific) (pontine) (progressive) (simple) (spinal) (subacute) (sympathetica) (toxic) 322.9
abacterial NEC (*see also* Meningitis, aseptic) 047.9
actinomycotic 039.8 *[320.7]*
adenoviral 049.1
Aerobacter acrogenes 320.82
anaerobes (cocci) (gram-negative) (gram-positive) (mixed) (NEC) 320.81
arbovirus NEC 066.9 *[321.2]*
specified type NEC 066.8 *[321.2]*
aseptic (acute) NEC 047.9
adenovirus 049.1
Coxsackievirus 047.0
due to
adenovirus 049.1
Coxsackievirus 047.0
ECHO virus 047.1
enterovirus 047.9
mumps 072.1
poliovirus (*see also* Poliomyelitis) 045.2 ✓5ᵗʰ *[321.2]*
ECHO virus 047.1
herpes (simplex) virus 054.72
zoster 053.0
leptospiral 100.81
lymphocytic choriomeningitis 049.0
noninfective 322.0
Bacillus pyocyaneus 320.89
bacterial NEC 320.9
anaerobic 320.81
gram-negative 320.82
anaerobic 320.81
Bacteroides (fragilis) (oralis) (melaninogenicus) 320.81
cancerous (M8000/6) 198.4
candidal 112.83
carcinomatous (M8010/6) 198.4
caseous (*see also* Tuberculosis, meninges) 013.0 ✓5ᵗʰ
cerebrospinal (acute) (chronic) (diplococcal) (endemic) (epidemic) (fulminant) (infectious) (malignant) (meningococcal) (sporadic) 036.0
carrier (suspected) of V02.59
chronic NEC 322.2
clear cerebrospinal fluid NEC 322.0
Clostridium (haemolyticum) (novyi) NEC 320.81
coccidioidomycosis 114.2
Coxsackievirus 047.0
cryptococcal 117.5 *[321.0]*
diplococcal 036.0
gram-negative 036.0
gram-positive 320.1
Diplococcus pneumoniae 320.1
due to
actinomycosis 039.8 *[320.7]*
adenovirus 049.1
coccidiomycosis 114.2
enterovirus 047.9
specified NEC 047.8
histoplasmosis (*see also* Histoplasmosis) 115.91
Listerosis 027.0 *[320.7]*

Meningitis — Menopause

Meningitis — continued
due to — continued
Lyme disease 088.81 [320.7]
moniliasis 112.83
mumps 072.1
neurosyphilis 094.2
nonbacterial organisms NEC 321.8
oidiomycosis 112.83
poliovirus (see also Poliomyelitis)
045.2 ✓5ᵗʰ [321.2]
preventive immunization, inoculation, or
vaccination 997.09 [321.8]
sarcoidosis 135 [321.4]
sporotrichosis 117.1 [321.1]
syphilis 094.2
acute 091.81
congenital 090.42
secondary 091.81
trypanosomiasis (see also Trypanosomiasis)
086.9 [321.3]
whooping cough 033.9 [320.7]
E. coli 320.82
ECHO virus 047.1
endothelial-leukocytic, benign, recurrent 047.9
Enterobacter aerogenes 320.82
enteroviral 047.9
specified type NEC 047.8
enterovirus 047.9
specified NEC 047.8
eosinophilic 322.1
epidemic NEC 036.0
Escherichia coli (E. coli) 320.82
Eubacterium 320.81
fibrinopurulent NEC 320.9
specified type NEC 320.89
Friedländer (bacillus) 320.82
fungal NEC 117.9 [321.1]
Fusobacterium 320.81
gonococcal 098.82
gram-negative bacteria NEC 320.82
anaerobic 320.81
cocci 036.0
specified NEC 320.82
gram-negative cocci NEC 036.0
specified NEC 320.82
gram-positive cocci NEC 320.9
H. influenzae 320.0
herpes (simplex) virus 054.72
zoster 053.0
infectious NEC 320.9
influenzal 320.0
Klebsiella pneumoniae 320.82
late effect — see Late, effect, meningitis
leptospiral (aseptic) 100.81
Listerella (monocytogenes) 027.0 [320.7]
Listeria monocytogenes 027.0 [320.7]
lymphocytic (acute) (benign) (serous) 049.0
choriomeningitis virus 049.0
meningococcal (chronic) 036.0
Mima polymorpha 320.82
Mollaret's 047.9
monilial 112.83
mumps (virus) 072.1
mycotic NEC 117.9 [321.1]
Neisseria 036.0
neurosyphilis 094.2
nonbacterial NEC (see also Meningitis, aseptic)
047.9
nonpyogenic NEC 322.0
oidiomycosis 112.83
ossificans 349.2
Peptococcus 320.81
Peptostreptococcus 320.81
pneumococcal 320.1
poliovirus (see also Poliomyelitis)
045.2 ✓5ᵗʰ [321.2]
Proprionibacterium 320.81
Proteus morganii 320.82
Pseudomonas (aeruginosa) (pyocyaneus) 320.82
purulent NEC 320.9
specified organism NEC 320.89
pyogenic NEC 320.9
specified organism NEC 320.89
Salmonella 003.21
septic NEC 320.9
specified organism NEC 320.89
serosa circumscripta NEC 322.0

Meningitis — continued
serous NEC (see also Meningitis, aseptic) 047.9
lymphocytic 049.0
syndrome 348.2
Serratia (marcescens) 320.82
specified organism NEC 320.89
sporadic cerebrospinal 036.0
sporotrichosis 117.1 [321.1]
staphylococcal 320.3
sterile 997.09
streptococcal (acute) 320.2
suppurative 320.9
specified organism NEC 320.89
syphilitic 094.2
acute 091.81
congenital 090.42
secondary 091.81
torula 117.5 [321.0]
traumatic (complication of injury) 958.8
Treponema (denticola) (Macrodenticum) 320.81
trypanosomiasis 086.1 [321.3]
tuberculous (see also Tuberculosis, meninges)
013.0 ✓5ᵗʰ
typhoid 002.0 [320.7]
Veillonella 320.81
Vibrio vulnificus 320.82
viral, virus NEC (see also Meningitis, aseptic)
047.9
Wallgren's (see also Meningitis, aseptic) 047.9
Meningocele (congenital) (spinal) (see also Spina
bifida) 741.9 ✓5ᵗʰ
acquired (traumatic) 349.2
cerebral 742.0
cranial 742.0
Meningocerebritis — see Meningoencephalitis
Meningococcemia (acute) (chronic) 036.2
Meningococcus, meningococcal (see also
condition) 036.9
adrenalitis, hemorrhagic 036.3
carditis 036.40
carrier (suspected) of V02.59
cerebrospinal fever 036.0
encephalitis 036.1
endocarditis 036.42
infection NEC 036.9
meningitis (cerebrospinal) 036.0
myocarditis 036.43
optic neuritis 036.81
pericarditis 036.41
septicemia (chronic) 036.2
Meningoencephalitis (see also Encephalitis)
323.9
acute NEC 048
bacterial, purulent, pyogenic, or septic — see
Meningitis
chronic NEC 094.1
diffuse NEC 094.1
diphasic 063.2
due to
actinomycosis 039.8 [320.7]
blastomycosis NEC (see also Blastomycosis)
116.0 [323.4]
free-living amebae 136.2
Listeria monocytogenes 027.0 [320.7]
Lyme disease 088.81 [320.7]
mumps 072.2
Naegleria (amebae) (gruberi) (organisms)
136.2
rubella 056.01
sporotrichosis 117.1 [321.1]
toxoplasmosis (acquired) 130.0
congenital (active) 771.2 [323.4]
Trypanosoma 086.1 [323.2]
epidemic 036.0
herpes 054.3
herpetic 054.3
H. influenzae 320.0
infectious (acute) 048
influenzal 320.0
late effect — see category 326
Listeria monocytogenes 027.0 [320.7]
lymphocytic (serous) 049.0
mumps 072.2
parasitic NEC 123.9 [323.4]
pneumococcal 320.1
primary amebic 136.2
rubella 056.01

Meningoencephalitis (see also Encephalitis) —
continued
serous 048
lymphocytic 049.0
specific 094.2
staphylococcal 320.3
streptococcal 320.2
syphilitic 094.2
toxic NEC 989.9 [323.7]
due to
carbon tetrachloride 987.8 [323.7]
hydroxyquinoline derivatives poisoning
961.3 [323.7]
lead 984.9 [323.7]
mercury 985.0 [323.7]
thallium 985.8 [323.7]
toxoplasmosis (acquired) 130.0
trypanosomic 086.1 [323.2]
tuberculous (see also Tuberculosis, meninges)
013.0 ✓5ᵗʰ
virus NEC 048
Meningoencephalocele 742.0
syphilitic 094.89
congenital 090.49
Meningoencephalomyelitis (see also
Meningoencephalitis) 323.9
acute NEC 048
disseminated (postinfectious) 136.9 [323.6]
postimmunization or postvaccination
323.5
due to
actinomycosis 039.8 [320.7]
torula 117.5 [323.4]
toxoplasma or toxoplasmosis (acquired)
130.0
congenital (active) 771.2 [323.4]
late effect — see category 326
Meningoencephalomyelopathy (see also
Meningoencephalomyelitis) 349.9
Meningoencephalopathy (see also
Meningoencephalitis) 348.3
Meningoencephalopoliomyelitis (see also
Poliomyelitis, bulbar) 045.0 ✓5ᵗʰ
late effect 138
Meningomyelitis (see also Meningoencephalitis)
323.9
blastomycotic NEC (see also Blastomycosis)
116.0 [323.4]
due to
actinomycosis 039.8 [320.7]
blastomycosis (see also Blastomycosis)
116.0 [323.4]
Meningococcus 036.0
sporotrichosis 117.1 [323.4]
torula 117.5 [323.4]
late effect — see category 326
lethargic 049.8
meningococcal 036.0
syphilitic 094.2
tuberculous (see also Tuberculosis, meninges)
013.0 ✓5ᵗʰ
Meningomyelocele (see also Spina bifida)
741.9 ✓5ᵗʰ
syphilitic 094.89
Meningomyeloneuritis — see
Meningoencephalitis
Meningoradiculitis — see Meningitis
Meningovascular — see condition
Meniscocytosis 282.60
Menkes' syndrome — see Syndrome, Menkes'
Menolipsis 626.0
Menometrorrhagia 626.2
Menopause, menopausal (symptoms) (syndrome)
627.2
arthritis (any site) NEC 716.3 ✓5ᵗʰ
artificial 627.4
bleeding 627.0
crisis 627.2
depression (see also Psychosis, affective)
296.2 ✓5ᵗʰ
agitated 296.2 ✓5ᵗʰ
recurrent episode 296.3 ✓5ᵗʰ
single episode 296.2 ✓5ᵗʰ

Menopause, menopausal — *continued*
- depression (*see also* Psychosis, affective) — *continued*
  - psychotic 296.2 ☑5ᵗʰ
    - recurrent episode 296.3 ☑5ᵗʰ
    - single episode 296.2 ☑5ᵗʰ
  - recurrent episode 296.3 ☑5ᵗʰ
  - single episode 296.2 ☑5ᵗʰ
  - melancholia (*see also* Psychosis, affective) 296.2 ☑5ᵗʰ
    - recurrent episode 296.3 ☑5ᵗʰ
    - single episode 296.2 ☑5ᵗʰ
- paranoid state 297.2
- paraphrenia 297.2
- postsurgical 627.4
- premature 256.31
  - postirradiation 256.2
  - postsurgical 256.2
- psychoneurosis 627.2
- psychosis NEC 298.8
- surgical 627.4
- toxic polyarthritis NEC 716.39

Menorrhagia (primary) 626.2
- climacteric 627.0
- menopausal 627.0
- postclimacteric 627.1
- postmenopausal 627.1
- preclimacteric 627.0
- premenopausal 627.0
- puberty (menses retained) 626.3

Menorrhalgia 625.3

Menoschesis 626.8

Menostaxis 626.2

Menses, retention 626.8

Menstrual — *see also* Menstruation
- cycle, irregular 626.4
- disorders NEC 626.9
- extraction V25.3
- fluid, retained 626.8
- molimen 625.4
- period, normal V65.5
- regulation V25.3

Menstruation
- absent 626.0
- anovulatory 628.0
- delayed 626.8
- difficult 625.3
- disorder 626.9
  - psychogenic 306.52
  - specified NEC 626.8
- during pregnancy 640.8 ☑5ᵗʰ
- excessive 626.2
- frequent 626.2
- infrequent 626.1
- irregular 626.4
- latent 626.8
- membranous 626.8
- painful (primary) (secondary) 625.3
  - psychogenic 306.52
- passage of clots 626.2
- precocious 626.8
- protracted 626.8
- retained 626.8
- retrograde 626.8
- scanty 626.1
- suppression 626.8
- vicarious (nasal) 625.8

Mentagra (*see also* Sycosis) 704.8

Mental — *see also* condition
- deficiency (*see also* Retardation, mental) 319
- deterioration (*see also* Psychosis) 298.9
- disorder (*see also* Disorder, mental) 300.9
- exhaustion 300.5
- insufficiency (congenital) (*see also* Retardation, mental) 319
- observation without need for further medical care NEC V71.09
- retardation (*see also* Retardation, mental) 319
- subnormality (*see also* Retardation, mental) 319
  - mild 317
  - moderate 318.0
  - profound 318.2
  - severe 318.1
- upset (*see also* Disorder, mental) 300.9

Meralgia paresthetica 355.1

Mercurial — *see* condition

Mercurialism NEC 985.0

Merergasia 300.9

MERFF 758.89

Merkel cell tumor — *see* Neoplasm, by site, malignant

Merocele (*see also* Hernia, femoral) 553.00

Meromelia 755.4
- lower limb 755.30
  - intercalary 755.32
    - femur 755.34
      - tibiofibular (complete) (incomplete) 755.33
    - fibula 755.37
    - metatarsal(s) 755.38
    - tarsal(s) 755.38
    - tibia 755.36
    - tibiofibular 755.35
  - terminal (complete) (partial) (transverse) 755.31
  - longitudinal 755.32
    - metatarsal(s) 755.38
    - phalange(s) 755.39
    - tarsal(s) 755.38
  - transverse 755.31
- upper limb 755.20
  - intercalary 755.22
    - carpal(s) 755.28
    - humeral 755.24
      - radioulnar (complete) (incomplete) 755.23
    - metacarpal(s) 755.28
    - phalange(s) 755.29
    - radial 755.26
    - radioulnar 755.25
    - ulnar 755.27
  - terminal (complete) (partial) (transverse) 755.21
  - longitudinal 755.22
    - carpal(s) 755.28
    - metacarpal(s) 755.28
    - phalange(s) 755.29
  - transverse 755.21

Merosmia 781.1

Merycism — *see also* Vomiting
- psychogenic 307.53

Merzbacher-Pelizaeus disease 330.0

Mesaortitis — *see* Aortitis

Mesarteritis — *see* Arteritis

Mesencephalitis (*see also* Encephalitis) 323.9
- late effect — *see* category 326

Mesenchymoma (M8990/1) — *see also* Neoplasm, connective tissue, uncertain behavior
- benign (M8990/0) — *see* Neoplasm, connective tissue, benign
- malignant (M8990/3) — *see* Neoplasm, connective tissue, malignant

Mesentery, mesenteric — *see* condition

Mesiodens, mesiodentes 520.1
- causing crowding 524.3

Mesio-occlusion 524.2

Mesocardia (with asplenia) 746.87

Mesocolon — *see* condition

Mesonephroma (malignant) (M9110/3) — *see also* Neoplasm, by site, malignant
- benign (M9110/0) — *see* Neoplasm, by site, benign

Mesophlebitis — *see* Phlebitis

Mesostromal dysgenesis 743.51

Mesothelioma (malignant) (M9050/3) — *see also* Neoplasm, by site, malignant
- benign (M9050/0) — *see* Neoplasm, by site, benign
- biphasic type (M9053/3) — *see also* Neoplasm, by site, malignant
  - benign (M9053/0) — *see* Neoplasm, by site, benign
- epithelioid (M9052/3) — *see also* Neoplasm, by site, malignant
  - benign (M9052/0) — *see* Neoplasm, by site, benign

Mesothelioma — *see also* Neoplasm, by site, malignant — *continued*
- fibrous (M9051/3) — *see also* Neoplasm, by site, malignant
  - benign (M9051/0) — *see* Neoplasm, by site, benign

Metabolism disorder 277.9
- specified type NEC 277.8

Metagonimiasis 121.5

Metagonimus infestation (small intestine) 121.5

Metal
- pigmentation (skin) 709.00
- polishers' disease 502

Metalliferous miners' lung 503

Metamorphopsia 368.14

Metaplasia
- bone, in skin 709.3
- breast 611.8
- cervix — *omit code*
- endometrium (squamous) 621.8
- intestinal, of gastric mucosa 537.89
- kidney (pelvis) (squamous) (*see also* Disease, renal) 593.89
- myelogenous 289.8
- myeloid (agnogenic) (megakaryocytic) 289.8
- spleen 289.59
- squamous cell
  - amnion 658.8 ☑5ᵗʰ
  - bladder 596.8
  - cervix — *see* condition
  - trachea 519.1
  - tracheobronchial tree 519.1
  - uterus 621.8
    - cervix — *see* condition

Metastasis, metastatic
- abscess — *see* Abscess
- calcification 275.40
- cancer, neoplasm, or disease
  - from specified site (M8000/3) — *see* Neoplasm, by site, malignant
  - to specified site (M8000/6) — *see* Neoplasm, by site, secondary
- deposits (in) (M8000/6) — *see* Neoplasm, by site, secondary
- pneumonia 038.8 [484.8]
- spread (to) (M8000/6) — *see* Neoplasm, by site, secondary

Metatarsalgia 726.70
- anterior 355.6
- due to Freiberg's disease 732.5
- Morton's 355.6

Metatarsus, metatarsal — *see also* condition
- abductus valgus (congenital) 754.60
- adductus varus (congenital) 754.53
- primus varus 754.52
- valgus (adductus) (congenital) 754.60
- varus (abductus) (congenital) 754.53
- primus 754.52

Methemoglobinemia 289.7
- acquired (with sulfhemoglobinemia) 289.7
- congenital 289.7
- enzymatic 289.7
- Hb-M disease 289.7
- hereditary 289.7
- toxic 289.7

Methemoglobinuria (*see also* Hemoglobinuria) 791.2

Methioninemia 270.4

Metritis (catarrhal) (septic) (suppurative) (*see also* Endometritis) 615.9
- blennorrhagic 098.16
  - chronic or duration of 2 months or over 098.36
- cervical (*see also* Cervicitis) 616.0
- gonococcal 098.16
  - chronic or duration of 2 months or over 098.36
- hemorrhagic 626.8
- puerperal, postpartum, childbirth 670 ☑5ᵗʰ
- tuberculous (*see also* Tuberculosis) 016.7 ☑5ᵗʰ

Metropathia hemorrhagica 626.8

Metroperitonitis (*see also* Peritonitis, pelvic, female) 614.5

☑4ᵗʰ Fourth-digit Required   ☑5ᵗʰ Fifth-digit Required   ▶◀ Revised Text   ● New Line   ▲ Revised Code

Metrorrhagia 626.6
arising during pregnancy — *see* Hemorrhage, pregnancy
postpartum NEC 666.2 ✓5ᵗʰ
primary 626.6
psychogenic 306.59
puerperal 666.2 ✓5ᵗʰ
Metrorrhexis — *see* Rupture, uterus
Metrosalpingitis (*see also* Salpingo-oophoritis) 614.2
Metrostaxis 626.6
Metrovaginitis (*see also* Endometritis) 615.9
gonococcal (acute) 098.16
chronic or duration of 2 months or over 098.36
Mexican fever — *see* Typhus, Mexican
Meyenburg-Altherr-Uehlinger syndrome 733.99
Meyer-Schwickerath and Weyers syndrome (dysplasia oculodentodigitalis) 759.89
Meynert's amentia (nonalcoholic) 294.0
alcoholic 291.1
Mibelli's disease 757.39
Mice, joint (*see also* Loose, body, joint) 718.1 ✓5ᵗʰ
knee 717.6
Micheli-Rietti syndrome (thalassemia minor) 282.4
Michotte's syndrome 721.5
Micrencephalon, micrencephaly 742.1
Microaneurysm, retina 362.14
diabetic 250.5 ✓5ᵗʰ [362.01]
Microangiopathy 443.9
diabetic (peripheral) 250.7 ✓5ᵗʰ [443.81]
retinal 250.5 ✓5ᵗʰ [362.01]
peripheral 443.9
diabetic 250.7 ✓5ᵗʰ [443.81]
retinal 362.18
diabetic 250.5 ✓5ᵗʰ [362.01]
thrombotic 446.6
Moschcowitz's (thrombotic thrombocytopenic purpura) 446.6
Microcalcification, mammographic 793.81
Microcephalus, microcephalic, microcephaly 742.1
due to toxoplasmosis (congenital) 771.2
Microcheilia 744.82
Microcolon (congenital) 751.5
Microcornea (congenital) 743.41
Microcytic — *see* condition
Microdontia 520.2
Microdrepanocytosis (thalassemia-Hb-S disease) 282.4
Microembolism
atherothrombotic — *see* Atheroembolism
retina 362.33
Microencephalon 742.1
Microfilaria streptocerca infestation 125.3
Microgastria (congenital) 750.7
Microgenia 524.0 ✓5ᵗʰ
Microgenitalia (congenital) 752.8
penis 752.64
Microglioma (M9710/3)
specified site — *see* Neoplasm, by site, malignant
unspecified site 191.9
Microglossia (congenital) 750.16
Micrognathia, micrognathism (congenital) 524.00
mandibular 524.04
alveolar 524.74
maxillary 524.03
alveolar 524.73
Microgyria (congenital) 742.2
Microinfarct, heart (*see also* Insufficiency, coronary) 411.89
Microlithiasis, alveolar, pulmonary 516.2
Micromyelia (congenital) 742.59
Micropenis 752.64
Microphakia (congenital) 743.36
Microphthalmia (congenital) (*see also* Microphthalmos) 743.10

Microphthalmos (congenital) 743.10
associated with eye and adnexal anomalies NEC 743.12
due to toxoplasmosis (congenital) 771.2
isolated 743.11
simple 743.11
syndrome 759.89
Micropsia 368.14
Microsporidiosis 136.8
Microsporon furfur infestation 111.0
Microsporosis (*see also* Dermatophytosis) 110.9
nigra 111.1
Microstomia (congenital) 744.84
Microthelia 757.6
Microthromboembolism — *see* Embolism
Microtia (congenital) (external ear) 744.23
Microtropia 378.34
Micturition
disorder NEC 788.69
psychogenic 306.53
frequency 788.41
psychogenic 306.53
nocturnal 788.43
painful 788.1
psychogenic 306.53
Middle
ear — *see* condition
lobe (right) syndrome 518.0
Midplane — *see* condition
Miescher's disease 709.3
cheilitis 351.8
granulomatosis disciformis 709.3
Miescher-Leder syndrome or granulomatosis 709.3
Mieten's syndrome 759.89
Migraine (idiopathic) 346.9 ✓5ᵗʰ
with aura 346.0 ✓5ᵗʰ
abdominal (syndrome) 346.2 ✓5ᵗʰ
allergic (histamine) 346.2 ✓5ᵗʰ
atypical 346.1 ✓5ᵗʰ
basilar 346.2 ✓5ᵗʰ
classical 346.0 ✓5ᵗʰ
common 346.1 ✓5ᵗʰ
hemiplegic 346.8 ✓5ᵗʰ
lower-half 346.2 ✓5ᵗʰ
menstrual 625.4
ophthalmic 346.8 ✓5ᵗʰ
ophthalmoplegic 346.8 ✓5ᵗʰ
retinal 346.2 ✓5ᵗʰ
variant 346.2 ✓5ᵗʰ
Migrant, social V60.0
Migratory, migrating — *see also* condition
person V60.0
testis, congenital 752.52
Mikulicz's disease or syndrome (dryness of mouth, absent or decreased lacrimation) 527.1
Milian atrophia blanche 701.3
Miliaria (crystallina) (rubra) (tropicalis) 705.1
apocrine 705.82
Miliary — *see* condition
Milium (*see also* Cyst, sebaceous) 706.2
colloid 709.3
eyelid 374.84
Milk
crust 690.11
excess secretion 676.6 ✓5ᵗʰ
fever, female 672 ✓5ᵗʰ
poisoning 988.8
retention 676.2 ✓5ᵗʰ
sickness 988.8
spots 423.1
Milkers' nodes 051.1
Milk-leg (deep vessels) 671.4 ✓5ᵗʰ
complicating pregnancy 671.3 ✓5ᵗʰ
nonpuerperal 451.19
puerperal, postpartum, childbirth 671.4 ✓5ᵗʰ
Milkman (-Looser) disease or syndrome (osteomalacia with pseudofractures) 268.2
Milky urine (*see also* Chyluria) 791.1
Millar's asthma (laryngismus stridulus) 478.75
Millard-Gubler paralysis or syndrome 344.89

Millard-Gubler-Foville paralysis 344.89
Miller's disease (osteomalacia) 268.2
Miller Fisher's syndrome 357.0
Milles' syndrome (encephalocutaneous angiomatosis) 759.6
Mills' disease 335.29
Millstone makers' asthma or lung 502
Milroy's disease (chronic hereditary edema) 757.0
Miners' — *see also* condition
asthma 500
elbow 727.2
knee 727.2
lung 500
nystagmus 300.89
phthisis (*see also* Tuberculosis) 011.4 ✓5ᵗʰ
tuberculosis (see also Tuberculosis) 011.4 ✓5ᵗʰ
Minkowski-Chauffard syndrome (*see also* Spherocytosis) 282.0
Minor — *see* condition
Minor's disease 336.1
Minot's disease (hemorrhagic disease, newborn) 776.0
Minot-von Willebrand (-Jürgens) disease or syndrome (angiohemophilia) 286.4
Minus (and plus) hand (intrinsic) 736.09
Miosis (persistent) (pupil) 379.42
Mirizzi's syndrome (hepatic duct stenosis) (*see also* Obstruction, biliary) 576.2
with calculus, cholelithiasis, or stones — *see* Choledocholithiasis
Mirror writing 315.09
secondary to organic lesion 784.69
Misadventure (prophylactic) (therapeutic) (*see also* Complications) 999.9
administration of insulin 962.3
infusion — *see* Complications, infusion
local applications (of fomentations, plasters, etc.) 999.9
burn or scald — *see* Burn, by site
medical care (early) (late) NEC 999.9
adverse effect of drugs or chemicals — *see* Table of Drugs and Chemicals
burn or scald — *see* Burn, by site
radiation NEC 990
radiotherapy NEC 990
surgical procedure (early) (late) — *see* Complications, surgical procedure
transfusion — *see* Complications, transfusion
vaccination or other immunological procedure — *see* Complications, vaccination
Misanthropy 301.7
Miscarriage — *see* Abortion, spontaneous
Mischief, malicious, child (*see also* Disturbance, conduct) 312.0 ✓5ᵗʰ
Misdirection
aqueous 365.83
Mismanagement, feeding 783.3
Misplaced, misplacement
kidney (*see also* Disease, renal) 593.0
congenital 753.3
organ or site, congenital NEC — *see* Malposition, congenital
Missed
abortion 632
delivery (at or near term) 656.4 ✓5ᵗʰ
labor (at or near term) 656.4 ✓5ᵗʰ
Missing — *see also* Absence
teeth (acquired) 525.10
congenital (see also Anodontia) 520.0
due to
caries 525.13
extraction 525.10
periodontal disease 525.12
specified NEC 525.19
trauma 525.11
vertebrae (congenital) 756.13
Misuse of drugs NEC (*see also* Abuse, drug, nondependent) 305.9 ✓5ᵗʰ
Mitchell's disease (erythromelalgia) 443.89
Mite(s)
diarrhea 133.8
grain (itch) 133.8

Mite(s) — *continued*
  hair follicle (itch) 133.8
  in sputum 133.8
Mitral — *see* condition
Mittelschmerz 625.2
Mixed — *see* condition
Mljet disease (mal de Meleda) 757.39
Mobile, mobility
  cecum 751.4
  coccyx 733.99
  excessive — *see* Hypermobility
  gallbladder 751.69
  kidney 593.0
    congenital 753.3
  organ or site, congenital NEC — *see*
    Malposition, congenital
  spleen 289.59
Mobitz heart block (atrioventricular) 426.10
  type I (Wenckebach's) 426.13
  type II 426.12
Möbius'
  disease 346.8 √5
  syndrome
    congenital oculofacial paralysis 352.6
    ophthalmoplegic migraine 346.8 √5
Moeller (-Barlow) disease (infantile scurvy) 267
  glossitis 529.4
Mohr's syndrome (types I and II) 759.89
Mola destruens (M9100/1) 236.1
Molarization, premolars 520.2
Molar pregnancy 631
  hydatidiform (delivered) (undelivered) 630
Mold(s)
  in vitreous 117.9
Molding, head (during birth) 767.3
Mole (pigmented) (M8720/0) — *see also*
  Neoplasm, skin, benign
  blood 631
  Breus' 631
  cancerous (M8720/3) — *see* Melanoma
  carneous 631
  destructive (M9100/1) 236.1
  ectopic — *see* Pregnancy, ectopic
  fleshy 631
  hemorrhagic 631
  hydatid, hydatidiform (benign) (complicating
    pregnancy) (delivered) (undelivered) (*see*
    also Hydatidiform mole) 630
    invasive (M9100/1) 236.1
    malignant (M9100/1) 236.1
    previous, affecting management of
      pregnancy V23.1
  invasive (hydatidiform) (M9100/1) 236.1
  malignant
    meaning
      malignant hydatidiform mole (9100/1)
        236.1
      melanoma (M8720/3) — *see* Melanoma
  nonpigmented (M8730/0) — *see* Neoplasm,
    skin, benign
  pregnancy NEC 631
  skin (M8720/0) — *see* Neoplasm, skin, benign
  tubal — *see* Pregnancy, tubal
  vesicular (*see also* Hydatidiform mole) 630
Molimen, molimina (menstrual) 625.4
Mollaret's meningitis 047.9
Mollities (cerebellar) (cerebral) 437.8
  ossium 268.2
Molluscum
  contagiosum 078.0
  epitheliale 078.0
  fibrosum (M8851/0) — *see* Lipoma, by site
  pendulum (M8851/0) — *see* Lipoma, by site
Mönckeberg's arteriosclerosis, degeneration,
  disease, or sclerosis (*see also*
  Arteriosclerosis, extremities) 440.20
Monday fever 504
Monday morning dyspnea or asthma 504
Mondini's malformation (cochlea) 744.05
Mondor's disease (thrombophlebitis of breast)
  451.89

Mongolian, mongolianism, mongolism,
  mongoloid 758.0
  spot 757.33
Monilethrix (congenital) 757.4
Monilia infestation — *see* Candidiasis
Moniliasis — *see also* Candidiasis
  neonatal 771.7
  vulvovaginitis 112.1
Monoarthritis 716.60
  ankle 716.67
  arm 716.62
    lower (and wrist) 716.63
    upper (and elbow) 716.62
  foot (and ankle) 716.67
  forearm (and wrist) 716.63
  hand 716.64
  leg 716.66
    lower 716.66
    upper 716.65
  pelvic region (hip) (thigh) 716.65
  shoulder (region) 716.61
  specified site NEC 716.68
Monoblastic — *see* condition
Monochromatism (cone) (rod) 368.54
Monocytic — *see* condition
Monocytosis (symptomatic) 288.8
Monofixation syndrome 378.34
Monomania (*see also* Psychosis) 298.9
Mononeuritis 355.9
  cranial nerve — *see* Disorder, nerve, cranial
  femoral nerve 355.2
  lateral
    cutaneous nerve of thigh 355.1
    popliteal nerve 355.3
  lower limb 355.8
    specified nerve NEC 355.79
  medial popliteal nerve 355.4
  median nerve 354.1
  multiplex 354.5
  plantar nerve 355.6
  posterior tibial nerve 355.5
  radial nerve 354.3
  sciatic nerve 355.0
  ulnar nerve 354.2
  upper limb 354.9
    specified nerve NEC 354.8
  vestibular 388.5
Mononeuropathy (*see also* Mononeuritis) 355.9
  diabetic NEC 250.6 √5 [355.9]
    lower limb 250.6 √5 [355.8]
    upper limb 250.6 √5 [354.9]
  iliohypogastric 355.79
  ilioinguinal 355.79
  obturator 355.79
  saphenous 355.79
Mononucleosis, infectious 075
  with hepatitis 075 [573.1]
Monoplegia 344.5
  brain (current episode) (*see also* Paralysis,
    brain) 437.8
    fetus or newborn 767.8
  cerebral (current episode) (*see also* Paralysis,
    brain) 437.8
  congenital or infantile (cerebral) (spastic)
    (spinal) 343.3
  embolic (current) (*see also* Embolism, brain)
    434.1 √5
    late effect — *see* Late effect(s) (of)
      cerebrovascular disease
  infantile (cerebral) (spastic) (spinal) 343.3
  lower limb 344.30
    affecting
      dominant side 344.31
      nondominant side 344.32
    due to late effect of cerebrovascular accident
      — *see* Late effect(s) (of)
      cerebrovascular accident
  newborn 767.8
  psychogenic 306.0
    specified as conversion reaction 300.11
  thrombotic (current) (*see also* Thrombosis,
    brain) 434.0 √5
    late effect — *see* Late effect(s) (of)
      cerebrovascular disease
  transient 781.4

Monoplegia — *continued*
  upper limb 344.40
    affecting
      dominant side 344.41
      nondominant side 344.42
    due to late effect of cerebrovascular accident
      — *see* Late effect(s) (of)
      cerebrovascular accident
Monorchism, monorchidism 752.8
Monster, monstrosity — *see* Anomaly
Monteggia's fracture (closed) 813.03
  open 813.13
Mood swings
  brief compensatory 296.99
  rebound 296.99
Moore's syndrome (*see also* Epilepsy) 345.5 √5
Mooren's ulcer (cornea) 370.07
Mooser-Neill reaction 081.0
Mooser bodies 081.0
Moral
  deficiency 301.7
  imbecility 301.7
Morax-Axenfeld conjunctivitis 372.03
Morbilli (*see also* Measles) 055.9
Morbus
  anglicus, anglorum 268.0
  Beigel 111.2
  caducus (*see also* Epilepsy) 345.9 √5
  caeruleus 746.89
  celiacus 579.0
  comitialis (see also Epilepsy) 345.9 √5
  cordis — *see also* Disease, heart
    valvulorum — *see* Endocarditis
  coxae 719.95
    tuberculous (*see also* Tuberculosis)
      015.1 √5
  hemorrhagicus neonatorum 776.0
  maculosus neonatorum 772.6
  renum 593.0
  senilis (*see also* Osteoarthrosis) 715.9 √5
Morel-Kraepelin disease (*see also* Schizophrenia)
  295.9 √5
Morel-Moore syndrome (hyperostosis frontalis
  interna) 733.3
Morel-Morgagni syndrome (hyperostosis frontalis
  interna) 733.3
Morgagni
  cyst, organ, hydatid, or appendage 752.8
    fallopian tube 752.11
  disease or syndrome (hyperostosis frontalis
    interna) 733.3
Morgagni-Adams-Stokes syndrome (syncope with
  heart block) 426.9
Morgagni-Stewart-Morel syndrome (hyperostosis
  frontalis interna) 733.3
Moria (*see also* Psychosis) 298.9
Morning sickness 643.0 √5
Moron 317
Morphea (guttate) (linear) 701.0
Morphine dependence (*see also* Dependence)
  304.0 √5
Morphinism (*see also* Dependence) 304.0 √5
Morphinomania (*see also* Dependence) 304.0 √5
Morphoea 701.0
Morquio (-Brailsford) (-Ullrich) disease or
  syndrome (mucopolysaccharidosis IV) 277.5
  kyphosis 277.5
Morris syndrome (testicular feminization) 257.8
Morsus humanus (open wound) — *see also*
  Wound, open, by site
  skin surface intact — *see* Contusion
Mortification (dry) (moist) (*see also* Gangrene)
  785.4
Morton's
  disease 355.6
  foot 355.6
  metatarsalgia (syndrome) 355.6
  neuralgia 355.6
  neuroma 355.6
  syndrome (metatarsalgia) (neuralgia) 355.6
  toe 355.6

√4 Fourth-digit Required   √5 Fifth-digit Required   ▶◀ Revised Text   ● New Line   ▲ Revised Code

Morvan's disease 336.0
Mosaicism, mosaic (chromosomal) 758.9
  autosomal 758.5
  sex 758.81
Moschcowitz's syndrome (thrombotic thrombocytopenic purpura) 446.6
Mother yaw 102.0
Motion sickness (from travel, any vehicle) (from roundabouts or swings) 994.6
Mottled teeth (enamel) (endemic) (nonendemic) 520.3
Mottling enamel (endemic) (nonendemic) (teeth) 520.3
Mouchet's disease 732.5
Mould(s) (in vitreous) 117.9
Moulders'
  bronchitis 502
  tuberculosis (see also Tuberculosis) 011.4 ✓5ᵗʰ
Mounier-Kuhn syndrome 494.0
  with acute exacerbation 494.1
Mountain
  fever — see Fever, mountain
  sickness 993.2
    with polycythemia, acquired 289.0
    acute 289.0
  tick fever 066.1
Mouse, joint (see also Loose, body, joint) 718.1 ✓5ᵗʰ
  knee 717.6
Mouth — see condition
Movable
  coccyx 724.71
  kidney (see also Disease, renal) 593.0
    congenital 753.3
  organ or site, congenital NEC — see Malposition, congenital
  spleen 289.59
Movement
  abnormal (dystonic) (involuntary) 781.0
  decreased fetal 655.7 ✓5ᵗʰ
  paradoxical facial 374.43
Moya Moya disease 437.5
Mozart's ear 744.29
Mucha's disease (acute parapsoriasis varioliformis) 696.2
Mucha-Haberman syndrome (acute parapsoriasis varioliformis) 696.2
Mu-chain disease 273.2
Mucinosis (cutaneous) (papular) 701.8
Mucocele
  appendix 543.9
  buccal cavity 528.9
  gallbladder (see also Disease, gallbladder) 575.3
  lacrimal sac 375.43
  orbit (eye) 376.81
  salivary gland (any) 527.6
  sinus (accessory) (nasal) 478.1
  turbinate (bone) (middle) (nasal) 478.1
  uterus 621.8
Mucocutaneous lymph node syndrome (acute) (febrile) (infantile) 446.1
Mucoenteritis 564.9
Mucolipidosis I, II, III 272.7
Mucopolysaccharidosis (types 1-6) 277.5
  cardiopathy 277.5 [425.7]
Mucormycosis (lung) 117.7
Mucositis — see also Inflammation by site
  necroticans agranulocytica 288.0
Mucous — see also condition
  patches (syphilitic) 091.3
    congenital 090.0
Mucoviscidosis 277.00
  with meconium obstruction 277.01
Mucus
  asphyxia or suffocation (see also Asphyxia, mucus) 933.1
    newborn 770.1
  in stool 792.1
  plug (see also Asphyxia, mucus) 933.1
    aspiration, of newborn 770.1

Mucus — continued
  plug (see also Asphyxia, mucus) — continued
    tracheobronchial 519.1
      newborn 770.1
Muguet 112.0
Mulberry molars 090.5
Mullerian mixed tumor (M8950/3) — see Neoplasm, by site, malignant
Multicystic kidney 753.19
Multilobed placenta — see Placenta, abnormal
Multinodular prostate 600.1
Multiparity V61.5
  affecting
    fetus or newborn 763.89
    management of
      labor and delivery 659.4 ✓5ᵗʰ
      pregnancy V23.3
  requiring contraceptive management (see also Contraception) V25.9
Multipartita placenta — see Placenta, abnormal
Multiple, multiplex — see also condition
  birth
    affecting fetus or newborn 761.5
    healthy liveborn — see Newborn, multiple
  digits (congenital) 755.00
    fingers 755.01
    toes 755.02
  organ or site NEC — see Accessory
  personality 300.14
  renal arteries 747.62
Mumps 072.9
  with complication 072.8
    specified type NEC 072.79
  encephalitis 072.2
  hepatitis 072.71
  meningitis (aseptic) 072.1
  meningoencephalitis 072.2
  oophoritis 072.79
  orchitis 072.0
  pancreatitis 072.3
  polyneuropathy 072.72
  vaccination, prophylactic (against) V04.6
Mumu (see also Infestation, filarial) 125.9
Münchausen syndrome 301.51
Münchmeyer's disease or syndrome (exostosis luxurians) 728.11
Mural — see condition
Murmur (cardiac) (heart) (nonorganic) (organic) 785.2
  abdominal 787.5
  aortic (valve) (see also Endocarditis, aortic) 424.1
  benign — omit code
  cardiorespiratory 785.2
  diastolic — see condition
  Flint (see also Endocarditis, aortic) 424.1
  functional — omit code
  Graham Steell (pulmonic regurgitation) (see also Endocarditis, pulmonary) 424.3
  innocent — omit code
  insignificant — omit code
  midsystolic 785.2
  mitral (valve) — see Stenosis, mitral
  physiologic — see condition
  presystolic, mitral — see Insufficiency, mitral
  pulmonic (valve) (see also Endocarditis, pulmonary) 424.3
  Still's (vibratory) — omit code
  systolic (valvular) — see condition
  tricuspid (valve) — see Endocarditis, tricuspid
  undiagnosed 785.2
  valvular — see condition
  vibratory — omit code
Murri's disease (intermittent hemoglobinuria) 283.2
Muscae volitantes 379.24
Muscle, muscular — see condition
Musculoneuralgia 729.1
Mushrooming hip 718.95
Mushroom workers' (pickers') lung 495.5
Mutism (see also Aphasia) 784.3
  akinetic 784.3
  deaf (acquired) (congenital) 389.7

Mutism (see also Aphasia) — continued
  elective (selective) 313.23
    adjustment reaction 309.83
  hysterical 300.11
Myà's disease (congenital dilation, colon) 751.3
Myalgia (intercostal) 729.1
  eosinophilia syndrome 710.5
  epidemic 074.1
    cervical 078.89
  psychogenic 307.89
  traumatic NEC 959.9
Myasthenia, myasthenic 358.0
  cordis — see Failure, heart
  gravis 358.0
    neonatal 775.2
    pseudoparalytica 358.0
  stomach 536.8
    psychogenic 306.4
  syndrome
    in
      botulism 005.1 [358.1]
      diabetes mellitus 250.6 ✓5ᵗʰ [358.1]
      hypothyroidism (see also Hypothyroidism) 244.9 [358.1]
      malignant neoplasm NEC 199.1 [358.1]
      pernicious anemia 281.0 [358.1]
      thyrotoxicosis (see also Thyrotoxicosis) 242.9 ✓5ᵗʰ [358.1]
Mycelium infection NEC 117.9
Mycetismus 988.1
Mycetoma (actinomycotic) 039.9
  bone 039.8
    mycotic 117.4
  foot 039.4
    mycotic 117.4
  madurae 039.9
    mycotic 117.4
  maduromycotic 039.9
    mycotic 117.4
  mycotic 117.4
  nocardial 039.9
Mycobacteriosis — see Mycobacterium
Mycobacterium, mycobacterial (infection) 031.9
  acid-fast (bacilli) 031.9
  anonymous (see also Mycobacterium, atypical) 031.9
  atypical (acid-fast bacilli) 031.9
    cutaneous 031.1
    pulmonary 031.0
      tuberculous (see also Tuberculosis, pulmonary) 011.9 ✓5ᵗʰ
    specified site NEC 031.8
  avium 031.0
    intracellulare complex bacteremia (MAC) 031.2
  balnei 031.1
  Battey 031.0
  cutaneous 031.1
  disseminated 031.2
    avium-intracellulare complex (DMAC) 031.2
  fortuitum 031.0
  intracellulare (battey bacillus) 031.0
  kakerifu 031.8
  kansasii 031.0
  kasongo 031.8
  leprae — see Leprosy
  luciflavum 031.0
  marinum 031.1
  pulmonary 031.0
    tuberculous (see also Tuberculosis, pulmonary) 011.9 ✓5ᵗʰ
  scrofulaceum 031.1
  tuberculosis (human, bovine) — see also Tuberculosis
    avian type 031.0
  ulcerans 031.1
  xenopi 031.0
Mycosis, mycotic 117.9
  cutaneous NEC 111.9
  ear 111.8 [380.15]
  fungoides (M9700/3) 202.1 ✓5ᵗʰ
  mouth 112.0
  pharynx 117.9
  skin NEC 111.9
  stomatitis 112.0
  systemic NEC 117.9

Mycosis, mycotic — *continued*
  tonsil 117.9
  vagina, vaginitis 112.1
Mydriasis (persistent) (pupil) 379.43
Myelatelia 742.59
Myelinoclasis, perivascular, acute
    (postinfectious) NEC 136.9 *[323.6]*
  postimmunization or postvaccinal 323.5
Myelinosis, central pontine 341.8
Myelitis (acute) (ascending) (cerebellar)
    (childhood) (chronic) (descending) (diffuse)
    (disseminated) (pressure) (progressive)
    (spinal cord) (subacute) (transverse) (*see also*
    Encephalitis) 323.9
  late effect — *see* category 326
  optic neuritis in 341.0
  postchickenpox 052.7
  postvaccinal 323.5
  syphilitic (transverse) 094.89
  tuberculous (*see also* Tuberculosis) 013.6 ✓5ᵗʰ
  virus 049.9
Myeloblastic — *see* condition
Myelocele (*see also* Spina bifida) 741.9 ✓5ᵗʰ
  with hydrocephalus 741.0 ✓5ᵗʰ
Myelocystocele (*see also* Spina bifida) 741.9 ✓5ᵗʰ
Myelocytic — *see* condition
Myelocytoma 205.1 ✓5ᵗʰ
Myelodysplasia (spinal cord) 742.59
  meaning myelodysplastic syndrome — *see*
    Syndrome, myelodysplastic
Myeloencephalitis — *see* Encephalitis
Myelofibrosis (osteosclerosis) 289.8
Myelogenous — *see* condition
Myeloid — *see* condition
Myelokathexis 288.0
Myeloleukodystrophy 330.0
Myelolipoma (M8870/0) — *see* Neoplasm, by site,
    benign
Myeloma (multiple) (plasma cell) (plasmacytic)
    (M9730/3) 203.0 ✓5ᵗʰ
  monostotic (M9731/1) 238.6
  solitary (M9731/1) 238.6
Myelomalacia 336.8
Myelomata, multiple (M9730/3) 203.0 ✓5ᵗʰ
Myelomatosis (M9730/3) 203.0 ✓5ᵗʰ
Myelomeningitis — *see* Meningoencephalitis
Myelomeningocele (spinal cord) (*see also* Spina
    bifida) 741.9 ✓5ᵗʰ
  fetal, causing fetopelvic disproportion 653.7 ✓5ᵗʰ
Myelo-osteo-musculodysplasia hereditaria
    756.89
Myelopathic — *see* condition
Myelopathy (spinal cord) 336.9
  cervical 721.1
  diabetic 250.6 ✓5ᵗʰ *[336.3]*
  drug-induced 336.8
  due to or with
    carbon tetrachloride 987.8 *[323.7]*
    degeneration or displacement, intervertebral
      disc 722.70
      cervical, cervicothoracic 722.71
      lumbar, lumbosacral 722.73
      thoracic, thoracolumbar 722.72
    hydroxyquinoline derivatives 961.3 *[323.7]*
    infection — *see* Encephalitis
    intervertebral disc disorder 722.70
      cervical, cervicothoracic 722.71
      lumbar, lumbosacral 722.73
      thoracic, thoracolumbar 722.72
    lead 984.9 *[323.7]*
    mercury 985.0 *[323.7]*
    neoplastic disease (*see also* Neoplasm, by
      site) 239.9 *[336.3]*
    pernicious anemia 281.0 *[336.3]*
    spondylosis 721.91
      cervical 721.1
      lumbar, lumbosacral 721.42
      thoracic 721.41
    thallium 985.8 *[323.7]*
  lumbar, lumbosacral 721.42
  necrotic (subacute) 336.1
  radiation-induced 336.8

Myelopathy — *continued*
  spondylogenic NEC 721.91
    cervical 721.1
    lumbar, lumbosacral 721.42
    thoracic 721.41
  thoracic 721.41
  toxic NEC 989.9 *[323.7]*
  transverse (*see also* Encephalitis) 323.9
  vascular 336.1
Myeloproliferative disease (M9960/1) 238.7
Myeloradiculitis (*see also* Polyneuropathy) 357.0
Myeloradiculodysplasia (spinal) 742.59
Myelosarcoma (M9930/3) 205.3 ✓5ᵗʰ
Myelosclerosis 289.8
  with myeloid metaplasia (M9961/1) 238.7
  disseminated, of nervous system 340
  megakaryocytic (M9961/1) 238.7
Myelosis (M9860/3) (*see also* Leukemia, myeloid)
    205.9 ✓5ᵗʰ
  acute (M9861/3) 205.0 ✓5ᵗʰ
  aleukemic (M9864/3) 205.8 ✓5ᵗʰ
  chronic (M9863/3) 205.1 ✓5ᵗʰ
  erythremic (M9840/3) 207.0 ✓5ᵗʰ
    acute (M9841/3) 207.0 ✓5ᵗʰ
  megakaryocytic (M9920/3) 207.2 ✓5ᵗʰ
  nonleukemic (chronic) 288.8
  subacute (M9862/3) 205.2 ✓5ᵗʰ
Myesthenia — *see* Myasthenia
Myiasis (cavernous) 134.0
  orbit 134.0 *[376.13]*
Myoadenoma, prostate 600.2
Myoblastoma
  granular cell (M9580/0) — *see also* Neoplasm,
    connective tissue, benign
    malignant (M9580/3) — *see* Neoplasm,
      connective tissue, malignant
  tongue (M9580/0) 210.1
Myocardial — *see* condition
Myocardiopathy (congestive) (constrictive)
    (familial) (hypertrophic nonobstructive)
    (idiopathic) (infiltrative) (obstructive)
    (primary) (restrictive) (sporadic) 425.4
  alcoholic 425.5
  amyloid 277.3 *[425.7]*
  beriberi 265.0 *[425.7]*
  cobalt-beer 425.5
  due to
    amyloidosis 277.3 *[425.7]*
    beriberi 265.0 *[425.7]*
    cardiac glycogenosis 271.0 *[425.7]*
    Chagas' disease 086.0
    Friedreich's ataxia 334.0 *[425.8]*
    influenza 487.8 *[425.8]*
    mucopolysaccharidosis 277.5 *[425.7]*
    myotonia atrophica 359.2 *[425.8]*
    progressive muscular dystrophy 359.1
      [425.8]
    sarcoidosis 135 *[425.8]*
  glycogen storage 271.0 *[425.7]*
  hypertrophic obstructive 425.1
  metabolic NEC 277.9 *[425.7]*
  nutritional 269.9 *[425.7]*
  obscure (African) 425.2
  postpartum 674.8 ✓5ᵗʰ
  secondary 425.9
  thyrotoxic (*see also* Thyrotoxicosis)
    242.9 ✓5ᵗʰ *[425.7]*
  toxic NEC 425.9
Myocarditis (fibroid) (interstitial) (old)
    (progressive) (senile) (with arteriosclerosis)
    429.0
  with
    rheumatic fever (conditions classifiable to
      390) 398.0
      active (*see also* Myocarditis, acute,
        rheumatic) 391.2
      inactive or quiescent (with chorea) 398.0
  active (nonrheumatic) 422.90
    rheumatic 391.2
      with chorea (acute) (rheumatic)
        (Sydenham's) 392.0
  acute or subacute (interstitial) 422.90
    due to Streptococcus (beta-hemolytic) 391.2
    idiopathic 422.91

Myocarditis — *continued*
  acute or subacute — *continued*
    rheumatic 391.2
      with chorea (acute) (rheumatic)
        (Sydenham's) 392.0
    specified type NEC 422.99
  aseptic of newborn 074.23
  bacterial (acute) 422.92
  chagasic 086.0
  chronic (interstitial) 429.0
  congenital 746.89
  constrictive 425.4
  Coxsackie (virus) 074.23
  diphtheritic 032.82
  due to or in
    Coxsackie (virus) 074.23
    diphtheria 032.82
    epidemic louse-borne typhus 080 *[422.0]*
    influenza 487.8 *[422.0]*
    Lyme disease 088.81 *[422.0]*
    scarlet fever 034.1 *[422.0]*
    toxoplasmosis (acquired) 130.3
    tuberculosis (*see also* Tuberculosis)
      017.9 *[422.0]*
    typhoid 002.0 *[422.0]*
    typhus NEC 081.9 *[422.0]*
  eosinophilic 422.91
  epidemic of newborn 074.23
  Fiedler's (acute) (isolated) (subacute) 422.91
  giant cell (acute) (subacute) 422.91
  gonococcal 098.85
  granulomatous (idiopathic) (isolated)
      (nonspecific) 422.91
  hypertensive (*see also* Hypertension, heart)
      402.90
  idiopathic 422.91
    granulomatous 422.91
  infective 422.92
  influenzal 487.8 *[422.0]*
  isolated (diffuse) (granulomatous) 422.91
  malignant 422.99
  meningococcal 036.43
  nonrheumatic, active 422.90
  parenchymatous 422.90
  pneumococcal (acute) (subacute) 422.92
  rheumatic (chronic) (inactive) (with chorea)
      398.0
    active or acute 391.2
      with chorea (acute) (rheumatic)
        (Sydenham's) 392.0
  septic 422.92
  specific (giant cell) (productive) 422.91
  staphylococcal (acute) (subacute) 422.92
  suppurative 422.92
  syphilitic (chronic) 093.82
  toxic 422.93
    rheumatic (*see also* Myocarditis, acute
      rheumatic) 391.2
  tuberculous (*see also* Tuberculosis)
      017.9 ✓5ᵗʰ *[422.0]*
  typhoid 002.0 *[422.0]*
  valvular — *see* Endocarditis
  viral, except Coxsackie 422.91
    Coxsackie 074.23
    of newborn (Coxsackie) 074.23
Myocardium, myocardial — *see* condition
Myocardosis (*see also* Cardiomyopathy) 425.4
Myoclonia (essential) 333.2
  epileptica 333.2
  Friedrich's 333.2
  massive 333.2
Myoclonic
  epilepsy, familial (progressive) 333.2
  jerks 333.2
Myoclonus (familial essential) (multifocal)
    (simplex) 333.2
  facial 351.8
  massive (infantile) 333.2
  pharyngeal 478.29
Myodiastasis 728.84
Myoendocarditis — *see also* Endocarditis
  acute or subacute 421.9
Myoepithelioma (M8982/0) — *see* Neoplasm, by
    site, benign
Myofascitis (acute) 729.1
  low back 724.2

Myofibroma (M8890/0) — *see also* Neoplasm, connective tissue, benign
  uterus (cervix) (corpus) (*see also* Leiomyoma) 218.9

Myofibrosis 728.2
  heart (*see also* Myocarditis) 429.0
  humeroscapular region 726.2
  scapulohumeral 726.2

Myofibrositis (*see also* Myositis) 729.1
  scapulohumeral 726.2

Myogelosis (occupational) 728.89

Myoglobinuria 791.3

Myoglobulinuria, primary 791.3

Myokymia — *see also* Myoclonus
  facial 351.8

Myolipoma (M8860/0)
  specified site — *see* Neoplasm, connective tissue, benign
  unspecified site 223.0

Myoma (M8895/0) — *see also* Neoplasm, connective tissue, benign
  cervix (stump) (uterus) (*see also* Leiomyoma) 218.9
  malignant (M8895/3) — *see* Neoplasm, connective tissue, malignant
  prostate 600.2
  uterus (cervix) (corpus) (*see also* Leiomyoma) 218.9
    in pregnancy or childbirth 654.1 ✓5ᵗʰ
      affecting fetus or newborn 763.89
      causing obstructed labor 660.2 ✓5ᵗʰ
        affecting fetus or newborn 763.1

Myomalacia 728.9
  cordis, heart (*see also* Degeneration, myocardial) 429.1

Myometritis (*see also* Endometritis) 615.9

Myometrium — *see* condition

Myonecrosis, clostridial 040.0

Myopathy 359.9
  alcoholic 359.4
  amyloid 277.3 [359.6]
  benign congenital 359.0
  central core 359.0
  centronuclear 359.0
  congenital (benign) 359.0
  critical illness 359.81 ●
  distal 359.1
  due to drugs 359.4
  endocrine 259.9 [359.5]
    specified type NEC 259.8 [359.5]
  extraocular muscles 376.82
  facioscapulohumeral 359.1
  in
    Addison's disease 255.4 [359.5]
    amyloidosis 277.3 [359.6]
    cretinism 243 [359.5]
    Cushing's syndrome 255.0 [359.5]
    disseminated lupus erythematosus 710.0 [359.6]
    giant cell arteritis 446.5 [359.6]
    hyperadrenocorticism NEC 255.3 [359.5]
    hyperparathyroidism 252.0 [359.5]
    hypopituitarism 253.2 [359.5]
    hypothyroidism (*see also* Hypothyroidism) 244.9 [359.5]
    malignant neoplasm NEC (M8000/3) 199.1 [359.6]
    myxedema (*see also* Myxedema) 244.9 [359.5]
    polyarteritis nodosa 446.0 [359.6]
    rheumatoid arthritis 714.0 [359.6]
    sarcoidosis 135 [359.6]
    scleroderma 710.1 [359.6]
    Sjögren's disease 710.2 [359.6]
    thyrotoxicosis (*see also* Thyrotoxicosis) 242.9 ✓5ᵗʰ [359.5]
  inflammatory 359.89 ▲
  intensive care (ICU) 359.81 ●
  limb-girdle 359.1
  myotubular 359.0
  necrotizing, acute 359.81 ●
  nemaline 359.0
  ocular 359.1
  oculopharyngeal 359.1
  of critical illness 359.81 ●

Myopathy — *continued*
  primary 359.89 ▲
  progressive NEC 359.89 ▲
  quadriplegic, acute 359.81 ●
  rod body 359.0
  scapulohumeral 359.1
  specified type NEC 359.89 ▲
  toxic 359.4

Myopericarditis (*see also* Pericarditis) 423.9

Myopia (axial) (congenital) (increased curvature or refraction, nucleus of lens) 367.1
  degenerative, malignant 360.21
  malignant 360.21
  progressive high (degenerative) 360.21

Myosarcoma (M8895/3) — *see* Neoplasm, connective tissue, malignant

Myosis (persistent) 379.42
  stromal (endolymphatic) (M8931/1) 236.0

Myositis 729.1
  clostridial 040.0
  due to posture 729.1
  epidemic 074.1
  fibrosa or fibrous (chronic) 728.2
    Volkmann's (complicating trauma) 958.6
  infective 728.0
  interstitial 728.81
  multiple — *see* Polymyositis
  occupational 729.1
  orbital, chronic 376.12
  ossificans 728.12
    circumscribed 728.12
    progressive 728.11
    traumatic 728.12
  progressive fibrosing 728.11
  purulent 728.0
  rheumatic 729.1
  rheumatoid 729.1
  suppurative 728.0
  syphilitic 095.6
  traumatic (old) 729.1

Myospasia impulsiva 307.23

Myotonia (acquisita) (intermittens) 728.85
  atrophica 359.2
  congenita 359.2
  dystrophica 359.2

Myotonic pupil 379.46

Myriapodiasis 134.1

Myringitis
  with otitis media — *see* Otitis media
  acute 384.00
    specified type NEC 384.09
  bullosa hemorrhagica 384.01
  bullous 384.01
  chronic 384.1

Mysophobia 300.29

Mytilotoxism 988.0

Myxadenitis labialis 528.5

Myxedema (adult) (idiocy) (infantile) (juvenile) (thyroid gland) (*see also* Hypothyroidism) 244.9
  circumscribed 242.9 ✓5ᵗʰ
  congenital 243
  cutis 701.8
  localized (pretibial) 242.9 ✓5ᵗʰ
  madness (acute) 293.0
    subacute 293.1
  papular 701.8
  pituitary 244.8
  postpartum 674.8 ✓5ᵗʰ
  pretibial 242.9 ✓5ᵗʰ
  primary 244.9

Myxochondrosarcoma (M9220/3) — *see* Neoplasm, cartilage, malignant

Myxofibroma (M8811/0) — *see also* Neoplasm, connective tissue, benign
  odontogenic (M9320/0) 213.1
    upper jaw (bone) 213.0

Myxofibrosarcoma (M8811/3) — *see* Neoplasm, connective tissue, malignant

Myxolipoma (M8852/0) (*see also* Lipoma, by site) 214.9

Myxoliposarcoma (M8852/3) — *see* Neoplasm, connective tissue, malignant

Myxoma (M8840/0) — *see also* Neoplasm, connective tissue, benign
  odontogenic (M9320/0) 213.1
    upper jaw (bone) 213.0

Myxosarcoma (M8840/3) — *see* Neoplasm, connective tissue, malignant

N

Naegeli's
  disease (hereditary hemorrhagic thrombasthenia) 287.1
  leukemia, monocytic (M9863/3) 205.1 ✓5ᵗʰ
  syndrome (incontinentia pigmenti) 757.33

Naffziger's syndrome 353.0

Naga sore (*see also* Ulcer, skin) 707.9

Nägele's pelvis 738.6
  with disproportion (fetopelvic) 653.0 ✓5ᵗʰ
    affecting fetus or newborn 763.1
    causing obstructed labor 660.1 ✓5ᵗʰ
      affecting fetus or newborn 763.1

Nager-de Reynier syndrome (dysostosis mandibularis) 756.0

Nail — *see also* condition
  biting 307.9
  patella syndrome (hereditary osteoonychodysplasia) 756.89

Nanism, nonosomia (*see also* Dwarfism) 259.4
  hypophyseal 253.3
  pituitary 253.3
  renis, renalis 588.0

Nanukayami 100.89

Napkin rash 691.0

Narcissism 301.81

Narcolepsy 347

Narcosis
  carbon dioxide (respiratory) 786.09
  due to drug
    correct substance properly administered 780.0
    overdose or wrong substance given or taken 977.9
      specified drug — *see* Table of Drugs and Chemicals

Narcotism (chronic) (*see also* listing under Dependence) 304.9 ✓5ᵗʰ
  acute
    correct substance properly administered 349.82
    overdose or wrong substance given or taken 967.8
      specified drug — *see* Table of Drugs and Chemicals

Narrow
  anterior chamber angle 365.02
  pelvis (inlet) (outlet) — *see* Contraction, pelvis

Narrowing
  artery NEC 447.1
    auditory, internal 433.8 ✓5ᵗʰ
    basilar 433.0 ✓5ᵗʰ
      with other precerebral artery 433.3 ✓5ᵗʰ
      bilateral 433.3 ✓5ᵗʰ
    carotid 433.1 ✓5ᵗʰ
      with other precerebral artery 433.3 ✓5ᵗʰ
      bilateral 433.3 ✓5ᵗʰ
    cerebellar 433.8 ✓5ᵗʰ
    choroidal 433.8 ✓5ᵗʰ
    communicating posterior 433.8 ✓5ᵗʰ
    coronary — *see also* Arteriosclerosis, coronary
      congenital 746.85
      due to syphilis 090.5
    hypophyseal 433.8 ✓5ᵗʰ
    pontine 433.8 ✓5ᵗʰ
    precerebral NEC 433.9 ✓5ᵗʰ
      multiple or bilateral 433.3 ✓5ᵗʰ
      specified NEC 433.8 ✓5ᵗʰ
    vertebral 433.2 ✓5ᵗʰ
      with other precerebral artery 433.3 ✓5ᵗʰ
      bilateral 433.3 ✓5ᵗʰ
  auditory canal (external) (*see also* Stricture, ear canal, acquired) 380.50
  cerebral arteries 437.0
  cicatricial — *see* Cicatrix

Narrowing — continued
congenital — see Anomaly, congenital
coronary artery — see Narrowing, artery,
coronary
ear, middle 385.22
Eustachian tube (see also Obstruction,
Eustachian tube) 381.60
eyelid 374.46
congenital 743.62
intervertebral disc or space NEC — see
Degeneration, intervertebral disc
joint space, hip 719.85
larynx 478.74
lids 374.46
congenital 743.62
mesenteric artery (with gangrene) 557.0
palate 524.8
palpebral fissure 374.46
retinal artery 362.13
ureter 593.3
urethra (see also Stricture, urethra) 598.9
Narrowness, abnormal, eyelid 743.62
Nasal — see condition
Nasolacrimal — see condition
Nasopharyngeal — see also condition
bursa 478.29
pituitary gland 759.2
torticollis 723.5
Nasopharyngitis (acute) (infective) (subacute) 460
chronic 472.2
due to external agent — see Condition,
respiratory, chronic, due to
due to external agent — see Condition,
respiratory, due to
septic 034.0
streptococcal 034.0
suppurative (chronic) 472.2
ulcerative (chronic) 472.2
Nasopharynx, nasopharyngeal — see condition
Natal tooth, teeth 520.6
Nausea (see also Vomiting) 787.02
with vomiting 787.01
epidemic 078.82
gravidarum — see Hyperemesis, gravidarum
marina 994.6
Navel — see condition
Neapolitan fever (see also Brucellosis) 023.9
Nearsightedness 367.1
Near-syncope 780.2
Nebécourt's syndrome 253.3
Nebula, cornea (eye) 371.01
congenital 743.43
interfering with vision 743.42
Necator americanus infestation 126.1
Necatoriasis 126.1
Neck — see condition
Necrencephalus (see also Softening, brain) 437.8
Necrobacillosis 040.3
Necrobiosis 799.8
brain or cerebral (see also Softening, brain)
437.8
lipoidica 709.3
diabeticorum 250.8 ✔5ᵗʰ [709.3]
Necrodermolysis 695.1
Necrolysis, toxic epidermal 695.1
due to drug
correct substance properly administered
695.1
overdose or wrong substance given or taken
977.9
specified drug — see Table of Drugs and
Chemicals
Necrophilia 302.89
Necrosis, necrotic
adrenal (capsule) (gland) 255.8
antrum, nasal sinus 478.1
aorta (hyaline) (see also Aneurysm, aorta)
441.9
cystic medial 441.00
abdominal 441.02
thoracic 441.01
thoracoabdominal 441.03
ruptured 441.5

Necrosis, necrotic — continued
arteritis 446.0
artery 447.5
aseptic, bone 733.40
femur (head) (neck) 733.42
medial condyle 733.43
humoral head 733.41
medial femoral condyle 733.43
specific site NEC 733.49
talus 733.44
avascular, bone NEC (see also Necrosis,
aseptic, bone) 733.40
bladder (aseptic) (sphincter) 596.8
bone (see also Osteomyelitis) 730.1 ✔5ᵗʰ
acute 730.0 ✔5ᵗʰ
aseptic or avascular 733.40
femur (head) (neck) 733.42
medial condyle 733.43
humoral head 733.41
medial femoral condyle 733.43
specified site NEC 733.49
talus 733.44
ethmoid 478.1
ischemic 733.40
jaw 526.4
marrow 289.8
Paget's (osteitis deformans) 731.0
tuberculous — see Tuberculosis, bone
brain (softening) (see also Softening, brain)
437.8
breast (aseptic) (fat) (segmental) 611.3
bronchus, bronchi 519.1
central nervous system NEC (see also
Softening, brain) 437.8
cerebellar (see also Softening, brain) 437.8
cerebral (softening) (see also Softening, brain)
437.8
cerebrospinal (softening) (see also Softening,
brain) 437.8
cornea (see also Keratitis) 371.40
cortical, kidney 583.6
cystic medial (aorta) 441.00
abdominal 441.02
thoracic 441.01
thoracoabdominal 441.03
dental 521.09
pulp 522.1
due to swallowing corrosive substance — see
Burn, by site
ear (ossicle) 385.24
esophagus 530.89
ethmoid (bone) 478.1
eyelid 374.50
fat, fatty (generalized) (see also Degeneration,
fatty) 272.8
breast (aseptic) (segmental) 611.3
intestine 569.89
localized — see Degeneration, by site, fatty
mesentery 567.8
omentum 567.8
pancreas 577.8
peritoneum 567.8
skin (subcutaneous) 709.3
newborn 778.1
femur (aseptic) (avascular) 733.42
head 733.42
medial condyle 733.43
neck 733.42
gallbladder (see also Cholecystitis, acute) 575.0
gangrenous 785.4
gastric 537.89
glottis 478.79
heart (myocardium) — see Infarct, myocardium
hepatic (see also Necrosis, liver) 570
hip (aseptic) (avascular) 733.42
intestine (acute) (hemorrhagic) (massive) 557.0
ischemic 785.4
jaw 526.4
kidney (bilateral) 583.9
acute 584.9
cortical 583.6
acute 584.6
with
abortion — see Abortion, by type,
with renal failure
ectopic pregnancy (see also
categories 633.0-633.9) 639.3

Necrosis, necrotic — continued
kidney — continued
cortical — continued
acute — continued
with — continued
molar pregnancy (see also
categories 630-632) 639.3
complicating pregnancy 646.2 ✔5ᵗʰ
affecting fetus or newborn 760.1
following labor and delivery 669.3 ✔5ᵗʰ
medullary (papillary) (see also Pyelitis)
590.80
in
acute renal failure 584.7
nephritis, nephropathy 583.7
papillary (see also Pyelitis) 590.80
in
acute renal failure 584.7
nephritis, nephropathy 583.7
tubular 584.5
with
abortion — see Abortion, by type, with
renal failure
ectopic pregnancy (see also categories
633.0-633.9) 639.3
molar pregnancy (see also categories
630-632) 639.3
complicating
abortion 639.3
ectopic or molar pregnancy 639.3
pregnancy 646.2 ✔5ᵗʰ
affecting fetus or newborn 760.1
following labor and delivery 669.3 ✔5ᵗʰ
traumatic 958.5
larynx 478.79
liver (acute) (congenital) (diffuse) (massive)
(subacute) 570
with
abortion — see Abortion, by type, with
specified complication NEC
ectopic pregnancy (see also categories
633.0-633.9) 639.8
molar pregnancy (see also categories 630-
632) 639.8
complicating pregnancy 646.7 ✔5ᵗʰ
affecting fetus or newborn 760.8
following
abortion 639.8
ectopic or molar pregnancy 639.8
obstetrical 646.7 ✔5ᵗʰ
postabortal 639.8
puerperal, postpartum 674.8 ✔5ᵗʰ
toxic 573.3
lung 513.0
lymphatic gland 683
mammary gland 611.3
mastoid (chronic) 383.1
mesentery 557.0
fat 567.8
mitral valve — see Insufficiency, mitral
myocardium, myocardial — see Infarct,
myocardium
nose (septum) 478.1
omentum 557.0
with mesenteric infarction 557.0
fat 567.8
orbit, orbital 376.10
ossicles, ear (aseptic) 385.24
ovary (see also Salpingo-oophoritis) 614.2
pancreas (aseptic) (duct) (fat) 577.8
acute 577.0
infective 577.0
papillary, kidney (see also Pyelitis) 590.80
peritoneum 557.0
with mesenteric infarction 557.0
fat 567.8
pharynx 462
in granulocytopenia 288.0
phosphorus 983.9
pituitary (gland) (postpartum) (Sheehan) 253.2
placenta (see also Placenta, abnormal)
656.7 ✔5ᵗʰ
pneumonia 513.0
pulmonary 513.0
pulp (dental) 522.1
pylorus 537.89
radiation — see Necrosis, by site

✔4ᵗʰ Fourth-digit Required   ✔5ᵗʰ Fifth-digit Required   ▶◀ Revised Text   ● New Line   ▲ Revised Code

Necrosis — Neonatorum

Necrosis, necrotic — *continued*
  radium — *see* Necrosis, by site
  renal — *see* Necrosis, kidney
  sclera 379.19
  scrotum 608.89
  skin or subcutaneous tissue 709.8
    due to burn — *see* Burn, by site
    gangrenous 785.4
  spine, spinal (column) 730.18
    acute 730.18
    cord 336.1
  spleen 289.59
  stomach 537.89
  stomatitis 528.1
  subcutaneous fat 709.3
    fetus or newborn 778.1
  subendocardial — *see* Infarct, myocardium
  suprarenal (capsule) (gland) 255.8
  teeth, tooth 521.09
  testis 608.89
  thymus (gland) 254.8
  tonsil 474.8
  trachea 519.1
  tuberculous NEC — *see* Tuberculosis
  tubular (acute) (anoxic) (toxic) 584.5
    due to a procedure 997.5
  umbilical cord, affecting fetus or newborn
    762.6
  vagina 623.8
  vertebra (lumbar) 730.18
    acute 730.18
    tuberculous (*see also* Tuberculosis)
      015.0 ✓5ᵗʰ [730.8] ✓5ᵗʰ
  vesical (aseptic) (bladder) 596.8
  x-ray — *see* Necrosis, by site

Necrospermia 606.0

Necrotizing angiitis 446.0

Negativism 301.7

Neglect (child) (newborn) NEC 995.52
  adult 995.84
  after or at birth 995.52
  hemispatial 781.8
  left-sided 781.8
  sensory 781.8
  visuospatial 781.8

Negri bodies 071

Neill-Dingwall syndrome (microcephaly and
  dwarfism) 759.89

Neisserian infection NEC — *see* Gonococcus

Nematodiasis NEC (*see also* Infestation,
  Nematode) 127.9
  ancylostoma (*see also* Ancylostomiasis) 126.9

Neoformans cryptococcus infection 117.5

Neonatal — *see also* condition
  teeth, tooth 520.6

Neonatorum — *see* condition

	Malignant			Benign	Uncertain Behavior	Unspecified
	Primary	**Secondary**	**Ca in situ**			
Neoplasm, neoplastic	199.1	199.1	234.9	229.9	238.9	239.9

Notes — 1. The list below gives the code numbers for neoplasms by anatomical site. For each site there are six possible code numbers according to whether the neoplasm in question is malignant, benign, in situ, of uncertain behavior, or of unspecified nature. The description of the neoplasm will often indicate which of the six columns is appropriate; e.g., malignant melanoma of skin, benign fibroadenoma of breast, carcinoma in situ of cervix uteri.

Where such descriptors are not present, the remainder of the Index should be consulted where guidance is given to the appropriate column for each morphological (histological) variety listed; e.g., Mesonephroma — see Neoplasm, malignant; Embryoma — see also Neoplasm, uncertain behavior; Disease, Bowen's — see Neoplasm, skin, in situ. However, the guidance in the Index can be overridden if one of the descriptors mentioned above is present; e.g., malignant adenoma of colon is coded to 153.9 and not to 211.3 as the adjective "malignant" overrides the Index entry "Adenoma — see also Neoplasm, benign."

*2. Sites marked with the sign * (e.g., face NEC*) should be classified to malignant neoplasm of skin of these sites if the variety of neoplasm is a squamous cell carcinoma or an epidermoid carcinoma, and to benign neoplasm of skin of these sites if the variety of neoplasm is a papilloma (any type).*

	Primary	Secondary	Ca in situ	Benign	Uncertain Behavior	Unspecified
abdomen, abdominal	195.2	198.89	234.8	229.8	238.8	239.8
cavity	195.2	198.89	234.8	229.8	238.8	239.8
organ	195.2	198.89	234.8	229.8	238.8	239.8
viscera	195.2	198.89	234.8	229.8	238.8	239.8
wall	173.5	198.2	232.5	216.5	238.2	239.2
connective tissue	171.5	198.89	—	215.5	238.1	239.2
abdominopelvic	195.8	198.89	234.8	229.8	238.8	239.8
accessory sinus — *see* Neoplasm, sinus						
acoustic nerve	192.0	198.4	—	225.1	237.9	239.7
acromion (process)	170.4	198.5	—	213.4	238.0	239.2
adenoid (pharynx) (tissue)	147.1	198.89	230.0	210.7	235.1	239.0
adipose tissue (*see also* Neoplasm, connective tissue)	171.9	198.89	—	215.9	238.1	239.2
adnexa (uterine)	183.9	198.82	233.3	221.8	236.3	239.5
adrenal (cortex) (gland) (medulla)	194.0	198.7	234.8	227.0	237.2	239.7
ala nasi (external)	173.3	198.2	232.3	216.3	238.2	239.2
alimentary canal or tract NEC	159.9	197.8	230.9	211.9	235.5	239.0
alveolar	143.9	198.89	230.0	210.4	235.1	239.0
mucosa	143.9	198.89	230.0	210.4	235.1	239.0
lower	143.1	198.89	230.0	210.4	235.1	239.0
upper	143.0	198.89	230.0	210.4	235.1	239.0
ridge or process	170.1	198.5	—	213.1	238.0	239.2
carcinoma	143.9	—	—	—	—	—
lower	143.1	—	—	—	—	—
upper	143.0	—	—	—	—	—
lower	170.1	198.5	—	213.1	238.0	239.2
mucosa	143.9	198.89	230.0	210.4	235.1	239.0
lower	143.1	198.89	230.0	210.4	235.1	239.0
upper	143.0	198.89	230.0	210.4	235.1	239.0
upper	170.0	198.5	—	213.0	238.0	239.2
sulcus	145.1	198.89	230.0	210.4	235.1	239.0
alveolus	143.9	198.89	230.0	210.4	235.1	239.0
lower	143.1	198.89	230.0	210.4	235.1	239.0
upper	143.0	198.89	230.0	210.4	235.1	239.0
ampulla of Vater	156.2	197.8	230.8	211.5	235.3	239.0
ankle NEC*	195.5	198.89	232.7	229.8	238.8	239.8
anorectum, anorectal (junction)	154.8	197.5	230.7	211.4	235.2	239.0
antecubital fossa or space*	195.4	198.89	232.6	229.8	238.8	239.8
antrum (Highmore) (maxillary)	160.2	197.3	231.8	212.0	235.9	239.1
pyloric	151.2	197.8	230.2	211.1	235.2	239.0
tympanicum	160.1	197.3	231.8	212.0	235.9	239.1
anus, anal	154.3	197.5	230.6	211.4	235.5	239.0
canal	154.2	197.5	230.5	211.4	233.5	239.0
contiguous sites with rectosigmoid junction or rectum	154.8	—	—	—	—	—
margin	173.5	198.2	232.5	216.5	238.2	239.2
skin	173.5	198.2	232.5	216.5	238.2	239.2
sphincter	154.2	197.5	230.5	211.4	235.5	239.0
aorta (thoracic)	171.4	198.89	—	215.4	238.1	239.2
abdominal	171.5	198.89	—	215.5	238.1	239.2
aortic body	194.6	198.89	—	227.6	237.3	239.7
aponeurosis	171.9	198.89	—	215.9	238.1	239.2
palmar	171.2	198.89	—	215.2	238.1	239.2
plantar	171.3	198.89	—	215.3	238.1	239.2
appendix	153.5	197.5	230.3	211.3	235.2	239.0
arachnoid (cerebral)	192.1	198.4	—	225.2	237.6	239.7
spinal	192.3	198.4	—	225.4	237.6	239.7

	Malignant					
	Primary	**Secondary**	**Ca in situ**	**Benign**	**Uncertain Behavior**	**Unspecified**
Neoplasm, neoplastic — *continued*						
areola (female)	174.0	198.81	233.0	217	238.3	239.3
male	175.0	198.81	233.0	217	238.3	239.3
arm NEC*	195.4	198.89	232.6	229.8	238.8	239.8
artery — *see* Neoplasm, connective tissue						
aryepiglottic fold	148.2	198.89	230.0	210.8	235.1	239.0
hypopharyngeal aspect	148.2	198.89	230.0	210.8	235.1	239.0
laryngeal aspect	161.1	197.3	231.0	212.1	235.6	239.1
marginal zone	148.2	198.89	230.0	210.8	235.1	239.0
arytenoid (cartilage)	161.3	197.3	231.0	212.1	235.6	239.1
fold — *see* Neoplasm, aryepiglottic						
atlas	170.2	198.5	—	213.2	238.0	239.2
atrium, cardiac	164.1	198.89	—	212.7	238.8	239.8
auditory						
canal (external) (skin)	173.2	198.2	232.2	216.2	238.2	239.2
internal	160.1	197.3	231.8	212.0	235.9	239.1
nerve	192.0	198.4	—	225.1	237.9	239.7
tube	160.1	197.3	231.8	212.0	235.9	239.1
opening	147.2	198.89	230.0	210.7	235.1	239.0
auricle, ear	173.2	198.2	232.2	216.2	238.2	239.2
cartilage	171.0	198.89	—	215.0	238.1	239.2
auricular canal (external)	173.2	198.2	232.2	216.2	238.2	239.2
internal	160.1	197.3	231.8	212.0	235.9	239.1
autonomic nerve or nervous system NEC	171.9	198.89	—	215.9	238.1	239.2
axilla, axillary	195.1	198.89	234.8	229.8	238.8	239.8
fold	173.5	198.2	232.5	216.5	238.2	239.2
back NEC*	195.8	198.89	232.5	229.8	238.8	239.8
Bartholin's gland	184.1	198.82	233.3	221.2	236.3	239.5
basal ganglia	191.0	198.3	—	225.0	237.5	239.6
basis pedunculi	191.7	198.3	—	225.0	237.5	239.6
bile or biliary (tract)	156.9	197.8	230.8	211.5	235.3	239.0
canaliculi (biliferi) (intrahepatic)	155.1	197.8	230.8	211.5	235.3	239.0
canals, interlobular	155.1	197.8	230.8	211.5	235.3	239.0
contiguous sites	156.8	—	—	—	—	—
duct or passage (common) (cystic) (extrahepatic)	156.1	197.8	230.8	211.5	235.3	239.0
contiguous sites with gallbladder	156.8	—	—	—	—	—
interlobular	155.1	197.8	230.8	211.5	235.3	239.0
intrahepatic	155.1	197.8	230.8	211.5	235.3	239.0
and extrahepatic	156.9	197.8	230.8	211.5	235.3	239.0
bladder (urinary)	188.9	198.1	233.7	223.3	236.7	239.4
contiguous sites	188.8	—	—	—	—	—
dome	188.1	198.1	233.7	223.3	236.7	239.4
neck	188.5	198.1	233.7	223.3	236.7	239.4
orifice	188.9	198.1	233.7	223.3	236.7	239.4
ureteric	188.6	198.1	233.7	223.3	236.7	239.4
urethral	188.5	198.1	233.7	223.3	236.7	239.4
sphincter	188.8	198.1	233.7	223.3	236.7	239.4
trigone	188.0	198.1	233.7	223.3	236.7	239.4
urachus	188.7	—	233.7	223.3	236.7	239.4
wall	188.9	198.1	233.7	223.3	236.7	239.4
anterior	188.3	198.1	233.7	223.3	236.7	239.4
lateral	188.2	198.1	233.7	223.3	236.7	239.4
posterior	188.4	198.1	233.7	223.3	236.7	239.4
blood vessel — *see* Neoplasm, connective tissue						
bone (periosteum)	170.9	198.5	—	213.9	238.0	239.2

Note — Carcinomas and adenocarcinomas, of any type other than intraosseous or odontogenic, of the sites listed under "Neoplasm, bone" should be considered as constituting metastatic spread from an unspecified primary site and coded to 198.5 for morbidity coding and to 199.1 for underlying cause of death coding.

acetabulum	170.6	198.5	—	213.6	238.0	239.2
acromion (process)	170.4	198.5	—	213.4	238.0	239.2
ankle	170.8	198.5	—	213.8	238.0	239.2
arm NEC	170.4	198.5	—	213.4	238.0	239.2
astragalus	170.8	198.5	—	213.8	238.0	239.2
atlas	170.2	198.5	—	213.2	238.0	239.2
axis	170.2	198.5	—	213.2	238.0	239.2
back NEC	170.2	198.5	—	213.2	238.0	239.2
calcaneus	170.8	198.5	—	213.8	238.0	239.2

✔4ᵗʰ Fourth-digit Required   ✔5ᵗʰ Fifth-digit Required   ▶◀ Revised Text   ● New Line   ▲ Revised Code

Neoplasm, neoplastic — continued	Malignant			Benign	Uncertain Behavior	Unspecified
	Primary	Secondary	Ca in situ	Benign	Uncertain Behavior	Unspecified
bone — continued						
calvarium	170.0	198.5	—	213.0	238.0	239.2
carpus (any)	170.5	198.5	—	213.5	238.0	239.2
cartilage NEC	170.9	198.5	—	213.9	238.0	239.2
clavicle	170.3	198.5	—	213.3	238.0	239.2
clivus	170.0	198.5	—	213.0	238.0	239.2
coccygeal vertebra	170.6	198.5	—	213.6	238.0	239.2
coccyx	170.6	198.5	—	213.6	238.0	239.2
costal cartilage	170.3	198.5	—	213.3	238.0	239.2
costovertebral joint	170.3	198.5	—	213.3	238.0	239.2
cranial	170.0	198.5	—	213.0	238.0	239.2
cuboid	170.8	198.5	—	213.8	238.0	239.2
cuneiform	170.9	198.5	—	213.9	238.0	239.2
ankle	170.8	198.5	—	213.8	238.0	239.2
wrist	170.5	198.5	—	213.5	238.0	239.2
digital	170.9	198.5	—	213.9	238.0	239.2
finger	170.5	198.5	—	213.5	238.0	239.2
toe	170.8	198.5	—	213.8	238.0	239.2
elbow	170.4	198.5	—	213.4	238.0	239.2
ethmoid (labyrinth)	170.0	198.5	—	213.0	238.0	239.2
face	170.0	198.5	—	213.0	238.0	239.2
lower jaw	170.1	198.5	—	213.1	238.0	239.2
femur (any part)	170.7	198.5	—	213.7	238.0	239.2
fibula (any part)	170.7	198.5	—	213.7	238.0	239.2
finger (any)	170.5	198.5	—	213.5	238.0	239.2
foot	170.8	198.5	—	213.8	238.0	239.2
forearm	170.4	198.5	—	213.4	238.0	239.2
frontal	170.0	198.5	—	213.0	238.0	239.2
hand	170.5	198.5	—	213.5	238.0	239.2
heel	170.8	198.5	—	213.8	238.0	239.2
hip	170.6	198.5	—	213.6	238.0	239.2
humerus (any part)	170.4	198.5	—	213.4	238.0	239.2
hyoid	170.0	198.5	—	213.0	238.0	239.2
ilium	170.6	198.5	—	213.6	238.0	239.2
innominate	170.6	198.5	—	213.6	238.0	239.2
intervertebral cartilage or disc	170.2	198.5	—	213.2	238.0	239.2
ischium	170.6	198.5	—	213.6	238.0	239.2
jaw (lower)	170.1	198.5	—	213.1	238.0	239.2
upper	170.0	198.5	—	213.0	238.0	239.2
knee	170.7	198.5	—	213.7	238.0	239.2
leg NEC	170.7	198.5	—	213.7	238.0	239.2
limb NEC	170.9	198.5	—	213.9	238.0	239.2
lower (long bones)	170.7	198.5	—	213.7	238.0	239.2
short bones	170.8	198.5	—	213.8	238.0	239.2
upper (long bones)	170.4	198.5	—	213.4	238.0	239.2
short bones	170.5	198.5	—	213.5	238.0	239.2
long	170.9	198.5	—	213.9	238.0	239.2
lower limbs NEC	170.7	198.5	—	213.7	238.0	239.2
upper limbs NEC	170.4	198.5	—	213.4	238.0	239.2
malar	170.0	198.5	—	213.0	238.0	239.2
mandible	170.1	198.5	—	213.1	238.0	239.2
marrow NEC	202.9 ✓5ᵗʰ	198.5	—	—	—	238.7
mastoid	170.0	198.5	—	213.0	238.0	239.2
maxilla, maxillary (superior)	170.0	198.5	—	213.0	238.0	239.2
inferior	170.1	198.5	—	213.1	238.0	239.2
metacarpus (any)	170.5	198.5	—	213.5	238.0	239.2
metatarsus (any)	170.8	198.5	—	213.8	238.0	239.2
navicular (ankle)	170.8	198.5	—	213.8	238.0	239.2
hand	170.5	198.5	—	213.5	238.0	239.2
nose, nasal	170.0	198.5	—	213.0	238.0	239.2
occipital	170.0	198.5	—	213.0	238.0	239.2
orbit	170.0	198.5	—	213.0	238.0	239.2
parietal	170.0	198.5	—	213.0	238.0	239.2
patella	170.8	198.5	—	213.8	238.0	239.2
pelvic	170.6	198.5	—	213.6	238.0	239.2

✓4ᵗʰ Fourth-digit Required   ✓5ᵗʰ Fifth-digit Required   ▶◀ Revised Text   ● New Line   ▲ Revised Code

| | Malignant | | | | | |
	Primary	Secondary	Ca in situ	Benign	Uncertain Behavior	Unspecified
Neoplasm, neoplastic — *continued*						
bone — *continued*						
phalanges	170.9	198.5	—	213.9	238.0	239.2
foot	170.8	198.5	—	213.8	238.0	239.2
hand	170.5	198.5	—	213.5	238.0	239.2
pubic	170.6	198.5	—	213.6	238.0	239.2
radius (any part)	170.4	198.5	—	213.4	238.0	239.2
rib	170.3	198.5	—	213.3	238.0	239.2
sacral vertebra	170.6	198.5	—	213.6	238.0	239.2
sacrum	170.6	198.5	—	213.6	238.0	239.2
scaphoid (of hand)	170.5	198.5	—	213.5	238.0	239.2
of ankle	170.8	198.5	—	213.8	238.0	239.2
scapula (any part)	170.4	198.5	—	213.4	238.0	239.2
sella turcica	170.0	198.5	—	213.0	238.0	239.2
short	170.9	198.5	—	213.9	238.0	239.2
lower limb	170.8	198.5	—	213.8	238.0	239.2
upper limb	170.5	198.5	—	213.5	238.0	239.2
shoulder	170.4	198.5	—	213.4	238.0	239.2
skeleton, skeletal NEC	170.9	198.5	—	213.9	238.0	239.2
skull	170.0	198.5	—	213.0	238.0	239.2
sphenoid	170.0	198.5	—	213.0	238.0	239.2
spine, spinal (column)	170.2	198.5	—	213.2	238.0	239.2
coccyx	170.6	198.5	—	213.6	238.0	239.2
sacrum	170.6	198.5	—	213.6	238.0	239.2
sternum	170.3	198.5	—	213.3	238.0	239.2
tarsus (any)	170.8	198.5	—	213.8	238.0	239.2
temporal	170.0	198.5	—	213.0	238.0	239.2
thumb	170.5	198.5	—	213.5	238.0	239.2
tibia (any part)	170.7	198.5	—	213.7	238.0	239.2
toe (any)	170.8	198.5	—	213.8	238.0	239.2
trapezium	170.5	198.5	—	213.5	238.0	239.2
trapezoid	170.5	198.5	—	213.5	238.0	239.2
turbinate	170.0	198.5	—	213.0	238.0	239.2
ulna (any part)	170.4	198.5	—	213.4	238.0	239.2
unciform	170.5	198.5	—	213.5	238.0	239.2
vertebra (column)	170.2	198.5	—	213.2	238.0	239.2
coccyx	170.6	198.5	—	213.6	238.0	239.2
sacrum	170.6	198.5	—	213.6	238.0	239.2
vomer	170.0	198.5	—	213.0	238.0	239.2
wrist	170.5	198.5	—	213.5	238.0	239.2
xiphoid process	170.3	198.5	—	213.3	238.0	239.2
zygomatic	170.0	198.5	—	213.0	238.0	239.2
book-leaf (mouth)	145.8	198.89	230.0	210.4	235.1	239.0
bowel — *see* Neoplasm, intestine						
brachial plexus	171.2	198.89	—	215.2	238.1	239.2
brain NEC	191.9	198.3	—	225.0	237.5	239.6
basal ganglia	191.0	198.3	—	225.0	237.5	239.6
cerebellopontine angle	191.6	198.3	—	225.0	237.5	239.6
cerebellum NOS	191.6	198.3	—	225.0	237.5	239.6
cerebrum	191.0	198.3	—	225.0	237.5	239.6
choroid plexus	191.5	198.3	—	225.0	237.5	239.6
contiguous sites	191.8	—	—	—	—	—
corpus callosum	191.8	198.3	—	225.0	237.5	239.6
corpus striatum	191.0	198.3	—	225.0	237.5	239.6
cortex (cerebral)	191.0	198.3	—	225.0	237.5	239.6
frontal lobe	191.1	198.3	—	225.0	237.5	239.6
globus pallidus	191.0	198.3	—	225.0	237.5	239.6
hippocampus	191.2	198.3	—	225.0	237.5	239.6
hypothalamus	191.0	198.3	—	225.0	237.5	239.6
internal capsule	191.0	198.3	—	225.0	237.5	239.6
medulla oblongata	191.7	198.3	—	225.0	237.5	239.6
meninges	192.1	198.4	—	225.2	237.6	239.7
midbrain	191.7	198.3	—	225.0	237.5	239.6
occipital lobe	191.4	198.3	—	225.0	237.5	239.6
parietal lobe	191.3	198.3	—	225.0	237.5	239.6
peduncle	191.7	198.3	—	225.0	237.5	239.6
pons	191.7	198.3	—	225.0	237.5	239.6

Ⱶ4ᵗ Fourth-digit Required   Ⱶ5ᵗ Fifth-digit Required   ▶◀ Revised Text   ● New Line   ▲ Revised Code

	Malignant					
	Primary	**Secondary**	**Ca in situ**	**Benign**	**Uncertain Behavior**	**Unspecified**
Neoplasm, neoplastic — *continued*						
brain NEC — *continued*						
stem	191.7	198.3	—	225.0	237.5	239.6
tapetum	191.8	198.3	—	225.0	237.5	239.6
temporal lobe	191.2	198.3	—	225.0	237.5	239.6
thalamus	191.0	198.3	—	225.0	237.5	239.6
uncus	191.2	198.3	—	225.0	237.5	239.6
ventricle (floor)	191.5	198.3	—	225.0	237.5	239.6
branchial (cleft) (vestiges)	146.8	198.89	230.0	210.6	235.1	239.0
breast (connective tissue) (female) (glandular tissue) (soft parts)	174.9	198.81	233.0	217	238.3	239.3
areola	174.0	198.81	233.0	217	238.3	239.3
male	175.0	198.81	233.0	217	238.3	239.3
axillary tail	174.6	198.81	233.0	217	238.3	239.3
central portion	174.1	198.81	233.0	217	238.3	239.3
contiguous sites	174.8	—	—	—	—	—
ectopic sites	174.8	198.81	233.0	217	238.3	239.3
inner	174.8	198.81	233.0	217	238.3	239.3
lower	174.8	198.81	233.0	217	238.3	239.3
lower-inner quadrant	174.3	198.81	233.0	217	238.3	239.3
lower-outer quadrant	174.5	198.81	233.0	217	238.3	239.3
male	175.9	198.81	233.0	217	238.3	239.3
areola	175.0	198.81	233.0	217	238.3	239.3
ectopic tissue	175.9	198.81	233.0	217	238.3	239.3
nipple	175.0	198.81	233.0	217	238.3	239.3
mastectomy site (skin)	173.5	198.2	—	—	—	—
specified as breast tissue	174.8	198.81	—	—	—	—
midline	174.8	198.81	233.0	217	238.3	239.3
nipple	174.0	198.81	233.0	217	238.3	239.3
male	175.0	198.81	233.0	217	238.3	239.3
outer	174.8	198.81	233.0	217	238.3	239.3
skin	173.5	198.2	232.5	216.5	238.2	239.2
tail (axillary)	174.6	198.81	233.0	217	238.3	239.3
upper	174.8	198.81	233.0	217	238.3	239.3
upper-inner quadrant	174.2	198.81	233.0	217	238.3	239.3
upper-outer quadrant	174.4	198.81	233.0	217	238.3	239.3
broad ligament	183.3	198.82	233.3	221.0	236.3	239.5
bronchiogenic, bronchogenic (lung)	162.9	197.0	231.2	212.3	235.7	239.1
bronchiole	162.9	197.0	231.2	212.3	235.7	239.1
bronchus	162.9	197.0	231.2	212.3	235.7	239.1
carina	162.2	197.0	231.2	212.3	235.7	239.1
contiguous sites with lung or trachea	162.8	—	—	—	—	—
lower lobe of lung	162.5	197.0	231.2	212.3	235.7	239.1
main	162.2	197.0	231.2	212.3	235.7	239.1
middle lobe of lung	162.4	197.0	231.2	212.3	235.7	239.1
upper lobe of lung	162.3	197.0	231.2	212.3	235.7	239.1
brow	173.3	198.2	232.3	216.3	238.2	239.2
buccal (cavity)	145.9	198.89	230.0	210.4	235.1	239.0
commissure	145.0	198.89	230.0	210.4	235.1	239.0
groove (lower) (upper)	145.1	198.89	230.0	210.4	235.1	239.0
mucosa	145.0	198.89	230.0	210.4	235.1	239.0
sulcus (lower) (upper)	145.1	198.89	230.0	210.4	235.1	239.0
bulbourethral gland	189.3	198.1	233.9	223.81	236.99	239.5
bursa — *see* Neoplasm, connective tissue						
buttock NEC*	195.3	198.89	232.5	229.8	238.8	239.8
calf*	195.5	198.89	232.7	229.8	238.8	239.8
calvarium	170.0	198.5	—	213.0	238.0	239.2
calyx, renal	189.1	198.0	233.9	223.1	236.91	239.5
canal						
anal	154.2	197.5	230.5	211.4	235.5	239.0
auditory (external)	173.2	198.2	232.2	216.2	238.2	239.2
auricular (external)	173.2	198.2	232.2	216.2	238.2	239.2
canaliculi, biliary (biliferi) (intrahepatic)	155.1	197.8	230.8	211.5	235.3	239.0
canthus (eye) (inner) (outer)	173.1	198.2	232.1	216.1	238.2	239.2
capillary — *see* Neoplasm, connective tissue						
caput coli	153.4	197.5	230.3	211.3	235.2	239.0
cardia (gastric)	151.0	197.8	230.2	211.1	235.2	239.0
cardiac orifice (stomach)	151.0	197.8	230.2	211.1	235.2	239.0

Neoplasm, brain — Neoplasm, cardiac orifice

▨**4ᵗʰ** Fourth-digit Required   ▨**5ᵗʰ** Fifth-digit Required   ▶◀ Revised Text   ● New Line   ▲ Revised Code

	Malignant			Benign	Uncertain Behavior	Unspecified
	Primary	Secondary	Ca in situ			
Neoplasm, neoplastic — *continued*						
cardio-esophageal junction	151.0	197.8	230.2	211.1	235.2	239.0
cardio-esophagus	151.0	197.8	230.2	211.1	235.2	239.0
carina (trachea) (bronchus)	162.2	197.0	231.2	212.3	235.7	239.1
carotid (artery)	171.0	198.89	—	215.0	238.1	239.2
body	194.5	198.89	—	227.5	237.3	239.7
carpus (any bone)	170.5	198.5	—	213.5	238.0	239.2
cartilage (articular) (joint) NEC — *see also* Neoplasm, bone	170.9	198.5	—	213.9	238.0	239.2
arytenoid	161.3	197.3	231.0	212.1	235.6	239.1
auricular	171.0	198.89	—	215.0	238.1	239.2
bronchi	162.2	197.3	—	212.3	235.7	239.1
connective tissue — *see* Neoplasm, connective tissue						
costal	170.3	198.5	—	213.3	238.0	239.2
cricoid	161.3	197.3	231.0	212.1	235.6	239.1
cuneiform	161.3	197.3	231.0	212.1	235.6	239.1
ear (external)	171.0	198.89	—	215.0	238.1	239.2
ensiform	170.3	198.5	—	213.3	238.0	239.2
epiglottis	161.1	197.3	231.0	212.1	235.6	239.1
anterior surface	146.4	198.89	230.0	210.6	235.1	239.0
eyelid	171.0	198.89	—	215.0	238.1	239.2
intervertebral	170.2	198.5	—	213.2	238.0	239.2
larynx, laryngeal	161.3	197.3	231.0	212.1	235.6	239.1
nose, nasal	160.0	197.3	231.8	212.0	235.9	239.1
pinna	171.0	198.89	—	215.0	238.1	239.2
rib	170.3	198.5	—	213.3	238.0	239.2
semilunar (knee)	170.7	198.5	—	213.7	238.0	239.2
thyroid	161.3	197.3	231.0	212.1	235.6	239.1
trachea	162.0	197.3	231.1	212.2	235.7	239.1
cauda equina	192.2	198.3	—	225.3	237.5	239.7
cavity						
buccal	145.9	198.89	230.0	210.4	235.1	239.0
nasal	160.0	197.3	231.8	212.0	235.9	239.1
oral	145.9	198.89	230.0	210.4	235.1	239.0
peritoneal	158.9	197.6	—	211.8	235.4	239.0
tympanic	160.1	197.3	231.8	212.0	235.9	239.1
cecum	153.4	197.5	230.3	211.3	235.2	239.0
central						
nervous system — *see* Neoplasm, nervous system						
white matter	191.0	198.3	—	225.0	237.5	239.6
cerebellopontine (angle)	191.6	198.3	—	225.0	237.5	239.6
cerebellum, cerebellar	191.6	198.3	—	225.0	237.5	239.6
cerebrum, cerebral (cortex) (hemisphere) (white matter)	191.0	198.3	—	225.0	237.5	239.6
meninges	192.1	198.4	—	225.2	237.6	239.7
peduncle	191.7	198.3	—	225.0	237.5	239.6
ventricle (any)	191.5	198.3	—	225.0	237.5	239.6
cervical region	195.0	198.89	234.8	229.8	238.8	239.8
cervix (cervical) (uteri) (uterus)	180.9	198.82	233.1	219.0	236.0	239.5
canal	180.0	198.82	233.1	219.0	236.0	239.5
contiguous sites	180.8	—	—	—	—	—
endocervix (canal) (gland)	180.0	198.82	233.1	219.0	236.0	239.5
exocervix	180.1	198.82	233.1	219.0	236.0	239.5
external os	180.1	198.82	233.1	219.0	236.0	239.5
internal os	180.0	198.82	233.1	219.0	236.0	239.5
nabothian gland	180.0	198.82	233.1	219.0	236.0	239.5
squamocolumnar junction	180.8	198.82	233.1	219.0	236.0	239.5
stump	180.8	198.82	233.1	219.0	236.0	239.5
cheek	195.0	198.89	234.8	229.8	238.8	239.8
external	173.3	198.2	232.3	216.3	238.2	239.2
inner aspect	145.0	198.89	230.0	210.4	235.1	239.0
internal	145.0	198.89	230.0	210.4	235.1	239.0
mucosa	145.0	198.89	230.0	210.4	235.1	239.0
chest (wall) NEC	195.1	198.89	234.8	229.8	238.8	239.8
chiasma opticum	192.0	198.4	—	225.1	237.9	239.7
chin	173.3	198.2	232.3	216.3	238.2	239.2
choana	147.3	198.89	230.0	210.7	235.1	239.0
cholangiole	155.1	197.8	230.8	211.5	235.3	239.0
choledochal duct	156.1	197.8	230.8	211.5	235.3	239.0

✔4ᵗʰ Fourth-digit Required　　✔5ᵗʰ Fifth-digit Required　　▶◀ Revised Text　　● New Line　　▲ Revised Code

| | Malignant | | | | | |
	Primary	Secondary	Ca in situ	Benign	Uncertain Behavior	Unspecified
Neoplasm, neoplastic — *continued*						
choroid	190.6	198.4	234.0	224.6	238.8	239.8
plexus	191.5	198.3	—	225.0	237.5	239.6
ciliary body	190.0	198.4	234.0	224.0	238.8	239.8
clavicle	170.3	198.5	—	213.3	238.0	239.2
clitoris	184.3	198.82	233.3	221.2	236.3	239.5
clivus	170.0	198.5	—	213.0	238.0	239.2
cloacogenic zone	154.8	197.5	230.7	211.4	235.5	239.0
coccygeal						
body or glomus	194.6	198.89	—	227.6	237.3	239.7
vertebra	170.6	198.5	—	213.6	238.0	239.2
coccyx	170.6	198.5	—	213.6	238.0	239.2
colon — *see also* Neoplasm, intestine, large						
and rectum	154.0	197.5	230.4	211.4	235.2	239.0
column, spinal — *see* Neoplasm, spine						
columnella	173.3	198.2	232.3	216.3	238.2	239.2
commissure						
labial, lip	140.6	198.89	230.0	210.4	235.1	239.0
laryngeal	161.0	197.3	231.0	212.1	235.6	239.1
common (bile) duct	156.1	197.8	230.8	211.5	235.3	239.0
concha	173.2	198.2	232.2	216.2	238.2	239.2
nose	160.0	197.3	231.8	212.0	235.9	239.1
conjunctiva	190.3	198.4	234.0	224.3	238.8	239.8
connective tissue NEC	171.9	198.89	—	215.9	238.1	239.2

Note — For neoplasms of connective tissue (blood vessel, bursa, fascia, ligament, muscle, peripheral nerves, sympathetic and parasympathetic nerves and ganglia, synovia, tendon, etc.) or of morphological types that indicate connective tissue, code according to the list under "Neoplasm, connective tissue"; for sites that do not appear in this list, code to neoplasm of that site; e.g.,

> *liposarcoma, shoulder 171.2*
> *leiomyosarcoma, stomach 151.9*
> *neurofibroma, chest wall 215.4*

Morphological types that indicate connective tissue appear in the proper place in the alphabetic index with the instruction "see Neoplasm, connective tissue..."

	Primary	Secondary	Ca in situ	Benign	Uncertain Behavior	Unspecified
abdomen	171.5	198.89	—	215.5	238.1	239.2
abdominal wall	171.5	198.89	—	215.5	238.1	239.2
ankle	171.3	198.89	—	215.3	238.1	239.2
antecubital fossa or space	171.2	198.89	—	215.2	238.1	239.2
arm	171.2	198.89	—	215.2	238.1	239.2
auricle (ear)	171.0	198.89	—	215.0	238.1	239.2
axilla	171.4	198.89	—	215.4	238.1	239.2
back	171.7	198.89	—	215.7	238.1	239.2
breast (female) (*see also* Neoplasm, breast)	174.9	198.81	233.0	217	238.3	239.3
male	175.9	198.81	233.0	217	238.3	239.3
buttock	171.6	198.89	—	215.6	238.1	239.2
calf	171.3	198.89	—	215.3	238.1	239.2
cervical region	171.0	198.89	—	215.0	238.1	239.2
cheek	171.0	198.89	—	215.0	238.1	239.2
chest (wall)	171.4	198.89	—	215.4	238.1	239.2
chin	171.0	198.89	—	215.0	238.1	239.2
contiguous sites	171.8	—	—	—	—	—
diaphragm	171.4	198.89	—	215.4	238.1	239.2
ear (external)	171.0	198.89	—	215.0	238.1	239.2
elbow	171.2	198.89	—	215.2	238.1	239.2
extrarectal	171.6	198.89	—	215.6	238.1	239.2
extremity	171.8	198.89	—	215.8	238.1	239.2
lower	171.3	198.89	—	215.3	238.1	239.2
upper	171.2	198.89	—	215.2	238.1	239.2
eyelid	171.0	198.89	—	215.0	238.1	239.2
face	171.0	198.89	—	215.0	238.1	239.2
finger	171.2	198.89	—	215.2	238.1	239.2
flank	171.7	198.89	—	215.7	238.1	239.2
foot	171.3	198.89	—	215.3	238.1	239.2
forearm	171.2	198.89	—	215.2	238.1	239.2
forehead	171.0	198.89	—	215.0	238.1	239.2
gluteal region	171.6	198.89	—	215.6	238.1	239.2
great vessels NEC	171.4	198.89	—	215.4	238.1	239.2
groin	171.6	198.89	—	215.6	238.1	239.2
hand	171.2	198.89	—	215.2	238.1	239.2
head	171.0	198.89	—	215.0	238.1	239.2

Neoplasm, choroid — Neoplasm, connective tissue

	Malignant				Uncertain Behavior	Unspecified
	Primary	Secondary	Ca in situ	Benign		
Neoplasm, neoplastic — *continued*						
connective tissue NEC — *continued*						
heel	171.3	198.89	—	215.3	238.1	239.2
hip	171.3	198.89	—	215.3	238.1	239.2
hypochondrium	171.5	198.89	—	215.5	238.1	239.2
iliopsoas muscle	171.6	198.89	—	215.5	238.1	239.2
infraclavicular region	171.4	198.89	—	215.4	238.1	239.2
inguinal (canal) (region)	171.6	198.89	—	215.6	238.1	239.2
intrathoracic	171.4	198.89	—	215.4	238.1	239.2
ischorectal fossa	171.6	198.89	—	215.6	238.1	239.2
jaw	143.9	198.89	230.0	210.4	235.1	239.0
knee	171.3	198.89	—	215.3	238.1	239.2
leg	171.3	198.89	—	215.3	238.1	239.2
limb NEC	171.9	198.89	—	215.8	238.1	239.2
lower	171.3	198.89	—	215.3	238.1	239.2
upper	171.2	198.89	—	215.2	238.1	239.2
nates	171.6	198.89	—	215.6	238.1	239.2
neck	171.0	198.89	—	215.0	238.1	239.2
orbit	190.1	198.4	234.0	224.1	238.8	239.8
pararectal	171.6	198.89	—	215.6	238.1	239.2
para-urethral	171.6	198.89	—	215.6	238.1	239.2
paravaginal	171.6	198.89	—	215.6	238.1	239.2
pelvis (floor)	171.6	198.89	—	215.6	238.1	239.2
pelvo-abdominal	171.8	198.89	—	215.8	238.1	239.2
perineum	171.6	198.89	—	215.6	238.1	239.2
perirectal (tissue)	171.6	198.89	—	215.6	238.1	239.2
periurethral (tissue)	171.6	198.89	—	215.6	238.1	239.2
popliteal fossa or space	171.3	198.89	—	215.3	238.1	239.2
presacral	171.6	198.89	—	215.6	238.1	239.2
psoas muscle	171.5	198.89	—	215.5	238.1	239.2
pterygoid fossa	171.0	198.89	—	215.0	238.1	239.2
rectovaginal septum or wall	171.6	198.89	—	215.6	238.1	239.2
rectovesical	171.6	198.89	—	215.6	238.1	239.2
retroperitoneum	158.0	197.6	—	211.8	235.4	239.0
sacrococcygeal region	171.6	198.89	—	215.6	238.1	239.2
scalp	171.0	198.89	—	215.0	238.1	239.2
scapular region	171.4	198.89	—	215.4	238.1	239.2
shoulder	171.2	198.89	—	215.2	238.1	239.2
skin (dermis) NEC	173.9	198.2	232.9	216.9	238.2	239.2
submental	171.0	198.89	—	215.0	238.1	239.2
supraclavicular region	171.0	198.89	—	215.0	238.1	239.2
temple	171.0	198.89	—	215.0	238.1	239.2
temporal region	171.0	198.89	—	215.0	238.1	239.2
thigh	171.3	198.89	—	215.3	238.1	239.2
thoracic (duct) (wall)	171.4	198.89	—	215.4	238.1	239.2
thorax	171.4	198.89	—	215.4	238.1	239.2
thumb	171.2	198.89	—	215.2	238.1	239.2
toe	171.3	198.89	—	215.3	238.1	239.2
trunk	171.7	198.89	—	215.7	238.1	239.2
umbilicus	171.5	198.89	—	215.5	238.1	239.2
vesicorectal	171.6	198.89	—	215.6	238.1	239.2
wrist	171.2	198.89	—	215.2	238.1	239.2
conus medullaris	192.2	198.3	—	225.3	237.5	239.7
cord (true) (vocal)	161.0	197.3	231.0	212.1	235.6	239.1
false	161.1	197.3	231.0	212.1	235.6	239.1
spermatic	187.6	198.82	233.6	222.8	236.6	239.5
spinal (cervical) (lumbar) (thoracic)	192.2	198.3	—	225.3	237.5	239.7
cornea (limbus)	190.4	198.4	234.0	224.4	238.8	239.8
corpus						
albicans	183.0	198.6	233.3	220	236.2	239.5
callosum, brain	191.8	198.3	—	225.0	237.5	239.6
cavernosum	187.3	198.82	233.5	222.1	236.6	239.5
gastric	151.4	197.8	230.2	211.1	235.2	239.0
penis	187.3	198.82	233.5	222.1	236.6	239.5
striatum, cerebrum	191.0	198.3	—	225.0	237.5	239.6
uteri	182.0	198.82	233.2	219.1	236.0	239.5
isthmus	182.1	198.82	233.2	219.1	236.0	239.5

Neoplasm, neoplastic — continued	Malignant			Benign	Uncertain Behavior	Unspecified
	Primary	Secondary	Ca in situ	Benign	Uncertain Behavior	Unspecified
cortex						
adrenal	194.0	198.7	234.8	227.0	237.2	239.7
cerebral	191.0	198.3	—	225.0	237.5	239.6
costal cartilage	170.3	198.5	—	213.3	238.0	239.2
costovertebral joint	170.3	198.5	—	213.3	238.0	239.2
Cowper's gland	189.3	198.1	233.9	223.81	236.99	239.5
cranial (fossa, any)	191.9	198.3	—	225.0	237.5	239.6
meninges	192.1	198.4	—	225.2	237.6	239.7
nerve (any)	192.0	198.4	—	225.1	237.9	239.7
craniobuccal pouch	194.3	198.89	234.8	227.3	237.0	239.7
craniopharyngeal (duct) (pouch)	194.3	198.89	234.8	227.3	237.0	239.7
cricoid	148.0	198.89	230.0	210.8	235.1	239.0
cartilage	161.3	197.3	231.0	212.1	235.6	239.1
cricopharynx	148.0	198.89	230.0	210.8	235.1	239.0
crypt of Morgagni	154.8	197.5	230.7	211.4	235.2	239.0
crystalline lens	190.0	198.4	234.0	224.0	238.8	239.8
cul-de-sac (Douglas')	158.8	197.6	—	211.8	235.4	239.0
cuneiform cartilage	161.3	197.3	231.0	212.1	235.6	239.1
cutaneous — see Neoplasm, skin						
cutis — see Neoplasm, skin						
cystic (bile) duct (common)	156.1	197.8	230.8	211.5	235.3	239.0
dermis — see Neoplasm, skin						
diaphragm	171.4	198.89	—	215.4	238.1	239.2
digestive organs, system, tube, or tract NEC	159.9	197.8	230.9	211.9	235.5	239.0
contiguous sites with peritoneum	159.8	—	—	—	—	—
disc, intervertebral	170.2	198.5	—	213.2	238.0	239.2
disease, generalized	199.0	199.0	234.9	229.9	238.9	199.0
disseminated	199.0	199.0	234.9	229.9	238.9	199.0
Douglas' cul-de-sac or pouch	158.8	197.6	—	211.8	235.4	239.0
duodenojejunal junction	152.8	197.4	230.7	211.2	235.2	239.0
duodenum	152.0	197.4	230.7	211.2	235.2	239.0
dura (cranial) (mater)	192.1	198.4	—	225.2	237.6	239.7
cerebral	192.1	198.4	—	225.2	237.6	239.7
spinal	192.3	198.4	—	225.4	237.6	239.7
ear (external)	173.2	198.2	232.2	216.2	238.2	239.2
auricle or auris	173.2	198.2	232.2	216.2	238.2	239.2
canal, external	173.2	198.2	232.2	216.2	238.2	239.2
cartilage	171.0	198.89	—	215.0	238.1	239.2
external meatus	173.2	198.2	232.2	216.2	238.2	239.2
inner	160.1	197.3	231.8	212.0	235.9	239.8 ▲
lobule	173.2	198.2	232.2	216.2	238.2	239.2
middle	160.1	197.3	231.8	212.0	235.9	239.8 ▲
contiguous sites with accessory sinuses or nasal cavities	160.8	—	—	—	—	—
skin	173.2	198.2	232.2	216.2	238.2	239.2
earlobe	173.2	198.2	232.2	216.2	238.2	239.2
ejaculatory duct	187.8	198.82	233.6	222.8	236.6	239.5
elbow NEC*	195.4	198.89	232.6	229.8	238.8	239.8
endocardium	164.1	198.89	—	212.7	238.8	239.8
endocervix (canal) (gland)	180.0	198.82	233.1	219.0	236.0	239.5
endocrine gland NEC	194.9	198.89	—	227.9	237.4	239.7
pluriglandular NEC	194.8	198.89	234.8	227.8	237.4	239.7
endometrium (gland) (stroma)	182.0	198.82	233.2	219.1	236.0	239.5
ensiform cartilage	170.3	198.5	—	213.3	238.0	239.2
enteric — see Neoplasm, intestine						
ependyma (brain)	191.5	198.3	—	225.0	237.5	239.6
epicardium	164.1	198.89	—	212.7	238.8	239.8
epididymis	187.5	198.82	233.6	222.3	236.6	239.5
epidural	192.9	198.4	—	225.9	237.9	239.7
epiglottis	161.1	197.3	231.0	212.1	235.6	239.1
anterior aspect or surface	146.4	198.89	230.0	210.6	235.1	239.0
cartilage	161.3	197.3	231.0	212.1	235.6	239.1
free border (margin)	146.4	198.89	230.0	210.6	235.1	239.0
junctional region	146.5	198.89	230.0	210.6	235.1	239.0
posterior (laryngeal) surface	161.1	197.3	231.0	212.1	235.6	239.1
suprahyoid portion	161.1	197.3	231.0	212.1	235.6	239.1
esophagogastric junction	151.0	197.8	230.2	211.1	235.2	239.0

▨4ᵗʰ Fourth-digit Required   ▨5ᵗʰ Fifth-digit Required   ▶◀ Revised Text   ● New Line   ▲ Revised Code

Neoplasm, neoplastic — continued	Malignant			Benign	Uncertain Behavior	Unspecified
	Primary	Secondary	Ca in situ	Benign	Uncertain Behavior	Unspecified
esophagus	150.9	197.8	230.1	211.0	235.5	239.0
abdominal	150.2	197.8	230.1	211.0	235.5	239.0
cervical	150.0	197.8	230.1	211.0	235.5	239.0
contiguous sites	150.8	—	—	—	—	—
distal (third)	150.5	197.8	230.1	211.0	235.5	239.0
lower (third)	150.5	197.8	230.1	211.0	235.5	239.0
middle (third)	150.4	197.8	230.1	211.0	235.5	239.0
proximal (third)	150.3	197.8	230.1	211.0	235.5	239.0
specified part NEC	150.8	197.8	230.1	211.0	235.5	239.0
thoracic	150.1	197.8	230.1	211.0	235.5	239.0
upper (third)	150.3	197.8	230.1	211.0	235.5	239.0
ethmoid (sinus)	160.3	197.3	231.8	212.0	235.9	239.1
bone or labyrinth	170.0	198.5	—	213.0	238.0	239.2
Eustachian tube	160.1	197.3	231.8	212.0	235.9	239.1
exocervix	180.1	198.82	233.1	219.0	236.0	239.5
external						
meatus (ear)	173.2	198.2	232.2	216.2	238.2	239.2
os, cervix uteri	180.1	198.82	233.1	219.0	236.0	239.5
extradural	192.9	198.4	—	225.9	237.9	239.7
extrahepatic (bile) duct	156.1	197.8	230.8	211.5	235.3	239.0
contiguous sites with gallbladder	156.8	—	—	—	—	—
extraocular muscle	190.1	198.4	234.0	224.1	238.8	239.8
extrarectal	195.3	198.89	234.8	229.8	238.8	239.8
extremity*	195.8	198.89	232.8	229.8	238.8	239.8
lower*	195.5	198.89	232.7	229.8	238.8	239.8
upper*	195.4	198.89	232.6	229.8	238.8	239.8
eye NEC	190.9	198.4	234.0	224.9	238.8	239.8
contiguous sites	190.8	—	—	—	—	—
specified sites NEC	190.8	198.4	234.0	224.8	238.8	239.8
eyeball	190.0	198.4	234.0	224.0	238.8	239.8
eyebrow	173.3	198.2	232.3	216.3	238.2	239.2
eyelid (lower) (skin) (upper)	173.1	198.2	232.1	216.1	238.2	239.2
cartilage	171.0	198.89	—	215.0	238.1	239.2
face NEC*	195.0	198.89	232.3	229.8	238.8	239.8
fallopian tube (accessory)	183.2	198.82	233.3	221.0	236.3	239.5
falx (cerebelli) (cerebri)	192.1	198.4	—	225.2	237.6	239.7
fascia — see also Neoplasm, connective tissue						
palmar	171.2	198.89	—	215.2	238.1	239.2
plantar	171.3	198.89	—	215.3	238.1	239.2
fatty tissue — see Neoplasm, connective tissue						
fauces, faucial NEC	146.9	198.89	230.0	210.6	235.1	239.0
pillars	146.2	198.89	230.0	210.6	235.1	239.0
tonsil	146.0	198.89	230.0	210.5	235.1	239.0
femur (any part)	170.7	198.5	—	213.7	238.0	239.2
fetal membrane	181	198.82	233.2	219.8	236.1	239.5
fibrous tissue — see Neoplasm, connective tissue						
fibula (any part)	170.7	198.5	—	213.7	238.0	239.2
filum terminale	192.2	198.3	—	225.3	237.5	239.7
finger NEC*	195.4	198.89	232.6	229.8	238.8	239.8
flank NEC*	195.8	198.89	232.5	229.8	238.8	239.8
follicle, nabothian	180.0	198.82	233.1	219.0	236.0	239.5
foot NEC*	195.5	198.89	232.7	229.8	238.8	239.8
forearm NEC*	195.4	198.89	232.6	229.8	238.8	239.8
forehead (skin)	173.3	198.2	232.3	216.3	238.2	239.2
foreskin	187.1	198.82	233.5	222.1	236.6	239.5
fornix						
pharyngeal	147.3	198.89	230.0	210.7	235.1	239.0
vagina	184.0	198.82	233.3	221.1	236.3	239.5
fossa (of)						
anterior (cranial)	191.9	198.3	—	225.0	237.5	239.6
cranial	191.9	198.3	—	225.0	237.5	239.6
ischiorectal	195.3	198.89	234.8	229.8	238.8	239.8
middle (cranial)	191.9	198.3	—	225.0	237.5	239.6
pituitary	194.3	198.89	234.8	227.3	237.0	239.7
posterior (cranial)	191.9	198.3	—	225.0	237.5	239.6
pterygoid	171.0	198.89	—	215.0	238.1	239.2

✓4ᵗʰ Fourth-digit Required   ✓5ᵗʰ Fifth-digit Required   ►◄ Revised Text   ● New Line   ▲ Revised Code

	Malignant					
	Primary	**Secondary**	**Ca in situ**	**Benign**	**Uncertain Behavior**	**Unspecified**
Neoplasm, neoplastic — *continued*						
fossa (of) — *continued*						
pyriform	148.1	198.89	230.0	210.8	235.1	239.0
Rosenmüller	147.2	198.89	230.0	210.7	235.1	239.0
tonsillar	146.1	198.89	230.0	210.6	235.1	239.0
fourchette	184.4	198.82	233.3	221.2	236.3	239.5
frenulum						
labii — *see* Neoplasm, lip, internal						
linguae	141.3	198.89	230.0	210.1	235.1	239.0
frontal						
bone	170.0	198.5	—	213.0	238.0	239.2
lobe, brain	191.1	198.3	—	225.0	237.5	239.6
meninges	192.1	198.4	—	225.2	237.6	239.7
pole	191.1	198.3	—	225.0	237.5	239.6
sinus	160.4	197.3	231.8	212.0	235.9	239.1
fundus						
stomach	151.3	197.8	230.2	211.1	235.2	239.0
uterus	182.0	198.82	233.2	219.1	236.0	239.5
gall duct (extrahepatic)	156.1	197.8	230.8	211.5	235.3	239.0
intrahepatic	155.1	197.8	230.8	211.5	235.3	239.0
gallbladder	156.0	197.8	230.8	211.5	235.3	239.0
contiguous sites with extrahepatic bile ducts	156.8	—	—	—	—	—
ganglia (*see also* Neoplasm, connective tissue)	171.9	198.89	—	215.9	238.1	239.2
basal	191.0	198.3	—	225.0	237.5	239.6
ganglion (*see also* Neoplasm, connective tissue)	171.9	198.89	—	215.9	238.1	239.2
cranial nerve	192.0	198.4	—	225.1	237.9	239.7
Gartner's duct	184.0	198.82	233.3	221.1	236.3	239.5
gastric — *see* Neoplasm, stomach						
gastrocolic	159.8	197.8	230.9	211.9	235.5	239.0
gastroesophageal junction	151.0	197.8	230.2	211.1	235.2	239.0
gastrointestinal (tract) NEC	159.9	197.8	230.9	211.9	235.5	239.0
generalized	199.0	199.0	234.9	229.9	238.9	199.0
genital organ or tract						
female NEC	184.9	198.82	233.3	221.9	236.3	239.5
contiguous sites	184.8	—	—	—	—	—
specified site NEC	184.8	198.82	233.3	221.8	236.3	239.5
male NEC	187.9	198.82	233.6	222.9	236.6	239.5
contiguous sites	187.8	—	—	—	—	—
specified site NEC	187.8	198.82	233.6	222.8	236.6	239.5
genitourinary tract						
female	184.9	198.82	233.3	221.9	236.3	239.5
male	187.9	198.82	233.6	222.9	236.6	239.5
gingiva (alveolar) (marginal)	143.9	198.89	230.0	210.4	235.1	239.0
lower	143.1	198.89	230.0	210.4	235.1	239.0
mandibular	143.1	198.89	230.0	210.4	235.1	239.0
maxillary	143.0	198.89	230.0	210.4	235.1	239.0
upper	143.0	198.89	230.0	210.4	235.1	239.0
gland, glandular (lymphatic) (system) — *see also* Neoplasm, lymph gland						
endocrine NEC	194.9	198.89	—	227.9	237.4	239.7
salivary — *see* Neoplasm, salivary, gland						
glans penis	187.2	198.82	233.5	222.1	236.6	239.5
globus pallidus	191.0	198.3	—	225.0	237.5	239.6
glomus						
coccygeal	194.6	198.89	—	227.6	237.3	239.7
jugularis	194.6	198.89	—	227.6	237.3	239.7
glosso-epiglottic fold(s)	146.4	198.89	230.0	210.6	235.1	239.0
glossopalatine fold	146.2	198.89	230.0	210.6	235.1	239.0
glossopharyngeal sulcus	146.1	198.89	230.0	210.6	235.1	239.0
glottis	161.0	197.3	231.0	212.1	235.6	239.1
gluteal region*	195.3	198.89	232.5	229.8	238.8	239.8
great vessels NEC	171.4	198.89	—	215.4	238.1	239.2
groin NEC*	195.3	198.89	232.5	229.8	238.8	239.8
gum	143.9	198.89	230.0	210.4	235.1	239.0
contiguous sites	143.8	—	—	—	—	—
lower	143.1	198.89	230.0	210.4	235.1	239.0
upper	143.0	198.89	230.0	210.4	235.1	239.0
hand NEC*	195.4	198.89	232.6	229.8	238.8	239.8

☑4ᵗʰ Fourth-digit Required   ☑5ᵗʰ Fifth-digit Required   ▶◀ Revised Text   ● New Line   ▲ Revised Code

	Malignant					
	Primary	**Secondary**	**Ca in situ**	**Benign**	**Uncertain Behavior**	**Unspecified**
Neoplasm, neoplastic — *continued*						
head NEC*	195.0	198.89	232.4	229.8	238.8	239.8
heart	164.1	198.89	—	212.7	238.8	239.8
contiguous sites with mediastinum or thymus	164.8	—	—	—	—	—
heel NEC*	195.5	198.89	232.7	229.8	238.8	239.8
helix	173.2	198.2	232.2	216.2	238.2	239.2
hematopoietic, hemopoietic tissue NEC	202.8 ✓5ᵗʰ	198.89	—	—	—	238.7
hemisphere, cerebral	191.0	198.3	—	225.0	237.5	239.6
hemorrhoidal zone	154.2	197.5	230.5	211.4	235.5	239.0
hepatic	155.2	197.7	230.8	211.5	235.3	239.0
duct (bile)	156.1	197.8	230.8	211.5	235.3	239.0
flexure (colon)	153.0	197.5	230.3	211.3	235.2	239.0
primary	155.0	—	—	—	—	—
hilus of lung	162.2	197.0	231.2	212.3	235.7	239.1
hip NEC*	195.5	198.89	232.7	229.8	238.8	239.8
hippocampus, brain	191.2	198.3	—	225.0	237.5	239.6
humerus (any part)	170.4	198.5	—	213.4	238.0	239.2
hymen	184.0	198.82	233.3	221.1	236.3	239.5
hypopharynx, hypopharyngeal NEC	148.9	198.89	230.0	210.8	235.1	239.0
contiguous sites	148.8	—	—	—	—	—
postcricoid region	148.0	198.89	230.0	210.8	235.1	239.0
posterior wall	148.3	198.89	230.0	210.8	235.1	239.0
pyriform fossa (sinus)	148.1	198.89	230.0	210.8	235.1	239.0
specified site NEC	148.8	198.89	230.0	210.8	235.1	239.0
wall	148.9	198.89	230.0	210.8	235.1	239.0
posterior	148.3	198.89	230.0	210.8	235.1	239.0
hypophysis	194.3	198.89	234.8	227.3	237.0	239.7
hypothalamus	191.0	198.3	—	225.0	237.5	239.6
ileocecum, ileocecal (coil) (junction) (valve)	153.4	197.5	230.3	211.3	235.2	239.0
ileum	152.2	197.4	230.7	211.2	235.2	239.0
ilium	170.6	198.5	—	213.6	238.0	239.2
immunoproliferative NEC	203.8 ✓5ᵗʰ	—	—	—	—	—
infraclavicular (region)*	195.1	198.89	232.5	229.8	238.8	239.8
inguinal (region)*	195.3	198.89	232.5	229.8	238.8	239.8
insula	191.0	198.3	—	225.0	237.5	239.6
insular tissue (pancreas)	157.4	197.8	230.9	211.7	235.5	239.0
brain	191.0	198.3	—	225.0	237.5	239.6
interarytenoid fold	148.2	198.89	230.0	210.8	235.1	239.0
hypopharyngeal aspect	148.2	198.89	230.0	210.8	235.1	239.0
laryngeal aspect	161.1	197.3	231.0	212.1	235.6	239.1
marginal zone	148.2	198.89	230.0	210.8	235.1	239.0
interdental papillae	143.9	198.89	230.0	210.4	235.1	239.0
lower	143.1	198.89	230.0	210.4	235.1	239.0
upper	143.0	198.89	230.0	210.4	235.1	239.0
internal						
capsule	191.0	198.3	—	225.0	237.5	239.6
os (cervix)	180.0	198.82	233.1	219.0	236.0	239.5
intervertebral cartilage or disc	170.2	198.5	—	213.2	238.0	239.2
intestine, intestinal	159.0	197.8	230.7	211.9	235.2	239.0
large	153.9	197.5	230.3	211.3	235.2	239.0
appendix	153.5	197.5	230.3	211.3	235.2	239.0
caput coli	153.4	197.5	230.3	211.3	235.2	239.0
cecum	153.4	197.5	230.3	211.3	235.2	239.0
colon	153.9	197.5	230.3	211.3	235.2	239.0
and rectum	154.0	197.5	230.4	211.4	235.2	239.0
ascending	153.6	197.5	230.3	211.3	235.2	239.0
caput	153.4	197.5	230.3	211.3	235.2	239.0
contiguous sites	153.8	—	—	—	—	—
descending	153.2	197.5	230.3	211.3	235.2	239.0
distal	153.2	197.5	230.3	211.3	235.2	239.0
left	153.2	197.5	230.3	211.3	235.2	239.0
pelvic	153.3	197.5	230.3	211.3	235.2	239.0
right	153.6	197.5	230.3	211.3	235.2	239.0
sigmoid (flexure)	153.3	197.5	230.3	211.3	235.2	239.0
transverse	153.1	197.5	230.3	211.3	235.2	239.0
contiguous sites	153.8	—	—	—	—	—

Neoplasm, neoplastic — *continued*	Malignant			Benign	Uncertain Behavior	Unspecified
	Primary	**Secondary**	**Ca in situ**	**Benign**	**Uncertain Behavior**	**Unspecified**
intestine, intestinal — *continued*						
large — *continued*						
hepatic flexure	153.0	197.5	230.3	211.3	235.2	239.0
ileocecum, ileocecal (coil) (valve)	153.4	197.5	230.3	211.3	235.2	239.0
sigmoid flexure (lower) (upper)	153.3	197.5	230.3	211.3	235.2	239.0
splenic flexure	153.7	197.5	230.3	211.3	235.2	239.0
small	152.9	197.4	230.7	211.2	235.2	239.0
contiguous sites	152.8	—	—	—	—	—
duodenum	152.0	197.4	230.7	211.2	235.2	239.0
ileum	152.2	197.4	230.7	211.2	235.2	239.0
jejunum	152.1	197.4	230.7	211.2	235.2	239.0
tract NEC	159.0	197.8	230.7	211.9	235.2	239.0
intra-abdominal	195.2	198.89	234.8	229.8	238.8	239.8
intracranial NEC	191.9	198.3	—	225.0	237.5	239.6
intrahepatic (bile) duct	155.1	197.8	230.8	211.5	235.3	239.0
intraocular	190.0	198.4	234.0	224.0	238.8	239.8
intraorbital	190.1	198.4	234.0	224.1	238.8	239.8
intrasellar	194.3	198.89	234.8	227.3	237.0	239.7
intrathoracic (cavity) (organs NEC)	195.1	198.89	234.8	229.8	238.8	239.8
contiguous sites with respiratory organs	165.8	—	—	—	—	—
iris	190.0	198.4	234.0	224.0	238.8	239.8
ischiorectal (fossa)	195.3	198.89	234.8	229.8	238.8	239.8
ischium	170.6	198.5	—	213.6	238.0	239.2
island of Reil	191.0	198.3	—	225.0	237.5	239.6
islands or islets of Langerhans	157.4	197.8	230.9	211.7	235.5	239.0
isthmus uteri	182.1	198.82	233.2	219.1	236.0	239.5
jaw	195.0	198.89	234.8	229.8	238.8	239.8
bone	170.1	198.5	—	213.1	238.0	239.2
carcinoma	143.9	—	—	—	—	—
lower	143.1	—	—	—	—	—
upper	143.0	—	—	—	—	—
lower	170.1	198.5	—	213.1	238.0	239.2
upper	170.0	198.5	—	213.0	238.0	239.2
carcinoma (any type) (lower) (upper)	195.0	—	—	—	—	—
skin	173.3	198.2	232.3	216.3	238.2	239.2
soft tissues	143.9	198.89	230.0	210.4	235.1	239.0
lower	143.1	198.89	230.0	210.4	235.1	239.0
upper	143.0	198.89	230.0	210.4	235.1	239.0
jejunum	152.1	197.4	230.7	211.2	235.2	239.0
joint NEC (*see also* Neoplasm, bone)	170.9	198.5	—	213.9	238.0	239.2
acromioclavicular	170.4	198.5	—	213.4	238.0	239.2
bursa or synovial membrane — *see* Neoplasm, connective tissue						
costovertebral	170.3	198.5	—	213.3	238.0	239.2
sternocostal	170.3	198.5	—	213.3	238.0	239.2
temporomandibular	170.1	198.5	—	213.1	238.0	239.2
junction						
anorectal	154.8	197.5	230.7	211.4	235.5	239.0
cardioesophageal	151.0	197.8	230.2	211.1	235.2	239.0
esophagogastric	151.0	197.8	230.2	211.1	235.2	239.0
gastroesophageal	151.0	197.8	230.2	211.1	235.2	239.0
hard and soft palate	145.5	198.89	230.0	210.4	235.1	239.0
ileocecal	153.4	197.5	230.3	211.3	235.2	239.0
pelvirectal	154.0	197.5	230.4	211.4	235.2	239.0
pelviureteric	189.1	198.0	233.9	223.1	236.91	239.5
rectosigmoid	154.0	197.5	230.4	211.4	235.2	239.0
squamocolumnar, of cervix	180.8	198.82	233.1	219.0	236.0	239.5
kidney (parenchyma)	189.0	198.0	233.9	223.0	236.91	239.5
calyx	189.1	198.0	233.9	223.1	236.91	239.5
hilus	189.1	198.0	233.9	223.1	236.91	239.5
pelvis	189.1	198.0	233.9	223.1	236.91	239.5
knee NEC*	195.5	198.89	232.7	229.8	238.8	239.8
labia (skin)	184.4	198.82	233.3	221.2	236.3	239.5
majora	184.1	198.82	233.3	221.2	236.3	239.5
minora	184.2	198.82	233.3	221.2	236.3	239.5
labial — *see also* Neoplasm, lip						
sulcus (lower) (upper)	145.1	198.89	230.0	210.4	235.1	239.0

✓4ᵗʰ Fourth-digit Required   ✓5ᵗʰ Fifth-digit Required   ▶◀ Revised Text   ● New Line   ▲ Revised Code

	Malignant					
	Primary	Secondary	Ca in situ	Benign	Uncertain Behavior	Unspecified
Neoplasm, neoplastic — *continued*						
labium (skin)	184.4	198.82	233.3	221.2	236.3	239.5
majus	184.1	198.82	233.3	221.2	236.3	239.5
minus	184.2	198.82	233.3	221.2	236.3	239.5
lacrimal						
canaliculi	190.7	198.4	234.0	224.7	238.8	239.8
duct (nasal)	190.7	198.4	234.0	224.7	238.8	239.8
gland	190.2	198.4	234.0	224.2	238.8	239.8
punctum	190.7	198.4	234.0	224.7	238.8	239.8
sac	190.7	198.4	234.0	224.7	238.8	239.8
Langerhans, islands or islets	157.4	197.8	230.9	211.7	235.5	239.0
laryngopharynx	148.9	198.89	230.0	210.8	235.1	239.0
larynx, laryngeal NEC	161.9	197.3	231.0	212.1	235.6	239.1
aryepiglottic fold	161.1	197.3	231.0	212.1	235.6	239.1
cartilage (arytenoid) (cricoid) (cuneiform) (thyroid)	161.3	197.3	231.0	212.1	235.6	239.1
commissure (anterior) (posterior)	161.0	197.3	231.0	212.1	235.6	239.1
contiguous sites	161.8	—	—	—	—	—
extrinsic NEC	161.1	197.3	231.0	212.1	235.6	239.1
meaning hypopharynx	148.9	198.89	230.0	210.8	235.1	239.0
interarytenoid fold	161.1	197.3	231.0	212.1	235.6	239.1
intrinsic	161.0	197.3	231.0	212.1	235.6	239.1
ventricular band	161.1	197.3	231.0	212.1	235.6	239.1
leg NEC*	195.5	198.89	232.7	229.8	238.8	239.8
lens, crystalline	190.0	198.4	234.0	224.0	238.8	239.8
lid (lower) (upper)	173.1	198.2	232.1	216.1	238.2	239.2
ligament — *see also* Neoplasm, connective tissue						
broad	183.3	198.82	233.3	221.0	236.3	239.5
Mackenrodt's	183.8	198.82	233.3	221.8	236.3	239.5
non-uterine — *see* Neoplasm, connective tissue						
round	183.5	198.82	—	221.0	236.3	239.5
sacro-uterine	183.4	198.82	—	221.0	236.3	239.5
uterine	183.4	198.82	—	221.0	236.3	239.5
utero-ovarian	183.8	198.82	233.3	221.8	236.3	239.5
uterosacral	183.4	198.82	—	221.0	236.3	239.5
limb*	195.8	198.89	232.8	229.8	238.8	239.8
lower*	195.5	198.89	232.7	229.8	238.8	239.8
upper*	195.4	198.89	232.6	229.8	238.8	239.8
limbus of cornea	190.4	198.4	234.0	224.4	238.8	239.8
lingual NEC (*see also* Neoplasm, tongue)	141.9	198.89	230.0	210.1	235.1	239.0
lingula, lung	162.3	197.0	231.2	212.3	235.7	239.1
lip (external) (lipstick area) (vermillion border)	140.9	198.89	230.0	210.0	235.1	239.0
buccal aspect — *see* Neoplasm, lip, internal						
commissure	140.6	198.89	230.0	210.4	235.1	239.0
contiguous sites	140.8	—	—	—	—	—
with oral cavity or pharynx	149.8	—	—	—	—	—
frenulum — *see* Neoplasm, lip, internal						
inner aspect — *see* Neoplasm, lip, internal						
internal (buccal) (frenulum) (mucosa) (oral)	140.5	198.89	230.0	210.0	235.1	239.0
lower	140.4	198.89	230.0	210.0	235.1	239.0
upper	140.3	198.89	230.0	210.0	235.1	239.0
lower	140.1	198.89	230.0	210.0	235.1	239.0
internal (buccal) (frenulum) (mucosa) (oral)	140.4	198.89	230.0	210.0	235.1	239.0
mucosa — *see* Neoplasm, lip, internal						
oral aspect — *see* Neoplasm, lip, internal						
skin (commissure) (lower) (upper)	173.0	198.2	232.0	216.0	238.2	239.2
upper	140.0	198.89	230.0	210.0	235.1	239.0
internal (buccal) (frenulum) (mucosa) (oral)	140.3	198.89	230.0	210.0	235.1	239.0
liver	155.2	197.7	230.8	211.5	235.3	239.0
primary	155.0	—	—	—	—	—
lobe						
azygos	162.3	197.0	231.2	212.3	235.7	239.1
frontal	191.1	198.3	—	225.0	237.5	239.6
lower	162.5	197.0	231.2	212.3	235.7	239.1
middle	162.4	197.0	231.2	212.3	235.7	239.1
occipital	191.4	198.3	—	225.0	237.5	239.6
parietal	191.3	198.3	—	225.0	237.5	239.6

☑4ᵗʰ Fourth-digit Required   ☑5ᵗʰ Fifth-digit Required   ▶◀ Revised Text   ● New Line   ▲ Revised Code

	Malignant					
	Primary	Secondary	Ca in situ	Benign	Uncertain Behavior	Unspecified
Neoplasm, neoplastic — *continued*						
lobe — *continued*						
temporal	191.2	198.3	—	225.0	237.5	239.6
upper	162.3	197.0	231.2	212.3	235.7	239.1
lumbosacral plexus	171.6	198.4	—	215.6	238.1	239.2
lung	162.9	197.0	231.2	212.3	235.7	239.1
azgos lobe	162.3	197.0	231.2	212.3	235.7	239.1
carina	162.2	197.0	231.2	212.3	235.7	239.1
contiguous sites with bronchus or trachea	162.8	—	—	—	—	—
hilus	162.2	197.0	231.2	212.3	235.7	239.1
lingula	162.3	197.0	231.2	212.3	235.7	239.1
lobe NEC	162.9	197.0	231.2	212.3	235.7	239.1
lower lobe	162.5	197.0	231.2	212.3	235.7	239.1
main bronchus	162.2	197.0	231.2	212.3	235.7	239.1
middle lobe	162.4	197.0	231.2	212.3	235.7	239.1
upper lobe	162.3	197.0	231.2	212.3	235.7	239.1
lymph, lymphatic						
channel NEC (*see also* Neoplasm, connective tissue)	171.9	198.89	—	215.9	238.1	239.2
gland (secondary)	—	196.9	—	229.0	238.8	239.8
abdominal	—	196.2	—	229.0	238.8	239.
aortic	—	196.2	—	229.0	238.8	239.8
arm	—	196.3	—	229.0	238.8	239.8
auricular (anterior) (posterior)	—	196.0	—	229.0	238.8	239.8
axilla, axillary	—	196.3	—	229.0	238.8	239.8
brachial	—	196.3	—	229.0	238.8	239.8
bronchial	—	196.1	—	229.0	238.8	239.8
bronchopulmonary	—	196.1	—	229.0	238.8	239.8
celiac	—	196.2	—	229.0	238.8	239.8
cervical	—	196.0	—	229.0	238.8	239.8
cervicofacial	—	196.0	—	229.0	238.8	239.8
Cloquet	—	196.5	—	229.0	238.8	239.8
colic	—	196.2	—	229.0	238.8	239.8
common duct	—	196.2	—	229.0	238.8	239.8
cubital	—	196.3	—	229.0	238.8	239.8
diaphragmatic	—	196.1	—	229.0	238.8	239.8
epigastric, inferior	—	196.6	—	229.0	238.8	239.8
epitrochlear	—	196.3	—	229.0	238.8	239.8
esophageal	—	196.1	—	229.0	238.8	239.8
face	—	196.0	—	229.0	238.8	239.8
femoral	—	196.5	—	229.0	238.8	239.8
gastric	—	196.2	—	229.0	238.8	239.8
groin	—	196.5	—	229.0	238.8	239.8
head	—	196.0	—	229.0	238.8	239.8
hepatic	—	196.2	—	229.0	238.8	239.8
hilar (pulmonary)	—	196.1	—	229.0	238.8	239.8
splenic	—	196.2	—	229.0	238.8	239.8
hypogastric	—	196.6	—	229.0	238.8	239.8
ileocolic	—	196.2	—	229.0	238.8	239.8
iliac	—	196.6	—	229.0	238.8	239.8
infraclavicular	—	196.3	—	229.0	238.8	239.8
inguina, inguinal	—	196.5	—	229.0	238.8	239.8
innominate	—	196.1	—	229.0	238.8	239.8
intercostal	—	196.1	—	229.0	238.8	239.8
intestinal	—	196.2	—	229.0	238.8	239.8
intra-abdominal	—	196.2	—	229.0	238.8	239.8
intrapelvic	—	196.6	—	229.0	238.8	239.8
intrathoracic	—	196.1	—	229.0	238.8	239.9
jugular	—	196.0	—	229.0	238.8	239.8
leg	—	196.5	—	229.0	238.8	239.8
limb						
lower	—	196.5	—	229.0	238.8	239.8
upper	—	196.3	—	229.0	238.8	239.8
lower limb	—	196.5	—	229.0	238.8	238.9
lumbar	—	196.2	—	229.0	238.8	239.8
mandibular	—	196.0	—	229.0	238.8	239.8
mediastinal	—	196.1	—	229.0	238.8	239.8
mesenteric (inferior) (superior)	—	196.2	—	229.0	238.8	239.8

	Malignant			Benign	Uncertain Behavior	Unspecified
	Primary	Secondary	Ca in situ			
Neoplasm, neoplastic — *continued*						
lymph, lymphatic — *continued*						
gland — *continued*						
midcolic	—	196.2	—	229.0	238.8	239.8
multiple sites in categories 196.0-196.6	—	196.8	—	229.0	238.8	239.8
neck	—	196.0	—	229.0	238.8	239.8
obturator	—	196.6	—	229.0	238.8	239.8
occipital	—	196.0	—	229.0	238.8	239.8
pancreatic	—	196.2	—	229.0	238.8	239.8
para-aortic	—	196.2	—	229.0	238.8	239.8
paracervical	—	196.6	—	229.0	238.8	239.8
parametrial	—	196.6	—	229.0	238.8	239.8
parasternal	—	196.1	—	229.0	238.8	239.8
parotid	—	196.0	—	229.0	238.8	239.8
pectoral	—	196.3	—	229.0	238.8	239.8
pelvic	—	196.6	—	229.0	238.8	239.8
peri-aortic	—	196.2	—	229.0	238.8	239.8
peripancreatic	—	196.2	—	229.0	238.8	239.8
popliteal	—	196.5	—	229.0	238.8	239.8
porta hepatis	—	196.2	—	229.0	238.8	239.8
portal	—	196.2	—	229.0	238.8	239.8
preauricular	—	196.0	—	229.0	238.8	239.8
prelaryngeal	—	196.0	—	229.0	238.8	239.8
presymphysial	—	196.6	—	229.0	238.8	239.8
pretracheal	—	196.0	—	229.0	238.8	239.8
primary (any site) NEC	202.9 √5ᵗʰ	—	—	—	—	—
pulmonary (hiler)	—	196.1	—	229.0	238.8	239.8
pyloric	—	196.2	—	229.0	238.8	239.8
retroperitoneal	—	196.2	—	229.0	238.8	239.8
retropharyngeal	—	196.0	—	229.0	238.8	239.8
Rosenmüller's	—	196.5	—	229.0	238.8	239.8
sacral	—	196.6	—	229.0	238.8	239.8
scalene	—	196.0	—	229.0	238.8	239.8
site NEC	—	196.9	—	229.0	238.8	239.8
splenic (hilar)	—	196.2	—	229.0	238.8	239.8
subclavicular	—	196.3	—	229.0	238.8	239.8
subinguinal	—	196.5	—	229.0	238.8	239.8
sublingual	—	196.0	—	229.0	238.8	239.8
submandibular	—	196.0	—	229.0	238.8	239.8
submaxillary	—	196.0	—	229.0	238.8	239.8
submental	—	196.0	—	229.0	238.8	239.8
subscapular	—	196.3	—	229.0	238.8	239.8
supraclavicular	—	196.0	—	229.0	238.8	239.8
thoracic	—	196.1	—	229.0	238.8	239.8
tibial	—	196.5	—	229.0	238.8	239.8
tracheal	—	196.1	—	229.0	238.8	239.8
tracheobronchial	—	196.1	—	229.0	238.8	239.8
upper limb	—	196.3	—	229.0	238.8	239.8
Virchow's	—	196.0	—	229.0	238.8	239.8
node — *see also* Neoplasm, lymph gland						
primary NEC	202.9 √5ᵗʰ	—	—	—	—	—
vessel (*see also* Neoplasm, connective tissue)	171.9	198.89	—	215.9	238.1	239.2
Nackenrodt's ligament	183.8	198.82	233.3	221.8	236.3	239.5
malar	170.0	198.5	—	213.0	238.0	239.2
region — *see* Neoplasm, cheek						
mammary gland — *see* Neoplasm, breast						
mandible	170.1	198.5	—	213.1	238.0	239.2
alveolar						
mucose	143.1	198.89	230.0	210.4	235.1	239.0
ridge or process	170.1	198.5	—	213.1	238.0	239.2
carcinoma	143.1	—	—	—	—	—
carcinoma	143.1	—	—	—	—	—
marrow (bone) NEC	202.9 √5ᵗʰ	198.5	—	—	—	238.7
mastectomy site (skin)	173.5	198.2	—	—	—	—
specified as breast tissue	174.8	198.81	—	—	—	—
mastoid (air cells) (antrum) (cavity)	160.1	197.3	231.8	212.0	235.9	239.1
bone or process	170.0	198.5	—	213.0	238.0	239.2

	Malignant					
	Primary	Secondary	Ca in situ	Benign	Uncertain Behavior	Unspecified
Neoplasm, neoplastic — *continued*						
maxilla, maxillary (superior)	170.0	198.5	—	213.0	238.0	239.2
alveolar						
mucosa	143.0	198.89	230.0	210.4	235.1	239.0
ridge or process	170.0	198.5	—	213.0	238.0	239.2
carcinoma	143.0	—	—	—	—	—
antrum	160.2	197.3	231.8	212.0	235.9	239.1
carcinoma	143.0	—	—	—	—	—
inferior — *see* Neoplasm, mandible						
sinus	160.2	197.3	231.8	212.0	235.9	239.1
meatus						
external (ear)	173.2	198.2	232.2	216.2	238.2	239.2
Meckel's diverticulum	152.3	197.4	230.7	211.2	235.2	239.0
mediastinum, mediastinal	164.9	197.1	—	212.5	235.8	239.8
anterior	164.2	197.1	—	212.5	235.8	239.8
contiguous sites with heart and thymus	164.8	—	—	—	—	—
posterior	164.3	197.1	—	212.5	235.8	239.8
medulla						
adrenal	194.0	198.7	234.8	227.0	237.2	239.7
oblongata	191.7	198.3	—	225.0	237.5	239.6
meibomian gland	173.1	198.2	232.1	216.1	238.2	239.2
melanoma — *see* Melanoma						
meninges (brain) (cerebral) (cranial) (intracranial)	192.1	198.4	—	225.2	237.6	239.7
spinal (cord)	192.3	198.4	—	225.4	237.6	239.7
meniscus, knee joint (lateral) (medial)	170.7	198.5	—	213.7	238.0	239.2
mesentery, mesenteric	158.8	197.6	—	211.8	235.4	239.0
mesoappendix	158.8	197.6	—	211.8	235.4	239.0
mesocolon	158.8	197.6	—	211.8	235.4	239.0
mesopharynx — *see* Neoplasm, oropharynx						
mesosalpinx	183.3	198.82	233.3	221.0	236.3	239.5
mesovarium	183.3	198.82	233.3	221.0	236.3	239.5
metacarpus (any bone)	170.5	198.5	—	213.5	238.0	239.2
metastatic NEC — *see also* Neoplasm, by site, secondary	—	199.1	—	—	—	—
metatarsus (any bone)	170.8	198.5	—	213.8	238.0	239.2
midbrain	191.7	198.3	—	225.0	237.5	239.6
milk duct — *see* Neoplasm, breast						
mons						
pubis	184.4	198.82	233.3	221.2	236.3	239.5
veneris	184.4	198.82	233.3	221.2	236.3	239.5
motor tract	192.9	198.4	—	225.9	237.9	239.7
brain	191.9	198.3	—	225.0	237.5	239.6
spinal	192.2	198.3	—	225.3	237.5	239.7
mouth	145.9	198.89	230.0	210.4	235.1	239.0
contiguous sites	145.8	—	—	—	—	—
floor	144.9	198.89	230.0	210.3	235.1	239.0
anterior portion	144.0	198.89	230.0	210.3	235.1	239.0
contiguous sites	144.8	—	—	—	—	—
lateral portion	144.1	198.89	230.0	210.3	235.1	239.0
roof	145.5	198.89	230.0	210.4	235.1	239.0
specified part NEC	145.8	198.89	230.0	210.4	235.1	239.0
vestibule	145.1	198.89	230.0	210.4	235.1	239.0
mucosa						
alveolar (ridge or process)	143.9	198.89	230.0	210.4	235.1	239.0
lower	143.1	198.89	230.0	210.4	235.1	239.0
upper	143.0	198.89	230.0	210.4	235.1	239.0
buccal	145.0	198.89	230.0	210.4	235.1	239.0
cheek	145.0	198.89	230.0	210.4	235.1	239.0
lip — *see* Neoplasm, lip, internal						
nasal	160.0	197.3	231.8	212.0	235.9	239.1
oral	145.0	198.89	230.0	210.4	235.1	239.0
Müllerian duct						
female	184.8	198.82	233.3	221.8	236.3	239.5
male	187.8	198.82	233.6	222.8	236.6	239.5
multiple sites NEC	199.0	199.0	234.9	229.9	238.9	199.0
muscle — *see also* Neoplasm, connective tissue						
extraocular	190.1	198.4	234.0	224.1	238.8	239.8
myocardium	164.1	198.89	—	212.7	238.8	239.8

✓4ᵗʰ Fourth-digit Required   ✓5ᵗʰ Fifth-digit Required   ▶◀ Revised Text   ● New Line   ▲ Revised Code

	Malignant					
	Primary	**Secondary**	**Ca in situ**	**Benign**	**Uncertain Behavior**	**Unspecified**
Neoplasm, neoplastic — *continued*						
myometrium	182.0	198.82	233.2	219.1	236.0	239.5
myopericardium	164.1	198.89	—	212.7	238.8	239.8
nabothian gland (follicle)	180.0	198.82	233.1	219.0	236.0	239.5
nail	173.9	198.2	232.9	216.9	238.2	239.2
finger	173.6	198.2	232.6	216.6	238.2	239.2
toe	173.7	198.2	232.7	216.7	238.2	239.2
nares, naris (anterior) (posterior)	160.0	197.3	231.8	212.0	235.9	239.1
nasal — *see* Neoplasm, nose						
nasolabial groove	173.3	198.2	232.3	216.3	238.2	239.2
nasolacrimal duct	190.7	198.4	234.0	224.7	238.8	239.8
nasopharynx, nasopharyngeal	147.9	198.89	230.0	210.7	235.1	239.0
contiguous sites	147.8	—	—	—	—	—
floor	147.3	198.89	230.0	210.7	235.1	239.0
roof	147.0	198.89	230.0	210.7	235.1	239.0
specified site NEC	147.8	198.89	230.0	210.7	235.1	239.0
wall	147.9	198.89	230.0	210.7	235.1	239.0
anterior	147.3	198.89	230.0	210.7	235.1	239.0
lateral	147.2	198.89	230.0	210.7	235.1	239.0
posterior	147.1	198.89	230.0	210.7	235.1	239.0
superior	147.0	198.89	230.0	210.7	235.1	239.0
nates	173.5	198.2	232.5	216.5	238.2	239.2
neck NEC*	195.0	198.89	234.8	229.8	238.8	239.8
nerve (autonomic) (ganglion) (parasympathetic) (peripheral) (sympathetic) — *see also* Neoplasm, connective tissue						
abducens	192.0	198.4	—	225.1	237.9	239.7
accessory (spinal)	192.0	198.4	—	225.1	237.9	239.7
acoustic	192.0	198.4	—	225.1	237.9	239.7
auditory	192.0	198.4	—	225.1	237.9	239.7
brachial	171.2	198.89	—	215.2	238.1	239.2
cranial (any)	192.0	198.4	—	225.1	237.9	239.7
facial	192.0	198.4	—	225.1	237.9	239.7
femoral	171.3	198.89	—	215.3	238.1	239.2
glossopharyngeal	192.0	198.4	—	225.1	237.9	239.7
hypoglossal	192.0	198.4	—	225.1	237.9	239.7
intercostal	171.4	198.89	—	215.4	238.1	239.2
lumbar	171.7	198.89	—	215.7	238.1	239.2
median	171.2	198.89	—	215.2	238.1	239.2
obturator	171.3	198.89	—	215.3	238.1	239.2
oculomotor	192.0	198.4	—	225.1	237.9	239.7
olfactory	192.0	198.4	—	225.1	237.9	239.7
optic	192.0	198.4	—	225.1	237.9	239.7
peripheral NEC	171.9	198.89	—	215.9	238.1	239.2
radial	171.2	198.89	—	215.2	238.1	239.2
sacral	171.6	198.89	—	215.6	238.1	239.2
sciatic	171.3	198.89	—	215.3	238.1	239.2
spinal NEC	171.9	198.89	—	215.9	238.1	239.2
trigeminal	192.0	198.4	—	225.1	237.9	239.7
trochlear	192.0	198.4	—	225.1	237.9	239.7
ulnar	171.2	198.89	—	215.2	238.1	239.2
vagus	192.0	198.4	—	225.1	237.9	239.7
nervous system (central) NEC	192.9	198.4	—	225.9	237.9	239.7
autonomic NEC	171.9	198.89	—	215.9	238.1	239.2
brain — *see also* Neoplasm, brain						
membrane or meninges	192.1	198.4	—	225.2	237.6	239.7
contiguous sites	192.8	—	—	—	—	—
parasympathetic NEC	171.9	198.89	—	215.9	238.1	239.2
sympathetic NEC	171.9	198.89	—	215.9	238.1	239.2
nipple (female)	174.0	198.81	233.0	217	238.3	239.3
male	175.0	198.81	233.0	217	238.3	239.3
nose, nasal	195.0	198.89	234.8	229.8	238.8	239.8
ala (external)	173.3	198.2	232.3	216.3	238.2	239.2
bone	170.0	198.5	—	213.0	238.0	239.2
cartilage	160.0	197.3	231.8	212.0	235.9	239.1
cavity	160.0	197.3	231.8	212.0	235.9	239.1
contiguous sites with accessory sinuses or middle ear	160.8	—	—	—	—	—
choana	147.3	198.89	230.0	210.7	235.1	239.0

Neoplasm, neoplastic — continued	Primary	Secondary	Ca in situ	Benign	Uncertain Behavior	Unspecified
nose, nasal — continued						
external (skin)	173.3	198.2	232.3	216.3	238.2	239.2
fossa	160.0	197.3	231.8	212.0	235.9	239.1
internal	160.0	197.3	231.8	212.0	235.9	239.1
mucosa	160.0	197.3	231.8	212.0	235.9	239.1
septum	160.0	197.3	231.8	212.0	235.9	239.1
posterior margin	147.3	198.89	230.0	210.7	235.1	239.0
sinus — see Neoplasm, sinus						
skin	173.3	198.2	232.3	216.3	238.2	239.2
turbinate (mucosa)	160.0	197.3	231.8	212.0	235.9	239.1
bone	170.0	198.5	—	213.0	238.0	239.2
vestibule	160.0	197.3	231.8	212.0	235.9	239.1
nostril	160.0	197.3	231.8	212.0	235.9	239.1
nucleus pulposus	170.2	198.5	—	213.2	238.0	239.2
occipital						
bone	170.0	198.5	—	213.0	238.0	239.2
lobe or pole, brain	191.4	198.3	—	225.0	237.5	239.6
odontogenic — see Neoplasm, jaw bone						
oesophagus — see Neoplasm, esophagus						
olfactory nerve or bulb	192.0	198.4	—	225.1	237.9	239.7
olive (brain)	191.7	198.3	—	225.0	237.5	239.6
omentum	158.8	197.6	—	211.8	235.4	239.0
operculum (brain)	191.0	198.3	—	225.0	237.5	239.6
optic nerve, chiasm, or tract	192.0	198.4	—	225.1	237.9	239.7
oral (cavity)	145.9	198.89	230.0	210.4	235.1	239.0
contiguous sites with lip or pharynx	149.8	—	—	—	—	—
ill-defined	149.9	198.89	230.0	210.4	235.1	239.0
mucosa	145.9	198.89	230.0	210.4	235.1	239.0
orbit	190.1	198.4	234.0	224.1	238.8	239.8
bone	170.0	198.5	—	213.0	238.0	239.2
eye	190.1	198.4	234.0	224.1	238.8	239.8
soft parts	190.1	198.4	234.0	224.1	238.8	239.8
organ of Zuckerkandl	194.6	198.89	—	227.6	237.3	239.7
oropharynx	146.9	198.89	230.0	210.6	235.1	239.0
branchial cleft (vestige)	146.8	198.89	230.0	210.6	235.1	239.0
contiguous sites	146.8	—	—	—	—	—
junctional region	146.5	198.89	230.0	210.6	235.1	239.0
lateral wall	146.6	198.89	230.0	210.6	235.1	239.0
pillars of fauces	146.2	198.89	230.0	210.6	235.1	239.0
posterior wall	146.7	198.89	230.0	210.6	235.1	239.0
specified part NEC	146.8	198.89	230.0	210.6	235.1	239.0
vallecula	146.3	198.89	230.0	210.6	235.1	239.0
os						
external	180.1	198.82	233.1	219.0	236.0	239.5
internal	180.0	198.82	233.1	219.0	236.0	239.5
ovary	183.0	198.6	233.3	220	236.2	239.5
oviduct	183.2	198.82	233.3	221.0	236.3	239.5
palate	145.5	198.89	230.0	210.4	235.1	239.0
hard	145.2	198.89	230.0	210.4	235.1	239.0
junction of hard and soft palate	145.5	198.89	230.0	210.4	235.1	239.0
soft	145.3	198.89	230.0	210.4	235.1	239.0
nasopharyngeal surface	147.3	198.89	230.0	210.7	235.1	239.0
posterior surface	147.3	198.89	230.0	210.7	235.1	239.0
superior surface	147.3	198.89	230.0	210.7	235.1	239.0
palatoglossal arch	146.2	198.89	230.0	210.6	235.1	239.0
palatopharyngeal arch	146.2	198.89	230.0	210.6	235.1	239.0
pallium	191.0	198.3	—	225.0	237.5	239.6
palpebra	173.1	198.2	232.1	216.1	238.2	239.2
pancreas	157.9	197.8	230.9	211.6	235.5	239.0
body	157.1	197.8	230.9	211.6	235.5	239.0
contiguous sites	157.8	—	—	—	—	—
duct (of Santorini) (of Wirsung)	157.3	197.8	230.9	211.6	235.5	239.0
ectopic tissue	157.8	197.8	230.9	211.6	235.5	239.0
head	157.0	197.8	230.9	211.6	235.5	239.0
islet cells	157.4	197.8	230.9	211.7	235.5	239.0

Neoplasm, nose — Neoplasm, pancreas

	Malignant					
	Primary	**Secondary**	**Ca in situ**	**Benign**	**Uncertain Behavior**	**Unspecified**
Neoplasm, neoplastic — *continued*						
pancreas — *continued*						
neck	157.8	197.8	230.9	211.6	235.5	239.0
tail	157.2	197.8	230.9	211.6	235.5	239.0
para-aortic body	194.6	198.89	—	227.6	237.3	239.7
paraganglion NEC	194.6	198.89	—	227.6	237.3	239.7
parametrium	183.4	198.82	—	221.0	236.3	239.5
paranephric	158.0	197.6	—	211.8	235.4	239.0
pararectal	195.3	198.89	—	229.8	238.8	239.8
parasagittal (region)	195.0	198.89	234.8	229.8	238.8	239.8
parasellar	192.9	198.4	—	225.9	237.9	239.7
parathyroid (gland)	194.1	198.89	234.8	227.1	237.4	239.7
paraurethral	195.3	198.89	—	229.8	238.8	239.8
gland	189.4	198.1	233.9	223.89	236.99	239.5
paravaginal	195.3	198.89	—	229.8	238.8	239.8
parenchyma, kidney	189.0	198.0	233.9	223.0	236.91	239.5
parietal						
bone	170.0	198.5	—	213.0	238.0	239.2
lobe, brain	191.3	198.3	—	225.0	237.5	239.6
paroophoron	183.3	198.82	233.3	221.0	236.3	239.5
parotid (duct) (gland)	142.0	198.89	230.0	210.2	235.0	239.0
parovarium	183.3	198.82	233.3	221.0	236.3	239.5
patella	170.8	198.5	—	213.8	238.0	239.2
peduncle, cerebral	191.7	198.3	—	225.0	237.5	239.6
pelvirectal junction	154.0	197.5	230.4	211.4	235.2	239.0
pelvis, pelvic	195.3	198.89	234.8	229.8	238.8	239.8
bone	170.6	198.5	—	213.6	238.0	239.2
floor	195.3	198.89	234.8	229.8	238.8	239.8
renal	189.1	198.0	233.9	223.1	236.91	239.5
viscera	195.3	198.89	234.8	229.8	238.8	239.8
wall	195.3	198.89	234.8	229.8	238.8	239.8
pelvo-abdominal	195.8	198.89	234.8	229.8	238.8	239.8
penis	187.4	198.82	233.5	222.1	236.6	239.5
body	187.3	198.82	233.5	222.1	236.6	239.5
corpus (cavernosum)	187.3	198.82	233.5	222.1	236.6	239.5
glans	187.2	198.82	233.5	222.1	236.6	239.5
skin NEC	187.4	198.82	233.5	222.1	236.6	239.5
periadrenal (tissue)	158.0	197.6	—	211.8	235.4	239.0
perianal (skin)	173.5	198.2	232.5	216.5	238.2	239.2
pericardium	164.1	198.89	—	212.7	238.8	239.8
perinephric	158.0	197.6	—	211.8	235.4	239.0
perineum	195.3	198.89	234.8	229.8	238.8	239.8
periodontal tissue NEC	143.9	198.89	230.0	210.4	235.1	239.0
periosteum — *see* Neoplasm, bone						
peripancreatic	158.0	197.6	—	211.8	235.4	239.0
peripheral nerve NEC	171.9	198.89	—	215.9	238.1	239.2
perirectal (tissue)	195.3	198.89	—	229.8	238.8	239.8
perirenal (tissue)	158.0	197.6	—	211.8	235.4	239.0
peritoneum, peritoneal (cavity)	158.9	197.6	—	211.8	235.4	239.0
contiguous sites	158.8	—	—	—	—	—
with digestive organs	159.8	—	—	—	—	—
parietal	158.8	197.6	—	211.8	235.4	239.0
pelvic	158.8	197.6	—	211.8	235.4	239.0
specified part NEC	158.8	197.6	—	211.8	235.4	239.0
peritonsillar (tissue)	195.0	198.89	234.8	229.8	238.8	239.8
periurethral tissue	195.3	198.89	—	229.8	238.8	239.8
phalanges	170.9	198.5	—	213.9	238.0	239.2
foot	170.8	198.5	—	213.8	238.0	239.2
hand	170.5	198.5	—	213.5	238.0	239.2
pharynx, pharyngeal	149.0	198.89	230.0	210.9	235.1	239.0
bursa	147.1	198.89	230.0	210.7	235.1	239.0
fornix	147.3	198.89	230.0	210.7	235.1	239.0
recess	147.2	198.89	230.0	210.7	235.1	239.0
region	149.0	198.89	230.0	210.9	235.1	239.0
tonsil	147.1	198.89	230.0	210.7	235.1	239.0
wall (lateral) (posterior)	149.0	198.89	230.0	210.9	235.1	239.0

✓4ᵗʰ Fourth-digit Required   ✓5ᵗʰ Fifth-digit Required   ▶◀ Revised Text   ● New Line   ▲ Revised Code

Neoplasm, neoplastic — continued	Malignant			Benign	Uncertain Behavior	Unspecified
	Primary	Secondary	Ca in situ	Benign	Uncertain Behavior	Unspecified
pia mater (cerebral) (cranial)	192.1	198.4	—	225.2	237.6	239.7
spinal	192.3	198.4	—	225.4	237.6	239.7
pillars of fauces	146.2	198.89	230.0	210.6	235.1	239.0
pineal (body) (gland)	194.4	198.89	234.8	227.4	237.1	239.7
pinna (ear) NEC	173.2	198.2	232.2	216.2	238.2	239.2
cartilage	171.0	198.89	—	215.0	238.1	239.2
piriform fossa or sinus	148.1	198.89	230.0	210.8	235.1	239.0
pituitary (body) (fossa) (gland) (lobe)	194.3	198.89	234.8	227.3	237.0	239.7
placenta	181	198.82	233.2	219.8	236.1	239.5
pleura, pleural (cavity)	163.9	197.2	—	212.4	235.8	239.1
contiguous sites	163.8	—	—	—	—	—
parietal	163.0	197.2	—	212.4	235.8	239.1
visceral	163.1	197.2	—	212.4	235.8	239.1
plexus						
brachial	171.2	198.89	—	215.2	238.1	239.2
cervical	171.0	198.89	—	215.0	238.1	239.2
choroid	191.5	198.3	—	225.0	237.5	239.6
lumbosacral	171.6	198.89	—	215.6	238.1	239.2
sacral	171.6	198.89	—	215.6	238.1	239.2
pluri-endocrine	194.8	198.89	234.8	227.8	237.4	239.7
pole						
frontal	191.1	198.3	—	225.0	237.5	239.6
occipital	191.4	198.3	—	225.0	237.5	239.6
pons (varolii)	191.7	198.3	—	225.0	237.5	239.6
popliteal fossa or space*	195.5	198.89	234.8	229.8	238.8	239.8
postcricoid (region)	148.0	198.89	230.0	210.8	235.1	239.0
posterior fossa (cranial)	191.6	198.3	—	225.0	237.5	239.6
postnasal space	147.9	198.89	230.0	210.7	235.1	239.0
prepuce	187.1	198.82	233.5	222.1	236.6	239.5
prepylorus	151.1	197.8	230.2	211.1	235.2	239.0
presacral (region)	195.3	198.89	—	229.8	238.8	239.8
prostate (gland)	185	198.82	233.4	222.2	236.5	239.5
utricle	189.3	198.1	233.9	223.81	236.99	239.5
pterygoid fossa	171.0	198.89	—	215.0	238.1	239.2
pubic bone	170.6	198.5	—	213.6	238.0	239.2
pudenda, pudendum (female)	184.4	198.82	233.3	221.2	236.3	239.5
pulmonary	162.9	197.0	231.2	212.3	235.7	239.1
putamen	191.0	198.3	—	225.0	237.5	239.6
pyloric						
antrum	151.2	197.8	230.2	211.1	235.2	239.0
canal	151.1	197.8	230.2	211.1	235.2	239.0
pylorus	151.1	197.8	230.2	211.1	235.2	239.0
pyramid (brain)	191.7	198.3	—	225.0	237.5	239.6
pyriform fossa or sinus	148.1	198.89	230.0	210.8	235.1	239.0
radius (any part)	170.4	198.5	—	213.4	238.0	239.2
Rathke's pouch	194.3	198.89	234.8	227.3	237.0	239.7
rectosigmoid (colon) (junction)	154.0	197.5	230.4	211.4	235.2	239.0
contiguous sites with anus or rectum	154.8	—	—	—	—	—
rectouterine pouch	158.8	197.6	—	211.8	235.4	239.0
rectovaginal septum or wall	195.3	198.89	234.8	229.8	238.8	239.8
rectovesical septum	195.3	198.89	234.8	229.8	238.8	239.8
rectum (ampulla)	154.1	197.5	230.4	211.4	235.2	239.0
and colon	154.0	197.5	230.4	211.4	235.2	239.0
contiguous sites with anus or rectosigmoid junction	154.8	—	—	—	—	—
renal	189.0	198.0	233.9	223.0	236.91	239.5
calyx	189.1	198.0	233.9	223.1	236.91	239.5
hilus	189.1	198.0	233.9	223.1	236.91	239.5
parenchyma	189.0	198.0	233.9	223.0	236.91	239.5
pelvis	189.1	198.0	233.9	223.1	236.91	239.5
respiratory						
organs or system NEC	165.9	197.3	231.9	212.9	235.9	239.1
contiguous sites with intrathoracic organs	165.8	—	—	—	—	—
specified sites NEC	165.8	197.3	231.8	212.8	235.9	239.1
tract NEC	165.9	197.3	231.9	212.9	235.9	239.1
upper	165.0	197.3	231.9	212.9	235.9	239.1
retina	190.5	198.4	234.0	224.5	238.8	239.8

Neoplasm, neoplastic — continued	Malignant			Benign	Uncertain Behavior	Unspecified
	Primary	Secondary	Ca in situ			
retrobulbar	190.1	198.4	—	224.1	238.8	239.8
retrocecal	158.0	197.6	—	211.8	235.4	239.0
retromolar (area) (triangle) (trigone)	145.6	198.89	230.0	210.4	235.1	239.0
retro-orbital	195.0	198.89	234.8	229.8	238.8	239.8
retroperitoneal (space) (tissue)	158.0	197.6	—	211.8	235.4	239.0
contiguous sites	158.8	—	—	—	—	—
retroperitoneum	158.0	197.6	—	211.8	235.4	239.0
contiguous sites	158.8	—	—	—	—	—
retropharyngeal	149.0	198.89	230.0	210.9	235.1	239.0
retrovesical (septum)	195.3	198.89	234.8	229.8	238.8	239.8
rhinencephalon	191.0	198.3	—	225.0	237.5	239.6
rib	170.3	198.5	—	213.3	238.0	239.2
Rosenmüller's fossa	147.2	198.89	230.0	210.7	235.1	239.0
round ligament	183.5	198.82	—	221.0	236.3	239.5
sacrococcyx, sacrococcygeal	170.6	198.5	—	213.6	238.0	239.2
region	195.3	198.89	234.8	229.8	238.8	239.8
sacrouterine ligament	183.4	198.82	—	221.0	236.3	239.5
sacrum, sacral (vertebra)	170.6	198.5	—	213.6	238.0	239.2
salivary gland or duct (major)	142.9	198.89	230.0	210.2	235.0	239.0
contiguous sites	142.8	—	—	—	—	—
minor NEC	145.9	198.89	230.0	210.4	235.1	239.0
parotid	142.0	198.89	230.0	210.2	235.0	239.0
pluriglandular	142.8	198.89	230.0	210.2	235.0	239.0
sublingual	142.2	198.89	230.0	210.2	235.0	239.0
submandibular	142.1	198.89	230.0	210.2	235.0	239.0
submaxillary	142.1	198.89	230.0	210.2	235.0	239.0
salpinx (uterine)	183.2	198.82	233.3	221.0	236.3	239.5
Santorini's duct	157.3	197.8	230.9	211.6	235.5	239.0
scalp	173.4	198.2	232.4	216.4	238.2	239.2
scapula (any part)	170.4	198.5	—	213.4	238.0	239.2
scapular region	195.1	198.89	234.8	229.8	238.8	239.8
scar NEC (see also Neoplasm, skin)	173.9	198.2	232.9	216.9	238.2	239.2
sciatic nerve	171.3	198.89	—	215.3	238.1	239.2
sclera	190.0	198.4	234.0	224.0	238.8	239.8
scrotum (skin)	187.7	198.82	233.6	222.4	236.6	239.5
sebaceous gland — see Neoplasm, skin						
sella turcica	194.3	198.89	234.8	227.3	237.0	239.7
bone	170.0	198.5	—	213.0	238.0	239.2
semilunar cartilage (knee)	170.7	198.5	—	213.7	238.0	239.2
seminal vesicle	187.8	198.82	233.6	222.8	236.6	239.5
septum						
nasal	160.0	197.3	231.8	212.0	235.9	239.1
posterior margin	147.3	198.89	230.0	210.7	235.1	239.0
rectovaginal	195.3	198.89	234.8	229.8	238.8	239.8
rectovesical	195.3	198.89	234.8	229.8	238.8	239.8
urethrovaginal	184.9	198.82	233.3	221.9	236.3	239.5
vesicovaginal	184.9	198.82	233.3	221.9	236.3	239.5
shoulder NEC*	195.4	198.89	232.6	229.8	238.8	239.8
sigmoid flexure (lower) (upper)	153.3	197.5	230.3	211.3	235.2	239.0
sinus (accessory)	160.9	197.3	231.8	212.0	235.9	239.1
bone (any)	170.0	198.5	—	213.0	238.0	239.2
contiguous sites with middle ear or nasal cavities	160.8	—	—	—	—	—
ethmoidal	160.3	197.3	231.8	212.0	235.9	239.1
frontal	160.4	197.3	231.8	212.0	235.9	239.1
maxillary	160.2	197.3	231.8	212.0	235.9	239.1
nasal, paranasal NEC	160.9	197.3	231.8	212.0	235.9	239.1
pyriform	148.1	198.89	230.0	210.8	235.1	239.0
sphenoidal	160.5	197.3	231.8	212.0	235.9	239.1
skeleton, skeletal NEC	170.9	198.5	—	213.9	238.0	239.2
Skene's gland	189.4	198.1	233.9	223.89	236.99	239.5
skin NEC	173.9	198.2	232.9	216.9	238.2	239.2
abdominal wall	173.5	198.2	232.5	216.5	238.2	239.2
ala nasi	173.3	198.2	232.3	216.3	238.2	239.2
ankle	173.7	198.2	232.7	216.7	238.2	239.2
antecubital space	173.6	198.2	232.6	216.6	238.2	239.2
anus	173.5	198.2	232.5	216.5	238.2	239.2

✓4ᵗʰ Fourth-digit Required   ✓5ᵗʰ Fifth-digit Required   ▶◀ Revised Text   ● New Line   ▲ Revised Code

	Malignant					
	Primary	**Secondary**	**Ca in situ**	**Benign**	**Uncertain Behavior**	**Unspecified**
Neoplasm, neoplastic — *continued*						
skin NEC — *continued*						
arm	173.6	198.2	232.6	216.6	238.2	239.2
auditory canal (external)	173.2	198.2	232.2	216.2	238.2	239.2
auricle (ear)	173.2	198.2	232.2	216.2	238.2	239.2
auricular canal (external)	173.2	198.2	232.2	216.2	238.2	239.2
axilla, axillary fold	173.5	198.2	232.5	216.5	238.2	239.2
back	173.5	198.2	232.5	216.5	238.2	239.2
breast	173.5	198.2	232.5	216.5	238.2	239.2
brow	173.3	198.2	232.3	216.3	238.2	239.2
buttock	173.5	198.2	232.5	216.5	238.2	239.2
calf	173.7	198.2	232.7	216.7	238.2	239.2
canthus (eye) (inner) (outer)	173.1	198.2	232.1	216.1	238.2	239.2
cervical region	173.4	198.2	232.4	216.4	238.2	239.2
cheek (external)	173.3	198.2	232.3	216.3	238.2	239.2
chest (wall)	173.5	198.2	232.5	216.5	238.2	239.2
chin	173.3	198.2	232.3	216.3	238.2	239.2
clavicular area	173.5	198.2	232.5	216.5	238.2	239.2
clitoris	184.3	198.82	233.3	221.2	236.3	239.5
columnella	173.3	198.2	232.3	216.3	238.2	239.2
concha	173.2	198.2	232.2	216.2	238.2	239.2
contiguous sites	173.8	—	—	—	—	—
ear (external)	173.2	198.2	232.2	216.2	238.2	239.2
elbow	173.6	198.2	232.6	216.6	238.2	239.2
eyebrow	173.3	198.2	232.3	216.3	238.2	239.2
eyelid	173.1	198.2	232.1	216.1	238.2	239.2
face NEC	173.3	198.2	232.3	216.3	238.2	239.2
female genital organs (external)	184.4	198.82	233.3	221.2	236.3	239.5
clitoris	184.3	198.82	233.3	221.2	236.3	239.5
labium NEC	184.4	198.82	233.3	221.2	236.3	239.5
majus	184.1	198.82	233.3	221.2	236.3	239.5
minus	184.2	198.82	233.3	221.2	236.3	239.5
pudendum	184.4	198.82	233.3	221.2	236.3	239.5
vulva	184.4	198.82	233.3	221.2	236.3	239.5
finger	173.6	198.2	232.6	216.6	238.2	239.2
flank	173.5	198.2	232.5	216.5	238.2	239.2
foot	173.7	198.2	232.7	216.7	238.2	239.2
forearm	173.6	198.2	232.6	216.6	238.2	239.2
forehead	173.3	198.2	232.3	216.3	238.2	239.2
glabella	173.3	198.2	232.3	216.3	238.2	239.2
gluteal region	173.5	198.2	232.5	216.5	238.2	239.2
groin	173.5	198.2	232.5	216.5	238.2	239.2
hand	173.6	198.2	232.6	216.6	238.2	239.2
head NEC	173.4	198.2	232.4	216.4	238.2	239.2
heel	173.7	198.2	232.7	216.7	238.2	239.2
helix	173.2	198.2	232.2	216.2	238.2	239.2
hip	173.7	198.2	232.7	216.7	238.2	239.2
infraclavicular region	173.5	198.2	232.5	216.5	238.2	239.2
inguinal region	173.5	198.2	232.5	216.5	238.2	239.2
jaw	173.3	198.2	232.3	216.3	238.2	239.2
knee	173.7	198.2	232.7	216.7	238.2	239.2
labia						
majora	184.1	198.82	233.3	221.2	236.3	239.5
minora	184.2	198.82	233.3	221.2	236.3	239.5
leg	173.7	198.2	232.7	216.7	238.2	239.2
lid (lower) (upper)	173.1	198.2	232.1	216.1	238.2	239.2
limb NEC	173.9	198.2	232.9	216.9	238.2	239.5
lower	173.7	198.2	232.7	216.7	238.2	239.2
upper	173.6	198.2	232.6	216.6	238.2	239.2
lip (lower) (upper)	173.0	198.2	232.0	216.0	238.2	239.2
male genital organs	187.9	198.82	233.6	222.9	236.6	239.5
penis	187.4	198.82	233.5	222.1	236.6	239.5
prepuce	187.1	198.82	233.5	222.1	236.6	239.5
scrotum	187.7	198.82	233.6	222.4	236.6	239.5
mastectomy site	173.5	198.2	—	—	—	—
specified as breast tissue	174.8	198.81	—	—	—	—
meatus, acoustic (external)	173.2	198.2	232.2	216.2	238.2	239.2

Neoplasm, skin — Neoplasm, skin

	Malignant					
	Primary	**Secondary**	**Ca in situ**	**Benign**	**Uncertain Behavior**	**Unspecified**
Neoplasm, neoplastic — *continued*						
skin NEC — *continued*						
melanoma — *see* Melanoma						
nates	173.5	198.2	232.5	216.5	238.2	239.0
neck	173.4	198.2	232.4	216.4	238.2	239.2
nose (external)	173.3	198.2	232.3	216.3	238.2	239.2
palm	173.6	198.2	232.6	216.6	238.2	239.2
palpebra	173.1	198.2	232.1	216.1	238.2	239.2
penis NEC	187.4	198.82	233.5	222.1	236.6	239.5
perianal	173.5	198.2	232.5	216.5	238.2	239.2
perineum	173.5	198.2	232.5	216.5	238.2	239.2
pinna	173.2	198.2	232.2	216.2	238.2	239.2
plantar	173.7	198.2	232.7	216.7	238.2	239.2
popliteal fossa or space	173.7	198.2	232.7	216.7	238.2	239.2
prepuce	187.1	198.82	233.5	222.1	236.6	239.5
pubes	173.5	198.2	232.5	216.5	238.2	239.2
sacrococcygeal region	173.5	198.2	232.5	216.5	238.2	239.2
scalp	173.4	198.2	232.4	216.4	238.2	239.2
scapular region	173.5	198.2	232.5	216.5	238.2	239.2
scrotum	187.7	198.82	233.6	222.4	236.6	239.5
shoulder	173.6	198.2	232.6	216.6	238.2	239.2
sole (foot)	173.7	198.2	232.7	216.7	238.2	239.2
specified sites NEC	173.8	198.2	232.8	216.8	232.8	239.2
submammary fold	173.5	198.2	232.5	216.5	238.2	239.2
supraclavicular region	173.4	198.2	232.4	216.4	238.2	239.2
temple	173.3	198.2	232.3	216.3	238.2	239.2
thigh	173.7	198.2	232.7	216.7	238.2	239.2
thoracic wall	173.5	198.2	232.5	216.5	238.2	239.2
thumb	173.6	198.2	232.6	216.6	238.2	239.2
toe	173.7	198.2	232.7	216.7	238.2	239.2
tragus	173.2	198.2	232.2	216.2	238.2	239.2
trunk	173.5	198.2	232.5	216.5	238.2	239.2
umbilicus	173.5	198.2	232.5	216.5	238.2	239.2
vulva	184.4	198.82	233.3	221.2	236.3	239.5
wrist	173.6	198.2	232.6	216.6	238.2	239.2
skull	170.0	198.5	—	213.0	238.0	239.2
soft parts or tissues — *see* Neoplasm, connective tissue						
specified site NEC	195.8	198.89	234.8	229.8	238.8	239.8
spermatic cord	187.6	198.82	233.6	222.8	236.6	239.5
sphenoid	160.5	197.3	231.8	212.0	235.9	239.1
bone	170.0	198.5	—	213.0	238.0	239.2
sinus	160.5	197.3	231.8	212.0	235.9	239.1
sphincter						
anal	154.2	197.5	230.5	211.4	235.5	239.0
of Oddi	156.1	197.8	230.8	211.5	235.3	239.0
spine, spinal (column)	170.2	198.5	—	213.2	238.0	239.2
bulb	191.7	198.3	—	225.0	237.5	239.6
coccyx	170.6	198.5	—	213.6	238.0	239.2
cord (cervical) (lumbar) (sacral) (thoracic)	192.2	198.3	—	225.3	237.5	239.7
dura mater	192.3	198.4	—	225.4	237.6	239.7
lumbosacral	170.2	198.5	—	213.2	238.0	239.2
membrane	192.3	198.4	—	225.4	237.6	239.7
meninges	192.3	198.4	—	225.4	237.6	239.7
nerve (root)	171.9	198.89	—	215.9	238.1	239.2
pia mater	192.3	198.4	—	225.4	237.6	239.7
root	171.9	198.89	—	215.9	238.1	239.2
sacrum	170.6	198.5	—	213.6	238.0	239.2
spleen, splenic NEC	159.1	197.8	230.9	211.9	235.5	239.0
flexure (colon)	153.7	197.5	230.3	211.3	235.2	239.0
stem, brain	191.7	198.3	—	225.0	237.5	239.6
Stensen's duct	142.0	198.89	230.0	210.2	235.0	239.0
sternum	170.3	198.5	—	213.3	238.0	239.2
stomach	151.9	197.8	230.2	211.1	235.2	239.0
antrum (pyloric)	151.2	197.8	230.2	211.1	235.2	239.0
body	151.4	197.8	230.2	211.1	235.2	239.0
cardia	151.0	197.8	230.2	211.1	235.2	239.0
cardiac orifice	151.0	197.8	230.2	211.1	235.2	239.0

	Malignant					
	Primary	Secondary	Ca in situ	Benign	Uncertain Behavior	Unspecified
Neoplasm, neoplastic — continued						
stomach — continued						
contiguous sites	151.8	—	—	—	—	—
corpus	151.4	197.8	230.2	211.1	235.2	239.0
fundus	151.3	197.8	230.2	211.1	235.2	239.0
greater curvature NEC	151.6	197.8	230.2	211.1	235.2	239.0
lesser curvature NEC	151.5	197.8	230.2	211.1	235.2	239.0
prepylorus	151.1	197.8	230.2	211.1	235.2	239.0
pylorus	151.1	197.8	230.2	211.1	235.2	239.0
wall NEC	151.9	197.8	230.2	211.1	235.2	239.0
anterior NEC	151.8	197.8	230.2	211.1	235.2	239.0
posterior NEC	151.8	197.8	230.2	211.1	235.2	239.0
stroma, endometrial	182.0	198.82	233.2	219.1	236.0	239.5
stump, cervical	180.8	198.82	233.1	219.0	236.0	239.5
subcutaneous (nodule) (tissue) NEC — see Neoplasm, connective tissue						
subdural	192.1	198.4	—	225.2	237.6	239.7
subglottis, subglottic	161.2	197.3	231.0	212.1	235.6	239.1
sublingual	144.9	198.89	230.0	210.3	235.1	239.0
gland or duct	142.2	198.89	230.0	210.2	235.0	239.0
submandibular gland	142.1	198.89	230.0	210.2	235.0	239.0
submaxillary gland or duct	142.1	198.89	230.0	210.2	235.0	239.0
submental	195.0	198.89	234.8	229.8	238.8	239.8
subpleural	162.9	197.0	—	212.3	235.7	239.1
substernal	164.2	197.1	—	212.5	235.8	239.8
sudoriferous, sudoriparous gland, site unspecified	173.9	198.2	232.9	216.9	238.2	239.2
specified site — see Neoplasm, skin						
supraclavicular region	195.0	198.89	234.8	229.8	238.8	239.8
supraglottis	161.1	197.3	231.0	212.1	235.6	239.1
suprarenal (capsule) (cortex) (gland) (medulla)	194.0	198.7	234.8	227.0	237.2	239.7
suprasellar (region)	191.9	198.3	—	225.0	237.5	239.6
sweat gland (apocrine) (eccrine), site unspecified	173.9	198.2	232.9	216.9	238.2	239.2
specified site — see Neoplasm, skin						
sympathetic nerve or nervous system NEC	171.9	198.89	—	215.9	238.1	239.2
symphysis pubis	170.6	198.5	—	213.6	238.0	239.2
synovial membrane — see Neoplasm, connective tissue						
tapetum, brain	191.8	198.3	—	225.0	237.5	239.6
tarsus (any bone)	170.8	198.5	—	213.8	238.0	239.2
temple (skin)	173.3	198.2	232.3	216.3	238.2	239.2
temporal						
bone	170.0	198.5	—	213.0	238.0	239.2
lobe or pole	191.2	198.3	—	225.0	237.5	239.6
region	195.0	198.89	234.8	229.8	238.8	239.8
skin	173.3	198.2	232.3	216.3	238.2	239.2
tendon (sheath) — see Neoplasm, connective tissue						
tentorium (cerebelli)	192.1	198.4	—	225.2	237.6	239.7
testis, testes (descended) (scrotal)	186.9	198.82	233.6	222.0	236.4	239.5
ectopic	186.0	198.82	233.6	222.0	236.4	239.5
retained	186.0	198.82	233.6	222.0	236.4	239.5
undescended	186.0	198.82	233.6	222.0	236.4	239.5
thalamus	191.0	198.3	—	225.0	237.5	239.6
thigh NEC*	195.5	198.89	234.8	229.8	238.8	239.8
thorax, thoracic (cavity) (organs NEC)	195.1	198.89	234.8	229.8	238.8	239.8
duct	171.4	198.89	—	215.4	238.1	239.2
wall NEC	195.1	198.89	234.8	229.8	238.8	239.8
throat	149.0	198.89	230.0	210.9	235.1	239.0
thumb NEC*	195.4	198.89	232.6	229.8	238.8	239.8
thymus (gland)	164.0	198.89	—	212.6	235.8	239.8
contiguous sites with heart and mediastinum	164.8	—	—	—	—	—
thyroglossal duct	193	198.89	234.8	226	237.4	239.7
thyroid (gland)	193	198.89	234.8	226	237.4	239.7
cartilage	161.3	197.3	231.0	212.1	235.6	239.1
tibia (any part)	170.7	198.5	—	213.7	238.0	239.2
toe NEC*	195.5	198.89	232.7	229.8	238.8	239.8
tongue	141.9	198.89	230.0	210.1	235.1	239.0
anterior (two-thirds) NEC	141.4	198.89	230.0	210.1	235.1	239.0
dorsal surface	141.1	198.89	230.0	210.1	235.1	239.0
ventral surface	141.3	198.89	230.0	210.1	235.1	239.0

✓4ᵗʰ Fourth-digit Required   ✓5ᵗʰ Fifth-digit Required   ▶◀ Revised Text   ● New Line   ▲ Revised Code

	Malignant			Benign	Uncertain Behavior	Unspecified
	Primary	Secondary	Ca in situ			
Neoplasm, neoplastic — *continued*						
tongue — *continued*						
base (dorsal surface)	141.0	198.89	230.0	210.1	235.1	239.0
border (lateral)	141.2	198.89	230.0	210.1	235.1	239.0
contiguous sites	141.8	—	—	—	—	—
dorsal surface NEC	141.1	198.89	230.0	210.1	235.1	239.0
fixed part NEC	141.0	198.89	230.0	210.1	235.1	239.0
foreamen cecum	141.1	198.89	230.0	210.1	235.1	239.0
frenulum linguae	141.3	198.89	230.0	210.1	235.1	239.0
junctional zone	141.5	198.89	230.0	210.1	235.1	239.0
margin (lateral)	141.2	198.89	230.0	210.1	235.1	239.0
midline NEC	141.1	198.89	230.0	210.1	235.1	239.0
mobile part NEC	141.4	198.89	230.0	210.1	235.1	239.0
posterior (third)	141.0	198.89	230.0	210.1	235.1	239.0
root	141.0	198.89	230.0	210.1	235.1	239.0
surface (dorsal)	141.1	198.89	230.0	210.1	235.1	239.0
base	141.0	198.89	230.0	210.1	235.1	239.0
ventral	141.3	198.89	230.0	210.1	235.1	239.0
tip	141.2	198.89	230.0	210.1	235.1	239.0
tonsil	141.6	198.89	230.0	210.1	235.1	239.0
tonsil	146.0	198.89	230.0	210.5	235.1	239.0
fauces, faucial	146.0	198.89	230.0	210.5	235.1	239.0
lingual	141.6	198.89	230.0	210.1	235.1	239.0
palatine	146.0	198.89	230.0	210.5	235.1	239.0
pharyngeal	147.1	198.89	230.0	210.7	235.1	239.0
pillar (anterior) (posterior)	146.2	198.89	230.0	210.6	235.1	239.0
tonsillar fossa	146.1	198.89	230.0	210.6	235.1	239.0
tooth socket NEC	143.9	198.89	230.0	210.4	235.1	239.0
trachea (cartilage) (mucosa)	162.0	197.3	231.1	212.2	235.7	239.1
contiguous sites with bronchus or lung	162.8	—	—	—	—	—
tracheobronchial	162.8	197.3	231.1	212.2	235.7	239.1
contiguous sites with lung	162.8	—	—	—	—	—
tragus	173.2	198.2	232.2	216.2	238.2	239.2
trunk NEC*	195.8	198.89	232.5	229.8	238.8	239.8
tubo-ovarian	183.8	198.82	233.3	221.8	236.3	239.5
tunica vaginalis	187.8	198.82	233.6	222.8	236.6	239.5
turbinate (bone)	170.0	198.5	—	213.0	238.0	239.2
nasal	160.0	197.3	231.8	212.0	235.9	239.1
tympanic cavity	160.1	197.3	231.8	212.0	235.9	239.1
ulna (any part)	170.4	198.5	—	213.4	238.0	239.2
umbilicus, umbilical	173.5	198.2	232.5	216.5	238.2	239.2
uncus, brain	191.2	198.3	—	225.0	237.5	239.6
unknown site or unspecified	199.1	199.1	234.9	229.9	238.9	239.9
urachus	188.7	198.1	233.7	223.3	236.7	239.4
ureter, ureteral	189.2	198.1	233.9	223.2	236.91	239.5
orifice (bladder)	188.6	198.1	233.7	223.3	236.7	239.4
ureter-bladder junction)	188.6	198.1	233.7	223.3	236.7	239.4
urethra, urethral (gland)	189.3	198.1	233.9	223.81	236.99	239.5
orifice, internal	188.5	198.1	233.7	223.3	236.7	239.4
urethrovaginal (septum)	184.9	198.82	233.3	221.9	236.3	239.5
urinary organ or system NEC	189.9	198.1	233.9	223.9	236.99	239.5
bladder — *see* Neoplasm, bladder						
contiguous sites	189.8	—	—	—	—	—
specified sites NEC	189.8	198.1	233.9	223.89	236.99	239.5
utero-ovarian	183.8	198.82	233.3	221.8	236.3	239.5
ligament	183.3	198.82	—	221.0	236.3	239.5
uterosacral ligament	183.4	198.82	—	221.0	236.3	239.5
uterus, uteri, uterine	179	198.82	233.2	219.9	236.0	239.5
adnexa NEC	183.9	198.82	233.3	221.8	236.3	239.5
contiguous sites	183.8	—	—	—	—	—
body	182.0	198.82	233.2	219.1	236.0	239.5
contiguous sites	182.8	—	—	—	—	—
cervix	180.9	198.82	233.1	219.0	236.0	239.5
tornu	182.0	198.82	233.2	219.1	236.0	239.5
corpus	182.0	198.82	233.2	219.1	236.0	239.5
endocervix (canal) (gland)	180.0	198.82	233.1	219.0	236.0	239.5
endometrium	182.0	198.82	233.2	219.1	236.0	239.5

✓4ᵗʰ Fourth-digit Required   ✓5ᵗʰ Fifth-digit Required   ▶◀ Revised Text   ● New Line   ▲ Revised Code

Neoplasm, tongue — Neoplasm, uterus

| | Malignant | | | | | |
	Primary	Secondary	Ca in situ	Benign	Uncertain Behavior	Unspecified
Neoplasm, neoplastic — *continued*						
uterus, uteri, uterine — *continued*						
exocervix	180.1	198.82	233.1	219.0	236.0	239.5
external os	180.1	198.82	233.1	219.0	236.0	239.5
fundus	182.0	198.82	233.2	219.1	236.0	239.5
internal os	180.0	198.82	233.1	219.0	236.0	239.5
isthmus	182.1	198.82	233.2	219.1	236.0	239.5
ligament	183.4	198.82	—	221.0	236.3	239.5
broad	183.3	198.82	233.3	221.0	236.3	239.5
round	183.5	198.82	—	221.0	236.3	239.5
lower segment	182.1	198.82	233.2	219.1	236.0	239.5
myometrium	182.0	198.82	233.2	219.1	236.0	239.5
squamocolumnar junction	180.8	198.82	233.1	219.0	236.0	239.5
tube	183.2	198.82	233.3	221.0	236.3	239.5
utricle, prostatic	189.3	198.1	233.9	223.81	236.99	239.5
uveal tract	190.0	198.4	234.0	224.0	238.8	239.8
uvula	145.4	198.89	230.0	210.4	235.1	239.0
vagina, vaginal (fornix) (vault) (wall)	184.0	198.82	233.3	221.1	236.3	239.5
vaginovesical	184.9	198.82	233.3	221.9	236.3	239.5
septum	194.9	198.82	233.3	221.9	236.3	239.5
vallecula (epiglottis)	146.3	198.89	230.0	210.6	235.1	239.0
vascular — *see* Neoplasm, connective tissue						
vas deferens	187.6	198.82	233.6	222.8	236.6	239.5
Vater's ampulla	156.2	197.8	230.8	211.5	235.3	239.0
vein, venous — *see* Neoplasm, connective tissue						
vena cava (abdominal) (inferior)	171.5	198.89	—	215.5	238.1	239.2
superior	171.4	198.89	—	215.4	238.1	239.2
ventricle (cerebral) (floor) (fourth) (lateral) (third)	191.5	198.3	—	225.0	237.5	239.6
cardiac (left) (right)	164.1	198.89	—	212.7	238.8	239.8
ventricular band of larynx	161.1	197.3	231.0	212.1	235.6	239.1
ventriculus — see Neoplasm, stomach						
vermillion border — *see* Neoplasm, lip						
vermis, cerebellum	191.6	198.3	—	225.0	237.5	239.6
vertebra (column)	170.2	198.5	—	213.2	238.0	239.2
coccyx	170.6	198.5	—	213.6	238.0	239.2
sacrum	170.6	198.5	—	213.6	238.0	239.2
vesical — *see* Neoplasm, bladder						
vesicle, seminal	187.8	198.82	233.6	222.8	236.6	239.5
vesicocervical tissue	184.9	198.82	233.3	221.9	236.3	239.5
vesicorectal	195.3	198.89	234.8	229.8	238.8	239.8
vesicovaginal	184.9	198.82	233.3	221.9	236.3	239.5
septum	184.9	198.82	233.3	221.9	236.3	239.5
vessel (blood) — *see* Neoplasm, connective tissue						
vestibular gland, greater	184.1	198.82	233.3	221.2	236.3	239.5
vestibule						
mouth	145.1	198.89	230.0	210.4	235.1	239.0
nose	160.0	197.3	231.8	212.0	235.9	239.1
Virchow's gland	—	196.0	—	229.0	238.8	239.8
viscera NEC	195.8	198.89	234.8	229.8	238.8	239.8
vocal cords (true)	161.0	197.3	231.0	212.1	235.6	239.1
false	161.1	197.3	231.0	212.1	235.6	239.1
vomer	170.0	198.5	—	213.0	238.0	239.2
vulva	184.4	198.82	233.3	221.2	236.3	239.5
vulvovaginal gland	184.4	198.82	233.3	221.2	236.3	239.5
Waldeyer's ring	149.1	198.89	230.0	210.9	235.1	239.0
Wharton's duct	142.1	198.89	230.0	210.2	235.0	239.0
white matter (central) (cerebral)	191.0	198.3	—	225.0	237.5	239.6
windpipe	162.0	197.3	231.1	212.2	235.7	239.1
Wirsung's duct	157.3	197.8	230.9	211.6	235.5	239.0
wolffian (body) (duct)						
female	184.8	198.82	233.3	221.8	236.3	239.5
male	187.8	198.82	233.6	222.8	236.6	239.5
womb — *see* Neoplasm, uterus						
wrist NEC*	195.4	198.89	232.6	229.8	238.8	239.8
xiphoid process	170.3	198.5	—	213.3	238.0	239.2
Zuckerkandl's organ	194.6	198.89	—	227.6	237.3	239.7

Neovascularization
- choroid 362.16
- ciliary body 364.42
- cornea 370.60
  - deep 370.63
  - localized 370.61
- iris 364.42
- retina 362.16
- subretinal 362.16

Nephralgia 788.0

Nephritis, nephritic (albuminuric) (azotemic) (congenital) (degenerative) (diffuse) (disseminated) (epithelial) (familial) (focal) (granulomatous) (hemorrhagic) (infantile) (nonsuppurative, excretory) (uremic) 583.9
- with
  - edema — see Nephrosis
  - lesion of
    - glomerulonephritis
      - hypocomplementemic persistent 583.2
        - with nephrotic syndrome 581.2
        - chronic 582.2
      - lobular 583.2
        - with nephrotic syndrome 581.2
        - chronic 582.2
      - membranoproliferative 583.2
        - with nephrotic syndrome 581.2
        - chronic 582.2
      - membranous 583.1
        - with nephrotic syndrome 581.1
        - chronic 582.1
      - mesangiocapillary 583.2
        - with nephrotic syndrome 581.2
        - chronic 582.2
      - mixed membranous and proliferative 583.2
        - with nephrotic syndrome 581.2
        - chronic 582.2
      - proliferative (diffuse) 583.0
        - with nephrotic syndrome 581.0
        - acute 580.0
        - chronic 582.0
      - rapidly progressive 583.4
        - acute 580.4
        - chronic 582.4
    - interstitial nephritis (diffuse) (focal) 583.89
      - with nephrotic syndrome 581.89
      - acute 580.89
      - chronic 582.89
    - necrotizing glomerulitis 583.4
      - acute 580.4
      - chronic 582.4
    - renal necrosis 583.9
      - cortical 583.6
      - medullary 583.7
    - specified pathology NEC 583.89
      - with nephrotic syndrome 581.89
      - acute 580.89
      - chronic 582.89
  - necrosis, renal 583.9
    - cortical 583.6
    - medullary (papillary) 583.7
  - nephrotic syndrome (see also Nephrosis) 581.9
  - papillary necrosis 583.7
  - specified pathology NEC 583.89
- acute 580.9
  - extracapillary with epithelial crescents 580.4
  - hypertensive (see also Hypertension, kidney) 403.90
  - necrotizing 580.4
  - poststreptococcal 580.0
  - proliferative (diffuse) 580.0
  - rapidly progressive 580.4
  - specified pathology NEC 580.89
- amyloid 277.3 [583.81]
  - chronic 277.3 [582.81]
- arteriolar (see also Hypertension, kidney) 403.90
- arteriosclerotic (see also Hypertension, kidney) 403.90
- ascending (see also Pyelitis) 590.80
- atrophic 582.9

Nephritis, nephritic — continued
- basement membrane NEC 583.89
  - with
    - pulmonary hemorrhage (Goodpasture's syndrome) 446.21 [583.81]
- calculous, calculus 592.0
- cardiac (see also Hypertension, kidney) 403.90
- cardiovascular (see also Hypertension, kidney) 403.90
- chronic 582.9
  - arteriosclerotic (see also Hypertension, kidney) 403.90
  - hypertensive (see also Hypertension, kidney) 403.90
- cirrhotic (see also Sclerosis, renal) 587
- complicating pregnancy, childbirth, or puerperium 646.2 ✓5ᵗʰ
  - with hypertension 642.1 ✓5ᵗʰ
  - affecting fetus or newborn 760.0
  - affecting fetus or newborn 760.1
- croupous 580.9
- desquamative — see Nephrosis
- due to
  - amyloidosis 277.3 [583.81]
    - chronic 277.3 [582.81]
  - arteriosclerosis (see also Hypertension, kidney) 403.90
  - diabetes mellitus 250.4 ✓5ᵗʰ [583.81]
    - with nephrotic syndrome 250.4 ✓5ᵗʰ [581.81]
  - diphtheria 032.89 [580.81]
  - gonococcal infection (acute) 098.19 [583.81]
    - chronic or duration of 2 months or over 098.39 [583.81]
  - gout 274.10
  - infectious hepatitis 070.9 [580.81]
  - mumps 072.79 [580.81]
  - specified kidney pathology NEC 583.89
    - acute 580.89
    - chronic 582.89
  - streptotrichosis 039.8 [583.81]
  - subacute bacterial endocarditis 421.0
  - systemic lupus erythematosus 710.0 [583.81]
    - chronic 710.0 [582.81]
  - typhoid fever 002.0 [580.81]
- endothelial 582.2
- end stage (chronic) (terminal) NEC 585
- epimembranous 581.1
- exudative 583.89
  - with nephrotic syndrome 581.89
  - acute 580.89
  - chronic 582.89
- gonococcal (acute) 098.19 [583.81]
  - chronic or duration of 2 months or over 098.39 [583.81]
- gouty 274.10
- hereditary (Alport's syndrome) 759.89
- hydremic — see Nephrosis
- hypertensive (see also Hypertension, kidney) 403.90
- hypocomplementemic persistent 583.2
  - with nephrotic syndrome 581.2
  - chronic 582.2
- immune complex NEC 583.89
- infective (see also Pyelitis) 590.80
- interstitial (diffuse) (focal) 583.89
  - with nephrotic syndrome 581.89
  - acute 580.89
  - chronic 582.89
- latent or quiescent — see Nephritis, chronic
- lead 984.9
  - specified type of lead — see Table of Drugs and Chemicals
- lobular 583.2
  - with nephrotic syndrome 581.2
  - chronic 582.2
- lupus 710.0 [583.81]
  - acute 710.0 [580.81]
  - chronic 710.0 [582.81]
- membranoproliferative 583.2
  - with nephrotic syndrome 581.2
  - chronic 582.2
- membranous 583.1
  - with nephrotic syndrome 581.1
  - chronic 582.1

Nephritis, nephritic — continued
- mesangiocapillary 583.2
  - with nephrotic syndrome 581.2
  - chronic 582.2
- minimal change 581.3
- mixed membranous and proliferative 583.2
  - with nephrotic syndrome 581.2
  - chronic 582.2
- necrotic, necrotizing 583.4
  - acute 580.4
  - chronic 582.4
- nephrotic — see Nephrosis
- old — see Nephritis, chronic
- parenchymatous 581.89
- polycystic 753.12
  - adult type (APKD) 753.13
  - autosomal dominant 753.13
  - autosomal recessive 753.14
  - childhood type (CPKD) 753.14
  - infantile type 753.14
- poststreptococcal 580.0
- pregnancy — see Nephritis, complicating pregnancy
- proliferative 583.0
  - with nephrotic syndrome 581.0
  - acute 580.0
  - chronic 582.0
- purulent (see also Pyelitis) 590.80
- rapidly progressive 583.4
  - acute 580.4
  - chronic 582.4
- salt-losing or salt-wasting (see also Disease, renal) 593.9
- saturnine 984.0
  - specified type of lead — see Table of Drugs and Chemicals
- septic (see also Pyelitis) 590.80
- specified pathology NEC 583.89
  - acute 580.89
  - chronic 582.89
- staphylococcal (see also Pyelitis) 590.80
- streptotrichosis 039.8 [583.81]
- subacute (see also Nephrosis) 581.9
- suppurative (see also Pyelitis) 590.80
- syphilitic (late) 095.4
  - congenital 090.5 [583.81]
  - early 091.69 [583.81]
- terminal (chronic) (end-stage) NEC 585
- toxic — see Nephritis, acute
- tubal, tubular — see Nephrosis, tubular
- tuberculous (see also Tuberculosis) 016.0 ✓5ᵗʰ [583.81]
- type II (Ellis) — see Nephrosis
- vascular — see Hypertension, kidney
- war 580.9

Nephroblastoma (M8960/3) 189.0
- epithelial (M8961/3) 189.0
- mesenchymal (M8962/3) 189.0

Nephrocalcinosis 275.49

Nephrocystitis, pustular (see also Pyelitis) 590.80

Nephrolithiasis (congenital) (pelvis) (recurrent) 592.0
- uric acid 274.11

Nephroma (M8960/3) 189.0
- mesoblastic (M8960/1) 236.9 ✓5ᵗʰ

Nephronephritis (see also Nephrosis) 581.9

Nephronopthisis 753.16

Nephropathy (see also Nephritis) 583.9
- with
  - exudative nephritis 583.89
  - interstitial nephritis (diffuse) (focal) 583.89
  - medullary necrosis 583.7
  - necrosis 583.9
    - cortical 583.6
    - medullary or papillary 583.7
  - papillary necrosis 583.7
  - specified lesion or cause NEC 583.89
- analgesic 583.89
  - with medullary necrosis, acute 584.7
- arteriolar (see also Hypertension, kidney) 403.90
- arteriosclerotic (see also Hypertension, kidney) 403.90
- complicating pregnancy 646.2 ✓5ᵗʰ
- diabetic 250.4 ✓5ᵗʰ [583.81]

Nephropathy (*see also* Nephritis) — *continued*
gouty 274.10
specified type NEC 274.19
hypercalcemic 588.8
hypertensive (*see also* Hypertension, kidney) 403.90
hypokalemic (vacuolar) 588.8
obstructive 593.89
congenital 753.20
phenacetin 584.7
phosphate-losing 588.0
potassium depletion 588.8
proliferative (*see also* Nephritis, proliferative) 583.0
protein-losing 588.8
salt-losing or salt-wasting (*see also* Disease, renal) 593.9
sickle-cell (*see also* Disease, sickle-cell) 282.60 *[583.81]*
toxic 584.5
vasomotor 584.5
water-losing 588.8
Nephroptosis (*see also* Disease, renal) 593.0
congenital (displaced) 753.3
Nephropyosis (*see also* Abscess, kidney) 590.2
Nephrorrhagia 593.81
Nephrosclerosis (arteriolar) (arteriosclerotic) (chronic) (hyaline) (*see also* Hypertension, kidney) 403.90
gouty 274.10
hyperplastic (arteriolar) (*see also* Hypertension, kidney) 403.90
senile (*see also* Sclerosis, renal) 587
Nephrosis, nephrotic (Epstein's) (syndrome) 581.9
with
lesion of
focal glomerulosclerosis 581.1
glomerulonephritis
endothelial 581.2
hypocomplementemic persistent 581.2
lobular 581.2
membranoproliferative 581.2
membranous 581.1
mesangiocapillary 581.2
minimal change 581.3
mixed membranous and proliferative 581.2
proliferative 581.0
segmental hyalinosis 581.1
specified pathology NEC 581.89
acute — *see* Nephrosis, tubular
anoxic — *see* Nephrosis, tubular
arteriosclerotic (*see also* Hypertension, kidney) 403.90
chemical — *see* Nephrosis, tubular
cholemic 572.4
complicating pregnancy, childbirth, or puerperium — *see* Nephritis, complicating pregnancy
diabetic 250.4 ✓5ᵗʰ *[581.81]*
hemoglobinuric — *see* Nephrosis, tubular
in
amyloidosis 277.3 *[581.81]*
diabetes mellitus 250.4 ✓5ᵗʰ *[581.81]*
epidemic hemorrhagic fever 078.6
malaria 084.9 *[581.81]*
polyarteritis 446.0 *[581.81]*
systemic lupus erythematosus 710.0 *[581.81]*
ischemic — *see* Nephrosis, tubular
lipoid 581.3
lower nephron — *see* Nephrosis, tubular
lupoid 710.0 *[581.81]*
lupus 710.0 *[581.81]*
malarial 084.9 *[581.81]*
minimal change 581.3
necrotizing — *see* Nephrosis, tubular
osmotic (sucrose) 588.8
polyarteritic 446.0 *[581.81]*
radiation 581.9
specified lesion or cause NEC 581.89
syphilitic 095.4
toxic — *see* Nephrosis, tubular

Nephrosis, nephrotic — *continued*
tubular (acute) 584.5
due to a procedure 997.5
radiation 581.9
Nephrosonephritis hemorrhagic (endemic) 078.6
Nephrostomy status V44.6
with complication 997.5
Nerve — *see* condition
Nerves 799.2
Nervous (*see also* condition) 799.2
breakdown 300.9
heart 306.2
stomach 306.4
tension 799.2
Nervousness 799.2
Nesidioblastoma (M8150/0) 211.7
pancreas 211.7
specified site NEC — *see* Neoplasm, by site, benign
unspecified site 211.7
Netherton's syndrome (ichthyosiform erythroderma) 757.1
Nettle rash 708.8
Nettleship's disease (urticaria pigmentosa) 757.33
Neumann's disease (pemphigus vegetans) 694.4
Neuralgia, neuralgic (acute) (*see also* Neuritis) 729.2
accessory (nerve) 352.4
acoustic (nerve) 388.5
ankle 355.8
anterior crural 355.8
anus 787.99
arm 723.4
auditory (nerve) 388.5
axilla 353.0
bladder 788.1
brachial 723.4
brain — *see* Disorder, nerve, cranial
broad ligament 625.9
cerebral — *see* Disorder, nerve, cranial
ciliary 346.2 ✓5ᵗʰ
cranial nerve — *see also* Disorder, nerve, cranial
fifth or trigeminal (*see also* Neuralgia, trigeminal) 350.1
ear 388.71
middle 352.1
facial 351.8
finger 354.9
flank 355.8
foot 355.8
forearm 354.9
Fothergill's (*see also* Neuralgia, trigeminal) 350.1
postherpetic 053.12
glossopharyngeal (nerve) 352.1
groin 355.8
hand 354.9
heel 355.8
Horton's 346.2 ✓5ᵗʰ
Hunt's 053.11
hypoglossal (nerve) 352.5
iliac region 355.8
infraorbital (*see also* Neuralgia, trigeminal) 350.1
inguinal 355.8
intercostal (nerve) 353.8
postherpetic 053.19
jaw 352.1
kidney 788.0
knee 355.8
loin 355.8
malarial (*see also* Malaria) 084.6
mastoid 385.89
maxilla 352.1
median thenar 354.1
metatarsal 355.6
middle ear 352.1
migrainous 346.2 ✓5ᵗʰ
Morton's 355.6
nerve, cranial — *see* Disorder, nerve, cranial
nose 352.0
occipital 723.8

Neuralgia, neuralgic (*see also* Neuritis) — *continued*
ophthalmic 377.30
postherpetic 053.19
optic (nerve) 377.30
penis 607.9
perineum 355.8
pleura 511.0
postherpetic NEC 053.19
geniculate ganglion 053.11
ophthalmic 053.19
trifacial 053.12
trigeminal 053.12
pubic region 355.8
radial (nerve) 723.4
rectum 787.99
sacroiliac joint 724.3
sciatic (nerve) 724.3
scrotum 608.9
seminal vesicle 608.9
shoulder 354.9
Sluder's 337.0
specified nerve NEC — *see* Disorder, nerve
spermatic cord 608.9
sphenopalatine (ganglion) 337.0
subscapular (nerve) 723.4
suprascapular (nerve) 723.4
testis 608.89
thenar (median) 354.1
thigh 355.8
tongue 352.5
trifacial (nerve) (*see also* Neuralgia, trigeminal) 350.1
trigeminal (nerve) 350.1
postherpetic 053.12
tympanic plexus 388.71
ulnar (nerve) 723.4
vagus (nerve) 352.3
wrist 354.9
writers' 300.89
organic 333.84
Neurapraxia — *see* Injury, nerve, by site
Neurasthenia 300.5
cardiac 306.2
gastric 306.4
heart 306.2
postfebrile 780.79
postviral 780.79
Neurilemmoma (M9560/0) — *see also* Neoplasm, connective tissue, benign
acoustic (nerve) 225.1
malignant (M9560/3) — *see also* Neoplasm, connective tissue, malignant
acoustic (nerve) 192.0
Neurilemmosarcoma (M9560/3) — *see* Neoplasm, connective tissue, malignant
Neurilemoma — *see* Neurilemmoma
Neurinoma (M9560/0) — *see* Neurilemmoma
Neurinomatosis (M9560/1) — *see also* Neoplasm, connective tissue, uncertain behavior
centralis 759.5
Neuritis (*see also* Neuralgia) 729.2
abducens (nerve) 378.54
accessory (nerve) 352.4
acoustic (nerve) 388.5
syphilitic 094.86
alcoholic 357.5
with psychosis 291.1
amyloid, any site 277.3 *[357.4]*
anterior crural 355.8
arising during pregnancy 646.4 ✓5ᵗʰ
arm 723.4
ascending 355.2
auditory (nerve) 388.5
brachial (nerve) NEC 723.4
due to displacement, intervertebral disc 722.0
cervical 723.4
chest (wall) 353.8
costal region 353.8
cranial nerve — *see also* Disorder, nerve, cranial
first or olfactory 352.0
second or optic 377.30
third or oculomotor 378.52
fourth or trochlear 378.53

Neuritis (see also Neuralgia) — continued
  cranial nerve — see also Disorder, nerve,
    cranial — continued
    fifth or trigeminal (see also Neuralgia,
      trigeminal) 350.1
    sixth or abducens 378.54
    seventh or facial 351.8
      newborn 767.5
    eighth or acoustic 388.5
    ninth or glossopharyngeal 352.1
    tenth or vagus 352.3
    eleventh or accessory 352.4
    twelfth or hypoglossal 352.5
  Déjérine-Sottas 356.0
  diabetic 250.6 ✔5ᵗʰ [357.2]
  diphtheritic 032.89 [357.4]
  due to
    beriberi 265.0 [357.4]
    displacement, prolapse, protrusion, or
      rupture of intervertebral disc 722.2
      cervical 722.0
      lumbar, lumbosacral 722.10
      thoracic, thoracolumbar 722.11
    herniation, nucleus pulposus 722.2
      cervical 722.0
      lumbar, lumbosacral 722.10
      thoracic, thoracolumbar 722.11
  endemic 265.0 [357.4]
  facial (nerve) 351.8
    newborn 767.5
  general — see Polyneuropathy
  geniculate ganglion 351.1
    due to herpes 053.11
  glossopharyngeal (nerve) 352.1
  gouty 274.89 [357.4]
  hypoglossal (nerve) 352.5
  ilioinguinal (nerve) 355.8
  in diseases classified elsewhere — see
    Polyneuropathy, in
  infectious (multiple) 357.0
  intercostal (nerve) 353.8
  interstitial hypertrophic progressive NEC 356.9
  leg 355.8
  lumbosacral NEC 724.4
  median (nerve) 354.1
    thenar 354.1
  multiple (acute) (infective) 356.9
    endemic 265.0 [357.4]
  multiplex endemica 265.0 [357.4]
  nerve root (see also Radiculitis) 729.2
  oculomotor (nerve) 378.52
  olfactory (nerve) 352.0
  optic (nerve) 377.30
    in myelitis 341.0
    meningococcal 036.81
  pelvic 355.8
  peripheral (nerve) — see also Neuropathy,
    peripheral
    complicating pregnancy or puerperium
      646.4 ✔5ᵗʰ
    specified nerve NEC — see Mononeuritis
  pneumogastric (nerve) 352.3
  postchickenpox 052.7
  postherpetic 053.19
  progressive hypertrophic interstitial NEC 356.9
  puerperal, postpartum 646.4 ✔5ᵗʰ
  radial (nerve) 723.4
  retrobulbar 377.32
    syphilitic 094.85
  rheumatic (chronic) 729.2
  sacral region 355.8
  sciatic (nerve) 724.3
    due to displacement of intervertebral disc
      722.10
  serum 999.5
  specified nerve NEC — see Disorder, nerve
  spinal (nerve) 355.9
    root (see also Radiculitis) 729.2
  subscapular (nerve) 723.4
  suprascapular (nerve) 723.4
  syphilitic 095.8
  thenar (median) 354.1
  thoracic NEC 724.4
  toxic NEC 357.7
  trochlear (nerve) 378.53
  ulnar (nerve) 723.4
  vagus (nerve) 352.3

Neuroangiomatosis, encephalofacial 759.6
Neuroastrocytoma (M9505/1) — see Neoplasm,
  by site, uncertain behavior
Neuro-avitaminosis 269.2
Neuroblastoma (M9500/3)
  olfactory (M9522/3) 160.0
  specified site — see Neoplasm, by site,
    malignant
  unspecified site 194.0
Neurochorioretinitis (see also Chorioretinitis)
  363.20
Neurocirculatory asthenia 306.2
Neurocytoma (M9506/0) — see Neoplasm, by
  site, benign
Neurodermatitis (circumscribed) (circumscripta)
  (local) 698.3
  atopic 691.8
  diffuse (Brocq) 691.8
  disseminated 691.8
  nodulosa 698.3
Neuroencephalomyelopathy, optic 341.0
Neuroepithelioma (M9503/3) — see also
  Neoplasm, by site, malignant
  olfactory (M9521/3) 160.0
Neurofibroma (M9540/0) — see also Neoplasm,
  connective tissue, benign
  melanotic (M9541/0) — see Neoplasm,
    connective tissue, benign
  multiple (M9540/1) 237.70
    type 1 237.71
    type 2 237.72
  plexiform (M9550/0) — see Neoplasm,
    connective tissue, benign
Neurofibromatosis (multiple) (M9540/1) 237.70
  acoustic 237.72
  malignant (M9540/3) — see Neoplasm,
    connective tissue, malignant
  type 1 237.71
  type 2 237.72
  von Recklinghausen's 237.71
Neurofibrosarcoma (M9540/3) — see Neoplasm,
  connective tissue, malignant
Neurogenic — see also condition
  bladder (atonic) (automatic) (autonomic)
    (flaccid) (hypertonic) (hypotonic) (inertia)
    (infranuclear) (irritable) (motor)
    (nonreflex) (nuclear) (paralysis) (reflex)
    (sensory) (spastic) (supranuclear)
    (uninhibited) 596.54
    with cauda equina syndrome 344.61
  bowel 564.81
  heart 306.2
Neuroglioma (M9505/1) — see Neoplasm, by site,
  uncertain behavior
Neurolabyrinthitis (of Dix and Hallpike) 386.12
Neurolathyrism 988.2
Neuroleprosy 030.1
Neuroleptic malignant syndrome 333.92
Neurolipomatosis 272.8
Neuroma (M9570/0) — see also Neoplasm,
  connective tissue, benign
  acoustic (nerve) (M9560/0) 225.1
  amputation (traumatic) — see also Injury,
    nerve, by site
    surgical complication (late) 997.61
  appendix 211.3
  auditory nerve 225.1
  digital 355.6
    toe 355.6
  interdigital (toe) 355.6
  intermetatarsal 355.6
  Morton's 355.6
  multiple 237.70
    type 1 237.71
    type 2 237.72
  nonneoplastic 355.9
    arm NEC 354.9
    leg NEC 355.8
    lower extremity NEC 355.8
    specified site NEC — see Mononeuritis, by
      site
    upper extremity NEC 354.9
  optic (nerve) 225.1
  plantar 355.6

Neuroma — see also Neoplasm, connective tissue,
  benign — continued
  plexiform (M9550/0) — see Neoplasm,
    connective tissue, benign
  surgical (nonneoplastic) 355.9
    arm NEC 354.9
    leg NEC 355.8
    lower extremity NEC 355.8
    upper extremity NEC 354.9
  traumatic — see also Injury, nerve, by site
    old — see Neuroma, nonneoplastic
Neuromyalgia 729.1
Neuromyasthenia (epidemic) 049.8
Neuromyelitis 341.8
  ascending 357.0
  optica 341.0
Neuromyopathy NEC 358.9
Neuromyositis 729.1
Neuronevus (M8725/0) — see Neoplasm, skin,
  benign
Neuronitis 357.0
  ascending (acute) 355.2
  vestibular 386.12
Neuroparalytic — see condition
Neuropathy, neuropathic (see also Disorder,
  nerve) 355.9
  acute motor 357.82   ●
  alcoholic 357.5
    with psychosis 291.1
  arm NEC 354.9
  autonomic (peripheral) — see Neuropathy,
    peripheral, autonomic
  axillary nerve 353.0
  brachial plexus 353.0
  cervical plexus 353.2
  chronic
    progressive segmentally demyelinating
      357.89   ▲
    relapsing demyelinating 357.89   ▲
  congenital sensory 356.2
  Déjérine-Sottas 356.0
  diabetic 250.6 ✔5ᵗʰ [357.2]
  entrapment 355.9
    iliohypogastric nerve 355.79
    ilioinguinal nerve 355.79
    lateral cutaneous nerve of thigh 355.1
    median nerve 354.0
    obturator nerve 355.79
    peroneal nerve 355.3
    posterior tibial nerve 355.5
    saphenous nerve 355.79
    ulnar nerve 354.2
  facial nerve 351.9
  hereditary 356.9
    peripheral 356.0
    sensory (radicular) 356.2
  hypertrophic
    Charcôt-Marie-Tooth 356.1
    Déjérine-Sottas 356.0
    interstitial 356.9
    Refsum 356.3
  intercostal nerve 354.8
  ischemic — see Disorder, nerve
  Jamaican (ginger) 357.7
  leg NEC 355.8
  lower extremity NEC 355.8
  lumbar plexus 353.1
  median nerve 354.1
  motor
    acute 357.82   ●
  multiple (acute) (chronic) (see also   ●
    Polyneuropathy) 356.9
  optic 377.39
    ischemic 377.41
    nutritional 377.33
    toxic 377.34
  peripheral (nerve) (see also Polyneuropathy)
    356.9
    arm NEC 354.9
    autonomic 337.9
      amyloid 277.3 [337.1]
      idiopathic 337.0
      in
        amyloidosis 277.3 [337.1]
        diabetes (mellitus) 250.6 ✔5ᵗʰ [337.1]
        diseases classified elsewhere 337.1

Neuropathy, neuropathic (*see also* Disorder, nerve) — *continued*
  peripheral (*see also* Polyneuropathy) — *continued*
    autonomic — *continued*
      in — *continued*
        gout 274.89 *[337.1]*
        hyperthyroidism 242.9 ✓5ᵗʰ *[337.1]*
    due to
      antitetanus scrum 357.6
      arsenic 357.7
      drugs 357.6
      lead 357.7
      organophosphate compounds 357.7
      toxic agent NEC 357.7
    hereditary 356.0
    idiopathic 356.9
      progresive 356.4
      specified type NEC 356.8
    in diseases classified elsewhere — *see* Polyneuropathy, in
    leg NEC 355.8
    lower extremity NEC 355.8
    upper extremity NEC 354.9
  plantar nerves 355.6
  progressive hypertrophic interstitial 356.9
  radicular NEC 729.2
    brachial 723.4
    cervical NEC 723.4
    hereditary sensory 356.2
    lumbar 724.4
    lumbosacral 724.4
    thoracic NEC 724.4
  sacral plexus 353.1
  sciatic 355.0
  spinal nerve NEC 355.9
    root (*see also* Radiculitis) 729.2
  toxic 357.7
  trigeminal sensory 350.8
  ulnar nerve 354.2
  upper extremity NEC 354.9
  uremic 585 *[357.4]*
  vitamin B$_{12}$ 266.2 *[357.4]*
    with anemia (pernicious) 281.0 *[357.4]*
      due to dietary deficiency 281.1 *[357.4]*

Neurophthisis — (*see also* Disorder, nerve peripheral) 356.9
  diabetic 250.6 ✓5ᵗʰ *[357.2]*

Neuropraxia — *see* Injury, nerve

Neuroretinitis 363.05
  syphilitic 094.85

Neurosarcoma (M9540/3) — *see* Neoplasm, connective tissue, malignant

Neurosclerosis — *see* Disorder, nerve

Neurosis, neurotic 300.9
  accident 300.16
  anancastic, anankastic 300.3
  anxiety (state) 300.00
    generalized 300.02
    panic type 300.01
  asthenic 300.5
  bladder 306.53
  cardiac (reflex) 306.2
  cardiovascular 306.2
  climacteric, unspecified type 627.2
  colon 306.4
  compensation 300.16
  compulsive, compulsion 300.3
  conversion 300.11
  craft 300.89
  cutaneous 306.3
  depersonalization 300.6
  depressive (reaction) (type) 300.4
  endocrine 306.6
  environmental 300.89
  fatigue 300.5
  functional (*see also* Disorder, psychosomatic) 306.9
  gastric 306.4
  gastrointestinal 306.4
  genitourinary 306.50
  heart 306.2
  hypochondriacal 300.7
  hysterical 300.10
    conversion type 300.11
    dissociative type 300.15

Neurosis, neurotic — *continued*
  impulsive 300.3
  incoordination 306.0
    larynx 306.1
    vocal cord 306.1
  intestine 306.4
  larynx 306.1
    hysterical 300.11
    sensory 306.1
  menopause, unspecified type 627.2
  mixed NEC 300.89
  musculoskeletal 306.0
  obsessional 300.3
    phobia 300.3
  obsessive-compulsive 300.3
  occupational 300.89
  ocular 306.7
  oral 307.0
  organ (*see also* Disorder, psychosomatic) 306.9
  pharynx 306.1
  phobic 300.20
  posttraumatic (acute) (situational) 308.3
    chronic 309.81
  psychasthenic (type) 300.89
  railroad 300.16
  rectum 306.4
  respiratory 306.1
  rumination 306.4
  senile 300.89
  sexual 302.70
  situational 300.89
  specified type NEC 300.89
  state 300.9
    with depersonalization episode 300.6
  stomach 306.4
  vasomotor 306.2
  visceral 306.4
  war 300.16

Neurospongioblastosis diffusa 759.5

Neurosyphilis (arrested) (early) (inactive) (late) (latent) (recurrent) 094.9
  with ataxia (cerebellar) (locomotor) (spastic) (spinal) 094.0
  acute meningitis 094.2
  aneurysm 094.89
  arachnoid (adhesive) 094.2
  arteritis (any artery) 094.89
  asymptomatic 094.3
  congenital 090.40
  dura (mater) 094.89
  general paresis 094.1
  gumma 094.9
  hemorrhagic 094.9
  juvenile (asymptomatic) (meningeal) 090.40
  leptomeninges (aseptic) 094.2
  meningeal 094.2
  meninges (adhesive) 094.2
  meningovascular (diffuse) 094.2
  optic atrophy 094.84
  parenchymatous (degenerative) 094.1
  paresis (*see also* Paresis, general) 094.1
  paretic (*see also* Paresis, general) 094.1
  relapse 094.9
  remission in (sustained) 094.9
  serological 094.3
  specified nature or site NEC 094.89
  tabes (dorsalis) 094.0
    juvenile 090.40
  tabetic 094.0
    juvenile 090.40
  taboparesis 094.1
    juvenile 090.40
  thrombosis 094.89
  vascular 094.89

Neurotic (*see also* Neurosis) 300.9
  excoriation 698.4
  psychogenic 306.3

Neurotmesis — *see* Injury, nerve, by site

Neurotoxemia — *see* Toxemia

Neuroclusion 524.2

Neutropenia, neutropenic (chronic) (cyclic) (drug-induced) (genetic) (idiopathic) (immune) (infantile) (malignant) (periodic) (pernicious) (primary) (splenic) (splenomegaly) (toxic) 288.0
  chronic hypoplastic 288.0

Neutropenia, neutropenic — *continued*
  congenital (nontransient) 288.0
  fever 288.0
  neonatal, transitory (isoimmune) (maternal transfer) 776.7

Neutrophilia, hereditary giant 288.2

Nevocarcinoma (M8720/3) — *see* Melanoma

Nevus (M8720/0) — *see also* Neoplasm, skin, benign

> Note — Except where otherwise indicated, varieties of nevus in the list below that are followed by a morphology code number (M----/0) should be coded by site as for "Neoplasm, skin, benign."

  acanthotic 702.8
  achromic (M8730/0)
  amelanotic (M8730/0)
  anemic, anemicus 709.09
  angiomatous (M9120/0) (*see also* Hemangioma) 228.00
  araneus 448.1
  avasculosus 709.09
  balloon cell (M8722/0)
  bathing trunk (M8761/1) 238.2
  blue (M8780/0)
    cellular (M8790/0)
    giant (M8790/0)
    Jadassohn's (M8780/0)
    malignant (M8780/3) — *see* Melanoma
  capillary (M9131/0) (*see also* Hemangioma) 228.00
  cavernous (M9121/0) (*see also* Hemangioma) 228.00
  cellular (M8720/0)
    blue (M8790/0)
  comedonicus 757.33
  compound (M8760/0)
  conjunctiva (M8720/0) 224.3
  dermal (M8750/0)
    and epidermal (M8760/0)
  epithelioid cell (and spindle cell) (M8770/0)
  flammeus 757.32
    osteohypertrophic 759.89
  hairy (M8720/0)
  halo (M8723/0)
  hemangiomatous (M9120/0) (*see also* Hemangioma) 228.00
  intradermal (M8750/0)
  intraepidermal (M8740/0)
  involuting (M8724/0)
  Jadassohn's (blue) (M8780/0)
  junction, junctional (M8740/0)
    malignant melanoma in (M8740/3) — *see* Melanoma
  juvenile (M8770/0)
  lymphatic (M9170/0) 228.1
  magnocellular (M8726/0)
    specified site — *see* Neoplasm, by site, benign
    unspecified site 224.0
  malignant (M8720/3) — *see* Melanoma
  meaning hemangioma (M9120/0) (*see also* Hemangioma) 228.00
  melanotic (pigmented) (M8720/0)
  multiplex 759.5
  nonneoplastic 448.1
  nonpigmented (M8730/0)
  nonvascular (M8720/0)
  oral mucosa, white sponge 750.26
  osteohypertrophic, flammeus 759.89
  papillaris (M8720/0)
  papillomatosus (M8720/0)
  pigmented (M8720/0)
    giant (M8761/1) — *see also* Neoplasm, skin, uncertain behavior
      malignant melanoma in (M8761/3) — *see* Melanoma
    systematicus 757.33
  pilosus (M8720/0)
  port wine 757.32
  sanguineous 757.32
  sebaceous (senile) 702.8
  senile 448.1
  spider 448.1
  spindle cell (and epithelioid cell) (M8770/0)

✓4ᵗʰ Fourth-digit Required   ✓5ᵗʰ Fifth-digit Required   ▶◀ Revised Text   ● New Line   ▲ Revised Code

Nevus — *see also* Neoplasm, skin, benign — *continued*
  stellar 448.1
  strawberry 757.32
  syringocystadenomatous papilliferous (M8406/0)
  unius lateris 757.33
  Unna's 757.32
  vascular 757.32
  verrucous 757.33
  white sponge (oral mucosa) 750.26
Newborn (infant) (liveborn)
  gestation
    24 completed weeks 765.22 ●
    25-26 completed weeks 765.23 ●
    27-28 completed weeks 765.24 ●
    29-30 completed weeks 765.25 ●
    31-32 completed weeks 765.26 ●
    33-34 completed weeks 765.27 ●
    35-36 completed weeks 765.28 ●
    37 or more completed weeks 765.29 ●
    less than 24 completed weeks 765.21 ●
    unspecified completed weeks 765.20 ●
  multiple NEC
    born in hospital (without mention of cesarean delivery or section) V37.00
      with cesarean delivery or section V37.01
    born outside hospital
      hospitalized V37.1
      not hospitalized V37.2
  mates all liveborn
    born in hospital (without mention of cesarean delivery or section) V34.00
      with cesarean delivery or section V34.01
    born outside hospital
      hospitalized V34.1
      not hospitalized V34.2
  mates all stillborn
    born in hospital (without mention of cesarean delivery or section) V35.00
      with cesarean delivery or section V35.01
    born outside hospital
      hospitalized V35.1
      not hospitalized V35.2
  mates liveborn and stillborn
    born in hospital (without mention of cesarean delivery or section) V36.00
      with cesarean delivery or section V36.01
    born outside hospital
      hospitalized V36.1
      not hospitalized V36.2
  single
    born in hospital (without mention of cesarean delivery or section) V30.00
      with cesarean delivery or section V30.01
    born outside hospital
      hospitalized V30.1
      not hospitalized V30.2
  twin NEC
    born in hospital (without mention of cesarean delivery or section) V33.00
      with cesarean delivery or section V33.01
    born outside hospital
      hospitalized V33.1
      not hospitalized V33.2
    mate liveborn
      born in hospital V31.0 ✓5ᵗʰ
      born outside hospital
        hospitalized V31.1
        not hospitalized V31.2
    mate stillborn
      born in hospital V32.0 ✓5ᵗʰ
      born outside hospital
        hospitalized V32.1
        not hospitalized V32.2
  unspecified as to single or multiple birth
    born in hospital (without mention of cesarean delivery or section) V39.00
      with cesarean delivery or section V39.01
    born outside hospital
      hospitalized V39.1
      not hospitalized V39.2
Newcastle's conjunctivitis or disease 077.8

Nezelof's syndrome (pure alymphocytosis) 279.13
Niacin (amide) deficiency 265.2
Nicolas-Durand-Favre disease (climatic bubo) 099.1
Nicolas-Favre disease (climatic bubo) 099.1
Nicotinic acid (amide) deficiency 265.2
Niemann-Pick disease (lipid histiocytosis) (splenomegaly) 272.7
Night
  blindness (*see also* Blindness, night) 368.60
    congenital 368.61
    vitamin A deficiency 264.5
  cramps 729.82
  sweats 780.8
  terrors, child 307.46
Nightmare 307.47
  REM-sleep type 307.47
Nipple — *see* condition
Nisbet's chancre 099.0
Nishimoto (-Takeuchi) disease 437.5
Nitritoid crisis or reaction — *see* Crisis, nitritoid
Nitrogen retention, extrarenal 788.9
Nitrosohemoglobinemia 289.8
Njovera 104.0
No
  diagnosis 799.9
  disease (found) V71.9
  room at the inn V65.0
Nocardiasis — *see* Nocardiosis
Nocardiosis 039.9
  with pneumonia 039.1
  lung 039.1
  specified type NEC 039.8
Nocturia 788.43
  psychogenic 306.53
Nocturnal — *see also* condition
  dyspnea (paroxysmal) 786.09
  emissions 608.89
  enuresis 788.36
    psychogenic 307.6
  frequency (micturition) 788.43
    psychogenic 306.53
Nodal rhythm disorder 427.89
Nodding of head 781.0
Node(s) — *see also* Nodule
  Heberden's 715.04
  larynx 478.79
  lymph — *see* condition
  milkers' 051.1
  Osler's 421.0
  rheumatic 729.89
  Schmorl's 722.30
    lumbar, lumbosacral 722.32
    specified region NEC 722.39
    thoracic, thoracolumbar 722.31
  singers' 478.5
  skin NEC 782.2
  tuberculous — *see* Tuberculosis, lymph gland
  vocal cords 478.5
Nodosities, Haygarth's 715.04
Nodule(s), nodular
  actinomycotic (*see also* Actinomycosis) 039.9
  arthritic — *see* Arthritis, nodosa
  cutaneous 782.2
  Haygarth's 715.04
  inflammatory — *see* Inflammation
  juxta-articular 102.7
    syphilitic 095.7
    yaws 102.7
  larynx 478.79
  lung, solitary 518.89
    emphysematous 492.8
  milkers' 051.1
  prostate 600.1
  rheumatic 729.89
  rheumatoid — *see* Arthritis, rheumatoid
  scrotum (inflammatory) 608.4
  singers' 478.5
  skin NEC 782.2
  solitary, lung 518.89
    emphysematous 492.8
  subcutaneous 782.2

Nodule(s), nodular — *continued*
  thyroid (gland) (nontoxic) (uninodular) 241.0
    with
      hyperthyroidism 242.1 ✓5ᵗʰ
      thyrotoxicosis 242.1 ✓5ᵗʰ
    toxic or with hyperthyroidism 242.1 ✓5ᵗʰ
    vocal cords 478.5
Noma (gangrenous) (hospital) (infective) 528.1
  auricle (*see also* Gangrene) 785.4
  mouth 528.1
  pudendi (*see also* Vulvitis) 616.10
  vulvae (*see also* Vulvitis) 616.10
Nomadism V60.0
Non-adherence
  artificial skin graft 996.55
  decellularized allodermis graft 996.55
Non-autoimmune hemolytic anemia NEC 283.10
Nonclosure — *see also* Imperfect, closure
  ductus
    arteriosus 747.0
    Botalli 747.0
  Eustachian valve 746.89
  foramen
    Botalli 745.5
    ovale 745.5
Noncompliance with medical treatment V15.81
Nondescent (congenital) — *see also* Malposition, congenital
  cecum 751.4
  colon 751.4
  testis 752.51
Nondevelopment
  brain 742.1
    specified part 742.2
  heart 746.89
  organ or site, congenital NEC — *see* Hypoplasia
Nonengagement
  head NEC 652.5 ✓5ᵗʰ
    in labor 660.1 ✓5ᵗʰ
      affecting fetus or newborn 763.1
Nonexanthematous tick fever 066.1
Nonexpansion, lung (newborn) NEC 770.4
Nonfunctioning
  cystic duct (*see also* Disease, gallbladder) 575.8
  gallbladder (*see also* Disease, gallbladder) 575.8
  kidney (*see also* Disease, renal) 593.9
  labyrinth 386.58
Nonhealing
  stump (surgical) 997.69
  wound, surgical 998.83
Nonimplantation of ovum, causing infertility 628.3
Noninsufflation, fallopian tube 628.2
Nonne-Milroy-Meige syndrome (chronic hereditary edema) 757.0
Nonovulation 628.0
Nonpatent fallopian tube 628.2
Nonpneumatization, lung NEC 770.4
Nonreflex bladder 596.54
  with cauda equina 344.61
Nonretention of food — *see* Vomiting
Nonrotation — *see* Malrotation
Nonsecretion, urine (*see also* Anuria) 788.5
  newborn 753.3
Nonunion
  fracture 733.82
  organ or site, congenital NEC — *see* Imperfect, closure
  symphysis pubis, congenital 755.69
  top sacrum, congenital 756.19
Nonviability 765.0 ✓5ᵗʰ
Nonvisualization, gallbladder 793.3
Nonvitalized tooth 522.9
Normal
  delivery — *see* category 650
  menses V65.5
  state (feared complaint unfounded) V65.5
Normoblastosis 289.8

Normocytic anemia (infectional) 285.9
   due to blood loss (chronic) 280.0
      acute 285.1
Norrie's disease (congenital) (progressive
   oculoacousticocerebral degeneration) 743.8
North American blastomycosis 116.0
Norwegian itch 133.0
Nose, nasal — *see* condition
Nosebleed 784.7
Nosomania 298.9
Nosophobia 300.29
Nostalgia 309.89
Notch of iris 743.46
Notched lip, congenital (*see also* Cleft, lip)
   749.10
Notching nose, congenital (tip) 748.1
Nothnagel's
   syndrome 378.52
   vasomotor acroparesthesia 443.89
Novy's relapsing fever (American) 087.1
Noxious
   foodstuffs, poisoning by
      fish 988.0
      fungi 988.1
      mushrooms 988.1
      plants (food) 988.2
      shellfish 988.0
      specified type NEC 988.8
      toadstool 988.1
   substances transmitted through placenta or
      breast milk 760.70
      alcohol 760.71
      anti-infective agents 760.74
      cocaine 760.75
      "crack" 760.75
      diethylstilbestrol (DES) 760.76
      hallucinogenic agents NEC 760.73
      medicinal agents NEC 760.79
      narcotics 760.72
      obstetric anesthetic or analgesic 763.5
      specified agent NEC 760.79
      suspected, affecting management of
         pregnancy 655.5 ✓5ᵗʰ
Nuchal hitch (arm) 652.8 ✓5ᵗʰ
Nucleus pulposus — *see* condition
Numbness 782.0
Nuns' knee 727.2
Nursemaid's
   elbow 832.0 ✓5ᵗʰ
   shoulder 831.0 ✓5ᵗʰ
Nutmeg liver 573.8
Nutrition, deficient or insufficient (particular
   kind of food) 269.9
   due to
      insufficient food 994.2
      lack of
         care (child) (infant) 995.52
            adult 995.84
         food 994.2
Nyctalopia (*see also* Blindness, night) 368.60
   vitamin A deficiency 264.5
Nycturia 788.43
   psychogenic 306.53
Nymphomania 302.89
Nystagmus 379.50
   associated with vestibular system disorders
      379.54
   benign paroxysmal positional 386.11
   central positional 386.2
   congenital 379.51
   deprivation 379.53
   dissociated 379.55
   latent 379.52
   miners' 300.89
   positional
      benign paroxysmal 386.11
      central 386.2
   specified NEC 379.56
   vestibular 379.54
   visual deprivation 379.53

✓4ᵗʰ Fourth-digit Required   ✓5ᵗʰ Fifth-digit Required   ▶◀ Revised Text   ● New Line   ▲ Revised Code

O

Oasthouse urine disease 270.2
Obermeyer's relapsing fever (European) 087.0
Obesity (constitutional) (exogenous) (familial)
(nutritional) (simple) 278.00
  adrenal 255.8
  due to hyperalimentation 278.00
  endocrine NEC 259.9
  endogenous 259.9
  Fröhlich's (adiposogenital dystrophy) 253.8
  glandular NEC 259.9
  hypothyroid (see also Hypothyroidism) 244.9
  morbid 278.01
  of pregnancy 646.1 ✓5ᵗʰ
  pituitary 253.8
  thyroid (see also Hypothyroidism) 244.9
Oblique — see also condition
  lie before labor, affecting fetus or newborn
    761.7
Obliquity, pelvis 738.6
Obliteration
  abdominal aorta 446.7
  appendix (lumen) 543.9
  artery 447.1
  ascending aorta 446.7
  bile ducts 576.8
    with calculus, choledocholithiasis, or stones
      — see Choledocholithiasis
    congenital 751.61
      jaundice from 751.61 [774.5]
  common duct 576.8
    with calculus, choledocholithiasis, or stones
      — see Choledocholithiasis
    congenital 751.61
  cystic duct 575.8
    with calculus, choledocholithiasis, or stones
      — see Choledocholithiasis
  disease, arteriolar 447.1
  endometrium 621.8
  eye, anterior chamber 360.34
  fallopian tube 628.2
  lymphatic vessel 457.1
    postmastectomy 457.0
  organ or site, congenital NEC — see Atresia
  placental blood vessels — see Placenta,
    abnormal
  supra-aortic branches 446.7
  ureter 593.89
  urethra 599.84
  vein 459.9
  vestibule (oral) 525.8
Observation (for) V71.9
  without need for further medical care V71.9
  accident NEC V71.4
    at work V71.3
  criminal V71.6
  deleterious agent ingestion V71.89
  disease V71.9
    cardiovascular V71.7
    heart V71.7
    mental V71.09
    specified condition NEC V71.89
  foreign body ingestion V71.89
  growth and development variations V21.8
  injuries (accidental) V71.4
    inflicted NEC V71.6
      during alleged rape or seduction V71.5
  malignant neoplasm, suspected V71.1
  postpartum
    immediately after delivery V24.0
    routine follow-up V24.2
  pregnancy
    high-risk V23.9
      specified problem NEC V23.8 ✓5ᵗʰ
    normal (without complication) V22.1
      with nonobstetric complication V22.2
      first V22.0
  rape or seduction, alleged V71.5
    injury during V71.5
  suicide attempt, alleged V71.89
  suspected (undiagnosed) (unproven)
    abuse V71.81
    cardiovascular disease V71.7
    child or wife battering victim V71.6
    concussion (cerebral) V71.6

Observation — continued
  suspected — continued
    condition NEC V71.89
      infant — see Observation, suspected,
        condition, newborn
    newborn V29.9
      cardiovascular disease V29.8
      congenital anomaly V29.8
      genetic V29.3
      infectious V29.0
      ingestion foreign object V29.8
      injury V29.8
      metabolic V29.3
      neoplasm V29.8
      neurological V29.1
      poison, poisoning V29.8
      respiratory V29.2
      specified NEC V29.8
    exposure   ●
      anthrax V71.82   ●
      biologic agent NEC V71.83   ●
    infectious disease not requiring isolation
      V71.89
    malignant neoplasm V71.1
    mental disorder V71.09
    neglect V71.81
    neoplasm
      benign V71.89
      malignant V71.1
    specified condition NEC V71.89
    tuberculosis V71.2
  tuberculosis, suspected V71.2
Obsession, obsessional 300.3
  ideas and mental images 300.3
  impulses 300.3
  neurosis 300.3
  phobia 300.3
  psychasthenia 300.3
  ruminations 300.3
  state 300.3
  syndrome 300.3
Obsessive-compulsive 300.3
  neurosis 300.3
  reaction 300.3
Obstetrical trauma NEC (complicating delivery)
  665.9 ✓5ᵗʰ
  with
    abortion — see Abortion, by type, with
      damage to pelvic organs
    ectopic pregnancy (see also categories
      633.0-633.9) 639.2
    molar pregnancy (see also categories 630-
      632) 639.2
  affecting fetus or newborn 763.89
  following
    abortion 639.2
    ectopic or molar pregnancy 639.2
Obstipation (see also Constipation) 564.00
  psychogenic 306.4
Obstruction, obstructed, obstructive
  airway NEC 519.8
    with
      allergic alveolitis NEC 495.9
      asthma NEC (see also Asthma) 493.9 ✓5ᵗʰ
      bronchiectasis 494.0
        with acute exacerbation 494.1
      bronchitis (chronic) (see also Bronchitis,
        with, obstruction) 491.20
      emphysema NEC 492.8
    chronic 496
      with
        allergic alveolitis NEC 495.5
        asthma NEC (see also Asthma)
          493.2 ✓5ᵗʰ
        bronchiectasis 494.0
          with acute exacerbation 494.1
        bronchitis (chronic) (see also
          Bronchitis, with, obstruction)
          491.20
        emphysema NEC 492.8
    due to
      bronchospasm 519.1
      foreign body 934.9
      inhalation of fumes or vapors 506.9
      laryngospasm 478.75

Obstruction, obstructed, obstructive —
  continued
  alimentary canal (see also Obstruction,
    intestine) 560.9
  ampulla of Vater 576.2
    with calculus, cholelithiasis, or stones — see
      Choledocholithiasis
  aortic (heart) (valve) (see also Stenosis, aortic)
    424.1
    rheumatic (see also Stenosis, aortic,
      rheumatic) 395.0
  aortoiliac 444.0
  aqueduct of Sylvius 331.4
    congenital 742.3
      with spina bifida (see also Spina bifida)
        741.0 ✓5ᵗʰ
  Arnold-Chiari (see also Spina bifida) 741.0 ✓5ᵗʰ
  artery (see also Embolism, artery) 444.9
    basilar (complete) (partial) (see also
      Occlusion, artery, basilar) 433.0 ✓5ᵗʰ
    carotid (complete) (partial) (see also
      Occlusion, artery, carotid) 433.1 ✓5ᵗʰ
    precerebral — see Occlusion, artery,
      precerebral NEC
    retinal (central) (see also Occlusion, retina)
      362.30
    vertebral (complete) (partial) (see also
      Occlusion, artery, vertebral) 433.2 ✓5ᵗʰ
  asthma (chronic) (with obstructive pulmonary
    disease) 493.2 ✓5ᵗʰ
  band (intestinal) 560.81
  bile duct or passage (see also Obstruction,
    biliary) 576.2
    congenital 751.61
      jaundice from 751.61 [774.5]
  biliary (duct) (tract) 576.2
    with calculus 574.51
      with cholecystitis (chronic) 574.41
        acute 574.31
    congenital 751.61
      jaundice from 751.61 [774.5]
    gallbladder 575.2
      with calculus 574.21
        with cholecystitis (chronic) 574.11
          acute 574.01
  bladder neck (acquired) 596.0
    congenital 753.6
  bowel (see also Obstruction, intestine) 560.9
  bronchus 519.1
  canal, ear (see also Stricture, ear canal,
    acquired) 380.50
  cardia 537.89
  caval veins (inferior) (superior) 459.2
  cecum (see also Obstruction, intestine) 560.9
  circulatory 459.9
  colon (see also Obstruction, intestine) 560.9
    sympathicotonic 560.89
  common duct (see also Obstruction, biliary)
    576.2
    congenital 751.61
  coronary (artery) (heart) — see also
    Arteriosclerosis, coronary
    acute (see also Infarct, myocardium)
      410.9 ✓5ᵗʰ
      without myocardial infarction 411.81
  cystic duct (see also Obstruction, gallbladder)
    575.2
    congenital 751.61
  device, implant, or graft — see Complications,
    due to (presence of) any device, implant,
    or graft classified to 996.0-996.5 NEC
  due to foreign body accidentally left in
    operation wound 998.4
  duodenum 537.3
    congenital 751.1
    due to
      compression NEC 537.3
      cyst 537.3
      intrinsic lesion or disease NEC 537.3
      scarring 537.3
      torsion 537.3
      ulcer 532.91
      volvulus 537.3
  ejaculatory duct 608.89
  endocardium 424.90
    arteriosclerotic 424.99
    specified cause, except rheumatic 424.99

✓4ᵗʰ Fourth-digit Required   ✓5ᵗʰ Fifth-digit Required   ►◄ Revised Text   ● New Line   ▲ Revised Code

Obstruction — Occlusion

Obstruction, obstructed, obstructive —
continued
esophagus 530.3
eustachian tube (complete) (partial) 381.60
  cartilaginous
    extrinsic 381.63
    intrinsic 381.62
  due to
    cholesteatoma 381.61
    osseous lesion NEC 381.61
    polyp 381.61
    osseous 381.61
fallopian tube (bilateral) 628.2
fecal 560.39
  with hernia — *see also* Hernia, by site, with
    obstruction
    gangrenous — *see* Hernia, by site, with
      gangrene
foramen of Monro (congenital) 742.3
  with spina bifida (*see also* Spina bifida)
    741.0 ✓5ᵗʰ
foreign body — *see* Foreign body
gallbladder 575.2
  with calculus, cholelithiasis, or stones
    574.21
    with cholecystitis (chronic) 574.11
      acute 574.01
  congenital 751.69
    jaundice from 751.69 [774.5]
gastric outlet 537.0
gastrointestinal (*see also* Obstruction,
  intestine) 560.9
glottis 478.79
hepatic 573.8
  duct (*see also* Obstruction, biliary) 576.2
    congenital 751.61
icterus (*see also* Obstruction, biliary) 576.8
  congenital 751.61
ileocecal coil (*see also* Obstruction, intestine)
  560.9
ileum (*see also* Obstruction, intestine) 560.9
iliofemoral (artery) 444.81
internal anastomosis — *see* Complications,
  mechanical, graft
intestine (mechanical) (neurogenic)
  (paroxysmal) (postinfectional) (reflex)
  560.9
  with
    adhesions (intestinal) (peritoneal) 560.81
    hernia — *see also* Hernia, by site, with
      obstruction
      gangrenous — *see* Hernia, by site,
        with gangrene
  adynamic (*see also* Ileus) 560.1
  by gallstone 560.31
  congenital or infantile (small) 751.1
    large 751.2
  due to
    Ascaris lumbricoides 127.0
    mural thickening 560.89
    procedure 997.4
      involving urinary tract 997.5
  impaction 560.39
  infantile — *see* Obstruction, intestine,
    congenital
  newborn
    due to
      fecaliths 777.1
      inspissated milk 777.2
      meconium (plug) 777.1
        in mucoviscidosis 277.01
      transitory 777.4
  specified cause NEC 560.89
  transitory, newborn 777.4
  volvulus 560.2
intracardiac ball valve prosthesis 996.02
jaundice (*see also* Obstruction, biliary) 576.8
  congenital 751.61
jejunum (*see also* Obstruction, intestine) 560.9
kidney 593.89
labor 660.9 ✓5ᵗʰ
  affecting fetus or newborn 763.1
  by
    bony pelvis (conditions classifiable to
      653.0-653.9) 660.1 ✓5ᵗʰ
    deep transverse arrest 660.3 ✓5ᵗʰ
    impacted shoulder 660.4 ✓5ᵗʰ

Obstruction, obstructed, obstructive —
continued
labor — *continued*
  by — *continued*
    locked twins 660.5 ✓5ᵗʰ
    malposition (fetus) (conditions classifiable
      to 652.0-652.9) 660.0 ✓5ᵗʰ
      head during labor 660.3 ✓5ᵗʰ
    persistent occipitoposterior position
      660.3 ✓5ᵗʰ
    soft tissue, pelvic (conditions classifiable
      to 654.0-654.9) 660.2 ✓5ᵗʰ
lacrimal
  canaliculi 375.53
  congenital 743.65
  punctum 375.52
  sac 375.54
lacrimonasal duct 375.56
  congenital 743.65
  neonatal 375.55
lacteal, with steatorrhea 579.2
laryngitis (*see also* Laryngitis) 464.01
larynx 478.79
  congenital 748.3
liver 573.8
  cirrhotic (*see also* Cirrhosis, liver) 571.5
lung 518.89
  with
    asthma — *see* Asthma
    bronchitis (chronic) 491.2 ✓5ᵗʰ
    emphysema NEC 492.8
  airway, chronic 496
  chronic NEC 496
    with
      asthma (chronic) (obstructive)
        493.2 ✓5ᵗʰ
  disease, chronic 496
    with
      asthma (chronic) (obstructive)
        493.2 ✓5ᵗʰ
  emphysematous 492.8
lymphatic 457.1
meconium
  fetus or newborn 777.1
    in mucoviscidosis 277.01
  newborn due to fecaliths 777.1
mediastinum 519.3
mitral (rheumatic) — *see* Stenosis, mitral
nasal 478.1
  duct 375.56
    neonatal 375.55
  sinus — *see* Sinusitis
nasolacrimal duct 375.56
  congenital 743.65
  neonatal 375.55
nasopharynx 478.29
nose 478.1
organ or site, congenital NEC — *see* Atresia
pancreatic duct 577.8
parotid gland 527.8
pelviureteral junction (*see also* Obstruction,
  ureter) 593.4
pharynx 478.29
portal (circulation) (vein) 452
prostate 600.9
  valve (urinary) 596.0
pulmonary
  valve (heart) (*see also* Endocarditis,
    pulmonary) 424.3
  vein, isolated 747.49
pyemic — *see* Septicemia
pylorus (acquired) 537.0
  congenital 750.5
  infantile 750.5
rectosigmoid (*see also* Obstruction, intestine)
  560.9
rectum 569.49
renal 593.89
respiratory 519.8
  chronic 496
retinal (artery) (vein) (central) (*see also*
  Occlusion, retina) 362.30
salivary duct (any) 527.8
  with calculus 527.5
sigmoid (*see also* Obstruction, intestine) 560.9
sinus (accessory) (nasal) (*see also* Sinusitis)
  473.9

Obstruction, obstructed, obstructive —
continued
Stensen's duct 527.8
stomach 537.89
  acute 536.1
  congenital 750.7
submaxillary gland 527.8
  with calculus 527.5
thoracic duct 457.1
thrombotic — *see* Thrombosis
tooth eruption 520.6
trachea 519.1
tracheostomy airway 519.09
tricuspid — *see* Endocarditis, tricuspid
upper respiratory, congenital 748.8
ureter (functional) 593.4
  congenital 753.20
  due to calculus 592.1
ureteropelvic junction, congenital 753.21
ureterovesical junction, congenital 753.22
urethra 599.6
  congenital 753.6
urinary (moderate) 599.6
  organ or tract (lower) 599.6
  prostatic valve 596.0
uropathy 599.6
uterus 621.8
vagina 623.2
valvular — *see* Endocarditis
vascular graft or shunt 996.1
  atherosclerosis — *see* Arteriosclerosis,
    coronary
  embolism 996.74
  occlusion NEC 996.74
  thrombus 996.74
vein, venous 459.2
  caval (inferior) (superior) 459.2
  thrombotic — *see* Thrombosis
vena cava (inferior) (superior) 459.2
ventricular shunt 996.2
vesical 596.0
vesicourethral orifice 596.0
vessel NEC 459.9

Obturator — *see* condition

Occlusal wear, teeth 521.1

Occlusion
anus 569.49
  congenital 751.2
  infantile 751.2
aortoiliac (chronic) 444.0
aqueduct of Sylvius 331.4
  congenital 742.3
    with spina bifida (*see also* Spina bifida)
      741.0 ✓5ᵗʰ
arteries of extremities, lower 444.22
  without thrombus or embolus (*see also*
    Arteriosclerosis, extremities) 440.20
  due to stricture or stenosis 447.1
  upper 444.21
    without thrombus or embolus (*see also*
      Arteriosclerosis, extremities) 440.20
    due to stricture or stenosis 447.1
artery NEC (*see also* Embolism, artery) 444.9
  auditory, internal 433.8 ✓5ᵗʰ
  basilar 433.0 ✓5ᵗʰ
    with other precerebral artery 433.3 ✓5ᵗʰ
    bilateral 433.3 ✓5ᵗʰ
  brain or cerebral (*see also* Infarct, brain)
    434.9 ✓5ᵗʰ
  carotid 433.1 ✓5ᵗʰ
    with other precerebral artery 433.3 ✓5ᵗʰ
    bilateral 433.3 ✓5ᵗʰ
  cerebellar (anterior inferior) (posterior
    inferior) (superior) 433.8 ✓5ᵗʰ
  cerebral (*see also* Infarct, brain) 434.9 ✓5ᵗʰ
  choroidal (anterior) 433.8 ✓5ᵗʰ
  communicating posterior 433.8 ✓5ᵗʰ
  coronary (thrombotic) (*see also* Infarct,
    myocardium) 410.9 ✓5ᵗʰ
    acute 410.9 ✓5ᵗʰ
      without myocardial infarction
        411.81
    healed or old 412
  hypophyseal 433.8 ✓5ᵗʰ
  iliac 444.81

Occlusion — *continued*
artery NEC (*see also* Embolism, artery) — *continued*
mesenteric (embolic) (thrombotic) (with gangrene) 557.0
pontine 433.8 ✓5ᵗʰ
precerebral NEC 433.9 ✓5ᵗʰ
late effect — *see* Late effect(s) (of) cerebrovascular disease
multiple or bilateral 433.3 ✓5ᵗʰ
puerperal, postpartum, childbirth 674.0 ✓5ᵗʰ
specified NEC 433.8 ✓5ᵗʰ
renal 593.81
retinal — *see* Occlusion, retina, artery
spinal 433.8 ✓5ᵗʰ
vertebral 433.2 ✓5ᵗʰ
with other precerebral artery 433.3 ✓5ᵗʰ
bilateral 433.3 ✓5ᵗʰ
basilar (artery) — *see* Occlusion, artery, basilar
bile duct (any) (*see also* Obstruction, biliary) 576.2
bowel (*see also* Obstruction, intestine) 560.9
brain (artery) (vascular) (*see also* Infarct, brain) 434.9 ✓5ᵗʰ
breast (duct) 611.8
carotid (artery) (common) (internal) — *see* Occlusion, artery, carotid
cerebellar (anterior inferior) (artery) (posterior inferior) (superior) 433.8 ✓5ᵗʰ
cerebral (artery) (*see also* Infarct, brain) 434.9 ✓5ᵗʰ
cerebrovascular (*see also* Infarct, brain) 434.9 ✓5ᵗʰ
diffuse 437.0
cervical canal (*see also* Stricture, cervix) 622.4
by falciparum malaria 084.0
cervix (uteri) (*see also* Stricture, cervix) 622.4
choanal 748.0
choroidal (artery) 433.8 ✓5ᵗʰ
colon (*see also* Obstruction, intestine) 560.9
communicating posterior artery 433.8 ✓5ᵗʰ
coronary (artery) (thrombotic) (*see also* Infarct, myocardium) 410.9 ✓5ᵗʰ
acute 410.9 ✓5ᵗʰ
without myocardial infarction 411.81
healed or old 412
without myocardial infarction 411.81
cystic duct (*see also* Obstruction, gallbladder) 575.2
congenital 751.69
embolic — *see* Embolism
fallopian tube 628.2
congenital 752.19
gallbladder (*see also* Obstruction, gallbladder) 575.2
congenital 751.69
jaundice from 751.69 [774.5]
gingiva, traumatic 523.8
hymen 623.3
congenital 752.42
hypophyseal (artery) 433.8 ✓5ᵗʰ
iliac artery 444.81
intestine (*see also* Obstruction, intestine) 560.9
kidney 593.89
lacrimal apparatus — *see* Stenosis, lacrimal
lung 518.89
lymph or lymphatic channel 457.1
mammary duct 611.8
mesenteric artery (embolic) (thrombotic) (with gangrene) 557.0
nose 478.1
congenital 748.0
organ or site, congenital NEC — *see* Atresia
oviduct 628.2
congenital 752.19
periodontal, traumatic 523.8
peripheral arteries (lower extremity) 444.22
without thrombus or embolus (*see also* Arteriosclerosis, extremities) 440.20
due to stricture or stenosis 447.1
upper extremity 444.21
without thrombus or embolus (*see also* Arteriosclerosis, extremities) 440.20
due to stricture or stenosis 447.1
pontine (artery) 433.8 ✓5ᵗʰ
posterior lingual, of mandibular teeth 524.2

Occlusion — *continued*
precerebral artery — *see* Occlusion, artery, precerebral NEC
puncta lacrimalia 375.52
pupil 364.74
pylorus (*see also* Stricture, pylorus) 537.0
renal artery 593.81
retina, retinal (vascular) 362.30
artery, arterial 362.30
branch 362.32
central (total) 362.31
partial 362.33
transient 362.34
tributary 362.32
vein 362.30
branch 362.36
central (total) 362.35
incipient 362.37
partial 362.37
tributary 362.36
spinal artery 433.8 ✓5ᵗʰ
stent
coronary 996.72
teeth (mandibular) (posterior lingual) 524.2
thoracic duct 457.1
tubal 628.2
ureter (complete) (partial) 593.4
congenital 753.29
urethra (*see also* Stricture, urethra) 598.9
congenital 753.6
uterus 621.8
vagina 623.2
vascular NEC 459.9
vein — *see* Thrombosis
vena cava (inferior) (superior) 453.2
ventricle (brain) NEC 331.4
vertebral (artery) — *see* Occlusion, artery, vertebral
vessel (blood) NEC 459.9
vulva 624.8
Occlusio pupillae 364.74
Occupational
problems NEC V62.2
therapy V57.21
Ochlophobia 300.29
Ochronosis (alkaptonuric) (congenital) (endogenous) 270.2
with chloasma of eyelid 270.2
Ocular muscle — *see also* condition
myopathy 359.1
torticollis 781.93
Oculoauriculovertebral dysplasia 756.0
Oculogyric
crisis or disturbance 378.87
psychogenic 306.7
Oculomotor syndrome 378.81
Oddi's sphincter spasm 576.5
Odelberg's disease (juvenile osteochondrosis) 732.1
Odontalgia 525.9
Odontoameloblastoma (M9311/0) 213.1
upper jaw (bone) 213.0
Odontoclasia 521.05
Odontoclasis 873.63
complicated 873.73
Odontodysplasia, regional 520.4
Odontogenesis imperfecta 520.5
Odontoma (M9280/0) 213.1
ameloblastic (M9311/0) 213.1
upper jaw (bone) 213.0
calcified (M9280/0) 213.1
upper jaw (bone) 213.0
complex (M9282/0) 213.1
upper jaw (bone) 213.0
compound (M9281/0) 213.1
upper jaw (bone) 213.0
fibroameloblastic (M9290/0) 213.1
upper jaw (bone) 213.0
follicular 526.0
upper jaw (bone) 213.0
Odontomyelitis (closed) (open) 522.0
Odontonecrosis 521.09
Odontorrhagia 525.8

Odontosarcoma, ameloblastic (M9290/3) 170.1
upper jaw (bone) 170.0
Odynophagia 787.2
Oesophagostomiasis 127.7
Oesophagostomum infestation 127.7
Oestriasis 134.0
Ogilvie's syndrome (sympathicotonic colon obstruction) 560.89
Oguchi's disease (retina) 368.61
Ohara's disease (*see also* Tularemia) 021.9
Oidiomycosis (*see also* Candidiasis) 112.9
Oidiomycotic meningitis 112.83
Oidium albicans infection (*see also* Candidiasis) 112.9
Old age 797
dementia (of) 290.0
Olfactory — *see* condition
Oligemia 285.9
Oligergasia (*see also* Retardation, mental) 319
Oligoamnios 658.0 ✓5ᵗʰ
affecting fetus or newborn 761.2
Oligoastrocytoma, mixed (M9382/3)
specified site — *see* Neoplasm, by site, malignant
unspecified site 191.9
Oligocythemia 285.9
Oligodendroblastoma (M9460/3)
specified site — *see* Neoplasm, by site, malignant
unspecified site 191.9
Oligodendroglioma (M9450/3)
anaplastic type (M9451/3)
specified site — *see* Neoplasm, by site, malignant
unspecified site 191.9
specified site — *see* Neoplasm, by site, malignant
unspecified site 191.9
Oligodendroma — *see* Oligodendroglioma
Oligodontia (*see also* Anodontia) 520.0
Oligoencephalon 742.1
Oligohydramnios 658.0 ✓5ᵗʰ
affecting fetus or newborn 761.2
due to premature rupture of membranes 658.1 ✓5ᵗʰ
affecting fetus or newborn 761.2
Oligohydrosis 705.0
Oligomenorrhea 626.1
Oligophrenia (*see also* Retardation, mental) 319
phenylpyruvic 270.1
Oligospermia 606.1
Oligotrichia 704.09
congenita 757.4
Oliguria 788.5
with
abortion — *see* Abortion, by type, with renal failure
ectopic pregnancy (*see also* categories 633.0-633.9) 639.3
molar pregnancy (*see also* categories 630-632) 639.3
complicating
abortion 639.3
ectopic or molar pregnancy 639.3
pregnancy 646.2 ✓5ᵗʰ
with hypertension — *see* Toxemia, of pregnancy
due to a procedure 997.5
following labor and delivery 669.3 ✓5ᵗʰ
heart or cardiac — *see* Failure, heart
puerperal, postpartum 669.3 ✓5ᵗʰ
specified due to a procedure 997.5
Ollier's disease (chondrodysplasia) 756.4
Omentitis (*see also* Peritonitis) 567.9
Omentocele (*see also* Hernia, omental) 553.8
Omentum, omental — *see* condition
Omphalitis (congenital) (newborn) 771.4
not of newborn 686.9
tetanus 771.3
Omphalocele 756.79
Omphalomesenteric duct, persistent 751.0

Omphalorrhagia, newborn 772.3
Omsk hemorrhagic fever 065.1
Onanism 307.9
Onchocerciasis 125.3
    eye 125.3 [360.13]
Onchocercosis 125.3
Oncocytoma (M8290/0) — see Neoplasm, by site,
    benign
Ondine's curse 348.8
Oneirophrenia (see also Schizophrenia) 295.4 ✓5ᵗʰ
Onychauxis 703.8
    congenital 757.5
Onychia (with lymphangitis) 681.9
    dermatophytic 110.1
    finger 681.02
    toe 681.11
Onychitis (with lymphangitis) 681.9
    finger 681.02
    toe 681.11
Onychocryptosis 703.0
Onychodystrophy 703.8
    congenital 757.5
Onychogryphosis 703.8
Onychogryposis 703.8
Onycholysis 703.8
Onychomadesis 703.8
Onychomalacia 703.8
Onychomycosis 110.1
    finger 110.1
    toe 110.1
Onycho-osteodysplasia 756.89
Onychophagy 307.9
Onychoptosis 703.8
Onychorrhexis 703.8
    congenital 757.5
Onychoschizia 703.8
Onychotrophia (see also Atrophy, nail) 703.8
O'nyong-nyong fever 066.3
Onyxis (finger) (toe) 703.0
Onyxitis (with lymphangitis) 681.9
    finger 681.02
    toe 681.11
Oophoritis (cystic) (infectional) (interstitial) (see
    also Salpingo-oophoritis) 614.2
    complicating pregnancy 646.6 ✓5ᵗʰ
    fetal (acute) 752.0
    gonococcal (acute) 098.19
        chronic or duration of 2 months or over
        098.39
    tuberculous (see also Tuberculosis) 016.6 ✓5ᵗʰ
Opacity, opacities
    cornea 371.00
        central 371.03
        congenital 743.43
            interfering with vision 743.42
        degenerative (see also Degeneration, cornea)
        371.40
        hereditary (see also Dystrophy, cornea)
        371.50
        inflammatory (see also Keratitis) 370.9
        late effect of trachoma (healed) 139.1
        minor 371.01
        peripheral 371.02
    enamel (fluoride) (nonfluoride) (teeth) 520.3
    lens (see also Cataract) 366.9
    snowball 379.22
    vitreous (humor) 379.24
        congenital 743.51
Opalescent dentin (hereditary) 520.5
Open, opening
    abnormal, organ or site, congenital — see
        Imperfect, closure
    angle with
        borderline intraocular pressure 365.01
        cupping of discs 365.01
    bite (anterior) (posterior) 524.2
    false — see Imperfect, closure
    wound — see Wound, open, by site

Operation
    causing mutilation of fetus 763.89
    destructive, on live fetus, to facilitate birth
        763.89
    for delivery, fetus or newborn 763.89
    maternal, unrelated to current delivery,
        affecting fetus or newborn 760.6
Operational fatigue 300.89
Operative — see condition
Operculitis (chronic) 523.4
    acute 523.3
Operculum, retina 361.32
    with detachment 361.01
Ophiasis 704.01
Ophthalmia (see also Conjunctivitis) 372.30
    actinic rays 370.24
    allergic (acute) 372.05
        chronic 372.14
    blennorrhagic (neonatorum) 098.40
    catarrhal 372.03
    diphtheritic 032.81
    Egyptian 076.1
    electric, electrica 370.24
    gonococcal (neonatorum) 098.40
    metastatic 360.11
    migraine 346.8 ✓5ᵗʰ
    neonatorum, newborn 771.6
        gonococcal 098.40
    nodosa 360.14
    phlyctenular 370.31
        with ulcer (see also Ulcer, cornea) 370.00
    sympathetic 360.11
Ophthalmitis — see Ophthalmia
Ophthalmocele (congenital) 743.66
Ophthalmoneuromyelitis 341.0
**Ophthalmopathy, infiltrative with
    thyrotoxicosis** 242.0 ✓5ᵗʰ
Ophthalmoplegia (see also Strabismus) 378.9
    anterior internuclear 378.86
    ataxia-areflexia syndrome 357.0
    bilateral 378.9
    diabetic 250.5 ✓5ᵗʰ [378.86]
    exophthalmic 242.0 ✓5ᵗʰ [376.22]
    external 378.55
        progressive 378.72
        total 378.56
    interna(l) (complete) (total) 367.52
    internuclear 378.86
    migraine 346.8 ✓5ᵗʰ
    painful 378.55
    Parinaud's 378.81
    progressive external 378.72
    supranuclear, progressive 333.0
    total (external) 378.56
        internal 367.52
    unilateral 378.9
Opisthognathism 524.00
Opisthorchiasis (felineus) (tenuicollis) (viverrini)
    121.0
Opisthotonos, opisthotonus 781.0
Opitz's disease (congestive splenomegaly) 289.51
Opiumism (see also Dependence) 304.0 ✓5ᵗʰ
Oppenheim's disease 358.8
Oppenheim-Urbach disease or syndrome
    (necrobiosis lipoidica diabeticorum)
    250.8 ✓5ᵗʰ [709.3]
Opsoclonia 379.59
Optic nerve — see condition
Orbit — see condition
Orchioblastoma (M9071/3) 186.9
Orchitis (nonspecific) (septic) 604.90
    with abscess 604.0
    blennorrhagic (acute) 098.13
        chronic or duration of 2 months or over
        098.33
    diphtheritic 032.89 [604.91]
    filarial 125.9 [604.91]
    gangrenous 604.99
    gonococcal (acute) 098.13
        chronic or duration of 2 months or over
        098.33
    mumps 072.0
    parotidea 072.0

Orchitis — continued
    suppurative 604.99
    syphilitic 095.8 [604.91]
    tuberculous (see also Tuberculosis)
        016.5 ✓5ᵗʰ [608.81]
Orf 051.2
Organic — see also condition
    heart — see Disease, heart
    insufficiency 799.8
Oriental
    bilharziasis 120.2
    schistosomiasis 120.2
    sore 085.1
Orifice — see condition
Origin, both great vessels from right ventricle
    745.11
Ormond's disease or syndrome 593.4
Ornithosis 073.9
    with
        complication 073.8
            specified NEC 073.7
        pneumonia 073.0
        pneumonitis (lobular) 073.0
Orodigitofacial dysostosis 759.89
Oropouche fever 066.3
Orotaciduria, oroticaciduria (congenital)
    (hereditary) (pyrimidine deficiency) 281.4
Oroya fever 088.0
Orthodontics V58.5
    adjustment V53.4
    aftercare V58.5
    fitting V53.4
Orthopnea 786.02
Orthoptic training V57.4
Os, uterus — see condition
Osgood-Schlatter
    disease 732.4
    osteochondrosis 732.4
Osler's
    disease (M9950/1) (polycythemia vera) 238.4
    nodes 421.0
Osler-Rendu disease (familial hemorrhagic
    telangiectasia) 448.0
Osler-Vaquez disease (M9950/1) (polycythemia
    vera) 238.4
Osler-Weber-Rendu syndrome (familial
    hemorrhagic telangiectasia) 448.0
Osmidrosis 705.89
Osseous — see condition
Ossification
    artery — see Arteriosclerosis
    auricle (ear) 380.39
    bronchus 519.1
    cardiac (see also Degeneration, myocardial)
        429.1
    cartilage (senile) 733.99
    coronary (artery) — see Arteriosclerosis,
        coronary
    diaphragm 728.10
    ear 380.39
        middle (see also Otosclerosis) 387.9
    falx cerebri 349.2
    fascia 728.10
    fontanel
        defective or delayed 756.0
        premature 756.0
    heart (see also Degeneration, myocardial) 429.1
        valve — see Endocarditis
    larynx 478.79
    ligament
        posterior longitudinal 724.8
            cervical 723.7
    meninges (cerebral) 349.2
        spinal 336.8
    multiple, eccentric centers 733.99
    muscle 728.10
        heterotopic, postoperative 728.13
    myocardium, myocardial (see also
        Degeneration, myocardial) 429.1
    penis 607.81
    periarticular 728.89
    sclera 379.16
    tendon 727.82

Ossification — *continued*
  trachea 519.1
  tympanic membrane (*see also*
    Tympanosclerosis) 385.00
  vitreous (humor) 360.44
Osteitis (*see also* Osteomyelitis) 730.2 ✓5ᵗʰ
  acute 730.0 ✓5ᵗʰ
  alveolar 526.5
  chronic 730.1 ✓5ᵗʰ
  condensans (ilii) 733.5
  deformans (Paget's) 731.0
    due to or associated with malignant
      neoplasm (*see also* Neoplasm, bone,
      malignant) 170.9 [731.1]
  due to yaws 102.6
  fibrosa NEC 733.29
    cystica (generalisata) 252.0
    disseminata 756.59
    osteoplastica 252.0
  fragilitans 756.51
  Garré's (sclerosing) 730.1 ✓5ᵗʰ
  infectious (acute) (subacute) 730.0 ✓5ᵗʰ
    chronic or old 730.1 ✓5ᵗʰ
  jaw (acute) (chronic) (lower) (neonatal)
    (suppurative) (upper) 526.4
  parathyroid 252.0
  petrous bone (*see also* Petrositis) 383.20
  pubis 733.5
  sclerotic, nonsuppurative 730.1 ✓5ᵗʰ
  syphilitic 095.5
  tuberculosa
    cystica (of Jüngling) 135
    multiplex cystoides 135
Osteoarthritica spondylitis (spine) (*see also*
  Spondylosis) 721.90
Osteoarthritis (*see also* Osteoarthrosis) 715.9 ✓5ᵗʰ
  distal interphalangeal 715.9 ✓5ᵗʰ
  hyperplastic 731.2
  interspinalis (*see also* Spondylosis) 721.90
  spine, spinal NEC (*see also* Spondylosis)
    721.90
Osteoarthropathy (*see also* Osteoarthrosis)
  715.9 ✓5ᵗʰ
  chronic idiopathic hypertrophic 757.39
  familial idiopathic 757.39
  hypertrophic pulmonary 731.2
    secondary 731.2
  idiopathic hypertrophic 757.39
  primary hypertrophic 731.2
  pulmonary hypertrophic 731.2
  secondary hypertrophic 731.2
Osteoarthrosis (degenerative) (hypertrophic)
  (rheumatoid) 715.9 ✓5ᵗʰ

> *Note — Use the following fifth-digit*
> *subclassification with category 715:*
>
>   *0   site unspecified*
>   *1   shoulder region*
>   *2   upper arm*
>   *3   forearm*
>   *4   hand*
>   *5   pelvic region and thigh*
>   *6   lower leg*
>   *7   ankle and foot*
>   *8   other specified sites except spine*
>   *9   multiple sites*

  Deformans alkaptonurica 270.2
  generalized 715.09
  juvenilis (Köhler's) 732.5
  localized 715.3 ✓5ᵗʰ
    idiopathic 715.1 ✓5ᵗʰ
    primary 715.1 ✓5ᵗʰ
    secondary 715.2 ✓5ᵗʰ
  multiple sites, not specified as generalized
    715.89
  polyarticular 715.09
  spine (*see also* Spondylosis) 721.90
  temporomandibular joint 524.69
Osteoblastoma (M9200/0) — *see* Neoplasm,
  bone, benign
Osteochondritis (*see also* Osteochondrosis) 732.9
  dissecans 732.7
    hip 732.7

Osteochondritis (*see also* Osteochondrosis) —
  continued
    ischiopubica 732.1
  multiple 756.59
  syphilitic (congenital) 090.0
Osteochondrodermodysplasia 756.59
Osteochondrodystrophy 277.5
  deformans 277.5
  familial 277.5
  fetalis 756.4
Osteochondrolysis 732.7
Osteochondroma (M9210/0) — *see also*
  Neoplasm, bone, benign
  multiple, congenital 756.4
Osteochondromatosis (M9210/1) 238.0
  synovial 727.82
Osteochondromyxosarcoma (M9180/3) — *see*
  Neoplasm, bone, malignant
Osteochondropathy NEC 732.9
Osteochondrosarcoma (M9180/3) — *see*
  Neoplasm, bone, malignant
Osteochondrosis 732.9
  acetabulum 732.1
  adult spine 732.8
  astragalus 732.5
  Blount's 732.4
  Buchanan's (juvenile osteochondrosis of iliac
    crest) 732.1
  Buchman's (juvenile osteochondrosis) 732.1
  Burns' 732.3
  calcaneus 732.5
  capitular epiphysis (femur) 732.1
  carpal
    lunate (wrist) 732.3
    scaphoid 732.3
  coxae juvenilis 732.1
  deformans juvenilis (coxae) (hip) 732.1
    Scheuermann's 732.0
    spine 732.0
    tibia 732.4
    vertebra 732.0
  Diaz's (astragalus) 732.5
  dissecans (knee) (shoulder) 732.7
  femoral capital epiphysis 732.1
  femur (head) (juvenile) 732.1
  foot (juvenile) 732.5
  Freiberg's (disease) (second metatarsal) 732.5
  Haas' 732.3
  Haglund's (os tibiale externum) 732.5
  hand (juvenile) 732.3
  head of
    femur 732.1
    humerus (juvenile) 732.3
  hip (juvenile) 732.1
  humerus (juvenile) 732.3
  iliac crest (juvenile) 732.1
  ilium (juvenile) 732.1
  ischiopubic synchondrosis 732.1
  Iselin's (osteochondrosis fifth metatarsal) 732.5
  juvenile, juvenilis 732.6
    arm 732.3
    capital femoral epiphysis 732.1
    capitellum humeri 732.3
    capitular epiphysis 732.1
    carpal scaphoid 732.3
    clavicle, sternal epiphysis 732.6
    coxae 732.1
    deformans 732.1
    foot 732.5
    hand 732.3
    hip and pelvis 732.1
    lower extremity, except foot 732.4
    lunate, wrist 732.3
    medial cuneiform bone 732.5
    metatarsal (head) 732.5
    metatarsophalangeal 732.5
    navicular, ankle 732.5
    patella 732.4
    primary patellar center (of Köhler) 732.4
    specified site NEC 732.6
    spine 732.0
    tarsal scaphoid 732.5
    tibia (epiphysis) (tuberosity) 732.4
    upper extremity 732.3
    vertebra (body) (Calvé) 732.0
      epiphyseal plates (of Scheuermann) 732.0

Osteochondrosis — *continued*
  Kienböck's (disease) 732.3
  Köhler's (disease) (navicular, ankle) 732.5
    patellar 732.4
    tarsal navicular 732.5
  Legg-Calvé-Perthes (disease) 732.1
  lower extremity (juvenile) 732.4
  lunate bone 732.3
  Mauclaire's 732.3
  metacarpal heads (of Mauclaire) 732.3
  metatarsal (fifth) (head) (second) 732.5
  navicular, ankle 732.5
  os calcis 732.5
  Osgood-Schlatter 732.4
  os tibiale externum 732.5
  Panner's 732.3
  patella (juvenile) 732.4
  patellar center
    primary (of Köhler) 732.4
    secondary (of Sinding-Larsen) 732.4
  pelvis (juvenile) 732.1
  Pierson's 732.1
  radial head (juvenile) 732.3
  Scheuermann's 732.0
  Sever's (calcaneum) 732.5
  Sinding-Larsen (secondary patellar center)
    732.4
  spine (juvenile) 732.0
    adult 732.8
  symphysis pubis (of Pierson) (juvenile) 732.1
  syphilitic (congenital) 090.0
  tarsal (navicular) (scaphoid) 732.5
  tibia (proximal) (tubercle) 732.4
  tuberculous — *see* Tuberculosis, bone
  ulna 732.3
  upper extremity (juvenile) 732.3
  van Neck's (juvenile osteochondrosis) 732.1
  vertebral (juvenile) 732.0
    adult 732.8
Osteoclastoma (M9250/1) 238.0
  malignant (M9250/3) — *see* Neoplasm, bone,
    malignant
Osteocopic pain 733.90
Osteodynia 733.90
Osteodystrophy
  azotemic 588.0
  chronica deformans hypertrophica 731.0
  congenital 756.50
    specified type NEC 756.59
  deformans 731.0
  fibrosa localisata 731.0
  parathyroid 252.0
  renal 588.0
Osteofibroma (M9262/0) — *see* Neoplasm, bone,
  benign
Osteofibrosarcoma (M9182/3) — *see* Neoplasm,
  bone, malignant
Osteogenesis imperfecta 756.51
Osteogenic — *see* condition
Osteoma (M9180/0) — *see also* Neoplasm, bone,
  benign
  osteoid (M9191/0) — *see also* Neoplasm, bone,
    benign
    giant (M9200/0) — *see* Neoplasm, bone,
      benign
Osteomalacia 268.2
  chronica deformans hypertrophica 731.0
  due to vitamin D deficiency 268.2
  infantile (*see also* Rickets) 268.0
  juvenile (*see also* Rickets) 268.0
  pelvis 268.2
  vitamin D-resistant 275.3
Osteomalacic bone 268.2
Osteomalacosis 268.2

Osteomyelitis — Otitis *(side tab)*

Osteomyelitis (general) (infective) (localized) (neonatal) (purulent) (pyogenic) (septic) (staphylococcal) (streptococcal) (suppurative) (with periostitis) 730.2 ✓5ᵗʰ

Note — Use the following fifth-digit subclassification with category 730:

0	site unspecified
1	shoulder region
2	upper arm
3	forearm
4	hand
5	pelvic region and thigh
6	lower leg
7	ankle and foot
8	other specified sites
9	multiple sites

acute or subacute 730.0 ✓5ᵗʰ
chronic or old 730.1 ✓5ᵗʰ
due to or associated with
  diabetes mellitus 250.8 ✓5ᵗʰ [731.8]
  tuberculosis (see also Tuberculosis, bone)
    015.9 ✓5ᵗʰ [730.8] ✓5ᵗʰ
    limb bones 015.5 ✓5ᵗʰ [730.8] ✓5ᵗʰ
    specified bones NEC
      015.7 ✓5ᵗʰ [730.8] ✓5ᵗʰ
    spine 015.0 ✓5ᵗʰ [730.8] ✓5ᵗʰ
    typhoid 002.0 [730.8] ✓5ᵗʰ
Garré's 730.1 ✓5ᵗʰ
jaw (acute) (chronic) (lower) (neonatal) (suppurative) (upper) 526.4
nonsuppurating 730.1 ✓5ᵗʰ
orbital 376.03
petrous bone (see also Petrositis) 383.20
Salmonella 003.24
sclerosing, nonsuppurative 730.1 ✓5ᵗʰ
sicca 730.1 ✓5ᵗʰ
syphilitic 095.5
  congenital 090.0 [730.8] ✓5ᵗʰ
tuberculous — see Tuberculosis, bone
typhoid 002.0 [730.8] ✓5ᵗʰ
Osteomyelofibrosis 289.8
Osteomyelosclerosis 289.8
Osteonecrosis 733.40 ▲
  meaning osteomyelitis 730.1 ✓5ᵗʰ ●
Osteo-onycho-arthro dysplasia 756.89
Osteo-onychodysplasia, hereditary 756.89
Osteopathia
  condensans disseminata 756.53
  hyperostotica multiplex infantilis 756.59
  hypertrophica toxica 731.2
  striata 756.4
Osteopathy resulting from poliomyelitis (see also Poliomyelitis) 045.9 ✓5ᵗʰ [730.7]
  familial dysplastic 731.2
Osteopecilia 756.53
Osteopenia 733.90
Osteoperiostitis (see also Osteomyelitis) 730.2 ✓5ᵗʰ
  ossificans toxica 731.2
  toxica ossificans 731.2
Osteopetrosis (familial) 756.52
Osteophyte — see Exostosis
Osteophytosis — see Exostosis
Osteopoikilosis 756.53
Osteoporosis (generalized) 733.00
  circumscripta 731.0
  disuse 733.03
  drug-induced 733.09
  idiopathic 733.02
  postmenopausal 733.01
  posttraumatic 733.7
  screening V82.81
  senile 733.01
  specified type NEC 733.09
Osteoporosis-osteomalacia syndrome 268.2
Osteopsathyrosis 756.51
Osteoradionecrosis, jaw 526.89
Osteosarcoma (M9180/3) — see also Neoplasm, bone, malignant
  chondroblastic (M9181/3) — see Neoplasm, bone, malignant

Osteosarcoma (M9180/3) — see also Neoplasm, bone, malignant — continued
  fibroblastic (M9182/3) — see Neoplasm, bone, malignant
  in Paget's disease of bone (M9184/3) — see Neoplasm, bone, malignant
  juxtacortical (M9190/3) — see Neoplasm, bone, malignant
  parosteal (M9190/3) — see Neoplasm, bone, malignant
  telangiectatic (M9183/3) — see Neoplasm, bone, malignant
Osteosclerosis 756.52
  fragilis (generalisata) 756.52
  myelofibrosis 289.8
Osteosclerotic anemia 289.8
Osteosis
  acromegaloid 757.39
  cutis 709.3
  parathyroid 252.0
  renal fibrocystic 588.0
Österreicher-Turner syndrome 756.89
Ostium
  atrioventriculare commune 745.69
  primum (arteriosum) (defect) (persistent) 745.61
  secundum (arteriosum) (defect) (patent) (persistent) 745.5
Ostrum-Furst syndrome 756.59
Otalgia 388.70
  otogenic 388.71
  referred 388.72
Othematoma 380.31
Otitic hydrocephalus 348.2
Otitis 382.9
  with effusion 381.4
    purulent 382.4
    secretory 381.4
    serous 381.4
    suppurative 382.4
  acute 382.9
  adhesive (see also Adhesions, middle ear) 385.10
  chronic 382.9
    with effusion 381.3
    mucoid, mucous (simple) 381.20
    purulent 382.3
    secretory 381.3
    serous 381.10
    suppurative 382.3
  diffuse parasitic 136.8
  externa (acute) (diffuse) (hemorrhagica) 380.10
    actinic 380.22
    candidal 112.82
    chemical 380.22
    chronic 380.23
      mycotic — see Otitis, externa, mycotic
      specified type NEC 380.23
    circumscribed 380.10
    contact 380.22
    due to
      erysipelas 035 [380.13]
      impetigo 684 [380.13]
      seborrheic dermatitis 690.10 [380.13]
    eczematoid 380.22
    furuncular 680.0 [380.13]
    infective 380.10
      chronic 380.16
    malignant 380.14
    mycotic (chronic) 380.15
      due to
        aspergillosis 117.3 [380.15]
        moniliasis 112.82
        otomycosis 111.8 [380.15]
    reactive 380.22
    specified type NEC 380.22
    tropical 111.8 [380.15]
  insidiosa (see also Otosclerosis) 387.9
  interna (see also Labyrinthitis) 386.30
  media (hemorrhagic) (staphylococcal) (streptococcal) 382.9
    acute 382.9
      with effusion 381.00
      allergic 381.04
        mucoid 381.05
        sanguineous 381.06

Otitis — continued
  media — continued
    acute — continued
      allergic — continued
        serous 381.04
      catarrhal 381.00
      exudative 381.00
      mucoid 381.02
        allergic 381.05
      necrotizing 382.00
        with spontaneous rupture of ear drum 382.01
        in
          influenza 487.8 [382.02]
          measles 055.2
          scarlet fever 034.1 [382.02]
      nonsuppurative 381.00
      purulent 382.00
        with spontaneous rupture of ear drum 382.01
      sanguineous 381.03
        allergic 381.06
      secretory 381.01
      seromucinous 381.02
      serous 381.01
        allergic 381.04
      suppurative 382.00
        with spontaneous rupture of ear drum 382.01
        due to
          influenza 487.8 [382.02]
          scarlet fever 034.1 [382.02]
      transudative 381.00
    adhesive (see also Adhesions, middle ear) 385.10
    allergic 381.4
      acute 381.04
        mucoid 381.05
        sanguineous 381.06
        serous 381.04
      chronic 381.3
    catarrhal 381.4
      acute 381.00
      chronic (simple) 381.10
    chronic 382.9
      with effusion 381.3
      adhesive (see also Adhesions, middle ear) 385.10
      allergic 381.3
      atticoantral, suppurative (with posterior or superior marginal perforation of ear drum) 382.2
      benign suppurative (with anterior perforation of ear drum) 382.1
      catarrhal 381.10
      exudative 381.3
      mucinous 381.20
      mucoid, mucous (simple) 381.20
      mucosanguineous 381.29
      nonsuppurative 381.3
      purulent 382.3
      secretory 381.3
      seromucinous 381.3
      serosanguineous 381.19
      serous (simple) 381.10
      suppurative 382.3
        atticoantral (with posterior or superior marginal perforation of ear drum) 382.2
        benign (with anterior perforation of ear drum) 382.1
      tuberculous (see also Tuberculosis) 017.4 ✓5ᵗʰ
      tubotympanic 382.1
      transudative 381.3
    exudative 381.4
      acute 381.00
      chronic 381.3
    fibrotic (see also Adhesions, middle ear) 385.10
    mucoid, mucous 381.4
      acute 381.02
      chronic (simple) 381.20
    mucosanguineous, chronic 381.29
    nonsuppurative 381.4
      acute 381.00
      chronic 381.3
    postmeasles 055.2

Otitis — *continued*
media — *continued*
purulent 382.4
acute 382.00
with spontaneous rupture of ear drum 382.01
chronic 382.3
sanguineous, acute 381.03
allergic 381.06
secretory 381.4
acute or subacute 381.01
chronic 381.3
seromucinous 381.4
acute or subacute 381.02
chronic 381.3
serosanguineous, chronic 381.19
serous 381.4
acute or subacute 381.01
chronic (simple) 381.10
subacute — *see* Otitis, media, acute
suppurative 382.4
acute 382.00
with spontaneous rupture of ear drum 382.01
chronic 382.3
atticoantral 382.2
benign 382.1
tuberculous (*see also* Tuberculosis) 017.4 ✓5ᵗʰ
tubotympanic 382.1
transudative 381.4
acute 381.00
chronic 381.3
tuberculous (*see also* Tuberculosis) 017.4 ✓5ᵗʰ
postmeasles 055.2
Otoconia 386.8
Otolith syndrome 386.19
Otomycosis 111.8 *[380.15]*
in
aspergillosis 117.3 *[380.15]*
moniliasis 112.82
Otopathy 388.9
Otoporosis (*see also* Otosclerosis) 387.9
Otorrhagia 388.69
traumatic — *see* nature of injury
Otorrhea 388.60
blood 388.69
cerebrospinal (fluid) 388.61
Otosclerosis (general) 387.9
cochlear (endosteal) 387.2
involving
otic capsule 387.2
oval window
nonobliterative 387.0
obliterative 387.1
round window 387.2
nonobliterative 387.0
obliterative 387.1
specified type NEC 387.8
Otospongiosis (*see also* Otosclerosis) 387.9
Otto's disease or pelvis 715.35
Outburst, aggressive (*see also* Disturbance, conduct) 312.0 ✓5ᵗʰ
in children and adolescents 313.9
Outcome of delivery
multiple birth NEC V27.9
all liveborn V27.5
all stillborn V27.7
some liveborn V27.6
unspecified V27.9
single V27.9
liveborn V27.0
stillborn V27.1
twins V27.9
both liveborn V27.2
both stillborn V27.4
one liveborn, one stillborn V27.3
Outlet — *see also* condition
syndrome (thoracic) 353.0
Outstanding ears (bilateral) 744.29
Ovalocytosis (congenital) (hereditary) (*see also* Elliptocytosis) 282.1

Ovarian — *see also* condition
pregnancy — *see* Pregnancy, ovarian
remnant syndrome 620.8
vein syndrome 593.4
Ovaritis (cystic) (*see also* Salpingo-oophoritis) 614.2
Ovary, ovarian — *see* condition
Overactive — *see also* Hyperfunction
bladder 596.51
eye muscle (*see also* Strabismus) 378.9
hypothalamus 253.8
thyroid (*see also* Thyrotoxicosis) 242.9 ✓5ᵗʰ
Overactivity, child 314.01
Overbite (deep) (excessive) (horizontal) (vertical) 524.2
Overbreathing (*see also* Hyperventilation) 786.01
Overconscientious personality 301.4
Overdevelopment — *see also* Hypertrophy
breast (female) (male) 611.1
nasal bones 738.0
prostate, congenital 752.8
Overdistention — *see* Distention
Overdose, overdosage (drug) 977.9
specified drug or substance — *see* Table of Drugs and Chemicals
Overeating 783.6
with obesity 278.0 ✓5ᵗʰ
nonorganic origin 307.51
Overexertion (effects) (exhaustion) 994.5
Overexposure (effects) 994.9
exhaustion 994.4
Overfeeding (*see also* Overeating) 783.6
Overgrowth, bone NEC 733.99
Overheated (effects) (places) — *see* Heat
Overinhibited child 313.0
Overjet 524.2
Overlaid, overlying (suffocation) 994.7
Overlapping toe (acquired) 735.8
congenital (fifth toe) 755.66
Overload
fluid 276.6
potassium (K) 276.7
sodium (Na) 276.0
Overnutrition (*see also* Hyperalimentation) 783.6
Overproduction — *see also* Hypersecretion
ACTH 255.3
cortisol 255.0
growth hormone 253.0
thyroid-stimulating hormone (TSH) 242.8 ✓5ᵗʰ
Overriding
aorta 747.21
finger (acquired) 736.29
congenital 755.59
toe (acquired) 735.8
congenital 755.66
Oversize
fetus (weight of 4500 grams or more) 766.0
affecting management of pregnancy 656.6 ✓5ᵗʰ
causing disproportion 653.5 ✓5ᵗʰ
with obstructed labor 660.1 ✓5ᵗʰ
affecting fetus or newborn 763.1
Overstimulation, ovarian 256.1
Overstrained 780.79
heart — *see* Hypertrophy, cardiac
Overweight (*see also* Obesity) 278.00
Overwork 780.79
Oviduct — *see* condition
Ovotestis 752.7
Ovulation (cycle)
failure or lack of 628.0
pain 625.2
Ovum
blighted 631
dropsical 631
pathologic 631
Owren's disease or syndrome (parahemophilia) (*see also* Defect, coagulation) 286.3
Oxalosis 271.8
Oxaluria 271.8

Ox heart — *see* Hypertrophy, cardiac
OX syndrome 758.6
Oxycephaly, oxycephalic 756.0
syphilitic, congenital 090.0
Oxyuriasis 127.4
Oxyuris vermicularis (infestation) 127.4
Ozena 472.0

P

Pacemaker syndrome 429.4
Pachyderma, pachydermia 701.8
laryngis 478.5
laryngitis 478.79
larynx (verrucosa) 478.79
Pachydermatitis 701.8
Pachydermatocele (congenital) 757.39
acquired 701.8
Pachydermatosis 701.8
Pachydermoperiostitis
secondary 731.2
Pachydermoperiostosis
primary idiopathic 757.39
secondary 731.2
Pachymeningitis (adhesive) (basal) (brain) (cerebral) (cervical) (chronic) (circumscribed) (external) (fibrous) (hemorrhagic) (hypertrophic) (internal) (purulent) (spinal) (suppurative) (*see also* Meningitis) 322.9
gonococcal 098.82
Pachyonychia (congenital) 757.5
acquired 703.8
Pachyperiosteodermia
primary or idiopathic 757.39
secondary 731.2
Pachyperiostosis
primary or idiopathic 757.39
secondary 731.2
Pacinian tumor (M9507/0) — *see* Neoplasm, skin, benign
Pads, knuckle or Garrod's 728.79
Paget's disease (osteitis deformans) 731.0
with infiltrating duct carcinoma of the breast (M8541/3) — *see* Neoplasm, breast, malignant
bone 731.0
osteosarcoma in (M9184/3) — *see* Neoplasm, bone, malignant
breast (M8540/3) 174.0
extramammary (M8542/3) — *see also* Neoplasm, skin, malignant
anus 154.3
skin 173.5
malignant (M8540/3)
breast 174.0
specified site NEC (M8542/3) — *see* Neoplasm, skin, malignant
unspecified site 174.0
mammary (M8540/3) 174.0
necrosis of bone 731.0
nipple (M8540/3) 174.0
osteitis deformans 731.0
Paget-Schroetter syndrome (intermittent venous claudication) 453.8
Pain(s)
abdominal 789.0 ✓5ᵗʰ
adnexa (uteri) 625.9
alimentary, due to vascular insufficiency 557.9
anginoid (*see also* Pain, precordial) 786.51anus 569.42
arch 729.5
arm 729.5
back (postural) 724.5
low 724.2
psychogenic 307.89
bile duct 576.9
bladder 788.9
bone 733.90
breast 611.71
psychogenic 307.89
broad ligament 625.9
cartilage NEC 733.90
cecum 789.0 ✓5ᵗʰ

Pain(s) — Palsy

☑4ᵗ Fourth-digit Required   ☑5ᵗ Fifth-digit Required   ▶◀ Revised Text   ● New Line   ▲ Revised Code

Palsy (see also Paralysis) — continued
  radial nerve (acute) 354.3
  seventh nerve 351.0
    newborn 767.5
  shaking (see also Parkinsonism) 332.0
  spastic (cerebral) (spinal) 343.9
    hemiplegic 343.1
  specified nerve NEC — see Disorder, nerve
  supranuclear NEC 356.8
    progressive 333.0
  ulnar nerve (tardy) 354.2
  wasting 335.21
Paltauf-Sternberg disease 201.9 ✓5ᵗʰ
Paludism — see Malaria
Panama fever 084.0
Panaris (with lymphangitis) 681.9
  finger 681.02
  toe 681.11
Panaritium (with lymphangitis) 681.9
  finger 681.02
  toe 681.11
Panarteritis (nodosa) 446.0
  brain or cerebral 437.4
Pancake heart 793.2
  with cor pulmonale (chronic) 416.9
Pancarditis (acute) (chronic) 429.89
  with
    rheumatic
      fever (active) (acute) (chronic) (subacute)
        391.8
        inactive or quiescent 398.99
  rheumatic, acute 391.8
  chronic or inactive 398.99
Pancoast's syndrome or tumor (carcinoma, pulmonary apex) (M8010/3) 162.3
Pancoast-Tobias syndrome (M8010/3) (carcinoma, pulmonary apex) 162.3
Pancolitis 556.6
Pancreas, pancreatic — see condition
Pancreatitis 577.0
  acute (edematous) (hemorrhagic) (recurrent) 577.0
  annular 577.0
  apoplectic 577.0
  calcercous 577.0
  chronic (infectious) 577.1
    recurrent 577.1
  cystic 577.2
  fibrous 577.8
  gangrenous 577.0
  hemorrhagic (acute) 577.0
  interstitial (chronic) 577.1
    acute 577.0
  malignant 577.0
  mumps 072.3
  painless 577.1
  recurrent 577.1
  relapsing 577.1
  subacute 577.0
  suppurative 577.0
  syphilitic 095.8
Pancreatolithiasis 577.8
Pancytolysis 289.9
Pancytopenia (acquired) 284.8
  with malformations 284.0
  congenital 284.0
Panencephalitis — see also Encephalitis
  subacute, sclerosing 046.2
Panhematopenia 284.8
  congenital 284.0
  constitutional 284.0
  splenic, primary 289.4
Panhemocytopenia 284.8
  congenital 284.0
  constitutional 284.0
Panhypogonadism 257.2
Panhypopituitarism 253.2
  prepubertal 253.3
Panic (attack) (state) 300.01
  reaction to exceptional stress (transient) 308.0
Panmyelopathy, familial constitutional 284.0
Panmyelophthisis 284.9
  acquired (secondary) 284.8

Panmyelophthisis — continued
  congenital 284.0
  idiopathic 284.9
Panmyelosis (acute) (M9951/1) 238.7
Panner's disease 732.3
  capitellum humeri 732.3
  head of humerus 732.3
  tarsal navicular (bone) (osteochondrosis) 732.5
Panneuritis endemica 265.0 [357.4]
Panniculitis 729.30
  back 724.8
  knee 729.31
  neck 723.6
  nodular, nonsuppurative 729.30
  sacral 724.8
  specified site NEC 729.39
Panniculus adiposus (abdominal) 278.1
Pannus 370.62
  allergic eczematous 370.62
  degenerativus 370.62
  keratic 370.62
  rheumatoid — see Arthritis, rheumatoid
  trachomatosus, trachomatous (active) 076.1 [370.62]
    late effect 139.1
Panophthalmitis 360.02
Panotitis — see Otitis media
Pansinusitis (chronic) (hyperplastic) (nonpurulent) (purulent) 473.8
  acute 461.8
  due to fungus NEC 117.9
  tuberculous (see also Tuberculosis) 012.8 ✓5ᵗʰ
Panuveitis 360.12
  sympathetic 360.11
Panvalvular disease — see Endocarditis, mitral
Papageienkrankheit 073.9
Papanicolaou smear
  cervix (screening test) V76.2
    as part of gynecological examination V72.3
    for suspected malignant neoplasm V76.2
      no disease found V71.1
    nonspecific abnormal finding 795.00 ▲
      atypical squamous cell changes of ●
        undetermined significance ●
        favor benign (ASCUS favor benign) ●
          795.01
        favor dysplasia (ASCUS favor ●
          dysplasia) 795.02 ●
      nonspecific finding NEC 795.09 ●
      unsatisfactory 795.09 ●
    other specified site — see also Screening, malignant neoplasm
      for suspected malignant neoplasm — see also Screening, malignant neoplasm
      no disease found V71.1
      nonspecific abnormal finding 795.1
    vagina V76.47
      following hysterectomy for malignant condition V67.01
Papilledema 377.00
  associated with
    decreased ocular pressure 377.02
    increased intracranial pressure 377.01
    retinal disorder 377.03
  choked disc 377.00
  infectional 377.00
Papillitis 377.31
  anus 569.49
  chronic lingual 529.4
  necrotizing, kidney 584.7
  optic 377.31
  rectum 569.49
  renal, necrotizing 584.7
  tongue 529.0
Papilloma (M8050/0) — see also Neoplasm, by site, benign

Note — Except where otherwise indicated, the morphological varieties of papilloma in the list below should be coded by site as for "Neoplasm, benign."

  acuminatum (female) (male) 078.1 ✓5ᵗʰ

Papilloma (M8050/0) — see also Neoplasm, by site, benign — continued
  bladder (urinary) (transitional cell) (M8120/1) 236.7
    benign (M8120/0) 223.3
  choroid plexus (M9390/0) 225.0
    anaplastic type (M9390/3) 191.5
    malignant (M9390/3) 191.5
  ductal (M8503/0)
  dyskeratotic (M8052/0)
  epidermoid (M8052/0)
  hyperkeratotic (M8052/0)
  intracystic (M8504/0)
  intraductal (M8503/0)
  inverted (M8053/0)
  keratotic (M8052/0)
  parakeratotic (M8052/0)
  pinta (primary) 103.0
  renal pelvis (transitional cell) (M8120/1) 236.99
    benign (M8120/0) 223.1
  Schneiderian (M8121/0)
    specified site — see Neoplasm, by site, benign
    unspecified site 212.0
  serous surface (M8461/0)
    borderline malignancy (M8461/1)
      specified site — see Neoplasm, by site, uncertain behavior
      unspecified site 236.2
    specified site — see Neoplasm, by site, benign
    unspecified site 220
  squamous (cell) (M8052/0)
  transitional (cell) (M8120/0)
    bladder (urinary) (M8120/1) 236.7
    inverted type (M8121/1) — see Neoplasm, by site, uncertain behavior
    renal pelvis (M8120/1) 236.91
    ureter (M8120/1) 236.91
  ureter (transitional cell) (M8120/1) 236.91
    benign (M8120/0) 223.2
  urothelial (M8120/1) — see Neoplasm, by site, uncertain behavior
  verrucous (M8051/0)
  villous (M8261/1) — see Neoplasm, by site, uncertain behavior
  yaws, plantar or palmar 102.1
Papillomata, multiple, of yaws 102.1
Papillomatosis (M8060/0) — see also Neoplasm, by site, benign
  confluent and reticulate 701.8
  cutaneous 701.8
  ductal, breast 610.1
  Gougerot-Carteaud (confluent reticulate) 701.8
  intraductal (diffuse) (M8505/0) — see Neoplasm, by site, benign
  subareolar duct (M8506/0) 217
Papillon-Léage and Psaume syndrome (orodigitofacial dysostosis) 759.89
Papule 709.8
  carate (primary) 103.0
  fibrous, of nose (M8724/0) 216.3
  pinta (primary) 103.0
Papulosis, malignant 447.8
Papyraceous fetus 779.89 ▲
  complicating pregnancy 646.0 ✓5ᵗʰ
Paracephalus 759.7
Parachute mitral valve 746.5
Paracoccidioidomycosis 116.1
  mucocutaneous-lymphangitic 116.1
  pulmonary 116.1
  visceral 116.1
Paracoccidiomycosis — see Paracoccidioidomycosis
Paracusis 388.40
Paradentosis 523.5
Paradoxical facial movements 374.43
Paraffinoma 999.9
Paraganglioma (M8680/1)
  adrenal (M8700/0) 227.0
    malignant (M8700/3) 194.0
  aortic body (M8691/1) 237.3
    malignant (M8691/3) 194.6
  carotid body (M8692/1) 237.3
    malignant (M8692/3) 194.5

✓4ᵗʰ Fourth-digit Required   ✓5ᵗʰ Fifth-digit Required   ▶◀ Revised Text   ● New Line   ▲ Revised Code

Paraganglioma — *continued*
  chromaffin (M8700/0) — *see also* Neoplasm, by
      site, benign
    malignant (M8700/3) — *see* Neoplasm, by
        site, malignant
  extra-adrenal (M8693/1)
    malignant (M8693/3)
      specified site — *see* Neoplasm, by site,
          malignant
      unspecified site 194.6
    specified site — *see* Neoplasm, by site,
        uncertain behavior
    unspecified site 237.3
  glomus jugulare (M8690/1) 237.3
    malignant (M8690/3) 194.6
  jugular (M8690/1) 237.3
    malignant (M8680/3)
      specified site — *see* Neoplasm, by site,
          malignant
      unspecified site 194.6
  nonchromaffin (M8693/1)
    malignant (M8693/3)
      specified site — *see* Neoplasm, by site,
          malignant
      unspecified site 194.6
    specified site — *see* Neoplasm, by site,
        uncertain behavior
    unspecified site 237.3
  parasympathetic (M8682/1)
    specified site — *see* Neoplasm, by site,
        uncertain behavior
    unspecified site 237.3
  specified site — *see* Neoplasm, by site,
      uncertain behavior
  sympathetic (M8681/1)
    specified site — *see* Neoplasm, by site,
        uncertain behavior
    unspecified site 237.3
  unspecified site 237.3

Parageusia 781.1
  psychogenic 306.7

Paragonimiasis 121.2

Paragranuloma, Hodgkin's (M9660/3) 201.0 ✓5ᵗʰ

Parahemophilia (*see also* Defect, coagulation)
    286.3

Parakeratosis 690.8
  psoriasiformis 696.2
  variegata 696.2

Paralysis, paralytic (complete) (incomplete) 344.9
  with
    broken
      back — *see* Fracture, vertebra, by site,
          with spinal cord injury
      neck — *see* Fracture, vertebra, cervical,
          with spinal cord injury
    fracture, vertebra — *see* Fracture, vertebra,
        by site, with spinal cord injury
    syphilis 094.89
  abdomen and back muscles 355.9
  abdominal muscles 355.9
  abducens (nerve) 378.54
  abductor 355.9
    lower extremity 355.8
    upper extremity 354.9
  accessory nerve 352.4
  accommodation 367.51
    hysterical 300.11
  acoustic nerve 388.5
  agitans 332.0
    arteriosclerotic 332.0
  alternating 344.89
    oculomotor 344.89
  amyotrophic 335.20
  ankle 355.8
  anterior serratus 355.9
  anus (sphincter) 569.49
  apoplectic (current episode) (*see also* Disease,
      cerebrovascular, acute) 436
    late effect — *see* Late effect(s) (of)
        cerebrovascular disease
  arm 344.40
    affecting
      dominant side 344.41
      nondominant side 344.42
    both 344.2
    due to old CVA — *see* category 438 ✓4ᵗʰ

Paralysis, paralytic — *continued*
  arm — *continued*
    hysterical 300.11
    late effect — *see* Late effect(s) (of)
        cerebrovascular disease
    psychogenic 306.0transient 781.4
      traumatic NEC (*see also* Injury, nerve,
          upper limb) 955.9
  arteriosclerotic (current episode) 437.0
    late effect — *see* Late effect(s) (of)
        cerebrovascular disease
  ascending (spinal), acute 357.0
  associated, nuclear 344.89
  asthenic bulbar 358.0
  ataxic NEC 334.9
    general 094.1
  athetoid 333.7
  atrophic 356.9
    infantile, acute (*see also* Poliomyelitis, with
        paralysis) 045.1 ✓5ᵗʰ
    muscle NEC 355.9
    progressive 335.21
    spinal (acute) (*see also* Poliomyelitis, with
        paralysis) 045.1 ✓5ᵗʰ
  attack (*see also* Disease, cerebrovascular,
      acute) 436
  axillary 353.0
  Babinski-Nageotte's 344.89
  Bell's 351.0
    newborn 767.5
  Benedikt's 344.89
  birth (injury) 767.7
    brain 767.0
    intracranial 767.0
    spinal cord 767.4
  bladder (sphincter) 596.53
    neurogenic 596.54
      with cauda equina syndrome 344.61
    puerperal, postpartum, childbirth 665.5 ✓5ᵗʰ
    sensory 344.61
      with cauda equina 344.61
    spastic 344.61
      with cauda equina 344.61
  bowel, colon, or intestine (*see also* Ileus) 560.1
  brachial plexus 353.0
    due to birth injury 767.6
    newborn 767.6
  brain
    congenital — *see* Palsy, cerebral
    current episode 437.8
    diplegia 344.2
    due to previous vascular lesion — *see*
        category 438 ✓4ᵗʰ
    hemiplegia 342.9
      due to previous vascular lesion — *see*
          category 438 ✓4ᵗʰ
      late effect — *see* Late effect(s) (of)
          cerebrovascular disease
    infantile — *see* Palsy, cerebral
    late effect — *see* Late effect(s) (of)
        cerebrovascular disease
    monoplegia — *see also* Monoplegia
      due to previous vascular lesion — *see*
          category 438 ✓4ᵗʰ
      late effect — *see* Late effect(s) (of)
          cerebrovascular disease
    paraplegia 344.1
    quadriplegia — *see* Quadriplegia
    syphilitic, congenital 090.49
    triplegia 344.89
  bronchi 519.1
  Brown-Séquard's 344.89
  bulbar (chronic) (progressive) 335.22
    infantile (*see also* Poliomyelitis, bulbar)
        045.0 ✓5ᵗʰ
    poliomyelitic (*see also* Poliomyelitis, bulbar)
        045.0 ✓5ᵗʰ
    pseudo 335.23
    supranuclear 344.89
  bulbospinal 358.0
  cardiac (*see also* Failure, heart) 428.9
  cerebral
    current episode 437.8
    spastic, infantile — *see* Palsy, cerebral
  cerebrocerebellar 437.8
    diplegic infantile 343.0

Paralysis, paralytic — *continued*
  cervical
    plexus 353.2
    sympathetic NEC 337.0
  Céstan-Chenais 344.89
  Charcôt-Marie-Tooth type 356.1
  childhood — *see* Palsy, cerebral
  Clark's 343.9
  colon (*see also* Ileus) 560.1
  compressed air 993.3
  compression
    arm NEC 354.9
    cerebral — *see* Paralysis, brain
    leg NEC 355.8
    lower extremity NEC 355.8
    upper extremity NEC 354.9
  congenital (cerebral) (spastic) (spinal) — *see*
      Palsy, cerebral
  conjugate movement (of eye) 378.81
    cortical (nuclear) (supranuclear) 378.81
  convergence 378.83
  cordis (*see also* Failure, heart) 428.9
  cortical (*see also* Paralysis, brain) 437.8
  cranial or cerebral nerve (*see also* Disorder,
      nerve, cranial) 352.9
  creeping 335.21
  crossed leg 344.89
  crutch 953.4
  deglutition 784.9
    hysterical 300.11
  dementia 094.1
  descending (spinal) NEC 335.9
  diaphragm (flaccid) 519.4
    due to accidental section of phrenic nerve
        during procedure 998.2
  digestive organs NEC 564.89
  diplegic — *see* Diplegia
  divergence (nuclear) 378.85
  divers' 993.3
  Duchenne's 335.22
  due to intracranial or spinal birth injury — *see*
      Palsy, cerebral
  embolic (current episode) (*see also* Embolism,
      brain) 434.1 ✓5ᵗʰ
    late effect — *see* Late effect(s) (of)
        cerebrovascular disease
  enteric (*see also* Ileus) 560.1
    with hernia — *see* Hernia, by site, with
        obstruction
  Erb's syphilitic spastic spinal 094.89
  Erb (-Duchenne) (birth) (newborn) 767.6
  esophagus 530.8 ✓5ᵗʰ
  essential, infancy (*see also* Poliomyelitis)
      045.9 ✓5ᵗʰ
  extremity
    lower — *see* Paralysis, leg
      spastic (hereditary) 343.3
        noncongenital or noninfantile 344.1
        transient (cause unknown) 781.4
    upper — *see* Paralysis, arm
  eye muscle (extrinsic) 378.55
    intrinsic 367.51
  facial (nerve) 351.0
    birth injury 767.5
    congenital 767.5
    following operation NEC 998.2
    newborn 767.5
  familial 359.3
    periodic 359.3
    spastic 334.1
  fauces 478.29
  finger NEC 354.9
  foot NEC 355.8
  gait 781.2
  gastric nerve 352.3
  gaze 378.81
  general 094.1
    ataxic 094.1
    insane 094.1
    juvenile 090.40
    progressive 094.1
    tabetic 094.1
  glossopharyngeal (nerve) 352.2
  glottis (*see also* Paralysis, vocal cord) 478.30
  gluteal 353.4
  Gubler (-Millard) 344.89
  hand 354.9
    hysterical 300.11

Paralysis, paralytic — *continued*
　hand — *continued*
　　psychogenic 306.0
　heart (*see also* Failure, heart) 428.9
　hemifacial, progressive 349.89
　hemiplegic — *see* Hemiplegia
　hyperkalemic periodic (familial) 359.3
　hypertensive (current episode) 437.8
　hypoglossal (nerve) 352.5
　hypokalemic periodic 359.3
　Hyrtl's sphincter (rectum) 569.49
　hysterical 300.11
　ileus (*see also* Ileus) 560.1
　infantile (*see also* Poliomyelitis) 045.9 ✓5ᵗʰ
　　atrophic acute 045.1 ✓5ᵗʰ
　　bulbar 045.0 ✓5ᵗʰ
　　cerebral — *see* Palsy, cerebral
　　paralytic 045.1 ✓5ᵗʰ
　　progressive acute 045.9 ✓5ᵗʰ
　　spastic — *see* Palsy, cerebral
　　spinal 045.9 ✓5ᵗʰ
　infective (*see also* Poliomyelitis) 045.9 ✓5ᵗʰ
　inferior nuclear 344.9
　insane, general or progressive 094.1
　internuclear 378.86
　interosseous 355.9
　intestine (*see also* Ileus) 560.1
　intracranial (current episode) (*see also*
　　Paralysis, brain) 437.8
　　due to birth injury 767.0
　iris 379.49
　　due to diphtheria (toxin) 032.81 [379.49]
　ischemic, Volkmann's (complicating trauma)
　　958.6
　Jackson's 344.8 ✓5ᵗʰ
　jake 357.7
　Jamaica ginger (jake) 357.7
　juvenile general 090.40
　Klumpke (-Déjérine) (birth) (newborn) 767.6
　labioglossal (laryngeal) (pharyngeal) 335.22
　Landry's 357.0
　laryngeal nerve (recurrent) (superior) (*see also*
　　Paralysis, vocal cord) 478.30
　larynx (*see also* Paralysis, vocal cord) 478.30
　　due to diphtheria (toxin) 032.3
　late effect
　　due to
　　　birth injury, brain or spinal (cord) — *see*
　　　　Palsy, cerebral
　　　edema, brain or cerebral — *see* Paralysis,
　　　　brain
　　　lesion
　　　　cerebrovascular — *see* category
　　　　　438 ✓4ᵗʰ
　　　　late effect — *see* Late effect(s) (of)
　　　　　cerebrovascular disease
　　　spinal (cord) — *see* Paralysis, spinal
　lateral 335.24
　lead 984.9
　　specified type of lead — *see* Table of Drugs
　　　and Chemicals
　left side — *see* Hemiplegia
　leg 344.30
　　affecting
　　　dominant side 344.31
　　　nondominant side 344.32
　　both (*see also* Paraplegia) 344.1
　　crossed 344.89
　　hysterical 300.11
　　psychogenic 306.0
　　transient or transitory 781.4
　　　traumatic NEC (*see also* Injury, nerve,
　　　　lower limb) 956.9
　levator palpebrae superioris 374.31
　limb NEC 344.5
　　all four — *see* Quadriplegia
　　quadriplegia — *see* Quadriplegia
　lip 528.5
　Lissauer's 094.1
　local 355.9
　lower limb — see also Paralysis, leg
　　both (*see also* Paraplegia) 344.1
　lung 518.89
　　newborn 770.89　　　　　　　▲
　median nerve 354.1
　medullary (tegmental) 344.89

Paralysis, paralytic — *continued*
　mesencephalic NEC 344.89
　　tegmental 344.89
　middle alternating 344.89
　Millard-Gubler-Foville 344.89
　monoplegic — *see* Monoplegia
　motor NEC 344.9
　　cerebral — *see* Paralysis, brain
　　spinal — *see* Paralysis, spinal
　multiple
　　cerebral — *see* Paralysis, brain
　　spinal — *see* Paralysis, spinal
　muscle (flaccid) 359.9
　　due to nerve lesion NEC 355.9
　　eye (extrinsic) 378.55
　　　intrinsic 367.51
　　　oblique 378.51
　　iris sphincter 364.8
　　ischemic (complicating trauma) (Volkmann's)
　　　958.6
　　pseudohypertrophic 359.1
　muscular (atrophic) 359.9
　　progressive 335.21
　musculocutaneous nerve 354.9
　musculospiral 354.9
　nerve — *see also* Disorder, nerve
　　third or oculomotor (partial) 378.51
　　　total 378.52
　　fourth or trochlear 378.53
　　sixth or abducens 378.54
　　seventh or facial 351.0
　　　birth injury 767.5
　　　due to
　　　　injection NEC 999.9
　　　　operation NEC 997.09
　　　newborn 767.5
　　accessory 352.4
　　auditory 388.5
　　birth injury 767.7
　　cranial or cerebral (*see also* Disorder, nerve,
　　　cranial) 352.9
　　facial 351.0
　　　birth injury 767.5
　　　newborn 767.5
　　laryngeal (*see also* Paralysis, vocal cord)
　　　478.30
　　newborn 767.7
　　phrenic 354.8
　　　newborn 767.7
　　radial 354.3
　　　birth injury 767.6
　　　newborn 767.6
　　syphilitic 094.89
　　traumatic NEC (*see also* Injury, nerve, by
　　　site) 957.9
　　trigeminal 350.9
　　ulnar 354.2
　newborn NEC 767.0
　normokalemic periodic 359.3
　obstetrical, newborn 767.7
　ocular 378.9
　oculofacial, congenital 352.6
　oculomotor (nerve) (partial) 378.51
　　alternating 344.89
　　external bilateral 378.55
　　total 378.52
　olfactory nerve 352.0
　palate 528.9
　palatopharyngolaryngeal 352.6
　paratrigeminal 350.9
　periodic (familial) (hyperkalemic) (hypokalemic)
　　(normokalemic) (secondary) 359.3
　peripheral
　　autonomic nervous system — *see*
　　　Neuropathy, peripheral, autonomic
　　nerve NEC 355.9
　peroneal (nerve) 355.3
　pharynx 478.29
　phrenic nerve 354.8
　plantar nerves 355.6
　pneumogastric nerve 352.3
　poliomyelitis (current) (*see also* Poliomyelitis,
　　with paralysis) 045.1 ✓5ᵗʰ
　　bulbar 045.0 ✓5ᵗʰ
　popliteal nerve 355.3
　pressure (*see also* Neuropathy, entrapment)
　　355.9

Paralysis, paralytic — *continued*
　progressive 335.21
　　atrophic 335.21
　　bulbar 335.22
　　general 094.1
　　hemifacial 349.89
　　infantile, acute (*see also* Poliomyelitis)
　　　045.9 ✓5ᵗʰ
　　multiple 335.20
　pseudobulbar 335.23
　pseudohypertrophic 359.1
　　muscle 359.1
　psychogenic 306.0
　pupil, pupillary 379.49
　quadriceps 355.8
　quadriplegic (*see also* Quadriplegia) 344.0
　radial nerve 354.3
　　birth injury 767.6
　rectum (sphincter) 569.49
　rectus muscle (eye) 378.55
　recurrent laryngeal nerve (*see also* Paralysis,
　　vocal cord) 478.30
　respiratory (muscle) (system) (tract) 786.09
　　center NEC 344.89
　　　fetus or newborn 770.89　　　　　▲
　　congenital 768.9
　　newborn 768.9
　right side — *see* Hemiplegia
　Saturday night 354.3
　saturnine 984.9
　　specified type of lead — *see* Table of Drugs
　　　and Chemicals
　sciatic nerve 355.0
　secondary — *see* Paralysis, late effect
　seizure (cerebral) (current episode) (*see also*
　　Disease, cerebrovascular, acute) 436
　　late effect — *see* Late effect(s) (of)
　　　cerebrovascular disease
　senile NEC 344.9
　serratus magnus 355.9
　shaking (*see also* Parkinsonism) 332.0
　shock (*see also* Disease, cerebrovascular, acute)
　　436
　　late effect — *see* Late effect(s) (of)
　　　cerebrovascular disease
　shoulder 354.9
　soft palate 528.9
　spasmodic — *see* Paralysis, spastic
　spastic 344.9
　　cerebral infantile — *see* Palsy, cerebral
　　congenital (cerebral) — *see* Palsy, cerebral
　　familial 334.1
　　hereditary 334.1
　　infantile 343.9
　　noncongenital or noninfantile, cerebral
　　　344.9
　　syphilitic 094.0
　　　spinal 094.89
　sphincter, bladder (*see also* Paralysis, bladder)
　　596.53
　spinal (cord) NEC 344.1
　　accessory nerve 352.4
　　acute (*see also* Poliomyelitis) 045.9 ✓5ᵗʰ
　　ascending acute 357.0
　　atrophic (acute) (*see also* Poliomyelitis, with
　　　paralysis) 045.1 ✓5ᵗʰ
　　　spastic, syphilitic 094.89
　　congenital NEC 343.9
　　hemiplegic — *see* Hemiplegia
　　hereditary 336.8
　　infantile (*see also* Poliomyelitis) 045.9 ✓5ᵗʰ
　　late effect NEC 344.89
　　monoplegic — *see* Monoplegia
　　nerve 355.9
　　progressive 335.10
　　quadriplegic — *see* Quadriplegia
　　spastic NEC 343.9
　　traumatic — *see* Injury, spinal, by site
　sternomastoid 352.4
　stomach 536.3
　　nerve 352.3
　stroke (current episode) (*see also* Disease,
　　cerebrovascular, acute) 436
　　late effect — *see* Late effect(s) (of)
　　　cerebrovascular disease
　subscapularis 354.8
　superior nuclear NEC 334.9

Paralysis — Paretic

Paralysis, paralytic — *continued*
supranuclear 356.8
sympathetic
cervical NEC 337.0
nerve NEC (*see also* Neuropathy, peripheral, autonomic) 337.9
nervous system — *see* Neuropathy, peripheral, autonomic
syndrome 344.9
specified NEC 344.89
syphilitic spastic spinal (Erb's) 094.89
tabetic general 094.1
thigh 355.8
throat 478.29
diphtheritic 032.0
muscle 478.29
thrombotic (current episode) (*see also* Thrombosis, brain) 434.0 ✓5ᵗʰ
late effect — *see* Late effect(s) (of) cerebrovascular disease
old — *see* category 438 ✓4ᵗʰ
thumb NEC 354.9
tick (-bite) 989.5
Todd's (postepileptic transitory paralysis) 344.89
toe 355.6
tongue 529.8
transient
arm or leg NEC 781.4
traumatic NEC (*see also* Injury, nerve, by site) 957.9
trapezius 352.4
traumatic, transient NEC (*see also* Injury, nerve, by site) 957.9
trembling (*see also* Parkinsonism) 332.0
triceps brachii 354.9
trigeminal nerve 350.9
trochlear nerve 378.53
ulnar nerve 354.2
upper limb — *see also* Paralysis, arm
both (*see also* Diplegia) 344.2
uremic — *see* Uremia
uveoparotitic 135
uvula 528.9
hysterical 300.11
postdiphtheritic 032.0
vagus nerve 352.3
vasomotor NEC 337.9
velum palati 528.9
vesical (*see also* Paralysis, bladder) 596.53
vestibular nerve 388.5
visual field, psychic 368.16
vocal cord 478.30
bilateral (partial) 478.33
complete 478.34
complete (bilateral) 478.34
unilateral (partial) 478.31
complete 478.32
Volkmann's (complicating trauma) 958.6
wasting 335.21
Weber's 344.89
wrist NEC 354.9
Paramedial orifice, urethrovesical 753.8
Paramenia 626.9
Parametritis (chronic) (*see also* Disease, pelvis, inflammatory) 614.4
acute 614.3
puerperal, postpartum, childbirth 670 ✓4ᵗʰ
Parametrium, parametric — *see* condition
Paramnesia (*see also* Amnesia) 780.99 ▲
Paramolar 520.1
causing crowding 524.3
Paramyloidosis 277.3
Paramyoclonus multiplex 333.2
Paramyotonia 359.2
congenita 359.2
Paraneoplastic syndrome — *see* condition
Parangi (*see also* Yaws) 102.9
Paranoia 297.1
alcoholic 291.5
querulans 297.8
senile 290.20
Paranoid
dementia (*see also* Schizophrenia) 295.3 ✓5ᵗʰ
praecox (acute) 295.3 ✓5ᵗʰ
senile 290.20

Paranoid — *continued*
personality 301.0
psychosis 297.9
alcoholic 291.5
climacteric 297.2
drug-induced 292.11
involutional 297.2
menopausal 297.2
protracted reactive 298.4
psychogenic 298.4
acute 298.3
senile 290.20
reaction (chronic) 297.9
acute 298.3
schizophrenia (acute) (*see also* Schizophrenia) 295.3 ✓5ᵗʰ
state 297.9
alcohol-induced 291.5
climacteric 297.2
drug-induced 292.11
due to or associated with
arteriosclerosis (cerebrovascular) 290.42
presenile brain disease 290.12
senile brain disease 290.20
involutional 297.2
menopausal 297.2
senile 290.20
simple 297.0
specified type NEC 297.8
tendencies 301.0
traits 301.0
trends 301.0
type, psychopathic personality 301.0
Paraparesis (*see also* Paralysis) 344.9
Paraphasia 784.3
Paraphilia (*see also* Deviation, sexual) 302.9
Paraphimosis (congenital) 605
chancroidal 099.0
Paraphrenia, paraphrenic (late) 297.2
climacteric 297.2
dementia (*see also* Schizophrenia) 295.3 ✓5ᵗʰ
involutional 297.2
menopausal 297.2
schizophrenia (acute) (*see also* Schizophrenia) 295.3 ✓5ᵗʰ
Paraplegia 344.1
with
broken back — *see* Fracture, vertebra, by site, with spinal cord injury
fracture, vertebra — *see* Fracture, vertebra, by site, with spinal cord injury
ataxic — *see* Degeneration, combined, spinal cord
brain (current episode) (*see also* Paralysis, brain) 437.8
cerebral (current episode) (*see also* Paralysis, brain) 437.8
congenital or infantile (cerebral) (spastic) (spinal) 343.0
cortical — *see* Paralysis, brain
familial spastic 334.1
functional (hysterical) 300.11
hysterical 300.11
infantile 343.0
late effect 344.1
Pott's (*see also* Tuberculosis) 015.0 ✓5ᵗʰ [730.88]
psychogenic 306.0
spastic
Erb's spinal 094.89
hereditary 334.1
not infantile or congenital 344.1
spinal (cord)
traumatic NEC — *see* Injury, spinal, by site
syphilitic (spastic) 094.89
traumatic NEC — *see* Injury, spinal, by site
Paraproteinemia 273.2
benign (familial) 273.1
monoclonal 273.1
secondary to malignant or inflammatory disease 273.1
Parapsoriasis 696.2
en plaques 696.2
guttata 696.2

Parapsoriasis — *continued*
lichenoides chronica 696.2
retiformis 696.2
varioliformis (acuta) 696.2
Parascarlatina 057.8
Parasitic — *see also* condition
disease NEC (*see also* Infestation, parasitic) 136.9
contact V01.89 ▲
exposure to V01.89 ▲
intestinal NEC 129
skin NEC 134.9
stomatitis 112.0
sycosis 110.0
beard 110.0
scalp 110.0
twin 759.4
Parasitism NEC 136.9
intestinal NEC 129
skin NEC 134.9
specified — *see* Infestation
Parasitophobia 300.29
Parasomnia 780.59
nonorganic origin 307.47
Paraspadias 752.69
Paraspasm facialis 351.8
Parathyroid gland — *see* condition
Parathyroiditis (autoimmune) 252.1
Parathyroprival tetany 252.1
Paratrachoma 077.0
Paratyphilitis (*see also* Appendicitis) 541
Paratyphoid (fever) — *see* Fever, paratyphoid
Paratyphus — *see* Fever, paratyphoid
Paraurethral duct 753.8
Para-urethritis 597.89
gonococcal (acute) 098.0
chronic or duration of 2 months or over 098.2
Paravaccinia NEC 051.9
milkers' node 051.1
Paravaginitis (*see also* Vaginitis) 616.10
Parencephalitis (*see also* Encephalitis) 323.9
late effect — *see* category 326
Parergasia 298.9
Paresis (*see also* Paralysis) 344.9
accommodation 367.51
bladder (spastic) (sphincter) (*see also* Paralysis, bladder) 596.53
tabetic 094.0
bowel, colon, or intestine (*see also* Ileus) 560.1
brain or cerebral — *see* Paralysis, brain
extrinsic muscle, eye 378.55
general 094.1
arrested 094.1
brain 094.1
cerebral 094.1
insane 094.1
juvenile 090.40
remission 090.49
progressive 094.1
remission (sustained) 094.1
tabetic 094.1
heart (*see also* Failure, heart) 428.9
infantile (*see also* Poliomyelitis) 045.9 ✓5ᵗʰ
insane 094.1
juvenile 090.40
late effect — *see* Paralysis, late effect
luetic (general) 094.1
peripheral progressive 356.9
pseudohypertrophic 359.1
senile NEC 344.9
stomach 536.3
syphilitic (general) 094.1
congenital 090.40
transient, limb 781.4
vesical (sphincter) NEC 596.53
Paresthesia (*see also* Disturbance, sensation) 782.0
Berger's (paresthesia of lower limb) 782.0
Bernhardt 355.1
Magnan's 782.0
Paretic — *see* condition

Parinaud's
conjunctivitis 372.02
oculoglandular syndrome 372.02
ophthalmoplegia 378.81
syndrome (paralysis of conjugate upward gaze) 378.81
Parkes Weber and Dimitri syndrome (encephalocutaneous angiomatosis) 759.6
Parkinson's disease, syndrome, or tremor — see Parkinsonism
Parkinsonism (arteriosclerotic) (idiopathic) (primary) 332.0
associated with orthostatic hypotension (idiopathic) (symptomatic) 333.0
due to drugs 332.1
secondary 332.1
syphilitic 094.82
Parodontitis 523.4
Parodontosis 523.5
Paronychia (with lymphangitis) 681.9
candidal (chronic) 112.3
chronic 681.9
candidal 112.3
finger 681.02
toe 681.11
finger 681.02
toe 681.11
tuberculous (primary) (see also Tuberculosis) 017.0 ✓5ᵗʰ
Parorexia NEC 307.52
hysterical 300.11
Parosmia 781.1
psychogenic 306.7
Parotid gland — see condition
Parotiditis (see also Parotitis) 527.2
epidemic 072.9
infectious 072.9
Parotitis 527.2
allergic 527.2
chronic 527.2
epidemic (see also Mumps) 072.9
infectious (see also Mumps) 072.9
noninfectious 527.2
nonspecific toxic 527.2
not mumps 527.2
postoperative 527.2
purulent 527.2
septic 527.2
suppurative (acute) 527.2
surgical 527.2
toxic 527.2
Paroxysmal — see also condition
dyspnea (nocturnal) 786.09
Parrot's disease (syphilitic osteochondritis) 090.0
Parrot fever 073.9
Parry's disease or syndrome (exophthalmic goiter) 242.0 ✓5ᵗʰ
Parry-Romberg syndrome 349.89
Parson's disease (exophthalmic goiter) 242.0 ✓5ᵗʰ
Parsonage-Aldren-Turner syndrome 353.5
Parsonage-Turner syndrome 353.5
Pars planitis 363.21
Particolored infant 757.39
Parturition — see Delivery
Passage
false, urethra 599.4
of sounds or bougies (see also Attention to artificial opening) V55.9
Passive — see condition
Pasteurella septica 027.2
Pasteurellosis (see also Infection, Pasteurella) 027.2
PAT (paroxysmal atrial tachycardia) 427.0
Patau's syndrome (trisomy D) 758.1
Patch
herald 696.3
Patches
mucous (syphilitic) 091.3
congenital 090.0
smokers' (mouth) 528.6
Patellar — see condition

Patellofemoral syndrome 719.46
Patent — see also Imperfect closure
atrioventricular ostium 745.69
canal of Nuck 752.41
cervix 622.5
complicating pregnancy 654.5 ✓5ᵗʰ
affecting fetus or newborn 761.0
ductus arteriosus or Botalli 747.0
Eustachian
tube 381.7
valve 746.89
foramen
Botalli 745.5
ovale 745.5
interauricular septum 745.5
interventricular septum 745.4
omphalomesenteric duct 751.0
os (uteri) — see Patent, cervix
ostium secundum 745.5
urachus 753.7
vitelline duct 751.0
Paternity testing V70.4
Paterson's syndrome (sideropenic dysphagia) 280.8
Paterson (-Brown) (-Kelly) syndrome (sideropenic dysphagia) 280.8
Paterson-Kelly syndrome or web (sideropenic dysphagia) 280.8
Pathologic, pathological — see also condition
asphyxia 799.0
drunkenness 291.4
emotionality 301.3
liar 301.7
personality 301.9
resorption, tooth 521.4
sexuality (see also Deviation, sexual) 302.9
Pathology (of) — see Disease
Patterned motor discharge, idiopathic (see also Epilepsy) 345.5 ✓5ᵗʰ
Patulous — see also Patent
anus 569.49
Eustachian tube 381.7
Pause, sinoatrial 427.81
Pavor nocturnus 307.46
Pavy's disease 593.6
Paxton's disease (white piedra) 111.2
Payr's disease or syndrome (splenic flexure syndrome) 569.89
Pearls
Elschnig 366.51
enamel 520.2
Pearl-workers' disease (chronic osteomyelitis) (see also Osteomyelitis) 730.1 ✓5ᵗʰ
Pectenitis 569.49
Pectenosis 569.49
Pectoral — see condition
Pectus
carinatum (congenital) 754.82
acquired 738.3
rachitic (see also Rickets) 268.0
excavatum (congenital) 754.81
acquired 738.3
rachitic (see also Rickets) 268.0
recurvatum (congenital) 754.81
acquired 738.3
Pedatrophia 261
Pederosis 302.2
Pediculosis (infestation) 132.9
capitis (head louse) (any site) 132.0
corporis (body louse) (any site) 132.1
eyelid 132.0 [373.6]
mixed (classifiable to more than one category in 132.0-132.2) 132.3
pubis (pubic louse) (any site) 132.2
vestimenti 132.1
vulvae 132.2
Pediculus (infestation) — see Pediculosis
Pedophilia 302.2
Peg-shaped teeth 520.2
Pel's crisis 094.0
Pel-Ebstein disease — see Disease, Hodgkin's
Pelade 704.01

Pelger-Huât anomaly or syndrome (hereditary hyposegmentation) 288.2
Peliosis (rheumatica) 287.0
Pelizaeus-Merzbacher
disease 330.0
sclerosis, diffuse cerebral 330.0
Pellagra (alcoholic or with alcoholism) 265.2
with polyneuropathy 265.2 [357.4]
Pellagra-cerebellar-ataxia-renal aminoaciduria syndrome 270.0
Pellegrini's disease (calcification, knee joint) 726.62
Pellegrini (-Stieda) disease or syndrome (calcification, knee joint) 726.62
Pellizzi's syndrome (pineal) 259.8
Pelvic — see also condition
congestion-fibrosis syndrome 625.5
kidney 753.3
Pelvioectasis 591
Pelviolithiasis 592.0
Pelviperitonitis
female (see also Peritonitis, pelvic, female) 614.5
male (see also Peritonitis) 567.2
Pelvis, pelvic — see also condition or type
infantile 738.6
Nägele's 738.6
obliquity 738.6
Robert's 755.69
Pemphigoid 694.5
benign, mucous membrane 694.60
with ocular involvement 694.61
bullous 694.5
cicatricial 694.60
with ocular involvement 694.61
juvenile 694.2
Pemphigus 694.4
benign 694.5
chronic familial 757.39
Brazilian 694.4
circinatus 694.0
congenital, traumatic 757.39
conjunctiva 694.61
contagiosus 684
erythematodes 694.4
erythematosus 694.4
foliaceus 694.4
frambesiodes 694.4
gangrenous (see also Gangrene) 785.4
malignant 694.4
neonatorum, newborn 684
ocular 694.61
papillaris 694.4
seborrheic 694.4
South American 694.4
syphilitic (congenital) 090.0
vegetans 694.4
vulgaris 694.4
wildfire 694.4
Pendred's syndrome (familial goiter with deaf-mutism) 243
Pendulous
abdomen 701.9
in pregnancy or childbirth 654.4 ✓5ᵗʰ
affecting fetus or newborn 763.89
breast 611.8
Penetrating wound — see also Wound, open, by site
with internal injury — see Injury, internal, by site, with open wound
eyeball 871.7
with foreign body (nonmagnetic) 871.6
magnetic 871.5
ocular (see also Penetrating wound, eyeball) 871.7
adnexa 870.3
with foreign body 870.4
orbit 870.3
with foreign body 870.4
Penetration, pregnant uterus by instrument
with
abortion — see Abortion, by type, with damage to pelvic organs

---

Penetration, pregnant uterus by instrument —
    continued
  with — *continued*
    ectopic pregnancy (*see also* categories
        633.0-633.9) 639.2
    molar pregnancy (*see also* categories 630-
        632) 639.2
  complication of delivery 665.1 ✔5ᵗʰ
    affecting fetus or newborn 763.89
  following
    abortion 639.2
    ectopic or molar pregnancy 639.2
Penfield's syndrome (*see also* Epilepsy)
    345.5 ✔5ᵗʰ
Penicilliosis of lung 117.3
Penis — *see* condition
Penitis 607.2
Penta X syndrome 758.81
Pentalogy (of Fallot) 745.2
Pentosuria (benign) (essential) 271.8
Peptic acid disease 536.8
Peregrinating patient V65.2
Perforated — *see* Perforation
Perforation, perforative (nontraumatic)
  antrum (*see also* Sinusitis, maxillary) 473.0
  appendix 540.0
    with peritoneal abscess 540.1
  atrial septum, multiple 745.5
  attic, ear 384.22
    healed 384.81
  bile duct, except cystic (*see also* Disease,
      biliary) 576.3
    cystic 575.4
  bladder (urinary) 596.6
    with
      abortion — *see* Abortion, by type, with
          damage to pelvic organs
      ectopic pregnancy (*see also* categories
          633.0-633.9) 639.2
      molar pregnancy (*see also* categories 630-
          632) 639.2
    following
      abortion 639.2
      ectopic or molar pregnancy 639.2
    obstetrical trauma 665.5 ✔5ᵗʰ
  bowel 569.83
    with
      abortion — *see* Abortion, by type, with
          damage to pelvic organs
      ectopic pregnancy (*see also* categories
          633.0-633.9) 639.2
      molar pregnancy (*see also* categories 630-
          632) 639.2
    fetus or newborn 777.6
    following
      abortion 639.2
      ectopic or molar pregnancy 639.2
    obstetrical trauma 665.5 ✔5ᵗʰ
  broad ligament
    with
      abortion — *see* Abortion, by type, with
          damage to pelvic organs
      ectopic pregnancy (*see also* categories
          633.0-633.9) 639.2
      molar pregnancy (*see also* categories 630-
          632) 639.2
    following
      abortion 639.2
      ectopic or molar pregnancy 639.2
    obstetrical trauma 665.6 ✔5ᵗʰ
  by
    device, implant, or graft — *see*
        Complications, mechanical
    foreign body left accidentally in operation
        wound 998.4
    instrument (any) during a procedure,
        accidental 998.2
  cecum 540.0
    with peritoneal abcess 540.1
  cervix (uteri) — *see also* Injury, internal, cervix
    with
      abortion — *see* Abortion, by type, with
          damage to pelvic organs
      ectopic pregnancy (*see also* categories
          633.0-633.9) 639.2

Perforation, perforative — *continued*
  cervix (uteri) — *see also* Injury, internal, cervix
      — *continued*
    with — *continued*
      molar pregnancy (*see also* categories 630-
          632) 639.2
    following
      abortion 639.2
      ectopic or molar pregnancy 639.2
    obstetrical trauma 665.3 ✔5ᵗʰ
  colon 569.83
  common duct (bile) 576.3
  cornea (*see also* Ulcer, cornea) 370.00
    due to ulceration 370.06
  cystic duct 575.4
  diverticulum (*see also* Diverticula) 562.10
    small intestine 562.00
  duodenum, duodenal (ulcer) — *see* Ulcer,
      duodenum, with perforation
  ear drum — *see* Perforation, tympanum
  enteritis — *see* Enteritis
  esophagus 530.4
  ethmoidal sinus (*see also* Sinusitis, ethmoidal)
      473.2
  foreign body (external site) — *see also* Wound,
      open, by site, complicated
    internal site, by ingested object — *see*
        Foreign body
  frontal sinus (*see also* Sinusitis, frontal) 473.1
  gallbladder or duct (*see also* Disease,
      gallbladder) 575.4
  gastric (ulcer) — *see* Ulcer, stomach, with
      perforation
  heart valve — *see* Endocarditis
  ileum (*see also* Perforation, intestine) 569.83
  instrumental
    external — *see* Wound, open, by site
    pregnant uterus, complicating delivery
        665.9 ✔5ᵗʰ
    surgical (accidental) (blood vessel) (nerve)
        (organ) 998.2
  intestine 569.83
    with
      abortion — *see* Abortion, by type, with
          damage to pelvic organs
      ectopic pregnancy (*see also* categories
          633.0-633.9) 639.2
      molar pregnancy (*see also* categories 630-
          632) 639.2
    fetus or newborn 777.6
    obstetrical trauma 665.5 ✔5ᵗʰ
    ulcerative NEC 569.83
  jejunum, jejunal 569.83
    ulcer — *see* Ulcer, gastrojejunal, with
        perforation
  mastoid (antrum) (cell) 383.89
  maxillary sinus (*see also* Sinusitis, maxillary)
      473.0
  membrana tympani — *see* Perforation,
      tympanum
  nasal
    septum 478.1
      congenital 748.1
      syphilitic 095.8
    sinus (*see also* Sinusitis) 473.9
      congenital 748.1
  palate (hard) 526.89
    soft 528.9
      syphilitic 095.8
        syphilitic 095.8
  palatine vault 526.89
    syphilitic 095.8
      congenital 090.5
  pelvic
    floor
      with
        abortion — *see* Abortion, by type, with
            damage to pelvic organs
        ectopic pregnancy (*see also* categories
            633.0-633.9) 639.2
        molar pregnancy (*see also* categories
            630-632) 639.2
      obstetrical trauma 664.1 ✔5ᵗʰ
    organ
      with
        abortion — *see* Abortion, by type, with
            damage to pelvic organs

Perforation, perforative — *continued*
  pelvic — *continued*
    organ — *continued*
      with — *continued*
        ectopic pregnancy (*see also* categories
            633.0-633.9) 639.2
        molar pregnancy (*see also* categories
            630-632) 639.2
      following
        abortion 639.2
        ectopic or molar pregnancy 639.2
      obstetrical trauma 665.5 ✔5ᵗʰ
  perineum — *see* Laceration, perineum
  periurethral tissue
    with
      abortion — *see* Abortion, by type, with
          damage to pelvic organs
      ectopic pregnancy (*see also* categories
          630-632) 639.2
      molar pregnancy (*see also* categories 630-
          632) 639.2
  pharynx 478.29
  pylorus, pyloric (ulcer) — *see* Ulcer, stomach,
      with perforation
  rectum 569.49
  sigmoid 569.83
  sinus (accessory) (chronic) (nasal) (*see also*
      Sinusitis) 473.9
  sphenoidal sinus (*see also* Sinusitis,
      sphenoidal) 473.3
  stomach (due to ulcer) — *see* Ulcer, stomach,
      with perforation
  surgical (accidental) (by instrument) (blood
      vessel) (nerve) (organ) 998.2
  traumatic
    external — *see* Wound, open, by site
    eye (*see also* Penetrating wound, ocular)
        871.7
    internal organ — *see* Injury, internal, by site
  tympanum (membrane) (persistent
      posttraumatic) (postinflammatory) 384.20
    with
      otitis media — *see* Otitis media
    attic 384.22
    central 384.21
    healed 384.81
    marginal NEC 384.23
    multiple 384.24
    pars flaccida 384.22
    total 384.25
    traumatic — *see* Wound, open, ear, drum
  typhoid, gastrointestinal 002.0
  ulcer — *see* Ulcer, by site, with perforation
  ureter 593.89
  urethra
    with
      abortion — *see* Abortion, by type, with
          damage to pelvic organs
      ectopic pregnancy (*see also* categories
          633.0-633.9) 639.2
      molar pregnancy (*see also* categories 630-
          632) 639.2
    following
      abortion 639.2
      ectopic or molar pregnancy 639.2
    obstetrical trauma 665.5 ✔5ᵗʰ
  uterus — *see also* Injury, internal, uterus
    with
      abortion — *see* Abortion, by type, with
          damage to pelvic organs
      ectopic pregnancy (*see also* categories
          633.0-633.9) 639.2
      molar pregnancy (*see also* categories 630-
          632) 639.2
    by intrauterine contraceptive device 996.32
    following
      abortion 639.2
      ectopic or molar pregnancy 639.2
    obstetrical trauma — *see* Injury, internal,
        uterus, obstetrical trauma
  uvula 528.9
    syphilitic 095.8
  vagina — *see* Laceration, vagina
  viscus NEC 799.8
    traumatic 868.00
      with open wound into cavity 868.10
Periadenitis mucosa necrotica recurrens 528.2

✔4ᵗʰ Fourth-digit Required   ✔5ᵗʰ Fifth-digit Required   ▶◀ Revised Text   ● New Line   ▲ Revised Code

Periangiitis 446.0
Periantritis 535.4 ✓5ᵗʰ
Periappendicitis (acute) (see also Appendicitis) 541
Periarteritis (disseminated) (infectious) (necrotizing) (nodosa) 446.0
Periarthritis (joint) 726.90
  Duplay's 726.2
  gonococcal 098.50
  humeroscapularis 726.2
  scapulohumeral 726.2
  shoulder 726.2
  wrist 726.4
Periarthrosis (angioneural) — see Periarthritis
Peribronchitis 491.9
  tuberculous (see also Tuberculosis) 011.3 ✓5ᵗʰ
Pericapsulitis, adhesive (shoulder) 726.0
Pericarditis (granular) (with decompensation) (with effusion) 423.9
  with
    rheumatic fever (conditions classifiable to 390)
      active (see also Pericarditis, rheumatic) 391.0
      inactive or quiescent 393
  actinomycotic 039.8 [420.0]
  acute (nonrheumatic) 420.90
    with chorea (acute) (rheumatic) (Sydenham's) 392.0
    bacterial 420.99
    benign 420.91
    hemorrhagic 420.90
    idiopathic 420.91
    infective 420.90
    nonspecific 420.91
    rheumatic 391.0
      with chorea (acute) (rheumatic) (Sydenham's) 392.0
    sicca 420.90
    viral 420.91
  adhesive or adherent (external) (internal) 423.1
    acute — see Pericarditis, acute
    rheumatic (external) (internal) 393
  amebic 006.8 [420.0]
  bacterial (acute) (subacute) (with serous or seropurulent effusion) 420.99
  calcareous 423.2
  cholesterol (chronic) 423.8
    acute 420.90
  chronic (nonrheumatic) 423.8
    rheumatic 393
  constrictive 423.2
  Coxsackie 074.21
  due to
    actinomycosis 039.8 [420.0]
    amebiasis 006.8 [420.0]
    Coxsackie (virus) 074.21
    histoplasmosis (see also Histoplasmosis) 115.93
    nocardiosis 039.8 [420.0]
    tuberculosis (see also Tuberculosis) 017.9 ✓5ᵗʰ [420.0]
  fibrinocaseous (see also Tuberculosis) 017.9 ✓5ᵗʰ [420.0]
  fibrinopurulent 420.99
  fibrinous — see Pericarditis, rheumatic
  fibropurulent 420.99
  fibrous 423.1
  gonococcal 098.83
  hemorrhagic 423.0
  idiopathic (acute) 420.91
  infective (acute) 420.90
  meningococcal 036.41
  neoplastic (chronic) 423.8
    acute 420.90
  nonspecific 420.91
  obliterans, obliterating 423.1
  plastic 423.1
  pneumococcal (acute) 420.99
  postinfarction 411.0
  purulent (acute) 420.99
  rheumatic (active) (acute) (with effusion) (with pneumonia) 391.0
    with chorea (acute) (rheumatic) (Sydenham's) 392.0
    chronic or inactive (with chorea) 393

Pericarditis — continued
  septic (acute) 420.99
  serofibrinous — see Pericarditis, rheumatic
  staphylococcal (acute) 420.99
  streptococcal (acute) 420.99
  suppurative (acute) 420.99
  syphilitic 093.81
  tuberculous (acute) (chronic) (see also Tuberculosis) 017.9 ✓5ᵗʰ [420.0]
  uremic 585 [420.0]
  viral (acute) 420.91
Pericardium, pericardial — see condition
Pericellulitis (see also Cellulitis) 682.9
Pericementitis 523.4
  acute 523.3
  chronic (suppurative) 523.4
Pericholecystitis (see also Cholecystitis) 575.10
Perichondritis
  auricle 380.00
    acute 380.01
    chronic 380.02
  bronchus 491.9
  ear (external) 380.00
    acute 380.01
    chronic 380.02
  larynx 478.71
    syphilitic 095.8
    typhoid 002.0 [478.71]
  nose 478.1
  pinna 380.00
    acute 380.01
    chronic 380.02
  trachea 478.9
Periclasia 523.5
Pericolitis 569.89
Pericoronitis (chronic) 523.4
  acute 523.3
Pericystitis (see also Cystitis) 595.9
Pericytoma (M9150/1) — see also Neoplasm, connective tissue, uncertain behavior
  benign (M9150/0) — see Neoplasm, connective tissue, benign
  malignant (M9150/3) — see Neoplasm, connective tissue, malignant
Peridacryocystitis, acute 375.32
Peridiverticulitis (see also Diverticulitis) 562.11
Periduodenitis 535.6 ✓5ᵗʰ
Periendocarditis (see also Endocarditis) 424.90
  acute or subacute 421.9
Periepididymitis (see also Epididymitis) 604.90
Perifolliculitis (abscedens) 704.8
  capitis, abscedens et suffodiens 704.8
  dissecting, scalp 704.8
  scalp 704.8
  superficial pustular 704.8
Perigastritis (acute) 535.0 ✓5ᵗʰ
Perigastrojejunitis (acute) 535.0 ✓5ᵗʰ
Perihepatitis (acute) 573.3
  chlamydial 099.56
  gonococcal 098.86
Peri-ileitis (subacute) 569.89
Perilabyrinthitis (acute) — see Labyrinthitis
Perimeningitis — see Meningitis
Perimetritis (see also Endometritis) 615.9
Perimetrosalpingitis (see also Salpingo-oophoritis) 614.2
Perinephric — see condition
Perinephritic — see condition
Perinephritis (see also Infection, kidney) 590.9
  purulent (see also Abscess, kidney) 590.2
Perineum, perineal — see condition
Perineuritis NEC 729.2
Periodic — see also condition
  disease (familial) 277.3
  edema 995.1
    hereditary 277.6
  fever 277.3
  paralysis (familial) 359.3
  peritonitis 277.3
  polyserositis 277.3
  somnolence 347

Periodontal
  cyst 522.8
  pocket 523.8
Periodontitis (chronic) (complex) (compound) (local) (simplex) 523.4
  acute 523.3
  apical 522.6
    acute (pulpal origin) 522.4
Periodontoclasia 523.5
Periodontosis 523.5
Periods — see also Menstruation
  heavy 626.2
  irregular 626.4
Perionychia (with lymphangitis) 681.9
  finger 681.02
  toe 681.11
Perioophoritis (see also Salpingo-oophoritis) 614.2
Periorchitis (see also Orchitis) 604.90
Periosteum, periosteal — see condition
Periostitis (circumscribed) (diffuse) (infective) 730.3 ✓5ᵗʰ

Note — Use the following fifth-digit subclassification with category 730:

  0   site unspecified
  1   shoulder region
  2   upper arm
  3   forearm
  4   hand
  5   pelvic region and thigh
  6   lower leg
  7   ankle and foot
  8   other specified sites
  9   multiple sites
---

  with osteomyelitis (see also Osteomyelitis) 730.2 ✓5ᵗʰ
    acute or subacute 730.0 ✓5ᵗʰ
    chronic or old 730.1 ✓5ᵗʰ
  albuminosa, albuminosus 730.3 ✓5ᵗʰ
  alveolar 526.5
  alveolodental 526.5
  dental 526.5
  gonorrheal 098.89
  hyperplastica, generalized 731.2
  jaw (lower) (upper) 526.4
  monomelic 733.99
  orbital 376.02
  syphilitic 095.5
    congenital 090.0 [730.8] ✓5ᵗʰ
    secondary 091.61
  tuberculous (see also Tuberculosis, bone) 015.9 ✓5ᵗʰ [730.8] ✓5ᵗʰ
  yaws (early) (hypertrophic) (late) 102.6
Periostosis (see also Periostitis) 730.3 ✓5ᵗʰ
  with osteomyelitis (see also Osteomyelitis) 730.2 ✓5ᵗʰ
    acute or subacute 730.0 ✓5ᵗʰ
    chronic or old 730.1 ✓5ᵗʰ
  hyperplastic 756.59
Periphlebitis (see also Phlebitis) 451.9
  lower extremity 451.2
    deep (vessels) 451.19
    superficial (vessels) 451.0
  portal 572.1
  retina 362.18
  superficial (vessels) 451.0
  tuberculous (see also Tuberculosis) 017.9 ✓5ᵗʰ
    retina 017.3 ✓5ᵗʰ [362.18]
Peripneumonia — see Pneumonia
Periproctitis 569.49
Periprostatitis (see also Prostatitis) 601.9
Perirectal — see condition
Perirenal — see condition
Perisalpingitis (see also Salpingo-oophoritis) 614.2
Perisigmoiditis 569.89
Perisplenitis (infectional) 289.59
Perispondylitis — see Spondylitis
Peristalsis reversed or visible 787.4

Peritendinitis (*see also* Tenosynovitis) 726.90
  adhesive (shoulder) 726.0
Perithelioma (M9150/1) — *see* Pericytoma
Peritoneum, peritoneal — *see also* condition
  equilibration test V56.32
Peritonitis (acute) (adhesive) (fibrinous)
    (hemorrhagic) (idiopathic) (localized)
    (perforative) (primary) (with adhesions) (with
    effusion) 567.9
  with or following
    abortion — *see* Abortion, by type, with
      sepsis
    abscess 567.2
    appendicitis 540.0
      with peritoneal abcess 540.1
    ectopic pregnancy (*see also* categories
      633.0-633.9) 639.0
    molar pregnancy (*see also* categories 630-
      632) 639.0
  aseptic 998.7
  bacterial 567.2
  bile, biliary 567.8
  chemical 998.7
  chlamydial 099.56
  chronic proliferative 567.8
  congenital NEC 777.6
  diaphragmatic 567.2
  diffuse NEC 567.2
  diphtheritic 032.83
  disseminated NEC 567.2
  due to
    bile 567.8
    foreign
      body or object accidentally left during a
        procedure (instrument) (sponge)
        (swab) 998.4
      substance accidentally left during a
        procedure (chemical) (powder) (talc)
        998.7
    talc 998.7
    urine 567.8
  fibrinopurulent 567.2
  fibrinous 567.2
  fibrocaseous (*see also* Tuberculosis) 014.0 ✔5ᵗʰ
  fibropurulent 567.2
  general, generalized (acute) 567.2
  gonococcal 098.86
  in infective disease NEC 136.9 *[567.0]*
  meconium (newborn) 777.6
  pancreatic 577.8
  paroxysmal, benign 277.3
  pelvic
    female (acute) 614.5
      chronic NEC 614.7
        with adhesions 614.6
      puerperal, postpartum, childbirth
        670 ✔4ᵗʰ
    male (acute) 567.2
  periodic (familial) 277.3
  phlegmonous 567.2
  pneumococcal 567.1
  postabortal 639.0
  proliferative, chronic 567.8
  puerperal, postpartum, childbirth 670 ✔4ᵗʰ
  purulent 567.2
  septic 567.2
  staphylococcal 567.2
  streptococcal 567.2
  subdiaphragmatic 567.2
  subphrenic 567.2
  suppurative 567.2
  syphilitic 095.2
    congenital 090.0 *[567.0]*
  talc 998.7
  tuberculous (*see also* Tuberculosis) 014.0 ✔5ᵗʰ
  urine 567.8
Peritonsillar — *see* condition
Peritonsillitis 475
Perityphlitis (*see also* Appendicitis) 541
Periureteritis 593.89
Periurethral — *see* condition
Periurethritis (gangrenous) 597.89
Periuterine — *see* condition
Perivaginitis (*see also* Vaginitis) 616.10
Perivasculitis, retinal 362.18

Perivasitis (chronic) 608.4
Periventricular leukomalacia 779.7
Perivesiculitis (seminal) (*see also* Vesiculitis)
  608.0
Perlèche 686.8
  due to
    moniliasis 112.0
    riboflavin deficiency 266.0
Pernicious — *see* condition
Pernio, perniosis 991.5
Persecution
  delusion 297.9
  social V62.4
Perseveration (tonic) 784.69
Persistence, persistent (congenital) 759.89
  anal membrane 751.2
  arteria stapedia 744.04
  atrioventricular canal 745.69
  bloody ejaculate 792.2
  branchial cleft 744.41
  bulbus cordis in left ventricle 745.8
  canal of Cloquet 743.51
  capsule (opaque) 743.51
  cilioretinal artery or vein 743.51
  cloaca 751.5
  communication — *see* Fistula, congenital
  convolutions
    aortic arch 747.21
    fallopian tube 752.19
    oviduct 752.19
    uterine tube 752.19
  double aortic arch 747.21
  ductus
    arteriosus 747.0
    Botalli 747.0
  fetal
    circulation 747.83 ▲
    form of cervix (uteri) 752.49
    hemoglobin (hereditary) ("Swiss variety")
      282.7
    pulmonary hypertension 747.83 ▲
  foramen
    Botalli 745.5
    ovale 745.5
  Gartner's duct 752.11
  hemoglobin, fetal (hereditary) (HPFH) 282.7
  hyaloid
    artery (generally incomplete) 743.51
    system 743.51
  hymen (tag)
    in pregnancy or childbirth 654.8 ✔5ᵗʰ
      causing obstructed labor 660.2 ✔5ᵗʰ
  lanugo 757.4
  left
    posterior cardinal vein 747.49
    root with right arch of aorta 747.21
    superior vena cava 747.49
  Meckel's diverticulum 751.0
  mesonephric duct 752.8
    fallopian tube 752.11
  mucosal disease (middle ear) (with posterior or
    superior marginal perforation of ear
    drum) 382.2
  nail(s), anomalous 757.5
  occiput, anterior or posterior 660.3 ✔5ᵗʰ
    fetus or newborn 763.1
  omphalomesenteric duct 751.0
  organ or site NEC — *see* Anomaly, specified
    type NEC
  ostium
    atrioventriculare commune 745.69
    primum 745.61
    secundum 745.5
  ovarian rests in fallopian tube 752.19
  pancreatic tissue in intestinal tract 751.5
  primary (deciduous)
    teeth 520.6
    vitreous hyperplasia 743.51
  pulmonary hypertension 747.83 ▲
  pupillary membrane 743.46
    iris 743.46
  Rhesus (Rh) titer 999.7
  right aortic arch 747.21
  sinus
    urogenitalis 752.8

Persistence, persistent — *continued*
  sinus — *continued*
    venosus with imperfect incorporation in
      right auricle 747.49
  thymus (gland) 254.8
    hyperplasia 254.0
  thyroglossal duct 759.2
  thyrolingual duct 759.2
  truncus arteriosus or communis 745.0
  tunica vasculosa lentis 743.39
  umbilical sinus 753.7
  urachus 753.7
  vegetative state 780.03
  vitelline duct 751.0
  wolffian duct 752.8
Person (with)
  admitted for clinical research, as participant or
    control subject V70.7
  awaiting admission to adequate facility
    elsewhere V63.2
    undergoing social agency investigation V63.8
  concern (normal) about sick person in family
    V61.49
  consulting on behalf of another V65.1
  feared
    complaint in whom no diagnosis was made
      V65.5
    condition not demonstrated V65.5
  feigning illness V65.2
  healthy, accompanying sick person V65.0
  living (in)
    alone V60.3
    boarding school V60.6
    residence remote from hospital or medical
      care facility V63.0
    residential institution V60.6
    without
      adequate
        financial resources V60.2
        housing (heating) (space) V60.1
      housing (permanent) (temporary) V60.0
      material resources V60.2
      person able to render necessary care
        V60.4
      shelter V60.0
  medical services in home not available V63.1
  on waiting list V63.2
    undergoing social agency investigation V63.8
  sick or handicapped in family V61.49
  "worried well" V65.5
Personality
  affective 301.10
  aggressive 301.3
  amoral 301.7
  anancastic, anankastic 301.4
  antisocial 301.7
  asocial 301.7
  asthenic 301.6
  avoidant 301.82
  borderline 301.83
  change 310.1
  compulsive 301.4
  cycloid 301.13
  cyclothymic 301.13
  dependent 301.6
  depressive (chronic) 301.12
  disorder, disturbance NEC 301.9
    with
      antisocial disturbance 301.7
      pattern disturbance NEC 301.9
      sociopathic disturbance 301.7
      trait disturbance 301.9
  dual 300.14
  dyssocial 301.7
  eccentric 301.89
    "haltlose" type 301.89
  emotionally unstable 301.59
  epileptoid 301.3
  explosive 301.3
  fanatic 301.0
  histrionic 301.50
  hyperthymic 301.11
  hypomanic 301.11
  hypothymic 301.12
  hysterical 301.50
  immature 301.89
  inadequate 301.6

Personality — *continued*
labile 301.59
masochistic 301.89
morally defective 301.7
multiple 300.14
narcissistic 301.81
obsessional 301.4
obsessive (-compulsive) 301.4
overconscientous 301.4
paranoid 301.0
passive (-dependent) 301.6
passive-aggressive 301.84
pathologic NEC 301.9
pattern defect or disturbance 301.9
pseudosocial 301.7
psychoinfantile 301.59
psychoneurotic NEC 301.89
psychopathic 301.9
  with
      amoral trend 301.7
      antisocial trend 301.7
      asocial trend 301.7
      pathologic sexuality (*see also* Deviation,
        sexual) 302.9
  mixed types 301.9
schizoid 301.20
  introverted 301.21
  schizotypal 301.22
  with sexual deviation (*see also* Deviation,
    sexual) 302.9
  antisocial 301.7
  dyssocial 301.7
type A 301.4
unstable (emotional) 301.59

Perthes' disease (capital femoral osteochondrosis)
  732.1
Pertussis (*see also* Whooping cough) 033.9
  vaccination, prophylactic (against) V03.6
Peruvian wart 088.0
Perversion, perverted
  appetite 307.52
    hysterical 300.11
  function
    pineal gland 259.8
    pituitary gland 253.9
      anterior lobe
        deficient 253.2
        excessive 253.1
      posterior lobe 253.6
    placenta — *see* Placenta, abnormal
  sense of smell or taste 781.1
  psychogenic 306.7
  sexual (*see also* Deviation, sexual) 302.9
Pervious, congenital — *see also* Imperfect,
    closure
  ductus arteriosus 747.0
Pes (congenital) (*see also* Talipes) 754.70
  abductus (congenital) 754.60
    acquired 736.79
  acquired NEC 736.79
    planus 734
  adductus (congenital) 754.79
    acquired 736.79
  cavus 754.71
    acquired 736.73
  planovalgus (congenital) 754.69
    acquired 736.79
  planus (acquired) (any degree) 734
    congenital 754.61
    rachitic 268.1
  valgus (congenital) 754.61
    acquired 736.79
  varus (congenital) 754.50
    acquired 736.79
Pest (*see also* Plague) 020.9
Pestis (*see also* Plague) 020.9
  bubonica 020.0
  fulminans 020.0
  minor 020.8
  pneumonica — *see* Plague, pneumonic
Petechia, petechiae 782.7
  fetus or newborn 772.6
Petechial
  fever 036.0
  typhus 081.9

Petges-Cléjat or Petges-Clégat syndrome
  (poikilodermatomyositis) 710.3
Petit's
  disease (*see also* Hernia, lumbar) 553.8
Petit mal (idiopathic) (*see also* Epilepsy)
  345.0 ✓5th
    status 345.2
Petrellidosis 117.6
Petrositis 383.20
  acute 383.21
  chronic 383.22
Peutz-Jeghers disease or syndrome 759.6
Peyronie's disease 607.89
Pfeiffer's disease 075
Phacentocele 379.32
  traumatic 921.3
Phacoanaphylaxis 360.19
Phacocele (old) 379.32
  traumatic 921.3
Phaehyphomycosis 117.8
Phagedena (dry) (moist) (*see also* Gangrene) 785.4
  arteriosclerotic 440.2 ✓5th [785.4]
  geometric 686.09
  penis 607.89
  senile 440.2 ✓5th [785.4]
  sloughing 785.4
  tropical (*see also* Ulcer, skin) 707.9
  vulva 616.50
Phagedenic — *see also* condition
  abscess — *see also* Abscess
    chancroid 099.0
  bubo NEC 099.8
  chancre 099.0
  ulcer (tropical) (*see also* Ulcer, skin) 707.9
Phagomania 307.52
Phakoma 362.89
Phantom limb (syndrome) 353.6
Pharyngeal — *see also* condition
  arch remnant 744.41
  pouch syndrome 279.11
Pharyngitis (acute) (catarrhal) (gangrenous)
    (infective) (malignant) (membranous)
    (phlegmonous) (pneumococcal)
    (pseudomembranous) (simple)
    (staphylococcal) (subacute) (suppurative)
    (ulcerative) (viral) 462
  with influenza, flu, or grippe 487.1
  aphthous 074.0
  atrophic 472.1
  chronic 472.1
  chlamydial 099.51
  coxsackie virus 074.0
  diphtheritic (membranous) 032.0
  follicular 472.1
  fusospirochetal 101
  gonococcal 098.6
  granular (chronic) 472.1
  herpetic 054.79
  hypertrophic 472.1
  infectional, chronic 472.1
  influenzal 487.1
  lymphonodular, acute 074.8
  septic 034.0
  streptococcal 034.0
  tuberculous (*see also* Tuberculosis) 012.8 ✓5th
  vesicular 074.0
Pharyngoconjunctival fever 077.2
Pharyngoconjunctivitis, viral 077.2
Pharyngolaryngitis (acute) 465.0
  chronic 478.9
  septic 034.0
Pharyngoplegia 478.29
Pharyngotonsillitis 465.8
  tuberculous 012.8 ✓5th
Pharyngotracheitis (acute) 465.8
  chronic 478.9
Pharynx, pharyngeal — *see* condition
Phase of life problem NEC V62.89
Phenomenon
  Arthus' — *see* Arthus' phenomenon
  flashback (drug) 292.89
  jaw-winking 742.8
  Jod-Basedow 242.8 ✓5th
  L. E. cell 710.0
  lupus erythematosus cell 710.0

Phenomenon — *continued*
  Pelger-Huët (hereditary hyposegmentation)
    288.2
  Raynaud's (paroxysmal digital cyanosis)
    (secondary) 443.0
  Reilly's (*see also* Neuropathy, peripheral,
    autonomic) 337.9
  vasomotor 780.2
  vasospastic 443.9
  vasovagal 780.2
  Wenckebach's, heart block (second degree)
    426.13
Phenylketonuria (PKU) 270.1
Phenylpyruvicaciduria 270.1
Pheochromoblastoma (M8700/3)
  specified site — *see* Neoplasm, by site,
    malignant
  unspecified site 194.0
Pheochromocytoma (M8700/0)
  malignant (M8700/3)
    specified site — *see* Neoplasm, by site,
      malignant
    unspecified site 194.0
  specified site — *see* Neoplasm, by site, benign
  unspecified site 227.0
Phimosis (congenital) 605
  chancroidal 099.0
  due to infection 605
Phlebectasia (*see also* Varicose, vein) 454.9
  congenital 747.6 ✓5th
  esophagus (*see also* Varix, esophagus) 456.1
    with hemorrhage (*see also* Varix, esophagus,
      bleeding) 456.0
Phlebitis (infective) (pyemic) (septic) (suppurative)
    451.9
  antecubital vein 451.82
  arm NEC 451.84
    axillary vein 451.89
    basilic vey 451.82
    deep 451.83
    superficial 451.82
  basilic vein 451.82
  blue 451.19
  brachial vein 451.83
  breast, superficial 451.89
  cavernous (venous) sinus — *see* Phlebitis,
    intracranial sinus
  cephalic vein 451.82
  cerebral (venous) sinus — *see* Phlebitis,
    intracranial sinus
  chest wall, superficial 451.89
  complicating pregnancy or puerperium
    671.9 ✓5th
    affecting fetus or newborn 760.3
  cranial (venous) sinus — *see* Phlebitis,
    intracranial sinus
  deep (vessels) 451.19
    femoral vein 451.11
    specified vessel NEC 451.19
  due to implanted device — *see* Complications,
    due to (presence of) any device, implant
    or graft classified to 996.0-996.5 NEC
  during or resulting from a procedure 997.2
  femoral vein (deep) 451.11
  femoropopliteal 451.0
  following infusion, perfusion, or transfusion
    999.2
  gouty 274.89 [451.9]
  hepatic veins 451.89
  iliac vein 451.81
  iliofemoral 451.11
  intracranial sinus (any) (venous) 325
    late effect — *see* category 326
    nonpyogenic 437.6
      in pregnancy or puerperium 671.5 ✓5th
  jugular vein 451.89
  lateral (venous) sinus — *see* Phlebitis,
    intracranial sinus
  leg 451.2
    deep (vessels) 451.19
      femoral vein 451.11
      specified vessel NEC 451.19
    superficial (vessels) 451.0
      femoral vein 451.11
  longitudinal sinus — *see* Phlebitis, intracranial
    sinus

Phlebitis — *continued*
  lower extremity 451.2
    deep (vessels) 451.19
      femoral vein 451.11
      specified vessel NEC 451.19
    superficial (vessels) 451.0
      femoral vein 451.11
    migrans, migrating (superficial) 453.1
  pelvic
    with
      abortion — *see* Abortion, by type, with
        sepsis
      ectopic pregnancy (*see also* categories
        633.0-633.9) 639.0
      molar pregnancy (*see also* categories 630-
        632) 639.0
    following
      abortion 639.0
      ectopic or molar pregnancy 639.0
    puerperal, postpartum 671.4 ☑5ᵗʰ
  popliteal vein 451.19
  portal (vein) 572.1
  postoperative 997.2
  pregnancy 671.9 ☑5ᵗʰ
    deep 671.3 ☑5ᵗʰ
    specified type NEC 671.5 ☑5ᵗʰ
    superficial 671.2 ☑5ᵗʰ
  puerperal, postpartum, childbirth 671.9 ☑5ᵗʰ
    deep 671.4 ☑5ᵗʰ
    lower extremities 671.2 ☑5ᵗʰ
    pelvis 671.4 ☑5ᵗʰ
    specified site NEC 671.5 ☑5ᵗʰ
    superficial 671.2 ☑5ᵗʰ
  radial vein 451.83
  retina 362.18
  saphenous (great) (long) 451.0
    accessory or small 451.0
  sinus (meninges) — *see* Phlebitis, intracranial
    sinus
  specified site NEC 451.89
  subclavian vein 451.89
  syphilitic 093.89
  tibial vein 451.19
  ulcer, ulcerative 451.9
    leg 451.2
      deep (vessels) 451.19
        femoral vein 451.11
        specified vessel NEC 451.19
      superficial (vessels) 451.0
        femoral vein 451.11
    lower extremity 451.2
      deep (vessels) 451.19
        femoral vein 451.11
        specified vessel NEC 451.19
      superficial (vessels) 451.0
  ulnar vein 451.83
  upper extremity — *see* Phlebitis, arm
  umbilicus 451.89
  uterus (septic) (*see also* Endometritis) 615.9
  varicose (leg) (lower extremity) (*see also*
    Varicose, vein) 454.1
Phlebofibrosis 459.89
Pheboliths 459.89
Phlebosclerosis 459.89
Phlebothrombosis — *see* Thrombosis
Phlebotomus fever 066.0
Phlegm, choked on 933.1
Phlegmasia
  alba dolens (deep vessels) 451.19
    complicating pregnancy 671.3 ☑5ᵗʰ
    nonpuerperal 451.19
    puerperal, postpartum, childbirth 671.4 ☑5ᵗʰ
  cerulea dolens 451.19
Phlegmon (*see also* Abscess) 682.9
  erysipelatous (*see also* Erysipelas) 035
  iliac 682.2
    fossa 540.1
  throat 478.29
Phlegmonous — *see* condition
Phlyctenulosis (allergic) (keratoconjuctivitis)
  (nontuberculous) 370.31
  cornea 370.31
    with ulcer (*see also* Ulcer, cornea) 370.00
  tuberculous (*see also* Tuberculosis) 017.3 ☑5ᵗʰ
    [370.31]

Phobia, phobic (reaction) 300.20
  animal 300.29
  isolated NEC 300.29
  obsessional 300.3
  simple NEC 300.29
  social 300.23
  specified NEC 300.29
  state 300.20
Phocas' disease 610.1
Phocomelia 755.4
  lower limb 755.32
    complete 755.33
    distal 755.35
    proximal 755.34
  upper limb 755.22
    complete 755.23
    distal 755.25
    proximal 755.24
Phoria (*see also* Heterophoria) 378.40
Phosphate-losing tubular disorder 588.0
Phosphatemia 275.3
Phosphaturia 275.3
Photoallergic response 692.72
Photocoproporphyria 277.1
Photodermatitis (sun) 692.72
  light other than sun 692.82
Photokeratitis 370.24
Photo-ophthalmia 370.24
Photophobia 368.13
Photopsia 368.15
Photoretinitis 363.31
Photoretinopathy 363.31
Photosensitiveness (sun) 692.72
  light other than sun 692.82
Photosensitization (sun) skin 692.72
  light other than sun 692.82
Phototoxic response 692.72
Phrenitis 323.9
Phrynoderma 264.8
Phthiriasis (pubis) (any site) 132.2
  with any infestation classifiable to 132.0, 132.1
    and 132.3
Phthirus infestation — *see* Phthiriasis
Phthisis (*see also* Tuberculosis) 011.9 ☑5ᵗʰ
  bulbi (infectional) 360.41
  colliers' 011.4 ☑5ᵗʰ
  cornea 371.05
  eyeball (due to infection) 360.41
  millstone makers' 011.4 ☑5ᵗʰ
  miners' 011.4 ☑5ᵗʰ
  potters' 011.4 ☑5ᵗʰ
  sandblasters' 011.4 ☑5ᵗʰ
  stonemasons' 011.4 ☑5ᵗʰ
Phycomycosis 117.7
Physalopteriasis 127.7
Physical therapy NEC V57.1
  breathing exercises V57.0
Physiological cup, optic papilla
  borderline, glaucoma suspect 365.00
  enlarged 377.14
  glaucomatous 377.14
Phytobezoar 938
  intestine 936
  stomach 935.2
Pian (*see also* Yaws) 102.9
Pianoma 102.1
Piarhemia, piarrhemia (*see also* Hyperlipemia)
  272.4
  bilharziasis 120.9
Pica 307.52
  hysterical 300.11
Pick's
  cerebral atrophy 331.1
    with dementia
      with behavioral disturbance 331.1
        [294.11]
      without behavioral disturbance 331.1
        [294.10]

Pick's — *continued*
  disease
    brain 331.1
      dementia in
        with behavioral disturbance 331.1
          [294.11]
        without behavioral disturbance 331.1
          [294.10]
    lipid histiocytosis 272.7
    liver (pericardial pseudocirrhosis of liver) 423.2
    pericardium (pericardial pseudocirrhosis of
      liver) 423.2
    polyserositis (pericardial pseudocirrhosis of
      liver) 423.2
  syndrome
    heart (pericardial pseudocirrhosis of liver)
      423.2
    liver (pericardial pseudocirrhosis of liver)
      423.2
  tubular adenoma (M8640/0)
    specified site — *see* Neoplasm, by site,
      benign
    unspecified site
      female 220
      male 222.0
Pick-Herxheimer syndrome (diffuse idiopathic
  cutaneous atrophy) 701.8
Pick-Niemann disease (lipid histiocytosis) 272.7
Pickwickian syndrome (cardiopulmonary obesity)
  278.8
Piebaldism, classic 709.09
Piedra 111.2
  beard 111.2
    black 111.3
    white 111.2
  black 111.3
  scalp 111.3
    black 111.3
    white 111.2
  white 111.2
Pierre Marie's syndrome (pulmonary
  hypertrophic osteoarthropathy) 731.2
Pierre Marie-Bamberger syndrome (hypertrophic
  pulmonary osteoarthropathy) 731.2
Pierre Mauriac's syndrome (diabetes-dwarfism-
  obesity) 258.1
Pierre Robin deformity or syndrome (congenital)
  756.0
Pierson's disease or osteochondrosis 732.1
Pigeon
  breast or chest (acquired) 738.3
    congenital 754.82
    rachitic (*see also* Rickets) 268.0
  breeders' disease or lung 495.2
  fanciers' disease or lung 495.2
  toe 735.8
Pigmentation (abnormal) 709.00
  anomaly 709.00
    congenital 757.33
    specified NEC 709.09
  conjunctiva 372.55
  cornea 371.10
    anterior 371.11
    posterior 371.13
    stromal 371.12
  lids (congenital) 757.33
    acquired 374.52
  limbus corneae 371.10
  metals 709.00
  optic papilla, congenital 743.57
  retina (congenital) (grouped) (nevoid) 743.53
    acquired 362.74
  scrotum, congenital 757.33
Piles — *see* Hemorrhoids
Pili
  annulati or torti (congenital) 757.4
  incarnati 704.8
Pill roller hand (intrinsic) 736.09
Pilomatrixoma (M8110/0) — *see* Neoplasm, skin,
  benign
Pilonidal — *see* condition
Pimple 709.8
PIN I (prostatic intraepithelial neoplasia
  I) 602.3

PIN II (prostatic intraepithelial neoplasia II) 602.3
PIN III (prostatic intraepithelial neoplasia III) 233.4
Pinched nerve — *see* Neuropathy, entrapment
Pineal body or gland — *see* condition
Pinealoblastoma (M9362/3) 194.4
Pinealoma (M9360/1) 237.1
  malignant (M9360/3) 194.4
Pineoblastoma (M9362/3) 194.4
Pineocytoma (M9361/1) 237.1
Pinguecula 372.51
Pinhole meatus (*see also* Stricture, urethra) 598.9
Pink
  disease 985.0
  eye 372.03
  puffer 492.8
Pinkus' disease (lichen nitidus) 697.1
Pinpoint
  meatus (*see also* Stricture, urethra) 598.9
  os uteri (*see also* Stricture, cervix) 622.4
Pinselhaare (congenital) 757.4
Pinta 103.9
  cardiovascular lesions 103.2
  chancre (primary) 103.0
  erythematous plaques 103.1
  hyperchromic lesions 103.1
  hyperkeratosis 103.1
  lesions 103.9
    cardiovascular 103.2
    hyperchromic 103.1
    intermediate 103.1
    late 103.2
    mixed 103.3
    primary 103.0
    skin (achromic) (cicatricial) (dyschromic) 103.2
      hyperchromic 103.1
      mixed (achromic and hyperchromic) 103.3
  papule (primary) 103.0
  skin lesions (achromic) (cicatricial) (dyschromic) 103.2
    hyperchromic 103.1
    mixed (achromic and hyperchromic) 103.3
  vitiligo 103.2
Pintid 103.0
Pinworms (disease) (infection) (infestation) 127.4
Piry fever 066.8
Pistol wound — *see* Gunshot wound
Pit, lip (mucus), congenital 750.25
Pitchers' elbow 718.82
Pithecoid pelvis 755.69
  with disproportion (fetopelvic) 653.2 ✓5ᵗʰ
    affecting fetus or newborn 763.1
    causing obstructed labor 660.1 ✓5ᵗʰ
Pithiatism 300.11
Pitted — *see also* Pitting
  teeth 520.4
Pitting (edema) (*see also* Edema) 782.3
  lip 782.3
  nail 703.8
    congenital 757.5
Pituitary gland — *see* condition
Pituitary snuff-takers' disease 495.8
Pityriasis 696.5
  alba 696.5
  capitis 690.11
  circinata (et maculata) 696.3
  Hebra's (exfoliative dermatitis) 695.89
  lichenoides et varioliformis 696.2
  maculata (et circinata) 696.3
  nigra 111.1
  pilaris 757.39
    acquired 701.1
    Hebra's 696.4
  rosea 696.3
  rotunda 696.3
  rubra (Hebra) 695.89
    pilaris 696.4
  sicca 690.18

Pityriasis — *continued*
  simplex 690.18
  specified type NEC 696.5
  streptogenes 696.5
  versicolor 111.0
    scrotal 111.0
Placenta, placental
  ablatio 641.2 ✓5ᵗʰ
    affecting fetus or newborn 762.1
  abnormal, abnormality 656.7 ✓5ᵗʰ
    with hemorrhage 641.8 ✓5ᵗʰ
      affecting fetus or newborn 762.1
    affecting fetus or newborn 762.2
  abruptio 641.2 ✓5ᵗʰ
    affecting fetus or newborn 762.1
  accessory lobe — *see* Placenta, abnormal
  accreta (without hemorrhage) 667.0 ✓5ᵗʰ
    with hemorrhage 666.0 ✓5ᵗʰ
  adherent (without hemorrhage) 667.0 ✓5ᵗʰ
    with hemorrhage 666.0 ✓5ᵗʰ
  apoplexy — *see* Placenta, separation
  battledore — *see* Placenta, abnormal
  bilobate — *see* Placenta, abnormal
  bipartita — *see* Placenta, abnormal
  carneous mole 631
  centralis — *see* Placenta, previa
  circumvallata — *see* Placenta, abnormal
  cyst (amniotic) — *see* Placenta, abnormal
  deficiency — *see* Placenta, insufficiency
  degeneration — *see* Placenta, insufficiency
  detachment (partial) (premature) (with hemorrhage) 641.2 ✓5ᵗʰ
    affecting fetus or newborn 762.1
  dimidiata — *see* Placenta, abnormal
  disease 656.7 ✓5ᵗʰ
    affecting fetus or newborn 762.2
  duplex — *see* Placenta, abnormal
  dysfunction — *see* Placenta, insufficiency
  fenestrata — *see* Placenta, abnormal
  fibrosis — *see* Placenta, abnormal
  fleshy mole 631
  hematoma — *see* Placenta, abnormal
  hemorrhage NEC — *see* Placenta, separation
  hormone disturbance or malfunction — *see* Placenta, abnormal
  hyperplasia — *see* Placenta, abnormal
  increta (without hemorrhage) 667.0 ✓5ᵗʰ
    with hemorrhage 666.0 ✓5ᵗʰ
  infarction 656.7 ✓5ᵗʰ
    affecting fetus or newborn 762.2
  insertion, vicious — *see* Placenta, previa
  insufficiency
    affecting
      fetus or newborn 762.2
      management of pregnancy 656.5 ✓5ᵗʰ
  lateral — *see* Placenta, previa
  low implantation or insertion — *see* Placenta, previa
  low-lying — *see* Placenta, previa
  malformation — *see* Placenta, abnormal
  malposition — *see* Placenta, previa
  marginalis, marginata — *see* Placenta, previa
  marginal sinus (hemorrhage) (rupture) 641.2 ✓5ᵗʰ
    affecting fetus or newborn 762.1
  membranacea — *see* Placenta, abnormal
  multilobed — *see* Placenta, abnormal
  multipartita — *see* Placenta, abnormal
  necrosis — *see* Placenta, abnormal
  percreta (without hemorrhage) 667.0 ✓5ᵗʰ
    with hemorrhage 666.0 ✓5ᵗʰ
  polyp 674.4 ✓5ᵗʰ
  previa (central) (centralis) (complete) (lateral) (marginal) (marginalis) (partial) (partialis) (total) (with hemorrhage) 641.1 ✓5ᵗʰ
    affecting fetus or newborn 762.0
    noted
      before labor, without hemorrhage (with cesarean delivery) 641.0 ✓5ᵗʰ
      during pregnancy (without hemorrhage) 641.0 ✓5ᵗʰ
    without hemorrhage (before labor and delivery) (during pregnancy) 641.0 ✓5ᵗʰ
  retention (with hemorrhage) 666.0 ✓5ᵗʰ
    fragments, complicating puerperium (delayed hemorrhage) 666.2 ✓5ᵗʰ

Placenta, placental — *continued*
  retention — *continued*
    fragments, complicating puerperium — *continued*
      without hemorrhage 667.1 ✓5ᵗʰ
    postpartum, puerperal 666.2 ✓5ᵗʰ
    without hemorrhage 667.0 ✓5ᵗʰ
  separation (normally implanted) (partial) (premature) (with hemorrhage) 641.2 ✓5ᵗʰ
    affecting fetus or newborn 762.1
  septuplex — *see* Placenta, abnormal
  small — *see* Placenta, insufficiency
  softening (premature) — *see* Placenta, abnormal
  spuria — *see* Placenta, abnormal
  succenturiata — *see* Placenta, abnormal
  syphilitic 095.8
  transfusion syndromes 762.3
  transmission of chemical substance — *see* Absorption, chemical, through placenta
  trapped (with hemorrhage) 666.0 ✓5ᵗʰ
    without hemorrhage 667.0 ✓5ᵗʰ
  trilobate — *see* Placenta, abnormal
  tripartita — *see* Placenta, abnormal
  triplex — *see* Placenta, abnormal
  varicose vessel — *see* Placenta, abnormal
  vicious insertion — *see* Placenta, previa
Placentitis
  affecting fetus or newborn 762.7
  complicating pregnancy 658.4 ✓5ᵗʰ
Plagiocephaly (skull) 754.0
Plague 020.9
  abortive 020.8
  ambulatory 020.8
  bubonic 020.0
  cellulocutaneous 020.1
  lymphatic gland 020.0
  pneumonic 020.5
    primary 020.3
    secondary 020.4
  pulmonary — *see* Plague, pneumonic
  pulmonic — *see* Plague, pneumonic
  septicemic 020.2
  tonsillar 020.9
    septicemic 020.2
  vaccination, prophylactic (against) V03.3
Planning, family V25.09
  contraception V25.9
  procreation V26.4
Plaque
  artery, arterial — *see* Arteriosclerosis
  calcareous — *see* Calcification
  Hollenhorst's (retinal) 362.33
  tongue 528.6
Plasma cell myeloma 203.0 ✓5ᵗʰ
Plasmacytoma, plasmocytoma (solitary) (M9731/1) 238.6
  benign (M9731/0) — *see* Neoplasm, by site, benign
  malignant (M9731/3) 203.8 ✓5ᵗʰ
Plasmacytosis 288.8
Plaster ulcer (*see also* Decubitus) 707.0
Platybasia 756.0
Platyonychia (congenital) 757.5
  acquired 703.8
Platypelloid pelvis 738.6
  with disproportion (fetopelvic) 653.2 ✓5ᵗʰ
    affecting fetus or newborn 763.1
    causing obstructed labor 660.1 ✓5ᵗʰ
      affecting fetus or newborn 763.1
  congenital 755.69
Platyspondylia 756.19
Plethora 782.62
  newborn 776.4
Pleura, pleural — *see* condition
Pleuralgia 786.52
Pleurisy (acute) (adhesive) (chronic) (costal) (diaphragmatic) (double) (dry) (fetid) (fibrinous) (fibrous) (interlobar) (latent) (lung) (old) (plastic) (primary) (residual) (sicca) (sterile) (subacute) (unresolved) (with adherent pleura) 511.0

Pleurisy — *continued*
with
effusion (without mention of cause) 511.9
bacterial, nontuberculous 511.1
nontuberculous NEC 511.9
bacterial 511.1
pneumococcal 511.1
specified type NEC 511.8
staphylococcal 511.1
streptococcal 511.1
tuberculous (*see also* Tuberculosis,
pleura) 012.0 ✓5ᵗʰ
primary, progressive 010.1 ✓5ᵗʰ
influenza, flu, or grippe 487.1
tuberculosis — *see* Pleurisy, tuberculous
encysted 511.8
exudative (*see also* Pleurisy, with effusion)
511.9
bacterial, nontuberculous 511.1
fibrinopurulent 510.9
with fistula 510.0
fibropurulent 510.9
with fistula 510.0
hemorrhagic 511.8
influenzal 487.1
pneumococcal 511.0
with effusion 511.1
purulent 510.9
with fistula 510.0
septic 510.9
with fistula 510.0
serofibrinous (*see also* Pleurisy, with effusion)
511.9
bacterial, nontuberculous 511.1
seropurulent 510.9
with fistula 510.0
serous (*see also* Pleurisy, with effusion) 511.9
bacterial, nontuberculous 511.1
staphylococcal 511.0
with effusion 511.1
streptococcal 511.0
with effusion 511.1
suppurative 510.9
with fistula 510.0
traumatic (post) (current) 862.29
with open wound into cavity 862.39
tuberculous (with effusion) (*see also*
Tuberculosis, pleura) 012.0 ✓5ᵗʰ
primary, progressive 010.1 ✓5ᵗʰ
Pleuritis sicca — *see* Pleurisy
Pleurobronchopneumonia (*see also* Pneumonia,
broncho-) 485
Pleurodynia 786.52
epidemic 074.1
viral 074.1
Pleurohepatitis 573.8
Pleuropericarditis (*see also* Pericarditis) 423.9
acute 420.90
Pleuropneumonia (acute) (bilateral) (double)
(septic) (*see also* Pneumonia) 486
chronic (*see also* Fibrosis, lung) 515
Pleurorrhea (*see also* Hydrothorax) 511.8
Plexitis, brachial 353.0
Plica
knee 727.83
polonica 132.0
tonsil 474.8
Plicae dysphonia ventricularis 784.49
Plicated tongue 529.5
congenital 750.13
Plug
bronchus NEC 519.1
meconium (newborn) NEC 777.1
mucus — *see* Mucus, plug
Plumbism 984.9
specified type of lead — *see* Table of Drugs and
Chemicals
Plummer's disease (toxic nodular goiter)
242.3 ✓5ᵗʰ
Plummer-Vinson syndrome (sideropenic
dysphagia) 280.8
Pluricarential syndrome of infancy 260
Plurideficiency syndrome of infancy 260

Plus (and minus) hand (intrinsic) 736.09
PMS 625.4
Pneumathemia — *see* Air, embolism, by type
Pneumatic drill or hammer disease 994.9
Pneumatocele (lung) 518.89
intracranial 348.8
tension 492.0
Pneumatosis
cystoides intestinalis 569.89
peritonei 568.89
pulmonum 492.8
Pneumaturia 599.84
Pneumoblastoma (M8981/3) — *see* Neoplasm,
lung, malignant
Pneumocephalus 348.8
Pneumococcemia 038.2
Pneumococcus, pneumococcal — *see* condition
Pneumoconiosis (due to) (inhalation of) 505
aluminum 503
asbestos 501
bagasse 495.1
bauxite 503
beryllium 503
carbon electrode makers' 503
coal
miners' (simple) 500
workers' (simple) 500
cotton dust 504
diatomite fibrosis 502
dust NEC 504
inorganic 503
lime 502
marble 502
organic NEC 504
fumes or vapors (from silo) 506.9
graphite 503
hard metal 503
mica 502
moldy hay 495.0
rheumatoid 714.81
silica NEC 502
and carbon 500
silicate NEC 502
talc 502
Pneumocystis carinii pneumonia 136.3
Pneumocystosis 136.3
with pneumonia 136.3
Pneumoenteritis 025
Pneumohemopericardium (*see also* Pericarditis)
423.9
Pneumohemothorax (*see also* Hemothorax) 511.8
traumatic 860.4
with open wound into thorax 860.5
Pneumohydropericardium (*see also* Pericarditis)
423.9
Pneumohydrothorax (*see also* Hydrothorax)
511.8
Pneumomediastinum 518.1
congenital 770.2
fetus or newborn 770.2
Pneumomycosis 117.9
Pneumonia (acute) (Alpenstich) (benign) (bilateral)
(brain) (cerebral) (circumscribed) (congestive
) (creeping) (delayed resolution) (double)
(epidemic) (fever) (flash) (fulminant) (fungoid)
(granulomatous) (hemorrhagic) (incipient)
(infantile) (infectious) (infiltration) (insular)
(intermittent) (latent) (lobe) (migratory)
(newborn) (organized) (overwhelming)
(primary) (progressive) (pseudolobar)
(purulent) (resolved) (secondary) (senile)
(septic) (suppurative) (terminal) (true)
(unresolved) (vesicular) 486
with influenza, flu, or grippe 487.0
adenoviral 480.0
adynamic 514
alba 090.0
allergic 518.3
alveolar — *see* Pneumonia, lobar
anaerobes 482.81
anthrax 022.1 [484.5]
apex, apical — *see* Pneumonia, lobar
ascaris 127.0 [484.8]

Pneumonia — *continued*
aspiration 507.0
due to
aspiration of microorganisms
bacterial 482.9
specified type NEC 482.89
specified organism NEC 483.8
bacterial NEC 482.89
viral 480.9
specified type NEC 480.8
food (regurgitated) 507.0
gastric secretions 507.0
milk 507.0
oils, essences 507.1
solids, liquids NEC 507.8
vomitus 507.0
newborn 770.1
asthenic 514
atypical (disseminated, focal) (primary) 486
with influenza 487.0
bacillus 482.9
specified type NEC 482.89
bacterial 482.9
specified type NEC 482.89
Bacteroides (fragilis) (oralis) (melaninogenicus)
482.81
basal, basic, basilar — *see* Pneumonia, lobar
broncho-, bronchial (confluent) (croupous)
(diffuse) (disseminated) (hemorrhagic)
(involving lobes) (lobar) (terminal) 485
with influenza 487.0
allergic 518.3
aspiration (*see also* Pneumonia, aspiration)
507.0
bacterial 482.9
specified type NEC 482.89
capillary 466.19
with bronchospasm or obstruction
466.19
chronic (*see also* Fibrosis, lung) 515
congenital (infective) 770.0
diplococcal 481
Eaton's agent 483.0
Escherichia coli (E. coli) 482.82
Friedländer's bacillus 482.0
Hemophilus influenzae 482.2
hiberno-vernal 083.0 [484.8]
hypostatic 514
influenzal 487.0
inhalation (*see also* Pneumonia, aspiration)
507.0
due to fumes or vapors (chemical) 506.0
Klebsiella 482.0
lipid 507.1
endogenous 516.8
Mycoplasma (pneumoniae) 483.0
ornithosis 073.0
pleuropneumonia-like organisms (PPLO)
483.0
pneumococcal 481
Proteus 482.83
pseudomonas 482.1
specified organism NEC 483.8
bacterial NEC 482.89
staphylococcal 482.40
aureus 482.41
specified type NEC 482.49
streptococcal — *see* Pneumonia,
streptococcal
typhoid 002.0 [484.8]
viral, virus (*see also* Pneumonia, viral) 480.9
butyrivibrio (fibriosolvens) 482.81
Candida 112.4
capillary 466.19
with bronchospasm or obstruction 466.19
caseous (*see also* Tuberculosis) 011.6 ✓5ᵗʰ
catarrhal — *see* Pneumonia, broncho-central —
see Pneumonia, lobar
Chlamydia, chlamydial 483.1
pneumoniae 483.1
psittaci 073.0
specified type NEC 483.1
trachomatis 483.1
cholesterol 516.8
chronic (*see also* Fibrosis, lung) 515
Clostridium (haemolyticum) (novyi) NEC 482.81
confluent — *see* Pneumonia, broncho-

Pneumonia — *continued*
  congenital (infective) 770.0
    aspiration 770.1
  croupous — *see* Pneumonia, lobar
  cytomegalic inclusion 078.5 *[484.1]*
  deglutition (*see also* Pneumonia, aspiration)
    507.0
  desquamative interstitial 516.8
  diffuse — *see* Pneumonia, broncho-
  diplococcal, diplococcus (broncho-) (lobar) 481
  disseminated (focal) — *see* Pneumonia,
    broncho-
  due to
    adenovirus 480.0
    Bacterium anitratum 482.83
    Chlamydia, chlamydial 483.1
      pneumoniae 483.1
      psittaci 073.0
      specified type NEC 483.1
      trachomatis 483.1
    coccidioidomycosis 114.0
    Diplococcus (pneumoniae) 481
    Eaton's agent 483.0
    Escherichia coli (E. coli) 482.82
    Friedländer's bacillus 482.0
    fumes or vapors (chemical) (inhalation)
      506.0
    fungus NEC 117.9 *[484.7]*
      coccidioidomycosis 114.0
    Hemophilus influenzae (H. influenzae) 482.2
    Herellea 482.83
    influenza 487.0
    Klebsiella pneumoniae 482.0
    Mycoplasma (pneumoniae) 483.0
    parainfluenza virus 480.2
    pleuropneumonia-like organism (PPLO)
      483.0
    Pneumococcus 481
    Pneumocystis carinii 136.3
    Proteus 482.83
    pseudomonas 482.1
    respiratory syncytial virus 480.1
    rickettsia 083.9 *[484.8]*
    specified
      bacteria NEC 482.89
      organism NEC 483.8
      virus NEC 480.8
    Staphylococcus 482.40
      aureus 482.41
      specified type NEC 482.49
    Streptococcus — *see also* Pneumonia,
      streptococcal
      pneumoniae 481
    virus (*see also* Pneumonia, viral) 480.9
  Eaton's agent 483.0
  embolic, embolism (*see also* Embolism,
    pulmonary) 415.1 ✓5ᵗʰ
  eosinophilic 518.3
  Escherichia coli (E. coli) 482.82
  Eubacterium 482.81
  fibrinous — *see* Pneumonia, lobar
  fibroid (chronic)(*see also* Fibrosis, lung) 515
  fibrous (*see also* Fibrosis, lung) 515
  Friedländer's bacillus 482.0
  Fusobacterium (nucleatum) 482.81
  gangrenous 513.0
  giant cell (*see also* Pneumonia, viral) 480.9
  gram-negative bacteria NEC 482.83
    anaerobic 482.81
  grippal 487.0
  Hemophilus influenzae (bronchial) (lobar) 482.2
  hypostatic (broncho-) (lobar) 514
  in
    actinomycosis 039.1
    anthrax 022.1 *[484.5]*
    aspergillosis 117.3 *[484.6]*
    candidiasis 112.4
    coccidioidomycosis 114.0
    cytomegalic inclusion disease 078.5 *[484.1]*
    histoplasmosis (*see also* Histoplasmosis)
      115.95
    infectious disease NEC 136.9 *[484.8]*
    measles 055.1
    mycosis, systemic NEC 117.9 *[484.7]*
    nocardiasis, nocardiosis 039.1
    ornithosis 073.0
    pneumocystosis 136.3

Pneumonia — *continued*
  in — *continued*
    psittacosis 073.0
    Q fever 083.0 *[484.8]*
    salmonellosis 003.22
    toxoplasmosis 130.4
    tularemia 021.2
    typhoid (fever) 002.0 *[484.8]*
    varicella 052.1
    whooping cough (*see also* Whooping cough)
      033.9 *[484.3]*
  infective, acquired prenatally 770.0
  influenzal (broncho) (lobar) (virus) 487.0
  inhalation (*see also* Pneumonia, aspiration)
    507.0
    fumes or vapors (chemical) 506.0
  interstitial 516.8
    with influenzal 487.0
    acute 136.3
    chronic (*see also* Fibrosis, lung) 515
    desquamative 516.8
    hypostatic 514
    lipoid 507.1
    lymphoid 516.8
    plasma cell 136.3
    pseudomonas 482.1
  intrauterine (infective) 770.0
    aspiration 770.1
  Klebsiella pneumoniae 482.0
  Legionnaires' 482.84
  lipid, lipoid (exogenous) (interstitial) 507.1
    endogenous 516.8
  lobar (diplococcal) (disseminated) (double)
    (interstitial) (pneumococcal, any type) 481
    with influenza 487.0
    bacterial 482.9
      specified type NEC 482.89
    chronic (*see also* Fibrosis, lung) 515
    Escherichia coli (E. coli) 482.82
    Friedländer's bacillus 482.0
    Hemophilus influenzae (H. influenzae) 482.2
    hypostatic 514
    influenzal 487.0
    Klebsiella 482.0
    ornithosis 073.0
    Proteus 482.83
    pseudomonas 482.1
    psittacosis 073.0
    specified organism NEC 483.8
      bacterial NEC 482.89
    staphylococcal 482.40
      aureus 482.41
      specified type NEC 482.49
    streptococcal — *see* Pneumonia,
      streptococcal
    viral, virus (*see also* Pneumonia, viral) 480.9
  lobular (confluent) — *see* Pneumonia, broncho-
  Löffler's 518.3
  massive — *see* Pneumonia, lobar
  meconium 770.1
  metastatic NEC 038.8 *[484.8]*
  Mycoplasma (pneumoniae) 483.0
  necrotic 513.0
  nitrogen dioxide 506.9
  orthostatic 514
  parainfluenza virus 480.2
  parenchymatous (*see also* Fibrosis, lung) 515
  passive 514
  patchy — *see* Pneumonia, broncho-
  Peptococcus 482.81
  Peptostreptococcus 482.81
  plasma cell 136.3
  pleurolobar — *see* Pneumonia, lobar
  pleuropneumonia-like organism (PPLO) 483.0
  pneumococcal (broncho) (lobar) 481
  Pneumocystis (carinii) 136.3
  postinfectional NEC 136.9 *[484.8]*
  postmeasles 055.1
  postoperative 997.3
  primary atypical 486
  Proprionibacterium 482.81
  Proteus 482.83
  pseudomonas 482.1
  psittacosis 073.0
  radiation 508.0
  respiratory syncytial virus 480.1
  resulting from a procedure 997.3
  rheumatic 390 *[517.1]*

Pneumonia — *continued*
  Salmonella 003.22
  segmented, segmental — *see* Pneumonia,
    broncho-
  Serratia (marcescens) 482.83
  specified
    bacteria NEC 482.89
    organism NEC 483.8
    virus NEC 480.8
  spirochetal 104.8 *[484.8]*
  staphylococcal (broncho) (lobar) 482.40
    aureus 482.41
    specified type NEC 482.49
  static, stasis 514
  streptococcal (broncho) (lobar) NEC 482.30
    Group
      A 482.31
      B 482.32
      specified NEC 482.39
    pneumoniae 481
    specified type NEC 482.39
  Streptococcus pneumoniae 481
  traumatic (complication) (early) (secondary)
    958.8
  tuberculous (any) (*see also* Tuberculosis)
    011.6 ✓5ᵗʰ
  tularemic 021.2
  TWAR agent 483.1
  varicella 052.1
  Veillonella 482.81
  viral, virus (broncho) (interstitial) (lobar) 480.9
    with influenza, flu, or grippe 487.0
    adenoviral 480.0
    parainfluenza 480.2
    respiratory syncytial 480.1
    specified type NEC 480.8
  white (congenital) 090.0

Pneumonic — *see* condition

Pneumonitis (acute) (primary) (*see also*
  Pneumonia) 486
  allergic 495.9
    specified type NEC 495.8
  aspiration 507.0
    due to fumes or gases 506.0
    newborn 770.1
    obstetric 668.0 ✓5ᵗʰ
  chemical 506.0
    due to fumes or gases 506.0
  cholesterol 516.8
  chronic (*see also* Fibrosis, lung) 515
  congenital rubella 771.0
  due to
    fumes or vapors 506.0
    inhalation
      food (regurgitated), milk, vomitus 507.0
      oils, essences 507.1
      saliva 507.0
      solids, liquids NEC 507.8
    toxoplasmosis (acquired) 130.4
      congenital (active) 771.2 *[484.8]*
  eosinophilic 518.3
  fetal aspiration 770.1
  hypersensitivity 495.9
  interstitial (chronic) (*see also* Fibrosis, lung)
    515
    lymphoid 516.8
  lymphoid, interstitial 516.8
  meconium 770.1
  postanesthetic
    correct substance properly administered
      507.0
    obstetric 668.0 ✓5ᵗʰ
    overdose or wrong substance given 968.4
      specified anesthetic — *see* Table of Drugs
        and Chemicals
  postoperative 997.3
    obstetric 668.0 ✓5ᵗʰ
  radiation 508.0
  rubella, congenital 771.0
  "ventilation" 495.7
  wood-dust 495.8

Pneumonoconiosis — *see* Pneumoconiosis

Pneumoparotid 527.8

Pneumopathy NEC 518.89
  alveolar 516.9
    specified NEC 516.8

Pneumopathy NEC — *continued*
  due to dust NEC 504
  parietoalveolar 516.9
    specified condition NEC 516.8
Pneumopericarditis (*see also* Pericarditis) 423.9
  acute 420.90
Pneumopericardium — *see also* Pericarditis
  congenital 770.2
  fetus or newborn 770.2
  traumatic (post) (*see also* Pneumothorax, traumatic) 860.0
    with open wound into thorax 860.1
Pneumoperitoneum 568.89
  fetus or newborn 770.2
Pneumophagia (psychogenic) 306.4
Pneumopleurisy, pneumopleuritis (*see also* Pneumonia) 486
Pneumopyopericardium 420.99
Pneumopyothorax (*see also* Pyopneumothorax) 510.9
  with fistula 510.0
Pneumorrhagia 786.3
  newborn 770.3
  tuberculous (*see also* Tuberculosis, pulmonary) 011.9
Pneumosiderosis (occupational) 503
Pneumothorax (acute) (chronic) 512.8
  congenital 770.2
  due to operative injury of chest wall or lung 512.1
    accidental puncture or laceration 512.1
  fetus or newborn 770.2
  iatrogenic 512.1
  postoperative 512.1
  spontaneous 512.8
    fetus or newborn 770.2
    tension 512.0
  sucking 512.8
    iatrogenic 512.1
    postoperative 512.1
  tense valvular, infectional 512.0
  tension 512.0
    iatrogenic 512.1
    postoperative 512.1
    spontaneous 512.0
  traumatic 860.0
    with
      hemothorax 860.4
        with open wound into thorax 860.5
      open wound into thorax 860.1
  tuberculous (*see also* Tuberculosis) 011.7
Pocket(s)
  endocardial (*see also* Endocarditis) 424.90
  periodontal 523.8
Podagra 274.9
Podencephalus 759.89
Poikilocytosis 790.09
Poikiloderma 709.09
  Civatte's 709.09
  congenital 757.33
  vasculare atrophicans 696.2
Poikilodermatomyositis 710.3
Pointed ear 744.29
Poise imperfect 729.9
Poisoned — *see* Poisoning
Poisoning (acute) — *see also* Table of Drugs and Chemicals
  Bacillus, B.
    aertrycke (*see also* Infection, Salmonella) 003.9
    botulinus 005.1
    cholerae (suis) (*see also* Infection, Salmonella) 003.9
    paratyphosus (*see also* Infection, Salmonella) 003.9
    suipestifer (*see also* Infection, Salmonella) 003.9
  bacterial toxins NEC 005.9
  berries, noxious 988.2
  blood (general) — *see* Septicemia
  botulism 005.1
  bread, moldy, mouldy — *see* Poisoning, food
  damaged meat — *see* Poisoning, food

Poisoning (acute) — *see also* Table of Drugs and Chemicals — *continued*
  death-cap (Amanita phalloides) (Amanita verna) 988.1
  decomposed food — *see* Poisoning, food
  diseased food — *see* Poisoning, food
  drug — *see* Table of Drugs and Chemicals
  epidemic, fish, meat, or other food — *see* Poisoning, food
  fava bean 282.2
  fish (bacterial) — *see also* Poisoning, food
    noxious 988.0
  food (acute) (bacterial) (diseased) (infected) NEC 005.9
    due to
      bacillus
        aertrycke (*see also* Poisoning, food, due to Salmonella) 003.9
        botulinus 005.1
        cereus 005.89
        choleraesuis (*see also* Poisoning, food, due to Salmonella) 003.9
        paratyphosus (*see also* Poisoning, food, due to Salmonella) 003.9
        suipestifer (*see also* Poisoning, food, due to Salmonella) 003.9
      Clostridium 005.3
        botulinum 005.1
        perfringens 005.2
        welchii 005.2
      Salmonella (aertrycke) (callinarum) (choleraesuis) (enteritidis) (paratyphi) (suipestifer) 003.9
        with
          gastroenteritis 003.0
          localized infection(s) (*see also* Infection, Salmonella) 003.20
          septicemia 003.1
          specified manifestation NEC 003.8
      specified bacterium NEC 005.89
      Staphylococcus 005.0
      Streptococcus 005.8
      Vibrio parahaemolyticus 005.4
      Vibrio vulnificus 005.81
    noxious or naturally toxic 988.0
      berries 988.2
      fish 988.0
      mushroom 988.1
      plants NEC 988.2
  ice cream — *see* Poisoning, food
  ichthyotoxism (bacterial) 005.9
  kreotoxism, food 005.9
  malarial — *see* Malaria
  meat — *see* Poisoning, food
  mushroom (noxious) 988.1
  mussel — *see also* Poisoning, food
    noxious 988.0
  noxious foodstuffs (*see also* Poisoning, food, noxious) 988.9
    specified type NEC 988.8
  plants, noxious 988.2
  pork — *see also* Poisoning, food
    specified NEC 988.8
    Trichinosis 124
  ptomaine — *see* Poisoning, food
  putrefaction, food — *see* Poisoning, food
  radiation 508.0
  Salmonella (*see also* Infection, Salmonella) 003.9
  sausage — *see also* Poisoning, food
    Trichinosis 124
  saxitoxin 988.0
  shellfish — *see also* Poisoning, food
    noxious 988.0
  Staphylococcus, food 005.0
  toxic, from disease NEC 799.8
  truffles — *see* Poisoning, food
  uremic — *see* Uremia
  uric acid 274.9
Poison ivy, oak, sumac or other plant dermatitis 692.6
Poker spine 720.0
Policeman's disease 729.2
Polioencephalitis (acute) (bulbar) (*see also* Poliomyelitis, bulbar) 045.0
  inferior 335.22

Polioencephalitis (*see also* Poliomyelitis, bulbar) — *continued*
  influenzal 487.8
  superior hemorrhagic (acute) (Wernicke's) 265.1
  Wernicke's (superior hemorrhagic) 265.1
Polioencephalomyelitis (acute) (anterior) (bulbar) (*see also* Polioencephalitis) 045.0
Polioencephalopathy, superior hemorrhagic 265.1
  with
    beriberi 265.0
    pellagra 265.2
Poliomeningoencephalitis — *see* Meningoencephalitis
Poliomyelitis (acute) (anterior) (epidemic) 045.9

> *Note* — Use the following fifth-digit subclassification with category 045:
>
> 0 poliovirus, unspecified type
> 1 poliovirus, type I
> 2 poliovirus, type II
> 3 poliovirus, type III

  with
    paralysis 045.1
      bulbar 045.0
  abortive 045.2
  ascending 045.9
    progressive 045.9
  bulbar 045.0
  cerebral 045.0
  chronic 335.21
  congenital 771.2
  contact V01.2
  deformities 138
  exposure to V01.2
  late effect 138
  nonepidemic 045.9
  nonparalytic 045.2
  old with deformity 138
  posterior, acute 053.19
  residual 138
  sequelae 138
  spinal, acute 045.9
  syphilitic (chronic) 094.89
  vaccination, prophylactic (against) V04.0
Poliosis (eyebrow) (eyelashes) 704.3
  circumscripta (congenital) 757.4
    acquired 704.3
  congenital 757.4
Pollakiuria 788.4
  psychogenic 306.53
Pollinosis 477.0
Pollitzer's disease (hidradenitis suppurativa) 705.83
Polyadenitis (*see also* Adenitis) 289.3
  malignant 020.0
Polyalgia 729.9
Polyangiitis (essential) 446.0
Polyarteritis (nodosa) (renal) 446.0
Polyarthralgia 719.49
  psychogenic 306.0
Polyarthritis, polyarthropathy NEC 716.59
  due to or associated with other specified conditions — *see* Arthritis, due to or associated with
  endemic (*see also* Disease, Kaschin-Beck) 716.0
  inflammatory 714.9
    specified type NEC 714.89
  juvenile (chronic) 714.30
    acute 714.31
  migratory — *see* Fever, rheumatic
  rheumatic 714.0
    fever (acute) — *see* Fever, rheumatic
Polycarential syndrome of infancy 260
Polychondritis (atrophic) (chronic) (relapsing) 733.99
Polycoria 743.46
Polycystic (congenital) (disease) 759.89
  degeneration, kidney — *see* Polycystic, kidney

Polycystic — continued
  kidney (congenital) 753.12
    adult type (APKD) 753.13
    autosomal dominant 753.13
    autosomal recessive 753.14
    childhood type (CPKD) 753.14
    infantile type 753.14
  liver 751.62
  lung 518.89
    congenital 748.4
  ovary, ovaries 256.4
  spleen 759.0
Polycythemia (primary) (rubra) (vera) (M9950/1) 238.4
  acquired 289.0
  benign 289.0
    familial 289.6
  due to
    donor twin 776.4
    fall in plasma volume 289.0
    high altitude 289.0
    maternal-fetal transfusion 776.4
    stress 289.0
  emotional 289.0
  erythropoietin 289.0
  familial (benign) 289.6
  Gaisböck's (hypertonica) 289.0
  high altitude 289.0
  hypertonica 289.0
  hypoxemic 289.0
  neonatorum 776.4
  nephrogenous 289.0
  relative 289.0
  secondary 289.0
  spurious 289.0
  stress 289.0
Polycytosis cryptogenica 289.0
Polydactylism, polydactyly 755.00
  fingers 755.01
  toes 755.02
Polydipsia 783.5
Polydystrophic oligophrenia 277.5
Polyembryoma (M9072/3) — see Neoplasm, by site, malignant
Polygalactia 676.6 ☑5ᵗʰ
Polyglandular
  deficiency 258.9
  dyscrasia 258.9
  dysfunction 258.9
  syndrome 258.8
Polyhydramnios (see also Hydramnios) 657 ☑5ᵗʰ
Polymastia 757.6
Polymenorrhea 626.2
Polymicrogyria 742.2
Polymyalgia 725
  arteritica 446.5
  rheumatica 725
Polymyositis (acute) (chronic) (hemorrhagic) 710.4
  with involvement of
    lung 710.4 [517.8]
    skin 710.3
  ossificans (generalisata) (progressiva) 728.19
  Wagner's (dermatomyositis) 710.3
Polyneuritis, polyneuritic (see also Polyneuropathy) 356.9
  alcoholic 357.5
    with psychosis 291.1
  cranialis 352.6
  diabetic 250.6 ☑5ᵗʰ [357.2]
  demyelinating, chronic inflammatory 357.81▲
  due to lack of vitamin NEC 269.2 [357.4]
  endemic 265.0 [357.4]
  erythredema 985.0
  febrile 357.0
  hereditary ataxic 356.3
  idiopathic, acute 357.0
  infective (acute) 357.0
  nutritional 269.9 [357.4]
  postinfectious 357.0
Polyneuropathy (peripheral) 356.9
  alcoholic 357.5
  amyloid 277.3 [357.4]
  arsenical 357.7
  critical illness 357.82

Polyneuropathy — continued
  diabetic 250.6 ☑5ᵗʰ [357.2]
  due to
    antitetanus serum 357.6
    arsenic 357.7
    drug or medicinal substance 357.6
      correct substance properly administered 357.6
      overdose or wrong substance given or taken 977.9
      specified drug — see Table of Drugs and Chemicals
    lack of vitamin NEC 269.2 [357.4]
    lead 357.7
    organophosphate compounds 357.7
    pellagra 265.2 [357.4]
    porphyria 277.1 [357.4]
    serum 357.6
    toxic agent NEC 357.7
  hereditary 356.0
  idiopathic 356.9
    progressive 356.4
  in
    amyloidosis 277.3 [357.4]
    avitaminosis 269.2 [357.4]
      specified NEC 269.1 [357.4]
    beriberi 265.0 [357.4]
    collagen vascular disease NEC 710.9 [357.1]
    deficiency
      B-complex NEC 266.2 [357.4]
      vitamin B 266.9 [357.4]
      vitamin B 266.1 [357.4]
    diabetes 250.6 ☑5ᵗʰ [357.2]
    diphtheria (see also Diphtheria) 032.89 [357.4]
    disseminated lupus erythematosus 710.0 [357.1]
    herpes zoster 053.13
    hypoglycemia 251.2 [357.4]
    malignant neoplasm (M8000/3) NEC 199.1 [357.3]
    mumps 072.72
    pellagra 265.2 [357.4]
    polyarteritis nodosa 446.0 [357.1]
    porphyria 277.1 [357.4]
    rheumatoid arthritis 714.0 [357.1]
    sarcoidosis 135 [357.4]
    uremia 585 [357.4]
  lead 357.7
  nutritional 269.9 [357.4]
    specified NEC 269.8 [357.4]
  postherpetic 053.13
  progressive 356.4
  sensory (hereditary) 356.2
Polyonychia 757.5
Polyopia 368.2
  refractive 368.15
Polyorchism, polyorchidism (three testes) 752.8
Polyrrhymenitis (peritoneal) (see also Polyserositis) 568.82
  pericardial 423.2
Polyostotic fibrous dysplasia 756.54
Polyotia 744.1
Polyp, polypus

Note — Polyps of organs or sites that do not appear in the list below should be coded to the residual category for diseases of the organ or site concerned.

  accessory sinus 471.8
  adenoid tissue 471.0
  adenomatous (M8210/0) — see also Neoplasm, by site, benign
    adenocarcinoma in (M8210/3) — see Neoplasm, by site, malignant
    carcinoma in (M8210/3) — see Neoplasm, by site, malignant
    multiple (M8221/0) — see Neoplasm, by site, benign
  antrum 471.8
  anus, anal (canal) (nonadenomatous) 569.0
    adenomatous 211.4
  Bartholin's gland 624.6
  bladder (M8120/1) 236.7
  broad ligament 620.8

Polyp, polypus — continued
  cervix (uteri) 622.7
    adenomatous 219.0
    in pregnancy or childbirth 654.6 ☑5ᵗʰ
      affecting fetus or newborn 763.89
      causing obstructed labor 660.2 ☑5ᵗʰ
    mucous 622.7
    nonneoplastic 622.7
  choanal 471.0
  cholesterol 575.6
  clitoris 624.6
  colon (M8210/0) (see also Polyp, adenomatous) 211.3
  corpus uteri 621.0
  dental 522.0
  ear (middle) 385.30
  endometrium 621.0
  ethmoidal (sinus) 471.8
  fallopian tube 620.8
  female genital organs NEC 624.8
  frontal (sinus) 471.8
  gallbladder 575.6
  gingiva 523.8
  gum 523.8
  labia 624.6
  larynx (mucous) 478.4
  malignant (M8000/3) — see Neoplasm, by site, malignant
  maxillary (sinus) 471.8
  middle ear 385.30
  myometrium 621.0
  nares
    anterior 471.9
    posterior 471.0
  nasal (mucous) 471.9
    cavity 471.0
    septum 471.9
  nasopharyngeal 471.0
  neoplastic (M8210/0) — see Neoplasm, by site, benign
  nose (mucous) 471.9
  oviduct 620.8
  paratubal 620.8
  pharynx 478.29
    congenital 750.29
  placenta, placental 674.4 ☑5ᵗʰ
  prostate 600.2
  pudenda 624.6
  pulp (dental) 522.0
  rectosigmoid 211.4
  rectum (nonadenomatous) 569.0
    adenomatous 211.4
  septum (nasal) 471.9
  sinus (accessory) (ethmoidal) (frontal) (maxillary) (sphenoidal) 471.8
  sphenoidal (sinus) 471.8
  stomach (M8210/0) 211.1
  tube, fallopian 620.8
  turbinate, mucous membrane 471.8
  ureter 593.89
  urethra 599.3
  uterine
    ligament 620.8
    tube 620.8
  uterus (body) (corpus) (mucous) 621.0
    in pregnancy or childbirth 654.1 ☑5ᵗʰ
      affecting fetus or newborn 763.89
      causing obstructed labor 660.2 ☑5ᵗʰ
  vagina 623.7
  vocal cord (mucous) 478.4
  vulva 624.6
Polyphagia 783.6
Polypoid — see condition
Polyposis — see also Polyp
  coli (adenomatous) (M8220/0) 211.3
    adenocarcinoma in (M8220/3) 153.9
    carcinoma in (M8220/3) 153.9
  familial (M8220/0) 211.3
  intestinal (adenomatous) (M8220/0) 211.3
  multiple (M8221/0) — see Neoplasm, by site, benign
Polyradiculitis (acute) 357.0
Polyradiculoneuropathy (acute) (segmentally demyelinating) 357.0
Polysarcia 278.00

Polyserositis (peritoneal) 568.82
   due to pericarditis 423.2
   paroxysmal (familial) 277.3
   pericardial 423.2
   periodic 277.3
   pleural — *see* Pleurisy
   recurrent 277.3
   tuberculous (*see also* Tuberculosis,
      polyserositis) 018.9 ✓5ᵗʰ
Polysialia 527.7
Polysplenia syndrome 759.0
Polythelia 757.6
Polytrichia (*see also* Hypertrichosis) 704.1
Polyunguia (congenital) 757.5
   acquired 703.8
Polyuria 788.42
Pompe's disease (glycogenosis II) 271.0
Pompholyx 705.81
Poncet's disease (tuberculous rheumatism) (*see*
   also Tuberculosis) 015.9 ✓5ᵗʰ
Pond fracture — *see* Fracture, skull, vault
Ponos 085.0
Pons, pontine — *see* condition
Poor
   contractions, labor 661.2 ✓5ᵗʰ
      affecting fetus or newborn 763.7
   fetal growth NEC 764.9 ✓5ᵗʰ
      affecting management of pregnancy
         656.5 ✓5ᵗʰ
   incorporation
      artificial skin graft 996.55
      decellularized allodermis graft 996.55
   obstetrical history V13.49 ●
      affecting management of current ●
         pregnancy V23.49 ●
         pre-term labor V23.41 ●
      pre-term labor V13.41 ●
   sucking reflex (newborn) 796.1
   vision NEC 369.9
Poradenitis, nostras 099.1
Porencephaly (congenital) (developmental) (true)
   742.4
   acquired 348.0
   nondevelopmental 348.0
   traumatic (post) 310.2
Porocephaliasis 134.1
Porokeratosis 757.39
   disseminated superficial actinic (DSAP) 692.75
Poroma, eccrine (M8402/0) — *see* Neoplasm,
   skin, benign
Porphyria (acute) (congenital) (constitutional)
   (erythropoietic) (familial) (hepatica)
   (idiopathic) (idiosyncratic) (intermittent)
   (latent) (mixed hepatic) (photosensitive)
   (South African genetic) (Swedish) 277.1
   acquired 277.1
   cutaneatarda
      hereditaria 277.1
      symptomatica 277.1
   due to drugs
      correct substance properly administered
         277.1
      overdose or wrong substance given or taken
         977.9
         specified drug — *see* Table of Drugs and
            Chemicals
   secondary 277.1
   toxic NEC 277.1
   variegata 277.1
Porphyrinuria (acquired) (congenital) (secondary)
   277.1
Porphyruria (acquired) (congenital) 277.1
Portal — *see* condition
Port wine nevus or mark 757.32
Posadas-Wernicke disease 114.9
Position
   fetus, abnormal (*see also* Presentation, fetal)
      652.9 ✓5ᵗʰ
   teeth, faulty 524.3
Positive
   culture (nonspecific) 795.39 ▲
      AIDS virus V08
      blood 790.7

Positive — *continued*
   culture — *continued*
      HIV V08
      human immunodeficiency virus V08
      nose 795.39 ▲
      skin lesion NEC 795.39 ▲
      spinal fluid 792.0
      sputum 795.39 ▲
      stool 792.1
      throat 795.39 ▲
      urine 791.9
      wound 795.39 ▲
   findings, anthrax 795.31 ●
   HIV V08
   human immunodeficiency virus (HIV) V08
   PPD 795.5
   serology
      AIDS virus V08
         inconclusive 795.71
      HIV V08
         inconclusive 795.71
      human immunodeficiency virus (HIV) V08
         inconclusive 795.71
      syphilis 097.1
         with signs or symptoms — *see* Syphilis,
            by site and stage
         false 795.6
   skin test 795.7
      tuberculin (without active tuberculosis)
         795.5
   VDRL 097.1
      with signs or symptoms — *see* Syphilis, by
         site and stage
      false 795.6
   Wassermann reaction 097.1
      false 795.6
Postcardiotomy syndrome 429.4
Postcaval ureter 753.4
Postcholecystectomy syndrome 576.0
Postclimacteric bleeding 627.1
Postcommissurotomy syndrome 429.4
Postconcussional syndrome 310.2
Postcontusional syndrome 310.2
Postcricoid region — *see* condition
Post-dates (pregnancy) — *see* Pregnancy
Postencephalitic — *see also* condition
   syndrome 310.8
Posterior — *see* condition
Posterolateral sclerosis (spinal cord) — *see*
   Degeneration, combined
Postexanthematous — *see* condition
Postfebrile — *see* condition
Postgastrectomy dumping syndrome 564.2
Posthemiplegic chorea 344.89
Posthemorrhagic anemia (chronic) 280.0
   acute 285.1
   newborn 776.5
Posthepatitis syndrome 780.79
Postherpetic neuralgia (intercostal) (syndrome)
   (zoster) 053.19
   geniculate ganglion 053.11
   ophthalmica 053.19
   trigeminal 053.12
Posthitis 607.1
Postimmunization complication or reaction —
   see Complications, vaccination
Postinfectious — *see* condition
Postinfluenzal syndrome 780.79
Postlaminectomy syndrome 722.80
   cervical, cervicothoracic 722.81
   kyphosis 737.12
   lumbar, lumbosacral 722.83
   thoracic, thoracolumbar 722.82
Postleukotomy syndrome 310.0
Postlobectomy syndrome 310.0
Postmastectomy lymphedema (syndrome) 457.0
Postmaturity, postmature (fetus or newborn)
   766.2
   affecting management of pregnancy
      post term pregnancy 645.1 ✓5ᵗʰ
      prolonged pregnancy 645.2 ✓5ᵗʰ
   syndrome 766.2

Postmeasles — *see also* condition
   complication 055.8
      specified NEC 055.79
Postmenopausal
   endometrium (atrophic) 627.8
      suppurative (see also Endometritis) 615.9
   hormone replacement V07.4
   status (age related) (natural) V49.81
Postnasal drip — *see* Sinusitis
Postnatal — *see* condition
Postoperative — *see also* condition
   confusion state 293.9
   psychosis 293.9
   status NEC (*see also* Status (post)) V45.89
Postpancreatectomy hyperglycemia 251.3
Postpartum — *see also* condition
   observation
      immediately after delivery V24.0
      routine follow-up V24.2
Postperfusion syndrome NEC 999.8
   bone marrow 996.85
Postpoliomyelitic — *see* condition
Postsurgery status NEC (*see also* Status (post))
   V45.89
Post-term (pregnancy) 645.1 ✓5ᵗʰ
   infant (294 days or more gestation) 766.2
Posttraumatic — *see* condition
Posttraumatic brain syndrome, nonpsychotic
   310.2
Post-typhoid abscess 002.0
Postures, hysterical 300.11
Postvaccinal reaction or complication — *see*
   Complications, vaccination
Postvagotomy syndrome 564.2
Postvalvulotomy syndrome 429.4
Postvasectomy sperm count V25.8
Potain's disease (pulmonary edema) 514
Potain's syndrome (gastrectasis with dyspepsia)
   536.1
Pott's
   curvature (spinal) (*see also* Tuberculosis)
      015.0 ✓5ᵗʰ *[737.43]*
   disease or paraplegia (*see also* Tuberculosis)
      015.0 ✓5ᵗʰ *[730.88]*
   fracture (closed) 824.4
      open 824.5
   gangrene 440.24
   osteomyelitis (*see also* Tuberculosis)
      015.0 ✓5ᵗʰ *[730.88]*
   spinal curvature (*see also* Tuberculosis)
      015.0 ✓5ᵗʰ *[737.43]*
   tumor, puffy (*see also* Osteomyelitis) 730.2 ✓5ᵗʰ
Potter's
   asthma 502
   disease 753.0
   facies 754.0
   lung 502
   syndrome (with renal agenesis) 753.0
Pouch
   bronchus 748.3
   Douglas' — *see* condition
   esophagus, esophageal (congenital) 750.4
      acquired 530.6
   gastric 537.1
   Hartmann's (abnormal sacculation of
      gallbladder neck) 575.8
      of intestine V44.3
         attention to V55.3
   pharynx, pharyngeal (congenital) 750.27
Poulet's disease 714.2
Poultrymen's itch 133.8
Poverty V60.2
Prader-Labhart-Willi-Fanconi syndrome
   (hypogenital dystrophy with diabetic
   tendency) 759.81
Prader-Willi syndrome (hypogenital dystrophy
   with diabetic tendency) 759.81
Preachers' voice 784.49
Pre-AIDS — *see* Human immunodeficiency virus
   (disease) (illness) (infection)
Preauricular appendage 744.1

Prebetalipoproteinemia (acquired) (essential) (familial) (hereditary) (primary) (secondary) 272.1
  with chylomicronemia 272.3

Precipitate labor 661.3 ✓5ᵗʰ
  affecting fetus or newborn 763.6

Preclimacteric bleeding 627.0
  menorrhagia 627.0

Precocious
  adrenarche 259.1
  menarche 259.1
  menstruation 626.8
  pubarche 259.1
  puberty NEC 259.1
  sexual development NEC 259.1
  thelarche 259.1

Precocity, sexual (constitutional) (cryptogenic) (female) (idiopathic) (male) NEC 259.1
  with adrenal hyperplasia 255.2

Precordial pain 786.51
  psychogenic 307.89

Predeciduous teeth 520.2

Prediabetes, prediabetic 790.2
  complicating pregnancy, childbirth, or puerperium 648.8 ✓5ᵗʰ
  fetus or newborn 775.8

Predislocation status of hip, at birth (see also Subluxation, congenital, hip) 754.32

Preeclampsia (mild) 642.4 ✓5ᵗʰ
  with pre-existing hypertension 642.7 ✓5ᵗʰ
  affecting fetus or newborn 760.0
  severe 642.5 ✓5ᵗʰ
  superimposed on pre-existing hypertensive disease 642.7 ✓5ᵗʰ

Preeruptive color change, teeth, tooth 520.8

Preexcitation 426.7
  atrioventricular conduction 426.7
  ventricular 426.7

Preglaucoma 365.00

Pregnancy (single) (uterine) (without sickness) V22.2

> Note — Use the following fifth-digit subclassification with categories 640-648, 651-676:
>
> 0 unspecified as to episode of care
> 1 delivered, with or without mention of antepartum condition
> 2 delivered, with mention of postpartum complication
> 3 antepartum condition or complication
> 4 postpartum condition or complication

  abdominal (ectopic) 633.00 ▲
    with intrauterine pregnancy 633.01 ●
      affecting fetus or newborn 761.4
  abnormal NEC 646.9 ✓5ᵗʰ
  ampullar — see Pregnancy, tubal
  broad ligament — see Pregnancy, cornual
  cervical — see Pregnancy, cornual
  combined (extrauterine and intrauterine) — see Pregnancy, cornual
  complicated (by)
    abnormal, abnormality NEC 646.9 ✓5ᵗʰ
      cervix 654.6 ✓5ᵗʰ
      cord (umbilical) 663.9 ✓5ᵗʰ
      glucose tolerance (conditions classifiable to 790.2) 648.8 ✓5ᵗʰ
      injury 648.9 ✓5ᵗʰ
        obstetrical NEC 665.9 ✓5ᵗʰ
      obstetrical trauma NEC 665.9 ✓5ᵗʰ
      pelvic organs or tissues NEC 654.9 ✓5ᵗʰ
      pelvis (bony) 653.0 ✓5ᵗʰ
      perineum or vulva 654.8 ✓5ᵗʰ
      placenta, placental (vessel) 656.7 ✓5ᵗʰ
      position
        cervix 654.4 ✓5ᵗʰ
        placenta 641.1 ✓5ᵗʰ
          without hemorrhage 641.0 ✓5ᵗʰ
        uterus 654.4 ✓5ᵗʰ

Pregnancy — continued
  complicated (by) — continued
    abnormal, abnormality NEC — continued
      size, fetus 653.5 ✓5ᵗʰ
      uterus (congenital) 654.0 ✓5ᵗʰ
    abscess or cellulitis
      bladder 646.6 ✓5ᵗʰ
      genitourinary tract (conditions classifiable to 590, 595, 597, 599.0, 614-616) 646.6 ✓5ᵗʰ
      kidney 646.6 ✓5ᵗʰ
      urinary tract NEC 646.6 ✓5ᵗʰ
    air embolism 673.0 ✓5ᵗʰ
    albuminuria 646.2 ✓5ᵗʰ
      with hypertension — see Toxemia, of pregnancy
    amnionitis 658.4 ✓5ᵗʰ
    amniotic fluid embolism 673.1 ✓5ᵗʰ
    anemia (conditions classifiable to 280-285) 648.2 ✓5ᵗʰ
    atrophy, yellow (acute) (liver) (subacute) 646.7 ✓5ᵗʰ
    bacilluria, asymptomatic 646.5 ✓5ᵗʰ
    bacteriuria, asymptomatic 646.5 ✓5ᵗʰ
    bicornis or bicornuate uterus 654.0 ✓5ᵗʰ
    bone and joint disorders (conditions classifiable to 720-724 or conditions affecting lower limbs classifiable to 711-719, 725-738) 648.7 ✓5ᵗʰ
    breech presentation 652.2 ✓5ᵗʰ
      with successful version 652.1 ✓5ᵗʰ
    cardiovascular disease (conditions classifiable to 390-398, 410-429) 648.6 ✓5ᵗʰ
      congenital (conditions classifiable to 745-747) 648.5 ✓5ᵗʰ
    cerebrovascular disorders (conditions classifiable to 430-434, 436-437) 674.0 ✓5ᵗʰ
    cervicitis (conditions classifiable to 616.0) 646.6 ✓5ᵗʰ
    chloasma (gravidarum) 646.8 ✓5ᵗʰ
    chorea (gravidarum) — see Eclampsia, pregnancy
    cholelithiasis 646.8 ✓5ᵗʰ   ●
    contraction, pelvis (general) 653.1 ✓5ᵗʰ
      inlet 653.2 ✓5ᵗʰ
      outlet 653.3 ✓5ᵗʰ
    convulsions (eclamptic) (uremic) 642.6 ✓5ᵗʰ
      with pre-existing hypertension 642.7 ✓5ᵗʰ
    current disease or condition (nonobstetric)
      abnormal glucose tolerance 648.8 ✓5ᵗʰ
      anemia 648.2 ✓5ᵗʰ
      bone and joint (lower limb) 648.7 ✓5ᵗʰ
      cardiovascular 648.6 ✓5ᵗʰ
        congenital 648.5 ✓5ᵗʰ
      cerebrovascular 674.0 ✓5ᵗʰ
      diabetic 648.0 ✓5ᵗʰ
      drug dependence 648.3 ✓5ᵗʰ
      genital organ or tract 646.6 ✓5ᵗʰ
      gonorrheal 647.1 ✓5ᵗʰ
      hypertensive 642.2 ✓5ᵗʰ
        renal 642.1 ✓5ᵗʰ
      infectious 647.9 ✓5ᵗʰ
        specified type NEC 647.8 ✓5ᵗʰ
      liver 646.7 ✓5ᵗʰ
      malarial 647.4 ✓5ᵗʰ
      nutritional deficiency 648.9 ✓5ᵗʰ
      parasitic NEC 647.8 ✓5ᵗʰ
      renal 646.2 ✓5ᵗʰ
        hypertensive 642.1 ✓5ᵗʰ
      rubella 647.5 ✓5ᵗʰ
      specified condition NEC 648.9 ✓5ᵗʰ
      syphilitic 647.0 ✓5ᵗʰ
      thyroid 648.1 ✓5ᵗʰ
      tuberculous 647.3 ✓5ᵗʰ
      urinary 646.6 ✓5ᵗʰ
      venereal 647.2 ✓5ᵗʰ
      viral NEC 647.6 ✓5ᵗʰ
    cystitis 646.6 ✓5ᵗʰ
    cystocele 654.4 ✓5ᵗʰ
    death of fetus (near term) 656.4 ✓5ᵗʰ
      early pregnancy (before 22 completed weeks gestation) 632
    deciduitis 646.6 ✓5ᵗʰ
    decreased fetal movements 655.7

Pregnancy — continued
  complicated (by) — continued
    diabetes (mellitus) (conditions classifiable to 250) 648.0 ✓5ᵗʰ
    disorders of liver 646.7 ✓5ᵗʰ
    displacement, uterus NEC 654.4 ✓5ᵗʰ
    disproportion — see Disproportion
    double uterus 654.0 ✓5ᵗʰ
    drug dependence (conditions classifiable to 304) 648.3 ✓5ᵗʰ
    dysplasia, cervix 654.6 ✓5ᵗʰ
    early onset of delivery (spontaneous) 644.2 ✓5ᵗʰ
    eclampsia, eclamptic (coma) (convulsions) (delirium) (nephritis) (uremia) 642.6 ✓5ᵗʰ
      with pre-existing hypertension 642.7 ✓5ᵗʰ
    edema 646.1 ✓5ᵗʰ
      with hypertension — see Toxemia, of pregnancy
    effusion, amniotic fluid 658.1 ✓5ᵗʰ
      delayed delivery following 658.2 ✓5ᵗʰ
    embolism
      air 673.0 ✓5ᵗʰ
      amniotic fluid 673.1 ✓5ᵗʰ
      blood-clot 673.2 ✓5ᵗʰ
      cerebral 674.0 ✓5ᵗʰ
      pulmonary NEC 673.2 ✓5ᵗʰ
      pyemic 673.3 ✓5ᵗʰ
      septic 673.3 ✓5ᵗʰ
    emesis (gravidarum) — see Pregnancy, complicated, vomiting
    endometritis (conditions classifiable to 615.0-615.9) 646.6 ✓5ᵗʰ
      decidual 646.6 ✓5ᵗʰ
    excessive weight gain NEC 646.1 ✓5ᵗʰ
    face presentation 652.4 ✓5ᵗʰ
    failure, fetal head to enter pelvic brim 652.5 ✓5ᵗʰ
    false labor (pains) 644.1 ✓5ᵗʰ
    fatigue 646.8 ✓5ᵗʰ
    fatty metamorphosis of liver 646.7 ✓5ᵗʰ
    fetal
      death (near term) 656.4 ✓5ᵗʰ
        early (before 22 completed weeks gestation) 632
      deformity 653.7 ✓5ᵗʰ
      distress 656.8 ✓5ᵗʰ
    fibroid (tumor) (uterus) 654.1 ✓5ᵗʰ
    footling presentation 652.8 ✓5ᵗʰ
      with successful version 652.1 ✓5ᵗʰ
    gallbladder disease 646.8 ✓5ᵗʰ   ●
    goiter 648.1 ✓5ᵗʰ
    gonococcal infection (conditions classifiable to 098) 647.1 ✓5ᵗʰ
    gonorrhea (conditions classifiable to 098) 647.1 ✓5ᵗʰ
    hemorrhage 641.9 ✓5ᵗʰ
      accidental 641.2 ✓5ᵗʰ
      before 22 completed weeks gestation NEC 640.9 ✓5ᵗʰ
      cerebrovascular 674.0 ✓5ᵗʰ
      due to
        afibrinogenemia or other coagulation defect (conditions classifiable to 286.0-286.9) 641.3 ✓5ᵗʰ
        leiomyoma, uterine 641.8 ✓5ᵗʰ
        marginal sinus (rupture) 641.2 ✓5ᵗʰ
        premature separation, placenta 641.2 ✓5ᵗʰ
        trauma 641.8 ✓5ᵗʰ
      early (before 22 completed weeks gestation) 640.9 ✓5ᵗʰ
      threatened abortion 640.0 ✓5ᵗʰ
      unavoidable 641.1 ✓5ᵗʰ
    hepatitis (acute) (malignant) (subacute) 646.7 ✓5ᵗʰ
      viral 647.6 ✓5ᵗʰ
    herniation of uterus 654.4 ✓5ᵗʰ
    high head at term 652.5 ✓5ᵗʰ
    hydatidiform mole (delivered) (undelivered) 630
    hydramnios 657 ✓5ᵗʰ
    hydrocephalic fetus 653.6 ✓5ᵗʰ
    hydrops amnii 657 ✓5ᵗʰ
    hydrorrhea 658.1 ✓5ᵗʰ
    hyperemesis (gravidarum) — see Hyperemesis, gravidarum

Pregnancy — *continued*
  complicated (by) — *continued*
    hypertension — *see* Hypertension, complicating pregnancy
    hypertensive
      heart and renal disease 642.2 ✓5ᵗʰ
      heart disease 642.2 ✓5ᵗʰ
      renal disease 642.2 ✓5ᵗʰ
    hyperthyroidism 648.1 ✓5ᵗʰ
    hypothyroidism 648.1 ✓5ᵗʰ
    hysteralgia 646.8 ✓5ᵗʰ
    icterus gravis 646.7 ✓5ᵗʰ
    incarceration, uterus 654.3 ✓5ᵗʰ
    incompetent cervix (os) 654.5 ✓5ᵗʰ
    infection 647.9 ✓5ᵗʰ
      amniotic fluid 658.4 ✓5ᵗʰ
      bladder 646.6 ✓5ᵗʰ
      genital organ (conditions classifiable to 614-616) 646.6 ✓5ᵗʰ
      kidney (conditions classifiable to 590.0-590.9) 646.6 ✓5ᵗʰ
      urinary (tract) 646.6 ✓5ᵗʰ
        asymptomatic 646.5 ✓5ᵗʰ
    infective and parasitic diseases NEC 647.8 ✓5ᵗʰ
    inflammation
      bladder 646.6 ✓5ᵗʰ
      genital organ (conditions classifiable to 614-616) 646.6 ✓5ᵗʰ
      urinary tract NEC 646.6 ✓5ᵗʰ
    insufficient weight gain 646.8 ✓5ᵗʰ
    intrauterine fetal death (near term) NEC 656.4 ✓5ᵗʰ
      early (before 22 completed weeks' gestation) 632
    malaria (conditions classifiable to 084) 647.4 ✓5ᵗʰ
    malformation, uterus (congenital) 654.0 ✓5ᵗʰ
    malnutrition (conditions classifiable to 260-269) 648.9 ✓5ᵗʰ
    malposition
      fetus — *see* Pregnancy, complicated, malpresentation
      uterus or cervix 654.4 ✓5ᵗʰ
    malpresentation 652.9 ✓5ᵗʰ
      with successful version 652.1 ✓5ᵗʰ
      in multiple gestation 652.6 ✓5ᵗʰ
      specified type NEC 652.8 ✓5ᵗʰ
    marginal sinus hemorrhage or rupture 641.2 ✓5ᵗʰ
    maternal obesity syndrome 646.1 ✓5ᵗʰ
    menstruation 640.8 ✓5ᵗʰ
    mental disorders (conditions classifiable to 290-303, 305-316, 317-319) 648.4 ✓5ᵗʰ
    mentum presentation 652.4 ✓5ᵗʰ
    missed
      abortion 632
      delivery (at or near term) 656.4 ✓5ᵗʰ
      labor (at or near term) 656.4 ✓5ᵗʰ
    necrosis
      genital organ or tract (conditions classifiable to 614-616) 646.6 ✓5ᵗʰ
      liver (conditions classifiable to 570) 646.7 ✓5ᵗʰ
      renal, cortical 646.2 ✓5ᵗʰ
    nephritis or nephrosis (conditions classifiable to 580-589) 646.2 ✓5ᵗʰ
      with hypertension 642.1 ✓5ᵗʰ
    nephropathy NEC 646.2 ✓5ᵗʰ
    neuritis (peripheral) 646.4 ✓5ᵗʰ
    nutritional deficiency (conditions classifiable to 260-269) 648.9 ✓5ᵗʰ
    oblique lie or presentation 652.3 ✓5ᵗʰ
      with successful version 652.1 ✓5ᵗʰ
    obstetrical trauma NEC 665.9 ✓5ᵗʰ
    oligohydramnios NEC 658.0 ✓5ᵗʰ
    onset of contractions before 37 weeks 644.0 ✓5ᵗʰ
    oversize fetus 653.5 ✓5ᵗʰ
    papyraceous fetus 646.0 ✓5ᵗʰ
    patent cervix 654.5 ✓5ᵗʰ
    pelvic inflammatory disease (conditions classifiable to 614-616) 646.6 ✓5ᵗʰ
    placenta, placental
      abnormality 656.7 ✓5ᵗʰ
      abruptio or ablatio 641.2 ✓5ᵗʰ
      detachment 641.2 ✓5ᵗʰ

Pregnancy — *continued*
  complicated (by) — *continued*
    placenta, placental — *continued*
      disease 656.7 ✓5ᵗʰ
      infarct 656.7 ✓5ᵗʰ
      low implantation 641.1 ✓5ᵗʰ
        without hemorrhage 641.0 ✓5ᵗʰ
      malformation 656.7 ✓5ᵗʰ
      malposition 641.1 ✓5ᵗʰ
        without hemorrhage 641.0 ✓5ᵗʰ
      marginal sinus hemorrhage 641.2 ✓5ᵗʰ
      previa 641.1 ✓5ᵗʰ
        without hemorrhage 641.0 ✓5ᵗʰ
      separation (premature) (undelivered) 641.2 ✓5ᵗʰ
    placentitis 658.4 ✓5ᵗʰ
    polyhydramnios 657 ✓5ᵗʰ
    postmaturity
      post term 645.1 ✓5ᵗʰ
      prolonged 645.2 ✓5ᵗʰ
    prediabetes 648.8 ✓5ᵗʰ
    pre-eclampsia (mild) 642.4 ✓5ᵗʰ
      severe 642.5 ✓5ᵗʰ
      superimposed on pre-existing hypertensive disease 642.7 ✓5ᵗʰ
    premature rupture of membranes 658.1 ✓5ᵗʰ
      with delayed delivery 658.2 ✓5ᵗʰ
    previous
      infertility V23.0
      nonobstetric condition V23.8 ✓5ᵗʰ
      poor obstetrical history V23.49   ▲
      premature delivery V23.41   ▲
      trophoblastic disease (conditions classifiable to 630) V23.1
    prolapse, uterus 654.4 ✓5ᵗʰ
    proteinuria (gestational) 646.2 ✓5ᵗʰ
      with hypertension — *see* Toxemia, of pregnancy
    pruritus (neurogenic) 646.8 ✓5ᵗʰ
    psychosis or psychoneurosis 648.4 ✓5ᵗʰ
    ptyalism 646.8 ✓5ᵗʰ
    pyelitis (conditions classifiable to 590.0-590.9) 646.6 ✓5ᵗʰ
    renal disease or failure NEC 646.2 ✓5ᵗʰ
      with secondary hypertension 642.1 ✓5ᵗʰ
      hypertensive 642.2 ✓5ᵗʰ
    retention, retained dead ovum 631
    retroversion, uterus 654.3 ✓5ᵗʰ
    Rh immunization, incompatibility, or sensitization 656.1 ✓5ᵗʰ
    rubella (conditions classifiable to 056) 647.5 ✓5ᵗʰ
    rupture
      amnion (premature) 658.1 ✓5ᵗʰ
        with delayed delivery 658.2 ✓5ᵗʰ
      marginal sinus (hemorrhage) 641.2 ✓5ᵗʰ
      membranes (premature) 658.1 ✓5ᵗʰ
        with delayed delivery 658.2 ✓5ᵗʰ
      uterus (before onset of labor) 665.0 ✓5ᵗʰ
    salivation (excessive) 646.8 ✓5ᵗʰ
    salpingo-oophoritis (conditions classifiable to 614.0-614.2) 646.6 ✓5ᵗʰ
    septicemia (conditions classifiable to 038.0-038.9) 647.8 ✓5ᵗʰ
      postpartum 670 ✓4ᵗʰ
      puerperal 670 ✓4ᵗʰ
    spasms, uterus (abnormal) 646.8 ✓5ᵗʰ
    specified condition NEC 646.8 ✓5ᵗʰ
    spurious labor pains 644.1 ✓5ᵗʰ
    superfecundation 651.9 ✓5ᵗʰ
    superfetation 651.9 ✓5ᵗʰ
    syphilis (conditions classifiable to 090-097) 647.0 ✓5ᵗʰ
    threatened
      abortion 640.0 ✓5ᵗʰ
      premature delivery 644.2 ✓5ᵗʰ
      premature labor 644.0 ✓5ᵗʰ
    thrombophlebitis (superficial) 671.2 ✓5ᵗʰ
      deep 671.3 ✓5ᵗʰ
    thrombosis 671.9 ✓5ᵗʰ
      venous (superficial) 671.2 ✓5ᵗʰ
        deep 671.3 ✓5ᵗʰ
    thyroid dysfunction (conditions classifiable to 240-246) 648.1 ✓5ᵗʰ
    thyroiditis 648.1 ✓5ᵗʰ
    thyrotoxicosis 648.1 ✓5ᵗʰ
    torsion of uterus 654.4 ✓5ᵗʰ

Pregnancy — *continued*
  complicated (by) — *continued*
    toxemia — *see* Toxemia, of pregnancy
    transverse lie or presentation 652.3 ✓5ᵗʰ
      with successful version 652.1 ✓5ᵗʰ
    tuberculosis (conditions classifiable to 010-018) 647.3 ✓5ᵗʰ
    tumor
      cervix 654.6 ✓5ᵗʰ
      ovary 654.4 ✓5ᵗʰ
      pelvic organs or tissue NEC 654.4 ✓5ᵗʰ
      uterus (body) 654.1 ✓5ᵗʰ
        cervix 654.6 ✓5ᵗʰ
      vagina 654.7 ✓5ᵗʰ
      vulva 654.8 ✓5ᵗʰ
    unstable lie 652.0 ✓5ᵗʰ
    uremia — *see* Pregnancy, complicated, renal disease
    urethritis 646.6 ✓5ᵗʰ
    vaginitis or vulvitis (conditions classifiable to 616.1) 646.6 ✓5ᵗʰ
    varicose
      placental vessels 656.7 ✓5ᵗʰ
      veins (legs) 671.0 ✓5ᵗʰ
        perineum 671.1 ✓5ᵗʰ
        vulva 671.1 ✓5ᵗʰ
    varicosity, labia or vulva 671.1 ✓5ᵗʰ
    venereal disease NEC (conditions classifiable to 099) 647.2 ✓5ᵗʰ
    viral disease NEC (conditions classifiable to 042, 050-055, 057-079) 647.6 ✓5ᵗʰ
    vomiting (incoercible) (pernicious) (persistent) (uncontrollable) (vicious) 643.9 ✓5ᵗʰ
      due to organic disease or other cause 643.8 ✓5ᵗʰ
      early — *see* Hyperemesis, gravidarum
      late (after 22 completed weeks gestation) 643.2 ✓5ᵗʰ
    young maternal age 659.8 ✓5ᵗʰ
  complications NEC 646.9 ✓5ᵗʰ
  cornual 633.80   ▲
    with intrauterine pregnancy 633.81   ●
    affecting fetus or newborn 761.4
  death, maternal NEC 646.9 ✓5ᵗʰ
  delivered — *see* Delivery
  ectopic (ruptured) NEC 633.90   ▲
    with intrauterine pregnancy 633.91   ●
    abdominal — *see* Pregnancy, abdominal
    affecting fetus or newborn 761.4
    combined (extrauterine and intrauterine) — *see* Pregnancy, cornual
    ovarian — *see* Pregnancy, ovarian
    specified type NEC 633.80   ▲
      with intrauterine pregnancy 633.81   ●
      affecting fetus or newborn 761.4
    tubal — *see* Pregnancy, tubal
  examination, pregnancy not confirmed V72.4
  extrauterine — *see* Pregnancy, ectopic
  fallopian — *see* Pregnancy, tubal
  false 300.11
    labor (pains) 644.1 ✓5ᵗʰ
  fatigue 646.8 ✓5ᵗʰ
  illegitimate V61.6
  incidental finding V22.2
  in double uterus 654.0 ✓5ᵗʰ
  interstitial — *see* Pregnancy, cornual
  intraligamentous — *see* Pregnancy, cornual
  intramural — *see* Pregnancy, cornual
  intraperitoneal — *see* Pregnancy, abdominal
  isthmian — *see* Pregnancy, tubal
  management affected by
    abnormal, abnormality
      fetus (suspected) 655.9 ✓5ᵗʰ
        specified NEC 655.8 ✓5ᵗʰ
      placenta 656.7 ✓5ᵗʰ
    advanced maternal age NEC 659.6 ✓5ᵗʰ
      multigravida 659.6 ✓5ᵗʰ
      primigravida 659.5 ✓5ᵗʰ
    antibodies (maternal)
      anti-c 656.1 ✓5ᵗʰ
      anti-d 656.1 ✓5ᵗʰ
      anti-e 656.1 ✓5ᵗʰ
      blood group (ABO) 656.2 ✓5ᵗʰ
        Rh(esus) 656.1 ✓5ᵗʰ
    elderly multigravida 659.6 ✓5ᵗʰ
    elderly primigravida 659.5 ✓5ᵗʰ

Pregnancy — *continued*
  management affected by — *continued*
    fetal (suspected)
      abnormality 655.9 ✓5ᵗʰ
        acid-base balance 656.8 ✓5ᵗʰ
        heart rate or rhythm 659.7 ✓5ᵗʰ
        specified NEC 655.8 ✓5ᵗʰ
      acidemia 656.3 ✓5ᵗʰ
      anencephaly 655.0 ✓5ᵗʰ
      bradycardia 659.7 ✓5ᵗʰ
      central nervous system malformation 655.0 ✓5ᵗʰ
      chromosomal abnormalities (conditions classifiable to 758.0-758.9) 655.1 ✓5ᵗʰ
      damage from
        drugs 655.5 ✓5ᵗʰ
          obstetric, anesthetic, or sedative 655.5 ✓5ᵗʰ
        environmental toxins 655.8 ✓5ᵗʰ
        intrauterine contraceptive device 655.8 ✓5ᵗʰ
      maternal
        alcohol addiction 655.4 ✓5ᵗʰ
        disease NEC 655.4 ✓5ᵗʰ
        drug use 655.5 ✓5ᵗʰ
        listeriosis 655.4 ✓5ᵗʰ
        rubella 655.3 ✓5ᵗʰ
        toxoplasmosis 655.4 ✓5ᵗʰ
        viral infection 655.3 ✓5ᵗʰ
      radiation 655.6 ✓5ᵗʰ
      death (near term) 656.4 ✓5ᵗʰ
        early (before 22 completed weeks' gestation) 632
      distress 656.8 ✓5ᵗʰ
      excessive growth 656.6 ✓5ᵗʰ
      growth retardation 656.5 ✓5ᵗʰ
      hereditary disease 655.2 ✓5ᵗʰ
      hydrocephalus 655.0 ✓5ᵗʰ
      intrauterine death 656.4 ✓5ᵗʰ
      poor growth 656.5 ✓5ᵗʰ
      spina bifida (with myelomeningocele) 655.0 ✓5ᵗʰ
    fetal-maternal hemorrhage 656.0 ✓5ᵗʰ
    hereditary disease in family (possibly) affecting fetus 655.2 ✓5ᵗʰ
    incompatibility, blood groups (ABO) 656.2 ✓5ᵗʰ
      rh(esus) 656.1 ✓5ᵗʰ
    insufficient prenatal care V23.7
    intrauterine death 656.4 ✓5ᵗʰ
    isoimmunization (ABO) 656.2 ✓5ᵗʰ
      rh(esus) 656.1 ✓5ᵗʰ
    large-for-dates fetus 656.6 ✓5ᵗʰ
    light-for-dates fetus 656.5 ✓5ᵗʰ
    meconium in liquor 656.8 ✓5ᵗʰ
    mental disorder (conditions classifiable to 290-303, 305-316, 317-319) 648.4 ✓5ᵗʰ
    multiparity (grand) 659.4 ✓5ᵗʰ
    poor obstetric history V23.49 ▲
      pre-term labor V23.41 ●
    postmaturity
      post term 645.1 ✓5ᵗʰ
      prolonged 645.2 ✓5ᵗʰ
    post term pregnancy 645.1 ✓5ᵗʰ
    previous
      abortion V23.2
        habitual 646.3 ✓5ᵗʰ
      cesarean delivery 654.2 ✓5ᵗʰ
      difficult delivery V23.49 ▲
      forceps delivery V23.49 ▲
      habitual abortions 646.3 ✓5ᵗʰ
      hemorrhage, antepartum or postpartum V23.49 ▲
      hydatidiform mole V23.1
      infertility V23.0
      malignancy NEC V23.8 ✓5ᵗʰ
      nonobstetrical conditions V23.8 ✓5ᵗʰ
      premature delivery V23.41 ▲
      trophoblastic disease (conditions in 630) V23.1
      vesicular mole V23.1
    prolonged pregnancy 645.2 ✓5ᵗʰ
    small-for-dates fetus 656.5 ✓5ᵗʰ
    young maternal age 659.8 ✓5ᵗʰ
  maternal death NEC 646.9 ✓5ᵗʰ

Pregnancy — *continued*
  mesometric (mural) — *see* Pregnancy, cornual
  molar 631
    hydatidiform (*see also* Hydatidiform mole) 630
      previous, affecting management of pregnancy V23.1
    previous, affecting management of pregnancy V23.49 ▲
  multiple NEC 651.9 ✓5ᵗʰ
    with fetal loss and retention of one or more fetus(es) 651.6 ✓5ᵗʰ
    affecting fetus or newborn 761.5
    specified type NEC 651.8 ✓5ᵗʰ
      with fetal loss and retention of one or more fetus(es) 651.6 ✓5ᵗʰ
  mural — *see* Pregnancy, cornual
  observation NEC V22.1
    first pregnancy V22.0
    high-risk V23.9
      specified problem NEC V23.8 ✓5ᵗʰ
  ovarian 633.20 ▲
    with intrauterine pregnancy 633.21 ●
    affecting fetus or newborn 761.4
  postmature
    post term 645.1 ✓5ᵗʰ
    prolonged 645.2 ✓5ᵗʰ
  post term 645.1 ✓5ᵗʰ
  prenatal care only V22.1
    first pregnancy V22.0
    high-risk V23.9
      specified problem NEC V23.8 ✓5ᵗʰ
  prolonged 645.2 ✓5ᵗʰ
  quadruplet NEC 651.2 ✓5ᵗʰ
    with fetal loss and retention of one or more fetus(es) 651.5 ✓5ᵗʰ
    affecting fetus or newborn 761.5
  quintuplet NEC 651.8 ✓5ᵗʰ
    with fetal loss and retention of one or more fetus(es) 651.6 ✓5ᵗʰ
    affecting fetus or newborn 761.5
  sextuplet NEC 651.8 ✓5ᵗʰ
    with fetal loss and retention of one or more fetus(es) 651.6 ✓5ᵗʰ
    affecting fetus or newborn 761.5
  spurious 300.11
  superfecundation NEC 651.9 ✓5ᵗʰ
    with fetal loss and retention of one or more fetus(es) 651.6 ✓5ᵗʰ
  superfetation NEC 651.9 ✓5ᵗʰ
    with fetal loss and retention of one or more fetus(es) 651.6 ✓5ᵗʰ
  supervision (of) (for) — *see also* Pregnancy, management affected by
    elderly
      multigravida V23.82
      primigravida V23.81
    high-risk V23.9
      insufficient prenatal care V23.7
      specified problem NEC V23.8 ✓5ᵗʰ
    multiparity V23.3
    normal NEC V22.1
      first V22.0
    poor
      obstetric history V23.49 ▲
        pre-term labor V23.41 ●
      reproductive history V23.5
    previous
      abortion V23.2
      hydatidiform mole V23.1
      infertility V23.0
      neonatal death V23.5
      stillbirth V23.5
      trophoblastic disease V23.1
      vesicular mole V23.1
    specified problem NEC V23.8 ✓5ᵗʰ
    young
      multigravida V23.84
      primigravida V23.83
  triplet NEC 651.1 ✓5ᵗʰ
    with fetal loss and retention of one or more fetus(es) 651.4 ✓5ᵗʰ
    affecting fetus or newborn 761.5
  tubal (with rupture) 633.10 ▲
    with intrauterine pregnancy 633.11 ●
    affecting fetus or newborn 761.4

Pregnancy — *continued*
  twin NEC 651.0 ✓5ᵗʰ
    with fetal loss and retention of one fetus 651.3 ✓5ᵗʰ
    affecting fetus or newborn 761.5
  unconfirmed V72.4
  undelivered (no other diagnosis) V22.2
    with false labor 644.1 ✓5ᵗʰ
    high-risk V23.9
      specified problem NEC V23.8 ✓5ᵗʰ
  unwanted NEC V61.7
Pregnant uterus — *see* condition
Preiser's disease (osteoporosis) 733.09
Prekwashiorkor 260
Preleukemia 238.7
Preluxation of hip, congenital (*see also* Subluxation, congenital, hip) 754.32
Premature — *see also* condition
  beats (nodal) 427.60
    atrial 427.61
    auricular 427.61
    postoperative 997.1
    specified type NEC 427.69
    supraventricular 427.61
    ventricular 427.69
  birth NEC 765.1 ✓5ᵗʰ
  closure
    cranial suture 756.0
    fontanel 756.0
    foramen ovale 745.8
  contractions 427.60
    atrial 427.61
    auricular 427.61
    auriculoventricular 427.61
    heart (extrasystole) 427.60
    junctional 427.60
    nodal 427.60
    postoperative 997.1
    ventricular 427.69
  ejaculation 302.75
  infant NEC 765.1 ✓5ᵗʰ
    excessive 765.0 ✓5ᵗʰ
    light-for-dates — *see* Light-for-dates
  labor 644.2 ✓5ᵗʰ
    threatened 644.0 ✓5ᵗʰ
  lungs 770.4
  menopause 256.31
  puberty 259.1
  rupture of membranes or amnion 658.1 ✓5ᵗʰ
    affecting fetus or newborn 761.1
    delayed delivery following 658.2 ✓5ᵗʰ
  senility (syndrome) 259.8
  separation, placenta (partial) — *see* Placenta, separation
  ventricular systole 427.69
Prematurity NEC 765.1 ✓5ᵗʰ
  extreme 765.0 ✓5ᵗʰ
Premenstrual syndrome 625.4
Premenstrual tension 625.4
Premolarization, cuspids 520.2
Premyeloma 273.1
Prenatal
  care, normal pregnancy V22.1
    first V22.0
  death, cause unknown — *see* Death, fetus
  screening — *see* Antenatal, screening
Prepartum — *see* condition
Preponderance, left or right ventricular 429.3
Prepuce — *see* condition
Presbycardia 797
  hypertensive (*see also* Hypertension, heart) 402.90
Presbycusis 388.01
Presbyesophagus 530.89
Presbyophrenia 310.1
Presbyopia 367.4
Prescription of contraceptives NEC V25.02
  diaphragm V25.02
  oral (pill) V25.01
    repeat V25.41
  repeat V25.40
    oral (pill) V25.41

Pregnancy — Prescription

*(left margin, vertical)* Presenile — Problem

Presenile — *see also* condition
- aging 259.8
- dementia (*see also* Dementia, presenile) 290.10

Presenility 259.8

Presentation, fetal
- abnormal 652.9 ✓5ᵗʰ
  - with successful version 652.1 ✓5ᵗʰ
    - before labor, affecting fetus or newborn 761.7
  - causing obstructed labor 660.0 ✓5ᵗʰ
    - affecting fetus or newborn, any, except breech 763.1
  - in multiple gestation (one or more) 652.6 ✓5ᵗʰ
  - specified NEC 652.8 ✓5ᵗʰ
- arm 652.7 ✓5ᵗʰ
  - causing obstructed labor 660.0 ✓5ᵗʰ
- breech (buttocks) (complete) (frank) 652.2 ✓5ᵗʰ
  - with successful version 652.1 ✓5ᵗʰ
    - before labor, affecting fetus or newborn 761.7
    - before labor, affecting fetus or newborn 761.7
- brow 652.4 ✓5ᵗʰ
  - causing obstructed labor 660.0 ✓5ᵗʰ
- buttocks 652.2 ✓5ᵗʰ
- chin 652.4 ✓5ᵗʰ
- complete 652.2 ✓5ᵗʰ
- compound 652.8 ✓5ᵗʰ
- cord 663.0 ✓5ᵗʰ
- extended head 652.4 ✓5ᵗʰ
- face 652.4 ✓5ᵗʰ
  - to pubes 652.8 ✓5ᵗʰ
- footling 652.8 ✓5ᵗʰ
- frank 652.2 ✓5ᵗʰ
- hand, leg, or foot NEC 652.8 ✓5ᵗʰ
- incomplete 652.8 ✓5ᵗʰ
- mentum 652.4 ✓5ᵗʰ
- multiple gestation (one fetus or more) 652.6 ✓5ᵗʰ
- oblique 652.3 ✓5ᵗʰ
  - with successful version 652.1 ✓5ᵗʰ
- shoulder 652.8 ✓5ᵗʰ
  - affecting fetus or newborn 763.1
- transverse 652.3 ✓5ᵗʰ
  - with successful version 652.1 ✓5ᵗʰ
- umbilical cord 663.0 ✓5ᵗʰ
- unstable 652.0 ✓5ᵗʰ

Prespondylolisthesis (congenital) (lumbosacral) 756.11

Pressure
- area, skin ulcer (*see also* Decubitus) 707.0
- atrophy, spine 733.99
- birth, fetus or newborn NEC 767.9
- brachial plexus 353.0
- brain 348.4
  - injury at birth 767.0
- cerebral — *see* Pressure, brain
- chest 786.59
- cone, tentorial 348.4
  - injury at birth 767.0
- funis — *see* Compression, umbilical cord
- hyposystolic (*see also* Hypotension) 458.9
- increased
  - intracranial 781.99
    - due to
      - benign intracranial hypertension 348.2
      - hydrocephalus — *see* hydrocephalus
      - injury at birth 767.8
  - intraocular 365.00
- lumbosacral plexus 353.1
- mediastinum 519.3
- necrosis (chronic) (skin) (*see also* Decubitus) 707.0
- nerve — *see* Compression, nerve
- paralysis (*see also* Neuropathy, entrapment) 355.9
- sore (chronic) (*see also* Decubitus) 707.0
- spinal cord 336.9
- ulcer (chronic) (*see also* Decubitus) 707.0
- umbilical cord — *see* Compression, umbilical cord
- venous, increased 459.89

Pre-syncope 780.2

Preterm infant NEC 765.1 ✓5ᵗʰ
- extreme 765.0 ✓5ᵗʰ

Priapism (penis) 607.3

Prickling sensation (*see also* Disturbance, sensation) 782.0

Prickly heat 705.1

Primary — *see* condition

Primigravida, elderly
- affecting
  - fetus or newborn 763.89
  - management of pregnancy, labor, and delivery 659.5 ✓5ᵗʰ

Primipara, old
- affecting
  - fetus or newborn 763.89
  - management of pregnancy, labor, and delivery 659.5 ✓5ᵗʰ

Primula dermatitis 692.6

Primus varus (bilateral) (metatarsus) 754.52

P.R.I.N.D. 436

Pringle's disease (tuberous sclerosis) 759.5

Prinzmetal's angina 413.1

Prinzmetal-Massumi syndrome (anterior chest wall) 786.52

Prizefighter ear 738.7

Problem (with) V49.9
- academic V62.3
- acculturation V62.4
- adopted child V61.29
- aged
  - in-law V61.3
  - parent V61.3
  - person NEC V61.8
- alcoholism in family V61.41
- anger reaction (*see also* Disturbance, conduct) 312.0 ✓5ᵗʰ
- behavior, child 312.9
- behavioral V40.9
  - specified NEC V40.3
- betting V69.3
- cardiorespiratory NEC V47.2
- care of sick or handicapped person in family or household V61.49
- career choice V62.2
- communication V40.1
- conscience regarding medical care V62.6
- delinquency (juvenile) 312.9
- diet, inappropriate V69.1
- digestive NEC V47.3
- ear NEC V41.3
- eating habits, inappropriate V69.1
- economic V60.2
  - affecting care V60.9
    - specified type NEC V60.8
- educational V62.3
- enuresis, child 307.6
- exercise, lack of V69.0
- eye NEC V41.1
- family V61.9
  - specified circumstance NEC V61.8
- fear reaction, child 313.0
- feeding (elderly) (infant) 783.3
  - newborn 779.3
  - nonorganic 307.50
- fetal, affecting management of pregnancy 656.9 ✓5ᵗʰ
  - specified type NEC 656.8 ✓5ᵗʰ
- financial V60.2
- foster child V61.29
  - specified NEC V41.8
- functional V41.9
  - specified type NEC V41.8
- gambling V69.3
- genital NEC V47.5
- head V48.9
  - deficiency V48.0
  - disfigurement V48.6
  - mechanical V48.2
  - motor V48.2
  - movement of V48.2
  - sensory V48.4
  - specified condition NEC V48.8
- hearing V41.2
- high-risk sexual behavior V69.2
- influencing health status NEC V49.89
- internal organ NEC V47.9
  - deficiency V47.0

Problem (with) — *continued*
- internal organ NEC — *continued*
  - mechanical or motor V47.1
- interpersonal NEC V62.81
- jealousy, child 313.3
- learning V40.0
- legal V62.5
- life circumstance NEC V62.89
- lifestyle V69.9
  - specified NEC V69.8
- limb V49.9
  - deficiency V49.0
  - disfigurement V49.4
  - mechanical V49.1
  - motor V49.2
  - movement, involving
    - musculoskeletal system V49.1
    - nervous system V49.2
  - sensory V49.3
  - specified condition NEC V49.5
- litigation V62.5
- living alone V60.3
- loneliness NEC V62.89
- marital V61.10
  - involving
    - divorce V61.0
    - estrangement V61.0
    - psychosexual disorder 302.9
    - sexual function V41.7
- mastication V41.6
- medical care, within family V61.49
- mental V40.9
  - specified NEC V40.2
- mental hygiene, adult V40.9
- multiparity V61.5
- nail biting, child 307.9
- neck V48.9
  - deficiency V48.1
  - disfigurement V48.7
  - mechanical V48.3
  - motor V48.3
  - movement V48.3
  - sensory V48.5
  - specified condition NEC V48.8
- neurological NEC 781.99
- none (feared complaint unfounded) V65.5
- occupational V62.2
- parent-child V61.20
- partner V61.10
- personal NEC V62.89
  - interpersonal conflict NEC V62.81
- personality (*see also* Disorder, personality) 301.9
- phase of life V62.89
- placenta, affecting managment of pregnancy 656.9 ✓5ᵗʰ
  - specified type NEC 656.8 ✓5ᵗʰ
- poverty V60.2
- presence of sick or handicapped person in family or household V61.49
- psychiatric 300.9
- psychosocial V62.9
  - specified type NEC V62.89
- relational NEC V62.81
- relationship, childhood 313.3
- religious or spiritual belief
  - other than medical care V62.89
  - regarding medical care V62.6
- self-damaging behavior V69.8
- sexual
  - behavior, high-risk V69.2
  - function NEC V41.7
- sibling relational V61.8
- sight V41.0
- sleep disorder, child 307.40
- smell V41.5
- speech V40.1
- spite reaction, child (*see also* Disturbance, conduct) 312.0 ✓5ᵗʰ
- spoiled child reaction (*see also* Disturbance, conduct) 312.1 ✓5ᵗʰ
- swallowing V41.6
- tantrum, child (*see also* Disturbance, conduct) 312.1 ✓5ᵗʰ
- taste V41.5
- thumb sucking, child 307.9
- tic, child 307.21

Problem (with) — *continued*
 trunk V48.9
  deficiency V48.1
  disfigurement• V48.7
  mechanical V48.3
  motor V48.3
  movement V48.3
  sensory V48.5
  specified condition NEC V48.8
 unemployment V62.0
 urinary NEC V47.4
 voice production V41.4
Procedure (surgical) not done NEC V64.3
 because of
  contraindication V64.1
  patient's decision V64.2
   for reasons of conscience or religion
    V62.6
  specified reason NEC V64.3
Procidentia
 anus (sphincter) 569.1
 rectum (sphincter) 569.1
 stomach 537.89
 uteri 618.1
Proctalgia 569.42
 fugax 564.6
 spasmodic 564.6
  psychogenic 307.89
Proctitis 569.49
 amebic 006.8
 chlamydial 099.52
 gonococcal 098.7
 granulomatous 555.1
 idiopathic 556.2
  with ulcerative sigmoiditis 556.3
 tuberculous (*see also* Tuberculosis) 014.8 ✓5ᵗʰ
 ulcerative (chronic) (nonspecific) 556.2
  with ulcerative sigmoiditis 556.3
Proctocele
 female (without uterine prolapse) 618.0
  with uterine prolapse 618.4
   complete 618.3
   incomplete 618.2
 male 569.49
Proctocolitis, idiopathic 556.2
 with ulcerative sigmoiditis 556.3
Proctoptosis 569.1
Proctosigmoiditis 569.89
 ulcerative (chronic) 556.3
Proctospasm 564.6
 psychogenic 306.4
Prodromal-AIDS — *see* Human immunodeficiency
  virus (disease) (illness) (infection)
Profichet's disease or syndrome 729.9
Progeria (adultorum) (syndrome) 259.8
Prognathism (mandibular) (maxillary) 524.00
Progonoma (melanotic) (M9363/0) — *see*
  Neoplasm, by site, benign
Progressive — *see* condition
Prolapse, prolapsed
 anus, anal (canal) (sphincter) 569.1
 arm or hand, complicating delivery 652.7 ✓5ᵗʰ
  causing obstructed labor 660.0 ✓5ᵗʰ
   affecting fetus or newborn 763.1
  fetus or newborn 763.1
 bladder (acquired) (mucosa) (sphincter)
  congenital (female) (male) 756.71
  female 618.0
  male 596.8
 breast implant (prosthetic) 996.54
 cecostomy 569.69
 cecum 569.89
 cervix, cervical (stump) (hypertrophied) 618.1
  anterior lip, obstructing labor 660.2 ✓5ᵗʰ
   affecting fetus or newborn 763.1
  congenital 752.49
  postpartal (old) 618.1
 ciliary body 871.1
 colon (pedunculated) 569.89
 colostomy 569.69
 conjunctiva 372.73
 cord — *see* Prolapse, umbilical cord
 disc (intervertebral) — *see* Displacement,
  intervertebral disc

Prolapse, prolapsed — *continued*
 duodenum 537.89
 eye implant (orbital) 996.59
  lens (ocular) 996.53
 fallopian tube 620.4
 fetal extremity, complicating delivery 652.8 ✓5ᵗʰ
  causing obstructed labor 660.0 ✓5ᵗʰ
  fetus or newborn 763.1
 funis — *see* Prolapse, umbilical cord
 gastric (mucosa) 537.89
 genital, female 618.9
  specified NEC 618.8
 globe 360.81
 ileostomy bud 569.69
 intervertebral disc — *see* Displacement,
  intervertebral disc
 intestine (small) 569.89
 iris 364.8
  traumatic 871.1
 kidney (*see also* Disease, renal) 593.0
  congenital 753.3
 laryngeal muscles or ventricle 478.79
 leg, complicating delivery 652.8 ✓5ᵗʰ
  causing obstructed labor 660.0 ✓5ᵗʰ
  fetus or newborn 763.1
 liver 573.8
 meatus urinarius 599.5
 mitral valve 424.0
 ocular lens implant 996.53
 organ or site, congenital NEC — *see*
  Malposition, congenital
 ovary 620.4
 pelvic (floor), female 618.8
 perineum, female 618.8
 pregnant uterus 654.4 ✓5ᵗʰ
 rectum (mucosa) (sphincter) 569.1
  due to Trichuris trichiuria 127.3
 spleen 289.59
 stomach 537.89
 umbilical cord
  affecting fetus or newborn 762.4
  complicating delivery 663.0 ✓5ᵗʰ
 ureter 593.89
  with obstruction 593.4
 ureterovesical orifice 593.89
 urethra (acquired) (infected) (mucosa) 599.5
  congenital 753.8
 uterovaginal 618.4
  complete 618.3
  incomplete 618.2
  specified NEC 618.8
 uterus (first degree) (second degree) (third
  degree) (complete) (without vaginal wall
  prolapse) 618.1
  with mention of vaginal wall prolapse — *see*
   Prolapse, uterovaginal
  congenital 752.3
  in pregnancy or childbirth 654.4 ✓5ᵗʰ
   affecting fetus or newborn 763.1
   causing obstructed labor 660.2 ✓5ᵗʰ
    affecting fetus or newborn 763.1
  postpartal (old) 618.1
 uveal 871.1
 vagina (anterior) (posterior) (vault) (wall)
  (without uterine prolapse) 618.0
  with uterine prolapse 618.4
   complete 618.3
   incomplete 618.2
  posthysterectomy 618.5
 vitreous (humor) 379.26
  traumatic 871.1
 womb — *see* Prolapse, uterus
Prolapsus, female 618.9
Proliferative — *see* condition
Prolinemia 270.8
Prolinuria 270.8
Prolonged, prolongation
 bleeding time (*see also* Defect, coagulation)
  790.92
  "idiopathic" (in von Willebrand's disease)
   286.4
 coagulation time (*see also* Defect, coagulation)
  790.92
 gestation syndrome 766.2
 labor 662.1 ✓5ᵗʰ
  affecting fetus or newborn 763.89
  first stage 662.0 ✓5ᵗʰ

Prolonged, prolongation — *continued*
 labor — *continued*
  second stage 662.2 ✓5ᵗʰ
 pregnancy 645.2 ✓5ᵗʰ
 PR interval 426.11
 prothrombin time (*see also* Defect, coagulation)
  790.92
 rupture of membranes (24 hours or more prior
  to onset of labor) 658.2 ✓5ᵗʰ
 uterine contractions in labor 661.4 ✓5ᵗʰ
  affecting fetus or newborn 763.7
Prominauris 744.29
Prominence
 auricle (ear) (congenital) 744.29
  acquired 380.32
 ischial spine or sacral promontory
  with disproportion (fetopelvic) 653.3 ✓5ᵗʰ
   affecting fetus or newborn 763.1
   causing obstructed labor 660.1 ✓5ᵗʰ
    affecting fetus or newborn 763.1
 nose (congenital) 748.1
  acquired 738.0
Pronation
 ankle 736.79
 foot 736.79
  congenital 755.67
Prophylactic
 administration of
  antibiotics V07.39
  antitoxin, any V07.2
  antivenin V07.2
  chemotherapeutic agent NEC V07.39
   fluoride V07.31
  diphtheria antitoxin V07.2
  gamma globulin V07.2
  immune sera (gamma globulin) V07.2
  RhoGAM V07.2
  tetanus antitoxin V07.2
 chemotherapy NEC V07.39
  fluoride V07.31
 immunotherapy V07.2
 measure V07.9
  specified type NEC V07.8
 postmenopausal hormone replacement V07.4
 sterilization V25.2
Proptosis (ocular) (*see also* Exophthalmos) 376.30
 thyroid 242.0 ✓5ᵗʰ
Propulsion
 eyeball 360.81
Prosecution, anxiety concerning V62.5
Prostate, prostatic — *see* condition
Prostatism 600.9
Prostatitis (congestive) (suppurative) 601.9
 acute 601.0
 cavitary 601.8
 chlamydial 099.54
 chronic 601.1
 diverticular 601.8
 due to Trichomonas (vaginalis) 131.03
 fibrous 600.9
 gonococcal (acute) 098.12
  chronic or duration of 2 months or over
   098.32
 granulomatous 601.8
 hypertrophic 600.0
 specified type NEC 601.8
 subacute 601.1
 trichomonal 131.03
 tuberculous (*see also* Tuberculosis)
  016.5 ✓5ᵗʰ [601.4]
Prostatocystitis 601.3
Prostatorrhea 602.8
Prostatoseminovesiculitis, trichomonal 131.03
Prostration 780.79
 heat 992.5
  anhydrotic 992.3
  due to
   salt (and water) depletion 992.4
   water depletion 992.3
 nervous 300.5
 newborn 779.89
 senile 797
Protanomaly 368.51

▲

Protanopia (anomalous trichromat) (complete) (incomplete) 368.51

Protein
deficiency 260
malnutrition 260
sickness (prophylactic) (therapeutic) 999.5

Proteinemia 790.99

Proteinosis
alveolar, lung or pulmonary 516.0
lipid 272.8
lipoid (of Urbach) 272.8

Proteinuria (see also Albuminuria) 791.0
Bence-Jones NEC 791.0
gestational 646.2 ✓5ᵗʰ
with hypertension — see Toxemia, of pregnancy
orthostatic 593.6
postural 593.6

Proteolysis, pathologic 286.6

Protocoproporphyria 277.1

Protoporphyria (erythrohepatic) (erythropoietic) 277.1

Protrusio acetabuli 718.65

Protrusion
acetabulum (into pelvis) 718.65
device, implant, or graft — see Complications, mechanical
ear, congenital 744.29
intervertebral disc — see Displacement, intervertebral disc
nucleus pulposus — see Displacement, intervertebral disc

Proud flesh 701.5

Prune belly (syndrome) 756.71

Prurigo (ferox) (gravis) (Hebra's) (hebrae) (mitis) (simplex) 698.2
agria 698.3
asthma syndrome 691.8
Besnier's (atopic dermatitis) (infantile eczema) 691.8
eczematodes allergicum 691.8
estivalis (Hutchinson's) 692.72
Hutchinson's 692.72
nodularis 698.3
psychogenic 306.3

Pruritus, pruritic 698.9
ani 698.0
psychogenic 306.3
conditions NEC 698.9
psychogenic 306.3
due to Onchocerca volvulus 125.3
ear 698.9
essential 698.9
genital organ(s) 698.1
psychogenic 306.3
gravidarum 646.8 ✓5ᵗʰ
hiemalis 698.8
neurogenic (any site) 306.3
perianal 698.0
psychogenic (any site) 306.3
scrotum 698.1
psychogenic 306.3
senile, senilis 698.8
Trichomonas 131.9
vulva, vulvae 698.1
psychogenic 306.3

Psammocarcinoma (M8140/3) — see Neoplasm, by site, malignant

Pseudarthrosis, pseudoarthrosis (bone) 733.82
joint following fusion V45.4

Pseudoacanthosis
nigricans 701.8

Pseudoaneurysm — see Aneurysm

Pseudoangina (pectoris) — see Angina

Pseudoangioma 452

Pseudo-Argyll-Robertson pupil 379.45

Pseudoarteriosus 747.89

Pseudoarthrosis — see Pseudarthrosis

Pseudoataxia 799.8

Pseudobursa 727.89

Pseudocholera 025

Pseudochromidrosis 705.89

Pseudocirrhosis, liver, pericardial 423.2

Pseudocoarctation 747.21

Pseudocowpox 051.1

Pseudocoxalgia 732.1

Pseudocroup 478.75

Pseudocyesis 300.11

Pseudocyst
lung 518.89
pancreas 577.2
retina 361.19

Pseudodementia 300.16

Pseudoelephantiasis neuroarthritica 757.0

Pseudoemphysema 518.89

Pseudoencephalitis
superior (acute) hemorrhagic 265.1

Pseudoerosion cervix, congenital 752.49

Pseudoexfoliation, lens capsule 366.11

Pseudofracture (idiopathic) (multiple) (spontaneous) (symmetrical) 268.2

Pseudoglanders 025

Pseudoglioma 360.44

Pseudogout — see Chondrocalcinosis

Pseudohallucination 780.1

Pseudohemianesthesia 782.0

Pseudohemophilia (Bernuth's) (hereditary) (type B) 286.4
type A 287.8
vascular 287.8

Pseudohermaphroditism 752.7
with chromosomal anomaly — see Anomaly, chromosomal
adrenal 255.2
female (without adrenocortical disorder) 752.7
with adrenocortical disorder 255.2
adrenal 255.2
male (without gonadal disorder) 752.7
with
adrenocortical disorder 255.2
cleft scrotum 752.7
feminizing testis 257.8
gonadal disorder 257.9
adrenal 255.2

Pseudohole, macula 362.54

Pseudo-Hurler's disease (mucolipidosis III) 272.7

Pseudohydrocephalus 348.2

Pseudohypertrophic muscular dystrophy (Erb's) 359.1

Pseudohypertrophy, muscle 359.1

Pseudohypoparathyroidism 275.49

Pseudoinfluenza 487.1

Pseudoinsomnia 307.49

Pseudoleukemia 288.8
infantile 285.8

Pseudomembranous — see condition

Pseudomeningocele (cerebral) (infective) (surgical) 349.2
spinal 349.2

Pseudomenstruation 626.8

Pseudomucinous
cyst (ovary) (M8470/0) 220
peritoneum 568.89

Pseudomyeloma 273.1

Pseudomyxoma peritonei (M8480/6) 197.6

Pseudoneuritis optic (nerve) 377.24
papilla 377.24
congenital 743.57

Pseudoneuroma — see Injury, nerve, by site

Pseudo-obstruction
intestine 564.89

Pseudopapilledema 377.24.

Pseudoparalysis
arm or leg 781.4
atonic, congenital 358.8

Pseudopelade 704.09

Pseudophakia V43.1

Pseudopolycythemia 289.0

Pseudopolyposis, colon 556.4

Pseudoporencephaly 348.0

Pseudopseudohypoparathyroidism 275.49

Pseudopsychosis 300.16

Pseudopterygium 372.52

Pseudoptosis (eyelid) 374.34

Pseudorabies 078.89

Pseudoretinitis, pigmentosa 362.65

Pseudorickets 588.0
senile (Pozzi's) 731.0

Pseudorubella 057.8

Pseudoscarlatina 057.8

Pseudosclerema 778.1

Pseudosclerosis (brain)
Jakob's 046.1
of Westphal (-Strümpell) (hepatolenticular degeneration) 275.1
spastic 046.1
with dementia
with behavioral disturbance 046.1 [294.11]
without behavioral disturbance 046.1 [294.10]

Pseudoseizure 780.39
non-psychiatric 780.39
psychiatric 300.11

Pseudotabes 799.8
diabetic 250.6 ✓5ᵗʰ [337.1]

Pseudotetanus (see also Convulsions) 780.39

Pseudotetany 781.7
hysterical 300.11

Pseudothalassemia 285.0

Pseudotrichinosis 710.3

Pseudotruncus arteriosus 747.29

Pseudotuberculosis, pasteurella (infection) 027.2

Pseudotumor
cerebri 348.2
orbit (inflammatory) 376.11

Pseudo-Turner's syndrome 759.89

Pseudoxanthoma elasticum 757.39

Psilosis (sprue) (tropical) 579.1
Monilia 112.89
nontropical 579.0
not sprue 704.00

Psittacosis 073.9

Psoitis 728.89

Psora NEC 696.1

Psoriasis 696.1
any type, except arthropathic 696.1
arthritic, arthropathic 696.0
buccal 528.6
flexural 696.1
follicularis 696.1
guttate 696.1
inverse 696.1
mouth 528.6
nummularis 696.1
psychogenic 316 [696.1]
punctata 696.1
pustular 696.1
rupioides 696.1
vulgaris 696.1

Psorospermiasis 136.4

Psorospermosis 136.4
follicularis (vegetans) 757.39

Psychalgia 307.80

Psychasthenia 300.89
compulsive 300.3
mixed compulsive states 300.3
obsession 300.3

Psychiatric disorder or problem NEC 300.9

Psychogenic — see also condition
factors associated with physical conditions 316

Psychoneurosis, psychoneurotic (see also Neurosis) 300.9
anxiety (state) 300.00
climacteric 627.2
compensation 300.16
compulsion 300.3
conversion hysteria 300.11
depersonalization 300.6
depressive type 300.4
dissociative hysteria 300.15

Psychoneurosis, psychoneurotic (*see also* Neurosis) — *continued*
  hypochondriacal 300.7
  hysteria 300.10
    conversion type 300.11
    dissociative type 300.15
  mixed NEC 300.89
  neurasthenic 300.5
  obsessional 300.3
  obsessive-compulsive 300.3
  occupational 300.89
  personality NEC 301.89
  phobia 300.20
  senile NEC 300.89

Psychopathic — *see also* condition
  constitution, posttraumatic 310.2
    with psychosis 293.9
  personality 301.9
    amoral trends 301.7
    antisocial trends 301.7
    asocial trends 301.7
    mixed types 301.7
  state 301.9

Psychopathy, sexual (*see also* Deviation, sexual) 302.9

Psychophysiologic, psychophysiological condition — *see* Reaction, psychophysiologic

Psychose passionelle 297.8

Psychosexual identity disorder 302.6
  adult-life 302.85
  childhood 302.6

Psychosis 298.9
  acute hysterical 298.1
  affecting management of pregnancy, childbirth, or puerperium 648.4 ✓5ᵗʰ
  affective NEC 296.90

> Note — Use the following fifth-digit subclassification with categories 296.0-296.6:
>
> 0   unspecified
> 1   mild
> 2   moderate
> 3   severe, without mention of psychotic behavior
> 4   severe, specified as with psychotic behavior
> 5   in partial or unspecified remission
> 6   in full remission

    drug-induced 292.84
    due to or associated with physical condition 293.83
    involutional 296.2 ✓5ᵗʰ
      recurrent episode 296.3 ✓5ᵗʰ
      single episode 296.2 ✓5ᵗʰ
    manic-depressive 296.80
      circular (alternating) 296.7
        currently depressed 296.5 ✓5ᵗʰ
        currently manic 296.4 ✓5ᵗʰ
      depressed type 296.2 ✓5ᵗʰ
        atypical 296.82
        recurrent episode 296.3 ✓5ᵗʰ
        single episode 296.2 ✓5ᵗʰ
      manic 296.0 ✓5ᵗʰ
        atypical 296.81
        recurrent episode 296.1 ✓5ᵗʰ
        single episode 296.0 ✓5ᵗʰ
      mixed type NEC 296.89
      specified type NEC 296.89
    senile 290.21
    specified type NEC 296.99
  alcoholic 291.9
    with
      anxiety 291.89
      delirium tremens 291.0
      delusions 291.5
      dementia 291.2
      hallucinosis 291.3
      mood disturbance 291.89
      jealousy 291.5
      paranoia 291.5
      persisting amnesia 291.1

Psychosis — *continued*
  alcoholic — *continued*
    with — *continued*
      sexual dysfunction 291.89
      sleep disturbance 291.89
    amnestic confabulatory 291.1
    delirium tremens 291.0
    hallucinosis 291.3
    Korsakoff's, Korsakov's, Korsakow's 291.1
    paranoid type 291.5
    pathological intoxication 291.4
    polyneuritic 291.1
    specified type NEC 291.89
  alternating (*see also* Psychosis, manic-depressive, circular) 296.7
  anergastic (*see also* Psychosis, organic) 294.9
  arteriosclerotic 290.40
    with
      acute confusional state 290.41
      delirium 290.41
      delusional features 290.42
      depressive features 290.43
    depressed type 290.43
    paranoid type 290.42
    simple type 290.40
    uncomplicated 290.40
  atypical 298.9
    depressive 296.82
    manic 296.81
  borderline (schizophrenia) (*see also* Schizophrenia) 295.5 ✓5ᵗʰ
    of childhood (*see also* Psychosis, childhood) 299.8 ✓5ᵗʰ
    prepubertal 299.8 ✓5ᵗʰ
  brief reactive 298.8
  childhood, with origin specific to 299.9 ✓5ᵗʰ

> Note — Use the following fifth-digit subclassification with category 299:
>
> 0   current or active state
> 1   residual state

    atypical 299.8 ✓5ᵗʰ
    specified type NEC 299.8 ✓5ᵗʰ
  circular (*see also* Psychosis, manic-depressive, circular) 296.7
  climacteric (*see also* Psychosis, involutional) 298.8
  confusional 298.9
    acute 293.0
    reactive 298.2
    subacute 293.1
  depressive (*see also* Psychosis, affective) 296.2 ✓5ᵗʰ
    atypical 296.82
    involutional 296.2 ✓5ᵗʰ
      recurrent episode 296.3 ✓5ᵗʰ
      single episode 296.2 ✓5ᵗʰ
    psychogenic 298.0
    reactive (emotional stress) (psychological trauma) 298.0
    recurrent episode 296.3 ✓5ᵗʰ
      with hypomania (bipolar II) 296.89
    single episode 296.2 ✓5ᵗʰ
  disintegrative (childhood) (*see also* Psychosis, childhood) 299.1 ✓5ᵗʰ
  drug 292.9
    with
      affective syndrome 292.84
      amnestic syndrome 292.83
      anxiety 292.89
      delirium 292.81
        withdrawal 292.0
      delusional syndrome 292.11
      dementia 292.82
      depressive state 292.84
      hallucinosis 292.12
      mood disturbance 292.84
      organic personality syndrome NEC 292.89
      sexual dysfunction 292.89
      sleep disturbance 292.89
      withdrawal syndrome (and delirium) 292.0
    affective syndrome 292.84
    delusional state 292.11
    hallucinatory state 292.12

Psychosis — *continued*
  drug — *continued*
    hallucinosis 292.12
    paranoid state 292.11
    specified type NEC 292.89
    withdrawal syndrome (and delirium) 292.0
  due to or associated with physical condition (*see also* Psychosis, organic) 293.9
  epileptic NEC 294.8
  excitation (psychogenic) (reactive) 298.1
  exhaustive (*see also* Reaction, stress, acute) 308.9
  hypomanic (*see also* Psychosis, affective) 296.0 ✓5ᵗʰ
    recurrent episode 296.1 ✓5ᵗʰ
    single episode 296.0 ✓5ᵗʰ
  hysterical 298.8
    acute 298.1
  incipient 298.8
    schizophrenic (*see also* Schizophrenia) 295.5 ✓5ᵗʰ
  induced 297.3
  infantile (*see also* Psychosis, childhood) 299.0 ✓5ᵗʰ
  infective 293.9
    acute 293.0
    subacute 293.1
  in pregnancy, childbirth, or puerperium 648.4 ✓5ᵗʰ
  interactional (childhood) (*see also* Psychosis, childhood) 299.1 ✓5ᵗʰ
  involutional 298.8
    depressive (*see also* Psychosis, affective) 296.2 ✓5ᵗʰ
      recurrent episode 296.3 ✓5ᵗʰ
      single episode 296.2 ✓5ᵗʰ
    melancholic 296.2 ✓5ᵗʰ
      recurrent episode 296.3 ✓5ᵗʰ
      single episode 296.2 ✓5ᵗʰ
    paranoid state 297.2
    paraphrenia 297.2
  Korsakoff's, Korakov's, Korsakow's (nonalcoholic) 294.0
    alcoholic 291.1
  mania (phase) (*see also* Psychosis, affective) 296.0 ✓5ᵗʰ
    recurrent episode 296.1 ✓5ᵗʰ
    single episode 296.0 ✓5ᵗʰ
  manic (*see also* Psychosis, affective) 296.0 ✓5ᵗʰ
    atypical 296.81
    recurrent episode 296.1 ✓5ᵗʰ
    single episode 296.0 ✓5ᵗʰ
  manic-depressive 296.80
    circular 296.7
      currently
        depressed 296.5 ✓5ᵗʰ
        manic 296.4 ✓5ᵗʰ
        mixed 296.6 ✓5ᵗʰ
    depressive 296.2 ✓5ᵗʰ
      recurrent episode 296.3 ✓5ᵗʰ
        with hypomania (bipolar II) 296.89
      single episode 296.2 ✓5ᵗʰ
    hypomanic 296.0 ✓5ᵗʰ
      recurrent episode 296.1 ✓5ᵗʰ
      single episode 296.0 ✓5ᵗʰ
    manic 296.0 ✓5ᵗʰ
      atypical 296.81
      recurrent episode 296.1 ✓5ᵗʰ
      single episode 296.0 ✓5ᵗʰ
    mixed NEC 296.89
    perplexed 296.89
    stuporous 296.89
  menopausal (*see also* Psychosis, involutional) 298.8
  mixed schizophrenic and affective (*see also* Schizophrenia) 295.7 ✓5ᵗʰ
  multi-infarct (cerebrovascular) (*see also* Psychosis, arteriosclerotic) 290.40
  organic NEC 294.9
    due to or associated with
      addiction
        alcohol (*see also* Psychosis, alcoholic) 291.9
        drug (*see also* Psychosis, drug) 292.9
      alcohol intoxication, acute (*see also* Psychosis, alcoholic) 291.9

Psychoneurosis — Psychosis

Psychosis — Puberty

Psychosis — *continued*
organic NEC — *continued*
  due to or associated with — *continued*
    alcoholism (*see also* Psychosis, alcoholic)
      291.9
    arteriosclerosis (cerebral) (*see also*
      Psychosis, arteriosclerotic) 290.40
    cerebrovascular disease
      acute (psychosis) 293.0
      arteriosclerotic (*see also* Psychosis,
        arteriosclerotic) 290.40
    childbirth — *see* Psychosis, puerperal
    dependence
      alcohol (*see also* Psychosis, alcoholic)
        291.9
      drug 292.9
    disease
      alcoholic liver (*see also* Psychosis,
        alcoholic) 291.9
      brain
        arteriosclerotic (*see also* Psychosis,
          arteriosclerotic) 290.40
        cerebrovascular
          acute (psychosis) 293.0
          arteriosclerotic (*see also* Psychosis,
            arteriosclerotic) 290.40
        endocrine or metabolic 293.9
          acute (psychosis) 293.0
          subacute (psychosis) 293.1
        Jakob-Creutzfeldt
          with behavioral disturbance 046.1
            [294.11]
          without behavioral disturbance
            046.1 [294.10]
      liver, alcoholic (*see also* Psychosis,
        alcoholic) 291.9
    disorder
      cerebrovascular
        acute (psychosis) 293.0
      endocrine or metabolic 293.9
        acute (psychosis) 293.0
        subacute (psychosis) 293.1
    epilepsy
      with behavioral disturbance
        345.9 ✓5ᵗʰ [294.11]
      without behavioral disturbance
        345.9 ✓5ᵗʰ [294.10]
      transient (acute) 293.0
    Huntington's chorea
      with behavioral disturbance
        333.4 [294.11]
      without behavioral disturbance
        333.4 [294.10]
    infection
      brain 293.9
        acute (psychosis) 293.0
        chronic 294.8
        subacute (psychosis) 293.1
      intracranial NEC 293.9
        acute (psychosis) 293.0
        chronic 294.8
        subacute (psychosis) 293.1
    intoxication
      alcoholic (acute) (*see also* Psychosis,
        alcoholic) 291.9
        pathological 291.4
      drug (*see also* Psychosis, drug) 292.2
    ischemia
      cerebrovascular (generalized) (*see also*
        Psychosis, arteriosclerotic)
        290.40
    Jakob-Creutzfeldt disease or syndrome
      with behavioral disturbance
        046.1 [294.11]
      without behavioral disturbance
        046.1 [294.10]
    multiple sclerosis
      with behavioral disturbance
        340 [294.11]
      without behavioral disturbance
        340 [294.10]
    physical condition NEC 293.9
      with
        delusions 293.81
        hallucinations 293.82

Psychosis — *continued*
organic NEC — *continued*
  due to or associated with — *continued*
    presenility 290.10
    puerperium — *see* Psychosis, puerperal
    sclerosis, multiple
      with behavioral disturbance
        340 [294.11]
      without behavioral disturbance
        340 [294.10]
    senility 290.20
    status epilepticus
      with behavioral disturbance
        345.3 ✓5ᵗʰ [294.11]
      without behavioral disturbance
        345.3 ✓5ᵗʰ [294.10]
    trauma
      brain (birth) (from electrical current)
        (surgical) 293.9
        acute (psychosis) 293.0
        chronic 294.8
        subacute (psychosis) 293.1
        unspecified physical condition
          294.9
    infective 293.9
      acute (psychosis) 293.0
      subacute 293.1
    posttraumatic 293.9
      acute 293.0
      subacute 293.1
    specified type NEC 294.8
    transient 293.9
      with
        anxiety 293.84
        delusions 293.81
        depression 293.83
        hallucinations 293.82
      depressive type 293.83
      hallucinatory type 293.82
      paranoid type 293.81
      specified type NEC 293.89
paranoic 297.1
paranoid (chronic) 297.9
  alcoholic 291.5
  chronic 297.1
  climacteric 297.2
  involuntional 297.2
  menopausal 297.2
  protracted reactive 298.4
  psychogenic 298.4
    acute 298.3
  schizophrenic (*see also* Schizophrenia)
    295.3 ✓5ᵗʰ
  senile 290.20
paroxysmal 298.9
  senile 290.20
polyneuritic, alcoholic 291.1
postoperative 293.9
postpartum — *see* Psychosis, puerperal
prepsychotic (*see also* Schizophrenia) 295.5 ✓5ᵗʰ
presbyophrenic (type) 290.8
presenile (*see also* Dementia, presenile) 290.10
prison 300.16
psychogenic 298.8
  depressive 298.0
  paranoid 298.4
    acute 298.3
puerperal
  specified type — *see* categories 295-298 ✓5ᵗʰ
  unspecified type 293.89
    acute 293.0
    chronic 293.89
    subacute 293.1
reactive (emotional stress) (psychological
    trauma) 298.8
  brief 298.8
  confusion 298.2
  depressive 298.0
  excitation 298.1
schizo-affective (depressed) (excited) (*see also*
    Schizophrenia) 295.7 ✓5ᵗʰ
schizophrenia, schizophrenic (*see also*
    Schizophrenia) 295.9 ✓5ᵗʰ
  borderline type 295.5 ✓5ᵗʰ
    of childhood (*see also* Psychosis,
      childhood) 299.8 ✓5ᵗʰ
  catatonic (excited) (withdrawn) 295.2 ✓5ᵗʰ

Psychosis — *continued*
schizophrenia, schizophrenic (*see also*
    Schizophrenia) — *continued*
  childhood type (*see also* Psychosis,
    childhood) 299.9 ✓5ᵗʰ
    hebephrenic 295.1 ✓5ᵗʰ
    incipient 295.5 ✓5ᵗʰ
    latent 295.5 ✓5ᵗʰ
    paranoid 295.3 ✓5ᵗʰ
    prepsychotic 295.5 ✓5ᵗʰ
    prodromal 295.5 ✓5ᵗʰ
    pseudoneurotic 295.5 ✓5ᵗʰ
    pseudopsychopathic 295.5 ✓5ᵗʰ
    schizophreniform 295.4 ✓5ᵗʰ
    simple 295.0 ✓5ᵗʰ
  schizophreniform 295.4 ✓5ᵗʰ
  senile NEC 290.20
    with
      delusional features 290.20
      depressive features 290.21
    depressed type 290.21
    paranoid type 290.20
    simple deterioration 290.20
    specified type — *see* categories 295-298 ✓5ᵗʰ
  shared 297.3
  situational (reactive) 298.8
  symbiotic (childhood) (*see also* Psychosis,
    childhood) 299.1 ✓5ᵗʰ
  toxic (acute) 293.9
Psychotic (*see also* condition) 298.9
  episode 298.9
    due to or associated with physical
      conditions (*see also* Psychosis,
      organic) 293.9
Pterygium (eye) 372.40
  central 372.43
  colli 744.5
  double 372.44
  peripheral (stationary) 372.41
    progressive 372.42
  recurrent 372.45
Ptilosis 374.55
Ptomaine (poisoning) (*see also* Poisoning, food)
    005.9
Ptosis (adiposa) 374.30
  breast 611.8
  cecum 569.89
  colon 569.89
  congenital (eyelid) 743.61
    specified site NEC — *see* Anomaly, specified
      type NEC
  epicanthus syndrome 270.2
  eyelid 374.30
    congenital 743.61
    mechanical 374.33
    myogenic 374.32
    paralytic 374.31
  gastric 537.5
  intestine 569.89
  kidney (*see also* Disease, renal) 593.0
    congenital 753.3
  liver 573.8
  renal (*see also* Disease, renal) 593.0
    congenital 753.3
  splanchnic 569.89
  spleen 289.59
  stomach 537.5
  viscera 569.89
Ptyalism 527.7
  hysterical 300.11
  periodic 527.2
  pregnancy 646.8 ✓5ᵗʰ
  psychogenic 306.4
Ptyalolithiasis 527.5
Pubalgia 848.8
Pubarche, precocious 259.1
Pubertas praecox 259.1
Puberty V21.1
  abnormal 259.9
  bleeding 626.3
  delayed 259.0
  precocious (constitutional) (cryptogenic)
    (idiopathic) NEC 259.1

Puberty — *continued*
precocious — *continued*
  due to
    adrenal
      cortical hyperfunction 255.2
      hyperplasia 255.2
    cortical hyperfunction 255.2
    ovarian hyperfunction 256.1
      estrogen 256.0
    pineal tumor 259.8
    testicular hyperfunction 257.0
premature 259.1
  due to
    adrenal cortical hyperfunction 255.2
    pineal tumor 259.8
    pituitary (anterior) hyperfunction 253.1

Puckering, macula 362.56

Pudenda, pudendum — *see* condition

Puente's disease (simple glandular cheilitis) 528.5

Puerperal
abscess
  areola 675.1 ✓5th
  Bartholin's gland 646.6 ✓5th
  breast 675.1 ✓5th
  cervix (uteri) 670 ✓4th
  fallopian tube 670 ✓4th
  genital organ 670 ✓4th
  kidney 646.6 ✓5th
  mammary 675.1 ✓5th
  mesosalpinx 670 ✓4th
  nabothian 646.6 ✓5th
  nipple 675.0 ✓5th
  ovary, ovarian 670 ✓4th
  oviduct 670 ✓4th
  parametric 670 ✓4th
  para-uterine 670 ✓4th
  pelvic 670 ✓4th
  perimetric 670 ✓4th
  periuterine 670 ✓4th
  retro-uterine 670 ✓4th
  subareolar 675.1 ✓5th
  suprapelvic 670 ✓4th
  tubal (ruptured) 670 ✓4th
  tubo-ovarian 670 ✓4th
  urinary tract NEC 646.6 ✓5th
  uterine, uterus 670 ✓4th
  vagina (wall) 646.6 ✓5th
  vaginorectal 646.6 ✓5th
  vulvovaginal gland 646.6 ✓5th
accident 674.9 ✓5th
adnexitis 670 ✓4th
afibrinogenemia, or other coagulation defect 666.3 ✓5th
albuminuria (acute) (subacute) 646.2 ✓5th
  pre-eclamptic 642.4 ✓5th
anemia (conditions classifiable to 280-285) 648.2 ✓5th
anuria 669.3 ✓5th
apoplexy 674.0 ✓5th
asymptomatic bacteriuria 646.5 ✓5th
atrophy, breast 676.3 ✓5th
blood dyscrasia 666.3 ✓5th
caked breast 676.2 ✓5th
cardiomyopathy 674.8 ✓5th
cellulitis — *see* Puerperal, abscess
cerebrovascular disorder (conditions classifiable to 430-434, 436-437) 674.0 ✓5th
cervicitis (conditions classifiable to 616.0) 646.6 ✓5th
coagulopathy (any) 666.3 ✓5th
complications 674.9 ✓5th
  specified type NEC 674.8 ✓5th
convulsions (eclamptic) (uremic) 642.6 ✓5th
  with pre-existing hypertension 642.7 ✓5th
cracked nipple 676.1 ✓5th
cystitis 646.6 ✓5th
cystopyelitis 646.6 ✓5th
deciduitis (acute) 670 ✓4th
delirium NEC 293.9
diabetes (mellitus) (conditions classifiable to 250) 648.0 ✓5th
disease 674.9 ✓5th
  breast NEC 676.3 ✓5th
    cerebrovascular (acute) 674.0 ✓5th

Puerperal — *continued*
disease — *continued*
  nonobstetric NEC (*see also* Pregnancy, complicated, current disease or condition) 648.9 ✓5th
  pelvis inflammatory 670 ✓4th
  renal NEC 646.2 ✓5th
  tubo-ovarian 670 ✓4th
  Valsuani's (progressive pernicious anemia) 648.2 ✓5th
disorder
  lactation 676.9 ✓5th
    specified type NEC 676.8 ✓5th
  nonobstetric NEC (*see also* Pregnancy, complicated, current disease or condition) 648.9 ✓5th
disruption
  cesarean wound 674.1 ✓5th
  episiotomy wound 674.2 ✓5th
  perineal laceration wound 674.2 ✓5th
drug dependence (conditions classifiable to 304) 648.3 ✓5th
eclampsia 642.6 ✓5th
  with pre-existing hypertension 642.7 ✓5th
embolism (pulmonary) 673.2 ✓5th
  air 673.0 ✓5th
  amniotic fluid 673.1 ✓5th
  blood-clot 673.2 ✓5th
  brain or cerebral 674.0 ✓5th
  cardiac 674.8 ✓5th
  fat 673.8 ✓5th
  intracranial sinus (venous) 671.5 ✓5th
  pyemic 673.3 ✓5th
  septic 673.3 ✓5th
  spinal cord 671.5 ✓5th
endometritis (conditions classifiable to 615.0-615.9) 670 ✓4th
endophlebitis — *see* Puerperal, phlebitis
endotrachelitis 646.6 ✓5th
engorgement, breasts 676.2 ✓5th
erysipelas 670 ✓4th
failure
  lactation 676.4 ✓5th
  renal, acute 669.3 ✓5th
fever 670 ✓4th
  meaning pyrexia (of unknown origin) 672 ✓4th
  meaning sepsis 670 ✓4th
fissure, nipple 676.1 ✓5th
fistula
  breast 675.1 ✓5th
  mammary gland 675.1 ✓5th
  nipple 675.0 ✓5th
galactophoritis 675.2 ✓5th
galactorrhea 676.6 ✓5th
gangrene
  gas 670 ✓4th
  uterus 670 ✓4th
gonorrhea (conditions classifiable to 098) 647.1 ✓5th
hematoma, subdural 674.0 ✓5th
hematosalpinx, infectional 670 ✓4th
hemiplegia, cerebral 674.0 ✓5th
hemorrhage 666.1 ✓5th
  brain 674.0 ✓5th
  bulbar 674.0 ✓5th
  cerebellar 674.0 ✓5th
  cerebral 674.0 ✓5th
  cortical 674.0 ✓5th
  delayed (after 24 hours) (uterine) 666.2 ✓5th
  extradural 674.0 ✓5th
  internal capsule 674.0 ✓5th
  intracranial 674.0 ✓5th
  intrapontine 674.0 ✓5th
  meningeal 674.0 ✓5th
  pontine 674.0 ✓5th
  subarachnoid 674.0 ✓5th
  subcortical 674.0 ✓5th
  subdural 674.0 ✓5th
  uterine, delayed 666.2 ✓5th
  ventricular 674.0 ✓5th
hemorrhoids 671.8 ✓5th
hepatorenal syndrome 674.8 ✓5th
hypertrophy
  breast 676.3 ✓5th
  mammary gland 676.3 ✓5th
induration breast (fibrous) 676.3 ✓5th

Puerperal — *continued*
infarction
  lung — *see* Puerperal, embolism
  pulmonary — *see* Puerperal, embolism
infection
  Bartholin's gland 646.6 ✓5th
  breast 675.2 ✓5th
    with nipple 675.9 ✓5th
      specified type NEC 675.8 ✓5th
  cervix 646.6 ✓5th
  endocervix 646.6 ✓5th
  fallopian tube 670 ✓4th
  generalized 670 ✓4th
  genital tract (major) 670 ✓4th
    minor or localized 646.6 ✓5th
  kidney (bacillus coli) 646.6 ✓5th
  mammary gland 675.2 ✓5th
    with nipple 675.9 ✓5th
      specified type NEC 675.8 ✓5th
  nipple 675.0 ✓5th
    with breast 675.9 ✓5th
      specified type NEC 675.8 ✓5th
  ovary 670 ✓4th
  pelvic 670 ✓4th
  peritoneum 670 ✓4th
  renal 646.6 ✓5th
  tubo-ovarian 670 ✓4th
  urinary (tract) NEC 646.6 ✓5th
    asymptomatic 646.5 ✓5th
  uterus, uterine 670 ✓4th
  vagina 646.6 ✓5th
inflammation — *see also* Puerperal, infection
  areola 675.1 ✓5th
  Bartholin's gland 646.6 ✓5th
  breast 675.2 ✓5th
  broad ligament 670 ✓4th
  cervix (uteri) 646.6 ✓5th
  fallopian tube 670 ✓4th
  genital organs 670 ✓4th
    localized 646.6 ✓5th
  mammary gland 675.2 ✓5th
  nipple 675.0 ✓5th
  ovary 670 ✓4th
  oviduct 670 ✓4th
  pelvis 670 ✓4th
  periuterine 670 ✓4th
  tubal 670 ✓4th
  vagina 646.6 ✓5th
  vein — *see* Puerperal, phlebitis
inversion, nipple 676.3 ✓5th
ischemia, cerebral 674.0 ✓5th
lymphangitis 670 ✓4th
  breast 675.2 ✓5th
malaria (conditions classifiable to 084) 647.4 ✓5th
malnutrition 648.9 ✓5th
mammillitis 675.0 ✓5th
mammitis 675.2 ✓5th
mania 296.0 ✓5th
  recurrent episode 296.1 ✓5th
  single episode 296.0 ✓5th
mastitis 675.2 ✓5th
  purulent 675.1 ✓5th
  retromammary 675.1 ✓5th
  submammary 675.1 ✓5th
melancholia 296.2 ✓5th
  recurrent episode 296.3 ✓5th
  single episode 296.2 ✓5th
mental disorder (conditions classifiable to 290-303, 305-316, 317-319) 648.4 ✓5th
metritis (septic) (suppurative) 670 ✓4th
metroperitonitis 670 ✓4th
metrorrhagia 666.2 ✓5th
metrosalpingitis 670 ✓4th
metrovaginitis 670 ✓4th
milk leg 671.4 ✓5th
monoplegia, cerebral 674.0 ✓5th
necrosis
  kidney, tubular 669.3 ✓5th
  liver (acute) (subacute) (conditions classifiable to 570) 674.8 ✓5th
  ovary 670 ✓4th
  renal cortex 669.3 ✓5th
nephritis or nephrosis (conditions classifiable to 580-589) 646.2 ✓5th
  with hypertension 642.1 ✓5th

Puerperal — Putrefaction, intestinal

Puerperal — *continued*
  nutritional deficiency (conditions classifiable to 260-269) 648.9 ✓5th
  occlusion, precerebral artery 674.0 ✓5th
  oliguria 669.3 ✓5th
  oophoritis 670 ✓5th
  ovaritis 670 ✓4th
  paralysis
    bladder (sphincter) 665.5 ✓5th
    cerebral 674.0 ✓5th
  paralytic stroke 674.0 ✓5th
  parametritis 670 ✓4th
  paravaginitis 646.6 ✓5th
  pelviperitonitis 670 ✓4th
  perimetritis 670 ✓4th
  perimetrosalpingitis 670 ✓4th
  perinephritis 646.6 ✓5th
  perioophoritis 670 ✓4th
  periphlebitis — *see* Puerperal, phlebitis
  perisalpingitis 670 ✓4th
  peritoneal infection 670 ✓4th
  peritonitis (pelvic) 670 ✓4th
  perivaginitis 646.6 ✓5th
  phlebitis 671.9 ✓5th
    deep 671.4 ✓5th
    intracranial sinus (venous) 671.5 ✓5th
    pelvic 671.4 ✓5th
    specified site NEC 671.5 ✓5th
    superficial 671.2 ✓5th
  phlegmasia alba dolens 671.4 ✓5th
  placental polyp 674.4 ✓5th
  pneumonia, embolic — *see* Puerperal, embolism
  prediabetes 648.8 ✓5th
  pre-eclampsia (mild) 642.4 ✓5th
    with pre-existing hypertension 642.7 ✓5th
    severe 642.5 ✓5th
  psychosis, unspecified (*see also* Psychosis, puerperal) 293.89
  pyelitis 646.6 ✓5th
  pyelocystitis 646.6 ✓5th
  pyelohydronephrosis 646.6 ✓5th
  pyelonephritis 646.6 ✓5th
  pyelonephrosis 646.6 ✓5th
  pyemia 670 ✓4th
  pyocystitis 646.6 ✓5th
  pyohemia 670 ✓4th
  pyometra 670 ✓4th
  pyonephritis 646.6 ✓5th
  pyonephrosis 646.6 ✓5th
  pyo-oophoritis 670 ✓4th
  pyosalpingitis 670 ✓4th
  pyosalpinx 670 ✓4th
  pyrexia (of unknown origin) 672 ✓5th
  renal
    disease NEC 646.2 ✓5th
    failure, acute 669.3 ✓5th
  retention
    decidua (fragments) (with delayed hemorrhage) 666.2 ✓5th
      without hemorrhage 667.1 ✓5th
    placenta (fragments) (with delayed hemorrhage) 666.2 ✓5th
      without hemorrhage 667.1 ✓5th
    secundines (fragments) (with delayed hemorrhage) 666.2 ✓5th
      without hemorrhage 667.1 ✓5th
  retracted nipple 676.0 ✓5th
  rubella (conditions classifiable to 056) 647.5 ✓5th
  salpingitis 670 ✓4th
  salpingo-oophoritis 670 ✓4th
  salpingo-ovaritis 670 ✓4th
  salpingoperitonitis 670 ✓4th
  sapremia 670 ✓4th
  secondary perineal tear 674.2 ✓5th
  sepsis (pelvic) 670 ✓4th
  septicemia 670 ✓4th
  subinvolution (uterus) 674.8 ✓5th
  sudden death (cause unknown) 674.9 ✓5th
  suppuration — *see* Puerperal, abscess
  syphilis (conditions classifiable to 090-097) 647.0 ✓5th
  tetanus 670 ✓4th
  thelitis 675.0 ✓5th
  thrombocytopenia 666.3 ✓5th
  thrombophlebitis (superficial) 671.2 ✓5th
    deep 671.4 ✓5th

Puerperal — *continued*
  thrombophlebitis — *continued*
    pelvic 671.4 ✓5th
    specified site NEC 671.5 ✓5th
  thrombosis (venous) — *see* Thrombosis, puerperal
  thyroid dysfunction (conditions classifiable to 240-246) 648.1 ✓5th
  toxemia (*see also* Toxemia, of pregnancy) 642.4 ✓5th
    eclamptic 642.6 ✓5th
      with pre-existing hypertension 642.7 ✓5th
    pre-eclamptic (mild) 642.4 ✓5th
      with
        convulsions 642.6 ✓5th
        pre-existing hypertension 642.7 ✓5th
      severe 642.5 ✓5th
  tuberculosis (conditions classifiable to 010-018) 647.3 ✓5th
  uremia 669.3 ✓5th
  vaginitis (conditions classifiable to 616.1) 646.6 ✓5th
  varicose veins (legs) 671.0 ✓5th
    vulva or perineum 671.1 ✓5th
  vulvitis (conditions classifiable to 616.1) 646.6 ✓5th
  vulvovaginitis (conditions classifiable to 616.1) 646.6 ✓5th
  white leg 671.4 ✓5th
Pulled muscle — *see* Sprain, by site
Pulmolithiasis 518.89
Pulmonary — *see* condition
Pulmonitis (unknown etiology) 486
Pulpitis (acute) (anachoretic) (chronic) (hyperplastic) (putrescent) (suppurative) (ulcerative) 522.0
Pulpless tooth 522.9
Pulse
  alternating 427.89
    psychogenic 306.2
  bigeminal 427.89
  fast 785.0
  feeble, rapid, due to shock following injury 958.4
  rapid 785.0
  slow 427.89
  strong 785.9
  trigeminal 427.89
  water-hammer (*see also* Insufficiency, aortic) 424.1
  weak 785.9
Pulseless disease 446.7
Pulsus
  alternans or trigeminy 427.89
    psychogenic 306.2
Punch drunk 310.2
Puncta lacrimalia occlusion 375.52
Punctiform hymen 752.49
Puncture (traumatic) — *see also* Wound, open, by site
  accidental, complicating surgery 998.2
  bladder, nontraumatic 596.6
  by
    device, implant, or graft — *see* Complications, mechanical
    foreign body
      internal organs — *see also* Injury, internal, by site
        by ingested object — *see* Foreign body
    left accidentally in operation wound 998.4
  instrument (any) during a procedure, accidental 998.2
  internal organs, abdomen, chest, or pelvis — *see* Injury, internal, by site
  kidney, nontraumatic 593.89
Pupil — *see* condition
Pupillary membrane 364.74
  persistent 743.46
Pupillotonia 379.46
  pseudotabetic 379.46
Purpura 287.2
  abdominal 287.0
  allergic 287.0

Purpura — *continued*
  anaphylactoid 287.0
  annularis telangiectodes 709.1
  arthritic 287.0
  autoerythrocyte sensitization 287.2
  autoimmune 287.0
  bacterial 287.0
  Bateman's (senile) 287.2
  capillary fragility (hereditary) (idiopathic) 287.8
  cryoglobulinemic 273.2
  devil's pinches 287.2
  fibrinolytic (*see also* Fibrinolysis) 286.6
  fulminans, fulminous 286.6
  gangrenous 287.0
  hemorrhagic (*see also* Purpura, thrombocytopenic) 287.3
    nodular 272.7
    nonthrombocytopenic 287.0
    thrombocytopenic 287.3
  Henoch's (purpura nervosa) 287.0
  Henoch-Schönlein (allergic) 287.0
  hypergammaglobulinemic (benign primary) (Waldenström's) 273.0
  idiopathic 287.3
    nonthrombocytopenic 287.0
    thrombocytopenic 287.3
  infectious 287.0
  malignant 287.0
  neonatorum 772.6
  nervosa 287.0
  newborn NEC 772.6
  nonthrombocytopenic 287.2
    hemorrhagic 287.0
    idiopathic 287.0
  nonthrombopenic 287.2
  peliosis rheumatica 287.0
  pigmentaria, progressiva 709.09
  posttransfusion 287.4
  primary 287.0
  primitive 287.0
  red cell membrane sensitivity 287.2
  rheumatica 287.0
  Schönlein (-Henoch) (allergic) 287.0
  scorbutic 267
  senile 287.2
  simplex 287.2
  symptomatica 287.0
  telangiectasia annularis 709.1
  thrombocytopenic (congenital) (essential) (hereditary) (idiopathic) (primary) (*see also* Thrombocytopenia) 287.3
    neonatal, transitory (*see also* Thrombocytopenia, neonatal transitory) 776.1
    puerperal, postpartum 666.3 ✓5th
    thrombotic 446.6
  thrombohemolytic (*see also* Fibrinolysis) 286.6
  thrombopenic (congenital) (essential) (*see also* Thrombocytopenia) 287.3
    thrombotic 446.6
      thrombocytic 446.6
      thrombocytopenic 446.6
  toxic 287.0
  variolosa 050.0
  vascular 287.0
  visceral symptoms 287.0
  Werlhof's (*see also* Purpura, thrombocytopenic) 287.3
Purpuric spots 782.7
Purulent — *see* condition
Pus
  absorption, general — *see* Septicemia
  in
    stool 792.1
    urine 791.9
  tube (rupture) (*see also* Salpingo-oophoritis) 614.2
Pustular rash 782.1
Pustule 686.9
  malignant 022.0
  nonmalignant 686.9
Putnam's disease (subacute combined sclerosis with pernicious anemia) 281.0 *[336.2]*
Putnam-Dana syndrome (subacute combined sclerosis with pernicious anemia) 281.0 *[336.2]*
Putrefaction, intestinal 569.89

✓4th Fourth-digit Required   ✓5th Fifth-digit Required   ▶◀ Revised Text   ● New Line   ▲ Revised Code

Putrescent pulp (dental) 522.1
Pyarthritis — *see* Pyarthrosis
Pyarthrosis (*see also* Arthritis, pyogenic) 711.0 ☑5ᵗʰ
   tuberculous — *see* Tuberculosis, joint
Pycnoepilepsy, pycnolepsy (idiopathic) (*see also* Epilepsy) 345.0 ☑5ᵗʰ
Pyelectasia 593.89
Pyelectasis 593.89
Pyelitis (congenital) (uremic) 590.80
  with
     abortion — *see* Abortion, by type, with specified complication NEC
     contracted kidney 590.00
     ectopic pregnancy (*see also* categories 633.0-633.9) 639.8
     molar pregnancy (*see also* categories 630-632) 639.8
  acute 590.10
    with renal medullary necrosis 590.11
  chronic 590.00
    with
      renal medullary necrosis 590.01
  complicating pregnancy, childbirth, or puerperium 646.6 ☑5ᵗʰ
    affecting fetus or newborn 760.1
  cystica 590.3
    following
      abortion 639.8
      ectopic or molar pregnancy 639.8
  gonococcal 098.19
    chronic or duration of 2 months or over 098.39
  tuberculous (*see also* Tuberculosis) 016.0 ☑5ᵗʰ [590.81]
Pyelocaliectasis 593.89
Pyelocystitis (*see also* Pyelitis) 590.80
Pyelohydronephrosis 591
Pyelonephritis (*see also* Pyelitis) 590.80
  acute 590.10
    with renal medullary necrosis 590.11
  chronic 590.00
  syphilitic (late) 095.4
  tuberculous (*see also* Tuberculosis) 016.0 ☑5ᵗʰ [590.81]
Pyelonephrosis (*see also* Pyelitis) 590.80
  chronic 590.00
Pyelophlebitis 451.89
Pyelo-ureteritis cystica 590.3
Pyemia, pyemic (purulent) (*see also* Septicemia) 038.9
  abscess — *see* Abscess
  arthritis (*see also* Arthritis, pyogenic) 711.0 ☑5ᵗʰ
  Bacillus coli 038.42
  embolism — *see* Embolism, pyemic
  fever 038.9
  infection 038.9
  joint (*see also* Arthritis, pyogenic) 711.0 ☑5ᵗʰ
  liver 572.1
  meningococcal 036.2
  newborn 771.81 ▲
  phlebitis — *see* Phlebitis
  pneumococcal 038.2
  portal 572.1
  postvaccinal 999.3
  specified organism NEC 038.8
  staphylococcal 038.10
    aureus 038.11
    specified organism NEC 038.19
  streptococcal 038.0
  tuberculous — *see* Tuberculosis, miliary
Pygopagus 759.4
Pykno-epilepsy, pyknolepsy (idiopathic) (*see also* Epilepsy) 345.0 ☑5ᵗʰ
Pyle (-Cohn) disease (craniometaphyseal dysplasia) 756.89
Pylephlebitis (suppurative) 572.1
Pylethrombophlebitis 572.1
Pylethrombosis 572.1
Pyloritis (*see also* Gastritis) 535.5 ☑5ᵗʰ
Pylorospasm (reflex) 537.81
  congenital or infantile 750.5
  neurotic 306.4
  newborn 750.5
  psychogenic 306.4
Pylorus, pyloric — *see* condition
Pyoarthrosis — *see* Pyarthrosis

Pyocele
  mastoid 383.00
  sinus (accessory) (nasal) (*see also* Sinusitis) 473.9
  turbinate (bone) 473.9
  urethra (*see also* Urethritis) 597.0
Pyococcal dermatitis 686.00
Pyococcide, skin 686.00
Pyocolpos (*see also* Vaginitis) 616.10
Pyocyaneus dermatitis 686.09
Pyocystitis (*see also* Cystitis) 595.9
Pyoderma, pyodermia 686.00
  gangrenosum 686.01
  specified type NEC 686.09
  vegetans 686.8
Pyodermatitis 686.00
  vegetans 686.8
Pyogenic — *see* condition
Pyohemia — *see* Septicemia
Pyohydronephrosis (*see also* Pyelitis) 590.80
Pyometra 615.9
Pyometritis (*see also* Endometritis) 615.9
Pyometrium (*see also* Endometritis) 615.9
Pyomyositis 728.0
  ossificans 728.19
  tropical (bungpagga) 040.81
Pyonephritis (*see also* Pyelitis) 590.80
  chronic 590.00
Pyonephrosis (congenital) (*see also* Pyelitis) 590.80
  acute 590.10
Pyo-oophoritis (*see also* Salpingo-oophoritis) 614.2
Pyo-ovarium (*see also* Salpingo-oophoritis) 614.2
Pyopericarditis 420.99
Pyopericardium 420.99
Pyophlebitis — *see* Phlebitis
Pyopneumopericardium 420.99
Pyopneumothorax (infectional) 510.9
  with fistula 510.0
  subdiaphragmatic (*see also* Peritonitis) 567.2
  subphrenic (*see also* Peritonitis) 567.2
  tuberculous (*see also* Tuberculosis, pleura) 012.0 ☑5ᵗʰ
Pyorrhea (alveolar) (alveolaris) 523.4
  degenerative 523.5
Pyosalpingitis (*see also* Salpingo-oophoritis) 614.2
Pyosalpinx (*see also* Salpingo-oophoritis) 614.2
Pyosepticemia — *see* Septicemia
Pyosis
  Corlett's (impetigo) 684
  Manson's (pemphigus contagiosus) 684
Pyothorax 510.9
  with fistula 510.0
  tuberculous (*see also* Tuberculosis, pleura) 012.0 ☑5ᵗʰ
Pyoureter 593.89
  tuberculous (*see also* Tuberculosis) 016.2 ☑5ᵗʰ
Pyramidopallidonigral syndrome 332.0
Pyrexia (of unknown origin) (P.U.O.) 780.6
  atmospheric 992.0
  during labor 659.2 ☑5ᵗʰ
  environmentally-induced newborn 778.4
  heat 992.0
  newborn, environmentally-induced 778.4
  puerperal 672 ☑4ᵗʰ
Pyroglobulinemia 273.8
Pyromania 312.33
Pyrosis 787.1
Pyrroloporphyria 277.1
Pyuria (bacterial) 791.9

Q

Q fever 083.0
  with pneumonia 083.0 [484.8]
Quadricuspid aortic valve 746.89
Quadrilateral fever 083.0

Quadriparesis — *see* Quadriplegia
Quadriplegia 344.00
  with fracture, vertebra (process) — *see* Fracture, vertebra, cervical, with spinal cord injury
  brain (current episode) 437.8
  C1-C4
    complete 344.01
    incomplete 344.02
  C5-C7
    complete 344.03
    incomplete 344.04
  cerebral (current episode) 437.8
  congenital or infantile (cerebral) (spastic) (spinal) 343.2
  cortical 437.8
  embolic (current episode) (*see also* Embolism, brain) 434.1 ☑5ᵗʰ
  infantile (cerebral) (spastic) (spinal) 343.2
  newborn NEC 767.0
  specified NEC 344.09
  thrombotic (current episode) (*see also* Thrombosis, brain) 434.0 ☑5ᵗʰ
  traumatic — *see* Injury, spinal, cervical
Quadruplet
  affected by maternal complications of pregnancy 761.5
  healthy liveborn — *see* Newborn, multiple
  pregnancy (complicating delivery) NEC 651.8 ☑5ᵗʰ
    with fetal loss and retention of one or more fetus(es) 651.5 ☑5ᵗʰ
Quarrelsomeness 301.3
Quartan
  fever 084.2
  malaria (fever) 084.2
Queensland fever 083.0
  coastal 083.0
  seven-day 100.89
Quervain's disease 727.04
  thyroid (subacute granulomatous thyroiditis) 245.1
Queyrat's erythroplasia (M8080/2)
  specified site — *see* Neoplasm, skin, in situ
  unspecified site 233.5
Quincke's disease or edema — *see* Edema, angioneurotic
Quinquaud's disease (acne decalvans) 704.09
Quinsy (gangrenous) 475
Quintan fever 083.1
Quintuplet
  affected by maternal complications of pregnancy 761.5
  healthy liveborn — *see* Newborn, multiple
  pregnancy (complicating delivery) NEC 651.2 ☑5ᵗʰ
    with fetal loss and retention of one or more fetus(es) 651.6 ☑5ᵗʰ
Quotidian
  fever 084.0
  malaria (fever) 084.0

R

Rabbia 071
Rabbit fever (*see also* Tularemia) 021.9
Rabies 071
  contact V01.5
  exposure to V01.5
  inoculation V04.5
    reaction — *see* Complications, vaccination
  vaccination, prophylactic (against) V04.5
Rachischisis (*see also* Spina bifida) 741.9 ☑5ᵗʰ
Rachitic — *see also* condition
  deformities of spine 268.1
  pelvis 268.1
    with disproportion (fetopelvic) 653.2 ☑5ᵗʰ
      affecting fetus or newborn 763.1
      causing obstructed labor 660.1 ☑5ᵗʰ
        affecting fetus or newborn 763.1
Rachitis, rachitism — *see also* Rickets
  acute 268.0
  fetalis 756.4

Rachitis, rachitism — *see also* Rickets —
  continued
  renalis 588.0
  tarda 268.0
Racket nail 757.5
Radial nerve — *see* condition
Radiation effects or sickness — *see also* Effect,
  adverse, radiation
  cataract 366.46
  dermatitis 692.82
    sunburn (*see also* Sunburn) 692.71
Radiculitis (pressure) (vertebrogenic) 729.2
  accessory nerve 723.4
  anterior crural 724.4
  arm 723.4
  brachial 723.4
  cervical NEC 723.4
  due to displacement of intervertebral disc —
    see Neuritis, due to, displacement
    intervertebral disc
  leg 724.4
  lumbar NEC 724.4
  lumbosacral 724.4
  rheumatic 729.2
  syphilitic 094.89
  thoracic (with visceral pain) 724.4
Radiculomyelitis 357.0
  toxic, due to
    Clostridium tetani 037
    Corynebacterium diphtheriae 032.89
Radiculopathy (*see also* Radiculitis) 729.2
Radioactive substances, adverse effect — *see*
  Effect, adverse, radioactive substance
Radiodermal burns (acute) (chronic)
  (occupational) — *see* Burn, by site
Radiodermatitis 692.82
Radionecrosis — *see* Effect, adverse, radiation
Radiotherapy session V58.0
Radium, adverse effect — *see* Effect, adverse,
  radioactive substance
Raeder-Harbitz syndrome (pulseless disease)
  446.7
Rage (*see also* Disturbance, conduct) 312.0 ✓5ᵗʰ
  meaning rabies 071
Rag sorters' disease 022.1
Raillietiniasis 123.8
Railroad neurosis 300.16
Railway spine 300.16
Raised — *see* Elevation
Raiva 071
Rake teeth, tooth 524.3
Rales 786.7
Ramifying renal pelvis 753.3
Ramsay Hunt syndrome (herpetic geniculate
  ganglionitis) 053.11
  meaning dyssynergia cerebellaris myoclonica
  334.2
Ranke's primary infiltration (*see also*
  Tuberculosis) 010.0 ✓5ᵗʰ
Ranula 527.6
  congenital 750.26
Rape — *see* Injury, by site
  alleged, observation or examination V71.5
Rapid
  feeble pulse, due to shock, following injury
    958.4
  heart (beat) 785.0
    psychogenic 306.2
  respiration 786.06
    psychogenic 306.1
  second stage (delivery) 661.3 ✓5ᵗʰ
    affecting fetus or newborn 763.6
  time-zone change syndrome 307.45
Rarefaction, bone 733.99
Rash 782.1
  canker 034.1
  diaper 691.0
  drug (internal use) 693.0
    contact 692.3
  ECHO 9 virus 078.89
  enema 692.89

Rash — *continued*
  food (*see also* Allergy, food) 693.1
  heat 705.1
  napkin 691.0
  nettle 708.8
  pustular 782.1
  rose 782.1
    epidemic 056.9
    of infants 057.8
  scarlet 034.1
  serum (prophylactic) (therapeutic) 999.5
  toxic 782.1
  wandering tongue 529.1
Rasmussen's aneurysm (*see also* Tuberculosis)
  011.2 ✓5ᵗʰ
Rat-bite fever 026.9
  due to Streptobacillus moniliformis 026.1 ✓5ᵗʰ
  spirochetal (morsus muris) 026.0 ✓5ᵗʰ
Rathke's pouch tumor (M9350/1) 237.0
Raymond (-Céstan) syndrome 433.8 ✓5ᵗʰ
Raynaud's
  disease or syndrome (paroxysmal digital
    cyanosis) 443.0
  gangrene (symmetric) 443.0 [785.4]
  phenomenon (paroxysmal digital cyanosis)
    (secondary) 443.0
RDS 769
Reaction
  acute situational maladjustment (*see also*
    Reaction, adjustment) 309.9
  adaptation (*see also* Reaction, adjustment)
    309.9
  adjustment 309.9
    with
      anxious mood 309.24
        with depressed mood 309.28
      conduct disturbance 309.3
        combined with disturbance of
          emotions 309.4
      depressed mood 309.0
        brief 309.0
          with anxious mood 309.28
        prolonged 309.1
      elective mutism 309.83
      mixed emotions and conduct 309.4
      mutism, elective 309.83
      physical symptoms 309.82
      predominant disturbance (of)
        conduct 309.3
        emotions NEC 309.29
          mixed 309.28
        mixed, emotions and conduct 309.4
        specified type NEC 309.89
      specific academic or work inhibition
        309.23
      withdrawal 309.83
    depressive 309.0
      with conduct disturbance 309.4
      brief 309.0
      prolonged 309.1
    specified type NEC 309.89
  adverse food NEC 995.7
  affective (*see also* Psychosis, affective) 296.90
    specified type NEC 296.99
  aggressive 301.3
    unsocialized (*see also* Disturbance, conduct)
      312.0 ✓5ᵗʰ
  allergic (*see also* Allergy) 995.3
    drug, medicinal substance, and biological —
      see Allergy, drug
    food — *see* Allergy, food
    serum 999.5
  anaphylactic — *see* Shock, anaphylactic
  anesthesia — *see* Anesthesia, complication
  anger 312.0 ✓5ᵗʰ
  antisocial 301.7
  antitoxin (prophylactic) (therapeutic) — *see*
    Complications, vaccination
  anxiety 300.00
  asthenic 300.5
  compulsive 300.3
  conversion (anesthetic) (autonomic)
    (hyperkinetic) (mixed paralytic)
    (paresthetic) 300.11
  deoxyribonuclease (DNA) (DNase)
    hypersensitivity NEC 287.2

Reaction — *continued*
  depressive 300.4
    acute 309.0
    affective (*see also* Psychosis, affective)
      296.2 ✓5ᵗʰ
      recurrent episode 296.3 ✓5ᵗʰ
      single episode 296.2 ✓5ᵗʰ
    brief 309.0
    manic (*see also* Psychosis, affective) 296.80
    neurotic 300.4
    psychoneurotic 300.4
    psychotic 298.0
  dissociative 300.15
  drug NEC (*see also* Table of Drugs and
    Chemicals) 995.2
    allergic — *see* Allergy, drug
    correct substance properly administered
      995.2
    obstetric anesthetic or analgesic NEC
      668.9 ✓5ᵗʰ
      affecting fetus or newborn 763.5
      specified drug — *see* Table of Drugs and
        Chemicals
    overdose or poisoning 977.9
      specified drug — *see* Table of Drugs and
        Chemicals
    specific to newborn 779.4
    transmitted via placenta or breast milk —
      see Absorption, drug, through
      placenta
    withdrawal NEC 292.0
      infant of dependent mother 779.5
    wrong substance given or taken in error
      977.9
      specified drug — *see* Table of Drugs and
        Chemicals
  dyssocial 301.7
  erysipeloid 027.1
  fear 300.20
    child 313.0
  fluid loss, cerebrospinal 349.0
  food — *see also* Allergy, food
    adverse NEC 995.7
    anaphylactic shock — *see* Anaphylactic
      shock, due to, food
  foreign
    body NEC 728.82
      in operative wound (inadvertently left)
        998.4
        due to surgical material intentionally
          left — *see* Complications, due to
          (presence of) any device, implant,
          or graft classified to 996.0-996.5
          NEC
    substance accidentally left during a
      procedure (chemical) (powder) (talc)
      998.7
      body or object (instrument) (sponge)
        (swab) 998.4
  graft-versus-host (GVH) 996.85
  grief (acute) (brief) 309.0
    prolonged 309.1
  gross stress (*see also* Reaction, stress, acute)
    308.9
  group delinquent (*see also* Disturbance,
    conduct) 312.2 ✓5ᵗʰ
  Herxheimer's 995.0
  hyperkinetic (*see also* Hyperkinesia) 314.9
  hypochondriacal 300.7
  hypoglycemic, due to insulin 251.0
    therapeutic misadventure 962.3
  hypomanic (*see also* Psychosis, affective)
    296.0 ✓5ᵗʰ
    recurrent episode 296.1 ✓5ᵗʰ
    single episode 296.0 ✓5ᵗʰ
  hysterical 300.10
    conversion type 300.11
    dissociative 300.15
  id (bacterial cause) 692.89
  immaturity NEC 301.89
    aggressive 301.3
    emotional instability 301.59
  immunization — *see* Complications,
    vaccination
  incompatibility
    blood group (ABO) (infusion) (transfusion)
      999.6

Reaction — *continued*
  incompatibility — *continued*
    Rh (factor) (infusion) (transfusion) 999.7
  inflammatory — *see* Infection
  infusion — *see* Complications, infusion
  inoculation (immune serum) — *see*
    Complications, vaccination
  insulin 995.2
  involutional
    paranoid 297.2
    psychotic (*see also* Psychosis, affective,
      depressive) 296.2 ✓5th
  leukemoid (lymphocytic) (monocytic)
    (myelocytic) 288.8
  LSD (*see also* Abuse, drugs, nondependent)
    305.3 ✓5th
  lumbar puncture 349.0
  manic-depressive (*see also* Psychosis, affective)
    296.80
    depressed 296.2 ✓5th
      recurrent episode 296.3 ✓5th
      single episode 296.2 ✓5th
    hypomanic 296.0 ✓5th
  neurasthenic 300.5
  neurogenic (*see also* Neurosis) 300.9
  neurotic NEC 300.9
  neurotic-depressive 300.4
  nitritoid — *see* Crisis, nitritoid
  obsessive (-compulsive) 300.3
  organic 293.9
    acute 293.0
    subacute 293.1
  overanxious, child or adolescent 313.0
  paranoid (chronic) 297.9
    acute 298.3
    climacteric 297.2
    involutional 297.2
    menopausal 297.2
    senile 290.20
    simple 297.0
  passive
    aggressive 301.84
    dependency 301.6
  personality (*see also* Disorder, personality)
    301.9
  phobic 300.20
  postradiation — *see* Effect, adverse, radiation
  psychogenic NEC 300.9
  psychoneurotic (*see also* Neurosis) 300.9
    anxiety 300.00
    compulsive 300.3
    conversion 300.11
    depersonalization 300.6
    depressive 300.4
    dissociative 300.15
    hypochondriacal 300.7
    hysterical 300.10
      conversion type 300.11
      dissociative type 300.15
    neurasthenic 300.5
    obsessive 300.3
    obsessive-compulsive 300.3
    phobic 300.20
    tension state 300.9
  psychophysiologic NEC (*see also* Disorder,
    psychosomatic) 306.9
    cardiovascular 306.2
    digestive 306.4
    endocrine 306.6
    gastrointestinal 306.4
    genitourinary 306.50
    heart 306.2
    hemic 306.8
    intestinal (large) (small) 306.4
    laryngeal 306.1
    lymphatic 306.8
    musculoskeletal 306.0
    pharyngeal 306.1
    respiratory 306.1
    skin 306.3
    special sense organs 306.7
  psychosomatic (*see also* Disorder,
    psychosomatic) 306.9
  psychotic (*see also* Psychosis) 298.9
    depressive 298.0
    due to or associated with physical condition
      (*see also* Psychosis, organic) 293.9

Reaction — *continued*
  psychotic (*see also* Psychosis) — *continued*
    involutional (*see also* Psychosis, affective)
      296.2 ✓5th
      recurrent episode 296.3 ✓5th
      single episode 296.2 ✓5th
  pupillary (myotonic) (tonic) 379.46
  radiation — *see* Effect, adverse, radiation
  runaway — *see also* Disturbance, conduct
    socialized 312.2 ✓5th
    undersocialized, unsocialized 312.1 ✓5th
  scarlet fever toxin — *see* Complications,
    vaccination
  schizophrenic (*see also* Schizophrenia)
    295.9 ✓5th
    latent 295.5 ✓5th
  serological for syphilis — *see* Serology for
    syphilis
  serum (prophylactic) (therapeutic) 999.5
    immediate 999.4
  situational (*see also* Reaction, adjustment)
    309.9
    acute, to stress 308.3
    adjustment (*see also* Reaction, adjustment)
      309.9
  somatization (*see also* Disorder, psychosomatic)
    306.9
  spinal puncture 349.0
  spite, child (*see also* Disturbance, conduct)
    312.0 ✓5th
  stress, acute 308.9
    with predominant disturbance (of)
      consciousness 308.1
      emotions 308.0
      mixed 308.4
      psychomotor 308.2
      specified type NEC 308.3
    bone or cartilage — *see* Fracture, stress
  surgical procedure — *see* Complications,
    surgical procedure
  tetanus antitoxin — *see* Complications,
    vaccination
  toxin-antitoxin — *see* Complications,
    vaccination
  transfusion (blood) (bone marrow)
    (lymphocytes) (allergic) — *see*
    Complications, transfusion
  tuberculin skin test, nonspecific (without active
    tuberculosis) 795.5
    positive (without active tuberculosis) 795.5
  ultraviolet — *see* Effect, adverse, ultraviolet
  undersocialized, unsocialized — *see also*
    Disturbance, conduct
    aggressive (type) 312.0 ✓5th
    unaggressive (type) 312.1 ✓5th
  vaccination (any) — *see* Complications,
    vaccination
  white graft (skin) 996.52
  withdrawing, child or adolescent 313.22
  x-ray — *see* Effect, adverse, x-rays
Reactive depression (*see also* Reaction,
  depressive) 300.4
  neurotic 300.4
  psychoneurotic 300.4
  psychotic 298.0
Rebound tenderness 789.6 ✓5th
Recalcitrant patient V15.81
Recanalization, thrombus — *see* Thrombosis
Recession, receding
  chamber angle (eye) 364.77
  chin 524.06
  gingival (generalized) (localized) (postinfective)
    (postoperative) 523.2
Recklinghausen's disease (M9540/1) 237.71
  bones (osteitis fibrosa cystica) 252.0
Recklinghausen-Applebaum disease
  (hemochromatosis) 275.0
Reclus' disease (cystic) 610.1
Recrudescent typhus (fever) 081.1
Recruitment, auditory 388.44
Rectalgia 569.42
Rectitis 569.49

Rectocele
  female (without uterine prolapse) 618.0
    with uterine prolapse 618.4
      complete 618.3
      incomplete 618.2
  in pregnancy or childbirth 654.4 ✓5th
    causing obstructed labor 660.2 ✓5th
      affecting fetus or newborn 763.1
  male 569.49
  vagina, vaginal (outlet) 618.0
Rectosigmoiditis 569.89
  ulcerative (chronic) 556.3
Rectosigmoid junction — *see* condition
Rectourethral — *see* condition
Rectovaginal — *see* condition
Rectovesical — *see* condition
Rectum, rectal — *see* condition
Recurrent — *see* condition
Red bugs 133.8
Red cedar asthma 495.8
Redness
  conjunctiva 379.93
  eye 379.93
  nose 478.1
Reduced ventilatory or vital capacity 794.2
Reduction
  function
    kidney (*see also* Disease, renal) 593.9
    liver 573.8
  ventilatory capacity 794.2
  vital capacity 794.2
Redundant, redundancy
  abdomen 701.9
  anus 751.5
  cardia 537.89
  clitoris 624.2
  colon (congenital) 751.5
  foreskin (congenital) 605
  intestine 751.5
  labia 624.3
  organ or site, congenital NEC — *see* Accessory
  panniculus (abdominal) 278.1
  prepuce (congenital) 605
  pylorus 537.89
  rectum 751.5
  scrotum 608.89
  sigmoid 751.5
  skin (of face) 701.9
    eyelids 374.30
  stomach 537.89
  uvula 528.9
  vagina 623.8
Reduplication — *see* Duplication
Referral
  adoption (agency) V68.89
  nursing care V63.8
  patient without examination or treatment
    V68.81
  social services V63.8
Reflex — *see also* condition
  blink, deficient 374.45
  hyperactive gag 478.29
  neurogenic bladder NEC 596.54
    atonic 596.54
      with cauda equina syndrome 344.61
  vasoconstriction 443.9
  vasovagal 780.2
Reflux
  esophageal 530.81
  esophagitis 530.11
  gastroesophageal 530.81
  mitral — *see* Insufficiency, mitral
  ureteral — *see* Reflux, vesicoureteral
  vesicoureteral 593.70
    with
      reflux nephropathy 593.73
        bilateral 593.72
        unilateral 593.71
Reformed gallbladder 576.0
Reforming, artificial openings (*see also*
  Attention to, artificial, opening) V55.9
Refractive error (*see also* Error, refractive) 367.9

✓4th Fourth-digit Required   ✓5th Fifth-digit Required   ►◄ Revised Text   ● New Line   ▲ Revised Code

Refsum's disease or syndrome (heredopathia
  atactica polyneuritiformis) 356.3
Refusal of
  food 307.59
    hysterical 300.11
    treatment because of, due to
      patient's decision NEC V64.2
      reason of conscience or religion V62.6
Regaud
  tumor (M8082/3) — see Neoplasm,
    nasopharynx, malignant
  type carcinoma (M8082/3) — see Neoplasm,
    nasopharynx, malignant
Regional — see condition
Regulation feeding (elderly) (infant) 783.3
  newborn 779.3
Regurgitated
  food, choked on 933.1
  stomach contents, choked on 933.1
Regurgitation
  aortic (valve) (see also Insufficiency, aortic)
    424.1
    congenital 746.4
    syphilitic 093.22
  food — see also Vomiting
    with reswallowing — see Rumination
    newborn 779.3
  gastric contents — see Vomiting
  heart — see Endocarditis
  mitral (valve) — see also Insufficiency, mitral
    congenital 746.6
  myocardial — see Endocarditis
  pulmonary (heart) (valve) (see also
    Endocarditis, pulmonary) 424.3
  stomach — see Vomiting
  tricuspid — see Endocarditis, tricuspid
  valve, valvular — see Endocarditis
  vesicoureteral — see Reflux, vesicoureteral
Rehabilitation V57.9
  multiple types V57.89
  occupational V57.21
  specified type NEC V57.89
  speech V57.3
  vocational V57.22
Reichmann's disease or syndrome
    (gastrosuccorrhea) 536.8
Reifenstein's syndrome (hereditary familial
    hypogonadism, male) 257.2
Reilly's syndrome or phenomenon (see also
    Neuropathy, peripheral, autonomic) 337.9
Reimann's periodic disease 277.3
Reinsertion, contraceptive device V25.42
Reiter's disease, syndrome, or urethritis
    099.3 [711.1] ✓5ᵗʰ
Rejection
  food, hysterical 300.11
  transplant 996.80
    bone marrow 996.85
    corneal 996.51
    organ (immune or nonimmune cause)
      996.80
      bone marrow 996.85
      heart 996.83
      intestines 996.87
      kidney 996.81
      liver 996.82
      lung 996.84
      pancreas 996.86
      specified NEC 996.89
    skin 996.52
      artificial 996.55
      decellularized allodermis 996.55
Relapsing fever 087.9
  Carter's (Asiatic) 087.0
  Dutton's (West African) 087.1
  Koch's 087.9
  louse-borne (epidemic) 087.0
  Novy's (American) 087.1
  Obermeyer's (European) 087.0
  Spirillum 087.9
  tick-borne (endemic) 087.1
Relaxation
  anus (sphincter) 569.49
    due to hysteria 300.11

Relaxation — continued
  arch (foot) 734
    congenital 754.61
  back ligaments 728.4
  bladder (sphincter) 596.59
  cardio-esophageal 530.89
  cervix (see also Incompetency, cervix) 622.5
  diaphragm 519.4
  inguinal rings — see Hernia, inguinal
  joint (capsule) (ligament) (paralytic) (see also
    Derangement, joint) 718.90
    congenital 755.8
  lumbosacral joint 724.6
  pelvic floor 618.8
  pelvis 618.8
  perineum 618.8
  posture 729.9
  rectum (sphincter) 569.49
  sacroiliac (joint) 724.6
  scrotum 608.89
  urethra (sphincter) 599.84
  uterus (outlet) 618.8
  vagina (outlet) 618.8
  vesical 596.59
Remains
  canal of Cloquet 743.51
  capsule (opaque) 743.51
Remittent fever (malarial) 084.6
Remnant
  canal of Cloquet 743.51
  capsule (opaque) 743.51
  cervix, cervical stump (acquired) (postoperative)
    622.8
  cystic duct, postcholecystectomy 576.0
  fingernail 703.8
    congenital 757.5
  meniscus, knee 717.5
  thyroglossal duct 759.2
  tonsil 474.8
    infected 474.00
  urachus 753.7
Remote effect of cancer — see condition
Removal (of)
  catheter (urinary) (indwelling) V53.6
    from artificial opening — see Attention to,
      artificial, opening
    non-vascular V58.82
    vascular V58.81
  cerebral ventricle (communicating) shunt
    V53.01
  device — see also Fitting (of)
    contraceptive V25.42
    fixation
      external V54.89 ▲
      internal V54.0
    traction V54.89 ▲
  dressing V58.3
  ileostomy V55.2
  Kirschner wire V54.89 ▲
  nonvascular catheter V58.82
  pin V54.0
  plaster cast V54.89 ▲
  plate (fracture) V54.0
  rod V54.0
  screw V54.0
  splint, external V54.89 ▲
  subdermal implantable contraceptive V25.43
  suture V58.3
  traction device, external V54.89 ▲
  vascular catheter V58.81
Ren
  arcuatus 753.3
  mobile, mobilis (see also Disease, renal) 593.0
    congenital 753.3
  unguliformis 753.3
Renal — see also condition
  glomerulohyalinosis-diabetic syndrome
    250.4 ✓5ᵗʰ [581.81]
Rendu-Osler-Weber disease or syndrome
    (familial hemorrhagic telangiectasia) 448.0
Reninoma (M8361/1) 236.91
Rénon-Delille syndrome 253.8

Repair
  pelvic floor, previous, in pregnancy or
    childbirth 654.4 ✓5ᵗʰ
    affecting fetus or newborn 763.89
  scarred tissue V51
**Replacement by artificial or mechanical device
  or prosthesis of** (see also Fitting (of))
  artificial skin V43.83
  bladder V43.5
  blood vessel V43.4
  breast V43.82
  eye globe V43.0
  heart V43.2
    valve V43.3
  intestine V43.89
  joint V43.60
    ankle V43.66
    elbow V43.62
    finger V43.69
    hip (partial) (total) V43.64
    knee V43.65
    shoulder V43.61
    specified NEC V43.69
    wrist V43.63
  kidney V43.89
  larynx V43.81
  lens V43.1
  limb(s) V43.7
  liver V43.89
  lung V43.89
  organ NEC V43.89
  pancreas V43.89
  skin (artificial) V43.83
  tissue NEC V43.89
Reprogramming
  cardiac pacemaker V53.31
Request for expert evidence V68.2
Reserve, decreased or low
  cardiac — see Disease, heart
  kidney (see also Disease, renal) 593.9
Residual — see also condition
  bladder 596.8
  foreign body — see Retention, foreign body
  state, schizophrenic (see also Schizophrenia)
    295.6 ✓5ᵗʰ
  urine 788.69
Resistance, resistant (to)

Note — use the following subclassification for
categories V09.5, V09.7, V09.8, V09.9:

  0   without mention of resistance to
       multiple drugs

  1   with resistance to multiple drugs
       V09.5   quinolones and
                fluoroquinolones
       V09.7   antimycobacterial agents
       V09.8   specified drugs NEC
       V09.9   unspecified drugs

  9   multiple sites

  drugs by microorganisms V09.9 ✓5ᵗʰ
    Amikacin V09.4
    aminoglycosides V09.4
    Amodiaquine V09.5 ✓5ᵗʰ
    Amoxicillin V09.0
    Ampicillin V09.0
    antimycobacterial agents V09.7 ✓5ᵗʰ ●
    Azithromycin V09.2
    Azlocillin V09.0
    Aztreonam V09.1
    B-lactam antibiotics V09.1
    bacampicillin V09.0
    Bacitracin V09.8 ✓5ᵗʰ
    Benznidazole V09.8 ✓5ᵗʰ
    Capreomycin V09.7 ✓5ᵗʰ
    Carbenicillin V09.0
    Cefaclor V09.1
    Cefadroxil V09.1
    Cefamandole V09.1
    Cefatetan V09.1
    Cefazolin V09.1
    Cefixime V09.1
    Cefonicid V09.1
    Cefoperazone V09.1
    Ceforanide V09.1

Resistance, resistant (to) — *continued*
  drugs by microorganisms — *continued*
    Cefotaxime V09.1
    Cefoxitin V09.1
    Ceftazidime V09.1
    Ceftizoxime V09.1
    Ceftriaxone V09.1
    Cefuroxime V09.1
    Cephalexin V09.1
    Cephaloglycin V09.1
    Cephaloridine V09.1
    Cephalosporins V09.1
    Cephalothin V09.1
    Cephapirin V09.1
    Cephradine V09.1
    Chloramphenicol V09.8 ✓5th
    Chloraquine V09.5 ✓5th
    Chlorguanide V09.8 ✓5th
    Chlorproguanil V09.8 ✓5th
    Chlortetracycline V09.3
    Cinoxacin V09.5 ✓5th
    Ciprofloxacin V09.5 ✓5th
    Clarithromycin V09.2
    Clindamycin V09.8 ✓5th
    Clioquinol V09.5 ✓5th
    Clofazimine V09.7 ✓5th
    Cloxacillin V09.0
    Cyclacillin V09.0
    Cycloserine V09.7 ✓5th
    Dapsone [DZ] V09.7 ✓5th
    Demeclocycline V09.3
    Dicloxacillin V09.0
    Doxycycline V09.3
    Enoxacin V09.5 ✓5th
    Erythromycin V09.2
    Ethambutol [EMB] V09.7 ✓5th
    Ethionamide [ETA] V09.7 ✓5th
    fluoroquinolones V09.5 ✓5th
    Gentamicin V09.4
    Halofantrine V09.8 ✓5th
    Imipenem V09.1
    Iodoquinol V09.5 ✓5th
    Isoniazid [INH] V09.7 ✓5th
    Kanamycin V09.4
    macrolides V09.2
    Mafenide V09.6
    Mefloquine V09.8 ✓5th
    Melasoprol V09.8 ✓5th
    Methacycline V09.3
    Methenamine V09.8 ✓5th
    Methicillin V09.0
    Metronidazole V09.8 ✓5th
    Mezlocillin V09.0
    Minocycline V09.3
    Nafcillin V09.0
    Nalidixic acid V09.5 ✓5th
    Natamycin V09.2
    Neomycin V09.4
    Netilmicin V09.4
    Nifurtimox V09.8 ✓5th
    Nimorazole V09.8 ✓5th
    Nitrofurantoin V09.8 ✓5th
    Norfloxacin V09.5 ✓5th
    Nystatin V09.2
    Ofloxacin V09.5 ✓5th
    Oleandomycin V09.2
    Oxacillin V09.0
    Oxytetracycline V09.3
    Para-amino salicylic acid [PAS] V09.7 ✓5th
    Paromomycin V09.4
    Penicillin (G) (V) (VK) V09.0
    penicillins V09.0
    Pentamidine V09.8 ✓5th
    Piperacillin V09.0
    Primaquine V09.5 ✓5th
    Proguanil V09.8 ✓5th
    Pyrazinamide [PZA] V09.7 ✓5th
    Pyrimethamine/sulfalene V09.8 ✓5th
    Pyrimethamine/sulfodoxine V09.8 ✓5th
    Quinacrine V09.5 ✓5th
    Quinidine V09.8 ✓5th
    Quinine V09.8 ✓5th
    quinolones V09.5 ✓5th
    Rifabutin V09.7 ✓5th
    Rifampin [RIF] V09.7 ✓5th
    Rifamycin V09.7 ✓5th
    Rolitetracycline V09.3

Resistance, resistant (to) — *continued*
  drugs by microorganisms — *continued*
    Specified drugs NEC V09.8 ✓5th
    Spectinomycin V09.8 ✓5th
    Spiramycin V09.2
    Streptomycin [SM] V09.4
    Sulfacetamide V09.6
    Sulfacytine V09.6
    Sulfadiazine V09.6
    Sulfadoxine V09.6
    Sulfamethoxazole V09.6
    Sulfapyridine V09.6
    Sulfasalizine V09.6
    Sulfasoxazone V09.6
    sulfonamides V09.6
    Sulfoxone V09.7 ✓5th
    tetracycline V09.3
    tetracyclines V09.3
    Thiamphenicol V09.8 ✓5th
    Ticarcillin V09.0
    Tinidazole V09.8 ✓5th
    Tobramycin V09.4
    Triamphenicol V09.8 ✓5th
    Trimethoprim V09.8 ✓5th
    Vancomycin V09.8 ✓5th

Resorption
  biliary 576.8
    purulent or putrid (*see also* Cholecystitis) 576.8
  dental (roots) 521.4
    alveoli 525.8
  septic — *see* Septicemia
  teeth (external) (internal) (pathological) (roots) 521.4

Respiration
  asymmetrical 786.09
  bronchial 786.09
  Cheyne-Stokes (periodic respiration) 786.04
  decreased, due to shock following injury 958.4
  disorder of 786.00
    psychogenic 306.1
    specified NEC 786.09
  failure 518.81
    acute 518.81
    acute and chronic 518.84
    chronic 518.83
    newborn 770.84 ▲
  insufficiency 786.09
    acute 518.82
    newborn NEC 770.89 ▲
  Kussmaul (air hunger) 786.09
  painful 786.52
  periodic 786.09
  poor 786.09
    newborn NEC 770.89 ▲
  sighing 786.7
    psychogenic 306.1
  wheezing 786.07

Respiratory — *see also* condition
  distress 786.09
    acute 518.82
    fetus or newborn NEC 770.89 ▲
    syndrome (newborn) 769
      adult (following shock, surgery, or trauma) 518.5
      specified NEC 518.82
  failure 518.81
    acute 518.81
    acute and chronic 518.8
    chronic 518.83

Respiratory syncytial virus (RSV) 079.6
  bronchiolitis 466.11
  pneumonia 480.1

Response
  photoallergic 692.72
  phototoxic 692.72

Rest, rests
  mesonephric duct 752.8
    fallopian tube 752.11
  ovarian, in fallopian tubes 752.19
  wolffian duct 752.8

Restless leg (syndrome) 333.99

Restlessness 799.2

Restoration of organ continuity from previous sterilization (tuboplasty) (vasoplasty) V26.0

Restriction of housing space V60.1

Restzustand, schizophrenic (*see also* Schizophrenia) 295.6 ✓5th

Retained — *see* Retention

Retardation
  development, developmental, specific (*see also* Disorder, development, specific) 315.9
  learning, specific 315.2
    arithmetical 315.1
    language (skills) 315.31
      expressive 315.31
      mixed receptive-expressive 315.32
    mathematics 315.1
    reading 315.00
      phonological 315.39
    written expression 315.2
  motor 315.4
  endochondral bone growth 733.91
  growth (physical) in childhood 783.43
    due to malnutrition 263.2
    fetal (intrauterine) 764.9 ✓5th
      affecting management of pregnancy 656.5 ✓5th
  intrauterine growth 764.9 ✓5th
    affecting management of pregnancy 656.5 ✓5th
  mental 319
    borderline V62.89
    mild, IQ 50-70 317
    moderate, IQ 35-49 318.0
    profound, IQ under 20 318.2
    severe, IQ 20-34 318.1
  motor, specific 315.4
  physical 783.43
    child 783.43
    due to malnutrition 263.2
    fetus (intrauterine) 764.9 ✓5th
      affecting management of pregnancy 656.5 ✓5th
  psychomotor NEC 307.9
  reading 315.00

Retching — *see* Vomiting

Retention, retained
  bladder NEC (*see also* Retention, urine) 788.20
    psychogenic 306.53
  carbon dioxide 276.2
  cyst — *see* Cyst
  dead
    fetus (after 22 completed weeks gestation) 656.4 ✓5th
      early fetal death (before 22 completed weeks gestation) 632
    ovum 631
  decidua (following delivery) (fragments) (with hemorrhage) 666.2 ✓5th
    without hemorrhage 667.1 ✓5th
  deciduous tooth 520.6
  dental root 525.3
  fecal (*see also* Constipation) 564.00
  fluid 276.6
  foreign body — *see also* Foreign body, retained
    bone 733.99
    current trauma — *see* Foreign body, by site or type
    middle ear 385.83
    muscle 729.6
    soft tissue NEC 729.6
  gastric 536.8
  membranes (following delivery) (with hemorrhage) 666.2 ✓5th
    with abortion — *see* Abortion, by type
    without hemorrhage 667.1 ✓5th
  menses 626.8
  milk (puerperal) 676.2 ✓5th
  nitrogen, extrarenal 788.9
  placenta (total) (with hemorrhage) 666.0 ✓5th
    with abortion — *see* Abortion, by type
    portions or fragments 666.2 ✓5th
      without hemorrhage 667.1 ✓5th
    without hemorrhage 667.0 ✓5th
  products of conception
    early pregnancy (fetal death before 22 completed weeks gestation) 632
    following
      abortion — *see* Abortion, by type

Retention, retained — *continued*
  products of conception — *continued*
    following — *continued*
      delivery 666.2 ✓5ᵗʰ
        with hemorrhage 666.2 ✓5ᵗʰ
        without hemorrhage 667.1 ✓5ᵗʰ
      secundines (following delivery) (with
        hemorrhage) 666.2 ✓5ᵗʰ
    with abortion — *see* Abortion, by type
    complicating puerperium (delayed
      hemorrhage) 666.2 ✓5ᵗʰ
      without hemorrhage 667.1 ✓5ᵗʰ
  smegma, clitoris 624.8
  urine NEC 788.20
    bladder, incomplete emptying 788.21
    psychogenic 306.53
    specified NEC 788.29
  water (in tissue) (*see also* Edema) 782.3
Reticulation, dust (occupational) 504
Reticulocytosis NEC 790.99
Reticuloendotheliosis
  acute infantile (M9722/3) 202.5 ✓5ᵗʰ
  leukemic (M9940/3) 202.4 ✓5ᵗʰ
  malignant (M9720/3) 202.3 ✓5ᵗʰ
  nonlipid (M9722/3) 202.5 ✓5ᵗʰ
Reticulohistiocytoma (giant cell) 277.8
Reticulohistiocytosis, multicentric 272.8
Reticulolymphosarcoma (diffuse) (M9613/3)
    200.8 ✓5ᵗʰ
  follicular (M9691/3) 202.0 ✓5ᵗʰ
  nodular (M9691/3) 202.0 ✓5ᵗʰ
Reticulosarcoma (M9640/3) 200.0 ✓5ᵗʰ
  nodular (M9642/3) 200.0 ✓5ᵗʰ
  pleomorphic cell type (M9641/3) 200.0 ✓5ᵗʰ
Reticulosis (skin)
  acute of infancy (M9722/3) 202.5 ✓5ᵗʰ
  histiocytic medullary (M9721/3) 202.3 ✓5ᵗʰ
  lipomelanotic 695.89
  malignant (M9720/3) 202.3 ✓5ᵗʰ
  Sézary's (M9701/3) 202.2 ✓5ᵗʰ
Retina, retinal — *see* condition
Retinitis (*see also* Chorioretinitis) 363.20
  albuminurica 585 [363.10]
  arteriosclerotic 440.8 [362.13]
  central angiospastic 362.41
  Coat's 362.12
  diabetic 250.5 ✓5ᵗʰ [362.01]
  disciformis 362.52
  disseminated 363.10
    metastatic 363.14
    neurosyphilitic 094.83
    pigment epitheliopathy 363.15
  exudative 362.12
  focal 363.00
    in histoplasmosis 115.92
      capsulatum 115.02
      duboisii 115.12
    juxtapapillary 363.05
    macular 363.06
    paramacular 363.06
    peripheral 363.08
    posterior pole NEC 363.07
  gravidarum 646.8 ✓5ᵗʰ
  hemorrhagica externa 362.12
  juxtapapillary (Jensen's) 363.05
  luetic — *see* Retinitis, syphilitic
  metastatic 363.14
  pigmentosa 362.74
  proliferans 362.29
  proliferating 362.29
  punctata albescens 362.76
  renal 585 [363.13]
  syphilitic (secondary) 091.51
    congenital 090.0 [363.13]
    early 091.51
    late 095.8 [363.13]
  syphilitica, central, recurrent 095.8 [363.13]
  tuberculous (*see also* Tuberculous)
    017.3 ✓5ᵗʰ [363.13]
Retinoblastoma (M9510/3) 190.5
  differentiated type (M9511/3) 190.5
  undifferentiated type (M9512/3) 190.5

Retinochoroiditis (*see also* Chorioretinitis)
    363.20
  central angiospastic 362.41
  disseminated 363.10
    metastatic 363.14
    neurosyphilitic 094.83
    pigment epitheliopathy 363.15
    syphilitic 094.83
  due to toxoplasmosis (acquired) (focal) 130.2
  focal 363.00
    in histoplasmosis 115.92
      capsulatum 115.02
      duboisii 115.12
    juxtapapillary (Jensen's) 363.05
    macular 363.06
    paramacular 363.06
    peripheral 363.08
    posterior pole NEC 363.07
  juxtapapillaris 363.05
  syphilitic (disseminated) 094.83
Retinopathy (background) 362.10
  arteriosclerotic 440.8 [362.13]
  atherosclerotic 440.8 [362.13]
  central serous 362.41
  circinate 362.10
  Coat's 362.12
  diabetic 250.5 ✓5ᵗʰ [362.01]
    proliferative 250.5 ✓5ᵗʰ [362.02]
  exudative 362.12
  hypertensive 362.11
  of prematurity 362.21
  pigmentary, congenital 362.74
  proliferative 362.29
    diabetic 250.5 [362.02]
    sickle-cell 282.60 [362.29]
  solar 363.31
Retinoschisis 361.10
  bullous 361.12
  congenital 743.56
  flat 361.11
  juvenile 362.73
Retractile testis 752.52
Retraction
  cervix (*see also* Retroversion, uterus) 621.6
  drum (membrane) 384.82
  eyelid 374.41
  finger 736.29
  head 781.0
  lid 374.41
  lung 518.89
  mediastinum 519.3
  nipple 611.79
    congenital 757.6
    puerperal, postpartum 676.0 ✓5ᵗʰ
  palmar fascia 728.6
  pleura (*see also* Pleurisy) 511.0
  ring, uterus (Bandl's) (pathological) 661.4 ✓5ᵗʰ
    affecting fetus or newborn 763.7
  sternum (congenital) 756.3
    acquired 738.3
    during respiration 786.9
  substernal 738.3
  supraclavicular 738.8
  syndrome (Duane's) 378.71
  uterus (*see also* Retroversion, uterus) 621.6
  valve (heart) — *see* Endocarditis
Retrobulbar — *see* condition
Retrocaval ureter 753.4
Retrocecal — *see also* condition
  appendix (congenital) 751.5
Retrocession — *see* Retroversion
Retrodisplacement — *see* Retroversion
Retroflection, retroflexion — *see* Retroversion
Retrognathia, retrognathism (mandibular)
  (maxillary) 524.06
Retrograde
  ejaculation 608.87
  menstruation 626.8
Retroiliac ureter 753.4
Retroperineal — *see* condition
Retroperitoneal — *see* condition
Retroperitonitis (*see also* Peritonitis) 567.9
Retropharyngeal — *see* condition
Retroplacental — *see* condition

Retroposition — *see* Retroversion
Retrosternal thyroid (congenital) 759.2
Retroversion, retroverted
  cervix (*see also* Retroversion, uterus) 621.6
  female NEC (*see also* Retroversion, uterus)
    621.6
  iris 364.70
  testis (congenital) 752.51
  uterus, uterine (acquired) (acute) (adherent)
    (any degree) (asymptomatic) (cervix)
    (postinfectional) (postpartal, old) 621.6
    congenital 752.3
    in pregnancy or childbirth 654.3 ✓5ᵗʰ
      affecting fetus or newborn 763.89
      causing obstructed labor 660.2 ✓5ᵗʰ
        affecting fetus or newborn 763.1
Retrusion, premaxilla (developmental) 524.04
Rett's syndrome 330.8
Reverse, reversed
  peristalsis 787.4
Reye's syndrome 331.81
Reye-Sheehan syndrome (postpartum pituitary
  necrosis) 253.2
Rh (factor)
  hemolytic disease 773.0
  incompatibility, immunization, or sensitization
    affecting management of pregnancy
      656.1 ✓5ᵗʰ
    fetus or newborn 773.0
    transfusion reaction 999.7
  negative mother, affecting fetus or newborn
    773.0
  titer elevated 999.7
  transfusion reaction 999.7
Rhabdomyolysis (idiopathic) 728.89
Rhabdomyoma (M8900/0) — *see also* Neoplasm,
  connective tissue, benign
  adult (M8904/0) — *see* Neoplasm, connective
    tissue, benign
  fetal (M8903/0) — *see* Neoplasm, connective
    tissue, benign
  glycogenic (M8904/0) — *see* Neoplasm,
    connective tissue, benign
Rhabdomyosarcoma (M8900/3) — *see also*
  Neoplasm, connective tissue, malignant
  alveolar (M8920/3) — *see* Neoplasm,
    connective tissue, malignant
  embryonal (M8910/3) — *see* Neoplasm,
    connective tissue, malignant
  mixed type (M8902/3) — *see* Neoplasm,
    connective tissue, malignant
  pleomorphic (M8901/3) — *see* Neoplasm,
    connective tissue, malignant
Rhabdosarcoma (M8900/3) — *see*
  Rhabdomyosarcoma
Rhesus (factor) (Rh) incompatibility — *see* Rh,
  incompatibility
Rheumaticosis — *see* Rheumatism
Rheumatism, rheumatic (acute NEC) 729.0
  adherent pericardium 393
  arthritis
    acute or subacute — *see* Fever, rheumatic
    chronic 714.0
      spine 720.0
  articular (chronic) NEC (*see also* Arthritis)
    716.9 ✓5ᵗʰ
    acute or subacute — *see* Fever, rheumatic
  back 724.9
  blennorrhagic 098.59
  carditis — *see* Disease, heart, rheumatic
  cerebral — *see* Fever, rheumatic
  chorea (acute) — *see* Chorea, rheumatic
  chronic NEC 729.0
  coronary arteritis 391.9
    chronic 398.99
  degeneration, myocardium (*see also*
    Degeneration, myocardium, with
    rheumatic fever) 398.0
  desert 114.0
  febrile — *see* Fever, rheumatic
  fever — *see* Fever, rheumatic
  gonococcal 098.59
  gout 274.0

Retention — Rheumatism

Rheumatism, rheumatic — *continued*
heart
disease (*see also* Disease, heart, rheumatic) 398.90
failure (chronic) (congestive) (inactive) 398.91
hemopericardium — *see* Rheumatic, pericarditis
hydropericardium — *see* Rheumatic, pericarditis
inflammatory (acute) (chronic) (subacute) — *see* Fever, rheumatic
intercostal 729.0
meaning Tietze's disease 733.6
joint (chronic) NEC (*see also* Arthritis) 716.9 ✓5ᵗʰ
acute — *see* Fever, rheumatic
mediastinopericarditis — *see* Rheumatic, pericarditis
muscular 729.0
myocardial degeneration (*see also* Degeneration, myocardium, with rheumatic fever) 398.0
myocarditis (chronic) (inactive) (with chorea) 398.0
active or acute 391.2
with chorea (acute) (rheumatic) (Sydenham's) 392.0
myositis 729.1
neck 724.9
neuralgic 729.0
neuritis (acute) (chronic) 729.2
neuromuscular 729.0
nodose — *see* Arthritis, nodosa
nonarticular 729.0
palindromic 719.30
ankle 719.37
elbow 719.32
foot 719.37
hand 719.34
hip 719.35
knee 719.36
multiple sites 719.39
pelvic region 719.35
shoulder (region) 719.31
specified site NEC 719.38
wrist 719.33
pancarditis, acute 391.8
with chorea (acute) (rheumatic) (Sydenham's) 392.0
chronic or inactive 398.99
pericarditis (active) (acute) (with effusion) (with pneumonia) 391.0
with chorea (acute) (rheumatic) (Sydenham's) 392.0
chronic or inactive 393
pericardium — *see* Rheumatic, pericarditis
pleuropericarditis — *see* Rheumatic, pericarditis
pneumonia 390 [517.1]
pneumonitis 390 [517.1]
pneumopericarditis — *see* Rheumatic, pericarditis
polyarthritis
acute or subacute — *see* Fever, rheumatic
chronic 714.0
polyarticular NEC (*see also* Arthritis) 716.9 ✓5ᵗʰ
psychogenic 306.0
radiculitis 729.2
sciatic 724.3
septic — *see* Fever, rheumatic
spine 724.9
subacute NEC 729.0
torticollis 723.5
tuberculous NEC (*see also* Tuberculosis) 015.9 ✓5ᵗʰ
typhoid fever 002.0
Rheumatoid — *see also* condition
lungs 714.81
Rhinitis (atrophic) (catarrhal) (chronic) (croupous) (fibrinous) (hyperplastic) (hypertrophic) (membranous) (purulent) (suppurative) (ulcerative) 472.0
with
hay fever (*see also* Fever, hay) 477.9
with asthma (bronchial) 493.0 ✓5ᵗʰ
sore throat — *see* Nasopharyngitis

Rhinitis — *continued*
acute 460
allergic (nonseasonal) (seasonal) (*see also* Fever, hay) 477.9
with asthma (*see also* Asthma) 493.0 ✓5ᵗʰ
due to food 477.1
granulomatous 472.0
infective 460
obstructive 472.0
pneumococcal 460
syphilitic 095.8
congenital 090.0
tuberculous (*see also* Tuberculosis) 012.8 ✓5ᵗʰ
vasomotor (*see also* Fever, hay) 477.9
Rhinoantritis (chronic) 473.0
acute 461.0
Rhinodacryolith 375.57
Rhinolalia (aperta) (clausa) (open) 784.49
Rhinolith 478.1
nasal sinus (*see also* Sinusitis) 473.9
Rhinomegaly 478.1
Rhinopharyngitis (acute) (subacute) (*see also* Nasopharyngitis) 460
chronic 472.2
destructive ulcerating 102.5
mutilans 102.5
Rhinophyma 695.3
Rhinorrhea 478.1
cerebrospinal (fluid) 349.81
paroxysmal (*see also* Fever, hay) 477.9
spasmodic (*see also* Fever, hay) 477.9
Rhinosalpingitis 381.50
acute 381.51
chronic 381.52
Rhinoscleroma 040.1
Rhinosporidiosis 117.0
Rhinovirus infection 079.3
Rhizomelique, pseudopolyarthritic 446.5
Rhoads and Bomford anemia (refractory) 284.9
Rhus
diversiloba dermatitis 692.6
radicans dermatitis 692.6
toxicodendron dermatitis 692.6
venenata dermatitis 692.6
verniciflua dermatitis 692.6
Rhythm
atrioventricular nodal 427.89
disorder 427.9
coronary sinus 427.89
ectopic 427.89
nodal 427.89
escape 427.89
heart, abnormal 427.9
fetus or newborn — *see* Abnormal, heart rate
idioventricular 426.89
accelerated 427.89
nodal 427.89
sleep, inversion 780.55
nonorganic origin 307.45
Rhytidosis facialis 701.8
Rib — *see also* condition
cervical 756.2
Riboflavin deficiency 266.0
Rice bodies (*see also* Loose, body, joint) 718.1 ✓5ᵗʰ
knee 717.6
Richter's hernia — *see* Hernia, Richter's
Ricinism 988.2
Rickets (active) (acute) (adolescent) (adult) (chest wall) (congenital) (current) (infantile) (intestinal) 268.0
celiac 579.0
fetal 756.4
hemorrhagic 267
hypophosphatemic with nephroticglycosuric dwarfism 270.0
kidney 588.0
late effect 268.1
renal 588.0
scurvy 267
vitamin D-resistant 275.3

Rickettsial disease 083.9
specified type NEC 083.8
Rickettsialpox 083.2
Rickettsiosis NEC 083.9
specified type NEC 083.8
tick-borne 082.9
specified type NEC 082.8
vesicular 083.2
Ricord's chancre 091.0
Riddoch's syndrome (visual disorientation) 368.16
Rider's
bone 733.99
chancre 091.0
Ridge, alveolus — *see also* condition
flabby 525.2
Ridged ear 744.29
Riedel's
disease (ligneous thyroiditis) 245.3
lobe, liver 751.69
struma (ligneous thyroiditis) 245.3
thyroiditis (ligneous) 245.3
Rieger's anomaly or syndrome (mesodermal dysgenesis, anterior ocular segment) 743.44
Riehl's melanosis 709.09
Rietti-Greppi-Micheli anemia or syndrome 282.4
Rieux's hernia — *see* Hernia, Rieux's
Rift Valley fever 066.3
Riga's disease (cachectic aphthae) 529.0
Riga-Fede disease (cachectic aphthae) 529.0
Riggs' disease (compound periodontitis) 523.4
Right middle lobe syndrome 518.0
Rigid, rigidity — *see also* condition
abdominal 789.4 ✓5ᵗʰ
articular, multiple congenital 754.89
back 724.8
cervix uteri
in pregnancy or childbirth 654.6 ✓5ᵗʰ
affecting fetus or newborn 763.89
causing obstructed labor 660.2 ✓5ᵗʰ
affecting fetus or newborn 763.1
hymen (acquired) (congenital) 623.3
nuchal 781.6
pelvic floor
in pregnancy or childbirth 654.4 ✓5ᵗʰ
affecting fetus or newborn 763.89
causing obstructed labor 660.2 ✓5ᵗʰ
affecting fetus or newborn 763.1
perineum or vulva
in pregnancy or childbirth 654.8 ✓5ᵗʰ
affecting fetus or newborn 763.89
causing obstructed labor 660.2 ✓5ᵗʰ
affecting fetus or newborn 763.1
spine 724.8
vagina
in pregnancy or childbirth 654.7 ✓5ᵗʰ
affecting fetus or newborn 763.89
causing obstructed labor 660.2 ✓5ᵗʰ
affecting fetus or newborn 763.1
Rigors 780.99 ▲
Riley-Day syndrome (familial dysautonomia) 742.8
Ring(s)
aorta 747.21
Bandl's, complicating delivery 661.4 ✓5ᵗʰ
affecting fetus or newborn 763.7
contraction, complicating delivery 661.4 ✓5ᵗʰ
affecting fetus or newborn 763.7
esophageal (congenital) 750.3
Fleischer (-Kayser) (cornea) 275.1 [371.14]
hymenal, tight (acquired) (congenital) 623.3
Kayser-Fleischer (cornea) 275.1 [371.14]
retraction, uterus, pathological 661.4 ✓5ᵗʰ
affecting fetus or newborn 763.7
Schatzki's (esophagus) (congenital) (lower) 750.3
acquired 530.3
Soemmering's 366.51
trachea, abnormal 748.3
vascular (congenital) 747.21
Vossius' 921.3
late effect 366.21

Rheumatism — Ring(s)

Ringed hair (congenital) 757.4
Ringing in the ear (*see also* Tinnitus) 388.30
Ringworm 110.9
  beard 110.0
  body 110.5
  Burmese 110.9
  corporeal 110.5
  foot 110.4
  groin 110.3
  hand 110.2
  honeycomb 110.0
  nails 110.1
  perianal (area) 110.3
  scalp 110.0
  specified site NEC 110.8
  Tokelau 110.5
Rise, venous pressure 459.89
Risk
  factor — *see* Problem
  suicidal 300.9
Ritter's disease (dermatitis exfoliativa
  neonatorum) 695.81
Rivalry, sibling 313.3
Rivalta's disease (cervicofacial actinomycosis)
  039.3
River blindness 125.3 *[360.13]*
Robert's pelvis 755.69
  with disproportion (fetopelvic) 653.0 ☑5th
    affecting fetus or newborn 763.1
    causing obstructed labor 660.1 ☑5th
      affecting fetus or newborn 763.1
Robin's syndrome 756.0
Robinson's (hidrotic) ectodermal dysplasia
  757.31
Robles' disease (onchocerciasis) 125.3 *[360.13]*
Rochalimea — *see* Rickettsial disease
Rocky Mountain fever (spotted) 082.0
Rodent ulcer (M8090/3) — *see also* Neoplasm,
  skin, malignant
  cornea 370.07
Roentgen ray, adverse effect — *see* Effect,
  adverse, x-ray
Roetheln 056.9
Roger's disease (congenital interventricular septal
  defect) 745.4
Rokitansky's
  disease (*see also* Necrosis, liver) 570
  tumor 620.2
Rokitansky-Aschoff sinuses (mucosal
  outpouching of gallbladder) (*see also*
  Disease, gallbladder) 575.8
Rokitansky-Kuster-Hauser syndrome (congenital
  absence vagina) 752.49
Rollet's chancre (syphilitic) 091.0
Rolling of head 781.0
Romano-Ward syndrome (prolonged Q-T interval)
  794.31
Romanus lesion 720.1
Romberg's disease or syndrome 349.89
Roof, mouth — *see* condition
Rosacea 695.3
  acne 695.3
  keratitis 695.3 *[370.49]*
Rosary, rachitic 268.0
Rose
  cold 477.0
  fever 477.0
  rash 782.1
    epidemic 056.9
    of infants 057.8
Rosen-Castleman-Liebow syndrome (pulmonary
  proteinosis) 516.0
Rosenbach's erysipelatoid or erysipeloid 027.1
Rosenthal's disease (factor XI deficiency) 286.2
Roseola 057.8
  infantum, infantilis 057.8
Rossbach's disease (hyperchlorhydria) 536.8
  psychogenic 306.4
Rössle-Urbach-Wiethe lipoproteinosis 272.8
Ross river fever 066.3

Rostan's asthma (cardiac) (*see also* Failure,
  ventricular, left) 428.1
Rot
  Barcoo (*see also* Ulcer, skin) 707.9
  knife-grinders' (*see also* Tuberculosis)
    011.4 ☑5th
Rot-Bernhardt disease 355.1
Rotation
  anomalous, incomplete or insufficient — *see*
    Malrotation
  cecum (congenital) 751.4
  colon (congenital) 751.4
  manual, affecting fetus or newborn 763.89
  spine, incomplete or insufficient 737.8
  tooth, teeth 524.3
  vertebra, incomplete or insufficient 737.8
Röteln 056.9
Roth's disease or meralgia 355.1
Roth-Bernhardt disease or syndrome 355.1
Rothmund (-Thomson) syndrome 757.33
Rotor's disease or syndrome (idiopathic
  hyperbilirubinemia) 277.4
Rotundum ulcus — *see* Ulcer, stomach
Round
  back (with wedging of vertebrae) 737.10
    late effect of rickets 268.1
  hole, retina 361.31
    with detachment 361.01
  ulcer (stomach) — *see* Ulcer, stomach
  worms (infestation) (large) NEC 127.0
Roussy-Lévy syndrome 334.3
Routine postpartum follow-up V24.2
Roy (-Jutras) syndrome (acropachyderma)
  757.39
Rubella (German measles) 056.9
  complicating pregnancy, childbirth, or
    puerperium 647.5 ☑5th
  complication 056.8
    neurological 056.00
      encephalomyelitis 056.01
      specified type NEC 056.09
    specified type NEC 056.79
  congenital 771.0
  contact V01.4
  exposure to V01.4
  maternal
    with suspected fetal damage affecting
      management of pregnancy 655.3 ☑5th
    affecting fetus or newborn 760.2
      manifest rubella in infant 771.0
  specified complications NEC 056.79
  vaccination, prophylactic (against) V04.3
Rubeola (measles) (*see also* Measles) 055.9
  complicated 055.8
  meaning rubella (*see also* Rubella) 056.9
  scarlatinosis 057.8
Rubeosis iridis 364.42
  diabetica 250.5 ☑5th *[364.42]*
Rubinstein-Taybi's syndrome (brachydactylia,
  short stature, and mental retardation)
  759.89
Rud's syndrome (mental deficiency, epilepsy, and
  infantilism) 759.89
Rudimentary (congenital) — *see also* Agenesis
  arm 755.22
  bone 756.9
  cervix uteri 752.49
  eye (*see also* Microphthalmos) 743.10
  fallopian tube 752.19
  leg 755.32
  lobule of ear 744.21
  patella 755.64
  respiratory organs in thoracopagus 759.4
  tracheal bronchus 748.3
  uterine horn 752.3
  uterus 752.3
    in male 752.7
    solid or with cavity 752.3
  vagina 752.49
Ruiter-Pompen (-Wyers) syndrome
  (angiokeratoma corporis diffusum) 272.7
Ruled out condition (*see also* Observation,
  suspected) V71.9

Rumination — *see also* Vomiting
  neurotic 300.3
  obsessional 300.3
  psychogenic 307.53
Runaway reaction — *see also* Disturbance,
  conduct
  socialized 312.2 ☑5th
  undersocialized, unsocialized 312.1 ☑5th
Runeberg's disease (progressive pernicious
  anemia) 281.0
Runge's syndrome (postmaturity) 766.2
Rupia 091.3
  congenital 090.0
  tertiary 095.9
Rupture, ruptured 553.9
  abdominal viscera NEC 799.8
    obstetrical trauma 665.5 ☑5th
  abscess (spontaneous) — *see* Abscess, by site
  amnion — *see* Rupture, membranes
  aneurysm — *see* Aneurysm
  anus (sphincter) — *see* Laceration, anus
  aorta, aortic 441.5
    abdominal 441.3
    arch 441.1
    ascending 441.1
    descending 441.5
      abdominal 441.3
      thoracic 441.1
    syphilitic 093.0
    thoracoabdominal 441.6
    thorax, thoracic 441.1
    transverse 441.1
    traumatic (thoracic) 901.0
      abdominal 902.0
    valve or cusp (*see also* Endocarditis, aortic)
      424.1
  appendix (with peritonitis) 540.0
    with peritoneal abscess 540.1
    traumatic — *see* Injury, internal,
      gastrointestinal tract
  arteriovenous fistula, brain (congenital) 430
  artery 447.2
    brain (*see also* Hemorrhage, brain) 431
    coronary (*see also* Infarct, myocardium)
      410.9 ☑5th
    heart (*see also* Infarct, myocardium)
      410.9 ☑5th
    pulmonary 417.8
    traumatic (complication) (*see also* Injury,
      blood vessel, by site) 904.9
  bile duct, except cystic (*see also* Disease,
    biliary) 576.3
    cystic 575.4
    traumatic — *see* Injury, internal, intra-
      abdominal
  bladder (sphincter) 596.6
    with
      abortion — *see* Abortion, by type, with
        damage to pelvic organs
      ectopic pregnancy (*see also* categories
        633.0-633.9) 639.2
      molar pregnancy (*see also* categories 630-
        632) 639.2
    following
      abortion 639.2
      ectopic or molar pregnancy 639.2
    nontraumatic 596.6
    obstetrical trauma 665.5 ☑5th
    spontaneous 596.6
    traumatic — *see* Injury, internal, bladder
  blood vessel (*see also* Hemorrhage) 459.0
    brain (*see also* Hemorrhage, brain) 431
    heart (*see also* Infarct, myocardium)
      410.9 ☑5th
    traumatic (complication) (*see also* Injury,
      blood vessel, by site) 904.9
  bone — *see* Fracture, by site
  bowel 569.89
    traumatic — *see* Injury, internal, intestine
  Bowman's membrane 371.31
  brain
    aneurysm (congenital) (*see also* Hemorrhage,
      subarachnoid) 430
    late effect — *see* Late effect(s) (of)
      cerebrovascular disease
    syphilitic 094.87

☑4th Fourth-digit Required   ☑5th Fifth-digit Required   ◄► Revised Text   ● New Line   ▲ Revised Code

Rupture, ruptured — *continued*
brain — *continued*
　hemorrhagic (*see also* Hemorrhage, brain) 431
　injury at birth 767.0
　syphilitic 094.89
capillaries 448.9
cardiac (*see also* Infarct, myocardium) 410.9 ✓5ᵗʰ
cartilage (articular) (current) — *see also* Sprain, by site
　knee — *see* Tear, meniscus
　semilunar — *see* Tear, meniscus
cecum (with peritonitis) 540.0
　with peritoneal abscess 540.1
　traumatic 863.89
　　with open wound into cavity 863.99
cerebral aneurysm (congenital) (*see also* Hemorrhage, subarachnoid) 430
　late effect — *see* Late effect(s) (of) cerebrovascular disease
cervix (uteri)
　with
　　abortion — *see* Abortion, by type, with damage to pelvic organs
　　ectopic pregnancy (*see also* categories 633.0-633.9) 639.2
　　molar pregnancy (*see also* categories 630-632) 639.2
　following
　　abortion 639.2
　　ectopic or molar pregnancy 639.2
　obstetrical trauma 665.3 ✓5ᵗʰ
　traumatic — *see* Injury, internal, cervix
chordae tendineae 429.5
choroid (direct) (indirect) (traumatic) 363.63
circle of Willis (*see also* Hemorrhage, subarachnoid) 430
　late effect — *see* Late effect(s) (of) cerebrovascular disease
colon 569.89
　traumatic — *see* Injury, internal, colon
cornea (traumatic) — *see also* Rupture, eye
　due to ulcer 370.00
coronary (artery) (thrombotic) (*see also* Infarct, myocardium) 410.9 ✓5ᵗʰ
corpus luteum (infected) (ovary) 620.1
cyst — *see* Cyst
cystic duct (*see also* Disease, gallbladder) 575.4
Descemet's membrane 371.33
　traumatic — *see* Rupture, eye
diaphragm — *see also* Hernia, diaphragm
　traumatic — *see* Injury, internal, diaphragm
diverticulum
　bladder 596.3
　intestine (large) (*see also* Diverticula) 562.10
　　small 562.00
duodenal stump 537.89
duodenum (ulcer) — *see* Ulcer, duodenum, with perforation
ear drum (*see also* Perforation, tympanum) 384.20
　with otitis media — *see* Otitis media
　traumatic — *see* Wound, open, ear
esophagus 530.4
　traumatic 862.22
　　with open wound into cavity 862.32
　　cervical region — *see* Wound, open, esophagus
eye (without prolapse of intraocular tissue) 871.0
　with
　　exposure of intraocular tissue 871.1
　　partial loss of intraocular tissue 871.2
　　prolapse of intraocular tissue 871.1
　due to burn 940.5
fallopian tube 620.8
　due to pregnancy — *see* Pregnancy, tubal
　traumatic — *see* Injury, internal, fallopian tube
fontanel 767.3
free wall (ventricle) (*see also* Infarct, myocardium) 410.9 ✓5ᵗʰ
gallbladder or duct (*see also* Disease, gallbladder) 575.4
　traumatic — *see* Injury, internal, gallbladder

Rupture, ruptured — *continued*
gastric (*see also* Rupture, stomach) 537.89
　vessel 459.0
globe (eye) (traumatic) — *see* Rupture, eye
graafian follicle (hematoma) 620.0
heart (auricle) (ventricle) (*see also* Infarct, myocardium) 410.9 ✓5ᵗʰ
　infectional 422.90
　traumatic — *see* Rupture, myocardium, traumatic
hymen 623.8
internal
　organ, traumatic — *see also* Injury, internal, by site
　　heart — *see* Rupture, myocardium, traumatic
　　kidney — *see* Rupture, kidney
　　liver — *see* Rupture, liver
　　spleen — *see* Rupture, spleen, traumatic
　　semilunar cartilage — *see* Tear, meniscus
intervertebral disc — *see* Displacement, intervertebral disc
　traumatic (current) — *see* Dislocation, vertebra
intestine 569.89
　traumatic — *see* Injury, internal, intestine
intracranial, birth injury 767.0
iris 364.76
　traumatic — *see* Rupture, eye
joint capsule — *see* Sprain, by site
kidney (traumatic) 866.03
　with open wound into cavity 866.13
　due to birth injury 767.8
　nontraumatic 593.89
lacrimal apparatus (traumatic) 870.2
lens (traumatic) 366.20
ligament — *see also* Sprain, by site
　with open wound — *see* Wound, open, by site
　old (*see also* Disorder, cartilage, articular) 718.0 ✓5ᵗʰ
liver (traumatic) 864.04
　with open wound into cavity 864.14
　due to birth injury 767.8
　nontraumatic 573.8
lymphatic (node) (vessel) 457.8
marginal sinus (placental) (with hemorrhage) 641.2 ✓5ᵗʰ
　affecting fetus or newborn 762.1
meaning hernia — *see* Hernia
membrana tympani (*see also* Perforation, tympanum) 384.20
　with otitis media — *see* Otitis media
　traumatic — *see* Wound, open, ear
membranes (spontaneous)
　artificial
　　delayed delivery following 658.3 ✓5ᵗʰ
　　　affecting fetus or newborn 761.1
　　　fetus or newborn 761.1
　delayed delivery following 658.2 ✓5ᵗʰ
　　affecting fetus or newborn 761.1
　premature (less than 24 hours prior to onset of labor) 658.1 ✓5ᵗʰ
　　affecting fetus or newborn 761.1
　delayed delivery following 658.2 ✓5ᵗʰ
　　affecting fetus or newborn 761.1
meningeal artery (*see also* Hemorrhage, subarachnoid) 430
　late effect — *see* Late effect(s) (of) cerebrovascular diseas
meniscus (knee) — *see* Tear, meniscus
　old (*see also* Derangement, meniscus) 717.5
　　site other than knee — *see* Disorder, cartilage, articular
　site other than knee — *see* Sprain, by site
mesentery 568.89
　traumatic — *see* Injury, internal, mesentery
mitral — *see* Insufficiency, mitral
muscle (traumatic) NEC — *see also* Sprain, by site
　with open wound — *see* Wound, open, by site
　nontraumatic 728.83
musculotendinous cuff (nontraumatic) (shoulder) 840.4

Rupture, ruptured — *continued*
mycotic aneurysm, causing cerebral hemorrhage (*see also* Hemorrhage, subarachnoid) 430
　late effect — *see* Late effect(s) (of) cerebrovascular disease
myocardium, myocardial (*see also* Infarct, myocardium) 410.9 ✓5ᵗʰ
　traumatic 861.03
　　with open wound into thorax 861.13
nontraumatic (meaning hernia) (*see also* Hernia, by site) 553.9
obstructed (*see also* Hernia, by site, with obstruction) 552.9
　gangrenous (*see also* Hernia, by site, with gangrene) 551.9
operation wound 998.32　　　　▲
　internal 998.31　　　　　　　●
ovary, ovarian 620.8
　corpus luteum 620.1
　follicle (graafian) 620.0
oviduct 620.8
　due to pregnancy — *see* Pregnancy, tubal
pancreas 577.8
　traumatic — *see* Injury, internal, pancreas
papillary muscle (ventricular) 429.6
pelvic
　floor, complicating delivery 664.1 ✓5ᵗʰ
　organ NEC — *see* Injury, pelvic, organs
penis (traumatic) — *see* Wound, open, penis
perineum 624.8
　during delivery (*see also* Laceration, perineum, complicating delivery) 664.4 ✓5ᵗʰ
pharynx (nontraumatic) (spontaneous) 478.29
pregnant uterus (before onset of labor) 665.0 ✓5ᵗʰ
prostate (traumatic) — *see* Injury, internal, prostate
pulmonary
　artery 417.8
　valve (heart) (*see also* Endocarditis, pulmonary) 424.3
　vein 417.8
　vessel 417.8
pupil, sphincter 364.75
pus tube (*see also* Salpingo-oophoritis) 614.2
pyosalpinx (*see also* Salpingo-oophoritis) 614.2
rectum 569.49
　traumatic — *see* Injury, internal, rectum
retina, retinal (traumatic) (without detachment) 361.30
　with detachment (*see also* Detachment, retina, with retinal defect) 361.00
rotator cuff (capsule) (traumatic) 840.4
　nontraumatic, complete 727.61
sclera 871.0
semilunar cartilage, knee (*see also* Tear, meniscus) 836.2
　old (*see also* Derangement, meniscus) 717.5
septum (cardiac) 410.8 ✓5ᵗʰ
sigmoid 569.89
　traumatic — *see* Injury, internal, colon, sigmoid
sinus of Valsalva 747.29
spinal cord — *see also* Injury, spinal, by site
　due to injury at birth 767.4
　fetus or newborn 767.4
　syphilitic 094.89
　traumatic — *see also* Injury, spinal, by site
　　with fracture — *see* Fracture, vertebra, by site, with spinal cord injury
spleen 289.59
　congenital 767.8
　due to injury at birth 767.8
　malarial 084.9
　nontraumatic 289.59
　spontaneous 289.59
　traumatic 865.04
　　with open wound into cavity 865.14
splenic vein 459.0
stomach 537.89
　due to injury at birth 767.8
　traumatic — *see* Injury, internal, stomach
　ulcer — *see* Ulcer, stomach, with perforation
synovium 727.50
　specified site NEC 727.59

✓4ᵗʰ Fourth-digit Required　　✓5ᵗʰ Fifth-digit Required　　▶◀ Revised Text　　● New Line　　▲ Revised Code

Rupture — Rupture

Rupture, ruptured — *continued*
  tendon (traumatic) — *see also* Sprain, by site
    with open wound — *see* Wound, open, by
      site
    Achilles 845.09
      nontraumatic 727.67
    ankle 845.09
      nontraumatic 727.68
    biceps (long bead) 840.8
      nontraumatic 727.62
    foot 845.10
      interphalangeal (joint) 845.13
      metatarsophalangeal (joint) 845.12
      nontraumatic 727.68
      specified site NEC 845.19
      tarsometatarsal (joint) 845.11
    hand 842.10
      carpometacarpal (joint) 842.11
      interphalangeal (joint) 842.13
      metacarpophalangeal (joint) 842.12
      nontraumatic 727.63
        extensors 727.63
        flexors 727.64
      specified site NEC 842.19
    nontraumatic 727.60
      specified site NEC 727.69
    patellar 844.8
      nontraumatic 727.66
    quadriceps 844.8
      nontraumatic 727.65
    rotator cuff (capsule) 840.4
      nontraumatic, complete 727.61
    wrist 842.00
      carpal (joint) 842.01
      nontraumatic 727.63
        extensors 727.63
        flexors 727.64
      radiocarpal (joint) (ligament) 842.02
      radioulnar (joint), distal 842.09
      specified site NEC 842.09
  testis (traumatic) 878.2
    complicated 878.3
    due to syphilis 095.8
  thoracic duct 457.8
  tonsil 474.8
  traumatic
    with open wound — *see* Wound, open, by
      site
    aorta — *see* Rupture, aorta, traumatic
    ear drum — *see* Wound, open, ear, drum
    external site — *see* Wound, open, by site
    eye 871.2
    globe (eye) — *see* Wound, open, eyeball
    internal organ (abdomen, chest, or pelvis) —
      see also Injury, internal, by site
      heart — *see* Rupture, myocardium,
        traumatic
      kidney — *see* Rupture, kidney
      liver — *see* Rupture, liver
      spleen — *see* Rupture, spleen, traumatic
    ligament, muscle, or tendon — *see also*
      Sprain, by site
      with open wound — *see* Wound, open, by
        site
    meaning hernia — *see* Hernia
  tricuspid (heart) (valve) — *see* Endocarditis,
    tricuspid
  tube, tubal 620.8
    abscess (*see also* Salpingo-oophoritis) 614.2
    due to pregnancy — *see* Pregnancy, tubal
  tympanum, tympanic (membrane) (*see also*
    Perforation, tympanum) 384.20
    with otitis media — *see* Otitis media
    traumatic — *see* Wound, open, ear, drum
  umbilical cord 663.8 ✓5ᵗʰ
    fetus or newborn 772.0
  ureter (traumatic) (*see also* Injury, internal,
    ureter) 867.2
    nontraumatic 593.89
  urethra 599.84
    with
      abortion — *see* Abortion, by type, with
        damage to pelvic organs
      ectopic pregnancy (*see also* categories
        633.0-633.9) 639.2
      molar pregnancy (*see also* categories 630-
        632) 639.2

Rupture, ruptured — *continued*
  urethra — *continued*
    following
      abortion 639.2
      ectopic or molar pregnancy 639.2
    obstetrical trauma 665.5 ✓5ᵗʰ
    traumatic — *see* Injury, internal urethra
  uterosacral ligament 620.8
  uterus (traumatic) — *see also* Injury, internal
    uterus
    affecting fetus or newborn 763.89
    during labor 665.1 ✓5ᵗʰ
    nonpuerperal, nontraumatic 621.8
    nontraumatic 621.8
    pregnant (during labor) 665.1 ✓5ᵗʰ
      before labor 665.0 ✓5ᵗʰ
  vagina 878.6
    complicated 878.7
    complicating delivery — *see* Laceration,
      vagina, complicating delivery
  valve, valvular (heart) — *see* Endocarditis
  varicose vein — *see* Varicose, vein
  varix — *see* Varix
  vena cava 459.0
  ventricle (free wall) (left) (*see also* Infarct,
    myocardium) 410.9 ✓5ᵗʰ
  vesical (urinary) 596.6
    traumatic — *see* Injury, internal, bladder
  vessel (blood) 459.0
    pulmonary 417.8
  viscus 799.8
  vulva 878.4
    complicated 878.5
    complicating delivery 664.0 ✓5ᵗʰ
Russell's dwarf (uterine dwarfism and
  craniofacial dysostosis) 759.89
Russell's dysentery 004.8
Russell (-Silver) syndrome (congenital
  hemihypertrophy and short stature) 759.89
Russian spring-summer type encephalitis 063.0
Rust's disease (tuberculous spondylitis)
  015.0 ✓5ᵗʰ *[720.81]*
Rustitskii's disease (multiple myeloma)
  (M9730/3) 203.0 ✓5ᵗʰ
Ruysch's disease (Hirschsprung's disease) 751.3
Rytand-Lipsitch syndrome (complete
  atrioventricular bloc) 426.0

S

Saber
  shin 090.5
  tibia 090.5
Sac, lacrimal — *see* condition
Saccharomyces infection (*see also* Candidiasis)
  112.9
Saccharopinuria 270.7
Saccular — *see* condition
Sacculation
  aorta (nonsyphilitic) (*see also* Aneurysm, aorta)
    441.9
    ruptured 441.5
    syphilitic 093.0
  bladder 596.3
  colon 569.89
  intralaryngeal (congenital) (ventricular) 748.3
  larynx (congenital) (ventricular) 748.3
  organ or site, congenital — *see* Distortion
  pregnant uterus, complicating delivery
    654.4 ☑5ᵗʰ
      affecting fetus or newborn 763.1
      causing obstructed labor 660.2 ☑5ᵗʰ
        affecting fetus or newborn 763.1
  rectosigmoid 569.89
  sigmoid 569.89
  ureter 593.89
  urethra 599.2
  vesical 596.3
Sachs (-Tay) disease (amaurotic familial idiocy)
  330.1
Sacks-Libman disease 710.0 [424.91]
Sacralgia 724.6
Sacralization
  fifth lumbar vertebra 756.15
  incomplete (vertebra) 756.15
Sacrodynia 724.6
Sacroiliac joint — *see* condition
Sacroiliitis NEC 720.2
Sacrum — *see* condition
Saddle
  back 737.8
  embolus, aorta 444.0
  nose 738.0
    congenital 754.0
    due to syphilis 090.5
Sadism (sexual) 302.84
Saemisch's ulcer 370.04
Saenger's syndrome 379.46
Sago spleen 277.3
Sailors' skin 692.74
Saint
  Anthony's fire (*see also* Erysipelas) 035
  Guy's dance — *see* Chorea
  Louis-type encephalitis 062.3
  triad (*see also* Hernia, diaphragm) 553.3
  Vitus' dance — *see* Chorea
Salicylism
  correct substance properly administered
    535.4 ☑5ᵗʰ
  overdose or wrong substance given or taken
    965.1
Salivary duct or gland — *see also* condition
  virus disease 078.5
Salivation (excessive) (*see also* Ptyalism) 527.7
Salmonella (aertrycke) (choleraesuis) (enteritidis)
    (gallinarum) (suipestifer) (typhimurium) (*see
    also* Infection, Salmonella) 003.9
  arthritis 003.23
  carrier (suspected) of V02.3
  meningitis 003.21
  osteomyelitis 003.24
  pneumonia 003.22
  septicemia 003.1
  typhosa 002.0
    carrier (suspected) of V02.1
Salmonellosis 003.0
  with pneumonia 003.22

Salpingitis (catarrhal) (fallopian tube) (nodular)
    (pseudofollicular) (purulent) (septic) (*see also*
    Salpingo-oophoritis) 614.2
  ear 381.50
    acute 381.51
    chronic 381.52
Salpingitis
  Eustachian (tube) 381.50
    acute 381.51
    chronic 381.52
  follicularis 614.1
  gonococcal (chronic) 098.37
    acute 098.17
  interstitial, chronic 614.1
  isthmica nodosa 614.1
  old — *see* Salpingo-oophoritis, chronic
  puerperal, postpartum, childbirth 670 ☑5ᵗʰ
  specific (chronic) 098.37
    acute 098.17
  tuberculous (acute) (chronic) (*see also*
    Tuberculosis) 016.6 ☑5ᵗʰ
  venereal (chronic) 098.37
    acute 098.17
Salpingocele 620.4
Salpingo-oophoritis (catarrhal) (purulent)
    (ruptured) (septic) (suppurative) 614.2
  acute 614.0
    with
      abortion — *see* Abortion, by type, with
        sepsis
      ectopic pregnancy (*see also* categories
        633-633.9) 639.0
      molar pregnancy (*see also* categories 630-
        632) 639.0
    following
      abortion 639.0
      ectopic or molar pregnancy 639.0
    gonococcal 098.17
    puerperal, postpartum, childbirth 670 ☑4ᵗʰ
    tuberculous (*see also* Tuberculosis)
      016.6 ☑5ᵗʰ
  chronic 614.1
    gonococcal 098.37
    tuberculous (*see also* Tuberculosis)
      016.6 ☑5ᵗʰ
  complicating pregnancy 646.6 ☑5ᵗʰ
    affecting fetus or newborn 760.8
  gonococcal (chronic) 098.37
    acute 098.17
  old — *see* Salpingo-oophoritis, chronic
  puerperal 670 ☑4ᵗʰ
  specific — *see* Salpingo-oophoritis, gonococcal
  subacute (*see also* Salpingo-oophoritis, acute)
    614.0
  tuberculous (acute) (chronic) (*see also*
    Tuberculosis) 016.6 ☑5ᵗʰ
  venereal — *see* Salpingo-oophoritis, gonococcal
Salpingo-ovaritis (*see also* Salpingooophoritis)
  614.2
Salpingoperitonitis (*see also* Salpingo-oophoritis)
  614.2
Salt-losing
  nephritis (*see also* Disease, renal) 593.9
  syndrome (*see also* Disease, renal) 593.9
Salt-rheum (*see also* Eczema) 692.9
Salzmann's nodular dystrophy 371.46
Sampson's cyst or tumor 617.1
Sandblasters'
  asthma 502
  lung 502
Sander's disease (paranoia) 297.1
Sandfly fever 066.0
Sandhoff's disease 330.1
Sanfilippo's syndrome (mucopolysaccharidosis
  III) 277.5
Sanger-Brown's ataxia 334.2
San Joaquin Valley fever 114.0
Sao Paulo fever or typhus 082.0
Saponification, mesenteric 567.8
Sapremia — *see* Septicemia
Sarcocele (benign)
  syphilitic 095.8
    congenital 090.5

Sarcoepiplocele (*see also* Hernia) 553.9
Sarcoepiplomphalocele (*see also* Hernia,
  umbilicus) 553.1
Sarcoid (any site) 135
  with lung involvement 135 [517.8]
  Boeck's 135
  Darier-Roussy 135
  Spiegler-Fendt 686.8
Sarcoidosis 135
  cardiac 135 [425.8]
  lung 135 [517.8]
Sarcoma (M8800/3) — *see also* Neoplasm,
    connective tissue, malignant
  alveolar soft part (M9581/3) — *see* Neoplasm,
    connective tissue, malignant
  ameloblastic (M9330/3) 170.1
    upper jaw (bone) 170.0
  botryoid (M8910/3) — *see* Neoplasm,
    connective tissue, malignant
  botryoides (M8910/3) — *see* Neoplasm,
    connective tissue, malignant
  cerebellar (M9480/3) 191.6
    circumscribed (arachnoidal) (M9471/3)
      191.6
  circumscribed (arachnoidal) cerebellar
    (M9471/3) 191.6
  clear cell, of tendons and aponeuroses
    (M9044/3) — *see* Neoplasm, connective
    tissue, malignant
  embryonal (M8991/3) — *see* Neoplasm,
    connective tissue, malignant
  endometrial (stromal) (M8930/3) 182.0
    isthmus 182.1
  endothelial (M9130/3) — *see also* Neoplasm,
    connective tissue, malignant
    bone (M9260/3) — *see* Neoplasm, bone,
      malignant
  epithelioid cell (M8804/3) — *see* Neoplasm,
    connective tissue, malignant
  Ewing's (M9260/3) — *see* Neoplasm, bone,
    malignant
  germinoblastic (diffuse) (M9632/3) 202.8 ☑5ᵗʰ
    follicular (M9697/3) 202.0 ☑5ᵗʰ
  giant cell (M8802/3) — *see also* Neoplasm,
    connective tissue, malignant
    bone (M9250/3) — *see* Neoplasm, bone,
      malignant
  glomoid (M8710/3) — *see* Neoplasm,
    connective tissue, malignant
  granulocytic (M9930/3) 205.3 ☑5ᵗʰ
  hemangioendothelial (M9130/3) — *see*
    Neoplasm, connective tissue, malignant
  hemorrhagic, multiple (M9140/3) — *see*
    Kaposi's, sarcoma
  Hodgkin's (M9662/3) 201.2 ☑5ᵗʰ
  immunoblastic (M9612/3) 200.8 ☑5ᵗʰ
  Kaposi's (M9140/3) — *see* Kaposi's, sarcoma
  Kupffer cell (M9124/3) 155.0
  leptomeningeal (M9530/3) — *see* Neoplasm,
    meninges, malignant
  lymphangioendothelial (M9170/3) — *see*
    Neoplasm, connective tissue, malignant
  lymphoblastic (M9630/3) 200.1 ☑5ᵗʰ
  lymphocytic (M9620/3) 200.1 ☑5ᵗʰ
  mast cell (M9740/3) 202.6 ☑5ᵗʰ
  melanotic (M8720/3) — *see* Melanoma
  meningeal (M9530/3) — *see* Neoplasm,
    meninges, malignant
  meningothelial (M9530/3) — *see* Neoplasm,
    meninges, malignant
  mesenchymal (M8800/3) — *see also* Neoplasm,
    connective tissue, malignant
    mixed (M8990/3) — *see* Neoplasm,
      connective tissue, malignant
  mesothelial (M9050/3) — *see* Neoplasm, by
    site, malignant
  monstrocellular (M9481/3)
    specified site — *see* Neoplasm, by site,
      malignant
    unspecified site 191.9
  myeloid (M9930/3) 205.3 ☑5ᵗʰ
  neurogenic (M9540/3) — *see* Neoplasm,
    connective tissue, malignant
  odontogenic (M9270/3) 170.1
    upper jaw (bone) 170.0
  osteoblastic (M9180/3) — *see* Neoplasm, bone,
    malignant

Sarcoma — *see also* Neoplasm, connective tissue, malignant — *continued*
  osteogenic (M9180/3) — *see also* Neoplasm, bone, malignant
    juxtacortical (M9190/3) — *see* Neoplasm, bone, malignant
    periosteal (M9190/3) — *see* Neoplasm, bone, malignant
    periosteal (M8812/3) — *see also* Neoplasm, bone, malignant
    osteogenic (M9190/3) — *see also* Neoplasm, bone, malignant
  plasma cell (M9731/3) 203.8 ✓5ᵗʰ
  pleomorphic cell (M8802/3) — *see* Neoplasm, connective tissue, malignant
  reticuloendothelial (M9720/3) 202.3 ✓5ᵗʰ
  reticulum cell (M9640/3) 200.0 ✓5ᵗʰ
    nodular (M9642/3) 200.0 ✓5ᵗʰ
    pleomorphic cell type (M9641/3) 200.0 ✓5ᵗʰ
  round cell (M8803/3) — *see* Neoplasm, connective tissue, malignant
  small cell (M8803/3) — *see* Neoplasm, connective tissue, malignant
  spindle cell (M8801/3) — *see* Neoplasm, connective tissue, malignant
  stromal (endometrial) (M8930/3) 182.0
    isthmus 182.1
  synovial (M9040/3) — *see also* Neoplasm, connective tissue, malignant
    biphasic type (M9043/3) — *see* Neoplasm, connective tissue, malignant
    epithelioid cell type (M9042/3) — *see* Neoplasm, connective tissue, malignant
    spindle cell type (M9041/3) — *see* Neoplasm, connective tissue, malignant

Sarcomatosis
  meningeal (M9539/3) — *see* Neoplasm, meninges, malignant
  specified site NEC (M8800/3) — *see* Neoplasm, connective tissue, malignant
  unspecified site (M8800/6) 171.9

Sarcosinemia 270.8
Sarcosporidiosis 136.5
Saturnine — *see* condition
Saturnism 984.9
  specified type of lead — *see* Table of Drugs and Chemicals
Satyriasis 302.89
Sauriasis — *see* Ichthyosis
Sauriderma 757.39
Sauriosis — *see* Ichthyosis
Savill's disease (epidemic exfoliative dermatitis) 695.89
SBE (subacute bacterial endocarditis) 421.0
Scabies (any site) 133.0
Scabs 782.8
Scaglietti-Dagnini syndrome (acromegalic macrospondylitis) 253.0
Scald, scalded — *see also* Burn, by site
  skin syndrome 695.1
Scalenus anticus (anterior) syndrome 353.0
Scales 782.8
Scalp — *see* condition
Scaphocephaly 756.0
Scaphoiditis, tarsal 732.5
Scapulalgia 733.90
Scapulohumeral myopathy 359.1
Scar, scarring (*see also* Cicatrix) 709.2
  adherent 709.2
  atrophic 709.2
  cervix
    in pregnancy or childbirth 654.6 ✓5ᵗʰ
      affecting fetus or newborn 763.89
      causing obstructed labor 660.2 ✓5ᵗʰ
        affecting fetus or newborn 763.1
  cheloid 701.4
  chorioretinal 363.30
    disseminated 363.35
    macular 363.32
    peripheral 363.34

Scar, scarring (*see also* Cicatrix) — *continued*
  chorioretinal — *continued*
    posterior pole NEC 363.33
  choroid (*see also* Scar, chorioretinal) 363.30
  compression, pericardial 423.9
  congenital 757.39
  conjunctiva 372.64
  cornea 371.00
    xerophthalmic 264.6
  due to previous cesarean delivery, complicating pregnancy or childbirth 654.2 ✓5ᵗʰ
    affecting fetus or newborn 763.89
  duodenal (bulb) (cap) 537.3
  hypertrophic 701.4
  keloid 701.4
  labia 624.4
  lung (base) 518.89
  macula 363.32
    disseminated 363.35
    peripheral 363.34
  muscle 728.89
  myocardium, myocardial 412
  painful 709.2
  papillary muscle 429.81
  posterior pole NEC 363.33
    macular — *see* Scar, macula
  postnecrotic (hepatic) (liver) 571.9
  psychic V15.49
  retina (*see also* Scar, chorioretinal) 363.30
  trachea 478.9
  uterus 621.8
    in pregnancy or childbirth NEC 654.9 ✓5ᵗʰ
      affecting fetus or newborn 763.89
      due to previous cesarean delivery 654.2 ✓5ᵗʰ
  vulva 624.4
Scarabiasis 134.1
Scarlatina 034.1
  anginosa 034.1
  maligna 034.1
  myocarditis, acute 034.1 [422.0]
    old (*see also* Myocarditis) 429.0
  otitis media 034.1 [382.02]
  ulcerosa 034.1
Scarlatinella 057.8
Scarlet fever (albuminuria) (angina) (convulsions) (lesions of lid) (rash) 034.1
Schamberg's disease, dermatitis, or dermatosis (progressive pigmentary dermatosis) 709.09
Schatzki's ring (esophagus) (lower) (congenital) 750.3
  acquired 530.3
Schaufenster krankheit 413.9
Schaumann's
  benign lymphogranulomatosis 135
  disease (sarcoidosis) 135
  syndrome (sarcoidosis) 135
Scheie's syndrome (mucopolysaccharidosis IS) 277.5
Schenck's disease (sporotrichosis) 117.1
Scheuermann's disease or osteochondrosis 732.0
Scheuthauer-Marie-Sainton syndrome (cleidocranialis dysostosis) 755.59
Schilder (-Flatau) disease 341.1
Schilling-type monocytic leukemia (M9890/3) 206.9 ✓5ᵗʰ
Schimmelbusch's disease, cystic mastitis, or hyperplasia 610.1
Schirmer's syndrome (encephalocutaneous angiomatosis) 759.6
Schistocelia 756.79
Schistoglossia 750.13
Schistosoma infestation — *see* Infestation, Schistosoma
Schistosomiasis 120.9
  Asiatic 120.2
  bladder 120.0
  chestermani 120.8
  colon 120.1
  cutaneous 120.3
  due to
    S. hematobium 120.0
    S. japonicum 120.2

Schistosomiasis — *continued*
  due to — *continued*
    S. mansoni 120.1
    S. mattheii 120.8
  eastern 120.2
  genitourinary tract 120.0
  intestinal 120.1
  lung 120.2
  Manson's (intestinal) 120.1
  Oriental 120.2
  pulmonary 120.2
  specified type NEC 120.8
  vesical 120.0
Schizencephaly 742.4
Schizo-affective psychosis (*see also* Schizophrenia) 295.7 ✓5ᵗʰ
Schizodontia 520.2
Schizoid personality 301.20
  introverted 301.21
  schizotypal 301.22
Schizophrenia, schizophrenic (reaction) 295.9 ✓5ᵗʰ

> *Note — Use the following fifth-digit subclassification with category 295:*
>
> | | |
> |---|---|
> | 0 | *unspecified* |
> | 1 | *subchronic* |
> | 2 | *chronic* |
> | 3 | *subchronic with acute exacerbation* |
> | 4 | *chronic with acute exacerbation* |
> | 5 | *in remission* |

  acute (attack) NEC 295.8 ✓5ᵗʰ
    episode 295.4 ✓5ᵗʰ
  atypical form 295.8 ✓5ᵗʰ
  borderline 295.5 ✓5ᵗʰ
  catalepsy 295.2 ✓5ᵗʰ
  catatonic (type) (acute) (excited) (withdrawn) 295.2 ✓5ᵗʰ
  childhood (type) (*see also* Psychosis, childhood) 299.9 ✓5ᵗʰ
  chronic NEC 295.6 ✓5ᵗʰ
  coenesthesiopathic 295.8 ✓5ᵗʰ
  cyclic (type) 295.7 ✓5ᵗʰ
  disorganized (type) 295.1 ✓5ᵗʰ
  flexibilitas cerea 295.2 ✓5ᵗʰ
  hebephrenic (type) (acute) 295.1 ✓5ᵗʰ
  incipient 295.5 ✓5ᵗʰ
  latent 295.5 ✓5ᵗʰ
  paranoid (type) (acute) 295.3 ✓5ᵗʰ
  paraphrenic (acute) 295.3 ✓5ᵗʰ
  prepsychotic 295.5 ✓5ᵗʰ
  primary (acute) 295.0 ✓5ᵗʰ
  prodromal 295.5 ✓5ᵗʰ
  pseudoneurotic 295.5 ✓5ᵗʰ
  pseudopsychopathic 295.5 ✓5ᵗʰ
  reaction 295.9 ✓5ᵗʰ
  residual (state) (type) 295.6 ✓5ᵗʰ
  restzustand 295.6 ✓5ᵗʰ
  schizo-affective (type) (depressed) (excited) 295.7 ✓5ᵗʰ
  schizophreniform type 295.4 ✓5ᵗʰ
  simple (type) (acute) 295.0 ✓5ᵗʰ
  simplex (acute) 295.0 ✓5ᵗʰ
  specified type NEC 295.8 ✓5ᵗʰ
  syndrome of childhood NEC (*see also* Psychosis, childhood) 299.9 ✓5ᵗʰ
  undifferentiated 295.9 ✓5ᵗʰ
    acute 295.8 ✓5ᵗʰ
    chronic 295.6 ✓5ᵗʰ
Schizothymia 301.20
  introverted 301.21
  schizotypal 301.22
Schlafkrankheit 086.5
Schlatter's tibia (osteochondrosis) 732.4
Schlatter-Osgood disease (osteochondrosis, tibial tubercle) 732.4
Schloffer's tumor (*see also* Peritonitis) 567.2
Schmidt's syndrome
  sphallo-pharyngo-laryngeal hemiplegia 352.6
  thyroid-adrenocortical insufficiency 258.1
  vagoaccessory 352.6

Schmincke
  carcinoma (M8082/3) — *see* Neoplasm,
    nasopharynx, malignant
  tumor (M8082/3) — *see* Neoplasm,
    nasopharynx, malignant
Schmitz (-Stutzer) dysentery 004.0
Schmorl's disease or nodes 722.30
  lumbar, lumbosacral 722.32
  specified region NEC 722.39
  thoracic, thoracolumbar 722.31
Schneider's syndrome 047.9
Schneiderian
  carcinoma (M8121/3)
    specified site — *see* Neoplasm, by site,
      malignant
    unspecified site 160.0
  papilloma (M8121/0)
    specified site — *see* Neoplasm, by site,
      benign
    unspecified site 212.0
Schoffer's tumor (*see also* Peritonitis) 567.2
Scholte's syndrome (malignant carcinoid) 259.2
Scholz's disease 330.0
Scholz (-Bielschowsky-Henneberg) syndrome
  330.0
Schönlein (-Henoch) disease (primary) (purpura)
  (rheumatic) 287.0
School examination V70.3
Schottmüller's disease (*see also* Fever,
  paratyphoid) 002.9
Schroeder's syndrome (endocrine-hypertensive)
  255.3
Schüller-Christian disease or syndrome (chronic
  histiocytosis X) 277.8
Schultz's disease or syndrome (agranulocytosis)
  288.0
Schultze's acroparesthesia, simple 443.89
Schwalbe-Ziehen-Oppenheimer disease 333.6
Schwannoma (M9560/0) — *see also* Neoplasm,
  connective tissue, benign
  malignant (M9560/3) — *see* Neoplasm,
    connective tissue, malignant
Schwartz (-Jampel) syndrome 756.89
Schwartz-Bartter syndrome (inappropriate
  secretion of antidiuretic hormone) 253.6
Schweninger-Buzzi disease (macular atrophy)
  701.3
Sciatic — *see* condition
Sciatica (infectional) 724.3
  due to
    displacement of intervertebral disc 722.10
    herniation, nucleus pulposus 722.10
Scimitar syndrome (anomalous venous drainage,
  right lung to inferior vena cava) 747.49
Sclera — *see* condition
Sclerectasia 379.11
Scleredema
  adultorum 710.1
  Buschke's 710.1
  newborn 778.1
Sclerema
  adiposum (newborn) 778.1
  adultorum 710.1
  edematosum (newborn) 778.1
  neonatorum 778.1
  newborn 778.1
Scleriasis — *see* Scleroderma
Scleritis 379.00
  with corneal involvement 379.05
  anterior (annular) (localized) 379.03
  brawny 379.06
  granulomatous 379.09
  posterior 379.07
  specified NEC 379.09
  suppurative 379.09
  syphilitic 095.0
  tuberculous (nodular) (*see also* Tuberculosis)
    017.3 ✓5ᵗʰ [379.09]
Sclerochoroiditis (*see also* Scleritis) 379.00
Scleroconjunctivitis (*see also* Scleritis) 379.00
Sclerocystic ovary (syndrome) 256.4

Sclerodactylia 701.0
Scleroderma, sclerodermia (acrosclerotic)
  (diffuse) (generalized) (progressive)
  (pulmonary) 710.1
  circumscribed 701.0
  linear 701.0
  localized (linear) 701.0
  newborn 778.1
Sclerokeratitis 379.05
  meaning sclerosing keratitis 370.54
  tuberculous (*see also* Tuberculosis)
    017.3 ✓5ᵗʰ [379.09]
Scleroma, trachea 040.1
Scleromalacia
  multiple 731.0
  perforans 379.04
Scleromyxedema 701.8
Scleroperikeratitis 379.05
Sclerose en plaques 340
Sclerosis, sclerotic
  adrenal (gland) 255.8
  Alzheimer's 331.0
    with dementia — *see* Alzheimer's, dementia
  amyotrophic (lateral) 335.20
  annularis fibrosi
    aortic 424.1
    mitral 424.0
  aorta, aortic 440.0
    valve (*see also* Endocarditis, aortic) 424.1
  artery, arterial, arteriolar, arteriovascular —
    see Arteriosclerosis
  ascending multiple 340
  Balo's (concentric) 341.1
  basilar — *see* Sclerosis, brain
  bone (localized) NEC 733.99
  brain (general) (lobular) 341.9
    Alzheimer's — *see* Alzheimer's, dementia
    artery, arterial 437.0
    atrophic lobar 331.0
      with dementia
        with behavioral disturbance 331.0
          [294.11]
        without behavioral disturbance 331.0
          [294.10]
    diffuse 341.1
      familial (chronic) (infantile) 330.0
      infantile (chronic) (familial) 330.0
      Pelizaeus-Merzbacher type 330.0
    disseminated 340
    hereditary 334.2
    infantile, (degenerative) (diffuse) 330.0
    insular 340
    Krabbe's 330.0
    miliary 340
    multiple 340
    Pelizaeus-Merzbacher 330.0
    progressive familial 330.0
    senile 437.0
    tuberous 759.5
  bulbar, progressive 340
  bundle of His 426.50
    left 426.3
    right 426.4
  cardiac — *see* Arteriosclerosis, coronary
  cardiorenal (*see also* Hypertension, cardiorenal)
    404.90
  cardiovascular (*see also* Disease,
    cardiovascular) 429.2
    renal (*see also* Hypertension, cardiorenal)
      404.90
  centrolobar, familial 330.0
  cerebellar — *see* Sclerosis, brain
  cerebral — *see* Sclerosis, brain
  cerebrospinal 340
    disseminated 340
    multiple 340
  cerebrovascular 437.0
  choroid 363.40
    diffuse 363.56
  combined (spinal cord) — *see also*
    Degeneration, combined
    multiple 340
  concentric, Balo's 341.1
  cornea 370.54
  coronary (artery) — *see* Arteriosclerosis,
    coronary

Sclerosis, sclerotic — *continued*
  corpus cavernosum
    female 624.8
    male 607.89
  Dewitzky's
    aortic 424.1
    mitral 424.0
  diffuse NEC 341.1
  disease, heart — *see* Arteriosclerosis, coronary
  disseminated 340
  dorsal 340
  dorsolateral (spinal cord) — *see* Degeneration,
    combined
  endometrium 621.8
  extrapyramidal 333.90
  eye, nuclear (senile) 366.16
  Friedreich's (spinal cord) 334.0
  funicular (spermatic cord) 608.89
  gastritis 535.4 ✓5ᵗʰ
  general (vascular) — *see* Arteriosclerosis
  gland (lymphatic) 457.8
  hepatic 571.9
  hereditary
    cerebellar 334.2
    spinal 334.0
  idiopathic cortical (Garré's) (*see also*
    Osteomyelitis) 730.1 ✓5ᵗʰ
  ilium, piriform 733.5
  insular 340
    pancreas 251.8
  Islands of Langerhans 251.8
  kidney — *see* Sclerosis, renal
  larynx 478.79
  lateral 335.24
    amyotrophic 335.20
    descending 335.24
    primary 335.24
    spinal 335.24
  liver 571.9
  lobar, atrophic (of brain) 331.0
    with dementia
      with behavioral disturbance 331.0
        [294.11]
      without behavioral disturbance 331.0
        [294.10]
  lung (*see also* Fibrosis, lung) 515
  mastoid 383.1
  mitral — *see* Endocarditis, mitral
  Mönckeberg's (medial) (*see also*
    Arteriosclerosis, extremities) 440.20
  multiple (brain stem) (cerebral) (generalized)
    (spinal cord) 340
  myocardium, myocardial — *see*
    Arteriosclerosis, coronary
  nuclear (senile), eye 366.16
  ovary 620.8
  pancreas 577.8
  penis 607.89
  peripheral arteries NEC (*see also*
    Arteriosclerosis, extremities) 440.20
  plaques 340
  pluriglandular 258.8
  polyglandular 258.8
  posterior (spinal cord) (syphilitic) 094.0
  posterolateral (spinal cord) — *see* Degeneration,
    combined
  prepuce 607.89
  primary lateral 335.24
  progressive systemic 710.1
  pulmonary (*see also* Fibrosis, lung) 515
    artery 416.0
    valve (heart) (*see also* Endocarditis,
      pulmonary) 424.3
  renal 587
    with
      cystine storage disease 270.0
      hypertension (*see also* Hypertension,
        kidney) 403.90
      hypertensive heart disease (conditions
        classifiable to 402) (*see also*
        Hypertension, cardiorenal) 404.90
      arteriolar (hyaline) (*see also* Hypertension,
        kidney) 403.90
      hyperplastic (*see also* Hypertension,
        kidney) 403.90
  retina (senile) (vascular) 362.17
  rheumatic
    aortic valve 395.9

Schmincke — Sclerosis

Sclerosis, sclerotic — continued
  rheumatic — continued
    mitral valve 394.9
  Schilder's 341.1
  senile — see Arteriosclerosis
  spinal (cord) (general) (progressive) (transverse)
    336.8
    ascending 357.0
    combined — see also Degeneration,
      combined
      multiple 340
      syphilitic 094.89
    disseminated 340
    dorsolateral — see Degeneration, combined
    hereditary (Friedreich's) (mixed form) 334.0
    lateral (amyotrophic) 335.24
    multiple 340
    posterior (syphilitic) 094.0
  stomach 537.89
  subendocardial, congenital 425.3
  systemic (progressive) 710.1
    with lung involvement 710.1 [517.2]
  tricuspid (heart) (valve) — see Endocarditis,
    tricuspid
  tuberous (brain) 759.5
  tympanic membrane (see also
    Tympanosclerosis) 385.00
  valve, valvular (heart) — see Endocarditis
  vascular — see Arteriosclerosis
  vein 459.89

Sclerotenonitis 379.07

Sclerotitis (see also Scleritis) 379.00
  syphilitic 095.0
  tuberculous (see also Tuberculosis)
    017.3 ✔5ᵗʰ [379.09]

Scoliosis (acquired) (postural) 737.30
  congenital 754.2
  due to or associated with
    Charcôt-Marie-Tooth disease 356.1 [737.43]
    mucopolysaccharidosis 277.5 [737.43]
    neurofibromatosis 237.71 [737.43]
    osteitis
      deformans 731.0 [737.43]
      fibrosa cystica 252.0 [737.43]
    osteoporosis (see also Osteoporosis) 733.00
      [737.43]
    poliomyelitis 138 [737.43]
    radiation 737.33
    tuberculosis (see also Tuberculosis)
      015.0 ✔5ᵗʰ [737.43]
  idiopathic 737.30
    infantile
      progressive 737.32
      resolving 737.31
  paralytic 737.39
  rachitic 268.1
  sciatic 724.3
  specified NEC 737.39
  thoracogenic 737.34
  tuberculous (see also Tuberculosis)
    015.0 ✔5ᵗʰ [737.43]

Scoliotic pelvis 738.6
  with disproportion (fetopelvic) 653.0 ✔5ᵗʰ
    affecting fetus or newborn 763.1
    causing obstructed labor 660.1 ✔5ᵗʰ
      affecting fetus or newborn 763.1

Scorbutus, scorbutic 267
  anemia 281.8

Scotoma (ring) 368.44
  arcuate 368.43
  Bjerrum 368.43
  blind spot area 368.42
  central 368.41
  centrocecal 368.41
  paracecal 368.42
  paracentral 368.41
  scintillating 368.12
  Seidel 368.43

Scratch — see Injury, superficial, by site

Screening (for) V82.9
  alcoholism V79.1
  anemia, deficiency NEC V78.1
    iron V78.0
  anomaly, congenital V82.89
  antenatal V28.9
    alphafetoprotein levels, raised V28.1

Screening (for) — continued
  antenatal — continued
    based on amniocentesis V28.2
      chromosomal anomalies V28.0
      raised alphafetoprotein levels V28.1
    fetal growth retardation using
      ultrasonics V28.4
    isoimmunization V28.5
    malformations using ultrasonics V28.3
    raised alphafetoprotein levels V28.1
    specified condition NEC V28.8
    Streptococcus B V28.6
  arterial hypertension V81.1
  arthropod-borne viral disease NEC V73.5
  asymptomatic bacteriuria V81.5
  bacterial
    conjunctivitis V74.4
    disease V74.9
      specified condition NEC V74.8
  bacteriuria, asymptomatic V81.5
  blood disorder NEC V78.9
    specified type NEC V78.8
  bronchitis, chronic V81.3
  brucellosis V74.8
  cancer — see Screening, malignant neoplasm
  cardiovascular disease NEC V81.2
  cataract V80.2
  Chagas' disease V75.3
  chemical poisoning V82.5
  cholera V74.0
  cholesterol level V77.91
  chromosomal
    anomalies
      by amniocentesis, antenatal V28.0
      maternal postnatal V82.4
    athletes V70.3
  condition
    cardiovascular NEC V81.2
    eye NEC V80.2
    genitourinary NEC V81.6
    neurological V80.0
    respiratory NEC V81.4
    skin V82.0
    specified NEC V82.89
  congenital
    anomaly V82.89
      eye V80.2
    dislocation of hip V82.3
    eye condition or disease V80.2
  conjunctivitis, bacterial V74.4
  contamination NEC (see also Poisoning) V82.5
  coronary artery disease V81.0
  cystic fibrosis V77.6
  deficiency anemia NEC V78.1
    iron V78.0
  dengue fever V73.5
  depression V79.0
  developmental handicap V79.9
    in early childhood V79.3
    specified type NEC V79.8
  diabetes mellitus V77.1
  diphtheria V74.3
  disease or disorder V82.9
    bacterial V74.9
      specified NEC V74.8
    blood V78.9
      specified type NEC V78.8
    blood-forming organ V78.9
      specified type NEC V78.8
    cardiovascular NEC V81.2
      hypertensive V81.1
      ischemic V81.0
    Chagas' V75.3
    chlamydial V73.98
      specified NEC V73.88
    ear NEC V80.3
    endocrine NEC V77.99
    eye NEC V80.2
    genitourinary NEC V81.6
    heart NEC V81.2
      hypertensive V81.1
      ischemic V81.0
    immunity NEC V77.99
    infectious NEC V75.9
    lipoid NEC V77.91
    mental V79.9
      specified type NEC V79.8

Screening (for) — continued
  disease or disorder — continued
    metabolic NEC V77.99
      inborn NEC V77.7
    neurological V80.0
    nutritional NEC V77.99
    rheumatic NEC V82.2
    rickettsial V75.0
    sickle-cell V78.2
      trait V78.2
    specified type NEC V82.89
    thyroid V77.0
    vascular NEC V81.2
      ischemic V81.0
    venereal V74.5
    viral V73.99
      arthropod-borne NEC V73.5
      specified type NEC V73.89
  dislocation of hip, congenital V82.3
  drugs in athletes V70.3
  emphysema (chronic) V81.3
  encephalitis, viral (mosquito or tick borne)
    V73.5
  endocrine disorder NEC V77.99
  eye disorder NEC V80.2
    congenital V80.2
  fever
    dengue V73.5
    hemorrhagic V73.5
    yellow V73.4
  filariasis V75.6
  galactosemia V77.4
  genitourinary condition NEC V81.6
  glaucoma V80.1
  gonorrhea V74.5
  gout V77.5
  Hansen's disease V74.2
  heart disease NEC V81.2
    hypertensive V81.1
    ischemic V81.0
  heavy metal poisoning V82.5
  heiminthiasis, intestinal V75.7
  hematopoietic malignancy V76.89
  hemoglobinopathies NEC V78.3
  hemorrhagic fever V73.5
  Hodgkin's disease V76.89
  hormones in athletes V70.3
  hypercholesterolemia V77.91
  hyperlipdemia V77.91
  hypertension V81.1
  immunity disorder NEC V77.99
  inborn errors of metabolism NEC V77.7
  infection
    bacterial V74.9
      specified type NEC V74.8
    mycotic V75.4
    parasitic NEC V75.8
  infectious disease V75.9
    specified type NEC V75.8
  ingestion of radioactive substance V82.5
  intestinal helminthiasis V75.7
  iron deficiency anemia V78.0
  ischemic heart disease V81.0
  lead poisoning V82.5
  leishmaniasis V75.2
  leprosy V74.2
  leptospirosis V74.8
  leukemia V76.89
  lipoid disorder NEC V77.91
  lymphoma V76.89
  malaria V75.1
  malignant neoplasm (of) V76.9
    bladder V76.3
    blood V76.89
    breast V76.10
      mammogram NEC V76.12
        for high-risk patient V76.11
      specified type NEC V76.19
    cervix V76.2
    colon V76.51
    colorectal V76.51
    hematopoietic system V76.89
    intestine V76.50
      colon V76.51
      small V76.52
    lymph (glands) V76.89
    nervous system V76.81

Screening (for) — *continued*
  malignant neoplasm (of) — *continued*
    oral cavity V76.42
    other specified neoplasm NEC V76.89
    ovary V76.46
    prostate V76.44
    rectum V76.41
    respiratory organs V76.0
    skin V76.43
    specified sites NEC V76.49
    testis V76.45
    vagina V76.47
      following hysterectomy for malignant
        condition V67.01
  maternal postnatal chromosomal anomalies
    V82.4
  malnutrition V77.2
  mammogram NEC V76.12
    for high-risk patient V76.11
  measles V73.2
  mental
    disorder V79.9
      specified type NEC V79.8
    retardation V79.2
  metabolic disorder NEC V77.99
  metabolic errors, inborn V77.7
  mucoviscidosis V77.6
  multiphasic V82.6
  mycosis V75.4
  mycotic infection V75.4
  nephropathy V81.5
  neurological condition V80.0
  nutritional disorder V77.99
  obesity V77.8
  osteoporosis V82.81
  parasitic infection NEC V75.8
  phenylketonuria V77.3
  plague V74.8
  poisoning
    chemical NEC V82.5
    contaminated water supply V82.5
      heavy metal V82.5
  poliomyelitis V73.0
  postnatal chromosomal anomalies, maternal
    V82.4
  prenatal — *see* Screening, antenatal
  pulmonary tuberculosis V74.1
  radiation exposure V82.5
  renal disease V81.5
  respiratory condition NEC V81.4
  rheumatic disorder NEC V82.2
  rheumatoid arthritis V82.1
  rickettsial disease V75.0
  rubella V73.3
  schistosomiasis V75.5
  senile macular lesions of eye V80.2
  sickle-cell anemia, disease, or trait V78.2
  skin condition V82.0
  sleeping sickness V75.3
  smallpox V73.1
  special V82.9
    specified condition NEC V82.89
  specified type NEC V82.89
  spirochetal disease V74.9
    specified type NEC V74.8
  stimulants in athletes V70.3
  syphilis V74.5
  tetanus V74.8
  thyroid disorder V77.0
  trachoma V73.6
  trypanosomiasis V75.3
  tuberculosis, pulmonary V74.1
  venereal disease V74.5
  viral encephalitis
    mosquito-borne V73.5
    tick-borne V73.5
  whooping cough V74.8
  worms, intestinal V75.7
  yaws V74.6
  yellow fever V73.4
Scrofula (*see also* Tuberculosis) 017.2 ✓5ᵗʰ
Scrofulide (primary) (*see also* Tuberculosis)
  017.0 ✓5ᵗʰ
Scrofuloderma, scrofulodermia (any site)
  (primary) (*see also* Tuberculosis) 017.0 ✓5ᵗʰ
Scrofulosis (universal) (*see also* Tuberculosis)
  017.2 ✓5ᵗʰ

Scrofulosis lichen (primary) (*see also*
  Tuberculosis) 017.0 ✓5ᵗʰ
Scrofulous — *see* condition
Scrotal tongue 529.5
  congenital 750.13
Scrotum — *see* condition
Scurvy (gum) (infantile) (rickets) (scorbutic) 267
Sea-blue histiocyte syndrome 272.7
Seabright-Bantam syndrome
  (pseudohypoparathyroidism) 275.49
Seasickness 994.6
Seatworm 127.4
Sebaceous
  cyst (*see also* Cyst, sebaceous) 706.2
  gland disease NEC 706.9
Sebocystomatosis 706.2
Seborrhea, seborrheic 706.3
  adiposa 706.3
  capitis 690.11
  congestiva 695.4
  corporis 706.3
  dermatitis 690.10
    infantile 690.12
  diathesis in infants 695.89
  eczema 690.18
    infantile 691.12 ✓5ᵗʰ
  keratosis 702.19
    inflamed 702.11
  nigricans 705.89
  sicca 690.18
  wart 702.19
    inflamed 702.11
Seckel's syndrome 759.89
Seclusion pupil 364.74
Seclusiveness, child 313.22
Secondary — *see also* condition
  neoplasm — *see* Neoplasm, by site, malignant,
    secondary
Secretan's disease or syndrome (posttraumatic
  edema) 782.3
Secretion
  antidiuretic hormone, inappropriate (syndrome)
    253.6
  catecholamine, by pheochromocytoma 255.6
  hormone
    antidiuretic, inappropriate (syndrome) 253.6
    by
      carcinoid tumor 259.2
      pheochromocytoma 255.6
    ectopic NEC 259.3
  urinary
    excessive 788.42
    suppression 788.5
Section
  cesarean
    affecting fetus or newborn 763.4
    post mortem, affecting fetus or newborn
      761.6
    previous, in pregnancy or childbirth
      654.2 ✓5ᵗʰ
      affecting fetus or newborn 763.89
  nerve, traumatic — *see* Injury, nerve, by site
Seeligmann's syndrome (ichthyosis congenita)
  757.1
Segmentation, incomplete (congenital) — *see
  also* Fusion
  bone NEC 756.9
  lumbosacral (joint) 756.15
  vertebra 756.15
    lumbosacral 756.15
Seizure 780.39
  akinetic (idiopathic) (*see also* Epilepsy)
    345.0 ✓5ᵗʰ
    psychomotor 345.4 ✓5ᵗʰ
  apoplexy, apoplectic (*see also* Disease,
    cerebrovascular, acute) 436
  atonic (*see also* Epilepsy) 345.0 ✓5ᵗʰ
  autonomic 300.11
  brain or cerebral (*see also* Disease,
    cerebrovascular, acute) 436
  convulsive (*see also* Convulsions) 780.39
  cortical (focal) (motor) (*see also* Epilepsy)
    345.5 ✓5ᵗʰ

Seizure — *continued*
  epilepsy, epileptic (cryptogenic) (*see also*
    Epilepsy) 345.9 ✓5ᵗʰ
  epileptiform, epileptoid 780.39
    focal (*see also* Epilepsy) 345.5 ✓5ᵗʰ
  febrile 780.31
  heart — *see* Disease, heart
  hysterical 300.11
  Jacksonian (focal) (*see also* Epilepsy) 345.5 ✓5ᵗʰ
    motor type 345.5 ✓5ᵗʰ
    sensory type 345.5 ✓5ᵗʰ
  newborn 779.0
  paralysis (*see also* Disease, cerebrovascular,
    acute) 436
  recurrent 780.39
    epileptic — *see* Epilepsy
  repetitive 780.39
    epileptic — *see* Epilepsy
  salaam (*see also* Epilepsy) 345.6 ✓5ᵗʰ
  uncinate (*see also* Epilepsy) 345.4 ✓5ᵗʰ
Self-mutilation 300.9
Semicoma 780.09
Semiconsciousness 780.09
Seminal
  vesicle — *see* condition
  vesiculitis (*see also* Vesiculitis) 608.0
Seminoma (M9061/3)
  anaplastic type (M9062/3)
    specified site — *see* Neoplasm, by site,
      malignant
    unspecified site 186.9
  specified site — *see* Neoplasm, by site,
    malignant
  spermatocytic (M9063/3)
    specified site — *see* Neoplasm, by site,
      malignant
    unspecified site 186.9
  unspecified site 186.9
Semliki Forest encephalitis 062.8
Senear-Usher disease or syndrome (pemphigus
  erythematosus) 694.4
Senecio jacobae dermatitis 692.6
Senectus 797
Senescence 797
Senile (*see also* condition) 797
  cervix (atrophic) 622.8
  degenerative atrophy, skin 701.3
  endometrium (atrophic) 621.8
  fallopian tube (atrophic) 620.3
  heart (failure) 797
  lung 492.8
  ovary (atrophic) 620.3
  syndrome 259.8
  vagina, vaginitis (atrophic) 627.3
  wart 702.0
Senility 797
  with
    acute confusional state 290.3
    delirium 290.3
    mental changes 290.9
    psychosis NEC (*see also* Psychosis, senile)
      290.20
  premature (syndrome) 259.8
Sensation
  burning (*see also* Disturbance, sensation)
    782.0
    tongue 529.6
  choking 784.9
  loss of (*see also* Disturbance, sensation) 782.0
  prickling (*see also* Disturbance, sensation)
    782.0
  tingling (*see also* Disturbance, sensation) 782.0
Sense loss (touch) (*see also* Disturbance,
  sensation) 782.0
  smell 781.1
  taste 781.1
Sensibility disturbance NEC (cortical) (deep)
  (vibratory) (*see also* Disturbance, sensation)
  782.0
Sensitive dentine 521.8
Sensitiver Beziehungswahn 297.8
Sensitivity, sensitization — *see also* Allergy
  autoerythrocyte 287.2
  carotid sinus 337.0

Screening — Sensitivity

Sensitivity, sensitization — *see also* Allergy —
　continued
　child (excessive) 313.21
　cold, autoimmune 283.0
　methemoglobin 289.7
　suxamethonium 289.8
　tuberculin, without clinical or radiological
　　symptoms 795.5

Sensory
　extinction 781.8
　neglect 781.8

Separation
　acromioclavicular — *see* Dislocation,
　　acromioclavicular
　anxiety, abnormal 309.21
　apophysis, traumatic — *see* Fracture, by site
　choroid 363.70
　　hemorrhagic 363.72
　　serous 363.71
　costochondral (simple) (traumatic) — *see*
　　Dislocation, costochondral
　epiphysis, epiphyseal
　　nontraumatic 732.9
　　　upper femoral 732.2
　　traumatic — *see* Fracture, by site
　fracture — *see* Fracture, by site
　infundibulum cardiac from right ventricle by a
　　partition 746.83
　joint (current) (traumatic) — *see* Dislocation, by
　　site
　placenta (normally implanted) — *see* Placenta,
　　separation
　pubic bone, obstetrical trauma 665.6 ☑5ᵗʰ
　retina, retinal (*see also* Detachment, retina)
　　361.9
　　layers 362.40
　　　sensory (*see also* Retinoschisis) 361.10
　　pigment epithelium (exudative) 362.42
　　　hemorrhagic 362.43
　sternoclavicular (traumatic) — *see* Dislocation,
　　sternoclavicular
　symphysis pubis, obstetrical trauma 665.6 ☑5ᵗʰ
　tracheal ring, incomplete (congenital) 748.3

Sepsis (generalized) (*see also* Septicemia) 038.9
　with
　　abortion — *see* Abortion, by type, with
　　　sepsis
　　ectopic pregnancy (*see also* categories
　　　633.0-633.9) 639.0
　　molar pregnancy (*see also* categories 630-
　　　632) 639.0
　buccal 528.3
　complicating labor 659.3 ☑5ᵗʰ
　dental (pulpal origin) 522.4
　female genital organ NEC 614.9
　fetus (intrauterine) 771.81　　　　　　▲
　following
　　abortion 639.0
　　ectopic or molar pregnancy 639.0
　　infusion, perfusion, or transfusion 999.3
　Friedländer's 038.49
　intraocular 360.00
　localized
　　in operation wound 998.59
　　skin (*see also* Abscess) 682.9
　malleus 024
　nadir 038.9
　newborn (organism unspecified) NEC 771.81▲
　oral 528.3
　puerperal, postpartum, childbirth (pelvic)
　　670 ☑4ᵗʰ
　resulting from infusion, injection, transfusion,
　　or vaccination 999.3
　severe 995.92　　　　　　　　　　　●
　skin, localized (*see also* Abscess) 682.9
　umbilical (newborn) (organism unspecified)
　　771.89　　　　　　　　　　　　▲
　　tetanus 771.3
　urinary 599.0

Septate — *see also* Septum

Septic — *see also* condition
　adenoids 474.01
　　and tonsils 474.02
　arm (with lymphangitis) 682.3
　embolus — *see* Embolism

Septic — *see also* condition — *continued*
　finger (with lymphangitis) 681.00
　foot (with lymphangitis) 682.7
　gallbladder (*see also* Cholecystitis) 575.8
　hand (with lymphangitis) 682.4
　joint (*see also* Arthritis, septic) 711.0 ☑5ᵗʰ
　kidney (*see also* Infection, kidney) 590.9
　leg (with lymphangitis) 682.6
　mouth 528.3
　nail 681.9
　　finger 681.02
　　toe 681.11
　shock (endotoxic) 785.59
　sore (*see also* Abscess) 682.9
　　throat 034.0
　　　milk-borne 034.0
　　　streptococcal 034.0
　spleen (acute) 289.59
　teeth (pulpal origin) 522.4
　throat 034.0
　thrombus — *see* Thrombosis
　toe (with lymphangitis) 681.0 ☑5ᵗʰ
　tonsils 474.00
　　and adenoids 474.02
　umbilical cord (newborn) (organism
　　unspecified) 771.89　　　　　　▲
　uterus (*see also* Endometritis) 615.9

Septicemia, septicemic (generalized)
　(suppurative) 038.9
　with
　　abortion — *see* Abortion, by type, with
　　　sepsis
　　ectopic pregnancy (*see also* categories
　　　633.0-633.9) 639.0
　　molar pregnancy (*see also* categories 630-
　　　632) 639.0
　Aerobacter aerogenes 038.49
　anaerobic 038.3
　anthrax 022.3
　Bacillus coli 038.42
　Bacteroides 038.3
　Clostridium 038.3
　complicating labor 659.3 ☑5ᵗʰ
　cryptogenic 038.9
　enteric gram-negative bacilli 038.40
　Enterobacter aerogenes 038.49
　Erysipelothrix (insidiosa) (rhusiopathiae) 027.1
　Escherichia coli 038.42
　following
　　abortion 639.0
　　ectopic or molar pregnancy 639.0
　　infusion, injection, transfusion, or
　　　vaccination 999.3
　Friedländer's (bacillus) 038.49
　gangrenous 038.9
　gonococcal 098.89
　gram-negative (organism) 038.40
　　anaerobic 038.3
　Hemophilus influenzae 038.41
　herpes (simplex) 054.5
　herpetic 054.5
　Listeria monocytogenes 027.0
　meningeal — *see* Meningitis
　meningococcal (chronic) (fulminating) 036.2
　navel, newborn (organism unspecified)
　　771.89　　　　　　　　　　　　▲
　newborn (organism unspecified) 771.81　▲
　plague 020.2
　pneumococcal 038.2
　postabortal 639.0
　postoperative 998.59
　Proteus vulgaris 038.49
　Pseudomonas (aeruginosa) 038.43
　puerperal, postpartum 670 ☑4ᵗʰ
　Salmonella (aertrycke) (callinarum)
　　(choleraesuis) (enteritidis) (suipestifer)
　　003.1
　Serratia 038.44
　Shigella (*see also* Dysentery, bacillary) 004.9
　specified organism NEC 038.8
　staphylococcal 038.10
　　aureus 038.11
　　specified organism NEC 038.19
　streptococcal (anaerobic) 038.0
　suipestifer 003.1

Septicemia, septicemic — *continued*
　umbilicus, newborn (organism unspecified)
　　771.89　　　　　　　　　　　　▲
　viral 079.99
　Yersinia enterocolitica 038.49

Septum, septate (congenital) — *see also*
　Anomaly, specified type NEC
　anal 751.2
　aqueduct of Sylvius 742.3
　　with spina bifida (*see also* Spina bifida)
　　　741.0 ☑5ᵗʰ
　hymen 752.49
　uterus (*see also* Double, uterus) 752.2
　vagina 752.49
　　in pregnancy or childbirth 654.7 ☑5ᵗʰ
　　　affecting fetus or newborn 763.89
　　　causing obstructed labor 660.2 ☑5ᵗʰ
　　　　affecting fetus or newborn 763.1

Sequestration
　lung (congenital) (extralobar) (intralobar) 748.5
　orbit 376.10
　pulmonary artery (congenital) 747.3

Sequestrum
　bone (*see also* Osteomyelitis) 730.1 ☑5ᵗʰ
　　jaw 526.4
　dental 525.8
　jaw bone 526.4
　sinus (accessory) (nasal) (*see also* Sinusitis) 473.9
　　maxillary 473.0

Sequoiosis asthma 495.8

Serology for syphilis
　doubtful
　　with signs or symptoms — *see* Syphilis, by
　　　site and stage
　　follow-up of latent syphilis — *see* Syphilis,
　　　latent
　false positive 795.6
　negative, with signs or symptoms — *see*
　　Syphilis, by site and stage
　positive 097.1
　　with signs or symptoms — *see* Syphilis, by
　　　site and stage
　　false 795.6
　　follow-up of latent syphilis — *see* Syphilis,
　　　latent
　　only finding — *see* Syphilis, latent
　reactivated 097.1

Seroma (postoperative) (non-infected) 998.13
　infected 998.51

Seropurulent — *see* condition

Serositis, multiple 569.89
　pericardial 423.2
　peritoneal 568.82
　pleural — *see* Pleurisy

Serotonin syndrome 333.99

Serous — *see* condition

Sertoli cell
　adenoma (M8640/0)
　　specified site — *see* Neoplasm, by site,
　　　benign
　　unspecified site
　　　female 220
　　　male 222.0
　carcinoma (M8640/3)
　　specified site — *see* Neoplasm, by site,
　　　malignant
　　unspecified site 186.9
　syndrome (germinal aplasia) 606.0
　tumor (M8640/0)
　　with lipid storage (M8641/0)
　　　specified site — *see* Neoplasm, by site,
　　　　benign
　　　unspecified site
　　　　female 220
　　　　male 222.0
　　specified site — *see* Neoplasm, by site,
　　　benign
　　unspecified site
　　　female 220
　　　male 222.0

Sertoli-Leydig cell tumor (M8631/0)
　specified site — *see* Neoplasm, by site, benign
　unspecified site
　　female 220
　　male 222.0

☑4ᵗʰ Fourth-digit Required　　☑5ᵗʰ Fifth-digit Required　　▶◀ Revised Text　　● New Line　　▲ Revised Code

Serum
allergy, allergic reaction 999.5
shock 999.4
arthritis 999.5 *[713.6]*
complication or reaction NEC 999.5
disease NEC 999.5
hepatitis 070.3 ☑5ᵗʰ
intoxication 999.5
jaundice (homologous) — *see* Hepatitis, viral
neuritis 999.5
poisoning NEC 999.5
rash NEC 999.5
reaction NEC 999.5
sickness NEC 999.5
Sesamoiditis 733.99
Seven-day fever 061
of
Japan 100.89
Queensland 100.89
Sever's disease or osteochondrosis (calcaneum) 732.5
Sex chromosome mosaics 758.81
Sextuplet
affected by maternal complications of pregnancy 761.5
healthy liveborn — *see* Newborn, multiple
pregnancy (complicating delivery) NEC 651.8 ☑5ᵗʰ
with fetal loss and retention of one or more fetus(es) 651.6 ☑5ᵗʰ
Sexual
anesthesia 302.72
deviation (*see also* Deviation, sexual) 302.9
disorder (*see also* Deviation, sexual) 302.9
frigidity (female) 302.72
function, disorder of (psychogenic) 302.70
specified type NEC 302.79
immaturity (female) (male) 259.0
impotence (psychogenic) 302.72
organic origin NEC 607.84
precocity (constitutional) (cryptogenic) (female) (idiopathic) (male) NEC 259.1
with adrenal hyperplasia 255.2
sadism 302.84
Sexuality, pathological (*see also* Deviation, sexual) 302.9
Sézary's disease, reticulosis, or syndrome (M9701/3) 202.2 ☑5ᵗʰ
Shadow, lung 793.1
Shaken infant syndrome 995.55
Shaking
head (tremor) 781.0
palsy or paralysis (*see also* Parkinsonism) 332.0
Shallowness, acetabulum 736.39
Shaver's disease or syndrome (bauxite pneumoconiosis) 503
Shearing
artificial skin graft 996.55
decellularized allodermis graft 996.55
Sheath (tendon) — *see* condition
Shedding
nail 703.8
teeth, premature, primary (deciduous) 520.6
Sheehan's disease or syndrome (postpartum pituitary necrosis) 253.2
Shelf, rectal 569.49
Shell
shock (current) (*see also* Reaction, stress, acute) 308.9
lasting state 300.16
teeth 520.5
Shield kidney 753.3
Shift, mediastinal 793.2
Shifting
pacemaker 427.89
sleep-work schedule (affecting sleep) 307.45
Shiga's
bacillus 004.0
dysentery 004.0
Shigella (dysentery) (*see also* Dysentery, bacillary) 004.9
carrier (suspected) of V02.3

Shigellosis (*see also* Dysentery, bacillary) 004.9
Shingles (*see also* Herpes, zoster) 053.9
eye NEC 053.29
Shin splints 844.9
Shipyard eye or disease 077.1
Shirodkar suture, in pregnancy 654.5 ☑5ᵗʰ
Shock 785.50
with
abortion — *see* Abortion, by type, with shock
ectopic pregnancy (*see also* categories 633.0-633.9) 639.5
molar pregnancy (*see also* categories 630-632) 639.5
allergic — *see* Shock, anaphylactic
anaclitic 309.21
anaphylactic 995.0
chemical — *see* Table of Drugs and Chemicals
correct medicinal substance properly administered 995.0
drug or medicinal substance
correct substance properly administered 995.0
overdose or wrong substance given or taken 977.9
specified drug — *see* Table of Drugs and Chemicals
following sting(s) 989.5
food — *see* Anaphylactic shock, due to, food
immunization 999.4
serum 999.4
anaphylactoid — *see* Shock, anaphylactic
anesthetic
correct substance properly administered 995.0
overdose or wrong substance given 968.4
specified anesthetic — *see* Table of Drugs and Chemicals
birth, fetus or newborn NEC 779.89 ▲
cardiogenic 785.51
chemical substance — *see* Table of Drugs and Chemicals
circulatory 785.59
complicating
abortion — *see* Abortion, by type, with shock
ectopic pregnancy (*see also* categories 633.0-633.9) 639.5
labor and delivery 669.1 ☑5ᵗʰ
molar pregnancy (*see also* categories 630-632) 639.5
culture 309.29
due to
drug 995.0
correct substance properly administered 995.0
overdose or wrong substance given or taken 977.9
specified drug — *see* Table of Drugs and Chemicals
food — *see* Anaphylactic shock, due to, food
during labor and delivery 669.1 ☑5ᵗʰ
electric 994.8
endotoxic 785.59
due to surgical procedure 998.0
following
abortion 639.5
ectopic or molar pregnancy 639.5
injury (immediate) (delayed) 958.4
labor and delivery 669.1 ☑5ᵗʰ
gram-negative 785.59
hematogenic 785.59
hemorrhagic
due to
disease 785.59
surgery (intraoperative) (postoperative) 998.0
trauma 958.4
hypovolemic NEC 785.59
surgical 998.0
traumatic 958.4
insulin 251.0
therapeutic misadventure 962.3
kidney 584.5
traumatic (following crushing) 958.5

Shock — *continued*
lightning 994.0
lung 518.5
nervous (*see also* Reaction, stress, acute) 308.9
obstetric 669.1 ☑5ᵗʰ
with
abortion — *see* Abortion, by type, with shock
ectopic pregnancy (*see also* categories 633.0-633.9) 639.5
molar pregnancy (*see also* categories 630-632) 639.5
following
abortion 639.5
ectopic or molar pregnancy 639.5
paralysis, paralytic (*see also* Disease, cerebrovascular, acute) 436
late effect — *see* Late effect(s) (of) cerebrovascular disease
pleural (surgical) 998.0
due to trauma 958.4
postoperative 998.0
with
abortion — *see* Abortion, by type, with shock
ectopic pregnancy (*see also* categories 633.0-633.9) 639.5
molar pregnancy (*see also* categories 630-632) 639.5
following
abortion 639.5
ectopic or molar pregnancy 639.5
psychic (*see also* Reaction, stress, acute) 308.9
past history (of) V15.49
psychogenic (*see also* Reaction, stress, acute) 308.9
septic 785.59
with
abortion — *see* Abortion, by type, with shock
ectopic pregnancy (categories 633.0-633.9) 639.5
molar pregnancy (*see also* categories 630-632) 639.5
due to
surgical procedure 998.0
transfusion NEC 999.8
bone marrow 996.85
following
abortion 639.5
ectopic or molar pregnancy 639.5
surgical procedure 998.0
transfusion NEC 999.8
bone marrow 996.85
spinal — *see also* Injury, spinal, by site
with spinal bone injury — *see* Fracture, vertebra, by site, with spinal cord injury
surgical 998.0
therapeutic misadventure NEC (*see also* Complications) 998.89
thyroxin 962.7
toxic 040.82 ▲
transfusion — *see* Complications, transfusion
traumatic (immediate) (delayed) 958.4
Shoemakers' chest 738.3
Short, shortening, shortness
Achilles tendon (acquired) 727.81
arm 736.89
congenital 755.20
back 737.9
bowel syndrome 579.3
breath 786.05
common bile duct, congenital 751.69
cord (umbilical) 663.4 ☑5ᵗʰ
affecting fetus or newborn 762.6
cystic duct, congenital 751.69
esophagus (congenital) 750.4
femur (acquired) 736.81
congenital 755.34
frenulum linguae 750.0
frenum, lingual 750.0
hamstrings 727.81
hip (acquired) 736.39
congenital 755.63
leg (acquired) 736.81
congenital 755.30

☑4ᵗʰ Fourth-digit Required   ☑5ᵗʰ Fifth-digit Required   ▶◀ Revised Text   ● New Line   ▲ Revised Code

Short, shortening, shortness — continued
  metatarsus (congenital) 754.79
    acquired 736.79
  organ or site, congenital NEC — see Distortion
  palate (congenital) 750.26
  P-R interval syndrome 426.81
  radius (acquired) 736.09
    congenital 755.26
  round ligament 629.8
  sleeper 307.49
  stature, constitutional (hereditary) 783.43
  tendon 727.81
    Achilles (acquired) 727.81
      congenital 754.79
    congenital 756.89
    thigh (acquired) 736.81
      congenital 755.34
    tibialis anticus 727.81
    umbilical cord 663.4 ✓5ᵗʰ
      affecting fetus or newborn 762.6
  urethra 599.84
  uvula (congenital) 750.26
  vagina 623.8
Shortsightedness 367.1
Shoshin (acute fulminating beriberi) 265.0
Shoulder — see condition
Shovel-shaped incisors 520.2
Shower, thromboembolic — see Embolism
Shunt (status)
  aortocoronary bypass V45.81
  arterial-venous (dialysis) V45.1
  arteriovenous, pulmonary (acquired) 417.0
    congenital 747.3
    traumatic (complication) 901.40
  cerebral ventricle (communicating) in situ
    V45.2
  coronary artery bypass V45.81
  surgical, prosthetic, with complications — see
    Complications, shunt
  vascular NEC V45.89
Shutdown
  renal 586
    with
      abortion — see Abortion, by type, with
        renal failure
      ectopic pregnancy (see also categories
        633.0-633.9) 639.3
      molar pregnancy (see also categories 630-
        632) 639.3
    complicating
      abortion 639.3
      ectopic or molar pregnancy 639.3
    following labor and delivery 669.3 ✓5ᵗʰ
Shwachman's syndrome 288.0
Shy-Drager syndrome (orthostatic hypotension
  with multisystem degeneration) 333.0
Sialadenitis (any gland) (chronic) (suppurative)
    527.2
  epidemic — see Mumps
Sialadenosis, periodic 527.2
Sialaporia 527.7
Sialectasia 527.8
Sialitis 527.2
Sialoadenitis (see also Sialadenitis) 527.2
Sioloangitis 527.2
Sialodochitis (fibrinosa) 527.2
Sialodocholithiasis 527.5
Sialolithiasis 527.5
Sialorrhea (see also Ptyalism) 527.7
  periodic 527.2
Sialosis 527.8
  rheumatic 710.2
Siamese twin 759.4
Sicard's syndrome 352.6
Sicca syndrome (keratoconjunctivitis) 710.2
Sick 799.9
  cilia syndrome 759.89
  or handicapped person in family V61.49
Sickle-cell
  anemia (see also Disease, sickle-cell) 282.60
  disease (see also Disease, sickle-cell) 282.60

Sickle-cell — continued
  hemoglobin
    C disease 282.63
    D disease 282.69
    E disease 282.69
  thalassemia 282.4
  trait 282.5
Sicklemia (see also Disease, sickle-cell) 282.60
  trait 282.5
Sickness
  air (travel) 994.6
  airplane 994.6
  alpine 993.2
  altitude 993.2
  Andes 993.2
  aviators' 993.2
  balloon 993.2
  car 994.6
  compressed air 993.3
  decompression 993.3
  green 280.9
  harvest 100.89
  milk 988.8
  morning 643.0 ✓5ᵗʰ
  motion 994.6
  mountain 993.2
    acute 289.0
  protein (see also Complications, vaccination)
    999.5
  radiation NEC 990
  roundabout (motion) 994.6
  sea 994.6
  serum NEC 999.5
  sleeping (African) 086.5
    by Trypanosoma 086.5
      gambiense 086.3
      rhodesiense 086.4
    Gambian 086.3
    late effect 139.8
    Rhodesian 086.4
  sweating 078.2
  swing (motion) 994.6
  train (railway) (travel) 994.6
  travel (any vehicle) 994.6
Sick sinus syndrome 427.81
Sideropenia (see also Anemia, iron deficiency)
    280.9
Siderosis (lung) (occupational) 503
  cornea 371.15
  eye (bulbi) (vitreous) 360.23
  lens 360.23
Siegal-Cattan-Mamou disease (periodic) 277.3
Siemens' syndrome
  ectodermal dysplasia 757.31
  keratosis follicularis spinulosa (decalvans)
    757.39
Sighing respiration 786.7
Sigmoid
  flexure — see condition
  kidney 753.3
Sigmoiditis — see Enteritis
Silfverskiöld's syndrome 756.5 ✓5ᵗʰ
Silicosis, silicotic (complicated) (occupational)
    (simple) 502
  fibrosis, lung (confluent) (massive)
    (occupational) 502
  non-nodular 503
  pulmonum 502
Silicotuberculosis (see also Tuberculosis)
    011.4 ✓5ᵗʰ
Silo fillers' disease 506.9
Silver's syndrome (congenital hemihypertrophy
  and short stature) 759.89
Silver wire arteries, retina 362.13
Silvestroni-Bianco syndrome (thalassemia
  minima) 282.4
Simian crease 757.2
Simmonds' cachexia or disease (pituitary
  cachexia) 253.2
Simons' disease or syndrome (progressive
  lipodystrophy) 272.6
Simple, simplex — see condition

Sinding-Larsen disease (juvenile osteopathia
  patellae) 732.4
Singapore hemorrhagic fever 065.4
Singers' node or nodule 478.5
Single
  atrium 745.69
  coronary artery 746.85
  umbilical artery 747.5
  ventricle 745.3
Singultus 786.8
  epidemicus 078.89
Sinus — see also Fistula
  abdominal 569.81
  arrest 426.6
  arrhythmia 427.89
  bradycardia 427.89
    chronic 427.81
  branchial cleft (external) (internal) 744.41
  coccygeal (infected) 685.1
    with abscess 685.0
  dental 522.7
  dermal (congenital) 685.1
    with abscess 685.0
  draining — see Fistula
  infected, skin NEC 686.9
  marginal, ruptured or bleeding 641.2 ✓5ᵗʰ
    affecting fetus or newborn 762.1
  pause 426.6
  pericranii 742.0
  pilonidal (infected) (rectum) 685.1
    with abscess 685.0
  preauricular 744.46
  rectovaginal 619.1
  sacrococcygeal (dermoid) (infected) 685.1
    with abscess 685.0
  skin
    infected NEC 686.9
    noninfected — see Ulcer, skin
  tachycardia 427.89
  tarsi syndrome 726.79
  testis 608.89
  tract (postinfectional) — see Fistula
  urachus 753.7
Sinuses, Rokitansky-Aschoff (see also Disease,
  gallbladder) 575.8
Sinusitis (accessory) (nasal) (hyperplastic)
    (nonpurulent) (purulent) (chronic) 473.9
  with influenza, flu, or grippe 487.1
  acute 461.9
    ethmoidal 461.2
    frontal 461.1
    maxillary 461.0
    specified type NEC 461.8
    sphenoidal 461.3
  allergic (see also Fever, hay) 477.9
  antrum — see Sinusitis, maxillary
  due to
    fungus, any sinus 117.9
    high altitude 993.1
  ethmoidal 473.2
    acute 461.2
  frontal 473.1
    acute 461.1
  influenzal 478.1
  maxillary 473.0
    acute 461.0
  specified site NEC 473.8
  sphenoidal 473.3
    acute 461.3
  syphilitic, any sinus 095.8
  tuberculous, any sinus (see also Tuberculosis)
    012.8 ✓5ᵗʰ
Sinusitis-bronchiectasis-situs inversus
  (syndrome) (triad) 759.3
Sipple's syndrome (medullary thyroid carcinoma-
  pheochromocytoma) 193
Sirenomelia 759.89
Siriasis 992.0
Sirkari's disease 085.0
SIRS (systemic inflammatory response
    syndrome) 995.90 ●
  due to ●
    infectious process 995.91 ●
      with organ dysfunction 995.92 ●
    non-infectious process 995.93 ●
      with organ dysfunction 995.94 ●

✓4ᵗʰ Fourth-digit Required   ✓5ᵗʰ Fifth-digit Required   ▶◀ Revised Text   ● New Line   ▲ Revised Code

Siti 104.0
Sitophobia 300.29
Situation, psychiatric 300.9
Situational
  disturbance (transient) (*see also* Reaction, adjustment) 309.9
    acute 308.3
  maladjustment, acute (*see also* Reaction, adjustment) 309.9
  reaction (*see also* Reaction, adjustment) 309.9
    acute 308.3
Situs inversus or transversus 759.3
  abdominalis 759.3
  thoracis 759.3
Sixth disease 057.8
Sjögren (-Gougerot) syndrome or disease (keratoconjunctivitis sicca) 710.2
  with lung involvement 710.2 [517.8]
Sjögren-Larsson syndrome (ichthyosis congenita) 757.1
Skeletal — *see* condition
Skene's gland — *see* condition
Skenitis (*see also* Urethritis) 597.89
  gonorrheal (acute) 098.0
    chronic or duration of 2 months or over 098.2
Skerljevo 104.0
Skevas-Zerfus disease 989.5
Skin — *see also* condition
  donor V59.1
  hidebound 710.9
SLAP lesion (superior glenoid labrum) 840.7
Slate-dressers' lung 502
Slate-miners' lung 502
Sleep
  disorder 780.50
    with apnea — *see* Apnea, sleep
    child 307.40
    nonorganic origin 307.40
      specified type NEC 307.49
  disturbance 780.50
    with apnea — *see* Apnea, sleep
    nonorganic origin 307.40
      specified type NEC 307.49
  drunkenness 307.47
  paroxysmal 347
  rhythm inversion 780.55
    nonorganic origin 307.45
  walking 307.46
    hysterical 300.13
Sleeping sickness 086.5
  late effect 139.8
Sleeplessness (*see also* Insomnia) 780.52
  menopausal 627.2
  nonorganic origin 307.41
Slipped, slipping
  epiphysis (postinfectional) 732.9
    traumatic (old) 732.9
      current — *see* Fracture, by site
    upper femoral (nontraumatic) 732.2
  intervertebral disc — *see* Displacement, intervertebral disc
  ligature, umbilical 772.3
  patella 717.89
  rib 733.99
  sacroiliac joint 724.6
  tendon 727.9
  ulnar nerve, nontraumatic 354.2
  vertebra NEC (*see also* Spondylolisthesis) 756.12
Slocumb's syndrome 255.3
Sloughing (multiple) (skin) 686.9
  abscess — *see* Abscess, by site
  appendix 543.9
  bladder 596.8
  fascia 728.9
  graft — *see* Complications, graft
  phagedena (*see also* Gangrene) 785.4
  reattached extremity (*see also* Complications, reattached extremity) 996.90
  rectum 569.49
  scrotum 608.89
  tendon 727.9

Sloughing — *continued*
  transplanted organ (*see also* Rejection, transplant, organ, by site) 996.80
  ulcer (*see also* Ulcer, skin) 707.9
Slow
  feeding newborn 779.3
  fetal, growth NEC 764.9 ✓5ᵗʰ
    affecting management of pregnancy 656.5 ✓5ᵗʰ
Slowing
  heart 427.89
  urinary stream 788.62
Sluder's neuralgia or syndrome 337.0
Slurred, slurring, speech 784.5
Small, smallness
  cardiac reserve — *see* Disease, heart
  for dates
    fetus or newborn 764.0 ✓5ᵗʰ
      with malnutrition 764.1 ✓5ᵗʰ
      affecting management of pregnancy 656.5 ✓5ᵗʰ
    infant, term 764.0 ✓5ᵗʰ
      with malnutrition 764.1 ✓5ᵗʰ
      affecting management of pregnancy 656.5 ✓5ᵗʰ
  introitus, vagina 623.3
  kidney, unknown cause 589.9
    bilateral 589.1
    unilateral 589.0
  ovary 620.8
  pelvis
    with disproportion (fetopelvic) 653.1 ✓5ᵗʰ
      affecting fetus or newborn 763.1
    causing obstructed labor 660.1 ✓5ᵗʰ
      affecting fetus or newborn 763.1
  placenta — *see* Placenta, insufficiency
  uterus 621.8
  white kidney 582.9
Small-for-dates (*see also* Light-for-dates) 764.0 ✓5ᵗʰ
  affecting management of pregnancy 656.5 ✓5ᵗʰ
Smallpox 050.9
  contact V01.3
  exposure to V01.3
  hemorrhagic (pustular) 050.0
  malignant 050.0
  modified 050.2
  vaccination
    complications — *see* Complications, vaccination
    prophylactic (against) V04.1
Smith's fracture (separation) (closed) 813.41
  open 813.51
Smith-Lemii Opitz syndrome (cerebrohepatorenal syndrome) 759.89
Smith-Strang disease (oasthouse urine) 270.2
Smokers'
  bronchitis 491.0
  cough 491.0
  syndrome (*see also* Abuse, drugs, nondependent) 305.1
  throat 472.1
  tongue 528.6
Smothering spells 786.09
Snaggle teeth, tooth 524.3
Snapping
  finger 727.05
  hip 719.65
  jaw 524.69
  knee 717.9
  thumb 727.05
Sneddon-Wilkinson disease or syndrome (subcorneal pustular dermatosis) 694.1
Sneezing 784.9
  intractable 478.1
Sniffing
  cocaine (*see also* Dependence) 304.2 ✓5ᵗʰ
  ether (*see also* Dependence) 304.6 ✓5ᵗʰ
  glue (airplane) (*see also* Dependence) 304.6 ✓5ᵗʰ
Snoring 786.09
Snow blindness 370.24
Snuffles (nonsyphilitic) 460
  syphilitic (infant) 090.0

Social migrant V60.0
Sodoku 026.0
Soemmering's ring 366.51
Soft — *see also* condition
  enlarged prostate 600.0
  nails 703.8
Softening
  bone 268.2
  brain (necrotic) (progressive) 434.9 ✓5ᵗʰ
    arteriosclerotic 437.0
    congenital 742.4
    embolic (*see also* Embolism, brain) 434.1 ✓5ᵗʰ
    hemorrhagic (*see also* Hemorrhage, brain) 431
    occlusive 434.9 ✓5ᵗʰ
    thrombotic (*see also* Thrombosis, brain) 434.0 ✓5ᵗʰ
  cartilage 733.92
  cerebellar — *see* Softening, brain
  cerebral — *see* Softening, brain
  cerebrospinal — *see* Softening, brain
  myocardial, heart (*see also* Degeneration, myocardial) 429.1
  nails 703.8
  spinal cord 336.8
  stomach 537.89
Solar fever 061
Soldier's
  heart 306.2
  patches 423.1
Solitary
  cyst
    bone 733.21
    kidney 593.2
  kidney (congenital) 753.0
  tubercle, brain (*see also* Tuberculosis, brain) 013.2 ✓5ᵗʰ
  ulcer, bladder 596.8
Somatization reaction, somatic reaction (*see also* Disorder, psychosomatic) 306.9
  disorder 300.81
Somatoform disorder 300.82
  atypical 300.82
  severe 300.81
  undifferentiated 300.82
Somnambulism 307.46
  hysterical 300.13
Somnolence 780.09
  nonorganic origin 307.43
  periodic 349.89
Sonne dysentery 004.3
Soor 112.0
Sore
  Delhi 085.1
  desert (*see also* Ulcer, skin) 707.9
  eye 379.99
  Lahore 085.1
  mouth 528.9
    canker 528.2
    due to dentures 528.9
  muscle 729.1
  Naga (*see also* Ulcer, skin) 707.9
  oriental 085.1
  pressure 707.0
    with gangrene 707.0 [785.4]
  skin NEC 709.9
  soft 099.0
  throat 462
    with influenza, flu, or grippe 487.1
    acute 462
    chronic 472.1
    clergyman's 784.49
    coxsackie (virus) 074.0
    diphtheritic 032.0
    epidemic 034.0
    gangrenous 462
    herpetic 054.79
    influenzal 487.1
    malignant 462
    purulent 462
    putrid 462
    septic 034.0
    streptococcal (ulcerative) 034.0
    ulcerated 462

✓4ᵗʰ Fourth-digit Required   ✓5ᵗʰ Fifth-digit Required   ▶◀ Revised Text   ● New Line   ▲ Revised Code

Sore — *continued*
> throat — *continued*
>> viral NEC 462
>>> Coxsackie 074.0
>> tropical (*see also* Ulcer, skin) 707.9
>> veldt (*see also* Ulcer, skin) 707.9

Sotos' syndrome (cerebral gigantism) 253.0

Sounds
> friction, pleural 786.7
> succussion, chest 786.7

South African cardiomyopathy syndrome 425.2

South American
> blastomycosis 116.1
> trypanosomiasis — *see* Trypanosomiasis

Southeast Asian hemorrhagic fever 065.4

Spacing, teeth, abnormal 524.3

Spade-like hand (congenital) 754.89

Spading nail 703.8
> congenital 757.5

Spanemia 285.9

Spanish collar 605

Sparganosis 123.5

Spasm, spastic, spasticity (*see also* condition) 781.0
> accommodation 367.53
> ampulla of Vater (*see also* Disease, gallbladder) 576.8
> anus, ani (sphincter) (reflex) 564.6
>> psychogenic 306.4
> artery NEC 443.9
>> basilar 435.0
>> carotid 435.8
>> cerebral 435.9
>>> specified artery NEC 435.8
>> retinal (*see also* Occlusion, retinal, artery) 362.30
>> vertebral 435.1
>> vertebrobasilar 435.3
> Bell's 351.0
> bladder (sphincter, external or internal) 596.8
> bowel 564.9
>> psychogenic 306.4
> bronchus, bronchiole 519.1
> cardia 530.0
> cardiac — *see* Angina
> carpopedal (*see also* Tetany) 781.7
> cecum 564.9
>> psychogenic 306.4
> cerebral (arteries) (vascular) 435.9
>> specified artery NEC 435.8
> cerebrovascular 435.9
> cervix, complicating delivery 661.4 ☑5ᵗʰ
>> affecting fetus or newborn 763.7
> ciliary body (of accommodation) 367.53
> colon 564.1
>> psychogenic 306.4
> common duct (*see also* Disease, biliary) 576.8
> compulsive 307.22
> conjugate 378.82
> convergence 378.84
> coronary (artery) — *see* Angina
> diaphragm (reflex) 786.8
>> psychogenic 306.1
> duodenum, duodenal (bulb) 564.89
> esophagus (diffuse) 530.5
>> psychogenic 306.4
> facial 351.8
> fallopian tube 620.8
> gait 781.2
> gastrointestinal (tract) 536.8
>> psychogenic 306.4
> glottis 478.75
>> hysterical 300.11
>> psychogenic 306.1
>>> specified as conversion reaction 300.11
>> reflex through recurrent laryngeal nerve 478.75
> habit 307.20
>> chronic 307.22
>> transient of childhood 307.21
> heart — *see* Angina
> hourglass — *see* Contraction, hourglass
> hysterical 300.11
> infantile (*see also* Epilepsy) 345.6 ☑5ᵗʰ
> internal oblique, eye 378.51

Spasm, spastic, spasticity (*see also* condition) — *continued*
> intestinal 564.9
>> psychogenic 306.4
> larynx, laryngeal 478.75
>> hysterical 300.11
>> psychogenic 306.1
>>> specified as conversion reaction 300.11
> levator palpebrae superioris 333.81
> lightning (*see also* Epilepsy) 345.6 ☑5ᵗʰ
> mobile 781.0
> muscle 728.85
>> back 724.8
>> psychogenic 306.0
> nerve, trigeminal 350.1
> nervous 306.0
> nodding 307.3
>> infantile (*see also* Epilepsy) 345.6 ☑5ᵗʰ
> occupational 300.89
> oculogyric 378.87
> ophthalmic artery 362.30
> orbicularis 781.0
> perineal 625.8
> peroneo-extensor (*see also* Flat, foot) 734
> pharynx (reflex) 478.29
>> hysterical 300.11
>> psychogenic 306.1
>>> specified as conversion reaction 300.11
> pregnant uterus, complicating delivery 661.4 ☑5ᵗʰ
> psychogenic 306.0
> pylorus 537.81
>> adult hypertrophic 537.0
>> congenital or infantile 750.5
>> psychogenic 306.4
> rectum (sphincter) 564.6
>> psychogenic 306.4
> retinal artery NEC (*see also* Occlusion, retina, artery) 362.30
> sacroiliac 724.6
> salaam (infantile) (*see also* Epilepsy) 345.6 ☑5ᵗʰ
> saltatory 781.0
> sigmoid 564.9
>> psychogenic 306.4
> sphincter of Oddi (*see also* Disease, gallbladder) 576.5
> stomach 536.8
>> neurotic 306.4
> throat 478.29
>> hysterical 300.11
>> psychogenic 306.1
>>> specified as conversion reaction 300.11
> tic 307.20
>> chronic 307.22
>> transient of childhood 307.21
> tongue 529.8
> torsion 333.6
> trigeminal nerve 350.1
>> postherpetic 053.12
> ureter 593.89
> urethra (sphincter) 599.84
> uterus 625.8
>> complicating labor 661.4 ☑5ᵗʰ
>>> affecting fetus or newborn 763.7
> vagina 625.1
>> psychogenic 306.51
> vascular NEC 443.9
> vasomotor NEC 443.9
> vein NEC 459.89
> vesical (sphincter, external or internal) 596.8
> viscera 789.0 ☑5ᵗʰ

Spasmodic — *see* condition

Spasmophilia (*see also* Tetany) 781.7

Spasmus nutans 307.3

Spastic — *see also* Spasm
> child 343.9

Spasticity — *see also* Spasm
> cerebral, child 343.9

Speakers' throat 784.49

Specific, specified — *see* condition

Speech
> defect, disorder, disturbance, impediment NEC 784.5
>> psychogenic 307.9
> therapy V57.3

Spells 780.39
> breath-holding 786.9

Spencer's disease (epidemic vomiting) 078.82

Spens' syndrome (syncope with heart block) 426.9

Spermatic cord — *see* condition

Spermatocele 608.1
> congenital 752.8

Spermatocystitis 608.4

Spermatocytoma (M9063/3)
> specified site — *see* Neoplasm, by site, malignant
> unspecified site 186.9

Spermatorrhea 608.89

Sperm counts
> fertility testing V26.21
> following sterilization reversal V26.22
> postvasectomy V25.8

Sphacelus (*see also* Gangrene) 785.4

Sphenoidal — *see* condition

Sphenoiditis (chronic) (*see also* Sinusitis, sphenoidal) 473.3

Sphenopalatine ganglion neuralgia 337.0

Sphericity, increased, lens 743.36

Spherocytosis (congenital) (familial) (hereditary) 282.0
> hemoglobin disease 282.7
> sickle-cell (disease) 282.60

Spherophakia 743.36

Sphincter — *see* condition

Sphincteritis, sphincter of Oddi (*see also* Cholecystitis) 576.8

Sphingolipidosis 272.7

Sphingolipodystrophy 272.7

Sphingomyelinosis 272.7

Spicule tooth 520.2

Spider
> finger 755.59
> nevus 448.1
> vascular 448.1

Spiegler-Fendt sarcoid 686.8

Spielmeyer-Stock disease 330.1

Spielmeyer-Vogt disease 330.1

Spina bifida (aperta) 741.9 ☑5ᵗʰ

> *Note — Use the following fifth-digit subclassification with category 741:*
>
> | | |
> |---|---|
> | *0* | *unspecified region* |
> | *1* | *cervical region* |
> | *2* | *dorsal [thoracic] region* |
> | *3* | *lumbar region* |

> with hydrocephalus 741.0 ☑5ᵗʰ
>> fetal (suspected), affecting management of pregnancy 655.0 ☑5ᵗʰ
> occulta 756.17

Spindle, Krukenberg's 371.13

Spine, spinal — *see* condition

Spiradenoma (eccrine) (M8403/0) — *see* Neoplasm, skin, benign

Spirillosis NEC (*see also* Fever, relapsing) 087.9

Spirillum minus 026.0

Spirillum obermeieri infection 087.0

Spirochetal — *see* condition

Spirochetosis 104.9
> arthritic, arthritica 104.9 [711.8] ☑5ᵗʰ
> bronchopulmonary 104.8
> icterohemorrhagica 100.0
> lung 104.8

Spitting blood (*see also* Hemoptysis) 786.3

Splanchnomegaly 569.89

Splanchnoptosis 569.89

Spleen, splenic — *see also* condition
> agenesis 759.0
> flexure syndrome 569.89
> neutropenia syndrome 288.0
> sequestration syndrome 282.60

Splenectasis (*see also* Splenomegaly) 789.2

Splenitis (interstitial) (malignant) (nonspecific) 289.59
  malarial (*see also* Malaria) 084.6
  tuberculous (*see also* Tuberculosis) 017.7 ✓5ᵗʰ
Splenocele 289.59
Splenomegalia — *see* Splenomegaly
Splenomegalic — *see* condition
Splenomegaly 789.2
  Bengal 789.2
  cirrhotic 289.51
  congenital 759.0
  congestive, chronic 289.51
  cryptogenic 789.2
  Egyptian 120.1
  Gaucher's (cerebroside lipidosis) 272.7
  idiopathic 789.2
  malarial (*see also* Malaria) 084.6
  neutropenic 288.0
  Niemann-Pick (lipid histiocytosis) 272.7
  siderotic 289.51
  syphilitic 095.8
    congenital 090.0
  tropical (Bengal) (idiopathic) 789.2
Splenopathy 289.50
Splenopneumonia — *see* Pneumonia
Splenoptosis 289.59
Splinter — *see* Injury, superficial, by site
Split, splitting
  heart sounds 427.89
  lip, congenital (*see also* Cleft, lip) 749.10
  nails 703.8
  urinary stream 788.61
Spoiled child reaction (*see also* Disturbance, conduct) 312.1 ✓5ᵗʰ
Spondylarthritis (*see also* Spondylosis) 721.90
Spondylarthrosis (*see also* Spondylosis) 721.90
Spondylitis 720.9
  ankylopoietica 720.0
  ankylosing (chronic) 720.0
  atrophic 720.9
    ligamentous 720.9
  chronic (traumatic) (*see also* Spondylosis) 721.90
  deformans (chronic) (*see also* Spondylosis) 721.90
  gonococcal 098.53
  gouty 274.0
  hypertrophic (*see also* Spondylosis) 721.90
  infectious NEC 720.9
  juvenile (adolescent) 720.0
  Kümmell's 721.7
  Marie-Strümpell (ankylosing) 720.0
  muscularis 720.9
  ossificans ligamentosa 721.6
  osteoarthritica (*see also* Spondylosis) 721.90
  posttraumatic 721.7
  proliferative 720.0
  rheumatoid 720.0
  rhizomelica 720.0
  sacroiliac NEC 720.2
  senescent (*see also* Spondylosis) 721.90
  senile (*see also* Spondylosis) 721.90
  static (*see also* Spondylosis) 721.90
  traumatic (chronic) (*see also* Spondylosis) 721.90
  tuberculous (*see also* Tuberculosis) 015.0 ✓5ᵗʰ [720.81]
  typhosa 002.0 [720.81]
Spondyloarthrosis (*see also* Spondylosis) 721.90
Spondylolisthesis (congenital) (lumbosacral) 756.12
  with disproportion (fetopelvic) 653.3 ✓5ᵗʰ
    affecting fetus or newborn 763.1
    causing obstructed labor 660.1 ✓5ᵗʰ
      affecting fetus or newborn 763.1
  acquired 738.4
  degenerative 738.4
  traumatic 738.4
    acute (lumbar) — *see* Fracture, vertebra, lumbar
    site other than lumbosacral — *see* Fracture, vertebra, by site
Spondylolysis (congenital) 756.11
  acquired 738.4
  cervical 756.19

Spondylolysis — *continued*
  lumbosacral region 756.11
    with disproportion (fetopelvic) 653.3 ✓5ᵗʰ
      affecting fetus or newborn 763.1
      causing obstructed labor 660.1 ✓5ᵗʰ
        affecting fetus or newborn 763.1
Spondylopathy
  inflammatory 720.9
    specified type NEC 720.89
  traumatic 721.7
Spondylose rhizomelique 720.0
Spondylosis 721.90
  with
    disproportion 653.3 ✓5ᵗʰ
      affecting fetus or newborn 763.1
      causing obstructed labor 660.1 ✓5ᵗʰ
        affecting fetus or newborn 763.1
    myelopathy NEC 721.91
  cervical, cervicodorsal 721.0
    with myelopathy 721.1
    inflammatory 720.9
  lumbar, lumbosacral 721.3
    with myelopathy 721.42
  sacral 721.3
    with myelopathy 721.42
  thoracic 721.2
    with myelopathy 721.41
  traumatic 721.7
Sponge
  divers' disease 989.5
  inadvertently left in operation wound 998.4
  kidney (medullary) 753.17
Spongioblastoma (M9422/3)
  multiforme (M9440/3)
    specified site — *see* Neoplasm, by site, malignant
    unspecified site 191.9
  polare (M9423/3)
    specified site — *see* Neoplasm, by site, malignant
    unspecified site 191.9
  primitive polar (M9443/3)
    specified site — *see* Neoplasm, by site, malignant
    unspecified site 191.9
  specified site — *see* Neoplasm, by site, malignant
  unspecified site 191.9
Spongiocytoma (M9400/3)
  specified site — *see* Neoplasm, by site, malignant
  unspecified site 191.9
Spongioneuroblastoma (M9504/3) — *see* Neoplasm, by site, malignant
Spontaneous — *see also* condition
  fracture — *see* Fracture, pathologic
Spoon nail 703.8
  congenital 757.5
Sporadic — *see* condition
Sporotrichosis (bones) (cutaneous) (disseminated) (epidermal) (lymphatic) (lymphocutaneous) (mucous membranes) (pulmonary) (skeletal) (visceral) 117.1
Sporotrichum schenckii infection 117.1
Spots, spotting
  atrophic (skin) 701.3
  Bitôt's (in the young child) 264.1
  café au lait 709.09
  cayenne pepper 448.1
  cotton wool (retina) 362.83
  de Morgan's (senile angiomas) 448.1
  Fúchs' black (myopic) 360.21
  intermenstrual
    irregular 626.6
    regular 626.5
  interpalpebral 372.53
  Koplik's 055.9
  liver 709.09
  Mongolian (pigmented) 757.33
  of pregnancy 641.9 ✓5ᵗʰ
  purpuric 782.7
  ruby 448.1
Spotted fever — *see* Fever, spotted

Sprain, strain (joint) (ligament) (muscle) (tendon) 848.9
  abdominal wall (muscle) 848.8
  Achilles tendon 845.09
  acromioclavicular 840.0
  ankle 845.00
    and foot 845.00
  anterior longitudinal, cervical 847.0
  arm 840.9
    upper 840.9
      and shoulder 840.9
  astragalus 845.00
  atlanto-axial 847.0
  atlanto-occipital 847.0
  atlas 847.0
  axis 847.0
  back (*see also* Sprain, spine) 847.9
  breast bone 848.40
  broad ligament — *see* Injury, internal, broad ligament
  calcaneofibular 845.02
  carpal 842.01
  carpometacarpal 842.11
  cartilage
    costal, without mention of injury to sternum 848.3
      involving sternum 848.42
    ear 848.8
    knee 844.9
      with current tear (*see also* Tear, meniscus) 836.2
    semilunar (knee) 844.8
      with current tear (*see also* Tear, meniscus) 836.2
    septal, nose 848.0
    thyroid region 848.2
    xiphoid 848.49
  cervical, cervicodorsal, cervicothoracic 847.0
  chondrocostal, without mention of injury to sternum 848.3
    involving sternum 848.42
  chondrosternal 848.42
  chronic (joint) — *see* Derangement, joint
  clavicle 840.9
  coccyx 847.4
  collar bone 840.9
  collateral, knee (medial) (tibial) 844.1
    lateral (fibular) 844.0
    recurrent or old 717.89
      lateral 717.81
      medial 717.82
  coracoacromial 840.8
  coracoclavicular 840.1
  coracohumeral 840.2
  coracoid (process) 840.9
  coronary, knee 844.8
  costal cartilage, without mention of injury to sternum 848.3
    involving sternum 848.42
  cricoarytenoid articulation 848.2
  cricothyroid articulation 848.2
  cruciate
    knee 844.2
    old 717.89
      anterior 717.83
      posterior 717.84
  deltoid
    ankle 845.01
    shoulder 840.8
  dorsal (spine) 847.1
  ear cartilage 848.8
  elbow 841.9
    and forearm 841.9
    specified site NEC 841.8
  femur (proximal end) 843.9
    distal end 844.9
  fibula (proximal end) 844.9
    distal end 845.00
  fibulocalcaneal 845.02
  finger(s) 842.10
  foot 845.10
    and ankle 845.00
  forearm 841.9
    and elbow 841.9
    specified site NEC 841.8
  glenoid (shoulder) (*see also* SLAP lesion) 840.8
  hand 842.10

Splenitis — Sprain, strain

Sprain, strain — *continued*
  hip 843.9
    and thigh 843.9
  humerus (proximal end) 840.9
    distal end 841.9
  iliofemoral 843.0
  infraspinatus 840.3
  innominate
    acetabulum 843.9
    pubic junction 848.5
    sacral junction 846.1
  internal
    collateral, ankle 845.01
    semilunar cartilage 844.8
      with current tear (*see also* Tear,
        meniscus) 836.2
      old 717.5
  interphalangeal
    finger 842.13
    toe 845.13
  ischiocapsular 843.1
  jaw (cartilage) (meniscus) 848.1
    old 524.69
  knee 844.9
    and leg 844.9
    old 717.5
      collateral
        lateral 717.81
        medial 717.82
      cruciate
        anterior 717.83
        posterior 717.84
  late effect — *see* Late, effects (of), sprain
  lateral collateral, knee 844.0
    old 717.81
  leg 844.9
    and knee 844.9
  ligamentum teres femoris 843.8
  low back 846.9
  lumbar (spine) 847.2
  lumbosacral 846.0
    chronic or old 724.6
  mandible 848.1
    old 524.69
  maxilla 848.1
  medial collateral, knee 844.1
    old 717.82
  meniscus
    jaw 848.1
      old 524.69
    knee 844.8
      with current tear (*see also* Tear,
        meniscus) 836.2
      old 717.5
    mandible 848.1
      old 524.69
    specified site NEC 848.8
  metacarpal 842.10
    distal 842.12
    proximal 842.11
  metacarpophalangeal 842.12
  metatarsal 845.10
  metatarsophalangeal 845.12
  midcarpal 842.19
  midtarsal 845.19
  multiple sites, except fingers alone or toes
      alone 848.8
  neck 847.0
  nose (septal cartilage) 848.0
  occiput from atlas 847.0
  old — *see* Derangement, joint
  orbicular, hip 843.8
  patella(r) 844.8
    old 717.89
  pelvis 848.5
  phalanx
    finger 842.10
    toe 845.10
  radiocarpal 842.02
  radiohumeral 841.2
  radioulnar 841.9
    distal 842.09
  radius, radial (proximal end) 841.9
    and ulna 841.9
      distal 842.09
    collateral 841.0
    distal end 842.00

Sprain, strain — *continued*
  recurrent — *see* Sprain, by site
  rib (cage), without mention of injury to sternum
      848.3
    involving sternum 848.42
  rotator cuff (capsule) 840.4
  round ligament — *see also* Injury, internal,
      round ligament
    femur 843.8
  sacral (spine) 847.3
  sacrococcygeal 847.3
  sacroiliac (region) 846.9
    chronic or old 724.6
    ligament 846.1
    specified site NEC 846.8
  sacrospinatus 846.2
  sacrospinous 846.2
  sacrotuberous 846.3
  scaphoid bone, ankle 845.00
  scapula(r) 840.9
  semilunar cartilage (knee) 844.8
    with current tear (*see also* Tear, meniscus)
      836.2
    old 717.5
  septal cartilage (nose) 848.0
  shoulder 840.9
    and arm, upper 840.9
    blade 840.9
    specified site NEC 848.8
  spine 847.9
    cervical 847.0
    coccyx 847.4
    dorsal 847.1
    lumbar 847.2
    lumbosacral 846.0
      chronic or old 724.6
    sacral 847.3
    sacroiliac (*see also* Sprain, sacroiliac) 846.9
      chronic or old 724.6
    thoracic 847.1
  sternoclavicular 848.41
  sternum 848.40
  subglenoid (*see also* SLAP lesion) 840.8
  subscapularis 840.5
  supraspinatus 840.6
  symphysis
    jaw 848.1
      old 524.69
    mandibular 848.1
      old 524.69
    pubis 848.5
  talofibular 845.09
  tarsal 845.10
  tarsometatarsal 845.11
  temporomandibular 848.1
    old 524.69
  teres
    ligamentum femoris 843.8
    major or minor 840.8
  thigh (proximal end) 843.9
    and hip 843.9
    distal end 844.9
  thoracic (spine) 847.1
  thorax 848.8
  thumb 842.10
  thyroid cartilage or region 848.2
  tibia (proximal end) 844.9
    distal end 845.00
  tibiofibular
    distal 845.03
    superior 844.3
  toe(s) 845.10
  trachea 848.8
  trapezoid 840.8
  ulna, ulnar (proximal end) 841.9
    collateral 841.1
    distal end 842.00
  ulnohumeral 841.3
  vertebrae (*see also* Sprain, spine) 847.9
    cervical, cervicodorsal, cervicothoracic 847.0
  wrist (cuneiform) (scaphoid) (semilunar) 842.00
  xiphoid cartilage 848.49

Sprengel's deformity (congenital) 755.52

Spring fever 309.23

Sprue 579.1
  celiac 579.0
  idiopathic 579.0

Sprue — *continued*
  meaning thrush 112.0
  nontropical 579.0
  tropical 579.1

Spur — *see also* Exostosis
  bone 726.91
    calcaneal 726.73
  calcaneal 726.73
  iliac crest 726.5
  nose (septum) 478.1
    bone 726.91
  septal 478.1

Spuria placenta — *see* Placenta, abnormal

Spurway's syndrome (brittle bones and blue
    sclera) 756.51

Sputum, abnormal (amount) (color) (excessive)
    (odor) (purulent) 786.4
  bloody 786.3

Squamous — *see also* condition
  cell metaplasia
    bladder 596.8
    cervix — *see* condition
  epithelium in
    cervical canal (congenital) 752.49
    uterine mucosa (congenital) 752.3
  metaplasia
    bladder 596.8
    cervix — *see* condition

Squashed nose 738.0
  congenital 754.0

Squeeze, divers' 993.3

Squint (*see also* Strabismus) 378.9
  accommodative (*see also* Esotropia) 378.00
  concomitant (*see also* Heterotropia) 378.30

Stab — *see also* Wound, open, by site
  internal organs — *see* Injury, internal, by site,
    with open wound

Staggering gait 781.2
  hysterical 300.11

Staghorn calculus 592.0

Stälh's
  ear 744.29
  pigment line (cornea) 371.11

Stälhi's pigment lines (cornea) 371.11

Stain
  port wine 757.32
  tooth, teeth (hard tissues) 521.7
    due to
      accretions 523.6
      deposits (betel) (black) (green) (materia
        alba) (orange) (tobacco) 523.6
      metals (copper) (silver) 521.7
      nicotine 523.6
      pulpal bleeding 521.7
      tobacco 523.6

Stammering 307.0

Standstill
  atrial 426.6
  auricular 426.6
  cardiac (*see also* Arrest, cardiac) 427.5
  sinoatrial 429.6
  sinus 426.6
  ventricular (*see also* Arrest, cardiac) 427.5

Stannosis 503

Stanton's disease (melioidosis) 025

Staphylitis (acute) (catarrhal) (chronic)
    (gangrenous) (membranous) (suppurative)
    (ulcerative) 528.3

Staphylococcemia 038.10
  aureus 038.11
  specified organism NEC 038.19

Staphylococcus, staphylococcal — *see* condition

Staphyloderma (skin) 686.00

Staphyloma 379.11
  anterior, localized 379.14
  ciliary 379.11
  cornea 371.73
  equatorial 379.13
  posterior 379.12
  posticum 379.12
  ring 379.15
  sclera NEC 379.11

Starch eating 307.52

Stargardt's disease 362.75
Starvation (inanition) (due to lack of food) 994.2
  edema 262
  voluntary NEC 307.1
Stasis
  bile (duct) (*see also* Disease, biliary) 576.8
  bronchus (*see also* Bronchitis) 490
  cardiac (*see also* Failure, heart) 428.0
  cecum 564.89
  colon 564.89
  dermatitis (*see also* Varix, with stasis
     dermatitis) 454.1
  duodenal 536.8
  eczema (*see also* Varix, with stasis dermatitis)
     454.1
  edema (*see also* Hypertension, venous) ●
     459.30 ●
  foot 991.4
  gastric 536.3
  ileocecal coil 564.89
  ileum 564.89
  intestinal 564.89
  jejunum 564.89
  kidney 586
  liver 571.9
    cirrhotic — *see* Cirrhosis, liver
  lymphatic 457.8
  pneumonia 514
  portal 571.9
  pulmonary 514
  rectal 564.89
  renal 586
    tubular 584.5
  stomach 536.3
  ulcer
    with varicose veins 454.0
    without varicose veins 459.81
  urine NEC (*see also* Retention, urine) 788.20
  venous 459.81
State
  affective and paranoid, mixed, organic
    psychotic 294.8
  agitated 307.9
    acute reaction to stress 308.2
  anxiety (neurotic) (*see also* Anxiety) 300.00
    specified type NEC 300.09
  apprehension (*see also* Anxiety) 300.00
    specified type NEC 300.09
  climacteric, female 627.2
    following induced menopause 627.4
  clouded
    epileptic (*see also* Epilepsy) 345.9 ✓5ᵗʰ
    paroxysmal (idiopathic) (*see also* Epilepsy)
     345.9 ✓5ᵗʰ
  compulsive (mixed) (with obsession) 300.3
  confusional 298.9
    acute 293.0
     with
      arteriosclerotic dementia 290.41
      presenile brain disease 290.11
      senility 290.3
     alcoholic 291.0
     drug-induced 292.81
    epileptic 293.0
    postoperative 293.9
    reactive (emotional stress) (psychological
     trauma) 298.2
    subacute 293.1
  constitutional psychopathic 301.9
  convulsive (*see also* Convulsions) 780.39
  depressive NEC 311
    induced by drug 292.84
    neurotic 300.4
  dissociative 300.15
  hallucinatory 780.1
    induced by drug 292.12
  hyperdynamic beta-adrenergic circulatory
    429.82
  locked-in 344.81
  menopausal 627.2
    artificial 627.4
    following induced menopause 627.4
  neurotic NEC 300.9
    with depersonalization episode 300.6
  obsessional 300.3
  oneiroid (*see also* Schizophrenia) 295.4 ✓5ᵗʰ
  panic 300.01

State — *continued*
  paranoid 297.9
    alcohol-induced 291.5
    arteriosclerotic 290.42
    climacteric 297.2
    drug-induced 292.11
    in
      presenile brain disease 290.12
      senile brain disease 290.20
    involutional 297.2
    menopausal 297.2
    senile 290.20
    simple 297.0
  postleukotomy 310.0
  pregnant (*see also* Pregnancy) V22.2
  psychogenic, twilight 298.2
  psychotic, organic (*see also* Psychosis, organic)
    294.9
    mixed paranoid and affective 294.8
    senile or presenile NEC 290.9
    transient NEC 293.9
     with
      anxiety 293.84
      delusions 293.81
      depression 293.83
      hallucinations 293.82
  residual schizophrenic (*see also* Schizophrenia)
    295.6 ✓5ᵗʰ
  tension (*see also* Anxiety) 300.9
  transient organic psychotic 293.9
    anxiety type 293.84
    depressive type 293.83
    hallucinatory type 293.83
    paranoid type 293.81
    specified type NEC 293.89
  twilight
    epileptic 293.0
    psychogenic 298.2
  vegetative (persistent) 780.03
Status (post)
  absence
    epileptic (*see also* Epilepsy) 345.2
    of organ, acquired (postsurgical) — *see*
     Absence, by site, acquired
  anastomosis of intestine (for bypass) V45.3
  angioplasty, percutaneous transluminal
    coronary V45.82
  anginosus 413.9
  ankle prosthesis V43.66
  aortocoronary bypass or shunt V45.81
  arthrodesis V45.4
  artificially induced condition NEC V45.89
  artificial opening (of) V44.9
    gastrointestinal tract NEC V44.4
    specified site NEC V44.8
    urinary tract NEC V44.6
    vagina V44.7
  aspirator V46.0
  asthmaticus (*see also* Asthma) 493.9 ✓5ᵗʰ
  breast implant removal V45.83
  cardiac
    device (in situ) V45.00
      carotid sinus V45.09
        fitting or adjustment V53.39
      defibrillator, automatic implantable
        V45.02
      pacemaker V45.01
        fitting or adjustmanet V53.31
  carotid sinus stimulator V45.09
  cataract extraction V45.61
  chemotherapy V66.2
    current V58.69
  colostomy V44.3
  contraceptive device V45.59
    intrauterine V45.51
    subdermal V45.52
  convulsivus idiopathicus (*see also* Epilepsy)
    345.3
  coronary artery bypass or shunt V45.81
  cystostomy V44.50
    appendico-vesicostomy V44.52
    cutaneous-vesicostomy V44.51
    specified type NEC V44.59
  defibrillator, automatic implant-able cardiac
    V45.02
  dental crowns V45.84
  dental fillings V45.84

Status — *continued*
  dental restoration V45.84
  dental sealant V49.82
  dialysis V45.1
  donor V59.9
  drug therapy or regimen V67.59
    high-risk medication NEC V67.51
  elbow prosthesis V43.62
  enterostomy V44.4
  epileptic, epilepticus (absence) (grand mal) (*see*
    also Epilepsy) 345.3
    focal motor 345.7 ✓5ᵗʰ
    partial 345.7 ✓5ᵗʰ
    petit mal 345.2
    psychomotor 345.7 ✓5ᵗʰ
    temporal lobe 345.7 ✓5ᵗʰ
  eye (adnexa) surgery V45.69
  filtering bleb (eye) (postglaucoma) V45.69
    with rupture or complication 997.99
    pastcataract extraction (complication)
     997.99
  finger joint prosthesis V43.69
  gastrostomy V44.1
  grand mal 345.3
  heart valve prosthesis V43.3
  hip prosthesis (joint) (partial) (total) V43.64
  ileostomy V44.2
  intestinal bypass V45.3
  intrauterine contraceptive device V45.51
  jejunostomy V44.4
  knee joint prosthesis V43.65
  lacunaris 437.8
  lacunosis 437.8
  low birth weight V21.30
    less than 500 grams V21.31
    500-999 grams V21.32
    1000-1499 grams V21.33
    1500-1999 grams V21.34
    2000-2500 grams V21.35
  lymphaticus 254.8
  malignant neoplasm, ablated or excised — *see*
    History, malignant neoplasm
  marmoratus 333.7
  nephrostomy V44.6
  neuropacemaker NEC V45.89
    brain V45.89
    carotid sinus V45.09
    neurologic NEC V45.89
  organ replacement
    by artificial or mechanical device or
     prosthesis of
     artery V43.4
     artificial skin V43.83
     bladder V43.5
     blood vessel V43.4
     breast V43.82
     eye globe V43.0
     heart V43.2
      valve V43.3
     intestine V43.89
     joint V43.60
      ankle V43.66
      elbow V43.62
      finger V43.69
      hip (partial) (total) V43.64
      knee V43.65
      shoulder V43.61
      specified NEC V43.69
      wrist V43.63
     kidney V43.89
     larynx V43.81
     lens V43.1
     limb(s) V43.7
     liver V43.89
     lung V43.89
     organ NEC V43.89
     pancreas V43.89
     skin (artificial) V43.83
     tissue NEC V43.89
     vein V43.4
    by organ transplant (heterologous)
     (homologous) — *see* Status, transplant
  pacemaker
    brain V45.89
    cardiac V45.01
    carotid sinus V45.09
    neurologic NEC V45.89

Status — *continued*
 pacemaker — *continued*
  specified site NEC V45.89
 percutaneous transluminal coronary
   angioplasty V45.82
 petit mal 345.2
 postcommotio cerebri 310.2
 postmenopausal (age related) (natural) V49.81
 postoperative NEC V45.89
 postpartum NEC V24.2
  care immediately following delivery V24.0
  routine follow-up V24.2
 postsurgical NEC V45.89
 renal dialysis V45.1
 respirator V46.1
 reversed jejunal transposition (for bypass)
   V45.3
 shoulder prosthesis V43.61
 shunt
  aortocoronary bypass V45.81
  arteriovenous (for dialysis) V45.1
  cerebrospinal fluid V45.2
  vascular NEC V45.89
   aortocoronary (bypass) V45.81
  ventricular (communicating) (for drainage)
    V45.2
 sterilization
  tubal ligation V26.51
  vasectomy V26.52
 subdermal contraceptive device V45.52
 thymicolymphaticus 254.8
 thymicus 254.8
 thymolymphaticus 254.8
 tooth extraction 525.10
 tracheostomy V44.0
 transplant
  blood vessel V42.89
  bone V42.4
   marrow V42.81
  cornea V42.5
  heart V42.1
   valve V42.2
  intestine V42.84
  kidney V42.0
  liver V42.7
  lung V42.6
  organ V42.9
   specified site NEC V42.89
  pancreas V42.83
  peripheral stem cells V42.82
  skin V42.3
  stem cells, peripheral V42.82
  tissue V42.9
   specified type NEC V42.89
  vessel, blood V42.89
 tubal ligation V26.51
 ureterostomy V44.6
 urethrostomy V44.6
 vagina, artificial V44.7
 vascular shunt NEC V45.89
  aortocoronary (bypass) V45.81
 vasectomy V26.52
 ventilator V46.1
 wrist prosthesis V43.63
Stave fracture — *see* Fracture, metacarpus,
  metacarpal bone(s)
Steal
 subclavian artery 435.2
 vertebral artery 435.1
Stealing, solitary, child problem (*see also*
  Disturbance, conduct) 312.1 ✔5ᵗʰ
Steam burn — *see* Burn, by site
Steatocystoma multiplex 706.2
Steatoma (infected) 706.2
 eyelid (cystic) 374.84
  infected 373.13
Steatorrhea (chronic) 579.8
 with lacteal obstruction 579.2
 idiopathic 579.0
  adult 579.0
  infantile 579.0
 pancreatic 579.4
 primary 579.0
 secondary 579.8
 specified cause NEC 579.8
 tropical 579.1

Steatosis 272.8
 heart (*see also* Degeneration, myocardial) 429.1
 kidney 593.89
 liver 571.8
Steele-Richardson (-Olszewski) Syndrome 333.0
Stein's syndrome (polycystic ovary) 256.4
Stein-Leventhal syndrome (polycystic ovary)
  256.4
Steinbrocker's syndrome (*see also* Neuropathy,
  peripheral, autonomic) 337.9
Steinert's disease 359.2
Stenocardia (*see also* Angina) 413.9
Stenocephaly 756.0
Stenosis (cicatricial) — *see also* Stricture
 ampulla of Vater 576.2
  with calculus, cholelithiasis, or stones — *see*
    Choledocholithiasis
 anus, anal (canal) (sphincter) 569.2
  congenital 751.2
 aorta (ascending) 747.22
  arch 747.10
  arteriosclerotic 440.0
  calcified 440.0
 aortic (valve) 424.1
  with
   mitral (valve)
    insufficiency or incompetence 396.2
    stenosis or obstruction 396.0
  atypical 396.0
  congenital 746.3
  rheumatic 395.0
   with
    insufficiency, incompetency or
      regurgitation 395.2
     with mitral (valve) disease 396.8
    mitral (valve)
     disease (stenosis) 396.0
     insufficiency or incompetence 396.2
     stenosis or obstruction 396.0
  specified cause, except rheumatic 424.1
  syphilitic 093.22
 aqueduct of Sylvius (congenital) 742.3
  with spina bifida (*see also* Spina bifida)
    741.0 ✔5ᵗʰ
  acquired 331.4
 artery NEC 447.1
  basilar — *see* Narrowing, artery, basilar
  carotid (common) (internal) — *see*
    Narrowing, artery, carotid
  celiac 447.4
  cerebral 437.0
   due to
    embolism (*see also* Embolism, brain)
      434.1 ✔5ᵗʰ
    thrombus (*see also* Thrombosis, brain)
      434.0 ✔5ᵗʰ
  precerebral — *see* Narrowing, artery,
    precerebral
  pulmonary (congenital) 747.3
   acquired 417.8
  renal 440.1
  vertebral — *see* Narrowing, artery, vertebral
 bile duct or biliary passage (*see also*
   Obstruction, biliary) 576.2
  congenital 751.61
 bladder neck (acquired) 596.0
  congenital 753.6
 brain 348.8
 bronchus 519.1
  syphilitic 095.8
 cardia (stomach) 537.89
  congenital 750.7
 cardiovascular (*see also* Disease,
   cardiovascular) 429.2
 carotid artery — *see* Narrowing, artery, carotid
 cervix, cervical (canal) 622.4
  congenital 752.49
  in pregnancy or childbirth 654.6 ✔5ᵗʰ
   affecting fetus or newborn 763.89
   causing obstructed labor 660.2 ✔5ᵗʰ
    affecting fetus or newborn 763.1
 colon (*see also* Obstruction, intestine) 560.9
  congenital 751.2
 colostomy 569.62
 common bile duct (*see also* Obstruction,
   biliary) 576.2
  congenital 751.61

Stenosis — *see also* Stricture — *continued*
 coronary (artery) —*see* Arteriosclerosis,
   coronary
 cystic duct (*see also* Obstruction, gallbladder)
   575.2
  congenital 751.61
 due to (presence of) any device, implant, or
   graft classifiable to 996.0-996.5 — *see*
   Complications, due to (presence of) any
   device, implant, or graft classified to
   996.0-996.5 NEC
 duodenum 537.3
  congenital 751.1
 ejaculatory duct NEC 608.89
 endocervical os — *see* Stenosis, cervix
 enterostomy 569.62
 esophagus 530.3
  congenital 750.3
  syphilitic 095.8
   congenital 090.5
 external ear canal 380.50
  secondary to
   inflammation 380.53
   surgery 380.52
   trauma 380.51
 gallbladder (*see also* Obstruction, gallbladder)
   575.2
 glottis 478.74
 heart valve (acquired) — *see also* Endocarditis
  congenital NEC 746.89
   aortic 746.3
   mitral 746.5
   pulmonary 746.02
   tricuspid 746.1
 hepatic duct (*see also* Obstruction, biliary)
   576.2
 hymen 623.3
 hypertrophic subaortic (idiopathic) 425.1
 infundibulum cardiac 746.83
 intestine (*see also* Obstruction, intestine) 560.9
  congenital (small) 751.1
   large 751.2
 lacrimal
  canaliculi 375.53
  duct 375.56
   congenital 743.65
  punctum 375.52
   congenital 743.65
  sac 375.54
   congenital 743.65
 lacrimonasal duct 375.56
  congenital 743.65
  neonatal 375.55
 larynx 478.74
  congenital 748.3
  syphilitic 095.8
   congenital 090.5
 mitral (valve) (chronic) (inactive) 394.0
  with
   aortic (valve)
    disease (insufficiency) 396.1
    insufficiency or incompetence 396.1
    stenosis or obstruction 396.0
   incompetency, insufficiency or
     regurgitation 394.2
    with aortic valve disease 396.8
  active or acute 391.1
   with chorea (acute) (rheumatic)
     (Sydenham's) 392.0
  congenital 746.5
  specified cause, except rheumatic 424.0
  syphilitic 093.21
 myocardium, myocardial (*see also*
   Degeneration, myocardial) 429.1
  hypertrophic subaortic (idiopathic) 425.1
 nares (anterior) (posterior) 478.1
  congenital 748.0
 nasal duct 375.56
  congenital 743.65
 nasolacrimal duct 375.56
  congenital 743.65
  neonatal 375.55
 organ or site, congenital NEC — *see* Atresia
 papilla of Vater 576.2
  with calculus, cholelithiasis, or stones — *see*
    Choledocholithiasis

Status — Stenosis *(side tab)*

Stenosis — *see also* Stricture — *continued*
  pulmonary (artery) (congenital) 747.3
    with ventricular septal defect, dextraposition
        of aorta and hypertrophy of right
        ventricle 745.2
    acquired 417.8
    infundibular 746.83
    in tetralogy of Fallot 745.2
    subvalvular 746.83
    valve (*see also* Endocarditis, pulmonary)
        424.3
      congenital 746.02
    vein 747.49
      acquired 417.8
    vessel NEC 417.8
  pulmonic (congenital) 746.02
    infundibular 746.83
    subvalvular 746.83
  pylorus (hypertrophic) 537.0
    adult 537.0
    congenital 750.5
    infantile 750.5
  rectum (sphincter) (*see also* Stricture, rectum)
      569.2
  renal artery 440.1
  salivary duct (any) 527.8
  sphincter of Oddi (*see also* Obstruction, biliary)
      576.2
  spinal 724.00
    cervical 723.0
    lumbar, lumbosacral 724.02
    nerve (root) NEC 724.9
    specified region NEC 724.09
    thoracic, thoracolumbar 724.01
  stomach, hourglass 537.6
  subaortic 746.81
    hypertrophic (idiopathic) 425.1
  supra (valvular)-aortic 747.22
  trachea 519.1
    congenital 748.3
    syphilitic 095.8
    tuberculous (*see also* Tuberculosis)
        012.8 ✓5ᵗʰ
  tracheostomy 519.02
  tricuspid (valve) (*see also* Endocarditis,
      tricuspid) 397.0
    congenital 746.1
    nonrheumatic 424.2
  tubal 628.2
  ureter (*see also* Stricture, ureter) 593.3
    congenital 753.29
  urethra (*see also* Stricture, urethra) 598.9
  vagina 623.2
    congenital 752.49
    in pregnancy or childbirth 654.7 ✓5ᵗʰ
      affecting fetus or newborn 763.89
      causing obstructed labor 660.2 ✓5ᵗʰ
        affecting fetus or newborn 763.1
  valve (cardiac) (heart) (*see also* Endocarditis)
      424.90
    congenital NEC 746.89
      aortic 746.3
      mitral 746.5
      pulmonary 746.02
      tricuspid 746.1
      urethra 753.6
  valvular (*see also* Endocarditis) 424.90
    congenital NEC 746.89
      urethra 753.6
  vascular graft or shunt 996.1
    atherosclerosis — *see* Arteriosclerosis,
        extremitites
    embolism 996.74
    occlusion NEC 996.74
    thrombus 996.74
  vena cava (inferior) (superior) 459.2
    congenital 747.49
  ventricular shunt 996.2
  vulva 624.8
Stercolith (*see also* Fecalith) 560.39
  appendix 543.9
Stercoraceous, stercoral ulcer 569.82
  anus or rectum 569.41
Stereopsis, defective
  with fusion 368.33
  without fusion 368.32
Stereotypes NEC 307.3

Sterility
  female — *see* Infertility, female
  male (*see also* Infertility, male) 606.9
Sterilization, admission for V25.2
  status
    tubal ligation V26.51
    vasectomy V26.52
Sternalgia (*see also* Angina) 413.9
Sternopagus 759.4
Sternum bifidum 756.3
Sternutation 784.9
Steroid
  effects (adverse) (iatrogenic)
    cushingoid
      correct substance properly administered
          255.0
      overdose or wrong substance given or
          taken 962.0
    diabetes
      correct substance properly administered
          251.8
      overdose or wrong substance given or
          taken 962.0
    due to
      correct substance properly administered
          255.8
      overdose or wrong substance given or
          taken 962.0
    fever
      correct substance properly administered
          780.6
      overdose or wrong substance given or
          taken 962.0
    withdrawal
      correct substance properly administered
          255.4
      overdose or wrong substance given or
          taken 962.0
  responder 365.03
Stevens-Johnson disease or syndrome
    (erythema multiforme exudativum) 695.1
Stewart-Morel syndrome (hyperostosis frontalis
    interna) 733.3
Sticker's disease (erythema infectiosum) 057.0
Sticky eye 372.03
Stieda's disease (calcification, knee joint) 726.62
Stiff
  back 724.8
  neck (*see also* Torticollis) 723.5
Stiff-man syndrome 333.91
Stiffness, joint NEC 719.50
  ankle 719.57
  back 724.8
  elbow 719.52
  finger 719.54
  hip 719.55
  knee 719.56
  multiple sites 719.59
  sacroiliac 724.6
  shoulder 719.51
  specified site NEC 719.58
  spine 724.9
  surgical fusion V45.4
  wrist 719.53
Stigmata, congenital syphilis 090.5
Still's disease or syndrome 714.30
Still-Felty syndrome (rheumatoid arthritis with
    splenomegaly and leukopenia) 714.1
Stillbirth, stillborn NEC 779.9
Stiller's disease (asthenia) 780.79
Stilling-Türk-Duane syndrome (ocular retraction
    syndrome) 378.71
Stimulation, ovary 256.1
Sting (animal) (bee) (fish) (insect) (jellyfish)
    (Portuguese man-o-war) (wasp) (venomous)
    989.5
  anaphylactic shock or reaction 989.5
  plant 692.6
Stippled epiphyses 756.59

Stitch
  abscess 998.59
  burst (in ▶external◀ operation wound)   ▲
      998.32
    internal 998.31   ●
  in back 724.5
Stojano's (subcostal) syndrome 098.86
Stokes' disease (exophthalmic goiter) 242.0 ✓5ᵗʰ
Stokes-Adams syndrome (syncope with heart
    block) 426.9
Stokvis' (-Talma) disease (enterogenous cyanosis)
    289.7
Stomach — *see* condition
Stoma malfunction
  colostomy 569.62
  cystostomy 997.5
  enterostomy 569.62
  gastrostomy 536.42
  ileostomy 569.62
  nephrostomy 997.5
  tracheostomy 519.02
  ureterostomy 997.5
Stomatitis 528.0
  angular 528.5
    due to dietary or vitamin deficiency 266.0
  aphthous 528.2
  candidal 112.0
  catarrhal 528.0
  denture 528.9
  diphtheritic (membranous) 032.0
  due to
    dietary deficiency 266.0
    thrush 112.0
    vitamin deficiency 266.0
  epidemic 078.4
  epizootic 078.4
  follicular 528.0
  gangrenous 528.1
  herpetic 054.2
  herpetiformis 528.2
  malignant 528.0
  membranous acute 528.0
  monilial 112.0
  mycotic 112.0
  necrotic 528.1
    ulcerative 101
  necrotizing ulcerative 101
  parasitic 112.0
  septic 528.0
  spirochetal 101
  suppurative (acute) 528.0
  ulcerative 528.0
    necrotizing 101
  ulceromembranous 101
  vesicular 528.0
    with exanthem 074.3
  Vincent's 101
Stomatocytosis 282.8
Stomatomycosis 112.0
Stomatorrhagia 528.9
Stone(s) — *see also* Calculus
  bladder 594.1
    diverticulum 594.0
  cystine 270.0
  heart syndrome (*see also* Failure, ventricular,
      left) 428.1
  kidney 592.0
  prostate 602.0
  pulp (dental) 522.2
  renal 592.0
  salivary duct or gland (any) 527.5
  ureter 592.1
  urethra (impacted) 594.2
  urinary (duct) (impacted) (passage) 592.9
    bladder 594.1
      diverticulum 594.0
    lower tract NEC 594.9
    specified site 594.8
  xanthine 277.2
Stonecutters' lung 502
  tuberculous (*see also* Tuberculosis) 011.4 ✓5ᵗʰ
Stonemasons'
  asthma, disease, or lung 502
    tuberculous (*see also* Tuberculosis)
        011.4 ✓5ᵗʰ

✓4ᵗʰ Fourth-digit Required   ✓5ᵗʰ Fifth-digit Required   ▶◀ Revised Text   ● New Line   ▲ Revised Code

Stonemasons' — Stricture *(side tab)*

Stonemasons' — *continued*
phthisis (*see also* Tuberculosis) 011.4 ✓5ᵗʰ
Stoppage
bowel (*see also* Obstruction, intestine) 560.9
heart (*see also* Arrest, cardiac) 427.5
intestine (*see also* Obstruction, intestine) 560.9
urine NEC (*see also* Retention, urine) 788.20
Storm, thyroid (apathetic) (*see also*
Thyrotoxicosis) 242.9 ✓5ᵗʰ
Strabismus (alternating) (congenital)
(nonparalytic) 378.9
concomitant (*see also* Heterotropia) 378.30
convergent (*see also* Esotropia) 378.00
divergent (*see also* Exotropia) 378.10
convergent (*see also* Esotropia) 378.00
divergent (*see also* Exotropia) 378.10
due to adhesions, scars — *see* Strabismus,
mechanical
in neuromuscular disorder NEC 378.73
intermittent 378.20
vertical 378.31
latent 378.40
convergent (esophoria) 378.41
divergent (exophoria) 378.42
vertical 378.43
mechanical 378.60
due to
Brown's tendon sheath syndrome 378.61
specified musculofascial disorder NEC
378.62
paralytic 378.50
third or oculomotor nerve (partial) 378.51
total 378.52
fourth or trochlear nerve 378.53
sixth or abducens nerve 378.54
specified type NEC 378.73
vertical (hypertropia) 378.31
Strain — *see also* Sprain, by site
eye NEC 368.13
heart — *see* Disease, heart
meaning gonorrhea — *see* Gonorrhea
physical NEC V62.89
postural 729.9
psychological NEC V62.89
Strands
conjunctiva 372.62
vitreous humor 379.25
Strangulation, strangulated 994.7
appendix 543.9
asphyxiation or suffocation by 994.7
bladder neck 596.0
bowel — *see* Strangulation, intestine
colon — *see* Strangulation, intestine
cord (umbilical) — *see* Compression, umbilical
cord
due to birth injury 767.8
food or foreign body (*see also* Asphyxia, food)
933.1
hemorrhoids 455.8
external 455.5
internal 455.2
hernia — *see also* Hernia, by site, with
obstruction
gangrenous — *see* Hernia, by site, with
gangrene
intestine (large) (small) 560.2
with hernia — *see also* Hernia, by site, with
obstruction
gangrenous — *see* Hernia, by site, with
gangrene
congenital (small) 751.1
large 751.2
mesentery 560.2
mucus (*see also* Asphyxia, mucus) 933.1
newborn 770.1
omentum 560.2
organ or site, congenital NEC — *see* Atresia
ovary 620.8
due to hernia 620.4
penis 607.89
foreign body 939.3
rupture (*see also* Hernia, by site, with
obstruction) 552.9
gangrenous (*see also* Hernia, by site, with
gangrene) 551.9

Strangulation, strangulated — *continued*
stomach, due to hernia (*see also* Hernia, by
site, with obstruction) 552.9
with gangrene (*see also* Hernia, by site, with
gangrene) 551.9
umbilical cord — *see* Compression, umbilical
cord
vesicourethral orifice 596.0
Strangury 788.1
Strawberry
gallbladder (*see also* Disease, gallbladder)
575.6
mark 757.32
tongue (red) (white) 529.3
Straw itch 133.8
Streak, ovarian 752.0
Strephosymbolia 315.01
secondary to organic lesion 784.69
Streptobacillary fever 026.1
Streptobacillus moniliformis 026.1
Streptococcemia 038.0
Streptococcicosis — *see* Infection, streptococcal
Streptococcus, streptococcal — *see* condition
Streptoderma 686.00
Streptomycosis — *see* Actinomycosis
Streptothricosis — *see* Actinomycosis
Streptothrix — *see* Actinomycosis
Streptotrichosis — *see* Actinomycosis
Stress
fracture — *see* Fracture, stress
polycythemia 289.0
reaction (gross) (*see also* Reaction, stress,
acute) 308.9
Stretching, nerve — *see* Injury, nerve, by site
Striae (albicantes) (atrophicae) (cutis distensae)
(distensae) 701.3
Striations of nails 703.8
Stricture (*see also* Stenosis) 799.8
ampulla of Vater 576.2
with calculus, cholelithiasis, or stones — *see*
Choledocholithiasis
anus (sphincter) 569.2
congenital 751.2
infantile 751.2
aorta (ascending) 747.22
arch 747.10
arteriosclerotic 440.0
calcified 440.0
aortic (valve) (*see also* Stenosis, aortic) 424.1
congenital 746.3
aqueduct of Sylvius (congenital) 742.3
with spina bifida (*see also* Spina bifida)
741.0 ✓5ᵗʰ
acquired 331.4
artery 447.1
basilar — *see* Narrowing, artery, basilar
carotid (common) (internal) — *see*
Narrowing, artery, carotid
celiac 447.4
cerebral 437.0
congenital 747.81
due to
embolism (*see also* Embolism, brain)
434.1 ✓5ᵗʰ
thrombus (*see also* Thrombosis, brain)
434.0 ✓5ᵗʰ
congenital (peripheral) 747.60
cerebral 747.81
coronary 746.85
gastrointestinal 747.61
lower limb 747.64
renal 747.62
retinal 743.58
specified NEC 747.69
spinal 747.82
umbilical 747.5
upper limb 747.63
coronary — *see* Arteriosclerosis, coronary
congenital 746.85
precerebral — *see* Narrowing, artery,
precerebral NEC
pulmonary (congenital) 747.3
acquired 417.8

Stricture (*see also* Stenosis) — *continued*
artery — *continued*
renal 440.1
vertebral — *see* Narrowing, artery, vertebral
auditory canal (congenital) (external) 744.02
acquired (*see also* Stricture, ear canal,
acquired) 380.50
bile duct or passage (any) (postoperative) (*see
also* Obstruction, biliary) 576.2
congenital 751.61
bladder 596.8
congenital 753.6
neck 596.0
congenital 753.6
bowel (*see also* Obstruction, intestine) 560.9
brain 348.8
bronchus 519.1
syphilitic 095.8
cardia (stomach) 537.89
congenital 750.7
cardiac — *see also* Disease, heart
orifice (stomach) 537.89
cardiovascular (*see also* Disease,
cardiovascular) 429.2
carotid artery — *see* Narrowing, artery, carotid
cecum (*see also* Obstruction, intestine) 560.9
cervix, cervical (canal) 622.4
congenital 752.49
in pregnancy or childbirth 654.6 ✓5ᵗʰ
affecting fetus or newborn 763.89
causing obstructed labor 660.2 ✓5ᵗʰ
affecting fetus or newborn 763.1
colon (*see also* Obstruction, intestine) 560.9
congenital 751.2
colostomy 569.62
common bile duct (*see also* Obstruction,
biliary) 576.2
congenital 751.61
coronary (artery) — *see* Arteriosclerosis,
coronary
congenital 746.85
cystic duct (*see also* Obstruction, gallbladder)
575.2
congenital 751.61
cystostomy 997.5
digestive organs NEC, congenital 751.8
duodenum 537.3
congenital 751.1
ear canal (external) (congenital) 744.02
acquired 380.50
secondary to
inflammation 380.53
surgery 380.52
trauma 380.51
ejaculatory duct 608.85
enterostomy 569.62
esophagus (corrosive) (peptic) 530.3
congenital 750.3
syphilitic 095.8
congenital 090.5
eustachian tube (*see also* Obstruction,
Eustachian tube) 381.60
congenital 744.24
fallopian tube 628.2
gonococcal (chronic) 098.37
acute 098.17
tuberculous (*see also* Tuberculosis)
016.6 ✓5ᵗʰ
gallbladder (*see also* Obstruction, gallbladder)
575.2
congenital 751.69
glottis 478.74
heart — *see also* Disease, heart
congenital NEC 746.89
valve — *see also* Endocarditis
congenital NEC 746.89
aortic 746.3
mitral 746.5
pulmonary 746.02
tricuspid 746.1
hepatic duct (*see also* Obstruction, biliary)
576.2
hourglass, of stomach 537.6
hymen 623.3
hypopharynx 478.29

Stricture (*see also* Stenosis) — *continued*
  intestine (*see also* Obstruction, intestine) 560.9
    congenital (small) 751.1
      large 751.2
    ischemic 557.1
  lacrimal
    canaliculi 375.53
      congenital 743.65
    punctum 375.52
      congenital 743.65
    sac 375.54
      congenital 743.65
  lacrimonasal duct 375.56
    congenital 743.65
    neonatal 375.55
  larynx 478.79
    congenital 748.3
    syphilitic 095.8
      congenital 090.5
  lung 518.89
  meatus
    ear (congenital) 744.02
      acquired (*see also* Stricture, ear canal, acquired) 380.50
    osseous (congenital) (ear) 744.03
      acquired (*see also* Stricture, ear canal, acquired) 380.50
    urinarius (*see also* Stricture, urethra) 598.9
      congenital 753.6
  mitral (valve) (*see also* Stenosis, mitral) 394.0
    congenital 746.5
    specified cause, except rheumatic 424.0
  myocardium, myocardial (*see also* Degeneration, myocardial) 429.1
    hypertrophic subaortic (idiopathic) 425.1
  nares (anterior) (posterior) 478.1
    congenital 748.0
  nasal duct 375.56
    congenital 743.65
    neonatal 375.55
  nasolacrimal duct 375.56
    congenital 743.65
    neonatal 375.55
  nasopharynx 478.29
    syphilitic 095.8
  nephrostomy 997.5
  nose 478.1
    congenital 748.0
  nostril (anterior) (posterior) 478.1
    congenital 748.0
  organ or site, congenital NEC — *see* Atresia
  osseous meatus (congenital) (ear) 744.03
    acquired (*see also* Stricture, ear canal, acquired) 380.50
  os uteri (*see also* Stricture, cervix) 622.4
  oviduct — *see* Stricture, fallopian tube
  pelviureteric junction 593.3
  pharynx (dilation) 478.29
  prostate 602.8
  pulmonary, pulmonic
    artery (congenital) 747.3
      acquired 417.8
      noncongenital 417.8
    infundibulum (congenital) 746.83
    valve (*see also* Endocarditis, pulmonary) 424.3
      congenital 746.02
    vein (congenital) 747.49
      acquired 417.8
    vessel NEC 417.8
  punctum lacrimale 375.52
    congenital 743.65
  pylorus (hypertrophic) 537.0
    adult 537.0
    congenital 750.5
    infantile 750.5
  rectosigmoid 569.89
  rectum (sphincter) 569.2
    congenital 751.2
    due to
      chemical burn 947.3
      irradiation 569.2
      lymphogranuloma venereum 099.1
    gonococcal 098.7
    inflammatory 099.1
    syphilitic 095.8

Stricture (*see also* Stenosis) — *continued*
  rectum — *continued*
    tuberculous (*see also* Tuberculosis) 014.8 ✓5ᵗʰ
  renal artery 440.1
  salivary duct or gland (any) 527.8
  sigmoid (flexure) (*see also* Obstruction, intestine) 560.9
  spermatic cord 608.85
  stoma (following) (of)
    colostomy 569.62
    cystostomy 997.5
    enterostomy 569.62
    gastrostomy 536.42
    ileostomy 569.62
    nephrostomy 997.5
    tracheostomy 519.02
    ureterostomy 997.5
  stomach 537.89
    congenital 750.7
    hourglass 537.6
  subaortic 746.81
    hypertrophic (acquired) (idiopathic) 425.1
  subglottic 478.74
  syphilitic NEC 095.8
  tendon (sheath) 727.81
  trachea 519.1
    congenital 748.3
    syphilitic 095.8
    tuberculous (*see also* Tuberculosis) 012.8 ✓5ᵗʰ
  tracheostomy 519.02
  tricuspid (valve) (*see also* Endocarditis, tricuspid) 397.0
    congenital 746.1
    nonrheumatic 424.2
  tunica vaginalis 608.85
  ureter (postoperative) 593.3
    congenital 753.29
    tuberculous (*see also* Tuberculosis) 016.2 ✓5ᵗʰ
  ureteropelvic junction 593.3
    congenital 753.21
  ureterovesical orifice 593.3
    congenital 753.22
  urethra (anterior) (meatal) (organic) (posterior) (spasmodic) 598.9
    associated with schistosomiasis (*see also* Schistosomiasis) 120.9 [598.01]
    congenital (valvular) 753.6
    due to
      infection 598.00
        syphilis 095.8 [598.01]
      trauma 598.1
    gonococcal 098.2 [598.01]
    gonorrheal 098.2 [598.01]
    infective 598.00
    late effect of injury 598.1
    postcatheterization 598.2
    postobstetric 598.1
    postoperative 598.2
    specified cause NEC 598.8
    syphilitic 095.8 [598.01]
    traumatic 598.1
    valvular, congenital 753.6
  urinary meatus (*see also* Stricture, urethra) 598.9
    congenital 753.6
  uterus, uterine 621.5
    os (external) (internal) — *see* Stricture, cervix
  vagina (outlet) 623.2
    congenital 752.49
  valve (cardiac) (heart) (*see also* Endocarditis) 424.90
    congenital (cardiac) (heart) NEC 746.89
      aortic 746.3
      mitral 746.5
      pulmonary 746.02
      tricuspid 746.1
      urethra 753.6
  valvular (*see also* Endocarditis) 424.90
  vascular graft or shunt 996.1
    atherosclerosis — *see* Arteriosclerosis, extremities
    embolism 996.74
    occlusion NEC 996.74
    thrombus 996.74

Stricture (*see also* Stenosis) — *continued*
  vas deferens 608.85
    congenital 752.8
  vein 459.2
  vena cava (inferior) (superior) NEC 459.2
    congenital 747.49
  ventricular shunt 996.2
  vesicourethral orifice 596.0
    congenital 753.6
  vulva (acquired) 624.8
Stridor 786.1
  congenital (larynx) 748.3
Stridulous — *see* condition
Strippling of nails 703.8
Stroke (*see also* Disease, cerebrovascular, acute) 436
  apoplectic (*see also* Disease, cerebrovascular, acute) 436
  brain (*see also* Disease, cerebrovascular, acute) 436
  epileptic — *see* Epilepsy
  healed or old V12.59
  heart — *see* Disease, heart
  heat 992.0
  iatrogenic 997.02
  in evolution 435.9
  late effect — *see* Late effect(s) (of) cerebrovascular disease
  lightning 994.0
  paralytic (*see also* Disease, cerebrovascular, acute) 436
  postoperative 997.02
  progressive 435.9
Stromatosis, endometrial (M8931/1) 236.0
Strong pulse 785.9
Strongyloides stercoralis infestation 127.2
Strongyloidiasis 127.2
Strongyloidosis 127.2
Strongylus (gibsoni) infestation 127.7
Strophulus (newborn) 779.89   ▲
  pruriginosus 698.2
Struck by lightning 994.0
Struma (*see also* Goiter) 240.9
  fibrosa 245.3
  Hashimoto (struma lymphomatosa) 245.2
  lymphomatosa 245.2
  nodosa (simplex) 241.9
    endemic 241.9
    multinodular 241.1
    sporadic 241.9
    toxic or with hyperthyroidism 242.3 ✓5ᵗʰ
      multinodular 242.2 ✓5ᵗʰ
      uninodular 242.1 ✓5ᵗʰ
    toxicosa 242.3 ✓5ᵗʰ
      multinodular 242.2 ✓5ᵗʰ
      uninodular 242.1 ✓5ᵗʰ
    uninodular 241.0
  ovarii (M9090/0) 220
    and carcinoid (M9091/1) 236.2
    malignant (M9090/3) 183.0
  Riedel's (ligneous thyroiditis) 245.3
  scrofulous (*see also* Tuberculosis) 017.2 ✓5ᵗʰ
  tuberculous (*see also* Tuberculosis) 017.2 ✓5ᵗʰ
    abscess 017.2 ✓5ᵗʰ
    adenitis 017.2 ✓5ᵗʰ
    lymphangitis 017.2 ✓5ᵗʰ
    ulcer 017.2 ✓5ᵗʰ
Strumipriva cachexia (*see also* Hypothyroidism) 244.9
Strümpell-Marie disease or spine (ankylosing spondylitis) 720.0
Strümpell-Westphal pseudosclerosis (hepatolenticular degeneration) 275.1
Stuart's disease (congenital factor X deficiency) (*see also* Defect, coagulation) 286.3
Stuart-Prower factor deficiency (congenital factor X deficiency) (*see also* Defect, coagulation) 286.3
Students' elbow 727.2
Stuffy nose 478.1
Stump — *see also* Amputation
  cervix, cervical (healed) 622.8

Stupor — Suppuration

Stupor 780.09
catatonic (*see also* Schizophrenia) 295.2 ✓5ᵗʰ
circular (*see also* Psychosis, manic-depressive, circular) 296.7
manic 296.89
manic-depressive (*see also* Psychosis, affective) 296.89
mental (anergic) (delusional) 298.9
psychogenic 298.8
reaction to exceptional stress (transient) 308.2
traumatic NEC — *see also* Injury, intracranial
with spinal (cord)
lesion — *see* Injury, spinal, by site
shock — *see* Injury, spinal, by site
Sturge (-Weber) (-Dimitri) disease or syndrome (encephalocutan-eous angiomatosis) 759.6
Sturge-Kalischer-Weber syndrome (encephalocutaneous angiomatosis) 759.6
Stuttering 307.0
Sty, stye 373.11
external 373.11
internal 373.12
meibomian 373.12
Subacidity, gastric 536.8
psychogenic 306.4
Subacute — *see* condition
Subarachnoid — *see* condition
Subclavian steal syndrome 435.2
Subcortical — *see* condition
Subcostal syndrome 098.86
nerve compression 354.8
Subcutaneous, subcuticular — *see* condition
Subdelirium 293.1
Subdural — *see* condition
Subendocardium — *see* condition
Subependymoma (M9383/1) 237.5
Suberosis 495.3
Subglossitis — *see* Glossitis
Subhemophilia 286.0
Subinvolution (uterus) 621.1
breast (postlactational) (postpartum) 611.8
chronic 621.1
puerperal, postpartum 674.8 ✓5ᵗʰ
Sublingual — *see* condition
Sublinguitis 527.2
Subluxation — *see also* Dislocation, by site
congenital NEC — *see also* Malposition, congenital
hip (unilateral) 754.32
with dislocation of other hip 754.35
bilateral 754.33
joint
lower limb 755.69
shoulder 755.59
upper limb 755.59
lower limb (joint) 755.69
shoulder (joint) 755.59
upper limb (joint) 755.59
lens 379.32
anterior 379.33
posterior 379.34
rotary, cervical region of spine — *see* Fracture, vertebra, cervical
Submaxillary — *see* condition
Submersion (fatal) (nonfatal) 994.1
Submissiveness (undue), in child 313.0
Submucous — *see* condition
Subnormal, subnormality
accommodation (*see also* Disorder, accommodation) 367.9
mental (*see also* Retardation, mental) 319
mild 317
moderate 318.0
profound 318.2
severe 318.1
temperature (accidental) 991.6
not associated with low environmental temperature 780.99
Subphrenic — *see* condition
Subscapular nerve — *see* condition
Subseptus uterus 752.3
Subsiding appendicitis 542

Substernal thyroid (*see also* Goiter) 240.9
congenital 759.2
Substitution disorder 300.11
Subtentorial — *see* condition
Subtertian
fever 084.0
malaria (fever) 084.0
Subthyroidism (acquired) (*see also* Hypothyroidism) 244.9
congenital 243
Succenturiata placenta — *see* Placenta, abnormal
Succussion sounds, chest 786.7
Sucking thumb, child 307.9
Sudamen 705.1
Sudamina 705.1
Sudanese kala-azar 085.0
Sudden
death, cause unknown (less than 24 hours) 798.1
during childbirth 669.9 ✓5ᵗʰ
infant 798.0
puerperal, postpartum 674.9 ✓5ᵗʰ
hearing loss NEC 388.2
heart failure (*see also* Failure, heart) 428.9
infant death syndrome 798.0
Sudeck's atrophy, disease, or syndrome 733.7
SUDS (Sudden unexplained death) 798.2
Suffocation (*see also* Asphyxia) 799.0
by
bed clothes 994.7
bunny bag 994.7
cave-in 994.7
constriction 994.7
drowning 994.1
inhalation
food or foreign body (*see also* Asphyxia, food or foreign body) 933.1
oil or gasoline (*see also* Asphyxia, food or foreign body) 933.1
overlying 994.7
plastic bag 994.7
pressure 994.7
strangulation 994.7
during birth 768.1
mechanical 994.7
Sugar
blood
high 790.2
low 251.2
in urine 791.5
Suicide, suicidal (attempted)
by poisoning — *see* Table of Drugs and Chemicals
risk 300.9
tendencies 300.9
trauma NEC (*see also* nature and site of injury) 959.9
Suipestifer infection (*see also* Infection, Salmonella) 003.9
Sulfatidosis 330.0
Sulfhemoglobinemia, sulphemoglobinemia (acquired) (congenital) 289.7
Sumatran mite fever 081.2
Summer — *see* condition
Sunburn 692.71
dermatitis 692.71
due to
other ultraviolet radiation 692.82
tanning bed 692.82
first degree 692.71
second degree 692.76
third degree 692.77
Sunken
acetabulum 718.85
fontanels 756.0
Sunstroke 992.0
Superfecundation 651.9 ✓5ᵗʰ
with fetal loss and retention of one or more fetus(es) 651.6 ✓5ᵗʰ
Superfetation 651.9 ✓5ᵗʰ
with fetal loss and retention of one or more fetus(es) 651.6 ✓5ᵗʰ

Superinvolution uterus 621.8
Supernumerary (congenital)
aortic cusps 746.89
auditory ossicles 744.04
bone 756.9
breast 757.6
carpal bones 755.56
cusps, heart valve NEC 746.89
mitral 746.5
pulmonary 746.09
digit(s) 755.00
finger 755.01
toe 755.02
ear (lobule) 744.1
fallopian tube 752.19
finger 755.01
hymen 752.49
kidney 753.3
lacrimal glands 743.64
lacrimonasal duct 743.65
lobule (ear) 744.1
mitral cusps 746.5
muscle 756.82
nipples 757.6
organ or site NEC — *see* Accessory
ossicles, auditory 744.04
ovary 752.0
oviduct 752.19
pulmonic cusps 746.09
rib 756.3
cervical or first 756.2
syndrome 756.2
roots (of teeth) 520.2
spinal vertebra 756.19
spleen 759.0
tarsal bones 755.67
teeth 520.1
causing crowding 524.3
testis 752.8
thumb 755.01
toe 755.02
uterus 752.2
vagina 752.49
vertebra 756.19
Supervision (of)
contraceptive method previously prescribed V25.40
intrauterine device V25.42
oral contraceptive (pill) V25.41
specified type NEC V25.49
subdermal implantable contraceptive V25.43
dietary (for) V65.3
allergy (food) V65.3
colitis V65.3
diabetes mellitus V65.3
food allergy intolerance V65.3
gastritis V65.3
hypercholesterolemia V65.3
hypoglycemia V65.3
intolerance (food) V65.3
obesity V65.3
specified NEC V65.3
lactation V24.1
pregnancy — *see* Pregnancy, supervision of
Supplemental teeth 520.1
causing crowding 524.3
Suppression
binocular vision 368.31
lactation 676.5 ✓5ᵗʰ
menstruation 626.8
ovarian secretion 256.39
renal 586
urinary secretion 788.5
urine 788.5
Suppuration, suppurative — *see also* condition
accessory sinus (chronic) (*see also* Sinusitis) 473.9
adrenal gland 255.8
antrum (chronic) (*see also* Sinusitis, maxillary) 473.0
bladder (*see also* Cystitis) 595.89
bowel 569.89
brain 324.0
late effect 326
breast 611.0
puerperal, postpartum 675.1 ✓5ᵗʰ
dental periosteum 526.5

▲

Suppuration, suppurative — *see also* condition
    — *continued*
  diffuse (skin) 686.00
  ear (middle) (*see also* Otitis media) 382.4
    external (*see also* Otitis, externa) 380.10
    internal 386.33
  ethmoidal (sinus) (chronic) (*see also* Sinusitis,
      ethmoidal) 473.2
  fallopian tube (*see also* Salpingo-oophoritis)
      614.2
  frontal (sinus) (chronic) (*see also* Sinusitis,
      frontal) 473.1
  gallbladder (*see also* Cholecystitis, acute) 575.0
  gum 523.3
  hernial sac — *see* Hernia, by site
  intestine 569.89
  joint (*see also* Arthritis, suppurative) 711.0 ✓5ᵗʰ
  labyrinthine 386.33
  lung 513.0
  mammary gland 611.0
    puerperal, postpartum 675.1 ✓5ᵗʰ
  maxilla, maxillary 526.4
    sinus (chronic) (*see also* Sinusitis, maxillary)
        473.0
  muscle 728.0
  nasal sinus (chronic) (*see also* Sinusitis) 473.9
  pancreas 577.0
  parotid gland 527.2
  pelvis, pelvic
    female (*see also* Disease, pelvis,
        inflammatory) 614.4
      acute 614.3
    male (*see also* Peritonitis) 567.2
  pericranial (*see also* Osteomyelitis) 730.2 ✓5ᵗʰ
  salivary duct or gland (any) 527.2
  sinus (nasal) (*see also* Sinusitis) 473.9
  sphenoidal (sinus) (chronic) (*see also* Sinusitis,
      sphenoidal) 473.3
  thymus (gland) 254.1
  thyroid (gland) 245.0
  tonsil 474.8
  uterus (*see also* Endometritis) 615.9
  vagina 616.10
  wound — *see also* Wound, open, by site,
      complicated
    dislocation — *see* Dislocation, by site,
        compound
    fracture — *see* Fracture, by site, open
    scratch or other superficial injury — *see*
        Injury, superficial, by site
Supraglottitis 464.50
  with obstruction 464.51
Suprapubic drainage 596.8
Suprarenal (gland) — *see* condition
Suprascapular nerve — *see* condition
Suprasellar — *see* condition
Supraspinatus syndrome 726.10
Surfer knots 919.8
  infected 919.9
Surgery
  cosmetic NEC V50.1
    following healed injury or operation V51
    hair transplant V50.0
  elective V50.9
    breast augmentation or reduction V50.1
    circumcision, ritual or routine (in absence of
        medical indication) V50.2
    cosmetic NEC V50.1
    ear piercing V50.3
    face-lift V50.1
    following healed injury or operation V51
    hair transplant V50.0
  not done because of
    contraindication V64.1
    patient's decision V64.2
    specified reason NEC V64.3
  plastic
    breast augmentation or reduction V50.1
    cosmetic V50.1
    face-lift V50.1
    following healed injury or operation V51
    repair of scarred tissue (following healed
        injury or operation) V51
    specified type NEC V50.8

Surgery — *continued*
  previous, in pregnancy or childbirth
    cervix 654.6 ✓5ᵗʰ
      affecting fetus or newborn 763.89
      causing obstructed labor 660.2 ✓5ᵗʰ
        affecting fetus or newborn 763.1
    pelvic soft tissues NEC 654.9 ✓5ᵗʰ
      affecting fetus or newborn 763.89
      causing obstructed labor 660.2 ✓5ᵗʰ
        affecting fetus or newborn 763.1
    perineum or vulva 654.8 ✓5ᵗʰ
    uterus NEC 654.9 ✓5ᵗʰ
      affecting fetus or newborn 763.89
      causing obstructed labor 660.2 ✓5ᵗʰ
        affecting fetus or newborn 763.1
      due to previous cesarean delivery
          654.2 ✓5ᵗʰ
    vagina 654.7 ✓5ᵗʰ
Surgical
  abortion — *see* Abortion, legal
  emphysema 998.81
  kidney (*see also* Pyelitis) 590.80
  operation NEC 799.9
  procedures, complication or misadventure —
      see Complications, surgical procedure
  shock 998.0
Suspected condition, ruled out (*see also*
    Observation, suspected) V71.9
  specified condition NEC V71.89
Suspended uterus, in pregnancy or childbirth
    654.4 ✓5ᵗʰ
  affecting fetus or newborn 763.89
  causing obstructed labor 660.2 ✓5ᵗʰ
    affecting fetus or newborn 763.1
Sutton's disease 709.09
Sutton and Gull's disease (arteriolar
    nephrosclerosis) (*see also* Hypertension,
    kidney) 403.90
Suture
  burst (in ▶external◀ operation wound)   ▲
      998.32
    internal 998.31   ●
  inadvertently left in operation wound 998.4
  removal V58.3
  Shirodkar, in pregnancy (with or without
      cervical incompetence) 654.5 ✓5ᵗʰ
Swab inadvertently left in operation wound
    998.4
Swallowed, swallowing
  difficulty (*see also* Dysphagia) 787.2
  foreign body NEC (*see also* Foreign body) 938
Swamp fever 100.89
Swan neck hand (intrinsic) 736.09
Sweat(s), sweating
  disease or sickness 078.2
  excessive 780.8
  fetid 705.89
  fever 078.2
  gland disease 705.9
    specified type NEC 705.89
  miliary 078.2
  night 780.8
Sweeley-Klionsky disease (angiokeratoma
    corporis diffusum) 272.7
Sweet's syndrome (acute febrile neutrophilic
    dermatosis) 695.89
Swelling
  abdominal (not referable to specific organ)
      789.3 ✓5ᵗʰ
  adrenal gland, cloudy 255.8
  ankle 719.07
  anus 787.99
  arm 729.81
  breast 611.72
  Calabar 125.2
  cervical gland 785.6
  cheek 784.2
  chest 786.6
  ear 388.8
  epigastric 789.3 ✓5ᵗʰ
  extremity (lower) (upper) 729.81
  eye 379.92
  female genital organ 625.8
  finger 729.81
  foot 729.81

Swelling — *continued*
  glands 785.6
  gum 784.2
  hand 729.81
  head 784.2
  inflammatory — *see* Inflammation
  joint (*see also* Effusion, joint) 719.0 ✓5ᵗʰ
    tuberculous — *see* Tuberculosis, joint
  kidney, cloudy 593.89
  leg 729.81
  limb 729.81
  liver 573.8
  lung 786.6
  lymph nodes 785.6
  mediastinal 786.6
  mouth 784.2
  muscle (limb) 729.81
  neck 784.2
  nose or sinus 784.2
  palate 784.2
  pelvis 789.3 ✓5ᵗʰ
  penis 607.83
  perineum 625.8
  rectum 787.99
  scrotum 608.86
  skin 782.2
  splenic (*see also* Splenomegaly) 789.2
  substernal 786.6
  superficial, localized (skin) 782.2
  testicle 608.86
  throat 784.2
  toe 729.81
  tongue 784.2
  tubular (*see also* Disease, renal) 593.9
  umbilicus 789.3 ✓5ᵗʰ
  uterus 625.8
  vagina 625.8
  vulva 625.8
  wandering, due to Gnathostoma (spinigerum)
      128.1
  white — *see* Tuberculosis, arthritis
Swift's disease 985.0
Swimmers'
  ear (acute) 380.12
  itch 120.3
Swimming in the head 780.4
Swollen — *see also* Swelling
  glands 785.6
Swyer-James syndrome (unilateral hyperlucent
    lung) 492.8
Swyer's syndrome (XY pure gonadal dysgenesis)
    752.7
Sycosis 704.8
  barbae (not parasitic) 704.8
  contagiosa 110.0
  lupoid 704.8
  mycotic 110.0
  parasitic 110.0
  vulgaris 704.8
Sydenham's chorea — *see* Chorea, Sydenham's
Sylvatic yellow fever 060.0
Sylvest's disease (epidemic pleurodynia) 074.1
Symblepharon 372.63
  congenital 743.62
Symonds' syndrome 348.2
Sympathetic — *see* condition
Sympatheticotonia (*see also* Neuropathy,
    peripheral, autonomic) 337.9
Sympathicoblastoma (M9500/3)
  specified site — *see* Neoplasm, by site,
      malignant
  unspecified site 194.0
Sympathicogonioma (M9500/3) — *see*
    Sympathicoblastoma
Sympathoblastoma (M9500/3) — *see*
    Sympathicoblastoma
Sympathogonioma (M9500/3) — *see*
    Sympathicoblastoma
Symphalangy (*see also* Syndactylism) 755.10
Symptoms, specified (general) NEC 780.99   ▲
  abdomen NEC 789.9
  bone NEC 733.90
  breast NEC 611.79
  cardiac NEC 785.9

Symptoms, specified NEC — *continued*
cardiovascular NEC 785.9
chest NEC 786.9
development NEC 783.9
digestive system NEC 787.99
eye NEC 379.99
gastrointestinal tract NEC 787.99
genital organs NEC
female 625.9
male 608.9
head and neck NEC 784.9
heart NEC 785.9
joint NEC 719.60
ankle 719.67
elbow 719.62
foot 719.67
hand 719.64
hip 719.65
knee 719.66
multiple sites 719.69
pelvic region 719.65
shoulder (region) 719.61
specified site NEC 719.68
wrist 719.63
larynx NEC 784.9
limbs NEC 729.89
lymphatic system NEC 785.9
menopausal 627.2
metabolism NEC 783.9
mouth NEC 528.9
muscle NEC 728.9
musculoskeletal NEC 781.99
limbs NEC 729.89
nervous system NEC 781.99
neurotic NEC 300.9
nutrition, metabolism, and development NEC 783.9
pelvis NEC 789.9
female 625.9
peritoneum NEC 789.9
respiratory system NEC 786.9
skin and integument NEC 782.9
subcutaneous tissue NEC 782.9
throat NEC 784.9
tonsil NEC 784.9
urinary system NEC 788.9
vascular NEC 785.9

Sympus 759.89

Synarthrosis 719.80
ankle 719.87
elbow 719.82
foot 719.87
hand 719.84
hip 719.85
knee 719.86
multiple sites 719.89
pelvic region 719.85
shoulder (region) 719.81
specified site NEC 719.88
wrist 719.83

Syncephalus 759.4

Synchondrosis 756.9
abnormal (congenital) 756.9
ischiopubic (van Neck's) 732.1

Synchysis (senile) (vitreous humor) 379.21
scintillans 379.22

Syncope (near) (pre-) 780.2
anginosa 413.9
bradycardia 427.89
cardiac 780.2
carotid sinus 337.0
complicating delivery 669.2 ☑5ᵗʰ
due to lumbar puncture 349.0
fatal 798.1
heart 780.2
heat 992.1
laryngeal 786.2
tussive 786.2
vasoconstriction 780.2
vasodepressor 780.2
vasomotor 780.2
vasovagal 780.2

Syncytial infarct — *see* Placenta, abnormal

Syndactylism, syndactyly (multiple sites) 755.10
fingers (without fusion of bone) 755.11
with fusion of bone 755.12

Syndactylism, syndactyly — *continued*
toes (without fusion of bone) 755.13
with fusion of bone 755.14

Syndrome — *see also* Disease
abdominal
acute 789.0 ☑5ᵗʰ
migraine 346.2 ☑5ᵗʰ
muscle deficiency 756.79
Abercrombie's (amyloid degeneration) 277.3
abnormal innervation 374.43
abstinence
alcohol 291.81
drug 292.0
Abt-Letterer-Siwe (acute histiocytosis X) (M9722/3) 202.5 ☑5ᵗʰ
Achard-Thiers (adrenogenital) 255.2
acid pulmonary aspiration 997.3
obstetric (Mendelson's) 668.0 ☑5ᵗʰ
acquired immune deficiency 042
acquired immunodeficiency 042
acrocephalosyndactylism 755.55
acute abdominal 789.0 ☑5ᵗʰ
acute chest 282.62   ●
acute coronary 411.1   ●
Adair-Dighton (brittle bones and blue sclera, deafness) 756.51
Adams-Stokes (-Morgagni) (syncope with heart block) 426.9
addisonian 255.4
Adie (-Holmes) (pupil) 379.46
adiposogenital 253.8
adrenal
hemorrhage 036.3
meningococcic 036.3
adrenocortical 255.3
adrenogenital (acquired) (congenital) 255.2
feminizing 255.2
iatrogenic 760.79
virilism (acquired) (congenital) 255.2
affective organic NEC 293.89
drug-induced 292.84
afferent loop NEC 537.89
African macroglobulinemia 273.3
Ahumada-Del Castillo (nonpuerperal galactorrhea and amenorrhea) 253.1
air blast concussion — *see* Injury, internal, by site
Albright (-Martin) (pseudohypoparathyroidism) 275.49
Albright-McCune-Sternberg (osteitis fibrosa disseminata) 756.59
alcohol withdrawal 291.81
Alder's (leukocyte granulation anomaly) 288.2
Aldrich (-Wiskott) (eczema-thrombocytopenia) 279.12
Alibert-Bazin (mycosis fungoides) (M9700/3) 202.1 ☑5ᵗʰ
Alice in Wonderland 293.89
Allen-Masters 620.6
Alligator baby (ichthyosis congenita) 757.1
Alport's (hereditary hematuria-nephropathy-deafness) 759.89
Alvarez (transient cerebral ischemia) 435.9
alveolar capillary block 516.3
Alzheimer's 331.0
with dementia — *see* Alzheimer's, dementia
amnestic (confabulatory) 294.0
alcoholic 291.1
drug-induced 292.83
posttraumatic 294.0
amotivational 292.89
amyostatic 275.1
amyotrophic lateral sclerosis 335.20
angina (*see also* Angina) 413.9
ankyloglossia superior 750.0
anterior
chest wall 786.52
compartment (tibial) 958.8
spinal artery 433.8 ☑5ᵗʰ
compression 721.1
tibial (compartment) 958.8
antibody deficiency 279.00
agammaglobulinemic 279.00
congenital 279.00
hypogammaglobulinemic 279.00
anticardiolipin antibody 795.79
antimongolism 758.3

Syndrome — *see also* Disease — *continued*
antiphospholipid antibody 795.79
Anton (-Babinski) (hemiasomatognosia) 307.9
anxiety (*see also* Anxiety) 300.00
organic 293.84
aortic
arch 446.7
bifurcation (occlusion) 444.0
ring 747.21
Apert's (acrocephalosyndactyly) 755.55
Apert-Gallais (adrenogenital) 255.2
aphasia-apraxia-alexia 784.69
"approximate answers" 300.16
arcuate ligament (-celiac axis) 447.4
arcus aortae 446.7
arc-welders' 370.24
argentaffin, argintaffinoma 259.2
Argonz-Del Castillo (nonpuerperal galactorrhea and amenorrhea) 253.1
Argyll Robertson's (syphilitic) 094.89
nonsyphilitic 379.45
arm-shoulder (*see also* Neuropathy, peripheral, autonomic) 337.9
Arnold-Chiari (*see also* Spina bifida) 741.0 ☑5ᵗʰ
type I 348.4
type II 741.0 ☑5ᵗʰ
type III 742.0
type IV 742.2
Arrillaga-Ayerza (pulmonary artery sclerosis with pulmonary hypertension) 416.0
arteriomesenteric duodenum occlusion 537.89
arteriovenous steal 996.73
arteritis, young female (obliterative brachiocephalic) 446.7
aseptic meningitis — *see* Meningitis, aseptic
Asherman's 621.5
asphyctic (*see also* Anxiety) 300.00
aspiration, of newborn, massive or meconium 770.1
ataxia-telangiectasia 334.8
Audry's (acropachyderma) 757.39
auriculotemporal 350.8
autosomal — *see also* Abnormal, autosomes NEC
deletion 758.3
Avellis' 344.89
Axenfeld's 743.44
Ayerza (-Arrillaga) (pulmonary artery sclerosis with pulmonary hypertension) 416.0
Baader's (erythema multiforme exudativum) 695.1
Baastrup's 721.5
Babinski (-Vaquez) (cardiovascular syphilis) 093.89
Babinski-Fröhlich (adiposogenital dystrophy) 253.8
Babinski-Nageotte 344.89
Bagratuni's (temporal arteritis) 446.5
Bakwin-Krida (craniometaphyseal dysplasia) 756.89
Balint's (psychic paralysis of visual disorientation) 368.16
Ballantyne (-Runge) (postmaturity) 766.2
ballooning posterior leaflet 424.0
Banti's — *see* Cirrhosis, liver
Bard-Pic's (carcinoma, head of pancreas) 157.0
Bardet-Biedl (obesity, polydactyly, and mental retardation) 759.89
Barlow's (mitral valve prolapse) 424.0
Barlow (-Möller) (infantile scurvy) 267
Baron Munchausen's 301.51
Barré-Guillain 357.0
Barré-Liéou (posterior cervical sympathetic) 723.2
Barrett's (chronic peptic ulcer of esophagus) 530.2
Bársony-Polgár (corkscrew esophagus) 530.5
Bársony-Teschendorf (corkscrew esophagus) 530.5
Bartter's (secondary hyperaldosteronism with juxtaglomerular hyperplasia) 255.1
Basedow's (exophthalmic goiter) 242.0 ☑5ᵗʰ
basilar artery 435.0
basofrontal 377.04
Bassen-Kornzweig (abetalipoproteinemia) 272.5
Batten-Steinert 359.2
battered
adult 995.81

Syndrome — *see also* Disease — *continued*
battered — *continued*
  baby or child 995.54
  spouse 995.81
Baumgarten-Cruveilhier (cirrhosis of liver) 571.5
Bearn-Kunkel (-Slater) (lupoid hepatitis) 571.49
Beau's (*see also* Degeneration, myocardial) 429.1
Bechterew-Strümpell-Marie (ankylosing spondylitis) 720.0
Beck's (anterior spinal artery occlusion) 433.8 ✔5ᵗʰ
Beckwith (-Wiedemann) 759.89
Behçet's 136.1
Bekhterev-Strümpell-Marie (ankylosing spondylitis) 720.0
Benedikt's 344.89
Béquez César (-Steinbrinck-Chédiak- Higashi) (congenital gigantism of peroxidase granules) 288.2
Bernard-Horner (*see also* Neuropathy, peripheral, autonomic) 337.9
Bernard-Sergent (acute adrenocortical insufficiency) 255.4
Bernhardt-Roth 355.1
Bernheim's (*see also* Failure, heart) 428.0
Bertolotti's (sacralization of fifth lumbar vertebra) 756.15
Besnier-Boeck-Schaumann (sarcoidosis) 135
Bianchi's (aphasia-apraxia-alexia syndrome) 784.69
Biedl-Bardet (obesity, polydactyly, and mental retardation) 759.89
Biemond's (obesity, polydactyly, and mental retardation) 759.89
big spleen 289.4
bilateral polycystic ovarian 256.4
Bing-Horton's 346.2 ✔5ᵗʰ
Biörck (-Thorson) (malignant carcinoid) 259.2
Blackfan-Diamond (congenital hypoplastic anemia) 284.0
black lung 500
black widow spider bite 989.5
bladder neck (*see also* Incontinence, urine) 788.30
blast (concussion) — *see* Blast, injury
blind loop (postoperative) 579.2
Bloch-Siemens (incontinentia pigmenti) 757.33
Bloch-Sulzberger (incontinentia pigmenti) 757.33
Bloom (-Machacek) (-Torre) 757.39
Blount-Barber (tibia vara) 732.4
blue
  bloater 491.2 ✔5ᵗʰ
  diaper 270.0
  drum 381.02
  sclera 756.51
  toe — *see* Atherosclerosis
Boder-Sedgwick (ataxia-telangiectasia) 334.8
Boerhaave's (spontaneous esophageal rupture) 530.4
Bonnevie-Ullrich 758.6
Bonnier's 386.19
Bouillaud's (rheumatic heart disease) 391.9
Bourneville (-Pringle) (tuberous sclerosis) 759.5
Bouveret (-Hoffmann) (paroxysmal tachycardia) 427.2
brachial plexus 353.0
Brachman-de Lange (Amsterdam dwarf, mental retardation, and brachycephaly) 759.89
bradycardia-tachycardia 427.81
Brailsford-Morquio (dystrophy) (mucopolysaccharidosis IV) 277.5
brain (acute) (chronic) (nonpsychotic) (organic) (with behavioral reaction) (with neurotic reaction) 310.9
  with
    presenile brain disease (*see also* Dementia, presenile) 290.10
    psychosis, psychotic reaction (*see also* Psychosis, organic) 294.9
  chronic alcoholic 291.2
  congenital (*see also* Retardation, mental) 319
  postcontusional 310.2
  posttraumatic
    nonpsychotic 310.2

brain — *continued*
  posttraumatic — *continued*
    psychotic 293.9
     acute 293.0
     chronic (*see also* Psychosis, organic) 294.8
     subacute 293.1
    psycho-organic (*see also* Syndrome, psycho-organic) 310.9
    psychotic (*see also* Psychosis, organic) 294.9
    senile (*see also* Dementia, senile) 290.0
branchial arch 744.41
Brandt's (acrodermatitis enteropathica) 686.8
Brennemann's 289.2
Briquet's 300.81
Brissaud-Meige (infantile myxedema) 244.9
broad ligament laceration 620.6
Brock's (atelectasis due to enlarged lymph nodes) 518.0
Brown's tendon sheath 378.61
Brown-Séquard 344.89
brown spot 756.59
Brugada 746.89
Brugsch's (acropachyderma) 757.39
bubbly lung 770.7
Buchem's (hyperostosis corticalis) 733.3
Budd-Chiari (hepatic vein thrombosis) 453.0
Büdinger-Ludloff-Läwen 717.89
bulbar 335.22
  lateral (*see also* Disease, cerebrovascular, acute) 436
Bullis fever 082.8
bundle of Kent (anomalous atrioventricular excitation) 426.7
Bürger-Grütz (essential familial hyperlipemia) 272.3
Burke's (pancreatic insufficiency and chronic neutropenia) 577.8
Burnett's (milk-alkali) 999.9
Burnier's (hypophyseal dwarfism) 253.3
burning feet 266.2
Bywaters' 958.5
Caffey's (infantile cortical hyperostosis) 756.59
Calvé-Legg-Perthes (osteochondrosis, femoral capital) 732.1
Caplan (-Colinet) syndrome 714.81
capsular thrombosis (*see also* Thrombosis, brain) 434.0 ✔5ᵗʰ
carcinogenic thrombophlebitis 453.1
carcinoid 259.2
cardiac asthma (*see also* Failure, ventricular, left) 428.1
cardiacos negros 416.0
cardiopulmonary obesity 278.8
cardiorenal (*see also* Hypertension, cardiorenal) 404.90
cardiorespiratory distress (idiopathic), newborn 769
cardiovascular renal (*see also* Hypertension, cardiorenal) 404.90
cardiovasorenal 272.7
Carini's (ichthyosis congenita) 757.1
carotid
  artery (internal) 435.8
  body or sinus 337.0
carpal tunnel 354.0
Carpenter's 759.89
Cassidy (-Scholte) (malignant carcinoid) 259.2
cat-cry 758.3
cauda equina 344.60
causalgia 355.9
  lower limb 355.71
  upper limb 354.4
cavernous sinus 437.6
celiac 579.0
  artery compression 447.4
  axis 447.4
cerebellomedullary malformation (*see also* Spina bifida) 741.0 ✔5ᵗʰ
cerebral gigantism 253.0
cerebrohepatorenal 759.89
cervical (root) (spine) NEC 723.8
  disc 722.71
  posterior, sympathetic 723.2
  rib 353.0
  sympathetic paralysis 337.0
  traumatic (acute) NEC 847.0

cervicobrachial (diffuse) 723.3
cervicocranial 723.2
cervicodorsal outlet 353.2
Céstan's 344.89
Céstan (-Raymond) 433.8 ✔5ᵗʰ
Céstan-Chenais 344.89
chancriform 114.1
Charcôt's (intermittent claudication) 443.9
  angina cruris 443.9
  due to atherosclerosis 440.21
Charcôt-Marie-Tooth 356.1
Charcôt-Weiss-Baker 337.0
Cheadle (-Möller) (-Barlow) (infantile scurvy) 267
Chédiak-Higashi (-Steinbrinck) (congenital gigantism of peroxidase granules) 288.2
chest wall 786.52
Chiari's (hepatic vein thrombosis) 453.0
Chiari-Frommel 676.6 ✔5ᵗʰ
chiasmatic 368.41
Chilaiditi's (subphrenic displacement, colon) 751.4
chondroectodermal dysplasia 756.55
chorea-athetosis-agitans 275.1
Christian's (chronic histiocytosis X) 277.8
chromosome 4 short arm deletion 758.3
Churg-Strauss 446.4
Clarke-Hadfield (pancreatic infantilism) 577.8
Claude's 352.6
Claude Bernard-Horner (*see also* Neuropathy, peripheral, autonomic) 337.9
Clérambault's
  automatism 348.8
  erotomania 297.8
Clifford's (postmaturity) 766.2
climacteric 627.2
Clouston's (hidrotic ectodermal dysplasia) 757.31
clumsiness 315.4
Cockayne's (microencephaly and dwarfism) 759.89
Cockayne-Weber (epidermolysis bullosa) 757.39
Cogan's (nonsyphilitic interstitial keratitis) 370.52
cold injury (newborn) 778.2
Collet (-Sicard) 352.6
combined immunity deficiency 279.2
compartment(al) (anterior) (deep) (posterior) (tibial) 958.8
  nontraumatic 729.9
compression 958.5
  cauda equina 344.60
    with neurogenic bladder 344.61
concussion 310.2
congenital
  affecting more than one system 759.7
    specified type NEC 759.89
  facial diplegia 352.6
  muscular hypertrophy-cerebral 759.89
congestion-fibrosis (pelvic) 625.5
conjunctivourethrosynovial 099.3
Conn (-Louis) (primary aldosteronism) 255.1
Conradi (-Hünermann) (chondrodysplasia calcificans congenita) 756.59
conus medullaris 336.8
Cooke-Apert-Gallais (adrenogenital) 255.2
Cornelia de Lange's (Amsterdam dwarf, mental retardation, and brachycephaly) 759.8 ✔5ᵗʰ
coronary insufficiency or intermediate 411.1
cor pulmonale 416.9
corticosexual 255.2
Costen's (complex) 524.60
costochondral junction 733.6
costoclavicular 353.0
costovertebral 253.0
Cotard's (paranoia) 297.1
craniovertebral 723.2
Creutzfeldt-Jakob 046.1
  with dementia
    with behavioral disturbance 046.1 *[294.11]*
    without behavioral disturbance 046.1 *[294.10]*
crib death 798.0
cricopharyngeal 787.2
cri-du-chat 758.3

Syndrome — *see also* Disease — *continued*
  Crigler-Najjar (congenital hyperbilirubinemia) 277.4
  crocodile tears 351.8
  Cronkhite-Canada 211.3
  croup 464.4
  CRST (cutaneous systemic sclerosis) 710.1
  crush 958.5
  crushed lung (*see also* Injury, internal, lung) 861.20
  Cruveilhier-Baumgarten (cirrhosis of liver) 571.5
  cubital tunnel 354.2
  Cuiffini-Pancoast (M8010/3) (carcinoma, pulmonary apex) 162.3
  Curschmann (-Batten) (-Steinert) 359.2
  Cushing's (iatrogenic) (idiopathic) (pituitary basophilism) (pituitary-dependent) 255.0
    overdose or wrong substance given or taken 962.0
  Cyriax's (slipping rib) 733.99
  cystic duct stump 576.0
  Da Costa's (neurocirculatory asthenia) 306.2
  Dameshek's (erythroblastic anemia) 282.4
  Dana-Putnam (subacute combined sclerosis with pernicious anemia) 281.0 [336.2]
  Danbolt (-Closs) (acrodermatitis enteropathica) 686.8
  Dandy-Walker (atresia, foramen of Magendie) 742.3
    with spina bifida (*see also* Spina bifida) 741.0 ✓5ᵗʰ
  Danlos' 756.83
  Davies-Colley (slipping rib) 733.99
  dead fetus 641.3 ✓5ᵗʰ
  defeminization 255.2
  defibrination (*see also* Fibrinolysis) 286.6
  Degos' 447.8
  Deiters' nucleus 386.19
  Déjérine-Roussy 348.8
  Déjérine-Thomas 333.0
  de Lange's (Amsterdam dwarf, mental retardation, and brachycephaly) (Cornelia) 759.89
  Del Castillo's (germinal aplasia) 606.0
  deletion chromosomes 758.3
  delusional
    induced by drug 292.11
  dementia-aphonia, of childhood (*see also* Psychosis, childhood) 299.1 ✓5ᵗʰ
  demyelinating NEC 341.9
  denial visual hallucination 307.9
  depersonalization 300.6
  Dercum's (adiposis dolorosa) 272.8
  de Toni-Fanconi (-Debré) (cystinosis) 270.0
  diabetes-dwarfism-obesity (juvenile) 258.1
  diabetes mellitus-hypertension-nephrosis 250.4 ✓5ᵗʰ [581.81]
  diabetes mellitus in newborn infant 775.1
  diabetes-nephrosis 250.4 ✓5ᵗʰ [581.81]
  diabetic amyotrophy 250.6 ✓5ᵗʰ [358.1]
  Diamond-Blackfan (congenital hypoplastic anemia) 284.0
  Diamond-Gardner (autoerythrocyte sensitization) 287.2
  DIC (diffuse or disseminated intravascular coagulopathy) (*see also* Fibrinolysis) 286.6
  diencephalohypophyseal NEC 253.8
  diffuse cervicobrachial 723.3
  diffuse obstructive pulmonary 496
  DiGeorge's (thymic hypoplasia) 279.11
  Dighton's 756.51
  Di Guglielmo's (erythremic myelosis) (M9841/3) 207.0 ✓5ᵗʰ
  disc — *see* Displacement, intervertebral disc
  discogenic — *see* Displacement, intervertebral disc
  disequilibrium 276.9
  disseminated platelet thrombosis 446.6
  Ditthomska 307.81
  Doan-Wiseman (primary splenic neutropenia) 288.0
  Döhle body-panmyelopathic 288.2
  Donohue's (leprechaunism) 259.8
  dorsolateral medullary (*see also* Disease, cerebrovascular, acute) 436
  double whammy 360.81

Syndrome — *see also* Disease — *continued*
  Down's (mongolism) 758.0
  Dresbach's (elliptocytosis) 282.1
  Dressler's (postmyocardial infarction) 411.0
    hemoglobinuria 283.2
  drug withdrawal, infant, of dependent mother 779.5
  dry skin 701.1
    eye 375.15
  DSAP (disseminated superficial actinic porokeratosis) 692.75
  Duane's (retraction) 378.71
  Duane-Stilling-Türk (ocular retraction syndrome) 378.71
  Dubin-Johnson (constitutional hyperbilirubinemia) 277.4
  Dubin-Sprinz (constitutional hyperbilirubinemia) 277.4
  Duchenne's 335.22
  due to abnormality
    autosomal NEC (*see also* Abnormal, autosomes NEC) 758.5
      13 758.1
      18 758.2
      21 or 22 758.0
      D 758.1
      E 758.2
      G 758.0
    chromosomal 758.89
      sex 758.81
  dumping 564.2
    nonsurgical 536.8
  Duplay's 726.2
  Dupré's (meningism) 781.6
  Dyke-Young (acquired macrocytic hemolytic anemia) 283.9
  dyspraxia 315.4
  dystocia, dystrophia 654.9 ✓5ᵗʰ
  Eagle-Barret 756.71
  Eales' 362.18
  Eaton-Lambert (*see also* Neoplasm, by site, malignant) 199.1 [358.1]
  Ebstein's (downward displacement, tricuspid valve into right ventricle) 746.2
  ectopic ACTH secretion 255.0
  eczema-thrombocytopenia 279.12
  Eddowes' (brittle bones and blue sclera) 756.51
  Edwards' 758.2
  efferent loop 537.89
  effort (aviators') (psychogenic) 306.2
  Ehlers-Danlos 756.83
  Eisenmenger's (ventricular septal defect) 745.4
  Ekbom's (restless legs) 333.99
  Ekman's (brittle bones and blue sclera) 756.51
  electric feet 266.2
  Elephant man 237.71
  Ellison-Zollinger (gastric hypersecretion with pancreatic islet cell tumor) 251.5
  Ellis-van Creveld (chondroectodermal dysplasia) 756.55
  embryonic fixation 270.2
  empty sella (turcica) 253.8
  endocrine-hypertensive 255.3
  Engel-von Recklinghausen (osteitis fibrosa cystica) 252.0
  enteroarticular 099.3
  entrapment — *see* Neuropathy, entrapment
  eosinophilia myalgia 710.5
  epidemic vomiting 078.82
  Epstein's — *see* Nephrosis
  Erb (-Oppenheim) — Goldflam 358.0
  Erdheim's (acromegalic macrospondylitis) 253.0
  Erlacher-Blount (tibia vara) 732.4
  erythrocyte fragmentation 283.19
  euthyroid sick 790.94
  Evans' (thrombocytopenic purpura) 287.3
  excess cortisol, iatrogenic 255.0
  exhaustion 300.5
  extrapyramidal 333.90
  eyelid-malar-mandible 756.0
  eye retraction 378.71
  Faber's (achlorhydric anemia) 280.9
  Fabry (-Anderson) (angiokeratoma corporis diffusum) 272.7
  facet 724.8
  Fallot's 745.2
  falx (*see also* Hemorrhage, brain) 431
  familial eczema-thrombocytopenia 279.12

Syndrome — *see also* Disease — *continued*
  Fanconi's (anemia) (congenital pancytopenia) 284.0
  Fanconi (-de Toni) (-Debré) (cystinosis) 270.0
  Farber (-Uzman) (disseminated lipogranulomatosis) 272.8
  fatigue NEC 300.5
    chronic 780.71
  faulty bowel habit (idiopathic megacolon) 564.7
  FDH (focal dermal hypoplasia) 757.39
  fecal reservoir 560.39
  Feil-Klippel (brevicollis) 756.16
  Felty's (rheumatoid arthritis with splenomegaly and leukopenia) 714.1
  fertile eunuch 257.2
  fetal alcohol 760.71
    late effect 760.71
  fibrillation-flutter 427.32
  fibrositis (periarticular) 729.0
  Fiedler's (acute isolated myocarditis) 422.91
  Fiessinger-Leroy (-Reiter) 099.3
  Fiessinger-Rendu (erythema multiforme exudativum) 695.1
  first arch 756.0
  Fisher's 357.0
  Fitz's (acute hemorrhagic pancreatitis) 577.0
  Fitz-Hugh and Curtis (gonococcal peritonitis) 098.86
  Flajani (-Basedow) (exophthalmic goiter) 242.0 ✓5ᵗʰ
  floppy
    infant 781.99
    valve (mitral) 424.0
  flush 259.2
  Foix-Alajouanine 336.1
  Fong's (hereditary osteo-onychodysplasia) 756.89
  foramen magnum 348.4
  Forbes-Albright (nonpuerperal amenorrhea and lactation associated with pituitary tumor) 253.1
  Foster-Kennedy 377.04
  Foville's (peduncular) 344.89
  fragile X 759.83
  Franceschetti's (mandibulofacial dysostosis) 756.0
  Fraser's 759.89
  Freeman-Sheldon 759.89
  Frey's (auriculotemporal) 350.8
  Friderichsen-Waterhouse 036.3
  Friedrich-Erb-Arnold (acropachyderma) 757.39
  Fröhlich's (adiposogenital dystrophy) 253.8
  Froin's 336.8
  Frommel-Chiari 676.6 ✓5ᵗʰ
  frontal lobe 310.0
  Fuller Albright's (osteitis fibrosa disseminata) 756.59
  functional
    bowel 564.9
    prepubertal castrate 752.8
  Gaisböck's (polycythemia hypertonica) 289.0
  ganglion (basal, brain) 333.90
    geniculi 351.1
  Ganser's, hysterical 300.16
  Gardner-Diamond (autoerythrocyte sensitization) 287.2
  gastroesophageal junction 530.0
  gastroesophageal laceration-hemorrhage 530.7
  gastrojejunal loop obstruction 537.89
  Gayet-Wernicke's (superior hemorrhagic polioencephalitis) 265.1
  Gee-Herter-Heubner (nontropical sprue) 579.0
  Gélineau's 347
  genito-anorectal 099.1
  Gerhardt's (vocal cord paralysis) 478.30
  Gerstmann's (finger agnosia) 784.69
  Gilbert's 277.4
  Gilford (-Hutchinson) (progeria) 259.8
  Gilles de la Tourette's 307.23
  Gillespie's (dysplasia oculodentodigitalis) 759.89
  Glénard's (enteroptosis) 569.89
  Glinski-Simmonds (pituitary cachexia) 253.2
  glucuronyl transferase 277.4
  glue ear 381.20
  Goldberg (-Maxwell) (-Morris) (testicular feminization) 257.8

Syndrome — *see also* Disease — *continued*
  Goldenhar's (oculoauriculovertebral dysplasia) 756.0
  Goldflam-Erb 358.0
  Goltz-Gorlin (dermal hypoplasia) 757.39
  Goodpasture's (pneumorenal) 446.21
  Gopalan's (burning feet) 266.2
  Gorlin-Chaudhry-Moss 759.89
  Gougerot (-Houwer) — Sjögren (keratoconjunctivitis sicca) 710.2
  Gougerot-Blum (pigmented purpuric lichenoid dermatitis) 709.1
  Gougerot-Carteaud (confluent reticulate papillomatosis) 701.8
  Gouley's (constrictive pericarditis) 423.2
  Gowers' (vasovagal attack) 780.2
  Gowers-Paton-Kennedy 377.04
  Gradenigo's 383.02
  gray or grey (chloramphenicol) (newborn) 779.4
  Greig's (hypertelorism) 756.0
  Gubler-Millard 344.89
  Guérin-Stern (arthrogryposis multiplex congenita) 754.89
  Guillain-Barré (-Strohl) 357.0
  Gunn's (jaw-winking syndrome) 742.8
  Günther's (congenital erythropoietic porphyria) 277.1
  gustatory sweating 350.8
  H_3O 759.81
  Hadfield-Clarke (pancreatic infantilism) 577.8
  Haglund-Läwen-Fründ 717.89
  hairless women 257.8
  Hallermann-Streiff 756.0
  Hallervorden-Spatz 333.0
  Hamman's (spontaneous mediastinal emphysema) 518.1
  Hamman-Rich (diffuse interstitial pulmonary fibrosis) 516.3
  Hand-Schüller-Christian (chronic histiocytosis X) 277.8
  hand-foot 282.61
  Hanot-Chauffard (-Troisier) (bronze diabetes) 275.0
  Harada's 363.22
  Hare's (M8010/3) (carcinoma, pulmonary apex) 162.3
  Harkavy's 446.0
  harlequin color change 779.89 ▲
  Harris' (organic hyperinsulinism) 251.1
  Hart's (pellagra-cerebellar ataxia-renal aminoaciduria) 270.0
  Hayem-Faber (achlorhydric anemia) 280.9
  Hayem-Widal (acquired hemolytic jaundice) 283.9
  Heberden's (angina pectoris) 413.9
  Hedinger's (malignant carcinoid) 259.2
  Hegglin's 288.2
  Heller's (infantile psychosis) (*see also* Psychosis, childhood) 299.1 ✔5ᵗʰ
  H.E.L.L.P 642.5 ✔5ᵗʰ
  hemolytic-uremic (adult) (child) 283.11
  Hench-Rosenberg (palindromic arthritis) (*see also* Rheumatism, palindromic) 719.3 ✔5ᵗʰ
  Henoch-Schönlein (allergic purpura) 287.0
  hepatic flexure 569.89
  hepatorenal 572.4
    due to a procedure 997.4
    following delivery 674.8 ✔5ᵗʰ
  hepatourologic 572.4
  Herrick's (hemoglobin S disease) 282.61
  Herter (-Gee) (nontropical sprue) 579.0
  Heubner-Herter (nontropical sprue) 579.0
  Heyd's (hepatorenal) 572.4
  HHHO 759.81
  Hilger's 337.0
  Hoffa (-Kastert) (liposynovitis prepatellaris) 272.8
  Hoffmann's 244.9 [359.5]
  Hoffmann-Bouveret (paroxysmal tachycardia) 427.2
  Hoffmann-Werdnig 335.0
  Holländer-Simons (progressive lipodystrophy) 272.6
  Holmes' (visual disorientation) 368.16
  Holmes-Adie 379.46
  Hoppe-Goldflam 358.0

Syndrome — *see also* Disease — *continued*
  Horner's (*see also* Neuropathy, peripheral, autonomic) 337.9
    traumatic — *see* Injury, nerve, cervical sympathetic
  hospital addiction 301.51
  Hunt's (herpetic geniculate ganglionitis) 053.11
    dyssynergia cerebellaris myoclonica 334.2
  Hunter (-Hurler) (mucopolysaccharidosis II) 277.5
  hunterian glossitis 529.4
  Hurler (-Hunter) (mucopolysaccharidosis II) 277.5
  Hutchinson's incisors or teeth 090.5
  Hutchinson-Boeck (sarcoidosis) 135
  Hutchinson-Gilford (progeria) 259.8
  hydralazine
    correct substance properly administered 695.4
    overdose or wrong substance given or taken 972.6
  hydraulic concussion (abdomen) (*see also* Injury, internal, abdomen) 868.00
  hyperabduction 447.8
  hyperactive bowel 564.9
  hyperaldosteronism with hypokalemic alkalosis (Bartter's) 255.1
  hypercalcemic 275.42
  hypercoagulation NEC 289.8
  hypereosinophilic (idiopathic) 288.3
  hyperkalemic 276.7
  hyperkinetic — *see also* Hyperkinesia
    heart 429.82
  hyperlipemia-hemolytic anemia-icterus 571.1
  hypermobility 728.5
  hypernatremia 276.0
  hyperosmolarity 276.0
  hypersomnia-bulimia 349.89
  hypersplenic 289.4
  hypersympathetic (*see also* Neuropathy, peripheral, autonomic) 337.9
  hypertransfusion, newborn 776.4
  hyperventilation, psychogenic 306.1
  hyperviscosity (of serum) NEC 273.3
    polycythemic 289.0
    sclerothymic 282.8
  hypoglycemic (familial) (neonatal) 251.2
    functional 251.1
  hypokalemic 276.8
  hypophyseal 253.8
  hypophyseothalamic 253.8
  hypopituitarism 253.2
  hypoplastic left heart 746.7
  hypopotassemia 276.8
  hyposmolality 276.1
  hypotension, maternal 669.2 ✔5ᵗʰ
  hypotonia-hypomentia-hypogonadism-obesity 759.81
  ICF (intravascular coagulation-fibrinolysis) (*see also* Fibrinolysis) 286.6
  idiopathic cardiorespiratory distress, newborn 769
  idiopathic nephrotic (infantile) 581.9
  Imerslund (-Gräsbeck) (anemia due to familial selective vitamin B_{12} malabsorption) 281.1
  immobility (paraplegic) 728.3
  immunity deficiency, combined 279.2
  impending coronary 411.1
  impingement
    shoulder 726.2
    vertebral bodies 724.4
  inappropriate secretion of antidiuretic hormone (ADH) 253.6
  incomplete
    mandibulofacial 756.0
  infant
    death, sudden (SIDS) 798.0
    Hercules 255.2
    of diabetic mother 775.0
    shaken 995.55
  infantilism 253.3
  inferior vena cava 459.2
  influenza-like 487.1
  inspissated bile, newborn 774.4
  intermediate coronary (artery) 411.1
  internal carotid artery (*see also* Occlusion, artery, carotid) 433.1 ✔5ᵗʰ

Syndrome — *see also* Disease — *continued*
  interspinous ligament 724.8
  intestinal
    carcinoid 259.2
    gas 787.3
    knot 560.2
  intravascular
    coagulation-fibrinolysis (ICF) (*see also* Fibrinolysis) 286.6
    coagulopathy (*see also* Fibrinolysis) 286.6
  inverted Marfan's 759.89
  IRDS (idiopathic respiratory distress, newborn) 769
  irritable
    bowel 564.1
    heart 306.2
    weakness 300.5
  ischemic bowel (transient) 557.9
    chronic 557.1
    due to mesenteric artery insufficiency 557.1
  Itsenko-Cushing (pituitary basophilism) 255.0
  IVC (intravascular coagulopathy) (*see also* Fibrinolysis) 286.6
  Ivemark's (asplenia with congenital heart disease) 759.0
  Jaccoud's 714.4
  Jackson's 344.89
  Jadassohn-Lewandowski (pachyonchia congenita) 757.5
  Jaffe-Lichtenstein (-Uehlinger) 252.0
  Jahnke's (encephalocutaneous angiomatosis) 759.6
  Jakob-Creutzfeldt 046.1
    with dementia
      with behavioral disturbance 046.1 [294.11]
      without behavioral disturbance 046.1 [294.10]
  Jaksch's (pseudoleukemia infantum) 285.8
  Jaksch-Hayem (-Luzet) (pseudoleukemia infantum) 285.8
  jaw-winking 742.8
  jejunal 564.2
  jet lag 307.45
  Jeune's (asphyxiating thoracic dystrophy of newborn) 756.4
  Job's (chronic granulomatous disease) 288.1
  Jordan's 288.2
  Joseph-Diamond-Blackfan (congenital hypoplastic anemia) 284.0
  Joubert 759.89
  jugular foramen 352.6
  Kahler's (multiple myeloma) (M9730/3) 203.0 ✔5ᵗʰ
  Kalischer's (encephalocutaneous angiomatosis) 759.6
  Kallmann's (hypogonadotropic hypogonadism with anosmia) 253.4
  Kanner's (autism) (*see also* Psychosis, childhood) 299.0 ✔5ᵗʰ
  Kartagener's (sinusitis, bronchiectasis, situs inversus) 759.3
  Kasabach-Merritt (capillary hemangioma associated with thrombocytopenic purpura) 287.3
  Kast's (dyschondroplasia with hemangiomas) 756.4
  Kaznelson's (congenital hypoplastic anemia) 284.0
  Kelly's (sideropenic dysphagia) 280.8
  Kimmelstiel-Wilson (intercapillary glomerulosclerosis) 250.4 ✔5ᵗʰ [581.81]
  Klauder's (erythema multiforme exudativum) 695.1
  Klein-Waardenburg (ptosis-epicanthus) 270.2
  Kleine-Levin 349.89
  Klinefelter's 758.7
  Klippel-Feil (brevicollis) 756.16
  Klippel-Trenaunay 759.89
  Klumpke (-Déjérine) (injury to brachial plexus at birth) 767.6
  Klüver-Bucy (-Terzian) 310.0
  Köhler-Pellegrini-Stieda (calcification, knee joint) 726.62
  König's 564.89
  Korsakoff's (nonalcoholic) 294.0
    alcoholic 291.1

✔4ᵗʰ Fourth-digit Required   ✔5ᵗʰ Fifth-digit Required   ▶◀ Revised Text   ● New Line   ▲ Revised Code

Syndrome — *see also* Disease — *continued*
Korsakoff (-Wernicke) (nonalcoholic) 294.0
    alcoholic 291.1
Kostmann's (infantile genetic agranulocytosis) 288.0
Krabbe's
    congenital muscle hypoplasia 756.89
    cutaneocerebral angioma 759.6
Kunkel (lupoid hepatitis) 571.49
labyrinthine 386.50
laceration, broad ligament 620.6
Langdon Down (mongolism) 758.0
Larsen's (flattened facies and multiple congenital dislocations) 755.8
lateral
    cutaneous nerve of thigh 355.1
    medullary (*see also* Disease, cerebrovascular acute) 436
Launois' (pituitary gigantism) 253.0
Launois-Cléret (adiposogenital dystrophy) 253.8
Laurence-Moon (-Bardet) — Biedl (obesity, polydactyly, and mental retardation) 759.89
Lawford's (encephalocutaneous angiomatosis) 759.6
lazy
    leukocyte 288.0
    posture 728.3
Lederer-Brill (acquired infectious hemolytic anemia) 283.19
Legg-Calvé-Perthes (osteochondrosis capital femoral) 732.1
Lennox's (*see also* Epilepsy) 345.0 ✓5ᵗʰ
lenticular 275.1
Léopold-Lévi's (paroxysmal thyroid instability) 242.9 ✓5ᵗʰ
Lepore hemoglobin 282.4
Léri-Weill 756.59
Leriche's (aortic bifurcation occlusion) 444.0
Lermoyez's (*see also* Disease, Ménière's) 386.00
Lesch-Nyhan (hypoxanthine-guanine-phosphoribosyltransferase deficiency) 277.2
Lev's (acquired complete heart block) 426.0
Levi's (pituitary dwarfism) 253.3
Lévy-Roussy 334.3
Lichtheim's (subacute combined sclerosis with pernicious anemia) 281.0 [336.2]
Li-Fraumeni 758.3
Lightwood's (renal tubular acidosis) 588.8
Lignac (-de Toni) (-Fanconi) (-Debré) (cystinosis) 270.0
Likoff's (angina in menopausal women) 413.9
liver-kidney 572.4
Lloyd's 258.1
lobotomy 310.0
Löffler's (eosinophilic pneumonitis) 518.3
Löfgren's (sarcoidosis) 135
long arm 18 or 21 deletion 758.3
Looser (-Debray) — Milkman (osteomalacia with pseudofractures) 268.2
Lorain-Levi (pituitary dwarfism) 253.3
Louis-Bar (ataxia-telangiectasia) 334.8
low
    atmospheric pressure 993.2
    back 724.2
        psychogenic 306.0
    output (cardiac) (*see also* Failure, heart) 428.9
Lowe's (oculocerebrorenal dystrophy) 270.8
Lowe-Terrey-MacLachlan (oculocerebrorenal dystrophy) 270.8
lower radicular, newborn 767.4
Lown (-Ganong)-Levine (short P-R interval, normal QRS complex, and supraventricular tachycardia) 426.81
Lucey-Driscoll (jaundice due to delayed conjugation) 774.30
Luetscher's (dehydration) 276.5
lumbar vertebral 724.4
Lutembacher's (atrial septal defect with mitral stenosis) 745.5
Lyell's (toxic epidermal necrolysis) 695.1
    due to drug
        correct substance properly administered 695.1
        overdose or wrong substance given or taken 977.9

Syndrome — *see also* Disease — *continued*
Lyell's — *continued*
    due to drug — *continued*
        overdose or wrong substance given or taken — *continued*
            specified drug — *see* Table of Drugs and Chemicals
MacLeod's 492.8
macrogenitosomia praecox 259.8
macroglobulinemia 273.3
Maffucci's (dyschondroplasia with hemangiomas) 756.4
Magenblase 306.4
magnesium-deficiency 781.7
malabsorption 579.9
    postsurgical 579.3
    spinal fluid 331.3
malignant carcinoid 259.2
Mallory-Weiss 530.7
mandibulofacial dysostosis 756.0
manic-depressive (*see also* Psychosis, affective) 296.80
Mankowsky's (familial dysplastic osteopathy) 731.2
maple syrup (urine) 270.3
Marable's (celiac artery compression) 447.4
Marchesani (-Weill) (brachymorphism and ectopia lentis) 759.89
Marchiafava-Bignami 341.8
Marchiafava-Micheli (paroxysmal nocturnal hemoglobinuria) 283.2
Marcus Gunn's (jaw-winking syndrome) 742.8
Marfan's (arachnodactyly) 759.82
    meaning congenital syphilis 090.49
    with luxation of lens 090.49 [379.32]
Marie's (acromegaly) 253.0
    primary or idiopathic (acropachyderma) 757.39
    secondary (hypertrophic pulmonary osteoarthropathy) 731.2
Markus-Adie 379.46
Maroteaux-Lamy (mucopolysaccharidosis VI) 277.5
Martin's 715.27
Martin-Albright (pseudohypoparathyroidism) 275.49
Martorell-Fabré (pulseless disease) 446.7
massive aspiration of newborn 770.1
Masters-Allen 620.6
mastocytosis 757.33
maternal hypotension 669.2 ✓5ᵗʰ
maternal obesity 646.1 ✓5ᵗʰ
May (-Hegglin) 288.2
McArdle (-Schmid) (-Pearson) (glycogenosis V) 271.0
McCune-Albright (osteitis fibrosa disseminata) 756.59
McQuarrie's (idiopathic familial hypoglycemia) 251.2
meconium
    aspiration 770.1
    plug (newborn) NEC 777.1
median arcuate ligament 447.4
mediastinal fibrosis 519.3
Meekeren-Ehlers-Danlos 756.83
Meige (blepharospasm-oromandibular dystonia) 333.82
    -Milroy (chronic hereditary edema) 757.0
MELAS 758.89
Melkersson (-Rosenthal) 351.8
Mende's (ptosis-epicanthus) 270.2
Mendelson's (resulting from a procedure) 997.3
    during labor 668.0 ✓5ᵗʰ
    obstetric 668.0 ✓5ᵗʰ
Ménétrier's (hypertrophic gastritis) 535.2 ✓5ᵗʰ
Ménière's (*see also* Disease, Ménière's) 386.00
meningo-eruptive 047.1
Menkes' 759.89
    glutamic acid 759.89
    maple syrup (urine) disease 270.3
menopause 627.2
    postartificial 627.4
menstruation 625.4
MERFF 758.89
mesenteric
    artery, superior 557.1
    vascular insufficiency (with gangrene) 557.1
metastatic carcinoid 259.2

Syndrome — *see also* Disease — *continued*
Meyenburg-Altherr-Uehlinger 733.99
Meyer-Schwickerath and Weyers (dysplasia oculodentodigitalis) 759.89
Micheli-Rietti (thalassemia minor) 282.4
Michotte's 721.5
micrognathia-glossoptosis 756.0
microphthalmos (congenital) 759.89
midbrain 348.8
middle
    lobe (lung) (right) 518.0
    radicular 353.0
Miescher's
    familial acanthosis nigricans 701.2
    granulomatosis disciformis 709.3
Mieten's 759.89
migraine 346.0 ✓5ᵗʰ
Mikity-Wilson (pulmonary dysmaturity) 770.7
Mikulicz's (dryness of mouth, absent or decreased lacrimation) 527.1
milk alkali (milk drinkers') 999.9
Milkman (-Looser) (osteomalacia with pseudofractures) 268.2
Millard-Gubler 344.89
Miller Fisher's 357.0
Milles' (encephalocutaneous angiomatosis) 759.6
Minkowski-Chauffard (*see also* Spherocytosis) 282.0
Mirizzi's (hepatic duct stenosis) 576.2
    with calculus, cholelithiasis, or stones — *see* Choledocholithiasis
mitral
    click (-murmur) 785.2
    valve prolapse 424.0
Möbius'
    congenital oculofacial paralysis 352.6
    ophthalmoplegic migraine 346.8 ✓5ᵗʰ
Mohr's (types I and II) 759.89
monofixation 378.34
Moore's (*see also* Epilepsy) 345.5 ✓5ᵗʰ
Morel-Moore (hyperostosis frontalis interna) 733.3
Morel-Morgagni (hyperostosis frontalis interna) 733.3
Morgagni (-Stewart-Morel) (hyperostosis frontalis interna) 733.3
Morgagni-Adams-Stokes (syncope with heart block) 426.9
Morquio (-Brailsford) (-Ullrich) (mucopolysaccharidosis IV) 277.5
Morris (testicular feminization) 257.8
Morton's (foot) (metatarsalgia) (metatarsal neuralgia) (neuralgia) (neuroma) (toe) 355.6
Moschcowitz (-Singer-Symmers) (thrombotic thrombocytopenic purpura) 446.6
Mounier-Kuhn 494.0
    with acute exacerbation 494.1
Mucha-Haberman (acute parapsoriasis varioliformis) 696.2
mucocutaneous lymph node (acute) (febrile) (infantile) (MCLS) 446.1
multiple
    deficiency 260
    operations 301.51
Munchausen's 301.51
Münchmeyer's (exostosis luxurians) 728.11
Murchison-Sanderson — *see* Disease, Hodgkin's
myasthenic — *see* Myasthenia, syndrome
myelodysplastic 238.7
myeloproliferative (chronic) (M9960/1) 238.7
myofascial pain NEC 729.1
Naffziger's 353.0
Nager-de Reynier (dysostosis mandibularis) 756.0
nail-patella (hereditary osteo-onychodysplasia) 756.89
Nebécourt's 253.3
Neill-Dingwall (microencephaly and dwarfism) 759.89
nephrotic (*see also* Nephrosis) 581.9
    diabetic 250.4 ✓5ᵗʰ [581.81]
Netherton's (ichthyosiform erythroderma) 757.1
neurocutaneous 759.6
neuroleptic mailgnant 333.92
Nezelof's (pure alymphocytosis) 279.13

Syndrome — *see also* Disease — *continued*
Niemann-Pick (lipid histiocytosis) 272.7
Nonne-Milroy-Meige (chronic hereditary edema) 757.0
nonsense 300.16
Noonan's 759.89
Nothnagel's
  ophthalmoplegia-cerebellar ataxia 378.52
  vasomotor acroparesthesia 443.89
nucleus ambiguous-hypoglossal 352.6
OAV (oculoauriculovertebral dysplasia) 756.0
obsessional 300.3
oculocutaneous 364.24
oculomotor 378.81
oculourethroarticular 099.3
Ogilvie's (sympathicotonic colon obstruction) 560.89
ophthalmoplegia-cerebellar ataxia 378.52
Oppenheim-Urbach (necrobiosis lipoidica diabeticorum) 250.8 ☑5ᵗʰ [709.3]
oral-facial-digital 759.89
organic
  affective NEC 293.83
    drug-induced 292.84
  anxiety 293.84
  delusional 293.81
    alcohol-induced 291.5
    drug-induced 292.11
    due to or associated with
      arteriosclerosis 290.42
      presenile brain disease 290.12
      senility 290.20
  depressive 293.83
    drug-induced 292.84
    due to or associated with
      arteriosclerosis 290.43
      presenile brain disease 290.13
      senile brain disease 290.21
  hallucinosis 293.82
    drug-induced 292.84
organic affective 293.83
  induced by drug 292.84
organic personality 310.1
  induced by drug 292.89
Ormond's 593.4
orodigitofacial 759.89
orthostatic hypotensive-dysautonomic dyskinetic 333.0
Osler-Weber-Rendu (familial hemorrhagic telangiectasia) 448.0
osteodermopathic hyperostosis 757.39
osteoporosis-osteomalacia 268.2
Österreicher-Turner (hereditary osteo-onychodysplasia) 756.89
Ostrum-Furst 756.59
otolith 386.19
otopalatodigital 759.89
outlet (thoracic) 353.0
ovarian remant 620.8
ovarian vein 593.4
Owren's (*see also* Defect, coagulation) 286.3
OX 758.6
pacemaker 429.4
Paget-Schroetter (intermittent venous claudication) 453.8
pain — *see* Pain
painful
  apicocostal vertebral (M8010/3) 162.3
  arc 726.19
  bruising 287.2
  feet 266.2
Pancoast's (carcinoma, pulmonary apex) (M8010/3) 162.3
panhypopituitary (postpartum) 253.2
papillary muscle 429.81
  with myocardial infarction 410.8 ☑5ᵗʰ
Papillon-Léage and Psaume (orodigitofacial dysostosis) 759.89
parabiotic (transfusion)
  donor (twin) 772.0
  recipient (twin) 776.4
paralysis agitans 332.0
paralytic 344.9
  specified type NEC 344.89
paraneoplastic — *see* condition
Parinaud's (paralysis of conjugate upward gaze) 378.81

Syndrome — *see also* Disease — *continued*
Parinaud's — *continued*
  oculoglandular 372.02
Parkes Weber and Dimitri (encephalocutaneous angiomatosis) 759.6
Parkinson's (*see also* Parkinsonism) 332.0
parkinsonian (*see also* Parkinsonism) 332.0
Parry's (exophthalmic goiter) 242.0 ☑5ᵗʰ
Parry-Romberg 349.89
Parsonage-Aldren-Turner 353.5
Parsonage-Turner 353.5
Patau's (trisomy D) 758.1
patellofemoral 719.46
Paterson (-Brown) (-Kelly) (sideropenic dysphagia) 280.8
Payr's (splenic flexure syndrome) 569.89
pectoral girdle 447.8
pectoralis minor 447.8
Pelger-Huët (hereditary hyposegmentation) 288.2
pellagra-cerebellar ataxia-renal aminoaciduria 270.0
Pellegrini-Stieda 726.62
pellagroid 265.2
Pellizzi's (pineal) 259.8
pelvic congestion (-fibrosis) 625.5
Pendred's (familial goiter with deaf-mutism) 243
Penfield's (*see also* Epilepsy) 345.5 ☑5ᵗʰ
Penta X 758.81
peptic ulcer — *see* Ulcer, peptic 533.9 ☑5ᵗʰ
perabduction 447.8
periodic 277.3
periurethral fibrosis 593.4
persistent fetal circulation 747.83 ▲
Petges-Cléjat (poikilodermatomyositis) 710.3
Peutz-Jeghers 759.6
Pfeiffer (acrocephalosyndactyly) 755.55
phantom limb 353.6
pharyngeal pouch 279.11
Pick's (pericardial pseudocirrhosis of liver) 423.2
  heart 423.2
  liver 423.2
Pick-Herxheimer (diffuse idiopathic cutaneous atrophy) 701.8
Pickwickian (cardiopulmonary obesity) 278.8
PIE (pulmonary infiltration with eosinophilia) 518.3
Pierre Marie-Bamberger (hypertrophic pulmonary osteoarthropathy) 731.2
Pierre Mauriac's (diabetes-dwarfism-obesity) 258.1
Pierre Robin 756.0
pigment dispersion, iris 364.53
pineal 259.8
pink puffer 492.8
pituitary 253.0
placental
  dysfunction 762.2
  insufficiency 762.2
  transfusion 762.3
plantar fascia 728.71
plica knee 727.83
Plummer-Vinson (sideropenic dysphagia) 280.8
pluricarential of infancy 260
plurideficiency of infancy 260
pluriglandular (compensatory) 258.8
polycarential of infancy 260
polyglandular 258.8
polysplenia 759.0
pontine 433.8 ☑5ᵗʰ
popliteal
  artery entrapment 447.8
  web 756.89
postartificial menopause 627.4
postcardiotomy 429.4
postcholecystectomy 576.0
postcommissurotomy 429.4
postconcussional 310.2
postcontusional 310.2
postencephalitic 310.8
posterior
  cervical sympathetic 723.2
  fossa compression 348.4
  inferior cerebellar artery (*see also* Disease, cerebrovascular, acute) 436
postgastrectomy (dumping) 564.2

Syndrome — *see also* Disease — *continued*
post-gastric surgery 564.2
posthepatitis 780.79
postherpetic (neuralgia) (zoster) 053.19
  geniculate ganglion 053.11
  ophthalmica 053.19
postimmunization — *see* Complications, vaccination
postinfarction 411.0
postinfluenza (asthenia) 780.79
postirradiation 990
postlaminectomy 722.80
  cervical, cervicothoracic 722.81
  lumbar, lumbosacral 722.83
  thoracic, thoracolumbar 722.82
postleukotomy 310.0
postlobotomy 310.0
postmastectomy lymphedema 457.0
postmature (of newborn) 766.2
postmyocardial infarction 411.0
postoperative NEC 998.9
  blind loop 579.2
postpartum panhypopituitary 253.2
postperfusion NEC 999.8
  bone marrow 996.85
postpericardiotomy 429.4
postphlebitic ►(asymptomatic)◄ 459.10 ▲
  with •
    complications NEC 459.19 •
    inflammation 459.12 •
      and ulcer 459.13 •
    stasis dermatitis 459.12 •
      with ulcer 459.13 •
    ulcer 459.11 •
      with inflammation 459.13 •
postpolio (myelitis) 138
postvagotomy 564.2
postvalvulotomy 429.4
postviral (asthenia) NEC 780.79
Potain's (gastrectasis with dyspepsia) 536.1
potassium intoxication 276.7
Potter's 753.0
Prader (-Labhart) -Willi (-Fanconi) 759.81
preinfarction 411.1
preleukemic 238.7
premature senility 259.8
premenstrual 625.4
premenstrual tension 625.4
pre ulcer 536.9
Prinzmetal-Massumi (anterior chest wall syndrome) 786.52
Profichet's 729.9
progeria 259.8
progressive pallidal degeneration 333.0
prolonged gestation 766.2
Proteus (dermal hypoplasia) 757.39
prune belly 756.71
prurigo-asthma 691.8
pseudocarpal tunnel (sublimis) 354.0
pseudohermaphroditism-virilism-hirsutism 255.2
pseudoparalytica 358.0
pseudo-Turner's 759.89
psycho-organic 293.9
  acute 293.0
  anxiety type 293.84
  depressive type 293.83
  hallucinatory type 293.82
  nonpsychotic severity 310.1
    specified focal (partial) NEC 310.8
  paranoid type 293.81
  specified type NEC 293.89
  subacute 293.1
pterygolymphangiectasia 758.6
ptosis-epicanthus 270.2
pulmonary 660.1 ☑5ᵗʰ
  arteriosclerosis 416.0
  hypoperfusion (idiopathic) 769
  renal (hemorrhagic) 446.21
pulseless 446.7
Putnam-Dana (subacute combined sclerosis with pernicious anemia) 281.0 [336.2]
pyloroduodenal 537.89
pyramidopallidonigral 332.0
pyriformis 355.0
Q-T interval prolongation 794.31
radicular NEC 729.2
  lower limbs 724.4

☑4ᵗʰ Fourth-digit Required   ☑5ᵗʰ Fifth-digit Required   ►◄ Revised Text   ● New Line   ▲ Revised Code

Syndrome — Syndrome

Syndrome — *see also* Disease — *continued*
  radicular NEC — *continued*
    upper limbs 723.4
      newborn 767.4
  Raeder-Harbitz (pulseless disease) 446.7
  Ramsay Hunt's
    dyssynergia cerebellaris myoclonica 334.2
    herpetic geniculate ganglionitis 053.11
  rapid time-zone change 307.45
  Raymond (-Céstan) 433.8 ✔5ᵗʰ
  Raynaud's (paroxysmal digital cyanosis) 443.0
  RDS (respiratory distress syndrome, newborn)
    769
  Refsum's (heredopathia atactica
    polyneuritiformis) 356.3
  Reichmann's (gastrosuccorrhea) 536.8
  Reifenstein's (hereditary familial hypogonadism,
    male) 257.2
  Reilly's (*see also* Neuropathy, peripheral,
    autonomic) 337.9
  Reiter's 099.3
  renal glomerulohyalinosis-diabetic
    250.4 ✔5ᵗʰ [581.81]
  Rendu-Osler-Weber (familial hemorrhagic
    telangiectasia) 448.0
  renofacial (congenital biliary fibroangiomatosis)
    753.0
  Rénon-Delille 253.8
  respiratory distress (idiopathic) (newborn) 769
    adult (following shock, surgery, or trauma)
      518.5
    specified NEC 518.82
  restless leg 333.99
  retraction (Duane's) 378.71
  retroperitoneal fibrosis 593.4
  Rett's 330.8
  Reye's 331.81
  Reye-Sheehan (postpartum pituitary necrosis)
    253.2
  Riddoch's (visual disorientation) 368.16
  Ridley's (*see also* Failure, ventricular, left)
    428.1
  Rieger's (mesodermal dysgenesis, anterior
    ocular segment) 743.44
  Rietti-Greppi-Micheli (thalassemia minor) 282.4
  right ventricular obstruction — *see* Failure,
    heart
  Riley-Day (familial dysautonomia) 742.8
  Robin's 756.0
  Rokitansky-Kuster-Hauser (congenital absence,
    vagina) 752.49
  Romano-Ward (prolonged Q-T interval) 794.31
  Romberg's 349.89
  Rosen-Castleman-Liebow (pulmonary
    proteinosis) 516.0
  rotator cuff, shoulder 726.10
  Roth's 355.1
  Rothmund's (congenital poikiloderma) 757.33
  Rotor's (idiopathic hyperbilirubinemia) 277.4
  Roussy-Lévy 334.3
  Roy (-Jutras) (acropachyderma) 757.39
  rubella (congenital) 771.0
  Rubinstein-Taybi's (brachydactylia, short
    stature, and mental retardation) 759.89
  Rud's (mental deficiency, epilepsy, and
    infantilism) 759.89
  Ruiter-Pompen (-Wyers) (angiokeratoma
    corporis diffusum) 272.7
  Runge's (postmaturity) 766.2
  Russell (-Silver) (congenital hemihypertrophy
    and short stature) 759.89
  Rytand-Lipsitch (complete atrioventricular
    block) 426.0
  sacralization-scoliosis-sciatica 756.15
  sacroiliac 724.6
  Saenger's 379.46
  salt
    depletion (*see also* Disease, renal) 593.9
      due to heat NEC 992.8
        causing heat exhaustion or prostration
          992.4
    low (*see also* Disease, renal) 593.9
  salt-losing (*see also* Disease, renal) 593.9
  Sanfilippo's (mucopolysaccharidosis III) 277.5
  Scaglietti-Dagnini (acromegalic
    macrospondylitis) 253.0
  scalded skin 695.1
  scalenus anticus (anterior) 353.0

Syndrome — *see also* Disease — *continued*
  scapulocostal 354.8
  scapuloperoneal 359.1
  scapulovertebral 723.4
  Schaumann's (sarcoidosis) 135
  Scheie's (mucopolysaccharidosis IS) 277.5
  Scheuthauer-Marie-Sainton (cleidocranialis
    dysostosis) 755.59
  Schirmer's (encephalocutaneous angiomatosis)
    759.6
  schizophrenic, of childhood NEC (*see also*
    Psychosis, childhood) 299.9 ✔5ᵗʰ
  Schmidt's
    sphallo-pharyngo-laryngeal hemiplegia 352.6
    thyroid-adrenocortical insufficiency 258.1
    vagoaccessory 352.6
  Schneider's 047.9
  Scholte's (malignant carcinoid) 259.2
  Scholz (-Bielschowsky-Henneberg) 330.0
  Schroeder's (endocrine-hypertensive) 255.3
  Schüller-Christian (chronic histiocytosis X)
    277.8
  Schultz's (agranulocytosis) 288.0
  Schwartz (-Jampel) 756.89
  Schwartz-Bartter (inappropriate secretion of
    antidiuretic hormone) 253.6
  Scimitar (anomalous venous drainage, right
    lung to inferior vena cava) 747.49
  sclerocystic ovary 256.4
  sea-blue histiocyte 272.7
  Seabright-Bantam
    (pseudohypoparathyroidism) 275.49
  Seckel's 759.89
  Secretan's (posttraumatic edema) 782.3
  secretoinhibitor (keratoconjunctivitis sicca)
    710.2
  Seeligmann's (ichthyosis congenita) 757.1
  Senear-Usher (pemphigus erythematosus)
    694.4
  senilism 259.8
  serotonin 333.99
  serous meningitis 348.2
  Sertoli cell (germinal aplasia) 606.0
  sex chromosome mosaic 758.81
  Sézary's (reticulosis) (M9701/3) 202.2 ✔5ᵗʰ
  shaken infant 995.55
  Shaver's (bauxite pneumoconiosis) 503
  Sheehan's (postpartum pituitary necrosis)
    253.2
  shock (traumatic) 958.4
    kidney 584.5
      following crush injury 958.5
    lung 518.5
    neurogenic 308.9
    psychic 308.9
  short
    bowel 579.3
    P-R interval 426.81
  shoulder-arm (*see also* Neuropathy, peripheral,
    autonomic) 337.9
  shoulder-girdle 723.4
  shoulder-hand (*see also* Neuropathy,
    peripheral, autonomic) 337.9
  Shwachman's 288.0
  Shy-Drager (orthostatic hypotension with
    multisystem degeneration) 333.0
  Sicard's 352.6
  sicca (keratoconjunctivitis) 710.2
  sick
    cell 276.1
    cilia 759.89
    sinus 427.81
  sideropenic 280.8
  Siemens'
    ectodermal dysplasia 757.31
    keratosis follicularis spinulosa (decalvans)
      757.39
  Silfverskiöld's (osteochondrodystrophy,
    extremities) 756.50
  Silver's (congenital hemihypertrophy and short
    stature) 759.89
  Silvestroni-Bianco (thalassemia minima) 282.4
  Simons' (progressive lipodystrophy) 272.6
  sinus tarsi 726.79
  sinusitis-bronchiectasis-situs inversus 759.3
  Sipple's (medullary thyroid carcinoma-
    pheochromocytoma) 193

Syndrome — *see also* Disease — *continued*
  Sjögren (-Gougerot) (keratoconjunctivitis sicca)
    710.2
    with lung involvement 710.2 [517.8]
  Sjögren-Larsson (ichthyosis congenita) 757.1
  Slocumb's 255.3
  Sluder's 337.0
  Smith-Lemli-Opitz (cerebrohepatorenal
    syndrome) 759.89
  smokers' 305.1
  Sneddon-Wilkinson (subcorneal pustular
    dermatosis) 694.1
  Sotos' (cerebral gigantism) 253.0
  South African cardiomyopathy 425.2
  spasmodic
    upward movement, eye(s) 378.82
    winking 307.20
  Spens' (syncope with heart block) 426.9
  spherophakia-brachymorphia 759.89
  spinal cord injury — *see also* Injury, spinal, by
    site
    with fracture, vertebra — *see* Fracture,
      vertebra, by site, with spinal cord
      injury
    cervical — *see* Injury, spinal, cervical
    fluid malabsorption (acquired) 331.3
  splenic
    agenesis 759.0
    flexure 569.89
    neutropenia 288.0
    sequestration 282.60
  Spurway's (brittle bones and blue sclera)
    756.51
  staphylococcal scalded skin 695.1
  Stein's (polycystic ovary) 256.4
  Stein-Leventhal (polycystic ovary) 256.4
  Steinbrocker's (*see also* Neuropathy,
    peripheral, autonomic) 337.9
  Stevens-Johnson (erythema multiforme
    exudativum) 695.1
  Stewart-Morel (hyperostosis frontalis interna)
    733.3
  stiff-man 333.91
  Still's (juvenile rheumatoid arthritis) 714.30
  Still-Felty (rheumatoid arthritis with
    splenomegaly and leukopenia) 714.1
  Stilling-Türk-Duane (ocular retraction
    syndrome) 378.71
  Stojano's (subcostal) 098.86
  Stokes (-Adams) (syncope with heart block)
    426.9
  Stokvis-Talma (enterogenous cyanosis) 289.7
  stone heart (*see also* Failure, ventricular, left)
    428.1
  straight-back 756.19
  stroke (*see also* Disease, cerebrovascular,
    acute) 436
    little 435.9
  Sturge-Kalischer-Weber (encephalotrigeminal
    angiomatosis) 759.6
  Sturge-Weber (-Dimitri) (encephalocutaneous
    angiomatosis) 759.6
  subclavian-carotid obstruction (chronic) 446.7
  subclavian steal 435.2
  subcoracoid-pectoralis minor 447.8
  subcostal 098.86
    nerve compression 354.8
  subperiosteal hematoma 267
  subphrenic interposition 751.4
  sudden infant death (SIDS) 798.0
  Sudeck's 733.7
  Sudeck-Leriche 733.7
  superior
    cerebellar artery (*see also* Disease,
      cerebrovascular, acute) 436
    mesenteric artery 557.1
    pulmonary sulcus (tumor) (M8010/3) 162.3
    vena cava 459.2
  suprarenal cortical 255.3
  supraspinatus 726.10
  swallowed blood 777.3
  sweat retention 705.1
  Sweet's (acute febrile neutrophilic dermatosis)
    695.89
  Swyer-James (unilateral hyperlucent lung)
    492.8
  Swyer's (XY pure gonadal dysgenesis) 752.7
  Symonds' 348.2

✔4ᵗʰ Fourth-digit Required   ✔5ᵗʰ Fifth-digit Required   ▶◀ Revised Text   ● New Line   ▲ Revised Code

Syndrome — *see also* Disease — *continued*
  sympathetic
    cervical paralysis 337.0
    pelvic 625.5
  syndactylic oxycephaly 755.55
  syphilitic-cardiovascular 093.89
  systemic
    fibrosclerosing 710.8
    inflammatory response (SIRS) 995.90 ●
      due to ●
        infectious process 995.91 ●
          with organ dysfunction 995.92 ●
        non-infectious process 995.93 ●
          with organ dysfunction 995.94 ●
  systolic click (-murmur) 785.2
  Tabagism 305.1
  tachycardia-bradycardia 427.81
  Takayasu (-Onishi) (pulseless disease) 446.7
  Tapia's 352.6
  tarsal tunnel 355.5
  Taussig-Bing (transposition, aorta and
      overriding pulmonary artery) 745.11
  Taybi's (otopalatodigital) 759.89
  Taylor's 625.5
  teething 520.7
  tegmental 344.89
  telangiectasis-pigmentation-cataract 757.33
  temporal 383.02
    lobectomy behavior 310.0
  temporomandibular joint-pain-dysfunction
      [TMJ] NEC 524.60
    specified NEC 524.69
  Terry's 362.21
  testicular feminization 257.8
  testis, nonvirilizing 257.8
  tethered (spinal) cord 742.59
  thalamic 348.8
  Thibierge-Weissenbach (cutaneous systemic
      sclerosis) 710.1
  Thiele 724.6
  thoracic outlet (compression) 353.0
  thoracogenous rheumatic (hypertrophic
      pulmonary osteoarthropathy) 731.2
  Thorn's (*see also* Disease, renal) 593.9
  Thorson-Biörck (malignant carcinoid) 259.2
  thrombopenia-hemangioma 287.3
  thyroid-adrenocortical insufficiency 258.1
  Tietze's 733.6
  time-zone (rapid) 307.45
  Tobias' (carcinoma, pulmonary apex)
      (M8010/3) 162.3
  toilet seat 926.0
  Tolosa-Hunt 378.55
  Toni-Fanconi (cystinosis) 270.0
  Touraine's (hereditary osteo-onychodysplasia)
      756.89
  Touraine-Solente-Golé (acropachyderma)
      757.39
  toxic
    oil 710.5
    shock 040.82 ▲
  transfusion
    fetal-maternal 772.0
    twin
      donor (infant) 772.0
      recipient (infant) 776.4
  Treacher Collins' (incomplete mandibulofacial
      dysostosis) 756.0
  trigeminal plate 259.8
  triple X female 758.81
  trisomy NEC 758.5
    13 or D₁ 758.1
    16-18 or E 758.2
    18 or E₃ 758.2
    20 758.5
    21 or G (mongolism) 758.0
    22 or G (mongolism) 758.0
    G 758.0
  Troisier-Hanot-Chauffard (bronze diabetes)
      275.0
  tropical wet feet 991.4
  Trousseau's (thrombophlebitis migrans visceral
      cancer) 453.1
  Türk's (ocular retraction syndrome) 378.71
  Turner's 758.6

Syndrome — *see also* Disease — *continued*
  Turner-Varny 758.6
  twin-to-twin transfusion 762.3
    recipient twin 776.4
  Uehlinger's (acropachyderma) 757.39
  Ullrich (-Bonnevie) (-Turner) 758.6
  Ullrich-Feichtiger 759.89
  underwater blast injury (abdominal) (*see also*
      Injury, internal, abdomen) 868.00
  universal joint, cervix 620.6
  Unverricht (-Lundborg) 333.2
  Unverricht-Wagner (dermatomyositis) 710.3
  upward gaze 378.81
  Urbach-Oppenheim (necrobiosis lipoidica
      diabeticorum) 250.8 ✓5ᵗʰ [709.3]
  Urbach-Wiethe (lipoid proteinosis) 272.8
  uremia, chronic 585
  urethral 597.81
  urethro-oculoarticular 099.3
  urethro-oculosynovial 099.3
  urohepatic 572.4
  uveocutaneous 364.24
  uveomeningeal, uveomeningitis 363.22
  vagohypoglossal 352.6
  vagovagal 780.2
  van Buchem's (hyperostosis corticalis) 733.3
  van der Hoeve's (brittle bones and blue sclera,
      deafness) 756.51
  van der Hoeve-Halbertsma-Waardenburg
      (ptosis-epicanthus) 270.2
  van der Hoeve-Waardenburg-Gualdi (ptosis-
      epicanthus) 270.2
  van Neck-Odelberg (juvenile osteochondrosis)
      732.1
  vanishing twin 651.33
  vascular splanchnic 557.0
  vasomotor 443.9
  vasovagal 780.2
  VATER 759.89
  Velo-cardio-facial 759.89 ●
    with chromosomal deletion 758.5 ●
  vena cava (inferior) (superior) (obstruction)
      459.2
  Verbiest's (claudicatio intermittens spinalis)
      435.1
  Vernet's 352.6
  vertebral
    artery 435.1
      compression 721.1
    lumbar 724.4
    steal 435.1
  vertebrogenic (pain) 724.5
  vertiginous NEC 386.9
  video display tube 723.8
  Villaret's 352.6
  Vinson-Plummer (sideropenic dysphagia) 280.8
  virilizing adrenocortical hyperplasia, congenital
      255.2
  virus, viral 079.99
  visceral larval migrans 128.0
  visual disorientation 368.16
  vitamin B₆ deficiency 266.1
  vitreous touch 997.99
  Vogt's (corpus striatum) 333.7
  Vogt-Koyanagi 364.24
  Volkmann's 958.6
  von Bechterew-Strümpell (ankylosing
      spondylitis) 720.0
  von Graefe's 378.72
  von Hippel-Lindau (angiomatosis
      retinocerebellosa) 759.6
  von Schroetter's (intermittent venous
      claudication) 453.8
  von Willebrand (-Jürgens) (angiohemophilia)
      286.4
  Waardenburg-Klein (ptosis epicanthus) 270.2
  Wagner (-Unverricht) (dermatomyositis) 710.3
  Waldenström's (macroglobulinemia) 273.3
  Waldenström-Kjellberg (sideropenic dysphagia)
      280.8
  Wallenberg's (posterior inferior cerebellar
      artery) (*see also* Disease, cerebrovascular,
      acute) 436
  Waterhouse (-Friderichsen) 036.3
  water retention 276.6
  Weber's 344.89
  Weber-Christian (nodular nonsuppurative
      panniculitis) 729.30

Syndrome — *see also* Disease — *continued*
  Weber-Cockayne (epidermolysis bullosa) 757.39
  Weber-Dimitri (encephalocutaneous
      angiomatosis) 759.6
  Weber-Gubler 344.89
  Weber-Leyden 344.89
  Weber-Osler (familial hemorrhagic
      telangiectasia) 448.0
  Wegener's (necrotizing respiratory
      granulomatosis) 446.4
  Weill-Marchesani (brachymorphism and ectopia
      lentis) 759.89
  Weingarten's (tropical eosinophilia) 518.3
  Weiss-Baker (carotid sinus syncope) 337.0
  Weissenbach-Thibierge (cutaneous systemic
      sclerosis) 710.1
  Werdnig-Hoffmann 335.0
  Werlhof-Wichmann (*see also* Purpura,
      thrombocytopenic) 287.3
  Wermer's (polyendocrine adenomatosis) 258.0
  Werner's (progeria adultorum) 259.8
  Wernicke's (nonalcoholic) (superior hemorrhagic
      polioencephalitis) 265.1
  Wernicke-Korsakoff (nonalcoholic) 294.0
    alcoholic 291.1
  Westphal-Strümpell (hepatolenticular
      degeneration) 275.1
  wet
    brain (alcoholic) 303.9 ✓5ᵗʰ
    feet (maceration) (tropical) 991.4
    lung
      adult 518.5
      newborn 770.6
  whiplash 847.0
  Whipple's (intestinal lipodystrophy) 040.2
  "whistling face" (craniocarpotarsal dystrophy)
      759.89
  Widal (-Abrami) (acquired hemolytic jaundice)
      283.9
  Wilkie's 557.1
  Wilkinson-Sneddon (subcorneal pustular
      dermatosis) 694.1
  Willan-Plumbe (psoriasis) 696.1
  Willebrand (-Jürgens) (angiohemophilia) 286.4
  Willi-Prader (hypogenital dystrophy with
      diabetic tendency) 759.81
  Wilson's (hepatolenticular degeneration) 275.1
  Wilson-Mikity 770.7
  Wiskott-Aldrich (eczema-thrombocytopenia)
      279.12
  withdrawal
    alcohol 291.81
    drug 292.0
      infant of dependent mother 779.5
  Woakes' (ethmoiditis) 471.1
  Wolff-Parkinson-White (anomalous
      atrioventricular excitation) 426.7
  Wright's (hyperabduction) 447.8
  X
    cardiac 413.9
    dysmetabolic 277.7
  xiphoidalgia 733.99
  XO 758.6
  XXX 758.81
  XXXXY 758.81
  XXY 758.7
  yellow vernix (placental dysfunction) 762.2
  Zahorsky's 074.0
  Zieve's (jaundice, hyperlipemia and hemolytic
      anemia) 571.1
  Zollinger-Ellison (gastric hypersecretion with
      pancreatic islet cell tumor) 251.5
  Zuelzer-Ogden (nutritional megaloblastic
      anemia) 281.2
Synechia (iris) (pupil) 364.70
  anterior 364.72
    peripheral 364.73
  intrauterine (traumatic) 621.5
  posterior 364.71
  vulvae, congenital 752.49
Synesthesia (*see also* Disturbance, sensation)
    782.0
Synodontia 520.2
Synophthalmus 759.89
Synorchidism 752.8
Synorchism 752.8

Syndrome — Synorchism

Synostosis — Syphilis

Synostosis (congenital) 756.59
  astragaloscaphoid 755.67
  radioulnar 755.53
  talonavicular (bar) 755.67
  tarsal 755.67
Synovial — *see* condition
Synovioma (M9040/3) — *see also* Neoplasm,
  connective tissue, malignant
  benign (M9040/0) — *see* Neoplasm, connective
    tissue, benign
Synoviosarcoma (M9040/3) — *see* Neoplasm,
  connective tissue, malignant
Synovitis 727.00
  chronic crepitant, wrist 727.2
  due to crystals — *see* Arthritis, due to crystals
  gonococcal 098.51
  gouty 274.0
  syphilitic 095.7
    congenital 090.0
  traumatic, current — *see* Sprain, by site
  tuberculous — *see* Tuberculosis, synovitis
  villonodular 719.20
    ankle 719.27
    elbow 719.22
    foot 719.27
    hand 719.24
    hip 719.25
    knee 719.26
    multiple sites 719.29
    pelvic region 719.25
    shoulder (region) 719.21
    specified site NEC 719.28
    wrist 719.23
Syphilide 091.3
  congenital 090.0
  newborn 090.0
  tubercular 095.8
    congenital 090.0
Syphilis, syphilitic (acquired) 097.9
  with lung involvement 095.1
  abdomen (late) 095.2
  acoustic nerve 094.86
  adenopathy (secondary) 091.4
  adrenal (gland) 095.8
    with cortical hypofunction 095.8
  age under 2 years NEC (*see also* Syphilis,
    congenital) 090.9 ✓5ᵗʰ
    acquired 097.9
  alopecia (secondary) 091.82
  anemia 095.8
  aneurysm (artery) (ruptured) 093.89
    aorta 093.0
    central nervous system 094.89
    congenital 090.5
  anus 095.8
    primary 091.1
    secondary 091.3
  aorta, aortic (arch) (abdominal) (insufficiency)
    (pulmonary) (regurgitation) (stenosis)
    (thoracic) 093.89
    aneurysm 093.0
  arachnoid (adhesive) 094.2
  artery 093.89
    cerebral 094.89
    spinal 094.89
  arthropathy (neurogenic) (tabetic) 094.0 [713.5]
  asymptomatic — *see* Syphilis, latent
  ataxia, locomotor (progressive) 094.0
  atrophoderma maculatum 091.3
  auricular fibrillation 093.89
  Bell's palsy 094.89
  bladder 095.8
  bone 095.5
    secondary 091.61
  brain 094.89
  breast 095.8
  bronchus 095.8
  bubo 091.0
  bulbar palsy 094.89
  bursa (late) 095.7
  cardiac decompensation 093.89
  cardiovascular (early) (late) (primary)
    (secondary) (tertiary) 093.9
    specified type and site NEC 093.89
  causing death under 2 years of age (*see also*
    Syphilis, congenital) 090.9 ✓5ᵗʰ
    stated to be acquired NEC 097.9

Syphilis, syphilitic — *continued*
  central nervous system (any site) (early) (late)
    (latent) (primary) (recurrent) (relapse)
    (secondary) (tertiary) 094.9
    with
      ataxia 094.0
      paralysis, general 094.1
        juvenile 090.40
      paresis (general) 094.1
        juvenile 090.40
      tabes (dorsalis) 094.0
        juvenile 090.40
      taboparesis 094.1
        juvenile 090.40
    aneurysm (ruptured) 094.87
    congenital 090.40
    juvenile 090.40
    remission in (sustained) 094.9
    serology doubtful, negative, or positive 094.9
    specified nature or site NEC 094.89
    vascular 094.89
  cerebral 094.89
    meningovascular 094.2
    nerves 094.89
    sclerosis 094.89
    thrombosis 094.89
  cerebrospinal 094.89
    tabetic 094.0
  cerebrovascular 094.89
  cervix 095.8
  chancre (multiple) 091.0
    extragenital 091.2
    Rollet's 091.0
  Charcôt's joint 094.0 [713.5]
  choked disc 094.89 [377.00]
  chorioretinitis 091.51
    congenital 090.0 [363.13]
    late 094.83
  choroiditis 091.51
    congenital 090.0 [363.13]
    late 094.83
    prenatal 090.0 [363.13]
  choroidoretinitis (secondary) 091.51
    congenital 090.0 [363.13]
    late 094.83
  ciliary body (secondary) 091.52
    late 095.8 [364.11]
  colon (late) 095.8
  combined sclerosis 094.89
  complicating pregnancy, childbirth or
    puerperium 647.0 ✓5ᵗʰ
    affecting fetus or newborn 760.2
  condyloma (latum) 091.3
  congenital 090.9 ✓5ᵗʰ
    with
      encephalitis 090.41
      paresis (general) 090.40
      tabes (dorsalis) 090.40
      taboparesis 090.40
    chorioretinitis, choroiditis 090.0 [363.13]
    early or less than 2 years after birth NEC
      090.2
      with manifestations 090.0
      latent (without manifestations) 090.1
        negative spinal fluid test 090.1
        serology, positive 090.1
      symptomatic 090.0
    interstitial keratitis 090.3
    juvenile neurosyphilis 090.40
    late or 2 years or more after birth NEC
      090.7 ✓5ᵗʰ
      chorioretinitis, choroiditis 090.5 [363.13]
      interstitial keratitis 090.3
      juvenile neurosyphilis NEC 090.40
      latent (without manifestations) 090.6 ✓5ᵗʰ
        negative spinal fluid test 090.6 ✓5ᵗʰ
        serology, positive 090.6 ✓5ᵗʰ
      symptomatic or with manifestations NEC
        090.5
        interstitial keratitis 090.3
  conjugal 097.9
    tabes 094.0
  conjunctiva 095.8 [372.10]
  contact V01.6
  cord, bladder 094.0
  cornea, late 095.8 [370.59]
  coronary (artery) 093.89
    sclerosis 093.89

Syphilis, syphilitic — *continued*
  coryza 095.8
    congenital 090.0
  cranial nerve 094.89
  cutaneous — *see* Syphilis, skin
  dacryocystitis 095.8
  degeneration, spinal cord 094.89
  d'emblée 095.8
  dementia 094.1
    paralytica 094.1
      juvenilis 090.40
  destruction of bone 095.5
  dilatation, aorta 093.0
  due to blood transfusion 097.9
  dura mater 094.89
  ear 095.8
    inner 095.8
      nerve (eighth) 094.86
      neurorecurrence 094.86
  early NEC 091.0
    cardiovascular 093.9
    central nervous system 094.9
      paresis 094.1
      tabes 094.0
    latent (without manifestations) (less than 2
      years after infection) 092.9
      negative spinal fluid test 092.9
      serological relapse following treatment
        092.0
      serology positive 092.9
    paresis 094.1
    relapse (treated, untreated) 091.7
    skin 091.3
    symptomatic NEC 091.89
      extragenital chancre 091.2
      primary, except extragenital chancre
        091.0
      secondary (*see also* Syphilis, secondary)
        091.3
        relapse (treated, untreated) 091.7
    tabes 094.0
    ulcer 091.3
  eighth nerve 094.86
  endemic, nonvenereal 104.0
  endocarditis 093.20
    aortic 093.22
    mitral 093.21
    pulmonary 093.24
    tricuspid 093.23
  epididymis (late) 095.8
  epiglottis 095.8
  epiphysitis (congenital) 090.0
  esophagus 095.8
  Eustachian tube 095.8
  exposure to V01.6
  eye 095.8 [363.13]
    neuromuscular mechanism 094.85
  eyelid 095.8 [373.5]
    with gumma 095.8 [373.5]
    ptosis 094.89
  fallopian tube 095.8
  fracture 095.5
  gallbladder (late) 095.8
  gastric 095.8
    crisis 094.0
    polyposis 095.8
  general 097.9
    paralysis 094.1
      juvenile 090.40
  genital (primary) 091.0
  glaucoma 095.8
  gumma (late) NEC 095.9
    cardiovascular system 093.9
    central nervous system 094.9
    congenital 090.5
    heart or artery 093.89
  heart 093.89
    block 093.89
    decompensation 093.89
    disease 093.89
    failure 093.89
    valve (*see also* Syphilis, endocarditis) 093.20
  hemianesthesia 094.89
  hemianopsia 095.8
  hemiparesis 094.89
  hemiplegia 094.89
  hepatic artery 093.89

Syphilis, syphilitic — *continued*
  hepatitis 095.3
  hepatomegaly 095.3
    congenital 090.0
  hereditaria tarda (*see also* Syphilis, congenital, late) 090.7 ✓5ᵗʰ
  hereditary (*see also* Syphilis, congenital) 090.9 ✓5ᵗʰ
    interstitial keratitis 090.3
  Hutchinson's teeth 090.5
  hyalitis 095.8
  inactive — *see* Syphilis, latent
  infantum NEC (*see also* Syphilis, congenital) 090.9 ✓5ᵗʰ
  inherited — *see* Syphilis, congenital
  internal ear 095.8
  intestine (late) 095.8
  iris, iritis (secondary) 091.52
    late 095.8 [364.11]
  joint (late) 095.8
  keratitis (congenital) (early) (interstitial) (late) (parenchymatous) (punctata profunda) 090.3
  kidney 095.4
  lacrimal apparatus 095.8
  laryngeal paralysis 095.8
  larynx 095.8
  late 097.0
    cardiovascular 093.9
    central nervous system 094.9
    latent or 2 years or more after infection (without manifestations) 096
      negative spinal fluid test 096
      serology positive 096
    paresis 094.1
    specified site NEC 095.8
    symptomatic or with symptoms 095.9
    tabes 094.0
  latent 097.1
    central nervous system 094.9
    date of infection unspecified 097.1
    early or less than 2 years after infection 092.9
    late or 2 years or more after infection 096
    serology
      doubtful
        follow-up of latent syphilis 097.1
          central nervous system 094 ✓4ᵗʰ
          date of infection unspecified 097.1
          early or less than 2 years after infection 092 ✓4ᵗʰ
          late or 2 years or more after infection 096
      positive, only finding 097.1
        date of infection unspecified 097.1
        early or less than 2 years after infection 097.1
        late or 2 years or more after infection 097.1
  lens 095.8
  leukoderma 091.3
    late 095.8
  lienis 095.8
  lip 091.3
    chancre 091.2
    late 095.8
    primary 091.2
  Lissauer's paralysis 094.1
  liver 095.3
    secondary 091.62
  locomotor ataxia 094.0
  lung 095.1
  lymphadenitis (secondary) 091.4
  lymph gland (early) (secondary) 091.4
    late 095.8
  macular atrophy of skin 091.3
    striated 095.8
  maternal, affecting fetus or newborn 760.2
    manifest syphilis in newborn — *see* Syphilis, congenital
  mediastinum (late) 095.8
  meninges (adhesive) (basilar) (brain) (spinal cord) 094.2
  meningitis 094.2
    acute 091.81
    congenital 090.42
  meningoencephalitis 094.2

Syphilis, syphilitic — *continued*
  meningovascular 094.2
    congenital 090.49
  mesarteritis 093.89
    brain 094.89
    spine 094.89
  middle ear 095.8
  mitral stenosis 093.21
  monoplegia 094.89
  mouth (secondary) 091.3
    late 095.8
  mucocutaneous 091.3
    late 095.8
  mucous
    membrane 091.3
      late 095.8
    patches 091.3
      congenital 090.0
  mulberry molars 090.5
  muscle 095.6
  myocardium 093.82
  myositis 095.6
  nasal sinus 095.8
  neonatorum NEC (*see also* Syphilis, congenital) 090.9 ✓5ᵗʰ
  nerve palsy (any cranial nerve) 094.89
  nervous system, central 094.9
  neuritis 095.8
    acoustic nerve 094.86
  neurorecidive of retina 094.83
  neuroretinitis 094.85
  newborn (*see also* Syphilis, congenital) 090.9 ✓5ᵗʰ
  nodular superficial 095.8
  nonvenereal, endemic 104.0
  nose 095.8
    saddle back deformity 090.5
    septum 095.8
      perforated 095.8
  occlusive arterial disease 093.89
  ophthalmic 095.8 [363.13]
  ophthalmoplegia 094.89
  optic nerve (atrophy) (neuritis) (papilla) 094.84
  orbit (late) 095.8
  orchitis 095.8
  organic 097.9
  osseous (late) 095.5
  osteochondritis (congenital) 090.0
  osteoporosis 095.5
  ovary 095.8
  oviduct 095.8
  palate 095.8
    gumma 095.8
    perforated 090.5
  pancreas (late) 095.8
  pancreatitis 095.8
  paralysis 094.89
    general 094.1
    juvenile 090.40
  paraplegia 094.89
  paresis (general) 094.1
    juvenile 090.40
  paresthesia 094.89
  Parkinson's disease or syndrome 094.82
  paroxysmal tachycardia 093.89
  pemphigus (congenital) 090.0
  penis 091.0
    chancre 091.0
    late 095.8
  pericardium 093.81
  perichondritis, larynx 095.8
  periosteum 095.5
    congenital 090.0
    early 091.61
    secondary 091.61
  peripheral nerve 095.8
  petrous bone (late) 095.5
  pharynx 095.8
    secondary 091.3
  pituitary (gland) 095.8
  placenta 095.8
  pleura (late) 095.8
  pneumonia, white 090.0
  pontine (lesion) 094.89
  portal vein 093.89
  primary NEC 091.2
    anal 091.1

Syphilis, syphilitic — *continued*
  primary NEC — *continued*
    and secondary (*see also* Syphilis, secondary) 091.9
    cardiovascular 093.9
    central nervous system 094.9
    extragenital chancre NEC 091.2
    fingers 091.2
    genital 091.0
    lip 091.2
    specified site NEC 091.2
    tonsils 091.2
  prostate 095.8
  psychosis (intracranial gumma) 094.89
  ptosis (eyelid) 094.89
  pulmonary (late) 095.1
    artery 093.89
  pulmonum 095.1
  pyelonephritis 095.4
  recently acquired, symptomatic NEC 091.89
  rectum 095.8
  respiratory tract 095.8
  retina
    late 094.83
    neurorecidive 094.83
  retrobulbar neuritis 094.85
  salpingitis 095.8
  sclera (late) 095.0
  sclerosis
    cerebral 094.89
    coronary 093.89
    multiple 094.89
    subacute 094.89
  scotoma (central) 095.8
  scrotum 095.8
  secondary (and primary) 091.9
    adenopathy 091.4
    anus 091.3
    bone 091.61
    cardiovascular 093.9
    central nervous system 094.9
    chorioretinitis, choroiditis 091.51
    hepatitis 091.62
    liver 091.62
    lymphadenitis 091.4
    meningitis, acute 091.81
    mouth 091.3
    mucous membranes 091.3
    periosteum 091.61
    periostitis 091.61
    pharynx 091.3
    relapse (treated) (untreated) 091.7
    skin 091.3
    specified form NEC 091.89
    tonsil 091.3
    ulcer 091.3
    viscera 091.69
    vulva 091.3
  seminal vesicle (late) 095.8
  seronegative
    with signs or symptoms — *see* Syphilis, by site and stage
  seropositive
    with signs or symptoms — *see* Syphilis, by site and stage
    follow-up of latent syphilis — *see* Syphilis, latent
    only finding — *see* Syphilis, latent
  seventh nerve (paralysis) 094.89
  sinus 095.8
  sinusitis 095.8
  skeletal system 095.5
  skin (early) (secondary) (with ulceration) 091.3
    late or tertiary 095.8
  small intestine 095.8
  spastic spinal paralysis 094.0
  spermatic cord (late) 095.8
  spinal (cord) 094.89
    with
      paresis 094.1
      tabes 094.0
  spleen 095.8
  splenomegaly 095.8
  spondylitis 095.5
  staphyloma 095.8
  stigmata (congenital) 090.5
  stomach 095.8
  synovium (late) 095.7

Syphilis, syphilitic — *continued*
  tabes dorsalis (early) (late) 094.0
    juvenile 090.40
  tabetic type 094.0
    juvenile 090.40
  taboparesis 094.1
    juvenile 090.40
  tachycardia 093.89
  tendon (late) 095.7
  tertiary 097.0
    with symptoms 095.8
    cardiovascular 093.9
    central nervous system 094.9
    multiple NEC 095.8
    specified site NEC 095.8
  testis 095.8
  thorax 095.8
  throat 095.8
  thymus (gland) 095.8
  thyroid (late) 095.8
  tongue 095.8
  tonsil (lingual) 095.8
    primary 091.2
    secondary 091.3
  trachea 095.8
  tricuspid valve 093.23
  tumor, brain 094.89
  tunica vaginalis (late) 095.8
  ulcer (any site) (early) (secondary) 091.3
    late 095.9
    perforating 095.9
      foot 094.0
  urethra (stricture) 095.8
  urogenital 095.8
  uterus 095.8
  uveal tract (secondary) 091.50
    late 095.8 [363.13]
  uveitis (secondary) 091.50
    late 095.8 [363.13]
  uvula (late) 095.8
    perforated 095.8
  vagina 091.0
    late 095.8
  valvulitis NEC 093.20
  vascular 093.89
    brain or cerebral 094.89
  vein 093.89
    cerebral 094.89
  ventriculi 095.8
  vesicae urinariae 095.8
  viscera (abdominal) 095.2
    secondary 091.69
  vitreous (hemorrhage) (opacities) 095.8
  vulva 091.0
    late 095.8
    secondary 091.3
Syphiloma 095.9
  cardiovascular system 093.9
  central nervous system 094.9
  circulatory system 093.9
  congenital 090.5
Syphilophobia 300.29
Syringadenoma (M8400/0) — *see also* Neoplasm,
    skin, benign
  papillary (M8406/0) — *see* Neoplasm, skin,
    benign
Syringobulbia 336.0
Syringocarcinoma (M8400/3) — *see* Neoplasm,
    skin, malignant
Syringocystadenoma (M8400/0) — *see also*
    Neoplasm, skin, benign
  papillary (M8406/0) — *see* Neoplasm, skin,
    benign
Syringocystoma (M8407/0) — *see* Neoplasm,
    skin, benign
Syringoma (M8407/0) — *see also* Neoplasm, skin,
    benign
  chondroid (M8940/0) — *see* Neoplasm, by site,
    benign
Syringomyelia 336.0
Syringomyelitis 323.9
  late effect — *see* category 326
Syringomyelocele (*see also* Spina bifida)
    741.9 ✓5ᵗʰ
Syringopontia 336.0

System, systemic — *see also* condition
  disease, combined — *see* Degeneration,
    combined
  fibrosclerosing syndrome 710.8
  inflammatory response syndrome (SIRS)
    995.90   ●
    due to   ●
      infectious process 995.91   ●
        with organ dsfunction 995.92   ●
      non-infectious process 995.93   ●
        with organ dysfunction 995.94   ●
  lupus erythematosus 710.0
    inhibitor 286.5

T

Tab — *see* Tag
Tabacism 989.8 ✓5ᵗʰ
Tabacosis 989.8 ✓5ᵗʰ
Tabardillo 080
  flea-borne 081.0
  louse-borne 080
Tabes, tabetic
  with
    central nervous system syphilis 094.0
    Charcôt's joint 094.0 [713.5]
    cord bladder 094.0
    crisis, viscera (any) 094.0
    paralysis, general 094.1
    paresis (general) 094.1
    perforating ulcer 094.0
  arthropathy 094.0 [713.5]
  bladder 094.0
  bone 094.0
  cerebrospinal 094.0
  congenital 090.40
  conjugal 094.0
  dorsalis 094.0
    neurosyphilis 094.0
  early 094.0
  juvenile 090.40
  latent 094.0
  mesenterica (*see also* Tuberculosis) 014.8 ✓5ᵗʰ
  paralysis insane, general 094.1
  peripheral (nonsyphilitic) 799.8
  spasmodic 094.0
    not dorsal or dorsalis 343.9
  syphilis (cerebrospinal) 094.0
Taboparalysis 094.1
Taboparesis (remission) 094.1
  with
    Charcôt's joint 094.1 [713.5]
    cord bladder 094.1
    perforating ulcer 094.1
  juvenile 090.40
Tachyalimentation 579.3
Tachyarrhythmia, tachyrhythmia — *see also*
    Tachycardia
  paroxysmal with sinus bradycardia 427.81
Tachycardia 785.0
  atrial 427.89
  auricular 427.89
  newborn 779.82   ●
  nodal 427.89
    nonparoxysmal atrioventricular 426.89
    nonparoxysmal atrioventricular (nodal) 426.89
  paroxysmal 427.2
    with sinus bradycardia 427.81
    atrial (PAT) 427.0
      psychogenic 316 [427.0]
    atrioventricular (AV) 427.0
      psychogenic 316 [427.0]
    essential 427.2
    junctional 427.0
    nodal 427.0
    psychogenic 316 [427.2]
      atrial 316 [427.0]
      supraventricular 316 [427.0]
      ventricular 316 [427.1]
    supraventricular 427.0
      psychogenic 316 [427.0]
    ventricular 427.1
      psychogenic 316 [427.1]
  postoperative 997.1
  psychogenic 306.2
  sick sinus 427.81

Tachycardia — *continued*
  sinoauricular 427.89
  sinus 427.89
  supraventricular 427.89
  ventricular (paroxysmal) 427.1
    psychogenic 316 [427.1]
Tachypnea 786.06
  hysterical 300.11
  newborn (idiopathic) (transitory) 770.6
  psychogenic 306.1
  transitory, of newborn 770.6
Taenia (infection) (infestation) (*see also*
    Infestation, taenia) 123.3
  diminuta 123.6
  echinococcal infestation (*see also*
    Echinococcus) 122.9
  nana 123.6
  saginata infestation 123.2
  solium (intestinal form) 123.0
    larval form 123.1
Taeniasis (intestine) (*see also* Infestation, Taenia)
    123.3
  saginata 123.2
  solium 123.0
Taenzer's disease 757.4
Tag (hypertrophied skin) (infected) 701.9
  adenoid 474.8
  anus 455.9
  endocardial (*see also* Endocarditis) 424.90
  hemorrhoidal 455.9
  hymen 623.8
  perineal 624.8
  preauricular 744.1
  rectum 455.9
  sentinel 455.9
  skin 701.9
    accessory 757.39
    anus 455.9
    congenital 757.39
    preauricular 744.1
    rectum 455.9
  tonsil 474.8
  urethra, urethral 599.84
  vulva 624.8
Tahyna fever 062.5
Takayasu (-Onishi) disease or syndrome
    (pulseless disease) 446.7
Talc granuloma 728.82
Talcosis 502
Talipes (congenital) 754.70
  acquired NEC 736.79
    planus 734
  asymmetric 754.79
    acquired 736.79
  calcaneovalgus 754.62
    acquired 736.76
  calcaneovarus 754.59
    acquired 736.76
  calcaneus 754.79
    acquired 736.76
  cavovarus 754.59
    acquired 736.75
  cavus 754.71
    acquired 736.73
  equinovalgus 754.69
    acquired 736.72
  equinovarus 754.51
    acquired 736.71
  equinus 754.79
    acquired, NEC 736.72
  percavus 754.71
    acquired 736.73
  planovalgus 754.69
    acquired 736.79
  planus (acquired) (any degree) 734
    congenital 754.61
    due to rickets 268.1
  valgus 754.60
    acquired 736.79
  varus 754.50
    acquired 736.79
Talma's disease 728.85
Tamponade heart (Rose's) (*see also* Pericarditis)
    423.9
Tanapox 078.89

Tangier disease (familial high-density lipoprotein deficiency) 272.5

Tank ear 380.12

Tantrum (childhood) (*see also* Disturbance, conduct) 312.1 ✓5ᵗʰ

Tapeworm (infection) (infestation) (*see also* Infestation, tapeworm) 123.9

Tapia's syndrome 352.6

Tarantism 297.8

Target-oval cell anemia 282.4

Tarlov's cyst 355.9

Tarral-Besnier disease (pityriasis rubra pilaris) 696.4

Tarsalgia 729.2

Tarsal tunnel syndrome 355.5

Tarsitis (eyelid) 373.00
  syphilitic 095.8 [373.00]
  tuberculous (*see also* Tuberculosis) 017.0 ✓5ᵗʰ [373.4]

Tartar (teeth) 523.6

Tattoo (mark) 709.09

Taurodontism 520.2

Taussig-Bing defect, heart, or syndrome (transposition, aorta and overriding pulmonary artery) 745.11

Tay's choroiditis 363.41

Tay-Sachs
  amaurotic familial idiocy 330.1
  disease 330.1

Taybi's syndrome (otopalatodigital) 759.89

Taylor's
  disease (diffuse idiopathic cutaneous atrophy) 701.8
  syndrome 625.5

Tear, torn (traumatic) — *see also* Wound, open, by site
  anus, anal (sphincter) 863.89
    with open wound in cavity 863.99
    complicating delivery 664.2 ✓5ᵗʰ
      with mucosa 664.3 ✓5ᵗʰ
    nontraumatic, nonpuerperal 565.0
  articular cartilage, old (*see also* Disorder, cartilage, articular) 718.0 ✓5ᵗʰ
  bladder
    with
      abortion — *see* Abortion, by type, with damage to pelvic organs
      ectopic pregnancy (*see also* categories 633.0-633.9) 639.2
      molar pregnancy (*see also* categories 630-632) 639.2
    following
      abortion 639.2
      ectopic or molar pregnancy 639.2
    obstetrical trauma 665.5 ✓5ᵗʰ
  bowel
    with
      abortion — *see* Abortion, by type, with damage to pelvic organs
      ectopic pregnancy (*see also* categories 633.0-633.9) 639.2
      molar pregnancy (*see also* categories 630-632) 639.2
    following
      abortion 639.2
      ectopic or molar pregnancy 639.2
    obstetrical trauma 665.5 ✓5ᵗʰ
  broad ligament
    with
      abortion — *see* Abortion, by type, with damage to pelvic organs
      ectopic pregnancy (*see also* categories 633.0-633.9) 639.2
      molar pregnancy (*see also* categories 630-632) 639.2
    following
      abortion 639.2
      ectopic or molar pregnancy 639.2
    obstetrical trauma 665.6 ✓5ᵗʰ
  bucket handle (knee) (meniscus) — *see* Tear, meniscus

Tear, torn — *see also* Wound, open, by site — *continued*
  capsule
    joint — *see* Sprain, by site
    spleen — *see* Laceration, spleen, capsule
  cartilage — *see also* Sprain, by site
    articular, old (*see also* Disorder, cartilage, articular) 718.0 ✓5ᵗʰ
    knee — *see* Tear, meniscus
    semilunar (knee) (current injury) — *see* Tear, meniscus
  cervix
    with
      abortion — *see* Abortion, by type, with damage to pelvic organs
      ectopic pregnancy (*see also* categories 633.0-633.9) 639.2
      molar pregnancy (*see also* categories 630-632) 639.2
    following
      abortion 639.2
      ectopic or molar pregnancy 639.2
    obstetrical trauma (current) 665.3 ✓5ᵗʰ
    old 622.3
  internal organ (abdomen, chest, or pelvis) — *see* Injury, internal, by site
  ligament — *see also* Sprain, by site
    with open wound — *see* Wound, open by site
  meniscus (knee) (current injury) 836.2
    bucket handle 836.0
      old 717.0
    lateral 836.1
      anterior horn 836.1
        old 717.42
      bucket handle 836.1
        old 717.41
      old 717.40
      posterior horn 836.1
        old 717.43
      specified site NEC 836.1
        old 717.49
    medial 836.0
      anterior horn 836.0
        old 717.1
      bucket handle 836.0
        old 717.0
      old 717.3
      posterior horn 836.0
        old 717.2
    old NEC 717.5
    site other than knee — *see* Sprain, by site
  muscle — *see also* Sprain, by site
    with open wound — *see* Wound, open by site
  pelvic
    floor, complicating delivery 664.1 ✓5ᵗʰ
    organ NEC
      with
        abortion — *see* Abortion, by type, with damage to pelvic organs
        ectopic pregnancy (*see also* categories 633.0-633.9) 639.2
        molar pregnancy (*see also* categories 630-632) 639.2
      following
        abortion 639.2
        ectopic or molar pregnancy 639.2
      obstetrical trauma 665.5 ✓5ᵗʰ
  perineum — *see also* Laceration, perineum
    obstetrical trauma 665.5 ✓5ᵗʰ
  periurethral tissue
    with
      abortion — *see* Abortion, by type, with damage to pelvic organs
      ectopic pregnancy (*see also* categories 633.0-633.9) 639.2
      molar pregnancy (*see also* categories 630-632) 639.2
    following
      abortion 639.2
      ectopic or molar pregnancy 639.2
    obstetrical trauma 665.5 ✓5ᵗʰ
  rectovaginal septum — *see* Laceration, rectovaginal septum
  retina, retinal (recent) (with detachment) 361.00

Tear, torn — *see also* Wound, open, by site — *continued*
  retina, retinal — *continued*
    without detachment 361.30
    dialysis (juvenile) (with detachment) 361.04
    giant (with detachment) 361.03
    horseshoe (without detachment) 361.32
    multiple (with detachment) 361.02
      without detachment 361.33
    old
      delimited (partial) 361.06
      partial 361.06
      total or subtotal 361.07
    partial (without detachment)
      giant 361.03
      multiple defects 361.02
      old (delimited) 361.06
      single defect 361.01
    round hole (without detachment) 361.31
    single defect (with detachment) 361.01
    total or subtotal (recent) 361.05
      old 361.07
  rotator cuff (traumatic) 840.4
    current injury 840.4
    degenerative 726.10
    nontraumatic 727.61
  semilunar cartilage, knee (*see also* Tear, meniscus) 836.2
    old 717.5
  tendon — *see also* Sprain, by site
    with open wound — *see* Wound, open by site
  tentorial, at birth 767.0
  umbilical cord
    affecting fetus or newborn 772.0
    complicating delivery 663.8 ✓5ᵗʰ
  urethra
    with
      abortion — *see* Abortion, by type, with damage to pelvic organs
      ectopic pregnancy (*see also* categories 633.0-633.9) 639.2
      molar pregnancy (*see also* categories 630-632) 639.2
    following
      abortion 639.2
      ectopic or molar pregnancy 639.2
    obstetrical trauma 665.5 ✓5ᵗʰ
  uterus — *see* Injury, internal, uterus
  vagina — *see* Laceration, vagina
  vessel, from catheter 998.2
  vulva, complicating delivery 664.0 ✓5ᵗʰ

Tear stone 375.57

Teeth, tooth — *see also* condition
  grinding 306.8

Teething 520.7
  syndrome 520.7

Tegmental syndrome 344.89

Telangiectasia, telangiectasis (verrucous) 448.9
  ataxic (cerebellar) 334.8
  familial 448.0
  hemorrhagic, hereditary (congenital) (senile) 448.0
  hereditary hemorrhagic 448.0
  retina 362.15
  spider 448.1

Telecanthus (congenital) 743.63

Telescoped bowel or intestine (*see also* Intussusception) 560.0

Teletherapy, adverse effect NEC 990

Telogen effluvium 704.02

Temperature
  body, high (of unknown origin) (*see also* Pyrexia) 780.6
  cold, trauma from 991.9
    newborn 778.2
    specified effect NEC 991.8
  high
    body (of unknown origin) (*see also* Pyrexia) 780.6
    trauma from — *see* Heat

Temper tantrum (childhood) (*see also* Disturbance, conduct) 312.1 ✓5ᵗʰ

Temple — *see* condition

Temporal — *see also* condition
lobe syndrome 310.0
**Temporomandibular joint-pain-dysfunction
syndrome** 524.60
Temporosphenoidal — *see* condition
Tendency
bleeding (*see also* Defect, coagulation) 286.9
homosexual, ego-dystonic 302.0
paranoid 301.0
suicide 300.9
Tenderness
abdominal (generalized) (localized) 789.6 ✓5ᵗʰ
rebound 789.6 ✓5ᵗʰ
skin 782.0
Tendinitis, tendonitis (*see also* Tenosynovitis)
726.90
Achilles 726.71
adhesive 726.90
shoulder 726.0
calcific 727.82
shoulder 726.11
gluteal 726.5
patellar 726.64
peroneal 726.79
pes anserinus 726.61
psoas 726.5
tibialis (anterior) (posterior) 726.72
trochanteric 726.5
Tendon — *see* condition
Tendosynovitis — *see* Tenosynovitis
Tendovaginitis — *see* Tenosynovitis
Tenesmus 787.99
rectal 787.99
vesical 788.9
Tenia — *see* Taenia
Teniasis — *see* Taeniasis
Tennis elbow 726.32
Tenonitis — *see also* Tenosynovitis
eye (capsule) 376.04
Tenontosynovitis — *see* Tenosynovitis
Tenontothecitis — *see* Tenosynovitis
Tenophyte 727.9
Tenosynovitis 727.00
adhesive 726.90
shoulder 726.0
ankle 727.06
bicipital (calcifying) 726.12
buttock 727.09
due to crystals — *see* Arthritis, due to crystals
elbow 727.09
finger 727.05
foot 727.06
gonococcal 098.51
hand 727.05
hip 727.09
knee 727.09
radial styloid 727.04
shoulder 726.10
adhesive 726.0
spine 720.1
supraspinatus 726.10
toe 727.06
tuberculous — *see* Tuberculosis, tenosynovitis
wrist 727.05
Tenovaginitis — *see* Tenosynovitis
Tension
arterial, high (*see also* Hypertension) 401.9
without diagnosis of hypertension 796.2
headache 307.81
intraocular (elevated) 365.00
nervous 799.2
ocular (elevated) 365.00
pneumothorax 512.0
iatrogenic 512.1
postoperative 512.1
spontaneous 512.0
premenstrual 625.4
state 300.9
Tentorium — *see* condition
Teratencephalus 759.89
Teratism 759.7
Teratoblastoma (malignant) (M9080/3) — *see*
Neoplasm, by site, malignant

Teratocarcinoma (M9081/3) — *see also*
Neoplasm, by site, malignant
liver 155.0
Teratoma (solid) (M9080/1) — *see also* Neoplasm,
by site, uncertain behavior
adult (cystic) (M9080/0) — *see* Neoplasm, by
site, benign
and embryonal carcinoma, mixed (M9081/3) —
see Neoplasm, by site, malignant
benign (M9080/0) — *see* Neoplasm, by site,
benign
combined with choriocarcinoma (M9101/3) —
see Neoplasm, by site, malignant
cystic (adult) (M9080/0) — *see* Neoplasm, by
site, benign
differentiated type (M9080/0) — *see* Neoplasm,
by site, benign
embryonal (M9080/3) — *see also* Neoplasm, by
site, malignant
liver 155.0
fetal
sacral, causing fetopelvic disproportion
653.7 ✓5ᵗʰ
immature (M9080/3) — *see* Neoplasm, by site,
malignant
liver (M9080/3) 155.0
adult, benign, cystic, differentiated type or
mature (M9080/0) 211.5
malignant (M9080/3) — *see also* Neoplasm, by
site, malignant
anaplastic type (M9082/3) — *see* Neoplasm,
by site, malignant
intermediate type (M9083/3) — *see*
Neoplasm, by site, malignant
liver (M9080/3) 155.0
trophoblastic (M9102/3)
specified site — *see* Neoplasm, by site,
malignant
unspecified site 186.9
undifferentiated type (M9082/3) — *see*
Neoplasm, by site, malignant
mature (M9080/0) — *see* Neoplasm, by site,
benign
ovary (M9080/0) 220
embryonal, immature, or malignant
(M9080/3) 183.0
suprasellar (M9080/3) — *see* Neoplasm, by
site, malignant
testis (M9080/3) 186.9
adult, benign, cystic, differentiated type or
mature (M9080/0) 222.0
undescended 186.0
Terminal care V66.7
Termination
anomalous — *see also* Malposition, congenital
portal vein 747.49
right pulmonary vein 747.42
pregnancy (legal) (therapeutic) (*see* Abortion,
legal) 635.9 ✓5ᵗʰ
fetus NEC 779.6
illegal (*see also* Abortion, illegal) 636.9 ✓5ᵗʰ
Ternidens diminutus infestation 127.7
Terrors, night (child) 307.46
Terry's syndrome 362.21
Tertiary — *see* condition
Tessellated fundus, retina (tigroid) 362.89
Test(s)
AIDS virus V72.6
adequacy
hemodialysis V56.31
peritoneal dialysis V56.32
allergen V72.7
bacterial disease NEC (*see also* Screening, by
name of disease) V74.9
basal metabolic rate V72.6
blood-alcohol V70.4
blood-drug V70.4
for therapeutic drug monitoring V58.83
developmental, infant or child V20.2
Dick V74.8
fertility V26.21
genetic V26.3
hearing V72.1
HIV V72.6
human immunodeficiency virus V72.6
Kveim V82.89

Test(s) — *continued*
laboratory V72.6
for medicolegal reason V70.4
Mantoux (for tuberculosis) V74.1
mycotic organism V75.4
parasitic agent NEC V75.8
paternity V70.4
peritoneal equilibration V56.32
pregnancy
positive V22.1
first pregnancy V22.0
unconfirmed V72.4
preoperative V72.84
cardiovascular V72.81
respiratory V72.82
specified NEC V72.83
procreative management NEC V26.29
sarcoidosis V82.89
Schick V74.3
Schultz-Charlton V74.8
skin, diagnostic
allergy V72.7
bacterial agent NEC (*see also* Screening, by
name of disease) V74.9
Dick V74.8
hypersensitivity V72.7
Kveim V82.89
Mantoux V74.1
mycotic organism V75.4
parasitic agent NEC V75.8
sarcoidosis V82.89
Schick V74.3
Schultz-Charlton V74.8
tuberculin V74.1
specified type NEC V72.8 ✓5ᵗʰ
tuberculin V74.1
vision V72.0
Wassermann
positive (*see also* Serology for syphilis,
positive) 097.1
false 795.6
Testicle, testicular, testis — *see also* condition
feminization (syndrome) 257.8
Tetanus, tetanic (cephalic) (convulsions) 037
with
abortion — *see* Abortion, by type, with
sepsis
ectopic pregnancy (*see also* categories
633.0-633.9) 639.0
molar pregnancy (*see* categories 630-632)
639.0
following
abortion 639.0
ectopic or molar pregnancy 639.0
inoculation V03.7
reaction (due to serum) — *see*
Complications, vaccination
neonatorum 771.3
puerperal, postpartum, childbirth 670 ✓4ᵗʰ
Tetany, tetanic 781.7
alkalosis 276.3
associated with rickets 268.0
convulsions 781.7
hysterical 300.11
functional (hysterical) 300.11
hyperkinetic 781.7
hysterical 300.11
hyperpnea 786.01
hysterical 300.11
psychogenic 306.1
hyperventilation 786.01
hysterical 300.11
psychogenic 306.1
hypocalcemic, neonatal 775.4
hysterical 300.11
neonatal 775.4
parathyroid (gland) 252.1
parathyroprival 252.1
postoperative 252.1
postthyroidectomy 252.1
pseudotetany 781.7
hysterical 300.11
psychogenic 306.1
specified as conversion reaction 300.11
Tetralogy of Fallot 745.2
Tetraplegia — *see* Quadriplegia

Thailand hemorrhagic fever 065.4

Thalassanemia 282.4

Thalassemia (alpha) (beta) (disease) (Hb-C) (Hb-D) (Hb-E) (Hb-H) (Hb-I) (Hb-S) (high fetal gene) (high fetal hemoglobin) (intermedia) (major) (minima) (minor) (mixed) (sickle-cell) (trait) (with other hemoglobinopathy) 282.4

Thalassemic variants 282.4

Thaysen-Gee disease (nontropical sprue) 579.0

Thecoma (M8600/0) 220
  malignant (M8600/3) 183.0

Thelarche, precocious 259.1

Thelitis 611.0
  puerperal, postpartum 675.0 ☑5ᵗʰ

Therapeutic — see condition

Therapy V57.9
  blood transfusion, without reported diagnosis V58.2
  breathing V57.0
  chemotherapy V58.1
    fluoride V07.31
    prophylactic NEC V07.39
  dialysis (intermittent) (treatment)
    extracorporeal V56.0
    peritoneal V56.8
    renal V56.0
    specified type NEC V56.8
  exercise NEC V57.1
    breathing V57.0
  extracorporeal dialysis (renal) V56.0
  fluoride prophylaxis V07.31
  hemodialysis V56.0
  long term oxygen therapy V46.2
  occupational V57.21
  orthoptic V57.4
  orthotic V57.81
  peritoneal dialysis V56.8
  physical NEC V57.1
  postmenopausal hormone replacement V07.4
  radiation V58.0
  speech V57.3
  vocational V57.22

Thermalgesia 782.0

Thermalgia 782.0

Thermanalgesia 782.0

Thermanesthesia 782.0

Thermic — see condition

Thermography (abnormal) 793.9
  breast 793.89

Thermoplegia 992.0

Thesaurismosis
  amyloid 277.3
  bilirubin 277.4
  calcium 275.40
  cystine 270.0
  glycogen (see also Disease, glycogen storage) 271.0
  kerasin 272.7
  lipoid 272.7
  melanin 255.4
  phosphatide 272.7
  urate 274.9

Thiaminic deficiency 265.1
  with beriberi 265.0

Thibierge-Weissenbach syndrome (cutaneous systemic sclerosis) 710.1

Thickened endometrium 793.5

Thickening
  bone 733.99
    extremity 733.99
  breast 611.79
  hymen 623.3
  larynx 478.79
  nail 703.8
    congenital 757.5
  periosteal 733.99
  pluera (see also Pleurisy) 511.0
  skin 782.8
  subepiglottic 478.79
  tongue 529.8
  valve, heart — see Endocarditis

Thiele syndrome 724.6

Thigh — see condition

Thinning vertebra (see also Osteoporosis) 733.00

Thirst, excessive 783.5
  due to deprivation of water 994.3

Thomsen's disease 359.2

Thomson's disease (congenital poikiloderma) 757.33

Thoracic — see also condition
  kidney 753.3
  outlet syndrome 353.0
  stomach — see Hernia, diaphragm

Thoracogastroschisis (congenital) 759.89

Thoracopagus 759.4

Thoracoschisis 756.3

Thorax — see condition

Thorn's syndrome (see also Disease, renal) 593.9

Thornwaldt's, Tornwaldt's
  bursitis (pharyngeal) 478.29
  cyst 478.26
  disease (pharyngeal bursitis) 478.29

Thorson-Biörck syndrome (malignant carcinoid) 259.2

Threadworm (infection) (infestation) 127.4

Threatened
  abortion or miscarriage 640.0 ☑5ᵗʰ
    with subsequent abortion (see also Abortion, spontaneous) 634.9 ☑5ᵗʰ
    affecting fetus 762.1
  labor 644.1 ☑5ᵗʰ
    affecting fetus or newborn 761.8
    premature 644.0 ☑5ᵗʰ
  miscarriage 640.0 ☑5ᵗʰ
    affecting fetus 762.1
  premature
    delivery 644.2 ☑5ᵗʰ
      affecting fetus or newborn 761.8
    labor 644.0 ☑5ᵗʰ
      before 22 completed weeks gestation 640.0 ☑5ᵗʰ

Three-day fever 066.0

Threshers' lung 495.0

Thrix annulata (congenital) 757.4

Throat — see condition

Thrombasthenia (Glanzmann's) (hemorrhagic) (hereditary) 287.1

Thromboangiitis 443.1
  obliterans (general) 443.1
    cerebral 437.1
    vessels
      brain 437.1
      spinal cord 437.1

Thromboarteritis — see Arteritis

Thromboasthenia (Glanzmann's) (hemorrhagic) (hereditary) 287.1

Thrombocytasthenia (Glanzmann's) 287.1

Thrombocythemia (essential) (hemorrhagic) (primary) (M9962/1) 238.7
  idiopathic (M9962/1) 238.7

Thrombocytopathy (dystrophic) (granulopenic) 287.1

Thrombocytopenia, thrombocytopenic 287.5
  with giant hemangioma 287.3
  amegakaryocytic, congenital 287.3
  congenital 287.3
  cyclic 287.3
  dilutional 287.4
  due to
    drugs 287.4
    extracorporeal circulation of blood 287.4
    massive blood transfusion 287.4
    platelet alloimmunization 287.4
  essential 287.3
  hereditary 287.3
  Kasabach-Merritt 287.3
  neonatal, transitory 776.1
    due to
      exchange transfusion 776.1
      idiopathic maternal thrombocytopenia 776.1
      isoimmunization 776.1
  primary 287.3
  puerperal, postpartum 666.3 ☑5ᵗʰ

Thrombocytopenia, thrombocytopenic — continued
  purpura (see also Purpura, thrombocytopenic) 287.3
    thrombotic 446.6
  secondary 287.4
  sex-linked 287.3

Thrombocytosis, essential 289.9

Thromboembolism — see Embolism

Thrombopathy (Bernard-Soulier) 287.1
  constitutional 286.4
  Willebrand-Jürgens (angiohemophilia) 286.4

Thrombopenia (see also Thrombocytopenia) 287.5

Thrombophlebitis 451.9
  antecubital vein 451.82
  antepartum (superficial) 671.2 ☑5ᵗʰ
    affecting fetus or newborn 760.3
    deep 671.3 ☑5ᵗʰ
  arm 451.89
    deep 451.83
    superficial 451.82
  breast, superficial 451.89
  cavernous (venous) sinus — see Thrombophlebitis, intracranial venous sinus
  cephalic vein 451.82
  cerebral (sinus) (vein) 325
    late effect — see category 326
    nonpyogenic 437.6
      in pregnancy or puerperium 671.5 ☑5ᵗʰ
      late effect — see Late effect(s) (of) cerebrovascular disease
  due to implanted device — see Complications, due to (presence of) any device, implant or graft classified to 996.0-996.5 NEC
  during or resulting from a procedure NEC 997.2
  femoral 451.11
  femoropopliteal 451.19
  following infusion, perfusion, or transfusion 999.2
  hepatic (vein) 451.89
  idiopathic, recurrent 453.1
  iliac vein 451.81
  iliofemoral 451.11
  intracranial venous sinus (any) 325
    late effect — see category 326
    nonpyogenic 437.6
      in pregnancy or puerperium 671.5 ☑5ᵗʰ
      late effect — see Late effect(s) (of) cerebrovascular disease
  jugular vein 451.89
  lateral (venous) sinus — see Thrombophlebitis, intracranial venous sinus
  leg 451.2
    deep (vessels) 451.19
      femoral vein 451.11
      specified vessel NEC 451.19
    superficial (vessels) 451.0
      femoral vein 451.11
  longitudinal (venous) sinus — see Thrombophlebitis, intracranial venous sinus
  lower extremity 451.2
    deep (vessels) 451.19
      femoral vein 451.11
      specified vessel NEC 451.19
    superficial (vessels) 451.0
  migrans, migrating 453.1
  pelvic
    with
      abortion — see Abortion, by type, with sepsis
      ectopic pregnancy — (see also categories 633.0-633.9) 639.0
      molar pregnancy — (see also categories 630-632) 639.0
    following
      abortion 639.0
      ectopic or molar pregnancy 639.0
    puerperal 671.4 ☑5ᵗʰ
  popliteal vein 451.19
  portal (vein) 572.1
  postoperative 997.2
  pregnancy (superficial) 671.2 ☑5ᵗʰ
    affecting fetus or newborn 760.3

Thrombophlebitis — *continued*
  pregnancy — *continued*
    deep 671.3 ✓5ᵗʰ
    puerperal, postpartum, childbirth (extremities)
      (superficial) 671.2 ✓5ᵗʰ
      deep 671.4 ✓5ᵗʰ
      pelvic 671.4 ✓5ᵗʰ
      specified site NEC 671.5 ✓5ᵗʰ
  radial vein 451.83
  saphenous (greater) (lesser) 451.0
  sinus (intracranial) — *see* Thrombophlebitis,
    intracranial venous sinus
  specified site NEC 451.89
  tibial vein 451.19

Thrombosis, thrombotic (marantic) (multiple)
  (progressive) (septic) (vein) (vessel) 453.9
  with childbirth or during the puerperium — *see*
    Thrombosis, puerperal, postpartum
  antepartum — *see* Thrombosis, pregnancy
  aorta, aortic 444.1
    abdominal 444.0
    bifurcation 444.0
    saddle 444.0
    terminal 444.0
    thoracic 444.1
    valve — *see* Endocarditis, aortic
  apoplexy (*see also* Thrombosis, brain)
    434.0 ✓5ᵗʰ
    late effect — *see* Late effect(s) (of)
      cerebrovascular disease
  appendix, septic — *see* Appendicitis, acute
  arteriolar-capillary platelet, disseminated 446.6
  artery, arteries (postinfectional) 444.9
    auditory, internal 433.8 ✓5ᵗʰ
    basilar (*see also* Occlusion, artery, basilar)
      433.0 ✓5ᵗʰ
    carotid (common) (internal) (*see also*
      Occlusion, artery, carotid) 433.1 ✓5ᵗʰ
      with other precerebral artery 433.3 ✓5ᵗʰ
    cerebellar (anterior inferior) (posterior
      inferior) (superior) 433.8 ✓5ᵗʰ
    cerebral (*see also* Thrombosis, brain)
      434.0 ✓5ᵗʰ
    choroidal (anterior) 433.8 ✓5ᵗʰ
    communicating posterior 433.8 ✓5ᵗʰ
    coronary (*see also* Infarct, myocardium)
      410.9 ✓5ᵗʰ
      without myocardial infarction 411.81
      due to syphilis 093.89
      healed or specified as old 412
    extremities 444.22
      lower 444.22
      upper 444.21
    femoral 444.22
    hepatic 444.89
    hypophyseal 433.8 ✓5ᵗʰ
    meningeal, anterior or posterior 433.8 ✓5ᵗʰ
    mesenteric (with gangrene) 557.0
    ophthalmic (*see also* Occlusion, retina)
      362.30
    pontine 433.8 ✓5ᵗʰ
    popliteal 444.22
    precerebral — *see* Occlusion, artery,
      precerebral NEC
    pulmonary 415.19
      iatrogenic 415.11
      postoperative 415.11
    renal 593.81
    retinal (*see also* Occlusion, retina) 362.30
    specified site NEC 444.89
    spinal, anterior or posterior 433.8 ✓5ᵗʰ
    traumatic (complication) (early) (*see also*
      Injury, blood vessel, by site) 904.9
    vertebral (*see also* Occlusion, artery,
      vertebral) 433.2 ✓5ᵗʰ
      with other precerebral artery 433.3 ✓5ᵗʰ
  atrial (endocardial) 424.90
    due to syphilis 093.89
  auricular (*see also* Infarct, myocardium)
    410.9 ✓5ᵗʰ
  axillary (vein) 453.8
  basilar (artery) (*see also* Occlusion, artery,
    basilar) 433.0 ✓5ᵗʰ
  bland NEC 453.9
  brain (artery) (stem) 434.0 ✓5ᵗʰ
    due to syphilis 094.89
    iatrogenic 997.02

Thrombosis, thrombotic — *continued*
  brain — *continued*
    late effect — *see* Late effect(s) (of)
      cerebrovascular disease
    postoperative 997.02
    puerperal, postpartum, childbirth 674.0 ✓5ᵗʰ
    sinus (*see also* Thrombosis, intracranial
      venous sinus) 325
  capillary 448.9
    arteriolar, generalized 446.6
  cardiac (*see also* Infarct, myocardium)
    410.9 ✓5ᵗʰ
    due to syphilis 093.89
    healed or specified as old 412
    valve — *see* Endocarditis
  carotid (artery) (common) (internal) (*see also*
    Occlusion, artery, carotid) 433.1 ✓5ᵗʰ
    with other precerebral artery 433.3 ✓5ᵗʰ
  cavernous sinus (venous) — *see* Thrombosis,
    intracranial venous sinus
  cerebellar artery (anterior inferior) (posterior
    inferior) (superior) 433.8 ✓5ᵗʰ
    late effect — *see* Late effect(s) (of)
      cerebrovascular disease
  cerebral (arteries) (*see also* Thrombosis, brain)
    434.0 ✓5ᵗʰ
    late effect — *see* Late effect(s) (of)
      cerebrovascular disese
  coronary (artery) (*see also* Infarct, myocardium)
    410.9 ✓5ᵗʰ
    without myocardial infarction 411.81
    due to syphilis 093.89
    healed or specified as old 412
  corpus cavernosum 607.82
  cortical (*see also* Thrombosis, brain) 434.0 ✓5ᵗʰ
  due to (presence of) any device, implant, or
    graft classifiable to 996.0-996.5— *see*
    Complications, due to (presence of) any
    device, implant, or graft classified to
    996.0-996.5 NEC
  effort 453.8
  endocardial — *see* Infarct, myocardium
  eye (*see also* Occlusion, retina) 362.30
  femoral (vein) (deep) 453.8
    with inflammation or phlebitis 451.11
    artery 444.22
  genital organ, male 608.83
  heart (chamber) (*see also* Infarct, myocardium)
    410.9 ✓5ᵗʰ
  hepatic (vein) 453.0
    artery 444.89
    infectional or septic 572.1
  iliac (vein) 453.8
    with inflammation or phlebitis 451.81
    artery (common) (external) (internal) 444.81
  inflammation, vein — *see* Thrombophlebitis
  internal carotid artery (*see also* Occlusion,
    artery, carotid) 433.1 ✓5ᵗʰ
    with other precerebral artery 433.3 ✓5ᵗʰ
  intestine (with gangrene) 557.0
  intracranial (*see also* Thrombosis, brain)
    434.0 ✓5ᵗʰ
    venous sinus (any) 325
      nonpyogenic origin 437.6
        in pregnancy or puerperium 671.5 ✓5ᵗʰ
  intramural (*see also* Infarct, myocardium)
    410.9 ✓5ᵗʰ
    without
      cardiac condition 429.89
      coronary artery disease 429.89
      myocardial infarction 429.89
    healed or specified as old 412
  jugular (bulb) 453.8
  kidney 593.81
    artery 593.81
  lateral sinus (venous) — *see* Thrombosis,
    intracranial venous sinus
  leg 453.8
    with inflammation or phlebitis — *see*
      Thrombophlebitis
    deep (vessels) 453.8
    superficial (vessels) 453.8
  liver (venous) 453.0
    artery 444.89
    infectional or septic 572.1
    portal vein 452
  longitudinal sinus (venous) — *see* Thrombosis,
    intracranial venous sinus

Thrombosis, thrombotic — *continued*
  lower extremity — *see* Thrombosis, leg
  lung 415.19
    iatrogenic 415.11
    postoperative 415.11
  marantic, dural sinus 437.6
  meninges (brain) (*see also* Thrombosis, brain)
    434.0 ✓5ᵗʰ
  mesenteric (artery) (with gangrene) 557.0
    vein (inferior) (superior) 557.0
  mitral — *see* Insufficiency, mitral
  mural (heart chamber) (*see also* Infarct,
    myocardium) 410.9 ✓5ᵗʰ
    without
      cardiac condition 429.89
      coronary artery disease 429.89
      myocardial infarction 429.89
    due to syphilis 093.89
    following myocardial infarction 429.79
    healed or specified as old 412
  omentum (with gangrene) 557.0
  ophthalmic (artery) (*see also* Occlusion, retina)
    362.30
  pampiniform plexus (male) 608.83
    female 620.8
  parietal (*see also* Infarct, myocardium)
    410.9 ✓5ᵗʰ
  penis, penile 607.82
  peripheral arteries 444.22
    lower 444.22
    upper 444.21
  platelet 446.6
  portal 452
    due to syphilis 093.89
    infectional or septic 572.1
  precerebral artery — *see also* Occlusion, artery,
    precerebral NEC
  pregnancy 671.9 ✓5ᵗʰ
    deep (vein) 671.3 ✓5ᵗʰ
    superficial (vein) 671.2 ✓5ᵗʰ
  puerperal, postpartum, childbirth 671.9 ✓5ᵗʰ
    brain (artery) 674.0 ✓5ᵗʰ
      venous 671.5 ✓5ᵗʰ
    cardiac 674.8 ✓5ᵗʰ
    cerebral (artery) 674.0 ✓5ᵗʰ
      venous 671.5 ✓5ᵗʰ
    deep (vein) 671.4 ✓5ᵗʰ
    intracranial sinus (nonpyogenic) (venous)
      671.5 ✓5ᵗʰ
    pelvic 671.4 ✓5ᵗʰ
    pulmonary (artery) 673.2 ✓5ᵗʰ
    specified site NEC 671.5 ✓5ᵗʰ
    superficial 671.2 ✓5ᵗʰ
  pulmonary (artery) (vein) 415.19
    iatrogenic 415.11
    postoperative 415.11
  renal (artery) 593.81
    vein 453.3
  resulting from presence of shunt or other
    internal prosthetic device — *see*
    Complications, due to (presence of) any
    device, implant, or graft classified to
    996.0-996.5 NEC
  retina, retinal (artery) 362.30
    arterial branch 362.32
    central 362.31
    partial 362.33
    vein
      central 362.35
      tributary (branch) 362.36
  scrotum 608.83
  seminal vesicle 608.83
  sigmoid (venous) sinus (*see* Thrombosis,
    intracranial venous sinus) 325
  silent NEC 453.9
  sinus, intracranial (venous) (any) (*see also*
    Thrombosis, intracranial venous sinus)
    325
  softening, brain (*see also* Thrombosis, brain)
    434.0 ✓5ᵗʰ
  specified site NEC 453.8
  spermatic cord 608.83
  spinal cord 336.1
    due to syphilis 094.89
    in pregnancy or puerperium 671.5 ✓5ᵗʰ
    pyogenic origin 324.1
      late effect — *see* category 326

✓4ᵗʰ Fourth-digit Required   ✓5ᵗʰ Fifth-digit Required   ►◄ Revised Text   ● New Line   ▲ Revised Code

Thrombosis, thrombotic — *continued*
spleen, splenic 289.59
artery 444.89
testis 608.83
traumatic (complication) (early) (*see also* Injury,
blood vessel, by site) 904.9
tricuspid — *see* Endocarditis, tricuspid
tunica vaginalis 608.83
umbilical cord (vessels) 663.6 ✓5ᵗʰ
affecting fetus or newborn 762.6
vas deferens 608.83
vena cava (inferior) (superior) 453.2
Thrombus — *see* Thrombosis
Thrush 112.0
newborn 771.7
Thumb — *see also* condition
gamekeeper's 842.12
sucking (child problem) 307.9
Thygeson's superficial punctate keratitis
370.21
Thymergasia (*see also* Psychosis, affective)
296.80
Thymitis 254.8
Thymoma (benign) (M8580/0) 212.6
malignant (M8580/3) 164.0
Thymus, thymic (gland) — *see* condition
Thyrocele (*see also* Goiter) 240.9
Thyroglossal — *see also* condition
cyst 759.2
duct, persistent 759.2
Thyroid (body) (gland) — *see also* condition
lingual 759.2
Thyroiditis 245.9
acute (pyogenic) (suppurative) 245.0
nonsuppurative 245.0
autoimmune 245.2
chronic (nonspecific) (sclerosing) 245.8
fibrous 245.3
lymphadenoid 245.2
lymphocytic 245.2
lymphoid 245.2
complicating pregnancy, childbirth, or
puerperium 648.1 ✓5ᵗʰ
de Quervain's (subacute granulomatous) 245.1
fibrous (chronic) 245.3
giant (cell) (follicular) 245.1
granulomatous (de Quervain's) (subacute)
245.1
Hashimoto's (struma lymphomatosa) 245.2
iatrogenic 245.4
invasive (fibrous) 245.3
ligneous 245.3
lymphocytic (chronic) 245.2
lymphoid 245.2
lymphomatous 245.2
pseudotuberculous 245.1
pyogenic 245.0
radiation 245.4
Riedel's (ligneous) 245.3
subacute 245.1
suppurative 245.0
tuberculous (*see also* Tuberculosis) 017.5 ✓5ᵗʰ
viral 245.1
woody 245.3
Thyrolingual duct, persistent 759.2
Thyromegaly 240.9
Thyrotoxic
crisis or storm (*see also* Thyrotoxicosis)
242.9 ✓5ᵗʰ
heart failure (*see also* Thyrotoxicosis)
242.9 ✓5ᵗʰ [425.7]
Thyrotoxicosis 242.9 ✓5ᵗʰ

> Note — Use the following fifth-digit
> subclassification with category 242:
>
> 0   without mention of thyrotoxic crisis
>   or storm
>
> 1   with mention of thyrotoxic crisis or
>   storm

with
goiter (diffuse) 242.0 ✓5ᵗʰ
adenomatous 242.3 ✓5ᵗʰ
multinodular 242.2 ✓5ᵗʰ

Thyrotoxicosis — *continued*
with — *continued*
goiter — *continued*
adenomatous — *continued*
uninodular 242.1 ✓5ᵗʰ
nodular 242.3 ✓5ᵗʰ
multinodular 242.2 ✓5ᵗʰ
uninodular 242.1 ✓5ᵗʰ
infiltrative
dermopathy 242.0 ✓5ᵗʰ
ophthalmopathy 242.0 ✓5ᵗʰ
thyroid acropachy 242.0 ✓5ᵗʰ
complicating pregnancy, childbirth, or
puerperium 648.1 ✓5ᵗʰ
due to
ectopic thyroid nodule 242.4 ✓5ᵗʰ
ingestion of (excessive) thyroid material
242.8 ✓5ᵗʰ
specified cause NEC 242.8 ✓5ᵗʰ
factitia 242.8 ✓5ᵗʰ
heart 242.9 ✓5ᵗʰ [425.7]
neonatal (transient) 775.3
TIA (transient ischemic attack) 435.9
with transient neurologic deficit 435.9
late effect — *see* Late effect(s) (of)
cerebrovascular disease
Tibia vara 732.4
Tic 307.20
breathing 307.20
child problem 307.21
compulsive 307.22
convulsive 307.20
degenerative (generalized) (localized) 333.3
facial 351.8
douloureux (*see also* Neuralgia, trigeminal)
350.1
atypical 350.2
habit 307.20
chronic (motor or vocal) 307.22
transient of childhood 307.21
lid 307.20
transient of childhood 307.21
motor-verbal 307.23
occupational 300.89
orbicularis 307.20
transient of childhood 307.21
organic origin 333.3
postchoreic — *see* Chorea
psychogenic 307.20
compulsive 307.22
salaam 781.0
spasm 307.20
chronic (motor or vocal) 307.22
transient of childhood 307.21
Tick (-borne) fever NEC 066.1
American mountain 066.1
Colorado 066.1
hemorrhagic NEC 065.3
Crimean 065.0
Kyasanur Forest 065.2
Omsk 065.1
mountain 066.1
nonxanthematous 066.1
Tick-bite fever NEC 066.1
African 087.1
Colorado (virus) 066.1
Rocky Mountain 082.0
Tick paralysis 989.5
Tics and spasms, compulsive 307.22
Tietze's disease or syndrome 733.6
Tight, tightness
anus 564.89
chest 786.59
fascia (lata) 728.9
foreskin (congenital) 605
hymen 623.3
introitus (acquired) (congenital) 623.3
rectal sphincter 564.89
tendon 727.81
Achilles (heel) 727.81
urethral sphincter 598.9
Tilting vertebra 737.9
Timidity, child 313.21
Tinea (intersecta) (tarsi) 110.9
amiantacea 110.0

Tinea — *continued*
asbestina 110.0
barbae 110.0
beard 110.0
black dot 110.0
blanca 111.2
capitis 110.0
corporis 110.5
cruris 110.3
decalvans 704.09
flava 111.0
foot 110.4
furfuracea 111.0
imbricata (Tokelau) 110.5
lepothrix 039.0
manuum 110.2
microsporic (*see also* Dermatophytosis) 110.9
nigra 111.1
nodosa 111.2
pedis 110.4
scalp 110.0
specified site NEC 110.8
sycosis 110.0
tonsurans 110.0
trichophytic (*see also* Dermatophytosis) 110.9
unguium 110.1
versicolor 111.0
Tingling sensation (*see also* Disturbance,
sensation) 782.0
Tin-miners' lung 503
Tinnitus (aurium) 388.30
audible 388.32
objective 388.32
subjective 388.31
Tipping pelvis 738.6
with disproportion (fetopelvic) 653.0 ✓5ᵗʰ
affecting fetus or newborn 763.1
causing obstructed labor 660.1 ✓5ᵗʰ
affecting fetus or newborn 763.1
Tiredness 780.79
Tissue — *see* condition
Tobacco
abuse (affecting health) NEC (*see also* Abuse,
drugs, nondependent) 305.1
heart 989.8 ✓5ᵗʰ
Tobias' syndrome (carcinoma, pulmonary apex)
(M8010/3) 162.3
Tocopherol deficiency 269.1
Todd's
cirrhosis — *see* Cirrhosis, biliary
paralysis (postepileptic transitory paralysis)
344.8 ✓5ᵗʰ
Toe — *see* condition
Toilet, artificial opening (*see also* Attention to,
artificial, opening) V55.9
Tokelau ringworm 110.5
Tollwut 071
Tolosa-Hunt syndrome 378.55
Tommaselli's disease
correct substance properly administered 599.7
overdose or wrong substance given or taken
961.4
Tongue — *see also* condition
worms 134.1
Tongue tie 750.0
Toni-Fanconi syndrome (cystinosis) 270.0
Tonic pupil 379.46
Tonsil — *see* condition
Tonsillitis (acute) (catarrhal) (croupous)
(follicular) (gangrenous) (infective) (lacunar)
(lingual) (malignant) (membranous)
(phlegmonous) (pneumococcal)
(pseudomembranous) (purulent) (septic)
(staphylococcal) (subacute) (suppurative)
(toxic) (ulcerative) (vesicular) (viral) 463
with influenza, flu, or grippe 487.1
chronic 474.00
diphtheritic (membranous) 032.0
hypertrophic 474.00
influenzal 487.1
parenchymatous 475
streptococcal 034.0
tuberculous (*see also* Tuberculosis) 012.8 ✓5ᵗʰ

Tonsillitis — continued
Vincent's 101
Tonsillopharyngitis 465.8
Tooth, teeth — see condition
Toothache 525.9
Topagnosis 782.0
Tophi (gouty) 274.0
ear 274.81
heart 274.82
specified site NEC 274.82
Torn — see Tear, torn
Tornwaldt's bursitis (disease) (pharyngeal bursitis) 478.29
cyst 478.26
Torpid liver 573.9
Torsion
accessory tube 620.5
adnexa (female) 620.5
aorta (congenital) 747.29
acquired 447.1
appendix epididymis 608.2
bile duct 576.8
with calculus, choledocholithiasis or stones — see Choledocholithiasis
congenital 751.69
bowel, colon, or intestine 560.2
cervix (see also Malposition, uterus) 621.6
duodenum 537.3
dystonia — see Dystonia, torsion
epididymis 608.2
appendix 608.2
fallopian tube 620.5
gallbladder (see also Disease, gallbladder) 575.8
congenital 751.69
gastric 537.89
hydatid of Morgagni (female) 620.5
kidney (pedicle) 593.89
Meckel's diverticulum (congenital) 751.0
mesentery 560.2
omentum 560.2
organ or site, congenital NEC — see Anomaly, specified type NEC
ovary (pedicle) 620.5
congenital 752.0
oviduct 620.5
penis 607.89
congenital 752.69
renal 593.89
spasm — see Dystonia, torsion
spermatic cord 608.2
spleen 289.59
testicle, testis 608.2
tibia 736.89
umbilical cord — see Compression, umbilical cord
uterus (see also Malposition, uterus) 621.6
Torticollis (intermittent) (spastic) 723.5
congenital 754.1
sternomastoid 754.1
due to birth injury 767.8
hysterical 300.11
ocular 781.93 •
psychogenic 306.0
specified as conversion reaction 300.11
rheumatic 723.5
rheumatoid 714.0
spasmodic 333.83
traumatic, current NEC 847.0
Tortuous
artery 447.1
fallopian tube 752.19
organ or site, congenital NEC — see Distortion
renal vessel, congenital 747.62
retina vessel (congenital) 743.58
acquired 362.17
ureter 593.4
urethra 599.84
vein — see Varicose, vein
Torula, torular (infection) 117.5
histolytica 117.5
lung 117.5
Torulosis 117.5

Torus
fracture
fibula 823.41 •
with tibia 823.42 •
radius 813.45 •
tibia 823.40 •
with fibula 823.42 •
mandibularis 526.81
palatinus 526.81
Touch, vitreous 997.99
Touraine's syndrome (hereditary osteo-onychodysplasia) 756.89
Touraine-Solente-Golé syndrome (acropachyderma) 757.39
Tourette's disease (motor-verbal tic) 307.23
Tower skull 756.0
with exophthalmos 756.0
Toxemia 799.8
with
abortion — see Abortion, by type, with toxemia
bacterial — see Septicemia
biliary (see also Disease, biliary) 576.8
burn — see Burn, by site
congenital NEC 779.89 ▲
eclamptic 642.6 ☑5ᵗʰ
with pre-existing hypertension 642.7 ☑5ᵗʰ
erysipelatous (see also Erysipelas) 035
fatigue 799.8
fetus or newborn NEC 779.89 ▲
food (see also Poisoning, food) 005.9
gastric 537.89
gastrointestinal 558.2
intestinal 558.2
kidney (see also Disease, renal) 593.9
lung 518.89
malarial NEC (see also Malaria) 084.6
maternal (of pregnancy), affecting fetus or newborn 760.0
myocardial — see Myocarditis, toxic
of pregnancy (mild) (pre-eclamptic) 642.4 ☑5ᵗʰ
with
convulsions 642.6 ☑5ᵗʰ
pre-existing hypertension 642.7 ☑5ᵗʰ
affecting fetus or newborn 760.0
severe 642.5 ☑5ᵗʰ
pre-eclamptic — see Toxemia, of pregnancy
puerperal, postpartum — see Toxemia, of pregnancy
pulmonary 518.89
renal (see also Disease, renal) 593.9
septic (see also Septicemia) 038.9
small intestine 558.2
staphylococcal 038.10
aureus 038.11
due to food 005.0
specified organism NEC 038.19
stasis 799.8
stomach 537.89
uremic (see also Uremia) 586
urinary 586
Toxemica cerebropathia psychica (nonalcoholic) 294.0
alcoholic 291.1
Toxic (poisoning) — see also condition
from drug or poison — see Table of Drugs and Chemicals
oil syndrome 710.5
shock syndrome 040.82 ▲
thyroid (gland) (see also Thyrotoxicosis) 242.9 ☑5ᵗʰ
Toxicemia — see Toxemia
Toxicity
dilantin
asymptomatic 796.0
symptomatic — see Table of Drugs and Chemicals
drug
asymptomatic 796.0
symptomatic — see Table of Drugs and Chemicals
fava bean 282.2
from drug or poison
asymptomatic 796.0
symptomatic — see Table of Drugs and Chemicals

Toxicosis (see also Toxemia) 799.8
capillary, hemorrhagic 287.0
Toxinfection 799.8
gastrointestinal 558.2
Toxocariasis 128.0
Toxoplasma infection, generalized 130.9
Toxoplasmosis (acquired) 130.9
with pneumonia 130.4
congenital, active 771.2
disseminated (multisystemic) 130.8
maternal
with suspected damage to fetus affecting management of pregnancy 655.4 ☑5ᵗʰ
affecting fetus or newborn 760.2
manifest toxoplasmosis in fetus or newborn 771.2
multiple sites 130.8
multisystemic disseminated 130.8
specified site NEC 130.7
Trabeculation, bladder 596.8
Trachea — see condition
Tracheitis (acute) (catarrhal) (infantile) (membranous) (plastic) (pneumococcal) (septic) (suppurative) (viral) 464.10
with
bronchitis 490
acute or subacute 466.0
chronic 491.8
tuberculosis — see Tuberculosis, pulmonary
laryngitis (acute) 464.20
with obstruction 464.21
chronic 476.1
tuberculous (see also Tuberculosis, larynx) 012.3 ☑5ᵗʰ
obstruction 464.11
chronic 491.8
with
bronchitis (chronic) 491.8
laryngitis (chronic) 476.1
due to external agent — see Condition, respiratory, chronic, due to
diphtheritic (membranous) 032.3
due to external agent — see Inflammation, respiratory, upper, due to
edematous 464.11
influenzal 487.1
streptococcal 034.0
syphilitic 095.8
tuberculous (see also Tuberculosis) 012.8 ☑5ᵗʰ
Trachelitis (nonvenereal) (see also Cervicitis) 616.0
trichomonal 131.09
Tracheobronchial — see condition
Tracheobronchitis (see also Bronchitis) 490
acute or subacute 466.0
with bronchospasm or obstruction 466.0
chronic 491.8
influenzal 487.1
senile 491.8
Tracheobronchomegaly (congenital) 748.3
Tracheobronchopneumonitis — see Pneumonia, broncho
Tracheocele (external) (internal) 519.1
congenital 748.3
Tracheomalacia 519.1
congenital 748.3
Tracheopharyngitis (acute) 465.8
chronic 478.9
due to external agent — see Condition, respiratory, chronic, due to
due to external agent — see Inflammation, respiratory, upper, due to
Tracheostenosis 519.1
congenital 748.3
Tracheostomy
attention to V55.0
complication 519.00
hemorrhage 519.09
infection 519.01
malfunctioning 519.02
obstruction 519.09
sepsis 519.01
status V44.0

Tracheostomy — *continued*
   stenosis 519.02

Trachoma, trachomatous 076.9
   active (stage) 076.1
   contraction of conjunctiva 076.1
   dubium 076.0
   healed or late effect 139.1
   initial (stage) 076.0
   Türck's (chronic catarrhal laryngitis) 476.0

Trachyphonia 784.49

Training
   orthoptic V57.4
   orthotic V57.81

Train sickness 994.6

Trait
   hemoglobin
      abnormal NEC 282.7
         with thalassemia 282.4
      C (*see also* Disease, hemoglobin, C) 282.7
         with elliptocytosis 282.7
      S (Hb-S) 282.5
   Lepore 282.4
      with other abnormal hemoglobin NEC 282.4
   paranoid 301.0
   sickle-cell 282.5
      with
         elliptocytosis 282.5
         spherocytosis 282.5

Traits, paranoid 301.0

Tramp V60.0

Trance 780.09
   hysterical 300.13

Transaminasemia 790.4

Transfusion, blood
   donor V59.01
      stem cells V59.02
   incompatible 999.6
   reaction or complication — *see* Complications,
      transfusion
   syndrome
      fetomaternal 772.0
      twin-to-twin
         blood loss (donor twin) 772.0
         recipient twin 776.4
   without reported diagnosis V58.2

Transient — *see also* condition
   alteration of awareness 780.02
   blindness 368.12
   deafness (ischemic) 388.02
   global amnesia 437.7
   person (homeless) NEC V60.0

Transitional, lumbosacral joint of vertebra
   756.19

Translocation
   autosomes NEC 758.5
      13-15 758.1
      16-18 758.2
      21 or 22 758.0
      balanced in normal individual 758.4
      D₁ 758.1
      E₃ 758.2
      G 758.0
   balanced autosomal in normal individual 758.4
   chromosomes NEC 758.89
   Down's syndrome 758.0

Translucency, iris 364.53

Transmission of chemical substances through
   the placenta (affecting fetus or newborn)
   760.70
   alcohol 760.71
   anti-infective agents 760.74
   cocaine 760.75
   "crack" 760.75
   diethylstilbestrol [DES] 760.76
   hallucinogenic agents 760.73
   medicinal agents NEC 760.79
   narcotics 760.72
   obstetric anesthetic or analgesic drug 763.5
   specified agent NEC 760.79
   suspected, affecting management of pregnancy
      655.5 ☑5ᵗʰ

Transplant(ed)
   bone V42.4
      marrow V42.81

Transplant(ed) — *continued*
   complication — *see also* Complications, due to
      (presence of) any device, implant, or graft
      classified to 996.0-996.5 NEC
      bone marrow 996.85
      corneal graft NEC 996.79
         infection or inflammation 996.69
         reaction 996.51
         rejection 996.51
      organ (failure) (immune or nonimmune
         cause) (infection) (rejection) 996.87
         bone marrow 996.85
         heart 996.83
         intestines 996.87
         kidney 996.81
         liver 996.82
         lung 996.84
         pancreas 996.86
         specified NEC 996.89
      skin NEC 996.79
         infection or inflammation 996.69
         rejection 996.52
            artificial 996.55
            decellularized allodermis 996.55
   cornea V42.5
   hair V50.0
   heart V42.1
      valve V42.2
   intestine V42.84
   kidney V42.0
   liver V42.7
   lung V42.6
   organ V42.9
      specified NEC V42.89
   pancreas V42.83
   peripheral stem cells V42.82
   skin V42.3
   stem cells, peripheral V42.82
   tissue V42.9
      specified NEC V42.89

Transplants, ovarian, endometrial 617.1

Transposed — *see* Transposition

Transposition (congenital) — *see also*
   Malposition, congenital
   abdominal viscera 759.3
   aorta (dextra) 745.11
   appendix 751.5
   arterial trunk 745.10
   colon 751.5
   great vessels (complete) 745.10
      both originating from right ventricle 745.11
      corrected 745.12
      double outlet right ventricle 745.11
      incomplete 745.11
      partial 745.11
      specified type NEC 745.19
   heart 746.87
      with complete transposition of viscera 759.3
   intestine (large) (small) 751.5
   pulmonary veins 747.49
   reversed jejunal (for bypass) (status) V45.3
   stomach 750.7
      with general transposition of viscera 759.3
   teeth, tooth 524.3
   vessels (complete) 745.10
      partial 745.11
   viscera (abdominal) (thoracic) 759.3

Trans-sexualism 302.50
   with
      asexual history 302.51
      heterosexual history 302.53
      homosexual history 302.52

Transverse — *see also* condition
   arrest (deep), in labor 660.3 ☑5ᵗʰ
      affecting fetus or newborn 763.1
   lie 652.3 ☑5ᵗʰ
      before labor, affecting fetus or newborn
         761.7
      causing obstructed labor 660.0 ☑5ᵗʰ
         affecting fetus or newborn 763.1
      during labor, affecting fetus or newborn
         763.1

Transvestism, transvestitism (transvestic
   fetishism) 302.3

Trapped placenta (with hemorrhage) 666.0 ☑5ᵗʰ
   without hemorrhage 667.0 ☑5ᵗʰ

Trauma, traumatism (*see also* Injury, by site)
   959.9
   birth — *see* Birth, injury NEC
   causing hemorrhage of pregnancy or delivery
      641.8 ☑5ᵗʰ
   complicating
      abortion — *see* Abortion, by type, with
         damage to pelvic organs
      ectopic pregnancy (*see also* categories
         633.0-633.9) 639.2
      molar pregnancy (*see also* categories 630-
         632) 639.2
   during delivery NEC 665.9 ☑5ᵗʰ
   following
      abortion 639.2
      ectopic or molar pregnancy 639.2
   maternal, during pregnancy, affecting fetus or
      newborn 760.5
   neuroma — *see* Injury, nerve, by site
   previous major, affecting management of
      pregnancy, childbirth, or puerperium
      V23.8 ☑5ᵗʰ
   psychic (current) — *see also* Reaction,
      adjustment
      previous (history) V15.49
   psychologic, previous (affecting health) V15.49
   transient paralysis — *see* Injury, nerve, by site

Traumatic — *see* condition

Treacher Collins' syndrome (incomplete facial
   dysostosis) 756.0

Treitz's hernia — *see* Hernia, Treitz's

Trematode infestation NEC 121.9

Trematodiasis NEC 121.9

Trembles 988.8

Trembling paralysis (*see also* Parkinsonism)
   332.0

Tremor 781.0
   essential (benign) 333.1
   familial 333.1
   flapping (liver) 572.8
   hereditary 333.1
   hysterical 300.11
   intention 333.1
   mercurial 985.0
   muscle 728.85
   Parkinson's (*see also* Parkinsonism) 332.0
   psychogenic 306.0
      specified as conversion reaction 300.11
   senilis 797
   specified type NEC 333.1

Trench
   fever 083.1
   foot 991.4
   mouth 101
   nephritis — *see* Nephritis, acute

Treponema pallidum infection (*see also* Syphilis)
   097.9

Treponematosis 102.9
   due to
      T. pallidum — *see* Syphilis
      T. pertenue (yaws) (*see also* Yaws) 102.9

Triad
   Kartagener's 759.3
   Reiter's (complete) (incomplete) 099.3
   Saint's (*see also* Hernia, diaphragm) 553.3

Trichiasis 704.2
   cicatricial 704.2
   eyelid 374.05
      with entropion (*see also* Entropion) 374.00

Trichinella spiralis (infection) (infestation) 124

Trichinelliasis 124

Trichinellosis 124

Trichiniasis 124

Trichinosis 124

Trichobezoar 938
   intestine 936
   stomach 935.2

Trichocephaliasis 127.3

Trichocephalosis 127.3

Trichocephalus infestation 127.3

Trichoclasis 704.2

Trichoepithelioma (M8100/0) — *see also* Neoplasm, skin, benign
  breast 217
  genital organ NEC — *see* Neoplasm, by site, benign
  malignant (M8100/3) — *see* Neoplasm, skin, malignant

Trichofolliculoma (M8101/0) — *see* Neoplasm, skin, benign

Tricholemmoma (M8102/0) — *see* Neoplasm, skin, benign

Trichomatosis 704.2

Trichomoniasis 131.9
  bladder 131.09
  cervix 131.09
  intestinal 007.3
  prostate 131.03
  seminal vesicle 131.09
  specified site NEC 131.8
  urethra 131.02
  urogenitalis 131.00
  vagina 131.01
  vulva 131.01
  vulvovaginal 131.01

Trichomycosis 039.0
  axillaris 039.0
  nodosa 111.2
  nodularis 111.2
  rubra 039.0

Trichonocardiosis (axillaris) (palmellina) 039.0

Trichonodosis 704.2

Trichophytid, trichophyton infection (*see also* Dermatophytosis) 110.9

Trichophytide — *see* Dermatophytosis

Trichophytobezoar 938
  intestine 936
  stomach 935.2

Trichophytosis — *see* Dermatophytosis

Trichoptilosis 704.2

Trichorrhexis (nodosa) 704.2

Trichosporosis nodosa 111.2

Trichostasis spinulosa (congenital) 757.4

Trichostrongyliasis (small intestine) 127.6

Trichostrongylosis 127.6

Trichostrongylus (instabilis) infection 127.6

Trichotillomania 312.39

Trichromat, anomalous (congenital) 368.59

Trichromatopsia, anomalous (congenital) 368.59

Trichuriasis 127.3

Trichuris trichiuria (any site) (infection) (infestation) 127.3

Tricuspid (valve) — *see* condition

Trifid — *see also* Accessory
  kidney (pelvis) 753.3
  tongue 750.13

Trigeminal neuralgia (*see also* Neuralgia, trigeminal) 350.1

Trigeminoencephaloangiomatosis 759.6

Trigeminy 427.89
  postoperative 997.1

Trigger finger (acquired) 727.03
  congenital 756.89

Trigonitis (bladder) (chronic) (pseudomembranous) 595.3
  tuberculous (*see also* Tuberculosis) 016.1 ✓5ᵗʰ

Trigonocephaly 756.0

Trihexosidosis 272.7

Trilobate placenta — *see* Placenta, abnormal

Trilocular heart 745.8

Tripartita placenta — *see* Placenta, abnormal

Triple — *see also* Accessory
  kidneys 753.3
  uteri 752.2
  X female 758.81

Triplegia 344.89
  congenital or infantile 343.8

Triplet
  affected by maternal complications of pregnancy 761.5
  healthy liveborn — *see* Newborn, multiple

Triplet — *continued*
  pregnancy (complicating delivery) NEC 651.1 ✓5ᵗʰ
    with fetal loss and retention of one or more fetus(es) 651.4 ✓5ᵗʰ

Triplex placenta — *see* Placenta, abnormal

Triplication — *see* Accessory

Trismus 781.0
  neonatorum 771.3
  newborn 771.3

Trisomy (syndrome) NEC 758.5
  13 (partial) 758.1
  16-18 758.2
  18 (partial) 758.2
  21 (partial) 758.0
  22 758.0
  autosomes NEC 758.5
  D₁ 758.1
  E₃ 758.2
  G (group) 758.0
  group D₁ 758.1
  group E 758.2
  group G 758.0

Tritanomaly 368.53

Tritanopia 368.53

Troisier-Hanot-Chauffard syndrome (bronze diabetes) 275.0

Trombidiosis 133.8

Trophedema (hereditary) 757.0
  congenital 757.0

Trophoblastic disease (*see also* Hydatidiform mole) 630
  previous, affecting management of pregnancy V23.1

Tropholymphedema 757.0

Trophoneurosis NEC 356.9
  arm NEC 354.9
  disseminated 710.1
  facial 349.89
  leg NEC 355.8
  lower extremity NEC 355.8
  upper extremity NEC 354.9

Tropical — *see also* condition
  maceration feet (syndrome) 991.4
  wet foot (syndrome) 991.4

Trouble — *see also* Disease
  bowel 569.9
  heart — *see* Disease, heart
  intestine 569.9
  kidney (*see also* Disease, renal) 593.9
  nervous 799.2
  sinus (*see also* Sinusitis) 473.9

Trousseau's syndrome (thrombophlebitis migrans) 453.1

Truancy, childhood — *see also* Disturbance, conduct
  socialized 312.2 ✓5ᵗʰ
  undersocialized, unsocialized 312.1 ✓5ᵗʰ

Truncus
  arteriosus (persistent) 745.0
  common 745.0
  communis 745.0

Trunk — *see* condition

Trychophytide — *see* Dermatophytosis

Trypanosoma infestation — *see* Trypanosomiasis

Trypanosomiasis 086.9
  with meningoencephalitis 086.9 [323.2]
  African 086.5
    due to Trypanosoma 086.5
      gambiense 086.3
      rhodesiense 086.4
  American 086.2
    with
      heart involvement 086.0
      other organ involvement 086.1
    without mention of organ involvement 086.2
  Brazilian — *see* Trypanosomiasis, American
  Chagas' — *see* Trypanosomiasis, American
  due to Trypanosoma
    cruzi — *see* Trypanosomiasis, American
    gambiense 086.3
    rhodesiense 086.4

Trypanosomiasis — *continued*
  gambiensis, Gambian 086.3
  North American — *see* Trypanosomiasis, American
  rhodesiensis, Rhodesian 086.4
  South American — *see* Trypanosomiasis, American

T-shaped incisors 520.2

Tsutsugamushi fever 081.2

Tube, tubal, tubular — *see also* condition
  ligation, admission for V25.2

Tubercle — *see also* Tuberculosis
  brain, solitary 013.2 ✓5ᵗʰ
  Darwin's 744.29
  epithelioid noncaseating 135
  Ghon, primary infection 010.0 ✓5ᵗʰ

Tuberculid, tuberculide (indurating) (lichenoid) (miliary) (papulonecrotic) (primary) (skin) (subcutaneous) (*see also* Tuberculosis) 017.0 ✓5ᵗʰ

Tuberculoma — *see also* Tuberculosis
  brain (any part) 013.2 ✓5ᵗʰ
  meninges (cerebral) (spinal) 013.1 ✓5ᵗʰ
  spinal cord 013.4 ✓5ᵗʰ

Tuberculosis, tubercular, tuberculous (calcification) (calcified) (caseous) (chromogenic acid-fast bacilli) (congenital) (degeneration) (disease) (fibrocaseous) (fistula) (gangrene) (interstitial) (isolated circumscribed lesions) (necrosis) (parenchymatous) (ulcerative) 011.9

Note — Use the following fifth-digit subclassification with categories 010-018:

0	*unspecified*
1	*bacteriological or histological examination not done*
2	*bacteriological or histological examination unknown (at present)*
3	*tubercle bacilli found (in sputum) by microscopy*
4	*tubercle bacilli not found (in sputum) by microscopy, but found by bacterial culture*
5	*tubercle bacilli not found by bacteriological exam-ination, but tuberculosis confirmed histologically*
6	*tubercle bacilli not found by bacteriological or histological examination, but tuberculosis confirmed by other methods [inoculation of animals]*

For tuberculous conditions specified as late effects or sequelae, see category 137.

---

  abdomen 014.8 ✓5ᵗʰ
    lymph gland 014.8 ✓5ᵗʰ
  abscess 011.9 ✓5ᵗʰ
    arm 017.9 ✓5ᵗʰ
    bone (*see also* Osteomyelitis, due to, tuberculosis) 015.9 ✓5ᵗʰ [730.8] ✓5ᵗʰ
      hip 015.1 ✓5ᵗʰ [730.85]
      knee 015.2 ✓5ᵗʰ [730.96]
      sacrum 015.0 ✓5ᵗʰ [730.88]
      specified site NEC 015.7 ✓5ᵗʰ [730.88]
      spinal 015.0 ✓5ᵗʰ [730.88]
      vertebra 015.0 ✓5ᵗʰ [730.88]
    brain 013.3 ✓5ᵗʰ
    breast 017.9 ✓5ᵗʰ
    Cowper's gland 016.5 ✓5ᵗʰ
    dura (mater) 013.8 ✓5ᵗʰ
      brain 013.3 ✓5ᵗʰ
      spinal cord 013.5 ✓5ᵗʰ
    epidural 013.8 ✓5ᵗʰ
      brain 013.3 ✓5ᵗʰ
      spinal cord 013.5 ✓5ᵗʰ
    frontal sinus — *see* Tuberculosis, sinus
    genital organs NEC 016.9 ✓5ᵗʰ
      female 016.7 ✓5ᵗʰ
      male 016.5 ✓5ᵗʰ
    genitourinary NEC 016.9 ✓5ᵗʰ
    gland (lymphatic) — *see* Tuberculosis, lymph gland
    hip 015.1 ✓5ᵗʰ

Tuberculosis, tubercular, tuberculous — *continued*

abscess — *continued*
  iliopsoas 015.0 ✓5ᵗʰ [730.88]
  intestine 014.8 ✓5ᵗʰ
  ischiorectal 014.8 ✓5ᵗʰ
  joint 015.9 ✓5ᵗʰ
    hip 015.1 ✓5ᵗʰ
    knee 015.2 ✓5ᵗʰ
    specified joint NEC 015.8 ✓5ᵗʰ
    vertebral 015.0 ✓5ᵗʰ [730.88]
  kidney 016.0 ✓5ᵗʰ [590.81]
  knee 015.2 ✓5ᵗʰ
  lumbar 015.0 ✓5ᵗʰ [730.88]
  lung 011.2 ✓5ᵗʰ
    primary, progressive 010.8 ✓5ᵗʰ
  meninges (cerebral) (spinal) 013.0 ✓5ᵗʰ
  pelvic 016.9 ✓5ᵗʰ
    female 016.7 ✓5ᵗʰ
    male 016.5 ✓5ᵗʰ
  perianal 014.8 ✓5ᵗʰ
    fistula 014.8 ✓5ᵗʰ
  perinephritic 016.0 ✓5ᵗʰ [590.81]
  perineum 017.9 ✓5ᵗʰ
  perirectal 014.8 ✓5ᵗʰ
  psoas 015.0 ✓5ᵗʰ [730.88]
  rectum 014.8 ✓5ᵗʰ
  retropharyngeal 012.8 ✓5ᵗʰ
  sacrum 015.0 ✓5ᵗʰ [730.88]
  scrofulous 017.2 ✓5ᵗʰ
  scrotum 016.5 ✓5ᵗʰ
  skin 017.0 ✓5ᵗʰ
    primary 017.0 ✓5ᵗʰ
  spinal cord 013.5 ✓5ᵗʰ
  spine or vertebra (column)
    015.0 ✓5ᵗʰ [730.88]
  strumous 017.2 ✓5ᵗʰ
  subdiaphragmatic 014.8 ✓5ᵗʰ
  testis 016.5 ✓5ᵗʰ
  thigh 017.9 ✓5ᵗʰ
  urinary 016.3 ✓5ᵗʰ
    kidney 016.0 ✓5ᵗʰ [590.81]
  uterus 016.7 ✓5ᵗʰ
accessory sinus — *see* Tuberculosis, sinus
Addison's disease 017.6 ✓5ᵗʰ
adenitis (*see also* Tuberculosis, lymph gland)
  017.2 ✓5ᵗʰ
adenoids 012.8 ✓5ᵗʰ
adenopathy (*see also* Tuberculosis, lymph
  gland) 017.2 ✓5ᵗʰ
  tracheobronchial 012.1 ✓5ᵗʰ
    primary progressive 010.8 ✓5ᵗʰ
adherent pericardium 017.9 ✓5ᵗʰ [420.0]
adnexa (uteri) 016.7 ✓5ᵗʰ
adrenal (capsule) (gland) 017.6 ✓5ᵗʰ
air passage NEC 012.8 ✓5ᵗʰ
alimentary canal 014.8 ✓5ᵗʰ
anemia 017.9 ✓5ᵗʰ
ankle (joint) 015.8 ✓5ᵗʰ
  bone 015.5 ✓5ᵗʰ [730.87]
anus 014.8 ✓5ᵗʰ
apex (*see also* Tuberculosis, pulmonary)
  011.9 ✓5ᵗʰ
apical (*see also* Tuberculosis, pulmonary)
  011.9 ✓5ᵗʰ
appendicitis 014.8 ✓5ᵗʰ
appendix 014.8 ✓5ᵗʰ
arachnoid 013.0 ✓5ᵗʰ
artery 017.9 ✓5ᵗʰ
arthritis (chronic) (synovial) 015.9 ✓5ᵗʰ [711.40]
  ankle 015.8 ✓5ᵗʰ [730.87]
  hip 015.1 ✓5ᵗʰ [711.45]
  knee 015.2 ✓5ᵗʰ [711.46]
  specified site NEC 015.8 ✓5ᵗʰ [711.48]
  spine or vertebra (column)
    015.0 ✓5ᵗʰ [720.81]
  wrist 015.8 ✓5ᵗʰ [730.83]
articular — *see* Tuberculosis, joint
ascites 014.0 ✓5ᵗʰ
asthma (*see also* Tuberculosis, pulmonary)
  011.9 ✓5ᵗʰ
axilla, axillary 017.2 ✓5ᵗʰ
  gland 017.2 ✓5ᵗʰ
bilateral (*see also* Tuberculosis, pulmonary)
  011.9 ✓5ᵗʰ
bladder 016.1 ✓5ᵗʰ

Tuberculosis, tubercular, tuberculous — *continued*

bone (*see also* Osteomyelitis, due to,
  tuberculosis) 015.9 ✓5ᵗʰ [730.8] ✓5ᵗʰ
  hip 015.1 ✓5ᵗʰ [730.85]
  knee 015.2 ✓5ᵗʰ [730.86]
  limb NEC 015.5 ✓5ᵗʰ [730.88]
  sacrum 015.0 ✓5ᵗʰ [730.88]
  specified site NEC 015.7 ✓5ᵗʰ [730.88]
  spinal or vertebral column 015.0
    ✓5ᵗʰ [730.88]
bowel 014.8 ✓5ᵗʰ
  miliary 018.9 ✓5ᵗʰ
brain 013.2 ✓5ᵗʰ
breast 017.9 ✓5ᵗʰ
broad ligament 016.7 ✓5ᵗʰ
bronchi, bronchial, bronchus 011.3 ✓5ᵗʰ
  ectasia, ectasis 011.5 ✓5ᵗʰ
  fistula 011.3 ✓5ᵗʰ
    primary, progressive 010.8 ✓5ᵗʰ
  gland 012.1 ✓5ᵗʰ
    primary, progressive 010.8 ✓5ᵗʰ
  isolated 012.2 ✓5ᵗʰ
  lymph gland or node 012.1 ✓5ᵗʰ
    primary, progressive 010.8 ✓5ᵗʰ
bronchiectasis 011.5 ✓5ᵗʰ
bronchitis 011.3 ✓5ᵗʰ
bronchopleural 012.0 ✓5ᵗʰ
bronchopneumonia, bronchopneumonic
  011.6 ✓5ᵗʰ
bronchorrhagia 011.3 ✓5ᵗʰ
bronchotracheal 011.3 ✓5ᵗʰ
  isolated 012.2 ✓5ᵗʰ
bronchus — *see* Tuberculosis, bronchi
bronze disease (Addison's) 017.6 ✓5ᵗʰ
buccal cavity 017.9 ✓5ᵗʰ
bulbourethral gland 016.5 ✓5ᵗʰ
bursa (*see also* Tuberculosis, joint) 015.9 ✓5ᵗʰ
cachexia NEC (*see also* Tuberculosis,
  pulmonary) 011.9 ✓5ᵗʰ
cardiomyopathy 017.9 ✓5ᵗʰ [425.8]
caries (*see also* Tuberculosis, bone)
  015.9 ✓5ᵗʰ [730.8] ✓5ᵗʰ
cartilage (*see also* Tuberculosis, bone)
  015.9 ✓5ᵗʰ [730.8] ✓5ᵗʰ
  intervertebral 015.0 ✓5ᵗʰ [730.88]
catarrhal (*see also* Tuberculosis, pulmonary)
  011.9 ✓5ᵗʰ
cecum 014.8 ✓5ᵗʰ
cellular tissue (primary) 017.0 ✓5ᵗʰ
cellulitis (primary) 017.0 ✓5ᵗʰ
central nervous system 013.9 ✓5ᵗʰ
  specified site NEC 013.8 ✓5ᵗʰ
cerebellum (current) 013.2 ✓5ᵗʰ
cerebral (current) 013.2 ✓5ᵗʰ
  meninges 013.0 ✓5ᵗʰ
cerebrospinal 013.6 ✓5ᵗʰ
  meninges 013.0 ✓5ᵗʰ
cerebrum (current) 013.2 ✓5ᵗʰ
cervical 017.2 ✓5ᵗʰ
  gland 017.2 ✓5ᵗʰ
  lymph nodes 017.2 ✓5ᵗʰ
cervicitis (uteri) 016.7 ✓5ᵗʰ
cervix 016.7 ✓5ᵗʰ
chest (*see also* Tuberculosis, pulmonary)
  011.9 ✓5ᵗʰ
childhood type or first infection 010.0 ✓5ᵗʰ
choroid 017.3 ✓5ᵗʰ [363.13]
choroiditis 017.3 ✓5ᵗʰ [363.13]
ciliary body 017.3 ✓5ᵗʰ [364.11]
colitis 014.8 ✓5ᵗʰ
colliers' 011.4 ✓5ᵗʰ
colliquativa (primary) 017.0 ✓5ᵗʰ
colon 014.8 ✓5ᵗʰ
  ulceration 014.8 ✓5ᵗʰ
complex, primary 010.0 ✓5ᵗʰ
complicating pregnancy, childbirth, or
  puerperium 647.3 ✓5ᵗʰ
  affecting fetus or newborn 760.2
congenital 771.2
conjunctiva 017.3 ✓5ᵗʰ [370.31]
connective tissue 017.9 ✓5ᵗʰ
  bone — *see* Tuberculosis, bone
contact V01.1
converter (tuberculin test) (without disease)
  795.5
cornea (ulcer) 017.3 ✓5ᵗʰ [370.31]
Cowper's gland 016.5 ✓5ᵗʰ

Tuberculosis, tubercular, tuberculous — *continued*

coxae 015.1 ✓5ᵗʰ [730.85]
coxalgia 015.1 ✓5ᵗʰ [730.85]
cul-de-sac of Douglas 014.8 ✓5ᵗʰ
curvature, spine 015.0 ✓5ᵗʰ [737.40]
cutis (colliquativa) (primary) 017.0 ✓5ᵗʰ
cyst, ovary 016.6 ✓5ᵗʰ
cystitis 016.1 ✓5ᵗʰ
dacryocystitis 017.3 ✓5ᵗʰ [375.32]
dactylitis 015.5 ✓5ᵗʰ
diarrhea 014.8 ✓5ᵗʰ
diffuse (*see also* Tuberculosis, miliary)
  018.9 ✓5ᵗʰ
  lung — *see* Tuberculosis, pulmonary
  meninges 013.0 ✓5ᵗʰ
digestive tract 014.8 ✓5ᵗʰ
disseminated (*see also* Tuberculosis, miliary)
  018.9 ✓5ᵗʰ
  meninges 013.0 ✓5ᵗʰ
duodenum 014.8 ✓5ᵗʰ
dura (mater) 013.9 ✓5ᵗʰ
  abscess 013.8 ✓5ᵗʰ
    cerebral 013.3 ✓5ᵗʰ
    spinal 013.5 ✓5ᵗʰ
dysentery 014.8 ✓5ᵗʰ
ear (inner) (middle) 017.4 ✓5ᵗʰ
  bone 015.6 ✓5ᵗʰ
  external (primary) 017.0 ✓5ᵗʰ
  skin (primary) 017.0 ✓5ᵗʰ
elbow 015.8 ✓5ᵗʰ
emphysema — *see* Tuberculosis, pulmonary
empyema 012.0 ✓5ᵗʰ
encephalitis 013.6 ✓5ᵗʰ
endarteritis 017.9 ✓5ᵗʰ
endocarditis (any valve) 017.9 ✓5ᵗʰ [424.91]
endocardium (any valve) 017.9 ✓5ᵗʰ [424.91]
endocrine glands NEC 017.9 ✓5ᵗʰ
endometrium 016.7 ✓5ᵗʰ
enteric, enterica 014.8 ✓5ᵗʰ
enteritis 014.8 ✓5ᵗʰ
enterocolitis 014.8 ✓5ᵗʰ
epididymis 016.4 ✓5ᵗʰ
epididymitis 016.4 ✓5ᵗʰ
epidural abscess 013.8 ✓5ᵗʰ
  brain 013.3 ✓5ᵗʰ
  spinal cord 013.5 ✓5ᵗʰ
epiglottis 012.3 ✓5ᵗʰ
episcleritis 017.3 ✓5ᵗʰ [379.00]
erythema (induratum) (nodosum) (primary)
  017.1 ✓5ᵗʰ
esophagus 017.8 ✓5ᵗʰ
Eustachian tube 017.4 ✓5ᵗʰ
exposure to V01.1
exudative 012.0 ✓5ᵗʰ
  primary, progressive 010.1 ✓5ᵗʰ
eye 017.3 ✓5ᵗʰ
  glaucoma 017.3 ✓5ᵗʰ [365.62]
eyelid (primary) 017.0 ✓5ᵗʰ
  lupus 017.0 ✓5ᵗʰ [373.4]
fallopian tube 016.6 ✓5ᵗʰ
fascia 017.9 ✓5ᵗʰ
fauces 012.8 ✓5ᵗʰ
finger 017.9 ✓5ᵗʰ
first infection 010.0 ✓5ᵗʰ
fistula, perirectal 014.8 ✓5ᵗʰ
Florida 011.6 ✓5ᵗʰ
foot 017.9 ✓5ᵗʰ
funnel pelvis 137.3
gallbladder 017.9 ✓5ᵗʰ
galloping (*see also* Tuberculosis, pulmonary)
  011.9 ✓5ᵗʰ
ganglionic 015.9 ✓5ᵗʰ
gastritis 017.9 ✓5ᵗʰ
gastrocolic fistula 014.8 ✓5ᵗʰ
gastroenteritis 014.8 ✓5ᵗʰ
gastrointestinal tract 014.8 ✓5ᵗʰ
general, generalized 018.9 ✓5ᵗʰ
  acute 018.0 ✓5ᵗʰ
  chronic 018.8 ✓5ᵗʰ
genital organs NEC 016.9 ✓5ᵗʰ
  female 016.7 ✓5ᵗʰ
  male 016.5 ✓5ᵗʰ
genitourinary NEC 016.9 ✓5ᵗʰ
genu 015.2 ✓5ᵗʰ
glandulae suprarenalis 017.6 ✓5ᵗʰ
glandular, general 017.2 ✓5ᵗʰ
glottis 012.3 ✓5ᵗʰ

✓4ᵗʰ Fourth-digit Required   ✓5ᵗʰ Fifth-digit Required   ▶◀ Revised Text   ● New Line   ▲ Revised Code

Tuberculosis, tubercular, tuberculous —
continued
grinders' 011.4 ✓5ᵗʰ
groin 017.2 ✓5ᵗʰ
gum 017.9 ✓5ᵗʰ
hand 017.9 ✓5ᵗʰ
heart 017.9 ✓5ᵗʰ [425.8]
hematogenous — *see* Tuberculosis, miliary
hemoptysis (*see also* Tuberculosis, pulmonary)
    011.9 ✓5ᵗʰ
hemorrhage NEC (*see also* Tuberculosis,
    pulmonary) 011.9 ✓5ᵗʰ
hemothorax 012.0 ✓5ᵗʰ
hepatitis 017.9 ✓5ᵗʰ
hilar lymph nodes 012.1 ✓5ᵗʰ
    primary, progressive 010.8 ✓5ᵗʰ
hip (disease) (joint) 015.1 ✓5ᵗʰ
    bone 015.1 ✓5ᵗʰ [730.85]
hydrocephalus 013.8 ✓5ᵗʰ
hydropneumothorax 012.0 ✓5ᵗʰ
hydrothorax 012.0 ✓5ᵗʰ
hypoadrenalism 017.6 ✓5ᵗʰ
hypopharynx 012.8 ✓5ᵗʰ
ileocecal (hyperplastic) 014.8 ✓5ᵗʰ
ileocolitis 014.8 ✓5ᵗʰ
ileum 014.8 ✓5ᵗʰ
iliac spine (superior) 015.0 ✓5ᵗʰ [730.88]
incipient NEC (*see also* Tuberculosis,
    pulmonary) 011.9 ✓5ᵗʰ
indurativa (primary) 017.1 ✓5ᵗʰ
infantile 010.0 ✓5ᵗʰ
infection NEC 011.9 ✓5ᵗʰ
    without clinical manifestation 010.0 ✓5ᵗʰ
infraclavicular gland 017.2 ✓5ᵗʰ
inguinal gland 017.2 ✓5ᵗʰ
inguinalis 017.2 ✓5ᵗʰ
intestine (any part) 014.8 ✓5ᵗʰ
iris 017.3 ✓5ᵗʰ [364.11]
iritis 017.3 ✓5ᵗʰ [364.11]
ischiorectal 014.8 ✓5ᵗʰ
jaw 015.7 ✓5ᵗʰ [730.88]
jejunum 014.8 ✓5ᵗʰ
joint 015.9 ✓5ᵗʰ
    hip 015.1 ✓5ᵗʰ
    knee 015.2 ✓5ᵗʰ
    specified site NEC 015.8 ✓5ᵗʰ
    vertebral 015.0 ✓5ᵗʰ [730.88]
keratitis 017.3 ✓5ᵗʰ [370.31]
    interstitial 017.3 ✓5ᵗʰ [370.59]
keratoconjunctivitis 017.3 ✓5ᵗʰ [370.31]
kidney 016.0 ✓5ᵗʰ
knee (joint) 015.2 ✓5ᵗʰ
kyphoscoliosis 015.0 ✓5ᵗʰ [737.43]
kyphosis 015.0 ✓5ᵗʰ [737.41]
lacrimal apparatus, gland 017.3 ✓5ᵗʰ
laryngitis 012.3 ✓5ᵗʰ
larynx 012.3 ✓5ᵗʰ
leptomeninges, leptomeningitis (cerebral)
    (spinal) 013.0 ✓5ᵗʰ
lichenoides (primary) 017.0 ✓5ᵗʰ
linguae 017.9 ✓5ᵗʰ
lip 017.9 ✓5ᵗʰ
liver 017.9 ✓5ᵗʰ
lordosis 015.0 ✓5ᵗʰ [737.42]
lung — *see* Tuberculosis, pulmonary
luposa 017.0 ✓5ᵗʰ
    eyelid 017.0 ✓5ᵗʰ [373.4]
lymphadenitis — *see* Tuberculosis, lymph
    gland
lymphangitis — *see* Tuberculosis, lymph gland
lymphatic (gland) (vessel) — *see* Tuberculosis,
    lymph gland
lymph gland or node (peripheral) 017.2 ✓5ᵗʰ
    abdomen 014.8 ✓5ᵗʰ
    bronchial 012.1 ✓5ᵗʰ
        primary, progressive 010.8 ✓5ᵗʰ
    cervical 017.2 ✓5ᵗʰ
    hilar 012.1 ✓5ᵗʰ
        primary, progressive 010.8 ✓5ᵗʰ
    intrathoracic 012.1 ✓5ᵗʰ
        primary, progressive 010.8 ✓5ᵗʰ
    mediastinal 012.1 ✓5ᵗʰ
        primary, progressive 010.8 ✓5ᵗʰ
    mesenteric 014.8 ✓5ᵗʰ
    peripheral 017.2 ✓5ᵗʰ
    retroperitoneal 014.8 ✓5ᵗʰ
    tracheobronchial 012.1 ✓5ᵗʰ
        primary, progressive 010.8 ✓5ᵗʰ

Tuberculosis, tubercular, tuberculous —
continued
malignant NEC (*see also* Tuberculosis,
    pulmonary) 011.9 ✓5ᵗʰ
mammary gland 017.9 ✓5ᵗʰ
marasmus NEC (*see also* Tuberculosis,
    pulmonary) 011.9 ✓5ᵗʰ
mastoiditis 015.6 ✓5ᵗʰ
maternal, affecting fetus or newborn 760.2
mediastinal (lymph) gland or node 012.1 ✓5ᵗʰ
    primary, progressive 010.8 ✓5ᵗʰ
mediastinitis 012.8 ✓5ᵗʰ
    primary, progressive 010.8 ✓5ᵗʰ
mediastinopericarditis 017.9 ✓5ᵗʰ [420.0]
mediastinum 012.8 ✓5ᵗʰ
    primary, progressive 010.8 ✓5ᵗʰ
medulla 013.9 ✓5ᵗʰ
    brain 013.2 ✓5ᵗʰ
    spinal cord 013.4 ✓5ᵗʰ
melanosis, Addisonian 017.6 ✓5ᵗʰ
membrane, brain 013.0 ✓5ᵗʰ
meninges (cerebral) (spinal) 013.0 ✓5ᵗʰ
meningitis (basilar) (brain) (cerebral)
    (cerebrospinal) (spinal) 013.0 ✓5ᵗʰ
meningoencephalitis 013.0 ✓5ᵗʰ
mesentery, mesenteric 014.8 ✓5ᵗʰ
    lymph gland or node 014.8 ✓5ᵗʰ
miliary (any site) 018.9 ✓5ᵗʰ
    acute 018.0 ✓5ᵗʰ
    chronic 018.8 ✓5ᵗʰ
    specified type NEC 018.8 ✓5ᵗʰ
millstone makers' 011.4 ✓5ᵗʰ
miners' 011.4 ✓5ᵗʰ
moulders' 011.4 ✓5ᵗʰ
mouth 017.9 ✓5ᵗʰ
multiple 018.9 ✓5ᵗʰ
    acute 018.0 ✓5ᵗʰ
    chronic 018.8 ✓5ᵗʰ
muscle 017.9 ✓5ᵗʰ
myelitis 013.6 ✓5ᵗʰ
myocarditis 017.9 ✓5ᵗʰ [422.0]
myocardium 017.9 ✓5ᵗʰ [422.0]
nasal (passage) (sinus) 012.8 ✓5ᵗʰ
nasopharynx 012.8 ✓5ᵗʰ
neck gland 017.2 ✓5ᵗʰ
nephritis 016.0 ✓5ᵗʰ [583.81] ✓5ᵗʰ
nerve 017.9 ✓5ᵗʰ
nose (septum) 012.8 ✓5ᵗʰ
ocular 017.3 ✓5ᵗʰ [377.39]
old NEC 137.0
    without residuals V12.01
omentum 014.8 ✓5ᵗʰ
oophoritis (acute) (chronic) 016.6 ✓5ᵗʰ
optic 017.3 ✓5ᵗʰ [377.39]
    nerve trunk 017.3 ✓5ᵗʰ [377.39]
    papilla, papillae 017.3 ✓5ᵗʰ [377.39]
orbit 017.3 ✓5ᵗʰ
orchitis 016.5 ✓5ᵗʰ [608.81]
organ, specified NEC 017.9 ✓5ᵗʰ
orificialis (primary) 017.0 ✓5ᵗʰ
osseous (*see also* Tuberculosis, bone)
    015.9 ✓5ᵗʰ [730.8] ✓5ᵗʰ
osteitis (*see also* Tuberculosis, bone)
    015.9 ✓5ᵗʰ [730.8] ✓5ᵗʰ
osteomyelitis (*see also* Tuberculosis, bone)
    015.9 ✓5ᵗʰ [730.8] ✓5ᵗʰ
otitis (media) 017.4 ✓5ᵗʰ
ovaritis (acute) (chronic) 016.6 ✓5ᵗʰ
ovary (acute) (chronic) 016.6 ✓5ᵗʰ
oviducts (acute) (chronic) 016.6 ✓5ᵗʰ
pachymeningitis 013.0 ✓5ᵗʰ
palate (soft) 017.9 ✓5ᵗʰ
pancreas 017.9 ✓5ᵗʰ
papulonecrotic (primary) 017.0 ✓5ᵗʰ
parathyroid glands 017.9 ✓5ᵗʰ
paronychia (primary) 017.0 ✓5ᵗʰ
parotid gland or region 017.9 ✓5ᵗʰ
pelvic organ NEC 016.9 ✓5ᵗʰ
    female 016.7 ✓5ᵗʰ
    male 016.5 ✓5ᵗʰ
pelvis (bony) 015.7 ✓5ᵗʰ [730.85]
penis 016.5 ✓5ᵗʰ
peribronchitis 011.3 ✓5ᵗʰ
pericarditis 017.9 ✓5ᵗʰ [420.0]
pericardium 017.9 ✓5ᵗʰ [420.0]
perichondritis, larynx 012.3 ✓5ᵗʰ
perineum 017.9 ✓5ᵗʰ

Tuberculosis, tubercular, tuberculous —
continued
periostitis (*see also* Tuberculosis, bone)
    015.9 ✓5ᵗʰ [730.8]
periphlebitis 017.9 ✓5ᵗʰ
    eye vessel 017.3 ✓5ᵗʰ [362.18]
    retina 017.3 ✓5ᵗʰ [362.18]
perirectal fistula 014.8 ✓5ᵗʰ
peritoneal gland 014.8 ✓5ᵗʰ
peritoneum 014.0 ✓5ᵗʰ
peritonitis 014.0 ✓5ᵗʰ
pernicious NEC (*see also* Tuberculosis,
    pulmonary) 011.9 ✓5ᵗʰ
pharyngitis 012.8 ✓5ᵗʰ
pharynx 012.8 ✓5ᵗʰ
phlyctenulosis (conjunctiva) 017.3 ✓5ᵗʰ [370.31]
phthisis NEC (*see also* Tuberculosis,
    pulmonary) 011.9 ✓5ᵗʰ
pituitary gland 017.9 ✓5ᵗʰ
placenta 016.7 ✓5ᵗʰ
pleura, pleural, pleurisy, pleuritis (fibrinous)
    (obliterative) (purulent) (simple plastic)
    (with effusion) 012.0 ✓5ᵗʰ
    primary, progressive 010.1 ✓5ᵗʰ
pneumonia, pneumonic 011.6 ✓5ᵗʰ
pneumothorax 011.7 ✓5ᵗʰ
polyserositis 018.9 ✓5ᵗʰ
    acute 018.0 ✓5ᵗʰ
    chronic 018.8 ✓5ᵗʰ
potters' 011.4 ✓5ᵗʰ
prepuce 016.5 ✓5ᵗʰ
primary 010.9 ✓5ᵗʰ
    complex 010.0 ✓5ᵗʰ
    complicated 010.8 ✓5ᵗʰ
        with pleurisy or effusion 010.1 ✓5ᵗʰ
    progressive 010.8 ✓5ᵗʰ
        with pleurisy or effusion 010.1 ✓5ᵗʰ
    skin 017.0 ✓5ᵗʰ
proctitis 014.8 ✓5ᵗʰ
prostate 016.5 ✓5ᵗʰ [601.4]
prostatitis 016.5 ✓5ᵗʰ [601.4]
pulmonaris (*see also* Tuberculosis, pulmonary)
    011.9 ✓5ᵗʰ
pulmonary (artery) (incipient) (malignant)
    (multiple round foci) (pernicious)
    (reinfection stage) 011.9 ✓5ᵗʰ
    cavitated or with cavitation 011.2 ✓5ᵗʰ
        primary, progressive 010.8 ✓5ᵗʰ
    childhood type or first infection 010.0 ✓5ᵗʰ
    chromogenic acid-fast bacilli 795.39   ▲
    fibrosis or fibrotic 011.4 ✓5ᵗʰ
    infiltrative 011.0 ✓5ᵗʰ
        primary, progressive 010.9 ✓5ᵗʰ
    nodular 011.1 ✓5ᵗʰ
    specified NEC 011.8 ✓5ᵗʰ
    sputum positive only 795.39   ▲
    status following surgical collapse of lung
        NEC 011.9 ✓5ᵗʰ
pyelitis 016.0 ✓5ᵗʰ [590.81]
pyelonephritis 016.0 ✓5ᵗʰ [590.81]
pyemia — *see* Tuberculosis, miliary
pyonephrosis 016.0 ✓5ᵗʰ
pyopneumothorax 012.0 ✓5ᵗʰ
pyothorax 012.0 ✓5ᵗʰ
rectum (with abscess) 014.8 ✓5ᵗʰ
    fistula 014.8 ✓5ᵗʰ
reinfection stage (*see also* Tuberculosis,
    pulmonary) 011.9 ✓5ᵗʰ
renal 016.0 ✓5ᵗʰ
renis 016.0 ✓5ᵗʰ
reproductive organ 016.7 ✓5ᵗʰ
respiratory NEC (*see also* Tuberculosis,
    pulmonary) 011.9 ✓5ᵗʰ
    specified site NEC 012.8 ✓5ᵗʰ
retina 017.3 ✓5ᵗʰ [363.13]
retroperitoneal (lymph gland or node) 014.8 ✓5ᵗʰ
    gland 014.8 ✓5ᵗʰ
retropharyngeal abscess 012.8 ✓5ᵗʰ
rheumatism 015.9 ✓5ᵗʰ
rhinitis 012.8 ✓5ᵗʰ
sacroiliac (joint) 015.8 ✓5ᵗʰ
sacrum 015.0 ✓5ᵗʰ [730.88]
salivary gland 017.9 ✓5ᵗʰ
salpingitis (acute) (chronic) 016.6 ✓5ᵗʰ
sandblasters' 011.4 ✓5ᵗʰ
sclera 017.3 ✓5ᵗʰ [379.09]
scoliosis 015.0 ✓5ᵗʰ [737.43]
scrofulous 017.2 ✓5ᵗʰ

✓4ᵗʰ Fourth-digit Required   ✓5ᵗʰ Fifth-digit Required   ▶◀ Revised Text   ● New Line   ▲ Revised Code

Tuberculosis, tubercular, tuberculous — *continued*
scrotum 016.5 ✓5ᵗʰ
seminal tract or vesicle 016.5 ✓5ᵗʰ *[608.81]*
senile NEC (*see also* Tuberculosis, pulmonary) 011.9 ✓5ᵗʰ
septic NEC (*see also* Tuberculosis, miliary) 018.9 ✓5ᵗʰ
shoulder 015.8 ✓5ᵗʰ
  blade 015.7 ✓5ᵗʰ *[730.8]* ✓5ᵗʰ
sigmoid 014.8 ✓5ᵗʰ
sinus (accessory) (nasal) 012.8 ✓5ᵗʰ
  bone 015.7 ✓5ᵗʰ *[730.88]*
  epididymis 016.4 ✓5ᵗʰ
skeletal NEC (*see also* Osteomyelitis, due to tuberculosis) 015.9 ✓5ᵗʰ *[730.8]* ✓5ᵗʰ
skin (any site) (primary) 017.0 ✓5ᵗʰ
small intestine 014.8 ✓5ᵗʰ
soft palate 017.9 ✓5ᵗʰ
spermatic cord 016.5 ✓5ᵗʰ
spinal
  column 015.0 ✓5ᵗʰ *[730.88]*
  cord 013.4 ✓5ᵗʰ
  disease 015.0 ✓5ᵗʰ *[730.88]*
  medulla 013.4 ✓5ᵗʰ
  membrane 013.0 ✓5ᵗʰ
  meninges 013.0 ✓5ᵗʰ
spine 015.0 ✓5ᵗʰ *[730.88]*
spleen 017.7 ✓5ᵗʰ
splenitis 017.7 ✓5ᵗʰ
spondylitis 015.0 ✓5ᵗʰ *[720.81]*
spontaneous pneumothorax — *see* Tuberculosis, pulmonary
sternoclavicular joint 015.8 ✓5ᵗʰ
stomach 017.9 ✓5ᵗʰ
stonemasons' 011.4 ✓5ᵗʰ
struma 017.2 ✓5ᵗʰ
subcutaneous tissue (cellular) (primary) 017.0 ✓5ᵗʰ
subcutis (primary) 017.0 ✓5ᵗʰ
subdeltoid bursa 017.9 ✓5ᵗʰ
submaxillary 017.9 ✓5ᵗʰ
  region 017.9 ✓5ᵗʰ
supraclavicular gland 017.2 ✓5ᵗʰ
suprarenal (capsule) (gland) 017.6 ✓5ᵗʰ
swelling, joint (*see also* Tuberculosis, joint) 015.9 ✓5ᵗʰ
symphysis pubis 015.7 ✓5ᵗʰ *[730.88]*
synovitis 015.9 ✓5ᵗʰ *[727.01]*
  hip 015.1 ✓5ᵗʰ *[727.01]*
  knee 015.2 ✓5ᵗʰ *[727.01]*
  specified site NEC 015.8 ✓5ᵗʰ *[727.01]*
  spine or vertebra 015.0 ✓5ᵗʰ *[727.01]*
systemic — *see* Tuberculosis, miliary
tarsitis (eyelid) 017.0 ✓5ᵗʰ *[373.4]*
  ankle (bone) 015.5 ✓5ᵗʰ *[730.87]*
tendon (sheath) — *see* Tuberculosis, tenosynovitis
tenosynovitis 015.9 ✓5ᵗʰ *[727.01]*
  hip 015.1 ✓5ᵗʰ *[727.01]*
  knee 015.2 ✓5ᵗʰ *[727.01]*
  specified site NEC 015.8 ✓5ᵗʰ *[727.01]*
  spine or vertebra 015.0 ✓5ᵗʰ *[727.01]*
testis 016.5 ✓5ᵗʰ *[608.81]*
throat 012.8 ✓5ᵗʰ
thymus gland 017.9 ✓5ᵗʰ
thyroid gland 017.5 ✓5ᵗʰ
toe 017.9 ✓5ᵗʰ
tongue 017.9 ✓5ᵗʰ
tonsil (lingual) 012.8 ✓5ᵗʰ
tonsillitis 012.8 ✓5ᵗʰ
trachea, tracheal 012.8 ✓5ᵗʰ
  gland 012.1 ✓5ᵗʰ
    primary, progressive 010.8 ✓5ᵗʰ
    isolated 012.2 ✓5ᵗʰ
tracheobronchial 011.3 ✓5ᵗʰ
  glandular 012.1 ✓5ᵗʰ
    primary, progressive 010.8 ✓5ᵗʰ
    isolated 012.2 ✓5ᵗʰ
  lymph gland or node 012.1 ✓5ᵗʰ
    primary, progressive 010.8 ✓5ᵗʰ
tubal 016.6 ✓5ᵗʰ
tunica vaginalis 016.5 ✓5ᵗʰ
typhlitis 014.8 ✓5ᵗʰ
ulcer (primary) (skin) 017.0 ✓5ᵗʰ
  bowel or intestine 014.8 ✓5ᵗʰ
  specified site NEC — *see* Tuberculosis, by site

Tuberculosis, tubercular, tuberculous — *continued*
unspecified site — *see* Tuberculosis, pulmonary
ureter 016.2 ✓5ᵗʰ
urethra, urethral 016.3 ✓5ᵗʰ
urinary organ or tract 016.3 ✓5ᵗʰ
  kidney 016.0 ✓5ᵗʰ
uterus 016.7 ✓5ᵗʰ
uveal tract 017.3 ✓5ᵗʰ *[363.13]*
uvula 017.9 ✓5ᵗʰ
vaccination, prophylactic (against) V03.2
vagina 016.7 ✓5ᵗʰ
vas deferens 016.5 ✓5ᵗʰ
vein 017.9 ✓5ᵗʰ
verruca (primary) 017.0 ✓5ᵗʰ
verrucosa (cutis) (primary) 017.0 ✓5ᵗʰ
vertebra (column) 015.0 ✓5ᵗʰ *[730.88]*
vesiculitis 016.5 ✓5ᵗʰ *[608.81]*
viscera NEC 014.8 ✓5ᵗʰ
vulva 016.7 ✓5ᵗʰ *[616.51]*
wrist (joint) 015.8 ✓5ᵗʰ
  bone 015.5 ✓5ᵗʰ *[730.83]*
Tuberculum
auriculae 744.29
occlusal 520.2
paramolare 520.2
Tuberous sclerosis (brain) 759.5
Tubo-ovarian — *see* condition
Tuboplasty, after previous sterilization V26.0
Tubotympanitis 381.10
Tularemia 021.9
  with
    conjunctivitis 021.3
    pneumonia 021.2
  bronchopneumonic 021.2
  conjunctivitis 021.3
  cryptogenic 021.1
  disseminated 021.8
  enteric 021.1
  generalized 021.8
  glandular 021.8
  intestinal 021.1
  oculoglandular 021.3
  ophthalmic 021.3
  pneumonia 021.2
  pulmonary 021.2
  specified NEC 021.8
  typhoidal 021.1
  ulceroglandular 021.0
  vaccination, prophylactic (against) V03.4
Tularensis conjunctivitis 021.3
Tumefaction — *see also* Swelling
  liver (*see also* Hypertrophy, liver) 789.1
Tumor (M8000/1) — *see also* Neoplasm, by site, unspecified nature
  Abrikossov's (M9580/0) — *see also* Neoplasm, connective tissue, benign
    malignant (M9580/3) — *see* Neoplasm, connective tissue, malignant
  acinar cell (M8550/1) — *see* Neoplasm, by site, uncertain behavior
  acinic cell (M8550/1) — *see* Neoplasm, by site, uncertain behavior
  adenomatoid (M9054/0) — *see also* Neoplasm, by site, benign
    odontogenic (M9300/0) 213.1
      upper jaw (bone) 213.0
  adnexal (skin) (M8390/0) — *see* Neoplasm, skin, benign
  adrenal
    cortical (benign) (M8370/0) 227.0
      malignant (M8370/3) 194.0
    rest (M8671/0) — *see* Neoplasm, by site, benign
  alpha cell (M8152/0)
    malignant (M8152/3)
      pancreas 157.4
      specified site NEC — *see* Neoplasm, by site, malignant
      unspecified site 157.4
    pancreas 211.7
    specified site NEC — *see* Neoplasm, by site, benign
    unspecified site 211.7
  aneurysmal (*see also* Aneurysm) 442.9

Tumor — *see also* Neoplasm, by site, unspecified nature — *continued*
  aortic body (M8691/1) 237.3
    malignant (M8691/3) 194.6
  argentaffin (M8241/1) — *see* Neoplasm, by site, uncertain behavior
  basal cell (M8090/1) — *see also* Neoplasm, skin, uncertain behavior
  benign (M8000/0) — *see* Neoplasm, by site, benign
  beta cell (M8151/0)
    malignant (M8151/3)
      pancreas 157.4
      specified site — *see* Neoplasm, by site, malignant
      unspecified site 157.4
    pancreas 211.7
    specified site NEC — *see* Neoplasm, by site, benign
    unspecified site 211.7
  blood — *see* Hematoma
  Brenner (M9000/0) 220
    borderline malignancy (M9000/1) 236.2
    malignant (M9000/3) 183.0
    proliferating (M9000/1) 236.2
  Brooke's (M8100/0) — *see* Neoplasm, skin, benign
  brown fat (M8880/0) — *see* Lipoma, by site
  Burkitt's (M9750/3) 200.2 ✓5ᵗʰ
  calcifying epithelial odontogenic (M9340/0) 213.1
    upper jaw (bone) 213.0
  carcinoid (M8240/1) — *see* Carcinoid
  carotid body (M8692/1) 237.3
    malignant (M8692/3) 194.5
  Castleman's (mediastinal lymph node hyperplasia) 785.6
  cells (M8001/1) — *see also* Neoplasm, by site, unspecified nature
    benign (M8001/0) — *see* Neoplasm, by site, benign
    malignant (M8001/3) — *see* Neoplasm, by site, malignant
    uncertain whether benign or malignant (M8001/1) — *see* Neoplasm, by site, uncertain nature
  cervix
    in pregnancy or childbirth 654.6 ✓5ᵗʰ
      affecting fetus or newborn 763.89
      causing obstructed labor 660.2 ✓5ᵗʰ
        affecting fetus or newborn 763.1
  chondromatous giant cell (M9230/0) — *see* Neoplasm, bone, benign
  chromaffin (M8700/0) — *see also* Neoplasm, by site, benign
    malignant (M8700/3) — *see* Neoplasm, by site, malignant
  Cock's peculiar 706.2
  Codman's (benign chondroblastoma) (M9230/0) — *see* Neoplasm, bone, benign
  dentigerous, mixed (M9282/0) 213.1
    upper jaw (bone) 213.0
  dermoid (M9084/0) — *see* Neoplasm, by site, benign
    with malignant transformation (M9084/3) 183.0
  desmoid (extra-abdominal) (M8821/1) — *see also* Neoplasm, connective tissue, uncertain behavior
    abdominal (M8822/1) — *see* Neoplasm, connective tissue, uncertain behavior
  embryonal (mixed) (M9080/1) — *see also* Neoplasm, by site, uncertain behavior
    liver (M9080/3) 155.0
  endodermal sinus (M9071/3)
    specified site — *see* Neoplasm, by site, malignant
    unspecified site
      female 183.0
      male 186.9
  epithelial
    benign (M8010/0) — *see* Neoplasm, by site, benign
    malignant (M8010/3) — *see* Neoplasm, by site, malignant
  Ewing's (M9260/3) — *see* Neoplasm, bone, malignant

Tuberculosis — Tumor

Tumor — *see also* Neoplasm, by site, unspecified
nature — *continued*
fatty — *see* Lipoma
fetal, causing disproportion 653.7 ✓5ᵗʰ
  causing obstructed labor 660.1 ✓5ᵗʰ
fibroid (M8890/0) — *see* Leiomyoma
G cell (M8153/1)
  malignant (M8153/3)
    pancreas 157.4
    specified site NEC — *see* Neoplasm, by site, malignant
    unspecified site 157.4
  specified site — *see* Neoplasm, by site, uncertain behavior
  unspecified site 235.5
giant cell (type) (M8003/1) — *see also* Neoplasm, by site, unspecified nature
  bone (M9250/1) 238.0
    malignant (M9250/3) — *see* Neoplasm, bone, malignant
    chondromatous (M9230/0) — *see* Neoplasm, bone, benign
  malignant (M8003/3) — *see* Neoplasm, by site, malignant
  peripheral (gingiva) 523.8
  soft parts (M9251/1) — *see also* Neoplasm, connective tissue, uncertain behavior
    malignant (M9251/3) — *see* Neoplasm, connective tissue, malignant
  tendon sheath 727.02
glomus (M8711/0) — *see also* Hemangioma, by site
  jugulare (M8690/1) 237.3
    malignant (M8690/3) 194.6
gonadal stromal (M8590/1) — *see* Neoplasm, by site, uncertain behavior
granular cell (M9580/0) — *see also* Neoplasm, connective tissue, benign
  malignant (M9580/3) — *see* Neoplasm, connective tissue, malignant
granulosa cell (M8620/1) 236.2
  malignant (M8620/3) 183.0
granulosa cell-theca cell (M8621/1) 236.2
  malignant (M8621/3) 183.0
Grawitz's (hypernephroma) (M8312/3) 189.0
hazard-crile (M8350/3) 193
hemorrhoidal — *see* Hemorrhoids
hilar cell (M8660/0) 220
Hürthle cell (benign) (M8290/0) 226
  malignant (M8290/3) 193
hydatid (*see also* Echinococcus) 122.9
hypernephroid (M8311/1) — *see also* Neoplasm, by site, uncertain behavior
interstitial cell (M8650/1) — *see also* Neoplasm, by site, uncertain behavior
  benign (M8650/0) — *see* Neoplasm, by site, benign
  malignant (M8650/3) — *see* Neoplasm, by site, malignant
islet cell (M8150/0)
  malignant (M8150/3)
    pancreas 157.4
    specified site — *see* Neoplasm, by site, malignant
    unspecified site 157.4
  pancreas 211.7
  specified site NEC — *see* Neoplasm, by site, benign
  unspecified site 211.7
juxtaglomerular (M8361/1) 236.91
Krukenberg's (M8490/6) 198.6
Leydig cell (M8650/1)
  benign (M8650/0)
    specified site — *see* Neoplasm, by site, benign
    unspecified site
      female 220
      male 222.0
  malignant (M8650/3)
    specified site — *see* Neoplasm, by site, malignant
    unspecified site
      female 183.0
      male 186.9
  specified site — *see* Neoplasm, by site, uncertain behavior

Tumor — *see also* Neoplasm, by site, unspecified
nature — *continued*
Leydig cell — *continued*
  unspecified site
    female 236.2
    male 236.4
lipid cell, ovary (M8670/0) 220
lipoid cell, ovary (M8670/0) 220
lymphomatous, benign (M9590/0) — *see also* Neoplasm, by site, benign
Malherbe's (M8110/0) — *see* Neoplasm, skin, benign
malignant (M8000/3) — *see also* Neoplasm, by site, malignant
  fusiform cell (type) (M8004/3) — *see* Neoplasm, by site, malignant
  giant cell (type) (M8003/3) — *see* Neoplasm, by site, malignant
  mixed NEC (M8940/3) — *see* Neoplasm, by site, malignant
  small cell (type) (M8002/3) — *see* Neoplasm, by site, malignant
  spindle cell (type) (M8004/3) — *see* Neoplasm, by site, malignant
mast cell (M9740/1) 238.5
  malignant (M9740/3) 202.6 ✓5ᵗʰ
melanotic, neuroectodermal (M9363/0) — *see* Neoplasm, by site, benign
Merkel cell — *see* Neoplasm, by site, malignant
mesenchymal
  malignant (M8800/3) — *see* Neoplasm, connective tissue, malignant
  mixed (M8990/1) — *see* Neoplasm, connective tissue, uncertain behavior
mesodermal, mixed (M8951/3) — *see also* Neoplasm, by site, malignant
  liver 155.0
mesonephric (M9110/1) — *see also* Neoplasm, by site, uncertain behavior
  malignant (M9110/3) — *see* Neoplasm, by site, malignant
metastatic
  from specified site (M8000/3) — *see* Neoplasm, by site, malignant
  to specified site (M8000/6) — *see* Neoplasm, by site, malignant, secondary
mixed NEC (M8940/0) — *see also* Neoplasm, by site, benign
  malignant (M8940/3) — *see* Neoplasm, by site, malignant
mucocarcinoid, malignant (M8243/3) — *see* Neoplasm, by site, malignant
mucoepidermoid (M8430/1) — *see* Neoplasm, by site, uncertain behavior
Mullerian, mixed (M8950/3) — *see* Neoplasm, by site, malignant
myoepithelial (M8982/0) — *see* Neoplasm, by site, benign
neurogenic olfactory (M9520/3) 160.0
nonencapsulated sclerosing (M8350/3) 193
odontogenic (M9270/1) 238.0
  adenomatoid (M9300/0) 213.1
    upper jaw (bone) 213.0
  benign (M9270/0) 213.1
    upper jaw (bone) 213.0
  calcifying epithelial (M9340/0) 213.1
    upper jaw (bone) 213.0
  malignant (M9270/3) 170.1
    upper jaw (bone) 170.0
  squamous (M9312/0) 213.1
    upper jaw (bone) 213.0
ovarian stromal (M8590/1) 236.2
ovary
  in pregnancy or childbirth 654.4 ✓5ᵗʰ
    affecting fetus or newborn 763.89
    causing obstructed labor 660.2 ✓5ᵗʰ
      affecting fetus or newborn 763.1
pacinian (M9507/0) — *see* Neoplasm, skin, benign
Pancoast's (M8010/3) 162.3
papillary — *see* Papilloma
pelvic, in pregnancy or childbirth 654.9 ✓5ᵗʰ
  affecting fetus or newborn 763.89
  causing obstructed labor 660.2 ✓5ᵗʰ
    affecting fetus or newborn 763.1
phantom 300.11

Tumor — *see also* Neoplasm, by site, unspecified
nature — *continued*
plasma cell (M9731/1) 238.6
  benign (M9731/0) — *see* Neoplasm, by site, benign
  malignant (M9731/3) 203.8 ✓5ᵗʰ
polyvesicular vitelline (M9071/3)
  specified site — *see* Neoplasm, by site, malignant
  unspecified site
    female 183.0
    male 186.9
Pott's puffy (*see also* Osteomyelitis) 730.2 ✓5ᵗʰ
Rathke's pouch (M9350/1) 237.0
regaud's (M8082/3) — *see* Neoplasm, nasopharynx, malignant
rete cell (M8140/0) 222.0
retinal anlage (M9363/0) — *see* Neoplasm, by site, benign
Rokitansky's 620.2
salivary gland type, mixed (M8940/0) — *see also* Neoplasm, by site, benign
  malignant (M8940/3) — *see* Neoplasm, by site, malignant
Sampson's 617.1
Schloffer's (*see also* Peritonitis) 567.2
Schmincke (M8082/3) — *see* Neoplasm, nasopharynx, malignant
sebaceous (*see also* Cyst, sebaceous) 706.2
secondary (M8000/6) — *see* Neoplasm, by site, secondary
Sertoli cell (M8640/0)
  with lipid storage (M8641/0)
    specified site — *see* Neoplasm, by site, benign
    unspecified site
      female 220
      male 222.0
  specified site — *see* Neoplasm, by site, benign
  unspecified site
    female 220
    male 222.0
Sertoli-Leydig cell (M8631/0)
  specified site, — *see* Neoplasm, by site, benign
  unspecified site
    female 220
    male 222.0
sex cord (-stromal) (M8590/1) — *see* Neoplasm, by site, uncertain behavior
skin appendage (M8390/0) — *see* Neoplasm, skin, benign
soft tissue
  benign (M8800/0) — *see* Neoplasm, connective tissue, benign
  malignant (M8800/3) — *see* Neoplasm, connective tissue, malignant
sternomastoid 754.1
superior sulcus (lung) (pulmonary) (syndrome) (M8010/3) 162.3
suprasulcus (M8010/3) 162.3
sweat gland (M8400/1) — *see also* Neoplasm, skin, uncertain behavior
  benign (M8400/0) — *see* Neoplasm, skin, benign
  malignant (M8400/3) — *see* Neoplasm, skin, malignant
syphilitic brain 094.89
  congenital 090.49
testicular stromal (M8590/1) 236.4
theca cell (M8600/0) 220
theca cell-granulosa cell (M8621/1) 236.2
theca-lutein (M8610/0) 220
turban (M8200/0) 216.4
uterus
  in pregnancy or childbirth 654.1 ✓5ᵗʰ
    affecting fetus or newborn 763.89
    causing obstructed labor 660.2 ✓5ᵗʰ
      affecting fetus or newborn 763.1
vagina
  in pregnancy or childbirth 654.7 ✓5ᵗʰ
    affecting fetus or newborn 763.89
    causing obstructed labor 660.2 ✓5ᵗʰ
      affecting fetus or newborn 763.1
varicose (*see also* Varicose, vein) 454.9
von Recklinghausen's (M9540/1) 237.71

✓4ᵗʰ Fourth-digit Required   ✓5ᵗʰ Fifth-digit Required   ►◄ Revised Text   ● New Line   ▲ Revised Code

Tumor — *see also* Neoplasm, by site, unspecified nature — *continued*
- vulva
  - in pregnancy or childbirth 654.8 ✓5ᵗʰ
    - affecting fetus or newborn 763.89
    - causing obstructed labor 660.2 ✓5ᵗʰ
      - affecting fetus or newborn 763.1
- Warthin's (salivary gland) (M8561/0) 210.2
- white — *see also* Tuberculosis, arthritis
- White-Darier 757.39
- Wilms' (nephroblastoma) (M8960/3) 189.0
- yolk sac (M9071/3)
  - specified site — *see* Neoplasm, by site, malignant
  - unspecified site
    - female 183.0
    - male 186.9

Tumorlet (M8040/1) — *see* Neoplasm, by site, uncertain behavior

Tungiasis 134.1

Tunica vasculosa lentis 743.39

Tunnel vision 368.45

Turban tumor (M8200/0) 216.4

Türck's trachoma (chronic catarrhal laryngitis) 476.0

Türk's syndrome (ocular retraction syndrome) 378.71

Turner's
- hypoplasia (tooth) 520.4
- syndrome 758.6
- tooth 520.4

Turner-Kieser syndrome (hereditary osteo-onychodysplasia) 756.89

Turner-Varny syndrome 758.6

Turricephaly 756.0

Tussis convulsiva (*see also* Whooping cough) 033.9

Twin
- affected by maternal complications of pregnancy 761.5
- conjoined 759.4
- healthy liveborn — *see* Newborn, twin
- pregnancy (complicating delivery) NEC 651.0 ✓5ᵗʰ
  - with fetal loss and retention of one fetus 651.3 ✓5ᵗʰ

Twinning, teeth 520.2

Twist, twisted
- bowel, colon, or intestine 560.2
- hair (congenital) 757.4
- mesentery 560.2
- omentum 560.2
- organ or site, congenital NEC — *see* Anomaly, specified type NEC
- ovarian pedicle 620.5
  - congenital 752.0
- umbilical cord — *see* Compression, umbilical cord

Twitch 781.0

Tylosis 700
- buccalis 528.6
- gingiva 523.8
- linguae 528.6
- palmaris et plantaris 757.39

Tympanism 787.3

Tympanites (abdominal) (intestine) 787.3

Tympanitis — *see* Myringitis

Tympanosclerosis 385.00
- involving
  - combined sites NEC 385.09
    - with tympanic membrane 385.03
  - tympanic membrane 385.01
    - with ossicles 385.02
      - and middle ear 385.03

Tympanum — *see* condition

Tympany
- abdomen 787.3
- chest 786.7

Typhlitis (*see also* Appendicitis) 541

Typhoenteritis 002.0

Typhogastric fever 002.0

Typhoid (abortive) (ambulant) (any site) (fever) (hemorrhagic) (infection) (intermittent) (malignant) (rheumatic) 002.0
- with pneumonia 002.0 [484.8]
- abdominal 002.0
- carrier (suspected) of V02.1
- cholecystitis (current) 002.0
- clinical (Widal and blood test negative) 002.0
- endocarditis 002.0 [421.1]
- inoculation reaction — *see* Complications, vaccination
- meningitis 002.0 [320.7]
- mesenteric lymph nodes 002.0
- myocarditis 002.0 [422.0]
- osteomyelitis (*see also* Osteomyelitis, due to, typhoid) 002.0 [730.8] ✓5ᵗʰ
- perichondritis, larynx 002.0 [478.71]
- pneumonia 002.0 [484.8]
- spine 002.0 [720.81]
- ulcer (perforating) 002.0
- vaccination, prophylactic (against) V03.1
- Widal negative 002.0

Typhomalaria (fever) (*see also* Malaria) 084.6

Typhomania 002.0

Typhoperitonitis 002.0

Typhus (fever) 081.9
- abdominal, abdominalis 002.0
- African tick 082.1
- amarillic (*see also* Fever, Yellow) 060.9
- brain 081.9
- cerebral 081.9
- classical 080
- endemic (flea-borne) 081.0
- epidemic (louse-borne) 080
- exanthematic NEC 080
- exanthematicus SAI 080
  - brillii SAI 081.1
  - Mexicanus SAI 081.0
  - pediculo vestimenti causa 080
  - typhus murinus 081.0
- flea-borne 081.0
- Indian tick 082.1
- Kenya tick 082.1
- louse-borne 080
- Mexican 081.0
  - flea-borne 081.0
  - louse-borne 080
  - tabardillo 080
- mite-borne 081.2
- murine 081.0
- North Asian tick-borne 082.2
- petechial 081.9
- Queensland tick 082.3
- rat 081.0
- recrudescent 081.1
- recurrent (*see also* Fever, relapsing) 087.9
- São Paulo 082.0
- scrub (China) (India) (Malaya) (New Guinea) 081.2
- shop (of Malaya) 081.0
- Siberian tick 082.2
- tick-borne NEC 082.9
- tropical 081.2
- vaccination, prophylactic (against) V05.8

Tyrosinemia 270.2
- neonatal 775.8

Tyrosinosis (Medes) (Sakai) 270.2

Tyrosinuria 270.2

Tyrosyluria 270.2

U

Uehlinger's syndrome (acropachyderma) 757.39

Uhl's anomaly or disease (hypoplasia of myocardium, right ventricle) 746.84

Ulcer, ulcerated, ulcerating, ulceration, ulcerative 707.9
- with gangrene 707.9 [785.4]
- abdomen (wall) (*see also* Ulcer, skin) 707.8
- ala, nose 478.1
- alveolar process 526.5
- amebic (intestine) 006.9
  - skin 006.6
- anastomotic — *see* Ulcer, gastrojejunal
- anorectal 569.41

Ulcer, ulcerated, ulcerating, ulceration, ulcerative — *continued*
- antral — *see* Ulcer, stomach
- anus (sphincter) (solitary) 569.41
  - varicose — *see* Varicose, ulcer, anus
- aphthous (oral) (recurrent) 528.2
  - genital organ(s)
    - female 616.8
    - male 608.89
  - mouth 528.2
- arm (*see also* Ulcer, skin) 707.8
- arteriosclerotic plaque — *see* Arteriosclerosis, by site
- artery NEC 447.2
  - without rupture 447.8
- atrophic NEC — *see* Ulcer, skin
- Barrett's (chronic peptic ulcer of esophagus) 530.2
- bile duct 576.8
- bladder (solitary) (sphincter) 596.8
  - bilharzial (*see also* Schistosomiasis) 120.9 [595.4]
  - submucosal (*see also* Cystitis) 595.1
  - tuberculous (*see also* Tuberculosis) 016.1 ✓5ᵗʰ
- bleeding NEC — *see* Ulcer, peptic, with hemorrhage
- bone 730.9 ✓5ᵗʰ
- bowel (*see also* Ulcer, intestine) 569.82
- breast 611.0
- bronchitis 491.8
- bronchus 519.1
- buccal (cavity) (traumatic) 528.9
- burn (acute) — *see* Ulcer, duodenum
- Buruli 031.1
- buttock (*see also* Ulcer, skin) 707.8
  - decubitus (*see also* Ulcer, decubitus) 707.0
- cancerous (M8000/3) — *see* Neoplasm, by site, malignant
- cardia — *see* Ulcer, stomach
- cardio-esophageal (peptic) 530.2
- cecum (*see also* Ulcer, intestine) 569.82
- cervix (uteri) (trophic) 622.0
  - with mention of cervicitis 616.0
- chancroidal 099.0
- chest (wall) (*see also* Ulcer, skin) 707.8
- Chiclero 085.4
- chin (pyogenic) (*see also* Ulcer, skin) 707.8
- chronic (cause unknown) — *see also* Ulcer, skin
  - penis 607.89
- Cochin-China 085.1
- colitis — *see* Colitis, ulcerative
- colon (*see also* Ulcer, intestine) 569.82
- conjunctiva (acute) (postinfectional) 372.00
- cornea (infectional) 370.00
  - with perforation 370.06
  - annular 370.02
  - catarrhal 370.01
  - central 370.03
  - dendritic 054.42
  - marginal 370.01
  - mycotic 370.05
  - phlyctenular, tuberculous (*see also* Tuberculosis) 017.3 ✓5ᵗʰ [370.31]
  - ring 370.02
  - rodent 370.07
  - serpent, serpiginous 370.04
  - superficial marginal 370.01
  - tuberculous (*see also* Tuberculosis) 017.3 ✓5ᵗʰ [370.31]
- corpus cavernosum (chronic) 607.89
- crural — *see* Ulcer, lower extremity
- Curling's — *see* Ulcer, duodenum
- Cushing's — *see* Ulcer, peptic
- cystitis (interstitial) 595.1
- decubitus (any site) 707.0
  - with gangrene 707.0 [785.4]
- dendritic 054.42
- diabetes, diabetic (mellitus) 250.8 ✓5ᵗʰ [707.9]
  - lower limb 250.8 ✓5ᵗʰ [707.10]
    - ankle 250.8 ✓5ᵗʰ [707.13]
    - calf 250.8 ✓5ᵗʰ [707.12]
    - foot 250.8 ✓5ᵗʰ [707.15]
    - heel 250.8 ✓5ᵗʰ [707.14]
    - knee 250.8 ✓5ᵗʰ [707.19]
    - specified site NEC 250.8 ✓5ᵗʰ [707.19]

Ulcer — Ulcer

Ulcer, ulcerated, ulcerating, ulceration, ulcerative — *continued*
- diabetes, diabetic — *continued*
  - lower limb — *continued*
    - thigh 250.8 ✓5 [707.11]
    - toes 250.8 ✓5 [707.15]
    - specified site NEC 250.8 ✓5 [707.8]
- Dieulafoy — *see* ▶Lesion, Dieulafoy◀
- due to
  - infection NEC — *see* Ulcer, skin
  - radiation, radium — *see* Ulcer, by site
  - trophic disturbance (any region) — *see* Ulcer, skin
  - x-ray — *see* Ulcer, by site
- duodenum, duodenal (eroded) (peptic) 532.9 ✓5

> *Note — Use the following fifth-digit subclassification with categories 531-534:*
> 0 *without mention of obstruction*
> 1 *with obstruction*

  - with
    - hemorrhage (chronic) 532.4 ✓5
      - and perforation 532.6 ✓5
    - perforation (chronic) 532.5 ✓5
      - and hemorrhage 532.6 ✓5
    - acute 532.3 ✓5
      - with
        - hemorrhage 532.0 ✓5
          - and perforation 532.2 ✓5
        - perforation 532.1 ✓5
          - and hemorrhage 532.2 ✓5
    - bleeding (recurrent) — *see* Ulcer, duodenum, with hemorrhage
    - chronic 532.7 ✓5
      - with
        - hemorrhage 532.4 ✓5
          - and perforation 532.6 ✓5
        - perforation 532.5 ✓5
          - and hemorrhage 532.6 ✓5
    - penetrating — *see* Ulcer, duodenum, with perforation
    - perforating — *see* Ulcer, duodenum, with perforation
- dysenteric NEC 009.0
- elusive 595.1
- endocarditis (any valve) (acute) (chronic) (subacute) 421.0
- enteritis — *see* Colitis, ulcerative
- enterocolitis 556.0
- epiglottis 478.79
- esophagus (peptic) 530.2
  - due to ingestion
    - aspirin 530.2
    - chemicals 530.2
    - medicinal agents 530.2
  - fungal 530.2
  - infectional 530.2
  - varicose (*see also* Varix, esophagus) 456.1
    - bleeding (*see also* Varix, esophagus, bleeding) 456.0
- eye NEC 360.00
  - dendritic 054.42
- eyelid (region) 373.01
- face (*see also* Ulcer, skin) 707.8
- fauces 478.29
- Fenwick (-Hunner) (solitary) (*see also* Cystitis) 595.1
- fistulous NEC — *see* Ulcer, skin
- foot (indolent) (*see also* Ulcer, lower extremity) 707.15
  - perforating 707.15
    - leprous 030.1
    - syphilitic 094.0
  - trophic 707.15
  - varicose 454.0
    - inflamed or infected 454.2
- frambesial, initial or primary 102.0
- gallbladder or duct 575.8
- gall duct 576.8
- gangrenous (*see also* Gangrene) 785.4
- gastric — *see* Ulcer, stomach
- gastrocolic — *see* Ulcer, gastrojejunal
- gastroduodenal — *see* Ulcer, peptic
- gastroesophageal — *see* Ulcer, stomach
- gastrohepatic — *see* Ulcer, stomach

Ulcer, ulcerated, ulcerating, ulceration, ulcerative — *continued*
- gastrointestinal — *see* Ulcer, gastrojejunal
- gastrojejunal (eroded) (peptic) 534.9

> *Note — Use the following fifth-digit subclassification with categories 531-534:*
> 0 *without mention of obstruction*
> 1 *with obstruction*

  - with
    - hemorrhage (chronic) 534.4 ✓5
      - and perforation 534.6 ✓5
    - perforation 534.5 ✓5
      - and hemorrhage 534.6 ✓5
    - acute 534.3 ✓5
      - with
        - hemorrhage 534.0 ✓5
          - and perforation 534.2 ✓5
        - perforation 534.1 ✓5
          - and hemorrhage 534.2 ✓5
    - bleeding (recurrent) — *see* Ulcer, gastrojejunal, with hemorrhage
    - chronic 534.7 ✓5
      - with
        - hemorrhage 534.4 ✓5
          - and perforation 534.6 ✓5
        - perforation 534.5 ✓5
          - and hemorrhage 534.6 ✓5
    - penetrating — *see* Ulcer, gastrojejunal, with perforation
    - perforating — *see* Ulcer, gastrojejunal, with perforation
- gastrojejunocolic — *see* Ulcer, gastrojejunal
- genital organ
  - female 629.8
  - male 608.89
- gingiva 523.8
- gingivitis 523.1
- glottis 478.79
- granuloma of pudenda 099.2
- groin (*see also* Ulcer, skin) 707.8
- gum 523.8
- gumma, due to yaws 102.4
- hand (*see also* Ulcer, skin) 707.8
- hard palate 528.9
- heel (*see also* Ulcer, lower extremity) 707.14
  - decubitus (*see also* Ulcer, decubitus) 707.0
- hemorrhoids 455.8
  - external 455.5
  - internal 455.2
- hip (*see also* Ulcer, skin) 707.8
  - decubitus (*see also* Ulcer, decubitus) 707.0
- Hunner's 595.1
- hypopharynx 478.29
- hypopyon (chronic) (subacute) 370.04
- hypostaticum — *see* Ulcer, varicose
- ileocolitis 556.1
- ileum (*see also* Ulcer, intestine) 569.82
- intestine, intestinal 569.82
  - with perforation 569.83
  - amebic 006.9
  - duodenal — *see* Ulcer, duodenum
  - granulocytopenic (with hemorrhage) 288.0
  - marginal 569.82
  - perforating 569.83
  - small, primary 569.82
  - stercoraceous 569.82
  - stercoral 569.82
  - tuberculous (*see also* Tuberculosis) 014.8 ✓5
  - typhoid (fever) 002.0
  - varicose 456.8
- ischemic 707.9
  - lower extremity (*see also* Ulcer, lower extremity) 707.10
    - ankle 707.13
    - calf 707.12
    - foot 707.15
    - heel 707.14
    - knee 707.19
    - specified site NEC 707.19
    - thigh 707.11
    - toes 707.15
- jejunum, jejunal — *see* Ulcer, gastrojejunal
- keratitis (*see also* Ulcer, cornea) 370.00
- knee — *see* Ulcer, lower extremity

Ulcer, ulcerated, ulcerating, ulceration, ulcerative — *continued*
- labium (majus) (minus) 616.50
- laryngitis (*see also* Laryngitis) 464.00
  - with obstruction 464.01
- larynx (aphthous) (contact) 478.79
  - diphtheritic 032.3
- leg — *see* Ulcer, lower extremity
- lip 528.5
- Lipschütz's 616.50
- lower extremity (atrophic) (chronic) (neurogenic) (perforating) (pyogenic) (trophic) (tropical) 707.10
  - with gangrene (*see also* Ulcer, lower extremity) 707.10 [785.4]
    - arteriosclerotic 440.24
  - ankle 707.13
  - arteriosclerotic 440.23
    - with gangrene 440.24
  - calf 707.12
  - decubitus 707.0
    - with gangrene 707.0 [785.4]
  - foot 707.15
  - heel 707.14
  - knee 707.19
  - specified site NEC 707.19
  - thigh 707.11
  - toes 707.15
  - varicose 454.0
    - inflamed or infected 454.2
- luetic — *see* Ulcer, syphilitic
- lung 518.89
  - tuberculous (*see also* Tuberculosis) 011.2 ✓5
- malignant (M8000/3) — *see* Neoplasm, by site, malignant
- marginal NEC — *see* Ulcer, gastrojejunal
- meatus (urinarius) 597.89
- Meckel's diverticulum 751.0
- Meleney's (chronic undermining) 686.09
- Mooren's (cornea) 370.07
- mouth (traumatic) 528.9
- mycobacterial (skin) 031.1
- nasopharynx 478.29
- navel cord (newborn) 771.4
- neck (*see also* Ulcer, skin) 707.8
  - uterus 622.0
- neurogenic NEC — *see* Ulcer, skin
- nose, nasal (infectional) (passage) 478.1
  - septum 478.1
    - varicose 456.8
  - skin — *see* Ulcer, skin
  - spirochetal NEC 104.8
- oral mucosa (traumatic) 528.9
- palate (soft) 528.9
- penetrating NEC — *see* Ulcer, peptic, with perforation
- penis (chronic) 607.89
- peptic (site unspecified) 533.9

> *Note — Use the following fifth-digit subclassification with categories 531-534:*
> 0 *without mention of obstruction*
> 1 *with obstruction*

  - with
    - hemorrhage 533.4 ✓5
      - and perforation 533.6 ✓5
    - perforation (chronic) 533.5 ✓5
      - and hemorrhage 533.6 ✓5
    - acute 533.3 ✓5
      - with
        - hemorrhage 533.0 ✓5
          - and perforation 533.2 ✓5
        - perforation 533.1 ✓5
          - and hemorrhage 533.2 ✓5
    - bleeding (recurrent) — *see* Ulcer, peptic, with hemorrhage
    - chronic 533.7 ✓5
      - with
        - hemorrhage 533.4 ✓5
          - and perforation 533.6 ✓5
        - perforation 533.5 ✓5
          - and hemorrhage 533.6 ✓5
    - penetrating — *see* Ulcer, peptic, with perforation

✓4 Fourth-digit Required   ✓5 Fifth-digit Required   ▶◀ Revised Text   ● New Line   ▲ Revised Code

Ulcer, ulcerated, ulcerating, ulceration, ulcerative — *continued*
 perforating NEC (*see also* Ulcer, peptic, with perforation) 533.5 ✓5ᵗʰ
  skin 707.9
 perineum (*see also* Ulcer, skin) 707.8
 peritonsillar 474.8
 phagedenic (tropical) NEC — *see* Ulcer, skin
 pharynx 478.29
 phlebitis — *see* Phlebitis
 plaster (*see also* Ulcer, decubitus) 707.0
 popliteal space — *see* Ulcer, lower extremity
 postpyloric — *see* Ulcer, duodenum
 prepuce 607.89
 prepyloric — *see* Ulcer, stomach
 pressure (*see also* Ulcer, decubitus) 707.0
 primary of intestine 569.82
  with perforation 569.83
 proctitis 556.2
  with ulcerative sigmoiditis 556.3
 prostate 601.8
 pseudopeptic — *see* Ulcer, peptic
 pyloric — *see* Ulcer, stomach
 rectosigmoid 569.82
  with perforation 569.83
 rectum (sphincter) (solitary) 569.41
  stercoraceous, stercoral 569.41
  varicose — *see* Varicose, ulcer, anus
 retina (*see also* Chorioretinitis) 363.20
 rodent (M8090/3) — *see also* Neoplasm, skin, malignant
  cornea 370.07
 round — *see* Ulcer, stomach
 sacrum (region) (*see also* Ulcer, skin) 707.8
 Saemisch's 370.04
 scalp (*see also* Ulcer, skin) 707.8
 sclera 379.09
 scrofulous (*see also* Tuberculosis) 017.2 ✓5ᵗʰ
 scrotum 608.89
  tuberculous (*see also* Tuberculosis) 016.5 ✓5ᵗʰ
  varicose 456.4
 seminal vesicle 608.89
 sigmoid 569.82
  with perforation 569.83
 skin (atrophic) (chronic) (neurogenic) (non-healing) (perforating) (pyogenic) (trophic) 707.9
  with gangrene 707.9 [785.4]
  amebic 006.6
  decubitus 707.0
   with gangrene 707.0 [785.4]
  in granulocytopenia 288.0
  lower extremity (*see also* Ulcer, lower extremity) 707.10
   with gangrene 707.10 [785.4]
    arteriosclerotic 440.24
   ankle 707.13
   arteriosclerotic 440.23
    with gangrene 440.24
   calf 707.12
   foot 707.15
   heel 707.14
   knee 707.19
   specified site NEC 707.19
   thigh 707.11
   toes 707.15
  mycobacterial 031.1
  syphilitic (early) (secondary) 091.3
  tuberculous (primary) (*see also* Tuberculosis) 017.0 ✓5ᵗʰ
  varicose — *see* Ulcer, varicose
 sloughing NEC — *see* Ulcer, skin
 soft palate 528.9
 solitary, anus or rectum (sphincter) 569.41
 sore throat 462
  streptococcal 034.0
 spermatic cord 608.89
 spine (tuberculous) 015.0 ✓5ᵗʰ [730.88]
 stasis (leg) (venous) 454.0
  inflamed or infected 454.2
  without varicose veins 459.81
 stercoral, stercoraceous 569.82
  with perforation 569.83
  anus or rectum 569.41
 stoma, stomal — *see* Ulcer, gastrojejunal

Ulcer, ulcerated, ulcerating, ulceration, ulcerative — *continued*
 stomach (eroded) (peptic) (round) 531.9

> Note — Use the following fifth-digit subclassification with categories 531-534:
>
> 0   without mention of obstruction
> 1   with obstruction

  with
   hemorrhage 531.4 ✓5ᵗʰ
    and perforation 531.6 ✓5ᵗʰ
   perforation (chronic) 531.5 ✓5ᵗʰ
    and hemorrhage 531.6 ✓5ᵗʰ
  acute 531.3 ✓5ᵗʰ
   with
    hemorrhage 531.0 ✓5ᵗʰ
     and perforation 531.2 ✓5ᵗʰ
    perforation 531.1 ✓5ᵗʰ
     and hemorrhage 531.2 ✓5ᵗʰ
  bleeding (recurrent) — *see* Ulcer, stomach, with hemorrhage
  chronic 531.7 ✓5ᵗʰ
   with
    hemorrhage 531.4 ✓5ᵗʰ
     and perforation 531.6 ✓5ᵗʰ
    perforation 531.5 ✓5ᵗʰ
     and hemorrhage 531.6 ✓5ᵗʰ
  penetrating — *see* Ulcer, stomach, with perforation
  perforating — *see* Ulcer, stomach, with perforation
 stomatitis 528.0
 stress — *see* Ulcer, peptic
 strumous (tuberculous) (*see also* Tuberculosis) 017.2 ✓5ᵗʰ
 submental (*see also* Ulcer, skin) 707.8
 submucosal, bladder 595.1
 syphilitic (any site) (early) (secondary) 091.3
  late 095.9
  perforating 095.9
   foot 094.0
 testis 608.89
 thigh — *see* Ulcer, lower extremity
 throat 478.29
  diphtheritic 032.0
 toe — *see* Ulcer, lower extremity
 tongue (traumatic) 529.0
 tonsil 474.8
  diphtheritic 032.0
 trachea 519.1
 trophic — *see* Ulcer, skin
 tropical NEC (*see also* Ulcer, skin) 707.9
 tuberculous — *see* Tuberculosis, ulcer
 tunica vaginalis 608.89
 turbinate 730.9 ✓5ᵗʰ
 typhoid (fever) 002.0
  perforating 002.0
 umbilicus (newborn) 771.4
 unspecified site NEC — *see* Ulcer, skin
 urethra (meatus) (*see also* Urethritis) 597.89
 uterus 621.8
  cervix 622.0
   with mention of cervicitis 616.0
  neck 622.0
   with mention of cervicitis 616.0
 vagina 616.8
 valve, heart 421.0
 varicose (lower extremity, any part) 454.0
  anus — *see* Varicose, ulcer, anus
  broad ligament 456.5
  esophagus (*see also* Varix, esophagus) 456.1
   bleeding (*see also* Varix, esophagus, bleeding) 456.0
  inflamed or infected 454.2
  nasal septum 456.8
  perineum 456.6
  rectum — *see* Varicose, ulcer, anus
  scrotum 456.4
  specified site NEC 456.8
  sublingual 456.3
  vulva 456.6
 vas deferens 608.89
 vesical (*see also* Ulcer, bladder) 596.8
 vulva (acute) (infectional) 616.50
  Behçet's syndrome 136.1 [616.51]

Ulcer, ulcerated, ulcerating, ulceration, ulcerative — *continued*
 vulva — *continued*
  herpetic 054.12
  tuberculous 016.7 ✓5ᵗʰ [616.51]
 vulvobuccal, recurring 616.50
 x-ray — *see* Ulcer, by site
 yaws 102.4
Ulcerosa scarlatina 034.1
Ulcus — *see also* Ulcer
 cutis tuberculosum (*see also* Tuberculosis) 017.0 ✓5ᵗʰ
 duodeni — *see* Ulcer, duodenum
 durum 091.0
  extragenital 091.2
 gastrojejunale — *see* Ulcer, gastrojejunal
 hypostaticum — *see* Ulcer, varicose
 molle (cutis) (skin) 099.0
 serpens corneae (pneumococcal) 370.04
 ventriculi — *see* Ulcer, stomach
Ulegyria 742.4
Ulerythema
 acneiforma 701.8
 centrifugum 695.4
 ophryogenes 757.4
Ullrich (-Bonnevie) (-Turner) syndrome 758.6
Ullrich-Feichtiger syndrome 759.89
Ulnar — *see* condition
Ulorrhagia 523.8
Ulorrhea 523.8
Umbilicus, umbilical — *see also* condition
 cord necrosis, affecting fetus or newborn 762.6
Unavailability of medical facilities (at) V63.9
 due to
  investigation by social service agency V63.8
  lack of services at home V63.1
  remoteness from facility V63.0
  waiting list V63.2
 home V63.1
 outpatient clinic V63.0
 specified reason NEC V63.8
Uncinaria americana infestion 126.1
Uncinariasis (*see also* Ancylostomiasis) 126.9
Unconscious, unconsciousness 780.09
Underdevelopment — *see also* Undeveloped
 sexual 259.0
Undernourishment 269.9
Undernutrition 269.9
Under observation — *see* Observation
Underweight 783.22
 for gestational age — *see* Light-for-dates
Underwood's disease (sclerema neonatorum) 778.1
Undescended — *see also* Malposition, congenital
 cecum 751.4
 colon 751.4
 testis 752.51
Undetermined diagnosis or cause 799.9
Undeveloped, undevelopment — *see also* Hypoplasia
 brain (congenital) 742.1
 cerebral (congenital) 742.1
 fetus or newborn 764.9 ✓5ᵗʰ
 heart 746.89
 lung 748.5
 testis 257.2
 uterus 259.0
Undiagnosed (disease) 799.9
Undulant fever (*see also* Brucellosis) 023.9
Unemployment, anxiety concerning V62.0
Unequal leg (acquired) (length) 736.81
 congenital 755.30
Unerupted teeth, tooth 520.6
Unextracted dental root 525.3
Unguis incarnatus 703.0
Unicornis uterus 752.3
Unicorporeus uterus 752.3
Uniformis uterus 752.3
Unilateral — *see also* condition
 development, breast 611.8
 organ or site, congenital NEC — *see* Agenesis

✓4ᵗʰ Fourth-digit Required   ✓5ᵗʰ Fifth-digit Required   ►◄ Revised Text   ● New Line   ▲ Revised Code

Unilateral — *see also* condition — *continued*
  vagina 752.49
Unilateralis uterus 752.3
Unilocular heart 745.8
Uninhibited bladder 596.54
  with cauda equina syndrome 344.61
  neurogenic — *see* Neurogenic, bladder 596.54
Union, abnormal — *see also* Fusion
  divided tendon 727.89
  larynx and trachea 748.3
Universal
  joint, cervix 620.6
  mesentery 751.4
Unknown
  cause of death 799.9
  diagnosis 799.9
Unna's disease (seborrheic dermatitis) 690.10
Unresponsiveness, adrenocorticotropin (ACTH) 255.4
Unsoundness of mind (*see also* Psychosis) 298.9
Unspecified cause of death 799.9
Unstable
  back NEC 724.9
  colon 569.89
  joint — *see* Instability, joint
  lie 652.0 ✓5ᵗʰ
    affecting fetus or newborn (before labor) 761.7
    causing obstructed labor 660.0 ✓5ᵗʰ
      affecting fetus or newborn 763.1
  lumbosacral joint (congenital) 756.19
    acquired 724.6
  sacroiliac 724.6
  spine NEC 724.9
Untruthfulness, child problem (*see also* Disturbance, conduct) 312.0 ✓5ᵗʰ
Unverricht (-Lundborg) disease, syndrome, or epilepsy 333.2
Unverricht-Wagner syndrome (dermatomyositis) 710.3
Upper respiratory — *see* condition
Upset
  gastric 536.8
    psychogenic 306.4
  gastrointestinal 536.8
    psychogenic 306.4
    virus (*see also* Enteritis, viral) 008.8
  intestinal (large) (small) 564.9
    psychogenic 306.4
  menstruation 626.9
  mental 300.9
  stomach 536.8
    psychogenic 306.4
Urachus — *see also* condition
  patent 753.7
  persistent 753.7
Uratic arthritis 274.0
Urbach's lipoid proteinosis 272.8
Urbach-Oppenheim disease or syndrome (necrobiosis lipoidica diabeticorum) 250.8 ✓5ᵗʰ *[709.3]*
Urbach-Wiethe disease or syndrome (lipoid proteinosis) 272.8
Urban yellow fever 060.1
Urea, blood, high — *see* Uremia
Uremia, uremic (absorption) (amaurosis) (amblyopia) (aphasia) (apoplexy) (coma) (delirium) (dementia) (dropsy) (dyspnea) (fever) (intoxication) (mania) (paralysis) (poisoning) (toxemia) (vomiting) 586
  with
    abortion — *see* Abortion, by type, with renal failure
    ectopic pregnancy (*see also* categories 633.0-633.9) 639.3
    hypertension (*see also* Hypertension, kidney) 403.91
    molar pregnancy (*see also* categories 630-632) 639.3
  chronic 585
  complicating
    abortion 639.3
    ectopic or molar pregnancy 639.3

Uremia, uremic — *continued*
  complicating — *continued*
    hypertension (*see also* Hypertension, kidney) 403.91
    labor and delivery 669.3 ✓5ᵗʰ
  congenital 779.89   ▲
  extrarenal 788.9
  hypertensive (chronic) (*see also* Hypertension, kidney) 403.91
  maternal NEC, affecting fetus or newborn 760.1
  neuropathy 585 *[357.4]*
  pericarditis 585 *[420.0]*
  prerenal 788.9
  pyelitic (*see also* Pyelitis) 590.80
Ureter, ureteral — *see* condition
Ureteralgia 788.0
Ureterectasis 593.89
Ureteritis 593.89
  cystica 590.3
  due to calculus 592.1
  gonococcal (acute) 098.19
    chronic or duration of 2 months or over 098.39
  nonspecific 593.89
Ureterocele (acquired) 593.89
  congenital 753.23
Ureterolith 592.1
Ureterolithiasis 592.1
Ureterostomy status V44.6
  with complication 997.5
Urethra, urethral — *see* condition
Urethralgia 788.9
Urethritis (abacterial) (acute) (allergic) (anterior) (chronic) (nonvenereal) (posterior) (recurrent) (simple) (subacute) (ulcerative) (undifferentiated) 597.80
  diplococcal (acute) 098.0
    chronic or duration of 2 months or over 098.2
  due to Trichomonas (vaginalis) 131.02
  gonococcal (acute) 098.0
    chronic or duration of 2 months or over 098.2
  nongonococcal (sexually transmitted) 099.40
    Chlamydia trachomatis 099.41
    Reiter's 099.3
    specified organism NEC 099.49
  nonspecific (sexually transmitted) (*see also* Urethritis, nongonococcal) 099.40
  not sexually transmitted 597.80
  Reiter's 099.3
  trichomonal or due to Trichomonas (vaginalis) 131.02
  tuberculous (*see also* Tuberculosis) 016.3 ✓5ᵗʰ
  venereal NEC (*see also* Urethritis, nongonococcal) 099.40
Urethrocele
  female 618.0
    with uterine prolapse 618.4
      complete 618.3
      incomplete 618.2
  male 599.5
Urethrolithiasis 594.2
Urethro-oculoarticular syndrome 099.3
Urethro-oculosynovial syndrome 099.3
Urethrorectal — *see* condition
Urethrorrhagia 599.84
Urethrorrhea 788.7
Urethrostomy status V44.6
  with complication 997.5
Urethrotrigonitis 595.3
Urethrovaginal — *see* condition
Urhidrosis, uridrosis 705.89
Uric acid
  diathesis 274.9
  in blood 790.6
Uricacidemia 790.6
Uricemia 790.6
Uricosuria 791.9

Urination
  frequent 788.41
  painful 788.1
Urine, urinary — *see also* condition
  abnormality NEC 788.69
  blood in (*see also* Hematuria) 599.7
  discharge, excessive 788.42
  enuresis 788.30
    nonorganic origin 307.6
  extravasation 788.8
  frequency 788.41
  incontinence 788.30
    active 788.30
    female 788.30
      stress 625.6
        and urge 788.33
    male 788.30
      stress 788.32
        and urge 788.33
    mixed (stress and urge) 788.33
    neurogenic 788.39
    nonorganic origin 307.6
    stress (female) 625.6
      male NEC 788.32
  intermittent stream 788.61
  pus in 791.9
  retention or stasis NEC 788.20
    bladder, incomplete emptying 788.21
    psychogenic 306.53
    specified NEC 788.29
  secretion
    deficient 788.5
    excessive 788.42
    frequency 788.41
  stream
    intermittent 788.61
    slowing 788.62
    splitting 788.61
    weak 788.62
Urinemia — *see* Uremia
Urinoma NEC 599.9
  bladder 596.8
  kidney 593.89
  renal 593.89
  ureter 593.89
  urethra 599.84
Uroarthritis, infectious 099.3
Urodialysis 788.5
Urolithiasis 592.9
Uronephrosis 593.89
Uropathy 599.9
  obstructive 599.6
Urosepsis 599.0
  meaning sepsis 038.9
  meaning urinary tract infection 599.0
Urticaria 708.9
  with angioneurotic edema 995.1
    hereditary 277.6
  allergic 708.0
  cholinergic 708.5
  chronic 708.8
  cold, familial 708.2
  dermatographic 708.3
  due to
    cold or heat 708.2
    drugs 708.0
    food 708.0
    inhalants 708.0
    plants 708.8
    serum 999.5
  factitial 708.3
  giant 995.1
    hereditary 277.6
  gigantea 995.1
    hereditary 277.6
  idiopathic 708.1
  larynx 995.1
    hereditary 277.6
  neonatorum 778.8
  nonallergic 708.1
  papulosa (Hebra) 698.2
  perstans hemorrhagica 757.39
  pigmentosa 757.33
  recurrent periodic 708.8
  serum 999.5
  solare 692.72

Urticaria — *continued*
  specified type NEC 708.8
  thermal (cold) (heat) 708.2
  vibratory 708.4
Urticarioides acarodermatitis 133.9
Use of
  nonprescribed drugs (*see also* Abuse, drugs,
      nondependent) 305.9 ✓5ᵗʰ
  patent medicines (*see also* Abuse, drugs,
      nondependent) 305.9 ✓5ᵗʰ
Usher-Senear disease (pemphigus erythematosus)
    694.4
Uta 085.5
Uterine size-date discrepancy 646.8 ✓5ᵗʰ
Uteromegaly 621.2
Uterovaginal — *see* condition
Uterovesical — *see* condition
Uterus — *see* condition
Utriculitis (utriculus prostaticus) 597.89
Uveal — *see* condition
Uveitis (anterior) (*see also* Iridocyclitis) 364.3
  acute or subacute 364.00
    due to or associated with
      gonococcal infection 098.41
      herpes (simplex) 054.44
        zoster 053.22
    primary 364.01
    recurrent 364.02
    secondary (noninfectious) 364.04
      infectious 364.03
  allergic 360.11
  chronic 364.10
    due to or associated with
      sarcoidosis 135 *[364.11]*
      tuberculosis (*see also* Tuberculosis)
        017.3 ✓5ᵗʰ *[364.11]*
  due to
    operation 360.11
    toxoplasmosis (acquired) 130.2
      congenital (active) 771.2
  granulomatous 364.10
  heterochromic 364.21
  lens-induced 364.23
  nongranulomatous 364.00
  posterior 363.20
    disseminated — *see* Chorioretinitis,
        disseminated
    focal — *see* Chorioretinitis, focal
  recurrent 364.02
  sympathetic 360.11
  syphilitic (secondary) 091.50
    congenital 090.0 *[363.13]*
    late 095.8 *[363.13]*
  tuberculous (*see also* Tuberculosis)
    017.3 ✓5ᵗʰ *[364.11]*
Uveoencephalitis 363.22
Uveokeratitis (*see also* Iridocyclitis) 364.3
Uveoparotid fever 135
Uveoparotitis 135
Uvula — *see* condition
Uvulitis (acute) (catarrhal) (chronic) (gangrenous)
    (membranous) (suppurative) (ulcerative)
    528.3

V

Vaccination
complication or reaction — *see* Complications, vaccination
not done (contraindicated) V64.0
  because of patient's decision V64.2
prophylactic (against) V05.9
  arthropod-borne viral
    disease NEC V05.1
    encephalitis V05.0
  chickenpox V05.4
  cholera (alone) V03.0
    with typhoid-paratyphoid (cholera + TAB) V06.0
  common cold V04.7
  diphtheria (alone) V03.5
    with
      poliomyelitis (DTP+ polio) V06.3
      tetanus V06.5
        pertussis combined (DTP) V06.1
      typhoid-paratyphoid (DTP + TAB) V06.2
  disease (single) NEC V05.9
    bacterial NEC V03.9
      specified type NEC V03.89
    combinations NEC V06.9
      specified type NEC V06.8
    specified type NEC V05.8
  encephalitis, viral, arthropod-borne V05.0
  Hemophilus influenzae, type B [Hib] V03.81
  hepatitis, viral V05.3
  influenza V04.8
    with
      Streptococcus pneumoniae [pneumococcus] V06.6
  lileieshmaniasis V05.2
  measles (alone) V04.2
    with mumps-rubella (MMR) V06.4
  mumps (alone) V04.6
    with measles and rubella (MMR) V06.4
  pertussis alone V03.6
  plague V03.3
  poliomyelitis V04.0
    with diphtheria-tetanus-pertussis (DTP + polio) V06.3
  rabies V04.5
  rubella (alone) V04.3
    with measles and mumps (MMR) V06.4
  smallpox V04.1
  Streptococcus pneumoniae [pneumococcus] V03.82
    with
      influenza V06.6
  tetanus toxoid (alone) V03.7
    with diphtheria [Td] V06.5
      with
        pertussis (DTP) V06.1
          with poliomyelitis (DTP+polio) V06.3
  tuberculosis (BCG) V03.2
  tularemia V03.4
  typhoid-paratyphoid (TAB) (alone) V03.1
    with diphtheria-tetanus-pertussis (TAB + DTP) V06.2
  varicella V05.4
  viral
    encephalitis, arthropod-borne V05.0
    hepatitis V05.3
  yellow fever V04.4

Vaccinia (generalized) 999.0
congenital 771.2
conjunctiva 999.3
eyelids 999.0 *[373.5]*
localized 999.3
nose 999.3
not from vaccination 051.0
  eyelid 051.0 *[373.5]*
sine vaccinatione 051.0
without vaccination 051.0

Vacuum
extraction of fetus or newborn 763.3
in sinus (accessory) (nasal) (*see also* Sinusitis) 473.9

Vagabond V60.0

Vagabondage V60.0

Vagabonds' disease 132.1

Vagina, vaginal — *see* condition

Vaginalitis (tunica) 608.4

Vaginismus (reflex) 625.1
functional 306.51
hysterical 300.11
psychogenic 306.51

Vaginitis (acute) (chronic) (circumscribed) (diffuse) (emphysematous) (Hemophilus vaginalis) (nonspecific) (nonvenereal) (ulcerative) 616.10
with
  abortion — *see* Abortion, by type, with sepsis
  ectopic pregnancy (*see also* categories 633.0-633.9) 639.0
  molar pregnancy (*see also* categories 630-632) 639.0
adhesive, congenital 752.49
atrophic, postmenopausal 627.3
bacterial 616.10
blennorrhagic (acute) 098.0
  chronic or duration of 2 months or over 098.2
candidal 112.1
chlamydial 099.53
complicating pregnancy or puerperium 646.6 ✔5ᵗʰ
  affecting fetus or newborn 760.8
congenital (adhesive) 752.49
due to
  C. albicans 112.1
  Trichomonas (vaginalis) 131.01
following
  abortion 639.0
  ectopic or molar pregnancy 639.0
gonococcal (acute) 098.0
  chronic or duration of 2 months or over 098.2
granuloma 099.2
Monilia 112.1
mycotic 112.1
pinworm 127.4 *[616.11]*
postirradiation 616.10
postmenopausal atrophic 627.3
senile (atrophic) 627.3
syphilitic (early) 091.0
  late 095.8
trichomonal 131.01
tuberculous (*see also* Tuberculosis) 016.7 ✔5ᵗʰ
venereal NEC 099.8

Vaginosis — *see* Vaginitis

Vagotonia 352.3

Vagrancy V60.0

Vallecula — *see* condition

Valley fever 114.0

Valsuani's disease (progressive pernicious anemia, puerperal) 648.2 ✔5ᵗʰ

Valve, valvular (formation) — *see also* condition
cerebral ventricle (communicating) in situ V45.2
cervix, internal os 752.49
colon 751.5
congenital NEC — *see* Atresia
formation, congenital NEC — *see* Atresia
heart defect — *see* Anomaly, heart, valve
ureter 753.29
  pelvic junction 753.21
  vesical orifice 753.22
urethra 753.6

Valvulitis (chronic) (*see also* Endocarditis) 424.90
rheumatic (chronic) (inactive) (with chorea) 397.9
  active or acute (aortic) (mitral) (pulmonary) (tricuspid) 391.1
syphilitic NEC 093.20
  aortic 093.22
  mitral 093.21
  pulmonary 093.24
  tricuspid 093.23

Valvulopathy — *see* Endocarditis

van Bogaert's leukoencephalitis (sclerosing) (subacute) 046.2

van Bogaert-Nijssen (-Peiffer) disease 330.0

van Buchem's syndrome (hyperostosis corticalis) 733.3

van Creveld-von Gierke disease (glycogenosis I) 271.0

van den Bergh's disease (enterogenous cyanosis) 289.7

van der Hoeve's syndrome (brittle bones and blue sclera, deafness) 756.51

van der Hoeve-Halbertsma-Waardenburg syndrome (ptosis-epicanthus) 270.2

van der Hoeve-Waardenburg-Gualdi syndrome (ptosis epicanthus) 270.2

Vanillism 692.89

Vanishing lung 492.0

van Neck (-Odelberg) disease or syndrome (juvenile osteochondrosis) 732.1

Vanishing twin 651.33

Vapor asphyxia or suffocation NEC 987.9
specified agent — *see* Table of Drugs and Chemicals

Vaquez's disease (M9950/1) 238.4

Vaquez-Osler disease (polycythemia vera) (M9950/1) 238.4

Variance, lethal ball, prosthetic heart valve 996.02

Variants, thalassemic 282.4

Variations in hair color 704.3

Varicella 052.9
with
  complication 052.8
    specified NEC 052.7
  pneumonia 052.1
  vaccination and inoculation (prophylactic) V05.4

Varices — *see* Varix

Varicocele (scrotum) (thrombosed) 456.4
ovary 456.5
perineum 456.6
spermatic cord (ulcerated) 456.4

Varicose
aneurysm (ruptured) (*see also* Aneurysm) 442.9
dermatitis (lower extremity) — *see* Varicose, vein, inflamed or infected
eczema — *see* Varicose, vein
phlebitis — *see* Varicose, vein, inflamed or infected
placental vessel — *see* Placenta, abnormal
tumor — *see* Varicose, vein
ulcer (lower extremity, any part) 454.0
  anus 455.8
    external 455.5
    internal 455.2
  esophagus (*see also* Varix, esophagus) 456.1
    bleeding (*see also* Varix, esophagus, bleeding) 456.0
  inflamed or infected 454.2
  nasal septum 456.8
  perineum 456.6
  rectum — *see* Varicose, ulcer, anus
  scrotum 456.4
  specified site NEC 456.8
vein (lower extremity) (ruptured) (*see also* Varix) 454.9
  with
    complications NEC 454.8 ●
    edema 454.8 ●
    inflammation or infection 454.1
      ulcerated 454.2
    pain 454.8 ●
    stasis dermatitis 454.1
      with ulcer 454.2
    swelling 454.8 ●
    ulcer 454.0
      inflamed or infected 454.2
  anus — *see* Hemorrhoids
  broad ligament 456.5
  congenital (peripheral) NEC 747.60
    gastrointestinal 747.61
    lower limb 747.64
    renal 747.62
    specified NEC 747.69
    upper limb 747.63

Varicose — Version *(vertical text in left margin)*

Varicose — *continued*
vein (*see also* Varix) — *continued*
esophagus (ulcerated) (*see also* Varix, esophagus) 456.1
bleeding (*see also* Varix, esophagus, bleeding) 456.0
inflamed or infected 454.1
with ulcer 454.2
in pregnancy or puerperium 671.0 ✓5ᵗʰ
vulva or perineum 671.1 ✓5ᵗʰ
nasal septum (with ulcer) 456.8
pelvis 456.5
perineum 456.6
in pregnancy, childbirth, or puerperium 671.1 ✓5ᵗʰ
rectum — *see* Hemorrhoids
scrotum (ulcerated) 456.4
specified site NEC 456.8
sublingual 456.3
ulcerated 454.0
inflamed or infected 454.2
umbilical cord, affecting fetus or newborn 762.6
urethra 456.8
vulva 456.6
in pregnancy, childbirth, or puerperium 671.1 ✓5ᵗʰ
vessel — *see also* Varix
placenta — *see* Placenta, abnormal
Varicosis, varicosities, varicosity (*see also* Varix) 454.9
Variola 050.9
hemorrhagic (pustular) 050.0
major 050.0
minor 050.1
modified 050.2
Varioloid 050.2
Variolosa, purpura 050.0
Varix (lower extremity) (ruptured) 454.9
with
complications NEC 454.8 ●
edema 454.8 ●
inflammation or infection 454.1
with ulcer 454.2
pain 454.8 ●
stasis dermatitis 454.1
with ulcer 454.2
swelling 454.8 ●
ulcer 454.0
with inflammation or infection 454.2
aneurysmal (*see also* Aneurysm) 442.9
anus — *see* Hemorrhoids
arteriovenous (congenital) (peripheral) NEC 747.60
gastrointestinal 747.61
lower limb 747.64
renal 747.62
specified NEC 747.69
spinal 747.82
upper limb 747.63
bladder 456.5
broad ligament 456.5
congenital (peripheral) NEC 747.60
esophagus (ulcerated) 456.1
bleeding 456.0
in
cirrhosis of liver 571.5 *[456.20]*
portal hypertension 572.3 *[456.20]*
congenital 747.69
in
cirrhosis of liver 571.5 *[456.21]*
with bleeding 571.5 *[456.20]*
portal hypertension 572.3 *[456.21]*
with bleeding 572.3 *[456.20]*
gastric 456.8
inflamed or infected 454.1
ulcerated 454.2
in pregnancy or puerperium 671.0 ✓5ᵗʰ
perineum 671.1 ✓5ᵗʰ
vulva 671.1 ✓5ᵗʰ
labia (majora) 456.6
orbit 456.8
congenital 747.69
ovary 456.5
papillary 448.1
pelvis 456.5

Varix — *continued*
perineum 456.6
in pregnancy or puerperium 671.1 ✓5ᵗʰ
pharynx 456.8
placenta — *see* Placenta, abnormal
prostate 456.8
rectum — *see* Hemorrhoids
renal papilla 456.8
retina 362.17
scrotum (ulcerated) 456.4
sigmoid colon 456.8
specified site NEC 456.8
spinal (cord) (vessels) 456.8
spleen, splenic (vein) (with phlebolith) 456.8
sublingual 456.3
ulcerated 454.0
inflamed or infected 454.2
umbilical cord, affecting fetus or newborn 762.6
uterine ligament 456.5
vocal cord 456.8
vulva 456.6
in pregnancy, childbirth, or puerperium 671.1 ✓5ᵗʰ
Vasa previa 663.5 ✓5ᵗʰ
affecting fetus or newborn 762.6
hemorrhage from, affecting fetus or newborn 772.0
Vascular — *see also* condition
loop on papilla (optic) 743.57
sheathing, retina 362.13
spasm 443.9
spider 448.1
Vascularity, pulmonary, congenital 747.3
Vascularization
choroid 362.16
cornea 370.60
deep 370.63
localized 370.61
retina 362.16
subretinal 362.16
Vasculitis 447.6
allergic 287.0
cryoglobulinemic 273.2
disseminated 447.6
kidney 447.8
leukocytoclastic 446.29
nodular 695.2
retinal 362.18
rheumatic — *see* Fever, rheumatic
Vas deferens — *see* condition
Vas deferentitis 608.4
Vasectomy, admission for V25.2
Vasitis 608.4
nodosa 608.4
scrotum 608.4
spermatic cord 608.4
testis 608.4
tuberculous (*see also* Tuberculosis) 016.5 ✓5ᵗʰ
tunica vaginalis 608.4
vas deferens 608.4
Vasodilation 443.9
Vasomotor — *see* condition
Vasoplasty, after previous sterilization V26.0
Vasoplegia, splanchnic (*see also* Neuropathy, peripheral, autonomic) 337.9
Vasospasm 443.9
cerebral (artery) 435.9
with transient neurologic deficit 435.9
nerve
arm NEC 354.9
autonomic 337.9
brachial plexus 353.0
cervical plexus 353.2
leg NEC 355.8
lower extremity NEC 355.8
peripheral NEC 355.9
spinal NEC 355.9
sympathetic 337.9
upper extremity NEC 354.9
peripheral NEC 443.9
retina (artery) (*see also* Occlusion, retinal, artery) 362.30
Vasospastic — *see* condition

Vasovagal attack (paroxysmal) 780.2
psychogenic 306.2
Vater's ampulla — *see* condition
VATER syndrome 759.89
Vegetation, vegetative
adenoid (nasal fossa) 474.2
consciousness (persistent) 780.03
endocarditis (acute) (any valve) (chronic) (subacute) 421.0
heart (mycotic) (valve) 421.0
state (persistent) 780.03
Veil
Jackson's 751.4
over face (causing asphyxia) 768.9
Vein, venous — *see* condition
Veldt sore (*see also* Ulcer, skin) 707.9
Velpeau's hernia — *see* Hernia, femoral
Venereal
balanitis NEC 099.8
bubo 099.1
disease 099.9
specified nature or type NEC 099.8
granuloma inguinale 099.2
lymphogranuloma (Durand-Nicolas-Favre), any site 099.1
salpingitis 098.37
urethritis (*see also* Urethritis, nongonococcal) 099.40
vaginitis NEC 099.8
warts 078.19
Vengefulness, in child (*see also* Disturbance, conduct) 312.0 ✓5ᵗʰ
Venofibrosis 459.89
Venom, venomous
bite or sting (animal or insect) 989.5
poisoning 989.5
Venous — *see* condition
Ventouse delivery NEC 669.5 ✓5ᵗʰ
affecting fetus or newborn 763.3
Ventral — *see* condition
Ventricle, ventricular — *see also* condition
escape 427.69
standstill (*see also* Arrest, cardiac) 427.5
Ventriculitis, cerebral (*see also* Meningitis) 322.9
Ventriculostomy status V45.2
Verbiest's syndrome (claudicatio intermittens spinalis) 435.1
Vernet's syndrome 352.6
Verneuil's disease (syphilitic bursitis) 095.7
Verruca (filiformis) 078.10
acuminata (any site) 078.11
necrogenica (primary) (*see also* Tuberculosis) 017.0 ✓5ᵗʰ
plana (juvenilis) 078.19
peruana 088.0
peruviana 088.0
plantaris 078.19
seborrheica 702.19
inflamed 702.11
senilis 702.0
tuberculosa (primary) (*see also* Tuberculosis) 017.0 ✓5ᵗʰ
venereal 078.19
viral NEC 078.10
Verrucosities (*see also* Verruca) 078.10
Verrucous endocarditis (acute) (any valve) (chronic) (subacute) 710.0 *[424.91]*
nonbacterial 710.0 *[424.91]*
Verruga
peruana 088.0
peruviana 088.0
Verse's disease (calcinosis intervertebralis) 275.49 *[722.90]*
Version
before labor, affecting fetus or newborn 761.7
cephalic (correcting previous malposition) 652.1 ✓5ᵗʰ
affecting fetus or newborn 763.1
cervix (*see also* Malposition, uterus) 621.6
uterus (postinfectional) (postpartal, old) (*see also* Malposition, uterus) 621.6
forward — *see* Anteversion, uterus
lateral — *see* Lateroversion, uterus

Vertebra, vertebral — *see* condition
Vertigo 780.4
   auditory 386.19
   aural 386.19
   benign paroxysmal positional 386.11
   central origin 386.2
   cerebral 386.2
   Dix and Hallpike (epidemic) 386.12
   endemic paralytic 078.81
   epidemic 078.81
      Dix and Hallpike 386.12
      Gerlier's 078.81
      Pedersen's 386.12
      vestibular neuronitis 386.12
   epileptic — *see* Epilepsy
   Gerlier's (epidemic) 078.81
   hysterical 300.11
   labyrinthine 386.10
   laryngeal 786.2
   malignant positional 386.2
   Ménière's (*see also* Disease, Ménière's) 386.00
   menopausal 627.2
   otogenic 386.19
   paralytic 078.81
   paroxysmal positional, benign 386.11
   Pedersen's (epidemic) 386.12
   peripheral 386.10
      specified type NEC 386.19
   positional
      benign paroxysmal 386.11
      malignant 386.2
Verumontanitis (chronic) (*see also* Urethritis) 597.89
Vesania (*see also* Psychosis) 298.9
Vesical — *see* condition
Vesicle
   cutaneous 709.8
   seminal — *see* condition
   skin 709.8
Vesicocolic — *see* condition
Vesicoperineal — *see* condition
Vesicorectal — *see* condition
Vesicourethrorectal — *see* condition
Vesicovaginal — *see* condition
Vesicular — *see* condition
Vesiculitis (seminal) 608.0
   amebic 006.8
   gonorrheal (acute) 098.14
      chronic or duration of 2 months or over 098.34
   trichomonal 131.09
   tuberculous (*see also* Tuberculosis) 016.5 ✓5ᵗʰ [608.81]
Vestibulitis (ear) (*see also* Labyrinthitis) 386.30
   nose (external) 478.1
   vulvar 616.10
Vestibulopathy, acute peripheral (recurrent) 386.12
Vestige, vestigial — *see also* Persistence
   branchial 744.41
   structures in vitreous 743.51
Vibriosis NEC 027.9
Vidal's disease (lichen simplex chronicus) 698.3
Video display tube syndrome 723.8
Vienna type encephalitis 049.8
Villaret's syndrome 352.6
Villous — *see* condition
VIN I (vulvar intraepithelial neoplasia I) 624.8
VIN II (vulvar intraepithelial neoplasia II) 624.8
VIN III (vulvar intraepithelial neoplasia III) 233.3
Vincent's
   angina 101
   bronchitis 101
   disease 101
   gingivitis 101
   infection (any site) 101
   laryngitis 101
   stomatitis 101
   tonsillitis 101
Vinson-Plummer syndrome (sideropenic dysphagia) 280.8

Viosterol deficiency (*see also* Deficiency, calciferol) 268.9
Virchow's disease 733.99
Viremia 790.8
Virilism (adrenal) (female) NEC 255.2
   with
      3-beta-hydroxysteroid dehydrogenase defect 255.2
      11-hydroxylase defect 255.2
      21-hydroxylase defect 255.2
      adrenal
         hyperplasia 255.2
         insufficiency (congenital) 255.2
      cortical hyperfunction 255.2
Virilization (female) (suprarenal) (*see also* Virilism) 255.2
   isosexual 256.4
Virulent bubo 099.0
Virus, viral — *see also* condition
   infection NEC (*see also* Infection, viral) 079.99
   septicemia 079.99
Viscera, visceral — *see* condition
Visceroptosis 569.89
Visible peristalsis 787.4
Vision, visual
   binocular, suppression 368.31
   blurred, blurring 368.8
      hysterical 300.11
   defect, defective (*see also* Impaired, vision) 369.9
   disorientation (syndrome) 368.16
   disturbance NEC (*see also* Disturbance, vision) 368.9
      hysterical 300.11
   examination V72.0
   field, limitation 368.40
   fusion, with defective steropsis 368.33
   hallucinations 368.16
   halos 368.16
   loss 369.9
      both eyes (*see also* Blindness, both eyes) 369.3
      complete (*see also* Blindness, both eyes) 369.00
      one eye 369.8
      sudden 368.16
   low (both eyes) 369.20
      one eye (other eye normal) (*see also* Impaired, vision) 369.70
         blindness, other eye 369.10
   perception, simultaneous without fusion 368.32
   tunnel 368.45
Vitality, lack or want of 780.79
   newborn 779.89   ▲
Vitamin deficiency NEC (*see also* Deficiency, vitamin) 269.2
Vitelline duct, persistent 751.0
Vitiligo 709.01
   due to pinta (carate) 103.2
   eyelid 374.53
   vulva 624.8
Vitium cordis — *see* Disease, heart
Vitreous — *see also* condition
   touch syndrome 997.99
Vocal cord — *see* condition
Vocational rehabilitation V57.22
Vogt's (Cecile) disease or syndrome 333.7
Vogt-Koyanagi syndrome 364.24
Vogt-Spielmeyer disease (amaurotic familial idiocy) 330.1
Voice
   change (*see also* Dysphonia) 784.49
   loss (*see also* Aphonia) 784.41
Volhard-Fahr disease (malignant nephrosclerosis) 403.00
Volhynian fever 083.1
Volkmann's ischemic contracture or paralysis (complicating trauma) 958.6
Voluntary starvation 307.1

Volvulus (bowel) (colon) (intestine) 560.2
   with
      hernia — *see also* Hernia, by site, with obstruction
         gangrenous — *see* Hernia, by site, with gangrene
      perforation 560.2
   congenital 751.5
   duodenum 537.3
   fallopian tube 620.5
   oviduct 620.5
   stomach (due to absence of gastrocolic ligament) 537.89
Vomiting 787.03
   with nausea 787.01
   allergic 535.4 ✓5ᵗʰ
   asphyxia 933.1
   bilious (cause unknown) 787.0
      following gastrointestinal surgery 564.3
   blood (*see also* Hematemesis) 578.0
   causing asphyxia, choking, or suffocation (*see also* Asphyxia, food) 933.1
   cyclical 536.2
      psychogenic 306.4
   epidemic 078.82
   fecal matter 569.89
   following gastrointestinal surgery 564.3
   functional 536.8
      psychogenic 306.4
   habit 536.2
   hysterical 300.11
   nervous 306.4
   neurotic 306.4
   newborn 779.3
   of or complicating pregnancy 643.9 ✓5ᵗʰ
      due to
         organic disease 643.8 ✓5ᵗʰ
         specific cause NEC 643.8 ✓5ᵗʰ
      early — *see* Hyperemesis, gravidarum
      late (after 22 completed weeks of gestation) 643.2 ✓5ᵗʰ
   pernicious or persistent 536.2
      complicating pregnancy — *see* Hyperemesis, gravidarum
      psychogenic 306.4
   physiological 787.0
   psychic 306.4
   psychogenic 307.54
   stercoral 569.89
   uncontrollable 536.2
      psychogenic 306.4
   uremic — *see* Uremia
   winter 078.82
von Bechterew (-Strumpell) disease or syndrome (ankylosing spondylitis) 720.0
von Bezold's abscess 383.01
von Economo's disease (encephalitis lethargica) 049.8
von Eulenburg's disease (congenital paramyotonia) 359.2
von Gierke's disease (glycogenosis I) 271.0
von Gies' joint 095.8
von Graefe's disease or syndrome 378.72
von Hippel (-Lindau) disease or syndrome (retinocerebral angiomatosis) 759.6
von Jaksch's anemia or disease (pseudoleukemia infantum) 285.8
von Recklinghausen's
   disease or syndrome (nerves) (skin) (M9540/1) 237.71
      bones (osteitis fibrosa cystica) 252.0
   tumor (M9540/1) 237.71
von Recklinghausen-Applebaum disease (hemochromatosis) 275.0
von Schroetter's syndrome (intermittent venous claudication) 453.8
von Willebrand (-Jürgens) (-Minot) disease or syndrome (angiohemophilia) 286.4
von Zambusch's disease (lichen sclerosus et atrophicus) 701.0
Voorhoeve's disease or dyschondroplasia 756.4
Vossius' ring 921.3
   late effect 366.21
Voyeurism 302.82

Vrolik's disease (osteogenesis imperfecta) 756.51
Vulva — *see* condition
Vulvismus 625.1
Vulvitis (acute) (allergic) (aphthous) (chronic) (gangrenous) (hypertrophic) (intertriginous) 616.10
  with
    abortion — *see* Abortion, by type, with sepsis
    ectopic pregnancy (*see also* categories 633.0-633.9) 639.0
    molar pregnancy (*see also* categories 630-632) 639.0
  adhesive, congenital 752.49
  blennorhagic (acute) 098.0
    chronic or duration of 2 months or over 098.2
  chlamydial 099.53
  complicating pregnancy or puerperium 646.6 ☑5ᵗʰ
  due to Ducrey's bacillus 099.0
  following
    abortion 639.0
    ectopic or molar pregnancy 639.0
  gonococcal (acute) 098.0
    chronic or duration of 2 months or over 098.2
  herpetic 054.11
  leukoplakic 624.0
  monilial 112.1
  puerperal, postpartum, childbirth 646.6 ☑5ᵗʰ
  syphilitic (early) 091.0
    late 095.8
  trichomonal 131.01
Vulvodynia 625.9
Vulvorectal — *see* condition
Vulvovaginitis (*see also* Vulvitis) 616.10
  amebic 006.8
  chlamydial 099.53
  gonococcal (acute) 098.0
    chronic or duration of 2 months or over 098.2
  herpetic 054.11
  monilial 112.1
  trichomonal (Trichomonas vaginalis) 131.01

W

Waardenburg's syndrome 756.89
  meaning ptosis-epicanthus 270.2
Waardenburg-Klein syndrome (ptosis-epicanthus) 270.2
Wagner's disease (colloid milium) 709.3
Wagner (-Unverricht) syndrome (dermatomyositis) 710.3
Waiting list, person on V63.2
  undergoing social agency investigation V63.8
Wakefulness disorder (*see also* Hypersomnia) 780.54
  nonorganic origin 307.43
Waldenström's
  disease (osteochondrosis, capital femoral) 732.1
  hepatitis (lupoid hepatitis) 571.49
  hypergammaglobulinemia 273.0
  macroglobulinemia 273.3
  purpura, hypergammaglobulinemic 273.0
  syndrome (macroglobulinemia) 273.3
Waldenström-Kjellberg syndrome (sideropenic dysphagia) 280.8
Walking
  difficulty 719.7 ☑5ᵗʰ
    psychogenic 307.9
  sleep 307.46
    hysterical 300.13
Wall, abdominal — *see* condition
Wallenberg's syndrome (posterior inferior cerebellar artery) (*see also* Disease, cerebrovascular, acute) 436
Wallgren's
  disease (obstruction of splenic vein with collateral circulation) 459.89
  meningitis (*see also* Meningitis, aseptic) 047.9

Wandering
  acetabulum 736.39
  gallbladder 751.69
  kidney, congenital 753.3
  organ or site, congenital NEC — *see* Malposition, congenital
  pacemaker (atrial) (heart) 427.89
  spleen 289.59
Wardrop's disease (with lymphangitis) 681.9
  finger 681.02
  toe 681.11
War neurosis 300.16
Wart (common) (digitate) (filiform) (infectious) (juvenile) (plantar) (viral) 078.10
  external genital organs (venereal) 078.19
  fig 078.19
  Hassall-Henle's (of cornea) 371.41
  Henle's (of cornea) 371.41
  juvenile 078.19
  moist 078.10
  Peruvian 088.0
  plantar 078.19
  prosector (*see also* Tuberculosis) 017.0 ☑5ᵗʰ
  seborrheic 702.19
    inflamed 702.11
  senile 702.0
  specified NEC 078.19
  syphilitic 091.3
  tuberculous (*see also* Tuberculosis) 017.0 ☑5ᵗʰ
  venereal (female) (male) 078.19
Warthin's tumor (salivary gland) (M8561/0) 210.2
Washerwoman's itch 692.4
Wassilieff's disease (leptospiral jaundice) 100.0
Wasting
  disease 799.4
    due to malnutrition 261
  extreme (due to malnutrition) 261
  muscular NEC 728.2
  palsy, paralysis 335.21
Water
  clefts 366.12
  deprivation of 994.3
  in joint (*see also* Effusion, joint) 719.0 ☑5ᵗʰ
  intoxication 276.6
  itch 120.3
  lack of 994.3
  loading 276.6
  on
    brain — *see* Hydrocephalus
    chest 511.8
  poisoning 276.6
Waterbrash 787.1
Water-hammer pulse (*see also* Insufficiency, aortic) 424.1
Waterhouse (-Friderichsen) disease or syndrome 036.3
Water-losing nephritis 588.8
Wax in ear 380.4
Waxy
  degeneration, any site 277.3
  disease 277.3
  kidney 277.3 [583.81]
  liver (large) 277.3
  spleen 277.3
Weak, weakness (generalized) 780.79
  arches (acquired) 734
    congenital 754.61
  bladder sphincter 596.59
    congenital 779.89 ▲
  eye muscle — *see* Strabismus
  foot (double) — *see* Weak, arches
  heart, cardiac (*see also* Failure, heart) 428.9
    congenital 746.9
  mind 317
  muscle 728.9
  myocardium (*see also* Failure, heart) 428.9
  newborn 779.89 ▲
  pelvic fundus 618.8
  pulse 785.9
  senile 797
  valvular — *see* Endocarditis
Wear, worn, tooth, teeth (approximal) (hard tissues) (interproximal) (occlusal) 521.1

Weather, weathered
  effects of
    cold NEC 991.9
      specified effect NEC 991.8
    hot (*see also* Heat) 992.9
    skin 692.74
Web, webbed (congenital) — *see also* Anomaly, specified type NEC
  canthus 743.63
  digits (*see also* Syndactylism) 755.10
  esophagus 750.3
  fingers (*see also* Syndactylism, fingers) 755.11
  larynx (glottic) (subglottic) 748.2
  neck (pterygium colli) 744.5
  Paterson-Kelly (sideropenic dysphagia) 280.8
  popliteal syndrome 756.89
  toes (*see also* Syndactylism, toes) 755.13
Weber's paralysis or syndrome 344.89
Weber-Christian disease or syndrome (nodular nonsuppurative panniculitis) 729.30
Weber-Cockayne syndrome (epidermolysis bullosa) 757.39
Weber-Dimitri syndrome 759.6
Weber-Gubler syndrome 344.89
Weber-Leyden syndrome 344.89
Weber-Osler syndrome (familial hemorrhagic telangiectasia) 448.0
Wedge-shaped or wedging vertebra (*see also* Osteoporosis) 733.00
Wegener's granulomatosis or syndrome 446.4
Wegner's disease (syphilitic osteochondritis) 090.0
Weight
  gain (abnormal) (excessive) 783.1
    during pregnancy 646.1 ☑5ᵗʰ
      insufficient 646.8 ☑5ᵗʰ
  less than 1000 grams at birth 765.0 ☑5ᵗʰ
  loss (cause unknown) 783.21
Weightlessness 994.9
Weil's disease (leptospiral jaundice) 100.0
Weill-Marchesani syndrome (brachymorphism and ectopia lentis) 759.89
Weingarten's syndrome (tropical eosinophilia) 518.3
Weir Mitchell's disease (erythromelalgia) 443.89
Weiss-Baker syndrome (carotid sinus syncope) 337.0
Weissenbach-Thibierge syndrome (cutaneous systemic sclerosis) 710.1
Wen (*see also* Cyst, sebaceous) 706.2
Wenckebach's phenomenon, heart block (second degree) 426.13
Werdnig-Hoffmann syndrome (muscular atrophy) 335.0
Werlhof's disease (*see also* Purpura, thrombocytopenic) 287.3
Werlhof-Wichmann syndrome (*see also* Purpura, thrombocytopenic) 287.3
Wermer's syndrome or disease (polyendocrine adenomatosis) 258.0
Werner's disease or syndrome (progeria adultorum) 259.8
Werner-His disease (trench fever) 083.1
Werner-Schultz disease (agranulocytosis) 288.0
Wernicke's encephalopathy, disease, or syndrome (superior hemorrhagic polioencephalitis) 265.1
Wernicke-Korsakoff syndrome or psychosis (nonalcoholic) 294.0
  alcoholic 291.1
Wernicke-Posadas disease (*see also* Coccidioidomycosis) 114.9
Wesselsbron fever 066.3
West African fever 084.8
West Nile fever 066.4 ▲
West Nile virus 066.4 ●
Westphal-Strümpell syndrome (hepatolenticular degeneration) 275.1
Wet
  brain (alcoholic) (*see also* Alcoholism) 303.9 ☑5ᵗʰ

Wound, open — *continued*
ear 872.8
  canal 872.02
    complicated 872.12
  complicated 872.9
  drum 872.61
    complicated 872.71
  external 872.00
    complicated 872.10
  multiple sites 872.69
    complicated 872.79
  ossicles (incus) (malleus) (stapes) 872.62
    complicated 872.72
  specified part NEC 872.69
    complicated 872.79
elbow 881.01
  with tendon involvement 881.21
  complicated 881.11
epididymis 878.2
  complicated 878.3
epigastric region 879.2
  complicated 879.3
epiglottis 874.01
  complicated 874.11
esophagus (cervical) 874.4
  complicated 874.5
  thoracic — *see* Injury, internal, esophagus
Eustachian tube 872.63
  complicated 872.73
extremity
  lower (multiple) NEC 894.0
    with tendon involvement 894.2
    complicated 894.1
  upper (multiple) NEC 884.0
    with tendon involvement 884.2
    complicated 884.1
eye(s) (globe) — *see* Wound, open, intraocular
eyeball NEC 871.9
  laceration (*see also* Laceration, eyeball) 871.4
  penetrating (*see also* Penetrating wound, eyeball) 871.7
eyebrow 873.42
  complicated 873.52
eyelid NEC 870.8
  laceration — *see* Laceration, eyelid
face 873.40
  complicated 873.50
  multiple sites 873.49
    complicated 873.59
  specified part NEC 873.49
    complicated 873.59
fallopian tube — *see* Injury, internal, fallopian tube
finger(s) (nail) (subungual) 883.0
  with tendon involvement 883.2
  complicated 883.1
flank 879.4
  complicated 879.5
foot (any part except toe(s) alone) 892.0
  with tendon involvement 892.2
  complicated 892.1
forearm 881.00
  with tendon involvement 881.20
  complicated 881.10
forehead 873.42
  complicated 873.52
genital organs (external) NEC 878.8
  complicated 878.9
  internal — *see* Injury, internal, by site
globe (eye) (*see also* Wound, open, eyeball) 871.9
groin 879.4
  complicated 879.5
gum(s) 873.62
  complicated 873.72
hand (except finger(s) alone) 882.0
  with tendon involvement 882.2
  complicated 882.1
head NEC 873.8
  with intracranial injury — *see* Injury, intracranial
    due to or associated with skull fracture — *see* Fracture, skull
  complicated 873.9
  scalp — *see* Wound, open, scalp

Wound, open — *continued*
heel 892.0
  with tendon involvement 892.2
  complicated 892.1
high-velocity (grease gun) — *see* Wound, open, complicated, by site
hip 890.0
  with tendon involvement 890.2
  complicated 890.1
hymen 878.6
  complicated 878.7
hypochondrium 879.4
  complicated 879.5
hypogastric region 879.2
  complicated 879.3
iliac (region) 879.4
  complicated 879.5
incidental to
  dislocation — *see* Dislocation, open, by site
  fracture — *see* Fracture, open, by site
  intracranial injury — *see* Injury, intracranial, with open intracranial wound
  nerve injury — *see* Injury, nerve, by site
inguinal region 879.4
  complicated 879.5
instep 892.0
  with tendon involvement 892.2
  complicated 892.1
interscapular region 876.0
  complicated 876.1
intracranial — *see* Injury, intracranial, with open intracranial wound
intraocular 871.9
  with
    partial loss (of intraocular tissue) 871.2
    prolapse or exposure (of intraocular tissue) 871.1
  aceration (*see also* Laceration, eyeball) 871.4
  penetrating 871.7
    with foreign body (nonmagnetic) 871.6
      magnetic 871.5
  without prolapse (of intraocular tissue) 871.0
iris (*see also* Wound, open, eyeball) 871.9
jaw (fracture not involved) 873.44
  with fracture — *see* Fracture, jaw
  complicated 873.54
knee 891.0
  with tendon involvement 891.2
  complicated 891.1
labium (majus) (minus) 878.4
  complicated 878.5
lacrimal apparatus, gland, or sac 870.8
  with laceration of eyelid 870.2
larynx 874.01
  with trachea 874.00
    complicated 874.10
  complicated 874.11
leg (multiple) 891.0
  with tendon involvement 891.2
  complicated 891.1
  lower 891.0
    with tendon involvement 891.2
    complicated 891.1
  thigh 890.0
    with tendon involvement 890.2
    complicated 890.1
  upper 890.0
    with tendon involvement 890.2
    complicated 890.1
lens (eye) (alone) (*see also* Cataract, traumatic) 366.20
  with involvement of other eye structures — *see* Wound, open, eyeball
limb
  lower (multiple) NEC 894.0
    with tendon involvement 894.2
    complicated 894.1
  upper (multiple) NEC 884.0
    with tendon involvement 884.2
    complicated 884.1
lip 873.43
  complicated 873.53
loin 876.0
  complicated 876.1

Wound, open — *continued*
lumbar region 876.0
  complicated 876.1
malar region 873.41
  complicated 873.51
mastoid region 873.49
  complicated 873.59
mediastinum — *see* Injury, internal, mediastinum
midthoracic region 875.0
  complicated 875.1
mouth 873.60
  complicated 873.70
  floor 873.64
    complicated 873.74
  multiple sites 873.69
    complicated 873.79
  specified site NEC 873.69
    complicated 873.79
multiple, unspecified site(s) 879.8

> Note — *Multiple open wounds of sites classifiable to the same four-digit category should be classified to that category unless they are in different limbs.*
>
> *Multiple open wounds of sites classifiable to different four-digit categories, or to different limbs, should be coded separately.*

  complicated 879.9
  lower limb(s) (one or both) (sites classifiable to more than one three-digit category in 890 to 893) 894.0
    with tendon involvement 894.2
    complicated 894.1
  upper limb(s) (one or both) (sites classifiable to more than one three-digit category in 880 to 883) 884.0
    with tendon involvement 884.2
    complicated 884.1
muscle — *see* Sprain, by site
nail
  finger(s) 883.0
    complicated 883.1
  thumb 883.0
    complicated 883.1
  toe(s) 893.0
    complicated 893.1
nape (neck) 874.8
  complicated 874.9
  specified part NEC 874.8
    complicated 874.9
nasal — *see also* Wound, open, nose
  cavity 873.22
    complicated 873.32
  septum 873.21
    complicated 873.31
  sinuses 873.23
    complicated 873.33
nasopharynx 873.22
  complicated 873.32
neck 874.8
  complicated 874.9
  nape 874.8
    complicated 874.9
  specified part NEC 874.8
    complicated 874.9
nerve — *see* Injury, nerve, by site
non-healing surgical 998.83
nose 873.20
  complicated 873.30
  multiple sites 873.29
    complicated 873.39
  septum 873.21
    complicated 873.31
  sinuses 873.23
    complicated 873.33
occipital region — *see* Wound, open, scalp
ocular NEC 871.9
  adnexa 870.9
    specified region NEC 870.8
  laceration (*see also* Laceration, ocular) 871.4
  muscle (extraocular) 870.3
    with foreign body 870.4
    eyelid 870.1
    intraocular — *see* Wound, open, eyeball

Wound, open — *continued*
  ocular NEC — *continued*
    penetrating (*see also* Penetrating wound,
      ocular) 871.7
  orbit 870.8
    penetrating 870.3
      with foreign body 870.4
  orbital region 870.9
  ovary — *see* Injury, internal, pelvic organs
  palate 873.65
    complicated 873.75
  palm 882.0
    with tendon involvement 882.2
    complicated 882.1
  parathyroid (gland) 874.2
    complicated 874.3
  parietal region — *see* Wound, open, scalp
  pelvic floor or region 879.6
    complicated 879.7
  penis 878.0
    complicated 878.1
  perineum 879.6
    complicated 879.7
  periocular area 870.8
    laceration of skin 870.0
  pharynx 874.4
    complicated 874.5
  pinna 872.01
    complicated 872.11
  popliteal space 891.0
    with tendon involvement 891.2
    complicated 891.1
  prepuce 878.0
    complicated 878.1
  pubic region 879.2
    complicated 879.3
  pudenda 878.8
    complicated 878.9
  rectovaginal septum 878.8
    complicated 878.9
  sacral region 877.0
    complicated 877.1
  sacroiliac region 877.0
    complicated 877.1
  salivary (ducts) (glands) 873.69
    complicated 873.79
  scalp 873.0
    complicated 873.1
  scalpel, fetus or newborn 767.8
  scapular region 880.01
    with tendon involvement 880.21
    complicated 880.11
    involving other sites of upper arm 880.09
      with tendon involvement 880.29
      complicated 880.19
  sclera — (*see also* Wound, open, intraocular)
    871.9
  scrotum 878.2
    complicated 878.3
  seminal vesicle — *see* Injury, internal, pelvic
    organs
  shin 891.0
    with tendon involvement 891.2
    complicated 891.1
  shoulder 880.00
    with tendon involvement 880.20
    complicated 880.10
    involving other sites of upper arm 880.09
      with tendon involvement 880.29
      complicated 880.19
  skin NEC 879.8
    complicated 879.9
  skull — *see also* Injury, intracranial, with open
    intracranial wound
    with skull fracture — *see* Fracture, skull
  spermatic cord (scrotal) 878.2
    complicated 878.3
    pelvic region — *see* Injury, internal,
      spermatic cord
  spinal cord — *see* Injury, spinal
  sternal region 875.0
    complicated 875.1
  subconjunctival — *see* Wound, open,
    intraocular
  subcutaneous NEC 879.8
    complicated 879.9
  submaxillary region 873.44
    complicated 873.54

Wound, open — *continued*
  submental region 873.44
    complicated 873.54
  subungual
    finger(s) (thumb) — *see* Wound, open, finger
    toe(s) — *see* Wound, open, toe
  supraclavicular region 874.8
    complicated 874.9
  supraorbital 873.42
    complicated 873.52
  surgical, non-healing 998.83
  temple 873.49
    complicated 873.59
  temporal region 873.49
    complicated 873.59
  testis 878.2
    complicated 878.3
  thigh 890.0
    with tendon involvement 890.2
    complicated 890.1
  thorax, thoracic (external) 875.0
    complicated 875.1
  throat 874.8
    complicated 874.9
  thumb (nail) (subungual) 883.0
    with tendon involvement 883.2
    complicated 883.1
  thyroid (gland) 874.2
    complicated 874.3
  toe(s) (nail) (subungual) 893.0
    with tendon involvement 893.2
    complicated 893.1
  tongue 873.64
    complicated 873.74
  tonsil — *see* Wound, open, neck
  trachea (cervical region) 874.02
    with larynx 874.00
      complicated 874.10
    complicated 874.12
    intrathoracic — *see* Injury, internal, trachea
  trunk (multiple) NEC 879.6
    complicated 879.7
    specified site NEC 879.6
      complicated 879.7
  tunica vaginalis 878.2
    complicated 878.3
  tympanic membrane 872.61
    complicated 872.71
  tympanum 872.61
    complicated 872.71
  umbilical region 879.2
    complicated 879.3
  ureter — *see* Injury, internal, ureter
  urethra — *see* Injury, internal, urethra
  uterus — *see* Injury, internal, uterus
  uvula 873.69
    complicated 873.79
  vagina 878.6
    complicated 878.7
  vas deferens — *see* Injury, internal, vas
    deferens
  vitreous (humor) 871.2
  vulva 878.4
    complicated 878.5
  wrist 881.02
    with tendon involvement 881.22
    complicated 881.12

Wright's syndrome (hyperabduction) 447.8
  pneumonia 390 [517.1]

Wringer injury — *see* Crush injury, by site

Wrinkling of skin 701.8

Wrist — *see also* condition
  drop (acquired) 736.05

Wrong drug (given in error) NEC 977.9
  specified drug or substance — *see* Table of
    Drugs and Chemicals

Wry neck — *see also* Torticollis
  congenital 754.1

Wuchereria infestation 125.0
  bancrofti 125.0
  Brugia malayi 125.1
  malayi 125.1

Wuchereriasis 125.0

Wuchereriosis 125.0

Wuchernde struma langhans (M8332/3) 193

X

Xanthelasma 272.2
  eyelid 272.2 [374.51]
  palpebrarum 272.2 [374.51]

Xanthelasmatosis (essential) 272.2

Xanthelasmoidea 757.33

Xanthine stones 277.2

Xanthinuria 277.2

Xanthofibroma (M8831/0) — *see* Neoplasm,
  connective tissue, benign

Xanthoma(s), xanthomatosis 272.2
  with
    hyperlipoproteinemia
      type I 272.3
      type III 272.2
      type IV 272.1
      type V 272.3
  bone 272.7
  craniohypophyseal 277.8
  cutaneotendinous 272.7
  diabeticorum 250.8 ✓5ᵗʰ [272.2]
  disseminatum 272.7
  eruptive 272.2
  eyelid 272.2 [374.51]
  familial 272.7
  hereditary 272.7
  hypercholesterinemic 272.0
  hypercholesterolemic 272.0
  hyperlipemic 272.4
  hyperlipidemic 272.4
  infantile 272.7
  joint 272.7
  juvenile 272.7
  multiple 272.7
  multiplex 272.7
  primary familial 272.7
  tendon (sheath) 272.7
  tuberosum 272.2
  tuberous 272.2
  tubo-eruptive 272.2

Xanthosis 709.09
  surgical 998.81

Xenophobia 300.29

Xeroderma (congenital) 757.39
  acquired 701.1
    eyelid 373.33
  eyelid 373.33
  pigmentosum 757.33
  vitamin A deficiency 264.8

Xerophthalmia 372.53
  vitamin A deficiency 264.7

Xerosis
  conjunctiva 372.53
    with Bitôt's spot 372.53
      vitamin A deficiency 264.1
    vitamin A deficiency 264.0
  cornea 371.40
    with corneal ulceration 370.00
      vitamin A deficiency 264.3
    vitamin A deficiency 264.2
  cutis 706.8
  skin 706.8

Xerostomia 527.7

Xiphodynia 733.90

Xiphoidalgia 733.90

Xiphoiditis 733.99

Xiphopagus 759.4

XO syndrome 758.6

X-ray
  effects, adverse, NEC 990
  of chest
    for suspected tuberculosis V71.2
    routine V72.5

XXX syndrome 758.81

XXXXY syndrome 758.81

XXY syndrome 758.7

Xyloketosuria 271.8

Xylosuria 271.8

Xylulosuria 271.8

XYY syndrome 758.81

✓4ᵗʰ Fourth-digit Required   ✓5ᵗʰ Fifth-digit Required   ▶◀ Revised Text   ● New Line   ▲ Revised Code

Y

Yawning 786.09
  psychogenic 306.1
Yaws 102.9
  bone or joint lesions 102.6
  butter 102.1
  chancre 102.0
  cutaneous, less than five years after infection
      102.2
  early (cutaneous) (macular) (maculopapular)
      (micropapular) (papular) 102.2
    frambeside 102.2
    skin lesions NEC 102.2
  eyelid 102.9 [373.4]
  ganglion 102.6
  gangosis, gangosa 102.5
  gumma, gummata 102.4
    bone 102.6
  gummatous
    frambeside 102.4
    osteitis 102.6
    periostitis 102.6
  hydrarthrosis 102.6
  hyperkeratosis (early) (late) (palmar) (plantar)
      102.3
  initial lesions 102.0
  joint lesions 102.6
  juxta-articular nodules 102.7
  late nodular (ulcerated) 102.4
  latent (without clinical manifestations) (with
      positive serology) 102.8
  mother 102.0
  mucosal 102.7
  multiple papillomata 102.1
  nodular, late (ulcerated) 102.4
  osteitis 102.6
  papilloma, papillomata (palmar) (plantar) 102.1
  periostitis (hypertrophic) 102.6
  ulcers 102.4
  wet crab 102.1
Yeast infection (*see also* Candidiasis) 112.9
Yellow
  atrophy (liver) 570
    chronic 571.8
    resulting from administration of blood,
        plasma, serum, or other biological
        substance (within 8 months of
        administration) — *see* Hepatitis, viral
  fever — *see* Fever, yellow
  jack (*see also* Fever, yellow) 060.9
  jaundice (*see also* Jaundice) 782.4
Yersinia septica 027.8

Z

Zagari's disease (xerostomia) 527.7
Zahorsky's disease (exanthema subitum) 057.8
  syndrome (herpangina) 074.0
Zenker's diverticulum (esophagus) 530.6
Ziehen-Oppenheim disease 333.6
Zieve's syndrome (jaundice, hyperlipemia, and
      hemolytic anemia) 571.1
Zika fever 066.3
Zollinger-Ellison syndrome (gastric
      hypersecretion with pancreatic islet cell
      tumor) 251.5
Zona (*see also* Herpes, zoster) 053.9
Zoophilia (erotica) 302.1
Zoophobia 300.29
Zoster (herpes) (*see also* Herpes, zoster) 053.9
Zuelzer (-Ogden) anemia or syndrome
      (nutritional megaloblastic anemia) 281.2
Zygodactyly (*see also* Syndactylism) 755.10
Zygomycosis 117.7
Zymotic — *see* condition

SECTION 2

Alphabetic Index to Poisoning and External Causes of Adverse Effects of Drugs and Other Chemical Substances

TABLE OF DRUGS AND CHEMICALS

This table contains a classification of drugs and other chemical substances to identify poisoning states and external causes of adverse effects.

Each of the listed substances in the table is assigned a code according to the poisoning classification (960-989). These codes are used when there is a statement of poisoning, overdose, wrong substance given or taken, or intoxication.

The table also contains a listing of external causes of adverse effects. An adverse effect is a pathologic manifestation due to ingestion or exposure to drugs or other chemical substances (e.g., dermatitis, hypersensitivity reaction, aspirin gastritis). The adverse effect is to be identified by the appropriate code found in Section 1, Index to Diseases and Injuries. An external cause code can then be used to identify the circumstances involved. The table headings pertaining to external causes are defined below:

> **Accidental poisoning (E850-E869)** — accidental overdose of drug, wrong substance given or taken, drug taken inadvertently, accidents in the usage of drugs and biologicals in medical and surgical procedures, and to show external causes of poisonings classifiable to 980-989.

> **Therapeutic use (E930-E949)** — a correct substance properly administered in therapeutic or prophylactic dosage as the external cause of adverse effects.

> **Suicide attempt (E950-E952)** — instances in which self-inflicted injuries or poisonings are involved.

> **Assault (E961-E962)** — injury or poisoning inflicted by another person with the intent to injure or kill.

> **Undetermined (E980-E982)** — to be used when the intent of the poisoning or injury cannot be determined whether it was intentional or accidental.

The American Hospital Formulary Service list numbers are included in the table to help classify new drugs not identified in the table by name. The AHFS list numbers are keyed to the continually revised American Hospital Formulary Service (AHFS).* These listings are found in the table under the main term **Drug.**

Excluded from the table are radium and other radioactive substances. The classification of adverse effects and complications pertaining to these substances will be found in Section 1, Index to Diseases and Injuries, and Section 3, Index to External Causes of Injuries.

Although certain substances are indexed with one or more subentries, the majority are listed according to one use or state. It is recognized that many substances may be used in various ways, in medicine and in industry, and may cause adverse effects whatever the state of the agent (solid, liquid, or fumes arising from a liquid). In cases in which the reported data indicates a use or state not in the table, or which is clearly different from the one listed, an attempt should be made to classify the substance in the form which most nearly expresses the reported facts.

*American Hospital Formulary Service, 2 vol. (Washington, D.C.: American Society of Hospital Pharmacists, 1959-)

	Poisoning	External Cause (E-Code)				
		Accident	Therapeutic Use	Suicide Attempt	Assault	Undetermined
1-propanol	980.3	E860.4	—	E950.9	E962.1	E980.9
2-propanol	980.2	E860.3	—	E950.9	E962.1	E980.9
2, 4-D (dichlorophenoxyacetic acid)	989.4	E863.5	—	E950.6	E962.1	E980.7
2, 4-toluene diisocyanate	983.0	E864.0	—	E950.7	E962.1	E980.6
2, 4, 5-T (trichlorophenoxyacetic acid)	989.2	E863.5	—	E950.6	E962.1	E980.7
14-hydroxydihydromorphinone	965.09	E850.2	E935.2	E950.0	E962.0	E980.0
ABOB	961.7	E857	E931.7	E950.4	E962.0	E980.4
Abrus (seed)	988.2	E865.3	—	E950.9	E962.1	E980.9
Absinthe	980.0	E860.1	—	E950.9	E962.1	E980.9
beverage	980.0	E860.0	—	E950.9	E962.1	E980.9
Acenocoumarin, acenocoumarol	964.2	E858.2	E934.2	E950.4	E962.0	E980.4
Acepromazine	969.1	E853.0	E939.1	E950.3	E962.0	E980.3
Acetal	982.8	E862.4	—	E950.9	E962.1	E980.9
Acetaldehyde (vapor)	987.8	E869.8	—	E952.8	E962.2	E982.8
liquid	989.89	E866.8	—	E950.9	E962.1	E980.9
Acetaminophen	965.4	E850.4	E935.4	E950.0	E962.0	E980.0
Acetaminosalol	965.1	E850.3	E935.3	E950.0	E962.0	E980.0
Acetanilid(e)	965.4	E850.4	E935.4	E950.0	E962.0	E980.0
Acetarsol, acetarsone	961.1	E857	E931.1	E950.4	E962.0	E980.4
Acetazolamide	974.2	E858.5	E944.2	E950.4	E962.0	E980.4
Acetic						
acid	983.1	E864.1	—	E950.7	E962.1	E980.6
with sodium acetate (ointment)	976.3	E858.7	E946.3	E950.4	E962.0	E980.4
irrigating solution	974.5	E858.5	E944.5	E950.4	E962.0	E980.4
lotion	976.2	E858.7	E946.2	E950.4	E962.0	E980.4
anhydride	983.1	E864.1	—	E950.7	E962.1	E980.6
ether (vapor)	982.8	E862.4	—	E950.9	E962.1	E980.9
Acetohexamide	962.3	E858.0	E932.3	E950.4	E962.0	E980.4
Acetomenaphthone	964.3	E858.2	E934.3	E950.4	E962.0	E980.4
Acetomorphine	965.01	E850.0	E935.0	E950.0	E962.0	E980.0
Acetone (oils) (vapor)	982.8	E862.4	—	E950.9	E962.1	E980.9
Acetophenazine (maleate)	969.1	E853.0	E939.1	E950.3	E962.0	E980.3
Acetophenetidin	965.4	E850.4	E935.4	E950.0	E962.0	E980.0
Acetophenone	982.0	E862.4	—	E950.9	E962.1	E980.9
Acetorphine	965.09	E850.2	E935.2	E950.0	E962.0	E980.0
Acetosulfone (sodium)	961.8	E857	E931.8	E950.4	E962.0	E980.4
Acetrizoate (sodium)	977.8	E858.8	E947.8	E950.4	E962.0	E980.4
Acetylcarbromal	967.3	E852.2	E937.3	E950.2	E962.0	E980.2
Acetylcholine (chloride)	971.0	E855.3	E941.0	E950.4	E962.0	E980.4
Acetylcysteine	975.5	E858.6	E945.5	E950.4	E962.0	E980.4
Acetyldigitoxin	972.1	E858.3	E942.1	E950.4	E962.0	E980.4
Acetyldihydrocodeine	965.09	E850.2	E935.2	E950.0	E962.0	E980.0
Acetyldihydrocodeinone	965.09	E850.2	E935.2	E950.0	E962.0	E980.0
Acetylene (gas) (industrial)	987.1	E868.1	—	E951.8	E962.2	E981.8
incomplete combustion of — see Carbon monoxide, fuel, utility						
tetrachloride (vapor)	982.3	E862.4	—	E950.9	E962.1	E980.9
Acetyliodosalicylic acid	965.1	E850.3	E935.3	E950.0	E962.0	E980.0
Acetylphenylhydrazine	965.8	E850.8	E935.8	E950.0	E962.0	E980.0
Acetylsalicylic acid	965.1	E850.3	E935.3	E950.0	E962.0	E980.0
Achromycin	960.4	E856	E930.4	E950.4	E962.0	E980.4
ophthalmic preparation	976.5	E858.7	E946.5	E950.4	E962.0	E980.4
topical NEC	976.0	E858.7	E946.0	E950.4	E962.0	E980.4
Acidifying agents	963.2	E858.1	E933.2	E950.4	E962.0	E980.4
Acids (corrosive) NEC	983.1	E864.1	—	E950.7	E962.1	E980.6
Aconite (wild)	988.2	E865.4	—	E950.9	E962.1	E980.9
Aconitine (liniment)	976.8	E858.7	E946.8	E950.4	E962.0	E980.4
Aconitum ferox	988.2	E865.4	—	E950.9	E962.1	E980.9
Acridine	983.0	E864.0	—	E950.7	E962.1	E980.6
vapor	987.8	E869.8	—	E952.8	E962.2	E982.8
Acriflavine	961.9	E857	E931.9	E950.4	E962.0	E980.4
Acrisorcin	976.0	E858.7	E946.0	E950.4	E962.0	E980.4
Acrolein (gas)	987.8	E869.8	—	E952.8	E962.2	E982.8
liquid	989.89	E866.8	—	E950.9	E962.1	E980.9
Actaea spicata	988.2	E865.4	—	E950.9	E962.1	E980.9
Acterol	961.5	E857	E931.5	E950.4	E962.0	E980.4
ACTH	962.4	E858.0	E932.4	E950.4	E962.0	E980.4
Acthar	962.4	E858.0	E932.4	E950.4	E962.0	E980.4
Actinomycin (C)(D)	960.7	E856	E930.7	E950.4	E962.0	E980.4
Adalin (acetyl)	967.3	E852.2	E937.3	E950.2	E962.0	E980.2
Adenosine (phosphate)	977.8	E858.8	E947.8	E950.4	E962.0	E980.4
Adhesives	989.89	E866.6	—	E950.9	E962.1	E980.9
ADH	962.5	E858.0	E932.5	E950.4	E962.0	E980.4
Adicillin	960.0	E856	E930.0	E950.4	E962.0	E980.4
Adiphenine	975.1	E855.6	E945.1	E950.4	E962.0	E980.4
Adjunct, pharmaceutical	977.4	E858.8	E947.4	E950.4	E962.0	E980.4
Adrenal (extract, cortex or medulla) (glucocorticoids) (hormones)						
(mineralocorticoids)	962.0	E858.0	E932.0	E950.4	E962.0	E980.4
ENT agent	976.6	E858.7	E946.6	E950.4	E962.0	E980.4
ophthalmic preparation	976.5	E858.7	E946.5	E950.4	E962.0	E980.4
topical NEC	976.0	E858.7	E946.0	E950.4	E962.0	E980.4
Adrenalin	971.2	E855.5	E941.2	E950.4	E962.0	E980.4

	Poisoning	External Cause (E-Code)				
		Accident	Therapeutic Use	Suicide Attempt	Assault	Undetermined
Adrenergic blocking agents	971.3	E855.6	E941.3	E950.4	E962.0	E980.4
Adrenergics	971.2	E855.5	E941.2	E950.4	E962.0	E980.4
Adrenochrome (derivatives)	972.8	E858.3	E942.8	E950.4	E962.0	E980.4
Adrenocorticotropic hormone	962.4	E858.0	E932.4	E950.4	E962.0	E980.4
Adrenocorticotropin	962.4	E858.0	E932.4	E950.4	E962.0	E980.4
Adriamycin	960.7	E856	E930.7	E950.4	E962.0	E980.4
Aerosol spray — *see* Sprays						
Aerosporin	960.8	E856	E930.8	E950.4	E962.0	E980.4
ENT agent	976.6	E858.7	E946.6	E950.4	E962.0	E980.4
ophthalmic preparation	976.5	E858.7	E946.5	E950.4	E962.0	E980.4
topical NEC	976.0	E858.7	E946.0	E950.4	E962.0	E980.4
Aethusa cynapium	988.2	E865.4	—	E950.9	E962.1	E980.9
Afghanistan black	969.6	E854.1	E939.6	E950.3	E962.0	E980.3
Aflatoxin	989.7	E865.9	—	E950.9	E962.1	E980.9
African boxwood	988.2	E865.4	—	E950.9	E962.1	E980.9
Agar (-agar)	973.3	E858.4	E943.3	E950.4	E962.0	E980.4
Agricultural agent NEC	989.89	E863.9	—	E950.6	E962.1	E980.7
Agrypnal	967.0	E851	E937.0	E950.1	E962.0	E980.1
Air contaminant(s), source or type not specified	987.9	E869.9	—	E952.9	E962.2	E982.9
specified type — *see* specific substance						
Akee	988.2	E865.4	—	E950.9	E962.1	E980.9
Akrinol	976.0	E858.7	E946.0	E950.4	E962.0	E980.4
Alantolactone	961.6	E857	E931.6	E950.4	E962.0	E980.4
Albamycin	960.8	E856	E930.8	E950.4	E962.0	E980.4
Albumin (normal human serum)	964.7	E858.2	E934.7	E950.4	E962.0	E980.4
Albuterol ●	975.7	E858.6	E945.7	E950.4	E962.0	E980.4
Alcohol	980.9	E860.9	—	E950.9	E962.1	E980.9
absolute	980.0	E860.1	—	E950.9	E962.1	E980.9
beverage	980.0	E860.0	E947.8	E950.9	E962.1	E980.9
amyl	980.3	E860.4	—	E950.9	E962.1	E980.9
antifreeze	980.1	E860.2	—	E950.9	E962.1	E980.9
butyl	980.3	E860.4	—	E950.9	E962.1	E980.9
dehydrated	980.0	E860.1	—	E950.9	E862.1	E980.9
beverage	980.0	E860.0	E947.8	E950.9	E962.1	E980.9
denatured	980.0	E860.1	—	E950.9	E962.1	E980.9
deterrents	977.3	E858.8	E947.3	E950.4	E962.0	E980.4
diagnostic (gastric function)	977.8	E858.8	E947.8	E950.4	E962.0	E980.4
ethyl	980.0	E860.1	—	E950.9	E962.1	E980.9
beverage	980.0	E860.0	E947.8	E950.9	E962.1	E980.9
grain	980.0	E860.1	—	E950.9	E962.1	E980.9
beverage	980.0	E860.0	E947.8	E950.9	E962.1	E980.9
industrial	980.9	E860.9	—	E950.9	E962.1	E980.9
isopropyl	980.2	E860.3	—	E950.9	E962.1	E980.9
methyl	980.1	E860.2	—	E950.9	E962.1	E980.9
preparation for consumption	980.0	E860.0	E947.8	E950.9	E962.1	E980.9
propyl	980.3	E860.4	—	E950.9	E962.1	E980.9
secondary	980.2	E860.3	—	E950.9	E962.1	E980.9
radiator	980.1	E860.2	—	E950.9	E962.1	E980.9
rubbing	980.2	E860.3	—	E950.9	E962.1	E980.9
specified type NEC	980.8	E860.8	—	E950.9	E962.1	E980.9
surgical	980.9	E860.9	—	E950.9	E962.1	E980.9
vapor (from any type of alcohol)	987.8	E869.8	—	E952.8	E962.2	E982.8
wood	980.1	E860.2	—	E950.9	E962.1	E980.9
Alcuronium chloride	975.2	E858.6	E945.2	E950.4	E962.0	E980.4
Aldactone	974.4	E858.5	E944.4	E950.4	E962.0	E980.4
Aldicarb	989.3	E863.2	—	E950.6	E962.1	E980.7
Aldomet	972.6	E858.3	E942.6	E950.4	E962.0	E980.4
Aldosterone	962.0	E858.0	E932.0	E950.4	E962.0	E980.4
Aldrin (dust)	989.2	E863.0	—	E950.6	E962.1	E980.7
Algeldrate	973.0	E858.4	E943.0	E950.4	E962.0	E980.4
Alidase	963.4	E858.1	E933.4	E950.4	E962.0	E980.4
Aliphatic thiocyanates	989.0	E866.8	—	E950.9	E962.1	E980.9
Alkaline antiseptic solution (aromatic)	976.6	E858.7	E946.6	E950.4	E962.0	E980.4
Alkalinizing agents (medicinal)	963.3	E858.1	E933.3	E950.4	E962.0	E980.4
Alkalis, caustic	983.2	E864.2	—	E950.7	E962.1	E980.6
Alkalizing agents (medicinal)	963.3	E858.1	E933.3	E950.4	E962.0	E980.4
Alka-seltzer	965.1	E850.3	E935.3	E950.0	E962.0	E980.0
Alkavervir	972.6	E858.3	E942.6	E950.4	E962.0	E980.4
Allegron	969.0	E854.0	E939.0	E950.3	E962.0	E980.3
Alleve — *see* Naproxen						
Allobarbital, allobarbitone	967.0	E851	E937.0	E950.1	E962.0	E980.1
Allopurinol	974.7	E858.5	E944.7	E950.4	E962.0	E980.4
Allylestrenol	962.2	E858.0	E932.2	E950.4	E962.0	E980.4
Allylisopropylacetylurea	967.8	E852.8	E937.8	E950.2	E962.0	E980.2
Allylisopropylmalonylurea	967.0	E851	E937.0	E950.1	E962.0	E980.1
Allyltribromide	967.3	E852.2	E937.3	E950.2	E962.0	E980.2
Aloe, aloes, aloin	973.1	E858.4	E943.1	E950.4	E962.0	E980.4
Alosetron	973.8	E858.4	E943.8	E950.4	E962.0	E980.4
Aloxidone	966.0	E855.0	E936.0	E950.4	E962.0	E980.4
Aloxiprin	965.1	E850.3	E935.3	E950.0	E962.0	E980.0
Alpha amylase	963.4	E858.1	E933.4	E950.4	E962.0	E980.4

		External Cause (E-Code)				
	Poisoning	Accident	Therapeutic Use	Suicide Attempt	Assault	Undetermined
Alphaprodine (hydrochloride)	965.09	E850.2	E935.2	E950.0	E962.0	E980.0
Alpha tocopherol	963.5	E858.1	E933.5	E950.4	E962.0	E980.4
Alseroxylon	972.6	E858.3	E942.6	E950.4	E962.0	E980.4
Alum (ammonium) (potassium)	983.2	E864.2	—	E950.7	E962.1	E980.6
medicinal (astringent) NEC	976.2	E858.7	E946.2	E950.4	E962.0	E980.4
Aluminium, aluminum (gel) (hydroxide)	973.0	E858.4	E943.0	E950.4	E962.0	E980.4
acetate solution	976.2	E858.7	E946.2	E950.4	E962.0	E980.4
aspirin	965.1	E850.3	E935.3	E950.0	E962.0	E980.0
carbonate	973.0	E858.4	E943.0	E950.4	E962.0	E980.4
glycinate	973.0	E858.4	E943.0	E950.4	E962.0	E980.4
nicotinate	972.2	E858.3	E942.2	E950.4	E962.0	E980.4
ointment (surgical) (topical)	976.3	E858.7	E946.3	E950.4	E962.0	E980.4
phosphate	973.0	E858.4	E943.0	E950.4	E962.0	E980.4
subacetate	976.2	E858.7	E946.2	E950.4	E962.0	E980.4
topical NEC	976.3	E858.7	E946.3	E950.4	E962.0	E980.4
Alurate	967.0	E851	E937.0	E950.1	E962.0	E980.1
Alverine (citrate)	975.1	E858.6	E945.1	E950.4	E962.0	E980.4
Alvodine	965.09	E850.2	E935.2	E950.0	E962.0	E980.0
Amanita phalloides	988.1	E865.5	—	E950.9	E962.1	E980.9
Amantadine (hydrochloride)	966.4	E855.0	E936.4	E950.4	E962.0	E980.4
Ambazone	961.9	E857	E931.9	E950.4	E962.0	E980.4
Ambenonium	971.0	E855.3	E941.0	E950.4	E962.0	E980.4
Ambutonium bromide	971.1	E855.4	E941.1	E950.4	E962.0	E980.4
Ametazole	977.8	E858.8	E947.8	E950.4	E962.0	E980.4
Amethocaine (infiltration) (topical)	968.5	E855.2	E938.5	E950.4	E962.0	E980.4
nerve block (peripheral) (plexus)	968.6	E855.2	E938.6	E950.4	E962.0	E980.4
spinal	968.7	E855.2	E938.7	E950.4	E962.0	E980.4
Amethopterin	963.1	E858.1	E933.1	E950.4	E962.0	E980.4
Amfepramone	977.0	E858.8	E947.0	E950.4	E962.0	E980.4
Amidon	965.02	E850.1	E935.1	E950.0	E962.0	E980.0
Amidopyrine	965.5	E850.5	E935.5	E950.0	E962.0	E980.0
Aminacrine	976.0	E858.7	E946.0	E950.4	E962.0	E980.4
Aminitrozole	961.5	E857	E931.5	E950.4	E962.0	E980.4
Aminoacetic acid	974.5	E858.5	E944.5	E950.4	E962.0	E980.4
Amino acids	974.5	E858.5	E944.5	E950.4	E962.0	E980.4
Aminocaproic acid	964.4	E858.2	E934.4	E950.4	E962.0	E980.4
Aminoethylisothiourium	963.8	E858.1	E933.8	E950.4	E962.0	E980.4
Aminoglutethimide	966.3	E855.0	E936.3	E950.4	E962.0	E980.4
Aminometradine	974.3	E858.5	E944.3	E950.4	E962.0	E980.4
Aminopentamide	971.1	E855.4	E941.1	E950.4	E962.0	E980.4
Aminophenazone	965.5	E850.5	E935.5	E950.0	E962.0	E980.0
Aminophenol	983.0	E864.0	—	E950.7	E962.1	E980.6
Aminophenylpyridone	969.5	E853.8	E939.5	E950.3	E962.0	E980.3
Aminophyllin	975.7	E858.6	E945.7	E950.4	E962.0	E980.4
Aminopterin	963.1	E858.1	E933.1	E950.4	E962.0	E980.4
Aminopyrine	965.5	E850.5	E935.5	E950.0	E962.0	E980.0
Aminosalicylic acid	961.8	E857	E931.8	E950.4	E962.0	E980.4
Amiphenazole	970.1	E854.3	E940.1	E950.4	E962.0	E980.4
Amiquinsin	972.6	E858.3	E942.6	E950.4	E962.0	E980.4
Amisometradine	974.3	E858.5	E944.3	E950.4	E962.0	E980.4
Amitriptyline	969.0	E854.0	E939.0	E950.3	E962.0	E980.3
Ammonia (fumes) (gas) (vapor)	987.8	E869.8	—	E952.8	E962.2	E982.8
liquid (household) NEC	983.2	E861.4	—	E950.7	E962.1	E980.6
spirit, aromatic	970.8	E854.3	E940.8	E950.4	E962.0	E980.4
Ammoniated mercury	976.0	E858.7	E946.0	E950.4	E962.0	E980.4
Ammonium						
carbonate	983.2	E864.2	—	E950.7	E962.1	E980.6
chloride (acidifying agent)	963.2	E858.1	E933.2	E950.4	E962.0	E980.4
expectorant	975.5	E858.6	E945.5	E950.4	E962.0	E980.4
compounds (household) NEC	983.2	E861.4	—	E950.7	E962.1	E980.6
fumes (any usage)	987.8	E869.8	—	E952.8	E962.2	E982.8
industrial	983.2	E864.2	—	E950.7	E962.1	E980.6
ichthyosulfonate	976.4	E858.7	E946.4	E950.4	E962.0	E980.4
mandelate	961.9	E857	E931.9	E950.4	E962.0	E980.4
Amobarbital	967.0	E851	E937.0	E950.1	E962.0	E980.1
Amodiaquin(e)	961.4	E857	E931.4	E950.4	E962.0	E980.4
Amopyroquin(e)	961.4	E857	E931.4	E950.4	E962.0	E980.4
Amphenidone	969.5	E853.8	E939.5	E950.3	E962.0	E980.3
Amphetamine	969.7	E854.2	E939.7	E950.3	E962.0	E980.3
Amphomycin	960.8	E856	E930.8	E950.4	E962.0	E980.4
Amphotericin B	960.1	E856	E930.1	E950.4	E962.0	E980.4
topical	976.0	E858.7	E946.0	E950.4	E962.0	E980.4
Ampicillin	960.0	E856	E930.0	E950.4	E962.0	E980.4
Amprotropine	971.1	E855.4	E941.1	E950.4	E962.0	E980.4
Amygdalin	977.8	E858.8	E947.8	E950.4	E962.0	E980.4
Amyl						
acetate (vapor)	982.8	E862.4	—	E950.9	E962.1	E980.9
alcohol	980.3	E860.4	—	E950.9	E962.1	E980.9
nitrite (medicinal)	972.4	E858.3	E942.4	E950.4	E962.0	E980.4
Amylase (alpha)	963.4	E858.1	E933.4	E950.4	E962.0	E980.4
Amylene hydrate	980.8	E860.8	—	E950.9	E962.1	E980.9

	Poisoning	External Cause (E-Code)				
		Accident	Therapeutic Use	Suicide Attempt	Assault	Undetermined
Amylobarbitone	967.0	E851	E937.0	E950.1	E962.0	E980.1
Amylocaine	968.9	E855.2	E938.9	E950.4	E962.0	E980.4
infiltration (subcutaneous)	968.5	E855.2	E938.5	E950.4	E962.0	E980.4
nerve block (peripheral) (plexus)	968.6	E855.2	E938.6	E950.4	E962.0	E980.4
spinal	968.7	E855.2	E938.7	E950.4	E962.0	E980.4
topical (surface)	968.5	E855.2	E938.5	E950.4	E962.0	E980.4
Amytal (sodium)	967.0	E851	E937.0	E950.1	E962.0	E980.1
Analeptics	970.0	E854.3	E940.0	E950.4	E962.0	E980.4
Analgesics	965.9	E850.9	E935.9	E950.0	E962.0	E980.0
aromatic NEC	965.4	E850.4	E935.4	E950.0	E962.0	E980.0
non-narcotic NEC	965.7	E850.7	E935.7	E950.0	E962.0	E980.0
specified NEC	965.8	E850.8	E935.8	E950.0	E962.0	E980.0
Anamirta cocculus	988.2	E865.3	—	E950.9	E962.1	E980.9
Ancillin	960.0	E856	E930.0	E950.4	E962.0	E980.4
Androgens (anabolic congeners)	962.1	E858.0	E932.1	E950.4	E962.0	E980.4
Androstalone	962.1	E858.0	E932.1	E950.4	E962.0	E980.4
Androsterone	962.1	E858.0	E932.1	E950.4	E962.0	E980.4
Anemone pulsatilla	988.2	E865.4	—	E950.9	E962.1	E980.9
Anesthesia, anesthetic (general) NEC	968.4	E855.1	E938.4	E950.4	E962.0	E980.4
block (nerve) (plexus)	968.6	E855.2	E938.6	E950.4	E962.0	E980.4
gaseous NEC	968.2	E855.1	E938.2	E950.4	E962.0	E980.4
halogenated hydrocarbon derivatives NEC	968.2	E855.1	E938.2	E950.4	E962.0	E980.4
infiltration (intradermal) (subcutaneous) (submucosal)	968.5	E855.2	E938.5	E950.4	E962.0	E980.4
intravenous	968.3	E855.1	E938.3	E950.4	E962.0	E980.4
local NEC	968.9	E855.2	E938.9	E950.4	E962.0	E980.4
nerve blocking (peripheral) (plexus)	968.6	E855.2	E938.6	E950.4	E962.0	E980.4
rectal NEC	968.3	E855.1	E938.3	E950.4	E962.0	E980.4
spinal	968.7	E855.2	E938.7	E950.4	E962.0	E980.4
surface	968.5	E855.2	E938.5	E950.4	E962.0	E980.4
topical	968.5	E855.2	E938.5	E950.4	E962.0	E980.4
Aneurine	963.5	E858.1	E933.5	E950.4	E962.0	E980.4
Angio-Conray	977.8	E858.8	E947.8	E950.4	E962.0	E980.4
Angiotensin	971.2	E855.5	E941.2	E950.4	E962.0	E980.4
Anhydrohydroxyprogesterone	962.2	E858.0	E932.2	E950.4	E962.0	E980.4
Anhydron	974.3	E858.5	E944.3	E950.4	E962.0	E980.4
Anileridine	965.09	E850.2	E935.2	E950.0	E962.0	E980.0
Aniline (dye) (liquid)	983.0	E864.0	—	E950.7	E962.1	E980.6
analgesic	965.4	E850.4	E935.4	E950.0	E962.0	E980.0
derivatives, therapeutic NEC	965.4	E850.4	E935.4	E950.0	E962.0	E980.0
vapor	987.8	E869.8	—	E952.8	E962.2	E982.8
Anisindione	964.2	E858.2	E934.2	E950.4	E962.0	E980.4
Aniscoropine	971.1	E855.4	E941.1	E950.4	E962.0	E980.4
Anorexic agents	977.0	E858.8	E947.0	E950.4	E962.0	E980.4
Ant (bite) (sting)	989.5	E905.5	—	E950.9	E962.1	E980.9
Antabuse	977.3	E858.8	E947.3	E950.4	E962.0	E980.4
Antacids	973.0	E858.4	E943.0	E950.4	E962.0	E980.4
Antazoline	963.0	E858.1	E933.0	E950.4	E962.0	E980.4
Anthelmintics	961.6	E857	E931.6	E950.4	E962.0	E980.4
Anthralin	976.4	E858.7	E946.4	E950.4	E962.0	E980.4
Anthramycin	960.7	E856	E930.7	E950.4	E962.0	E980.4
Antiadrenergics	971.3	E855.6	E941.3	E950.4	E962.0	E980.4
Antiallergic agents	963.0	E858.1	E933.0	E950.4	E962.0	E980.4
Antianemic agents NEC	964.1	E858.2	E934.1	E950.4	E962.0	E980.4
Antiaris toxicaria	988.2	E865.4	—	E950.9	E962.1	E980.9
Antiarteriosclerotic agents	972.2	E858.3	E942.2	E950.4	E962.0	E980.4
Antiasthmatics	975.7	E858.6	E945.7	E950.4	E962.0	E980.4
Antibiotics	960.9	E856	E930.9	E950.4	E962.0	E980.4
antifungal	960.1	E856	E930.1	E950.4	E962.0	E980.4
antimycobacterial	960.6	E856	E930.6	E950.4	E962.0	E980.4
antineoplastic	960.7	E856	E930.7	E950.4	E962.0	E980.4
cephalosporin (group)	960.5	E856	E930.5	E950.4	E962.0	E980.4
chloramphenicol (group)	960.2	E856	E930.2	E950.4	E962.0	E980.4
macrolides	960.3	E856	E930.3	E950.4	E962.0	E980.4
specified NEC	960.8	E856	E930.8	E950.4	E962.0	E980.4
tetracycline (group)	960.4	E856	E930.4	E950.4	E962.0	E980.4
Anticancer agents NEC	963.1	E858.1	E933.1	E950.4	E962.0	E980.4
antibiotics	960.7	E856	E930.7	E950.4	E962.0	E980.4
Anticholinergics	971.1	E855.4	E941.1	E950.4	E962.0	E980.4
Anticholinesterase (organophosphorus) (reversible)	971.0	E855.3	E941.0	E950.4	E962.0	E980.4
Anticoagulants	964.2	E858.2	E934.2	E950.4	E962.0	E980.4
antagonists	964.5	E858.2	E934.5	E950.4	E962.0	E980.4
Anti-common cold agents NEC	975.6	E858.6	E945.6	E950.4	E962.0	E980.4
Anticonvulsants NEC	966.3	E855.0	E936.3	E950.4	E962.0	E980.4
Antidepressants	969.0	E854.0	E939.0	E950.3	E962.0	E980.3
Antidiabetic agents	962.3	E858.0	E932.3	E950.4	E962.0	E980.4
Antidiarrheal agents	973.5	E858.4	E943.5	E950.4	E962.0	E980.4
Antidiuretic hormone	962.5	E858.0	E932.5	E950.4	E962.0	E980.4
Antidotes NEC	977.2	E858.8	E947.2	E950.4	E962.0	E980.4
Antiemetic agents	963.0	E858.1	E933.0	E950.4	E962.0	E980.4
Antiepilepsy agent NEC	966.3	E855.0	E936.3	E950.4	E962.0	E980.4
Antifertility pills	962.2	E858.0	E932.2	E950.4	E962.0	E980.4

✔4ᵗʰ Fourth-digit Required   ✔5ᵗʰ Fifth-digit Required   ▶◀ Revised Text   ● New Line   ▲ Revised Code

	Poisoning	External Cause (E-Code)				
		Accident	Therapeutic Use	Suicide Attempt	Assault	Undetermined
Antiflatulents	973.8	E858.4	E943.8	E950.4	E962.0	E980.4
Antifreeze	989.89	E866.8	—	E950.9	E962.1	E980.9
alcohol	980.1	E860.2	—	E950.9	E962.1	E980.9
ethylene glycol	982.8	E862.4	—	E950.9	E962.1	E980.9
Antifungals (nonmedicinal) (sprays)	989.4	E863.6	—	E950.6	E962.1	E980.7
medicinal NEC	961.9	E857	E931.9	E950.4	E962.0	E980.4
antibiotic	960.1	E856	E930.1	E950.4	E962.0	E980.4
topical	976.0	E858.7	E946.0	E950.4	E962.0	E980.4
Antigastric secretion agents	973.0	E858.4	E943.0	E950.4	E962.0	E980.4
Anthelmintics	961.6	E857	E931.6	E950.4	E962.0	E980.4
Antihemophilic factor (human)	964.7	E858.2	E934.7	E950.4	E962.0	E980.4
Antihistamine	963.0	E858.1	E933.0	E950.4	E962.0	E980.4
Antihypertensive agents NEC	972.6	E858.3	E942.6	E950.4	E962.0	E980.4
Anti-infectives NEC	961.9	E857	E931.9	E950.4	E962.0	E980.4
antibiotics	960.9	E856	E930.9	E950.4	E962.0	E980.4
specified NEC	960.8	E856	E930.8	E950.4	E962.0	E980.4
anthelmintic	961.6	E857	E931.6	E950.4	E962.0	E980.4
antimalarial	961.4	E857	E931.4	E950.4	E962.0	E980.4
antimycobacterial NEC	961.8	E857	E931.8	E950.4	E962.0	E980.4
antibiotics	960.6	E856	E930.6	E950.4	E962.0	E980.4
antiprotozoal NEC	961.5	E857	E931.5	E950.4	E962.0	E980.4
blood	961.4	E857	E931.4	E950.4	E962.0	E980.4
antiviral	961.7	E857	E931.7	E950.4	E962.0	E980.4
arsenical	961.1	E857	E931.1	E950.4	E962.0	E980.4
ENT agents	976.6	E858.7	E946.6	E950.4	E962.0	E980.4
heavy metals NEC	961.2	E857	E931.2	E950.4	E962.0	E980.4
local	976.0	E858.7	E946.0	E950.4	E962.0	E980.4
ophthalmic preparation	976.5	E858.7	E946.5	E950.4	E962.0	E980.4
topical NEC	976.0	E858.7	E946.0	E950.4	E962.0	E980.4
Anti-inflammatory agents (topical)	976.0	E858.7	E946.0	E950.4	E962.0	E980.4
Antiknock (tetraethyl lead)	984.1	E862.1	—	E950.9	E962.1	E980.9
Antilipemics	972.2	E858.3	E942.2	E950.4	E962.0	E980.4
Antimalarials	961.4	E857	E931.4	E950.4	E962.0	E980.4
Antimony (compounds) (vapor) NEC	985.4	E866.2	—	E950.9	E962.1	E980.9
anti-infectives	961.2	E857	E931.2	E950.4	E962.0	E980.4
pesticides (vapor)	985.4	E863.4	—	E950.6	E962.2	E980.7
potassium tartrate	961.2	E857	E931.2	E950.4	E962.0	E980.4
tartrated	961.2	E857	E931.2	E950.4	E962.0	E980.4
Antimuscarinic agents	971.1	E855.4	E941.1	E950.4	E962.0	E980.4
Antimycobacterials NEC	961.8	E857	E931.8	E950.4	E962.0	E980.4
antibiotics	960.6	E856	E930.6	E950.4	E962.0	E980.4
Antineoplastic agents	963.1	E858.1	E933.1	E950.4	E962.0	E980.4
antibiotics	960.7	E856	E930.7	E950.4	E962.0	E980.4
Anti-Parkinsonism agents	966.4	E855.0	E936.4	E950.4	E962.0	E980.4
Antiphlogistics	965.69	E850.6	E935.6	E950.0	E962.0	E980.0
Antiprotozoals NEC	961.5	E857	E931.5	E950.4	E962.0	E980.4
blood	961.4	E857	E931.4	E950.4	E962.0	E980.4
Antipruritics (local)	976.1	E858.7	E946.1	E950.4	E962.0	E980.4
Antipsychotic agents NEC	969.3	E853.8	E939.3	E950.3	E962.0	E980.3
Antipyretics	965.9	E850.9	E935.9	E950.0	E962.0	E980.0
specified NEC	965.8	E850.8	E935.8	E950.0	E962.0	E980.0
Antipyrine	965.5	E850.5	E935.5	E950.0	E962.0	E980.0
Antirabies serum (equine)	979.9	E858.8	E949.9	E950.4	E962.0	E980.4
Antirheumatics	965.69	E850.6	E935.6	E950.0	E962.0	E980.0
Antiseborrheics	976.4	E858.7	E946.4	E950.4	E962.0	E980.4
Antiseptics (external) (medicinal)	976.0	E858.7	E946.0	E950.4	E962.0	E980.4
Antistine	963.0	E858.1	E933.0	E950.4	E962.0	E980.4
Antithyroid agents	962.8	E858.0	E932.8	E950.4	E962.0	E980.4
Antitoxin, any	979.9	E858.8	E949.9	E950.4	E962.0	E980.4
Antituberculars	961.8	E857	E931.8	E950.4	E962.0	E980.4
antibiotics	960.6	E856	E930.6	E950.4	E962.0	E980.4
Antitussives	975.4	E858.6	E945.4	E950.4	E962.0	E980.4
Antivaricose agents (sclerosing)	972.7	E858.3	E942.7	E950.4	E962.0	E980.4
Antivenin (crotaline) (spider-bite)	979.9	E858.8	E949.9	E950.4	E962.0	E980.4
Antivert	963.0	E858.1	E933.0	E950.4	E962.0	E980.4
Antivirals NEC	961.7	E857	E931.7	E950.4	E962.0	E980.4
Ant poisons — *see* Pesticides						
Antrol	989.4	E863.4	—	E950.6	E962.1	E980.7
fungicide	989.4	E863.6	—	E950.6	E962.1	E980.7
Apomorphine hydrochloride (emetic)	973.6	E858.4	E943.6	E950.4	E962.0	E980.4
Appetite depressants, central	977.0	E858.8	E947.0	E950.4	E962.0	E980.4
Apresoline	972.6	E858.3	E942.6	E950.4	E962.0	E980.4
Aprobarbital, aprobarbitone	967.0	E851	E937.0	E950.1	E962.0	E980.1
Apronalide	967.8	E852.8	E937.8	E950.2	E962.0	E980.2
Aqua fortis	983.1	E864.1	—	E950.7	E962.1	E980.6
Arachis oil (topical)	976.3	E858.7	E946.3	E950.4	E962.0	E980.4
cathartic	973.2	E858.4	E943.2	E950.4	E962.0	E980.4
Aralen	961.4	E857	E931.4	E950.4	E962.0	E980.4
Arginine salts	974.5	E858.5	E944.5	E950.4	E962.0	E980.4
Argyrol	976.0	E858.7	E946.0	E950.4	E962.0	E980.4
ENT agent	976.6	E858.7	E946.6	E950.4	E962.0	E980.4

✓4ᵗʰ Fourth-digit Required   ✓5ᵗʰ Fifth-digit Required   ►◄ Revised Text   ● New Line   ▲ Revised Code

	Poisoning	External Cause (E-Code)				
		Accident	Therapeutic Use	Suicide Attempt	Assault	Undetermined
Argyrol — *continued*						
ophthalmic preparation	976.5	E858.7	E946.5	E950.4	E962.0	E980.4
Aristocort	962.0	E858.0	E932.0	E950.4	E962.0	E980.4
ENT agent	976.6	E858.7	E946.6	E950.4	E962.0	E980.4
ophthalmic preparation	976.5	E858.7	E946.5	E950.4	E962.0	E980.4
topical NEC	976.0	E858.7	E946.0	E950.4	E962.0	E980.4
Aromatics, corrosive	983.0	E864.0	—	E950.7	E962.1	E980.6
disinfectants	983.0	E861.4	—	E950.7	E962.1	E980.6
Arsenate of lead (insecticide)	985.1	E863.4	—	E950.8	E962.1	E980.8
herbicide	985.1	E863.5	—	E950.8	E962.1	E980.8
Arsenic, arsenicals (compounds) (dust) (fumes) (vapor) NEC	985.1	E866.3	—	E950.8	E962.1	E980.8
anti-infectives	961.1	E857	E931.1	E950.4	E962.0	E980.4
pesticide (dust) (fumes)	985.1	E863.4	—	E950.8	E962.1	E980.8
Arsine (gas)	985.1	E866.3	—	E950.8	E962.1	E980.8
Arsphenamine (silver)	961.1	E857	E931.1	E950.4	E962.0	E980.4
Arsthinol	961.1	E857	E931.1	E950.4	E962.0	E980.4
Artane	971.1	E855.4	E941.1	E950.4	E962.0	E980.4
Arthropod (venomous) NEC	989.5	E905.5	—	E950.9	E962.1	E980.9
Asbestos	989.81	E866.8	—	E950.9	E962.1	E980.9
Ascaridole	961.6	E857	E931.6	E950.4	E962.0	E980.4
Ascorbic acid	963.5	E858.1	E933.5	E950.4	E962.0	E980.4
Asiaticoside	976.0	E858.7	E946.0	E950.4	E962.0	E980.4
Aspidium (oleoresin)	961.6	E857	E931.6	E950.4	E962.0	E980.4
Aspirin	965.1	E850.3	E935.3	E950.0	E962.0	E980.0
Astringents (local)	976.2	E858.7	E946.2	E950.4	E962.0	E980.4
Atabrine	961.3	E857	E931.3	E950.4	E962.0	E980.4
Ataractics	969.5	E853.8	E939.5	E950.3	E962.0	E980.3
Atonia drug, intestinal	973.3	E858.4	E943.3	E950.4	E962.0	E980.4
Atophan	974.7	E858.5	E944.7	E950.4	E962.0	E980.4
Atropine	971.1	E855.4	E941.1	E950.4	E962.0	E980.4
Attapulgite	973.5	E858.4	E943.5	E950.4	E962.0	E980.4
Attenuvax	979.4	E858.8	E949.4	E950.4	E962.0	E980.4
Aureomycin	960.4	E856	E930.4	E950.4	E962.0	E980.4
ophthalmic preparation	976.5	E858.7	E946.5	E950.4	E962.0	E980.4
topical NEC	976.0	E858.7	E946.0	E950.4	E962.0	E980.4
Aurothioglucose	965.69	E850.6	E935.6	E950.0	E962.0	E980.0
Aurothioglycanide	965.69	E850.6	E935.6	E950.0	E962.0	E980.0
Aurothiomalate	965.69	E850.6	E935.6	E950.0	E962.0	E980.0
Automobile fuel	981	E862.1	—	E950.9	E962.1	E980.9
Autonomic nervous system agents NEC	971.9	E855.9	E941.9	E950.4	E962.0	E980.4
Avlosulfon	961.8	E857	E931.8	E950.4	E962.0	E980.4
Avomine	967.8	E852.8	E937.8	E950.2	E962.0	E980.2
Azacyclonol	969.5	E853.8	E939.5	E950.3	E962.0	E980.3
Azapetine	971.3	E855.6	E941.3	E950.4	E962.0	E980.4
Azaribine	963.1	E858.1	E933.1	E950.4	E962.0	E980.4
Azaserine	960.7	E856	E930.7	E950.4	E962.0	E980.4
Azathioprine	963.1	E858.1	E933.1	E950.4	E962.0	E980.4
Azosulfamide	961.0	E857	E931.0	E950.4	E962.0	E980.4
Azulfidine	961.0	E857	E931.0	E950.4	E962.0	E980.4
Azuresin	977.8	E858.8	E947.8	E950.4	E962.0	E980.4
Bacimycin	976.0	E858.7	E946.0	E950.4	E962.0	E980.4
ophthalmic preparation	976.5	E858.7	E946.5	E950.4	E962.0	E980.4
Bacitracin	960.8	E856	E930.8	E950.4	E962.0	E980.4
ENT agent	976.6	E858.7	E946.6	E950.4	E962.0	E980.4
ophthalmic preparation	976.5	E858.7	E946.5	E950.4	E962.0	E980.4
topical NEC	976.0	E858.7	E946.0	E950.4	E962.0	E980.4
Baking soda	963.3	E858.1	E933.3	E950.4	E962.0	E980.4
BAL	963.8	E858.1	E933.8	E950.4	E962.0	E980.4
Bamethan (sulfate)	972.5	E858.3	E942.5	E950.4	E962.0	E980.4
Bamipine	963.0	E858.1	E933.0	E950.4	E962.0	E980.4
Baneberry	988.2	E865.4	—	E950.9	E962.1	E980.9
Banewort	988.2	E865.4	—	E950.9	E962.1	E980.9
Barbenyl	967.0	E851	E937.0	E950.1	E962.0	E980.1
Barbital, barbitone	967.0	E851	E937.0	E950.1	E962.0	E980.1
Barbiturates, barbituric acid	967.0	E851	E937.0	E950.1	E962.0	E980.1
anesthetic (intravenous)	968.3	E855.1	E938.3	E950.4	E962.0	E980.4
Barium (carbonate) (chloride) (sulfate)	985.8	E866.4	—	E950.9	E962.1	E980.9
diagnostic agent	977.8	E858.8	E947.8	E950.4	E962.0	E980.4
pesticide	985.8	E863.4	—	E950.6	E962.1	E980.7
rodenticide	985.8	E863.7	—	E950.6	E962.1	E980.7
Barrier cream	976.3	E858.7	E946.3	E950.4	E962.0	E980.4
Battery acid or fluid	983.1	E864.1	—	E950.7	E962.1	E980.6
Bay rum	980.8	E860.8	—	E950.9	E962.1	E980.9
BCG vaccine	978.0	E858.8	E948.0	E950.4	E962.0	E980.4
Bearsfoot	988.2	E865.4	—	E950.9	E962.1	E980.9
Beclamide	966.3	E855.0	E936.3	E950.4	E962.0	E980.4
Bee (sting) (venom)	989.5	E905.3	—	E950.9	E962.1	E980.9
Belladonna (alkaloids)	971.1	E855.4	E941.1	E950.4	E962.0	E980.4
Bemegride	970.0	E854.3	E940.0	E950.4	E962.0	E980.4
Benactyzine	969.8	E855.8	E939.8	E950.3	E962.0	E980.3
Benadryl	963.0	E858.1	E933.0	E950.4	E962.0	E980.4

☑4ᵗʰ Fourth-digit Required   ☑5ᵗʰ Fifth-digit Required   ▶◀ Revised Text   ● New Line   ▲ Revised Code

	Poisoning	External Cause (E-Code)				
		Accident	Therapeutic Use	Suicide Attempt	Assault	Undetermined
Bendrofluazide	974.3	E858.5	E944.3	E950.4	E962.0	E980.4
Bendroflumethiazide	974.3	E858.5	E944.3	E950.4	E962.0	E980.4
Benemid	974.7	E858.5	E944.7	E950.4	E962.0	E980.4
Benethamine penicillin G	960.0	E856	E930.0	E950.4	E962.0	E980.4
Benisone	976.0	E858.7	E946.0	E950.4	E962.0	E980.4
Benoquin	976.8	E858.7	E946.8	E950.4	E962.0	E980.4
Benoxinate	968.5	E855.2	E938.5	E950.4	E962.0	E980.4
Bentonite	976.3	E858.7	E946.3	E950.4	E962.0	E980.4
Benzalkonium (chloride)	976.0	E858.7	E946.0	E950.4	E962.0	E980.4
ophthalmic preparation	976.5	E858.7	E946.5	E950.4	E962.0	E980.4
Benzamidosalicylate (calcium)	961.8	E857	E931.8	E950.4	E962.0	E980.4
Benzathine penicillin	960.0	E856	E930.0	E950.4	E962.0	E980.4
Benzcarbimine	963.1	E858.1	E933.1	E950.4	E962.0	E980.4
Benzedrex	971.2	E855.5	E941.2	E950.4	E962.0	E980.4
Benzedrine (amphetamine)	969.7	E854.2	E939.7	E950.3	E962.0	E980.3
Benzene (acetyl) (dimethyl) (methyl) (solvent) (vapor)	982.0	E862.4	—	E950.9	E962.1	E980.9
hexachloride (gamma) (insecticide) (vapor)	989.2	E863.0	—	E950.6	E962.1	E980.7
Benzethonium	976.0	E858.7	E946.0	E950.4	E962.0	E980.4
Benzhexol (chloride)	966.4	E855.0	E936.4	E950.4	E962.0	E980.4
Benzilonium	971.1	E855.4	E941.1	E950.4	E962.0	E980.4
Benzin(e) — see Ligroin						
Benziodarone	972.4	E858.3	E942.4	E950.4	E962.0	E980.4
Benzocaine	968.5	E855.2	E938.5	E950.4	E962.0	E980.4
Benzodiapin	969.4	E853.2	E939.4	E950.3	E962.0	E980.3
Benzodiazepines (tranquilizers) NEC	969.4	E853.2	E939.4	E950.3	E962.0	E980.3
Benzoic acid (with salicylic acid) (anti-infective)	976.0	E858.7	E946.0	E950.4	E962.0	E980.4
Benzoin	976.3	E858.7	E946.3	E950.4	E962.0	E980.4
Benzol (vapor)	982.0	E862.4	—	E950.9	E962.1	E980.9
Benzomorphan	965.09	E850.2	E935.2	E950.0	E962.0	E980.0
Benzonatate	975.4	E858.6	E945.4	E950.4	E962.0	E980.4
Benzothiadiazides	974.3	E858.5	E944.3	E950.4	E962.0	E980.4
Benzoylpas	961.8	E857	E931.8	E950.4	E962.0	E980.4
Benzperidol	969.5	E853.8	E939.5	E950.3	E962.0	E980.3
Benzphetamine	977.0	E858.8	E947.0	E950.4	E962.0	E980.4
Benzpyrinium	971.0	E855.3	E941.0	E950.4	E962.0	E980.4
Benzquinamide	963.0	E858.1	E933.0	E950.4	E962.0	E980.4
Benzthiazide	974.3	E858.5	E944.3	E950.4	E962.0	E980.4
Benztropine	971.1	E855.4	E941.1	E950.4	E962.0	E980.4
Benzyl						
acetate	982.8	E862.4	—	E950.9	E962.1	E980.9
benzoate (anti-infective)	976.0	E858.7	E946.0	E950.4	E962.0	E980.4
morphine	965.09	E850.2	E935.2	E950.0	E962.0	E980.0
penicillin	960.0	E856	E930.0	E950.4	E962.0	E980.4
Bephenium hydroxynapthoate	961.6	E857	E931.6	E950.4	E962.0	E980.4
Bergamot oil	989.89	E866.8	—	E950.9	E962.1	E980.9
Berries, poisonous	988.2	E865.3	—	E950.9	E962.1	E980.9
Beryllium (compounds) (fumes)	985.3	E866.4	—	E950.9	E962.1	E980.9
Beta-carotene	976.3	E858.7	E946.3	E950.4	E962.0	E980.4
Beta-Chlor	967.1	E852.0	E937.1	E950.2	E962.0	E980.2
Betamethasone	962.0	E858.0	E932.0	E950.4	E962.0	E980.4
topical	976.0	E858.7	E946.0	E950.4	E962.0	E980.4
Betazole	977.8	E858.8	E947.8	E950.4	E962.0	E980.4
Bethanechol	971.0	E855.3	E941.0	E950.4	E962.0	E980.4
Bethanidine	972.6	E858.3	E942.6	E950.4	E962.0	E980.4
Betula oil	976.3	E858.7	E946.3	E950.4	E962.0	E980.4
Bhang	969.6	E854.1	E939.6	E950.3	E962.0	E980.3
Bialamicol	961.5	E857	E931.5	E950.4	E962.0	E980.4
Bichloride of mercury — see Mercury, chloride						
Bichromates (calcium) (crystals) (potassium) (sodium)	983.9	E864.3	—	E950.7	E962.1	E980.6
fumes	987.8	E869.8	—	E952.8	E962.2	E982.8
Biguanide derivatives, oral	962.3	E858.0	E932.3	E950.4	E962.0	E980.4
Biligrafin	977.8	E858.8	E947.8	E950.4	E962.0	E980.4
Bilopaque	977.8	E858.8	E947.8	E950.4	E962.0	E980.4
Bioflavonoids	972.8	E858.3	E942.8	E950.4	E962.0	E980.4
Biological substance NEC	979.9	E858.8	E949.9	E950.4	E962.0	E980.4
Biperiden	966.4	E855.0	E936.4	E950.4	E962.0	E980.4
Bisacodyl	973.1	E858.4	E943.1	E950.4	E962.0	E980.4
Bishydroxycoumarin	964.2	E858.2	E934.2	E950.4	E962.0	E980.4
Bismarsen	961.1	E857	E931.1	E950.4	E962.0	E980.4
Bismuth (compounds) NEC	985.8	E866.4	—	E950.9	E962.1	E980.9
anti-infectives	961.2	E857	E931.2	E950.4	E962.0	E980.4
subcarbonate	973.5	E858.4	E943.5	E950.4	E962.0	E980.4
sulfarsphenamine	961.1	E857	E931.1	E950.4	E962.0	E980.4
Bithionol	961.6	E857	E931.6	E950.4	E962.0	E980.4
Bitter almond oil	989.0	E866.8	—	E950.9	E962.1	E980.9
Bittersweet	988.2	E865.4	—	E950.9	E962.1	E930.9
Black						
flag	989.4	E863.4	—	E950.6	E962.1	E980.7
henbane	988.2	E865.4	—	E950.9	E962.1	E980.9
leaf (40)	989.4	E863.4	—	E950.6	E962.1	E980.7
widow spider (bite)	989.5	E905.1	—	E950.9	E962.1	E980.9

	Poisoning	External Cause (E-Code)				
		Accident	Therapeutic Use	Suicide Attempt	Assault	Undetermined
Black — *continued*						
widow spider — *continued*						
antivenin	979.9	E858.8	E949.9	E950.4	E962.0	E980.4
Blast furnace gas (carbon monoxide from)	986	E868.8	—	E952.1	E962.2	E982.1
Bleach NEC	983.9	E864.3	—	E950.7	E962.1	E980.6
Bleaching solutions	983.9	E864.3	—	E950.7	E962.1	E980.6
Bleomycin (sulfate)	960.7	E856	E930.7	E950.4	E962.0	E980.4
Blockain	968.9	E855.2	E938.9	E950.4	E962.0	E980.4
infiltration (subcutaneous)	968.5	E855.2	E938.5	E950.4	E962.0	E980.4
nerve block (peripheral) (plexus)	968.6	E855.2	E938.6	E950.4	E962.0	E980.4
topical (surface)	968.5	E855.2	E938.5	E950.4	E962.0	E980.4
Blood (derivatives) (natural) (plasma) (whole)	964.7	E858.2	E934.7	E950.4	E962.0	E980.4
affecting agent	964.9	E858.2	E934.9	E950.4	E962.0	E980.4
specified NEC	964.8	E858.2	E934.8	E950.4	E962.0	E980.4
substitute (macromolecular)	964.8	E858.2	E934.8	E950.4	E962.0	E980.4
Blue velvet	965.09	E850.2	E935.2	E950.0	E962.0	E980.0
Bone meal	989.89	E866.5	—	E950.9	E962.1	E980.9
Bonine	963.0	E858.1	E933.0	E950.4	E962.0	E980.4
Boracic acid	976.0	E858.7	E946.0	E950.4	E962.0	E980.4
ENT agent	976.6	E858.7	E946.6	E950.4	E962.0	E980.4
ophthalmic preparation	976.5	E858.7	E946.5	E950.4	E962.0	E980.4
Borate (cleanser) (sodium)	989.6	E861.3	—	E950.9	E962.1	E980.9
Borax (cleanser)	989.6	E861.3	—	E950.9	E962.1	E980.9
Boric acid	976.0	E858.7	E946.0	E950.4	E962.0	E980.4
ENT agent	976.6	E858.7	E946.6	E950.4	E962.0	E980.4
ophthalmic preparation	976.5	E858.7	E946.5	E950.4	E962.0	E980.4
Boron hydride NEC	989.89	E866.8	—	E950.9	E962.1	E980.9
fumes or gas	987.8	E869.8	—	E952.8	E962.2	E982.8
Brake fluid vapor	987.8	E869.8	—	E952.8	E962.2	E982.8
Brass (compounds) (fumes)	985.8	E866.4	—	E950.9	E962.1	E980.9
Brasso	981	E861.3	—	E950.9	E962.1	E980.9
Bretylium (tosylate)	972.6	E858.3	E942.6	E950.4	E962.0	E980.4
Brevital (sodium)	968.3	E855.1	E938.3	E950.4	E962.0	E980.4
British antilewisite	963.8	E858.1	E933.8	E950.4	E962.0	E980.4
Bromal (hydrate)	967.3	E852.2	E937.3	E950.2	E962.0	E980.2
Bromelains	963.4	E858.1	E933.4	E950.4	E962.0	E980.4
Bromides NEC	967.3	E852.2	E937.3	E950.2	E962.0	E980.2
Bromine (vapor)	987.8	E869.8	—	E952.8	E962.2	E982.8
compounds (medicinal)	967.3	E852.2	E937.3	E950.2	E962.0	E980.2
Bromisovalum	967.3	E852.2	E937.3	E950.2	E962.0	E980.2
Bromobenzyl cyanide	987.5	E869.3	—	E952.8	E962.2	E982.8
Bromodiphenhydramine	963.0	E858.1	E933.0	E950.4	E962.0	E980.4
Bromoform	967.3	E852.2	E937.3	E950.2	E962.0	E980.2
Bromophenol blue reagent	977.8	E858.8	E947.8	E950.4	E962.0	E980.4
Bromosalicylhydroxamic acid	961.8	E857	E931.8	E950.4	E962.0	E980.4
Bromo-seltzer	965.4	E850.4	E935.4	E950.0	E962.0	E980.0
Brompheniramine	963.0	E858.1	E933.0	E950.4	E962.0	E980.4
Bromural	967.3	E852.2	E937.3	E950.2	E962.0	E980.2
Brown spider (bite) (venom)	989.5	E905.1	—	E950.9	E962.1	E980.9
Brucia	988.2	E865.3	—	E950.9	E962.1	E980.9
Brucine	989.1	E863.7	—	E950.6	E962.1	E980.7
Brunswick green — *see* Copper						
Bruten — *see* Ibuprofen						
Bryonia (alba) (dioica)	988.2	E865.4	—	E950.9	E962.1	E980.9
Buclizine	969.5	E853.8	E939.5	E950.3	E962.0	E980.3
Bufferin	965.1	E850.3	E935.3	E950.0	E962.0	E980.0
Bufotenine	969.6	E854.1	E939.6	E950.3	E962.0	E980.3
Buphenine	971.2	E855.5	E941.2	E950.4	E962.0	E980.4
Bupivacaine	968.9	E855.2	E938.9	E950.4	E962.0	E980.4
infiltration (subcutaneous)	968.5	E855.2	E938.5	E950.4	E962.0	E980.4
nerve block (peripheral) (plexus)	968.6	E855.2	E938.6	E950.4	E962.0	E980.4
Busulfan	963.1	E858.1	E933.1	E950.4	E962.0	E980.4
Butabarbital (sodium)	967.0	E851	E937.0	E950.1	E962.0	E980.1
Butabarbitone	967.0	E851	E937.0	E950.1	E962.0	E980.1
Butabarpal	967.0	E851	E937.0	E950.1	E962.0	E980.1
Butacaine	968.5	E855.2	E938.5	E950.4	E962.0	E980.4
Butallylonal	967.0	E851	E937.0	E950.1	E962.0	E980.1
Butane (distributed in mobile container)	987.0	E868.0	—	E951.1	E962.2	E981.1
distributed through pipes	987.0	E867	—	E951.0	E962.2	E981.0
incomplete combustion of — *see* Carbon monoxide, butane						
Butanol	980.3	E860.4	—	E950.9	E962.1	E980.9
Butanone	982.8	E862.4	—	E950.9	E962.1	E980.9
Butaperazine	969.1	E853.0	E939.1	E950.3	E962.0	E980.3
Butazolidin	965.5	E850.5	E935.5	E950.0	E962.0	E980.0
Butethal	967.0	E851	E937.0	E950.1	E962.0	E980.1
Butethamate	971.1	E855.4	E941.1	E950.4	E962.0	E980.4
Buthalitone (sodium)	968.3	E855.1	E938.3	E950.4	E962.0	E980.4
Butisol (sodium)	967.0	E851	E937.0	E950.1	E962.0	E980.1
Butobarbital, butobarbitone	967.0	E851	E937.0	E950.1	E962.0	E980.1
Butriptyline	969.0	E854.0	E939.0	E950.3	E962.0	E980.3
Buttercups	988.2	E865.4	—	E950.9	E962.1	E980.9

	Poisoning	External Cause (E-Code)				
		Accident	Therapeutic Use	Suicide Attempt	Assault	Undetermined
Butter of antimony — *see* Antimony						
Butyl						
acetate (secondary)	982.8	E862.4	—	E950.9	E962.1	E980.9
alcohol	980.3	E860.4	—	E950.9	E962.1	E980.9
carbinol	980.8	E860.8	—	E950.9	E962.1	E980.9
carbitol	982.8	E862.4	—	E950.9	E962.1	E980.9
cellosolve	982.8	E862.4	—	E950.9	E962.1	E980.9
chloral (hydrate)	967.1	E852.0	E937.1	E950.2	E962.0	E980.2
formate	982.8	E862.4	—	E950.9	E962.1	E980.9
scopolammonium bromide	971.1	E855.4	E941.1	E950.4	E962.0	E980.4
Butyn	968.5	E855.2	E938.5	E950.4	E962.0	E980.4
Butyrophenone (-based tranquilizers)	969.2	E853.1	E939.2	E950.3	E962.0	E980.3
Cacodyl, cacodylic acid — *see* Arsenic						
Cactinomycin	960.7	E856	E930.7	E950.4	E962.0	E980.4
Cade oil	976.4	E858.7	E946.4	E950.4	E962.0	E980.4
Cadmium (chloride) (compounds) (dust) (fumes) (oxide)	985.5	E866.4	—	E950.9	E962.1	E980.9
sulfide (medicinal) NEC	976.4	E858.7	E946.4	E950.4	E962.0	E980.4
Caffeine	969.7	E854.2	E939.7	E950.3	E962.0	E980.3
Calabar bean	988.2	E865.4	—	E950.9	E962.1	E980.9
Caladium seguinium	988.2	E865.4	—	E950.9	E962.1	E980.9
Calamine (liniment) (lotion)	976.3	E858.7	E946.3	E950.4	E962.0	E980.4
Calciferol	963.5	E858.1	E933.5	E950.4	E962.0	E980.4
Calcium (salts) NEC	974.5	E858.5	E944.5	E950.4	E962.0	E980.4
acetylsalicylate	965.1	E850.3	E935.3	E950.0	E962.0	E980.0
benzamidosalicylate	961.8	E857	E931.8	E950.4	E962.0	E980.4
carbaspirin	965.1	E850.3	E935.3	E950.0	E962.0	E980.0
carbimide (citrated)	977.3	E858.8	E947.3	E950.4	E962.0	E980.4
carbonate (antacid)	973.0	E858.4	E943.0	E950.4	E962.0	E980.4
cyanide (citrated)	977.3	E858.8	E947.3	E950.4	E962.0	E980.4
dioctyl sulfosuccinate	973.2	E858.4	E943.2	E950.4	E962.0	E980.4
disodium edathamil	963.8	E858.1	E933.8	E950.4	E962.0	E980.4
disodium edetate	963.8	E858.1	E933.8	E950.4	E962.0	E980.4
EDTA	963.8	E858.1	E933.8	E950.4	E962.0	E980.4
hydrate, hydroxide	983.2	E864.2	—	E950.7	E962.1	E980.6
mandelate	961.9	E857	E931.9	E950.4	E962.0	E980.4
oxide	983.2	E864.2	—	E950.7	E962.1	E980.6
Calomel — *see* Mercury, chloride						
Caloric agents NEC	974.5	E858.5	E944.5	E950.4	E962.0	E980.4
Calusterone	963.1	E858.1	E933.1	E950.4	E962.0	E980.4
Camoquin	961.4	E857	E931.4	E950.4	E962.0	E980.4
Camphor (oil)	976.1	E858.7	E946.1	E950.4	E962.0	E980.4
Candeptin	976.0	E858.7	E946.0	E950.4	E962.0	E980.4
Candicidin	976.0	E858.7	E946.0	E950.4	E962.0	E980.4
Cannabinols	969.6	E854.1	E939.6	E950.3	E962.0	E980.3
Cannabis (derivatives) (indica) (sativa)	969.6	E854.1	E939.6	E950.3	E962.0	E980.3
Canned heat	980.1	E860.2	—	E950.9	E962.1	E980.9
Cantharides, cantharidin, cantharis	976.8	E858.7	E946.8	E950.4	E962.0	E980.4
Capillary agents	972.8	E858.3	E942.8	E950.4	E962.0	E980.4
Capreomycin	960.6	E856	E930.6	E950.4	E962.0	E980.4
Captodiame, captodiamine	969.5	E853.8	E939.5	E950.3	E962.0	E980.3
Caramiphen (hydrochloride)	971.1	E855.4	E941.1	E950.4	E962.0	E980.4
Carbachol	971.0	E855.3	E941.0	E950.4	E962.0	E980.4
Carbacrylamine resins	974.5	E858.5	E944.5	E950.4	E962.0	E980.4
Carbamate (sedative)	967.8	E852.8	E937.8	E950.2	E962.0	E980.2
herbicide	989.3	E863.5	—	E950.6	E962.1	E980.7
insecticide	989.3	E863.2	—	E950.6	E962.1	E980.7
Carbamazepine	966.3	E855.0	E936.3	E950.4	E962.0	E980.4
Carbamic esters	967.8	E852.8	E937.8	E950.2	E962.0	E980.2
Carbamide	974.4	E858.5	E944.4	E950.4	E962.0	E980.4
topical	976.8	E858.7	E946.8	E950.4	E962.0	E980.4
Carbamylcholine chloride	971.0	E855.3	E941.0	E950.4	E962.0	E980.4
Carbarsone	961.1	E857	E931.1	E950.4	E962.0	E980.4
Carbaryl	989.3	E863.2	—	E950.6	E962.1	E980.7
Carbaspirin	965.1	E850.3	E935.3	E950.0	E962.0	E980.0
Carbazochrome	972.8	E858.3	E942.8	E950.4	E962.0	E980.4
Carbenicillin	960.0	E856	E930.0	E950.4	E962.0	E980.4
Carbenoxolone	973.8	E858.4	E943.8	E950.4	E962.0	E980.4
Carbetapentane	975.4	E858.6	E945.4	E950.4	E962.0	E980.4
Carbimazole	962.8	E858.0	E932.8	E950.4	E962.0	E980.4
Carbinol	980.1	E860.2	—	E950.9	E962.1	E980.9
Carbinoxamine	963.0	E858.1	E933.0	E950.4	E962.0	E980.4
Carbitol	982.8	E862.4	—	E950.9	E962.1	E980.9
Carbocaine	968.9	E855.2	E938.9	E950.4	E962.0	E980.4
infiltration (subcutaneous)	968.5	E855.2	E938.5	E950.4	E962.0	E980.4
nerve block (peripheral) (plexus)	968.6	E855.2	E938.6	E950.4	E962.0	E980.4
topical (surface)	968.5	E855.2	E938.5	E950.4	E962.0	E980.4
Carbol-fuchsin solution	976.0	E858.7	E946.0	E950.4	E962.0	E980.4
Carbolic acid (*see also* Phenol)	983.0	E864.0	—	E950.7	E962.1	E980.6
Carbomycin	960.8	E856	E930.8	E950.4	E962.0	E980.4
Carbon						
bisulfide (liquid) (vapor)	982.2	E862.4	—	E950.9	E962.1	E980.9

	Poisoning	External Cause (E-Code)				
		Accident	Therapeutic Use	Suicide Attempt	Assault	Undetermined
Carbon — *continued*						
dioxide (gas)	987.8	E869.8	—	E952.8	E962.2	E982.8
disulfide (liquid) (vapor)	982.2	E862.4	—	E950.9	E962.1	E980.9
monoxide (from incomplete combustion of) (in) NEC	986	E868.9	—	E952.1	E962.2	E982.1
blast furnace gas	986	E868.8	—	E952.1	E962.2	E982.1
butane (distributed in mobile container)	986	E868.0	—	E951.1	E962.2	E981.1
distributed through pipes	986	E867	—	E951.0	E962.2	E981.0
charcoal fumes	986	E868.3	—	E952.1	E962.2	E982.1
coal						
gas (piped)	986	E867	—	E951.0	E962.2	E981.0
solid (in domestic stoves, fireplaces)	986	E868.3	—	E952.1	E962.2	E982.1
coke (in domestic stoves, fireplaces)	986	E868.3	—	E952.1	E962.2	E982.1
exhaust gas (motor) not in transit	986	E868.2	—	E952.0	E962.2	E982.0
combustion engine, any not in watercraft	986	E868.2	—	E952.0	E962.2	E982.0
farm tractor, not in transit	986	E868.2	—	E952.0	E962.2	E982.0
gas engine	986	E868.2	—	E952.0	E962.2	E982.0
motor pump	986	E868.2	—	E952.0	E962.2	E982.0
motor vehicle, not in transit	986	E868.2	—	E952.0	E962.2	E982.0
fuel (in domestic use)	986	E868.3	—	E952.1	E962.2	E982.1
gas (piped)	986	E867	—	E951.0	E962.2	E981.0
in mobile container	986	E868.0	—	E951.1	E962.2	E981.1
utility	986	E868.1	—	E951.8	E962.2	E981.1
in mobile container	986	E868.0	—	E951.1	E962.2	E981.1
piped (natural)	986	E867	—	E951.0	E962.2	E981.0
illuminating gas	986	E868.1	—	E951.8	E962.2	E981.8
industrial fuels or gases, any	986	E868.8	—	E952.1	E962.2	E982.1
kerosene (in domestic stoves, fireplaces)	986	E868.3	—	E952.1	E962.2	E982.1
kiln gas or vapor	986	E868.8	—	E952.1	E962.2	E982.1
motor exhaust gas, not in transit	986	E868.2	—	E952.0	E962.2	E982.0
piped gas (manufactured) (natural)	986	E867	—	E951.0	E962.2	E981.0
producer gas	986	E868.8	—	E952.1	E962.2	E982.1
propane (distributed in mobile container)	986	E868.0	—	E951.1	E962.2	E981.1
distributed through pipes	986	E867	—	E951.0	E962.2	E981.0
specified source NEC	986	E868.8	—	E952.1	E962.2	E982.1
stove gas	986	E868.1	—	E951.8	E962.2	E981.8
piped	986	E867	—	E951.0	E962.2	E981.0
utility gas	986	E868.1	—	E951.8	E962.2	E981.8
piped	986	E867	—	E951.0	E962.2	E981.0
water gas	986	E868.1	—	E951.8	E962.2	E981.8
wood (in domestic stoves, fireplaces)	986	E868.3	—	E952.1	E962.2	E982.1
tetrachloride (vapor) NEC	987.8	E869.8	—	E952.8	E962.2	E982.8
liquid (cleansing agent) NEC	982.1	E861.3	—	E950.9	E962.1	E980.9
solvent	982.1	E862.4	—	E950.9	E962.1	E980.9
Carbonic acid (gas)	987.8	E869.8	—	E952.8	E962.2	E982.8
anhydrase inhibitors	974.2	E858.5	E944.2	E950.4	E962.0	E980.4
Carbowax	976.3	E858.7	E946.3	E950.4	E962.0	E980.4
Carbrital	967.0	E851	E937.0	E950.1	E962.0	E980.1
Carbromal (derivatives)	967.3	E852.2	E937.3	E950.2	E962.0	E980.2
Cardiac						
depressants	972.0	E858.3	E942.0	E950.4	E962.0	E980.4
rhythm regulators	972.0	E858.3	E942.0	E950.4	E962.0	E980.4
Cardiografin	977.8	E858.8	E947.8	E950.4	E962.0	E980.4
Cardio-green	977.8	E858.8	E947.8	E950.4	E962.0	E980.4
Cardiotonic glycosides	972.1	E858.3	E942.1	E950.4	E962.0	E980.4
Cardiovascular agents NEC	972.9	E858.3	E942.9	E950.4	E962.0	E980.4
Cardrase	974.2	E858.5	E944.2	E950.4	E962.0	E980.4
Carfusin	976.0	E858.7	E946.0	E950.4	E962.0	E980.4
Carisoprodol	968.0	E855.1	E938.0	E950.4	E962.0	E980.4
Carmustine	963.1	E858.1	E933.1	E950.4	E962.0	E980.4
Carotene	963.5	E858.1	E933.5	E950.4	E962.0	E980.4
Carphenazine (maleate)	969.1	E853.0	E939.1	E950.3	E962.0	E980.3
Carter's Little Pills	973.1	E858.4	E943.1	E950.4	E962.0	E980.4
Cascara (sagrada)	973.1	E858.4	E943.1	E950.4	E962.0	E980.4
Cassava	988.2	E865.4	—	E950.9	E962.1	E980.9
Castellani's paint	976.0	E858.7	E946.0	E950.4	E962.0	E980.4
Castor						
bean	988.2	E865.3	—	E950.9	E962.1	E980.9
oil	973.1	E858.4	E943.1	E950.4	E962.0	E980.4
Caterpillar (sting)	989.5	E905.5	—	E950.9	E962.1	E980.9
Catha (edulis)	970.8	E854.3	E940.8	E950.4	E962.0	E980.4
Cathartics NEC	973.3	E858.4	E943.3	E950.4	E962.0	E980.4
contact	973.1	E858.4	E943.1	E950.4	E962.0	E980.4
emollient	973.2	E858.4	E943.2	E950.4	E962.0	E980.4
intestinal irritants	973.1	E858.4	E943.1	E950.4	E962.0	E980.4
saline	973.3	E858.4	E943.3	E950.4	E962.0	E980.4
Cathomycin	960.8	E856	E930.8	E950.4	E962.0	E980.4
Caustic(s)	983.9	E864.4	—	E950.7	E962.1	E980.6
alkali	983.2	E864.2	—	E950.7	E962.1	E980.6
hydroxide	983.2	E864.2	—	E950.7	E962.1	E980.6

☑4ᵗʰ Fourth-digit Required   ☑5ᵗʰ Fifth-digit Required   ▶◀ Revised Text   ● New Line   ▲ Revised Code

	Poisoning		External Cause (E-Code)			
		Accident	Therapeutic Use	Suicide Attempt	Assault	Undetermined
Caustic(s) — *continued*						
potash	983.2	E864.2	—	E950.7	E962.1	E980.6
soda	983.2	E864.2	—	E950.7	E962.1	E980.6
specified NEC	983.9	E864.3	—	E950.7	E962.1	E980.6
Ceepryn	976.0	E858.7	E946.0	E950.4	E962.0	E980.4
ENT agent	976.6	E858.7	E946.6	E950.4	E962.0	E980.4
lozenges	976.6	E858.7	E946.6	E950.4	E962.0	E980.4
Celestone	962.0	E858.0	E932.0	E950.4	E962.0	E980.4
topical	976.0	E858.7	E946.0	E950.4	E962.0	E980.4
Cellosolve	982.8	E862.4	—	E950.9	E962.1	E980.9
Cell stimulants and proliferants	976.8	E858.7	E946.8	E950.4	E962.0	E980.4
Cellulose derivatives, cathartic	973.3	E858.4	E943.3	E950.4	E962.0	E980.4
nitrates (topical)	976.3	E858.7	E946.3	E950.4	E962.0	E980.4
Centipede (bite)	989.5	E905.4	—	E950.9	E962.1	E980.9
Central nervous system						
depressants	968.4	E855.1	E938.4	E950.4	E962.0	E980.4
anesthetic (general) NEC	968.4	E855.1	E938.4	E950.4	E962.0	E980.4
gases NEC	968.2	E855.1	E938.2	E950.4	E962.0	E980.4
intravenous	968.3	E855.1	E938.3	E950.4	E962.0	E980.4
barbiturates	967.0	E851	E937.0	E950.1	E962.0	E980.1
bromides	967.3	E852.2	E937.3	E950.2	E962.0	E980.2
cannabis sativa	969.6	E854.1	E939.6	E950.3	E962.0	E980.3
chloral hydrate	967.1	E852.0	E937.1	E950.2	E962.0	E980.2
hallucinogenics	969.6	E854.1	E939.6	E950.3	E962.0	E980.3
hypnotics	967.9	E852.9	E937.9	E950.2	E962.0	E980.2
specified NEC	967.8	E852.8	E937.8	E950.2	E962.0	E980.2
muscle relaxants	968.0	E855.1	E938.0	E950.4	E962.0	E980.4
paraldehyde	967.2	E852.1	E937.2	E950.2	E962.0	E980.2
sedatives	967.9	E852.9	E937.9	E950.2	E962.0	E980.2
mixed NEC	967.6	E852.5	E937.6	E950.2	E962.0	E980.2
specified NEC	967.8	E852.8	E937.8	E950.2	E962.0	E980.2
muscle-tone depressants	968.0	E855.1	E938.0	E950.4	E962.0	E980.4
stimulants	970.9	E854.3	E940.9	E950.4	E962.0	E980.4
amphetamines	969.7	E854.2	E939.7	E950.3	E962.0	E980.3
analeptics	970.0	E854.3	E940.0	E950.4	E962.0	E980.4
antidepressants	969.0	E854.0	E939.0	E950.3	E962.0	E980.3
opiate antagonists	970.1	E854.3	E940.0	E950.4	E962.0	E980.4
specified NEC	970.8	E854.3	E940.8	E950.4	E962.0	E980.4
Cephalexin	960.5	E856	E930.5	E950.4	E962.0	E980.4
Cephaloglycin	960.5	E856	E930.5	E950.4	E962.0	E980.4
Cephaloridine	960.5	E856	E930.5	E950.4	E962.0	E980.4
Cephalosporins NEC	960.5	E856	E930.5	E950.4	E962.0	E980.4
N (adicillin)	960.0	E856	E930.0	E950.4	E962.0	E980.4
Cephalothin (sodium)	960.5	E856	E930.5	E950.4	E962.0	E980.4
Cerbera (odallam)	988.2	E865.4	—	E950.9	E962.1	E980.9
Cerberin	972.1	E858.3	E942.1	E950.4	E962.0	E980.4
Cerebral stimulants	970.9	E854.3	E940.9	E950.4	E962.0	E980.4
psychotherapeutic	969.7	E854.2	E939.7	E950.3	E962.0	E980.3
specified NEC	970.8	E854.3	E940.8	E950.4	E962.0	E980.4
Cetalkonium (chloride)	976.0	E858.7	E946.0	E950.4	E962.0	E980.4
Cetoxime	963.0	E858.1	E933.0	E950.4	E962.0	E980.4
Cetrimide	976.2	E858.7	E946.2	E950.4	E962.0	E980.4
Cetylpyridinium	976.0	E858.7	E946.0	E950.4	E962.0	E980.4
ENT agent	976.6	E858.7	E946.6	E950.4	E962.0	E980.4
lozenges	976.6	E858.7	E946.6	E950.4	E962.0	E980.4
Cevadilla — *see* Sabadilla						
Cevitamic acid	963.5	E858.1	E933.5	E950.4	E962.0	E980.4
Chalk, precipitated	973.0	E858.4	E943.0	E950.4	E962.0	E980.4
Charcoal						
fumes (carbon monoxide)	986	E868.3	—	E952.1	E962.2	E982.1
industrial	986	E868.8	—	E952.1	E962.2	E982.1
medicinal (activated)	973.0	E858.4	E943.0	E950.4	E962.0	E980.4
Chelating agents NEC	977.2	E858.8	E947.2	E950.4	E962.0	E980.4
Chelidonium majus	988.2	E865.4	—	E950.9	E962.1	E980.9
Chemical substance	989.9	E866.9	—	E950.9	E962.1	E980.9
specified NEC	989.89	E866.8	—	E950.9	E962.1	E980.9
Chemotherapy, antineoplastic	963.1	E858.1	E933.1	E950.4	E962.0	E980.4
Chenopodium (oil)	961.6	E857	E931.6	E950.4	E962.0	E980.4
Cherry laurel	988.2	E865.4	—	E950.9	E962.1	E980.9
Chiniofon	961.3	E857	E931.3	E950.4	E962.0	E980.4
Chlophedianol	975.4	E858.6	E945.4	E950.4	E962.0	E980.4
Chloral (betaine) (formamide) (hydrate)	967.1	E852.0	E937.1	E950.2	E962.0	E980.2
Chloralamide	967.1	E852.0	E937.1	E950.2	E962.0	E980.2
Chlorambucil	963.1	E858.1	E933.1	E950.4	E962.0	E980.4
Chloramphenicol	960.2	E856	E930.2	E950.4	E962.0	E980.4
ENT agent	976.6	E858.7	E946.6	E950.4	E962.0	E980.4
ophthalmic preparation	976.5	E858.7	E946.5	E950.4	E962.0	E980.4
topical NEC	976.0	E858.7	E946.0	E950.4	E962.0	E980.4
Chlorate(s) (potassium) (sodium) NEC	983.9	E864.3	—	E950.7	E962.1	E980.6
herbicides	989.4	E863.5	—	E950.6	E962.1	E980.7

	Poisoning	External Cause (E-Code)				
		Accident	Therapeutic Use	Suicide Attempt	Assault	Undetermined
Chlorcylizine	963.0	E858.1	E933.0	E950.4	E962.0	E980.4
Chlordan(e) (dust)	989.2	E863.0	—	E950.6	E962.1	E980.7
Chlordantoin	976.0	E858.7	E946.0	E950.4	E962.0	E980.4
Chlordiazepoxide	969.4	E853.2	E939.4	E950.3	E962.0	E980.3
Chloresium	976.8	E858.7	E946.8	E950.4	E962.0	E980.4
Chlorethiazol	967.1	E852.0	E937.1	E950.2	E962.0	E980.2
Chlorethyl — see Ethyl, chloride						
Chloretone	967.1	E852.0	E937.1	E950.2	E962.0	E980.2
Chlorex	982.3	E862.4	—	E950.9	E962.1	E980.9
Chlorhexadol	967.1	E852.0	E937.1	E950.2	E962.0	E980.2
Chlorhexidine (hydrochloride)	976.0	E858.7	E946.0	E950.4	E962.0	E980.4
Chlorhydroxyquinolin	976.0	E858.7	E946.0	E950.4	E962.0	E980.4
Chloride of lime (bleach)	983.9	E864.3	—	E950.7	E962.1	E980.6
Chlorinated						
camphene	989.2	E863.0	—	E950.6	E962.1	E980.7
diphenyl	989.89	E866.8	—	E950.9	E962.1	E980.9
hydrocarbons NEC	989.2	E863.0	—	E950.6	E962.1	E980.7
solvent	982.3	E862.4	—	E950.9	E962.1	E980.9
lime (bleach)	983.9	E864.3	—	E950.7	E962.1	E980.6
naphthalene — see Naphthalene						
pesticides NEC	989.2	E863.0	—	E950.6	E962.1	E980.7
soda — see Sodium, hypochlorite						
Chlorine (fumes) (gas)	987.6	E869.8	—	E952.8	E962.2	E982.8
bleach	983.9	E864.3	—	E950.7	E962.1	E980.6
compounds NEC	983.9	E864.3	—	E950.7	E962.1	E980.6
disinfectant	983.9	E861.4	—	E950.7	E962.1	E980.6
releasing agents NEC	983.9	E864.3	—	E950.7	E962.1	E980.6
Chlorisondamine	972.3	E858.3	E942.3	E950.4	E962.0	E980.4
Chlormadinone	962.2	E858.0	E932.2	E950.4	E962.0	E980.4
Chlormerodrin	974.0	E858.5	E944.0	E950.4	E962.0	E980.4
Chlormethiazole	967.1	E852.0	E937.1	E950.2	E962.0	E980.2
Chlormethylenecycline	960.4	E856	E930.4	E950.4	E962.0	E980.4
Chlormezanone	969.5	E853.8	E939.5	E950.3	E962.0	E980.3
Chloroacetophenone	987.5	E869.3	—	E952.8	E962.2	E982.8
Chloroaniline	983.0	E864.0	—	E950.7	E962.1	E980.6
Chlorobenzene, chlorobenzol	982.0	E862.4	—	E950.9	E962.1	E980.9
Chlorobutanol	967.1	E852.0	E937.1	E950.2	E962.0	E980.2
Chlorodinitrobenzene	983.0	E864.0	—	E950.7	E962.1	E980.6
dust or vapor	987.8	E869.8	—	E952.8	E962.2	E982.8
Chloroethane — see Ethyl, chloride						
Chloroform (fumes) (vapor)	987.8	E869.8	—	E952.8	E962.2	E982.8
anesthetic (gas)	968.2	E855.1	E938.2	E950.4	E962.0	E980.4
liquid NEC	968.4	E855.1	E938.4	E950.4	E962.0	E980.4
solvent	982.3	E862.4	—	E950.9	E962.1	E980.9
Chloroguanide	961.4	E857	E931.4	E950.4	E962.0	E980.4
Chloromycetin	960.2	E856	E930.2	E950.4	E962.0	E980.4
ENT agent	976.6	E858.7	E946.6	E950.4	E962.0	E980.4
ophthalmic preparation	976.5	E858.7	E946.5	E950.4	E962.0	E980.4
otic solution	976.6	E858.7	E946.6	E950.4	E962.0	E980.4
topical NEC	976.0	E858.7	E946.0	E950.4	E962.0	E980.4
Chloronitrobenzene	983.0	E864.0	—	E950.7	E962.1	E980.6
dust or vapor	987.8	E869.8	—	E952.8	E962.2	E982.8
Chlorophenol	983.0	E864.0	—	E950.7	E962.1	E980.6
Chlorophenothane	989.2	E863.0	—	E950.6	E962.1	E980.7
Chlorophyll (derivatives)	976.8	E858.7	E946.8	E950.4	E962.0	E980.4
Chloropicrin (fumes)	987.8	E869.8	—	E952.8	E962.2	E982.8
fumigant	989.4	E863.8	—	E950.6	E962.1	E980.7
fungicide	989.4	E863.6	—	E950.6	E962.1	E980.7
pesticide (fumes)	989.4	E863.4	—	E950.6	E962.1	E980.7
Chloroprocaine	968.9	E855.2	E938.9	E950.4	E962.0	E980.4
infiltration (subcutaneous)	968.5	E855.2	E938.5	E950.4	E962.0	E980.4
nerve block (peripheral) (plexus)	968.6	E855.2	E938.6	E950.4	E962.0	E980.4
Chloroptic	976.5	E858.7	E946.5	E950.4	E962.0	E980.4
Chloropurine	963.1	E858.1	E933.1	E950.4	E962.0	E980.4
Chloroquine (hydrochloride) (phosphate)	961.4	E857	E931.4	E950.4	E962.0	E980.4
Chlorothen	963.0	E858.1	E933.0	E950.4	E962.0	E980.4
Chlorothiazide	974.3	E858.5	E944.3	E950.4	E962.0	E980.4
Chlorotrianisene	962.2	E858.0	E932.2	E950.4	E962.0	E980.4
Chlorovinyldichloroarsine	985.1	E866.3	—	E950.8	E962.1	E980.8
Chloroxylenol	976.0	E858.7	E946.0	E950.4	E962.0	E980.4
Chlorphenesin (carbamate)	968.0	E855.1	E938.0	E950.4	E962.0	E980.4
topical (antifungal)	976.0	E858.7	E946.0	E950.4	E962.0	E980.4
Chlorpheniramine	963.0	E858.1	E933.0	E950.4	E962.0	E980.4
Chlorphenoxamine	966.4	E855.0	E936.4	E950.4	E962.0	E980.4
Chlorphentermine	977.0	E858.8	E947.0	E950.4	E962.0	E980.4
Chlorproguanil	961.4	E857	E931.4	E950.4	E962.0	E980.4
Chlorpromazine	969.1	E853.0	E939.1	E950.3	E962.0	E980.3
Chlorpropamide	962.3	E858.0	E932.3	E950.4	E962.0	E980.4
Chlorprothixene	969.3	E853.8	E939.3	E950.3	E962.0	E980.3
Chlorquinaldol	976.0	E858.7	E946.0	E950.4	E962.0	E980.4

Chlorcylizine — Chlorquinaldol

		External Cause (E-Code)				
	Poisoning	Accident	Therapeutic Use	Suicide Attempt	Assault	Undetermined
Chlortetracycline	960.4	E856	E930.4	E950.4	E962.0	E980.4
Chlorthalidone	974.4	E858.5	E944.4	E950.4	E962.0	E980.4
Chlortrianisene	962.2	E858.0	E932.2	E950.4	E962.0	E980.4
Chlor-Trimeton	963.0	E858.1	E933.0	E950.4	E962.0	E980.4
Chlorzoxazone	968.0	E855.1	E938.0	E950.4	E962.0	E980.4
Choke damp	987.8	E869.8	—	E952.8	E962.2	E982.8
Cholebrine	977.8	E858.8	E947.8	E950.4	E962.0	E980.4
Cholera vaccine	978.2	E858.8	E948.2	E950.4	E962.0	E980.4
Cholesterol-lowering agents	972.2	E858.3	E942.2	E950.4	E962.0	E980.4
Cholestyramine (resin)	972.2	E858.3	E942.2	E950.4	E962.0	E980.4
Cholic acid	973.4	E858.4	E943.4	E950.4	E962.0	E980.4
Choline						
dihydrogen citrate	977.1	E858.8	E947.1	E950.4	E962.0	E980.4
salicylate	965.1	E850.3	E935.3	E950.0	E962.0	E980.0
theophyllinate	974.1	E858.5	E944.1	E950.4	E962.0	E980.4
Cholinergics	971.0	E855.3	E941.0	E950.4	E962.0	E980.4
Cholografin	977.8	E858.8	E947.8	E950.4	E962.0	E980.4
Chorionic gonadotropin	962.4	E858.0	E932.4	E950.4	E962.0	E980.4
Chromates	983.9	E864.3	—	E950.7	E962.1	E980.6
dust or mist	987.8	E869.8	—	E952.8	E962.2	E982.8
lead	984.0	E866.0	—	E950.9	E962.1	E980.9
paint	984.0	E861.5	—	E950.9	E962.1	E980.9
Chromic acid	983.9	E864.3	—	E950.7	E962.1	E980.6
dust or mist	987.8	E869.8	—	E952.8	E962.2	E982.8
Chromium	985.6	E866.4	—	E950.9	E962.1	E980.9
compounds — see Chromates						
Chromonar	972.4	E858.3	E942.4	E950.4	E962.0	E980.4
Chromyl chloride	983.9	E864.3	—	E950.7	E962.1	E980.6
Chrysarobin (ointment)	976.4	E858.7	E946.4	E950.4	E962.0	E980.4
Chrysazin	973.1	E858.4	E943.1	E950.4	E962.0	E980.4
Chymar	963.4	E858.1	E933.4	E950.4	E962.0	E980.4
ophthalmic preparation	976.5	E858.7	E946.5	E950.4	E962.0	E980.4
Chymotrypsin	963.4	E858.1	E933.4	E950.4	E962.0	E980.4
ophthalmic preparation	976.5	E858.7	E946.5	E950.4	E962.0	E980.4
Cicuta maculata or virosa	988.2	E865.4	—	E950.9	E962.1	E980.9
Cigarette lighter fluid	981	E862.1	—	E950.9	E962.1	E980.9
Cinchocaine (spinal)	968.7	E855.2	E938.7	E950.4	E962.0	E980.4
topical (surface)	968.5	E855.2	E938.5	E950.4	E962.0	E980.4
Cinchona	961.4	E857	E931.4	E950.4	E962.0	E980.4
Cinchonine alkaloids	961.4	E857	E931.4	E950.4	E962.0	E980.4
Cinchophen	974.7	E858.5	E944.7	E950.4	E962.0	E980.4
Cinnarizine	963.0	E858.1	E933.0	E950.4	E962.0	E980.4
Citanest	968.9	E855.2	E938.9	E950.4	E962.0	E980.4
infiltration (subcutaneous)	968.5	E855.2	E938.5	E950.4	E962.0	E980.4
nerve block (peripheral) (plexus)	968.6	E855.2	E938.6	E950.4	E962.0	E980.4
Citric acid	989.89	E866.8	—	E950.9	E962.1	E980.9
Citrovorum factor	964.1	E858.2	E934.1	E950.4	E962.0	E980.4
Claviceps purpurea	988.2	E865.4	—	E950.9	E962.1	E980.9
Cleaner, cleansing agent NEC	989.89	E861.3	—	E950.9	E962.1	E980.9
of paint or varnish	982.8	E862.9	—	E950.9	E962.1	E980.9
Clematis vitalba	988.2	E865.4	—	E950.9	E962.1	E980.9
Clemizole	963.0	E858.1	E933.0	E950.4	E962.0	E980.4
penicillin	960.0	E856	E930.0	E950.4	E962.0	E980.4
Clidinium	971.1	E855.4	E941.1	E950.4	E962.0	E980.4
Clindamycin	960.8	E856	E930.8	E950.4	E962.0	E980.4
Cliradon	965.09	E850.2	E935.2	E950.0	E962.0	E980.0
Clocortolone	962.0	E858.0	E932.0	E950.4	E962.0	E980.4
Clofedanol	975.4	E858.6	E945.4	E950.4	E962.0	E980.4
Clofibrate	972.2	E858.3	E942.2	E950.4	E962.0	E980.4
Clomethiazole	967.1	E852.0	E937.1	E950.2	E962.0	E980.2
Clomiphene	977.8	E858.8	E947.8	E950.4	E962.0	E980.4
Clonazepam	969.4	E853.2	E939.4	E950.3	E962.0	E980.3
Clonidine	972.6	E858.3	E942.6	E950.4	E962.0	E980.4
Clopamide	974.3	E858.5	E944.3	E950.4	E962.0	E980.4
Clorazepate	969.4	E853.2	E939.4	E950.3	E962.0	E980.3
Clorexolone	974.4	E858.5	E944.4	E950.4	E962.0	E980.4
Clorox (bleach)	983.9	E864.3	—	E950.7	E962.1	E980.6
Clortermine	977.0	E858.8	E947.0	E950.4	E962.0	E980.4
Clotrimazole	976.0	E858.7	E946.0	E950.4	E962.0	E980.4
Cloxacillin	960.0	E856	E930.0	E950.4	E962.0	E980.4
Coagulants NEC	964.5	E858.2	E934.5	E950.4	E962.0	E980.4
Coal (carbon monoxide from) — see also Carbon, monoxide, coal						
oil — see Kerosene						
tar NEC	983.0	E864.0	—	E950.7	E962.1	E980.6
fumes	987.8	E869.8	—	E952.8	E962.2	E982.8
medicinal (ointment)	976.4	E858.7	E946.4	E950.4	E962.0	E980.4
analgesics NEC	965.5	E850.5	E935.5	E950.0	E962.0	E980.0
naphtha (solvent)	981	E862.0	—	E950.9	E962.1	E980.9
Cobalt (fumes) (industrial)	985.8	E866.4	—	E950.9	E962.1	E980.9
Cobra (venom)	989.5	E905.0	—	E950.9	E962.1	E980.9

Chlortetracycline — Cobra

	Poisoning	External Cause (E-Code)				
		Accident	**Therapeutic Use**	**Suicide Attempt**	**Assault**	**Undetermined**
Coca (leaf)	970.8	E854.3	E940.8	E950.4	E962.0	E980.4
Cocaine (hydrochloride) (salt)	970.8 ▲	E854.3 ▲	E940.8 ▲	E950.4	E962.0	E980.4
topical anesthetic ●	968.5	E855.2	E938.5	E950.4	E962.0	E980.4
Coccidioidin	977.8	E858.8	E947.8	E950.4	E962.0	E980.4
Cocculus indicus	988.2	E865.3	—	E950.9	E962.1	E980.9
Cochineal	989.89	E866.8	—	E950.9	E962.1	E980.9
medicinal products	977.4	E858.8	E947.4	E950.4	E962.0	E980.4
Codeine	965.09	E850.2	E935.2	E950.0	E962.0	E980.0
Coffee	989.89	E866.8	—	E950.9	E962.1	E980.9
Cogentin	971.1	E855.4	E941.1	E950.4	E962.0	E980.4
Coke fumes or gas (carbon monoxide)	986	E868.3	—	E952.1	E962.2	E982.1
industrial use	986	E868.8	—	E952.1	E962.2	E982.1
Colace	973.2	E858.4	E943.2	E950.4	E962.0	E980.4
Colchicine	974.7	E858.5	E944.7	E950.4	E962.0	E980.4
Colchicum	988.2	E865.3	—	E950.9	E962.1	E980.9
Cold cream	976.3	E858.7	E946.3	E950.4	E962.0	E980.4
Colestipol	972.2	E858.3	E942.2	E950.4	E962.0	E980.4
Colistimethate	960.8	E856	E930.8	E950.4	E962.0	E980.4
Colistin	960.8	E856	E930.8	E950.4	E962.0	E980.4
Collagenase	976.8	E858.7	E946.8	E950.4	E962.0	E980.4
Collagen	977.8	E866.8	E947.8	E950.9	E962.1	E980.9
Collodion (flexible)	976.3	E858.7	E946.3	E950.4	E962.0	E980.4
Colocynth	973.1	E858.4	E943.1	E950.4	E962.0	E980.4
Coloring matter — *see* Dye(s)						
Combustion gas — *see* Carbon, monoxide						
Compazine	969.1	E853.0	E939.1	E950.3	E962.0	E980.3
Compound						
42 (warfarin)	989.4	E863.7	—	E950.6	E962.1	E980.7
269 (endrin)	989.2	E863.0	—	E950.6	E962.1	E980.7
497 (dieldrin)	989.2	E863.0	—	E950.6	E962.1	E980.7
1080 (sodium fluoroacetate)	989.4	E863.7	—	E950.6	E962.1	E980.7
3422 (parathion)	989.3	E863.1	—	E950.6	E962.1	E980.7
3911 (phorate)	989.3	E863.1	—	E950.6	E962.1	E980.7
3956 (toxaphene)	989.2	E863.0	—	E950.6	E962.1	E980.7
4049 (malathion)	989.3	E863.1	—	E950.6	E962.1	E980.7
4124 (dicapthon)	989.4	E863.4	—	E950.6	E962.1	E980.7
E (cortisone)	962.0	E858.0	E932.0	E950.4	E962.0	E980.4
F (hydrocortisone)	962.0	E858.0	E932.0	E950.4	E962.0	E980.4
Congo red	977.8	E858.8	E947.8	E950.4	E962.0	E980.4
Coniine, conine	965.7	E850.7	E935.7	E950.0	E962.0	E980.0
Conium (maculatum)	988.2	E865.4	—	E950.9	E962.1	E980.9
Conjugated estrogens (equine)	962.2	E858.0	E932.2	E950.4	E962.0	E980.4
Contac	975.6	E858.6	E945.6	E950.4	E962.0	E980.4
Contact lens solution	976.5	E858.7	E946.5	E950.4	E962.0	E980.4
Contraceptives (oral)	962.2	E858.0	E932.2	E950.4	E962.0	E980.4
vaginal	976.8	E858.7	E946.8	E950.4	E962.0	E980.4
Contrast media (roentgenographic)	977.8	E858.8	E947.8	E950.4	E962.0	E980.4
Convallaria majalis	988.2	E865.4	—	E950.9	E962.1	E980.9
Copper (dust) (fumes) (salts) NEC	985.8	E866.4	—	E950.9	E962.1	E980.9
arsenate, arsenite	985.1	E866.3	—	E950.8	E962.1	E980.8
insecticide	985.1	E863.4	—	E950.8	E962.1	E980.8
emetic	973.6	E858.4	E943.6	E950.4	E962.0	E980.4
fungicide	985.8	E863.6	—	E950.6	E962.1	E980.7
insecticide	985.8	E863.4	—	E950.6	E962.1	E980.7
oleate	976.0	E858.7	E946.0	E950.4	E962.0	E980.4
sulfate	983.9	E864.3	—	E950.7	E962.1	E980.6
fungicide	983.9	E863.6	—	E950.7	E962.1	E980.6
cupric	973.6	E858.4	E943.6	E950.4	E962.0	E980.4
cuprous	983.9	E864.3	—	E950.7	E962.1	E980.6
Copperhead snake (bite) (venom)	989.5	E905.0	—	E950.9	E962.1	E980.9
Coral (sting)	989.5	E905.6	—	E950.9	E962.1	E980.9
snake (bite) (venom)	989.5	E905.0	—	E950.9	E962.1	E980.9
Cordran	976.0	E858.7	E946.0	E950.4	E962.0	E980.4
Corn cures	976.4	E858.7	E946.4	E950.4	E962.0	E980.4
Cornhusker's lotion	976.3	E858.7	E946.3	E950.4	E962.0	E980.4
Corn starch	976.3	E858.7	E946.3	E950.4	E962.0	E980.4
Corrosive	983.9	E864.4	—	E950.7	E962.1	E980.6
acids NEC	983.1	E864.1	—	E950.7	E962.1	E980.6
aromatics	983.0	E864.0	—	E950.7	E962.1	E980.6
disinfectant	983.0	E861.4	—	E950.7	E962.1	E980.6
fumes NEC	987.9	E869.9	—	E952.9	E962.2	E982.9
specified NEC	983.9	E864.3	—	E950.7	E962.1	E980.6
sublimate — *see* Mercury, chloride						
Cortate	962.0	E858.0	E932.0	E950.4	E962.0	E980.4
Cort-Dome	962.0	E858.0	E932.0	E950.4	E962.0	E980.4
ENT agent	976.6	E858.7	E946.6	E950.4	E962.0	E980.4
ophthalmic preparation	976.5	E858.7	E946.5	E950.4	E962.0	E980.4
topical NEC	976.0	E858.7	E946.0	E950.4	E962.0	E980.4
Cortef	962.0	E858.0	E932.0	E950.4	E962.0	E980.4
ENT agent	976.6	E858.7	E946.6	E950.4	E962.0	E980.4
ophthalmic preparation	976.5	E858.7	E946.5	E950.4	E962.0	E980.4

✓4ᵗʰ Fourth-digit Required   ✓5ᵗʰ Fifth-digit Required   ▶◀ Revised Text   ● New Line   ▲ Revised Code

	Poisoning	External Cause (E-Code)				
		Accident	Therapeutic Use	Suicide Attempt	Assault	Undetermined
Cortef — *continued*						
topical NEC	976.0	E858.7	E946.0	E950.4	E962.0	E980.4
Corticosteroids (fluorinated)	962.0	E858.0	E932.0	E950.4	E962.0	E980.4
ENT agent	976.6	E858.7	E946.6	E950.4	E962.0	E980.4
ophthalmic preparation	976.5	E858.7	E946.5	E950.4	E962.0	E980.4
topical NEC	976.0	E858.7	E946.0	E950.4	E962.0	E980.4
Corticotropin	962.4	E858.0	E932.4	E950.4	E962.0	E980.4
Cortisol	962.0	E858.0	E932.0	E950.4	E962.0	E980.4
ENT agent	976.6	E858.7	E946.6	E950.4	E962.0	E980.4
ophthalmic preparation	976.5	E858.7	E946.5	E950.4	E962.0	E980.4
topical NEC	976.0	E858.7	E946.0	E950.4	E962.0	E980.4
Cortisone derivatives (acetate)	962.0	E858.0	E932.0	E950.4	E962.0	E980.4
ENT agent	976.6	E858.7	E946.6	E950.4	E962.0	E980.4
ophthalmic preparation	976.5	E858.7	E946.5	E950.4	E962.0	E980.4
topical NEC	976.0	E858.7	E946.0	E950.4	E962.0	E980.4
Cortogen	962.0	E858.0	E932.0	E950.4	E962.0	E980.4
ENT agent	976.6	E858.7	E946.6	E950.4	E962.0	E980.4
ophthalmic preparation	976.5	E858.7	E946.5	E950.4	E962.0	E980.4
Cortone	962.0	E858.0	E932.0	E950.4	E962.0	E980.4
ENT agent	976.6	E858.7	E946.6	E950.4	E962.0	E980.4
ophthalmic preparation	976.5	E858.7	E946.5	E950.4	E962.0	E980.4
Cortril	962.0	E858.0	E932.0	E950.4	E962.0	E980.4
ENT agent	976.6	E858.7	E946.6	E950.4	E962.0	E980.4
ophthalmic preparation	976.5	E858.7	E946.5	E950.4	E962.0	E980.4
topical NEC	976.0	E858.7	E946.0	E950.4	E962.0	E980.4
Cosmetics	989.89	E866.7	—	E950.9	E962.1	E980.9
Cosyntropin	977.8	E858.8	E947.8	E950.4	E962.0	E980.4
Cotarnine	964.5	E858.2	E934.5	E950.4	E962.0	E980.4
Cottonseed oil	976.3	E858.7	E946.3	E950.4	E962.0	E980.4
Cough mixtures (antitussives)	975.4	E858.6	E945.4	E950.4	E962.0	E980.4
containing opiates	965.09	E850.2	E935.2	E950.0	E962.0	E980.0
expectorants	975.5	E858.6	E945.5	E950.4	E962.0	E980.4
Coumadin	964.2	E858.2	E934.2	E950.4	E962.0	E980.4
rodenticide	989.4	E863.7	—	E950.6	E962.1	E980.7
Coumarin	964.2	E858.2	E934.2	E950.4	E962.0	E980.4
Coumetarol	964.2	E858.2	E934.2	E950.4	E962.0	E980.4
Cowbane	988.2	E865.4	—	E950.9	E962.1	E980.9
Cozyme	963.5	E858.1	E933.5	E950.4	E962.0	E980.4
Crack ●	970.8	E854.3	E940.8	E950.4	E962.0	E980.4
Creolin	983.0	E864.0	—	E950.7	E962.1	E980.6
disinfectant	983.0	E861.4	—	E950.7	E962.1	E980.6
Creosol (compound)	983.0	E864.0	—	E950.7	E962.1	E980.6
Creosote (beechwood) (coal tar)	983.0	E864.0	—	E950.7	E962.1	E980.6
medicinal (expectorant)	975.5	E858.6	E945.5	E950.4	E962.0	E980.4
syrup	975.5	E858.6	E945.5	E950.4	E962.0	E980.4
Cresol	983.0	E864.0	—	E950.7	E962.1	E980.6
disinfectant	983.0	E861.4	—	E950.7	E962.1	E980.6
Cresylic acid	983.0	E864.0	—	E950.7	E962.1	E980.6
Cropropamide	965.7	E850.7	E935.7	E950.0	E962.0	E980.0
with crotethamide	970.0	E854.3	E940.0	E950.4	E962.0	E980.4
Crotamiton	976.0	E858.7	E946.0	E950.4	E962.0	E980.4
Crotethamide	965.7	E850.7	E935.7	E950.0	E962.0	E980.0
with cropropamide	970.0	E854.3	E940.0	E950.4	E962.0	E980.4
Croton (oil)	973.1	E858.4	E943.1	E950.4	E962.0	E980.4
chloral	967.1	E852.0	E937.1	E950.2	E962.0	E980.2
Crude oil	981	E862.1	—	E950.9	E962.1	E980.9
Cryogenine	965.8	E850.8	E935.8	E950.0	E962.0	E980.0
Cryolite (pesticide)	989.4	E863.4	—	E950.6	E962.1	E980.7
Cryptenamine	972.6	E858.3	E942.6	E950.4	E962.0	E980.4
Crystal violet	976.0	E858.7	E946.0	E950.4	E962.0	E980.4
Cuckoopint	988.2	E865.4	—	E950.9	E962.1	E980.9
Cumetharol	964.2	E858.2	E934.2	E950.4	E962.0	E980.4
Cupric sulfate	973.6	E858.4	E943.6	E950.4	E962.0	E980.4
Cuprous sulfate	983.9	E864.3	—	E950.7	E962.1	E980.6
Curare, curarine	975.2	E858.6	E945.2	E950.4	E962.0	E980.4
Cyanic acid — *see* Cyanide(s)						
Cyanide(s) (compounds) (hydrogen) (potassium) (sodium) NEC	989.0	E866.8	—	E950.9	E962.1	E980.9
dust or gas (inhalation) NEC	987.7	E869.8	—	E952.8	E962.2	E982.8
fumigant	989.0	E863.8	—	E950.6	E962.1	E980.7
mercuric — *see* Mercury						
pesticide (dust) (fumes)	989.0	E863.4	—	E950.6	E962.1	E980.7
Cyanocobalamin	964.1	E858.2	E934.1	E950.4	E962.0	E980.4
Cyanogen (chloride) (gas) NEC	987.8	E869.8	—	E952.8	E962.2	E982.8
Cyclaine	968.5	E855.2	E938.5	E950.4	E962.0	E980.4
Cyclamen europaeum	988.2	E865.4	—	E950.9	E962.1	E980.9
Cyclandelate	972.5	E858.3	E942.5	E950.4	E962.0	E980.4
Cyclazocine	965.09	E850.2	E935.2	E950.0	E962.0	E980.0
Cyclizine	963.0	E858.1	E933.0	E950.4	E962.0	E980.4
Cyclobarbital, cyclobarbitone	967.0	E851	E937.0	E950.1	E962.0	E980.1
Cycloguanil	961.4	E857	E931.4	E950.4	E962.0	E980.4
Cyclohexane	982.0	E862.4	—	E950.9	E962.1	E980.9

Cortef — Cyclohexane

	Poisoning	Accident	Therapeutic Use	Suicide Attempt	Assault	Undetermined
				External Cause (E-Code)		
Cyclohexanol	980.8	E860.8	—	E950.9	E962.1	E980.9
Cyclohexanone	982.8	E862.4	—	E950.9	E962.1	E980.9
Cyclomethycaine	968.5	E855.2	E938.5	E950.4	E962.0	E980.4
Cyclopentamine	971.2	E855.5	E941.2	E950.4	E962.0	E980.4
Cyclopenthiazide	974.3	E858.5	E944.3	E950.4	E962.0	E980.4
Cyclopentolate	971.1	E855.4	E941.1	E950.4	E962.0	E980.4
Cyclophosphamide	963.1	E858.1	E933.1	E950.4	E962.0	E980.4
Cyclopropane	968.2	E855.1	E938.2	E950.4	E962.0	E980.4
Cycloserine	960.6	E856	E930.6	E950.4	E962.0	E980.4
Cyclothiazide	974.3	E858.5	E944.3	E950.4	E962.0	E980.4
Cycrimine	966.4	E855.0	E936.4	E950.4	E962.0	E980.4
Cymarin	972.1	E858.3	E942.1	E950.4	E962.0	E980.4
Cyproheptadine	963.0	E858.1	E933.0	E950.4	E962.0	E980.4
Cyprolidol	969.0	E854.0	E939.0	E950.3	E962.0	E980.3
Cytarabine	963.1	E858.1	E933.1	E950.4	E962.0	E980.4
Cytisus						
laburnum	988.2	E865.4	—	E950.9	E962.1	E980.9
scoparius	988.2	E865.4	—	E950.9	E962.1	E980.9
Cytomel	962.7	E858.0	E932.7	E950.4	E962.0	E980.4
Cytosine (antineoplastic)	963.1	E858.1	E933.1	E950.4	E962.0	E980.4
Cytoxan	963.1	E858.1	E933.1	E950.4	E962.0	E980.4
Dacarbazine	963.1	E858.1	E933.1	E950.4	E962.0	E980.4
Dactinomycin	960.7	E856	E930.7	E950.4	E962.0	E980.4
DADPS	961.8	E857	E931.8	E950.4	E962.0	E980.4
Dakin's solution (external)	976.0	E858.7	E946.0	E950.4	E962.0	E980.4
Dalmane	969.4	E853.2	E939.4	E950.3	E962.0	E980.3
DAM	977.2	E858.8	E947.2	E950.4	E962.0	E980.4
Danilone	964.2	E858.2	E934.2	E950.4	E962.0	E980.4
Danthron	973.1	E858.4	E943.1	E950.4	E962.0	E980.4
Dantrolene	975.2	E858.6	E945.2	E950.4	E962.0	E980.4
Daphne (gnidium) (mezereum)	988.2	E865.4	—	E950.9	E962.1	E980.9
berry	988.2	E865.3	—	E950.9	E962.1	E980.9
Dapsone	961.8	E857	E931.8	E950.4	E962.0	E980.4
Daraprim	961.4	E857	E931.4	E950.4	E962.0	E980.4
Darnel	988.2	E865.3	—	E950.9	E962.1	E980.9
Darvon	965.8	E850.8	E935.8	E950.0	E962.0	E980.0
Daunorubicin	960.7	E856	E930.7	E950.4	E962.0	E980.4
DBI	962.3	E858.0	E932.3	E950.4	E962.0	E980.4
D-Con (rodenticide)	989.4	E863.7	—	E950.6	E962.1	E980.7
DDS	961.8	E857	E931.8	E950.4	E962.0	E980.4
DDT	989.2	E863.0	—	E950.6	E962.1	E980.7
Deadly nightshade	988.2	E865.4	—	E950.9	E962.1	E980.9
berry	988.2	E865.3	—	E950.9	E962.1	E980.9
Deanol	969.7	E854.2	E939.7	E950.3	E962.0	E980.3
Debrisoquine	972.6	E858.3	E942.6	E950.4	E962.0	E980.4
Decaborane	989.89	E866.8	—	E950.9	E962.1	E980.9
fumes	987.8	E869.8	—	E952.8	E962.2	E982.8
Decadron	962.0	E858.0	E932.0	E950.4	E962.0	E980.4
ENT agent	976.6	E858.7	E946.6	E950.4	E962.0	E980.4
ophthalmic preparation	976.5	E858.7	E946.5	E950.4	E962.0	E980.4
topical NEC	976.0	E858.7	E946.0	E950.4	E962.0	E980.4
Decahydronaphthalene	982.0	E862.4	—	E950.9	E962.1	E980.9
Decalin	982.0	E862.4	—	E950.9	E962.1	E980.9
Decamethonium	975.2	E858.6	E945.2	E950.4	E962.0	Undetermined
Decholin	973.4	E858.4	E943.4	E950.4	E962.0	E980.4
sodium (diagnostic)	977.8	E858.8	E947.8	E950.4	E962.0	E980.4
Declomycin	960.4	E856	E930.4	E950.4	E962.0	E980.4
Deferoxamine	963.8	E858.1	E933.8	E950.4	E962.0	E980.4
Dehydrocholic acid	973.4	E858.4	E943.4	E950.4	E962.0	E980.4
DeKalin	982.0	E862.4	—	E950.9	E962.1	E980.9
Delalutin	962.2	E858.0	E932.2	E950.4	E962.0	E980.4
Delphinium	988.2	E865.3	—	E950.9	E962.1	E980.9
Deltasone	962.0	E858.0	E932.0	E950.4	E962.0	E980.4
Deltra	962.0	E858.0	E932.0	E950.4	E962.0	E980.4
Delvinal	967.0	E851	E937.0	E950.1	E962.0	E980.1
Demecarium (bromide)	971.0	E855.3	E941.0	E950.4	E962.0	E980.4
Demeclocycline	960.4	E856	E930.4	E950.4	E962.0	E980.4
Demecolcine	963.1	E858.1	E933.1	E950.4	E962.0	E980.4
Demelanizing agents	976.8	E858.7	E946.8	E950.4	E962.0	E980.4
Demerol	965.09	E850.2	E935.2	E950.0	E962.0	E980.0
Demethylchlortetracycline	960.4	E856	E930.4	E950.4	E962.0	E980.4
Demethyltetracycline	960.4	E856	E930.4	E950.4	E962.0	E980.4
Demeton	989.3	E863.1	—	E950.6	E962.1	E980.7
Demulcents	976.3	E858.7	E946.3	E950.4	E962.0	E980.4
Demulen	962.2	E858.0	E932.2	E950.4	E962.0	E980.4
Denatured alcohol	980.0	E860.1	—	E950.9	E962.1	E980.9
Dendrid	976.5	E858.7	E946.5	E950.4	E962.0	E980.4
Dental agents, topical	976.7	E858.7	E946.7	E950.4	E962.0	E980.4
Deodorant spray (feminine hygiene)	976.8	E858.7	E946.8	E950.4	E962.0	E980.4
Deoxyribonuclease	963.4	E858.1	E933.4	E950.4	E962.0	E980.4

Cyclohexanol — Deoxyribonuclease

		External Cause (E-Code)				
	Poisoning	Accident	Therapeutic Use	Suicide Attempt	Assault	Undetermined
Depressants						
appetite, central	977.0	E858.8	E947.0	E950.4	E962.0	E980.4
cardiac	972.0	E858.3	E942.0	E950.4	E962.0	E980.4
central nervous system (anesthetic)	968.4	E855.1	E938.4	E950.4	E962.0	E980.4
psychotherapeutic	969.5	E853.9	E939.5	E950.3	E962.0	E980.3
Dequalinium	976.0	E858.7	E946.0	E950.4	E962.0	E980.4
Dermolate	976.2	E858.7	E946.2	E950.4	E962.0	E980.4
DES	962.2	E858.0	E932.2	E950.4	E962.0	E980.4
Desenex	976.0	E858.7	E946.0	E950.4	E962.0	E980.4
Deserpidine	972.6	E858.3	E942.6	E950.4	E962.0	E980.4
Desipramine	969.0	E854.0	E939.0	E950.3	E962.0	E980.3
Deslanoside	972.1	E858.3	E942.1	E950.4	E962.0	E980.4
Desocodeine	965.09	E850.2	E935.2	E950.0	E962.0	E980.0
Desomorphine	965.09	E850.2	E935.2	E950.0	E962.0	E980.0
Desonide	976.0	E858.7	E946.0	E950.4	E962.0	E980.4
Desoxycorticosterone derivatives	962.0	E858.0	E932.0	E950.4	E962.0	E980.4
Desoxyephedrine	969.7	E854.2	E939.7	E950.3	E962.0	E980.3
DET	969.6	E854.1	E939.6	E950.3	E962.0	E980.3
Detergents (ingested) (synthetic)	989.6	E861.0	—	E950.9	E962.1	E980.9
external medication	976.2	E858.7	E946.2	E950.4	E962.0	E980.4
Deterrent, alcohol	977.3	E858.8	E947.3	E950.4	E962.0	E980.4
Detrothyronine	962.7	E858.0	E932.7	E950.4	E962.0	E980.4
Dettol (external medication)	976.0	E858.7	E946.0	E950.4	E962.0	E980.4
Dexamethasone	962.0	E858.0	E932.0	E950.4	E962.0	E980.4
ENT agent	976.6	E858.7	E946.6	E950.4	E962.0	E980.4
ophthalmic preparation	976.5	E858.7	E946.5	E950.4	E962.0	E980.4
topical NEC	976.0	E858.7	E946.0	E950.4	E962.0	E980.4
Dexamphetamine	969.7	E854.2	E939.7	E950.3	E962.0	E980.3
Dexedrine	969.7	E854.2	E939.7	E950.3	E962.0	E980.3
Dexpanthenol	963.5	E858.1	E933.5	E950.4	E962.0	E980.4
Dextran	964.8	E858.2	E934.8	E950.4	E962.0	E980.4
Dextriferron	964.0	E858.2	E934.0	E950.4	E962.0	E980.4
Dextroamphetamine	969.7	E854.2	E939.7	E950.3	E962.0	E980.3
Dextro calcium pantothenate	963.5	E858.1	E933.5	E950.4	E962.0	E980.4
Dextromethorphan	975.4	E858.6	E945.4	E950.4	E962.0	E980.4
Dextromoramide	965.09	E850.2	E935.2	E950.0	E962.0	E980.0
Dextro pantothenyl alcohol	963.5	E858.1	E933.5	E950.4	E962.0	E980.4
topical	976.8	E858.7	E946.8	E950.4	E962.0	E980.4
Dextropropoxyphene (hydrochloride)	965.8	E850.8	E935.8	E950.0	E962.0	E980.0
Dextrorphan	965.09	E850.2	E935.2	E950.0	E962.0	E980.0
Dextrose NEC	974.5	E858.5	E944.5	E950.4	E962.0	E980.4
Dextrothyroxin	962.7	E858.0	E932.7	E950.4	E962.0	E980.4
DFP	971.0	E855.3	E941.0	E950.4	E962.0	E980.4
DHE-45	972.9	E858.3	E942.9	E950.4	E962.0	E980.4
Diabinese	962.3	E858.0	E932.3	E950.4	E962.0	E980.4
Diacetyl monoxime	977.2	E858.8	E947.2	E950.4	E962.0	E980.4
Diacetylmorphine	965.01	E850.0	E935.0	E950.0	E962.0	E980.0
Diagnostic agents	977.8	E858.8	E947.8	E950.4	E962.0	E980.4
Dial (soap)	976.2	E858.7	E946.2	E950.4	E962.0	E980.4
sedative	967.0	E851	E937.0	E950.1	E962.0	E980.1
Diallylbarbituric acid	967.0	E851	E937.0	E950.1	E962.0	E980.1
Diaminodiphenylsulfone	961.8	E857	E931.8	E950.4	E962.0	E980.4
Diamorphine	965.01	E850.0	E935.0	E950.0	E962.0	E980.0
Diamox	974.2	E858.5	E944.2	E950.4	E962.0	E980.4
Diamthazole	976.0	E858.7	E946.0	E950.4	E962.0	E980.4
Diaphenylsulfone	961.8	E857	E931.8	E950.4	E962.0	E980.4
Diasone (sodium)	961.8	E857	E931.8	E950.4	E962.0	E980.4
Diazepam	969.4	E853.2	E939.4	E950.3	E962.0	E980.3
Diazinon	989.3	E863.1	—	E950.6	E962.1	E980.7
Diazomethane (gas)	987.8	E869.8	—	E952.8	E962.2	E982.8
Diazoxide	972.5	E858.3	E942.5	E950.4	E962.0	E980.4
Dibenamine	971.3	E855.6	E941.3	E950.4	E962.0	E980.4
Dibenzheptropine	963.0	E858.1	E933.0	E950.4	E962.0	E980.4
Dibenzyline	971.3	E855.6	E941.3	E950.4	E962.0	E980.4
Diborane (gas)	987.8	E869.8	—	E952.8	E962.2	E982.8
Dibromomannitol	963.1	E858.1	E933.1	E950.4	E962.0	E980.4
Dibucaine (spinal)	968.7	E855.2	E938.7	E950.4	E962.0	E980.4
topical (surface)	968.5	E855.2	E938.5	E950.4	E962.0	E980.4
Dibunate sodium	975.4	E858.6	E945.4	E950.4	E962.0	E980.4
Dibutoline	971.1	E855.4	E941.1	E950.4	E962.0	E980.4
Dicapthon	989.4	E863.4	—	E950.6	E962.1	E980.7
Dichloralphenazone	967.1	E852.0	E937.1	E950.2	E962.0	E980.2
Dichlorodifluoromethane	987.4	E869.2	—	E952.8	E962.2	E982.8
Dichloroethane	982.3	E862.4	—	E950.9	E962.1	E980.9
Dichloroethylene	982.3	E862.4	—	E950.9	E962.1	E980.9
Dichloroethyl sulfide	987.8	E869.8	—	E952.8	E962.2	E982.8
Dichlorohydrin	982.3	E862.4	—	E950.9	E962.1	E980.9
Dichloromethane (solvent) (vapor)	982.3	E862.4	—	E950.9	E962.1	E980.9
Dichlorophen(e)	961.6	E857	E931.6	E950.4	E962.0	E980.4
Dichlorphenamide	974.2	E858.5	E944.2	E950.4	E962.0	E980.4
Dichlorvos	989.3	E863.1	—	E950.6	E962.1	E980.7

✓4ᵗʰ Fourth-digit Required   ✓5ᵗʰ Fifth-digit Required   ▶◀ Revised Text   ● New Line   ▲ Revised Code

		External Cause (E-Code)				
	Poisoning	Accident	Therapeutic Use	Suicide Attempt	Assault	Undetermined
Diclofenac sodium	965.69	E850.6	E935.6	E950.0	E962.0	E980.0
Dicoumarin, dicumarol	964.2	E858.2	E934.2	E950.4	E962.0	E980.4
Dicyanogen (gas)	987.8	E869.8	—	E952.8	E962.2	E982.8
Dicyclomine	971.1	E855.4	E941.1	E950.4	E962.0	E980.4
Dieldrin (vapor)	989.2	E863.0	—	E950.6	E962.1	E980.7
Dienestrol	962.2	E858.0	E932.2	E950.4	E962.0	E980.4
Dietetics	977.0	E858.8	E947.0	E950.4	E962.0	E980.4
Diethazine	966.4	E855.0	E936.4	E950.4	E962.0	E980.4
Diethyl						
barbituric acid	967.0	E851	E937.0	E950.1	E962.0	E980.1
carbamazine	961.6	E857	E931.6	E950.4	E962.0	E980.4
carbinol	980.8	E860.8	—	E950.9	E962.1	E980.9
carbonate	982.8	E862.4	—	E950.9	E962.1	E980.9
ether (vapor) — see Ether(s)						
propion	977.0	E858.8	E947.0	E950.4	E962.0	E980.4
stilbestrol	962.2	E858.0	E932.2	E950.4	E962.0	E980.4
Diethylene						
dioxide	982.8	E862.4	—	E950.9	E962.1	E980.9
glycol (monoacetate) (monoethyl ether)	982.8	E862.4	—	E950.9	E962.1	E980.9
Diethylsulfone-diethylmethane	967.8	E852.8	E937.8	E950.2	E962.0	E980.2
Difencloxazine	965.09	E850.2	E935.2	E950.0	E962.0	E980.0
Diffusin	963.4	E858.1	E933.4	E950.4	E962.0	E980.4
Diflos	971.0	E855.3	E941.0	E950.4	E962.0	E980.4
Digestants	973.4	E858.4	E943.4	E950.4	E962.0	E980.4
Digitalin(e)	972.1	E858.3	E942.1	E950.4	E962.0	E980.4
Digitalis glycosides	972.1	E858.3	E942.1	E950.4	E962.0	E980.4
Digitoxin	972.1	E858.3	E942.1	E950.4	E962.0	E980.4
Digoxin	972.1	E858.3	E942.1	E950.4	E962.0	E980.4
Dihydrocodeine	965.09	E850.2	E935.2	E950.0	E962.0	E980.0
Dihydrocodeinone	965.09	E850.2	E935.2	E950.0	E962.0	E980.0
Dihydroergocristine	972.9	E858.3	E942.9	E950.4	E962.0	E980.4
Dihydroergotamine	972.9	E858.3	E942.9	E950.4	E962.0	E980.4
Dihydroergotoxine	972.9	E858.3	E942.9	E950.4	E962.0	E980.4
Dihydrohydroxycodeinone	965.09	E850.2	E935.2	E950.0	E962.0	E980.0
Dihydrohydroxymorphinone	965.09	E850.2	E935.2	E950.0	E962.0	E980.0
Dihydroisocodeine	965.09	E850.2	E935.2	E950.0	E962.0	E980.0
Dihydromorphine	965.09	E850.2	E935.2	E950.0	E962.0	E980.0
Dihydromorphinone	965.09	E850.2	E935.2	E950.0	E962.0	E980.0
Dihydrostreptomycin	960.6	E856	E930.6	E950.4	E962.0	E980.4
Dihydrotachysterol	962.6	E858.0	E932.6	E950.4	E962.0	E980.4
Dihydroxyanthraquinone	973.1	E858.4	E943.1	E950.4	E962.0	E980.4
Dihydroxycodeinone	965.09	E850.2	E935.2	E950.0	E962.0	E980.0
Diiodohydroxyquin	961.3	E857	E931.3	E950.4	E962.0	E980.4
topical	976.0	E858.7	E946.0	E950.4	E962.0	E980.4
Diiodohydroxyquinoline	961.3	E857	E931.3	E950.4	E962.0	E980.4
Dilantin	966.1	E855.0	E936.1	E950.4	E962.0	E980.4
Dilaudid	965.09	E850.2	E935.2	E950.0	E962.0	E980.0
Diloxanide	961.5	E857	E931.5	E950.4	E962.0	E980.4
Dimefline	970.0	E854.3	E940.0	E950.4	E962.0	E980.4
Dimenhydrinate	963.0	E858.1	E933.0	E950.4	E962.0	E980.4
Dimercaprol	963.8	E858.1	E933.8	E950.4	E962.0	E980.4
Dimercaptopropanol	963.8	E858.1	E933.8	E950.4	E962.0	E980.4
Dimetane	963.0	E858.1	E933.0	E950.4	E962.0	E980.4
Dimethicone	976.3	E858.7	E946.3	E950.4	E962.0	E980.4
Dimethindene	963.0	E858.1	E933.0	E950.4	E962.0	E980.4
Dimethisoquin	968.5	E855.2	E938.5	E950.4	E962.0	E980.4
Dimethisterone	962.2	E858.0	E932.2	E950.4	E962.0	E980.4
Dimethoxanate	975.4	E858.6	E945.4	E950.4	E962.0	E980.4
Dimethyl						
arsine, arsinic acid — see Arsenic						
carbinol	980.2	E860.3	—	E950.9	E962.1	E980.9
diguanide	962.3	E858.0	E932.3	E950.4	E962.0	E980.4
ketone	982.8	E862.4	—	E950.9	E962.1	E980.9
vapor	987.8	E869.8	—	E952.8	E962.2	E982.8
meperidine	965.09	E850.2	E935.2	E950.0	E962.0	E980.0
parathion	989.3	E863.1	—	E950.6	E962.1	E980.7
polysiloxane	973.8	E858.4	E943.8	E950.4	E962.0	E980.4
sulfate (fumes)	987.8	E869.8	—	E952.8	E962.2	E982.8
liquid	983.9	E864.3	—	E950.7	E962.1	E980.6
sulfoxide NEC	982.8	E862.4	—	E950.9	E962.1	E980.9
medicinal	976.4	E858.7	E946.4	E950.4	E962.0	E980.4
triptamine	969.6	E854.1	E939.6	E950.3	E962.0	E980.3
tubocurarine	975.2	E858.6	E945.2	E950.4	E962.0	E980.4
Dindevan	964.2	E858.2	E934.2	E950.4	E962.0	E980.4
Dinitro (-ortho-) cresol (herbicide) (spray)	989.4	E863.5	—	E950.6	E962.1	E980.7
insecticide	989.4	E863.4	—	E950.6	E962.1	E980.7
Dinitrobenzene	983.0	E864.0	—	E950.7	E962.1	E980.6
vapor	987.8	E869.8	—	E952.8	E962.2	E982.8
Dinitro-orthocresol (herbicide)	989.4	E863.5	—	E950.6	E962.1	E980.7
insecticide	989.4	E863.4	—	E950.6	E962.1	E980.7

4ᵗʰ Fourth-digit Required   5ᵗʰ Fifth-digit Required   ▶◀ Revised Text   ● New Line   ▲ Revised Code

		External Cause (E-Code)				
	Poisoning	Accident	Therapeutic Use	Suicide Attempt	Assault	Undetermined
Dinitrophenol (herbicide) (spray)	989.4	E863.5	—	E950.6	E962.1	E980.7
insecticide	989.4	E863.4	—	E950.6	E962.1	E980.7
Dinoprost	975.0	E858.6	E945.0	E950.4	E962.0	E980.4
Dioctyl sulfosuccinate (calcium) (sodium)	973.2	E858.4	E943.2	E950.4	E962.0	E980.4
Diodoquin	961.3	E857	E931.3	E950.4	E962.0	E980.4
Dione derivatives NEC	966.3	E855.0	E936.3	E950.4	E962.0	E980.4
Dionin	965.09	E850.2	E935.2	E950.0	E962.0	E980.0
Dioxane	982.8	E862.4	—	E950.9	E962.1	E980.9
Dioxin — see Herbicide						
Dioxyline	972.5	E858.3	E942.5	E950.4	E962.0	E980.4
Dipentene	982.8	E862.4	—	E950.9	E962.1	E980.9
Diphemanil	971.1	E855.4	E941.1	E950.4	E962.0	E980.4
Diphenadione	964.2	E858.2	E934.2	E950.4	E962.0	E980.4
Diphenhydramine	963.0	E858.1	E933.0	E950.4	E962.0	E980.4
Diphenidol	963.0	E858.1	E933.0	E950.4	E962.0	E980.4
Diphenoxylate	973.5	E858.4	E943.5	E950.4	E962.0	E980.4
Diphenylchloroarsine	985.1	E866.3	—	E950.8	E962.1	E980.8
Diphenylhydantoin (sodium)	966.1	E855.0	E936.1	E950.4	E962.0	E980.4
Diphenylpyraline	963.0	E858.1	E933.0	E950.4	E962.0	E980.4
Diphtheria						
antitoxin	979.9	E858.8	E949.9	E950.4	E962.0	E980.4
toxoid	978.5	E858.8	E948.5	E950.4	E962.0	E980.4
with tetanus toxoid	978.9	E858.8	E948.9	E950.4	E962.0	E980.4
with pertussis component	978.6	E858.8	E948.6	E950.4	E962.0	E980.4
vaccine	978.5	E858.8	E948.5	E950.4	E962.0	E980.4
Dipipanone	965.09	E850.2	E935.2	E950.0	E962.0	E980.0
Diplovax	979.5	E858.8	E949.5	E950.4	E962.0	E980.4
Diprophylline	975.1	E858.6	E945.1	E950.4	E962.0	E980.4
Dipyridamole	972.4	E858.3	E942.4	E950.4	E962.0	E980.4
Dipyrone	965.5	E850.5	E935.5	E950.0	E962.0	E980.0
Diquat	989.4	E863.5	—	E950.6	E962.1	E980.7
Disinfectant NEC	983.9	E861.4	—	E950.7	E962.1	E980.6
alkaline	983.2	E861.4	—	E950.7	E962.1	E980.6
aromatic	983.0	E861.4	—	E950.7	E962.1	E980.6
Disipal	966.4	E855.0	E936.4	E950.4	E962.0	E980.4
Disodium edetate	963.8	E858.1	E933.8	E950.4	E962.0	E980.4
Disulfamide	974.4	E858.5	E944.4	E950.4	E962.0	E980.4
Disulfanilamide	961.0	E857	E931.0	E950.4	E962.0	E980.4
Disulfiram	977.3	E858.8	E947.3	E950.4	E962.0	E980.4
Dithiazanine	961.6	E857	E931.6	E950.4	E962.0	E980.4
Dithioglycerol	963.8	E858.1	E933.8	E950.4	E962.0	E980.4
Dithranol	976.4	E858.7	E946.4	E950.4	E962.0	E980.4
Diucardin	974.3	E858.5	E944.3	E950.4	E962.0	E980.4
Diupres	974.3	E858.5	E944.3	E950.4	E962.0	E980.4
Diuretics NEC	974.4	E858.5	E944.4	E950.4	E962.0	E980.4
carbonic acid anhydrase inhibitors	974.2	E858.5	E944.2	E950.4	E962.0	E980.4
mercurial	974.0	E858.5	E944.0	E950.4	E962.0	E980.4
osmotic	974.4	E858.5	E944.4	E950.4	E962.0	E980.4
purine derivatives	974.1	E858.5	E944.1	E950.4	E962.0	E980.4
saluretic	974.3	E858.5	E944.3	E950.4	E962.0	E980.4
Diuril	974.3	E858.5	E944.3	E950.4	E962.0	E980.4
Divinyl ether	968.2	E855.1	E938.2	E950.4	E962.0	E980.4
D-lysergic acid diethylamide	969.6	E854.1	E939.6	E950.3	E962.0	E980.3
DMCT	960.4	E856	E930.4	E950.4	E962.0	E980.4
DMSO	982.8	E862.4	—	E950.9	E962.1	E980.9
DMT	969.6	E854.1	E939.6	E950.3	E962.0	E980.3
DNOC	989.4	E863.5	—	E950.6	E962.1	E980.7
DOCA	962.0	E858.0	E932.0	E950.4	E962.0	E980.4
Dolophine	965.02	E850.1	E935.1	E950.0	E962.0	E980.0
Doloxene	965.8	E850.8	E935.8	E950.0	E962.0	E980.0
DOM	969.6	E854.1	E939.6	E950.3	E962.0	E980.3
Domestic gas — see Gas, utility						
Domiphen (bromide) (lozenges)	976.6	E858.7	E946.6	E950.4	E962.0	E980.4
Dopa (levo)	966.4	E855.0	E936.4	E950.4	E962.0	E980.4
Dopamine	971.2	E855.5	E941.2	E950.4	E962.0	E980.4
Doriden	967.5	E852.4	E937.5	E950.2	E962.0	E980.2
Dormiral	967.0	E851	E937.0	E950.1	E962.0	E980.1
Dormison	967.8	E852.8	E937.8	E950.2	E962.0	E980.2
Dornase	963.4	E858.1	E933.4	E950.4	E962.0	E980.4
Dorsacaine	968.5	E855.2	E938.5	E950.4	E962.0	E980.4
Dothiepin hydrochloride	969.0	E854.0	E939.0	E950.3	E962.0	E980.3
Doxapram	970.0	E854.3	E940.0	E950.4	E962.0	E980.4
Doxepin	969.0	E854.0	E939.0	E950.3	E962.0	E980.3
Doxorubicin	960.7	E856	E930.7	E950.4	E962.0	E980.4
Doxycycline	960.4	E856	E930.4	E950.4	E962.0	E980.4
Doxylamine	963.0	E858.1	E933.0	E950.4	E962.0	E980.4
Dramamine	963.0	E858.1	E933.0	E950.4	E962.0	E980.4
Drano (drain cleaner)	983.2	E864.2	—	E950.7	E962.1	E980.6
Dromoran	965.09	E850.2	E935.2	E950.0	E962.0	E980.0
Dromostanolone	962.1	E858.0	E932.1	E950.4	E962.0	E980.4
Droperidol	969.2	E853.1	E939.2	E950.3	E962.0	E980.3

✓4ᵗʰ Fourth-digit Required   ✓5ᵗʰ Fifth-digit Required   ►◄ Revised Text   ● New Line   ▲ Revised Code

		External Cause (E-Code)				
	Poisoning	Accident	Therapeutic Use	Suicide Attempt	Assault	Undetermined
Drug	977.9	E858.9	E947.9	E950.5	E962.0	E980.5
specified NEC	977.8	E858.8	E947.8	E950.4	E962.0	E980.4
AHFS List						
4:00 antihistamine drugs	963.0	E858.1	E933.0	E950.4	E962.0	E980.4
8:04 amebacides	961.5	E857	E931.5	E950.4	E962.0	E980.4
arsenical anti-infectives	961.1	E857	E931.1	E950.4	E962.0	E980.4
quinoline derivatives	961.3	E857	E931.3	E950.4	E962.0	E980.4
8:08 anthelmintics	961.6	E857	E931.6	E950.4	E962.0	E980.4
quinoline derivatives	961.3	E857	E931.3	E950.4	E962.0	E980.4
8:12.04 antifungal antibiotics	960.1	E856	E930.1	E950.4	E962.0	E980.4
8:12.06 cephalosporins	960.5	E856	E930.5	E950.4	E962.0	E980.4
8:12.08 chloramphenicol	960.2	E856	E930.2	E950.4	E962.0	E980.4
8:12.12 erythromycins	960.3	E856	E930.3	E950.4	E962.0	E980.4
8:12.16 penicillins	960.0	E856	E930.0	E950.4	E962.0	E980.4
8:12.20 streptomycins	960.6	E856	E930.6	E950.4	E962.0	E980.4
8:12.24 tetracyclines	960.4	E856	E930.4	E950.4	E962.0	E980.4
8:12.28 other antibiotics	960.8	E856	E930.8	E950.4	E962.0	E980.4
antimycobacterial	960.6	E856	E930.6	E950.4	E962.0	E980.4
macrolides	960.3	E856	E930.3	E950.4	E962.0	E980.4
8:16 antituberculars	961.8	E857	E931.8	E950.4	E962.0	E980.4
antibiotics	960.6	E856	E930.6	E950.4	E962.0	E980.4
8:18 antivirals	961.7	E857	E931.7	E950.4	E962.0	E980.4
8:20 plasmodicides (antimalarials)	961.4	E857	E931.4	E950.4	E962.0	E980.4
8:24 sulfonamides	961.0	E857	E931.0	E950.4	E962.0	E980.4
8:26 sulfones	961.8	E857	E931.8	E950.4	E962.0	E980.4
8:28 treponemicides	961.2	E857	E931.2	E950.4	E962.0	E980.4
8:32 trichomonacides	961.5	E857	E931.5	E950.4	E962.0	E980.4
quinoline derivatives	961.3	E857	E931.3	E950.4	E962.0	E980.4
nitrofuran derivatives	961.9	E857	E931.9	E950.4	E962.0	E980.4
8:36 urinary germicides	961.9	E857	E931.9	E950.4	E962.0	E980.4
quinoline derivatives	961.3	E857	E931.3	E950.4	E962.0	E980.4
8:40 other anti-infectives	961.9	E857	E931.9	E950.4	E962.0	E980.4
10:00 antineoplastic agents	963.1	E858.1	E933.1	E950.4	E962.0	E980.4
antibiotics	960.7	E856	E930.7	E950.4	E962.0	E980.4
progestogens	962.2	E858.0	E932.2	E950.4	E962.0	E980.4
12:04 parasympathomimetic (cholinergic) agents	971.0	E855.3	E941.0	E950.4	E962.0	E980.4
12:08 parasympatholytic (cholinergic-blocking) agents	971.1	E855.4	E941.1	E950.4	E962.0	E980.4
12:12 Sympathomimetic (adrenergic) agents	971.2	E855.5	E941.2	E950.4	E962.0	E980.4
12:16 sympatholytic (adrenergic-blocking) agents	971.3	E855.6	E941.3	E950.4	E962.0	E980.4
12:20 skeletal muscle relaxants						
central nervous system muscle-tone depressants	968.0	E855.1	E938.0	E950.4	E962.0	E980.4
myoneural blocking agents	975.2	E858.6	E945.2	E950.4	E962.0	E980.4
16:00 blood derivatives	964.7	E858.2	E934.7	E950.4	E962.0	E980.4
20:04 antianemia drugs	964.1	E858.2	E934.1	E950.4	E962.0	E980.4
20:04.04 iron preparations	964.0	E858.2	E934.0	E950.4	E962.0	E980.4
20:04.08 liver and stomach preparations	964.1	E858.2	E934.1	E950.4	E962.0	E980.4
20:12.04 anticoagulants	964.2	E858.2	E934.2	E950.4	E962.0	E980.4
20:12.08 antiheparin agents	964.5	E858.2	E934.5	E950.4	E962.0	E980.4
20:12.12 coagulants	964.5	E858.2	E934.5	E950.4	E962.0	E980.4
20:12.16 hemostatics NEC	964.5	E858.2	E934.5	E950.4	E962.0	E980.4
capillary active drugs	972.8	E858.3	E942.8	E950.4	E962.0	E980.4
24:04 cardiac drugs	972.9	E858.3	E942.9	E950.4	E962.0	E980.4
cardiotonic agents	972.1	E858.3	E942.1	E950.4	E962.0	E980.4
rhythm regulators	972.0	E858.3	E942.0	E950.4	E962.0	E980.4
24:06 antilipemic agents	972.2	E858.3	E942.2	E950.4	E962.0	E980.4
thyroid derivatives	962.7	E858.0	E932.7	E950.4	E962.0	E980.4
24:08 hypotensive agents	972.6	E858.3	E942.6	E950.4	E962.0	E980.4
adrenergic blocking agents	971.3	E855.6	E941.3	E950.4	E962.0	E980.4
ganglion blocking agents	972.3	E858.3	E942.3	E950.4	E962.0	E980.4
vasodilators	972.5	E858.3	E942.5	E950.4	E962.0	E980.4
24:12 vasodilating agents NEC	972.5	E858.3	E942.5	E950.4	E962.0	E980.4
coronary	972.4	E858.3	E942.4	E950.4	E962.0	E980.4
nicotinic acid derivatives	972.2	E858.3	E942.2	E950.4	E962.0	E980.4
24:16 sclerosing agents	972.7	E858.3	E942.7	E950.4	E962.0	E980.4
28:04 general anesthetics	968.4	E855.1	E938.4	E950.4	E962.0	E980.4
gaseous anesthetics	968.2	E855.1	E938.2	E950.4	E962.0	E980.4
halothane	968.1	E855.1	E938.1	E950.4	E962.0	E980.4
intravenous anesthetics	968.3	E855.1	E938.3	E950.4	E962.0	E980.4
28:08 analgesics and antipyretics	965.9	E850.9	E935.9	E950.0	E962.0	E980.0
antirheumatics	965.69	E850.6	E935.6	E950.0	E962.0	E980.0
aromatic analgesics	965.4	E850.4	E935.4	E950.0	E962.0	E980.0
non-narcotic NEC	965.7	E850.7	E935.7	E950.0	E962.0	E980.0
opium alkaloids	965.00	E850.2	E935.2	E950.0	E962.0	E980.0
heroin	965.01	E850.0	E935.0	E950.0	E962.0	E980.0
methadone	965.02	E850.1	E935.1	E950.0	E962.0	E980.0
specified type NEC	965.09	E850.2	E935.2	E950.0	E962.0	E980.0
pyrazole derivatives	965.5	E850.5	E935.5	E950.0	E962.0	E980.0
salicylates	965.1	E850.3	E935.3	E950.0	E962.0	E980.0
specified NEC	965.8	E850.8	E935.8	E950.0	E962.0	E980.0
28:10 narcotic antagonists	970.1	E854.3	E940.1	E950.4	E962.0	E980.4

☑4ᵗʰ Fourth-digit Required   ☑5ᵗʰ Fifth-digit Required   ▶◀ Revised Text   ● New Line   ▲ Revised Code

Drug	Poisoning	External Cause (E-Code)				
		Accident	Therapeutic Use	Suicide Attempt	Assault	Undetermined
Drug — *continued*						
28:12 anticonvulsants	966.3	E855.0	E936.3	E950.4	E962.0	E980.4
barbiturates	967.0	E851	E937.0	E950.1	E962.0	E980.1
benzodiazepine-based tranquilizers	969.4	E853.2	E939.4	E950.3	E962.0	E980.3
bromides	967.3	E852.2	E937.3	E950.2	E962.0	E980.2
hydantoin derivatives	966.1	E855.0	E936.1	E950.4	E962.0	E980.4
oxazolidine (derivatives)	966.0	E855.0	E936.0	E950.4	E962.0	E980.4
succinimides	966.2	E855.0	E936.2	E950.4	E962.0	E980.4
28:16.04 antidepressants	969.0	E854.0	E939.0	E950.3	E962.0	E980.3
28:16.08 tranquilizers	969.5	E853.9	E939.5	E950.3	E962.0	E980.3
benzodiazepine-based	969.4	E853.2	E939.4	E950.3	E962.0	E980.3
butyrophenone-based	969.2	E853.1	E939.2	E950.3	E962.0	E980.3
major NEC	969.3	E853.8	E939.3	E950.3	E962.0	E980.3
phenothiazine-based	969.1	E853.0	E939.1	E950.3	E962.0	E980.3
28:16.12 other psychotherapeutic agents	969.8	E855.8	E939.8	E950.3	E962.0	E980.3
28:20 respiratory and cerebral stimulants	970.9	E854.3	E940.9	E950.4	E962.0	E980.4
analeptics	970.0	E854.3	E940.0	E950.4	E962.0	E980.4
anorexigenic agents	977.0	E858.8	E947.0	E950.4	E962.0	E980.4
psychostimulants	969.7	E854.2	E939.7	E950.3	E962.0	E980.3
specified NEC	970.8	E854.3	E940.8	E950.4	E962.0	E980.4
28:24 sedatives and hypnotics	967.9	E852.9	E937.9	E950.2	E962.0	E980.2
barbiturates	967.0	E851	E937.0	E950.1	E962.0	E980.1
benzodiazepine-based tranquilizers	969.4	E853.2	E939.4	E950.3	E962.0	E980.3
chloral hydrate (group)	967.1	E852.0	E937.1	E950.2	E962.0	E980.2
glutethamide group	967.5	E852.4	E937.5	E950.2	E962.0	E980.2
intravenous anesthetics	968.3	E855.1	E938.3	E950.4	E962.0	E980.4
methaqualone (compounds)	967.4	E852.3	E937.4	E950.2	E962.0	E980.2
paraldehyde	967.2	E852.1	E937.2	E950.2	E962.0	E980.2
phenothiazine-based tranquilizers	969.1	E853.0	E939.1	E950.3	E962.0	E980.3
specified NEC	967.8	E852.8	E937.8	E950.2	E962.0	E980.2
thiobarbiturates	968.3	E855.1	E938.3	E950.4	E962.0	E980.4
tranquilizer NEC	969.5	E853.9	E939.5	E950.3	E962.0	E980.3
36:04 to 36:88 diagnostic agents	977.8	E858.8	E947.8	E950.4	E962.0	E980.4
40:00 electrolyte, caloric, and water balance agents NEC	974.5	E858.5	E944.5	E950.4	E962.0	E980.4
40:04 acidifying agents	963.2	E858.1	E933.2	E950.4	E962.0	E980.4
40:08 alkalinizing agents	963.3	E858.1	E933.3	E950.4	E962.0	E980.4
40:10 ammonia detoxicants	974.5	E858.5	E944.5	E950.4	E962.0	E980.4
40:12 replacement solutions	974.5	E858.5	E944.5	E950.4	E962.0	E980.4
plasma expanders	964.8	E858.2	E934.8	E950.4	E962.0	E980.4
40:16 sodium-removing resins	974.5	E858.5	E944.5	E950.4	E962.0	E980.4
40:18 potassium-removing resins	974.5	E858.5	E944.5	E950.4	E962.0	E980.4
40:20 caloric agents	974.5	E858.5	E944.5	E950.4	E962.0	E980.4
40:24 salt and sugar substitutes	974.5	E858.5	E944.5	E950.4	E962.0	E980.4
40:28 diuretics NEC	974.4	E858.5	E944.4	E950.4	E962.0	E980.4
carbonic acid anhydrase inhibitors	974.2	E858.5	E944.2	E950.4	E962.0	E980.4
mercurials	974.0	E858.5	E944.0	E950.4	E962.0	E980.4
purine derivatives	974.1	E858.5	E944.1	E950.4	E962.0	E980.4
saluretics	974.3	E858.5	E944.3	E950.4	E962.0	E980.4
thiazides	974.3	E858.5	E944.3	E950.4	E962.0	E980.4
40:36 irrigating solutions	974.5	E858.5	E944.5	E950.4	E962.0	E980.4
40:40 uricosuric agents	974.7	E858.5	E944.7	E950.4	E962.0	E980.4
44:00 enzymes	963.4	E858.1	E933.4	E950.4	E962.0	E980.4
fibrinolysis-affecting agents	964.4	E858.2	E934.4	E950.4	E962.0	E980.4
gastric agents	973.4	E858.4	E943.4	E950.4	E962.0	E980.4
48:00 expectorants and cough preparations						
antihistamine agents	963.0	E858.1	E933.0	E950.4	E962.0	E980.4
antitussives	975.4	E858.6	E945.4	E950.4	E962.0	E980.4
codeine derivatives	965.09	E850.2	E935.2	E950.0	E962.0	E980.0
expectorants	975.5	E858.6	E945.5	E950.4	E962.0	E980.4
narcotic agents NEC	965.09	E850.2	E935.2	E950.0	E962.0	E980.0
52:04 anti-infectives (EENT)						
ENT agent	976.6	E858.7	E946.6	E950.4	E962.0	E980.4
ophthalmic preparation	976.5	E858.7	E946.5	E950.4	E962.0	E980.4
52:04.04 antibiotics (EENT)						
ENT agent	976.6	E858.7	E946.6	E950.4	E962.0	E980.4
ophthalmic preparation	976.5	E858.7	E946.5	E950.4	E962.0	E980.4
52:04.06 antivirals (EENT)						
ENT agent	976.6	E858.7	E946.6	E950.4	E962.0	E980.4
ophthalmic preparation	976.5	E858.7	E946.5	E950.4	E962.0	E980.4
52:04.08 sulfonamides (EENT)						
ENT agent	976.6	E858.7	E946.6	E950.4	E962.0	E980.4
ophthalmic preparation	976.5	E858.7	E946.5	E950.4	E962.0	E980.4
52:04.12 miscellaneous anti-infectives (EENT)						
ENT agent	976.6	E858.7	E946.6	E950.4	E962.0	E980.4
ophthalmic preparation	976.5	E858.7	E946.5	E950.4	E962.0	E980.4
52:08 anti-inflammatory agents (EENT)						
ENT agent	976.6	E858.7	E946.6	E950.4	E962.0	E980.4
ophthalmic preparation	976.5	E858.7	E946.5	E950.4	E962.0	E980.4
52:10 carbonic anhydrase inhibitors	974.2	E858.5	E944.2	E950.4	E962.0	E980.4
52:12 contact lens solutions	976.5	E858.7	E946.5	E950.4	E962.0	E980.4

✓4ᵗ Fourth-digit Required ✓5ᵗ Fifth-digit Required ►◄ Revised Text ● New Line ▲ Revised Code

Drug — continued	Poisoning	Accident	Therapeutic Use	Suicide Attempt	Assault	Undetermined
52:16 local anesthetics (EENT)	968.5	E855.2	E938.5	E950.4	E962.0	E980.4
52:20 miotics	971.0	E855.3	E941.0	E950.4	E962.0	E980.4
52:24 mydriatics						
adrenergics	971.2	E855.5	E941.2	E950.4	E962.0	E980.4
anticholinergics	971.1	E855.4	E941.1	E950.4	E962.0	E980.4
antimuscarinics	971.1	E855.4	E941.1	E950.4	E962.0	E980.4
parasympatholytics	971.1	E855.4	E941.1	E950.4	E962.0	E980.4
spasmolytics	971.1	E855.4	E941.1	E950.4	E962.0	E980.4
sympathomimetics	971.2	E855.5	E941.2	E950.4	E962.0	E980.4
52:28 mouth washes and gargles	976.6	E858.7	E946.6	E950.4	E962.0	E980.4
52:32 vasoconstrictors (EENT)	971.2	E855.5	E941.2	E950.4	E962.0	E980.4
52:36 unclassified agents (EENT)						
ENT agent	976.6	E858.7	E946.6	E950.4	E962.0	E980.4
ophthalmic preparation	976.5	E858.7	E946.5	E950.4	E962.0	E980.4
56:04 antacids and adsorbents	973.0	E858.4	E943.0	E950.4	E962.0	E980.4
56:08 antidiarrhea agents	973.5	E858.4	E943.5	E950.4	E962.0	E980.4
56:10 antiflatulents	973.8	E858.4	E943.8	E950.4	E962.0	E980.4
56:12 cathartics NEC	973.3	E858.4	E943.3	E950.4	E962.0	E980.4
emollients	973.2	E858.4	E943.2	E950.4	E962.0	E980.4
irritants	973.1	E858.4	E943.1	E950.4	E962.0	E980.4
56:16 digestants	973.4	E858.4	E943.4	E950.4	E962.0	E980.4
56:20 emetics and antiemetics						
antiemetics	963.0	E858.1	E933.0	E950.4	E962.0	E980.4
emetics	973.6	E858.4	E943.6	E950.4	E962.0	E980.4
56:24 lipotropic agents	977.1	E858.8	E947.1	E950.4	E962.0	E980.4
56:40 miscellaneous G.I. drugs	973.8	E858.4	E943.8	E950.4	E962.0	E980.4
60:00 gold compounds	965.69	E850.6	E935.6	E950.0	E962.0	E980.0
64:00 heavy metal antagonists	963.8	E858.1	E933.8	E950.4	E962.0	E980.4
68:04 adrenals	962.0	E858.0	E932.0	E950.4	E962.0	E980.4
68:08 androgens	962.1	E858.0	E932.1	E950.4	E962.0	E980.4
68:12 contraceptives, oral	962.2	E858.0	E932.2	E950.4	E962.0	E980.4
68:16 estrogens	962.2	E858.0	E932.2	E950.4	E962.0	E980.4
68:18 gonadotropins	962.4	E858.0	E932.4	E950.4	E962.0	E980.4
68:20 insulins and antidiabetic agents	962.3	E858.0	E932.3	E950.4	E962.0	E980.4
68:20.08 insulins	962.3	E858.0	E932.3	E950.4	E962.0	E980.4
68:24 parathyroid	962.6	E858.0	E932.6	E950.4	E962.0	E980.4
68:28 pituitary (posterior)	962.5	E858.0	E932.5	E950.4	E962.0	E980.4
anterior	962.4	E858.0	E932.4	E950.4	E962.0	E980.4
68:32 progestogens	962.2	E858.0	E932.2	E950.4	E962.0	E980.4
68:34 other corpus luteum						
hormones NEC	962.2	E858.0	E932.2	E950.4	E962.0	E980.4
68:36 thyroid and antithyroid						
antithyroid	962.8	E858.0	E932.8	E950.4	E962.0	E980.4
thyroid (derivatives)	962.7	E858.0	E932.7	E950.4	E962.0	E980.4
72:00 local anesthetics NEC	968.9	E855.2	E938.9	E950.4	E962.0	E980.4
topical (surface)	968.5	E855.2	E938.5	E950.4	E962.0	E980.4
infiltration (intradermal) (subcutaneous) (submucosal)	968.5	E855.2	E938.5	E950.4	E962.0	E980.4
nerve blocking (peripheral) (plexus) (regional)	968.6	E855.2	E938.6	E950.4	E962.0	E980.4
spinal	968.7	E855.2	E938.7	E950.4	E962.0	E980.4
76:00 oxytocics	975.0	E858.6	E945.0	E950.4	E962.0	E980.4
78:00 radioactive agents	990	—	—	—	—	—
80:04 serums NEC	979.9	E858.8	E949.9	E950.4	E962.0	E980.4
immune gamma globulin (human)	964.6	E858.2	E934.6	E950.4	E962.0	E980.4
80:08 toxoids NEC	978.8	E858.8	E948.8	E950.4	E962.0	E980.4
diphtheria	978.5	E858.8	E948.5	E950.4	E962.0	E980.4
and tetanus	978.9	E858.8	E948.9	E950.4	E962.0	E980.4
with pertussis component	978.6	E858.8	E948.6	E950.4	E962.0	E980.4
tetanus	978.4	E858.8	E948.4	E950.4	E962.0	E980.4
and diphtheria	978.9	E858.8	E948.9	E950.4	E962.0	E980.4
with pertussis component	978.6	E858.8	E948.6	E950.4	E962.0	E980.4
80:12 vaccines	979.9	E858.8	E949.9	E950.4	E962.0	E980.4
bacterial NEC	978.8	E858.8	E948.8	E950.4	E962.0	E980.4
with						
other bacterial components	978.9	E858.8	E948.9	E950.4	E962.0	E980.4
pertussis component	978.6	E858.8	E948.6	E950.4	E962.0	E980.4
viral and rickettsial components	979.7	E858.8	E949.7	E950.4	E962.0	E980.4
rickettsial NEC	979.6	E858.8	E949.6	E950.4	E962.0	E980.4
with						
bacterial component	979.7	E858.8	E949.7	E950.4	E962.0	E980.4
pertussis component	978.6	E858.8	E948.6	E950.4	E962.0	E980.4
viral component	979.7	E858.8	E949.7	E950.4	E962.0	E980.4
viral NEC	979.6	E858.8	E949.6	E950.4	E962.0	E980.4
with						
bacterial component	979.7	E858.8	E949.7	E950.4	E962.0	E980.4
pertussis component	978.6	E858.8	E948.6	E950.4	E962.0	E980.4
rickettsial component	979.7	E858.8	E949.7	E950.4	E962.0	E980.4
84:04.04 antibiotics (skin and mucous membrane)	976.0	E858.7	E946.0	E950.4	E962.0	E980.4
84:04.08 fungicides (skin and mucous membrane)	976.0	E858.7	E946.0	E950.4	E962.0	E980.4
84:04.12 scabicides and pediculicides (skin and mucous membrane)	976.0	E858.7	E946.0	E950.4	E962.0	E980.4

✔4ᵗʰ Fourth-digit Required   ✔5ᵗʰ Fifth-digit Required   ▶◀ Revised Text   ● New Line   ▲ Revised Code

		External Cause (E-Code)				
	Poisoning	**Accident**	**Therapeutic Use**	**Suicide Attempt**	**Assault**	**Undetermined**
Drug — *continued*						
84:04.16 miscellaneous local anti-infectives (skin and mucous membrane)	976.0	E858.7	E946.0	E950.4	E962.0	E980.4
84:06 anti-inflammatory agents (skin and mucous membrane)	976.0	E858.7	E946.0	E950.4	E962.0	E980.4
84:08 antipruritics and local anesthetics						
antipruritics	976.1	E858.7	E946.1	E950.4	E962.0	E980.4
local anesthetics	968.5	E855.2	E938.5	E950.4	E962.0	E980.4
84:12 astringents	976.2	E858.7	E946.2	E950.4	E962.0	E980.4
84:16 cell stimulants and proliferants	976.8	E858.7	E946.8	E950.4	E962.0	E980.4
84:20 detergents	976.2	E858.7	E946.2	E950.4	E962.0	E980.4
84:24 emollients, demulcents, and protectants	976.3	E858.7	E946.3	E950.4	E962.0	E980.4
84:28 keratolytic agents	976.4	E858.7	E946.4	E950.4	E962.0	E980.4
84:32 keratoplastic agents	976.4	E858.7	E946.4	E950.4	E962.0	E980.4
84:36 miscellaneous agents (skin and mucous membrane)	976.8	E858.7	E946.8	E950.4	E962.0	E980.4
86:00 spasmolytic agents	975.1	E858.6	E945.1	E950.4	E962.0	E980.4
antiasthmatics	975.7	E858.6	E945.7	E950.4	E962.0	E980.4
papaverine	972.5	E858.3	E942.5	E950.4	E962.0	E980.4
theophylline	974.1	E858.5	E944.1	E950.4	E962.0	E980.4
88:04 vitamin A	963.5	E858.1	E933.5	E950.4	E962.0	E980.4
88:08 vitamin B complex	963.5	E858.1	E933.5	E950.4	E962.0	E980.4
hematopoietic vitamin	964.1	E858.2	E934.1	E950.4	E962.0	E980.4
nicotinic acid derivatives	972.2	E858.3	E942.2	E950.4	E962.0	E980.4
88:12 vitamin C	963.5	E858.1	E933.5	E950.4	E962.0	E980.4
88:16 vitamin D	963.5	E858.1	E933.5	E950.4	E962.0	E980.4
88:20 vitamin E	963.5	E858.1	E933.5	E950.4	E962.0	E980.4
88:24 vitamin K activity	964.3	E858.2	E934.3	E950.4	E962.0	E980.4
88:28 multivitamin preparations	963.5	E858.1	E933.5	E950.4	E962.0	E980.4
92:00 unclassified therapeutic agents	977.8	E858.8	E947.8	E950.4	E962.0	E980.4
Duboisine	971.1	E855.4	E941.1	E950.4	E962.0	E980.4
Dulcolax	973.1	E858.4	E943.1	E950.4	E962.0	E980.4
Duponol (C) (EP)	976.2	E858.7	E946.2	E950.4	E962.0	E980.4
Durabolin	962.1	E858.0	E932.1	E950.4	E962.0	E980.4
Dyclone	968.5	E855.2	E938.5	E950.4	E962.0	E980.4
Dyclonine	968.5	E855.2	E938.5	E950.4	E962.0	E980.4
Dydrogesterone	962.2	E858.0	E932.2	E950.4	E962.0	E980.4
Dyes NEC	989.89	E866.8	—	E950.9	E962.1	E980.9
diagnostic agents	977.8	E858.8	E947.8	E950.4	E962.0	E980.4
pharmaceutical NEC	977.4	E858.8	E947.4	E950.4	E962.0	E980.4
Dyfols	971.0	E855.3	E941.0	E950.4	E962.0	E980.4
Dymelor	962.3	E858.0	E932.3	E950.4	E962.0	E980.4
Dynamite	989.89	E866.8	—	E950.9	E962.1	E980.9
fumes	987.8	E869.8	—	E952.8	E962.2	E982.8
Dyphylline	975.1	E858.6	E945.1	E950.4	E962.0	E980.4
Ear preparations	976.6	E858.7	E946.6	E950.4	E962.0	E980.4
Echothiopate, ecothiopate	971.0	E855.3	E941.0	E950.4	E962.0	E980.4
Ectylurea	967.8	E852.8	E937.8	E950.2	E962.0	E980.2
Edathamil disodium	963.8	E858.1	E933.8	E950.4	E962.0	E980.4
Edecrin	974.4	E858.5	E944.4	E950.4	E962.0	E980.4
Edetate, disodium (calcium)	963.8	E858.1	E933.8	E950.4	E962.0	E980.4
Edrophonium	971.0	E855.3	E941.0	E950.4	E962.0	E980.4
Elase	976.8	E858.7	E946.8	E950.4	E962.0	E980.4
Elaterium	973.1	E858.4	E943.1	E950.4	E962.0	E980.4
Elder	988.2	E865.4	—	E950.9	E962.1	E980.9
berry (unripe)	988.2	E865.3	—	E950.9	E962.1	E980.9
Electrolytes NEC	974.5	E858.5	E944.5	E950.4	E962.0	E980.4
Electrolytic agent NEC	974.5	E858.5	E944.5	E950.4	E962.0	E980.4
Embramine	963.0	E858.1	E933.0	E950.4	E962.0	E980.4
Emetics	973.6	E858.4	E943.6	E950.4	E962.0	E980.4
Emetine (hydrochloride)	961.5	E857	E931.5	E950.4	E962.0	E980.4
Emollients	976.3	E858.7	E946.3	E950.4	E962.0	E980.4
Emylcamate	969.5	E853.8	E939.5	E950.3	E962.0	E980.3
Encyprate	969.0	E854.0	E939.0	E950.3	E962.0	E980.3
Endocaine	968.5	E855.2	E938.5	E950.4	E962.0	E980.4
Endrin	989.2	E863.0	—	E950.6	E962.1	E980.7
Enflurane	968.2	E855.1	E938.2	E950.4	E962.0	E980.4
Enovid	962.2	E858.0	E932.2	E950.4	E962.0	E980.4
ENT preparations (anti-infectives)	976.6	E858.7	E946.6	E950.4	E962.0	E980.4
Enzodase	963.4	E858.1	E933.4	E950.4	E962.0	E980.4
Enzymes NEC	963.4	E858.1	E933.4	E950.4	E962.0	E980.4
Epanutin	966.1	E855.0	E936.1	E950.4	E962.0	E980.4
Ephedra (tincture)	971.2	E855.5	E941.2	E950.4	E962.0	E980.4
Ephedrine	971.2	E855.5	E941.2	E950.4	E962.0	E980.4
Epiestriol	962.2	E858.0	E932.2	E950.4	E962.0	E980.4
Epilim — *see* Sodium Valproate						
Epinephrine	971.2	E855.5	E941.2	E950.4	E962.0	E980.4
Epsom sait	973.3	E858.4	E943.3	E950.4	E962.0	E980.4
Equanil	969.5	E853.8	E939.5	E950.3	E962.0	E980.3
Equisetum (diuretic)	974.4	E858.5	E944.4	E950.4	E962.0	E980.4
Ergometrine	975.0	E858.6	E945.0	E950.4	E962.0	E980.4
Ergonovine	975.0	E858.6	E945.0	E950.4	E962.0	E980.4

Drug — Ergonovine

	Poisoning	External Cause (E-Code)				
		Accident	Therapeutic Use	Suicide Attempt	Assault	Undetermined
Ergot NEC	988.2	E865.4	—	E950.9	E962.1	E980.9
medicinal (alkaloids)	975.0	E858.6	E945.0	E950.4	E962.0	E980.4
Ergotamine (tartrate) (for migraine) NEC	972.9	E858.3	E942.9	E950.4	E962.0	E980.4
Ergotrate	975.0	E858.6	E945.0	E950.4	E962.0	E980.4
Erythrityl tetranitrate	972.4	E858.3	E942.4	E950.4	E962.0	E980.4
Erythrol tetranitrate	972.4	E858.3	E942.4	E950.4	E962.0	E980.4
Erythromycin	960.3	E856	E930.3	E950.4	E962.0	E980.4
ophthalmic preparation	976.5	E858.7	E946.5	E950.4	E962.0	E980.4
topical NEC	976.0	E858.7	E946.0	E950.4	E962.0	E980.4
Eserine	971.0	E855.3	E941.0	E950.4	E962.0	E980.4
Eskabarb	967.0	E851	E937.0	E950.1	E962.0	E980.1
Eskalith	969.8	E855.8	E939.8	E950.3	E962.0	E980.3
Estradiol (cypionate) (dipropionate) (valerate)	962.2	E858.0	E932.2	E950.4	E962.0	E980.4
Estriol	962.2	E858.0	E932.2	E950.4	E962.0	E980.4
Estrogens (with progestogens)	962.2	E858.0	E932.2	E950.4	E962.0	E980.4
Estrone	962.2	E858.0	E932.2	E950.4	E962.0	E980.4
Etafedrine	971.2	E855.5	E941.2	E950.4	E962.0	E980.4
Ethacrynate sodium	974.4	E858.5	E944.4	E950.4	E962.0	E980.4
Ethacrynic acid	974.4	E858.5	E944.4	E950.4	E962.0	E980.4
Ethambutol	961.8	E857	E931.8	E950.4	E962.0	E980.4
Ethamide	974.2	E858.5	E944.2	E950.4	E962.0	E980.4
Ethamivan	970.0	E854.3	E940.0	E950.4	E962.0	E980.4
Ethamsylate	964.5	E858.2	E934.5	E950.4	E962.0	E980.4
Ethanol	980.0	E860.1	—	E950.9	E962.1	E980.9
beverage	980.0	E860.0	—	E950.9	E962.1	E980.9
Ethchlorvynol	967.8	E852.8	E937.8	E950.2	E962.0	E980.2
Ethebenecid	974.7	E858.5	E944.7	E950.4	E962.0	E980.4
Ether(s) (diethyl) (ethyl) (vapor)	987.8	E869.8	—	E952.8	E962.2	E982.8
anesthetic	968.2	E855.1	E938.2	E950.4	E962.0	E980.4
petroleum — see Ligroin						
solvent	982.8	E862.4	—	E950.9	E962.1	E980.9
Ethidine chloride (vapor)	987.8	E869.8	—	E952.8	E962.2	E982.8
liquid (solvent)	982.3	E862.4	—	E950.9	E962.1	E980.9
Ethinamate	967.8	E852.8	E937.8	E950.2	E962.0	E980.2
Ethinylestradiol	962.2	E858.0	E932.2	E950.4	E962.0	E980.4
Ethionamide	961.8	E857	E931.8	E950.4	E962.0	E980.4
Ethisterone	962.2	E858.0	E932.2	E950.4	E962.0	E980.4
Ethobral	967.0	E851	E937.0	E950.1	E962.0	E980.1
Ethocaine (infiltration) (topical)	968.5	E855.2	E938.5	E950.4	E962.0	E980.4
nerve block (peripheral) (plexus)	968.6	E855.2	E938.6	E950.4	E962.0	E980.4
spinal	968.7	E855.2	E938.7	E950.4	E962.0	E980.4
Ethoheptazine (citrate)	965.7	E850.7	E935.7	E950.0	E962.0	E980.0
Ethopropazine	966.4	E855.0	E936.4	E950.4	E962.0	E980.4
Ethosuximide	966.2	E855.0	E936.2	E950.4	E962.0	E980.4
Ethotoin	966.1	E855.0	E936.1	E950.4	E962.0	E980.4
Ethoxazene	961.9	E857	E931.9	E950.4	E962.0	E980.4
Ethoxzolamide	974.2	E858.5	E944.2	E950.4	E962.0	E980.4
Ethyl						
acetate (vapor)	982.8	E862.4	—	E950.9	E962.1	E980.9
alcohol	980.0	E860.1	—	E950.9	E962.1	E980.9
beverage	980.0	E860.0	—	E950.9	E962.1	E980.9
aldehyde (vapor)	987.8	E869.8	—	E952.8	E962.2	E982.8
liquid	989.89	E866.8	—	E950.9	E962.1	E980.9
aminobenzoate	968.5	E855.2	E938.5	E950.4	E962.0	E980.4
biscoumacetate	964.2	E858.2	E934.2	E950.4	E962.0	E980.4
bromide (anesthetic)	968.2	E855.1	E938.2	E950.4	E962.0	E980.4
carbamate (antineoplastic)	963.1	E858.1	E933.1	E950.4	E962.0	E980.4
carbinol	980.3	E860.4	—	E950.9	E962.1	E980.9
chaulmoograte	961.8	E857	E931.8	E950.4	E962.0	E980.4
chloride (vapor)	987.8	E869.8	—	E952.8	E962.2	E982.8
anesthetic (local)	968.5	E855.2	E938.5	E950.4	E962.0	E980.4
inhaled	968.2	E855.1	E938.2	E950.4	E962.0	E980.4
solvent	982.3	E862.4	—	E950.9	E962.1	E980.9
estranol	962.1	E858.0	E932.1	E950.4	E962.0	E980.4
ether — see Ether(s)						
formate (solvent) NEC	982.8	E862.4	—	E950.9	E962.1	E980.9
iodoacetate	987.5	E869.3	—	E952.8	E962.2	E982.8
lactate (solvent) NEC	982.8	E862.4	—	E950.9	E962.1	E980.9
methylcarbinol	980.8	E860.8	—	E950.9	E962.1	E980.9
morphine	965.09	E850.2	E935.2	E950.0	E962.0	E980.0
Ethylene (gas)	987.1	E869.8	—	E952.8	E962.2	E982.8
anesthetic (general)	968.2	E855.1	E938.2	E950.4	E962.0	E980.4
chlorohydrin (vapor)	982.3	E862.4	—	E950.9	E962.1	E980.9
dichloride (vapor)	982.3	E862.4	—	E950.9	E962.1	E980.9
glycol(s) (any) (vapor)	982.8	E862.4	—	E950.9	E962.1	E980.9
Ethylidene						
chloride NEC	982.3	E862.4	—	E950.9	E962.1	E980.9
diethyl ether	982.8	E862.4	—	E950.9	E962.1	E980.9
Ethynodiol	962.2	E858.0	E932.2	E950.4	E962.0	E980.4
Etidocaine	968.9	E855.2	E938.9	E950.4	E962.0	E980.4
infiltration (subcutaneous)	968.5	E855.2	E938.5	E950.4	E962.0	E980.4

Ergot NEC — Etidocaine

✓4ᵗʰ Fourth-digit Required   ✓5ᵗʰ Fifth-digit Required   ▶◀ Revised Text   ● New Line   ▲ Revised Code

		External Cause (E-Code)				
	Poisoning	**Accident**	**Therapeutic Use**	**Suicide Attempt**	**Assault**	**Undetermined**
Etidocaine — *continued*						
nerve (peripheral) (plexus)	968.6	E855.2	E938.6	E950.4	E962.0	E980.4
Etilfen	967.0	E851	E937.0	E950.1	E962.0	E980.1
Etomide	965.7	E850.7	E935.7	E950.0	E962.0	E980.0
Etorphine	965.09	E850.2	E935.2	E950.0	E962.0	E980.0
Etoval	967.0	E851	E937.0	E950.1	E962.0	E980.1
Etryptamine	969.0	E854.0	E939.0	E950.3	E962.0	E980.3
Eucaine	968.5	E855.2	E938.5	E950.4	E962.0	E980.4
Eucalyptus (oil) NEC	975.5	E858.6	E945.5	E950.4	E962.0	E980.4
Eucatropine	971.1	E855.4	E941.1	E950.4	E962.0	E980.4
Eucodal	965.09	E850.2	E935.2	E950.0	E962.0	E980.0
Euneryl	967.0	E851	E937.0	E950.1	E962.0	E980.1
Euphthalmine	971.1	E855.4	E941.1	E950.4	E962.0	E980.4
Eurax	976.0	E858.7	E946.0	E950.4	E962.0	E980.4
Euresol	976.4	E858.7	E946.4	E950.4	E962.0	E980.4
Euthroid	962.7	E858.0	E932.7	E950.4	E962.0	E980.4
Evans blue	977.8	E858.8	E947.8	E950.4	E962.0	E980.4
Evipal	967.0	E851	E937.0	E950.1	E962.0	E980.1
sodium	968.3	E855.1	E938.3	E950.4	E962.0	E980.4
Evipan	967.0	E851	E937.0	E950.1	E962.0	E980.1
sodium	968.3	E855.1	E938.3	E950.4	E962.0	E980.4
Exalgin	965.4	E850.4	E935.4	E950.0	E962.0	E980.0
Excipients, pharmaceutical	977.4	E858.8	E947.4	E950.4	E962.0	E980.4
Exhaust gas — *see* Carbon, monoxide						
Ex-Lax (phenolphthalein)	973.1	E858.4	E943.1	E950.4	E962.0	E980.4
Expectorants	975.5	E858.6	E945.5	E950.4	E962.0	E980.4
External medications (skin) (mucous membrane)	976.9	E858.7	E946.9	E950.4	E962.0	E980.4
dental agent	976.7	E858.7	E946.7	E950.4	E962.0	E980.4
ENT agent	976.6	E858.7	E946.6	E950.4	E962.0	E980.4
ophthalmic preparation	976.5	E858.7	E946.5	E950.4	E962.0	E980.4
specified NEC	976.8	E858.7	E946.8	E950.4	E962.0	E980.4
Eye agents (anti-infective)	976.5	E858.7	E946.5	E950.4	E962.0	E980.4
Factor IX complex (human)	964.5	E858.2	E934.5	E950.4	E962.0	E980.4
Fecal softeners	973.2	E858.4	E943.2	E950.4	E962.0	E980.4
Fenbutrazate	977.0	E858.8	E947.0	E950.4	E962.0	E980.4
Fencamfamin	970.8	E854.3	E940.8	E950.4	E962.0	E980.4
Fenfluramine	977.0	E858.8	E947.0	E950.4	E962.0	E980.4
Fenoprofen	965.61	E850.6	E935.6	E950.0	E962.0	E980.0
Fentanyl	965.09	E850.2	E935.2	E950.0	E962.0	E980.0
Fentazin	969.1	E853.0	E939.1	E950.3	E962.0	E980.3
Fenticlor, fentichlor	976.0	E858.7	E946.0	E950.4	E962.0	E980.4
Fer de lance (bite) (venom)	989.5	E905.0	—	E950.9	E962.1	E980.9
Ferric — *see* Iron						
Ferrocholinate	964.0	E858.2	E934.0	E950.4	E962.0	E980.4
Ferrous fumarate, gluconate, lactate, salt NEC, sulfate (medicinal)	964.0	E858.2	E934.0	E950.4	E962.0	E980.4
Ferrum — *see* Iron						
Fertilizers NEC	989.89	E866.5	—	E950.9	E962.1	E980.4
with herbicide mixture	989.4	E863.5	—	E950.6	E962.1	E980.7
Fibrinogen (human)	964.7	E858.2	E934.7	E950.4	E962.0	E980.4
Fibrinolysin	964.4	E858.2	E934.4	E950.4	E962.0	E980.4
Fibrinolysis-affecting agents	964.4	E858.2	E934.4	E950.4	E962.0	E980.4
Filix mas	961.6	E857	E931.6	E950.4	E962.0	E980.4
Fiorinal	965.1	E850.3	E935.3	E950.0	E962.0	E980.0
Fire damp	987.1	E869.8	—	E952.8	E962.2	E982.8
Fish, nonbacterial or noxious	988.0	E865.2	—	E950.9	E962.1	E980.9
shell	988.0	E865.1	—	E950.9	E962.1	E980.9
Flagyl	961.5	E857	E931.5	E950.4	E962.0	E980.4
Flavoxate	975.1	E858.6	E945.1	E950.4	E962.0	E980.4
Flaxedil	975.2	E858.6	E945.2	E950.4	E962.0	E980.4
Flaxseed (medicinal)	976.3	E858.7	E946.3	E950.4	E962.0	E980.4
Florantyrone	973.4	E858.4	E943.4	E950.4	E962.0	E980.4
Floraquin	961.3	E857	E931.3	E950.4	E962.0	E980.4
Florinef	962.0	E858.0	E932.0	E950.4	E962.0	E980.4
ENT agent	976.6	E858.7	E946.6	E950.4	E962.0	E980.4
ophthalmic preparation	976.5	E858.7	E946.5	E950.4	E962.0	E980.4
topical NEC	976.0	E858.7	E946.0	E950.4	E962.0	E980.4
Flowers of sulfur	976.4	E858.7	E946.4	E950.4	E962.0	E980.4
Floxuridine	963.1	E858.1	E933.1	E950.4	E962.0	E980.4
Flucytosine	961.9	E857	E931.9	E950.4	E962.0	E980.4
Fludrocortisone	962.0	E858.0	E932.0	E950.4	E962.0	E980.4
ENT agent	976.6	E858.7	E946.6	E950.4	E962.0	E980.4
ophthalmic preparation	976.5	E858.7	E946.5	E950.4	E962.0	E980.4
topical NEC	976.0	E858.7	E946.0	E950.4	E962.0	E980.4
Flumethasone	976.0	E858.7	E946.0	E950.4	E962.0	E980.4
Flumethiazide	974.3	E858.5	E944.3	E950.4	E962.0	E980.4
Flumidin	961.7	E857	E931.7	E950.4	E962.0	E980.4
Flunitrazepam	969.4	E853.2	E939.4	E950.3	E962.0	E980.3 ▲
Fluocinolone	976.0	E858.7	E946.0	E950.4	E962.0	E980.4
Fluocortolone	962.0	E858.0	E932.0	E950.4	E962.0	E980.4
Fluohydrocortisone	962.0	E858.0	E932.0	E950.4	E962.0	E980.4
ENT agent	976.6	E858.7	E946.6	E950.4	E962.0	E980.4

✓4ᵗʰ Fourth-digit Required   ✓5ᵗʰ Fifth-digit Required   ▶◀ Revised Text   ● New Line   ▲ Revised Code

		External Cause (E-Code)				
	Poisoning	Accident	Therapeutic Use	Suicide Attempt	Assault	Undetermined
Fluohydrocortisone — *continued*						
ophthalmic preparation	976.5	E858.7	E946.5	E950.4	E962.0	E980.4
topical NEC	976.0	E858.7	E946.0	E950.4	E962.0	E980.4
Fluonid	976.0	E858.7	E946.0	E950.4	E962.0	E980.4
Fluopromazine	969.1	E853.0	E939.1	E950.3	E962.0	E980.3
Fluoracetate	989.4	E863.7	—	E950.6	E962.1	E980.7
Fluorescein (sodium)	977.8	E858.8	E947.8	E950.4	E962.0	E980.4
Fluoride(s) (pesticides) (sodium) NEC	989.4	E863.4	—	E950.6	E962.1	E980.7
hydrogen — *see* Hydrofluoric acid						
medicinal	976.7	E858.7	E946.7	E950.4	E962.0	E980.4
not pesticide NEC	983.9	E864.4	—	E950.7	E962.1	E980.6
stannous	976.7	E858.7	E946.7	E950.4	E962.0	E980.4
Fluorinated corticosteroids	962.0	E858.0	E932.0	E950.4	E962.0	E980.4
Fluorine (compounds) (gas)	987.8	E869.8	—	E952.8	E962.2	E982.8
salt — *see* Fluoride(s)						
Fluoristan	976.7	E858.7	E946.7	E950.4	E962.0	E980.4
Fluoroacetate	989.4	E863.7	—	E950.6	E962.1	E980.7
Fluorodeoxyuridine	963.1	E858.1	E933.1	E950.4	E962.0	E980.4
Fluorometholone (topical) NEC	976.0	E858.7	E946.0	E950.4	E962.0	E980.4
ophthalmic preparation	976.5	E858.7	E946.5	E950.4	E962.0	E980.4
Fluorouracil	963.1	E858.1	E933.1	E950.4	E962.0	E980.4
Fluothane	968.1	E855.1	E938.1	E950.4	E962.0	E980.4
Fluoxetine hydrochloride	969.0	E854.0	E939.0	E950.3	E962.0	E980.3
Fluoxymesterone	962.1	E858.0	E932.1	E950.4	E962.0	E980.4
Fluphenazine	969.1	E853.0	E939.1	E950.3	E962.0	E980.3
Fluprednisolone	962.0	E858.0	E932.0	E950.4	E962.0	E980.4
Flurandrenolide	976.0	E858.7	E946.0	E950.4	E962.0	E980.4
Flurazepam (hydrochloride)	969.4	E853.2	E939.4	E950.3	E962.0	E980.3
Flurbiprofen	965.61	E850.6	E935.6	E950.0	E962.0	E980.0
Flurobate	976.0	E858.7	E946.0	E950.4	E962.0	E980.4
Flurothyl	969.8	E855.8	E939.8	E950.3	E962.0	E980.3
Fluroxene	968.2	E855.1	E938.2	E950.4	E962.0	E980.4
Folacin	964.1	E858.2	E934.1	E950.4	E962.0	E980.4
Folic acid	964.1	E858.2	E934.1	E950.4	E962.0	E980.4
Follicle stimulating hormone	962.4	E858.0	E932.4	E950.4	E962.0	E980.4
Food, foodstuffs, nonbacterial or noxious	988.9	E865.9	—	E950.9	E962.1	E980.9
berries, seeds	988.2	E865.3	—	E950.9	E962.1	E980.9
fish	988.0	E865.2	—	E950.9	E962.1	E980.9
mushrooms	988.1	E865.5	—	E950.9	E962.1	E980.9
plants	988.2	E865.9	—	E950.9	E962.1	E980.9
specified type NEC	988.2	E865.4	—	E950.9	E962.1	E980.9
shellfish	988.0	E865.1	—	E950.9	E962.1	E980.9
specified NEC	988.8	E865.8	—	E950.9	E962.1	E980.9
Fool's parsley	988.2	E865.4	—	E950.9	E962.1	E980.9
Formaldehyde (solution)	989.89	E861.4	—	E950.9	E962.1	E980.9
fungicide	989.4	E863.6	—	E950.6	E962.1	E980.7
gas or vapor	987.8	E869.8	—	E952.8	E962.2	E982.8
Formalin	989.89	E861.4	—	E950.9	E962.1	E980.9
fungicide	989.4	E863.6	—	E950.6	E962.1	E980.7
vapor	987.8	E869.8	—	E952.8	E962.2	E982.8
Formic acid	983.1	E864.1	—	E950.7	E962.1	E980.6
vapor	987.8	E869.8	—	E952.8	E962.2	E982.8
Fowler's solution	985.1	E866.3	—	E950.8	E962.1	E980.8
Foxglove	988.2	E865.4	—	E950.9	E962.1	E980.9
Fox green	977.8	E858.8	E947.8	E950.4	E962.0	E980.4
Framycetin	960.8	E856	E930.8	E950.4	E962.0	E980.4
Frangula (extract)	973.1	E858.4	E943.1	E950.4	E962.0	E980.4
Frei antigen	977.8	E858.8	E947.8	E950.4	E962.0	E980.4
Freons	987.4	E869.2	—	E952.8	E962.2	E982.8
Fructose	974.5	E858.5	E944.5	E950.4	E962.0	E980.4
Frusemide	974.4	E858.5	E944.4	E950.4	E962.0	E980.4
FSH	962.4	E858.0	E932.4	E950.4	E962.0	E980.4
Fuel						
automobile	981	E862.1	—	E950.9	E962.1	E980.9
exhaust gas, not in transit	986	E868.2	—	E952.0	E962.2	E982.0
vapor NEC	987.1	E869.8	—	E952.8	E962.2	E982.8
gas (domestic use) — *see also* Carbon, monoxide, fuel						
utility	987.1	E868.1	—	E951.8	E962.2	E981.8
incomplete combustion of — *see* Carbon, monoxide, fuel, utility						
in mobile container	987.0	E868.0	—	E951.1	E962.2	E981.1
piped (natural)	987.1	E867	—	E951.0	E962.2	E981.0
industrial, incomplete combustion	986	E868.3	—	E952.1	E962.2	E982.1
Fugillin	960.8	E856	E930.8	E950.4	E962.0	E980.4
Fulminate of mercury	985.0	E866.1	—	E950.9	E962.1	E980.9
Fulvicin	960.1	E856	E930.1	E950.4	E962.0	E980.4
Fumadil	960.8	E856	E930.8	E950.4	E962.0	E980.4
Fumagillin	960.8	E856	E930.8	E950.4	E962.0	E980.4
Fumes (from)	987.9	E869.9	—	E952.9	E962.2	E982.9
carbon monoxide — *see* Carbon, monoxide						
charcoal (domestic use)	986	E868.3	—	E952.1	E962.2	E982.1

Fluohydrocortisone — Fumes

		External Cause (E-Code)				
	Poisoning	Accident	Therapeutic Use	Suicide Attempt	Assault	Undetermined
Fumes — *continued*						
chloroform — *see* Chloroform						
coke (in domestic stoves, fireplaces)	986	E868.3	—	E952.1	E962.2	E982.1
corrosive NEC	987.8	E869.8	—	E952.8	E962.2	E982.8
ether — *see* Ether(s)						
freons	987.4	E869.2	—	E952.8	E962.2	E982.8
hydrocarbons	987.1	E869.8	—	E952.8	E962.2	E982.8
petroleum (liquefied)	987.0	E868.0	—	E951.1	E962.2	E981.1
distributed through pipes (pure or mixed with air)	987.0	E867	—	E951.0	E962.2	E981.0
lead — *see* Lead						
metals — *see* specified metal						
nitrogen dioxide	987.2	E869.0	—	E952.8	E962.2	E982.8
pesticides — *see* Pesticides						
petroleum (liquefied)	987.0	E868.0	—	E951.1	E962.2	E981.1
distributed through pipes (pure or mixed with air)	987.0	E867	—	E951.0	E962.2	E981.0
polyester	987.8	E869.8	—	E952.8	E962.2	E982.8
specified source other (*see also* substance specified)	987.8	E869.8	—	E952.8	E962.2	E982.8
sulfur dioxide	987.3	E869.1	—	E952.8	E962.2	E982.8
Fumigants	989.4	E863.8	—	E950.6	E962.1	E980.7
Fungi, noxious, used as food	988.1	E865.5	—	E950.9	E962.1	E980.9
Fungicides (*see also* Antifungals)	989.4	E863.6	—	E950.6	E962.1	E980.7
Fungizone	960.1	E856	E930.1	E950.4	E962.0	E980.4
topical	976.0	E858.7	E946.0	E950.4	E962.0	E980.4
Furacin	976.0	E858.7	E946.0	E950.4	E962.0	E980.4
Furadantin	961.9	E857	E931.9	E950.4	E962.0	E980.4
Furazolidone	961.9	E857	E931.9	E950.4	E962.0	E980.4
Furnace (coal burning) (domestic), gas from	986	E868.3	—	E952.1	E962.2	E982.1
industrial	986	E868.8	—	E952.1	E962.2	E982.1
Furniture polish	989.89	E861.2	—	E950.9	E962.1	E980.9
Furosemide	974.4	E858.5	E944.4	E950.4	E962.0	E980.4
Furoxone	961.9	E857	E931.9	E950.4	E962.0	E980.4
Fusel oil (amyl) (butyl) (propyl)	980.3	E860.4	—	E950.9	E962.1	E980.9
Fusidic acid	960.8	E856	E930.8	E950.4	E962.0	E980.4
Gallamine	975.2	E858.6	E945.2	E950.4	E962.0	E980.4
Gallotannic acid	976.2	E858.7	E946.2	E950.4	E962.0	E980.4
Gamboge	973.1	E858.4	E943.1	E950.4	E962.0	E980.4
Gamimune	964.6	E858.2	E934.6	E950.4	E962.0	E980.4
Gamma-benzene hexachloride (vapor)	989.2	E863.0	—	E950.6	E962.1	E980.7
Gamma globulin	964.6	E858.2	E934.6	E950.4	E962.0	E980.4
Gamma Hydroxy Butyrate (GHB)	968.4	E855.1	E938.4	E950.4	E962.0	E980.4
Gamulin	964.6	E858.2	E934.6	E950.4	E962.0	E980.4
Ganglionic blocking agents	972.3	E858.3	E942.3	E950.4	E962.0	E980.4
Ganja	969.6	E854.1	E939.6	E950.3	E962.0	E980.3
Garamycin	960.8	E856	E930.8	E950.4	E962.0	E980.4
ophthalmic preparation	976.5	E858.7	E946.5	E950.4	E962.0	E980.4
topical NEC	976.0	E858.7	E946.0	E950.4	E962.0	E980.4
Gardenal	967.0	E851	E937.0	E950.1	E962.0	E980.1
Gardepanyl	967.0	E851	E937.0	E950.1	E962.0	E980.1
Gas	987.9	E869.9	—	E952.9	E962.2	E982.9
acetylene	987.1	E868.1	—	E951.8	E962.2	E981.8
incomplete combustion of — *see* Carbon, monoxide, fuel, utility						
air contaminants, source or type not specified	987.9	E869.9	—	E952.9	E962.2	E982.9
anesthetic (general) NEC	968.2	E855.1	E938.2	E950.4	E962.0	E980.4
blast furnace	986	E868.8	—	E952.1	E962.2	E982.1
butane — *see* Butane						
carbon monoxide — *see* Carbon, monoxide						
chlorine	987.6	E869.8	—	E952.8	E962.2	E982.8
coal — *see* Carbon, monoxide, coal						
cyanide	987.7	E869.8	—	E952.8	E962.2	E982.8
dicyanogen	987.8	E869.8	—	E952.8	E962.2	E982.8
domestic — *see* Gas, utility						
exhaust — *see* Carbon, monoxide, exhaust gas						
from wood- or coal-burning stove or fireplace	986	E868.3	—	E952.1	E962.2	E982.1
fuel (domestic use) — *see also* Carbon, monoxide, fuel						
industrial use	986	E868.8	—	E952.1	E962.2	E982.1
utility	987.1	E868.1	—	E951.8	E962.2	E981.8
incomplete combustion of — *see* Carbon, monoxide, fuel, utility						
in mobile container	987.0	E868.0	—	E951.1	E962.2	E981.1
piped (natural)	987.1	E867	—	E951.0	E962.2	E981.0
garage	986	E868.2	—	E952.0	E962.2	E982.0
hydrocarbon NEC	987.1	E869.8	—	E952.8	E962.2	E982.8
incomplete combustion of — *see* Carbon, monoxide, fuel, utility						
liquefied (mobile container)	987.0	E868.0	—	E951.1	E962.2	E981.1
piped	987.0	E867	—	E951.0	E962.2	E981.0
hydrocyanic acid	987.7	E869.8	—	E952.8	E962.2	E982.8
illuminating — *see* Gas, utility						
incomplete combustion, any — *see* Carbon, monoxide						
kiln	986	E868.8	—	E952.1	E962.2	E982.1
lacrimogenic	987.5	E869.3	—	E952.8	E962.2	E982.8
marsh	987.1	E869.8	—	E952.8	E962.2	E982.8

		External Cause (E-Code)				
	Poisoning	Accident	Therapeutic Use	Suicide Attempt	Assault	Undetermined
Gas — *continued*						
motor exhaust, not in transit	986	E868.8	—	E952.1	E962.2	E982.1
mustard — *see* Mustard, gas						
natural	987.1	E867	—	E951.0	E962.2	E981.0
nerve (war)	987.9	E869.9	—	E952.9	E962.2	E982.9
oils	981	E862.1	—	E950.9	E962.1	E980.9
petroleum (liquefied) (distributed in mobile containers)	987.0	E868.0	—	E951.1	E962.2	E981.1
piped (pure or mixed with air)	987.0	E867	—	E951.1	E962.2	E981.1
piped (manufactured) (natural) NEC	987.1	E867	—	E951.0	E962.2	E981.0
producer	986	E868.8	—	E952.1	E962.2	E982.1
propane — *see* Propane						
refrigerant (freon)	987.4	E869.2	—	E952.8	E962.2	E982.8
not freon	987.9	E869.9	—	E952.9	E962.2	E982.9
sewer	987.8	E869.8	—	E952.8	E962.2	E982.8
specified source NEC (*see also* substance specified)	987.8	E869.8	—	E952.8	E962.2	E982.8
stove — *see* Gas, utility						
tear	987.5	E869.3	—	E952.8	E962.2	E982.8
utility (for cooking, heating, or lighting) (piped) NEC	987.1	E868.1	—	E951.8	E962.2	E981.8
incomplete combustion of — *see* Carbon, monoxide, fuel, utilty						
in mobile container	987.0	E868.0	—	E951.1	E962.2	E981.1
piped (natural)	987.1	E867	—	E951.0	E962.2	E981.0
water	987.1	E868.1	—	E951.8	E962.2	E981.8
incomplete combustion of — *see* Carbon, monoxide, fuel, utility						
Gaseous substance — *see* Gas						
Gasoline, gasolene	981	E862.1	—	E950.9	E962.1	E980.9
vapor	987.1	E869.8	—	E952.8	E962.2	E982.8
Gastric enzymes	973.4	E858.4	E943.4	E950.4	E962.0	E980.4
Gastrografin	977.8	E858.8	E947.8	E950.4	E962.0	E980.4
Gastrointestinal agents	973.9	E858.4	E943.9	E950.4	E962.0	E980.4
specified NEC	973.8	E858.4	E943.8	E950.4	E962.0	E980.4
Gaultheria procumbens	988.2	E865.4	—	E950.9	E962.1	E980.9
Gelatin (intravenous)	964.8	E858.2	E934.8	E950.4	E962.0	E980.4
absorbable (sponge)	964.5	E858.2	E934.5	E950.4	E962.0	E980.4
Gelfilm	976.8	E858.7	E946.8	E950.4	E962.0	E980.4
Gelfoam	964.5	E858.2	E934.5	E950.4	E962.0	E980.4
Gelsemine	970.8	E854.3	E940.8	E950.4	E962.0	E980.4
Gelsemium (sempervirens)	988.2	E865.4	—	E950.9	E962.1	E980.9
Gemonil	967.0	E851	E937.0	E950.1	E962.0	E980.1
Gentamicin	960.8	E856	E930.8	E950.4	E962.0	E980.4
ophthalmic preparation	976.5	E858.7	E946.5	E950.4	E962.0	E980.4
topical NEC	976.0	E858.7	E946.0	E950.4	E962.0	E980.4
Gentian violet	976.0	E858.7	E946.0	E950.4	E962.0	E980.4
Gexane	976.0	E858.7	E946.0	E950.4	E962.0	E980.4
Gila monster (venom)	989.5	E905.0	—	E950.9	E962.1	E980.9
Ginger, Jamaica	989.89	E866.8	—	E950.9	E962.1	E980.9
Gitalin	972.1	E858.3	E942.1	E950.4	E962.0	E980.4
Gitoxin	972.1	E858.3	E942.1	E950.4	E962.0	E980.4
Glandular extract (medicinal) NEC	977.9	E858.9	E947.9	E950.5	E962.0	E980.5
Glaucarubin	961.5	E857	E931.5	E950.4	E962.0	E980.4
Globin zinc insulin	962.3	E858.0	E932.3	E950.4	E962.0	E980.4
Glucagon	962.3	E858.0	E932.3	E950.4	E962.0	E980.4
Glucochloral	967.1	E852.0	E937.1	E950.2	E962.0	E980.2
Glucocorticoids	962.0	E858.0	E932.0	E950.4	E962.0	E980.4
Glucose	974.5	E858.5	E944.5	E950.4	E962.0	E980.4
oxidase reagent	977.8	E858.8	E947.8	E950.4	E962.0	E980.4
Glucosulfone sodium	961.8	E857	E931.8	E950.4	E962.0	E980.4
Glue(s)	989.89	E866.6	—	E950.9	E962.1	E980.9
Glutamic acid (hydrochloride)	973.4	E858.4	E943.4	E950.4	E962.0	E980.4
Glutathione	963.8	E858.1	E933.8	E950.4	E962.0	E980.4
Glutethimide (group)	967.5	E852.4	E937.5	E950.2	E962.0	E980.2
Glycerin (lotion)	976.3	E858.7	E946.3	E950.4	E962.0	E980.4
Glycerol (topical)	976.3	E858.7	E946.3	E950.4	E962.0	E980.4
Glyceryl						
guaiacolate	975.5	E858.6	E945.5	E950.4	E962.0	E980.4
triacetate (topical)	976.0	E858.7	E946.0	E950.4	E962.0	E980.4
trinitrate	972.4	E858.3	E942.4	E950.4	E962.0	E980.4
Glycine	974.5	E858.5	E944.5	E950.4	E962.0	E980.4
Glycobiarsol	961.1	E857	E931.1	E950.4	E962.0	E980.4
Glycols (ether)	982.8	E862.4	—	E950.9	E962.1	E980.9
Glycopyrrolate	971.1	E855.4	E941.1	E950.4	E962.0	E980.4
Glymidine	962.3	E858.0	E932.3	E950.4	E962.0	E980.4
Gold (compounds) (salts)	965.69	E850.6	E935.6	E950.0	E962.0	E980.0
Golden sulfide of antimony	985.4	E866.2	—	E950.9	E962.1	E980.9
Goldylocks	988.2	E865.4	—	E950.9	E962.1	E980.9
Gonadal tissue extract	962.9	E858.0	E932.9	E950.4	E962.0	E980.4
female	962.2	E858.0	E932.2	E950.4	E962.0	E980.4
male	962.1	E858.0	E932.1	E950.4	E962.0	E980.4
Gonadotropin	962.4	E858.0	E932.4	E950.4	E962.0	E980.4
Grain alcohol	980.0	E860.1	—	E950.9	E962.1	E980.9
beverage	980.0	E860.0	—	E950.9	E962.1	E980.9
Gramicidin	960.8	E856	E930.8	E950.4	E962.0	E980.4

Gas — Gramicidin

Gratiola officinalis — Homatropine

	Poisoning	External Cause (E-Code)				
		Accident	Therapeutic Use	Suicide Attempt	Assault	Undetermined
Gratiola officinalis	988.2	E865.4	—	E950.9	E962.1	E980.9
Grease	989.89	E866.8	—	E950.9	E962.1	E980.9
Green hellebore	988.2	E865.4	—	E950.9	E962.1	E980.9
Green soap	976.2	E858.7	E946.2	E950.4	E962.0	E980.4
Grifulvin	960.1	E856	E930.1	E950.4	E962.0	E980.4
Griseofulvin	960.1	E856	E930.1	E950.4	E962.0	E980.4
Growth hormone	962.4	E858.0	E932.4	E950.4	E962.0	E980.4
Guaiacol	975.5	E858.6	E945.5	E950.4	E962.0	E980.4
Guaiac reagent	977.8	E858.8	E947.8	E950.4	E962.0	E980.4
Guaifenesin	975.5	E858.6	E945.5	E950.4	E962.0	E980.4
Guaiphenesin	975.5	E858.6	E945.5	E950.4	E962.0	E980.4
Guanatol	961.4	E857	E931.4	E950.4	E962.0	E980.4
Guanethidine	972.6	E858.3	E942.6	E950.4	E962.0	E980.4
Guano	989.89	E866.5	—	E950.9	E962.1	E980.9
Guanochlor	972.6	E858.3	E942.6	E950.4	E962.0	E980.4
Guanoctine	972.6	E858.3	E942.6	E950.4	E962.0	E980.4
Guanoxan	972.6	E858.3	E942.6	E950.4	E962.0	E980.4
Hair treatment agent NEC	976.4	E858.7	E946.4	E950.4	E962.0	E980.4
Halcinonide	976.0	E858.7	E946.0	E950.4	E962.0	E980.4
Halethazole	976.0	E858.7	E946.0	E950.4	E962.0	E980.4
Hallucinogens	969.6	E854.1	E939.6	E950.3	E962.0	E980.3
Haloperidol	969.2	E853.1	E939.2	E950.3	E962.0	E980.3
Haloprogin	976.0	E858.7	E946.0	E950.4	E962.0	E980.4
Halotex	976.0	E858.7	E946.0	E950.4	E962.0	E980.4
Halothane	968.1	E855.1	E938.1	E950.4	E962.0	E980.4
Halquinols	976.0	E858.7	E946.0	E950.4	E962.0	E980.4
Harmonyl	972.6	E858.3	E942.6	E950.4	E962.0	E980.4
Hartmann's solution	974.5	E858.5	E944.5	E950.4	E962.0	E980.4
Hashish	969.6	E854.1	E939.6	E950.3	E962.0	E980.3
Hawaiian wood rose seeds	969.6	E854.1	E939.6	E950.3	E962.0	E980.3
Headache cures, drugs, powders NEC	977.9	E858.9	E947.9	E950.5	E962.0	E980.9
Heavenly Blue (morning glory)	969.6	E854.1	E939.6	E950.3	E962.0	E980.3
Heavy metal antagonists	963.8	E858.1	E933.8	E950.4	E962.0	E980.4
anti-infectives	961.2	E857	E931.2	E950.4	E962.0	E980.4
Hedaquinium	976.0	E858.7	E946.0	E950.4	E962.0	E980.4
Hedge hyssop	988.2	E865.4	—	E950.9	E962.1	E980.9
Heet	976.8	E858.7	E946.8	E950.4	E962.0	E980.4
Helenin	961.6	E857	E931.6	E950.4	E962.0	E980.4
Hellebore (black) (green) (white)	988.2	E865.4	—	E950.9	E962.1	E980.9
Hemlock	988.2	E865.4	—	E950.9	E962.1	E980.9
Hemostatics	964.5	E858.2	E934.5	E950.4	E962.0	E980.4
capillary active drugs	972.8	E858.3	E942.8	E950.4	E962.0	E980.4
Henbane	988.2	E865.4	—	E950.9	E962.1	E980.9
Heparin (sodium)	964.2	E858.2	E934.2	E950.4	E962.0	E980.4
Heptabarbital, heptabarbitone	967.0	E851	E937.0	E950.1	E962.0	E980.1
Heptachlor	989.2	E863.0	—	E950.6	E962.1	E980.7
Heptalgin	965.09	E850.2	E935.2	E950.0	E962.0	E980.0
Herbicides	989.4	E863.5	—	E950.6	E962.1	E980.7
Heroin	965.01	E850.0	E935.0	E950.0	E962.0	E980.0
Herplex	976.5	E858.7	E946.5	E950.4	E962.0	E980.4
HES	964.8	E858.2	E934.8	E950.4	E962.0	E980.4
Hetastarch	964.8	E858.2	E934.8	E950.4	E962.0	E980.4
Hexachlorocyclohexane	989.2	E863.0	—	E950.6	E962.1	E980.7
Hexachlorophene	976.2	E858.7	E946.2	E950.4	E962.0	E980.4
Hexadimethrine (bromide)	964.5	E858.2	E934.5	E950.4	E962.0	E980.4
Hexafluorenium	975.2	E858.6	E945.2	E950.4	E962.0	E980.4
Hexa-germ	976.2	E858.7	E946.2	E950.4	E962.0	E980.4
Hexahydrophenol	980.8	E860.8	—	E950.9	E962.1	E980.9
Hexalin	980.8	E860.8	—	E950.9	E962.1	E980.9
Hexamethonium	972.3	E858.3	E942.3	E950.4	E962.0	E980.4
Hexamethyleneamine	961.9	E857	E931.9	E950.4	E962.0	E980.4
Hexamine	961.9	E857	E931.9	E950.4	E962.0	E980.4
Hexanone	982.8	E862.4	—	E950.9	E962.1	E980.9
Hexapropymate	967.8	E852.8	E937.8	E950.2	E962.0	E980.2
Hexestrol	962.2	E858.0	E932.2	E950.4	E962.0	E980.4
Hexethal (sodium)	967.0	E851	E937.0	E950.1	E962.0	E980.1
Hexetidine	976.0	E858.7	E946.0	E950.4	E962.0	E980.4
Hexobarbital, hexobarbitone	967.0	E851	E937.0	E950.1	E962.0	E980.1
sodium (anesthetic)	968.3	E855.1	E938.3	E950.4	E962.0	E980.4
soluble	968.3	E855.1	E938.3	E950.4	E962.0	E980.4
Hexocyclium	971.1	E855.4	E941.1	E950.4	E962.0	E980.4
Hexoestrol	962.2	E858.0	E932.2	E950.4	E962.0	E980.4
Hexone	982.8	E862.4	—	E950.9	E962.1	E980.9
Hexylcaine	968.5	E855.2	E938.5	E950.4	E962.0	E980.4
Hexylresorcinol	961.6	E857	E931.6	E950.4	E962.0	E980.4
Hinkle's pills	973.1	E858.4	E943.1	E950.4	E962.0	E980.4
Histalog	977.8	E858.8	E947.8	E950.4	E962.0	E980.4
Histamine (phosphate)	972.5	E858.3	E942.5	E950.4	E962.0	E980.4
Histoplasmin	977.8	E858.8	E947.8	E950.4	E962.0	E980.4
Holly berries	988.2	E865.3	—	E950.9	E962.1	E980.9
Homatropine	971.1	E855.4	E941.1	E950.4	E962.0	E980.4

✓4ᵗʰ Fourth-digit Required   ✓5ᵗʰ Fifth-digit Required   ▶◀ Revised Text   ● New Line   ▲ Revised Code

	Poisoning	External Cause (E-Code)				
		Accident	Therapeutic Use	Suicide Attempt	Assault	Undetermined
Homo-tet	964.6	E858.2	E934.6	E950.4	E962.0	E980.4
Hormones (synthetic substitute) NEC	962.9	E858.0	E932.9	E950.4	E962.0	E980.4
adrenal cortical steroids	962.0	E858.0	E932.0	E950.4	E962.0	E980.4
antidiabetic agents	962.3	E858.0	E932.3	E950.4	E962.0	E980.4
follicle stimulating	962.4	E858.0	E932.4	E950.4	E962.0	E980.4
gonadotropic	962.4	E858.0	E932.4	E950.4	E962.0	E980.4
growth	962.4	E858.0	E932.4	E950.4	E962.0	E980.4
ovarian (substitutes)	962.2	E858.0	E932.2	E950.4	E962.0	E980.4
parathyroid (derivatives)	962.6	E858.0	E932.6	E950.4	E962.0	E980.4
pituitary (posterior)	962.5	E858.0	E932.5	E950.4	E962.0	E980.4
anterior	962.4	E858.0	E932.4	E950.4	E962.0	E980.4
thyroid (derivative)	962.7	E858.0	E932.7	E950.4	E962.0	E980.4
Hornet (sting)	989.5	E905.3	—	E950.9	E962.1	E980.9
Horticulture agent NEC	989.4	E863.9	—	E950.6	E962.1	E980.7
Hyaluronidase	963.4	E858.1	E933.4	E950.4	E962.0	E980.4
Hyazyme	963.4	E858.1	E933.4	E950.4	E962.0	E980.4
Hycodan	965.09	E850.2	E935.2	E950.0	E962.0	E980.0
Hydantoin derivatives	966.1	E855.0	E936.1	E950.4	E962.0	E980.4
Hydeltra	962.0	E858.0	E932.0	E950.4	E962.0	E980.4
Hydergine	971.3	E855.6	E941.3	E950.4	E962.0	E980.4
Hydrabamine penicillin	960.0	E856	E930.0	E950.4	E962.0	E980.4
Hydralazine, hydrallazine	972.6	E858.3	E942.6	E950.4	E962.0	E980.4
Hydrargaphen	976.0	E858.7	E946.0	E950.4	E962.0	E980.4
Hydrazine	983.9	E864.3	—	E950.7	E962.1	E980.6
Hydriodic acid	975.5	E858.6	E945.5	E950.4	E962.0	E980.4
Hydrocarbon gas	987.1	E869.8	—	E952.8	E962.2	E982.8
incomplete combustion of — *see* Carbon, monoxide, fuel, utility						
liquefied (mobile container)	987.0	E868.0	—	E951.1	E962.2	E981.1
piped (natural)	987.0	E867	—	E951.0	E962.2	E981.0
Hydrochloric acid (liquid)	983.1	E864.1	—	E950.7	E962.1	E980.6
medicinal	973.4	E858.4	E943.4	E950.4	E962.0	E980.4
vapor	987.8	E869.8	—	E952.8	E962.2	E982.8
Hydrochlorothiazide	974.3	E858.5	E944.3	E950.4	E962.0	E980.4
Hydrocodone	965.09	E850.2	E935.2	E950.0	E962.0	E980.0
Hydrocortisone	962.0	E858.0	E932.0	E950.4	E962.0	E980.4
ENT agent	976.6	E858.7	E946.6	E950.4	E962.0	E980.4
ophthalmic preparation	976.5	E858.7	E946.5	E950.4	E962.0	E980.4
topical NEC	976.0	E858.7	E946.0	E950.4	E962.0	E980.4
Hydrocortone	962.0	E858.0	E932.0	E950.4	E962.0	E980.4
ENT agent	976.6	E858.7	E946.6	E950.4	E962.0	E980.4
ophthalmic preparation	976.5	E858.7	E946.5	E950.4	E962.0	E980.4
topical NEC	976.0	E858.7	E946.0	E950.4	E962.0	E980.4
Hydrocyanic acid — *see* Cyanide(s)						
Hydroflumethiazide	974.3	E858.5	E944.3	E950.4	E962.0	E980.4
Hydrofluoric acid (liquid)	983.1	E864.1	—	E950.7	E962.1	E980.6
vapor	987.8	E869.8	—	E952.8	E962.2	E982.8
Hydrogen	987.8	E869.8	—	E952.8	E962.2	E982.8
arsenide	985.1	E866.3	—	E950.8	E962.1	E980.8
arseniureted	985.1	E866.3	—	E950.8	E962.1	E980.8
cyanide (salts)	989.0	E866.8	—	E950.9	E962.1	E980.9
gas	987.7	E869.8	—	E952.8	E962.2	E982.8
fluoride (liquid)	983.1	E864.1	—	E950.7	E962.1	E980.6
vapor	987.8	E869.8	—	E952.8	E962.2	E982.8
peroxide (solution)	976.6	E858.7	E946.6	E950.4	E962.0	E980.4
phosphureted	987.8	E869.8	—	E952.8	E962.2	E982.8
sulfide (gas)	987.8	E869.8	—	E952.8	E962.2	E982.8
arseniureted	985.1	E866.3	—	E950.8	E962.1	E980.8
sulfureted	987.8	E869.8	—	E952.8	E962.2	E982.8
Hydromorphinol	965.09	E850.2	E935.2	E950.0	E962.0	E980.0
Hydromorphinone	965.09	E850.2	E935.2	E950.0	E962.0	E980.0
Hydromorphone	965.09	E850.2	E935.2	E950.0	E962.0	E980.0
Hydromox	974.3	E858.5	E944.3	E950.4	E962.0	E980.4
Hydrophilic lotion	976.3	E858.7	E946.3	E950.4	E962.0	E980.4
Hydroquinone	983.0	E864.0	—	E950.7	E962.1	E980.6
vapor	987.8	E869.8	—	E952.8	E962.2	E982.8
Hydrosulfuric acid (gas)	987.8	E869.8	—	E952.8	E962.2	E982.8
Hydrous wool fat (lotion)	976.3	E858.7	E946.3	E950.4	E962.0	E980.4
Hydroxide, caustic	983.2	E864.2	—	E950.7	E962.1	E980.6
Hydroxocobalamin	964.1	E858.2	E934.1	E950.4	E962.0	E980.4
Hydroxyamphetamine	971.2	E855.5	E941.2	E950.4	E962.0	E980.4
Hydroxychloroquine	961.4	E857	E931.4	E950.4	E962.0	E980.4
Hydroxydihydrocodeinone	965.09	E850.2	E935.2	E950.0	E962.0	E980.0
Hydroxyethyl starch	964.8	E858.2	E934.8	E950.4	E962.0	E980.4
Hydroxyphenamate	969.5	E853.8	E939.5	E950.3	E962.0	E980.3
Hydroxyphenylbutazone	965.5	E850.5	E935.5	E950.0	E962.0	E980.0
Hydroxyprogesterone	962.2	E858.0	E932.2	E950.4	E962.0	E980.4
Hydroxyquinoline derivatives	961.3	E857	E931.3	E950.4	E962.0	E980.4
Hydroxystilbamidine	961.5	E857	E931.5	E950.4	E962.0	E980.4
Hydroxyurea	963.1	E858.1	E933.1	E950.4	E962.0	E980.4
Hydroxyzine	969.5	E853.8	E939.5	E950.3	E962.0	E980.3
Hyoscine (hydrobromide)	971.1	E855.4	E941.1	E950.4	E962.0	E980.4

Homo-tet — Hyoscine

✓4ᵗʰ Fourth-digit Required   ✓5ᵗʰ Fifth-digit Required   ▶◀ Revised Text   ● New Line   ▲ Revised Code

	Poisoning	External Cause (E-Code)				
		Accident	Therapeutic Use	Suicide Attempt	Assault	Undetermined
Hyoscyamine	971.1	E855.4	E941.1	E950.4	E962.0	E980.4
Hyoscyamus (albus) (niger)	988.2	E865.4	—	E950.9	E962.1	E980.9
Hypaque	977.8	E858.8	E947.8	E950.4	E962.0	E980.4
Hypertussis	964.6	E858.2	E934.6	E950.4	E962.0	E980.4
Hypnotics NEC	967.9	E852.9	E937.9	E950.2	E962.0	E980.2
Hypochlorites — *see* Sodium, hypochlorite						
Hypotensive agents NEC	972.6	E858.3	E942.6	E950.4	E962.0	E980.4
Ibufenac	965.69	E850.6	E935.6	E950.0	E962.0	E980.0
Ibuprofen	965.61	E850.6	E935.6	E950.0	E962.0	E980.0
ICG	977.8	E858.8	E947.8	E950.4	E962.0	E980.4
Ichthammol	976.4	E858.7	E946.4	E950.4	E962.0	E980.4
Ichthyol	976.4	E858.7	E946.4	E950.4	E962.0	E980.4
Idoxuridine	976.5	E858.7	E946.5	E950.4	E962.0	E980.4
IDU	976.5	E858.7	E946.5	E950.4	E962.0	E980.4
Iletin	962.3	E858.0	E932.3	E950.4	E962.0	E980.4
Ilex	988.2	E865.4	—	E950.9	E962.1	E980.9
Illuminating gas — *see* Gas, utility						
Ilopan	963.5	E858.1	E933.5	E950.4	E962.0	E980.4
Ilotycin	960.3	E856	E930.3	E950.4	E962.0	E980.4
ophthalmic preparation	976.5	E858.7	E946.5	E950.4	E962.0	E980.4
topical NEC	976.0	E858.7	E946.0	E950.4	E962.0	E980.4
Imipramine	969.0	E854.0	E939.0	E950.3	E962.0	E980.3
Immu-G	964.6	E858.2	E934.6	E950.4	E962.0	E980.4
Immuglobin	964.6	E858.2	E934.6	E950.4	E962.0	E980.4
Immune serum globulin	964.6	E858.2	E934.6	E950.4	E962.0	E980.4
Immunosuppressive agents	963.1	E858.1	E933.1	E950.4	E962.0	E980.4
Immu-tetanus	964.6	E858.2	E934.6	E950.4	E962.0	E980.4
Indandione (derivatives)	964.2	E858.2	E934.2	E950.4	E962.0	E980.4
Inderal	972.0	E858.3	E942.0	E950.4	E962.0	E980.4
Indian						
hemp	969.6	E854.1	E939.6	E950.3	E962.0	E980.3
tobacco	988.2	E865.4	—	E950.9	E962.1	E980.9
Indigo carmine	977.8	E858.8	E947.8	E950.4	E962.0	E980.4
Indocin	965.69	E850.6	E935.6	E950.0	E962.0	E980.0
Indocyanine green	977.8	E858.8	E947.8	E950.4	E962.0	E980.4
Indomethacin	965.69	E850.6	E935.6	E950.0	E962.0	E980.0
Industrial						
alcohol	980.9	E860.9	—	E950.9	E962.1	E980.9
fumes	987.8	E869.8	—	E952.8	E962.2	E982.8
solvents (fumes) (vapors)	982.8	E862.9	—	E950.9	E962.1	E980.9
Influenza vaccine	979.6	E858.8	E949.6	E950.4	E962.0	E982.8
Ingested substances NEC	989.9	E866.9	—	E950.9	E962.1	E980.9
INH (isoniazid)	961.8	E857	E931.8	E950.4	E962.0	E980.4
Inhalation, gas (noxious) — *see* Gas						
Ink	989.89	E866.8	—	E950.9	E962.1	E980.9
Innovar	967.6	E852.5	E937.6	E950.2	E962.0	E980.2
Inositol niacinate	972.2	E858.3	E942.2	E950.4	E962.0	E980.4
Inproquone	963.1	E858.1	E933.1	E950.4	E962.0	E980.4
Insect (sting), venomous	989.5	E905.5	—	E950.9	E962.1	E980.9
Insecticides (*see also* Pesticides)	989.4	E863.4	—	E950.6	E962.1	E980.7
chlorinated	989.2	E863.0	—	E950.6	E962.1	E980.7
mixtures	989.4	E863.3	—	E950.6	E962.1	E980.7
organochlorine (compounds)	989.2	E863.0	—	E950.6	E962.1	E980.7
organophosphorus (compounds)	989.3	E863.1	—	E950.6	E962.1	E980.7
Insular tissue extract	962.3	E858.0	E932.3	E950.4	E962.0	E980.4
Insulin (amorphous) (globin) (isophane) (Lente) (NPH) (protamine) (Semilente) (Ultralente) (zinc)	962.3	E858.0	E932.3	E950.4	E962.0	E980.4
Intranarcon	968.3	E855.1	E938.3	E950.4	E962.0	E980.4
Inulin	977.8	E858.8	E947.8	E950.4	E962.0	E980.4
Invert sugar	974.5	E858.5	E944.5	E950.4	E962.0	E980.4
Iodide NEC (*see also* Iodine)	976.0	E858.7	E946.0	E950.4	E962.0	E980.4
mercury (ointment)	976.0	E858.7	E946.0	E950.4	E962.0	E980.4
methylate	976.0	E858.7	E946.0	E950.4	E962.0	E980.4
potassium (expectorant) NEC	975.5	E858.6	E945.5	E950.4	E962.0	E980.4
Iodinated glycerol	975.5	E858.6	E945.5	E950.4	E962.0	E980.4
Iodine (antiseptic, external) (tincture) NEC	976.0	E858.7	E946.0	E950.4	E962.0	E980.4
diagnostic	977.8	E858.8	E947.8	E950.4	E962.0	E980.4
for thyroid conditions (antithyroid)	962.8	E858.0	E932.8	E950.4	E962.0	E980.4
vapor	987.8	E869.8	—	E952.8	E962.2	E982.8
Iodized oil	977.8	E858.8	E947.8	E950.4	E962.0	E980.4
Iodobismitol	961.2	E857	E931.2	E950.4	E962.0	E980.4
Iodochlorhydroxyquin	961.3	E857	E931.3	E950.4	E962.0	E980.4
topical	976.0	E858.7	E946.0	E950.4	E962.0	E980.4
Iodoform	976.0	E858.7	E946.0	E950.4	E962.0	E980.4
Iodopanoic acid	977.8	E858.8	E947.8	E950.4	E962.0	E980.4
Iodophthalein	977.8	E858.8	E947.8	E950.4	E962.0	E980.4
Ion exchange resins	974.5	E858.5	E944.5	E950.4	E962.0	E980.4
Iopanoic acid	977.8	E858.8	E947.8	E950.4	E962.0	E980.4
Iophendylate	977.8	E858.8	E947.8	E950.4	E962.0	E980.4
Iothiouracil	962.8	E858.0	E932.8	E950.4	E962.0	E980.4
Ipecac	973.6	E858.4	E943.6	E950.4	E962.0	E980.4

	Poisoning	External Cause (E-Code)				
		Accident	Therapeutic Use	Suicide Attempt	Assault	Undetermined
Ipecacuanha	973.6	E858.4	E943.6	E950.4	E962.0	E980.4
Ipodate	977.8	E858.8	E947.8	E950.4	E962.0	E980.4
Ipral	967.0	E851	E937.0	E950.1	E962.0	E980.1
Ipratropium ●	975.1	E858.6	E945.1	E950.4	E962.0	E980.4
Iproniazid	969.0	E854.0	E939.0	E950.3	E962.0	E980.3
Iron (compounds) (medicinal) (preparations)	964.0	E858.2	E934.0	E950.4	E962.0	E980.4
dextran	964.0	E858.2	E934.0	E950.4	E962.0	E980.4
nonmedicinal (dust) (fumes) NEC	985.8	E866.4	—	E950.9	E962.1	E980.9
Irritant drug	977.9	E858.9	E947.9	E950.5	E962.0	E980.5
Ismelin	972.6	E858.3	E942.6	E950.4	E962.0	E980.4
Isoamyl nitrite	972.4	E858.3	E942.4	E950.4	E962.0	E980.4
Isobutyl acetate	982.8	E862.4	—	E950.9	E962.1	E980.9
Isocarboxazid	969.0	E854.0	E939.0	E950.3	E962.0	E980.3
Isoephedrine	971.2	E855.5	E941.2	E950.4	E962.0	E980.4
Isoetharine	971.2	E855.5	E941.2	E950.4	E962.0	E980.4
Isofluorophate	971.0	E855.3	E941.0	E950.4	E962.0	E980.4
Isoniazid (INH)	961.8	E857	E931.8	E950.4	E962.0	E980.4
Isopentaquine	961.4	E857	E931.4	E950.4	E962.0	E980.4
Isophane insulin	962.3	E858.0	E932.3	E950.4	E962.0	E980.4
Isopregnenone	962.2	E858.0	E932.2	E950.4	E962.0	E980.4
Isoprenaline	971.2	E855.5	E941.2	E950.4	E962.0	E980.4
Isopropamide	971.1	E855.4	E941.1	E950.4	E962.0	E980.4
Isopropanol	980.2	E860.3	—	E950.9	E962.1	E980.9
topical (germicide)	976.0	E858.7	E946.0	E950.4	E962.0	E980.4
Isopropyl						
acetate	982.8	E862.4	—	E950.9	E962.1	E980.9
alcohol	980.2	E860.3	—	E950.9	E962.1	E980.9
topical (germicide)	976.0	E858.7	E946.0	E950.4	E962.0	E980.4
ether	982.8	E862.4	—	E950.9	E962.1	E980.9
Isoproterenol	971.2	E855.5	E941.2	E950.4	E962.0	E980.4
Isosorbide dinitrate	972.4	E858.3	E942.4	E950.4	E962.0	E980.4
Isothipendyl	963.0	E858.1	E933.0	E950.4	E962.0	E980.4
Isoxazolyl penicillin	960.0	E856	E930.0	E950.4	E962.0	E980.4
Isoxsuprine hydrochloride	972.5	E858.3	E942.5	E950.4	E962.0	E980.4
I-thyroxine sodium	962.7	E858.0	E932.7	E950.4	E962.0	E980.4
Jaborandi (pilocarpus) (extract)	971.0	E855.3	E941.0	E950.4	E962.0	E980.4
Jalap	973.1	E858.4	E943.1	E950.4	E962.0	E980.4
Jamaica						
dogwood (bark)	965.7	E850.7	E935.7	E950.0	E962.0	E980.0
ginger	989.89	E866.8	—	E950.9	E962.1	E980.9
Jatropha	988.2	E865.4	—	E950.9	E962.1	E980.9
curcas	988.2	E865.3	—	E950.9	E962.1	E980.9
Jectofer	964.0	E858.2	E934.0	E950.4	E962.0	E980.4
Jellyfish (sting)	989.5	E905.6	—	E950.9	E962.1	E980.9
Jequirity (bean)	988.2	E865.3	—	E950.9	E962.1	E980.9
Jimson weed	988.2	E865.4	—	E950.9	E962.1	E980.9
seeds	988.2	E865.3	—	E950.9	E962.1	E980.9
Juniper tar (oil) (ointment)	976.4	E858.7	E946.4	E950.4	E962.0	E980.4
Kallikrein	972.5	E858.3	E942.5	E950.4	E962.0	E980.4
Kanamycin	960.6	E856	E930.6	E950.4	E962.0	E980.4
Kantrex	960.6	E856	E930.6	E950.4	E962.0	E980.4
Kaolin	973.5	E858.4	E943.5	E950.4	E962.0	E980.4
Karaya (gum)	973.3	E858.4	E943.3	E950.4	E962.0	E980.4
Kemithal	968.3	E855.1	E938.3	E950.4	E962.0	E980.4
Kenacort	962.0	E858.0	E932.0	E950.4	E962.0	E980.4
Keratolytics	976.4	E858.7	E946.4	E950.4	E962.0	E980.4
Keratoplastics	976.4	E858.7	E946.4	E950.4	E962.0	E980.4
Kerosene, kerosine (fuel) (solvent) NEC	981	E862.1	—	E950.9	E962.1	E980.9
insecticide	981	E863.4	—	E950.6	E962.1	E980.7
vapor	987.1	E869.8	—	E952.8	E962.2	E982.8
Ketamine	968.3	E855.1	E938.3	E950.4	E962.0	E980.4
Ketobemidone	965.09	E850.2	E935.2	E950.0	E962.0	E980.0
Ketols	982.8	E862.4	—	E950.9	E962.1	E980.9
Ketone oils	982.8	E862.4	—	E950.9	E962.1	E980.9
Ketoprofen	965.61	E850.6	E935.6	E950.0	E962.0	E980.0
Kiln gas or vapor (carbon monoxide)	986	E868.8	—	E952.1	E962.2	E982.1
Konsyl	973.3	E858.4	E943.3	E950.4	E962.0	E980.4
Kosam seed	988.2	E865.3	—	E950.9	E962.1	E980.9
Krait (venom)	989.5	E905.0	—	E950.9	E962.1	E980.9
Kwell (insecticide)	989.2	E863.0	—	E950.6	E962.1	E980.7
anti-infective (topical)	976.0	E858.7	E946.0	E950.4	E962.0	E980.4
Laburnum (flowers) (seeds)	988.2	E865.3	—	E950.9	E962.1	E980.9
leaves	988.2	E865.4	—	E950.9	E962.1	E980.9
Lacquers	989.89	E861.6	—	E950.9	E962.1	E980.9
Lacrimogenic gas	987.5	E869.3	—	E952.8	E962.2	E982.8
Lactic acid	983.1	E864.1	—	E950.7	E962.1	E980.6
Lactobacillus acidophilus	973.5	E858.4	E943.5	E950.4	E962.0	E980.4
Lactoflavin	963.5	E858.1	E933.5	E950.4	E962.0	E980.4
Lactuca (virosa) (extract)	967.8	E852.8	E937.8	E950.2	E962.0	E980.2
Lactucarium	967.8	E852.8	E937.8	E950.2	E962.0	E980.2
Laevulose	974.5	E858.5	E944.5	E950.4	E962.0	E980.4

✔4ᵗʰ Fourth-digit Required   ✔5ᵗʰ Fifth-digit Required   ▶◀ Revised Text   ● New Line   ▲ Revised Code

		External Cause (E-Code)				
	Poisoning	Accident	Therapeutic Use	Suicide Attempt	Assault	Undetermined
Lanatoside (C)	972.1	E858.3	E942.1	E950.4	E962.0	E980.4
Lanolin (lotion)	976.3	E858.7	E946.3	E950.4	E962.0	E980.4
Largactil	969.1	E853.0	E939.1	E950.3	E962.0	E980.3
Larkspur	988.2	E865.3	—	E950.9	E962.1	E980.9
Laroxyl	969.0	E854.0	E939.0	E950.3	E962.0	E980.3
Lasix	974.4	E858.5	E944.4	E950.4	E962.0	E980.4
Latex	989.82	E866.8	—	E950.9	E962.1	E980.9
Lathyrus (seed)	988.2	E865.3	—	E950.9	E962.1	E980.9
Laudanum	965.09	E850.2	E935.2	E950.0	E962.0	E980.0
Laudexium	975.2	E858.6	E945.2	E950.4	E962.0	E980.4
Laurel, black or cherry	988.2	E865.4	—	E950.9	E962.1	E980.9
Laurolinium	976.0	E858.7	E946.0	E950.4	E962.0	E980.4
Lauryl sulfoacetate	976.2	E858.7	E946.2	E950.4	E962.0	E980.4
Laxatives NEC	973.3	E858.4	E943.3	E950.4	E962.0	E980.4
emollient	973.2	E858.4	E943.2	E950.4	E962.0	E980.4
L-dopa	966.4	E855.0	E936.4	E950.4	E962.0	E980.4
Lead (dust) (fumes) (vapor) NEC	984.9	E866.0	—	E950.9	E962.1	E980.9
acetate (dust)	984.1	E866.0	—	E950.9	E962.1	E980.9
anti-infectives	961.2	E857	E931.2	E950.4	E962.0	E980.4
antiknock compound (tetraethyl)	984.1	E862.1	—	E950.9	E962.1	E980.9
arsenate, arsenite (dust) (insecticide) (vapor)	985.1	E863.4	—	E950.8	E962.1	E980.8
herbicide	985.1	E863.5	—	E950.8	E962.1	E980.8
carbonate	984.0	E866.0	—	E950.9	E962.1	E980.9
paint	984.0	E861.5	—	E950.9	E962.1	E980.9
chromate	984.0	E866.0	—	E950.9	E962.1	E980.9
paint	984.0	E861.5	—	E950.9	E962.1	E980.9
dioxide	984.0	E866.0	—	E950.9	E962.1	E980.9
inorganic (compound)	984.0	E866.0	—	E950.9	E962.1	E980.9
paint	984.0	E861.5	—	E950.9	E962.1	E980.9
iodide	984.0	E866.0	—	E950.9	E962.1	E980.9
pigment (paint)	984.0	E861.5	—	E950.9	E962.1	E980.9
monoxide (dust)	984.0	E866.0	—	E950.9	E962.1	E980.9
paint	984.0	E861.5	—	E950.9	E962.1	E980.9
organic	984.1	E866.0	—	E950.9	E962.1	E980.9
oxide	984.0	E866.0	—	E950.9	E962.1	E980.9
paint	984.0	E861.5	—	E950.9	E962.1	E980.9
paint	984.0	E861.5	—	E950.9	E962.1	E980.9
salts	984.0	E866.0	—	E950.9	E962.1	E980.9
specified compound NEC	984.8	E866.0	—	E950.9	E962.1	E980.9
tetra-ethyl	984.1	E862.1	—	E950.9	E962.1	E980.9
Lebanese red	969.6	E854.1	E939.6	E950.3	E962.0	E980.3
Lente Iletin (insulin)	962.3	E858.0	E932.3	E950.4	E962.0	E980.4
Leptazol	970.0	E854.3	E940.0	E950.4	E962.0	E980.4
Leritine	965.09	E850.2	E935.2	E950.0	E962.0	E980.0
Letter	962.7	E858.0	E932.7	E950.4	E962.0	E980.4
Lettuce opium	967.8	E852.8	E937.8	E950.2	E962.0	E980.2
Leucovorin (factor)	964.1	E858.2	E934.1	E950.4	E962.0	E980.4
Leukeran	963.1	E858.1	E933.1	E950.4	E962.0	E980.4
Levalbuterol ●	975.7	E858.6	E945.7	E950.4	E962.0	E980.4
Levallorphan	970.1	E854.3	E940.1	E950.4	E962.0	E980.4
Levanil	967.8	E852.8	E937.8	E950.2	E962.0	E980.2
Levarterenol	971.2	E855.5	E941.2	E950.4	E962.0	E980.4
Levodopa	966.4	E855.0	E936.4	E950.4	E962.0	E980.4
Levo-dromoran	965.09	E850.2	E935.2	E950.0	E962.0	E980.0
Levoid	962.7	E858.0	E932.7	E950.4	E962.0	E980.4
Levo-iso-methadone	965.02	E850.1	E935.1	E950.0	E962.0	E980.0
Levomepromazine	967.8	E852.8	E937.8	E950.2	E962.0	E980.2
Levoprome	967.8	E852.8	E937.8	E950.2	E962.0	E980.2
Levopropoxyphene	975.4	E858.6	E945.4	E950.4	E962.0	E980.4
Levorphan, levophanol	965.09	E850.2	E935.2	E950.0	E962.0	E980.0
Levothyroxine (sodium)	962.7	E858.0	E932.7	E950.4	E962.0	E980.4
Levsin	971.1	E855.4	E941.1	E950.4	E962.0	E980.4
Levulose	974.5	E858.5	E944.5	E950.4	E962.0	E980.4
Lewisite (gas)	985.1	E866.3	—	E950.8	E962.1	E980.8
Librium	969.4	E853.2	E939.4	E950.3	E962.0	E980.3
Lidex	976.0	E858.7	E946.0	E950.4	E962.0	E980.4
Lidocaine (infiltration) (topical)	968.5	E855.2	E938.5	E950.4	E962.0	E980.4
nerve block (peripheral) (plexus)	968.6	E855.2	E938.6	E950.4	E962.0	E980.4
spinal	968.7	E855.2	E938.7	E950.4	E962.0	E980.4
Lighter fluid	981	E862.1	—	E950.9	E962.1	E980.9
Lignocaine (infiltration) (topical)	968.5	E855.2	E938.5	E950.4	E962.0	E980.4
nerve block (peripheral) (plexus)	968.6	E855.2	E938.6	E950.4	E962.0	E980.4
spinal	968.7	E855.2	E938.7	E950.4	E962.0	E980.4
Ligroin(e) (solvent)	981	E862.0	—	E950.9	E962.1	E980.9
vapor	987.1	E869.8	—	E952.8	E962.2	E982.8
Ligustrum vulgare	988.2	E865.3	—	E950.9	E962.1	E980.9
Lily of the valley	988.2	E865.4	—	E950.9	E962.1	E980.9
Lime (chloride)	983.2	E864.2	—	E950.7	E962.1	E980.6
solution, sulferated	976.4	E858.7	E946.4	E950.4	E962.0	E980.4
Limonene	982.8	E862.4	—	E950.9	E962.1	E980.9
Lincomycin	960.8	E856	E930.8	E950.4	E962.0	E980.4

		External Cause (E-Code)				
	Poisoning	Accident	Therapeutic Use	Suicide Attempt	Assault	Undetermined
Lindane (insecticide) (vapor)	989.2	E863.0	—	E950.6	E962.1	E980.7
anti-infective (topical)	976.0	E858.7	E946.0	E950.4	E962.0	E980.4
Liniments NEC	976.9	E858.7	E946.9	E950.4	E962.0	E980.4
Linoleic acid	972.2	E858.3	E942.2	E950.4	E962.0	E980.4
Liothyronine	962.7	E858.0	E932.7	E950.4	E962.0	E980.4
Liotrix	962.7	E858.0	E932.7	E950.4	E962.0	E980.4
Lipancreatin	973.4	E858.4	E943.4	E950.4	E962.0	E980.4
Lipo-Lutin	962.2	E858.0	E932.2	E950.4	E962.0	E980.4
Lipotropic agents	977.1	E858.8	E947.1	E950.4	E962.0	E980.4
Liquefied petroleum gases	987.0	E868.0	—	E951.1	E962.2	E981.1
piped (pure or mixed with air)	987.0	E867	—	E951.0	E962.2	E981.0
Liquid petrolatum	973.2	E858.4	E943.2	E950.4	E962.0	E980.4
substance	989.9	E866.9	—	E950.9	E962.1	E980.9
specified NEC	989.89	E866.8	—	E950.9	E962.1	E980.9
Lirugen	979.4	E858.8	E949.4	E950.4	E962.0	E980.4
Lithane	969.8	E855.8	E939.8	E950.3	E962.0	E980.3
Lithium	985.8	E866.4	—	E950.9	E962.1	E980.9
carbonate	969.8	E855.8	E939.8	E950.3	E962.0	E980.3
Lithonate	969.8	E855.8	E939.8	E950.3	E962.0	E980.3
Liver (extract) (injection) (preparations)	964.1	E858.2	E934.1	E950.4	E962.0	E980.4
Lizard (bite) (venom)	989.5	E905.0	—	E950.9	E962.1	E980.9
LMD	964.8	E858.2	E934.8	E950.4	E962.0	E980.4
Lobelia	988.2	E865.4	—	E950.9	E962.1	E980.9
Lobeline	970.0	E854.3	E940.0	E950.4	E962.0	E980.4
Locorten	976.0	E858.7	E946.0	E950.4	E962.0	E980.4
Lolium temulentum	988.2	E865.3	—	E950.9	E962.1	E980.9
Lomotil	973.5	E858.4	E943.5	E950.4	E962.0	E980.4
Lomustine	963.1	E858.1	E933.1	E950.4	E962.0	E980.4
Lophophora williamsii	969.6	E854.1	E939.6	E950.3	E962.0	E980.3
Lorazepam	969.4	E853.2	E939.4	E950.3	E962.0	E980.3
Lotions NEC	976.9	E858.7	E946.9	E950.4	E962.0	E980.4
Lotronex	973.8	E858.4	E943.8	E950.4	E962.0	E980.4
Lotusate	967.0	E851	E937.0	E950.1	E962.0	E980.1
Lowila	976.2	E858.7	E946.2	E950.4	E962.0	E980.4
Loxapine	969.3	E853.8	E939.3	E950.3	E962.0	E980.3
Lozenges (throat)	976.6	E858.7	E946.6	E950.4	E962.0	E980.4
LSD (25)	969.6	E854.1	E939.6	E950.3	E962.0	E980.3
Lubricating oil NEC	981	E862.2	—	E950.9	E962.1	E980.9
Lucanthone	961.6	E857	E931.6	E950.4	E962.0	E980.4
Luminal	967.0	E851	E937.0	E950.1	E962.0	E980.1
Lung irritant (gas) NEC	987.9	E869.9	—	E952.9	E962.2	E982.9
Lutocylol	962.2	E858.0	E932.2	E950.4	E962.0	E980.4
Lutromone	962.2	E858.0	E932.2	E950.4	E962.0	E980.4
Lututrin	975.0	E858.6	E945.0	E950.4	E962.0	E980.4
Lye (concentrated)	983.2	E864.2	—	E950.7	E962.1	E980.6
Lygranum (skin test)	977.8	E858.8	E947.8	E950.4	E962.0	E980.4
Lymecycline	960.4	E856	E930.4	E950.4	E962.0	E980.4
Lymphogranuloma venereum antigen	977.8	E858.8	E947.8	E950.4	E962.0	E980.4
Lynestrenol	962.2	E858.0	E932.2	E950.4	E962.0	E980.4
Lyovac Sodium Edecrin	974.4	E858.5	E944.4	E950.4	E962.0	E980.4
Lypressin	962.5	E858.0	E932.5	E950.4	E962.0	E980.4
Lysergic acid (amide) (diethylamide)	969.6	E854.1	E939.6	E950.3	E962.0	E980.3
Lysergide	969.6	E854.1	E939.6	E950.3	E962.0	E980.3
Lysine vasopressin	962.5	E858.0	E932.5	E950.4	E962.0	E980.4
Lysol	983.0	E864.0	—	E950.7	E962.1	E980.6
Lytta (vitatta)	976.8	E858.7	E946.8	E950.4	E962.0	E980.4
Mace	987.5	E869.3	—	E952.8	E962.2	E982.8
Macrolides (antibiotics)	960.3	E856	E930.3	E950.4	E962.0	E980.4
Mafenide	976.0	E858.7	E946.0	E950.4	E962.0	E980.4
Magaldrate	973.0	E858.4	E943.0	E950.4	E962.0	E980.4
Magic mushroom	969.6	E854.1	E939.6	E950.3	E962.0	E980.3
Magnamycin	960.8	E856	E930.8	E950.4	E962.0	E980.4
Magnesia magma	973.0	E858.4	E943.0	E950.4	E962.0	E980.4
Magnesium (compounds) (fumes) NEC	985.8	E866.4	—	E950.9	E962.1	E980.9
antacid	973.0	E858.4	E943.0	E950.4	E962.0	E980.4
carbonate	973.0	E858.4	E943.0	E950.4	E962.0	E980.4
cathartic	973.3	E858.4	E943.3	E950.4	E962.0	E980.4
citrate	973.3	E858.4	E943.3	E950.4	E962.0	E980.4
hydroxide	973.0	E858.4	E943.0	E950.4	E962.0	E980.4
oxide	973.0	E858.4	E943.0	E950.4	E962.0	E980.4
sulfate (oral)	973.3	E858.4	E943.3	E950.4	E962.0	E980.4
intravenous	966.3	E855.0	E936.3	E950.4	E962.0	E980.4
trisilicate	973.0	E858.4	E943.0	E950.4	E962.0	E980.4
Malathion (insecticide)	989.3	E863.1	—	E950.6	E962.1	E980.7
Male fern (oleoresin)	961.6	E857	E931.6	E950.4	E962.0	E980.4
Mandelic acid	961.9	E857	E931.9	E950.4	E962.0	E980.4
Manganese compounds (fumes) NEC	985.2	E866.4	—	E950.9	E962.1	E980.9
Mannitol (diuretic) (medicinal) NEC	974.4	E858.5	E944.4	E950.4	E962.0	E980.4
hexanitrate	972.4	E858.3	E942.4	E950.4	E962.0	E980.4
mustard	963.1	E858.1	E933.1	E950.4	E962.0	E980.4

		External Cause (E-Code)				
	Poisoning	Accident	Therapeutic Use	Suicide Attempt	Assault	Undetermined
Mannomustine	963.1	E858.1	E933.1	E950.4	E962.0	E980.4
MAO inhibitors	969.0	E854.0	E939.0	E950.3	E962.0	E980.3
Mapharsen	961.1	E857	E931.1	E950.4	E962.0	E980.4
Marcaine	968.9	E855.2	E938.9	E950.4	E962.0	E980.4
infiltration (subcutaneous)	968.5	E855.2	E938.5	E950.4	E962.0	E980.4
nerve block (peripheral) (plexus)	968.6	E855.2	E938.6	E950.4	E962.0	E980.4
Marezine	963.0	E858.1	E933.0	E950.4	E962.0	E980.4
Marihuana, marijuana (derivatives)	969.6	E854.1	E939.6	E950.3	E962.0	E980.3
Marine animals or plants (sting)	989.5	E905.6	—	E950.9	E962.1	E980.9
Marplan	969.0	E854.0	E939.0	E950.3	E962.0	E980.3
Marsh gas	987.1	E869.8	—	E952.8	E962.2	E982.8
Marsilid	969.0	E854.0	E939.0	E950.3	E962.0	E980.3
Matulane	963.1	E858.1	E933.1	E950.4	E962.0	E980.4
Mazindol	977.0	E858.8	E947.0	E950.4	E962.0	E980.4
Meadow saffron	988.2	E865.3	—	E950.9	E962.1	E980.9
Measles vaccine	979.4	E858.8	E949.4	E950.4	E962.0	E980.4
Meat, noxious or nonbacterial	988.8	E865.0	—	E950.9	E962.1	E980.9
Mebanazine	969.0	E854.0	E939.0	E950.3	E962.0	E980.3
Mebaral	967.0	E851	E937.0	E950.1	E962.0	E980.1
Mebendazole	961.6	E857	E931.6	E950.4	E962.0	E980.4
Mebeverine	975.1	E858.6	E945.1	E950.4	E962.0	E980.4
Mebhydroline	963.0	E858.1	E933.0	E950.4	E962.0	E980.4
Mebrophenhydramine	963.0	E858.1	E933.0	E950.4	E962.0	E980.4
Mebutamate	969.5	E853.8	E939.5	E950.3	E962.0	E980.3
Mecamylamine (chloride)	972.3	E858.3	E942.3	E950.4	E962.0	E980.4
Mechlorethamine hydrochloride	963.1	E858.1	E933.1	E950.4	E962.0	E980.4
Meclizene (hydrochloride)	963.0	E858.1	E933.0	E950.4	E962.0	E980.4
Meclofenoxate	970.0	E854.3	E940.0	E950.4	E962.0	E980.4
Meclozine (hydrochloride)	963.0	E858.1	E933.0	E950.4	E962.0	E980.4
Medazepam	969.4	E853.2	E939.4	E950.3	E962.0	E980.3
Medicine, medicinal substance	977.9	E858.9	E947.9	E950.5	E962.0	E980.5
specified NEC	977.8	E858.8	E947.8	E950.4	E962.0	E980.4
Medinal	967.0	E851	E937.0	E950.1	E962.0	E980.1
Medomin	967.0	E851	E937.0	E950.1	E962.0	E980.1
Medroxyprogesterone	962.2	E858.0	E932.2	E950.4	E962.0	E980.4
Medrysone	976.5	E858.7	E946.5	E950.4	E962.0	E980.4
Mefenamic acid	965.7	E850.7	E935.7	E950.0	E962.0	E980.0
Megahallucinogen	969.6	E854.1	E939.6	E950.3	E962.0	E980.3
Megestrol	962.2	E858.0	E932.2	E950.4	E962.0	E980.4
Meglumine	977.8	E858.8	E947.8	E950.4	E962.0	E980.4
Meladinin	976.3	E858.7	E946.3	E950.4	E962.0	E980.4
Melanizing agents	976.3	E858.7	E946.3	E950.4	E962.0	E980.4
Melarsoprol	961.1	E857	E931.1	E950.4	E962.0	E980.4
Melia azedarach	988.2	E865.3	—	E950.9	E962.1	E980.9
Mellaril	969.1	E853.0	E939.1	E950.3	E962.0	E980.3
Meloxine	976.3	E858.7	E946.3	E950.4	E962.0	E980.4
Melphalan	963.1	E858.1	E933.1	E950.4	E962.0	E980.4
Menadiol sodium diphosphate	964.3	E858.2	E934.3	E950.4	E962.0	E980.4
Menadione (sodium bisulfite)	964.3	E858.2	E934.3	E950.4	E962.0	E980.4
Menaphthone	964.3	E858.2	E934.3	E950.4	E962.0	E980.4
Meningococcal vaccine	978.8	E858.8	E948.8	E950.4	E962.0	E980.4
Menningovax-C	978.8	E858.8	E948.8	E950.4	E962.0	E980.4
Menotropins	962.4	E858.0	E932.4	E950.4	E962.0	E980.4
Menthol NEC	976.1	E858.7	E946.1	E950.4	E962.0	E980.4
Mepacrine	961.3	E857	E931.3	E950.4	E962.0	E980.4
Meparfynol	967.8	E852.8	E937.8	E950.2	E962.0	E980.2
Mepazine	969.1	E853.0	E939.1	E950.3	E962.0	E980.3
Mepenzolate	971.1	E855.4	E941.1	E950.4	E962.0	E980.4
Meperidine	965.09	E850.2	E935.2	E950.0	E962.0	E980.0
Mephenamin(e)	966.4	E855.0	E936.4	E950.4	E962.0	E980.4
Mephenesin (carbamate)	968.0	E855.1	E938.0	E950.4	E962.0	E980.4
Mephenoxalone	969.5	E853.8	E939.5	E950.3	E962.0	E980.3
Mephentermine	971.2	E855.5	E941.2	E950.4	E962.0	E980.4
Mephenytoin	966.1	E855.0	E936.1	E950.4	E962.0	E980.4
Mephobarbital	967.0	E851	E937.0	E950.1	E962.0	E980.1
Mepiperphenidol	971.1	E855.4	E941.1	E950.4	E962.0	E980.4
Mepivacaine	968.9	E855.2	E938.9	E950.4	E962.0	E980.4
infiltration (subcutaneous)	968.5	E855.2	E938.5	E950.4	E962.0	E980.4
nerve block (peripheral) (plexus)	968.6	E855.2	E938.6	E950.4	E962.0	E980.4
topical (surface)	968.5	E855.2	E938.5	E950.4	E962.0	E980.4
Meprednisone	962.0	E858.0	E932.0	E950.4	E962.0	E980.4
Meprobam	969.5	E853.8	E939.5	E950.3	E962.0	E980.3
Meprobamate	969.5	E853.8	E939.5	E950.3	E962.0	E980.3
Mepyramine (maleate)	963.0	E858.1	E933.0	E950.4	E962.0	E980.4
Meralluride	974.0	E858.5	E944.0	E950.4	E962.0	E980.4
Merbaphen	974.0	E858.5	E944.0	E950.4	E962.0	E980.4
Merbromin	976.0	E858.7	E946.0	E950.4	E962.0	E980.4
Mercaptomerin	974.0	E858.5	E944.0	E950.4	E962.0	E980.4
Mercaptopurine	963.1	E858.1	E933.1	E950.4	E962.0	E980.4
Mercumatilin	974.0	E858.5	E944.0	E950.4	E962.0	E980.4
Mercuramide	974.0	E858.5	E944.0	E950.4	E962.0	E980.4

✓4ᵗʰ Fourth-digit Required   ✓5ᵗʰ Fifth-digit Required   ▶◀ Revised Text   ● New Line   ▲ Revised Code

	Poisoning	External Cause (E-Code)				
		Accident	Therapeutic Use	Suicide Attempt	Assault	Undetermined
Mercuranin	976.0	E858.7	E946.0	E950.4	E962.0	E980.4
Mercurochrome	976.0	E858.7	E946.0	E950.4	E962.0	E980.4
Mercury, mercuric, mercurous (compounds) (cyanide) (fumes) (nonmedicinal) (vapor) NEC	985.0	E866.1	—	E950.9	E962.1	E980.9
ammoniated	976.0	E858.7	E946.0	E950.4	E962.0	E980.4
anti-infective	961.2	E857	E931.2	E950.4	E962.0	E980.4
topical	976.0	E858.7	E946.0	E950.4	E962.0	E980.4
chloride (antiseptic) NEC	976.0	E858.7	E946.0	E950.4	E962.0	E980.4
fungicide	985.0	E863.6	—	E950.6	E962.1	E980.7
diuretic compounds	974.0	E858.5	E944.0	E950.4	E962.0	E980.4
fungicide	985.0	E863.6	—	E950.6	E962.1	E980.7
organic (fungicide)	985.0	E863.6	—	E950.6	E962.1	E980.7
Merethoxylline	974.0	E858.5	E944.0	E950.4	E962.0	E980.4
Mersalyl	974.0	E858.5	E944.0	E950.4	E962.0	E980.4
Merthiolate (topical)	976.0	E858.7	E946.0	E950.4	E962.0	E980.4
ophthalmic preparation	976.5	E858.7	E946.5	E950.4	E962.0	E980.4
Meruvax	979.4	E858.8	E949.4	E950.4	E962.0	E980.4
Mescal buttons	969.6	E854.1	E939.6	E950.3	E962.0	E980.3
Mescaline (salts)	969.6	E854.1	E939.6	E950.3	E962.0	E980.3
Mesoridazine besylate	969.1	E853.0	E939.1	E950.3	E962.0	E980.3
Mestanolone	962.1	E858.0	E932.1	E950.4	E962.0	E980.4
Mestranol	962.2	E858.0	E932.2	E950.4	E962.0	E980.4
Metacresylacetate	976.0	E858.7	E946.0	E950.4	E962.0	E980.4
Metaldehyde (snail killer) NEC	989.4	E863.4	—	E950.6	E962.1	E980.7
Metals (heavy) (nonmedicinal) NEC	985.9	E866.4	—	E950.9	E962.1	E980.9
dust, fumes, or vapor NEC	985.9	E866.4	—	E950.9	E962.1	E980.9
light NEC	985.9	E866.4	—	E950.9	E962.1	E980.9
dust, fumes, or vapor NEC	985.9	E866.4	—	E950.9	E962.1	E980.9
pesticides (dust) (vapor)	985.9	E863.4	—	E950.6	E962.1	E980.7
Metamucil	973.3	E858.4	E943.3	E950.4	E962.0	E980.4
Metaphen	976.0	E858.7	E946.0	E950.4	E962.0	E980.4
Metaproterenol	975.1	E858.6	E945.1	E950.4	E962.0	E980.4
Metaraminol	972.8	E858.3	E942.8	E950.4	E962.0	E980.4
Metaxalone	968.0	E855.1	E938.0	E950.4	E962.0	E980.4
Metformin	962.3	E858.0	E932.3	E950.4	E962.0	E980.4
Methacycline	960.4	E856	E930.4	E950.4	E962.0	E980.4
Methadone	965.02	E850.1	E935.1	E950.0	E962.0	E980.0
Methallenestril	962.2	E858.0	E932.2	E950.4	E962.0	E980.4
Methamphetamine	969.7	E854.2	E939.7	E950.3	E962.0	E980.3
Methandienone	962.1	E858.0	E932.1	E950.4	E962.0	E980.4
Methandriol	962.1	E858.0	E932.1	E950.4	E962.0	E980.4
Methandrostenolone	962.1	E858.0	E932.1	E950.4	E962.0	E980.4
Methane gas	987.1	E869.8	—	E952.8	E962.2	E982.8
Methanol	980.1	E860.2	—	E950.9	E962.1	E980.9
vapor	987.8	E869.8	—	E952.8	E962.2	E982.8
Methantheline	971.1	E855.4	E941.1	E950.4	E962.0	E980.4
Methaphenilene	963.0	E858.1	E933.0	E950.4	E962.0	E980.4
Methapyrilene	963.0	E858.1	E933.0	E950.4	E962.0	E980.4
Methaqualone (compounds)	967.4	E852.3	E937.4	E950.2	E962.0	E980.2
Metharbital, metharbitone	967.0	E851	E937.0	E950.1	E962.0	E980.1
Methazolamide	974.2	E858.5	E944.2	E950.4	E962.0	E980.4
Methdilazine	963.0	E858.1	E933.0	E950.4	E962.0	E980.4
Methedrine	969.7	E854.2	E939.7	E950.3	E962.0	E980.3
Methenamine (mandelate)	961.9	E857	E931.9	E950.4	E962.0	E980.4
Methenolone	962.1	E858.0	E932.1	E950.4	E962.0	E980.4
Methergine	975.0	E858.6	E945.0	E950.4	E962.0	E980.4
Methiacil	962.8	E858.0	E932.8	E950.4	E962.0	E980.4
Methicillin (sodium)	960.0	E856	E930.0	E950.4	E962.0	E980.4
Methimazole	962.8	E858.0	E932.8	E950.4	E962.0	E980.4
Methionine	977.1	E858.8	E947.1	E950.4	E962.0	E980.4
Methisazone	961.7	E857	E931.7	E950.4	E962.0	E980.4
Methitural	967.0	E851	E937.0	E950.1	E962.0	E980.1
Methixene	971.1	E855.4	E941.1	E950.4	E962.0	E980.4
Methobarbital, methobarbitone	967.0	E851	E937.0	E950.1	E962.0	E980.1
Methocarbamol	968.0	E855.1	E938.0	E950.4	E962.0	E980.4
Methohexital, methohexitone (sodium)	968.3	E855.1	E938.3	E950.4	E962.0	E980.4
Methoin	966.1	E855.0	E936.1	E950.4	E962.0	E980.4
Methopholine	965.7	E850.7	E935.7	E950.0	E962.0	E980.0
Methorate	975.4	E858.6	E945.4	E950.4	E962.0	E980.4
Methoserpidine	972.6	E858.3	E942.6	E950.4	E962.0	E980.4
Methotrexate	963.1	E858.1	E933.1	E950.4	E962.0	E980.4
Methotrimeprazine	967.8	E852.8	E937.8	E950.2	E962.0	E980.2
Methoxa-Dome	976.3	E858.7	E946.3	E950.4	E962.0	E980.4
Methoxamine	971.2	E855.5	E941.2	E950.4	E962.0	E980.4
Methoxsalen	976.3	E858.7	E946.3	E950.4	E962.0	E980.4
Methoxybenzyl penicillin	960.0	E856	E930.0	E950.4	E962.0	E980.4
Methoxychlor	989.2	E863.0	—	E950.6	E962.1	E980.7
Methoxyflurane	968.2	E855.1	E938.2	E950.4	E962.0	E980.4
Methoxyphenamine	971.2	E855.5	E941.2	E950.4	E962.0	E980.4
Methoxypromazine	969.1	E853.0	E939.1	E950.3	E962.0	E980.3
Methoxypsoralen	976.3	E858.7	E946.3	E950.4	E962.0	E980.4

Mercuranin — Methoxypsoralen

	Poisoning	External Cause (E-Code)				
		Accident	Therapeutic Use	Suicide Attempt	Assault	Undetermined
Methscopolamine (bromide)	971.1	E855.4	E941.1	E950.4	E962.0	E980.4
Methsuximide	966.2	E855.0	E936.2	E950.4	E962.0	E980.4
Methyclothiazide	974.3	E858.5	E944.3	E950.4	E962.0	E980.4
Methyl						
acetate	982.8	E862.4	—	E950.9	E962.1	E980.9
acetone	982.8	E862.4	—	E950.9	E962.1	E980.9
alcohol	980.1	E860.2	—	E950.9	E962.1	E980.9
amphetamine	969.7	E854.2	E939.7	E950.3	E962.0	E980.3
androstanolone	962.1	E858.0	E932.1	E950.4	E962.0	E980.4
atropine	971.1	E855.4	E941.1	E950.4	E962.0	E980.4
benzene	982.0	E862.4	—	E950.9	E962.1	E980.9
bromide (gas)	987.8	E869.8	—	E952.8	E962.2	E982.8
fumigant	987.8	E863.8	—	E950.6	E962.2	E980.7
butanol	980.8	E860.8	—	E950.9	E962.1	E980.9
carbinol	980.1	E860.2	—	E950.9	E962.1	E980.9
cellosolve	982.8	E862.4	—	E950.9	E962.1	E980.9
cellulose	973.3	E858.4	E943.3	E950.4	E962.0	E980.4
chloride (gas)	987.8	E869.8	—	E952.8	E962.2	E982.8
cyclohexane	982.8	E862.4	—	E950.9	E962.1	E980.9
cyclohexanone	982.8	E862.4	—	E950.9	E962.1	E980.9
dihydromorphinone	965.09	E850.2	E935.2	E950.0	E962.0	E980.0
ergometrine	975.0	E858.6	E945.0	E950.4	E962.0	E980.4
ergonovine	975.0	E858.6	E945.0	E950.4	E962.0	E980.4
ethyl ketone	982.8	E862.4	—	E950.9	E962.1	E980.9
hydrazine	983.9	E864.3	—	E950.7	E962.1	E980.6
isobutyl ketone	982.8	E862.4	—	E950.9	E962.1	E980.9
morphine NEC	965.09	E850.2	E935.2	E950.0	E962.0	E980.0
parafynol	967.8	E852.8	E937.8	E950.2	E962.0	E980.2
parathion	989.3	E863.1	—	E950.6	E962.1	E980.7
pentynol NEC	967.8	E852.8	E937.8	E950.2	E962.0	E980.2
peridol	969.2	E853.1	E939.2	E950.3	E962.0	E980.3
phenidate	969.7	E854.2	E939.7	E950.3	E962.0	E980.3
prednisolone	962.0	E858.0	E932.0	E950.4	E962.0	E980.4
ENT agent	976.6	E858.7	E946.6	E950.4	E962.0	E980.4
ophthalmic preparation	976.5	E858.7	E946.5	E950.4	E962.0	E980.4
topical NEC	976.0	E858.7	E946.0	E950.4	E962.0	E980.4
propylcarbinol	980.8	E860.8	—	E950.9	E962.1	E980.9
rosaniline NEC	976.0	E858.7	E946.0	E950.4	E962.0	E980.4
salicylate NEC	976.3	E858.7	E946.3	E950.4	E962.0	E980.4
sulfate (fumes)	987.8	E869.8	—	E952.8	E962.2	E982.8
liquid	983.9	E864.3	—	E950.7	E962.1	E980.6
sulfonal	967.8	E852.8	E937.8	E950.2	E962.0	E980.2
testosterone	962.1	E858.0	E932.1	E950.4	E962.0	E980.4
thiouracil	962.8	E858.0	E932.8	E950.4	E962.0	E980.4
Methylated spirit	980.0	E860.1	—	E950.9	E962.1	E980.9
Methyldopa	972.6	E858.3	E942.6	E950.4	E962.0	E980.4
Methylene						
blue	961.9	E857	E931.9	E950.4	E962.0	E980.4
chloride or dichloride (solvent) NEC	982.3	E862.4	—	E950.9	E962.1	E980.9
Methylhexabital	967.0	E851	E937.0	E950.1	E962.0	E980.1
Methylparaben (ophthalmic)	976.5	E858.7	E946.5	E950.4	E962.0	E980.4
Methyprylon	967.5	E852.4	E937.5	E950.2	E962.0	E980.2
Methysergide	971.3	E855.6	E941.3	E950.4	E962.0	E980.4
Metoclopramide	963.0	E858.1	E933.0	E950.4	E962.0	E980.4
Metofoline	965.7	E850.7	E935.7	E950.0	E962.0	E980.0
Metopon	965.09	E850.2	E935.2	E950.0	E962.0	E980.0
Metronidazole	961.5	E857	E931.5	E950.4	E962.0	E980.4
Metycaine	968.9	E855.2	E938.9	E950.4	E962.0	E980.4
infiltration (subcutaneous)	968.5	E855.2	E938.5	E950.4	E962.0	E980.4
nerve block (peripheral) (plexus)	968.6	E855.2	E938.6	E950.4	E962.0	E980.4
topical (surface)	968.5	E855.2	E938.5	E950.4	E962.0	E980.4
Metyrapone	977.8	E858.8	E947.8	E950.4	E962.0	E980.4
Mevinphos	989.3	E863.1	—	E950.6	E962.1	E980.7
Mezereon (berries)	988.2	E865.3	—	E950.9	E962.1	E980.9
Micatin	976.0	E858.7	E946.0	E950.4	E962.0	E980.4
Miconazole	976.0	E858.7	E946.0	E950.4	E962.0	E980.4
Midol	965.1	E850.3	E935.3	E950.0	E962.0	E980.0
Mifepristone	962.9	E858.0	E932.9	E950.4	E962.0	E980.4
Milk of magnesia	973.0	E858.4	E943.0	E950.4	E962.0	E980.4
Millipede (tropical) (venomous)	989.5	E905.4	—	E950.9	E962.1	E980.9
Miltown	969.5	E853.8	E939.5	E950.3	E962.0	E980.3
Mineral						
oil (medicinal)	973.2	E858.4	E943.2	E950.4	E962.0	E980.4
nonmedicinal	981	E862.1	—	E950.9	E962.1	E980.9
topical	976.3	E858.7	E946.3	E950.4	E962.0	E980.4
salts NEC	974.6	E858.5	E944.6	E950.4	E962.0	E980.4
spirits	981	E862.0	—	E950.9	E962.1	E980.9
Minocycline	960.4	E856	E930.4	E950.4	E962.0	E980.4
Mithramycin (antineoplastic)	960.7	E856	E930.7	E950.4	E962.0	E980.4
Mitobronitol	963.1	E858.1	E933.1	E950.4	E962.0	E980.4
Mitomycin (antineoplastic)	960.7	E856	E930.7	E950.4	E962.0	E980.4

Methscopolamine — Mitomycin

☑4ᵗʰ Fourth-digit Required   ☑5ᵗʰ Fifth-digit Required   ▶◀ Revised Text   ● New Line   ▲ Revised Code

	Poisoning	External Cause (E-Code)				
		Accident	Therapeutic Use	Suicide Attempt	Assault	Undetermined
Mitotane	963.1	E858.1	E933.1	E950.4	E962.0	E980.4
Moderil	972.6	E858.3	E942.6	E950.4	E962.0	E980.4
Mogadon — see Nitrazepam						
Molindone	969.3	E853.8	E939.3	E950.3	E962.0	E980.3
Monistat	976.0	E858.7	E946.0	E950.4	E962.0	E980.4
Monkshood	988.2	E865.4	—	E950.9	E962.1	E980.9
Monoamine oxidase inhibitors	969.0	E854.0	E939.0	E950.3	E962.0	E980.3
Monochlorobenzene	982.0	E862.4	—	E950.9	E962.1	E980.9
Monosodium glutamate	989.89	E866.8	—	E950.9	E962.1	E980.9
Monoxide, carbon — see Carbon, monoxide						
Moperone	969.2	E853.1	E939.2	E950.3	E962.0	E980.3
Morning glory seeds	969.6	E854.1	E939.6	E950.3	E962.0	E980.3
Moroxydine (hydrochloride)	961.7	E857	E931.7	E950.4	E962.0	E980.4
Morphazinamide	961.8	E857	E931.8	E950.4	E962.0	E980.4
Morphinans	965.09	E850.2	E935.2	E950.0	E962.0	E980.0
Morphine NEC	965.09	E850.2	E935.2	E950.0	E962.0	E980.0
antagonists	970.1	E854.3	E940.1	E950.4	E962.0	E980.4
Morpholinylethylmorphine	965.09	E850.2	E935.2	E950.0	E962.0	E980.0
Morrhuate sodium	972.7	E858.3	E942.7	E950.4	E962.0	E980.4
Moth balls (see also Pesticides)	989.4	E863.4	—	E950.6	E962.1	E980.7
naphthalene	983.0	E863.4	—	E950.7	E962.1	E980.6
Motor exhaust gas — see Carbon, monoxide, exhaust gas						
Mouth wash	976.6	E858.7	E946.6	E950.4	E962.0	E980.4
Mucolytic agent	975.5	E858.6	E945.5	E950.4	E962.0	E980.4
Mucomyst	975.5	E858.6	E945.5	E950.4	E962.0	E980.4
Mucous membrane agents (external)	976.9	E858.7	E946.9	E950.4	E962.0	E980.4
specified NEC	976.8	E858.7	E946.8	E950.4	E962.0	E980.4
Mumps						
immune globulin (human)	964.6	E858.2	E934.6	E950.4	E962.0	E980.4
skin test antigen	977.8	E858.8	E947.8	E950.4	E962.0	E980.4
vaccine	979.6	E858.8	E949.6	E950.4	E962.0	E980.4
Mumpsvax	979.6	E858.8	E949.6	E950.4	E962.0	E980.4
Muriatic acid — see Hydrochloric acid						
Muscarine	971.0	E855.3	E941.0	E950.4	E962.0	E980.4
Muscle affecting agents NEC	975.3	E858.6	E945.3	E950.4	E962.0	E980.4
oxytocic	975.0	E858.6	E945.0	E950.4	E962.0	E980.4
relaxants	975.3	E858.6	E945.3	E950.4	E962.0	E980.4
central nervous system	968.0	E855.1	E938.0	E950.4	E962.0	E980.4
skeletal	975.2	E858.6	E945.2	E950.4	E962.0	E980.4
smooth	975.1	E858.6	E945.1	E950.4	E962.0	E980.4
Mushrooms, noxious	988.1	E865.5	—	E950.9	E962.1	E980.9
Mussel, noxious	988.0	E865.1	—	E950.9	E962.1	E980.9
Mustard (emetic)	973.6	E858.4	E943.6	E950.4	E962.0	E980.4
gas	987.8	E869.8	—	E952.8	E962.2	E982.8
nitrogen	963.1	E858.1	E933.1	E950.4	E962.0	E980.4
Mustine	963.1	E858.1	E933.1	E950.4	E962.0	E980.4
M-vac	979.4	E858.8	E949.4	E950.4	E962.0	E980.4
Mycifradin	960.8	E856	E930.8	E950.4	E962.0	E980.4
topical	976.0	E858.7	E946.0	E950.4	E962.0	E980.4
Mycitracin	960.8	E856	E930.8	E950.4	E962.0	E980.4
ophthalmic preparation	976.5	E858.7	E946.5	E950.4	E962.0	E980.4
Mycostatin	960.1	E856	E930.1	E950.4	E962.0	E980.4
topical	976.0	E858.7	E946.0	E950.4	E962.0	E980.4
Mydriacyl	971.1	E855.4	E941.1	E950.4	E962.0	E980.4
Myelobromal	963.1	E858.1	E933.1	E950.4	E962.0	E980.4
Myleran	963.1	E858.1	E933.1	E950.4	E962.0	E980.4
Myochrysin(e)	965.69	E850.6	E935.6	E950.0	E962.0	E980.0
Myoneural blocking agents	975.2	E858.6	E945.2	E950.4	E962.0	E980.4
Myristica fragrans	988.2	E865.3	—	E950.9	E962.1	E980.9
Myristicin	988.2	E865.3	—	E950.9	E962.1	E980.9
Mysoline	966.3	E855.0	E936.3	E950.4	E962.0	E980.4
Nafcillin (sodium)	960.0	E856	E930.0	E950.4	E962.0	E980.4
Nail polish remover	982.8	E862.4	—	E950.9	E962.1	E908.9
Nalidixic acid	961.9	E857	E931.9	E950.4	E962.0	E980.4
Nalorphine	970.1	E854.3	E940.1	E950.4	E962.0	E980.4
Naloxone	970.1	E854.3	E940.1	E950.4	E962.0	E980.4
Nandrolone (decanoate) (phenproprioate)	962.1	E858.0	E932.1	E950.4	E962.0	E980.4
Naphazoline	971.2	E855.5	E941.2	E950.4	E962.0	E980.4
Naphtha (painter's) (petroleum)	981	E862.0	—	E950.9	E962.1	E980.9
solvent	981	E862.0	—	E950.9	E962.1	E980.9
vapor	987.1	E869.8	—	E952.8	E962.2	E982.8
Naphthalene (chlorinated)	983.0	E864.0	—	E950.7	E962.1	E980.6
insecticide or moth repellent	983.0	E863.4	—	E950.7	E962.1	E980.6
vapor	987.8	E869.8	—	E952.8	E962.2	E982.8
Naphthol	983.0	E864.0	—	E950.7	E962.1	E980.6
Naphthylamine	983.0	E864.0	—	E950.7	E962.1	E980.6
Naprosyn — see Naproxen						
Naproxen	965.61	E850.6	E935.6	E950.0	E962.0	E980.0
Narcotic (drug)	967.9	E852.9	E937.9	E950.2	E962.0	E980.2
analgesic NEC	965.8	E850.8	E935.8	E950.0	E962.0	E980.0
antagonist	970.1	E854.3	E940.1	E950.4	E962.0	E980.4

☑4ᵗʰ Fourth-digit Required   ☑5ᵗʰ Fifth-digit Required   ▶◀ Revised Text   ● New Line   ▲ Revised Code

Mitotane — Narcotic

	External Cause (E-Code)					
	Poisoning	**Accident**	**Therapeutic Use**	**Suicide Attempt**	**Assault**	**Undetermined**
Narcotic — *continued*						
specified NEC	967.8	E852.8	E937.8	E950.2	E962.0	E980.2
Narcotine	975.4	E858.6	E945.4	E950.4	E962.0	E980.4
Nardil	969.0	E854.0	E939.0	E950.3	E962.0	E980.3
Natrium cyanide — *see* Cyanide(s)						
Natural						
blood (product)	964.7	E858.2	E934.7	E950.4	E962.0	E980.4
gas (piped)	987.1	E867	—	E951.0	E962.2	E981.0
incomplete combustion	986	E867	—	E951.0	E962.2	E981.0
Nealbarbital, nealbarbitone	967.0	E851	E937.0	E950.1	E962.0	E980.1
Nectadon	975.4	E858.6	E945.4	E950.4	E962.0	E980.4
Nematocyst (sting)	989.5	E905.6	—	E950.9	E962.1	E980.9
Nembutal	967.0	E851	E937.0	E950.1	E962.0	E980.1
Neoarsphenamine	961.1	E857	E931.1	E950.4	E962.0	E980.4
Neocinchophen	974.7	E858.5	E944.7	E950.4	E962.0	E980.4
Neomycin	960.8	E856	E930.8	E950.4	E962.0	E980.4
ENT agent	976.6	E858.7	E946.6	E950.4	E962.0	E980.4
ophthalmic preparation	976.5	E858.7	E946.5	E950.4	E962.0	E980.4
topical NEC	976.0	E858.7	E946.0	E950.4	E962.0	E980.4
Neonal	967.0	E851	E937.0	E950.1	E962.0	E980.1
Neoprontosil	961.0	E857	E931.0	E950.4	E962.0	E980.4
Neosalvarsan	961.1	E857	E931.1	E950.4	E962.0	E980.4
Neosilversalvarsan	961.1	E857	E931.1	E950.4	E962.0	E980.4
Neosporin	960.8	E856	E930.8	E950.4	E962.0	E980.4
ENT agent	976.6	E858.7	E946.6	E950.4	E962.0	E980.4
opthalmic preparation	976.5	E858.7	E946.5	E950.4	E962.0	E980.4
topical NEC	976.0	E858.7	E946.0	E950.4	E962.0	E980.4
Neostigmine	971.0	E855.3	E941.0	E950.4	E962.0	E980.4
Neraval	967.0	E851	E937.0	E950.1	E962.0	E980.1
Neravan	967.0	E851	E937.0	E950.1	E962.0	E980.1
Nerium oleander	988.2	E865.4	—	E950.9	E962.1	E980.9
Nerve gases (war)	987.9	E869.9	—	E952.9	E962.2	E982.9
Nesacaine	968.9	E855.2	E938.9	E950.4	E962.0	E980.4
infiltration (subcutaneous)	968.5	E855.2	E938.5	E950.4	E962.0	E980.4
nerve block (peripheral) (plexus)	968.6	E855.2	E938.6	E950.4	E962.0	E980.4
Neurobarb	967.0	E851	E937.0	E950.1	E962.0	E980.1
Neuroleptics NEC	969.3	E853.8	E939.3	E950.3	E962.0	E980.3
Neuroprotective agent	977.8	E858.8	E947.8	E950.4	E962.0	E980.4
Neutral spirits	980.0	E860.1	—	E950.9	E962.1	E980.9
beverage	980.0	E860.0	—	E950.9	E962.1	E980.9
Niacin, niacinamide	972.2	E858.3	E942.2	E950.4	E962.0	E980.4
Nialamide	969.0	E854.0	E939.0	E950.3	E962.0	E980.3
Nickle (carbonyl) (compounds) (fumes) (tetracarbonyl) (vapor)	985.8	E866.4	—	E950.9	E962.1	E980.9
Niclosamide	961.6	E857	E931.6	E950.4	E962.0	E980.4
Nicomorphine	965.09	E850.2	E935.2	E950.0	E962.0	E980.0
Nicotinamide	972.2	E858.3	E942.2	E950.4	E962.0	E980.4
Nicotine (insecticide) (spray) (sulfate) NEC	989.4	E863.4	—	E950.6	E962.1	E980.7
not insecticide	989.89	E866.8	—	E950.9	E962.1	E980.9
Nicotinic acid (derivatives)	972.2	E858.3	E942.2	E950.4	E962.0	E980.4
Nicotinyl alcohol	972.2	E858.3	E942.2	E950.4	E962.0	E980.4
Nicoumalone	964.2	E858.2	E934.2	E950.4	E962.0	E980.4
Nifenazone	965.5	E850.5	E935.5	E950.0	E962.0	E980.0
Nifuraldezone	961.9	E857	E931.9	E950.4	E962.0	E980.4
Nightshade (deadly)	988.2	E865.4	—	E950.9	E962.1	E980.9
Nikethamide	970.0	E854.3	E940.0	E950.4	E962.0	E980.4
Nilstat	960.1	E856	E930.1	E950.4	E962.0	E980.4
topical	976.0	E858.7	E946.0	E950.4	E962.0	E980.4
Nimodipine	977.8	E858.8	E947.8	E950.4	E962.0	E980.4
Niridazole	961.6	E857	E931.6	E950.4	E962.0	E980.4
Nisentil	965.09	E850.2	E935.2	E950.0	E962.0	E980.0
Nitrates	972.4	E858.3	E942.4	E950.4	E962.0	E980.4
Nitrazepam	969.4	E853.2	E939.4	E950.3	E962.0	E980.3
Nitric						
acid (liquid)	983.1	E864.1	—	E950.7	E962.1	E980.6
vapor	987.8	E869.8	—	E952.8	E962.2	E982.8
oxide (gas)	987.2	E869.0	—	E952.8	E962.2	E982.8
Nitrite, amyl (medicinal) (vapor)	972.4	E858.3	E942.4	E950.4	E962.0	E980.4
Nitroaniline	983.0	E864.0	—	E950.7	E962.1	E980.6
vapor	987.8	E869.8	—	E952.8	E962.2	E982.8
Nitrobenzene, nitrobenzol	983.0	E864.0	—	E950.7	E962.1	E980.6
vapor	987.8	E869.8	—	E952.8	E962.2	E982.8
Nitrocellulose	976.3	E858.7	E946.3	E950.4	E962.0	E980.4
Nitrofuran derivatives	961.9	E857	E931.9	E950.4	E962.0	E980.4
Nitrofurantoin	961.9	E857	E931.9	E950.4	E962.0	E980.4
Nitrofurazone	976.0	E858.7	E946.0	E950.4	E962.0	E980.4
Nitrogen (dioxide) (gas) (oxide)	987.2	E869.0	—	E952.8	E962.2	E982.8
mustard (antineoplastic)	963.1	E858.1	E933.1	E950.4	E962.0	E980.4
Nitroglycerin, nitroglycerol (medicinal)	972.4	E858.3	E942.4	E950.4	E962.0	E980.4
nonmedicinal	989.89	E866.8	—	E950.9	E962.1	E980.9
fumes	987.8	E869.8	—	E952.8	E962.2	E982.8
Nitrohydrochloric acid	983.1	E864.1	—	E950.7	E962.1	E980.6

	Poisoning	External Cause (E-Code)				
		Accident	Therapeutic Use	Suicide Attempt	Assault	Undetermined
Nitromersol	976.0	E858.7	E946.0	E950.4	E962.0	E980.4
Nitronaphthalene	983.0	E864.0	—	E950.7	E962.2	E980.6
Nitrophenol	983.0	E864.0	—	E950.7	E962.2	E980.6
Nitrothiazol	961.6	E857	E931.6	E950.4	E962.0	E980.4
Nitrotoluene, nitrotoluol	983.0	E864.0	—	E950.7	E962.1	E980.6
vapor	987.8	E869.8	—	E952.8	E962.2	E982.8
Nitrous	968.2	E855.1	E938.2	E950.4	E962.0	E980.4
acid (liquid)	983.1	E864.1	—	E950.7	E962.1	E980.6
fumes	987.2	E869.0	—	E952.8	E962.2	E982.8
oxide (anesthetic) NEC	968.2	E855.1	E938.2	E950.4	E962.0	E980.4
Nitrozone	976.0	E858.7	E946.0	E950.4	E962.0	E980.4
Noctec	967.1	E852.0	E937.1	E950.2	E962.0	E980.2
Noludar	967.5	E852.4	E937.5	E950.2	E962.0	E980.2
Noptil	967.0	E851	E937.0	E950.1	E962.0	E980.1
Noradrenalin	971.2	E855.5	E941.2	E950.4	E962.0	E980.4
Noramidopyrine	965.5	E850.5	E935.5	E950.0	E962.0	E980.0
Norepinephrine	971.2	E855.5	E941.2	E950.4	E962.0	E980.4
Norethandrolone	962.1	E858.0	E932.1	E950.4	E962.0	E980.4
Norethindrone	962.2	E858.0	E932.2	E950.4	E962.0	E980.4
Norethisterone	962.2	E858.0	E932.2	E950.4	E962.0	E980.4
Norethynodrel	962.2	E858.0	E932.2	E950.4	E962.0	E980.4
Norlestrin	962.2	E858.0	E932.2	E950.4	E962.0	E980.4
Norlutin	962.2	E858.0	E932.2	E950.4	E962.0	E980.4
Normison — *see* Benzodiazepines						
Normorphine	965.09	E850.2	E935.2	E950.0	E962.0	E980.0
Nortriptyline	969.0	E854.0	E939.0	E950.3	E962.0	E980.3
Noscapine	975.4	E858.6	E945.4	E950.4	E962.0	E980.4
Nose preparations	976.6	E858.7	E946.6	E950.4	E962.0	E980.4
Novobiocin	960.8	E856	E930.8	E950.4	E962.0	E980.4
Novocain (infiltration) (topical)	968.5	E855.2	E938.5	E950.4	E962.0	E980.4
nerve block (peripheral) (plexus)	968.6	E855.2	E938.6	E950.4	E962.0	E980.4
spinal	968.7	E855.2	E938.7	E950.4	E962.0	E980.4
Noxythiolin	961.9	E857	E931.9	E950.4	E962.0	E980.4
NPH Iletin (insulin)	962.3	E858.0	E932.3	E950.4	E962.0	E980.4
Numorphan	965.09	E850.2	E935.2	E950.0	E962.0	E980.0
Nunol	967.0	E851	E937.0	E950.1	E962.0	E980.1
Nupercaine (spinal anesthetic)	968.7	E855.2	E938.7	E950.4	E962.0	E980.4
topical (surface)	968.5	E855.2	E938.5	E950.4	E962.0	E980.4
Nutmeg oil (liniment)	976.3	E858.7	E946.3	E950.4	E962.0	E980.4
Nux vomica	989.1	E863.7	—	E950.6	E962.1	E980.7
Nydrazid	961.8	E857	E931.8	E950.4	E962.0	E980.4
Nylidrin	971.2	E855.5	E941.2	E950.4	E962.0	E980.4
Nystatin	960.1	E856	E930.1	E950.4	E962.0	E980.4
topical	976.0	E858.7	E946.0	E950.4	E962.0	E980.4
Nytol	963.0	E858.2	E934.2	E950.4	E962.0	E980.4
Oblivion	967.8	E852.8	E937.8	E950.2	E962.0	E980.2
Octyl nitrite	972.4	E858.3	E942.4	E950.4	E962.0	E980.4
Oestradiol (cypionate) (dipropionate) (valerate)	962.2	E858.0	E932.2	E950.4	E962.0	E980.4
Oestriol	962.2	E858.0	E932.2	E950.4	E962.0	E980.4
Oestrone	962.2	E858.0	E932.2	E950.4	E962.0	E980.4
Oil (of) NEC	989.89	E866.8	—	E950.9	E962.1	E980.9
bitter almond	989.0	E866.8	—	E950.9	E962.1	E980.9
camphor	976.1	E858.7	E946.1	E950.4	E962.0	E980.4
colors	989.89	E861.6	—	E950.9	E962.1	E980.9
fumes	987.8	E869.8	—	E952.8	E962.2	E982.8
lubricating	981	E862.2	—	E950.9	E962.1	E980.9
specified source, other — *see* substance specified						
vitriol (liquid)	983.1	E864.1	—	E950.7	E962.1	E980.6
fumes	987.8	E869.8	—	E952.8	E962.2	E982.8
wintergreen (bitter) NEC	976.3	E858.7	E946.3	E950.4	E962.0	E980.4
Ointments NEC	976.9	E858.7	E946.9	E950.4	E962.0	E980.4
Oleander	988.2	E865.4	—	E950.9	E962.1	E980.9
Oleandomycin	960.3	E856	E930.3	E950.4	E962.0	E980.4
Oleovitamin A	963.5	E858.1	E933.5	E950.4	E962.0	E980.4
Oleum ricini	973.1	E858.4	E943.1	E950.4	E962.0	E980.4
Olive oil (medicinal) NEC	973.2	E858.4	E943.2	E950.4	E962.0	E980.4
OMPA	989.3	E863.1	—	E950.6	E962.1	E980.7
Oncovin	963.1	E858.1	E933.1	E950.4	E962.0	E980.4
Ophthaine	968.5	E855.2	E938.5	E950.4	E962.0	E980.4
Ophthetic	968.5	E855.2	E938.5	E950.4	E962.0	E980.4
Opiates, opioids, opium NEC	965.00	E850.2	E935.2	E950.0	E962.0	E980.0
antagonists	970.1	E854.3	E940.1	E950.4	E962.0	E980.4
Oracon	962.2	E858.0	E932.2	E950.4	E962.0	E980.4
Oragrafin	977.8	E858.8	E947.8	E950.4	E962.0	E980.4
Oral contraceptives	962.2	E858.0	E932.2	E950.4	E962.0	E980.4
Orciprenaline	975.1	E858.6	E945.1	E950.4	E962.0	E980.4
Organidin	975.5	E858.6	E945.5	E950.4	E962.0	E980.4
Organophosphates	989.3	E863.1	—	E950.6	E962.1	E980.7
Orimune	979.5	E858.8	E949.5	E950.4	E962.0	E980.4
Orinase	962.3	E858.0	E932.3	E950.4	E962.0	E980.4
Orphenadrine	966.4	E855.0	E936.4	E950.4	E962.0	E980.4

Nitromersol — Orphenadrine

Ortal — Para-aminosalicylic acid

	Poisoning	External Cause (E-Code)				
		Accident	Therapeutic Use	Suicide Attempt	Assault	Undetermined
Ortal (sodium)	967.0	E851	E937.0	E950.1	E962.0	E980.1
Orthoboric acid	976.0	E858.7	E946.0	E950.4	E962.0	E980.4
ENT agent	976.6	E858.7	E946.6	E950.4	E962.0	E980.4
ophthalmic preparation	976.5	E858.7	E946.5	E950.4	E962.0	E980.4
Orthocaine	968.5	E855.2	E938.5	E950.4	E962.0	E980.4
Ortho-Novum	962.2	E858.0	E932.2	E950.4	E962.0	E980.4
Orthotolidine (reagent)	977.8	E858.8	E947.8	E950.4	E962.0	E980.4
Osmic acid (liquid)	983.1	E864.1	—	E950.7	E962.1	E980.6
fumes	987.8	E869.8	—	E952.8	E962.2	E982.8
Osmotic diuretics	974.4	E858.5	E944.4	E950.4	E962.0	E980.4
Ouabain	972.1	E858.3	E942.1	E950.4	E962.0	E980.4
Ovarian hormones (synthetic substitutes)	962.2	E858.0	E932.2	E950.4	E962.0	E980.4
Ovral	962.2	E858.0	E932.2	E950.4	E962.0	E980.4
Ovulation suppressants	962.2	E858.0	E932.2	E950.4	E962.0	E980.4
Ovulen	962.2	E858.0	E932.2	E950.4	E962.0	E980.4
Oxacillin (sodium)	960.0	E856	E930.0	E950.4	E962.0	E980.4
Oxalic acid	983.1	E864.1	—	E950.7	E962.1	E980.6
Oxanamide	969.5	E853.8	E939.5	E950.3	E962.0	E980.3
Oxandrolone	962.1	E858.0	E932.1	E950.4	E962.0	E980.4
Oxaprozin	965.61	E850.6	E935.6	E950.0	E962.0	E980.0
Oxazepam	969.4	E853.2	E939.4	E950.3	E962.0	E980.3
Oxazolidine derivatives	966.0	E855.0	E936.0	E950.4	E962.0	E980.4
Ox bile extract	973.4	E858.4	E943.4	E950.4	E962.0	E980.4
Oxedrine	971.2	E855.5	E941.2	E950.4	E962.0	E980.4
Oxeladin	975.4	E858.6	E945.4	E950.4	E962.0	E980.4
Oxethazaine NEC	968.5	E855.2	E938.5	E950.4	E962.0	E980.4
Oxidizing agents NEC	983.9	E864.3	—	E950.7	E962.1	E980.6
Oxolinic acid	961.3	E857	E931.3	E950.4	E962.0	E980.4
Oxophenarsine	961.1	E857	E931.1	E950.4	E962.0	E980.4
Oxsoralen	976.3	E858.7	E946.3	E950.4	E962.0	E980.4
Oxtriphylline	975.7	E858.6	E945.7	E950.4	E962.0	E980.4
Oxybuprocaine	968.5	E855.2	E938.5	E950.4	E962.0	E980.4
Oxybutynin	975.1	E858.6	E945.1	E950.4	E962.0	E980.4
Oxycodone	965.09	E850.2	E935.2	E950.0	E962.0	E980.0
Oxygen	987.8	E869.8	—	E952.8	E962.2	E982.8
Oxylone	976.0	E858.7	E946.0	E950.4	E962.0	E980.4
ophthalmic preparation	976.5	E858.7	E946.5	E950.4	E962.0	E980.4
Oxymesterone	962.1	E858.0	E932.1	E950.4	E962.0	E980.4
Oxymetazoline	971.2	E855.5	E941.2	E950.4	E962.0	E980.4
Oxymetholone	962.1	E858.0	E932.1	E950.4	E962.0	E980.4
Oxymorphone	965.09	E850.2	E935.2	E950.0	E962.0	E980.0
Oxypertine	969.0	E854.0	E939.0	E950.3	E962.0	E980.3
Oxyphenbutazone	965.5	E850.5	E935.5	E950.0	E962.0	E980.0
Oxyphencyclimine	971.1	E855.4	E941.1	E950.4	E962.0	E980.4
Oxyphenisatin	973.1	E858.4	E943.1	E950.4	E962.0	E980.4
Oxyphenonium	971.1	E855.4	E941.1	E950.4	E962.0	E980.4
Oxyquinoline	961.3	E857	E931.3	E950.4	E962.0	E980.4
Oxytetracycline	960.4	E856	E930.4	E950.4	E962.0	E980.4
Oxytocics	975.0	E858.6	E945.0	E950.4	E962.0	E980.4
Oxytocin	975.0	E858.6	E945.0	E950.4	E962.0	E980.4
Ozone	987.8	E869.8	—	E952.8	E962.2	E982.8
PABA	976.3	E858.7	E946.3	E950.4	E962.0	E980.4
Packed red cells	964.7	E858.2	E934.7	E950.4	E962.0	E980.4
Paint NEC	989.89	E861.6	—	E950.9	E962.1	E980.9
cleaner	982.8	E862.9	—	E950.9	E962.1	E980.9
fumes NEC	987.8	E869.8	—	E952.8	E962.1	E982.8
lead (fumes)	984.0	E861.5	—	E950.9	E962.1	E980.9
solvent NEC	982.8	E862.9	—	E950.9	E962.1	E980.9
stripper	982.8	E862.9	—	E950.9	E962.1	E980.9
Palfium	965.09	E850.2	E935.2	E950.0	E962.0	E980.0
Palivizumab	979.9	E858.8	E949.6	E950.4	E962.0	E980.4
Paludrine	961.4	E857	E931.4	E950.4	E962.0	E980.4
PAM	977.2	E855.8	E947.2	E950.4	E962.0	E980.4
Pamaquine (naphthoate)	961.4	E857	E931.4	E950.4	E962.0	E980.4
Pamprin	965.1	E850.3	E935.3	E950.0	E962.0	E980.0
Panadol	965.4	E850.4	E935.4	E950.0	E962.0	E980.0
Pancreatic dornase (mucolytic)	963.4	E858.1	E933.4	E950.4	E962.0	E980.4
Pancreatin	973.4	E858.4	E943.4	E950.4	E962.0	E980.4
Pancrelipase	973.4	E858.4	E943.4	E950.4	E962.0	E980.4
Pangamic acid	963.5	E858.1	E933.5	E950.4	E962.0	E980.4
Panthenol	963.5	E858.1	E933.5	E950.4	E962.0	E980.4
topical	976.8	E858.7	E946.8	E950.4	E962.0	E980.4
Pantopaque	977.8	E858.8	E947.8	E950.4	E962.0	E980.4
Pantopon	965.00	E850.2	E935.2	E950.0	E962.0	E980.0
Pantothenic acid	963.5	E858.1	E933.5	E950.4	E962.0	E980.4
Panwarfin	964.2	E858.2	E934.2	E950.4	E962.0	E980.4
Papain	973.4	E858.4	E943.4	E950.4	E962.0	E980.4
Papaverine	972.5	E858.3	E942.5	E950.4	E962.0	E980.4
Para-aminobenzoic acid	976.3	E858.7	E946.3	E950.4	E962.0	E980.4
Para-aminophenol derivatives	965.4	E850.4	E935.4	E950.0	E962.0	E980.0
Para-aminosalicylic acid (derivatives)	961.8	E857	E931.8	E950.4	E962.0	E980.4

	Poisoning	External Cause (E-Code)				
		Accident	Therapeutic Use	Suicide Attempt	Assault	Undetermined
Paracetaldehyde (medicinal)	967.2	E852.1	E937.2	E950.2	E962.0	E980.2
Paracetamol	965.4	E850.4	E935.4	E950.0	E962.0	E980.0
Paracodin	965.09	E850.2	E935.2	E950.0	E962.0	E980.0
Paradione	966.0	E855.0	E936.0	E950.4	E962.0	E980.4
Paraffin(s) (wax)	981	E862.3	—	E950.9	E962.1	E980.9
liquid (medicinal)	973.2	E858.4	E943.2	E950.4	E962.0	E980.4
nonmedicinal (oil)	981	E962.1	—	E950.9	E962.1	E980.9
Paraldehyde (medicinal)	967.2	E852.1	E937.2	E950.2	E962.0	E980.2
Paramethadione	966.0	E855.0	E936.0	E950.4	E962.0	E980.4
Paramethasone	962.0	E858.0	E932.0	E950.4	E962.0	E980.4
Paraquat	989.4	E863.5	—	E950.6	E962.1	E980.7
Parasympatholytics	971.1	E855.4	E941.1	E950.4	E962.0	E980.4
Parasympathomimetics	971.0	E855.3	E941.0	E950.4	E962.0	E980.4
Parathion	989.3	E863.1	—	E950.6	E962.1	E980.7
Parathormone	962.6	E858.0	E932.6	E950.4	E962.0	E980.4
Parathyroid (derivatives)	962.6	E858.0	E932.6	E950.4	E962.0	E980.4
Paratyphoid vaccine	978.1	E858.8	E948.1	E950.4	E962.0	E980.4
Paredrine	971.2	E855.5	E941.2	E950.4	E962.0	E980.4
Paregoric	965.00	E850.2	E935.2	E950.0	E962.0	E980.0
Pargyline	972.3	E858.3	E942.3	E950.4	E962.0	E980.4
Paris green	985.1	E866.3	—	E950.8	E962.1	E980.8
insecticide	985.1	E863.4	—	E950.8	E962.1	E980.8
Parnate	969.0	E854.0	E939.0	E950.3	E962.0	E980.3
Paromomycin	960.8	E856	E930.8	E950.4	E962.0	E980.4
Paroxypropione	963.1	E858.1	E933.1	E950.4	E962.0	E980.4
Parzone	965.09	E850.2	E935.2	E950.0	E962.0	E980.0
PAS	961.8	E857	E931.8	E950.4	E962.0	E980.4
PCBs	981	E862.3	—	E950.9	E962.1	E980.9
PCP (pentachlorophenol)	989.4	E863.6	—	E950.6	E962.1	E980.7
herbicide	989.4	E863.5	—	E950.6	E962.1	E980.7
insecticide	989.4	E863.4	—	E950.6	E962.1	E980.7
phencyclidine	968.3	E855.1	E938.3	E950.4	E962.0	E980.4
Peach kernel oil (emulsion)	973.2	E858.4	E943.2	E950.4	E962.0	E980.4
Peanut oil (emulsion) NEC	973.2	E858.4	E943.2	E950.4	E962.0	E980.4
topical	976.3	E858.7	E946.3	E950.4	E962.0	E980.4
Pearly Gates (morning glory seeds)	969.6	E854.1	E939.6	E950.3	E962.0	E980.3
Pecazine	969.1	E853.0	E939.1	E950.3	E962.0	E980.3
Pecilocin	960.1	E856	E930.1	E950.4	E962.0	E980.4
Pectin (with kaolin) NEC	973.5	E858.4	E943.5	E950.4	E962.0	E980.4
Pelletierine tannate	961.6	E857	E931.6	E950.4	E962.0	E980.4
Pemoline	969.7	E854.2	E939.7	E950.3	E962.0	E980.3
Pempidine	972.3	E858.3	E942.3	E950.4	E962.0	E980.4
Penamecillin	960.0	E856	E930.0	E950.4	E962.0	E980.4
Penethamate hydriodide	960.0	E856	E930.0	E950.4	E962.0	E980.4
Penicillamine	963.8	E858.1	E933.8	E950.4	E962.0	E980.4
Penicillin (any type)	960.0	E856	E930.0	E950.4	E962.0	E980.4
Penicillinase	963.4	E858.1	E933.4	E950.4	E962.0	E980.4
Pentachlorophenol (fungicide)	989.4	E863.6	—	E950.6	E962.1	E980.7
herbicide	989.4	E863.5	—	E950.6	E962.1	E980.7
insecticide	989.4	E863.4	—	E950.6	E962.1	E980.7
Pentaerythritol	972.4	E858.3	E942.4	E950.4	E962.0	E980.4
chloral	967.1	E852.0	E937.1	E950.2	E962.0	E980.2
tetranitrate NEC	972.4	E858.3	E942.4	E950.4	E962.0	E980.4
Pentagastrin	977.8	E858.8	E947.8	E950.4	E962.0	E980.4
Pentalin	982.3	E862.4	—	E950.9	E962.1	E980.9
Pentamethonium (bromide)	972.3	E858.3	E942.3	E950.4	E962.0	E980.4
Pentamidine	961.5	E857	E931.5	E950.4	E962.0	E980.4
Pentanol	980.8	E860.8	—	E950.9	E962.1	E980.9
Pentaquine	961.4	E857	E931.4	E950.4	E962.0	E980.4
Pentazocine	965.8	E850.8	E935.8	E950.0	E962.0	E980.0
Penthienate	971.1	E855.4	E941.1	E950.4	E962.0	E980.4
Pentobarbital, pentobarbitone (sodium)	967.0	E851	E937.0	E950.1	E962.0	E980.1
Pentolinium (tartrate)	972.3	E858.3	E942.3	E950.4	E962.0	E980.4
Pentothal	968.3	E855.1	E938.3	E950.4	E962.0	E980.4
Pentylenetetrazol	970.0	E854.3	E940.0	E950.4	E962.0	E980.4
Pentylsalicylamide	961.8	E857	E931.8	E950.4	E962.0	E980.4
Pepsin	973.4	E858.4	E943.4	E950.4	E962.0	E980.4
Peptavlon	977.8	E858.8	E947.8	E950.4	E962.0	E980.4
Percaine (spinal)	968.7	E855.2	E938.7	E950.4	E962.0	E980.4
topical (surface)	968.5	E855.2	E938.5	E950.4	E962.0	E980.4
Perchloroethylene (vapor)	982.3	E862.4	—	E950.9	E962.1	E980.9
medicinal	961.6	E857	E931.6	E950.4	E962.0	E980.4
Percodan	965.09	E850.2	E935.2	E950.0	E962.0	E980.0
Percogesic	965.09	E850.2	E935.2	E950.0	E962.0	E980.0
Percorten	962.0	E858.0	E932.0	E950.4	E962.0	E980.4
Pergonal	962.4	E858.0	E932.4	E950.4	E962.0	E980.4
Perhexiline	972.4	E858.3	E942.4	E950.4	E962.0	E980.4
Periactin	963.0	E858.1	E933.0	E950.4	E962.0	E980.4
Periclor	967.1	E852.0	E937.1	E950.2	E962.0	E980.2
Pericyazine	969.1	E853.0	E939.1	E950.3	E962.0	E980.3
Peritrate	972.4	E858.3	E942.4	E950.4	E962.0	E980.4

▨4ᵗʰ Fourth-digit Required   ▨5ᵗʰ Fifth-digit Required   ▶◀ Revised Text   ● New Line   ▲ Revised Code

		External Cause (E-Code)				
	Poisoning	Accident	Therapeutic Use	Suicide Attempt	Assault	Undetermined
Permanganates NEC	983.9	E864.3	—	E950.7	E962.1	E980.6
potassium (topical)	976.0	E858.7	E946.0	E950.4	E962.0	E980.4
Pernocton	967.0	E851	E937.0	E950.1	E962.0	E980.1
Pernoston	967.0	E851	E937.0	E950.1	E962.0	E980.1
Peronin(e)	965.09	E850.2	E935.2	E950.0	E962.0	E980.0
Perphenazine	969.1	E853.0	E939.1	E950.3	E962.0	E980.3
Pertofrane	969.0	E854 ✓4ᵗʰ	E939.0	E950.3	E962.0	E980.3
Pertussis						
immune serum (human)	964.6	E858.2	E934.6	E950.4	E962.0	E980.4
vaccine (with diphtheria toxoid) (with tetanus toxoid)	978.6	E858.8	E948.6	E950.4	E962.0	E980.4
Peruvian balsam	976.8	E858.7	E946.8	E950.4	E962.0	E980.4
Pesticides (dust) (fumes) (vapor)	989.4	E863.4	—	E950.6	E962.1	E980.7
arsenic	985.1	E863.4	—	E950.8	E962.1	E980.8
chlorinated	989.2	E863.0	—	E950.6	E962.1	E980.7
cyanide	989.0	E863.4	—	E950.6	E962.1	E980.7
kerosene	981	E863.4	—	E950.6	E962.1	E980.7
mixture (of compounds)	989.4	E863.3	—	E950.6	E962.1	E980.7
naphthalene	983.0	E863.4	—	E950.7	E962.1	E980.6
organochlorine (compounds)	989.2	E863.0	—	E950.6	E962.1	E980.7
petroleum (distillate) (products) NEC	981	E863.4	—	E950.6	E962.1	E980.7
specified ingredient NEC	989.4	E863.4	—	E950.6	E962.1	E980.7
strychnine	989.1	E863.4	—	E950.6	E962.1	E980.7
thallium	985.8	E863.7	—	E950.6	E962.1	E980.7
Pethidine (hydrochloride)	965.09	E850.2	E935.2	E950.0	E962.0	E980.0
Petrichloral	967.1	E852.0	E937.1	E950.2	E962.0	E980.2
Petrol	981	E862.1	—	E950.9	E962.1	E980.9
vapor	987.1	E869.8	—	E952.8	E962.2	E982.8
Petrolatum (jelly) (ointment)	976.3	E858.7	E946.3	E950.4	E962.0	E980.4
hydrophilic	976.3	E858.7	E946.3	E950.4	E962.0	E980.4
liquid	973.2	E858.4	E943.2	E950.4	E962.0	E980.4
topical	976.3	E858.7	E946.3	E950.4	E962.0	E980.4
nonmedicinal	981	E862.1	—	E950.9	E962.1	E980.9
Petroleum (cleaners) (fuels) (products) NEC	981	E862.1		E950.9	E962.1	E980.9
benzin(e) — *see* Ligroin						
ether — *see* Ligroin						
jelly — *see* Petrolatum						
naphtha — *see* Ligroin						
pesticide	981	E863.4	—	E950.6	E962.1	E980.7
solids	981	E862.3	—	E950.9	E962.1	E980.9
solvents	981	E862.0	—	E950.9	E962.1	E980.9
vapor	987.1	E869.8	—	E952.8	E962.2	E982.8
Peyote	969.6	E854.1	E939.6	E950.3	E962.0	E980.3
Phanodorm, phanodorn	967.0	E851	E937.0	E950.1	E962.0	E980.1
Phanquinone, phanquone	961.5	E857	E931.5	E950.4	E962.0	E980.4
Pharmaceutical excipient or adjunct	977.4	E858.8	E947.4	E950.4	E962.0	E980.4
Phenacemide	966.3	E855.0	E936.3	E950.4	E962.0	E980.4
Phenacetin	965.4	E850.4	E935.4	E950.0	E962.0	E980.0
Phenadoxone	965.09	E850.2	E935.2	E950.0	E962.0	E980.0
Phenaglycodol	969.5	E853.8	E939.5	E950.3	E962.0	E980.3
Phenantoin	966.1	E855.0	E936.1	E950.4	E962.0	E980.4
Phenaphthazine reagent	977.8	E858.8	E947.8	E950.4	E962.0	E980.4
Phenazocine	965.09	E850.2	E935.2	E950.0	E962.0	E980.0
Phenazone	965.5	E850.5	E935.5	E950.0	E962.0	E980.0
Phenazopyridine	976.1	E858.7	E946.1	E950.4	E962.0	E980.4
Phenbenicillin	960.0	E856	E930.0	E950.4	E962.0	E980.4
Phenbutrazate	977.0	E858.8	E947.0	E950.4	E962.0	E980.4
Phencyclidine	968.3	E855.1	E938.3	E950.4	E962.0	E980.4
Phendimetrazine	977.0	E858.8	E947.0	E950.4	E962.0	E980.4
Phenelzine	969.0	E854.0	E939.0	E950.3	E962.0	E980.3
Phenergan	967.8	E852.8	E937.8	E950.2	E962.0	E980.2
Phenethicillin (potassium)	960.0	E856	E930.0	E950.4	E962.0	E980.4
Phenetsal	965.1	E850.3	E935.3	E950.0	E962.0	E980.0
Pheneturide	966.3	E855.0	E936.3	E950.4	E962.0	E980.4
Phenformin	962.3	E858.0	E932.3	E950.4	E962.0	E980.4
Phenglutarimide	971.1	E855.4	E941.1	E950.4	E962.0	E980.4
Phenicarbazide	965.8	E850.8	E935.8	E950.0	E962.0	E980.0
Phenindamine (tartrate)	963.0	E858.1	E933.0	E950.4	E962.0	E980.4
Phenindione	964.2	E858.2	E934.2	E950.4	E962.0	E980.4
Pheniprazine	969.0	E854.0	E939.0	E950.3	E962.0	E980.3
Pheniramine (maleate)	963.0	E858.1	E933.0	E950.4	E962.0	E980.4
Phenmetrazine	977.0	E858.8	E947.0	E950.4	E962.0	E980.4
Phenobal	967.0	E851	E937.0	E950.1	E962.0	E980.1
Phenobarbital	967.0	E851	E937.0	E950.1	E962.0	E980.1
Phenobarbitone	967.0	E851	E937.0	E950.1	E962.0	E980.1
Phenoctide	976.0	E858.7	E946.0	E950.4	E962.0	E980.4
Phenol (derivatives) NEC	983.0	E864.0	—	E950.7	E962.1	E980.6
disinfectant	983.0	E864.0	—	E950.7	E962.1	E980.6
pesticide	989.4	E863.4	—	E950.6	E962.1	E980.7
red	977.8	E858.8	E947.8	E950.4	E962.0	E980.4
Phenolphthalein	973.1	E858.4	E943.1	E950.4	E962.0	E980.4
Phenolsulfonphthalein	977.8	E858.8	E947.8	E950.4	E962.0	E980.4

✓4ᵗʰ Fourth-digit Required   ✓5ᵗʰ Fifth-digit Required   ►◄ Revised Text   ● New Line   ▲ Revised Code

	Poisoning	External Cause (E-Code)				
		Accident	Therapeutic Use	Suicide Attempt	Assault	Undetermined
Phenomorphan	965.09	E850.2	E935.2	E950.0	E962.0	E980.0
Phenonyl	967.0	E851	E937.0	E950.1	E962.0	E980.1
Phenoperidine	965.09	E850.2	E935.2	E950.0	E962.0	E980.0
Phenoquin	974.7	E858.5	E944.7	E950.4	E962.0	E980.4
Phenothiazines (tranquilizers) NEC	969.1	E853.0	E939.1	E950.3	E962.0	E980.3
insecticide	989.3	E863.4	—	E950.6	E962.1	E980.7
Phenoxybenzamine	971.3	E855.6	E941.3	E950.4	E962.0	E980.4
Phenoxymethyl penicillin	960.0	E856	E930.0	E950.4	E962.0	E980.4
Phenprocoumon	964.2	E858.2	E934.2	E950.4	E962.0	E980.4
Phensuximide	966.2	E855.0	E936.2	E950.4	E962.0	E980.4
Phentermine	977.0	E858.8	E947.0	E950.4	E962.0	E980.4
Phentolamine	971.3	E855.6	E941.3	E950.4	E962.0	E980.4
Phenyl						
butazone	965.5	E850.5	E935.5	E950.0	E962.0	E980.0
enediamine	983.0	E864.0	—	E950.7	E962.1	E980.6
hydrazine	983.0	E864.0	—	E950.7	E962.1	E980.6
antineoplastic	963.1	E858.1	E933.1	E950.4	E962.0	E980.4
mercuric compounds — see Mercury						
salicylate	976.3	E858.7	E946.3	E950.4	E962.0	E980.4
Phenylephrin	971.2	E855.5	E941.2	E950.4	E962.0	E980.4
Phenylethylbiguanide	962.3	E858.0	E932.3	E950.4	E962.0	E980.4
Phenylpropanolamine	971.2	E855.5	E941.2	E950.4	E962.0	E980.4
Phenylsulfthion	989.3	E863.1	—	E950.6	E962.1	E980.7
Phenyramidol, phenyramidon	965.7	E850.7	E935.7	E950.0	E962.0	E980.0
Phenytoin	966.1	E855.0	E936.1	E950.4	E962.0	E980.4
pHisoHex	976.2	E858.7	E946.2	E950.4	E962.0	E980.4
Pholcodine	965.09	E850.2	E935.2	E950.0	E962.0	E980.0
Phorate	989.3	E863.1	—	E950.6	E962.1	E980.7
Phosdrin	989.3	E863.1	—	E950.6	E962.1	E980.7
Phosgene (gas)	987.8	E869.8	—	E952.8	E962.2	E982.8
Phosphate (tricresyl)	989.89	E866.8	—	E950.9	E962.1	E980.9
organic	989.3	E863.1	—	E950.6	E962.1	E980.7
solvent	982.8	E862.4	—	E950.9	E926.1	E980.9
Phosphine	987.8	E869.8	—	E952.8	E962.2	E982.8
fumigant	987.8	E863.8	—	E950.6	E962.2	E980.7
Phospholine	971.0	E855.3	E941.0	E950.4	E962.0	E980.4
Phosphoric acid	983.1	E864.1	—	E950.7	E962.1	E980.6
Phosphorus (compounds) NEC	983.9	E864.3	—	E950.7	E962.1	E980.6
rodenticide	983.9	E863.7	—	E950.7	E962.1	E980.6
Phthalimidoglutarimide	967.8	E852.8	E937.8	E950.2	E962.0	E980.2
Phthalylsulfathiazole	961.0	E857	E931.0	E950.4	E962.0	E980.4
Phylloquinone	964.3	E858.2	E934.3	E950.4	E962.0	E980.4
Physeptone	965.02	E850.1	E935.1	E950.0	E962.0	E980.0
Physostigma venenosum	988.2	E865.4	—	E950.9	E962.1	E980.9
Physostigmine	971.0	E855.3	E941.0	E950.4	E962.0	E980.4
Phytolacca decandra	988.2	E865.4	—	E950.9	E962.1	E980.9
Phytomenadione	964.3	E858.2	E934.3	E950.4	E962.0	E980.4
Phytonadione	964.3	E858.2	E934.3	E950.4	E962.0	E980.4
Picric (acid)	983.0	E864.0	—	E950.7	E962.1	E980.6
Picrotoxin	970.0	E854.3	E940.0	E950.4	E962.0	E980.4
Pilocarpine	971.0	E855.3	E941.0	E950.4	E962.0	E980.4
Pilocarpus (jaborandi) extract	971.0	E855.3	E941.0	E950.4	E962.0	E980.4
Pimaricin	960.1	E856	E930.1	E950.4	E962.0	E980.4
Piminodine	965.09	E850.2	E935.2	E950.0	E962.0	E980.0
Pine oil, pinesol (disinfectant)	983.9	E861.4	—	E950.7	E962.1	E980.6
Pinkroot	961.6	E857	E931.6	E950.4	E962.0	E980.4
Pipadone	965.09	E850.2	E935.2	E950.0	E962.0	E980.0
Pipamazine	963.0	E858.1	E933.0	E950.4	E962.0	E980.4
Pipazethate	975.4	E858.6	E945.4	E950.4	E962.0	E980.4
Pipenzolate	971.1	E855.4	E941.1	E950.4	E962.0	E980.4
Piperacetazine	969.1	E853.0	E939.1	E950.3	E962.0	E980.3
Piperazine NEC	961.6	E857	E931.6	E950.4	E962.0	E980.4
estrone sulfate	962.2	E858.0	E932.2	E950.4	E962.0	E980.4
Piper cubeba	988.2	E865.4	—	E950.9	E962.1	E980.9
Piperidione	975.4	E858.6	E945.4	E950.4	E962.0	E980.4
Piperidolate	971.1	E855.4	E941.1	E950.4	E962.0	E980.4
Piperocaine	968.9	E855.2	E938.9	E950.4	E962.0	E980.4
infiltration (subcutaneous)	968.5	E855.2	E938.5	E950.4	E962.0	E980.4
nerve block (peripheral) (plexus)	968.6	E855.2	E938.6	E950.4	E962.0	E980.4
topical (surface)	968.5	E855.2	E938.5	E950.4	E962.0	E980.4
Pipobroman	963.1	E858.1	E933.1	E950.4	E962.0	E980.4
Pipradrol	970.8	E854.3	E940.8	E950.4	E962.0	E980.4
Piscidia (bark) (erythrina)	965.7	E850.7	E935.7	E950.0	E962.0	E980.0
Pitch	983.0	E864.0	—	E950.7	E962.1	E980.6
Pitkin's solution	968.7	E855.2	E938.7	E950.4	E962.0	E980.4
Pitocin	975.0	E858.6	E945.0	E950.4	E962.0	E980.4
Pitressin (tannate)	962.5	E858.0	E932.5	E950.4	E962.0	E980.4
Pituitary extracts (posterior)	962.5	E858.0	E932.5	E950.4	E962.0	E980.4
anterior	962.4	E858.0	E932.4	E950.4	E962.0	E980.4
Pituitrin	962.5	E858.0	E932.5	E950.4	E962.0	E980.4
Placental extract	962.9	E858.0	E932.9	E950.4	E962.0	E980.4

Phenomorphan — Placental extract

		External Cause (E-Code)				
	Poisoning	Accident	Therapeutic Use	Suicide Attempt	Assault	Undetermined
Placidyl	967.8	E852.8	E937.8	E950.2	E962.0	E980.2
Plague vaccine	978.3	E858.8	E948.3	E950.4	E962.0	E980.4
Plant foods or fertilizers NEC	989.89	E866.5	—	E950.9	E962.1	E980.9
mixed with herbicides	989.4	E863.5	—	E950.6	E962.1	E980.7
Plants, noxious, used as food	988.2	E865.9	—	E950.9	E962.1	E980.9
berries and seeds	988.2	E865.3	—	E950.9	E962.1	E980.9
specified type NEC	988.2	E865.4	—	E950.9	E962.1	E980.9
Plasma (blood)	964.7	E858.2	E934.7	E950.4	E962.0	E980.4
expanders	964.8	E858.2	E934.8	E950.4	E962.0	E980.4
Plasmanate	964.7	E858.2	E934.7	E950.4	E962.0	E980.4
Plegicil	969.1	E853.0	E939.1	E950.3	E962.0	E980.3
Podophyllin	976.4	E858.7	E946.4	E950.4	E962.0	E980.4
Podophyllum resin	976.4	E858.7	E946.4	E950.4	E962.0	E980.4
Poison NEC	989.9	E866.9	—	E950.9	E962.1	E980.9
Poisonous berries	988.2	E865.3	—	E950.9	E962.1	E980.9
Pokeweed (any part)	988.2	E865.4	—	E950.9	E962.1	E980.9
Poldine	971.1	E855.4	E941.1	E950.4	E962.0	E980.4
Poliomyelitis vaccine	979.5	E858.8	E949.5	E950.4	E962.0	E980.4
Poliovirus vaccine	979.5	E858.8	E949.5	E950.4	E962.0	E980.4
Polish (car) (floor) (furniture) (metal) (silver)	989.89	E861.2	—	E950.9	E962.1	E980.9
abrasive	989.89	E861.3	—	E950.9	E962.1	E980.9
porcelain	989.89	E861.3	—	E950.9	E962.1	E980.9
Poloxalkol	973.2	E858.4	E943.2	E950.4	E962.0	E980.4
Polyaminostyrene resins	974.5	E858.5	E944.5	E950.4	E962.0	E980.4
Polychlorinated biphenyl — *see* PCBs						
Polycycline	960.4	E856	E930.4	E950.4	E962.0	E980.4
Polyester resin hardener	982.8	E862.4	—	E950.9	E962.1	E980.9
fumes	987.8	E869.8	—	E952.8	E962.2	E982.8
Polyestradiol (phosphate)	962.2	E858.0	E932.2	E950.4	E962.0	E980.4
Polyethanolamine alkyl sulfate	976.2	E858.7	E946.2	E950.4	E962.0	E980.4
Polyethylene glycol	976.3	E858.7	E946.3	E950.4	E962.0	E980.4
Polyferose	964.0	E858.2	E934.0	E950.4	E962.0	E980.4
Polymyxin B	960.8	E856	E930.8	E950.4	E962.0	E980.4
ENT agent	976.6	E858.7	E946.6	E950.4	E962.0	E980.4
ophthalmic preparation	976.5	E858.7	E946.5	E950.4	E962.0	E980.4
topical NEC	976.0	E858.7	E946.0	E950.4	E962.0	E980.4
Polynoxylin(e)	976.0	E858.7	E946.0	E950.4	E962.0	E980.4
Polyoxymethyleneurea	976.0	E858.7	E946.0	E950.4	E962.0	E980.4
Polytetrafluoroethylene (inhaled)	987.8	E869.8	—	E952.8	E962.2	E982.8
Polythiazide	974.3	E858.5	E944.3	E950.4	E962.0	E980.4
Polyvinylpyrrolidone	964.8	E858.2	E934.8	E950.4	E962.0	E980.4
Pontocaine (hydrochloride) (infiltration) (topical)	968.5	E855.2	E938.5	E950.4	E962.0	E980.4
nerve block (peripheral) (plexus)	968.6	E855.2	E938.6	E950.4	E962.0	E980.4
spinal	968.7	E855.2	E938.7	E950.4	E962.0	E980.4
Pot	969.6	E854.1	E939.6	E950.3	E962.0	E980.3
Potash (caustic)	983.2	E864.2	—	E950.7	E962.1	E980.6
Potassic saline injection (lactated)	974.5	E858.5	E944.5	E950.4	E962.0	E980.4
Potassium (salts) NEC	974.5	E858.5	E944.5	E950.4	E962.0	E980.4
aminosalicylate	961.8	E857	E931.8	E950.4	E962.0	E980.4
arsenite (solution)	985.1	E866.3	—	E950.8	E962.1	E980.8
bichromate	983.9	E864.3	—	E950.7	E962.1	E980.6
bisulfate	983.9	E864.3	—	E950.7	E962.1	E980.6
bromide (medicinal) NEC	967.3	E852.2	E937.3	E950.2	E962.0	E980.2
carbonate	983.2	E864.2	—	E950.7	E962.1	E980.6
chlorate NEC	983.9	E864.3	—	E950.7	E962.1	E980.6
cyanide — *see* Cyanide						
hydroxide	983.2	E864.2	—	E950.7	E962.1	E980.6
iodide (expectorant) NEC	975.5	E858.6	E945.5	E950.4	E962.0	E980.4
nitrate	989.89	E866.8	—	E950.9	E962.1	E980.9
oxalate	983.9	E864.3	—	E950.7	E962.1	E980.6
perchlorate NEC	977.8	E858.8	E947.8	E950.4	E962.0	E980.4
antithyroid	962.8	E858.0	E932.8	E950.4	E962.0	E980.4
permanganate	976.0	E858.7	E946.0	E950.4	E962.0	E980.4
nonmedicinal	983.9	E864.3	—	E950.7	E962.1	E980.6
Povidone-iodine (anti-infective) NEC	976.0	E858.7	E946.0	E950.4	E962.0	E980.4
Practolol	972.0	E858.3	E942.0	E950.4	E962.0	E980.4
Pralidoxime (chloride)	977.2	E858.8	E947.2	E950.4	E962.0	E980.4
Pramoxine	968.5	E855.2	E938.5	E950.4	E962.0	E980.4
Prazosin	972.6	E858.3	E942.6	E950.4	E962.0	E980.4
Prednisolone	962.0	E858.0	E932.0	E950.4	E962.0	E980.4
ENT agent	976.6	E858.7	E946.6	E950.4	E962.0	E980.4
ophthalmic preparation	976.5	E858.7	E946.5	E950.4	E962.0	E980.4
topical NEC	976.0	E858.7	E946.0	E950.4	E962.0	E980.4
Prednisone	962.0	E858.0	E932.0	E950.4	E962.0	E980.4
Pregnanediol	962.2	E858.0	E932.2	E950.4	E962.0	E980.4
Pregneninolone	962.2	E858.0	E932.2	E950.4	E962.0	E980.4
Preludin	977.0	E858.8	E947.0	E950.4	E962.0	E980.4
Premarin	962.2	E858.0	E932.2	E950.4	E962.0	E980.4
Prenylamine	972.4	E858.3	E942.4	E950.4	E962.0	E980.4
Preparation H	976.8	E858.7	E946.8	E950.4	E962.0	E980.4
Preservatives	989.89	E866.8	—	E950.9	E962.1	E980.9

		External Cause (E-Code)				
	Poisoning	**Accident**	**Therapeutic Use**	**Suicide Attempt**	**Assault**	**Undetermined**
Pride of China	988.2	E865.3	—	E950.9	E962.1	E980.9
Prilocaine	968.9	E855.2	E938.9	E950.4	E962.0	E980.4
infiltration (subcutaneous)	968.5	E855.2	E938.5	E950.4	E962.0	E980.4
nerve block (peripheral) (plexus)	968.6	E855.2	E938.6	E950.4	E962.0	E980.4
Primaquine	961.4	E857	E931.4	E950.4	E962.0	E980.4
Primidone	966.3	E855.0	E936.3	E950.4	E962.0	E980.4
Primula (veris)	988.2	E865.4	—	E950.9	E962.1	E980.9
Prinadol	965.09	E850.2	E935.2	E950.0	E962.0	E980.0
Priscol, Priscoline	971.3	E855.6	E941.3	E950.4	E962.0	E980.4
Privet	988.2	E865.4	—	E950.9	E962.1	E980.9
Privine	971.2	E855.5	E941.2	E950.4	E962.0	E980.4
Pro-Banthine	971.1	E855.4	E941.1	E950.4	E962.0	E980.4
Probarbital	967.0	E851	E937.0	E950.1	E962.0	E980.1
Probenecid	974.7	E858.5	E944.7	E950.4	E962.0	E980.4
Procainamide (hydrochloride)	972.0	E858.3	E942.0	E950.4	E962.0	E980.4
Procaine (hydrochloride) (infiltration) (topical)	968.5	E855.2	E938.5	E950.4	E962.0	E980.4
nerve block (peripheral) (plexus)	968.6	E855.2	E938.6	E950.4	E962.0	E980.4
penicillin G	960.0	E856	E930.0	E950.4	E962.0	E980.4
spinal	968.7	E855.2	E938.7	E950.4	E962.0	E980.4
Procalmidol	969.5	E853.8	E939.5	E950.3	E962.0	E980.3
Procarbazine	963.1	E858.1	E933.1	E950.4	E962.0	E980.4
Prochlorperazine	969.1	E853.0	E939.1	E950.3	E962.0	E980.3
Procyclidine	966.4	E855.0	E936.4	E950.4	E962.0	E980.4
Producer gas	986	E868.8	—	E952.1	E962.2	E982.1
Profenamine	966.4	E855.0	E936.4	E950.4	E962.0	E980.4
Profenil	975.1	E858.6	E945.1	E950.4	E962.0	E980.4
Progesterones	962.2	E858.0	E932.2	E950.4	E962.0	E980.4
Progestin	962.2	E858.0	E932.2	E950.4	E962.0	E980.4
Progestogens (with estrogens)	962.2	E858.0	E932.2	E950.4	E962.0	E980.4
Progestone	962.2	E858.0	E932.2	E950.4	E962.0	E980.4
Proguanil	961.4	E857	E931.4	E950.4	E962.0	E980.4
Prolactin	962.4	E858.0	E932.4	E950.4	E962.0	E980.4
Proloid	962.7	E858.0	E932.7	E950.4	E962.0	E980.4
Proluton	962.2	E858.0	E932.2	E950.4	E962.0	E980.4
Promacetin	961.8	E857	E931.8	E950.4	E962.0	E980.4
Promazine	969.1	E853.0	E939.1	E950.3	E962.0	E980.3
Promedol	965.09	E850.2	E935.2	E950.0	E962.0	E980.0
Promethazine	967.8	E852.8	E937.8	E950.2	E962.0	E980.2
Promin	961.8	E857	E931.8	E950.4	E962.0	E980.4
Pronestyl (hydrochloride)	972.0	E858.3	E942.0	E950.4	E962.0	E980.4
Pronetalol, pronethalol	972.0	E858.3	E942.0	E950.4	E962.0	E980.4
Prontosil	961.0	E857	E931.0	E950.4	E962.0	E980.4
Propamidine isethionate	961.5	E857	E931.5	E950.4	E962.0	E980.4
Propanal (medicinal)	967.8	E852.8	E937.8	E950.2	E962.0	E980.2
Propane (gas) (distributed in mobile container)	987.0	E868.0	—	E951.1	E962.2	E981.1
distributed through pipes	987.0	E867	—	E951.0	E962.2	E981.0
incomplete combustion of — *see* Carbon monoxide, Propane						
Propanidid	968.3	E855.1	E938.3	E950.4	E962.0	E980.4
Propanol	980.3	E860.4	—	E950.9	E962.1	E980.9
Propantheline	971.1	E855.4	E941.1	E950.4	E962.0	E980.4
Proparacaine	968.5	E855.2	E938.5	E950.4	E962.0	E980.4
Propatyl nitrate	972.4	E858.3	E942.4	E950.4	E962.0	E980.4
Propicillin	960.0	E856	E930.0	E950.4	E962.0	E980.4
Propiolactone (vapor)	987.8	E869.8	—	E952.8	E962.2	E982.8
Propiomazine	967.8	E852.8	E937.8	E950.2	E962.0	E980.2
Propionaldehyde (medicinal)	967.8	E852.8	E937.8	E950.2	E962.0	E980.2
Propionate compound	976.0	E858.7	E946.0	E950.4	E962.0	E980.4
Propion gel	976.0	E858.7	E946.0	E950.4	E962.0	E980.4
Propitocaine	968.9	E855.2	E938.9	E950.4	E962.0	E980.4
infiltration (subcutaneous)	968.5	E855.2	E938.5	E950.4	E962.0	E980.4
nerve block (peripheral) (plexus)	968.6	E855.2	E938.6	E950.4	E962.0	E980.4
Propoxur	989.3	E863.2	—	E950.6	E962.1	E980.7
Propoxycaine	968.9	E855.2	E938.9	E950.4	E962.0	E980.4
infiltration (subcutaneous)	968.5	E855.2	E938.5	E950.4	E962.0	E980.4
nerve block (peripheral) (plexus)	968.6	E855.2	E938.6	E950.4	E962.0	E980.4
topical (surface)	968.5	E855.2	E938.5	E950.4	E962.0	E980.4
Propoxyphene (hydrochloride)	965.8	E850.8	E935.8	E950.0	E962.0	E980.0
Propranolol	972.0	E858.3	E942.0	E950.4	E962.0	E980.4
Propyl						
alcohol	980.3	E860.4	—	E950.9	E962.1	E980.9
carbinol	980.3	E860.4	—	E950.9	E962.1	E980.9
hexadrine	971.2	E855.5	E941.2	E950.4	E962.0	E980.4
iodone	977.8	E858.8	E947.8	E950.4	E962.0	E980.4
thiouracil	962.8	E858.0	E932.8	E950.4	E962.0	E980.4
Propylene	987.1	E869.8	—	E952.8	E962.2	E982.8
Propylparaben (ophthalmic)	976.5	E858.7	E946.5	E950.4	E962.0	E980.4
Proscillaridin	972.1	E858.3	E942.1	E950.4	E962.0	E980.4
Prostaglandins	975.0	E858.6	E945.0	E950.4	E962.0	E980.4
Prostigmin	971.0	E855.3	E941.0	E950.4	E962.0	E980.4
Protamine (sulfate)	964.5	E858.2	E934.5	E950.4	E962.0	E980.4
zinc insulin	962.3	E858.0	E932.3	E950.4	E962.0	E980.4

▨4ᵗ Fourth-digit Required   ▨5ᵗ Fifth-digit Required   ▶◀ Revised Text   ● New Line   ▲ Revised Code

		External Cause (E-Code)				
	Poisoning	Accident	Therapeutic Use	Suicide Attempt	Assault	Undetermined
Protectants (topical)	976.3	E858.7	E946.3	E950.4	E962.0	E980.4
Protein hydrolysate	974.5	E858.5	E944.5	E950.4	E962.0	E980.4
Prothiaden — *see* Dothiepin hydrochloride						
Prothionamide	961.8	E857	E931.8	E950.4	E962.0	E980.4
Prothipendyl	969.5	E853.8	E939.5	E950.3	E962.0	E980.3
Protokylol	971.2	E855.5	E941.2	E950.4	E962.0	E980.4
Protopam	977.2	E858.8	E947.2	E950.4	E962.0	E980.4
Protoveratrine(s) (A) (B)	972.6	E858.3	E942.6	E950.4	E962.0	E980.4
Protriptyline	969.0	E854.0	E939.0	E950.3	E962.0	E980.3
Provera	962.2	E858.0	E932.2	E950.4	E962.0	E980.4
Provitamin A	963.5	E858.1	E933.5	E950.4	E962.0	E980.4
Proxymetacaine	968.5	E855.2	E938.5	E950.4	E962.0	E980.4
Proxyphylline	975.1	E858.6	E945.1	E950.4	E962.0	E980.4
Prozac — *see* Fluoxetine hydrochloride						
Prunus						
laurocerasus	988.2	E865.4	—	E950.9	E962.1	E980.9
virginiana	988.2	E865.4	—	E950.9	E962.1	E980.9
Prussic acid	989.0	E866.8	—	E950.9	E962.1	E980.9
vapor	987.7	E869.8	—	E952.8	E962.2	E982.8
Pseudoephedrine	971.2	E855.5	E941.2	E950.4	E962.0	E980.4
Psilocin	969.6	E854.1	E939.6	E950.3	E962.0	E980.3
Psilocybin	969.6	E854.1	E939.6	E950.3	E962.0	E980.3
PSP	977.8	E858.8	E947.8	E950.4	E962.0	E980.4
Psychedelic agents	969.6	E854.1	E939.6	E950.3	E962.0	E980.3
Psychodysleptics	969.6	E854.1	E939.6	E950.3	E962.0	E980.3
Psychostimulants	969.7	E854.2	E939.7	E950.3	E962.0	E980.3
Psychotherapeutic agents	969.9	E855.9	E939.9	E950.3	E962.0	E980.3
antidepressants	969.0	E854.0	E939.0	E950.3	E962.0	E980.3
specified NEC	969.8	E855.8	E939.8	E950.3	E962.0	E980.3
tranquilizers NEC	969.5	E853.9	E939.5	E950.3	E962.0	E980.3
Psychotomimetic agents	969.6	E854.1	E939.6	E950.3	E962.0	E980.3
Psychotropic agents	969.9	E854.8	E939.9	E950.3	E962.0	E980.3
specified NEC	969.8	E854.8	E939.8	E950.3	E962.0	E980.3
Psyllium	973.3	E858.4	E943.3	E950.4	E962.0	E980.4
Pteroylglutamic acid	964.1	E858.2	E934.1	E950.4	E962.0	E980.4
Pteroyltriglutamate	963.1	E858.1	E933.1	E950.4	E962.0	E980.4
PTFE	987.8	E869.8	—	E952.8	E962.2	E982.8
Pulsatilla	988.2	E865.4	—	E950.9	E962.1	E980.9
Purex (bleach)	983.9	E864.3	—	E950.7	E962.1	E980.6
Purine diuretics	974.1	E858.5	E944.1	E950.4	E962.0	E980.4
Purinethol	963.1	E858.1	E933.1	E950.4	E962.0	E980.4
PVP	964.8	E858.2	E934.8	E950.4	E962.0	E980.4
Pyrabital	965.7	E850.7	E935.7	E950.0	E962.0	E980.0
Pyramidon	965.5	E850.5	E935.5	E950.0	E962.0	E980.0
Pyrantel (pamoate)	961.6	E857	E931.6	E950.4	E962.0	E980.4
Pyrathiazine	963.0	E858.1	E933.0	E950.4	E962.0	E980.4
Pyrazinamide	961.8	E857	E931.8	E950.4	E962.0	E980.4
Pyrazinoic acid (amide)	961.8	E857	E931.8	E950.4	E962.0	E980.4
Pyrazole (derivatives)	965.5	E850.5	E935.5	E950.0	E962.0	E980.0
Pyrazolone (analgesics)	965.5	E850.5	E935.5	E950.0	E962.0	E980.0
Pyrethrins, pyrethrum	989.4	E863.4	—	E950.6	E962.1	E980.7
Pyribenzamine	963.0	E858.1	E933.0	E950.4	E962.0	E980.4
Pyridine (liquid) (vapor)	982.0	E862.4	—	E950.9	E962.1	E980.9
aldoxime chloride	977.2	E858.8	E947.2	E950.4	E962.0	E980.4
Pyridium	976.1	E858.7	E946.1	E950.4	E962.0	E980.4
Pyridostigmine	971.0	E855.3	E941.0	E950.4	E962.0	E980.4
Pyridoxine	963.5	E858.1	E933.5	E950.4	E962.0	E980.4
Pyrilamine	963.0	E858.1	E933.0	E950.4	E962.0	E980.4
Pyrimethamine	961.4	E857	E931.4	E950.4	E962.0	E980.4
Pyrogallic acid	983.0	E864.0	—	E950.7	E962.1	E980.6
Pyroxylin	976.3	E858.7	E946.3	E950.4	E962.0	E980.4
Pyrrobutamine	963.0	E858.1	E933.0	E950.4	E962.0	E980.4
Pyrrocitine	968.5	E855.2	E938.5	E950.4	E962.0	E980.4
Pyrvinium (pamoate)	961.6	E857	E931.6	E950.4	E962.0	E980.4
PZI	962.3	E858.0	E932.3	E950.4	E962.0	E980.4
Quaalude	967.4	E852.3	E937.4	E950.2	E962.0	E980.2
Quaternary ammonium derivatives	971.1	E855.4	E941.1	E950.4	E962.0	E980.4
Quicklime	983.2	E864.2	—	E950.7	E962.1	E980.6
Quinacrine	961.3	E857	E931.3	E950.4	E962.0	E980.4
Quinaglute	972.0	E858.3	E942.0	E950.4	E962.0	E980.4
Quinalbarbitone	967.0	E851	E937.0	E950.1	E962.0	E980.1
Quinestradiol	962.2	E858.0	E932.2	E950.4	E962.0	E980.4
Quinethazone	974.3	E858.5	E944.3	E950.4	E962.0	E980.4
Quinidine (gluconate) (polygalacturonate) (salts) (sulfate)	972.0	E858.3	E942.0	E950.4	E962.0	E980.4
Quinine	961.4	E857	E931.4	E950.4	E962.0	E980.4
Quiniobine	961.3	E857	E931.3	E950.4	E962.0	E980.4
Quinolines	961.3	E857	E931.3	E950.4	E962.0	E980.4
Quotane	968.5	E855.2	E938.5	E950.4	E962.0	E980.4
Rabies						
immune globulin (human)	964.6	E858.2	E934.6	E950.4	E962.0	E980.4
vaccine	979.1	E858.8	E949.1	E950.4	E962.0	E980.4

	Poisoning	External Cause (E-Code)				
		Accident	Therapeutic Use	Suicide Attempt	Assault	Undetermined
Racemoramide	965.09	E850.2	E935.2	E950.0	E962.0	E980.0
Racemorphan	965.09	E850.2	E935.2	E950.0	E962.0	E980.0
Radiator alcohol	980.1	E860.2	—	E950.9	E962.1	E980.9
Radio-opaque (drugs) (materials)	977.8	E858.8	E947.8	E950.4	E962.0	E980.4
Ranunculus	988.2	E865.4	—	E950.9	E962.1	E980.9
Rat poison	989.4	E863.7	—	E950.6	E962.1	E980.7
Rattlesnake (venom)	989.5	E905.0	—	E950.9	E962.1	E980.9
Raudixin	972.6	E858.3	E942.6	E950.4	E962.0	E980.4
Rautensin	972.6	E858.3	E942.6	E950.4	E962.0	E980.4
Rautina	972.6	E858.3	E942.6	E950.4	E962.0	E980.4
Rautotal	972.6	E858.3	E942.6	E950.4	E962.0	E980.4
Rauwiloid	972.6	E858.3	E942.6	E950.4	E962.0	E980.4
Rauwoldin	972.6	E858.3	E942.6	E950.4	E962.0	E980.4
Rauwolfia (alkaloids)	972.6	E858.3	E942.6	E950.4	E962.0	E980.4
Realgar	985.1	E866.3	—	E950.8	E962.1	E980.8
Red cells, packed	964.7	E858.2	E934.7	E950.4	E962.0	E980.4
Reducing agents, industrial NEC	983.9	E864.3	—	E950.7	E962.1	E980.6
Refrigerant gas (freon)	987.4	E869.2	—	E952.8	E962.2	E982.8
not freon	987.9	E869.9	—	E952.9	E962.2	E982.9
Regroton	974.4	E858.5	E944.4	E950.4	E962.0	E980.4
Rela	968.0	E855.1	E938.0	E950.4	E962.0	E980.4
Relaxants, skeletal muscle (autonomic)	975.2	E858.6	E945.2	E950.4	E962.0	E980.4
central nervous system	968.0	E855.1	E938.0	E950.4	E962.0	E980.4
Renese	974.3	E858.5	E944.3	E950.4	E962.0	E980.4
Renografin	977.8	E858.8	E947.8	E950.4	E962.0	E980.4
Replacement solutions	974.5	E858.5	E944.5	E950.4	E962.0	E980.4
Rescinnamine	972.6	E858.3	E942.6	E950.4	E962.0	E980.4
Reserpine	972.6	E858.3	E942.6	E950.4	E962.0	E980.4
Resorcin, resorcinol	976.4	E858.7	E946.4	E950.4	E962.0	E980.4
Respaire	975.5	E858.6	E945.5	E950.4	E962.0	E980.4
Respiratory agents NEC	975.8	E858.6	E945.8	E950.4	E962.0	E980.4
Retinoic acid	976.8	E858.7	E946.8	E950.4	E962.0	E980.4
Retinol	963.5	E858.1	E933.5	E950.4	E962.0	E980.4
Rh (D) immune globulin (human)	964.6	E858.2	E934.6	E950.4	E962.0	E980.4
Rhodine	965.1	E850.3	E935.3	E950.0	E962.0	E980.0
RhoGAM	964.6	E858.2	E934.6	E950.4	E962.0	E980.4
Riboflavin	963.5	E858.1	E933.5	E950.4	E962.0	E980.4
Ricin	989.89	E866.8	—	E950.9	E962.1	E980.9
Ricinus communis	988.2	E865.3	—	E950.9	E962.1	E980.9
Rickettsial vaccine NEC	979.6	E858.8	E949.6	E950.4	E962.0	E980.4
with viral and bacterial vaccine	979.7	E858.8	E949.7	E950.4	E962.0	E980.4
Rifampin	960.6	E856	E930.6	E950.4	E962.0	E980.4
Rimifon	961.8	E857	E931.8	E950.4	E962.0	E980.4
Ringer's injection (lactated)	974.5	E858.5	E944.5	E950.4	E962.0	E980.4
Ristocetin	960.8	E856	E930.8	E950.4	E962.0	E980.4
Ritalin	969.7	E854.2	E939.7	E950.3	E962.0	E980.3
Roach killers — see Pesticides						
Rocky Mountain spotted fever vaccine	979.6	E858.8	E949.6	E950.4	E962.0	E980.4
Rodenticides	989.4	E863.7	—	E950.6	E962.1	E980.7
Rohypnol	969.4	E853.2	E939.4	E950.3	E962.0	E980.3 ▲
Rolaids	973.0	E858.4	E943.0	E950.4	E962.0	E980.4
Rolitetracycline	960.4	E856	E930.4	E950.4	E962.0	E980.4
Romilar	975.4	E858.6	E945.4	E950.4	E962.0	E980.4
Rose water ointment	976.3	E858.7	E946.3	E950.4	E962.0	E980.4
Rotenone	989.4	E863.7	—	E950.6	E962.1	E980.7
Rotoxamine	963.0	E858.1	E933.0	E950.4	E962.0	E980.4
Rough-on-rats	989.4	E863.7	—	E950.6	E962.1	E980.7
RU486	962.9	E858.0	E932.9	E950.4	E962.0	E980.4
Rubbing alcohol	980.2	E860.3	—	E950.9	E962.1	E980.9
Rubella virus vaccine	979.4	E858.8	E949.4	E950.4	E962.0	E980.4
Rubelogen	979.4	E858.8	E949.4	E950.4	E962.0	E980.4
Rubeovax	979.4	E858.8	E949.4	E950.4	E962.0	E980.4
Rubidomycin	960.7	E856	E930.7	E950.4	E962.0	E980.4
Rue	988.2	E865.4	—	E950.9	E962.1	E980.9
Ruta	988.2	E865.4	—	E950.9	E962.1	E980.9
Sabadilla (medicinal)	976.0	E858.7	E946.0	E950.4	E962.0	E980.4
pesticide	989.4	E863.4	—	E950.6	E962.1	E980.7
Sabin oral vaccine	979.5	E858.8	E949.5	E950.4	E962.0	E980.4
Saccharated iron oxide	964.0	E858.2	E934.0	E950.4	E962.0	E980.4
Saccharin	974.5	E858.5	E944.5	E950.4	E962.0	E980.4
Safflower oil	972.2	E858.3	E942.2	E950.4	E962.0	E980.4
Salbutamol sulfate	975.7	E858.6	E945.7	E950.4	E962.0	E980.4
Salicylamide	965.1	E850.3	E935.3	E950.0	E962.0	E980.0
Salicylate(s)	965.1	E850.3	E935.3	E950.0	E962.0	E980.0
methyl	976.3	E858.7	E946.3	E950.4	E962.0	E980.4
theobromine calcium	974.1	E858.5	E944.1	E950.4	E962.0	E980.4
Salicylazosulfapyridine	961.0	E857	E931.0	E950.4	E962.0	E980.4
Salicylhydroxamic acid	976.0	E858.7	E946.0	E950.4	E962.0	E980.4
Salicylic acid (keratolytic) NEC	976.4	E858.7	E946.4	E950.4	E962.0	E980.4
congeners	965.1	E850.3	E935.3	E950.0	E962.0	E980.0
salts	965.1	E850.3	E935.3	E950.0	E962.0	E980.0

✓4th Fourth-digit Required   ✓5th Fifth-digit Required   ►◄ Revised Text   ● New Line   ▲ Revised Code

		External Cause (E-Code)				
	Poisoning	Accident	Therapeutic Use	Suicide Attempt	Assault	Undetermined
Saliniazid	961.8	E857	E931.8	E950.4	E962.0	E980.4
Salol	976.3	E858.7	E946.3	E950.4	E962.0	E980.4
Salt (substitute) NEC	974.5	E858.5	E944.5	E950.4	E962.0	E980.4
Saluretics	974.3	E858.5	E944.3	E950.4	E962.0	E980.4
Saluron	974.3	E858.5	E944.3	E950.4	E962.0	E980.4
Salvarsan 606 (neosilver) (silver)	961.1	E857	E931.1	E950.4	E962.0	E980.4
Sambucus canadensis	988.2	E865.4	—	E950.9	E962.1	E980.9
berry	988.2	E865.3	—	E950.9	E962.1	E980.9
Sandril	972.6	E858.3	E942.6	E950.4	E962.0	E980.4
Sanguinaria canadensis	988.2	E865.4	—	E950.9	E962.1	E980.9
Saniflush (cleaner)	983.9	E861.3	—	E950.7	E962.1	E980.6
Santonin	961.6	E857	E931.6	E950.4	E962.0	E980.4
Santyl	976.8	E858.7	E946.8	E950.4	E962.0	E980.4
Sarkomycin	960.7	E856	E930.7	E950.4	E962.0	E980.4
Saroten	969.0	E854.0	E939.0	E950.3	E962.0	E980.3
Saturnine — *see* Lead						
Savin (oil)	976.4	E858.7	E946.4	E950.4	E962.0	E980.4
Scammony	973.1	E858.4	E943.1	E950.4	E962.0	E980.4
Scarlet red	976.8	E858.7	E946.8	E950.4	E962.0	E980.4
Scheele's green	985.1	E866.3	—	E950.8	E962.1	E980.8
insecticide	985.1	E863.4	—	E950.8	E962.1	E980.8
Schradan	989.3	E863.1	—	E950.6	E962.1	E980.7
Schweinfurt(h) green	985.1	E866.3	—	E950.8	E962.1	E980.8
insecticide	985.1	E863.4	—	E950.8	E962.1	E980.8
Scilla — *see* Squill						
Sclerosing agents	972.7	E858.3	E942.7	E950.4	E962.0	E980.4
Scopolamine	971.1	E855.4	E941.1	E950.4	E962.0	E980.4
Scouring powder	989.89	E861.3	—	E950.9	E962.1	E980.9
Sea						
anemone (sting)	989.5	E905.6	—	E950.9	E962.1	E980.9
cucumber (sting)	989.5	E905.6	—	E950.9	E962.1	E980.9
snake (bite) (venom)	989.5	E905.0	—	E950.9	E962.1	E980.9
urchin spine (puncture)	989.5	E905.6	—	E950.9	E962.1	E980.9
Secbutabarbital	967.0	E851	E937.0	E950.1	E962.0	E980.1
Secbutabarbitone	967.0	E851	E937.0	E950.1	E962.0	E980.1
Secobarbital	967.0	E851	E937.0	E950.1	E962.0	E980.1
Seconal	967.0	E851	E937.0	E950.1	E962.0	E980.1
Secretin	977.8	E858.8	E947.8	E950.4	E962.0	E980.4
Sedatives, nonbarbiturate	967.9	E852.9	E937.9	E950.2	E962.0	E980.2
specified NEC	967.8	E852.8	E937.8	E950.2	E962.0	E980.2
Sedormid	967.8	E852.8	E937.8	E950.2	E962.0	E980.2
Seed (plant)	988.2	E865.3	—	E950.9	E962.1	E980.9
disinfectant or dressing	989.89	E866.5	—	E950.9	E962.1	E980.9
Selenium (fumes) NEC	985.8	E866.4	—	E950.9	E962.1	E980.9
disulfide or sulfide	976.4	E858.7	E946.4	E950.4	E962.0	E980.4
Selsun	976.4	E858.7	E946.4	E950.4	E962.0	E980.4
Senna	973.1	E858.4	E943.1	E950.4	E962.0	E980.4
Septisol	976.2	E858.7	E946.2	E950.4	E962.0	E980.4
Serax	969.4	E853.2	E939.4	E950.3	E962.0	E980.3
Serenesil	967.8	E852.8	E937.8	E950.2	E962.0	E980.2
Serenium (hydrochloride)	961.9	E857	E931.9	E950.4	E962.0	E980.4
Sernyl	968.3	E855.1	E938.3	E950.4	E962.0	E980.4
Serotonin	977.8	E858.8	E947.8	E950.4	E962.0	E980.4
Serpasil	972.6	E858.3	E942.6	E950.4	E962.0	E980.4
Sewer gas	987.8	E869.8	—	E952.8	E962.2	E982.8
Shampoo	989.6	E861.0	—	E950.9	E962.1	E980.9
Shellfish, nonbacterial or noxious	988.0	E865.1	—	E950.9	E962.1	E980.9
Silicones NEC	989.83	E866.8	E947.8	E950.9	E962.1	E980.9
Silvadene	976.0	E858.7	E946.0	E950.4	E962.0	E980.4
Silver (compound) (medicinal) NEC	976.0	E858.7	E946.0	E950.4	E962.0	E980.4
anti-infectives	976.0	E858.7	E946.0	E950.4	E962.0	E980.4
arsphenamine	961.1	E857	E931.1	E950.4	E962.0	E980.4
nitrate	976.0	E858.7	E946.0	E950.4	E962.0	E980.4
ophthalmic preparation	976.5	E858.7	E946.5	E950.4	E962.0	E980.4
toughened (keratolytic)	976.4	E858.7	E946.4	E950.4	E962.0	E980.4
nonmedicinal (dust)	985.8	E866.4	—	E950.9	E962.1	E980.9
protein (mild) (strong)	976.0	E858.7	E946.0	E950.4	E962.0	E980.4
salvarsan	961.1	E857	E931.1	E950.4	E962.0	E980.4
Simethicone	973.8	E858.4	E943.8	E950.4	E962.0	E980.4
Sinequan	969.0	E854.0	E939.0	E950.3	E962.0	E980.3
Singoserp	972.6	E858.3	E942.6	E950.4	E962.0	E980.4
Sintrom	964.2	E858.2	E934.2	E950.4	E962.0	E980.4
Sitosterols	972.2	E858.3	E942.2	E950.4	E962.0	E980.4
Skeletal muscle relaxants	975.2	E858.6	E945.2	E950.4	E962.0	E980.4
Skin						
agents (external)	976.9	E858.7	E946.9	E950.4	E962.0	E980.4
specified NEC	976.8	E858.7	E946.8	E950.4	E962.0	E980.4
test antigen	977.8	E858.8	E947.8	E950.4	E962.0	E980.4
Sleep-eze	963.0	E858.1	E933.0	E950.4	E962.0	E980.4
Sleeping draught (drug) (pill) (tablet)	967.9	E852.9	E937.9	E950.2	E962.0	E980.2
Smallpox vaccine	979.0	E858.8	E949.0	E950.4	E962.0	E980.4

		External Cause (E-Code)				
	Poisoning	Accident	Therapeutic Use	Suicide Attempt	Assault	Undetermined
Smelter fumes NEC	985.9	E866.4	—	E950.9	E962.1	E980.9
Smog	987.3	E869.1	—	E952.8	E962.2	E982.8
Smoke NEC	987.9	E869.9	—	E952.9	E962.2	E982.9
Smooth muscle relaxant	975.1	E858.6	E945.1	E950.4	E962.0	E980.4
Snail killer	989.4	E863.4	—	E950.6	E962.1	E980.7
Snake (bite) (venom)	989.5	E905.0	—	E950.9	E962.1	E980.9
Snuff	989.89	E866.8	—	E950.9	E962.1	E980.9
Soap (powder) (product)	989.6	E861.1	—	E950.9	E962.1	E980.9
medicinal, soft	976.2	E858.7	E946.2	E950.4	E962.0	E980.4
Soda (caustic)	983.2	E864.2	—	E950.7	E962.1	E980.6
bicarb	963.3	E858.1	E933.3	E950.4	E962.0	E980.4
chlorinated — *see* Sodium, hypochlorite						
Sodium						
acetosulfone	961.8	E857	E931.8	E950.4	E962.0	E980.4
acetrizoate	977.8	E858.8	E947.8	E950.4	E962.0	E980.4
amytal	967.0	E851	E937.0	E950.1	E962.0	E980.1
arsenate — *see* Arsenic						
bicarbonate	963.3	E858.1	E933.3	E950.4	E962.0	E980.4
bichromate	983.9	E864.3	—	E950.7	E962.1	E980.6
biphosphate	963.2	E858.1	E933.2	E950.4	E962.0	E980.4
bisulfate	983.9	E864.3	—	E950.7	E962.1	E980.6
borate (cleanser)	989.6	E861.3	—	E950.9	E962.1	E980.9
bromide NEC	967.3	E852.2	E937.3	E950.2	E962.0	E980.2
cacodylate (nonmedicinal) NEC	978.8	E858.8	E948.8	E950.4	E962.0	E980.4
anti-infective	961.1	E857	E931.1	E950.4	E962.0	E980.4
herbicide	989.4	E863.5	—	E950.6	E962.1	E980.7
calcium edetate	963.8	E858.1	E933.8	E950.4	E962.0	E980.4
carbonate NEC	983.2	E864.2	—	E950.7	E962.1	E980.6
chlorate NEC	983.9	E864.3	—	E950.7	E962.1	E980.6
herbicide	983.9	E863.5	—	E950.7	E962.1	E980.6
chloride NEC	974.5	E858.5	E944.5	E950.4	E962.0	E980.4
chromate	983.9	E864.3	—	E950.7	E962.1	E980.6
citrate	963.3	E858.1	E933.3	E950.4	E962.0	E980.4
cyanide — *see* Cyanide(s)						
cyclamate	974.5	E858.5	E944.5	E950.4	E962.0	E980.4
diatrizoate	977.8	E858.8	E947.8	E950.4	E962.0	E980.4
dibunate	975.4	E858.6	E945.4	E950.4	E962.0	E980.4
dioctyl sulfosuccinate	973.2	E858.4	E943.2	E950.4	E962.0	E980.4
edetate	963.8	E858.1	E933.8	E950.4	E962.0	E980.4
ethacrynate	974.4	E858.5	E944.4	E950.4	E962.0	E980.4
fluoracetate (dust) (rodenticide)	989.4	E863.7	—	E950.6	E962.1	E980.7
fluoride — *see* Fluoride(s)						
free salt	974.5	E858.5	E944.5	E950.4	E962.0	E980.4
glucosulfone	961.8	E857	E931.8	E950.4	E962.0	E980.4
hydroxide	983.2	E864.2	—	E950.7	E962.1	E980.6
hypochlorite (bleach) NEC	983.9	E864.3	—	E950.7	E962.1	E980.6
disinfectant	983.9	E861.4	—	E950.7	E962.1	E980.6
medicinal (anti-infective) (external)	976.0	E858.7	E946.0	E950.4	E962.0	E980.4
vapor	987.8	E869.8	—	E952.8	E962.2	E982.8
hyposulfite	976.0	E858.7	E946.0	E950.4	E962.0	E980.4
indigotindisulfonate	977.8	E858.8	E947.8	E950.4	E962.0	E980.4
iodide	977.8	E858.8	E947.8	E950.4	E962.0	E980.4
iothalamate	977.8	E858.8	E947.8	E950.4	E962.0	E980.4
iron edetate	964.0	E858.2	E934.0	E950.4	E962.0	E980.4
lactate	963.3	E858.1	E933.3	E950.4	E962.0	E980.4
lauryl sulfate	976.2	E858.7	E946.2	E950.4	E962.0	E980.4
L-triiodothyronine	962.7	E858.0	E932.7	E950.4	E962.0	E980.4
metrizoate	977.8	E858.8	E947.8	E950.4	E962.0	E980.4
monofluoracetate (dust) (rodenticide)	989.4	E863.7	—	E950.6	E962.1	E980.7
morrhuate	972.7	E858.3	E942.7	E950.4	E962.0	E980.4
nafcillin	960.0	E856	E930.0	E950.4	E962.0	E980.4
nitrate (oxidizing agent)	983.9	E864.3	—	E950.7	E962.1	E980.6
nitrite (medicinal)	972.4	E858.3	E942.4	E950.4	E962.0	E980.4
nitroferricyanide	972.6	E858.3	E942.6	E950.4	E962.0	E980.4
nitroprusside	972.6	E858.3	E942.6	E950.4	E962.0	E980.4
para-aminohippurate	977.8	E858.8	E947.8	E950.4	E962.0	E980.4
perborate (nonmedicinal) NEC	989.89	E866.8	—	E950.9	E962.1	E980.9
medicinal	976.6	E858.7	E946.6	E950.4	E962.0	E980.4
soap	989.6	E861.1	—	E950.9	E962.1	E980.9
percarbonate — *see* Sodium, perborate						
phosphate	973.3	E858.4	E943.3	E950.4	E962.0	E980.4
polystyrene sulfonate	974.5	E858.5	E944.5	E950.4	E962.0	E980.4
propionate	976.0	E858.7	E946.0	E950.4	E962.0	E980.4
psylliate	972.7	E858.3	E942.7	E950.4	E962.0	E980.4
removing resins	974.5	E858.5	E944.5	E950.4	E962.0	E980.4
salicylate	965.1	E850.3	E935.3	E950.0	E962.0	E980.0
sulfate	973.3	E858.4	E943.3	E950.4	E962.0	E980.4
sulfoxone	961.8	E857	E931.8	E950.4	E962.0	E980.4
tetradecyl sulfate	972.7	E858.3	E942.7	E950.4	E962.0	E980.4
thiopental	968.3	E855.1	E938.3	E950.4	E962.0	E980.4
thiosalicylate	965.1	E850.3	E935.3	E950.0	E962.0	E980.0

Smelter fumes — Sodium

✓4ᵗʰ Fourth-digit Required ✓5ᵗʰ Fifth-digit Required ▶◀ Revised Text ● New Line ▲ Revised Code

		External Cause (E-Code)				
	Poisoning	Accident	Therapeutic Use	Suicide Attempt	Assault	Undetermined
Sodium — *continued*						
thiosulfate	976.0	E858.7	E946.0	E950.4	E962.0	E980.4
tolbutamide	977.8	E858.8	E947.8	E950.4	E962.0	E980.4
tyropanoate	977.8	E858.8	E947.8	E950.4	E962.0	E980.4
valproate	966.3	E855.0	E936.3	E950.4	E962.0	E980.4
Solanine	977.8	E858.8	E947.8	E950.4	E962.0	E980.4
Solanum dulcamara	988.2	E865.4	—	E950.9	E962.1	E980.9
Solapsone	961.8	E857	E931.8	E950.4	E962.0	E980.4
Solasulfone	961.8	E857	E931.8	E950.4	E962.0	E980.4
Soldering fluid	983.1	E864.1	—	E950.7	E962.1	E980.6
Solid substance	989.9	E866.9	—	E950.9	E962.1	E980.9
specified NEC	989.9	E866.8	—	E950.9	E962.1	E980.9
Solvents, industrial	982.8	E862.9	—	E950.9	E962.1	E980.9
naphtha	981	E862.0	—	E950.9	E962.1	E980.9
petroleum	981	E862.0	—	E950.9	E962.1	E980.9
specified NEC	982.8	E862.4	—	E950.9	E962.1	E980.9
Soma	968.0	E855.1	E938.0	E950.4	E962.0	E980.4
Somatotropin	962.4	E858.0	E932.4	E950.4	E962.0	E980.4
Sominex	963.0	E858.1	E933.0	E950.4	E962.0	E980.4
Somnos	967.1	E852.0	E937.1	E950.2	E962.0	E980.2
Somonal	967.0	E851	E937.0	E950.1	E962.0	E980.1
Soneryl	967.0	E851	E937.0	E950.1	E962.0	E980.1
Soothing syrup	977.9	E858.9	E947.9	E950.5	E962.0	E980.5
Sopor	967.4	E852.3	E937.4	E950.2	E962.0	E980.2
Soporific drug	967.9	E852.9	E937.9	E950.2	E962.0	E980.2
specified type NEC	967.8	E852.8	E937.8	E950.2	E962.0	E980.2
Sorbitol NEC	977.4	E858.8	E947.4	E950.4	E962.0	E980.4
Sotradecol	972.7	E858.3	E942.7	E950.4	E962.0	E980.4
Spacoline	975.1	E858.6	E945.1	E950.4	E962.0	E980.4
Spanish fly	976.8	E858.7	E946.8	E950.4	E962.0	E980.4
Sparine	969.1	E853.0	E939.1	E950.3	E962.0	E980.3
Sparteine	975.0	E858.6	E945.0	E950.4	E962.0	E980.4
Spasmolytics	975.1	E858.6	E945.1	E950.4	E962.0	E980.4
anticholinergics	971.1	E855.4	E941.1	E950.4	E962.0	E980.4
Spectinomycin	960.8	E856	E930.8	E950.4	E962.0	E980.4
Speed	969.7	E854.2	E939.7	E950.3	E962.0	E980.3
Spermicides	976.8	E858.7	E946.8	E950.4	E962.0	E980.4
Spider (bite) (venom)	989.5	E905.1	—	E950.9	E962.1	E980.9
antivenin	979.9	E858.8	E949.9	E950.4	E962.0	E980.4
Spigelia (root)	961.6	E857	E931.6	E950.4	E962.0	E980.4
Spiperone	969.2	E853.1	E939.2	E950.3	E962.0	E980.3
Spiramycin	960.3	E856	E930.3	E950.4	E962.0	E980.4
Spirilene	969.5	E853.8	E939.5	E950.3	E962.0	E980.3
Spirit(s) (neutral) NEC	980.0	E860.1	—	E950.9	E962.1	E980.9
beverage	980.0	E860.0	—	E950.9	E962.1	E980.9
industrial	980.9	E860.9	—	E950.9	E962.1	E980.9
mineral	981	E862.0	—	E950.9	E962.1	E980.9
of salt — *see* Hydrochloric acid						
surgical	980.9	E860.9	—	E950.9	E962.1	E980.9
Spironolactone	974.4	E858.5	E944.4	E950.4	E962.0	E980.4
Sponge, absorbable (gelatin)	964.5	E858.2	E934.5	E950.4	E962.0	E980.4
Sporostacin	976.0	E858.7	E946.0	E950.4	E962.0	E980.4
Sprays (aerosol)	989.89	E866.8	—	E950.9	E962.1	E980.9
cosmetic	989.89	E866.7	—	E950.9	E962.1	E980.9
medicinal NEC	977.9	E858.9	E947.9	E950.5	E962.0	E980.5
pesticides — *see* Pesticides						
specified content — *see* substance specified						
Spurge flax	988.2	E865.4	—	E950.9	E962.1	E980.9
Spurges	988.2	E865.4	—	E950.9	E962.1	E980.9
Squill (expectorant) NEC	975.5	E858.6	E945.5	E950.4	E962.0	E980.4
rat poison	989.4	E863.7	—	E950.6	E962.1	E980.7
Squirting cucumber (cathartic)	973.1	E858.4	E943.1	E950.4	E962.0	E980.4
Stains	989.89	E866.8	—	E950.9	E962.1	E980.9
Stannous — *see also* Tin						
fluoride	976.7	E858.7	E946.7	E950.4	E962.0	E980.4
Stanolone	962.1	E858.0	E932.1	E950.4	E962.0	E980.4
Stanozolol	962.1	E858.0	E932.1	E950.4	E962.0	E980.4
Staphisagria or stavesacre (pediculicide)	976.0	E858.7	E946.0	E950.4	E962.0	E980.4
Stelazine	969.1	E853.0	E939.1	E950.3	E962.0	E980.3
Stemetil	969.1	E853.0	E939.1	E950.3	E962.0	E980.3
Sterculia (cathartic) (gum)	973.3	E858.4	E943.3	E950.4	E962.0	E980.4
Sternutator gas	987.8	E869.8	—	E952.8	E962.2	E982.8
Steroids NEC	962.0	E858.0	E932.0	E950.4	E962.0	E980.4
ENT agent	976.6	E858.7	E946.6	E950.4	E962.0	E980.4
ophthalmic preparation	976.5	E858.7	E946.5	E950.4	E962.0	E980.4
topical NEC	976.0	E858.7	E946.0	E950.4	E962.0	E980.4
Stibine	985.8	E866.4	—	E950.9	E962.1	E980.9
Stibophen	961.2	E857	E931.2	E950.4	E962.0	E980.4
Stilbamide, stilbamidine	961.5	E857	E931.5	E950.4	E962.0	E980.4
Stilbestrol	962.2	E858.0	E932.2	E950.4	E962.0	E980.4

		External Cause (E-Code)				
	Poisoning	**Accident**	**Therapeutic Use**	**Suicide Attempt**	**Assault**	**Undetermined**
Stimulants (central nervous system)	970.9	E854.3	E940.9	E950.4	E962.0	E980.4
analeptics	970.0	E854.3	E940.0	E950.4	E962.0	E980.4
opiate antagonist	970.1	E854.3	E940.1	E950.4	E962.0	E980.4
psychotherapeutic NEC	969.0	E854.0	E939.0	E950.3	E962.0	E980.3
specified NEC	970.8	E854.3	E940.8	E950.4	E962.0	E980.4
Storage batteries (acid) (cells)	983.1	E864.1	—	E950.7	E962.1	E980.6
Stovaine	968.9	E855.2	E938.9	E950.4	E962.0	E980.4
infiltration (subcutaneous)	968.5	E855.2	E938.5	E950.4	E962.0	E980.4
nerve block (peripheral) (plexus)	968.6	E855.2	E938.6	E950.4	E962.0	E980.4
spinal	968.7	E855.2	E938.7	E950.4	E962.0	E980.4
topical (surface)	968.5	E855.2	E938.5	E950.4	E962.0	E980.4
Stovarsal	961.1	E857	E931.1	E950.4	E962.0	E980.4
Stove gas — *see* Gas, utility						
Stoxil	976.5	E858.7	E946.5	E950.4	E962.0	E980.4
STP	969.6	E854.1	E939.6	E950.3	E962.0	E980.3
Stramonium (medicinal) NEC	971.1	E855.4	E941.1	E950.4	E962.0	E980.4
natural state	988.2	E865.4	—	E950.9	E962.1	E980.9
Streptodornase	964.4	E858.2	E934.4	E950.4	E962.0	E980.4
Streptoduocin	960.6	E856	E930.6	E950.4	E962.0	E980.4
Streptokinase	964.4	E858.2	E934.4	E950.4	E962.0	E980.4
Streptomycin	960.6	E856	E930.6	E950.4	E962.0	E980.4
Streptozocin	960.7	E856	E930.7	E950.4	E962.0	E980.4
Stripper (paint) (solvent)	982.8	E862.9	—	E950.9	E962.1	E980.9
Strobane	989.2	E863.0	—	E950.6	E962.1	E980.7
Strophanthin	972.1	E858.3	E942.1	E950.4	E962.0	E980.4
Strophanthus hispidus or kombe	988.2	E865.4	—	E950.9	E962.1	E980.9
Strychnine (rodenticide) (salts)	989.1	E863.7	—	E950.6	E962.1	E980.7
medicinal NEC	970.8	E854.3	E940.8	E950.4	E962.0	E980.4
Strychnos (ignatii) — *see* Strychnine						
Styramate	968.0	E855.1	E938.0	E950.4	E962.0	E980.4
Styrene	983.0	E864.0	—	E950.7	E962.1	E980.6
Succinimide (anticonvulsant)	966.2	E855.0	E936.2	E950.4	E962.0	E980.4
mercuric — *see* Mercury						
Succinylcholine	975.2	E858.6	E945.2	E950.4	E962.0	E980.4
Succinylsulfathiazole	961.0	E857	E931.0	E950.4	E962.0	E980.4
Sucrose	974.5	E858.5	E944.5	E950.4	E962.0	E980.4
Sulfacetamide	961.0	E857	E931.0	E950.4	E962.0	E980.4
ophthalmic preparation	976.5	E858.7	E946.5	E950.4	E962.0	E980.4
Sulfachlorpyridazine	961.0	E857	E931.0	E950.4	E962.0	E980.4
Sulfacytine	961.0	E857	E931.0	E950.4	E962.0	E980.4
Sulfadiazine	961.0	E857	E931.0	E950.4	E962.0	E980.4
silver (topical)	976.0	E858.7	E946.0	E950.4	E962.0	E980.4
Sulfadimethoxine	961.0	E857	E931.0	E950.4	E962.0	E980.4
Sulfadimidine	961.0	E857	E931.0	E950.4	E962.0	E980.4
Sulfaethidole	961.0	E857	E931.0	E950.4	E962.0	E980.4
Sulfafurazole	961.0	E857	E931.0	E950.4	E962.0	E980.4
Sulfaguanidine	961.0	E857	E931.0	E950.4	E962.0	E980.4
Sulfamerazine	961.0	E857	E931.0	E950.4	E962.0	E980.4
Sulfameter	961.0	E857	E931.0	E950.4	E962.0	E980.4
Sulfamethizole	961.0	E857	E931.0	E950.4	E962.0	E980.4
Sulfamethoxazole	961.0	E857	E931.0	E950.4	E962.0	E980.4
Sulfamethoxydiazine	961.0	E857	E931.0	E950.4	E962.0	E980.4
Sulfamethoxypyridazine	961.0	E857	E931.0	E950.4	E962.0	E980.4
Sulfamethylthiazole	961.0	E857	E931.0	E950.4	E962.0	E980.4
Sulfamylon	976.0	E858.7	E946.0	E950.4	E962.0	E980.4
Sulfan blue (diagnostic dye)	977.8	E858.8	E947.8	E950.4	E962.0	E980.4
Sulfanilamide	961.0	E857	E931.0	E950.4	E962.0	E980.4
Sulfanilylguanidine	961.0	E857	E931.0	E950.4	E962.0	E980.4
Sulfaphenazole	961.0	E857	E931.0	E950.4	E962.0	E980.4
Sulfaphenylthiazole	961.0	E857	E931.0	E950.4	E962.0	E980.4
Sulfaproxyline	961.0	E857	E931.0	E950.4	E962.0	E980.4
Sulfapyridine	961.0	E857	E931.0	E950.4	E962.0	E980.4
Sulfapyrimidine	961.0	E857	E931.0	E950.4	E962.0	E980.4
Sulfarsphenamine	961.1	E857	E931.1	E950.4	E962.0	E980.4
Sulfasalazine	961.0	E857	E931.0	E950.4	E962.0	E980.4
Sulfasomizole	961.0	E857	E931.0	E950.4	E962.0	E980.4
Sulfasuxidine	961.0	E857	E931.0	E950.4	E962.0	E980.4
Sulfinpyrazone	974.7	E858.5	E944.7	E950.4	E962.0	E980.4
Sulfisoxazole	961.0	E857	E931.0	E950.4	E962.0	E980.4
ophthalmic preparation	976.5	E858.7	E946.5	E950.4	E962.0	E980.4
Sulfomyxin	960.8	E856	E930.8	E950.4	E962.0	E980.4
Sulfonal	967.8	E852.8	E937.8	E950.2	E962.0	E980.2
Sulfonamides (mixtures)	961.0	E857	E931.0	E950.4	E962.0	E980.4
Sulfones	961.8	E857	E931.8	E950.4	E962.0	E980.4
Sulfonethylmethane	967.8	E852.8	E937.8	E950.2	E962.0	E980.2
Sulfonmethane	967.8	E852.8	E937.8	E950.2	E962.0	E980.2
Sulfonphthal, sulfonphthol	977.8	E858.8	E947.8	E950.4	E962.0	E980.4
Sulfonylurea derivatives, oral	962.3	E858.0	E932.3	E950.4	E962.0	E980.4
Sulfoxone	961.8	E857	E931.8	E950.4	E962.0	E980.4
Sulfur, sulfureted, sulfuric, sulfurous, sulfuryl (compounds) NEC	989.89	E866.8	—	E950.9	E962.1	E980.9
acid	983.1	E864.1	—	E950.7	E962.1	E980.6

✓4ᵗʰ Fourth-digit Required   ✓5ᵗʰ Fifth-digit Required   ▶◀ Revised Text   ● New Line   ▲ Revised Code

	Poisoning	External Cause (E-Code)				
		Accident	Therapeutic Use	Suicide Attempt	Assault	Undetermined
Sulfur, sulfureted, sulfuric, sulfurous, sulfuryl NEC — *continued*						
dioxide	987.3	E869.1	—	E952.8	E962.2	E982.8
ether — *see* Ether(s)						
hydrogen	987.8	E869.8	—	E952.8	E962.2	E982.8
medicinal (keratolytic) (ointment) NEC	976.4	E858.7	E946.4	E950.4	E962.0	E980.4
pesticide (vapor)	989.4	E863.4	—	E950.6	E962.1	E980.7
vapor NEC	987.8	E869.8	—	E952.8	E962.2	E982.8
Sulkowitch's reagent	977.8	E858.8	E947.8	E950.4	E962.0	E980.4
Sulph — *see also* Sulf-						
Sulphadione	961.8	E857	E931.8	E950.4	E962.0	E980.4
Sulthiame, sultiame	966.3	E855.0	E936.3	E950.4	E962.0	E980.4
Superinone	975.5	E858.6	E945.5	E950.4	E962.0	E980.4
Suramin	961.5	E857	E931.5	E950.4	E962.0	E980.4
Surfacaine	968.5	E855.2	E938.5	E950.4	E962.0	E980.4
Surital	968.3	E855.1	E938.3	E950.4	E962.0	E980.4
Sutilains	976.8	E858.7	E946.8	E950.4	E962.0	E980.4
Suxamethonium (bromide) (chloride) (iodide)	975.2	E858.6	E945.2	E950.4	E962.0	E980.4
Suxethonium (bromide)	975.2	E858.6	E945.2	E950.4	E962.0	E980.4
Sweet oil (birch)	976.3	E858.7	E946.3	E950.4	E962.0	E980.4
Sym-dichloroethyl ether	982.3	E862.4	—	E950.9	E962.1	E980.9
Sympatholytics	971.3	E855.6	E941.3	E950.4	E962.0	E980.4
Sympathomimetics	971.2	E855.5	E941.2	E950.4	E962.0	E980.4
Synagis	979.6 ▲	E858.8	E949.6	E950.4	E962.0	E980.4
Synalar	976.0	E858.7	E946.0	E950.4	E962.0	E980.4
Synthroid	962.7	E858.0	E932.7	E950.4	E962.0	E980.4
Syntocinon	975.0	E858.6	E945.0	E950.4	E962.0	E950.4
Syrosingopine	972.6	E858.3	E942.6	E950.4	E962.0	E980.4
Systemic agents (primarily)	963.9	E858.1	E933.9	E950.4	E962.0	E980.4
specified NEC	963.8	E858.1	E933.8	E950.4	E962.0	E980.4
Tablets (*see also* specified substance)	977.9	E858.9	E947.9	E950.5	E962.0	E980.5
Tace	962.2	E858.0	E932.2	E950.4	E962.0	E980.4
Tacrine	971.0	E855.3	E941.0	E950.4	E962.0	E980.4
Talbutal	967.0	E851	E937.0	E950.1	E962.0	E980.1
Talc	976.3	E858.7	E946.3	E950.4	E962.0	E980.4
Talcum	976.3	E858.7	E946.3	E950.4	E962.0	E980.4
Tandearil, tanderil	965.5	E850.5	E935.5	E950.0	E962.0	E980.0
Tannic acid	983.1	E864.1	—	E950.7	E962.1	E980.6
medicinal (astringent)	976.2	E858.7	E946.2	E950.4	E962.0	E980.4
Tannin — *see* Tannic acid						
Tansy	988.2	E865.4	—	E950.9	E962.1	E980.9
TAO	960.3	E856	E930.3	E950.4	E962.0	E980.4
Tapazole	962.8	E858.0	E932.8	E950.4	E962.0	E980.4
Tar NEC	983.0	E864.0	—	E950.7	E962.1	E980.6
camphor — *see* Naphthalene						
fumes	987.8	E869.8	—	E952.8	E962.2	E982.8
Taractan	969.3	E853.8	E939.3	E950.3	E962.0	E980.3
Tarantula (venomous)	989.5	E905.1	—	E950.9	E962.1	E980.9
Tartar emetic (anti-infective)	961.2	E857	E931.2	E950.4	E962.0	E980.4
Tartaric acid	983.1	E864.1	—	E950.7	E962.1	E980.6
Tartrated antimony (anti-infective)	961.2	E857	E931.2	E950.4	E962.0	E980.4
TCA — *see* Trichloroacetic acid						
TDI	983.0	E864.0	—	E950.7	E962.1	E980.6
vapor	987.8	E869.8	—	E952.8	E962.2	E982.8
Tear gas	987.5	E869.3	—	E952.8	E962.2	E982.8
Teclothiazide	974.3	E858.5	E944.3	E950.4	E962.0	E980.4
Tegretol	966.3	E855.0	E936.3	E950.4	E962.0	E980.4
Telepaque	977.8	E858.8	E947.8	E950.4	E962.0	E980.4
Tellurium	985.8	E866.4	—	E950.9	E962.1	E980.9
fumes	985.8	E866.4	—	E950.9	E962.1	E980.9
TEM	963.1	E858.1	E933.1	E950.4	E962.0	E980.4
Temazepan — *see* Benzodiazepines						
TEPA	963.1	E858.1	E933.1	E950.4	E962.0	E980.4
TEPP	989.3	E863.1	—	E950.6	E962.1	E980.7
Terbutaline	971.2	E855.5	E941.2	E950.4	E962.0	E980.4
Teroxalene	961.6	E857	E931.6	E950.4	E962.0	E980.4
Terpin hydrate	975.5	E858.6	E945.5	E950.4	E962.0	E980.4
Terramycin	960.4	E856	E930.4	E950.4	E962.0	E980.4
Tessalon	975.4	E858.6	E945.4	E950.4	E962.0	E980.4
Testosterone	962.1	E858.0	E932.1	E950.4	E962.0	E980.4
Tetanus (vaccine)	978.4	E858.8	E948.4	E950.4	E962.0	E980.4
antitoxin	979.9	E858.8	E949.9	E950.4	E962.0	E980.4
immune globulin (human)	964.6	E858.2	E934.6	E950.4	E962.0	E980.4
toxoid	978.4	E858.8	E948.4	E950.4	E962.0	E980.4
with diphtheria toxoid	978.9	E858.8	E948.9	E950.4	E962.0	E980.4
with pertussis	978.6	E858.8	E948.6	E950.4	E962.0	E980.4
Tetrabenazine	969.5	E853.8	E939.5	E950.3	E962.0	E980.3
Tetracaine (infiltration) (topical)	968.5	E855.2	E938.5	E950.4	E962.0	E980.4
nerve block (peripheral) (plexus)	968.6	E855.2	E938.6	E950.4	E962.0	E980.4
spinal	968.7	E855.2	E938.7	E950.4	E962.0	E980.4
Tetrachlorethylene — *see* Tetrachloroethylene						
Tetrachlormethiazide	974.3	E858.5	E944.3	E950.4	E962.0	E980.4

✓4ᵗʰ Fourth-digit Required   ✓5ᵗʰ Fifth-digit Required   ▶◀ Revised Text   ● New Line   ▲ Revised Code

Sulfur — Tetrachlormethiazide

Table of Drugs and Chemicals — Titanium

Substance	Poisoning	Accident	Therapeutic Use	Suicide Attempt	Assault	Undetermined
Tetrachloroethane (liquid) (vapor)	982.3	E862.4	—	E950.9	E962.1	E980.9
paint or varnish	982.3	E861.6	—	E950.9	E962.1	E980.9
Tetrachloroethylene (liquid) (vapor)	982.3	E862.4	—	E950.9	E962.1	E980.9
medicinal	961.6	E857	E931.6	E950.4	E962.0	E980.4
Tetrachloromethane — see Carbon, tetrachloride						
Tetracycline	960.4	E856	E930.4	E950.4	E962.0	E980.4
ophthalmic preparation	976.5	E858.7	E946.5	E950.4	E962.0	E980.4
topical NEC	976.0	E858.7	E946.0	E950.4	E962.0	E980.4
Tetraethylammonium chloride	972.3	E858.3	E942.3	E950.4	E962.0	E980.4
Tetraethyl lead (antiknock compound)	984.1	E862.1	—	E950.9	E962.1	E980.9
Tetraethyl pyrophosphate	989.3	E863.1	—	E950.6	E962.1	E980.7
Tetraethylthiuram disulfide	977.3	E858.8	E947.3	E950.4	E962.0	E980.4
Tetrahydroaminoacridine	971.0	E855.3	E941.0	E950.4	E962.0	E980.4
Tetrahydrocannabinol	969.6	E854.1	E939.6	E950.3	E962.0	E980.3
Tetrahydronaphthalene	982.0	E862.4	—	E950.9	E962.1	E980.9
Tetrahydrozoline	971.2	E855.5	E941.2	E950.4	E962.0	E980.4
Tetralin	982.0	E862.4	—	E950.9	E962.1	E980.9
Tetramethylthiuram (disulfide) NEC	989.4	E863.6	—	E950.6	E962.1	E980.7
medicinal	976.2	E858.7	E946.2	E950.4	E962.0	E980.4
Tetronal	967.8	E852.8	E937.8	E950.2	E962.0	E980.2
Tetryl	983.0	E864.0	—	E950.7	E962.1	E980.6
Thalidomide	967.8	E852.8	E937.8	E950.2	E962.0	E980.2
Thallium (compounds) (dust) NEC	985.8	E866.4	—	E950.9	E962.1	E980.9
pesticide (rodenticide)	985.8	E863.7	—	E950.6	E962.1	E980.7
THC	969.6	E854.1	E939.6	E950.3	E962.0	E980.3
Thebacon	965.09	E850.2	E935.2	E950.0	E962.0	E980.0
Thebaine	965.09	E850.2	E935.2	E950.0	E962.0	E980.0
Theobromine (calcium salicylate)	974.1	E858.5	E944.1	E950.4	E962.0	E980.4
Theophylline (diuretic)	974.1	E858.5	E944.1	E950.4	E962.0	E980.4
ethylenediamine	975.7	E858.6	E945.7	E950.4	E962.0	E980.4
Thiabendazole	961.6	E857	E931.6	E950.4	E962.0	E980.4
Thialbarbital, thialbarbitone	968.3	E855.1	E938.3	E950.4	E962.0	E980.4
Thiamine	963.5	E858.1	E933.5	E950.4	E962.0	E980.4
Thiamylal (sodium)	968.3	E855.1	E938.3	E950.4	E962.0	E980.4
Thiazesim	969.0	E854.0	E939.0	E950.3	E962.0	E980.3
Thiazides (diuretics)	974.3	E858.5	E944.3	E950.4	E962.0	E980.4
Thiethylperazine	963.0	E858.1	E933.0	E950.4	E962.0	E980.4
Thimerosal (topical)	976.0	E858.7	E946.0	E950.4	E962.0	E980.4
ophthalmic preparation	976.5	E858.7	E946.5	E950.4	E962.0	E980.4
Thioacetazone	961.8	E857	E931.8	E950.4	E962.0	E980.4
Thiobarbiturates	968.3	E855.1	E938.3	E950.4	E962.0	E980.4
Thiobismol	961.2	E857	E931.2	E950.4	E962.0	E980.4
Thiocarbamide	962.8	E858.0	E932.8	E950.4	E962.0	E980.4
Thiocarbarsone	961.1	E857	E931.1	E950.4	E962.0	E980.4
Thiocarlide	961.8	E857	E931.8	E950.4	E962.0	E980.4
Thioguanine	963.1	E858.1	E933.1	E950.4	E962.0	E980.4
Thiomercaptomerin	974.0	E858.5	E944.0	E950.4	E962.0	E980.4
Thiomerin	974.0	E858.5	E944.0	E950.4	E962.0	E980.4
Thiopental, thiopentone (sodium)	968.3	E855.1	E938.3	E950.4	E962.0	E980.4
Thiopropazate	969.1	E853.0	E939.1	E950.3	E962.0	E980.3
Thioproperazine	969.1	E853.0	E939.1	E950.3	E962.0	E980.3
Thioridazine	969.1	E853.0	E939.1	E950.3	E962.0	E980.3
Thio-TEPA, thiotepa	963.1	E858.1	E933.1	E950.4	E962.0	E980.4
Thiothixene	969.3	E853.8	E939.3	E950.3	E962.0	E980.3
Thiouracil	962.8	E858.0	E932.8	E950.4	E962.0	E980.4
Thiourea	962.8	E858.0	E932.8	E950.4	E962.0	E980.4
Thiphenamil	971.1	E855.4	E941.1	E950.4	E962.0	E980.4
Thiram NEC	989.4	E863.6	—	E950.6	E962.1	E980.7
medicinal	976.2	E858.7	E946.2	E950.4	E962.0	E980.4
Thonzylamine	963.0	E858.1	E933.0	E950.4	E962.0	E980.4
Thorazine	969.1	E853.0	E939.1	E950.3	E962.0	E980.3
Thornapple	988.2	E865.4	—	E950.9	E962.1	E980.9
Throat preparation (lozenges) NEC	976.6	E858.7	E946.6	E950.4	E962.0	E980.4
Thrombin	964.5	E858.2	E934.5	E950.4	E962.0	E980.4
Thrombolysin	964.4	E858.2	E934.4	E950.4	E962.0	E980.4
Thymol	983.0	E864.0	—	E950.7	E962.1	E980.6
Thymus extract	962.9	E858.0	E932.9	E950.4	E962.0	E980.4
Thyroglobulin	962.7	E858.0	E932.7	E950.4	E962.0	E980.4
Thyroid (derivatives) (extract)	962.7	E858.0	E932.7	E950.4	E962.0	E980.4
Thyrolar	962.7	E858.0	E932.7	E950.4	E962.0	E980.4
Thyrothrophin, thyrotropin	977.8	E858.8	E947.8	E950.4	E962.0	E980.4
Thyroxin(e)	962.7	E858.0	E932.7	E950.4	E962.0	E980.4
Tigan	963.0	E858.1	E933.0	E950.4	E962.0	E980.4
Tigloidine	968.0	E855.1	E938.0	E950.4	E962.0	E980.4
Tin (chloride) (dust) (oxide) NEC	985.8	E866.4	—	E950.9	E962.1	E980.9
anti-infectives	961.2	E857	E931.2	E950.4	E962.0	E980.4
Tinactin	976.0	E858.7	E946.0	E950.4	E962.0	E980.4
Tincture, iodine — see Iodine						
Tindal	969.1	E853.0	E939.1	E950.3	E962.0	E980.3
Titanium (compounds) (vapor)	985.8	E866.4	—	E950.9	E962.1	E980.9
ointment	976.3	E858.7	E946.3	E950.4	E962.0	E980.4

Tetrachloroethane — Titanium

Titroid — Triethylenephosphoramide

	Poisoning	External Cause (E-Code)				
		Accident	Therapeutic Use	Suicide Attempt	Assault	Undetermined
Titroid	962.7	E858.0	E932.7	E950.4	E962.0	E980.4
TMTD — *see* Tetramethylthiuram disulfide						
TNT	989.89	E866.8	—	E950.9	E962.1	E980.9
fumes	987.8	E869.8	—	E952.8	E962.2	E982.8
Toadstool	988.1	E865.5	—	E950.9	E962.1	E980.9
Tobacco NEC	989.84	E866.8	—	E950.9	E962.1	E980.9
Indian	988.2	E865.4	—	E950.9	E962.1	E980.9
smoke, second-hand	987.8	E869.4	—	—	—	—
Tocopherol	963.5	E858.1	E933.5	E950.4	E962.0	E980.4
Tocosamine	975.0	E858.6	E945.0	E950.4	E962.0	E980.4
Tofranil	969.0	E854.0	E939.0	E950.3	E962.0	E980.3
Toilet deodorizer	989.89	E866.8	—	E950.9	E962.1	E980.9
Tolazamide	962.3	E858.0	E932.3	E950.4	E962.0	E980.4
Tolazoline	971.3	E855.6	E941.3	E950.4	E962.0	E980.4
Tolbutamide	962.3	E858.0	E932.3	E950.4	E962.0	E980.4
sodium	977.8	E858.8	E947.8	E950.4	E962.0	E980.4
Tolmetin	965.69	E850.6	E935.6	E950.0	E962.0	E980.0
Tolnaftate	976.0	E858.7	E946.0	E950.4	E962.0	E980.4
Tolpropamine	976.1	E858.7	E946.1	E950.4	E962.0	E980.4
Tolserol	968.0	E855.1	E938.0	E950.4	E962.0	E980.4
Toluene (liquid) (vapor)	982.0	E862.4	—	E950.9	E962.1	E980.9
diisocyanate	983.0	E864.0	—	E950.7	E962.1	E980.6
Toluidine	983.0	E864.0	—	E950.7	E962.1	E980.6
vapor	987.8	E869.8	—	E952.8	E962.2	E982.8
Toluol (liquid) (vapor)	982.0	E862.4	—	E950.9	E962.1	E980.9
Tolylene-2, 4-diisocyanate	983.0	E864.0	—	E950.7	E962.1	E980.6
Tonics, cardiac	972.1	E858.3	E942.1	E950.4	E962.0	E980.4
Toxaphene (dust) (spray)	989.2	E863.0	—	E950.6	E962.1	E980.7
Toxoids NEC	978.8	E858.8	E948.8	E950.4	E962.0	E980.4
Tractor fuel NEC	981	E862.1	—	E950.9	E962.1	E980.9
Tragacanth	973.3	E858.4	E943.3	E950.4	E962.0	E980.4
Tramazoline	971.2	E855.5	E941.2	E950.4	E962.0	E980.4
Tranquilizers	969.5	E853.9	E939.5	E950.3	E962.0	E980.3
benzodiazepine-based	969.4	E853.2	E939.4	E950.3	E962.0	E980.3
butyrophenone-based	969.2	E853.1	E939.2	E950.3	E962.0	E980.3
major NEC	969.3	E853.8	E939.3	E950.3	E962.0	E980.3
phenothiazine-based	969.1	E853.0	E939.1	E950.3	E962.0	E980.3
specified NEC	969.5	E853.8	E939.5	E950.3	E962.0	E980.3
Trantoin	961.9	E857	E931.9	E950.4	E962.0	E980.4
Tranxene	969.4	E853.2	E939.4	E950.3	E962.0	E980.3
Tranylcypromine (sulfate)	969.0	E854.0	E939.0	E950.3	E962.0	E980.3
Trasentine	975.1	E858.6	E945.1	E950.4	E962.0	E980.4
Travert	974.5	E858.5	E944.5	E950.4	E962.0	E980.4
Trecator	961.8	E857	E931.8	E950.4	E962.0	E980.4
Tretinoin	976.8	E858.7	E946.8	E950.4	E962.0	E980.4
Triacetin	976.0	E858.7	E946.0	E950.4	E962.0	E980.4
Triacetyloleandomycin	960.3	E856	E930.3	E950.4	E962.0	E980.4
Triamcinolone	962.0	E858.0	E932.0	E950.4	E962.0	E980.4
ENT agent	976.6	E858.7	E946.6	E950.4	E962.0	E980.4
ophthalmic preparation	976.5	E858.7	E946.5	E950.4	E962.0	E980.4
topical NEC	976.0	E858.7	E946.0	E950.4	E962.0	E980.4
Triamterene	974.4	E858.5	E944.4	E950.4	E962.0	E980.4
Triaziquone	963.1	E858.1	E933.1	E950.4	E962.0	E980.4
Tribromacetaldehyde	967.3	E852.2	E937.3	E950.2	E962.0	E980.2
Tribromoethanol	968.2	E855.1	E938.2	E950.4	E962.0	E980.4
Tribromomethane	967.3	E852.2	E937.3	E950.2	E962.0	E980.2
Trichlorethane	982.3	E862.4	—	E950.9	E962.1	E980.9
Trichlormethiazide	974.3	E858.5	E944.3	E950.4	E962.0	E980.4
Trichloroacetic acid	983.1	E864.1	—	E950.7	E962.1	E980.6
medicinal (keratolytic)	976.4	E858.7	E946.4	E950.4	E962.0	E980.4
Trichloroethanol	967.1	E852.0	E937.1	E950.2	E962.0	E980.2
Trichloroethylene (liquid) (vapor)	982.3	E862.4	—	E950.9	E962.1	E980.9
anesthetic (gas)	968.2	E855.1	E938.2	E950.4	E962.0	E980.4
Trichloroethyl phosphate	967.1	E852.0	E937.1	E950.2	E962.0	E980.2
Trichlorofluoromethane NEC	987.4	E869.2	—	E952.8	E962.2	E982.8
Trichlorotriethylamine	963.1	E858.1	E933.1	E950.4	E962.0	E980.4
Trichomonacides NEC	961.5	E857	E931.5	E950.4	E962.0	E980.4
Trichomycin	960.1	E856	E930.1	E950.4	E962.0	E980.4
Triclofos	967.1	E852.0	E937.1	E950.2	E962.0	E980.2
Tricresyl phosphate	989.89	E866.8	—	E950.9	E962.1	E980.9
solvent	982.8	E862.4	—	E950.9	E962.1	E980.9
Tricyclamol	966.4	E855.0	E936.4	E950.4	E962.0	E980.4
Tridesilon	976.0	E858.7	E946.0	E950.4	E962.0	E980.4
Tridihexethyl	971.1	E855.4	E941.1	E950.4	E962.0	E980.4
Tridione	966.0	E855.0	E936.0	E950.4	E962.0	E980.4
Triethanolamine NEC	983.2	E864.2	—	E950.7	E962.1	E980.6
detergent	983.2	E861.0	—	E950.7	E962.1	E980.6
trinitrate	972.4	E858.3	E942.4	E950.4	E962.0	E980.4
Triethanomelamine	963.1	E858.1	E933.1	E950.4	E962.0	E980.4
Triethylene melamine	963.1	E858.1	E933.1	E950.4	E962.0	E980.4
Triethylenephosphoramide	963.1	E858.1	E933.1	E950.4	E962.0	E980.4

		External Cause (E-Code)				
	Poisoning	Accident	Therapeutic Use	Suicide Attempt	Assault	Undetermined
Triethylenethiophosphoramide	963.1	E858.1	E933.1	E950.4	E962.0	E980.4
Trifluoperazine	969.1	E853.0	E939.1	E950.3	E962.0	E980.3
Trifluperidol	969.2	E853.1	E939.2	E950.3	E962.0	E980.3
Triflupromazine	969.1	E853.0	E939.1	E950.3	E962.0	E980.3
Trihexyphenidyl	971.1	E855.4	E941.1	E950.4	E962.0	E980.4
Triiodothyronine	962.7	E858.0	E932.7	E950.4	E962.0	E980.4
Trilene	968.2	E855.1	E938.2	E950.4	E962.0	E980.4
Trimeprazine	963.0	E858.1	E933.0	E950.4	E962.0	E980.4
Trimetazidine	972.4	E858.3	E942.4	E950.4	E962.0	E980.4
Trimethadione	966.0	E855.0	E936.0	E950.4	E962.0	E980.4
Trimethaphan	972.3	E858.3	E942.3	E950.4	E962.0	E980.4
Trimethidinium	972.3	E858.3	E942.3	E950.4	E962.0	E980.4
Trimethobenzamide	963.0	E858.1	E933.0	E950.4	E962.0	E980.4
Trimethylcarbinol	980.8	E860.8	—	E950.9	E962.1	E980.9
Trimethylpsoralen	976.3	E858.7	E946.3	E950.4	E962.0	E980.4
Trimeton	963.0	E858.1	E933.0	E950.4	E962.0	E980.4
Trimipramine	969.0	E854.0	E939.0	E950.3	E962.0	E980.3
Trimustine	963.1	E858.1	E933.1	E950.4	E962.0	E980.4
Trinitrin	972.4	E858.3	E942.4	E950.4	E962.0	E980.4
Trinitrophenol	983.0	E864.0	—	E950.7	E962.1	E980.6
Trinitrotoluene	989.89	E866.8	—	E950.9	E962.1	E980.9
fumes	987.8	E869.8	—	E952.8	E962.2	E982.8
Trional	967.8	E852.8	E937.8	E950.2	E962.0	E980.2
Trioxide of arsenic — *see* Arsenic						
Trioxsalen	976.3	E858.7	E946.3	E950.4	E962.0	E980.4
Tripelennamine	963.0	E858.1	E933.0	E950.4	E962.0	E980.4
Triperidol	969.2	E853.1	E939.2	E950.3	E962.0	E980.3
Triprolidine	963.0	E858.1	E933.0	E950.4	E962.0	E980.4
Trisoralen	976.3	E858.7	E946.3	E950.4	E962.0	E980.4
Troleandomycin	960.3	E856	E930.3	E950.4	E962.0	E980.4
Trolnitrate (phosphate)	972.4	E858.3	E942.4	E950.4	E962.0	E980.4
Trometamol	963.3	E858.1	E933.3	E950.4	E962.0	E980.4
Tromethamine	963.3	E858.1	E933.3	E950.4	E962.0	E980.4
Tronothane	968.5	E855.2	E938.5	E950.4	E962.0	E980.4
Tropicamide	971.1	E855.4	E941.1	E950.4	E962.0	E980.4
Troxidone	966.0	E855.0	E936.0	E950.4	E962.0	E980.4
Tryparsamide	961.1	E857	E931.1	E950.4	E962.0	E980.4
Trypsin	963.4	E858.1	E933.4	E950.4	E962.0	E980.4
Tryptizol	969.0	E854.0	E939.0	E950.3	E962.0	E980.3
Tuaminoheptane	971.2	E855.5	E941.2	E950.4	E962.0	E980.4
Tuberculin (old)	977.8	E858.8	E947.8	E950.4	E962.0	E980.4
Tubocurare	975.2	E858.6	E945.2	E950.4	E962.0	E980.4
Tubocurarine	975.2	E858.6	E945.2	E950.4	E962.0	E980.4
Turkish green	969.6	E854.1	E939.6	E950.3	E962.0	E980.3
Turpentine (spirits of) (liquid) (vapor)	982.8	E862.4	—	E950.9	E962.1	E980.9
Tybamate	969.5	E853.8	E939.5	E950.3	E962.0	E980.3
Tyloxapol	975.5	E858.6	E945.5	E950.4	E962.0	E980.4
Tymazoline	971.2	E855.5	E941.2	E950.4	E962.0	E980.4
Typhoid vaccine	978.1	E858.8	E948.1	E950.4	E962.0	E980.4
Typhus vaccine	979.2	E858.8	E949.2	E950.4	E962.0	E980.4
Tyrothricin	976.0	E858.7	E946.0	E950.4	E962.0	E980.4
ENT agent	976.6	E858.7	E946.6	E950.4	E962.0	E980.4
ophthalmic preparation	976.5	E858.7	E946.5	E950.4	E962.0	E980.4
Undecenoic acid	976.0	E858.7	E946.0	E950.4	E962.0	E980.4
Undecylenic acid	976.0	E858.7	E946.0	E950.4	E962.0	E980.4
Unna's boot	976.3	E858.7	E946.3	E950.4	E962.0	E980.4
Uracil mustard	963.1	E858.1	E933.1	E950.4	E962.0	E980.4
Uramustine	963.1	E858.1	E933.1	E950.4	E962.0	E980.4
Urari	975.2	E858.6	E945.2	E950.4	E962.0	E980.4
Urea	974.4	E858.5	E944.4	E950.4	E962.0	E980.4
topical	976.8	E858.7	E946.8	E950.4	E962.0	E980.4
Urethan(e) (antineoplastic)	963.1	E858.1	E933.1	E950.4	E962.0	E980.4
Urginea (maritima) (scilla) — *see* Squill						
Uric acid metabolism agents NEC	974.7	E858.5	E944.7	E950.4	E962.0	E980.4
Urokinase	964.4	E858.2	E934.4	E950.4	E962.0	E980.4
Urokon	977.8	E858.8	E947.8	E950.4	E962.0	E980.4
Urotropin	961.9	E857	E931.9	E950.4	E962.0	E980.4
Urtica	988.2	E865.4	—	E950.9	E962.1	E980.9
Utility gas — *see* Gas, utility						
Vaccine NEC	979.9	E858.8	E949.9	E950.4	E962.0	E980.4
bacterial NEC	978.8	E858.8	E948.8	E950.4	E962.0	E980.4
with						
other bacterial component	978.9	E858.8	E948.9	E950.4	E962.0	E980.4
pertussis component	978.6	E858.8	E948.6	E950.4	E962.0	E980.4
viral-rickettsial component	979.7	E858.8	E949.7	E950.4	E962.0	E980.4
mixed NEC	978.9	E858.8	E948.9	E950.4	E962.0	E980.4
BCG	978.0	E858.8	E948.0	E950.4	E962.0	E980.4
cholera	978.2	E858.8	E948.2	E950.4	E962.0	E980.4
diphtheria	978.5	E858.8	E948.5	E950.4	E962.0	E980.4
influenza	979.6	E858.8	E949.6	E950.4	E962.0	E980.4
measles	979.4	E858.8	E949.4	E950.4	E962.0	E980.4

Triethylenethiophosphoramide — Vaccine

▪4ᵗʰ Fourth-digit Required   ▪5ᵗʰ Fifth-digit Required   ▶◀ Revised Text   ● New Line   ▲ Revised Code

	Poisoning	External Cause (E-Code)				
		Accident	Therapeutic Use	Suicide Attempt	Assault	Undetermined
Vaccine NEC — *continued*						
meningococcal	978.8	E858.8	E948.8	E950.4	E962.0	E980.4
mumps	979.6	E858.8	E949.6	E950.4	E962.0	E980.4
paratyphoid	978.1	E858.8	E948.1	E950.4	E962.0	E980.4
pertussis (with diphtheria toxoid) (with tetanus toxoid)	978.6	E858.8	E948.6	E950.4	E962.0	E980.4
plague	978.3	E858.8	E948.3	E950.4	E962.0	E980.4
poliomyelitis	979.5	E858.8	E949.5	E950.4	E962.0	E980.4
poliovirus	979.5	E858.8	E949.5	E950.4	E962.0	E980.4
rabies	979.1	E858.8	E949.1	E950.4	E962.0	E980.4
respiratory syncytial virus	979.6 ▲	E858.8	E949.6	E950.4	E962.0	E980.4
rickettsial NEC	979.6	E858.8	E949.6	E950.4	E962.0	E980.4
with						
bacterial component	979.7	E858.8	E949.7	E950.4	E962.0	E980.4
pertussis component	978.6	E858.8	E948.6	E950.4	E962.0	E980.4
viral component	979.7	E858.8	E949.7	E950.4	E962.0	E980.4
Rocky mountain spotted fever	979.6	E858.8	E949.6	E950.4	E962.0	E980.4
rotavirus	979.6	E858.8	E949.6	E950.4	E962.0	E980.4
rubella virus	979.4	E858.8	E949.4	E950.4	E962.0	E980.4
sabin oral	979.5	E858.8	E949.5	E950.4	E962.0	E980.4
smallpox	979.0	E858.8	E949.0	E950.4	E962.0	E980.4
tetanus	978.4	E858.8	E948.4	E950.4	E962.0	E980.4
typhoid	978.1	E858.8	E948.1	E950.4	E962.0	E980.4
typhus	979.2	E858.8	E949.2	E950.4	E962.0	E980.4
viral NEC	979.6	E858.8	E949.6	E950.4	E962.0	E980.4
with						
bacterial component	979.7	E858.8	E949.7	E950.4	E962.0	E980.4
pertussis component	978.6	E858.8	E948.6	E950.4	E962.0	E980.4
rickettsial component	979.7	E858.8	E949.7	E950.4	E962.0	E980.4
yellow fever	979.3	E858.8	E949.3	E950.4	E962.0	E980.4
Vaccinia immune globulin (human)	964.6	E858.2	E934.6	E950.4	E962.0	E980.4
Vaginal contraceptives	976.8	E858.7	E946.8	E950.4	E962.0	E980.4
Valethamate	971.1	E855.4	E941.1	E950.4	E962.0	E980.4
Valisone	976.0	E858.7	E946.0	E950.4	E962.0	E980.4
Valium	969.4	E853.2	E939.4	E950.3	E962.0	E980.3
Valmid	967.8	E852.8	E937.8	E950.2	E962.0	E980.2
Vanadium	985.8	E866.4	—	E950.9	E962.1	E980.9
Vancomycin	960.8	E856	E930.8	E950.4	E962.0	E980.4
Vapor (*see also* Gas)	987.9	E869.9	—	E952.9	E962.2	E982.9
kiln (carbon monoxide)	986	E868.8	—	E952.1	E962.2	E982.1
lead — *see* Lead						
specified source NEC (*see also* specific substance)	987.8	E869.8	—	E952.8	E962.2	E982.8
Varidase	964.4	E858.2	E934.4	E950.4	E962.0	E980.4
Varnish	989.89	E861.6	—	E950.9	E962.1	E980.9
cleaner	982.8	E862.9	—	E950.9	E962.1	E980.9
Vaseline	976.3	E858.7	E946.3	E950.4	E962.0	E980.4
Vasodilan	972.5	E858.3	E942.5	E950.4	E962.0	E980.4
Vasodilators NEC	972.5	E858.3	E942.5	E950.4	E962.0	E980.4
coronary	972.4	E858.3	E942.4	E950.4	E962.0	E980.4
Vasopressin	962.5	E858.0	E932.5	E950.4	E962.0	E980.4
Vasopressor drugs	962.5	E858.0	E932.5	E950.4	E962.0	E980.4
Venom, venomous (bite) (sting)	989.5	E905.9	—	E950.9	E962.1	E980.9
arthropod NEC	989.5	E905.5	—	E950.9	E962.1	E980.9
bee	989.5	E905.3	—	E950.9	E962.1	E980.9
centipede	989.5	E905.4	—	E950.9	E962.1	E980.9
hornet	989.5	E905.3	—	E950.9	E962.1	E980.9
lizard	989.5	E905.0	—	E950.9	E962.1	E980.9
marine animals or plants	989.5	E905.6	—	E950.9	E962.1	E980.9
millipede (tropical)	989.5	E905.4	—	E950.9	E962.1	E980.9
plant NEC	989.5	E905.7	—	E950.9	E962.1	E980.9
marine	989.5	E905.6	—	E950.9	E962.1	E980.9
scorpion	989.5	E905.2	—	E950.9	E962.1	E980.9
snake	989.5	E905.0	—	E950.9	E962.1	E980.9
specified NEC	989.5	E905.8	—	E950.9	E962.1	E980.9
spider	989.5	E905.1	—	E950.9	E962.1	E980.9
wasp	989.5	E905.3	—	E950.9	E962.1	E980.9
Veramon	967.0	E851	E937.0	E950.1	E962.0	E980.1
Veratrum						
album	988.2	E865.4	—	E950.9	E962.1	E980.9
alkaloids	972.6	E858.3	E942.6	E950.4	E962.0	E980.4
viride	988.2	E865.4	—	E950.9	E962.1	E980.9
Verdigris (*see also* Copper)	985.8	E866.4	—	E950.9	E962.1	E980.9
Veronal	967.0	E851	E937.0	E950.1	E962.0	E980.1
Veroxil	961.6	E857	E931.6	E950.4	E962.0	E980.4
Versidyne	965.7	E850.7	E935.7	E950.0	E962.0	E980.0
Viagra	972.5	E858.3	E942.5	E950.4	E962.0	E980.4
Vienna						
green	985.1	E866.3	—	E950.8	E962.1	E980.8
insecticide	985.1	E863.4	—	E950.6	E962.1	E980.7
red	989.89	E866.8	—	E950.9	E962.1	E980.9
pharmaceutical dye	977.4	E858.8	E947.4	E950.4	E962.0	E980.4
Vinbarbital, vinbarbitone	967.0	E851	E937.0	E950.1	E962.0	E980.1

▨ 4ᵗʰ Fourth-digit Required   ▨ 5ᵗʰ Fifth-digit Required   ▶◀ Revised Text   ● New Line   ▲ Revised Code

Vaccine — Vinbarbital

		External Cause (E-Code)				
	Poisoning	Accident	Therapeutic Use	Suicide Attempt	Assault	Undetermined
Vinblastine	963.1	E858.1	E933.1	E950.4	E962.0	E980.4
Vincristine	963.1	E858.1	E933.1	E950.4	E962.0	E980.4
Vinesthene, vinethene	968.2	E855.1	E938.2	E950.4	E962.0	E980.4
Vinyl						
bital	967.0	E851	E937.0	E950.1	E962.0	E980.1
ether	968.2	E855.1	E938.2	E950.4	E962.0	E980.4
Vioform	961.3	E857	E931.3	E950.4	E962.0	E980.4
topical	976.0	E858.7	E946.0	E950.4	E962.0	E980.4
Viomycin	960.6	E856	E930.6	E950.4	E962.0	E980.4
Viosterol	963.5	E858.1	E933.5	E950.4	E962.0	E980.4
Viper (venom)	989.5	E905.0	—	E950.9	E962.1	E980.9
Viprynium (embonate)	961.6	E857	E931.6	E950.4	E962.0	E980.4
Virugon	961.7	E857	E931.7	E950.4	E962.0	E980.4
Visine	976.5	E858.7	E946.5	E950.4	E962.0	E980.4
Vitamins NEC	963.5	E858.1	E933.5	E950.4	E962.0	E980.4
B_{12}	964.1	E858.2	E934.1	E950.4	E962.0	E980.4
hematopoietic	964.1	E858.2	E934.1	E950.4	E962.0	E980.4
K	964.3	E858.2	E934.3	E950.4	E962.0	E980.4
Vleminckx's solution	976.4	E858.7	E946.4	E950.4	E962.0	E980.4
Voltaren — *see* Diclofenac sodium						
Ventolin — *see* Salbutamol sulfate						
Warfarin (potassium) (sodium)	964.2	E858.2	E934.2	E950.4	E962.0	E980.4
rodenticide	989.4	E863.7	—	E950.6	E962.1	E980.7
Wasp (sting)	989.5	E905.3	—	E950.9	E962.1	E980.9
Water						
balance agents NEC	974.5	E858.5	E944.5	E950.4	E962.0	E980.4
gas	987.1	E868.1	—	E951.8	E962.2	E981.8
incomplete combustion of — *see* Carbon, monoxide, fuel, utility						
hemlock	988.2	E865.4	—	E950.9	E962.1	E980.9
moccasin (venom)	989.5	E905.0	—	E950.9	E962.1	E980.9
Wax (paraffin) (petroleum)	981	E862.3	—	E950.9	E962.1	E980.9
automobile	989.89	E861.2	—	E950.9	E962.1	E980.9
floor	981	E862.0	—	E950.9	E962.1	E980.9
Weed killers NEC	989.4	E863.5	—	E950.6	E962.1	E980.7
Welldorm	967.1	E852.0	E937.1	E950.2	E962.0	E980.2
White						
arsenic — *see* Arsenic						
hellebore	988.2	E865.4	—	E950.9	E962.1	E980.9
lotion (keratolytic)	976.4	E858.7	E946.4	E950.4	E962.0	E980.4
spirit	981	E862.0	—	E950.9	E962.1	E980.9
Whitewashes	989.89	E861.6	—	E950.9	E962.1	E980.9
Whole blood	964.7	E858.2	E934.7	E950.4	E962.0	E980.4
Wild						
black cherry	988.2	E865.4	—	E950.9	E962.1	E980.9
poisonous plants NEC	988.2	E865.4	—	E950.9	E962.1	E980.9
Window cleaning fluid	989.89	E861.3	—	E950.9	E962.1	E980.9
Wintergreen (oil)	976.3	E858.7	E946.3	E950.4	E962.0	E980.4
Witch hazel	976.2	E858.7	E946.2	E950.4	E962.0	E980.4
Wood						
alcohol	980.1	E860.2	—	E950.9	E962.1	E980.9
spirit	980.1	E860.2	—	E950.9	E962.1	E980.9
Woorali	975.2	E858.6	E945.2	E950.4	E962.0	E980.4
Wormseed, American	961.6	E857	E931.6	E950.4	E962.0	E980.4
Xanthine diuretics	974.1	E858.5	E944.1	E950.4	E962.0	E980.4
Xanthocillin	960.0	E856	E930.0	E950.4	E962.0	E980.4
Xanthotoxin	976.3	E858.7	E946.3	E950.4	E962.0	E980.4
Xylene (liquid) (vapor)	982.0	E862.4	—	E950.9	E962.1	E980.9
Xylocaine (infiltration) (topical)	968.5	E855.2	E938.5	E950.4	E962.0	E980.4
nerve block (peripheral) (plexus)	968.6	E855.2	E938.6	E950.4	E962.0	E980.4
spinal	968.7	E855.2	E938.7	E950.4	E962.0	E980.4
Xylol (liquid) (vapor)	982.0	E862.4	—	E950.9	E962.1	E980.9
Xylometazoline	971.2	E855.5	E941.2	E950.4	E962.0	E980.4
Yellow						
fever vaccine	979.3	E858.8	E949.3	E950.4	E962.0	E980.4
jasmine	988.2	E865.4	—	E950.9	E962.1	E980.9
Yew	988.2	E865.4	—	E950.9	E962.1	E980.9
Zactane	965.7	E850.7	E935.7	E950.0	E962.0	E980.0
Zaroxolyn	974.3	E858.5	E944.3	E950.4	E962.0	E980.4
Zephiran (topical)	976.0	E858.7	E946.0	E950.4	E962.0	E980.4
ophthalmic preparation	976.5	E858.7	E946.5	E950.4	E962.0	E980.4
Zerone	980.1	E860.2	—	E950.9	E962.1	E980.9
Zinc (compounds) (fumes) (salts) (vapor) NEC	985.8	E866.4	—	E950.9	E962.1	E980.9
anti-infectives	976.0	E858.7	E946.0	E950.4	E962.0	E980.4
antivaricose	972.7	E858.3	E942.7	E950.4	E962.0	E980.4
bacitracin	976.0	E858.7	E946.0	E950.4	E962.0	E980.4
chloride	976.2	E858.7	E946.2	E950.4	E962.0	E980.4
gelatin	976.3	E858.7	E946.3	E950.4	E962.0	E980.4
oxide	976.3	E858.7	E946.3	E950.4	E962.0	E980.4
peroxide	976.0	E858.7	E946.0	E950.4	E962.0	E980.4
pesticides	985.8	E863.4	—	E950.6	E962.1	E980.7
phosphide (rodenticide)	985.8	E863.7	—	E950.6	E962.1	E980.7

Vinblastine — Zinc

	Poisoning	External Cause (E-Code)				
		Accident	Therapeutic Use	Suicide Attempt	Assault	Undetermined
Zinc NEC — *continued*						
stearate	976.3	E858.7	E946.3	E950.4	E962.0	E980.4
sulfate (antivaricose)	972.7	E858.3	E942.7	E950.4	E962.0	E980.4
ENT agent	976.6	E858.7	E946.6	E950.4	E962.0	E980.4
ophthalmic solution	976.5	E858.7	E946.5	E950.4	E962.0	E980.4
topical NEC	976.0	E858.7	E946.0	E950.4	E962.0	E980.4
undecylenate	976.0	E858.7	E946.0	E950.4	E962.0	E980.4
Zoxazolamine	968.0	E855.1	E938.0	E950.4	E962.0	E980.4
Zygadenus (venenosus)	988.2	E865.4	—	E950.9	E962.1	E980.9

Zinc — Zygadenus

SECTION 3
Alphabetic Index to External Causes of Injury and Poisoning (E Code)

This section contains the index to the codes which classify environmental events, circumstances, and other conditions as the cause of injury and other adverse effects. Where a code from the section Supplementary Classification of External Causes of Injury and Poisoning (E800-E998) is applicable, it is intended that the E code shall be used in addition to a code from the main body of the classification, Chapters 1 to 17.

The alphabetic index to the E codes is organized by main terms which describe the *accident, circumstance, event,* or *specific agent* which caused the injury or other adverse effect.

Note — Transport accidents (E800-E848) include accidents involving:
> *aircraft and spacecraft (E840-E845)*
> *watercraft (E830-E838)*
> *motor vehicle (E810-E825)*
> *railway (E800-E807)*
> *other road vehicles (E826-E829)*

For definitions and examples related to transport accidents — see Volume 1 code categories E800-E848.

The fourth-digit subdivisions for use with categories E800-E848 to identify the injured person are found at the end of this section.

For identifying the place in which an accident or poisoning occurred (circumstances classifiable to categories E850-E869 and E880-E928) — see the listing in this section under "Accident, occurring."

See the Table of Drugs and Chemicals (Section 2 of this volume) for identifying the specific agent involved in drug overdose or a wrong substance given or taken in error, and for intoxication or poisoning by a drug or other chemical substance.

The specific adverse effect, reaction, or localized toxic effect to a correct drug or substance properly administered in therapeutic or prophylactic dosage should be classified according to the nature of the adverse effect (e.g., allergy, dermatitis, tachycardia) listed in Section 1 of this volume.

A

Abandonment
  causing exposure to weather conditions — see Exposure
  child, with intent to injure or kill E968.4
  helpless person, infant, newborn E904.0
    with intent to injure or kill E968.4

Abortion, criminal, injury to child E968.8

Abuse (alleged) (suspected)
  adult
    by
      child E967.4
      ex-partner E967.3
      ex-spouse E967.3
      father E967.0
      grandchild E967.7
      grandparent E967.6
      mother E967.2
      non-related caregiver E967.8
      other relative E967.7
      other specified person E967.1
      partner E967.3
      sibling E967.5
      spouse E967.3
      stepfather E967.0
      stepmother E967.2
      unspecified person E967.9
  child
    by
      boyfriend of parent or guardian E967.0
      child E967.4
      father E967.0
      female partner of parent or guardian E967.2
      girlfriend of parent or guardian E967.2
      grandchild E967.7
      grandparent E967.6
      male partner of parent or guardian E967.2
      mother E967.2
      non-related caregiver E967.8
      other relative E967.7
      other specified person(s) E967.1
      sibling E967.5
      stepfather E967.0
      stepmother E967.2
      unspecified person E967.9

Accident (to) E928.9
  aircraft (in transit) (powered) E841 ✓4ᵗʰ
    at landing, take-off E840 ✓4ᵗʰ
    due to, caused by cataclysm — see categories E908 ✓4ᵗʰ, E909 ✓4ᵗʰ
    late effect of E929.1
    unpowered (see also Collision, aircraft, unpowered) E842 ✓4ᵗʰ
    while alighting, boarding E843 ✓4ᵗʰ
  amphibious vehicle
    on
      land — see Accident, motor vehicle
      water — see Accident, watercraft
  animal, ridden NEC E828 ✓4ᵗʰ
  animal-drawn vehicle NEC E827 ✓4ᵗʰ
  balloon (see also Collision, aircraft, unpowered) E842 ✓4ᵗʰ
  caused by, due to
    abrasive wheel (metalworking) E919.3
    animal NEC E906.9
      being ridden (in sport or transport) E828 ✓4ᵗʰ
    avalanche NEC E909.2
    band saw E919.4
    bench saw E919.4
    bore, earth-drilling or mining (land) (seabed) E919.1
    bulldozer E919.7
    cataclysmic
      earth surface movement or eruption E909.9
      storm E908.9
    chain
      hoist E919.2
        agricultural operations E919.0
        mining operations E919.1
      saw E920.1
    circular saw E919.4

Accident (to) — continued
  caused by, due to — continued
    cold (excessive) (see also Cold, exposure to) E901.9
    combine E919.0
    conflagration — see Conflagration
    corrosive liquid, substance NEC E924.1
    cotton gin E919.8
    crane E919.2
      agricultural operations E919.0
      mining operations E919.1
    cutting or piercing instrument (see also Cut) E920.9
    dairy equipment E919.8
    derrick E919.2
      agricultural operations E919.0
      mining operations E919.1
    drill E920.1
      earth (land) (seabed) E919.1
      hand (powered) E920.1
        not powered E920.4
      metalworking E919.3
      woodworking E919.4
    earth(-)
      drilling machine E919.1
      moving machine E919.7
      scraping machine E919.7
    electric
      current (see also Electric shock) E925.9
      motor — see also Accident, machine, by type of machine
        current (of) — see Electric shock
    elevator (building) (grain) E919.2
      agricultural operations E919.0
      mining operations E919.1
    environmental factors NEC E928.9
    excavating machine E919.7
    explosive material (see also Explosion) E923.9
    farm machine E919.0
    fire, flames — see also Fire
      conflagration — see Conflagration
    firearm missile — see Shooting
    forging (metalworking) machine E919.3
    forklift (truck) E919.2
      agricultural operations E919.0
      mining operations E919.1
    gas turbine E919.5
    harvester E919.0
    hay derrick, mower, or rake E919.0
    heat (excessive) (see also Heat) E900.9
    hoist (see also Accident, caused by, due to, lift) E919.2
      chain — see Accident, caused by, due to, chain
      shaft E919.1
    hot
      liquid E924.0
        caustic or corrosive E924.1
      object (not producing fire or flames) E924.8
      substance E924.9
        caustic or corrosive E924.1
        liquid (metal) NEC E924.0
        specified type NEC E924.8
    human bite E928.3
    ignition — see Ignition
    internal combustion engine E919.5
    landslide NEC E909.2
    lathe (metalworking) E919.3
      turnings E920.8
      woodworking E919.4
    lift, lifting (appliances) E919.2
      agricultural operations E919.0
      mining operations E919.1
      shaft E919.1
    lightning NEC E907
    machine, machinery — see also Accident, machine
      drilling, metal E919.3
      manufacturing, for manufacture of
        beverages E919.8
        clothing E919.8
        foodstuffs E919.8
        paper E919.8
        textiles E919.8

Accident (to) — continued
  caused by, due to — continued
    machine, machinery — see also Accident, machine — continued
      milling, metal E919.3
      moulding E919.4
      power press, metal E919.3
      printing E919.8
      rolling mill, metal E919.3
      sawing, metal E919.3
      specified type NEC E919.8
      spinning E919.8
      weaving E919.8
    natural factor NEC E928.9
    overhead plane E919.4
    plane E920.4
      overhead E919.4
    powered
      hand tool NEC E920.1
      saw E919.4
        hand E920.1
    printing machine E919.8
    pulley (block) E919.2
      agricultural operations E919.0
      mining operations E919.1
      transmission E919.6
    radial saw E919.4
    radiation — see Radiation
    reaper E919.0
    road scraper E919.7
      when in transport under its own power — see categories E810-E825 ✓4ᵗʰ
    roller coaster E919.8
    sander E919.4
    saw E920.4
      band E919.4
      bench E919.4
      chain E920.1
      circular E919.4
      hand E920.4
        powered E920.1
      powered, except hand E919.4
      radial E919.4
    sawing machine, metal E919.3
    shaft
      hoist E919.1
      lift E919.1
      transmission E919.6
    shears E920.4
      hand E920.4
        powered E920.1
      mechanical E919.3
    shovel E920.4
      steam E919.7
    spinning machine E919.8
    steam — see also Burning, steam
      engine E919.5
      shovel E919.7
    thresher E919.0
    thunderbolt NEC E907
    tractor E919.0
      when in transport under its own power — see categories E810-E825 ✓4ᵗʰ
    transmission belt, cable, chain, gear, pinion, pulley, shaft E919.6
    turbine (gas) (water driven) E919.5
    under-cutter E919.1
    weaving machine E919.8
    winch E919.2
      agricultural operations E919.0
      mining operations E919.1
  diving E883.0
    with insufficient air supply E913.2
  glider (hang) (see also Collision, aircraft, unpowered) E842 ✓4ᵗʰ
  hovercraft
    on
      land — see Accident, motor vehicle
      water — see Accident, watercraft
  ice yacht (see also Accident, vehicle NEC) E848
  in
    medical, surgical procedure
      as, or due to misadventure — see Misadventure

Accident (to) — *continued*
  in — *continued*
    medical, surgical procedure — *continued*
      causing an abnormal reaction or later
        complication without mention of
        misadventure — *see* Reaction,
        abnormal
    kite carrying a person (*see also* Collision,
      aircraft, unpowered) E842 ☑4ᵗʰ
    land yacht (*see also* Accident, vehicle NEC)
      E848
    late effect of — *see* Late effect
    launching pad E845 ☑4ᵗʰ
    machine, machinery (*see also* Accident, caused
      by, due to, by specific type of machine)
      E919.9
      agricultural including animal-powered
        E919.0
      earth-drilling E919.1
      earth moving or scraping E919.7
      excavating E919.7
      involving transport under own power on
        highway or transport vehicle — *see*
        categories E810-E825 ☑4ᵗʰ,
        E840-E845 ☑4ᵗʰ
      lifting (appliances) E919.2
      metalworking E919.3
      mining E919.1
      prime movers, except electric motors E919.5
        electric motors — *see* Accident, machine,
        by specific type of machine
      recreational E919.8
      specified type NEC E919.8
      transmission E919.6
      watercraft (deck) (engine room) (galley)
        (laundry) (loading) E836 ☑4ᵗʰ
      woodworking or forming E919.4
    motor vehicle (on public highway) (traffic)
      E819 ☑4ᵗʰ
      due to cataclysm — *see* categories
        E908 ☑4ᵗʰ, E909 ☑4ᵗʰ
      involving
        collision (*see also* Collision, motor vehicle)
        E812 ☑4ᵗʰ
      nontraffic, not on public highway — *see*
        categories E820-E825 ☑4ᵗʰ
      not involving collision — *see* categories
        E816-E819 ☑4ᵗʰ
    nonmotor vehicle NEC E829 ☑4ᵗʰ
      nonroad — *see* Accident, vehicle NEC
      road, except pedal cycle, animal-drawn
        vehicle, or animal being ridden
        E829 ☑4ᵗʰ
    nonroad vehicle NEC — *see* Accident, vehicle
      NEC
    not elsewhere classifiable involving
      cable car (not on rails) E847
        on rails E829 ☑4ᵗʰ
      coal car in mine E846
      hand truck — *see* Accident, vehicle NEC
      logging car E846
      sled(ge), meaning snow or ice vehicle E848
      tram, mine or quarry E846
      truck
        mine or quarry E846
        self-propelled, industrial E846
        station baggage E846
      tub, mine or quarry E846
      vehicle NEC E848
        snow and ice E848
        used only on industrial premises E846
      wheelbarrow E848
    occurring (at) (in)
      apartment E849.0
      baseball field, diamond E849.4
      construction site, any E849.3
      dock E849.8
        yard E849.3
      dormitory E849.7
      factory (building) (premises) E849.3
      farm E849.1
        buildings E849.1
        house E849.0
      football field E849.4
      forest E849.8
      garage (place of work) E849.3
        private (home) E849.0

Accident (to) — *continued*
  occurring (at) (in) — *continued*
    gravel pit E849.2
    gymnasium E849.4
    highway E849.5
    home (private) (residential) E849.0
      institutional E849.7
    hospital E849.7
    hotel E849.6
    house (private) (residential) E849.0
      movie E849.6
      public E849.6
    institution, residential E849.7
    jail E849.7
    mine E849.2
    motel E849.6
    movie house E849.6
    office (building) E849.6
    orphanage E849.7
    park (public) E849.4
      mobile home E849.8
      trailer E849.8
    parking lot or place E849.8
    place
      industrial NEC E849.3
      parking E849.8
      public E849.8
        specified place NEC E849.5
      recreational NEC E849.4
      sport NEC E849.4
    playground (park) (school) E849.4
    prison E849.6
    public building NEC E849.6
    quarry E849.2
    railway
      line NEC E849.8
      yard E849.3
    residence
      home (private) E849.0
    resort (beach) (lake) (mountain) (seashore)
      (vacation) E849.4
    restaurant E849.6
    sand pit E849.2
    school (building) (private) (public) (state)
      E849.6
      reform E849.7
      riding E849.4
    seashore E849.8
      resort E849.4
    shop (place of work) E849.3
      commercial E849.6
    skating rink E849.4
    sports palace E849.4
    stadium E849.4
    store E849.6
    street E849.5
    swimming pool (public) E849.4
      private home or garden E849.0
    tennis court E849.4
    theatre, theater E849.6
    trailer court E849.8
    tunnel E849.8
      under construction E849.2
    warehouse E849.3
    yard
      dock E849.3
      industrial E849.3
      private (home) E849.0
      railway E849.3
  off-road type motor vehicle (not on public
    highway) NEC E821 ☑4ᵗʰ
    on public highway — *see* categories
      E810-E819 ☑4ᵗʰ
  pedal cycle E826 ☑4ᵗʰ
  railway E807 ☑4ᵗʰ
    due to cataclysm — *see* categories
      E908 ☑4ᵗʰ, E909 ☑4ᵗʰ
    involving
      avalanche E909.2
      burning by engine, locomotive, train (*see
        also* Explosion, railway engine)
        E803 ☑4ᵗʰ
      collision (*see also* Collision, railway)
        E800 ☑4ᵗʰ
      derailment (*see also* Derailment, railway)
        E802 ☑4ᵗʰ

Accident (to) — *continued*
  railway — *continued*
    involving — *continued*
      explosion (*see also* Explosion, railway
        engine) E803 ☑4ᵗʰ
      fall (*see also* Fall, from, railway rolling
        stock) E804 ☑4ᵗʰ
      fire (*see also* Explosion, railway engine)
        E803 ☑4ᵗʰ
      hitting by, being struck by
        object falling in, on, from, rolling
          stock, train, vehicle E806 ☑4ᵗʰ
        rolling stock, train, vehicle E805 ☑4ᵗʰ
      overturning, railway rolling stock, train,
        vehicle (*see also* Derailment,
        railway) E802 ☑4ᵗʰ
      running off rails, railway (*see also*
        Derailment, railway) E802 ☑4ᵗʰ
      specified circumstances NEC E806 ☑4ᵗʰ
      train or vehicle hit by
        avalanche E909 ☑4ᵗʰ
        falling object (earth, rock, tree) E806 ☑4ᵗʰ
          due to cataclysm — *see* categories
            E908 ☑4ᵗʰ, E909 ☑4ᵗʰ
        landslide E909 ☑4ᵗʰ
  roller skate E885.1
  scooter (nonmotorized) E885.0 ●
  skateboard E885.2
  ski(ing) E885.3
    jump E884.9
    lift or tow (with chair or gondola) E847
  snow vehicle, motor driven (not on public
    highway) E820 ☑4ᵗʰ
    on public highway — *see* categories E810-
      E819 ☑4ᵗʰ
  snowboard E885.4
  spacecraft E845 ☑4ᵗʰ
  specified cause NEC E928.8
  street car E829 ☑4ᵗʰ
  traffic NEC E819 ☑4ᵗʰ
  vehicle NEC (with pedestrian) E848
    battery powered
      airport passenger vehicle E846
      truck (baggage) (mail) E846
    powered commercial or industrial (with
      other vehicle or object within
      commercial or industrial premises)
      E846
  watercraft E838 ☑4ᵗʰ
    with
      drowning or submersion resulting from
        accident other than to watercraft
        E832 ☑4ᵗʰ
        accident to watercraft E830 ☑4ᵗʰ
      injury, except drowning or submersion,
        resulting from
        accident other than to watercraft —
          see categories E833-E838 ☑4ᵗʰ
        accident to watercraft E831 ☑4ᵗʰ
    due to, caused by cataclysm — *see*
      categories E908 ☑4ᵗʰ, E909 ☑4ᵗʰ
    machinery E836 ☑4ᵗʰ

Acid throwing E961

Acosta syndrome E902.0

Aeroneurosis E902.1

Aero-otitis media — *see* Effects of, air pressure

Aerosinusitis — *see* Effects of, air pressure

After-effect, late — *see* Late effect

Air
  blast
    in
      terrorism E979.2
      war operations E993 ●
  embolism (traumatic) NEC E928.9
    in
      infusion or transfusion E874.1
      perfusion E874.2
  sickness E903

Alpine sickness E902.0

Altitude sickness — *see* Effects of, air pressure

Anaphylactic shock, anaphylaxis (*see also* Table
  of Drugs and Chemicals) E947.9
  due to bite or sting (venomous) — *see* Bite,
    venomous

Andes disease E902.0

Apoplexy
  heat — *see* Heat

Arachnidism E905.1

Arson E968.0

Asphyxia, asphyxiation
  by
    chemical
      in
        terrorism E979.7
        war operations E997.2
    explosion — *see* Explosion
    food (bone) (regurgitated food) (seed) E911
    foreign object, except food E912
    fumes
      in
        terrorism (chemical weapons) E979.7
        war operations E997.2
    gas — *see also* Table of Drugs and Chemicals
      in
        terrorism E979.7
        war operations E997.2
      legal
        execution E978
        intervention (tear) E972
      tear E972
    mechanical means (*see also* Suffocation) E913.9
  from
    conflagration — *see* Conflagration
    fire — *see also* Fire E899
      in
        terrorism E979.3
        war operations E990.9
    ignition — *see* Ignition

Aspiration
  foreign body — *see* Foreign body, aspiration
  mucus, not of newborn (with asphyxia, obstruction respiratory passage, suffocation) E912
  phlegm (with asphyxia, obstruction respiratory passage, suffocation) E912
  vomitus (with asphyxia, obstruction respiratory passage, suffocation) (*see also* Foreign body, aspiration, food) E911

Assassination (attempt) (*see also* Assault) E968.9

Assault (homicidal) (by) (in) E968.9
  acid E961
    swallowed E962.1
  air gun E968.6
  BB gun E968.6
  bite NEC E968.8
    of human being E968.7
  bomb ((placed in) car or house) E965.8
    antipersonnel E965.5
    letter E965.7
    petrol E965.7
  brawl (hand) (fists) (foot) E960.0
  burning, burns (by fire) E968.0
    acid E961
      swallowed E962.1
    caustic, corrosive substance E961
      swallowed E962.1
    chemical from swallowing caustic, corrosive substance NEC E962.1
    hot liquid E968.3
    scalding E968.3
    vitriol E961
      swallowed E962.1
  caustic, corrosive substance E961
    swallowed E962.1
  cut, any part of body E966
  dagger E966
  drowning E964
  explosive(s) E965.9
    bomb (*see also* Assault, bomb) E965.8
    dynamite E965.8
  fight (hand) (fists) (foot) E960.0
    with weapon E968.9
      blunt or thrown E968.2
      cutting or piercing E966
      firearm — *see* Shooting, homicide
  fire E968.0
  firearm(s) — *see* Shooting, homicide

Assault — *continued*
  garrotting E963
  gunshot (wound) — *see* Shooting, homicide
  hanging E963
  injury NEC E968.9
  knife E966
  late effect of E969
  ligature E963
  poisoning E962.9
    drugs or medicinals E962.0
    gas(es) or vapors, except drugs and medicinals E962.2
    solid or liquid substances, except drugs and medicinals E962.1
  puncture, any part of body E966
  pushing
    before moving object, train, vehicle E968.5
    from high place E968.1
  rape E960.1
  scalding E968.3
  shooting — *see* Shooting, homicide
  sodomy E960.1
  stab, any part of body E966
  strangulation E963
  submersion E964
  suffocation E963
  transport vehicle E968.5
  violence NEC E968.9
  vitriol E961
    swallowed E962.1
  weapon E968.9
    blunt or thrown E968.2
    cutting or piercing E966
    firearm — *see* Shooting, homicide
  wound E968.9
    cutting E966
    gunshot — *see* Shooting, homicide
    knife E966
    piercing E966
    puncture E966
    stab E966

Attack by animal NEC E906.9

Avalanche E909.2
  falling on or hitting
    motor vehicle (in motion) (on public highway) E909.2
    railway train E909.2

Aviators' disease E902.1

B

Barotitis, barodontalgia, barosinusitis, barotrauma (otitic) (sinus) — *see* Effects of, air pressure

Battered
  baby or child (syndrome) — *see* Abuse, child; category E967
  person other than baby or child — *see* Assault

Bayonet wound (*see also* Cut, by bayonet) E920.3
  in
    legal intervention E974
    terrorism E979.8
    war operations E995

Bean in nose E912

Bed set on fire NEC E898.0

Beheading (by guillotine)
  homicide E966
  legal execution E978

Bending, injury in E927

Bends E902.0

Bite
  animal (nonvenomous) NEC E906.5
    other specified (except arthropod) E906.3
    venomous NEC E905.9
  arthropod (nonvenomous) NEC E906.4
    venomous — *see* Sting
  black widow spider E905.1
  cat E906.3
  centipede E905.4
  cobra E905.0
  copperhead snake E905.0
  coral snake E905.0
  dog E906.0
  fer de lance E905.0
  gila monster E905.0

Bite — *continued*
  human being
    accidental E928.3
    assault E968.7
  insect (nonvenomous) E906.4
    venomous — *see* Sting
  krait E905.0
  late effect of — *see* Late effect
  lizard E906.2
    venomous E905.0
  mamba E905.0
  marine animal
    nonvenomous E906.3
      snake E906.2
    venomous E905.6
      snake E905.0
  millipede E906.4
    venomous E905.4
  moray eel E906.3
  rat E906.1
  rattlesnake E905.0
  rodent, except rat E906.3
  serpent — *see* Bite, snake
  shark E906.3
  snake (venomous) E905.0
    nonvenomous E906.2
    sea E905.0
  spider E905.1
    nonvenomous E906.4
  tarantula (venomous) E905.1
  venomous NEC E905.9
    by specific animal — *see category* E905
  viper E905.0
  water moccasin E905.0

Blast (air)
  from nuclear explosion E996
  in
    terrorism E979.2
      from nuclear explosion E979.5
      underwater E979.0
    war operations E993
      from nuclear explosion E996
      underwater E992
  underwater E992

Blizzard E908.3

Blow E928.9
  by law-enforcing agent, police (on duty) E975
    with blunt object (baton) (nightstick) (stave) (truncheon) E973

Blowing up (*see also* Explosion) E923.9

Brawl (hand) (fists) (foot) E960.0

Breakage (accidental)
  cable of cable car not on rails E847
  ladder (causing fall) E881.0
  part (any) of
    animal-drawn vehicle E827
    ladder (causing fall) E881.0
    motor vehicle
      in motion (on public highway) E818
        not on public highway E825
    nonmotor road vehicle, except animal-drawn vehicle or pedal cycle E829
    off-road type motor vehicle (not on public highway) NEC E821
      on public highway E818
    pedal cycle E826
    scaffolding (causing fall) E881.1
    snow vehicle, motor-driven (not on public highway) E820
      on public highway E818
    vehicle NEC — *see* Accident, vehicle

Broken
  glass
    fall on E888.0
    injury by E920.8
  power line (causing electric shock) E925.1

Bumping against, into (accidentally)
  object (moving) E917.9
    caused by crowd E917.1
      with subsequent fall E917.6
    furniture E917.3
      with subsequent fall E917.7
    in
      running water E917.2
      sports E917.0
        with subsequent fall E917.5

Bumping against, into — *continued*
  object — *continued*
    stationary E917.4
      with subsequent fall E917.8
    person(s) E917.9
      with fall E886.9
        in sports E886.0
      as, or caused by, a crowd E917.1
        with subsequent fall E917.6
      in sports E917.0
        with fall E886.0

Burning, burns (accidental) (by) (from) (on) E899
  acid (any kind) E924.1
    swallowed — *see* Table of Drugs and Chemicals
  bedclothes (*see also* Fire, specified NEC) E898.0
  blowlamp (*see also* Fire, specified NEC) E898.1
  blowtorch (*see also* Fire, specified NEC) E898.1
  boat, ship, watercraft — *see* categories E830 ☑4ᵗʰ, E831 ☑4ᵗʰ, E837 ☑4ᵗʰ
  bonfire (controlled) E897
    uncontrolled E892
  candle (*see also* Fire, specified NEC) E898.1
  caustic liquid, substance E924.1
    swallowed — *see* Table of Drugs and Chemicals
  chemical E924.1
    from swallowing caustic, corrosive substance — *see* Table of Drugs and Chemicals
    in
      terrorism E979.7
      war operations E997.2
  cigar(s) or cigarette(s) (*see also* Fire, specified NEC) E898.1
  clothes, clothing, nightdress — *see* Ignition, clothes
    with conflagration — *see* Conflagration
  conflagration — *see* Conflagration
  corrosive liquid, substance E924.1
    swallowed — *see* Table of Drugs and Chemicals
  electric current (*see also* Electric shock) E925.9
  fire, flames (*see also* Fire) E899
  flare, Verey pistol E922.8
  heat
    from appliance (electrical) E924.8
    in local application, or packing during medical or surgical procedure E873.5
  homicide (attempt) (*see also* Assault, burning) E968.0
  hot
    liquid E924.0
      caustic or corrosive E924.1
    object (not producing fire or flames) E924.8
    substance E924.9
      caustic or corrosive E924.1
      liquid (metal) NEC E924.0
      specified type NEC E924.8
    tap water E924.2
  ignition — *see* Ignition
    clothes, clothing, nightdress — *see also* Ignition, clothes
      with conflagration — *see* Conflagration
    highly inflammable material (benzine) (fat) (gasoline) (kerosene) (paraffin) (petrol) E894
  inflicted by other person
    stated as
      homicidal, intentional (*see also* Assault, burning) E968.0
      undetermined whether accidental or intentional (*see also* Burn, stated as undetermined whether accidental or intentional) E988.1
  internal, from swallowed caustic, corrosive liquid, substance — *see* Table of Drugs and Chemicals
  in
    terrorism E979.3
      from nuclear explosion E979.5
      petrol bomb E979.3

Burning, burns — *continued*
  in — *continued*
    war operations (from fire-producing device or conventional weapon) E990.9
      from nuclear explosion E996
      petrol bomb E990.0
  lamp (*see also* Fire, specified NEC) E898.1
  late effect of NEC E929.4
  lighter (cigar) (cigarette) (*see also* Fire, specified NEC) E898.1
  lightning E907
  liquid (boiling) (hot) (molten) E924.0
    caustic, corrosive (external) E924.1
      swallowed — *see* Table of Drugs and Chemicals
  local application of externally applied substance in medical or surgical care E873.5
  machinery — *see* Accident, machine
  matches (*see also* Fire, specified NEC) E898.1
  medicament, externally applied E873.5
  metal, molten E924.0
  object (hot) E924.8
    producing fire or flames — *see* Fire
  oven (electric) (gas) E924.8
  pipe (smoking) (*see also* Fire, specified NEC) E898.1
  radiation — *see* Radiation
  railway engine, locomotive, train (*see also* Explosion, railway engine) E803 ☑4ᵗʰ
  self-inflicted (unspecified whether accidental or intentional) E988.1
    caustic or corrosive substance NEC E988.7
    stated as intentional, purposeful E958.1
      caustic or corrosive substance NEC E958.7
    stated as undetermined whether accidental or intentional E988.1
      caustic or corrosive substance NEC E988.7
  steam E924.0
    pipe E924.8
  substance (hot) E924.9
    boiling or molten E924.0
    caustic, corrosive (external) E924.1
      swallowed — *see* Table of Drugs and Chemicals
  suicidal (attempt) NEC E958.1
    caustic substance E958.7
    late effect of E959
  tanning bed E926.2
  therapeutic misadventure
    overdose of radiation E873.2
  torch, welding (*see also* Fire, specified NEC) E898.1
  trash fire (*see also* Burning, bonfire) E897
  vapor E924.0
  vitriol E924.1
  x-rays E926.3
    in medical, surgical procedure — *see* Misadventure, failure, in dosage, radiation

Butted by animal E906.8

Cachexia, lead or saturnine E866.0
  from pesticide NEC (*see also* Table of Drugs and Chemicals) E863.4
Caisson disease E902.2
Capital punishment (any means) E978
Car sickness E903
Casualty (not due to war) NEC E928.9
  terrorism E979.8
  war (*see also* War operations) E995
Cat
  bite E906.3
  scratch E906.8
Cataclysmic (any injury)
  earth surface movement or eruption E909.9
    specified type NEC E909.8
  storm or flood resulting from storm E908.9
    specified type NEC E909.8
Catching fire — *see* Ignition

Caught
  between
    objects (moving) (stationary and moving) E918
    and machinery — *see* Accident, machine
  by cable car, not on rails E847
  in
    machinery (moving parts of) — *see*, Accident, machine
    object E918
Cave-in (causing asphyxia, suffocation (by pressure)) (*see also* Suffocation, due to, cave-in) E913.3
  with injury other than asphyxia or suffocation E916
    with asphyxia or suffocation (*see also* Suffocation, due to, cave-in) E913.3
  struck or crushed by E916
    with asphyxia or suffocation (*see also* Suffocation, due to, cave-in) E913.3
Change(s) in air pressure — *see also* Effects of, air pressure
  sudden, in aircraft (ascent) (descent) (causing aeroneurosis or aviators' disease) E902.1
Chilblains E901.0
  due to manmade conditions E901.1
Choking (on) (any object except food or vomitus) E912
  apple E911
  bone E911
  food, any type (regurgitated) E911
  mucus or phlegm E912
  seed E911
Civil insurrection — *see* War operations
Cloudburst E908.8
Cold, exposure to (accidental) (excessive) (extreme) (place) E901.9
  causing chilblains or immersion foot E901.0
  due to
    manmade conditions E901.1
    specified cause NEC E901.8
    weather (conditions) E901.0
  late effect of NEC E929.5
  self-inflicted (undetermined whether accidental or intentional) E988.3
    suicidal E958.3
  suicide E958.3
Colic, lead, painter's, or saturnine — *see* category E866 ☑4ᵗʰ
Collapse
  building (moveable) E916
    burning ▶(uncontrolled fire)◀ E891.8
      in terrorism E979.3
      private E890.8
  dam E909.3
  due to heat — *see* Heat
  machinery — *see* Accident, machine
  man-made structure E909.3
  postoperative NEC E878.9
  structure, burning NEC E891.8
    burning (uncontrolled fire)
      in terrorism E979.3

Collision (accidental)

> *Note* — *In the case of collisions between different types of vehicles, persons and objects, priority in classification is in the following order:*
>
> > *Aircraft*
> >
> > *Watercraft*
> >
> > *Motor vehicle*
> >
> > *Railway vehicle*
> >
> > *Pedal cycle*
> >
> > *Animal-drawn vehicle*
> >
> > *Animal being ridden*
> >
> > *Streetcar or other nonmotor road vehicle*
> >
> > *Other vehicle*
> >
> > *Pedestrian or person using pedestrian conveyance*
> >
> > *Object (except where falling from or set in motion by vehicle etc. listed above)*
>
> *In the listing below, the combinations are listed only under the vehicle etc. having priority. For definitions, see Volume 1, page 247.*

aircraft (with object or vehicle) (fixed) (movable) (moving) E841 ✓4th
  with
    person (while landing, taking off) (without accident to aircraft) E844 ✓4th
    powered (in transit) (with unpowered aircraft) E841 ✓4th
    while landing, taking off E840 ✓4th
    unpowered E842 ✓4th
    while landing, taking off E840 ✓4th
animal being ridden (in sport or transport) E828 ✓4th
  and
    animal (being ridden) (herded) (unattended) E828 ✓4th
    nonmotor road vehicle, except pedal cycle or animal-drawn vehicle E828 ✓4th
    object (fallen) (fixed) (movable) (moving) not falling from or set in motion by vehicle of higher priority E828 ✓4th
    pedestrian (conveyance or vehicle) E828 ✓4th
animal-drawn vehicle E827 ✓4th
  and
    animal (being ridden) (herded) (unattended) E827 ✓4th
    nonmotor road vehicle, except pedal cycle E827 ✓4th
    object (fallen) (fixed) (movable) (moving) not falling from or set in motion by vehicle of higher priority E827 ✓4th
    pedestrian (conveyance or vehicle) E827 ✓4th
    streetcar E827 ✓4th
motor vehicle (on public highway) (traffic accident) E812 ✓4th
  after leaving, running off, public highway (without antecedent collision) (without re-entry) E816 ✓4th
  with antecedent collision on public highway — *see* categories E810-E815 ✓4th
  with re-entrance collision with another motor vehicle E811 ✓4th
  and
    abutment (bridge) (overpass) E815 ✓4th
    animal (herded) (unattended) E815 ✓4th
    carrying person, property E813 ✓4th
    animal-drawn vehicle E813 ✓4th
    another motor vehicle (abandoned) (disabled) (parked) (stalled) (stopped) E812 ✓4th

Collision — *continued*
  motor vehicle — *continued*
    and — *continued*
      another motor vehicle — *continued*
        with, involving re-entrance (on same roadway) (across median strip) E811 ✓4th
      any object, person, or vehicle off the public highway resulting from a noncollision motor vehicle nontraffic accident E816 ✓4th
      avalanche, fallen or not moving E815 ✓4th
        falling E909 ✓4th
      boundary fence E815 ✓4th
      culvert E815 ✓4th
      fallen
        stone E815 ✓4th
        tree E815 ✓4th
      falling E909.2
      guard post or guard rail E815 ✓4th
      inter-highway divider E815 ✓4th
      landslide, fallen or not moving E815 ✓4th
        moving E909 ✓4th
      machinery (road) E815 ✓4th
      moving E909.2
      nonmotor road vehicle NEC E813 ✓4th
      object (any object, person, or vehicle off the public highway resulting from a noncollision motor vehicle nontraffic accident) E815 ✓4th
        off, normally not on, public highway resulting from a noncollision motor vehicle traffic accident E816 ✓4th
      pedal cycle E813 ✓4th
      pedestrian (conveyance) E814 ✓4th
      person (using pedestrian conveyance) E814 ✓4th
      post or pole (lamp) (light) (signal) (telephone) (utility) E815 ✓4th
      railway rolling stock, train, vehicle E810 ✓4th
      safety island E815 ✓4th
      street car E813 ✓4th
      traffic signal, sign, or marker (temporary) E815 ✓4th
      tree E815 ✓4th
      tricycle E813 ✓4th
      wall of cut made for road E815 ✓4th
    due to cataclysm — *see* categories E908 ✓4th, E909 ✓4th
    not on public highway, nontraffic accident E822 ✓4th
    and
      animal (carrying person, property) (herded) (unattended) E822 ✓4th
      animal-drawn vehicle E822 ✓4th
      another motor vehicle (moving), except off-road motor vehicle E822 ✓4th
        stationary E823 ✓4th
      avalanche, fallen, not moving E823 ✓4th
        moving E909 ✓4th
      landslide, fallen, not moving E823 ✓4th
        moving E909 ✓4th
      nonmotor vehicle (moving) E822 ✓4th
        stationary E823 ✓4th
      object (fallen) (normally) (fixed) (movable but not in motion) (stationary) E823 ✓4th
        moving, except when falling from, set in motion by, aircraft or cataclysm E822 ✓4th
      pedal cycle (moving) E822 ✓4th
        stationary E823 ✓4th
      pedestrian (conveyance) E822 ✓4th
      person (using pedestrian conveyance) E822 ✓4th
      railway rolling stock, train, vehicle (moving) E822 ✓4th
        stationary E823 ✓4th
      road vehicle (any) (moving) E822 ✓4th
        stationary E823 ✓4th
      tricycle (moving) E822 ✓4th
        stationary E823 ✓4th
    moving E909.2

Collision — *continued*
  off-road type motor vehicle (not on public highway) E821 ✓4th
  and
    animal (being ridden) (-drawn vehicle) E821 ✓4th
    another off-road motor vehicle, except snow vehicle E821 ✓4th
    other motor vehicle, not on public highway E821 ✓4th
    other object or vehicle NEC, fixed or movable, not set in motion by aircraft, motor vehicle on highway, or snow vehicle, motor driven E821 ✓4th
    pedal cycle E821 ✓4th
    pedestrian (conveyance) E821 ✓4th
    railway train E821 ✓4th
  on public highway — *see* Collision, motor vehicle
  pedal cycle E826 ✓4th
  and
    animal (carrying person, property) (herded) (unherded) E826 ✓4th
    animal-drawn vehicle E826 ✓4th
    another pedal cycle E826 ✓4th
    nonmotor road vehicle E826 ✓4th
    object (fallen) (fixed) (movable) (moving) not falling from or set in motion by aircraft, motor vehicle, or railway train NEC E826 ✓4th
    pedestrian (conveyance) E826 ✓4th
    person (using pedestrian conveyance) E826 ✓4th
    street car E826 ✓4th
  pedestrian(s) (conveyance) E917.9
  with fall E886.9
    in sports E886.0
  and
    crowd, human stampede E917.1
      with subsequent fall E917.6
    furniture E917.3
      with subsequent fall E917.7
    machinery — *see* Accident, machine
    object (fallen) (moving) not falling from NEC, fixed or set in motion by any vehicle classifiable to E800-E848 E917.9
      with subsequent fall E917.6
      caused by a crowd E917.1
        with subsequent fall E917.6
      furniture E917.3
        with subsequent fall E917.7
      in
        running water E917.2
          with drowning or submersion — *see* Submersion
        sports E917.0
          with subsequent fall E917.5
        stationary E917.4
          with subsequent fall E917.8
    vehicle, nonmotor, nonroad E848
  in
    running water E917.2
      with drowning or submersion — *see* Submersion
    sports E917.0
      with fall E886.0
  person(s) (using pedestrian conveyance) (*see also* Collision, pedestrian) E917.9
  railway (rolling stock) (train) (vehicle) (with (subsequent) derailment, explosion, fall or fire) E800 ✓4th
  with antecedent derailment E802 ✓4th
  and
    animal (carrying person) (herded) (unattended) E801 ✓4th
    another railway train or vehicle E800 ✓4th
    buffers E801 ✓4th
    fallen tree on railway E801 ✓4th
    farm machinery, nonmotor (in transport) (stationary) E801 ✓4th
    gates E801 ✓4th
    nonmotor vehicle E801 ✓4th

Collision — Cut

Collision — *continued*
  railway — *continued*
    and — *continued*
      object (fallen) (fixed) (movable) (moving)
        not falling from, set in motion by,
        aircraft or motor vehicle NEC
        E801 ✓4th
      pedal cycle E801 ✓4th
      pedestrian (conveyance) E805 ✓4th
      person (using pedestrian conveyance)
        E805 ✓4th
      platform E801 ✓4th
      rock on railway E801 ✓4th
      street car E801 ✓4th
  snow vehicle, motor-driven (not on public
    highway) E820 ✓4th
    and
      animal (being ridden) (-drawn vehicle)
        E820 ✓4th
      another off-road motor vehicle E820 ✓4th
      other motor vehicle, not on public
        highway E820 ✓4th
      other object or vehicle NEC, fixed or
        movable, not set in motion by
        aircraft or motor vehicle on highway
        E820 ✓4th
      pedal cycle E820 ✓4th
      pedestrian (conveyance) E820 ✓4th
      railway train E820 ✓4th
    on public highway — *see* Collision, motor
      vehicle
  street car(s) E829 ✓4th
    and
      animal, herded, not being ridden,
        unattended E829 ✓4th
      nonmotor road vehicle NEC E829 ✓4th
      object (fallen) (fixed) (movable) (moving)
        not falling from or set in motion by
        aircraft, animal-drawn vehicle,
        animal being ridden, motor vehicle,
        pedal cycle, or railway train
        E829 ✓4th
      pedestrian (conveyance) E829 ✓4th
      person (using pedestrian conveyance)
        E829 ✓4th
  vehicle
    animal-drawn — *see* Collision, animal-
      drawn vehicle
    motor — *see* Collision, motor vehicle
    nonmotor
      nonroad E848
      and
        another nonmotor, nonroad vehicle
        E848
        object (fallen) (fixed) (movable)
          (moving) not falling from or
          set in motion by aircraft,
          animal-drawn vehicle, animal
          being ridden, motor vehicle,
          nonmotor road vehicle, pedal
          cycle, railway train, or
          streetcar E848
      road, except animal being ridden, animal-
        drawn vehicle, or pedal cycle
        E829 ✓4th
        and
          animal, herded, not being ridden,
            unattended E829 ✓4th
          another nonmotor road vehicle,
            except animal being ridden,
            animal-drawn vehicle, or
            pedal cycle E829 ✓4th
          object (fallen) (fixed) (movable)
            (moving) not falling from or
            set in motion by, aircraft,
            animal-drawn vehicle, animal
            being ridden, motor vehicle,
            pedal cycle, or railway train
            E829 ✓4th
          pedestrian (conveyance) E829 ✓4th
          person (using pedestrian
            conveyance) E829 ✓4th
          vehicle, nonmotor, nonroad
            E829 ✓4th

Collision — *continued*
  watercraft E838 ✓4th
    and
      person swimming or water skiing
        E838 ✓4th
    causing
      drowning, submersion E830 ✓4th
      injury except drowning, submersion
        E831 ✓4th
Combustion, spontaneous — *see* Ignition
Complication of medical or surgical procedure
  or treatment
  as an abnormal reaction — *see* Reaction,
    abnormal
  delayed, without mention of misadventure —
    see Reaction, abnormal
  due to misadventure — *see* Misadventure
Compression
  divers' squeeze E902.2
  trachea by
    food E911
    foreign body, except food E912
Conflagration
  building or structure, except private dwelling
    (barn) (church) (convalescent or
    residential home) (factory) (farm
    outbuilding) (hospital) (hotel) (institution
    (educational) (domitory) (residential))
    (school) (shop) (store) (theatre) E891.9
    with or causing (injury due to)
      accident or injury NEC E891.9
        specified circumstance NEC E891.8
      burns, burning E891.3
      carbon monoxide E891.2
      fumes E891.2
        polyvinylchloride (PVC) or similar
          material E891.1
      smoke E891.2
    causing explosion E891.0
    in terrorism E979.3
  not in building or structure E892
  private dwelling (apartment) (boarding house)
    (camping place) (caravan) (farmhouse)
    (home (private)) (house) (lodging house)
    (private garage) (rooming house)
    (tenement) E890.9
    with or causing (injury due to)
      accident or injury NEC E890.9
        specified circumstance NEC E890.8
      burns, burning E890.3
      carbon monoxide E890.2
      fumes E890.2
        polyvinylchloride (PVC) or similar
          material E890.1
      smoke E890.2
    causing explosion E890.0
Contact with
  dry ice E901.1
  liquid air, hydrogen, nitrogen E901.1
Cramp(s)
  Heat — *see* Heat
  swimmers (*see also* category E910 ✓4th) E910.2
    not in recreation or sport E910.3
Cranking (car) (truck) (bus) (engine), injury by
  E917.9
Crash
  aircraft (in transit) (powered) E841 ✓4th
    at landing, take-off E840 ✓4th
    in
      terrorism E979.1
      war operations E994
    on runway NEC E840 ✓4th
    stated as
      homicidal E968.8
      suicidal E958.6
      undetermined whether accidental or
        intentional E988.6
    unpowered E842 ✓4th
  glider E842 ✓4th
  motor vehicle — *see also* Accident, motor
    vehicle
    homicidal E968.5
    suicidal E958.5
    undetermined whether accidental or
      intentional E988.5

Crushed (accidentally) E928.9
  between
    boat(s), ship(s), watercraft (and dock or pier)
      (without accident to watercraft)
      E838 ✓4th
      after accident to, or collision, watercraft
        E831 ✓4th
    objects (moving) (stationary and moving)
      E918
  by
    avalanche NEC E909.2
    boat, ship, watercraft after accident to,
      collision, watercraft E831 ✓4th
    cave-in E916
      with asphyxiation or suffocation (*see also*
        Suffocation, due to, cave-in) E913.3
    crowd, human stampede E917.1
    falling
      aircraft (*see also* Accident, aircraft)
        E841 ✓4th
      in
        terrorism E979.1
        war operations E994
      earth, material E916
        with asphyxiation or suffocation (*see
          also* Suffocation, due to, cave-in)
          E913.3
      object E916
        on ship, watercraft E838 ✓4th
        while loading, unloading watercraft
          E838 ✓4th
    landslide NEC E909.2
    lifeboat after abandoning ship E831 ✓4th
    machinery — *see* Accident, machine
    railway rolling stock, train, vehicle (part of)
      E805 ✓4th
    street car E829 ✓4th
    vehicle NEC — *see* Accident, vehicle NEC
  in
    machinery — *see* Accident, machine
    object E918
    transport accident — *see* categories E800-
      E848 ✓4th
  late effect of NEC E929.9
Cut, cutting (any part of body) (accidental)
  E920.9
  by
    arrow E920.8
    axe E920.4
    bayonet (*see also* Bayonet wound) E920.3
    blender E920.2
    broken glass E920.8
      following fall E888.0
    can opener E920.4
      powered E920.2
    chisel E920.4
    circular saw E919.4
    cutting or piercing instrument — *see also*
      category E920 ✓4th
      following fall E888.0
      late effect of E929.8
    dagger E920.3
    dart E920.8
    drill — *see* Accident, caused by drill
    edge of stiff paper E920.8
    electric
      beater E920.2
      fan E920.2
      knife E920.2
      mixer E920.2
    fork E920.4
    garden fork E920.4
    hand saw or tool (not powered) E920.4
      powered E920.1
    hedge clipper E920.4
      powered E920.1
    hoe E920.4
    ice pick E920.4
    knife E920.3
      electric E920.2
    lathe turnings E920.8
    lawn mower E920.4
      powered E920.0
      riding E919.8
    machine — *see* Accident, machine
    meat
      grinder E919.8

Cut, cutting — *continued*
  by — *continued*
    meat — *continued*
      slicer E919.8
    nails E920.8
    needle E920.4
      hypodermic E920.5
    object, edged, pointed, sharp — *see* category
      E920 [✓4th]
      following fall E888.0
    paper cutter E920.4
    piercing instrument — *see also* category
      E920 [✓4th]
      late effect of E929.8
    pitchfork E920.4
    powered
      can opener E920.2
      garden cultivator E920.1
        riding E919.8
      hand saw E920.1
      hand tool NEC E920.1
      hedge clipper E920.1
      household appliance or implement
        E920.2
      lawn mower (hand) E920.0
        riding E919.8
      rivet gun E920.1
      staple gun E920.1
    rake E920.4
    saw
      circular E919.4
      hand E920.4
    scissors E920.4
    screwdriver E920.4
    sewing machine (electric) (powered) E920.2
      not powered E920.4
    shears E920.4
    shovel E920.4
    spade E920.4
    splinters E920.8
    sword E920.3
    tin can lid E920.8
    wood slivers E920.8
  homicide (attempt) E966
  inflicted by other person
    stated as
      intentional, homicidal E966
      undetermined whether accidental or
        intentional E986
  late effect of NEC E929.8
  legal
    execution E978
    intervention E974
  self-inflicted (unspecified whether accidental or
    intentional) E986
    stated as intentional, purposeful E956
    stated as undetermined whether accidental or
      intentional E986
  suicidal (attempt) E956
  terrorism E979.8
  war operations E995
Cyclone E908.1

<hr>

D

Death due to injury occurring one year or more
  previous — *see* Late effect
Decapitation (accidental circumstances) NEC
  E928.9
  homicidal E966
  legal execution (by guillotine) E978
Deprivation — *see also* Privation
  homicidal intent E968.4
Derailment (accidental)
  railway (rolling stock) (train) (vehicle) (with
    subsequent collision) E802 [✓4th]
    with
      collision (antecedent) (*see also* Collision,
        railway) E800 [✓4th]
      explosion (subsequent) (without
        antecedent collision) E802 [✓4th]
        antecedent collision E803 [✓4th]
      fall (without collision (antecedent))
        E802 [✓4th]

Derailment — *continued*
  railway — *continued*
    with — *continued*
      fire (without collision (antecedent))
        E802 [✓4th]
    street car E829 [✓4th]
Descent
  parachute (voluntary) (without accident to
    aircraft) E844 [✓4th]
    due to accident to aircraft — *see* categories
      E840-E842 [✓4th]
Desertion
  child, with intent to injure or kill E968.4
  helpless person, infant, newborn E904.0
    with intent to injure or kill E968.4
Destitution — *see* Privation
Disability, late effect or sequela of injury — *see*
  Late effect
Disease
  Andes E902.0
  aviators' E902.1
  caisson E902.2
  range E902.0
Divers' disease, palsy, paralysis, squeeze
  E902.0
Dog bite E906.0
Dragged by
  cable car (not on rails) E847
    on rails E829 [✓4th]
  motor vehicle (on highway) E814 [✓4th]
    not on highway, nontraffic accident E825 [✓4th]
  street car E829 [✓4th]
Drinking poison (accidental) — *see* Table of
  Drugs and Chemicals
Drowning — *see* Submersion
Dust in eye E914

<hr>

E

Earth falling (on) (with asphyxia or suffocation
  (by pressure)) (*see also* Suffocation, due to,
  cave-in) E913.3
  as, or due to, a cataclysm (involving any
    transport vehicle) — *see* categories
    E908 [✓4th], E909 [✓4th]
  not due to cataclysmic action E913.3
    motor vehicle (in motion) (on public
      highway) E810 [✓4th]
      not on public highway E825 [✓4th]
    nonmotor road vehicle NEC E829 [✓4th]
    pedal cycle E826 [✓4th]
    railway rolling stock, train, vehicle E806 [✓4th]
    street car E829 [✓4th]
  struck or crushed by E916
    with asphyxiation or suffocation E913.3
    with injury other than asphyxia,
      suffocation E916
Earthquake (any injury) E909.0
Effect(s) (adverse) of
  air pressure E902.9
    at high altitude E902.9
      in aircraft E902.1
      residence or prolonged visit (causing
        conditions classifiable to E902.0)
        E902.0
    due to
      diving E902.2
      specified cause NEC E902.8
    in aircraft E902.1
  cold, excessive (exposure to) (*see also* Cold,
    exposure to) E901.9
  heat (excessive) (*see also* Heat) E900.9
  hot
    place — *see* Heat
    weather E900.0
  insulation — *see* Heat
  late — *see* Late effect of
  motion E903
  nuclear explosion or weapon
    in
      terrorism E979.5
      war operations (blast) (fireball) (heat)
        (radiation) (direct) (secondary)
        E996

Effect(s) (adverse) of — *continued*
  radiation — *see* Radiation
  terrorism, secondary E979.9
  travel E903
Electric shock, electrocution (accidental) (from
  exposed wire, faulty appliance, high voltage
  cable, live rail, open socket) (by) (in) E925.9
  appliance or wiring
    domestic E925.0
    factory E925.2
    farm (building) E925.8
      house E925.0
    home E925.0
    industrial (conductor) (control apparatus)
      (transformer) E925.2
    outdoors E925.8
    public building E925.8
    residential institution E925.8
    school E925.8
    specified place NEC E925.8
  caused by other person
    stated as
      intentional, homicidal E968.8
      undetermined whether accidental or
        intentional E988.4
  electric power generating plant, distribution
    station E925.1
  homicidal (attempt) E968.8
  legal execution E978
  lightning E907
  machinery E925.9
    domestic E925.0
    factory E925.2
    farm E925.8
    home E925.0
  misadventure in medical or surgical procedure
    in electroshock therapy E873.4
  self-inflicted (undetermined whether accidental
    or intentional) E988.4
    stated as intentional E958.4
  stated as undetermined whether accidental or
    intentional E988.4
  suicidal (attempt) E958.4
  transmission line E925.1
Electrocution — *see* Electric shock
Embolism
  air (traumatic) NEC — *see* Air, embolism
Encephalitis
  lead or saturnine E866.0
    from pesticide NEC E863.4
Entanglement
  in
    bedclothes, causing suffocation E913.0
    wheel of pedal cycle E826 [✓4th]
Entry of foreign body, material, any — *see*
  Foreign body
Execution, legal (any method) E978
Exhaustion
  cold — *see* Cold, exposure to
  due to excessive exertion E927
  heat — *see* Heat
Explosion (accidental) (in) (of) (on) E923.9
  acetylene E923.2
  aerosol can E921.8
  aircraft (in transit) (powered) E841 [✓4th]
    at landing, take-off E840 [✓4th]
    in
      terrorism E979.1
      war operations E994
    unpowered E842 [✓4th]
  air tank (compressed) (in machinery) E921.1
  anesthetic gas in operating theatre E923.2
  automobile tire NEC E921.8
    causing transport accident — *see* categories
      E810-E825 [✓4th]
  blasting (cap) (materials) E923.1
  boiler (machinery), not on transport vehicle
    E921.0
    steamship — *see* Explosion, watercraft
  bomb E923.8
    in
      terrorism E979.2
      war operations E993
        after cessation of hostilities E998
        atom, hydrogen or nuclear E996

Cut — Explosion

Explosion — *continued*
  bomb — *continued*
    in — *continued*
      war operations — *continued*
        injury by fragments from E991.9
          antipersonnel bomb E991.3
  butane E923.2
  caused by
    other person
      stated as
        intentional, homicidal — *see* Assault,
          explosive
        undetermined whether accidental or
          homicidal E985.5
  coal gas E923.2
  detonator E923.1
  dyamite E923.1
  explosive (material) NEC E923.9
    gas(es) E923.2
    missile E923.8
      in
        terrorism E979.2
        war operations E993
          injury by fragments from E991.9
            antipersonnel bomb E991.3
    used in blasting operations E923.1
  fire-damp E923.2
  fireworks E923.0
  gas E923.2
    cylinder (in machinery) E921.1
    pressure tank (in machinery) E921.1
  gasoline (fumes) (tank) not in moving motor
    vehicle E923.2
  grain store (military) (munitions) E923.8
  grenade E923.8
    in
      terrorism E979.2
      war operations E993
        injury by fragments from E991.9
  homicide (attempt) — *see* Assault, explosive
  hot water heater, tank (in machinery) E921.0
  in mine (of explosive gases) NEC E923.2
  late effect of NEC E929.8
  machinery — *see also* Accident, machine
    pressure vessel — *see* Explosion, pressure
      vessel
  methane E923.2
  missile E923.8
    in
      terrorism E979.2
      war operations E993
        injury by fragments from E991.9
  motor vehicle (part of)
    in motion (on public highway) E818 ✓4th
      not on public highway E825 ✓4th
  munitions (dump) (factory) E923.8
    in
      terrorism E979.2
      war operations E993
  of mine E923.8
    in
      terrorism
        at sea or in harbor E979.0
        land E979.2
        marine E979.0
      war operations
        after cessation of hostilities E998
        at sea or in harbor E992
        land E993
          after cessation of hostilities E998
          injury by fragments from E991.9
        marine E992
  own weapons
    in
      terrorism (*see also* Suicide) E979.2
      war operations E993
        injury by fragments from E991.9
          antipersonnel bomb E991.3
      injury by fragments from E991.9
        antipersonnel bomb E991.3
  pressure
    cooker E921.8
    gas tank (in machinery) E921.1
    vessel (in machinery) E921.9
      on transport vehicle — *see* categories
        E800-E848 ✓4th
      specified type NEC E921.8

Explosion — *continued*
  propane E923.2
  railway engine, locomotive, train (boiler) (with
    subsequent collision, derailment, fall)
    E803 ✓4th
    with
      collision (antecedent) (*see also* Collision,
        railway) E800 ✓4th
      derailment (antecedent) E802 ✓4th
      fire (without antecedent collision or
        derailment) E803 ✓4th
  secondary fire resulting from — *see* Fire
  self-inflicted (unspecified whether accidental or
    intentional) E985.5
    stated as intentional, purposeful E955.5
  shell (artillery) E923.8
    in
      terrorism E979.2
      war operations E993
        injury by fragments from E991.9
  stated as undetermined whether caused
    accidentally or purposely inflicted E985.5
  steam or water lines (in machinery) E921.0
  suicide (attempted) E955.5
  terrorism — *see* Terrorism, explosion
  torpedo E923.8
    in
      terrorism E979.0
      war operations E992
  transport accident — *see* categories
    E800-E848 ✓4th
  war operations — *see* War operations,
    explosion
  watercraft (boiler) E837 ✓4th
    causing drowning, submersion (after
      jumping from watercraft) E830 ✓4th
Exposure (weather) (conditions) (rain) (wind)
  E904.3
  with homicidal intent E968.4
  excessive E904.3
    cold (*see also* Cold, exposure to) E901.9
      self-inflicted — *see* Cold, exposure to,
        self-inflicted
    heat (*see also* Heat) E900.9
  fire — *see* Fire
  helpless person, infant, newborn due to
    abandonment or neglect E904.0
  noise E928.1
  prolonged in deep-freeze unit or refrigerator
    E901.1
  radiation — *see* Radiation
  resulting from transport accident — *see*
    categories E800-E848 ✓4th
  smoke from, due to
    fire — *see* Fire
    tobacco, second-hand E869.4
  vibration E928.2

F

Fall, falling (accidental) E888.9
  building E916
    burning E891.8
      private E890.8
  down
    escalator E880.0
    ladder E881.0
      in boat, ship, watercraft E833 ✓4th
    staircase E880.9
    stairs, steps — *see* Fall, from, stairs
  earth (with asphyxia or suffocation (by
    pressure)) (*see also* Earth, falling) E913.3
  from, off
    aircraft (at landing, take-off) (in-transit)
      (while alighting, boarding) E843 ✓4th
      resulting from accident to aircraft — *see*
        categories E840-E842 ✓4th
    animal (in sport or transport) E828 ✓4th
    animal-drawn vehicle E827 ✓4th
    balcony E882
    bed E884.4
    bicycle E826 ✓4th
    boat, ship, watercraft (into water) E832 ✓4th
      after accident to, collision, fire on
        E830 ✓4th
      and subsequently struck by (part of)
        boat E831 ✓4th

Fall, falling — *continued*
  from, off — *continued*
    boat, ship, watercraft — *continued*
      and subsequently struck by (part of) boat
        E831 ✓4th
      burning, crushed, sinking E830 ✓4th
        and subsequently struck by (part of)
          boat E831 ✓4th
    bridge E882
    building E882
      burning ▶(uncontrolled fire)◀ E891.8
        in terrorism E979.3
      private E890.8
    bunk in boat, ship, watercraft E834 ✓4th
      due to accident to watercraft E831 ✓4th
    cable car (not on rails) E847
      on rails E829 ✓4th
    car — *see* Fall from motor vehicle
    chair E884.2
    cliff E884.1
    commode E884.6
    curb (sidewalk) E880.1
    elevation aboard ship E834 ✓4th
      due to accident to ship E831 ✓4th
    embankment E884.9
    escalator E880.0
    fire escape E882
    flagpole E882
    furniture NEC E884.5
    gangplank (into water) (*see also* Fall, from,
      boat) E832 ✓4th
      to deck, dock E834 ✓4th
    hammock on ship E834 ✓4th
      due to accident to watercraft E831 ✓4th
    haystack E884.9
    high place NEC E884.9
      stated as undetermined whether
        accidental or intentional — *see*
        Jumping, from, high place
    horse (in sport or transport) E828 ✓4th
    in-line skates E885.1
    ladder E881.0
      in boat, ship, watercraft E833 ✓4th
      due to accident to watercraft E831 ✓4th
    machinery — *see also* Accident, machine
      not in operation E884.9
    motor vehicle (in motion) (on public
      highway) E818 ✓4th
      not on public highway E825 ✓4th
        stationary, except while alighting,
          boarding, entering, leaving
          E884.9
        while alighting, boarding, entering,
          leaving E824 ✓4th
      stationary, except while alighting,
        boarding, entering, leaving E884.9
      while alighting, boarding, entering,
        leaving, except off-road type motor
        vehicle E817 ✓4th
      off-road type — *see* Fall, from, off-road
        type motor vehicle
    nonmotor road vehicle (while alighting,
      boarding) NEC E829 ✓4th
      stationary, except while alighting,
        boarding, entering, leaving E884.9
    off road type motor vehicle (not on public
      highway) NEC E821 ✓4th
      on public highway E818 ✓4th
        while alighting, boarding, entering,
          leaving E817 ✓4th
    snow vehicle — *see* Fall from snow
      vehicle, motor-driven
  one
    deck to another on ship E834 ✓4th
      due to accident to ship E831 ✓4th
    level to another NEC E884.9
      boat, ship, or watercraft E834 ✓4th
        due to accident to watercraft
          E831 ✓4th
  pedal cycle E826 ✓4th
  playground equipment E884.0
  railway rolling stock, train, vehicle, (while
    alighting, boarding) E804 ✓4th
    with
      collision (*see also* Collision, railway)
        E800 ✓4th

Explosion — Fall (side tab)

Fall, falling — *continued*
from, off — *continued*
   railway rolling stock, train, vehicle —
      continued
      with — *continued*
         derailment (*see also* Derailment,
           railway) E802 ✓4th
         explosion (*see also* Explosion, railway
           engine) E803 ✓4th
   rigging (aboard ship) E834 ✓4th
      due to accident to watercraft E831 ✓4th
   roller skates E885.1
   scaffolding E881.1
   scooter (nonmotorized) E885.0
   sidewalk (curb) E880.1
      moving E885.9
   skateboard E885.2
   skis E885.3
   snow vehicle, motor-driven (not on public
      highway) E820 ✓4th
      on public highway E818 ✓4th
         while alighting, boarding, entering,
           leaving E817 ✓4th
   snowboard E885.4
   stairs, step E880.9
      boat, ship, watercraft E833 ✓4th
         due to accident to watercraft E831 ✓4th
      motor bus, motor vehicle — *see* Fall,
         from, motor vehicle, while alighting,
         boarding
      street car E829 ✓4th
   stationary vehicle NEC E884.9
   stepladder E881.0
   street car (while boarding, alighting)
      E829 ✓4th
      stationary, except while boarding or
         alighting F884.9 ✓4th
   structure NEC E882
      burning ▶(uncontrolled fire)◀ E891.8
         in terrorism E979.3
   table E884.9
   toilet E884.6
   tower E882
   tree E884.9
   turret E882
   vehicle NEC — *see also* Accident, vehicle
      NEC
      stationary E884.9
   viaduct E882
   wall E882
   wheelchair E884.3
   window E882
in, on
   aircraft (at landing, take-off) (in-transit)
      E843 ✓4th
      resulting from accident to aircraft — *see*
         categories E840-E842 ✓4th
   boat, ship, watercraft E835 ✓4th
      due to accident to watercraft E831 ✓4th
      one level to another NEC E834 ✓4th
      on ladder, stairs E833 ✓4th
   cutting or piercing instrument or machine
      E888.0
   deck (of boat, ship, watercraft) E835 ✓4th
      due to accident to watercraft E831 ✓4th
   escalator E880.0
   gangplank E835 ✓4th
   glass, broken E888.0
   knife E888.0
   ladder E881.0
      in boat, ship, watercraft E833 ✓4th
         due to accident to watercraft E831 ✓4th
   object
      edged, pointed or sharp E888.0
      other E888.1
   pitchfork E888.0
   railway rolling stock, train, vehicle (while
      alighting, boarding) E804 ✓4th
      with
         collision (*see also* Collision, railway)
           E800 ✓4th
         derailment (*see also* Derailment,
           railway) E802 ✓4th
         explosion (*see also* Explosion, railway
           engine) E803 ✓4th
   scaffolding E881.1
   scissors E888.0

Fall, falling — *continued*
in, on — *continued*
   staircase, stairs, steps (*see also* Fall, from,
      stairs) E880.9
   street car E829 ✓4th
   water transport (*see also* Fall, in, boat)
      E835 ✓4th
into
   cavity E883.9
   dock E883.9
      from boat, ship, watercraft (*see also* Fall,
         from, boat) E832 ✓4th
   hold (of ship) E834 ✓4th
      due to accident to watercraft E831 ✓4th
   hole E883.9
   manhole E883.2
   moving part of machinery — *see* Accident,
      machine
   opening in surface NEC E883.9
   pit E883.9
   quarry E883.9
   shaft E883.9
   storm drain E883.2
   tank E883.9
   water (with drowning or submersion) E910.9
   well E883.1
late effect of NEC E929.3
object (*see also* Hit by, object, falling) E916
other E888.8
over
   animal E885.9
   cliff E884.1
   embankment E884.9
   small object E885
overboard (*see also* Fall, from, boat) E832 ✓4th
resulting in striking against object E888.1
   sharp E888.0
rock E916
same level NEC E888.9
   aircraft (any kind) E843 ✓4th
      resulting from accident to aircraft — *see*
         categories E840-E842 ✓4th
   boat, ship, watercraft E835 ✓4th
      due to accident to, collision, watercraft
         E831 ✓4th
   from
      collision, pushing, shoving, by or with
         other person(s) E886.9
         as, or caused by, a crowd E917.6
           in sports E886.0
      scooter (nonmotorized) E885.0
      slipping stumbling, tripping E885
snowslide E916
   as avalanche E909.2
stone E916
through
   hatch (on ship) E834 ✓4th
      due to accident to watercraft E831 ✓4th
   roof E882
   window E882
timber E916
while alighting from, boarding, entering, leaving
   aircraft (any kind) E843 ✓4th
   motor bus, motor vehicle — *see* Fall, from,
      motor vehicle, while alighting,
      boarding
   nonmotor road vehicle NEC E829 ✓4th
   railway train E804 ✓4th
   street car E829 ✓4th

Fallen on by
   animal (horse) (not being ridden) E906.8
      being ridden (in sport or transport) E828 ✓4th

Fell or jumped from high place, so stated —
   see Jumping, from, high place

Felo-de-se (*see also* Suicide) E958.9

Fever
   heat — *see* Heat
   thermic — *see* Heat

Fight (hand) (fist) (foot) (*see also* Assault, fight)
   E960.0

Fire (accidental) (caused by great heat from
   appliance (electrical), hot object or hot
   substance) (secondary, resulting from
   explosion) E899
   conflagration — *see* Conflagration

Fire — *continued*
   controlled, normal (in brazier, fireplace,
      furnace, or stove) (charcoal) (coal) (coke)
      (electric) (gas) (wood)
      bonfire E897
      brazier, not in building or structure E897
      in building or structure, except private
         dwelling (barn) (church) (convalescent
         or residential home) (factory) (farm
         outbuilding) (hospital) (hotel)
         (institution (educational) (dormitory)
         (residential)) (private garage) (school)
         (shop) (store) (theatre) E896
      in private dwelling (apartment) (boarding
         house) (camping place) (caravan)
         (farmhouse) (home (private)) (house)
         (lodging house) (rooming house)
         (tenement) E895
      not in building or structure E897
      trash E897
   forest (uncontrolled) E892
   grass (uncontrolled) E892
   hay (uncontrolled) E892
   homicide (attempt) E968.0
      late effect of E969
   in, of, on, starting in E892
      aircraft (in transit) (powered) E841 ✓4th
         at landing, take-off E840 ✓4th
         stationary E892
         unpowered (balloon) (glider) E842 ✓4th
      balloon E842 ✓4th
      boat, ship, watercraft — *see* categories
         E830 ✓4th, E831 ✓4th, E837 ✓4th
      building or structure, except private dwelling
         (barn) (church) (convalescent or
         residential home) (factory) (farm
         outbuilding) (hospital) (hotel)
         (institution (educational) (dormitory)
         (residential)) (school) (shop) (store)
         (theatre) (*see also* Conflagration,
         building or structure, except private
         dwelling) E891.9
      forest (uncontrolled) E892
      glider E842 ✓4th
      grass (uncontrolled) E892
      hay (uncontrolled) E892
      lumber (uncontrolled) E892
      machinery — *see* Accident, machine
      mine (uncontrolled) E892
      motor vehicle (in motion) (on public
         highway) E818 ✓4th
         not on public highway E825 ✓4th
         stationary E892
      prairie (uncontrolled) E892
      private dwelling (apartment) (boarding
         house) (camping place) (caravan)
         (farmhouse) (home (private)) (house)
         (lodging house) (private garage)
         (rooming house) (tenement) (*see also*
         Conflagration, private dwelling) E890.9
      railway rolling stock, train, vehicle (*see also*
         Explosion, railway engine) E803 ✓4th
         stationary E892
      room NEC E898.1
      street car (in motion) E829 ✓4th
         stationary E892
      terrorism (by fire-producing device)
         E979.3
         fittings or furniture (burning building)
           (uncontrolled fire) E979.3
         from nuclear explosion E979.5
      transport vehicle, stationary NEC E892
      tunnel (uncontrolled) E892
      war operations (by fire-producing device or
         conventional weapon) E990.9
         from nuclear explosion E996
         petrol bomb E990.0
   late effect of NEC E929.4
   lumber (uncontrolled) E892
   mine (uncontrolled) E892
   prairie (uncontrolled) E892
   self-inflicted (unspecified whether accidental or
      intentional) E988.1
      stated as intentional, purposeful E958.1
   specified NEC E898.1
      with
         conflagration — *see* Conflagration

*(side tab)* Fall — Fire

Fire — *continued*
  specified — *continued*
    with — *continued*
      ignition (of)
        clothing — *see* Ignition, clothes
        highly inflammable material (benzene)
          (fat) (gasoline) (kerosene)
          (paraffin) (petrol) E894
  started by other person
    stated as
      with intent to injure or kill E968.0
      undetermined whether or not with intent
        to injure or kill E988.1
  suicide (attempted) E958.1
    late effect of E959
  tunnel (uncontrolled) E892
Fireball effects from nuclear explosion
  in
    terrorism E979.5
    war operations E996
Fireworks (explosion) E923.0
Flash burns from explosion (*see also* Explosion)
  E923.9
Flood (any injury) (resulting from storm) E908.2
  caused by collapse of dam or manmade
    structure E909.3
Forced landing (aircraft) E840 ✓4ᵗʰ
Foreign body, object or material (entrance into
  (accidental))
  air passage (causing injury) E915
    with asphyxia, obstruction, suffocation E912
      food or vomitus E911
    nose (with asphyxia, obstruction,
      suffocation) E912
      causing injury without asphyxia,
        obstruction, suffocation E915
  alimentary canal (causing injury) (with
    obstruction) E915
    with asphyxia, obstruction respiratory
      passage, suffocation E912
      food E911
    mouth E915
      with asphyxia, obstruction, suffocation
        E912
        food E911
    pharynx E915
      with asphyxia, obstruction, suffocation
        E912
        food E911
  aspiration (with asphyxia, obstruction
    respiratory passage, suffocation) E912
    causing injury without asphyxia, obstruction
      respiratory passage, suffocation E915
    food (regurgitated) (vomited) E911
      causing injury without asphyxia,
        obstruction respiratory passage,
        suffocation E915
    mucus (not of newborn) E912
    phlegm E912
  bladder (causing injury or obstruction) E915
  bronchus, bronchi — *see* Foreign body, air
    passages
  conjunctival sac E914
  digestive system — *see* Foreign body,
    alimentary canal
  ear (causing injury or obstruction) E915
  esophagus (causing injury or obstruction) (*see
    also* Foreign body, alimentary canal)
    E915
  eye (any part) E914
  eyelid E914
  hairball (stomach) (with obstruction) E915
  ingestion — *see* Foreign body, alimentary canal
  inhalation — *see* Foreign body, aspiration
  intestine (causing injury or obstruction) E915
  iris E914
  lacrimal apparatus E914
  larynx — *see* Foreign body, air passage
  late effect of NEC E929.8
  lung — *see* Foreign body, air passage
  mouth — *see* Foreign body, alimentary canal,
    mouth
  nasal passage — *see* Foreign body, air passage,
    nose
  nose — *see* Foreign body, air passage, nose
  ocular muscle E914

Foreign body, object or material — *continued*
  operation wound (left in) — *see* Misadventure,
    foreign object
  orbit E914
  pharynx — *see* Foreign body, alimentary canal,
    pharynx
  rectum (causing injury or obstruction) E915
  stomach (hairball) (causing injury or
    obstruction) E915
  tear ducts or glands E914
  trachea — *see* Foreign body, air passage
  urethra (causing injury or obstruction) E915
  vagina (causing injury or obstruction) E915
Found dead, injured
  from exposure (to) — *see* Exposure
  on
    public highway E819 ✓4ᵗʰ
    railway right of way E807 ✓4ᵗʰ
Fracture (circumstances unknown or unspecified)
  E887
  due to specified external means — *see* manner
    of accident
  late effect of NEC E929.3
  occuring in water transport NEC E835 ✓4ᵗʰ
Freezing — *see* Cold, exposure to
Frostbite E901.0
  due to manmade conditions E901.1
Frozen — *see* Cold, exposure to

G

Garrotting, homicidal (attempted) E963
Gored E906.8
Gunshot wound (*see also* Shooting) E922.9

H

Hailstones, injury by E904.3
Hairball (stomach) (with obstruction) E915
Hanged himself (*see also* Hanging, self-inflicted)
  E983.0
Hang gliding E842 ✓4ᵗʰ
Hanging (accidental) E913.8
  caused by other person
    in accidental circumstances E913.8
    stated as
      intentional, homicidal E963
      undetermined whether accidental or
        intentional E983.0
  homicide (attempt) E963
  in bed or cradle E913.0
  legal execution E978
  self-inflicted (unspecified whether accidental or
    intentional) E983.0
    in accidental circumstances E913.8
    stated as intentional, purposeful E953.0
  stated as undetermined whether accidental or
    intentional E983.0
  suicidal (attempt) E953.0
Heat (apoplexy) (collapse) (cramps) (effects of)
  (excessive) (exhaustion) (fever) (prostration)
  (stroke) E900.9
  due to
    manmade conditions (as listed in E900.1,
      except boat, ship, watercraft) E900.1
    weather (conditions) E900.0
  from
    electric heating appartus causing burning
      E924.8
    nuclear explosion
      in
        terrorism E979.5
        war operations E996
  generated in, boiler, engine, evaporator, fire
    room of boat, ship, watercraft E838 ✓4ᵗʰ
  inappropriate in local application or packing in
    medical or surgical procedure E873.5
  late effect of NEC E989
Hemorrhage
  delayed following medical or surgical treatment
    without mention of misadventure — *see*
    Reaction, abnormal
  during medical or surgical treatment as
    misadventure — *see* Misadventure, cut

High
  altitude, effects E902.9
  level of radioactivity, effects — *see* Radiation
  pressure effects — *see also* Effects of, air
    pressure
    from rapid descent in water (causing caisson
      or divers' disease, palsy, or paralysis)
      E902.2
  temperature, effects — *see* Heat
Hit, hitting (accidental) by
  aircraft (propeller) (without accident to aircraft)
    E844 ✓4ᵗʰ
    unpowered E842 ✓4ᵗʰ
  avalanche E909.2
  being thrown against object in or part of
    motor vehicle (in motion) (on public
      highway) E818 ✓4ᵗʰ
      not on public highway E825 ✓4ᵗʰ
    nonmotor road vehicle NEC E829 ✓4ᵗʰ
    street car E829 ✓4ᵗʰ
  boat, ship, watercraft
    after fall from watercraft E838 ✓4ᵗʰ
      damaged, involved in accident E831 ✓4ᵗʰ
    while swimming, water skiing E838 ✓4ᵗʰ
  bullet (*see also* Shooting) E922.9
    from air gun E922.4
    in
      terrorism E979.4
      war operations E991.2
        rubber E991.0
  flare, Verey pistol (*see also* Shooting) E922.8
  hailstones E904.3
  landslide E909.2
  law-enforcing agent (on duty) E975
    with blunt object (baton) (night stick) (stave)
      (truncheon) E973
  machine — *see* Accident, machine
  missile
    firearm (*see also* Shooting) E922.9
    in
      terrorism — *see* Terrorism, mission
      war operations — *see* War operations,
        missile
  motor vehicle (on public highway) (traffic
    accident) E814 ✓4ᵗʰ
    not on public highway, nontraffic accident
      E822 ✓4ᵗʰ
  nonmotor road vehicle NEC E829 ✓4ᵗʰ
  object
    falling E916
      from, in, on
        aircraft E844 ✓4ᵗʰ
          due to accident to aircraft — *see*
            categories E840-E842 ✓4ᵗʰ
          unpowered E842 ✓4ᵗʰ
        boat, ship, watercraft E838 ✓4ᵗʰ
          due to accident to watercraft
          E831 ✓4ᵗʰ
        building E916
          burning (uncontrolled fire)
          E891.8
            in terrorism E979.3
            private E890.8
        cataclysmic
          earth surface movement or eruption
          E909.9
          storm E908.9
        cave-in E916
          with asphyxiation or suffocation
          (*see also* Suffocation, due to,
          cave-in) E913.3
        earthquake E909.0
        motor vehicle (in motion) (on public
          highway) E818 ✓4ᵗʰ
          not on public highway E825 ✓4ᵗʰ
          stationary E916
        nonmotor road vehicle NEC E829 ✓4ᵗʰ
        pedal cycle E826 ✓4ᵗʰ
        railway rolling stock, train, vehicle
          E806 ✓4ᵗʰ
        street car E829 ✓4ᵗʰ
        structure, burning NEC E891.8
        vehicle, stationary E916
    moving NEC — *see* Striking against, object
    projected NEC — *see* Striking against, object

Hit, hitting — *continued*
  object — *continued*
    set in motion by
      compressed air or gas, spring, striking,
        throwing — *see* Striking against,
        object
      explosion — *see* Explosion
    thrown into, on, or towards
      motor vehicle (in motion) (on public
        highway) E818 ✓4th
        not on public highway E825 ✓4th
      nonmotor road vehicle NEC E829 ✓4th
      pedal cycle E826 ✓4th
      street car E829 ✓4th
    off-road type motor vehicle (not on public
      highway) E821 ✓4th
    on public highway E814 ✓4th
  other person(s) E917.9
    with blunt or thrown object E917.9
      in sports E917.0
        with subsequent fall E917.5
      intentionally, homicidal E968.2
    as, or caused by, a crowd E917.1
      with subsequent fall E917.6
      in sports E917.0
  pedal cycle E826 ✓4th
  police (on duty) E975
    with blunt object (baton) (nightstick) (stave)
      (truncheon) E973
  railway, rolling stock, train, vehicle (part of)
    E805 ✓4th
  shot — *see* Shooting
  snow vehicle, motor-driven (not on public
    highway) E820 ✓4th
    on public highway E814 ✓4th
  street car E829 ✓4th
  vehicle NEC — *see* Accident, vehicle NEC
Homicide, homicidal (attempt) (justifiable) (*see also* Assault) E968.9
Hot
  liquid, object, substance, accident caused by —
    see also Accident, caused by, hot, by type
    of substance
    late effect of E929.8
  place, effects — *see* Heat
  weather, effects E900.0
Humidity, causing problem E904.3
Hunger E904.1
  resulting from
    abandonment or neglect E904.0
    transport accident — *see* categories E800-
      E848 ✓4th
Hurricane (any injury) E908.0
Hypobarism, hypobaropathy — *see* Effects of, air
  pressure
Hypothermia — *see* Cold, exposure to

I

Ictus
  caloris — *see* Heat
  solaris E900.0
Ignition (accidental)
  anesthetic gas in operating theatre E923.2
  bedclothes
    with
      conflagration — *see* Conflagration
      ignition (of)
        clothing — *see* Ignition, clothes
        highly inflammable material (benzine)
          (fat) (gasoline) (kerosene)
          (paraffin) (petrol) E894
  benzine E894
  clothes, clothing (from controlled fire) (in
    building) E893.9
    with conflagration — *see* Conflagration
    from
      bonfire E893.2
      highly inflammable material E894
      sources or material as listed in E893.8
      trash fire E893.2
      uncontrolled fire — *see* Conflagration

Ignition — *continued*
  clothes, clothing — *continued*
    in
      private dwelling E893.0
      specified building or structure, except
        private dwelling E893.1
    not in building or structure E893.2
  explosive material — *see* Explosion
  fat E894
  gasoline E894
  kerosene E894
  material
    explosive — *see* Explosion
    highly inflammable E894
      with conflagration — *see* Conflagration
      with explosion E923.2
  nightdress — *see* Ignition, clothes
  paraffin E894
  petrol E894
Immersion — *see* Submersion
Implantation of quills of porcupine E906.8
Inanition (from) E904.9
  hunger — *see* Lack of, food
  resulting from homicidal intent E968.4
  thirst — *see* Lack of, water
Inattention after, at birth E904.0
  homicidal, infanticidal intent E968.4
Infanticide (*see also* Assault)
Ingestion
  foreign body (causing injury) (with obstruction)
    — *see* Foreign body, alimentary canal
  poisonous substance NEC — *see* Table of
    Drugs and Chemicals
Inhalation
  excessively cold substance, manmade E901.1
  foreign body — *see* Foreign body, aspiration
  liquid air, hydrogen, nitrogen E901.1
  mucus, not of newborn (with asphyxia,
    obstruction respiratory passage,
    suffocation) E912
  phlegm (with asphyxia, obstruction respiratory
    passage, suffocation) E912
  poisonous gas — *see* Table of Drugs and
    Chemicals
  smoke from, due to
    fire — *see* Fire
    tobacco, second-hand E869.4
  vomitus (with asphyxia, obstruction respiratory
    passage, suffocation) E911
Injury, injured (accidental(ly)) NEC E928.9
  by, caused by, from
    air rifle (BB gun) E922.4
    animal (not being ridden) NEC E906.9
      being ridden (in sport or transport)
        E828 ✓4th
    assault (*see also* Assault) E968.9
    avalanche E909.2
    bayonet (*see also* Bayonet wound) E920.3
    being thrown against some part of, or object
      in
      motor vehicle (in motion) (on public
        highway) E818 ✓4th
        not on public highway E825 ✓4th
      nonmotor road vehicle NEC E829 ✓4th
      off-road motor vehicle NEC E821 ✓4th
      railway train E806 ✓4th
      snow vehicle, motor-driven E820 ✓4th
      street car E829 ✓4th
    bending E927
    broken glass E920.8
    bullet — *see* Shooting
    cave-in (*see also* Suffocation, due to, cave-
      in) E913.3
      earth surface movement or eruption
        E909.9
      earthquake E909.0
      flood E908.2
      hurricane E908.0
      landslide E909.2
      storm E908.9
      without asphyxiation or suffocation E916
    cloudburst E908.8
    cutting or piercing instrument (*see also* Cut)
      E920.9
    cyclone E908.1
    earth surface movement or eruption E909.9

Injury, injured — *continued*
  by, caused by, from — *continued*
    earthquake E909 ✓4th
    electric current (*see also* Electric shock)
      E925.9
    explosion (*see also* Explosion) E923.9
    fire — *see* Fire
    flare, Verey pistol E922.8
    flood E908
    foreign body — *see* Foreign body
    hailstones E904.3
    hurricane E908
    landslide E909 ✓4th
    law-enforcing agent, police, in course of legal
      intervention — *see* Legal intervention
    lightning E907
    live rail or live wire — *see* Electric shock
    machinery — *see also* Accident, machine
      aircraft, without accident to aircraft
        E844 ✓4th
      boat, ship, watercraft (deck) (engine
        room) (galley) (laundry) (loading)
        E836 ✓4th
    missile
      explosive E923.8
      firearm — *see* Shooting
      in
        terrorism — *see* Terrorism, missile ●
        war operations — *see* War
          operations, missile
    moving part of motor vehicle (in motion) (on
      public highway) E818 ✓4th
      not on public highway, nontraffic
        accident E825 ✓4th
      while alighting, boarding, entering,
        leaving — *see* Fall, from, motor
        vehicle, while alighting, boarding
    nail E920.8
    needle (sewing) E920.4
      hypodermic E920.5
    noise E928.1
    object
      fallen on
        motor vehicle (in motion) (on public
          highway) E818 ✓4th
          not on public highway E825 ✓4th
      falling — *see* Hit by, object, falling
    paintball gun E922.5 ●
    radiation — *see* Radiation
    railway rolling stock, train, vehicle (part of)
      E805 ✓4th
      door or window E806 ✓4th
    rotating propeller, aircraft E844 ✓4th
    rough landing of off-road type motor vehicle
      (after leaving ground or rough terrain)
      E821 ✓4th
    snow vehicle E820 ✓4th
    saber (*see also* Wound, saber) E920.3
    shot — *see* Shooting
    sound waves E928.1
    splinter or sliver, wood E920.8
    straining E927
    street car (door) E829 ✓4th
    suicide (attempt) E958.9
    sword E920.3
    terrorism — *see* Terrorism ●
    third rail — *see* Electric shock
    thunderbolt E907
    tidal wave E909.4
      caused by storm E908.0
    tornado E908.1
    torrential rain E908.2
    twisting E927
    vehicle NEC — *see* Accident, vehicle NEC
    vibration E928.2
    volcanic eruption E909.1
    weapon burst, in war operations E993
    weightlessness (in spacecraft, real or
      simulated) E928.0
    wood splinter or sliver E920.8
  due to
    civil insurrection — *see* War operations
      occurring after cessation of hostilities
      E998
    terrorism — *see* Terrorism ●

(side tab) **Hit — Injury**

Injury — Late effect

Injury, injured — *continued*
  due to — *continued*
    war operations — *see* War operations
      occurring after cessation of hostilities
      E998
  homicidal (*see also* Assault) E968.9
  in, on
    civil insurrection — *see* War operations
    fight E960.0
    parachute descent (voluntary) (without
      accident to aircraft) E844 ✓4ᵗʰ
      with accident to aircraft — *see* categories
      E840-E842 ✓4ᵗʰ
    public highway E819 ✓4ᵗʰ
    railway right of way E807 ✓4ᵗʰ
    terrorism — *see* Terrorism ●
    war operations — *see* War operations
  inflicted (by)
    in course of arrest (attempted), suppression
      of disturbance, maintenance of order,
      by law enforcing agents — *see* Legal
      intervention
    law-enforcing agent (on duty) — *see* Legal
      intervention
    other person
      stated as
        accidental E928.9
        homicidal, intentional — *see* Assault
        undetermined whether accidental or
          intentional — *see* Injury, stated
          as undetermined
    police (on duty) — *see* Legal intervention
  late effect of E929.9
  purposely (inflicted) by other person(s) — *see*
    Assault
  self-inflicted (unspecified whether accidental or
    intentional) E988.9
    stated as
      accidental E928.9
      intentionally, purposely E958.9
  specified cause NEC E928.8
  stated as
    undetermined whether accidentally or
      purposely inflicted (by) E988.9
      cut (any part of body) E986
      cutting or piercing instrument
        (classifiable to E920) E986
      drowning E984
      explosive(s) (missile) E985.5
      falling from high place E987.9
        manmade structure, except residential
          E987.1
        natural site E987.2
        residential premises E987.0
      hanging E983.0
      knife E986
      late effect of E989
      puncture (any part of body) E986
      shooting — *see* Shooting, stated as
        undetermined whether accidental or
        intentional
      specified means NEC E988.8
      stab (any part of body) E986
      strangulation — *see* Suffocation, stated as
        undetermined whether accidental or
        intentional
      submersion E984
      suffocation — *see* Suffocation, stated as
        undetermined whether accidental or
        intentional
  to child due to criminal abortion E968.8

Insufficient nourishment — *see also* Lack of,
  food
  homicidal intent E968.4

Insulation, effects — *see* Heat

Interruption of respiration by
  food lodged in esophagus E911
  foreign body, except food, in esophagus E912

Intervention, legal — *see* Legal intervention

Intoxication, drug or poison — *see* Table of
  Drugs and Chemicals

Irradiation — *see* Radiation

J

Jammed (accidentally)
  between objects (moving) (stationary and
    moving) E918
  in object E918

Jumped or fell from high place, so stated —
  see Jumping, from, high place, stated as
  in undetermined circumstances

Jumping
  before train, vehicle or other moving object
    (unspecified whether accidental or
    intentional) E988.0
    stated as
      intentional, purposeful E958.0
      suicidal (attempt) E958.0
  from
    aircraft
      by parachute (voluntarily) (without
        accident to aircraft) E844 ✓4ᵗʰ
      due to accident to aircraft — *see*
        categories E840-E842 ✓4ᵗʰ
    boat, ship, watercraft (into water)
      after accident to, fire on, watercraft
        E830 ✓4ᵗʰ
        and subsequently struck by (part of)
          boat E831 ✓4ᵗʰ
      burning, crushed, sinking E830 ✓4ᵗʰ
        and subsequently struck by (part of)
          boat E831 ✓4ᵗʰ
      voluntarily, without accident (to boat)
        with injury other than drowning or
          submersion E883.0
    building ▶— *see also* Jumping, from, high
      place◀
      burning ▶(uncontrolled fire)◀ E891.8
        in terrorism E979.3 ●
        private E890.8
    cable car (not on rails) E847
      on rails E829 ✓4ᵗʰ
    high place
      in accidental circumstances or in sport —
        see categories E880-E884 ✓4ᵗʰ
      stated as
        with intent to injure self E957.9
          man-made structures NEC E957.1
          natural sites E957.2
          residential premises E957.0
        in undetermined circumstances
          E987.9
          man-made structures NEC E987.1
          natural sites E987.2
          residential premises E987.0
        suicidal (attempt) E957.9
          man-made structures NEC E957.1
          natural sites E957.1
          residential premises E957.0
    motor vehicle (in motion) (on public
      highway) — *see* Fall, from, motor
      vehicle
    nonmotor road vehicle NEC E829 ✓4ᵗʰ
    street car E829 ✓4ᵗʰ
    structure ▶— *see also* Jumping, from, high
      place◀
      burning NEC (uncontrolled fire) ●
        E891.8 ●
        in terrorism E979.3 ●
  into water
    with injury other than drowning or
      submersion E883.0
    drowning or submersion — *see*
      Submersion
  from, off, watercraft — *see* Jumping, from,
    boat

Justifiable homicide — *see* Assault

K

Kicked by
  animal E906.8
  person(s) (accidentally) E917.9
    with intent to injure or kill E960.0
    as, or caused by a crowd E917.1
      with subsequent fall E917.6
    in fight E960.0

Kicked by — *continued*
  person(s) — *continued*
    in sports E917.0
      with subsequent fall E917.5

Kicking against
  object (moving) E917.9
    in sports E917.0
      with subsequent fall E917.5
    stationary E917.4
      with subsequent fall E917.8
  person — *see* Striking against, person

Killed, killing (accidentally) NEC (*see also* Injury)
  E928.9
  in
    action — *see* War operations
    brawl, fight (hand) (fists) (foot) E960.0
      by weapon — *see also* Assault
        cutting, piercing E966
        firearm — *see* Shooting, homicide
  self
    stated as
      accident E928.9
      suicide — *see* Suicide
    unspecified whether accidental or suicidal
      E988.9

Knocked down (accidentally) (by) NEC E928.9
  animal (not being ridden) E906.8
    being ridden (in sport or transport) E828 ✓4ᵗʰ
  blast from explosion (*see also* Explosion)
    E923.9
  crowd, human stampede E917.6
  late effect of — *see* Late effect
  person (accidentally) E917.9
    in brawl, fight E960.0
    in sports E917.5
  transport vehicle — *see* vehicle involved under
    Hit by
  while boxing E917.5

L

Laceration NEC E928.9

Lack of
  air (refrigerator or closed place), suffocation by
    E913.2
  care (helpless person) (infant) (newborn) E904.0
    homicidal intent E968.4
  food except as result of transport accident
    E904.1
    helpless person, infant, newborn due to
      abandonment or neglect E904.0
  water except as result of transport accident
    E904.2
    helpless person, infant, newborn due to
      abandonment or neglect E904.0

Landslide E909.2
  falling on, hitting
    motor vehicle (any) (in motion) (on or off
      public highway) E909.2
    railway rolling stock, train, vehicle E909.2

Late effect of
  accident NEC (accident classifiable to E928.9)
    E929.9
    specified NEC (accident classifiable to E910-
      E928.8) E929.8
  assault E969
  fall, accidental (accident classifiable to E880-
    E888) E929.3
  fire, accident caused by (accident classifiable to
    E890-E899) E929.4
  homicide, attempt (any means) E969
  injury due to terrorism E999.1 ●
  injury undetermined whether accidentally or
    purposely inflicted (injury classifiable to
    E980-E988) E989
  legal intervention (injury classifiable to E970-
    E976) E977
  medical or surgical procedure, test or therapy
    as, or resulting in, or from
      abnormal or delayed reaction or
        complication — *see* Reaction,
        abnormal
      misadventure — *see* Misadventure
  motor vehicle accident (accident classifiable to
    E810-E825) E929.0

Late effect of — *continued*

natural or environmental factor, accident due to (accident classifiable to E900-E909) E929.5

poisoning, accidental (accident classifiable to E850-E858, E860-E869) E929.2

suicide, attempt (any means) E959

transport accident NEC (accident classifiable to E800-E807, E826-E838, E840-E848) E929.1

war operations, injury due to (injury classifiable to E990-E998) E999.0 ▲

Launching pad accident E845 ✓4ᵗʰ

Legal

execution, any method E978

intervention (by) (injury from) E976

baton E973

bayonet E974

blow E975

blunt object (baton) (nightstick) (stave) (truncheon) E973

cutting or piercing instrument E974

dynamite E971

execution, any method E973

explosive(s) (shell) E971

firearm(s) E970

gas (asphyxiation) (poisoning) (tear) E972

grenade E971

late effect of E977

machine gun E970

manhandling E975

mortar bomb E971

nightstick E973

revolver E970

rifle E970

specified means NEC E975

stabbing E974

stave E973

truncheon E973

Lifting, injury in E927

Lightning (shock) (stroke) (struck by) E907

Liquid (noncorrosive) in eye E914

corrosive E924.1

Loss of control

motor vehicle (on public highway) (without antecedent collision) E816 ✓4ᵗʰ

with

antecedent collision on public highway — *see* Collision, motor vehicle

involving any object, person or vehicle not on public highway E816 ✓4ᵗʰ

on public highway — *see* Collision, motor vehicle

not on public highway, nontraffic accident E825 ✓4ᵗʰ

with antecedent collision — *see* Collision, motor vehicle, not on public highway

off-road type motor vehicle (not on public highway) E821 ✓4ᵗʰ

on public highway — *see* Loss of control, motor vehicle

snow vehicle, motor-driven (not on public highway) E820 ✓4ᵗʰ

on public highway — *see* Loss of control, motor vehicle

Lost at sea E832 ✓4ᵗʰ

with accident to watercraft E830 ✓4ᵗʰ

in war operations E995

Low

pressure, effects — *see* Effects of, air pressure

temperature, effects — *see* Cold, exposure to

Lying before train, vehicle or other moving object (unspecified whether accidental or intentional) E988.0

stated as intentional, purposeful, suicidal (attempt) E958.0

Lynching (*see also* Assault) E968.9

M

Malfunction, atomic power plant in water transport E838 ✓4ᵗʰ

Mangled (accidentally) NEC E928.9

Manhandling (in brawl, fight) E960.0

legal intervention E975

Manslaughter (nonaccidental) — *see* Assault

Marble in nose E912

Mauled by animal E906.8

Medical procedure, complication of

delayed or as an abnormal reaction

without mention of misadventure — *see* Reaction, abnormal

due to or as a result of misadventure — *see* Misadventure

Melting of fittings and furniture in burning ●

in terrorism E979.3 ●

Minamata disease E865.2

Misadventure(s) to patient(s) during surgical or medical care E876.9

contaminated blood, fluid, drug or biological substance (presence of agents and toxins as listed in E875) E875.9

administered (by) NEC E875.9

infusion E875.0

injection E875.1

specified means NEC E875.2

transfusion E875.0

vaccination E875.1

cut, cutting, puncture, perforation or hemorrhage (accidental) (inadvertent) (inappropriate) (during) E870.9

aspiration of fluid or tissue (by puncture or catheterization, except heart) E870.5

biopsy E870.8

needle (aspirating) E870.5

blood sampling E870.5

catheterization E870.5

heart E870.6

dialysis (kidney) E870.2

endoscopic examination E870.4

enema E870.7

infusion E870.1

injection E870.3

lumbar puncture E870.5

needle biopsy E870.5

paracentesis, abdominal E870.5

perfusion E870.2

specified procedure NEC E870.8

surgical operation E870.0

thoracentesis E870.5

transfusion E870.1

vaccination E870.3

excessive amount of blood or other fluid during transfusion or infusion E873.0

failure

in dosage E873.9

electroshock therapy E873.4

inappropriate temperature (too hot or too cold) in local application and packing E873.5

infusion

excessive amount of fluid E873.0

incorrect dilution of fluid E873.1

insulin-shock therapy E873.4

nonadministration of necessary drug or medicinal E873.6

overdose — *see also* Overdose

radiation, in therapy E873.2

radiation

inadvertent exposure of patient (receiving radiation for test or therapy) E873.3

not receiving radiation for test or therapy — *see* Radiation

overdose E873.2

specified procedure NEC E873.8

transfusion

excessive amount of blood E873.0

mechanical, of instrument or apparatus (during procedure) E874.9

aspiration of fluid or tissue (by puncture or catheterization, except of heart) E874.4

biopsy E874.8

needle (aspirating) E874.4

blood sampling E874.4

catheterization E874.4

heart E874.5

Misadventure(s) to patient(s) during surgical or medical care — *continued*

failure — *continued*

mechanical, of instrument or apparatus — *continued*

dialysis (kidney) E874.2

endoscopic examination E874.3

enema E874.8

infusion E874.1

injection E874.8

lumbar puncture E874.4

needle biopsy E874.4

paracentesis, abdominal E874.4

perfusion E874.2

specified procedure NEC E874.8

surgical operation E874.0

thoracentesis E874.4

transfusion E874.1

vaccination E874.8

sterile precautions (during procedure) E872.9

aspiration of fluid or tissue (by puncture or catheterization, except heart) E872.5

biopsy E872.8

needle (aspirating) E872.5

blood sampling E872.5

catheterization E872.5

heart E872.6

dialysis (kidney) E872.2

endoscopic examination E872.4

enema E872.8

infusion E872.1

injection E872.3

lumbar puncture E872.5

needle biopsy E872.5

paracentesis, abdominal E872.5

perfusion E872.2

removal of catheter or packing E872.8

specified procedure NEC E872.8

surgical operation E872.0

thoracentesis E872.5

transfusion E872.1

vaccination E872.3

suture or ligature during surgical procedure E876.2

to introduce or to remove tube or instrument E876.4

foreign object left in body — *see* Misadventure, foreign object

foreign object left in body (during procedure) E871.9

aspiration of fluid or tissue (by puncture or catheterization, except heart) E871.5

biopsy E871.8

needle (aspirating) E871.5

blood sampling E871.5

catheterization E871.5

heart E871.6

dialysis (kidney) E871.2

endoscopic examination E871.4

enema E871.8

infusion E871.1

injection E871.3

lumbar puncture E871.5

needle biopsy E871.5

paracentesis, abdominal E871.5

perfusion E871.2

removal of catheter or packing E871.7

specified procedure NEC E871.8

surgical operation E871.0

thoracentesis E871.5

transfusion E871.1

vaccination E871.3

hemorrhage — *see* Misadventure, cut

inadvertent exposure of patient to radiation (being received for test or therapy) E873.3

inappropriate

operation performed E876.5

temperature (too hot or too cold) in local application or packing E873.5

infusion — *see also* Misadventure, by specific type, infusion

excessive amount of fluid E873.0

incorrect dilution of fluid E873.1

wrong fluid E876.1

mismatched blood in transfusion E876.0

Misadventure(s) to patient(s) during surgical or medical care — *continued*
 nonadministration of necessary drug or medicinal E873.6
 overdose — *see also* Overdose
 radiation, in therapy E873.2
 perforation — *see* Misadventure, cut
 performance of inappropriate operation E876.5
 puncture — *see* Misadventure, cut
 specified type NEC E876.8
  failure
   suture or ligature during surgical operation E876.2
   to introduce or to remove tube or instrument E876.4
    foreign object left in body E871.9
  infusion of wrong fluid E876.1
  performance of inappropriate operation E876.5
  transfusion of mismatched blood E876.0
  wrong
   fluid in infusion E876.1
   placement of endotracheal tube during anesthetic procedure E876.3
 transfusion — *see also* Misadventure, by specific type, transfusion
  excessive amount of blood E873.0
  mismatched blood E876.0
 wrong
  drug given in error — *see* Table of Drugs and Chemicals
  fluid in infusion E876.1
  placement of endotracheal tube during anesthetic procedure E876.3
Motion (effects) E903
 sickness E903
Mountain sickness E902.0
Mucus aspiration or inhalation, not of newborn (with asphyxia, obstruction respiratory passage, suffocation) E912
Mudslide of cataclysmic nature E909.2
Murder (attempt) (*see also* Assault) E968.9

N

Nail, injury by E920.8
Needlestick (sewing needle) E920.4
 hypodermic E920.5
Neglect — *see also* Privation
 criminal E968.4
 homicidal intent E968.4
Noise (causing injury) (pollution) E928.1

O

Object
 falling
  from, in, on, hitting
   aircraft E844 ✓4th
    due to accident to aircraft — *see* categories E840-E842 ✓4th
   machinery — *see also* Accident, machine
    not in operation E916
   motor vehicle (in motion) (on public highway) E818 ✓4th
    not on public highway E825 ✓4th
    stationary E916
   nonmotor road vehicle NEC E829 ✓4th
   pedal cycle E826 ✓4th
   person E916
   railway rolling stock, train, vehicle E806 ✓4th
   street car E829 ✓4th
   watercraft E838 ✓4th
    due to accident to watercraft E831 ✓4th
 set in motion by
  accidental explosion of pressure vessel — *see* category E921 ✓4th
  firearm — *see* category E922 ✓4th
  machine(ry) — *see* Accident, machine
  transport vehicle — *see* categories E800-E848 ✓4th

Object — *continued*
 thrown from, in, on, towards
  aircraft E844 ✓4th
  cable car (not on rails) E847
   on rails E829 ✓4th
  motor vehicle (in motion) (on public highway) E818 ✓4th
   not on public highway E825 ✓4th
  nonmotor road vehicle NEC E829 ✓4th
  pedal cycle E826 ✓4th
  street car E829 ✓4th
  vehicle NEC — *see* Accident, vehicle NEC
Obstruction
 air passages, larynx, respiratory passages
  by
   external means NEC — *see* Suffocation
   food, any type (regurgitated) (vomited) E911
   material or object, except food E912
   mucus E912
   phlegm E912
   vomitus E911
 digestive tract, except mouth or pharynx
  by
   food, any type E915
   foreign body (any) E915
 esophagus
  food E911
  foreign body, except food E912
  without asphyxia or obstruction of respiratory passage E915
 mouth or pharynx
  by
   food, any type E911
   material or object, except food E912
 respiration — *see* Obstruction, air passages
Oil in eye E914
Overdose
 anesthetic (drug) — *see* Table of Drugs and Chemicals
 drug — *see* Table of Drugs and Chemicals
Overexertion (lifting) (pulling) (pushing) E927
Overexposure (accidental) (to)
 cold (*see also* Cold, exposure to) E901.9
  due to manmade conditions E901.1
 heat (*see also* Heat) E900.9
 radiation — *see* Radiation
 radioactivity — *see* Radiation
 sun, except sunburn E900.0
 weather — *see* Exposure
 wind — *see* Exposure
Overheated (*see also* Heat) E900.9
Overlaid E913.0
Overturning (accidental)
 animal-drawn vehicle E827 ✓4th
 boat, ship, watercraft
  causing
   drowning, submersion E830 ✓4th
   injury except drowning, submersion E831 ✓4th
 machinery — *see* Accident, machine
 motor vehicle (*see also* Loss of control, motor vehicle) E816 ✓4th
  with antecedent collision on public highway — *see* Collision, motor vehicle
  not on public highway, nontraffic accident E825 ✓4th
   with antecedent collision — *see* Collision, motor vehicle, not on public highway
 nonmotor road vehicle NEC E829 ✓4th
 off-road type motor vehicle — *see* Loss of control, off-road type motor vehicle
 pedal cycle E826 ✓4th
 railway rolling stock, train, vehicle (*see also* Derailment, railway) E802 ✓4th
 street car E829 ✓4th
 vehicle NEC — *see* Accident, vehicle NEC

P

Palsy, divers' E902.2
Parachuting (voluntary) (without accident to aircraft) E844 ✓4th

Parachuting — *continued*
 due to accident to aircraft — *see* categories E840-E842 ✓4th
Paralysis
 divers' E902.2
 lead or saturnine E866.0
  from pesticide NEC E863.4
Pecked by bird E906.8
Phlegm aspiration or inhalation (with asphyxia, obstruction respiratory passage, suffocation) E912
Piercing (*see also* Cut) E920.9
Pinched
 between objects (moving) (stationary and moving) E918
 in object E918
Pinned under
 machine(ry) — *see* Accident, machine
Place of occurrence of accident — *see* Accident (to), occurring (at) (in)
Plumbism E866.0
 from insecticide NEC E863.4
Poisoning (accidental) (by) — *see also* Table of Drugs and Chemicals
 carbon monoxide
  generated by
   aircraft in transit E844 ✓4th
   motor vehicle
    in motion (on public highway) E818 ✓4th
    not on public highway E825 ✓4th
   watercraft (in transit) (not in transit) E838 ✓4th
 caused by injection of poisons or toxins into or through skin by plant thorns, spines, or other mechanism E905.7
  marine or sea plants E905.6
 fumes or smoke due to
  conflagration — *see* Conflagration
  explosion or fire — *see* Fire
  ignition — *see* Ignition
 gas
  in legal intervention E972
  legal execution, by E978
  on watercraft E838 ✓4th
  used as anesthetic — *see* Table of Drugs and Chemicals
 in
  terrorism (chemical weapons) E979.7   ●
  war operations E997.2
 late effect of — *see* Late effect
 legal
  execution E978
  intervention
   by gas E972
Pressure, external, causing asphyxia, suffocation (*see also* Suffocation) E913.9
Privation E904.9
 food (*see also* Lack of, food) E904.1
 helpless person, infant, newborn due to abandonment or neglect E904.0
 late effect of NEC E929.5
 resulting from transport accident — *see* categories E800-E848 ✓4th
 water (*see also* Lack of, water) E904.2
Projected objects, striking against or struck by — *see* Striking against, object
Prolonged stay in
 high altitude (causing conditions as listed in E902.0) E902.0
 weightless environment E928.0
Prostration
 heat — *see* Heat
Pulling, injury in E927
Puncture, puncturing (*see also* Cut) E920.9
 by
  plant thorns or spines E920.8
   toxic reaction E905.7
    marine or sea plants E905.6
  sea-urchin spine E905.6

✓4th Fourth-digit Required   ▶◀ Revised Text   ● New Line   ▲ Revised Code

Pushing (injury in) (overexertion) E927
  by other person(s) (accidental) E917.9
    as, or caused by, a crowd, human stampede
      E917.1
      with subsequent fall E917.6
    before moving vehicle or object
      stated as
        intentional, homicidal E968.5
        undetermined whether accidental or
          intentional E988.8
  from
    high place
      in accidental circum-stances — *see*
        categories E880-E884 ✓4ᵗʰ
      stated as
        intentional, homicidal E968.1
        undetermined whether accidental or
          intentional E987.9
          man-made structure, except
            residential E987.1
          natural site E987.2
          residential E987.0
    motor vehicle (*see also* Fall, from, motor
      vehicle) E818 ✓4ᵗʰ
      stated as
        intentional, homicidal E968.5
        undetermined whether accidental or
          intentional E988.8
  in sports E917.0
    with fall E886.0
    with fall E886.9
      in sports E886.0

R

Radiation (exposure to) E926.9
  abnormal reaction to medical test or therapy
    E879.2
  arc lamps E926.2
  atomic power plant (malfunction) NEC E926.9
    in water transport E838 ✓4ᵗʰ
  electromagnetic, ionizing E926.3
  gamma rays E926.3
    in
      terrorism (from or following nuclear
        explosion) (direct) (secondary)
        E979.5
        laser E979.8
      war operations (from or following nuclear
        explosion) (direct) (secondary) E996
        laser(s) E997.0
    water transport E838 ✓4ᵗʰ
  inadvertent exposure of patient (receiving test
    or therapy) E873.3
  infrared (heaters and lamps) E926.1
    excessive heat E900.1
  ionized, ionizing (particles, artificially
    accelerated) E926.8
    electromagnetic E926.3
  isotopes, radioactive — *see* Radiation,
    radioactive isotopes
  laser(s) E926.4
    in
      terrorism E979.8
      war operations E997.0
    misadventure in medical care — *see*
      Misadventure, failure, in dosage,
      radiation
  late effect of NEC E929.8
    excessive heat from — *see* Heat
  light sources (visible) (ultraviolet) E926.2
  misadventure in medical or surgical procedure
    — *see* Misadventure, failure, in dosage,
    radiation
  overdose (in medical or surgical procedure)
    E873.2
  radar E926.0
  radioactive isotopes E926.5
    atomic power plant malfunction E926.5
      in water transport E838 ✓4ᵗʰ
    misadventure in medical or surgical
      treatment — *see* Misadventure, failure,
      in dosage, radiation
  radiobiologicals — *see* Radiation, radioactive
    isotopes
  radiofrequency E926.0

Radiation — *continued*
  radiopharmaceuticals — *see* Radiation,
    radioactive isotopes
  radium NEC E926.9
  sun E926.2
    excessive heat from E900.0
  tanning bed E926.2
  welding arc or torch E926.2
    excessive heat from E900.1
  x-rays (hard) (soft) E926.3
    misadventure in medical or surgical
      treatment — *see* Misadventure, failure,
      in dosage, radiation
Rape E960.1
Reaction, abnormal to or following (medical or
  surgical procedure) E879.9
  amputation (of limbs) E878.5
  anastomosis (arteriovenous) (blood vessel)
    (gastrojejunal) (skin) (tendon) (natural,
    artificial material, tissue) E878.2
    external stoma, creation of E878.3
  aspiration (of fluid) E879.4
    tissue E879.8
  biopsy E879.8
  blood
    sampling E879.7
    transfusion
      procedure E879.8
  bypass — *see* Reaction, abnormal, anastomosis
  catheterization
    cardiac E879.0
    urinary E879.6
  colostomy E878.3
  cystostomy E878.3
  dialysis (kidney) E879.1
  drugs or biologicals — *see* Table of Drugs and
    Chemicals
  duodenostomy E878.3
  electroshock therapy E879.3
  formation of external stoma E878.3
  gastrostomy E878.3
  graft — *see* Reaction, abnormal, anastomosis
  hypothermia E879.8
  implant, implantation (of)
    artificial
      internal device (cardiac pacemaker)
        (electrodes in brain) (heart valve
        prosthesis) (orthopedic) E878.1
    material or tissue (for anastomosis or
      bypass) E878.2
      with creation of external stoma E878.3
    natural tissues (for anastomosis or bypass)
      E878.2
      as transplantion — *see* Reaction,
        abnormal, transplant
      with creation of external stoma E878.3
  infusion
    procedure E879.8
  injection
    procedure E879.8
  insertion of gastric or duodenal sound E879.5
  insulin-shock therapy E879.3
  lumbar puncture E879.4
  perfusion E879.1
  procedures other than surgical operation (*see
    also* Reaction, abnormal, by
    specific type of procedure) E879.9
    specified procedure NEC E879.8
  radiological procedure or therapy E879.2
  removal of organ (partial) (total) NEC E878.6
    with
      anastomosis, bypass or graft E878.2
      formation of external stoma E878.3
      implant of artificial internal device
        E878.1
      transplant(ation)
        partial organ E878.4
        whole organ E878.0
  sampling
    blood E879.7
    fluid NEC E879.4
    tissue E879.8
  shock therapy E879.3
  surgical operation (*see also* Reaction,
    abnormal, by specified type of operation)
    E878.9

Reaction, abnormal to or following — *continued*
  surgical operation (*see also* Reaction,
    abnormal, by specified type of operation)
    — *continued*
    restorative NEC E878.4
      with
        anastomosis, bypass or graft E878.2
        fomation of external stoma E878.3
        implant(ation) — *see* Reaction,
          abnormal, implant
        transplant(ation) — *see* Reaction,
          abnormal, transplant
    specified operation NEC E878.8
  thoracentesis E879.4
  transfusion
    procedure E879.8
  transplant, transplantation (heart) (kidney)
    (liver) E878.0
    partial organ E878.4
  ureterostomy E878.3
  vaccination E879.8
Reduction in
  atmospheric pressure — *see also* Effects of, air
    pressure
    while surfacing from
      deep water diving causing caisson or
        divers' disease, palsy or paralysis
        E902.2
      underground E902.8
Residual (effect) — *see* Late effect
Rock falling on or hitting (accidentally)
  motor vehicle (in motion) (on public highway)
    E818 ✓4ᵗʰ
    not on public highway E825 ✓4ᵗʰ
  nonmotor road vehicle NEC E829 ✓4ᵗʰ
  pedal cycle E826 ✓4ᵗʰ
  person E916
  railway rolling stock, train, vehicle E806 ✓4ᵗʰ
Running off, away
  animal (being ridden) (in sport or transport)
    E829 ✓4ᵗʰ
    not being ridden E906.8
  animal-drawn vehicle E827 ✓4ᵗʰ
  rails, railway (*see also* Derailment) E802 ✓4ᵗʰ
  roadway
    motor vehicle (without antecedent collision)
      E816 ✓4ᵗʰ
      nontraffic accident E825 ✓4ᵗʰ
        with antecedent collision — *see*
          Collision, motor vehicle, not on
          public highway
      with
        antecedent collision — *see* Collision
          motor vehicle
        subsequent collision
          involving any object, person or
            vehicle not on public highway
            E816 ✓4ᵗʰ
          on public highway E811 ✓4ᵗʰ
    nonmotor road vehicle NEC E829 ✓4ᵗʰ
    pedal cycle E826 ✓4ᵗʰ
Run over (accidentally) (by)
  animal (not being ridden) E906.8
    being ridden (in sport or transport) E828 ✓4ᵗʰ
  animal-drawn vehicle E827 ✓4ᵗʰ
  machinery — *see* Accident, machine
  motor vehicle (on public highway) — *see* Hit by,
    motor vehicle
  nonmotor road vehicle NEC E829 ✓4ᵗʰ
  railway train E805 ✓4ᵗʰ
  street car E829 ✓4ᵗʰ
  vehicle NEC E848

S

Saturnism E866.0
  from insecticide NEC E863.4
Scald, scalding (accidental) (by) (from) (in) E924.0
  acid — *see* Scald, caustic
  boiling tap water E924.2
  caustic or corrosive liquid, substance E924.1
    swallowed — *see* Table of Drugs and
      Chemicals
  homicide (attempt) — *see* Assault, burning

Scald, scalding — *continued*
inflicted by other person
stated as
intentional or homicidal E968.3
undetermined whether accidental or
intentional E988.2
late effect of NEC E929.8
liquid (boiling) (hot) E924.0
local application of externally applied
substance in medical or surgical care
E873.5
molten metal E924.0
self-inflicted (unspecified whether accidental or
intentional) E988.2
stated as intentional, purposeful E958.2
stated as undetermined whether accidental or
intentional E988.2
steam E924.0
tap water (boiling) E924.2
transport accident — *see* catagories E800-E848
vapor E924.0
Scratch, cat E906.8
Sea
sickness E903
Self-mutilation — *see* Suicide
Sequelae (of) •
in •
terrorism E999.1 •
war operations E999.0 •
Shock
anaphylactic (*see also* Table of Drugs and
Chemicals) E947.9
due to
bite (venomous) — *see* Bite, venomous
NEC
sting — *see* Sting
electric (*see also* Electric shock) E925.9
from electric appliance or current (*see also*
Electric shock) E925.9
Shooting, shot (accidental(ly)) E922.9
air gun E922.4
BB gun E922.4
hand gun (pistol) (revolver) E922.0
himself (*see also* Shooting, self-inflicted)
E985.4
hand gun (pistol) (revolver) E985.0
military firearm, except hand gun E985.3
hand gun (pistol) (revolver) E985.0
rifle (hunting) E985.2
military E985.3
shotgun (automatic) E985.1
specified firearm NEC E985.4
Verey pistol E985.4
homicide (attempt) E965.4
air gun E968.6
BB gun E968.6
hand gun (pistol) (revolver) E965.0
military firearm, except hand gun E965.3
hand gun (pistol) (revolver) E965.0
paintball gun E965.4 •
rifle (hunting) E965.2
military E965.3
shotgun (automatic) E965.1
specified firearm NEC E965.4
Verey pistol E965.4
inflicted by other person
in accidental circumstances E922.9
hand gun (pistol) (revolver) E922.0
military firearm, except hand gun E922.3
hand gun (pistol) (revolver) E922.0
rifle (hunting) E922.2
military E922.3
shotgun (automatic) E922.1
specified firearm NEC E922.8
Verey pistol E922.8
stated as
intentional, homicidal E965.4
hand gun (pistol) (revolver) E965.0
military firearm, except hand gun
E965.3
hand gun (pistol) (revolver) E965.0
paintball gun E965.4 •
rifle (hunting) E965.2
military E965.3
shotgun (automatic) E965.1
specified firearm E965.4

Shooting, shot — *continued*
inflicted by other person — *continued*
stated as — *continued*
intentional, homicidal — *continued*
Verey pistol E965.4
undetermined whether accidental or
intentional E985.4
air gun E985.6
BB gun E985.6
hand gun (pistol) (revolver) E985.0
military firearm, except hand gun
E985.3
hand gun (pistol) (revolver) E985.0
paintball gun E985.7 •
rifle (hunting) E985.2
shotgun (automatic) E985.1
specified firearm NEC E985.4
Verey pistol E985.4
in
terrorism — *see* Terrorism, shooting •
war operations — *see* War operations,
shooting
legal
execution E978
intervention E970
military firearm, except hand gun E922.3
hand gun (pistol) (revolver) E922.0
paintball gun E922.5 •
rifle (hunting) E922.2
military E922.3
self-inflicted (unspecified whether accidental or
intentional) E985.4
air gun E985.6
BB gun E985.6
hand gun (pistol) (revolver) E985.0
military firearm, except hand gun E985.3
hand gun (pistol) (revolver) E985.0
paintball gun E985.7 •
rifle (hunting) E985.2
military E985.3
shotgun (automatic) E985.1
specified firearm NEC E985.4
stated as
accidental E922.9
hand gun (pistol) (revolver) E922.0
military firearm, except hand gun
E922.3
hand gun (pistol) (revolver) E922.0
paintball gun E922.5 •
rifle (hunting) E922.2
military E922.3
shotgun (automatic) E922.1
specified firearm NEC E922.8
Verey pistol E922.8
intentional, purposeful E955.4
hand gun (pistol) (revolver) E955.0
military firearm, except hand gun
E955.3
hand gun (pistol) (revolver) E955.0
paintball gun E955.7 •
rifle (hunting) E955.2
military E955.3
shotgun (automatic) E955.1
specified firearm NEC E955.4
Verey pistol E955.4
shotgun (automatic) E922.1
specified firearm NEC E922.8
stated as undetermined whether accidental or
intentional E985.4
hand gun (pistol) (revolver) E985.0
military firearm, except hand gun E985.3
hand gun (pistol) (revolver) E985.0
paintball gun E985.7 •
rifle (hunting) E985.2
military E985.3
shotgun (automatic) E985.1
specified firearm NEC E985.4
Verey pistol E985.4
suicidal (attempt) E955.4
air gun E955.6
BB gun E955.6
hand gun (pistol) (revolver) E955.0
military firearm, except hand gun E955.3
hand gun (pistol) (revolver) E955.0
paintball gun E955.7 •
rifle (hunting) E955.2
military E955.3

Shooting, shot — *continued*
suicidal — *continued*
shotgun (automatic) E955.1
specified firearm NEC E955.4
Verey pistol E955.4
Verey pistol E922.8
Shoving (accidentally) by other person (*see also*
Pushing by other person) E917.9
Sickness
air E903
alpine E902.0
car E903
motion E903
mountain E902.0
sea E903
travel E903
Sinking (accidental)
boat, ship, watercraft (causing drowning,
submersion) E830 [✔4ᵗʰ]
causing injury except drowning, submersion
E831 [✔4ᵗʰ]
Siriasis E900.0
Skydiving E844 [✔4ᵗʰ]
Slashed wrists (*see also* Cut, self-inflicted) E986
Slipping (accidental)
on
deck (of boat, ship, watercraft) (icy) (oily)
(wet) E835 [✔4ᵗʰ]
ice E885
ladder of ship E833 [✔4ᵗʰ]
due to accident to watercraft E831 [✔4ᵗʰ]
mud E885
oil E885
snow E885
stairs of ship E833 [✔4ᵗʰ]
due to accident to watercraft E831 [✔4ᵗʰ]
surface
slippery E885
wet E885
Sliver, wood, injury by E920.8
Smouldering building or structure in •
terrorism E979.3 •
Smothering, smothered (*see also* Suffocation)
E913.9
Sodomy (assault) E960.1
Solid substance in eye (any part) or adnexa E914
Sound waves (causing injury) E928.1
Splinter, injury by E920.8
Stab, stabbing E966
accidental — *see* Cut
Starvation E904.1
helpless person, infant, newborn — *see* Lack of
food
homicidal intent E968.4
late effect of NEC E929.5
resulting from accident connected with
transport — *see* catagories E800-E848
Stepped on
by
animal (not being ridden) E906.8
being ridden (in sport or transport)
E828 [✔4ᵗʰ]
crowd E917.1
person E917.9
in sports E917.0
in sports E917.0
Stepping on
object (moving) E917.9
in sports E917.0
with subsequent fall E917.5
stationary E917.4
with subsequent fall E917.8
person E917.9
as, or caused by a crowd E917.1
with subsequent fall E917.6
in sports E917.0
Sting E905.9
ant E905.5
bee E905.3
caterpillar E905.5
coral E905.6
hornet E905.3
insect NEC E905.5
jellyfish E905.6

Sting — *continued*
  marine animal or plant E905.6
  nematocysts E905.6
  scorpion E905.2
  sea anemone E905.6
  sea cucumber E905.6
  wasp E905.3
  yellow jacket E905.3
Storm E908.9
  specified type NEC E908.8
Straining, injury in E927
Strangling — *see* Suffocation
Strangulation — *see* Suffocation
Strenuous movements (in recreational or other activities) E927
Striking against
  bottom (when jumping or diving into water) E883.0
  object (moving) E917.9
    caused by crowd E917.1
      with subsequent fall E917.6
    furniture E917.3
      with subsequent fall E917.7
    in
      running water E917.2
        with drowning or submersion — *see* Submersion
      sports E917.0
        with subsequent fall E917.5
    stationary E917.4
      with subsequent fall E917.8
  person(s) E917.9
    with fall E886.9
      in sports E886.0
    as, or caused by, a crowd E917.1
      with subsequent fall E917.6
        in sports E917.0
          with fall E886.0
Stroke
  heat — *see* Heat
  lightning E907
Struck by — *see also* Hit by
  bullet
    in
      terrorism E979.4
      war operations E991.2
        rubber E991.0
  lightning E907
  missile
    in terrorism — *see* Terrorism, missile
  object
    falling
      from, in, on
        building
          burning (uncontrolled fire)
            in terrorism E979.3
  thunderbolt E907
Stumbling over animal, carpet, curb, rug or (small) object (with fall) E885
  without fall — *see* Striking against, object
Submersion (accidental) E910.8
  boat, ship, watercraft (causing drowning, submersion) E830 ✓4ᵗʰ
    causing injury except drowning, submersion E831 ✓4ᵗʰ
  by other person
    in accidental circumstances — *see category* E910 ✓4ᵗʰ
    intentional, homicidal E964
    stated as undetermined whether due to accidental or intentional E984
  due to
    accident
      machinery — *see* Accident, machine
      to boat, ship, watercraft E830 ✓4ᵗʰ
      transport — *see categories* E800-E848 ✓4ᵗʰ
    avalanche E909.2
    cataclysmic
      earth surface movement or eruption E909.9
      storm E908.9
    cloudburst E908.8
    cyclone E908.1

Submersion — *continued*
  due to — *continued*
    fall
      from
        boat, ship, watercraft (not involved in accident) E832 ✓4ᵗʰ
          burning, crushed E830 ✓4ᵗʰ
          involved in accident, collision E830 ✓4ᵗʰ
        gangplank (into water) E832 ✓4ᵗʰ
        overboard NEC E832 ✓4ᵗʰ
    flood E908.2
    hurricane E908.0
    jumping into water E910.8
      from boat, ship, watercraft
        burning, crushed, sinking E830 ✓4ᵗʰ
        involved in accident, collision E830 ✓4ᵗʰ
        not involved in accident, for swim E910.2
    in recreational activity (without diving equipment) E910.2
      with or using diving equipment E910.1
    to rescue another person E910.3
  homicide (attempt) E964
  in
    bathtub E910.4
    specified activity, not sport, transport or recreational E910.3
    sport or recreational activity (without diving equipment) E910.2
      with or using diving equipment E910.1
      water skiing E910.0
    swimming pool NEC E910.8
    terrorism E979.8
    war operations E995
    water transport E832 ✓4ᵗʰ
      due to accident to boat, ship, watercraft E830 ✓4ᵗʰ
  landslide E909.2
    overturning boat, ship, watercraft E909.2
    sinking boat, ship, watercraft E909.2
    submersion boat, ship, watercraft E909.2
    tidal wave E909.4
      caused by storm E908.0
    torrential rain E908.2
  late effect of NEC E929.8
  quenching tank E910.8
  self-inflicted (unspecified whether accidental or intentional) E984
    in accidental circumstances — *see category* E910 ✓4ᵗʰ
    stated as intentional, purposeful E954
  stated as undetermined whether accidental or intentional E984
  suicidal (attempted) E954
  while
    attempting rescue of another person E910.3
    engaged in
      marine salvage E910.3
      underwater construction or repairs E910.3
    fishing, not from boat E910.2
    hunting, not from boat E910.2
    ice skating E910.2
    pearl diving E910.3
    placing fishing nets E910.3
    playing in water E910.2
    scuba diving E910.1
      nonrecreational E910.3
    skin diving E910.1
    snorkel diving E910.2
    spear fishing underwater E910.1
    surfboarding E910.2
    swimming (swimming pool) E910.2
    wading (in water) E910.2
    water skiing E910.0
Sucked
  into
    jet (aircraft) E844 ✓4ᵗʰ
Suffocation (accidental) (by external means) (by pressure) (mechanical) E913.9
  caused by other person
    in accidental circumstances — *see category* E913 ✓4ᵗʰ

Suffocation — *continued*
  caused by other person — *continued*
    stated as
      intentional, homicidal E963
      undetermined whether accidental or intentional E983.9
        by, in
          hanging E983.0
          plastic bag E983.1
          specified means NEC E983.8
  due to, by
    avalanche E909.2
    bedclothes E913.0
    bib E913.0
    blanket E913.0
    cave-in E913.3
      caused by cataclysmic earth surface movement or eruption E909.9
    conflagration — *see* Conflagration
    explosion — *see* Explosion
    falling earth, other substance E913.3
    fire — *see* Fire
    food, any type (ingestion) (inhalation) (regurgitated) (vomited) E911
    foreign body, except food (ingestion) (inhalation) E912
    ignition — *see* Ignition
    landslide E909.2
    machine(ry) — *see* Accident, machine
    material, object except food entering by nose or mouth, ingested, inhaled E912
    mucus (aspiration) (inhalation), not of newborn E912
    phlegm (aspiration) (inhalation) E912
    pillow E913.0
    plastic bag — *see* Suffocation, in, plastic bag
    sheet (plastic) E913.0
    specified means NEC E913.8
    vomitus (aspiration) (inhalation) E911
  homicidal (attempt) E963
  in
    airtight enclosed place E913.2
    baby carriage E913.0
    bed E913.0
    closed place E913.2
    cot, cradle E913.0
    perambulator E913.0
    plastic bag (in accidental circumstances) E913.1
      homicidal, purposely inflicted by other person E963
      self-inflicted (unspecified whether accidental or intentional) E983.1
        in accidental circumstances E913.1
        intentional, suicidal E953.1
      stated as undetermined whether accidentally or purposely inflicted E983.1
      suicidal, purposely self-inflicted E953.1
    refrigerator E913.2
  self-inflicted — *see also* Suffocation, stated as undetermined whether accidental or intentional E953.9
    in accidental circumstances — *see category* E913 ✓4ᵗʰ
    stated as intentional, purposeful — *see* Suicide, suffocation
  stated as undetermined whether accidental or intentional E983.9
    by, in
      hanging E983.0
      plastic bag E983.1
      specified means NEC E983.8
  suicidal — *see* Suicide, suffocation
Suicide, suicidal (attempted) (by) E958.9
  burning, burns E958.1
  caustic substance E958.7
    poisoning E950.7
    swallowed E950.7
  cold, extreme E958.3
  cut (any part of body) E956
  cutting or piercing instrument (classifiable to E920) E956
  drowning E954
  electrocution E958.4
  explosive(s) (classifiable to E923) E955.5
  fire E958.1

Sting — Suicide

Suicide, suicidal — *continued*
  firearm (classifiable to E922) — *see* Shooting, suicidal
  hanging E953.0
  jumping
    before moving object, train, vehicle E958.0
    from high place — *see* Jumping, from, high place, stated as, suicidal
  knife E956
  late effect of E959
  motor vehicle, crashing of E958.5
  poisoning — *see* Table of Drugs and Chemicals
  puncture (any part of body) E956
  scald E958.2
  shooting — *see* Shooting, suicidal
  specified means NEC E958.8
  stab (any part of body) E956
  strangulation — *see* Suicide, suffocation
  submersion E954
  suffocation E953.9
    by, in
      hanging E953.0
      plastic bag E953.1
      specified means NEC E953.8
  wound NEC E958.9

Sunburn E926.2

Sunstroke E900.0

Supersonic waves (causing injury) E928.1

Surgical procedure, complication of
  delayed or as an abnormal reaction without mention of misadventure — *see* Reaction, abnormal
  due to or as a result of misadventure — *see* Misadventure

Swallowed, swallowing
  foreign body — *see* Foreign body, alimentary canal
  poison — *see* Table of Drugs and Chemicals substance
    caustic — *see* Table of Drugs and Chemicals
    corrosive — *see* Table or drugs and chemicals
    poisonous — *see* Table of Drugs and Chemicals

Swimmers cramp (*see also* category E910 ✓4ᵗʰ) E910.2
  not in recreation or sport E910.3

Syndrome, battered
  baby or child — *see* Abuse, child
  wife — *see* Assault

T

Tackle in sport E886.0

Terrorism (injury) (by) (in) E979.8
  air blast E979.2
  aircraft burned, destroyed, exploded, shot down E979.1
    used as a weapon E979.1
  anthrax E979.6
  asphyxia from
    chemical (weapons) E979.7
    fire, conflagration (caused by fire-producing device) E979.3
      from nuclear explosion E979.5
    gas or fumes E979.7
  bayonet E979.8
  biological agents E979.6
  blast (air) (effects) E979.2
    from nuclear explosion E979.5
    underwater E979.0
  bomb (antipersonnel) (mortar) (explosion) (fragments) E979.2
  bullet(s) (from carbine, machine gun, pistol, rifle, shotgun) E979.4
  burn from
    chemical E979.7
    fire, conflagration (caused by fire-producing device) E979.3
      from nuclear explosion E979.5
    gas E979.7
  burning aircraft E979.1
  chemical E979.7
  cholera E979.6
  conflagration E979.3
  crushed by falling aircraft E979.1

Terrorism — *continued*
  depth-charge E979.0
  destruction of aircraft E979.1
  disability, as sequelae one year or more after injury E999.1
  drowning E979.8
  effect
    of nuclear weapon (direct) (secondary) E979.5
    secondary NEC E979.9
    sequelae E999.1
  explosion (artillery shell) (breech-block) (cannon block) E979.2
    aircraft E979.1
    bomb (antipersonnel) (mortar) E979.2
      nuclear (atom) (hydrogen) E979.5
    depth-charge E979.0
    grenade E979.2
    injury by fragments from E979.2
    land-mine E979.2
    marine weapon E979.0
    mine (land) E979.2
      at sea or in harbor E979.0
      marine E979.0
    missile (explosive) NEC E979.2
    munitions (dump) (factory) E979.2
    nuclear (weapon) E979.5
      other direct and secondary effects of E979.5
    sea-based artillery shell E979.0
    torpedo E979.0
  exposure to ionizing radiation from nuclear explosion E979.5
  falling aircraft E979.1
  fire or fire-producing device E979.3
  firearms E979.4
  fireball effects from nuclear explosion E979.5
  fragments from artillery shell, bomb NEC, grenade, guided missile, land-mine, rocket, shell, shrapnel E979.2
  gas or fumes E979.7
  grenade (explosion) (fragments) E979.2
  guided missile (explosion) (fragments) E979.2
    nuclear E979.5
  heat from nuclear explosion E979.5
  hot substances E979.3
  hydrogen cyanide E979.7
  land-mine (explosion) (fragments) E979.2
  laser(s) E979.8
  late effect of E999.1
  lewisite E979.7
  lung irritant (chemical) (fumes) (gas) E979.7
  marine mine E979.0
  mine E979.2
    at sea E979.0
    in harbor E979.0
    land (explosion) (fragments) E979.2
    marine E979.0
  missile (explosion) (fragments) (guided) E979.2
    marine E979.0
    nuclear E979.5
  mortar bomb (explosion) (fragments) E979.2
  mustard gas E979.7
  nerve gas E979.7
  nuclear weapons E979.5
  pellets (shotgun) E979.4
  petrol bomb E979.3
  piercing object E979.8
  phosgene E979.7
  poisoning (chemical) (fumes) (gas) E979.7
  radiation, ioninizing from nuclear explosion E979.5
  rocket (explosion) (fragments) E979.2
  saber, sabre E979.8
  sarin E979.7
  screening smoke E979.7
  sequelae effect (of) E999.1
  shell (aircraft) (artillery) (cannon) (land-based) (explosion) (fragments) E979.2
    sea-based E979.0
  shooting E979.4
    bullet(s) E979.4
    pellet(s) (rifle) (shotgun) E979.4
  shrapnel E979.2

Terrorism — *continued*
  smallpox E979.7
  stabbing object(s) E979.8
  submersion E979.8
  torpedo E979.0
  underwater blast E979.0
  vesicant (chemical) (fumes) (gas) E979.7
  weapon burst E979.2

Thermic fever E900.9

Thermoplegia E900.9

Thirst — *see also* Lack of water
  resulting from accident connected with transport — *see* categories E800-E848 ✓4ᵗʰ

Thrown (accidently)
  against object in or part of vehicle
    by motion of vehicle
      aircraft E844 ✓4ᵗʰ
      boat, ship, watercraft E838 ✓4ᵗʰ
      motor vehicle (on public highway) E818 ✓4ᵗʰ
        not on public highway E825 ✓4ᵗʰ
        off-road type (not on public highway) E821 ✓4ᵗʰ
          on public highway E818 ✓4ᵗʰ
        snow vehicle E820 ✓4ᵗʰ
          on public high-way E818 ✓4ᵗʰ
      nonmotor road vehicle NEC E829 ✓4ᵗʰ
      railway rolling stock, train, vehicle E806 ✓4ᵗʰ
      street car E829 ✓4ᵗʰ
  from
    animal (being ridden) (in sport or transport) E828 ✓4ᵗʰ
    high place, homicide (attempt) E968.1
    machinery — *see* Accident, machine
    vehicle NEC — *see* Accident, vehicle NEC
  off — *see* Thrown, from
  overboard (by motion of boat, ship, watercraft) E832 ✓4ᵗʰ
    by accident to boat, ship, watercraft E830 ✓4ᵗʰ

Thunderbolt NEC E907

Tidal wave (any injury) E909.4
  caused by storm E908.0

Took
  overdose of drug — *see* Table of Drugs and Chemicals
  poison — *see* Table of Drugs and Chemicals

Tornado (any injury) E908.1

Torrential rain (any injury) E908.2

Traffic accident NEC E819 ✓4ᵗʰ

Trampled by animal E906.8
  being ridden (in sport or transport) E828 ✓4ᵗʰ

Trapped (accidently)
  between
    objects (moving) (stationary and moving) E918
  by
    door of
      elevator E918
      motor vehicle (on public highway) (while alighting, boarding) — *see* Fall, from, motor vehicle, while alighting
      railway train (underground) E806 ✓4ᵗʰ
      street car E829 ✓4ᵗʰ
      subway train E806 ✓4ᵗʰ
  in object E918

Travel (effects) E903
  sickness E903

Tree
  falling on or hitting E916
    motor vehicle (in motion) (on public highway) E818 ✓4ᵗʰ
      not on public highway E825 ✓4ᵗʰ
    nonmotor road vehicle NEC E829 ✓4ᵗʰ
    pedal cycle E826 ✓4ᵗʰ
    person E916
    railway rolling stock, train, vehicle E806 ✓4ᵗʰ
    street car E829 ✓4ᵗʰ

Trench foot E901.0

Tripping over animal, carpet, curb, rug, or small object (with fall) E885
  without fall — *see* Striking against, object

✓4ᵗʰ Fourth-digit Required   ▶◀ Revised Text   ● New Line   ▲ Revised Code

Tsunami E909.4
Twisting, injury in E927

V

Violence, nonaccidental (*see also* Assault)
　　E968.9
Volcanic eruption (any injury) E909.1
Vomitus in air passages (with asphyxia,
　　obstruction or suffocation) E911

W

War operations (during hostilities) (injury) (by) (in)
　　E995
　after cessation of hostilities, injury due to E998
　air blast E993
　aircraft burned, destroyed, exploded, shot
　　　down E994
　asphyxia from
　　chemical E997.2
　　fire, conflagration (caused by fire producing
　　　　device or conventional weapon) E990.9
　　　from nuclear explosion E996
　　　petrol bomb E990.0
　　fumes E997.2
　　gas E997.2
　battle wound NEC E995
　bayonet E995
　biological warfare agents E997.1
　blast (air) (effects) E993
　　from nuclear explosion E996
　　underwater E992
　bomb (mortar) (explosion) E993
　　after cessation of hostilities E998
　　fragments, injury by E991.9
　　　antipersonnel E991.3
　bullet(s) (from carbine, machine gun, pistol,
　　　rifle, shotgun) E991.2
　　rubber E991.0
　burn from
　　chemical E997.2
　　fire, conflagration (caused by fire-producing
　　　　device or conventional weapon) E990.9
　　　from nuclear explosion E996
　　　petrol bomb E990.0
　　gas E997.2
　burning aircraft E994
　chemical E997.2
　chlorine E997.2
　conventional warfare, specified from NEC E995
　crushing by falling aircraft E994
　depth charge E992
　destruction of aircraft E994
　disability as sequela one year or more after
　　　injury E999.0　　　　　　　　　　　　▲
　drowning E995
　effect (direct) (secondary) nuclear weapon E996
　explosion (artillery shell) (breech block) (cannon
　　　shell) E993
　　after cessation of hostilities of bomb, mine
　　　　placed in war E998
　　aircraft E994
　　bomb (mortar) E993
　　　atom E996
　　　hydrogen E996
　　　injury by fragments from E991.9
　　　　antipersonnel E991.3
　　　nuclear E996
　　depth charge E992
　　injury by fragments from E991.9
　　　antipersonnel E991.3
　　marine weapon E992
　　mine
　　　at sea or in harbor E992
　　　land E993
　　　　injury by fragments from E991.9
　　　marine E992
　　munitions (accidental) (being used in war)
　　　　(dump) (factory) E993
　　nuclear (weapon) E996
　　own weapons (accidental) E993
　　　injury by fragments from E991.9
　　　　antipersonnel E991.3
　　sea-based artillery shell E992
　　torpedo E992

War operations — *continued*
　exposure to ionizing radiation from nuclear
　　　explosion E996
　falling aircraft E994
　fire or fire-producing device E990.9
　　petrol bomb E990.0
　fireball effects from nuclear explosion E996
　fragments from
　　antipersonnel bomb E991.3
　　artillery shell, bomb NEC, grenade, guided
　　　　missile, land mine, rocket, shell,
　　　　shrapnel E991.9
　fumes E997.2
　gas E997.2
　grenade (explosion) E993
　　fragments, injury by E991.9
　guided missile (explosion) E993
　　fragments, injury by E991.9
　　nuclear E996
　heat from nuclear explosion E996
　injury due to, but occurring after cessation of
　　　hostilities E998
　lacrimator (gas) (chemical) E997.2
　land mine (explosion) E993
　　after cessation of hostilities E998
　　fragments, injury by E991.9
　laser(s) E997.0
　late effect of E999.0　　　　　　　　　　　▲
　lewisite E997.2
　lung irritant (chemical) (fumes) (gas) E997.2
　marine mine E992
　mine
　　after cessation of hostilities E998
　　at sea E992
　　in harbor E992
　　land (explosion) E993
　　　fragments, injury by E991.9
　　marine E992
　missile (guided) (explosion) E993
　　fragments, injury by E991.9
　　marine E992
　　nuclear E996
　mortar bomb (explosion) E993
　　fragments, injury by E991.9
　mustard gas E997.2
　nerve gas E997.2
　phosgene E997.2
　poisoning (chemical) (fumes) (gas) E997.2
　radiation, ionizing from nuclear explosion E996
　rocket (explosion) E993
　　fragments, injury by E991.9
　saber, sabre E995
　screening smoke E997.8
　shell (aircraft) (artillery) (cannon) (land based)
　　　(explosion) E993
　　fragments, injury by E991.9
　　sea-based E992
　shooting E991.2
　　after cessation of hostilities E998
　　bullet(s) E991.2
　　　rubber E991.0
　　pellet(s) (rifle) E991.1
　　shrapnel E991.9
　　submersion E995
　　torpedo E992
　unconventional warfare, except by nuclear
　　　weapon E997.9
　　biological (warfare) E997.1
　　gas, fumes, chemicals E997.2
　　laser(s) E997.0
　　specified type NEC E997.8
　underwater blast E992
　vesicant (chemical) (fumes) (gas) E997.2
　weapon burst E993
Washed
　away by flood — *see* Flood
　away by tidal wave — *see* Tidal wave
　off road by storm (transport vehicle) E908.9
　overboard E832
Weather exposure — *see also* Exposure
　cold E901.0
　hot E900.0
Weightlessness (causing injury) (effects of) (in
　　spacecraft, real or simulated) E928.0

Wound (accidental) NEC (*see also* Injury) E928.9
　battle (*see also* War operations) E995
　bayonet E920.3
　　in
　　　legal intervention E974
　　　war operations E995
　gunshot — *see* Shooting
　incised — *see* Cut
　saber, sabre E920.3
　　in war operations E995

▪⁴ᵗʰ Fourth-digit Required　　　　　◄► Revised Text　　　　　● New Line　　　　　▲ Revised Code

Railway Accidents (E800-E807)

The following fourth-digit subdivisions are for use with categories E800-E807 to identify the injured person:

.0   **Railway employee**
Any person who by virtue of his employment in connection with a railway, whether by the railway company or not, is at increased risk of involvement in a railway accident, such as:

        catering staff on train
        postal staff on train
        driver
        railway fireman
        guard
        shunter
        porter

        sleeping car attendant

.1   **Passenger on railway**
Any authorized person traveling on a train, except a railway employee
EXCLUDES   intending passenger waiting at station (.8)
                  unauthorized rider on railway vehicle (.8)

.2   **Pedestrian**
See definition (r), Vol. 1, page 248

.3   **Pedal cyclist**
See definition (p), Vol. 1, page 248

.8   **Other specified person**
Intending passenger waiting at station
Unauthorized rider on railway vehicle

.9   **Unspecified person**

Motor Vehicle Traffic and Nontraffic Accidents (E810-E825)

The following fourth-digit subdivisions are for use with categories E810-E819 and E820-E825 to identify the injured person:

.0   **Driver of motor vehicle other than motorcycle**
See definition (1), Vol. 1, page 248

.1   **Passenger in motor vehicle other than motorcycle**
See definition (1), Vol. 1, page 248

.2   **Motorcyclist**
See definition (1), Vol. 1, page 248

.3   **Passenger on motorcycle**
See definition (1), Vol. 1, page 248

.4   **Occupant of streetcar**

.5   **Rider of animal; occupant of animal-drawn vehicle**

.6   **Pedal cyclist**
See definition (p), Vol. 1, page 248

.7   **Pedestrian**
See definition (r), Vol. 1, page 248

.8   **Other specified person**
Occupant of vehicle other than above
Person in railway train involved in accident
Unauthorized rider of motor vehicle

.9   **Unspecified person**

Index to External Causes

Fourth-digit Required   ▶◀ Revised Text   ● New Line   ▲ Revised Code

Other Road Vehicle Accidents (E826-E829)

(animal-drawn vehicle, streetcar, pedal cycle, and other nonmotor road vehicle accidents)

The following fourth-digit subdivisions are for use with categories E826-E829 to identify the injured person:

.0 **Pedestrian**
See definition (r), Vol. 1, page 248

.1 **Pedal cyclist** (does not apply to codes E827, E828, E829)
See definition (p), Vol. 1, page 248

.2 **Rider of animal** (does not apply to code E829)

.3 **Occupant of animal-drawn vehicle** (does not apply to codes E828, E829)

.4 **Occupant of streetcar**

.8 **Other specified person**

.9 **Unspecified person**

Water Transport Accidents (E830-E838)

The following fourth-digit subdivisions are for use with categories E830-E838 to identify the injured person:

.0 **Occupant of small boat, unpowered**

.1 **Occupant of small boat, powered**
See definition (t), Vol. 1, page 248

   EXCLUDES   water skier (.4)

.2 **Occupant of other watercraft — crew**
Persons:

   engaged in operation of watercraft

   providing passenger services [cabin attendants, ship's physician, catering personnel]

   working on ship during voyage in other capacity [musician in band, operators of shops and beauty parlors]

.3 **Occupant of other watercraft — other than crew**
Passenger
Occupant of lifeboat, other than crew, after abandoning ship

.4 **Water skier**

.5 **Swimmer**

.6 **Dockers, stevedores**
Longshoreman employed on the dock in loading and unloading ships

.8 **Other specified person**
Immigration and custom officials on board ship
Persons:

   accompanying passenger or member of crew visiting boat

Pilot (guiding ship into port)

.9 **Unspecified person**

Air and Space Transport Accidents (E840-E845)

The following fourth-digit subdivisions are for use with categories E840-E845 to identify the injured person:

.0 **Occupant of spacecraft**

.1 **Occupant of military aircraft, any**

Crew
Passenger (civilian)
(military)
Troops
} in military aircraft [air force] [army] [national guard] [navy]

EXCLUDES occupants of aircraft operated under jurisdiction of police departments (.5)
parachutist (.7)

.2 **Crew of commercial aircraft (powered) in surface to surface transport**

.3 **Other occupant of commercial aircraft (powered) in surface to surface transport**

Flight personnel:
not part of crew
on familiarization flight

Passenger on aircraft

.4 **Occupant of commercial aircraft (powered) in surface to air transport**

Occupant [crew] [passenger] of aircraft (powered) engaged in activities, such as:

air drops of emergency supplies
air drops of parachutists, except from military craft
crop dusting
lowering of construction material [bridge or telephone pole]
sky writing

.5 **Occupant of other powered aircraft**

Occupant [crew] [passenger] of aircraft (powered) engaged in activities, such as:

aerial spraying (crops) (fire retardants)
aerobatic flying
aircraft racing
rescue operation
storm surveillance
traffic suveillance

Occupant of private plane NOS

.6 **Occupant of unpowered aircraft, except parachutist**
Occupant of aircraft classifiable to E842

.7 **Parachutist (military) (other)**
Person making voluntary descent

EXCLUDES person making descent after accident to aircraft (.1-.6)

.8 **Ground crew, airline employee**
Persons employed at airfields (civil) (military) or launching pads, not occupants of aircraft

.9 **Other person**

---

1. INFECTIOUS AND PARASITIC DISEASES (001–139)

Note: Categories for "late effects" of infectious and parasitic diseases are to be found at 137–139.

INCLUDES   diseases generally recognized as communicable or transmissible as well as a few diseases of unknown but possibly infectious origin

EXCLUDES   *acute respiratory infections (460-466)*
carrier or suspected carrier of infectious organism (V02.0-V02.9)
certain localized infections
influenza (487.0-487.8)

INTESTINAL INFECTIOUS DISEASES (001–009)

EXCLUDES   *helminthiases (120.0-129)*

✓4th **001 Cholera**

DEF: An acute infectious enteritis caused by a potent enterotoxin elaborated by *Vibrio cholerae*; the vibrio produces a toxin in the intestinal tract that changes the permeability of the mucosa leading to diarrhea and dehydration.

001.0 Due to Vibrio cholerae

001.1 Due to Vibrio cholerae el tor

001.9 Cholera, unspecified

✓4th **002 Typhoid and paratyphoid fevers**

DEF: Typhoid fever: an acute generalized illness caused by *Salmonella typhi*; notable clinical features are fever, headache, abdominal pain, cough, toxemia, leukopenia, abnormal pulse, rose spots on the skin, bacteremia, hyperplasia of intestinal lymph nodes, mesenteric lymphadenopathy, and Peyer's patches in the intestines.

DEF: Paratyphoid fever: a prolonged febrile illness, much like typhoid but usually less severe; caused by salmonella serotypes other than *S. typhi*, especially *S. enteritidis* serotypes paratyphi A and B and S. *choleraesuis*.

002.0 Typhoid fever
Typhoid (fever) (infection) [any site]

002.1 Paratyphoid fever A

002.2 Paratyphoid fever B

002.3 Paratyphoid fever C

002.9 Paratyphoid fever, unspecified

✓4th **003 Other salmonella infections**

INCLUDES   infection or food poisoning by Salmonella [any serotype]

DEF: Infections caused by a genus of gram-negative, anaerobic bacteria of the family *Enterobacteriaceae*; affecting warm-blooded animals, like humans; major symptoms are enteric fevers, acute gastroenteritis and septicemia.

003.0 Salmonella gastroenteritis
Salmonellosis

003.1 Salmonella septicemia

✓5th **003.2 Localized salmonella infections**

003.20 Localized salmonella infection, unspecified

003.21 Salmonella meningitis

003.22 Salmonella pneumonia

003.23 Salmonella arthritis

003.24 Salmonella osteomyelitis

003.29 Other

003.8 Other specified salmonella infections

003.9 Salmonella infection, unspecified

✓4th **004 Shigellosis**

INCLUDES   bacillary dysentery

DEF: Acute infectious dysentery caused by the genus *Shigella*, of the family *Enterobacteriaceae*; affecting the colon causing the release of blood-stained stools with accompanying tenesmus, abdominal cramps and fever.

004.0 Shigella dysenteriae
Infection by group A Shigella (Schmitz) (Shiga)

004.1 Shigella flexneri
Infection by group B Shigella

004.2 Shigella boydii
Infection by group C Shigella

004.3 Shigella sonnei
Infection by group D Shigella

004.8 Other specified Shigella infections

004.9 Shigellosis, unspecified

✓4th **005 Other food poisoning (bacterial)**

EXCLUDES   *salmonella infections (003.0-003.9)*
toxic effect of:
food contaminants (989.7)
noxious foodstuffs (988.0-988.9)

DEF: Enteritis caused by ingesting contaminated foods and characterized by diarrhea, abdominal pain, vomiting; symptoms may be mild or life threatening.

005.0 Staphylococcal food poisoning
Staphylococcal toxemia specified as due to food

005.1 Botulism
Food poisoning due to Clostridium botulinum

005.2 Food poisoning due to Clostridium perfringens [C. welchii]
Enteritis necroticans

005.3 Food poisoning due to other Clostridia

005.4 Food poisoning due to Vibrio parahaemolyticus

✓5th **005.8 Other bacterial food poisoning**

EXCLUDES   *salmonella food poisoning (003.0-003.9)*

005.81 Food poisoning due to Vibrio vulnificus

005.89 Other bacterial food poisoning
Food poisoning due to Bacillus cereus

005.9 Food poisoning, unspecified

✓4th **006 Amebiasis**

INCLUDES   infection due to Entamoeba histolytica

EXCLUDES   *amebiasis due to organisms other than Entamoeba histolytica (007.8)*

DEF: Infection of the large intestine caused by *Entamoeba histolytica*; usually asymptomatic but symptoms may range from mild diarrhea to profound life-threatening dysentery. Extraintestinal complications include hepatic abscess, which may rupture into the lung, pericardium or abdomen, causing life-threatening infections.

006.0 Acute amebic dysentery without mention of abscess
Acute amebiasis

006.1 Chronic intestinal amebiasis without mention of abscess
Chronic: Chronic:
amebiasis   amebic dysentery

006.2 Amebic nondysenteric colitis
DEF: *Entamoeba histolytica* infection with inflamed colon but no dysentery.

006.3 Amebic liver abscess
Hepatic amebiasis

006.4 Amebic lung abscess
Amebic abscess of lung (and liver)

006.5 Amebic brain abscess
Amebic abscess of brain (and liver) (and lung)

006.6 Amebic skin ulceration
Cutaneous amebiasis

006.8 Amebic infection of other sites
Amebic: Ameboma
appendicitis
balanitis

EXCLUDES   *specific infections by free-living amebae (136.2)*

006.9 Amebiasis, unspecified
Amebiasis NOS

✓4th **007 Other protozoal intestinal diseases**

INCLUDES   protozoal: protozoal:
colitis   dysentery
diarrhea

007.0 Balantidiasis
Infection by Balantidium coli

007.1 Giardiasis
Infection by Giardia lamblia   Lambliasis

✓4th ✓5th Additional Digit Required   Unspecified Code   Other Specified Code   Manifestation Code   ▶◀ Revised Text   ● New Code   ▲ Revised Code Title

007.2　Coccidiosis
Infection by Isospora belli and Isospora hominis
Isosporiasis

007.3　Intestinal trichomoniasis
DEF: Colitis, diarrhea, or dysentery caused by the protozoa *Trichomonas*.

007.4　Cryptosporidiosis
DEF: An intestinal infection by protozoan parasites causing intractable diarrhea in patients with AIDS and other immunosuppressed individuals.

007.5　Cyclosporiasis
DEF: An infection of the small intestine by the protozoal organism, *Cyclospora caytenanesis,* spread to humans though ingestion of contaminated water or food. Symptoms include watery diarrhea with frequent explosive bowel movements, loss of appetite, loss of weight, bloating, increased gas, stomach cramps, nausea, vomiting, muscle aches, low grade fever, and fatigue.

007.8　Other specified protozoal intestinal diseases
Amebiasis due to organisms other than Entamoeba histolytica

007.9　Unspecified protozoal intestinal disease
Flagellate diarrhea
Protozoal dysentery NOS

√4ᵗʰ 008　Intestinal infections due to other organisms
INCLUDES　any condition classifiable to 009.0-009.3 with mention of the responsible organisms
EXCLUDES　*food poisoning by these organisms (005.0-005.9)*

√5ᵗʰ 008.0　Escherichia coli [E. coli]

008.00　E. coli, unspecified
E. coli enteritis NOS

008.01　Enteropathogenic E. coli
DEF: E. coli causing inflammation of intestines.

008.02　Enterotoxigenic E. coli
DEF: A toxic reaction to E. coli of the intestinal mucosa, causing voluminous watery secretions.

008.03　Enteroinvasive E. coli
DEF: E. coli infection penetrating intestinal mucosa.

008.04　Enterohemorrhagic E. coli
DEF: E. coli infection penetrating the intestinal mucosa, producing microscopic ulceration and bleeding.

008.09　Other intestinal E. coli infections
008.1　Arizona group of paracolon bacilli
008.2　Aerobacter aerogenes
Enterobacter aeogenes
008.3　Proteus (mirabilis) (morganii)

√5ᵗʰ 008.4　Other specified bacteria
008.41　Staphylococcus
Staphylococcal enterocolitis
008.42　Pseudomonas
008.43　Campylobacter
008.44　Yersinia enterocolitica
008.45　Clostridium difficile
Pseudomembranous colitis
DEF: An overgrowth of a species of bacterium that is a part of the normal colon flora in human infants and sometimes in adults; produces a toxin that causes pseudomembranous enterocolitis; typically is seen in patients undergoing antibiotic therapy.

008.46　Other anaerobes
Anaerobic enteritis NOS
Bacteroides (fragilis)
Gram-negative anaerobes

008.47　Other gram-negative bacteria
Gram-negative enteritis NOS
EXCLUDES　*gram-negative anaerobes (008.46)*

008.49　Other
008.5　Bacterial enteritis, unspecified

√5ᵗʰ 008.6　Enteritis due to specified virus
008.61　Rotavirus
008.62　Adenovirus
008.63　Norwalk virus
Norwalk-like agent
008.64　Other small round viruses [SRVs]
Small round virus NOS
008.65　Calicivirus
DEF: Enteritis due to a subgroup of *Picornaviruses.*
008.66　Astrovirus
008.67　Enterovirus NEC
Coxsackie virus　Echovirus
EXCLUDES　*poliovirus (045.0-045.9)*
008.69　Other viral enteritis
Torovirus

008.8　Other organism, not elsewhere classified
Viral:
enteritis NOS
gastroenteritis
EXCLUDES　*influenza with involvement of gastrointestinal tract (487.8)*

√4ᵗʰ 009　Ill-defined intestinal infections
EXCLUDES　*diarrheal disease or intestinal infection due to specified organism (001.0-008.8)*
diarrhea following gastrointestinal surgery (564.4)
intestinal malabsorption (579.0-579.9)
ischemic enteritis (557.0-557.9)
other noninfectious gastroenteritis and colitis (558.1-558.9)
regional enteritis (555.0-555.9)
ulcerative colitis (556)

009.0　Infectious colitis, enteritis, and gastroenteritis
Colitis
Enteritis 　} septic
Gastroenteritis

Dysentery:
NOS
catarrhal
hemorrhagic

DEF: Colitis: An inflammation of mucous membranes of the colon.

DEF: Enteritis: An inflammation of mucous membranes of the small intestine.

DEF: Gastroenteritis: An inflammation of mucous membranes of stomach and intestines.

009.1　Colitis, enteritis, and gastroenteritis of presumed infectious origin
EXCLUDES　*colitis NOS (558.9)*
enteritis NOS (558.9)
gastroenteritis NOS (558.9)

009.2　Infectious diarrhea
Diarrhea:
dysenteric
epidemic
Infectious diarrheal disease NOS

009.3　Diarrhea of presumed infectious origin
EXCLUDES　*diarrhea NOS (787.91)*

N　Newborn Age: 0　　　　P　Pediatric Age: 0-17　　　　M　Maternity Age: 12-55　　　　A　Adult Age: 15-124　　　　MSP　Medicare Secondary Payer

TUBERCULOSIS (010-018)

INCLUDES   infection by Mycobacterium tuberculosis
(human) (bovine)

EXCLUDES   *congenital tuberculosis (771.2)*
late effects of tuberculosis (137.0-137.4)

The following fifth-digit subclassification is for use with
categories 010-018:

   0 unspecified
   1 bacteriological or histological examination not
      done
   2 bacteriological or histological examination
      unknown (at present)
   3 tubercle bacilli found (in sputum) by
      microscopy
   4 tubercle bacilli not found (in sputum) by
      microscopy, but found by bacterial culture
   5 tubercle bacilli not found by bacteriological
      examination, but tuberculosis confirmed
      histologically
   6 tubercle bacilli not found by bacteriological or
      histological examination but tuberculosis
      confirmed by other methods [inoculation of
      animals]

DEF: An infection by *Mycobacterium tuberculosis* causing the formation of
small, rounded nodules, called tubercles, that can disseminate throughout the
body via lymph and blood vessels. Localized tuberculosis is most often seen
in the lungs.

✓4th **010 Primary tuberculous infection**
   DEF: Tuberculosis of the lungs occurring when the patient is first infected.

§ ✓5th **010.0   Primary tuberculous infection**
      EXCLUDES   *nonspecific reaction to tuberculin skin*
                  test without active tuberculosis
                  (795.5)
                  positive PPD (795.5)
                  positive tuberculin skin test without
                  active tuberculosis (795.5)
      DEF: Hilar or paratracheal lymph node enlargement in pulmonary
      tuberculosis.

§ ✓5th **010.1   Tuberculous pleurisy in primary progressive
            tuberculosis**
      DEF: Inflammation and exudation in the lining of the tubercular
      lung.

§ ✓5th **010.8   Other primary progressive tuberculosis**
      EXCLUDES   *tuberculous erythema nodosum (017.1)*

§ ✓5th **010.9   Primary tuberculous infection, unspecified**

✓4th **011 Pulmonary tuberculosis**
      Use additional code to identify any associated silicosis (502)

§ ✓5th **011.0   Tuberculosis of lung, infiltrative**
§ ✓5th **011.1   Tuberculosis of lung, nodular**
§ ✓5th **011.2   Tuberculosis of lung with cavitation**
§ ✓5th **011.3   Tuberculosis of bronchus**
      EXCLUDES   *isolated bronchial tuberculosis (012.2)*
§ ✓5th **011.4   Tuberculous fibrosis of lung**
§ ✓5th **011.5   Tuberculous bronchiectasis**
§ ✓5th **011.6   Tuberculous pneumonia [any form]**
      DEF: Inflammatory pulmonary reaction to tuberculous cells.
§ ✓5th **011.7   Tuberculous pneumothorax**
      DEF: Spontaneous rupture of damaged tuberculous pulmonary
      tissue.
§ ✓5th **011.8   Other specified pulmonary tuberculosis**
§ ✓5th **011.9   Pulmonary tuberculosis, unspecified**
      Respiratory tuberculosis NOS
      Tuberculosis of lung NOS

✓4th **012 Other respiratory tuberculosis**
      EXCLUDES   *respiratory tuberculosis, unspecified (011.9)*

§ ✓5th **012.0   Tuberculous pleurisy**
      Tuberculosis of pleura
      Tuberculous empyema
      Tuberculous hydrothorax
      EXCLUDES   *pleurisy with effusion without mention*
                  of cause (511.9)
                  tuberculous pleurisy in primary
                  progressive tuberculosis (010.1)
      DEF: Inflammation and exudation in the lining of the tubercular
      lung.

§ ✓5th **012.1   Tuberculosis of intrathoracic lymph nodes**
      Tuberculosis of lymph nodes:
         hilar
         mediastinal
         tracheobronchial
      Tuberculous tracheobronchial adenopathy
      EXCLUDES   *that specified as primary (010.0-010.9)*

§ ✓5th **012.2   Isolated tracheal or bronchial tuberculosis**

§ ✓5th **012.3   Tuberculous laryngitis**
      Tuberculosis of glottis

§ ✓5th **012.8   Other specified respiratory tuberculosis**
      Tuberculosis of:
         mediastinum
         nasopharynx
         nose (septum)
         sinus [any nasal]

✓4th **013 Tuberculosis of meninges and central nervous system**
§ ✓5th **013.0   Tuberculous meningitis**
      Tuberculosis of meninges (cerebral) (spinal)
      Tuberculous:
         leptomeningitis
         meningoencephalitis
      EXCLUDES   *tuberculoma of meninges (013.1)*

§ ✓5th **013.1   Tuberculoma of meninges**
§ ✓5th **013.2   Tuberculoma of brain**
      Tuberculosis of brain (current disease)
§ ✓5th **013.3   Tuberculous abscess of brain**
§ ✓5th **013.4   Tuberculoma of spinal cord**
§ ✓5th **013.5   Tuberculous abscess of spinal cord**
§ ✓5th **013.6   Tuberculous encephalitis or myelitis**
§ ✓5th **013.8   Other specified tuberculosis of central nervous
            system**
§ ✓5th **013.9   Unspecified tuberculosis of central nervous
            system**
      Tuberculosis of central nervous system NOS

✓4th **014 Tuberculosis of intestines, peritoneum, and mesenteric
         glands**
§ ✓5th **014.0   Tuberculous peritonitis**
      Tuberculous ascites
      DEF: Tuberculous inflammation of the membrane lining the
      abdomen.

§ ✓5th **014.8   Other**
      Tuberculosis (of):
         anus
         intestine (large) (small)
         mesenteric glands
         rectum
         retroperitoneal (lymph nodes)
      Tuberculous enteritis

§ Requires fifth-digit. See beginning of section 010–018 for codes and definitions.

✓4th ✓5th Additional Digit Required   Unspecified Code   Other Specified Code   Manifestation Code   ▶◀ Revised Text   ● New Code   ▲ Revised Code Title

2003 ICD•9•CM   Volume 1 — 3

✓4ᵗʰ **015 Tuberculosis of bones and joints**
Use additional code to identify manifestation, as:
tuberculous:
arthropathy (711.4)
necrosis of bone (730.8)
osteitis (730.8)
osteomyelitis (730.8)
synovitis (727.01)
tenosynovitis (727.01)

§ ✓5ᵗʰ **015.0 Vertebral column**
Pott's disease
Use additional code to identify manifestation, as:
curvature of spine [Pott's] (737.4)
kyphosis (737.4)
spondylitis (720.81)

§ ✓5ᵗʰ **015.1 Hip**

§ ✓5ᵗʰ **015.2 Knee**

§ ✓5ᵗʰ **015.5 Limb bones**
Tuberculous dactylitis

§ ✓5ᵗʰ **015.6 Mastoid**
Tuberculous mastoiditis

§ ✓5ᵗʰ **015.7 Other specified bone**

§ ✓5ᵗʰ **015.8 Other specified joint**

§ ✓5ᵗʰ **015.9 Tuberculosis of unspecified bones and joints**

✓4ᵗʰ **016 Tuberculosis of genitourinary system**

§ ✓5ᵗʰ **016.0 Kidney**
Renal tuberculosis
Use additional code to identify manifestation, as:
tuberculous:
nephropathy (583.81)
pyelitis (590.81)
pyelonephritis (590.81)

§ ✓5ᵗʰ **016.1 Bladder**

§ ✓5ᵗʰ **016.2 Ureter**

§ ✓5ᵗʰ **016.3 Other urinary organs**

§ ✓5ᵗʰ **016.4 Epididymis**   ♂

§ ✓5ᵗʰ **016.5 Other male genital organs**   ♂
Use additional code to identify manifestation, as:
tuberculosis of:
prostate (601.4)
seminal vesicle (608.81)
testis (608.81)

§ ✓5ᵗʰ **016.6 Tuberculous oophoritis and salpingitis**   ♀

§ ✓5ᵗʰ **016.7 Other female genital organs**   ♀
Tuberculous:
cervicitis
endometritis

§ ✓5ᵗʰ **016.9 Genitourinary tuberculosis, unspecified**

✓4ᵗʰ **017 Tuberculosis of other organs**

§ ✓5ᵗʰ **017.0 Skin and subcutaneous cellular tissue**
Lupus: Tuberculosis:
exedens   cutis
vulgaris   lichenoides
Scrofuloderma   papulonecrotica
Tuberculosis: verrucosa cutis
colliquativa
EXCLUDES *lupus erythematosus (695.4)*
disseminated (710.0)
lupus NOS (710.0)
nonspecific reaction to tuberculin skin
test without active tuberculosis
(795.5)
positive PPD (795.5)
positive tuberculin skin test without
active tuberculosis (795.5)

§ ✓5ᵗʰ **017.1 Erythema nodosum with hypersensitivity reaction in tuberculosis**
Bazin's disease
Erythema:
induratum
nodosum, tuberculous
Tuberculosis indurativa
EXCLUDES *erythema nodosum NOS (695.2)*
DEF: Tender, inflammatory, bilateral nodules appearing on the shins and thought to be an allergic reaction to tuberculotoxin.

§ ✓5ᵗʰ **017.2 Peripheral lymph nodes**
Scrofula
Scrofulous abscess
Tuberculous adenitis
EXCLUDES *tuberculosis of lymph nodes:*
bronchial and mediastinal (012.1)
mesenteric and retroperitoneal
(014.8)
tuberculous tracheobronchial
adenopathy (012.1)
DEF: Scrofula: Old name for tuberculous cervical lymphadenitis.

§ ✓5ᵗʰ **017.3 Eye**
Use additional code to identify manifestation, as:
tuberculous:
chorioretinitis, disseminated (363.13)
episcleritis (379.09)
interstitial keratitis (370.59)
iridocyclitis, chronic (364.11)
keratoconjunctivitis (phlyctenular) (370.31)

§ ✓5ᵗʰ **017.4 Ear**
Tuberculosis of ear
Tuberculous otitis media
EXCLUDES *tuberculous mastoiditis (015.6)*

§ ✓5ᵗʰ **017.5 Thyroid gland**

§ ✓5ᵗʰ **017.6 Adrenal glands**
Addison's disease, tuberculous

§ ✓5ᵗʰ **017.7 Spleen**

§ ✓5ᵗʰ **017.8 Esophagus**

§ ✓5ᵗʰ **017.9 Other specified organs**
Use additional code to identify manifestation, as:
tuberculosis of:
endocardium [any valve] (424.91)
myocardium (422.0)
pericardium (420.0)

✓4ᵗʰ **018 Miliary tuberculosis**
INCLUDES tuberculosis:
disseminated
generalized
miliary, whether of a single specified site,
multiple sites, or unspecified site
polyserositis
DEF: A form of tuberculosis caused by caseous material carried through the bloodstream planting seedlike tubercles in various body organs.

§ ✓5ᵗʰ **018.0 Acute miliary tuberculosis**

§ ✓5ᵗʰ **018.8 Other specified miliary tuberculosis**

§ ✓5ᵗʰ **018.9 Miliary tuberculosis, unspecified**

ZOONOTIC BACTERIAL DISEASES (020-027)

✓4ᵗʰ **020 Plague**
INCLUDES infection by Yersinia [Pasteurella] pestis

020.0 Bubonic
DEF: Most common acute and severe form of plague characterized by lymphadenopathy (buboes), chills, fever and headache.

020.1 Cellulocutaneous
DEF: Plague characterized by inflammation and necrosis of skin.

---

§ Requires fifth-digit. See beginning of section 010–018 for codes and definitions.

N   Newborn Age: 0   P   Pediatric Age: 0-17   M   Maternity Age: 12-55   A   Adult Age: 15-124   MSP   Medicare Secondary Payer

020.2 Septicemic

DEF: Plague characterized by massive infection in the bloodstream.

020.3 Primary pneumonic

DEF: Plague characterized by massive pulmonary infection.

020.4 Secondary pneumonic

DEF: Lung infection as a secondary complication of plague.

020.5 Pneumonic, unspecified

020.8 Other specified types of plague

Abortive plague   Pestis minor
Ambulatory plague

020.9 Plague, unspecified

√4ᵗʰ 021 Tularemia

INCLUDES   deerfly fever
infection by Francisella [Pasteurella] tularensis
rabbit fever

DEF: A febrile disease transmitted by the bites of deer flies, fleas and ticks, by inhalations of aerosolized *F. tuarensis* or by ingestion of contaminated food or water; patients quickly develop fever, chills, weakness, headache, backache and malaise.

021.0 Ulceroglandular tularemia

DEF: Lesions occur at the site *Francisella tularensis;* organism enters body, usually the fingers or hands.

021.1 Enteric tularemia

Tularemia: Tularemia:
  cryptogenic   typhoidal
  intestinal

021.2 Pulmonary tularemia

Bronchopneumonic tularemia

021.3 Oculoglandular tularemia

DEF: Painful conjunctival infection by *Francisella tularensis* organism with possible corneal, preauricular lymph, or lacrimal involvement.

021.8 Other specified tularemia

Tularemia:
  generalized or disseminated
  glandular

021.9 Unspecified tularemia

√4ᵗʰ 022 Anthrax

DEF: An infectious bacterial disease usually transmitted by contact with infected animals or their discharges or products; it is classified by primary routes of inoculation as cutaneous, gastrointestinal and by inhalation.

022.0 Cutaneous anthrax

Malignant pustule

022.1 Pulmonary anthrax

Respiratory anthrax
Wool-sorters' disease

022.2 Gastrointestinal anthrax

022.3 Anthrax septicemia

022.8 Other specified manifestations of anthrax

022.9 Anthrax, unspecified

√4ᵗʰ 023 Brucellosis

INCLUDES   fever:
  Malta
  Mediterranean
  undulant

DEF: An infectious disease caused by gram-negative, *aerobic coccobacilli* organisms; it is transmitted to humans through contact with infected tissue or dairy products; fever, sweating, weakness and aching are symptoms of the disease.

023.0 Brucella melitensis

DEF: Infection from direct or indirect contact with infected sheep or goats.

023.1 Brucella abortus

DEF: Infection from direct or indirect contact with infected cattle.

023.2 Brucella suis

DEF: Infection from direct or indirect contact with infected swine.

023.3 Brucella canis

DEF: Infection from direct or indirect contact with infected dogs.

023.8 Other brucellosis

Infection by more than one organism

023.9 Brucellosis, unspecified

024 Glanders

Infection by:
  Actinobacillus mallei
  Malleomyces mallei
  Pseudomonas mallei
Farcy
Malleus

DEF: Equine infection causing mucosal inflammation and skin ulcers in humans.

025 Melioidosis

Infection by:
  Malleomyces pseudomallei
  Pseudomonas pseudomallei
  Whitmore's bacillus
Pseudoglanders

DEF: Rare infection caused by *Pseudomonas pseudomallei;* clinical symptoms range from localized infection to fatal septicemia.

√4ᵗʰ 026 Rat-bite fever

026.0 Spirillary fever

Rat-bite fever due to Spirillum minor [S. minus]
Sodoku

026.1 Streptobacillary fever

Epidemic arthritic erythema
Haverhill fever
Rat-bite fever due to Streptobacillus moniliformis

026.9 Unspecified rat-bite fever

√4ᵗʰ 027 Other zoonotic bacterial diseases

027.0 Listeriosis

Infection ⎫
Septicemia ⎬ by Listeria monocytogenes

Use additional code to identify manifestation, as meningitis (320.7)

EXCLUDES   congenital listeriosis (771.2)

027.1 Erysipelothrix infection

Erysipeloid (of Rosenbach)
Infection ⎫ by Erysipelothrix insidiosa
Septicemia ⎬   [E. rhusiopathiae]

DEF: Usually associated with handling of fish, meat, or poultry; symptoms range from localized inflammation to septicemia.

027.2 Pasteurellosis

Pasteurella pseudotuberculosis infection
Mesenteric adenitis ⎫ by Pasteurella
Septic infection (cat bite) ⎬   multocida [P.
  (dog bite) ⎭   septica]

EXCLUDES   infection by:
  Francisella [Pasteurella] tularensis
    (021.0-021.9)
  Yersinia [Pasteurella] pestis (020.0-
    020.9)

DEF: Swelling, abscesses, or septicemia from *Pasteurella multocida*, commonly transmitted to humans by a dog or cat scratch.

027.8 Other specified zoonotic bacterial diseases

027.9 Unspecified zoonotic bacterial disease

✓4ᵗʰ
✓5ᵗʰ Additional Digit Required   Unspecified Code   Other Specified Code   Manifestation Code   ►◄ Revised Text   ● New Code   ▲ Revised Code Title

2003 ICD•9•CM   **Volume 1 — 5**

Infectious and Parasitic Diseases 030–036.9

OTHER BACTERIAL DISEASES (030-041)

EXCLUDES   bacterial venereal diseases (098.0-099.9)
bartonellosis (088.0)

√4th **030 Leprosy**

INCLUDES   Hansen's disease
infection by Mycobacterium leprae

030.0 Lepromatous [type L]
Lepromatous leprosy (macular) (diffuse) (infiltrated) (nodular) (neuritic)

DEF: Infectious disseminated leprosy bacilli with lesions and deformities.

030.1 Tuberculoid [type T]
Tuberculoid leprosy (macular) (maculoanesthetic) (major) (minor) (neuritic)

DEF: Relatively benign, self-limiting leprosy with neuralgia and scales.

030.2 Indeterminate [group I]
Indeterminate [uncharacteristic] leprosy (macular) (neuritic)

DEF: Uncharacteristic leprosy, frequently an early manifestation.

030.3 Borderline [group B]
Borderline or dimorphous leprosy (infiltrated) (neuritic)

DEF: Transitional form of leprosy, neither lepromatous nor tuberculoid.

030.8 Other specified leprosy

030.9 Leprosy, unspecified

√4th **031 Diseases due to other mycobacteria**

031.0 Pulmonary
Battey disease
Infection by Mycobacterium:
avium
intracellulare [Battey bacillus]
kansasii

031.1 Cutaneous
Buruli ulcer
Infection by Mycobacterium:
marinum [M. balnei]
ulcerans

031.2 Disseminated
Disseminated mycobacterium avium-intracellulare complex (DMAC)
Mycobacterium avium-intracellulare complex (MAC) bacteremia

DEF: Disseminated mycobacterium avium-intracellulare complex (DMAC): A serious systemic form of MAC commonly observed in patients in the late course of AIDS.

DEF: Mycobacterium avium-intracellulare complex (MAC) bacterium: Human pulmonary disease, lymphadenitis in children and systemic disease in immunocompromised individuals caused by a slow growing, gram-positive, aerobic organism.

031.8 Other specified mycobacterial diseases

031.9 Unspecified diseases due to mycobacteria
Atypical mycobacterium infection NOS

√4th **032 Diphtheria**

INCLUDES   infection by Corynebacterium diphtheriae

032.0 Faucial diphtheria
Membranous angina, diphtheritic

DEF: Diphtheria of the throat.

032.1 Nasopharyngeal diphtheria

032.2 Anterior nasal diphtheria

032.3 Laryngeal diphtheria
Laryngotracheitis, diphtheritic

√5th **032.8 Other specified diphtheria**

032.81 Conjunctival diphtheria
Pseudomembranous diphtheritic conjunctivitis

032.82 Diphtheritic myocarditis

032.83 Diphtheritic peritonitis

032.84 Diphtheritic cystitis

032.85 Cutaneous diphtheria

032.89 Other

032.9 Diphtheria, unspecified

√4th **033 Whooping cough**

INCLUDES   pertussis
Use additional code to identify any associated pneumonia (484.3)

DEF: An acute, highly contagious respiratory tract infection caused by *Bordetella pertussis* and *B. bronchiseptica*; characteristic paroxysmal cough.

033.0 Bordetella pertussis [B. pertussis]

033.1 Bordetella parapertussis [B. parapertussis]

033.8 Whooping cough due to other specified organism
Bordetella bronchiseptica [B. bronchiseptica]

033.9 Whooping cough, unspecified organism

√4th **034 Streptococcal sore throat and scarlet fever**

034.0 Streptococcal sore throat

Septic:	Streptococcal:
angina	laryngitis
sore throat	pharyngitis
Streptococcal:	tonsillitis
angina	

034.1 Scarlet fever
Scarlatina

EXCLUDES   parascarlatina (057.8)

DEF: Streptococcal infection and fever with red rash spreading from trunk.

035 Erysipelas

EXCLUDES   postpartum or puerperal erysipelas (670)

DEF: An acute superficial cellulitis involving the dermal lymphatics; it is often caused by group A streptococci.

√4th **036 Meningococcal infection**

036.0 Meningococcal meningitis
Cerebrospinal fever (meningococcal)
Meningitis:
cerebrospinal
epidemic

036.1 Meningococcal encephalitis

036.2 Meningococcemia
Meningococcal septicemia

036.3 Waterhouse-Friderichsen syndrome, meningococcal
Meningococcal hemorrhagic adrenalitis
Meningococcic adrenal syndrome
Waterhouse-Friderichsen syndrome NOS

√5th **036.4 Meningococcal carditis**

036.40 Meningococcal carditis, unspecified

036.41 Meningococcal pericarditis

DEF: Meningococcal infection of the outer membrane of the heart.

036.42 Meningococcal endocarditis

DEF: Meningococcal infection of the membranes lining the cavities of the heart.

036.43 Meningococcal myocarditis

DEF: Meningococcal infection of the muscle of the heart.

√5th **036.8 Other specified meningococcal infections**

036.81 Meningococcal optic neuritis

036.82 Meningococcal arthropathy

036.89 Other

036.9 Meningococcal infection, unspecified
Meningococcal infection NOS

N   Newborn Age: 0   P   Pediatric Age: 0-17   M   Maternity Age: 12-55   A   Adult Age: 15-124   MSP   Medicare Secondary Payer

037 Tetanus

> EXCLUDES   tetanus:
> complicating:
> abortion (634-638 with .0, 639.0)
> ectopic or molar pregnancy (639.0)
> neonatorum (771.3)
> puerperal (670)

DEF: An acute, often fatal, infectious disease caused by the anaerobic, spore-forming bacillus *Clostridium tetani*; the bacillus most often enters the body through a contaminated wound, burns, surgical wounds, or cutaneous ulcers. Symptoms include lockjaw, spasms, seizures, and paralysis.

√4th 038 Septicemia

> EXCLUDES   bacteremia (790.7)
> during labor (659.3)
> following ectopic or molar pregnancy (639.0)
> following infusion, injection, transfusion, or vaccination (999.3)
> postpartum, puerperal (670)
> ▶septicemia (sepsis) of newborn (771.81)◀
> that complicating abortion (634-638 with .0, 639.0)

DEF: A systemic disease associated with the presence and persistence of pathogenic microorganisms or their toxins in the blood.

038.0 Streptococcal septicemia

√5th 038.1 Staphylococcal septicemia

    038.10 Staphylococcal septicemia, unspecified

    038.11 Staphylococcus aureus septicemia

    038.19 Other staphylococcal septicemia

038.2 Pneumococcal septicemia [Streptococcus pneumoniae septicemia]

038.3 Septicemia due to anaerobes

    Septicemia due to bacteroides

> EXCLUDES   gas gangrene (040.0)
> that due to anaerobic streptococci (038.0)

DEF: Infection of blood by microorganisms that thrive without oxygen.

√5th 038.4 Septicemia due to other gram-negative organisms

DEF: Infection of blood by microorganisms categorized as gram-negative by Gram's method of staining for identification of bacteria.

    038.40 Gram-negative organism, unspecified

      Gram-negative septicemia NOS

    038.41 Hemophilus influenzae [H. influenzae]

    038.42 Escherichia coli [E. coli]

    038.43 Pseudomonas

    038.44 Serratia

    038.49 Other

038.8 Other specified septicemias

> EXCLUDES   septicemia (due to):
> anthrax (022.3)
> gonococcal (098.89)
> herpetic (054.5)
> meningococcal (036.2)
> septicemic plague (020.2)

038.9 Unspecified septicemia

    Septicemia NOS

> EXCLUDES   bacteremia NOS (790.7)

√4th 039 Actinomycotic infections

> INCLUDES   actinomycotic mycetoma
> infection by Actinomycetales, such as species of Actinomyces, Actinomadura, Nocardia, Streptomyces
> maduromycosis (actinomycotic)
> schizomycetoma (actinomycotic)

DEF: Inflammatory lesions and abscesses at site of infection by *Actinomyces israelii*.

039.0 Cutaneous

    Erythrasma

    Trichomycosis axillaris

039.1 Pulmonary

    Thoracic actinomycosis

039.2 Abdominal

039.3 Cervicofacial

039.4 Madura foot

> EXCLUDES   madura foot due to mycotic infection (117.4)

039.8 Of other specified sites

039.9 Of unspecified site

    Actinomycosis NOS   Nocardiosis NOS

    Maduromycosis NOS

√4th 040 Other bacterial diseases

> EXCLUDES   bacteremia NOS (790.7)
> bacterial infection NOS (041.9)

040.0 Gas gangrene

    Gas bacillus infection or gangrene

    Infection by Clostridium:

      histolyticum

      oedematiens

      perfringens [welchii]

      septicum

      sordellii

    Malignant edema

    Myonecrosis, clostridial

    Myositis, clostridial

040.1 Rhinoscleroma

DEF: Growths on the nose and nasopharynx caused by *Klebsiella rhinoscleromatis*.

040.2 Whipple's disease

    Intestinal lipodystrophy

040.3 Necrobacillosis

DEF: Infection with *Fusobacterium necrophorum* causing abscess or necrosis.

√5th 040.8 Other specified bacterial diseases

    040.81 Tropical pyomyositis

    040.82 Toxic shock syndrome

      Use additional code to identify the organism

    040.89 Other

√4th 041 Bacterial infection in conditions classified elsewhere and of unspecified site

Note: This category is provided to be used as an additional code to identify the bacterial agent in diseases classified elsewhere. This category will also be used to classify bacterial infections of unspecified nature or site.

> EXCLUDES   bacteremia NOS (790.7)
> septicemia (038.0-038.9)

√5th 041.0 Streptococcus

    041.00 Streptococcus, unspecified

    041.01 Group A

    041.02 Group B

    041.03 Group C

    041.04 Group D [Enterococcus]

    041.05 Group G

    041.09 Other Streptococcus

√5th 041.1 Staphylococcus

    041.10 Staphylococcus, unspecified

    041.11 Staphylococcus aureus

    041.19 Other Staphylococcus

041.2 Pneumococcus

041.3 Friedländer's bacillus

    Infection by Klebsiella pneumoniae

041.4 Escherichia coli [E. coli]

041.5 Hemophilus influenzae [H. influenzae]

041.6 Proteus (mirabilis) (morganii)

041.7 Pseudomonas

√4th √5th   Additional Digit Required   Unspecified Code   Other Specified Code   Manifestation Code   ▶◀ Revised Text   ● New Code   ▲ Revised Code Title

✓5th 041.8 Other specified bacterial infections

041.81 Mycoplasma
Eaton's agent
Pleuropneumonia-like organisms [PPLO]

041.82 Bacillus fragilis

041.83 Clostridium perfringens

041.84 Other anaerobes
Bacteroides (fragilis)
Gram-negative anaerobes
> EXCLUDES   *Helicobacter pylori (041.86)*

041.85 Other gram-negative organisms
Aerobacter aerogenes
Gram-negative bacteria NOS
Mima polymorpha
Serratia
> EXCLUDES   *gram-negative anaerobes (041.84)*

041.86 Helicobacter pylori (H. pylori)

041.89 Other specified bacteria

041.9 Bacterial infection, unspecified

HUMAN IMMUNODEFICIENCY VIRUS (HIV) INFECTION (042)

042 Human immunodeficiency virus [HIV] disease
Acquired immune deficiency syndrome
Acquired immunodeficiency syndrome
AIDS
AIDS-like syndrome
AIDS-related complex
ARC
HIV infection, symptomatic
Use additional code(s) to identify all manifestations of HIV.
Use additional code to identify HIV-2 infection (079.53).
> EXCLUDES   *asymptomatic HIV infection status (V08)*
> *exposure to HIV virus (V01.7)*
> *nonspecific serologic evidence of HIV (795.71)*

POLIOMYELITIS AND OTHER NON-ARTHROPOD-BORNE VIRAL DISEASES OF CENTRAL NERVOUS SYSTEM (045-049)

✓4th 045 Acute poliomyelitis
> EXCLUDES   *late effects of acute poliomyelitis (138)*

The following fifth-digit subclassification is for use with category 045:

  0 poliovirus, unspecified type
  1 poliovirus type I
  2 poliovirus type II
  3 poliovirus type III

✓5th 045.0 Acute paralytic poliomyelitis specified as bulbar
Infantile paralysis (acute)
Poliomyelitis (acute) } specified as bulbar
(anterior)

Polioencephalitis (acute) (bulbar)
Polioencephalomyelitis (acute) (anterior) (bulbar)

DEF: Acute paralytic infection occurring where the brain merges with the spinal cord; affecting breathing, swallowing, and heart rate.

✓5th 045.1 Acute poliomyelitis with other paralysis
Paralysis: Paralysis:
acute atrophic, spinal   infantile, paralytic
Poliomyelitis (acute)
anterior   } with paralysis except bulbar
epidemic

DEF: Paralytic infection affecting peripheral or spinal nerves.

✓5th 045.2 Acute nonparalytic poliomyelitis
Poliomyelitis (acute)
anterior   } specified as nonparalytic
epidemic

DEF: Nonparalytic infection causing pain, stiffness, and paresthesias.

✓5th 045.9 Acute poliomyelitis, unspecified
Infantile paralysis
Poliomyelitis (acute) } unspecified whether paralytic or nonparalytic
anterior
epidemic

✓4th 046 Slow virus infection of central nervous system

046.0 Kuru
DEF: A chronic, progressive, fatal nervous system disorder; clinical symptoms include cerebellar ataxia, trembling, spasticity and progressive dementia.

046.1 Jakob-Creutzfeldt disease
Subacute spongiform encephalopathy
DEF: Communicable, progressive spongiform encephalopathy thought to be caused by an infectious particle known as a "prion" (proteinaceous infection particle). This is a progressive, fatal disease manifested principally by mental deterioration.

046.2 Subacute sclerosing panencephalitis
Dawson's inclusion body encephalitis
Van Bogaert's sclerosing leukoencephalitis
DEF: Progressive viral infection causing cerebral dysfunction, blindness, dementia, and death (SSPE).

046.3 Progressive multifocal leukoencephalopathy
Multifocal leukoencephalopathy NOS
DEF: Infection affecting cerebral cortex in patients with weakened immune systems.

046.8 Other specified slow virus infection of central nervous system

046.9 Unspecified slow virus infection of central nervous system

✓4th 047 Meningitis due to enterovirus
> INCLUDES   meningitis:
> abacterial
> aseptic
> viral
> EXCLUDES   meningitis due to:
> *adenovirus (049.1)*
> *arthropod-borne virus (060.0-066.9)*
> *leptospira (100.81)*
> *virus of:*
>   *herpes simplex (054.72)*
>   *herpes zoster (053.0)*
>   *lymphocytic choriomeningitis (049.0)*
>   *mumps (072.1)*
>   *poliomyelitis (045.0-045.9)*
> *any other infection specifically classified elsewhere*

047.0 Coxsackie virus

047.1 ECHO virus
Meningo-eruptive syndrome

047.8 Other specified viral meningitis

047.9 Unspecified viral meningitis
Viral meningitis NOS

048 Other enterovirus diseases of central nervous system
Boston exanthem

✓4th 049 Other non-arthropod-borne viral diseases of central nervous system
> EXCLUDES   *late effects of viral encephalitis (139.0)*

049.0 Lymphocytic choriomeningitis
Lymphocytic:
meningitis (serous) (benign)
meningoencephalitis (serous) (benign)

049.1 Meningitis due to adenovirus
DEF: Inflammation of lining of brain caused by Arenaviruses and usually occurring in adults in fall and winter months.

049.8 Other specified non-arthropod-borne viral diseases of central nervous system

Encephalitis:
- acute:
  - inclusion body
  - necrotizing
- epidemic
- lethargica
- Rio Bravo
- von Economo's disease

049.9 Unspecified non-arthropod-borne viral diseases of central nervous system

Viral encephalitis NOS

VIRAL DISEASES ACCOMPANIED BY EXANTHEM (050-057)

EXCLUDES   *arthropod-borne viral diseases (060.0-066.9)*
Boston exanthem (048)

√4th **050 Smallpox**

050.0 Variola major

Hemorrhagic (pustular) smallpox
Malignant smallpox
Purpura variolosa

DEF: Form of smallpox known for its high mortality; exists only in laboratories.

050.1 Alastrim

Variola minor

DEF: Mild form of smallpox known for its low mortality rate.

050.2 Modified smallpox

Varioloid

DEF: Mild form occurring in patients with history of infection or vaccination.

050.9 Smallpox, unspecified

√4th **051 Cowpox and paravaccinia**

051.0 Cowpox

Vaccinia not from vaccination

EXCLUDES   *vaccinia (generalized) (from vaccination) (999.0)*

DEF: A disease contracted by milking infected cows; vesicles usually appear on the fingers, may spread to hands and adjacent areas and usually disappear without scarring; other associated features of the disease may include local edema, lymphangitis and regional lymphadenitis with or without fever.

051.1 Pseudocowpox

Milkers' node

DEF: Hand lesions and mild fever in dairy workers caused by exposure to paravaccinia.

051.2 Contagious pustular dermatitis

Ecthyma contagiosum
Orf

DEF: Skin eruptions caused by exposure to poxvirus-infected sheep or goats.

051.9 Paravaccinia, unspecified

√4th **052 Chickenpox**

DEF: Contagious infection by varicella-zoster virus causing rash with pustules and fever.

052.0 Postvaricella encephalitis

Postchickenpox encephalitis

052.1 Varicella (hemorrhagic) pneumonitis
052.7 With other specified complications
052.8 With unspecified complication
052.9 Varicella without mention of complication

Chickenpox NOS
Varicella NOS

√4th **053 Herpes zoster**

INCLUDES   shingles
zona

DEF: Self-limiting infection by varicella-zoster virus causing unilateral eruptions and neuralgia along affected nerves.

053.0 With meningitis

DEF: Varicella-zoster virus infection causing inflammation of the lining of the brain and/or spinal cord.

√5th **053.1 With other nervous system complications**

053.10 With unspecified nervous system complication

053.11 Geniculate herpes zoster

Herpetic geniculate ganglionitis

DEF: Unilateral eruptions and neuralgia along the facial nerve geniculum affecting face and outer and middle ear.

053.12 Postherpetic trigeminal neuralgia

DEF: Severe oral or nasal pain following a herpes zoster infection.

053.13 Postherpetic polyneuropathy

DEF: Multiple areas of pain following a herpes zoster infection.

053.19 Other

√5th **053.2 With ophthalmic complications**

053.20 Herpes zoster dermatitis of eyelid

Herpes zoster ophthalmicus

053.21 Herpes zoster keratoconjunctivitis
053.22 Herpes zoster iridocyclitis
053.29 Other

√5th **053.7 With other specified complications**

053.71 Otitis externa due to herpes zoster
053.79 Other

053.8 With unspecified complication
053.9 Herpes zoster without mention of complication

Herpes zoster NOS

√4th **054 Herpes simplex**

EXCLUDES   *congenital herpes simplex (771.2)*

054.0 Eczema herpeticum

Kaposi's varicelliform eruption

DEF: Herpes simplex virus invading site of preexisting skin inflammation.

√5th **054.1 Genital herpes**

054.10 Genital herpes, unspecified

Herpes progenitalis

054.11 Herpetic vulvovaginitis ♀
054.12 Herpetic ulceration of vulva ♀
054.13 Herpetic infection of penis ♂
054.19 Other

054.2 Herpetic gingivostomatitis
054.3 Herpetic meningoencephalitis

Herpes encephalitis
Simian B disease

DEF: Inflammation of the brain and its lining; caused by infection of herpes simplex 1 in adults and simplex 2 in newborns.

√5th **054.4 With ophthalmic complications**

054.40 With unspecified ophthalmic complication

054.41 Herpes simplex dermatitis of eyelid
054.42 Dendritic keratitis
054.43 Herpes simplex disciform keratitis
054.44 Herpes simplex iridocyclitis
054.49 Other

054.5 Herpetic septicemia

√4th Additional Digit Required   √5th
Unspecified Code   Other Specified Code   Manifestation Code   ▶◀ Revised Text   ● New Code   ▲ Revised Code Title

2003 ICD•9•CM   **Volume 1 — 9**

Infectious and Parasitic Diseases 054.6–063.2

054.6   **Herpetic whitlow**
Herpetic felon
DEF: A primary infection of the terminal segment of a finger by herpes simplex; intense itching and pain start the disease, vesicles form, and tissue ultimately is destroyed.

√5th **054.7**   **With other specified complications**
054.71 Visceral herpes simplex
054.72 Herpes simplex meningitis
054.73 Herpes simplex otitis externa
054.79 Other
054.8   **With unspecified complication**
054.9   **Herpes simplex without mention of complication**

√4th **055 Measles**
INCLUDES	morbilli
	rubeola

055.0   **Postmeasles encephalitis**
055.1   **Postmeasles pneumonia**
055.2   **Postmeasles otitis media**
√5th **055.7**   **With other specified complications**
055.71 Measles keratoconjunctivitis
Measles keratitis
055.79 Other
055.8   **With unspecified complication**
055.9   **Measles without mention of complication**

√4th **056 Rubella**
INCLUDES	German measles
EXCLUDES	congenital rubella (771.0)

DEF: Acute but usually benign togavirus infection causing fever, sore throat, and rash; associated with complications to fetus as a result of maternal infection.

√5th **056.0**   **With neurological complications**
056.00 With unspecified neurological complication
056.01 Encephalomyelitis due to rubella
Encephalitis } due to
Meningoencephalitis } rubella
056.09 Other
√5th **056.7**   **With other specified complications**
056.71 Arthritis due to rubella
056.79 Other
056.8   **With unspecified complications**
056.9   **Rubella without mention of complication**

√4th **057 Other viral exanthemata**
DEF: Skin eruptions or rashes and fever caused by viruses, including poxviruses.

057.0   **Erythema infectiosum [fifth disease]**
DEF: A moderately contagious, benign, epidemic disease, usually seen in children, and of probable viral etiology; a red macular rash appears on the face and may spread to the limbs and trunk.

057.8   **Other specified viral exanthemata**
Dukes (-Filatow) disease
Exanthema subitum [sixth disease]
Fourth disease
Parascarlatina
Pseudoscarlatina
Roseola infantum
057.9   **Viral exanthem, unspecified**

ARTHROPOD-BORNE VIRAL DISEASES (060-066)

Use additional code to identify any associated meningitis (321.2)
EXCLUDES	late effects of viral encephalitis (139.0)

√4th **060 Yellow fever**
DEF: Fever and jaundice from infection by mosquito-borne virus of genus Flavivirus.

060.0   **Sylvatic**
Yellow fever:
jungle
sylvan
DEF: Yellow fever transmitted from animal to man, via mosquito.

060.1   **Urban**
DEF: Yellow fever transmitted from man to man, via mosquito.

060.9   **Yellow fever, unspecified**

061 Dengue
Breakbone fever
EXCLUDES	hemorrhagic fever caused by dengue virus (065.4)

DEF: Acute, self-limiting infection by mosquito-borne virus characterized by fever and generalized aches

√4th **062 Mosquito-borne viral encephalitis**
062.0   **Japanese encephalitis**
Japanese B encephalitis
DEF: Flavivirus causing inflammation of the brain, and Russia, with a wide range of clinical manifestations

062.1   **Western equine encephalitis**
DEF: Alphavirus WEE infection causing inflammation of the brain, found in areas west of the Mississippi; transmitted horse to mosquito to man.

062.2   **Eastern equine encephalitis**
EXCLUDES	Venezuelan equine encephalitis (066.2)

DEF: Alphavirus EEE causing inflammation of the brain and spinal cord, found as far north as Canada and south into South America and Mexico; transmitted horse to mosquito to man.

062.3   **St. Louis encephalitis**
DEF: Epidemic form caused by Flavivirus and transmitted by mosquito, and characterized by fever, difficulty in speech, and headache.

062.4   **Australian encephalitis**
Australian arboencephalitis
Australian X disease
Murray Valley encephalitis
DEF: Flavivirus causing inflammation of the brain, occurring in Australia and New Guinea.

062.5   **California virus encephalitis**
Encephalitis: Tahyna fever
   California
   La Crosse
DEF: Bunya virus causing inflammation of the brain.

062.8   **Other specified mosquito-borne viral encephalitis**
Encephalitis by Ilheus virus
EXCLUDES	▶West Nile virus (066.4)◀

062.9   **Mosquito-borne viral encephalitis, unspecified**

√4th **063 Tick-borne viral encephalitis**
INCLUDES	diphasic meningoencephalitis

063.0   **Russian spring-summer [taiga] encephalitis**
063.1   **Louping ill**
DEF: Inflammation of brain caused by virus transmitted sheep to tick to man; incidence usually limited to British Isles.

063.2   **Central European encephalitis**
DEF: Inflammation of brain caused by virus transmitted by tick; limited to central Europe and presenting with two distinct phases.

063.8 Other specified tick-borne viral encephalitis
Langat encephalitis
Powassan encephalitis

063.9 Tick-borne viral encephalitis, unspecified

064 Viral encephalitis transmitted by other and unspecified arthropods
Arthropod-borne viral encephalitis, vector unknown
Negishi virus encephalitis
EXCLUDES *viral encephalitis NOS (049.9)*

√4ᵗʰ **065 Arthropod-borne hemorrhagic fever**

065.0 Crimean hemorrhagic fever [CHF Congo virus]
Central Asian hemorrhagic fever

065.1 Omsk hemorrhagic fever

065.2 Kyasanur Forest disease

065.3 Other tick-borne hemorrhagic fever

065.4 Mosquito-borne hemorrhagic fever
Chikungunya hemorrhagic fever
Dengue hemorrhagic fever
EXCLUDES *Chikungunya fever (066.3)*
dengue (061)
yellow fever (060.0-060.9)

065.8 Other specified arthropod-borne hemorrhagic fever
Mite-borne hemorrhagic fever

065.9 Arthropod-borne hemorrhagic fever, unspecified
Arbovirus hemorrhagic fever NOS

√4ᵗʰ **066 Other arthropod-borne viral diseases**

066.0 Phlebotomus fever
Changuinola fever
Sandfly fever
DEF: Sandfly-borne viral infection occurring in Asia, Middle East and South America.

066.1 Tick-borne fever
Nairobi sheep disease
Tick fever:
American mountain
Colorado
Kemerovo
Quaranfil

066.2 Venezuelan equine fever
Venezuelan equine encephalitis
DEF: Alphavirus VEE infection causing inflammation of the brain, usually limited to South America, Mexico, and Florida; transmitted horse to mosquito to man.

066.3 Other mosquito-borne fever

Fever (viral):	Fever (viral):
Bunyamwera	Oropouche
Bwamba	Pixuna
Chikungunya	Rift valley
Guama	Ross river
Mayaro	Wesselsbron
Mucambo	Zika
O'Nyong-Nyong	

EXCLUDES *dengue (061)*
yellow fever (060.0-060.9)

● **066.4 West Nile fever**
West Nile encephalitis
West Nile encephalomyelitis
West Nile virus

066.8 Other specified arthropod-borne viral diseases
Chandipura fever　　Piry fever

066.9 Arthropod-borne viral disease, unspecified
Arbovirus infection NOS

OTHER DISEASES DUE TO VIRUSES AND CHLAMYDIAE (070-079)

√4ᵗʰ **070 Viral hepatitis**
INCLUDES viral hepatitis (acute) (chronic)
EXCLUDES *cytomegalic inclusion virus hepatitis (078.5)*

DEF: Hepatitis A: HAV infection is self-limiting with flu like symptoms; transmission, fecal-oral.

DEF: Hepatitis B: HBV infection can be chronic and systemic; transmission, bodily fluids.

DEF: Hepatitis C: HCV infection can be chronic and systemic; transmission, blood transfusion and unidentified agents.

DEF: Hepatitis D (delta): HDV occurs only in the presence of hepatitis B virus.

DEF: Hepatitis E: HEV is epidemic form; transmission and nature under investigation.

070.0 Viral hepatitis A with hepatic coma

070.1 Viral hepatitis A without mention of hepatic coma
Infectious hepatitis

The following fifth-digit subclassification is for use with categories 070.2 and 070.3:
　0 **acute or unspecified, without mention of hepatitis delta**
　1 **acute or unspecified, with hepatitis delta**
　2 **chronic, without mention of hepatitis delta**
　3 **chronic, with hepatitis delta**

√5ᵗʰ **070.2 Viral hepatitis B with hepatic coma**

√5ᵗʰ **070.3 Viral hepatitis B without mention of hepatic coma**
Serum hepatitis

√5ᵗʰ **070.4 Other specified viral hepatitis with hepatic coma**

070.41 Acute or unspecified hepatitis C with hepatic coma

070.42 Hepatitis delta without mention of active hepatitis B disease with hepatic coma
Hepatitis delta with hepatitis B carrier state

070.43 Hepatitis E with hepatic coma

070.44 Chronic hepatitis C with hepatic coma

070.49 Other specified viral hepatitis with hepatic coma

√5ᵗʰ **070.5 Other specified viral hepatitis without mention of hepatic coma**

070.51 Acute or unspecified hepatitis C without mention of hepatic coma

070.52 Hepatitis delta without mention of active hepatititis B disease or hepatic coma

070.53 Hepatitis E without mention of hepatic coma

070.54 Chronic hepatitis C without mention of hepatic coma

070.59 Other specified viral hepatitis without mention of hepatic coma

070.6 Unspecified viral hepatitis with hepatic coma

070.9 Unspecified viral hepatitis without mention of hepatic coma
Viral hepatitis NOS

071 Rabies
Hydrophobia
Lyssa
DEF: Acute infectious disease of the CNS caused by a rhabdovirus; usually spread by virus-laden saliva from bites by infected animals; it progresses from fever, restlessness, and extreme excitability, to hydrophobia, seizures, confusion and death.

√4ᵗʰ **072 Mumps**
DEF: Acute infectious disease caused by paramyxovirus; usually seen in children less than 15 years of age; salivary glands are typically enlarged, and other organs, such as testes, pancreas and meninges, are often involved.

072.0 Mumps orchitis　　　♂

072.1 Mumps meningitis

√4ᵗʰ / √5ᵗʰ Additional Digit Required　　Unspecified Code　　Other Specified Code　　Manifestation Code　　►◄ Revised Text　　● New Code　　▲ Revised Code Title

2003 ICD•9•CM　　　　October 2002 • Volume 1 — 11

Infectious and Parasitic Diseases 072.2–078.2

072.2   Mumps encephalitis
     Mumps meningoencephalitis

072.3   Mumps pancreatitis

√5ᵗʰ **072.7   Mumps with other specified complications**

     072.71 Mumps hepatitis

     072.72 Mumps polyneuropathy

     072.79 Other

072.8   Mumps with unspecified complication

072.9   Mumps without mention of complication
     Epidemic parotitis
     Infectious parotitis

073   Ornithosis

     INCLUDES   parrot fever
                  psittacosis

     DEF: *Chlamydia psittaci* infection often transmitted from birds to humans.

073.0   With pneumonia
     Lobular pneumonitis due to ornithosis

073.7   With other specified complications

073.8   With unspecified complication

073.9   Ornithosis, unspecified

√4ᵗʰ **074   Specific diseases due to Coxsackie virus**

     EXCLUDES   *Coxsackie virus:*
                infection NOS (079.2)
                meningitis (047.0)

074.0   Herpangina
     Vesicular pharyngitis

     DEF: Acute infectious coxsackie virus infection causing throat lesions, fever, and vomiting; generally affects children in summer.

074.1   Epidemic pleurodynia
     Bornholm disease   Epidemic:
     Devil's grip   myalgia
                        myositis

     DEF: Paroxysmal pain in chest, accompanied by fever and usually limited to children and young adults; caused by coxsackie virus.

√5ᵗʰ **074.2   Coxsackie carditis**

     074.20 Coxsackie carditis, unspecified

     074.21 Coxsackie pericarditis

         DEF: Coxsackie infection of the outer lining of the heart.

     074.22 Coxsackie endocarditis

         DEF: Coxsackie infection within the heart's cavities.

     074.23 Coxsackie myocarditis
         Aseptic myocarditis of newborn

         DEF: Coxsackie infection of the muscle of the heart.

074.3   Hand, foot, and mouth disease
     Vesicular stomatitis and exanthem

     DEF: Mild coxsackie infection causing lesions on hands, feet and oral mucosa; most commonly seen in preschool children.

074.8   Other specified diseases due to Coxsackie virus
     Acute lymphonodular pharyngitis

075   Infectious mononucleosis
     Glandular fever   Pfeiffer's disease
     Monocytic angina

     DEF: Acute infection by Epstein-Barr virus causing fever, sore throat, enlarged lymph glands and spleen, and fatigue; usually seen in teens and young adults.

√4ᵗʰ **076   Trachoma**

     EXCLUDES   *late effect of trachoma (139.1)*

     DEF: A chronic infectious disease of the cornea and conjunctiva caused by a strain of the bacteria *Chlamydia trachomatis*; the infection can cause photophobia, pain, excessive tearing and sometimes blindness.

076.0   Initial stage
     Trachoma dubium

076.1   Active stage
     Granular conjunctivitis (trachomatous)
     Trachomatous
         follicular conjunctivitis
         pannus

076.9   Trachoma, unspecified
     Trachoma NOS

√4ᵗʰ **077   Other diseases of conjunctiva due to viruses and Chlamydiae**

     EXCLUDES   *ophthalmic complications of viral diseases classified elsewhere*

077.0   Inclusion conjunctivitis
     Paratrachoma
     Swimming pool conjunctivitis

     EXCLUDES   *inclusion blennorrhea (neonatal) (771.6)*

     DEF: Pus in conjunctiva caused by *Chlamydiae trachomatis* infection.

077.1   Epidemic keratoconjunctivitis
     Shipyard eye

     DEF: Highly contagious corneal or conjunctival infection caused by adenovirus type 8; symptoms include inflammation and corneal infiltrates.

077.2   Pharyngoconjunctival fever
     Viral pharyngoconjunctivitis

077.3   Other adenoviral conjunctivitis
     Acute adenoviral follicular conjunctivitis

077.4   Epidemic hemorrhagic conjunctivitis
     Apollo:
         conjunctivitis
         disease
     Conjunctivitis due to enterovirus type 70
     Hemorrhagic conjunctivitis (acute) (epidemic)

077.8   Other viral conjunctivitis
     Newcastle conjunctivitis

√5ᵗʰ **077.9   Unspecified diseases of conjunctiva due to viruses and Chlamydiae**

     DEF: A genus of the family *Chlamydiaceae; C. psittaci* causes psittacosis in man and ornithosis in birds, and *C. trachomatis* causes trachoma, conjunctivitis, lymphogranuloma venereum, pneumonitis and pneumonia.

     077.98 Due to Chlamydiae

     077.99 Due to viruses
         Viral conjunctivitis NOS

√4ᵗʰ **078   Other diseases due to viruses and Chlamydiae**

     EXCLUDES   *viral infection NOS (079.0-079.9)*
                viremia NOS (790.8)

078.0   Molluscum contagiosum

     DEF: Benign poxvirus infection causing small bumps on the skin or conjunctiva; transmitted by close contact.

√5ᵗʰ **078.1   Viral warts**
     Viral warts due to human papilloma virus

     DEF: A keratotic papilloma of the epidermis caused by the human papilloma virus; the superficial vegetative lesions last for varying durations and eventually regress spontaneously.

     078.10 Viral warts, unspecified
         Condyloma NOS
         Verruca:
              NOS
              Vulgaris
         Warts (infectious)

     078.11 Condyloma acuminatum

         DEF: Clusters of mucosa or epidermal lesions on external genitalia; viral infection is sexually transmitted.

     078.19 Other specified viral warts
         Genital warts NOS
         Verruca:
              plana
              plantaris

078.2   Sweating fever
     Miliary fever
     Sweating disease

     DEF: A viral infection characterized by profuse sweating; various papular, vesicular and other eruptions cause the blockage of sweat glands.

N Newborn Age: 0   P Pediatric Age: 0-17   M Maternity Age: 12-55   A Adult Age: 15-124   MSP Medicare Secondary Payer

078.3 Cat-scratch disease
     Benign lymphoreticulosis (of inoculation)
     Cat-scratch fever

078.4 Foot and mouth disease
     Aphthous fever
     Epizootic:
        aphthae
        stomatitis

DEF: Ulcers on oral mucosa, legs, and feet after exposure to infected animal.

078.5 Cytomegaloviral disease
     Cytomegalic inclusion disease
     Salivary gland virus disease
     Use additional code to identify manifestation, as:
        cytomegalic inclusion virus:
           hepatitis (573.1)
           pneumonia (484.1)
     EXCLUDES *congenital cytomegalovirus infection (771.1)*

DEF: A herpes virus inclusion associated with serious disease morbidity including fever, leukopenia, pneumonia, retinitis, hepatitis and organ transplant; often leads to syndromes such as hepatomegaly, splenomegaly and thrombocytopenia; a common post-transplant complication for organ transplant recipients.

078.6 Hemorrhagic nephrosonephritis
     Hemorrhagic fever:
        epidemic
        Korean
        Russian
        with renal syndrome

DEF: Viral infection causing kidney dysfunction and bleeding disorders.

078.7 Arenaviral hemorrhagic fever
     Hemorrhagic fever:
        Argentine
        Bolivian
        Junin virus
        Machupo virus

√5th **078.8 Other specified diseases due to viruses and Chlamydiae**
     EXCLUDES *epidemic diarrhea (009.2)*
                     lymphogranuloma venereum (099.1)

     078.81 Epidemic vertigo
     078.82 Epidemic vomiting syndrome
        Winter vomiting disease
     078.88 Other specified diseases due to Chlamydiae
     078.89 Other specified diseases due to viruses
        Epidemic cervical myalgia
        Marburg disease
        Tanapox

√4th **079 Viral and chlamydial infection in conditions classified elsewhere and of unspecified site**
     Note: This category is provided to be used as an additional code to identify the viral agent in diseases classifiable elsewhere. This category will also be used to classify virus infection of unspecified nature or site.

079.0 Adenovirus
079.1 ECHO virus
     DEF: An "orphan" enteric RNA virus, certain serotypes of which are associated with human disease, especially aseptic meningitis.

079.2 Coxsackie virus
     DEF: A heterogenous group of viruses associated with aseptic meningitis, myocarditis, pericarditis, and acute onset juvenile diabetes.

079.3 Rhinovirus
     DEF: Rhinoviruses affect primarily the upper respiratory tract. Over 100 distinct types infect humans.

079.4 Human papillomavirus
     DEF: Viral infection caused by the genus *Papillomavirus* causing cutaneous and genital warts, including verruca vulgaris and condyloma acuminatum; certain types are associated with cervical dysplasia, cancer and other genital malignancies.

√5th **079.5 Retrovirus**
     EXCLUDES *human immunodeficiency virus, type 1 [HIV-1] (042)*
                     human T-cell lymphotrophic virus, type III [HTLV-III] (042)
                     lymphadenopathy-associated virus [LAV] (042)

DEF: A large group of RNA viruses that carry reverse transcriptase and include the leukoviruses and lentiviruses.

     079.50 Retrovirus, unspecified
     079.51 Human T-cell lymphotrophic virus, type I [HTLV-I]
     079.52 Human T-cell lymphotrophic virus, type II [HTLV-II]
     079.53 Human immunodeficiency virus, type 2 [HIV-2]
     079.59 Other specified retrovirus

079.6 Respiratory syncytial virus (RSV)
     DEF: The major respiratory pathogen of young children, causing severe bronchitis and bronchopneumonia, and minor infection in adults.

√5th **079.8 Other specified viral and chlamydial infections**
     079.81 Hantavirus
        DEF: An infection caused by the Muerto Canyon virus whose primary rodent reservoir is the deer mouse Peromyscus maniculatus; commonly characterized by fever, myalgias, headache, cough and rapid respiratory failure.

     079.88 Other specified chlamydial infection
     079.89 Other specified viral infection

√5th **079.9 Unspecified viral and chlamydial infections**
     EXCLUDES *viremia NOS (790.8)*
     079.98 Unspecified chlamydial infection
        Chlamydial infections NOS
     079.99 Unspecified viral infection
        Viral infections NOS

RICKETTSIOSES AND OTHER ARTHROPOD-BORNE DISEASES (080-088)

     EXCLUDES *arthropod-borne viral diseases (060.0-066.9)*

080 Louse-borne [epidemic] typhus
     Typhus (fever):   Typhus (fever):
        classical   exanthematic NOS
        epidemic   louse-borne

DEF: *Rickettsia prowazekii*; causes severe headache, rash, high fever.

√4th **081 Other typhus**
     081.0 Murine [endemic] typhus
        Typhus (fever):   Typhus (fever):
        endemic   flea-borne

        DEF: Milder typhus caused by *Rickettsia typhi (mooseri)*; transmitted by rat flea.

     081.1 Brill's disease
        Brill-Zinsser disease
        Recrudescent typhus (fever)

     081.2 Scrub typhus
        Japanese river fever   Mite-borne typhus
        Kedani fever   Tsutsugamushi

        DEF: Typhus caused by *Rickettsia tsutsugamushi* transmitted by chigger.

     081.9 Typhus, unspecified
        Typhus (fever) NOS

√4th √5th Additional Digit Required   Unspecified Code   Other Specified Code   Manifestation Code   ▶◀ Revised Text   ● New Code   ▲ Revised Code Title

2003 ICD•9•CM   **Volume 1 — 13**

✓4th **082 Tick-borne rickettsioses**

082.0 Spotted fevers
Rocky mountain spotted fever
Sao Paulo fever

082.1 Boutonneuse fever
African tick typhus   Marseilles fever
India tick typhus   Mediterranean tick fever
Kenya tick typhus

082.2 North Asian tick fever
Siberian tick typhus

082.3 Queensland tick typhus

✓5th **082.4 Ehrlichiosis**

082.40 Ehrlichiosis, unspecified

082.41 Ehrlichiosis chaffeensis [E. chaffeensis]
DEF: A febrile illness caused by bacterial infection, also called human monocytic ehrlichiosis (HME). Causal organism is *Ehrlichia chaffeensis,* transmitted by the Lone Star tick, *Amblyomma americanum.* Symptoms include fever, chills, myalgia, nausea, vomiting, diarrhea, confusion, and severe headache occurring one week after a tick bite. Clinical findings are lymphadenopathy, rash, thrombocytopenia, leukopenia, and abnormal liver function tests

082.49 Other ehrlichiosis

082.8 Other specified tick-borne rickettsioses
Lone star fever

082.9 Tick-borne rickettsiosis, unspecified
Tick-borne typhus NOS

✓4th **083 Other rickettsioses**

083.0 Q fever
DEF: Infection of *Coxiella burnetii* usually acquired through airborne organisms.

083.1 Trench fever
Quintan fever   Wolhynian fever

083.2 Rickettsialpox
Vesicular rickettsiosis
DEF: Infection of *Rickettsia akari* usually acquired through a mite bite.

083.8 Other specified rickettsioses

083.9 Rickettsiosis, unspecified

✓4th **084 Malaria**
Note: Subcategories 084.0-084.6 exclude the listed conditions with mention of pernicious complications (084.8-084.9).
EXCLUDES *congenital malaria (771.2)*
DEF: Mosquito-borne disease causing high fever and prostration and cataloged by species of *Plasmodium: P. falciparum, P. malariae, P. ovale,* and *P. vivax.*

084.0 Falciparum malaria [malignant tertian]
Malaria (fever):
by Plasmodium falciparum
subtertian

084.1 Vivax malaria [benign tertian]
Malaria (fever) by Plasmodium vivax

084.2 Quartan malaria
Malaria (fever) by Plasmodium malariae
Malariae malaria

084.3 Ovale malaria
Malaria (fever) by Plasmodium ovale

084.4 Other malaria
Monkey malaria

084.5 Mixed malaria
Malaria (fever) by more than one parasite

084.6 Malaria, unspecified
Malaria (fever) NOS

084.7 Induced malaria
Therapeutically induced malaria
EXCLUDES *accidental infection from syringe, blood transfusion, etc. (084.0-084.6, above, according to parasite species)*
transmission from mother to child during delivery (771.2)

084.8 Blackwater fever
Hemoglobinuric: Malarial hemoglobinuria
fever (bilious)
malaria
DEF: Severe hemic and renal complication of *Plasmodium falciparum* infection.

084.9 Other pernicious complications of malaria
Algid malaria
Cerebral malaria
Use additional code to identify complication, as:
malarial:
hepatitis (573.2)
nephrosis (581.81)

✓4th **085 Leishmaniasis**

085.0 Visceral [kala-azar]
Dumdum fever
Infection by Leishmania:
donovani
infantum
Leishmaniasis:
dermal, post-kala-azar
Mediterranean
visceral (Indian)

085.1 Cutaneous, urban
Aleppo boil   Leishmaniasis, cutaneous:
Baghdad boil   dry form
Delhi boil   late
Infection by Leishmania   recurrent
tropica (minor)   ulcerating
               Oriental sore

085.2 Cutaneous, Asian desert
Infection by Leishmania tropica major
Leishmaniasis, cutaneous:
acute necrotizing
rural
wet form
zoonotic form

085.3 Cutaneous, Ethiopian
Infection by Leishmania ethiopica
Leishmaniasis, cutaneous:
diffuse
lepromatous

085.4 Cutaneous, American
Chiclero ulcer
Infection by Leishmania mexicana
Leishmaniasis tegumentaria diffusa

085.5 Mucocutaneous (American)
Espundia
Infection by Leishmania braziliensis
Uta

085.9 Leishmaniasis, unspecified

✓4th **086 Trypanosomiasis**
Use additional code to identify manifestations, as:
trypanosomiasis:
encephalitis (323.2)
meningitis (321.3)

086.0 Chagas' disease with heart involvement
American trypanosomiasis   ⎤
Infection by Trypanosoma ⎬ with heart
cruzi   ⎦ involvement

Any condition classifiable to 086.2 with heart involvement

086.1 Chagas' disease with other organ involvement

American trypanosomiasis
Infection by Trypanosoma cruzi
} with involvement of organ other than heart

Any condition classifiable to 086.2 with involvement of organ other than heart

086.2 Chagas' disease without mention of organ involvement
American trypanosomiasis
Infection by Trypanosoma cruzi

086.3 Gambian trypanosomiasis
Gambian sleeping sickness
Infection by Trypanosoma gambiense

086.4 Rhodesian trypanosomiasis
Infection by Trypanosoma rhodesiense
Rhodesian sleeping sickness

086.5 African trypanosomiasis, unspecified
Sleeping sickness NOS

086.9 Trypanosomiasis, unspecified

✓4ᵗʰ 087 Relapsing fever
     INCLUDES   recurrent fever

DEF: Infection by *Borrelia*; symptoms are episodic and include fever and arthralgia.

087.0 Louse-borne
087.1 Tick-borne
087.9 Relapsing fever, unspecified

✓4ᵗʰ 088 Other arthropod-borne diseases

088.0 Bartonellosis
Carrión's disease   Verruga peruana
Oroya fever

✓5ᵗʰ 088.8 Other specified arthropod-borne diseases

088.81 Lyme disease
Erythema chronicum migrans

DEF: A recurrent multisystem disorder caused by the spirochete *Borrelia burgdorferi* with the carrier being the tick *Ixodes dammini*; the disease begins with lesions of erythema chronicum migrans; it is followed by arthritis of the large joints, myalgia, malaise, and neurological and cardiac manifestations.

088.82 Babesiosis
Babesiasis

DEF: A tick-borne disease caused by infection of *Babesia*, characterized by fever, malaise, listlessness, severe anemia and hemoglobinuria.

088.89 Other
088.9 Arthropod-borne disease, unspecified

SYPHILIS AND OTHER VENEREAL DISEASES (090-099)

     EXCLUDES   nonvenereal endemic syphilis (104.0)
                       urogenital trichomoniasis (131.0)

✓4ᵗʰ 090 Congenital syphilis

DEF: Infection by spirochete *Treponema pallidum* acquired in utero from the infected mother.

090.0 Early congenital syphilis, symptomatic
Congenital syphilitic: Congenital syphilitic:
   choroiditis   splenomegaly
   coryza (chronic)   Syphilitic (congenital):
   hepatomegaly   epiphysitis
   mucous patches   osteochondritis
   periostitis   pemphigus
Any congenital syphilitic condition specified as early or manifest less than two years after birth

090.1 Early congenital syphilis, latent
Congenital syphilis without clinical manifestations, with positive serological reaction and negative spinal fluid test, less than two years after birth

090.2 Early congenital syphilis, unspecified
Congenital syphilis NOS, less than two years after birth

090.3 Syphilitic interstitial keratitis
Syphilitic keratitis:
   parenchymatous
   punctata profunda
     EXCLUDES   interstitial keratitis NOS (370.50)

✓5ᵗʰ 090.4 Juvenile neurosyphilis
Use additional code to identify any associated mental disorder

DEF: *Treponema pallidum* infection involving the nervous system.

090.40 Juvenile neurosyphilis, unspecified
Congenital neurosyphilis
Dementia paralytica juvenilis
Juvenile:
   general paresis
   tabes
   taboparesis

090.41 Congenital syphilitic encephalitis
DEF: Congenital *Treponema pallidum* infection involving the brain.

090.42 Congenital syphilitic meningitis
DEF: Congenital *Treponema pallidum* infection involving the lining of the brain and/or spinal cord.

090.49 Other
090.5 Other late congenital syphilis, symptomatic
Gumma due to congenital syphilis
Hutchinson's teeth
Syphilitic saddle nose
Any congenital syphilitic condition specified as late or manifest two years or more after birth

090.6 Late congenital syphilis, latent
Congenital syphilis without clinical manifestations, with positive serological reaction and negative spinal fluid test, two years or more after birth

090.7 Late congenital syphilis, unspecified
Congenital syphilis NOS, two years or more after birth

090.9 Congenital syphilis, unspecified

✓4ᵗʰ 091 Early syphilis, symptomatic
     EXCLUDES   early cardiovascular syphilis (093.0-093.9)
                       early neurosyphilis (094.0-094.9)

091.0 Genital syphilis (primary)
Genital chancre

DEF: Genital lesion at the site of initial infection by *Treponema pallidum*.

091.1 Primary anal syphilis
DEF: Anal lesion at the site of initial infection by *Treponema pallidum*.

091.2 Other primary syphilis
Primary syphilis of: Primary syphilis of:
   breast   lip
   fingers   tonsils

DEF: Lesion at the site of initial infection by *Treponema pallidum*.

091.3 Secondary syphilis of skin or mucous membranes
Condyloma latum   Secondary syphilis of:
Secondary syphilis of: skin
   anus   tonsils
   mouth   vulva
   pharynx

DEF: Transitory or chronic lesions following initial syphilis infection.

091.4 Adenopathy due to secondary syphilis
Syphilitic adenopathy (secondary)
Syphilitic lymphadenitis (secondary)

✓4ᵗʰ / ✓5ᵗʰ Additional Digit Required   Unspecified Code   Other Specified Code   Manifestation Code   ▶◀ Revised Text   ● New Code   ▲ Revised Code Title

2003 ICD•9•CM   **Volume 1 — 15**

√5th **091.5 Uveitis due to secondary syphilis**
091.50 Syphilitic uveitis, unspecified
091.51 Syphilitic chorioretinitis (secondary)
DEF: Inflammation of choroid and retina as a secondary infection.

091.52 Syphilitic iridocyclitis (secondary)
DEF: Inflammation of iris and ciliary body as a secondary infection.

√5th **091.6 Secondary syphilis of viscera and bone**
091.61 Secondary syphilitic periostitis
DEF: Inflammation of outer layers of bone as a secondary infection.

091.62 Secondary syphilitic hepatitis
Secondary syphilis of liver
091.69 Other viscera
091.7 Secondary syphilis, relapse
Secondary syphilis, relapse (treated) (untreated)
√5th **091.8 Other forms of secondary syphilis**
091.81 Acute syphilitic meningitis (secondary)
DEF: Sudden, severe inflammation of the lining of the brain and/or spinal cord as a secondary infection.

091.82 Syphilitic alopecia
DEF: Hair loss following initial syphilis infection.

091.89 Other
091.9 Unspecified secondary syphilis
√4th **092 Early syphilis, latent**
INCLUDES syphilis (acquired) without clinical manifestations, with positive serological reaction and negative spinal fluid test, less than two years after infection

092.0 Early syphilis, latent, serological relapse after treatment
092.9 Early syphilis, latent, unspecified
√4th **093 Cardiovascular syphilis**
093.0 Aneurysm of aorta, specified as syphilitic
Dilatation of aorta, specified as syphilitic
093.1 Syphilitic aortitis
DEF: Inflammation of the aorta - the main artery leading from the heart.

√5th **093.2 Syphilitic endocarditis**
DEF: Inflammation of the tissues lining the cavities of the heart.

093.20 Valve, unspecified
Syphilitic ostial coronary disease
093.21 Mitral valve
093.22 Aortic valve
Syphilitic aortic incompetence or stenosis
093.23 Tricuspid valve
093.24 Pulmonary valve
√5th **093.8 Other specified cardiovascular syphilis**
093.81 Syphilitic pericarditis
DEF: Inflammation of the outer lining of the heart.

093.82 Syphilitic myocarditis
DEF: Inflammation of the muscle of the heart.

093.89 Other
093.9 Cardiovascular syphilis, unspecified

√4th **094 Neurosyphilis**
Use additional code to identify any associated mental disorder
094.0 Tabes dorsalis
Locomotor ataxia (progressive)
Posterior spinal sclerosis (syphilitic)
Tabetic neurosyphilis
Use additional code to identify manifestation, as:
neurogenic arthropathy [Charcot's joint disease] (713.5)
DEF: Progressive degeneration of nerves associated with long-term syphilis; causing pain, wasting away, incontinence, and ataxia.

094.1 General paresis
Dementia paralytica
General paralysis (of the insane) (progressive)
Paretic neurosyphilis
Taboparesis
DEF: Degeneration of brain associated with long-term syphilis, causing loss of brain function, progressive dementia, and paralysis.

094.2 Syphilitic meningitis
Meningovascular syphilis
EXCLUDES acute syphilitic meningitis (secondary) (091.81)
DEF: Inflammation of the lining of the brain and/or spinal cord.

094.3 Asymptomatic neurosyphilis
√5th **094.8 Other specified neurosyphilis**
094.81 Syphilitic encephalitis
094.82 Syphilitic Parkinsonism
DEF: Decreased motor function, tremors, and muscular rigidity.

094.83 Syphilitic disseminated retinochoroiditis
DEF: Inflammation of retina and choroid due to neurosyphilis.

094.84 Syphilitic optic atrophy
DEF: Degeneration of the eye and its nerves due to neurosyphilis.

094.85 Syphilitic retrobulbar neuritis
DEF: Inflammation of the posterior optic nerve due to neurosyphilis.

094.86 Syphilitic acoustic neuritis
DEF: Inflammation of acoustic nerve due to neurosyphilis.

094.87 Syphilitic ruptured cerebral aneurysm
094.89 Other
094.9 Neurosyphilis, unspecified
Gumma (syphilitic)
Syphilis (early) (late) } of central nervous
Syphiloma } system NOS

√4th **095 Other forms of late syphilis, with symptoms**
INCLUDES gumma (syphilitic)
syphilis, late, tertiary, or unspecified stage
095.0 Syphilitic episcleritis
095.1 Syphilis of lung
095.2 Syphilitic peritonitis
095.3 Syphilis of liver
095.4 Syphilis of kidney
095.5 Syphilis of bone
095.6 Syphilis of muscle
Syphilitic myositis
095.7 Syphilis of synovium, tendon, and bursa
Syphilitic: Syphilitic:
bursitis   synovitis
095.8 Other specified forms of late symptomatic syphilis
EXCLUDES cardiovascular syphilis (093.0-093.9)
neurosyphilis (094.0-094.9)

N Newborn Age: 0   P Pediatric Age: 0-17   M Maternity Age: 12-55   A Adult Age: 15-124   MSP Medicare Secondary Payer

095.9 Late symptomatic syphilis, unspecified

096 Late syphilis, latent

Syphilis (acquired) without clinical manifestations, with positive serological reaction and negative spinal fluid test, two years or more after infection

√4th 097 Other and unspecified syphilis

097.0 Late syphilis, unspecified

097.1 Latent syphilis, unspecified

Positive serological reaction for syphilis

097.9 Syphilis, unspecified

Syphilis (acquired) NOS

> **EXCLUDES** syphilis NOS causing death under two years of age (090.9)

√4th 098 Gonococcal infections

DEF: *Neisseria gonorrhoeae* infection generally acquired in utero or in sexual congress.

098.0 Acute, of lower genitourinary tract

Gonococcal: Gonorrhea (acute):
Bartholinitis (acute)   NOS
urethritis (acute)   genitourinary (tract) NOS
vulvovaginitis (acute)

√5th 098.1 Acute, of upper genitourinary tract

098.10 Gonococcal infection (acute) of upper genitourinary tract, site unspecified

098.11 Gonococcal cystitis (acute)
Gonorrhea (acute) of bladder

098.12 Gonococcal prostatitis (acute)   ♂

098.13 Gonococcal epididymo-orchitis (acute)   ♂
Gonococcal orchitis (acute)
DEF: Acute inflammation of the testes.

098.14 Gonococcal seminal vesiculitis (acute)   ♂
Gonorrhea (acute) of seminal vesicle

098.15 Gonococcal cervicitis (acute)   ♀
Gonorrhea (acute) of cervix

098.16 Gonococcal endometritis (acute)   ♀
Gonorrhea (acute) of uterus

098.17 Gonococcal salpingitis, specified as acute ♀
DEF: Acute inflammation of the fallopian tubes.

098.19 Other

098.2 Chronic, of lower genitourinary tract

Gonococcal:
Bartholinitis
urethritis   } specified as chronic or
vulvovaginitis   with duration of
Gonorrhea: two months or
NOS   more
genitourinary (tract)

Any condition classifiable to 098.0 specified as chronic or with duration of two months or more

√5th 098.3 Chronic, of upper genitourinary tract

> **INCLUDES** any condition classifiable to 098.1 stated as chronic or with a duration of two months or more

098.30 Chronic gonococcal infection of upper genitourinary tract, site unspecified

098.31 Gonococcal cystitis, chronic
Any condition classifiable to 098.11, specified as chronic
Gonorrhea of bladder, chronic

098.32 Gonococcal prostatitis, chronic   ♂
Any condition classifiable to 098.12, specified as chronic

098.33 Gonococcal epididymo-orchitis, chronic   ♂
Any condition classifiable to 098.13, specified as chronic
Chronic gonococcal orchitis
DEF: Chronic inflammation of the testes.

098.34 Gonococcal seminal vesiculitis, chronic   ♂
Any condition classifiable to 098.14, specified as chronic
Gonorrhea of seminal vesicle, chronic

098.35 Gonococcal cervicitis, chronic   ♀
Any condition classifiable to 098.15, specified as chronic
Gonorrhea of cervix, chronic

098.36 Gonococcal endometritis, chronic   ♀
Any condition classifiable to 098.16, specified as chronic
DEF: Chronic inflammation of the uterus.

098.37 Gonococcal salpingitis (chronic)   ♀
DEF: Chronic inflammation of the fallopian tubes.

098.39 Other

√5th 098.4 Gonococcal infection of eye

098.40 Gonococcal conjunctivitis (neonatorum)
Gonococcal ophthalmia (neonatorum)
DEF: Inflammation and infection of conjunctiva present at birth.

098.41 Gonococcal iridocyclitis
DEF: Inflammation and infection of iris and ciliary body.

098.42 Gonococcal endophthalmia
DEF: Inflammation and infection of the contents of the eyeball.

098.43 Gonococcal keratitis
DEF: Inflammation and infection of the cornea.

098.49 Other

√5th 098.5 Gonococcal infection of joint

098.50 Gonococcal arthritis
Gonococcal infection of joint NOS

098.51 Gonococcal synovitis and tenosynovitis

098.52 Gonococcal bursitis
DEF: Inflammation of the sac-like cavities in a joint.

098.53 Gonococcal spondylitis

098.59 Other
Gonococcal rheumatism

098.6 Gonococcal infection of pharynx

098.7 Gonococcal infection of anus and rectum
Gonococcal proctitis

√5th 098.8 Gonococcal infection of other specified sites

098.81 Gonococcal keratosis (blennorrhagica)
DEF: Pustular skin lesions caused by *Neisseria gonorrhoeae.*

098.82 Gonococcal meningitis
DEF: Inflammation of the lining of the brain and/or spinal cord.

098.83 Gonococcal pericarditis
DEF: Inflammation of the outer lining of the heart.

098.84 Gonococcal endocarditis
DEF: Inflammation of the tissues lining the cavities of the heart.

098.85 Other gonococcal heart disease

098.86 Gonococcal peritonitis
DEF: Inflammation of the membrane lining the abdomen.

098.89 Other
Gonococcemia

√4th
√5th Additional Digit Required   Unspecified Code   Other Specified Code   Manifestation Code   ►◄ Revised Text   ● New Code   ▲ Revised Code Title

2003 ICD•9•CM   **Volume 1 — 17**

✓4th **099 Other venereal diseases**

099.0 Chancroid

Bubo (inguinal):   Chancre:
chancroidal   Ducrey's
due to Hemophilus   simple
ducreyi   soft
                 Ulcus molle (cutis) (skin)

DEF: A sexually transmitted disease caused by *Haemophilus ducreyi*; it is identified by a painful primary ulcer at the site of inoculation (usually on the external genitalia) with related lymphadenitis.

099.1 Lymphogranuloma venereum

Climatic or tropical bubo
(Durand-) Nicolas-Favre disease
Esthiomene
Lymphogranuloma inguinale

DEF: Sexually transmitted infection of *Chlamydia trachomatis* causing skin lesions.

099.2 Granuloma inguinale

Donovanosis   Granuloma venereum
Granuloma pudendi   Pudendal ulcer
(ulcerating)

DEF: Chronic, sexually transmitted infection of *Calymmatobacterium granulomatis,* resulting in progressive, anogenital skin ulcers.

099.3 Reiter's disease

Reiter's syndrome
Use additional code for associated:
arthropathy (711.1)
conjunctivitis (372.33)

DEF: A symptom complex of unknown etiology consisting of urethritis, conjunctivitis, arthritis and myocutaneous lesions. It occurs most commonly in young men and patients with HIV and may precede or follow AIDS. Also a form of reactive arthritis.

✓5th **099.4 Other nongonococcal urethritis [NGU]**

099.40 Unspecified
Nonspecific urethritis

099.41 Chlamydia trachomatis

099.49 Other specified organism

✓5th **099.5 Other venereal diseases due to Chlamydia trachomatis**

EXCLUDES   *Chlamydia trachomatis infection of conjunctiva (076.0-076.9, 077.0, 077.9)*
Lymphogranuloma venereum (099.1)

DEF: Venereal diseases caused by *Chlamydia trachomatis* at other sites besides the urethra (e.g., pharynx, anus and rectum, conjunctiva and peritoneum).

099.50 Unspecified site

099.51 Pharynx

099.52 Anus and rectum

099.53 Lower genitourinary sites
EXCLUDES   *urethra (099.41)*
Use additional code to specify site of infection, such as:
bladder (595.4)
cervix (616.0)
vagina and vulva (616.11)

099.54 Other genitourinary sites
Use additional code to specify site of infection, such as:
pelvic inflammatory disease NOS (614.9)
testis and epididymis (604.91)

099.55 Unspecified genitourinary site

099.56 Peritoneum
Perihepatitis

099.59 Other specified site

099.8 Other specified venereal diseases

099.9 Venereal disease, unspecified

OTHER SPIROCHETAL DISEASES (100-104)

✓4th **100 Leptospirosis**

DEF: An infection of any spirochete of the genus Leptospire in blood. This zoonosis is transmitted to humans most often by exposure with contaminated animal tissues or water and less often by contact with urine. Patients present with flulike symptoms, the most common being muscle aches involving the thighs and low back. Treatment is with hydration and antibiotics.

100.0 Leptospirosis icterohemorrhagica
Leptospiral or spirochetal jaundice (hemorrhagic)
Weil's disease

✓5th **100.8 Other specified leptospiral infections**

100.81 Leptospiral meningitis (aseptic)

100.89 Other
Fever: Infection by Leptospira:
Fort Bragg   australis
pretibial   bataviae
swamp   pyrogenes

100.9 Leptospirosis, unspecified

101 Vincent's angina

Acute necrotizing ulcerative: Trench mouth
gingivitis   Vincent's:
stomatitis   gingivitis
Fusospirochetal pharyngitis   infection [any site]
Spirochetal stomatitis

DEF: Painful ulceration with edema and hypermic patches of the oropharyngeal and throat membranes; it is caused by spreading of acute ulcerative gingivitis.

✓4th **102 Yaws**

INCLUDES   frambesia
pian

DEF: An infectious, endemic, tropical disease caused by *Treponema pertenue*; it usually affects persons 15 years old or younger; a primary cutaneous lesion develops, then a granulomatous skin eruption, and occasionally lesions that destroy skin and bone.

102.0 Initial lesions
Chancre of yaws
Frambesia, initial or primary
Initial frambesial ulcer
Mother yaw

102.1 Multiple papillomata and wet crab yaws
Butter yaws   Plantar or palmar
Frambesioma   papilloma of yaws
Pianoma

102.2 Other early skin lesions
Cutaneous yaws, less than five years after infection
Early yaws (cutaneous) (macular) (papular)
(maculopapular) (micropapular)
Frambeside of early yaws

102.3 Hyperkeratosis
Ghoul hand
Hyperkeratosis, palmar or plantar (early) (late) due to yaws
Worm-eaten soles

DEF: Overgrowth of the skin of the palms or bottoms of the feet, due to yaws.

102.4 Gummata and ulcers
Gummatous frambeside
Nodular late yaws (ulcerated)

DEF: Rubbery lesions and areas of dead skin caused by yaws.

102.5 Gangosa
Rhinopharyngitis mutilans

DEF: Massive, mutilating lesions of the nose and oral cavity caused by yaws.

102.6 Bone and joint lesions

Goundou
Gumma, bone
Gummatous osteitis or periostitis } of yaws (late)

Hydrarthrosis
Osteitis
Periostitis (hypertrophic) } of yaws (early) (late)

102.7 Other manifestations

Juxta-articular nodules of yaws
Mucosal yaws

102.8 Latent yaws

Yaws without clinical manifestations, with positive serology

102.9 Yaws, unspecified

✓4th **103 Pinta**

DEF: A chronic form of treponematosis, endemic in areas of tropical America; it is identified by the presence of red, violet, blue, coffee-colored or white spots on the skin.

103.0 Primary lesions

Chancre (primary)
Papule (primary)
Pintid } of pinta [carate]

103.1 Intermediate lesions

Erythematous plaques
Hyperchromic lesions
Hyperkeratosis } of pinta [carate]

103.2 Late lesions

Cardiovascular lesions
Skin lesions:
  achromic
  cicatricial
  dyschromic
Vitiligo } of pinta [carate]

103.3 Mixed lesions

Achromic and hyperchromic skin lesions of pinta [carate]

103.9 Pinta, unspecified

✓4th **104 Other spirochetal infection**

104.0 Nonvenereal endemic syphilis

Bejel
Njovera

DEF: *Treponema pallidum, T. pertenue,* or *T. carateum* infection transmitted non-sexually, causing lesions on mucosa and skin.

104.8 Other specified spirochetal infections

EXCLUDES   *relapsing fever (087.0-087.9)*
                syphilis (090.0-097.9)

104.9 Spirochetal infection, unspecified

MYCOSES (110-118)

Use additional code to identify manifestation as:
  arthropathy (711.6)
  meningitis (321.0-321.1)
  otitis externa (380.15)

EXCLUDES   *infection by Actinomycetales, such as species of Actinomyces, Actinomadura, Nocardia, Streptomyces (039.0-039.9)*

✓4th **110 Dermatophytosis**

INCLUDES   infection by species of Epidermophyton, Microsporum, and Trichophyton
                 tinea, any type except those in 111

DEF: Superficial infection of the skin caused by a parasitic fungus.

110.0 Of scalp and beard

Kerion   Trichophytic tinea
Sycosis, mycotic   [black dot tinea], scalp

110.1 Of nail

Dermatophytic onychia   Tinea unguium
Onychomycosis

110.2 Of hand

Tinea manuum

110.3 Of groin and perianal area

Dhobie itch   Tinea cruris
Eczema marginatum

110.4 Of foot

Athlete's foot   Tinea pedis

110.5 Of the body

Herpes circinatus   Tinea imbricata [Tokelau]

110.6 Deep seated dermatophytosis

Granuloma trichophyticum
Majocchi's granuloma

110.8 Of other specified sites

110.9 Of unspecified site

Favus NOS   Ringworm NOS
Microsporic tinea NOS

✓4th **111 Dermatomycosis, other and unspecified**

111.0 Pityriasis versicolor

Infection by Malassezia [Pityrosporum] furfur
Tinea flava
Tinea versicolor

111.1 Tinea nigra

Infection by Cladosporium species
Keratomycosis nigricans
Microsporosis nigra
Pityriasis nigra
Tinea palmaris nigra

111.2 Tinea blanca

Infection by Trichosporon (beigelii) cutaneum
White piedra

111.3 Black piedra

Infection by Piedraia hortai

111.8 Other specified dermatomycoses

111.9 Dermatomycosis, unspecified

✓4th **112 Candidiasis**

INCLUDES   infection by Candida species
               moniliasis

EXCLUDES   *neonatal monilial infection (771.7)*

DEF: Fungal infection caused by *Candida;* usually seen in mucous membranes or skin.

112.0 Of mouth

Thrush (oral)

112.1 Of vulva and vagina   ♀

Candidal vulvovaginitis   Monilial vulvovaginitis

112.2 Of other urogenital sites

Candidal balanitis

112.3 Of skin and nails

Candidal intertrigo   Candidal perionyxis
Candidal onychia   [paronychia]

112.4 Of lung

Candidal pneumonia

112.5 Disseminated

Systemic candidiasis

✓5th **112.8 Of other specified sites**

112.81 Candidal endocarditis

112.82 Candidal otitis externa

Otomycosis in moniliasis

112.83 Candidal meningitis

112.84 Candidal esophagitis

112.85 Candidal enteritis

112.89 Other

112.9 Of unspecified site

Infectious and Parasitic Diseases 102.6–112.9

✓4th ✓5th   Additional Digit Required   Unspecified Code   Other Specified Code   Manifestation Code   ▶◀ Revised Text   ● New Code   ▲ Revised Code Title

2003 ICD•9•CM   **Volume 1 — 19**

✓4ᵗʰ **114 Coccidioidomycosis**

> INCLUDES   infection by Coccidioides (immitis)
> Posada-Wernicke disease

DEF: A fungal disease caused by inhalation of dust particles containing arthrospores of *Coccidioides immitis*; a self-limited respiratory infection; the primary form is known as San Joaquin fever, desert fever or valley fever.

114.0 Primary coccidioidomycosis (pulmonary)
Acute pulmonary coccidioidomycosis
Coccidioidomycotic pneumonitis
Desert rheumatism
Pulmonary coccidioidomycosis
San Joaquin Valley fever
DEF: Acute, self-limiting *Coccidioides immitis* infection of the lung.

114.1 Primary extrapulmonary coccidioidomycosis
Chancriform syndrome
Primary cutaneous coccidioidomycosis
DEF: Acute, self-limiting *Coccidioides immitis* infection in non-pulmonary site.

114.2 Coccidioidal meningitis
DEF: *Coccidioides immitis* infection of the lining of the brain and/or spinal cord.

114.3 Other forms of progressive coccidioidomycosis
Coccidioidal granuloma
Disseminated coccidioidomycosis

114.4 Chronic pulmonary coccidioidomycosis

114.5 Pulmonary coccidioidomycosis, unspecified

114.9 Coccidioidomycosis, unspecified

✓4ᵗʰ **115 Histoplasmosis**

> The following fifth-digit subclassification is for use with category 115:
>
> **0 without mention of manifestation**
> **1 meningitis**
> **2 retinitis**
> **3 pericarditis**
> **4 endocarditis**
> **5 pneumonia**
> **9 other**

✓5ᵗʰ **115.0 Infection by Histoplasma capsulatum**
American histoplasmosis
Darling's disease
Reticuloendothelial cytomycosis
Small form histoplasmosis
DEF: Infection resulting from inhalation of fungal spores, causing acute pneumonia, an influenza-like illness, or a disseminated disease of the reticuloendothelial system. In immunocompromised patients it can reactivate, affecting lungs, meninges, heart, peritoneum and adrenals.

✓5ᵗʰ **115.1 Infection by Histoplasma duboisii**
African histoplasmosis
Large form histoplasmosis

✓5ᵗʰ **115.9 Histoplasmosis, unspecified**
Histoplasmosis NOS

✓4ᵗʰ **116 Blastomycotic infection**

116.0 Blastomycosis
Blastomycotic dermatitis
Chicago disease
Cutaneous blastomycosis
Disseminated blastomycosis
Gilchrist's disease
Infection by Blastomyces [Ajellomyces] dermatitidis
North American blastomycosis
Primary pulmonary blastomycosis

116.1 Paracoccidioidomycosis
Brazilian blastomycosis
Infection by Paracoccidioides [Blastomyces] brasiliensis
Lutz-Splendore-Almeida disease
Mucocutaneous-lymphangitic paracoccidioidomycosis
Pulmonary paracoccidioidomycosis
South American blastomycosis
Visceral paracoccidioidomycosis

116.2 Lobomycosis
Infections by Loboa [Blastomyces] loboi
Keloidal blastomycosis
Lobo's disease

✓4ᵗʰ **117 Other mycoses**

117.0 Rhinosporidiosis
Infection by Rhinosporidium seeberi

117.1 Sporotrichosis
Cutaneous sporotrichosis
Disseminated sporotrichosis
Infection by Sporothrix [Sporotrichum] schenckii
Lymphocutaneous sporotrichosis
Pulmonary sporotrichosis
Sporotrichosis of the bones

117.2 Chromoblastomycosis
Chromomycosis
Infection by Cladosporidium carrionii, Fonsecaea compactum, Fonsecaea pedrosoi, Phialophora verrucosa

117.3 Aspergillosis
Infection by Aspergillus species, mainly A. fumigatus, A. flavus group, A. terreus group

117.4 Mycotic mycetomas
Infection by various genera and species of Ascomycetes and Deuteromycetes, such as Acremonium [Cephalosporium] falciforme, Neotestudina rosatii, Madurella grisea, Madurella mycetomii, Pyrenochaeta romeroi, Zopfia [Leptosphaeria] senegalensis
Madura foot, mycotic
Maduromycosis, mycotic
> EXCLUDES   *actinomycotic mycetomas (039.0-039.9)*

117.5 Cryptococcosis
Busse-Buschke's disease
European cryptococcosis
Infection by Cryptococcus neoformans
Pulmonary cryptococcosis
Systemic cryptococcosis
Torula

117.6 Allescheriosis [Petriellidosis]
Infections by Allescheria [Petriellidium] boydii [Monosporium apiospermum]
> EXCLUDES   *mycotic mycetoma (117.4)*

117.7 Zygomycosis [Phycomycosis or Mucormycosis]
Infection by species of Absidia, Basidiobolus, Conidiobolus, Cunninghamella, Entomophthora, Mucor, Rhizopus, Saksenaea

117.8 Infection by dematiacious fungi, [Phaehyphomycosis]
Infection by dematiacious fungi, such as Cladosporium trichoides [bantianum], Dreschlera hawaiiensis, Phialophora gougerotii, Phialophora jeanselmi

117.9 Other and unspecified mycoses

118 Opportunistic mycoses
Infection of skin, subcutaneous tissues, and/or organs by a wide variety of fungi generally considered to be pathogenic to compromised hosts only (e.g., infection by species of Alternaria, Dreschlera, Fusarium)

HELMINTHIASES (120-129)

✓4th 120 Schistosomiasis [bilharziasis]

DEF: Infection caused by *Schistosoma*, a genus of flukes or trematode parasites.

120.0 Schistosoma haematobium
Vesical schistosomiasis NOS

120.1 Schistosoma mansoni
Intestinal schistosomiasis NOS

120.2 Schistosoma japonicum
Asiatic schistosomiasis NOS
Katayama disease or fever

120.3 Cutaneous
Cercarial dermatitis
Infection by cercariae of Schistosoma
Schistosome dermatitis
Swimmers' itch

120.8 Other specified schistosomiasis
Infection by Schistosoma:
bovis
intercalatum
mattheii
spindale
Schistosomiasis chestermani

120.9 Schistosomiasis, unspecified
Blood flukes NOS
Hemic distomiasis

✓4th 121 Other trematode infections

121.0 Opisthorchiasis
Infection by:
cat liver fluke
Opisthorchis (felineus) (tenuicollis) (viverrini)

121.1 Clonorchiasis
Biliary cirrhosis due to clonorchiasis
Chinese liver fluke disease
Hepatic distomiasis due to Clonorchis sinensis
Oriental liver fluke disease

121.2 Paragonimiasis
Infection by Paragonimus
Lung fluke disease (oriental)
Pulmonary distomiasis

121.3 Fascioliasis
Infection by Fasciola:
gigantica
hepatica
Liver flukes NOS
Sheep liver fluke infection

121.4 Fasciolopsiasis
Infection by Fasciolopsis (buski)
Intestinal distomiasis

121.5 Metagonimiasis
Infection by Metagonimus yokogawai

121.6 Heterophyiasis
Infection by:
Heterophyes heterophyes
Stellantchasmus falcatus

121.8 Other specified trematode infections
Infection by:
Dicrocoelium dendriticum
Echinostoma ilocanum
Gastrodiscoides hominis

121.9 Trematode infection, unspecified
Distomiasis NOS
Fluke disease NOS

✓4th 122 Echinococcosis
INCLUDES echinococciasis
hydatid disease
hydatidosis

DEF: Infection caused by larval forms of tapeworms of the genus *Echinococcus.*

122.0 Echinococcus granulosus infection of liver
122.1 Echinococcus granulosus infection of lung

122.2 Echinococcus granulosus infection of thyroid
122.3 Echinococcus granulosus infection, other
122.4 Echinococcus granulosus infection, unspecified
122.5 Echinococcus multilocularis infection of liver
122.6 Echinococcus multilocularis infection, other
122.7 Echinococcus multilocularis infection, unspecified
122.8 Echinococcosis, unspecified, of liver
122.9 Echinococcosis, other and unspecified

✓4th 123 Other cestode infection

123.0 Taenia solium infection, intestinal form
Pork tapeworm (adult) (infection)

123.1 Cysticercosis
Cysticerciasis
Infection by Cysticercus cellulosae [larval form of Taenia solium]

123.2 Taenia saginata infection
Beef tapeworm (infection)
Infection by Taeniarhynchus saginatus

123.3 Taeniasis, unspecified

123.4 Diphyllobothriasis, intestinal
Diphyllobothrium (adult) (latum) (pacificum) infection
Fish tapeworm (infection)

123.5 Sparganosis [larval diphyllobothriasis]
Infection by:
Diphyllobothrium larvae
Sparganum (mansoni) (proliferum)
Spirometra larvae

123.6 Hymenolepiasis
Dwarf tapeworm (infection)
Hymenolepis (diminuta) (nana) infection
Rat tapeworm (infection)

123.8 Other specified cestode infection
Diplogonoporus (grandis)
Dipylidium (caninum) } infection
Dog tapeworm (infection)

123.9 Cestode infection, unspecified
Tapeworm (infection) NOS

124 Trichinosis
Trichinella spiralis infection
Trichinellosis
Trichiniasis

DEF: Infection by *Trichinella spiralis*, the smallest of the parasitic nematodes.

✓4th 125 Filarial infection and dracontiasis

125.0 Bancroftian filariasis
Chyluria
Elephantiasis
Infection } due to Wuchereria bancrofti
Lymphadenitis
Lymphangitis

Wuchereriasis

125.1 Malayan filariasis
Brugia filariasis
Chyluria
Elephantiasis } due to Brugia [Wuchereria] malayi
Infection
Lymphadenitis
Lymphangitis

125.2 Loiasis
Eyeworm disease of Africa   Loa loa infection

125.3 Onchocerciasis
Onchocerca volvulus infection
Onchocercais

125.4 Dipetalonemiasis
Infection by:
Acanthocheilonema perstans
Dipetalonema perstans

125.5 Mansonella ozzardi infection
Filariasis ozzardi

Infectious and Parasitic Diseases 125.6–133.9

125.6　Other specified filariasis
　　Dirofilaria infection
　　Infection by:
　　　　Acanthocheilonema streptocerca
　　　　Dipetalonema streptocerca

125.7　Dracontiasis
　　Guinea-worm infection
　　Infection by Dracunculus medinensis

125.9　Unspecified filariasis

✓4th **126　Ancylostomiasis and necatoriasis**
　　INCLUDES　cutaneous larva migrans due to Ancylostoma
　　　　hookworm (disease) (infection)
　　　　uncinariasis

126.0　Ancylostoma duodenale

126.1　Necator americanus

126.2　Ancylostoma braziliense

126.3　Ancylostoma ceylanicum

126.8　Other specified Ancylostoma

126.9　Ancylostomiasis and necatoriasis, unspecified
　　Creeping eruption NOS
　　Cutaneous larva migrans NOS

✓4th **127　Other intestinal helminthiases**
127.0　Ascariasis
　　Ascaridiasis
　　Infection by Ascaris lumbricoides
　　Roundworm infection

127.1　Anisakiasis
　　Infection by Anisakis larva

127.2　Strongyloidiasis
　　Infection by Strongyloides stercoralis
　　EXCLUDES　trichostrongyliasis (127.6)

127.3　Trichuriasis
　　Infection by Trichuris trichiura
　　Trichocephaliasis
　　Whipworm (disease) (infection)

127.4　Enterobiasis
　　Infection by Enterobius vermicularis
　　Oxyuriasis
　　Oxyuris vermicularis infection
　　Pinworm (disease) (infection)
　　Threadworm infection

127.5　Capillariasis
　　Infection by Capillaria philippinensis
　　EXCLUDES　infection by Capillaria hepatica (128.8)

127.6　Trichostrongyliasis
　　Infection by Trichostrongylus species

127.7　Other specified intestinal helminthiasis
　　Infection by:
　　　　Oesophagostomum apiostomum and related
　　　　　　species
　　　　Ternidens diminutus
　　　　other specified intestinal helminth
　　　　Physalopteriasis

127.8　Mixed intestinal helminthiasis
　　Infection by intestinal helminths classified to more
　　　　than one of the categories 120.0-127.7
　　Mixed helminthiasis NOS

127.9　Intestinal helminthiasis, unspecified

✓4th **128　Other and unspecified helminthiases**
128.0　Toxocariasis
　　Larva migrans visceralis
　　Toxocara (canis) (cati) infection
　　Visceral larva migrans syndrome

128.1　Gnathostomiasis
　　Infection by Gnathostoma spinigerum and related
　　　　species

128.8　Other specified helminthiasis
　　Infection by:
　　　　Angiostrongylus cantonensis
　　　　Capillaria hepatica
　　　　other specified helminth

128.9　Helminth infection, unspecified
　　Helminthiasis NOS
　　Worms NOS

129　Intestinal parasitism, unspecified

OTHER INFECTIOUS AND PARASITIC DISEASES (130–136)

✓4th **130　Toxoplasmosis**
　　INCLUDES　infection by toxoplasma gondii
　　　　toxoplasmosis (acquired)
　　EXCLUDES　congenital toxoplasmosis (771.2)

130.0　Meningoencephalitis due to toxoplasmosis
　　Encephalitis due to acquired toxoplasmosis

130.1　Conjunctivitis due to toxoplasmosis

130.2　Chorioretinitis due to toxoplasmosis
　　Focal retinochoroiditis due to acquired
　　　　toxoplasmosis

130.3　Myocarditis due to toxoplasmosis

130.4　Pneumonitis due to toxoplasmosis

130.5　Hepatitis due to toxoplasmosis

130.7　Toxoplasmosis of other specified sites

130.8　Multisystemic disseminated toxoplasmosis
　　Toxoplasmosis of multiple sites

130.9　Toxoplasmosis, unspecified

✓4th **131　Trichomoniasis**
　　INCLUDES　infection due to Trichomonas (vaginalis)

✓5th **131.0　Urogenital trichomoniasis**
131.00　Urogenital trichomoniasis, unspecified
　　Fluor (vaginalis)　　⎫　trichomonal or due
　　Leukorrhea　　　　 ⎬　to Trichomonas
　　　(vaginalis)　　　⎭　(vaginalis)

　　DEF: *Trichomonas vaginalis* infection of reproductive and
　　urinary organs, transmitted through coitus.

131.01　Trichomonal vulvovaginitis　　　　　　♀
　　Vaginitis, trichomonal or due to
　　　　Trichomonas (vaginalis)

　　DEF: *Trichomonas vaginalis* infection of vulva and
　　vagina; often asymptomatic, transmitted through coitus.

131.02　Trichomonal urethritis
　　DEF: *Trichomonas vaginalis* infection of the urethra.

131.03　Trichomonal prostatitis　　　　　　　♂
　　DEF: *Trichomonas vaginalis* infection of the prostate.

131.09　Other

131.8　Other specified sites
　　EXCLUDES　intestinal (007.3)

131.9　Trichomoniasis, unspecified

✓4th **132　Pediculosis and phthirus infestation**
132.0　Pediculus capitis [head louse]

132.1　Pediculus corporis [body louse]

132.2　Phthirus pubis [pubic louse]
　　Pediculus pubis

132.3　Mixed infestation
　　Infestation classifiable to more than one of the
　　　　categories 132.0-132.2

132.9　Pediculosis, unspecified

✓4th **133　Acariasis**
133.0　Scabies
　　Infestation by Sarcoptes scabiei
　　Norwegian scabies
　　Sarcoptic itch

133.8　Other acariasis
　　Chiggers
　　Infestation by:
　　　　Demodex folliculorum
　　　　Trombicula

133.9　Acariasis, unspecified
　　Infestation by mites NOS

☑4ᵗʰ **134 Other infestation**

134.0 Myiasis

Infestation by:
Dermatobia (hominis)
fly larvae
Gasterophilus (intestinalis)
maggots
Oestrus ovis

134.1 Other arthropod infestation

Infestation by:
chigoe
sand flea
Tunga penetrans
Jigger disease
Tungiasis
Scarabiasis

134.2 Hirudiniasis

Hirudiniasis (external) (internal)
Leeches (aquatic) (land)

134.8 Other specified infestations

134.9 Infestation, unspecified

Infestation (skin) NOS
Skin parasites NOS

135 Sarcoidosis

Besnier-Boeck-Schaumann disease
Lupoid (miliary) of Boeck
Lupus pernio (Besnier)
Lymphogranulomatosis, benign (Schaumann's)
Sarcoid (any site):
NOS
Boeck
Darier-Roussy
Uveoparotid fever

DEF: A chronic, granulomatous reticulosis (abnormal increase in cells), affecting any organ or tissue; acute form has high rate of remission; chronic form is progressive.

☑4ᵗʰ **136 Other and unspecified infectious and parasitic diseases**

136.0 Ainhum

Dactylolysis spontanea

DEF: A disease affecting the toes, especially the fifth digit, and sometimes the fingers, especially seen in black adult males; it is characterized by a linear constriction around the affected digit leading to spontaneous amputation of the distal part of the digit.

136.1 Behçet's syndrome

DEF: A chronic inflammatory disorder of unknown etiology involving the small blood vessels; it is characterized by recurrent aphthous ulceration of the oral and pharyngeal mucous membranes and the genitalia, skin lesions, severe uvetis, retinal vascularitis and optic atrophy.

136.2 Specific infections by free-living amebae

Meningoencephalitis due to Naegleria

136.3 Pneumocystosis

Pneumonia due to Pneumocystis carinii

DEF: *Pneumocystis carinii* fungus causing pneumonia in immunocompromised patients; a leading cause of death among AIDS patients.

136.4 Psorospermiasis

136.5 Sarcosporidiosis

Infection by Sarcocystis lindemanni

DEF: Sarcocystis infection causing muscle cysts of intestinal inflammation.

136.8 Other specified infectious and parasitic diseases

Candiru infestation

136.9 Unspecified infectious and parasitic diseases

Infectious disease NOS
Parasitic disease NOS

LATE EFFECTS OF INFECTIOUS AND PARASITIC DISEASES (137-139)

☑4ᵗʰ **137 Late effects of tuberculosis**

Note: This category is to be used to indicate conditions classifiable to 010-018 as the cause of late effects, which are themselves classified elsewhere. The "late effects" include those specified as such, as sequelae, or as due to old or inactive tuberculosis, without evidence of active disease.

137.0 Late effects of respiratory or unspecified tuberculosis

137.1 Late effects of central nervous system tuberculosis

137.2 Late effects of genitourinary tuberculosis

137.3 Late effects of tuberculosis of bones and joints

137.4 Late effects of tuberculosis of other specified organs

138 Late effects of acute poliomyelitis

Note: This category is to be used to indicate conditions classifiable to 045 as the cause of late effects, which are themselves classified elsewhere. The "late effects" include conditions specified as such, or as sequelae, or as due to old or inactive poliomyelitis, without evidence of active disease.

☑4ᵗʰ **139 Late effects of other infectious and parasitic diseases**

Note: This category is to be used to indicate conditions classifiable to categories 001-009, 020-041, 046-136 as the cause of late effects, which are themselves classified elsewhere. The "late effects" include conditions specified as such; they also include sequela of diseases classifiable to the above categories if there is evidence that the disease itself is no longer present.

139.0 Late effects of viral encephalitis

Late effects of conditions classifiable to 049.8-049.9, 062-064

139.1 Late effects of trachoma

Late effects of conditions classifiable to 076

139.8 Late effects of other and unspecified infectious and parasitic diseases

---

☑4ᵗʰ
☑5ᵗʰ Additional Digit Required   Unspecified Code   Other Specified Code   Manifestation Code   ▶◀ Revised Text   ● New Code   ▲ Revised Code Title

2003 ICD•9•CM   Volume 1 — 23

2. NEOPLASMS (140-239)

Notes:

1. Content

This chapter contains the following broad groups:

140-195   Malignant neoplasms, stated or presumed to be primary, of specified sites, except of lymphatic and hematopoietic tissue

196-198   Malignant neoplasms, stated or presumed to be secondary, of specified sites

199   Malignant neoplasms, without specification of site

200-208   Malignant neoplasms, stated or presumed to be primary, of lymphatic and hematopoietic tissue

210-229   Benign neoplasms

230-234   Carcinoma in situ

235-238   Neoplasms of uncertain behavior [see Note at beginning of section]

239   Neoplasms of unspecified nature

2. Functional activity

All neoplasms are classified in this chapter, whether or not functionally active. An additional code from Chapter 3 may be used to identify such functional activity associated with any neoplasm, e.g.:

catecholamine-producing malignant pheochromocytoma of adrenal:

code 194.0, additional code 255.6

basophil adenoma of pituitary with Cushing's syndrome:

code 227.3, additional code 255.0

3. Morphology [Histology]

For those wishing to identify the histological type of neoplasms, a comprehensive coded nomenclature, which comprises the morphology rubrics of the ICD-Oncology, is given in Appendix A.

4. Malignant neoplasms overlapping site boundaries

Categories 140-195 are for the classification of primary malignant neoplasms according to their point of origin. A malignant neoplasm that overlaps two or more subcategories within a three-digit rubric and whose point of origin cannot be determined should be classified to the subcategory .8 "Other."

For example, "carcinoma involving tip and ventral surface of tongue" should be assigned to 141.8. On the other hand, "carcinoma of tip of tongue, extending to involve the ventral surface" should be coded to 141.2, as the point of origin, the tip, is known. Three subcategories (149.8, 159.8, 165.8) have been provided for malignant neoplasms that overlap the boundaries of three-digit rubrics within certain systems.

Overlapping malignant neoplasms that cannot be classified as indicated above should be assigned to the appropriate subdivision of category 195 (Malignant neoplasm of other and ill-defined sites).

DEF: An abnormal growth, such as a tumor. Morphology determines behavior, i.e., whether it will remain intact (benign) or spread to adjacent tissue (malignant). The term mass is not synonymous with neoplasm, as it is often used to describe cysts and thickenings such as those occurring with hematoma or infection.

MALIGNANT NEOPLASM OF LIP, ORAL CAVITY, AND PHARYNX (140-149)

$\boxed{\textit{EXCLUDES}}$ carcinoma in situ (230.0)

√4th **140 Malignant neoplasm of lip**

$\boxed{\textit{EXCLUDES}}$ skin of lip (173.0)

140.0   Upper lip, vermilion border

Upper lip: Upper lip:
NOS   lipstick area
external

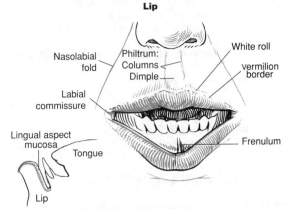

Lip

140.1   Lower lip, vermilion border

Lower lip: Lower lip:
NOS   lipstick area
external

140.3   Upper lip, inner aspect

Upper lip: Upper lip:
buccal aspect   mucosa
frenulum   oral aspect

140.4   Lower lip, inner aspect

Lower lip: Lower lip:
buccal aspect   mucosa
frenulum   oral aspect

140.5   Lip, unspecified, inner aspect

Lip, not specified whether upper or lower:
buccal aspect
frenulum
mucosa
oral aspect

140.6   Commissure of lip

Labial commissure

140.8   Other sites of lip

Malignant neoplasm of contiguous or overlapping sites of lip whose point of origin cannot be determined

140.9   Lip, unspecified, vermilion border

Lip, not specified as upper or lower:
NOS
external
lipstick area

√4th **141 Malignant neoplasm of tongue**

141.0   Base of tongue

Dorsal surface of base of tongue
Fixed part of tongue NOS

141.1   Dorsal surface of tongue

Anterior two-thirds of tongue, dorsal surface
Dorsal tongue NOS
Midline of tongue

$\boxed{\textit{EXCLUDES}}$ dorsal surface of base of tongue (141.0)

Tongue

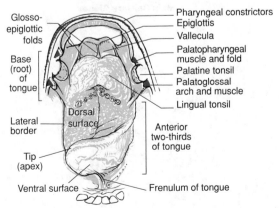

√4th / √5th Additional Digit Required   Unspecified Code   Other Specified Code   Manifestation Code   ▶◀ Revised Text   ● New Code   ▲ Revised Code Title

2003 ICD•9•CM   **Volume 1 — 25**

141.2   Tip and lateral border of tongue

141.3   Ventral surface of tongue
Anterior two-thirds of tongue, ventral surface
Frenulum linguae

141.4   Anterior two-thirds of tongue, part unspecified
Mobile part of tongue NOS

141.5   Junctional zone
Border of tongue at junction of fixed and mobile
parts at insertion of anterior tonsillar pillar

141.6   Lingual tonsil

141.8   Other sites of tongue
Malignant neoplasm of contiguous or overlapping
sites of tongue whose point of origin cannot be
determined

141.9   Tongue, unspecified
Tongue NOS

✓4th **142   Malignant neoplasm of major salivary glands**
INCLUDES   salivary ducts
EXCLUDES   *malignant neoplasm of minor salivary glands:*
NOS (145.9)
buccal mucosa (145.0)
soft palate (145.3)
tongue (141.0-141.9)
tonsil, palatine (146.0)

142.0   Parotid gland

142.1   Submandibular gland
Submaxillary gland

142.2   Sublingual gland

142.8   Other major salivary glands
Malignant neoplasm of contiguous or overlapping
sites of salivary glands and ducts whose point
of origin cannot be determined

142.9   Salivary gland, unspecified
Salivary gland (major) NOS

✓4th **143   Malignant neoplasm of gum**
INCLUDES   alveolar (ridge) mucosa
gingiva (alveolar) (marginal)
interdental papillae
EXCLUDES   *malignant odontogenic neoplasms (170.0-170.1)*

143.0   Upper gum

143.1   Lower gum

143.8   Other sites of gum
Malignant neoplasm of contiguous or overlapping
sites of gum whose point of origin cannot be
determined

143.9   Gum, unspecified

✓4th **144   Malignant neoplasm of floor of mouth**

144.0   Anterior portion
Anterior to the premolar-canine junction

144.1   Lateral portion

Main Salivary Glands

Mouth

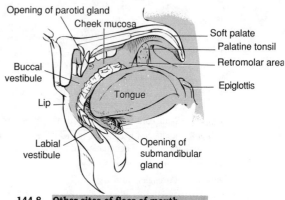

144.8   Other sites of floor of mouth
Malignant neoplasm of contiguous or overlapping
sites of floor of mouth whose point of origin
cannot be determined

144.9   Floor of mouth, part unspecified

✓4th **145   Malignant neoplasm of other and unspecified parts of
mouth**
EXCLUDES   *mucosa of lips (140.0-140.9)*

145.0   Cheek mucosa
Buccal mucosa
Cheek, inner aspect

145.1   Vestibule of mouth
Buccal sulcus (upper) (lower)
Labial sulcus (upper) (lower)

145.2   Hard palate

145.3   Soft palate
EXCLUDES   *nasopharyngeal [posterior] [superior]*
surface of soft palate (147.3)

145.4   Uvula

145.5   Palate, unspecified
Junction of hard and soft palate
Roof of mouth

145.6   Retromolar area

145.8   Other specified parts of mouth
Malignant neoplasm of contiguous or overlapping
sites of mouth whose point of origin cannot be
determined

145.9   Mouth, unspecified
Buccal cavity NOS
Minor salivary gland, unspecified site
Oral cavity NOS

✓4th **146   Malignant neoplasm of oropharynx**

146.0   Tonsil
Tonsil: Tonsil:
NOS   palatine
faucial
EXCLUDES   *lingual tonsil (141.6)*
pharyngeal tonsil (147.1)

146.1   Tonsillar fossa

146.2   Tonsillar pillars (anterior) (posterior)
Faucial pillar   Palatoglossal arch
Glossopalatine fold   Palatopharyngeal arch

146.3   Vallecula
Anterior and medial surface of the
pharyngoepiglottic fold

146.4   Anterior aspect of epiglottis
Epiglottis, free border [margin]
Glossoepiglottic fold(s)
EXCLUDES   *epiglottis:*
NOS (161.1)
suprahyoid portion (161.1)

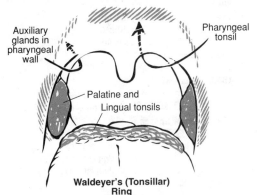

Waldeyer's (Tonsillar) Ring

Auxiliary glands in pharyngeal wall
Pharyngeal tonsil
Palatine and Lingual tonsils
Waldeyer's (Tonsillar) Ring

146.5 Junctional region
Junction of the free margin of the epiglottis, the aryepiglottic fold, and the pharyngoepiglottic fold

146.6 Lateral wall of oropharynx

146.7 Posterior wall of oropharynx

146.8 Other specified sites of oropharynx
Branchial cleft
Malignant neoplasm of contiguous or overlapping sites of oropharynx whose point of origin cannot be determined

146.9 Oropharynx, unspecified

✓4th **147 Malignant neoplasm of nasopharynx**

147.0 Superior wall
Roof of nasopharynx

147.1 Posterior wall
Adenoid
Pharyngeal tonsil

147.2 Lateral wall
Fossa of Rosenmüller
Opening of auditory tube
Pharyngeal recess

147.3 Anterior wall
Floor of nasopharynx
Nasopharyngeal [posterior] [superior] surface of soft palate
Posterior margin of nasal septum and choanae

147.8 Other specified sites of nasopharynx
Malignant neoplasm of contiguous or overlapping sites of nasopharynx whose point of origin cannot be determined

147.9 Nasopharynx, unspecified
Nasopharyngeal wall NOS

✓4th **148 Malignant neoplasm of hypopharynx**

148.0 Postcricoid region

148.1 Pyriform sinus
Pyriform fossa

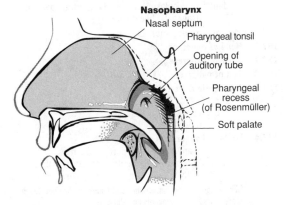

Nasopharynx

Nasal septum
Pharyngeal tonsil
Opening of auditory tube
Pharyngeal recess (of Rosenmüller)
Soft palate

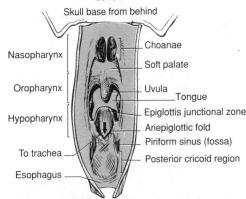

Hypopharynx

Skull base from behind
Nasopharynx
Oropharynx
Hypopharynx
To trachea
Esophagus
Choanae
Soft palate
Uvula
Tongue
Epiglottis junctional zone
Ariepiglottic fold
Piriform sinus (fossa)
Posterior cricoid region

148.2 Aryepiglottic fold, hypopharyngeal aspect
Aryepiglottic fold or interarytenoid fold:
NOS
marginal zone
EXCLUDES   *aryepiglottic fold or interarytenoid fold, laryngeal aspect (161.1)*

148.3 Posterior hypopharyngeal wall

148.8 Other specified sites of hypopharynx
Malignant neoplasm of contiguous or overlapping sites of hypopharynx whose point of origin cannot be determined

148.9 Hypopharynx, unspecified
Hypopharyngeal wall NOS
Hypopharynx NOS

✓4th **149 Malignant neoplasm of other and ill-defined sites within the lip, oral cavity, and pharynx**

149.0 Pharynx, unspecified

149.1 Waldeyer's ring

149.8 Other
Malignant neoplasms of lip, oral cavity, and pharynx whose point of origin cannot be assigned to any one of the categories 140-148
EXCLUDES   *"book leaf" neoplasm [ventral surface of tongue and floor of mouth] (145.8)*

149.9 Ill-defined

MALIGNANT NEOPLASM OF DIGESTIVE ORGANS AND PERITONEUM (150-159)
EXCLUDES   *carcinoma in situ (230.1-230.9)*

✓4th **150 Malignant neoplasm of esophagus**

150.0 Cervical esophagus

150.1 Thoracic esophagus

150.2 Abdominal esophagus
EXCLUDES   *adenocarcinoma (151.0)*
cardio-esophageal junction (151.0)

150.3 Upper third of esophagus
Proximal third of esophagus

150.4 Middle third of esophagus

150.5 Lower third of esophagus
Distal third of esophagus
EXCLUDES   *adenocarcinoma (151.0)*
cardio-esophageal junction (151.0)

150.8 Other specified part
Malignant neoplasm of contiguous or overlapping sites of esophagus whose point of origin cannot be determined

150.9 Esophagus, unspecified

✓4th **151 Malignant neoplasm of stomach**

151.0 Cardia
Cardiac orifice   Cardio-esophageal junction
EXCLUDES   *squamous cell carcinoma (150.2, 150.5)*

✓4th ✓5th Additional Digit Required   Unspecified Code   Other Specified Code   Manifestation Code   ▶◀ Revised Text   ● New Code   ▲ Revised Code Title

2003 ICD•9•CM   **Volume 1 — 27**

Neoplasms 146.5–151.0

Neoplasms 151.1–157.4

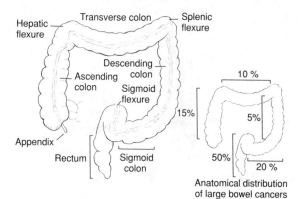

Colon

Anatomical distribution of large bowel cancers

151.1 **Pylorus**
Prepylorus   Pyloric canal

151.2 **Pyloric antrum**
Antrum of stomach NOS

151.3 **Fundus of stomach**

151.4 **Body of stomach**

151.5 **Lesser curvature, unspecified**
Lesser curvature, not classifiable to 151.1-151.4

151.6 **Greater curvature, unspecified**
Greater curvature, not classifiable to 151.0-151.4

151.8 **Other specified sites of stomach**
Anterior wall, not classifiable to 151.0-151.4
Posterior wall, not classifiable to 151.0-151.4
Malignant neoplasm of contiguous or overlapping
sites of stomach whose point of origin cannot
be determined

151.9 **Stomach, unspecified**
Carcinoma ventriculi Gastric cancer

✓4ᵗʰ 152 **Malignant neoplasm of small intestine, including duodenum**
152.0 **Duodenum**
152.1 **Jejunum**
152.2 **Ileum**
EXCLUDES *ileocecal valve (153.4)*
152.3 **Meckel's diverticulum**
152.8 **Other specified sites of small intestine**
Duodenojejunal junction
Malignant neoplasm of contiguous or overlapping
sites of small intestine whose point of origin
cannot be determined
152.9 **Small intestine, unspecified**

✓4ᵗʰ 153 **Malignant neoplasm of colon**
153.0 **Hepatic flexure**
153.1 **Transverse colon**
153.2 **Descending colon**
Left colon
153.3 **Sigmoid colon**
Sigmoid (flexure)
EXCLUDES *rectosigmoid junction (154.0)*
153.4 **Cecum**
Ileocecal valve
153.5 **Appendix**
153.6 **Ascending colon**
Right colon
153.7 **Splenic flexure**
153.8 **Other specified sites of large intestine**
Malignant neoplasm of contiguous or overlapping
sites of colon whose point of origin cannot be
determined
EXCLUDES *ileocecal valve (153.4)*
rectosigmoid junction (154.0)
153.9 **Colon, unspecified**
Large intestine NOS

✓4ᵗʰ 154 **Malignant neoplasm of rectum, rectosigmoid junction, and anus**
154.0 **Rectosigmoid junction**
Colon with rectum
Rectosigmoid (colon)
154.1 **Rectum**
Rectal ampulla
154.2 **Anal canal**
Anal sphincter
EXCLUDES *skin of anus (172.5, 173.5)*
154.3 **Anus, unspecified**
EXCLUDES *anus:*
margin (172.5, 173.5)
skin (172.5, 173.5)
perianal skin (172.5, 173.5)
154.8 **Other**
Anorectum
Cloacogenic zone
Malignant neoplasm of contiguous or overlapping
sites of rectum, rectosigmoid junction, and
anus whose point of origin cannot be
determined

✓4ᵗʰ 155 **Malignant neoplasm of liver and intrahepatic bile ducts**
155.0 **Liver, primary**
Carcinoma:
hepatocellular
liver cell
liver, specified as primary
Hepatoblastoma
155.1 **Intrahepatic bile ducts**
Canaliculi biliferi   Intrahepatic:
Interlobular: biliary passages
bile ducts   canaliculi
biliary canals   gall duct
EXCLUDES *hepatic duct (156.1)*
155.2 **Liver, not specified as primary or secondary**

✓4ᵗʰ 156 **Malignant neoplasm of gallbladder and extrahepatic bile ducts**
156.0 **Gallbladder**
156.1 **Extrahepatic bile ducts**
Biliary duct or passage NOS
Common bile duct
Cystic duct
Hepatic duct
Sphincter of Oddi
156.2 **Ampulla of Vater**
DEF: Malignant neoplasm in the area of dilation at the juncture of
the common bile and pancreatic ducts near the opening into the
lumen of the duodenum.
156.8 **Other specified sites of gallbladder and
extrahepatic bile ducts**
Malignant neoplasm of contiguous or overlapping
sites of gallbladder and extrahepatic bile ducts
whose point of origin cannot be determined
156.9 **Biliary tract, part unspecified**
Malignant neoplasm involving both intrahepatic and
extrahepatic bile ducts

✓4ᵗʰ 157 **Malignant neoplasm of pancreas**
157.0 **Head of pancreas**
157.1 **Body of pancreas**
157.2 **Tail of pancreas**
157.3 **Pancreatic duct**
Duct of:
Santorini
Wirsung
157.4 **Islets of Langerhans**
Islets of Langerhans, any part of pancreas
Use additional code to identify any functional
activity
DEF: Malignant neoplasm within the structures of the pancreas that
produce insulin, somatostatin and glucagon.

N Newborn Age: 0   **P** Pediatric Age: 0-17   **M** Maternity Age: 12-55   **A** Adult Age: 15-124   **MSP** Medicare Secondary Payer

Retroperitoneum and Peritoneum

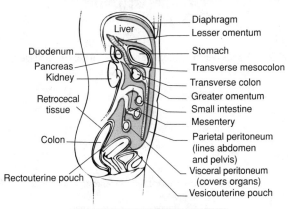

157.8   **Other specified sites of pancreas**
    Ectopic pancreatic tissue
    Malignant neoplasm of contiguous or overlapping
       sites of pancreas whose point of origin cannot
       be determined

157.9   **Pancreas, part unspecified**

✓4ᵗʰ 158 **Malignant neoplasm of retroperitoneum and peritoneum**

158.0   **Retroperitoneum**
    Periadrenal tissue
    Perinephric tissue
    Perirenal tissue
    Retrocecal tissue

158.8   **Specified parts of peritoneum**
    Cul-de-sac (of Douglas)
    Mesentery
    Mesocolon
    Omentum
    Peritoneum:
      parietal
      pelvic
    Rectouterine pouch
    Malignant neoplasm of contiguous or overlapping
       sites of retroperitoneum and peritoneum whose
       point of origin cannot be determined

158.9   **Peritoneum, unspecified**

✓4ᵗʰ 159 **Malignant neoplasm of other and ill-defined sites within the digestive organs and peritoneum**

159.0   **Intestinal tract, part unspecified**
    Intestine NOS

159.1   **Spleen, not elsewhere classified**
    Angiosarcoma ⎫
    Fibrosarcoma ⎬ of spleen
           ⎭
      EXCLUDES *Hodgkin's disease (201.0-201.9)*
                 lymphosarcoma (200.1)
                 reticulosarcoma (200.0)

159.8   **Other sites of digestive system and intra-abdominal organs**
    Malignant neoplasm of digestive organs and
       peritoneum whose point of origin cannot be
       assigned to any one of the categories 150-158
      EXCLUDES *anus and rectum (154.8)*
                 cardio-esophageal junction (151.0)
                 colon and rectum (154.0)

159.9   **Ill-defined**
    Alimentary canal or tract NOS
    Gastrointestinal tract NOS
      EXCLUDES *abdominal NOS (195.2)*
                 intra-abdominal NOS (195.2)

MALIGNANT NEOPLASM OF RESPIRATORY AND INTRATHORACIC ORGANS (160-165)
    EXCLUDES *carcinoma in situ (231.0-231.9)*

✓4ᵗʰ 160 **Malignant neoplasm of nasal cavities, middle ear, and accessory sinuses**

160.0   **Nasal cavities**
    Cartilage of nose   Septum of nose
    Conchae, nasal   Vestibule of nose
    Internal nose
      EXCLUDES *nasal bone (170.0)*
                 nose NOS (195.0)
                 olfactory bulb (192.0)
                 posterior margin of septum and
                    choanae (147.3)
                 skin of nose (172.3, 173.3)
                 turbinates (170.0)

160.1   **Auditory tube, middle ear, and mastoid air cells**
    Antrum tympanicum Tympanic cavity
    Eustachian tube
      EXCLUDES *auditory canal (external) (172.2, 173.2)*
                 bone of ear (meatus) (170.0)
                 cartilage of ear (171.0)
                 ear (external) (skin) (172.2, 173.2)

160.2   **Maxillary sinus**
    Antrum (Highmore) (maxillary)

160.3   **Ethmoidal sinus**

160.4   **Frontal sinus**

160.5   **Sphenoidal sinus**

160.8   **Other**
    Malignant neoplasm of contiguous or overlapping
       sites of nasal cavities, middle ear, and
       accessory sinuses whose point of origin cannot
       be determined

160.9   **Accessory sinus, unspecified**

✓4ᵗʰ 161 **Malignant neoplasm of larynx**

161.0   **Glottis**
    Intrinsic larynx
    Laryngeal commissure (anterior) (posterior)
    True vocal cord
    Vocal cord NOS

161.1   **Supraglottis**
    Aryepiglottic fold or interarytenoid fold, laryngeal
       aspect
    Epiglottis (suprahyoid portion) NOS
    Extrinsic larynx
    False vocal cords
    Posterior (laryngeal) surface of epiglottis
    Ventricular bands
      EXCLUDES *anterior aspect of epiglottis (146.4)*
                 aryepiglottic fold or interarytenoid fold:
                    NOS (148.2)
                    hypopharyngeal aspect (148.2)
                    marginal zone (148.2)

161.2   **Subglottis**

161.3   **Laryngeal cartilages**
    Cartilage: Cartilage:
      arytenoid   cuneiform
      cricoid   thyroid

161.8   **Other specified sites of larynx**
    Malignant neoplasm of contiguous or overlapping
       sites of larynx whose point of origin cannot be
       determined

161.9   **Larynx, unspecified**

✓4ᵗʰ 162 **Malignant neoplasm of trachea, bronchus, and lung**

162.0   **Trachea**
    Cartilage ⎫
    Mucosa   ⎬ of trachea
           ⎭

162.2   **Main bronchus**
    Carina
    Hilus of lung

✓4ᵗʰ
✓5ᵗʰ
  Additional Digit Required   Unspecified Code   Other Specified Code   Manifestation Code   ▶◀ Revised Text   ● New Code   ▲ Revised Code Title

2003 ICD•9•CM   **Volume 1 — 29**

162.3   **Upper lobe, bronchus or lung**

162.4   **Middle lobe, bronchus or lung**

162.5   **Lower lobe, bronchus or lung**

162.8   **Other parts of bronchus or lung**
Malignant neoplasm of contiguous or overlapping sites of bronchus or lung whose point of origin cannot be determined

162.9   **Bronchus and lung, unspecified**

✓4ᵗʰ **163 Malignant neoplasm of pleura**

163.0   **Parietal pleura**

163.1   **Visceral pleura**

163.8   **Other specified sites of pleura**
Malignant neoplasm of contiguous or overlapping sites of pleura whose point of origin cannot be determined

163.9   **Pleura, unspecified**

✓4ᵗʰ **164 Malignant neoplasm of thymus, heart, and mediastinum**

164.0   **Thymus**

164.1   **Heart**
Endocardium
Epicardium
Myocardium
Pericardium
EXCLUDES *great vessels (171.4)*

164.2   **Anterior mediastinum**

164.3   **Posterior mediastinum**

164.8   **Other**
Malignant neoplasm of contiguous or overlapping sites of thymus, heart, and mediastinum whose point of origin cannot be determined

164.9   **Mediastinum, part unspecified**

✓4ᵗʰ **165 Malignant neoplasm of other and ill-defined sites within the respiratory system and intrathoracic organs**

165.0   **Upper respiratory tract, part unspecified**

165.8   **Other**
Malignant neoplasm of respiratory and intrathoracic organs whose point of origin cannot be assigned to any one of the categories 160-164

165.9   **Ill-defined sites within the respiratory system**
Respiratory tract NOS
EXCLUDES *intrathoracic NOS (195.1)*
thoracic NOS (195.1)

Skull

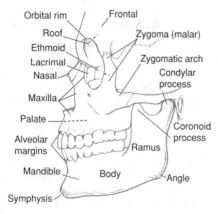

Orbital rim
Frontal
Roof
Zygoma (malar)
Ethmoid
Lacrimal
Zygomatic arch
Nasal
Condylar process
Maxilla
Palate
Coronoid process
Alveolar margins
Ramus
Mandible
Body
Angle
Symphysis

MALIGNANT NEOPLASM OF BONE, CONNECTIVE TISSUE, SKIN, AND BREAST (170-176)

EXCLUDES *carcinoma in situ:*
breast (233.0)
skin (232.0-232.9)

✓4ᵗʰ **170 Malignant neoplasm of bone and articular cartilage**
INCLUDES cartilage (articular) (joint)
periosteum
EXCLUDES *bone marrow NOS (202.9)*
cartilage:
ear (171.0)
eyelid (171.0)
larynx (161.3)
nose (160.0)
synovia (171.0-171.9)

170.0   **Bones of skull and face, except mandible**

Bone:	Bone:
ethmoid	sphenoid
frontal	temporal
malar	zygomatic
nasal	Maxilla (superior)
occipital	Turbinate
orbital	Upper jaw bone
parietal	Vomer

EXCLUDES *carcinoma, any type except*
intraosseous or odontogenic:
maxilla, maxillary (sinus) (160.2)
upper jaw bone (143.0)
jaw bone (lower) (170.1)

170.1   **Mandible**
Inferior maxilla
Jaw bone NOS
Lower jaw bone
EXCLUDES *carcinoma, any type except*
intraosseous or odontogenic:
jaw bone NOS (143.9)
lower (143.1)
upper jaw bone (170.0)

170.2   **Vertebral column, excluding sacrum and coccyx**
Spinal column   Vertebra
Spine
EXCLUDES *sacrum and coccyx (170.6)*

170.3   **Ribs, sternum, and clavicle**
Costal cartilage
Costovertebral joint
Xiphoid process

170.4   **Scapula and long bones of upper limb**
Acromion
Bones NOS of upper limb
Humerus
Radius
Ulna

170.5   **Short bones of upper limb**

Carpal	Scaphoid (of hand)
Cuneiform, wrist	Semilunar or lunate
Metacarpal	Trapezium
Navicular, of hand	Trapezoid
Phalanges of hand	Unciform
Pisiform	

170.6   **Pelvic bones, sacrum, and coccyx**

Coccygeal vertebra	Pubic bone
Ilium	Sacral vertebra
Ischium	

170.7   **Long bones of lower limb**
Bones NOS of lower limb
Femur
Fibula
Tibia

170.8   **Short bones of lower limb**

Astragalus [talus]	Navicular (of ankle)
Calcaneus	Patella
Cuboid	Phalanges of foot
Cuneiform, ankle	Tarsal
Metatarsal	

170.9   **Bone and articular cartilage, site unspecified**

☑4ᵗʰ **171** **Malignant neoplasm of connective and other soft tissue**

INCLUDES   blood vessel
bursa
fascia
fat
ligament, except uterine
muscle
peripheral, sympathetic, and parasympathetic
    nerves and ganglia
synovia
tendon (sheath)

EXCLUDES   *cartilage (of):*
    articular (170.0-170.9)
    larynx (161.3)
    nose (160.0)
connective tissue:
    breast (174.0-175.9)
    internal organs—code to malignant neoplasm
        of the site [e.g., leiomyosarcoma of
        stomach, 151.9]
    heart (164.1)
    uterine ligament (183.4)

171.0   **Head, face, and neck**

Cartilage of:	Cartilage of:
ear	eyelid

171.2   **Upper limb, including shoulder**

Arm	Forearm
Finger	Hand

171.3   **Lower limb, including hip**

Foot	Thigh
Leg	Toe
Popliteal space	

171.4   **Thorax**

Axilla	Great vessels
Diaphragm	

EXCLUDES   *heart (164.1)*
mediastinum (164.2-164.9)
thymus (164.0)

171.5   **Abdomen**

Abdominal wall
Hypochondrium

EXCLUDES   *peritoneum (158.8)*
retroperitoneum (158.0)

171.6   **Pelvis**

Buttock	Inguinal region
Groin	Perineum

EXCLUDES   *pelvic peritoneum (158.8)*
retroperitoneum (158.0)
uterine ligament, any (183.3-183.5)

171.7   **Trunk, unspecified**

Back NOS
Flank NOS

171.8   **Other specified sites of connective and other soft tissue**

Malignant neoplasm of contiguous or overlapping
    sites of connective tissue whose point of origin
    cannot be determined

171.9   **Connective and other soft tissue, site unspecified**

☑4ᵗʰ **172** **Malignant melanoma of skin**

INCLUDES   melanocarcinoma
melanoma (skin) NOS

EXCLUDES   *skin of genital organs (184.0-184.9, 187.1-187.9)*
sites other than skin—code to malignant
    neoplasm of the site

DEF: Malignant neoplasm of melanocytes; most common in skin, may involve oral cavity, esophagus, anal canal, vagina, leptomeninges or conjunctiva.

172.0   **Lip**

EXCLUDES   *vermilion border of lip (140.0-140.1, 140.9)*

172.1   **Eyelid, including canthus**

172.2   **Ear and external auditory canal**

Auricle (ear)
Auricular canal, external
External [acoustic] meatus
Pinna

172.3   **Other and unspecified parts of face**

Cheek (external)	Forehead
Chin	Nose, external
Eyebrow	Temple

172.4   **Scalp and neck**

172.5   **Trunk, except scrotum**

Axilla	Perianal skin
Breast	Perineum
Buttock	Umbilicus
Groin	

EXCLUDES   *anal canal (154.2)*
anus NOS (154.3)
scrotum (187.7)

172.6   **Upper limb, including shoulder**

Arm	Forearm
Finger	Hand

172.7   **Lower limb, including hip**

Ankle	Leg
Foot	Popliteal area
Heel	Thigh
Knee	Toe

172.8   **Other specified sites of skin**

Malignant melanoma of contiguous or overlapping
    sites of skin whose point of origin cannot be
    determined

172.9   **Melanoma of skin, site unspecified**

☑4ᵗʰ **173** **Other malignant neoplasm of skin**

INCLUDES   malignant neoplasm of:
    sebaceous glands
    sudoriferous, sudoriparous glands
    sweat glands

EXCLUDES   *Kaposi's sarcoma (176.0-176.9)*
malignant melanoma of skin (172.0-172.9)
skin of genital organs (184.0-184.9, 187.1-187.9)

173.0   **Skin of lip**

EXCLUDES   *vermilion border of lip (140.0-140.1, 140.9)*

173.1   **Eyelid, including canthus**

EXCLUDES   *cartilage of eyelid (171.0)*

173.2   **Skin of ear and external auditory canal**

Auricle (ear)
Auricular canal, external
External meatus
Pinna

EXCLUDES   *cartilage of ear (171.0)*

173.3   **Skin of other and unspecified parts of face**

Cheek, external	Forehead
Chin	Nose, external
Eyebrow	Temple

173.4   **Scalp and skin of neck**

☑4ᵗʰ
☑5ᵗʰ Additional Digit Required   Unspecified Code   Other Specified Code   Manifestation Code   ▶◀ Revised Text   ● New Code   ▲ Revised Code Title

Neoplasms 173.5–183.2

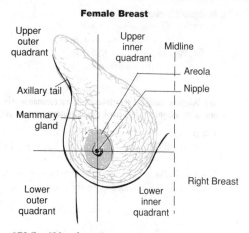

Female Breast

173.5   **Skin of trunk, except scrotum**
Axillary fold   Skin of:
Perianal skin   buttock
Skin of: chest wall
   abdominal wall   groin
   anus   perineum
   back   Umbilicus
   breast

> **EXCLUDES**   *anal canal (154.2)*
> *anus NOS (154.3)*
> *skin of scrotum (187.7)*

173.6   **Skin of upper limb, including shoulder**
Arm   Forearm
Finger   Hand

173.7   **Skin of lower limb, including hip**
Ankle   Leg
Foot   Popliteal area
Heel   Thigh
Knee   Toe

173.8   **Other specified sites of skin**
Malignant neoplasm of contiguous or overlapping sites of skin whose point of origin cannot be determined

173.9   **Skin, site unspecified**

√4ᵗʰ   174   **Malignant neoplasm of female breast**
> **INCLUDES**   breast (female)
> connective tissue
> soft parts
> Paget's disease of:
>   breast
>   nipple

> **EXCLUDES**   *skin of breast (172.5, 173.5)*

174.0   **Nipple and areola**   ♀
174.1   **Central portion**   ♀
174.2   **Upper-inner quadrant**   ♀
174.3   **Lower-inner quadrant**   ♀
174.4   **Upper-outer quadrant**   ♀
174.5   **Lower-outer quadrant**   ♀
174.6   **Axillary tail**   ♀
174.8   **Other specified sites of female breast**   ♀
Ectopic sites
Inner breast
Lower breast
Malignant neoplasm of contiguous or overlapping sites of breast whose point of origin cannot be determined
Midline of breast
Outer breast
Upper breast

174.9   **Breast (female), unspecified**   ♀

√4ᵗʰ   175   **Malignant neoplasm of male breast**
> **EXCLUDES**   *skin of breast (172.5, 173.5)*

175.0   **Nipple and areola**   ♂
175.9   **Other and unspecified sites of male breast**   ♂
Ectopic breast tissue, male

√4ᵗʰ   176   **Kaposi's sarcoma**
176.0   **Skin**
176.1   **Soft tissue**
> **INCLUDES**   blood vessel
> connective tissue
> fascia
> ligament
> lymphatic(s) NEC
> muscle

> **EXCLUDES**   *lymph glands and nodes (176.5)*

176.2   **Palate**
176.3   **Gastrointestinal sites**
176.4   **Lung**
176.5   **Lymph nodes**
176.8   **Other specified sites**
> **INCLUDES**   oral cavity NEC

176.9   **Unspecified**
Viscera NOS

MALIGNANT NEOPLASM OF GENITOURINARY ORGANS (179-189)
> **EXCLUDES**   *carcinoma in situ (233.1-233.9)*

179   **Malignant neoplasm of uterus, part unspecified**   ♀

√4ᵗʰ   180   **Malignant neoplasm of cervix uteri**
> **INCLUDES**   invasive malignancy [carcinoma]
> **EXCLUDES**   *carcinoma in situ (233.1)*

180.0   **Endocervix**   ♀
Cervical canal NOS   Endocervical gland
Endocervical canal
180.1   **Exocervix**   ♀
180.8   **Other specified sites of cervix**   ♀
Cervical stump
Squamocolumnar junction of cervix
Malignant neoplasm of contiguous or overlapping sites of cervix uteri whose point of origin cannot be determined
180.9   **Cervix uteri, unspecified**   ♀

181   **Malignant neoplasm of placenta**   ♀
Choriocarcinoma NOS
Chorioepithelioma NOS
> **EXCLUDES**   *chorioadenoma (destruens) (236.1)*
> *hydatidiform mole (630)*
>   *malignant (236.1)*
> *invasive mole (236.1)*
> *male choriocarcinoma NOS (186.0-186.9)*

√4ᵗʰ   182   **Malignant neoplasm of body of uterus**
> **EXCLUDES**   *carcinoma in situ (233.2)*

182.0   **Corpus uteri, except isthmus**   ♀
Cornu   Fundus
Endometrium   Myometrium
182.1   **Isthmus**   ♀
Lower uterine segment
182.8   **Other specified sites of body of uterus**   ♀
Malignant neoplasm of contiguous or overlapping sites of body of uterus whose point of origin cannot be determined
> **EXCLUDES**   *uterus NOS (179)*

√4ᵗʰ   183   **Malignant neoplasm of ovary and other uterine adnexa**
> **EXCLUDES**   *Douglas' cul-de-sac (158.8)*

183.0   **Ovary**   ♀
Use additional code to identify any functional activity
183.2   **Fallopian tube**   ♀
Oviduct   Uterine tube

183.3 Broad ligament ♀
     Mesovarium   Parovarian region

183.4 Parametrium ♀
     Uterine ligament NOS   Uterosacral ligament

183.5 Round ligament ♀

183.8 Other specified sites of uterine adnexa ♀
     Tubo-ovarian
     Utero-ovarian
     Malignant neoplasm of contiguous or overlapping
        sites of ovary and other uterine adnexa whose
        point of origin cannot be determined

183.9 Uterine adnexa, unspecified ♀

✓4ᵗʰ 184 Malignant neoplasm of other and unspecified female genital organs
     EXCLUDES   *carcinoma in situ (233.3)*

184.0 Vagina ♀
     Gartner's duct   Vaginal vault

184.1 Labia majora ♀
     Greater vestibular [Bartholin's] gland

184.2 Labia minora ♀

184.3 Clitoris ♀

184.4 Vulva, unspecified ♀
     External female genitalia NOS
     Pudendum

184.8 Other specified sites of female genital organs ♀
     Malignant neoplasm of contiguous or overlapping
        sites of female genital organs whose point of
        origin cannot be determined

184.9 Female genital organ, site unspecified ♀
     Female genitourinary tract NOS

185 Malignant neoplasm of prostate ♂
     EXCLUDES   *seminal vesicles (187.8)*

✓4ᵗʰ 186 Malignant neoplasm of testis
     Use additional code to identify any functional activity

186.0 Undescended testis ♂
     Ectopic testis   Retained testis

186.9 Other and unspecified testis ♂
     Testis: Testis:
       NOS   scrotal
       descended

✓4ᵗʰ 187 Malignant neoplasm of penis and other male genital organs

187.1 Prepuce ♂
     Foreskin

187.2 Glans penis ♂

187.3 Body of penis ♂
     Corpus cavernosum

187.4 Penis, part unspecified ♂
     Skin of penis NOS

187.5 Epididymis ♂

187.6 Spermatic cord ♂
     Vas deferens

187.7 Scrotum ♂
     Skin of scrotum

187.8 Other specified sites of male genital organs ♂
     Seminal vesicle
     Tunica vaginalis
     Malignant neoplasm of contiguous or overlapping
        sites of penis and other male genital organs
        whose point of origin cannot be determined

187.9 Male genital organ, site unspecified ♂
     Male genital organ or tract NOS

✓4ᵗʰ 188 Malignant neoplasm of bladder
     EXCLUDES   *carcinoma in situ (233.7)*

188.0 Trigone of urinary bladder

188.1 Dome of urinary bladder

188.2 Lateral wall of urinary bladder

188.3 Anterior wall of urinary bladder

188.4 Posterior wall of urinary bladder

188.5 Bladder neck
     Internal urethral orifice

188.6 Ureteric orifice

188.7 Urachus

188.8 Other specified sites of bladder
     Malignant neoplasm of contiguous or overlapping
        sites of bladder whose point of origin cannot be
        determined

188.9 Bladder, part unspecified
     Bladder wall NOS

✓4ᵗʰ 189 Malignant neoplasm of kidney and other and unspecified urinary organs

189.0 Kidney, except pelvis
     Kidney NOS
     Kidney parenchyma

189.1 Renal pelvis
     Renal calyces
     Ureteropelvic junction

189.2 Ureter
     EXCLUDES   *ureteric orifice of bladder (188.6)*

189.3 Urethra
     EXCLUDES   *urethral orifice of bladder (188.5)*

189.4 Paraurethral glands

189.8 Other specified sites of urinary organs
     Malignant neoplasm of contiguous or overlapping
        sites of kidney and other urinary organs whose
        point of origin cannot be determined

189.9 Urinary organ, site unspecified
     Urinary system NOS

MALIGNANT NEOPLASM OF OTHER AND UNSPECIFIED SITES (190-199)

     EXCLUDES   *carcinoma in situ (234.0-234.9)*

✓4ᵗʰ 190 Malignant neoplasm of eye
     EXCLUDES   *carcinoma in situ (234.0)*
                 eyelid (skin) (172.1, 173.1)
                    cartilage (171.0)
                 optic nerve (192.0)
                 orbital bone (170.0)

190.0 Eyeball, except conjunctiva, cornea, retina, and choroid
     Ciliary body   Sclera
     Crystalline lens   Uveal tract
     Iris

190.1 Orbit
     Connective tissue of orbit   Retrobulbar
     Extraocular muscle
     EXCLUDES   *bone of orbit (170.0)*

190.2 Lacrimal gland

190.3 Conjunctiva

190.4 Cornea

190.5 Retina

190.6 Choroid

190.7 Lacrimal duct
     Lacrimal sac
     Nasolacrimal duct

190.8 Other specified sites of eye
     Malignant neoplasm of contiguous or overlapping
        sites of eye whose point of origin cannot be
        determined

190.9 Eye, part unspecified

✓4ᵗʰ 191 Malignant neoplasm of brain
     EXCLUDES   *cranial nerves (192.0)*
                 retrobulbar area (190.1)

191.0 Cerebrum, except lobes and ventricles
     Basal ganglia   Globus pallidus
     Cerebral cortex   Hypothalamus
     Corpus striatum   Thalamus

191.1 Frontal lobe

✓4ᵗʰ / ✓5ᵗʰ Additional Digit Required   Unspecified Code   Other Specified Code   Manifestation Code   ▶◀ Revised Text   ● New Code   ▲ Revised Code Title

Brain

Fourth ventricle

Cerebrum

Corpus callosum

Thalamus

Hypothalamus

Hypophysis

Pons

Cerebellum

Medulla oblongata

Midsagittal Section (between hemispheres)

191.2 Temporal lobe
Hippocampus   Uncus

191.3 Parietal lobe

191.4 Occipital lobe

191.5 Ventricles
Choroid plexus   Floor of ventricle

191.6 Cerebellum NOS
Cerebellopontine angle

191.7 Brain stem
Cerebral peduncle   Midbrain
Medulla oblongata   Pons

191.8 Other parts of brain
Corpus callosum
Tapetum
Malignant neoplasm of contiguous or overlapping sites of brain whose point of origin cannot be determined

191.9 Brain, unspecified
Cranial fossa NOS

✓4ᵗʰ **192 Malignant neoplasm of other and unspecified parts of nervous system**
EXCLUDES   *peripheral, sympathetic, and parasympathetic nerves and ganglia (171.0-171.9)*

192.0 Cranial nerves
Olfactory bulb

192.1 Cerebral meninges
Dura (mater)   Meninges NOS
Falx (cerebelli) (cerebri)   Tentorium

192.2 Spinal cord
Cauda equina

192.3 Spinal meninges

192.8 Other specified sites of nervous system
Malignant neoplasm of contiguous or overlapping sites of other parts of nervous system whose point of origin cannot be determined

192.9 Nervous system, part unspecified
Nervous system (central) NOS
EXCLUDES   *meninges NOS (192.1)*

193 Malignant neoplasm of thyroid gland
Sipple's syndrome
Thyroglossal duct
Use additional code to identify any functional activity

✓4ᵗʰ **194 Malignant neoplasm of other endocrine glands and related structures**
Use additional code to identify any functional activity
EXCLUDES   *islets of Langerhans (157.4)*
ovary (183.0)
testis (186.0-186.9)
thymus (164.0)

194.0 Adrenal gland
Adrenal cortex   Suprarenal gland
Adrenal medulla

194.1 Parathyroid gland

194.3 Pituitary gland and craniopharyngeal duct
Craniobuccal pouch   Rathke's pouch
Hypophysis   Sella turcica

194.4 Pineal gland

194.5 Carotid body

194.6 Aortic body and other paraganglia
Coccygeal body   Para-aortic body
Glomus jugulare

194.8 Other
Pluriglandular involvement NOS
Note: If the sites of multiple involvements are known, they should be coded separately.

194.9 Endocrine gland, site unspecified

✓4ᵗʰ **195 Malignant neoplasm of other and ill-defined sites**
INCLUDES   malignant neoplasms of contiguous sites, not elsewhere classified, whose point of origin cannot be determined
EXCLUDES   *malignant neoplasm:*
lymphatic and hematopoietic tissue (200.0-208.9)
secondary sites (196.0-198.8)
unspecified site (199.0-199.1)

195.0 Head, face, and neck
Cheek NOS   Nose NOS
Jaw NOS   Supraclavicular region NOS

195.1 Thorax
Axilla   Intrathoracic NOS
Chest (wall) NOS

195.2 Abdomen
Intra-abdominal NOS

195.3 Pelvis
Groin
Inguinal region NOS
Presacral region
Sacrococcygeal region
Sites overlapping systems within pelvis, as:
rectovaginal (septum)
rectovesical (septum)

195.4 Upper limb

195.5 Lower limb

195.8 Other specified sites
Back NOS   Trunk NOS
Flank NOS

✓4ᵗʰ **196 Secondary and unspecified malignant neoplasm of lymph nodes**
EXCLUDES   *any malignant neoplasm of lymph nodes, specified as primary (200.0-202.9)*
Hodgkin's disease (201.0-201.9)
lymphosarcoma (200.1)
reticulosarcoma (200.0)
other forms of lymphoma (202.0-202.9)

196.0 Lymph nodes of head, face, and neck
Cervical   Scalene
Cervicofacial   Supraclavicular

196.1 Intrathoracic lymph nodes
Bronchopulmonary   Mediastinal
Intercostal   Tracheobronchial

196.2 Intra-abdominal lymph nodes
Intestinal   Retroperitoneal
Mesenteric

196.3 Lymph nodes of axilla and upper limb
Brachial   Infraclavicular
Epitrochlear   Pectoral

196.5 Lymph nodes of inguinal region and lower limb
Femoral   Popliteal
Groin   Tibial

196.6 Intrapelvic lymph nodes
Hypogastric   Obturator
Iliac   Parametrial

196.8 Lymph nodes of multiple sites

196.9 Site unspecified
Lymph nodes NOS

Lymph Nodes

- Head, neck, and face
- Thoracic ducts empty into
- Left subclavian vein
- Intrathoracic
- Axillary and upper limb
- Intraabdominal
- Thoracic duct (transmits lymph through diaphragm using one-way valves)
- Cisterna chyli
- Nodes generally accompany large blood vessels
- Intrapelvic
- Inguinal and lower limb

✓4ᵗʰ **197 Secondary malignant neoplasm of respiratory and digestive systems**

> **EXCLUDES** *lymph node metastasis (196.0-196.9)*

197.0 Lung
Bronchus

197.1 Mediastinum

197.2 Pleura

197.3 Other respiratory organs
Trachea

197.4 Small intestine, including duodenum

197.5 Large intestine and rectum

197.6 Retroperitoneum and peritoneum

197.7 Liver, specified as secondary

197.8 Other digestive organs and spleen

✓4ᵗʰ **198 Secondary malignant neoplasm of other specified sites**

> **EXCLUDES** *lymph node metastasis (196.0-196.9)*

198.0 Kidney

198.1 Other urinary organs

198.2 Skin
Skin of breast

198.3 Brain and spinal cord

198.4 Other parts of nervous system
Meninges (cerebral) (spinal)

198.5 Bone and bone marrow

198.6 Ovary ♀

198.7 Adrenal gland
Suprarenal gland

✓5ᵗʰ **198.8 Other specified sites**

198.81 Breast

> **EXCLUDES** *skin of breast (198.2)*

198.82 Genital organs

198.89 Other

> **EXCLUDES** *retroperitoneal lymph nodes (196.2)*

✓4ᵗʰ **199 Malignant neoplasm without specification of site**

199.0 Disseminated
Carcinomatosis
Generalized:
  cancer   unspecified site
  malignancy   (primary)
  Multiple cancer   (secondary)

199.1 Other
Cancer   unspecified site
Carcinoma   (primary)
Malignancy   (secondary)

MALIGNANT NEOPLASM OF LYMPHATIC AND HEMATOPOIETIC TISSUE (200-208)

> **EXCLUDES** *secondary neoplasm of:*
> *bone marrow (198.5)*
> *spleen (197.8)*
> *secondary and unspecified neoplasm of lymph nodes (196.0-196.9)*

The following fifth-digit subclassification is for use with categories 200-202:

  0 **unspecified site, extranodal and solid organ sites**
  1 **lymph nodes of head, face, and neck**
  2 **intrathoracic lymph nodes**
  3 **intra-abdominal lymph nodes**
  4 **lymph nodes of axilla and upper limb**
  5 **lymph nodes of inguinal region and lower limb**
  6 **intrapelvic lymph nodes**
  7 **spleen**
  8 **lymph nodes of multiple sites**

✓4ᵗʰ **200 Lymphosarcoma and reticulosarcoma**

§ ✓5ᵗʰ **200.0 Reticulosarcoma**
Lymphoma (malignant):
  histiocytic (diffuse):
    nodular
    pleomorphic cell type
  reticulum cell type
Reticulum cell sarcoma:
  NOS
  pleomorphic cell type

> **DEF:** Malignant lymphoma of primarily histolytic cells; commonly originates in reticuloendothelium of lymph nodes.

§ ✓5ᵗʰ **200.1 Lymphosarcoma**
Lymphoblastoma (diffuse)
Lymphoma (malignant):
  lymphoblastic (diffuse)
  lymphocytic (cell type) (diffuse)
  lymphosarcoma type
Lymphosarcoma:
  NOS
  diffuse NOS
  lymphoblastic (diffuse)
  lymphocytic (diffuse)
  prolymphocytic

> **EXCLUDES** *lymphosarcoma:*
> *follicular or nodular (202.0)*
> *mixed cell type (200.8)*
> *lymphosarcoma cell leukemia (207.8)*

> **DEF:** Malignant lymphoma created from anaplastic lymphoid cells resembling lymphocytes or lymphoblasts.

§ ✓5ᵗʰ **200.2 Burkitt's tumor or lymphoma**
Malignant lymphoma, Burkitt's type

> **DEF:** Large osteolytic lesion most common in jaw or as abdominal mass; usually found in central Africa but reported elsewhere.

§ ✓5ᵗʰ **200.8 Other named variants**
Lymphoma (malignant):
  lymphoplasmacytoid type
  mixed lymphocytic-histiocytic (diffuse)
Lymphosarcoma, mixed cell type (diffuse)
Reticulolymphosarcoma (diffuse)

✓4ᵗʰ **201 Hodgkin's disease**

> **DEF:** Painless, progressive enlargement of lymph nodes, spleen and general lymph tissue; symptoms include anorexia, lassitude, weight loss, fever, pruritis, night sweats, anemia.

§ ✓5ᵗʰ **201.0 Hodgkin's paragranuloma**

§ ✓5ᵗʰ **201.1 Hodgkin's granuloma**

§ ✓5ᵗʰ **201.2 Hodgkin's sarcoma**

§ ✓5ᵗʰ **201.4 Lymphocytic-histiocytic predominance**

---

§ Requires fifth-digit. See beginning of section 200–208 for codes and definitions.

✓4ᵗʰ / ✓5ᵗʰ Additional Digit Required   Unspecified Code   Other Specified Code   Manifestation Code   ▶◀ Revised Text   ● New Code   ▲ Revised Code Title

Neoplasms 197–201.4

§ ✓5ᵗʰ **201.5　Nodular sclerosis**
　　　　Hodgkin's disease, nodular sclerosis:
　　　　　NOS
　　　　　cellular phase

§ ✓5ᵗʰ **201.6　Mixed cellularity**

§ ✓5ᵗʰ **201.7　Lymphocytic depletion**
　　　　Hodgkin's disease, lymphocytic depletion:
　　　　　NOS
　　　　　diffuse fibrosis
　　　　　reticular type

§ ✓5ᵗʰ **201.9　Hodgkin's disease, unspecified**
　　　　Hodgkin's:　　　　Malignant:
　　　　　disease NOS　　　lymphogranuloma
　　　　　lymphoma NOS　　lymphogranulomatosis

✓4ᵗʰ **202　Other malignant neoplasms of lymphoid and histiocytic tissue**

§ ✓5ᵗʰ **202.0　Nodular lymphoma**
　　　　Brill-Symmers disease
　　　　Lymphoma:
　　　　　follicular (giant)
　　　　　lymphocytic, nodular
　　　　Lymphosarcoma:
　　　　　follicular (giant)
　　　　　nodular
　　　　Reticulosarcoma, follicular or nodular

　　　　DEF: Lymphomatous cells clustered into nodules within the lymph node; usually occurs in older adults and may involve all nodes and possibly extranodal sites.

§ ✓5ᵗʰ **202.1　Mycosis fungoides**
　　　　DEF: Type of cutaneous T-cell lymphoma; may evolve into generalized lymphoma; formerly thought to be of fungoid origin.

§ ✓5ᵗʰ **202.2　Sézary's disease**
　　　　DEF: Type of cutaneous T-cell lymphoma with erythroderma, intense pruritus, peripheral lymphadenopathy, abnormal hyperchromatic mononuclear cells in skin, lymph nodes and peripheral blood.

§ ✓5ᵗʰ **202.3　Malignant histiocytosis**
　　　　Histiocytic medullary reticulosis
　　　　Malignant:
　　　　　reticuloendotheliosis
　　　　　reticulosis

§ ✓5ᵗʰ **202.4　Leukemic reticuloendotheliosis**
　　　　Hairy-cell leukemia
　　　　DEF: Chronic leukemia with large, mononuclear cells with "hairy" appearance in marrow, spleen, liver, blood.

§ ✓5ᵗʰ **202.5　Letterer-Siwe disease**
　　　　Acute:
　　　　　differentiated progressive histiocytosis
　　　　　histiocytosis X (progressive)
　　　　　infantile reticuloendotheliosis
　　　　　reticulosis of infancy
　　　　　　EXCLUDES　*Hand-Schüller-Christian disease (277.8)*
　　　　　　　　　　　　　histiocytosis (acute) (chronic) (277.8)
　　　　　　　　　　　　　histiocytosis X (chronic) (277.8)

　　　　DEF: A recessive reticuloendotheliosis of early childhood, with a hemorrhagic tendency, eczema-like skin eruption, hepato-splenomegaly, including lymph node enlargement, and progressive anemia; it is often a fatal disease with no established cause.

§ ✓5ᵗʰ **202.6　Malignant mast cell tumors**
　　　　Malignant:　　　　Mast cell sarcoma
　　　　　mastocytoma　　Systemic tissue mast
　　　　　mastocytosis　　　cell disease
　　　　　　EXCLUDES　*mast cell leukemia (207.8)*

§ ✓5ᵗʰ **202.8　Other lymphomas**
　　　　Lymphoma (malignant):
　　　　　NOS
　　　　　diffuse
　　　　　　EXCLUDES　*benign lymphoma (229.0)*

§ ✓5ᵗʰ **202.9　Other and unspecified malignant neoplasms of lymphoid and histiocytic tissue**
　　　　Malignant neoplasm of bone marrow NOS

✓4ᵗʰ **203　Multiple myeloma and immunoproliferative neoplasms**

　　　　The following fifth-digit subclassification is for use with category 203:
　　　　　0　without mention of remission
　　　　　1　in remission

✓5ᵗʰ **203.0　Multiple myeloma**
　　　　Kahler's disease　　　Myelomatosis
　　　　　　EXCLUDES　*solitary myeloma (238.6)*

✓5ᵗʰ **203.1　Plasma cell leukemia**
　　　　Plasmacytic leukemia

✓5ᵗʰ **203.8　Other immunoproliferative neoplasms**

✓4ᵗʰ **204　Lymphoid leukemia**
　　　　INCLUDES　leukemia:
　　　　　　　　　　　lymphatic
　　　　　　　　　　　lymphoblastic
　　　　　　　　　　　lymphocytic
　　　　　　　　　　　lymphogenous

　　　　The following fifth-digit subclassification is for use with category 204:
　　　　　0　without mention of remission
　　　　　1　in remission

✓5ᵗʰ **204.0　Acute**
　　　　　　EXCLUDES　*acute exacerbation of chronic lymphoid leukemia (204.1)*

✓5ᵗʰ **204.1　Chronic**

✓5ᵗʰ **204.2　Subacute**

✓5ᵗʰ **204.8　Other lymphoid leukemia**
　　　　Aleukemic leukemia:　Aleukemic leukemia:
　　　　　lymphatic　　　　　lymphoid
　　　　　lymphocytic

✓5ᵗʰ **204.9　Unspecified lymphoid leukemia**

✓4ᵗʰ **205　Myeloid leukemia**
　　　　INCLUDES　leukemia:
　　　　　　　　　　　granulocytic
　　　　　　　　　　　myeloblastic
　　　　　　　　　　　myelocytic
　　　　　　　　　　　myelogenous
　　　　　　　　　　　myelomonocytic
　　　　　　　　　　　myelosclerotic
　　　　　　　　　　　myelosis

　　　　The following fifth-digit subclassification is for use with category 205:
　　　　　0　without mention of remission
　　　　　1　in remission

✓5ᵗʰ **205.0　Acute**
　　　　Acute promyelocytic leukemia
　　　　　　EXCLUDES　*acute exacerbation of chronic myeloid leukemia (205.1)*

✓5ᵗʰ **205.1　Chronic**
　　　　Eosinophilic leukemia
　　　　Neutrophilic leukemia

✓5ᵗʰ **205.2　Subacute**

✓5ᵗʰ **205.3　Myeloid sarcoma**
　　　　Chloroma
　　　　Granulocytic sarcoma

§ Requires fifth-digit. See beginning of section 200–208 for codes and definitions.

√5th **205.8 Other myeloid leukemia**

Aleukemic leukemia: Aleukemic leukemia:
    granulocytic   myeloid
    myelogenous   Aleukemic myelosis

√5th **205.9 Unspecified myeloid leukemia**

√4th **206 Monocytic leukemia**

INCLUDES   leukemia:
      histiocytic
      monoblastic
      monocytoid

The following fifth-digit subclassification is for use with category 206:

   0 without mention of remission
   1 in remission

√5th **206.0 Acute**

EXCLUDES   *acute exacerbation of chronic monocytic leukemia (206.1)*

√5th **206.1 Chronic**

√5th **206.2 Subacute**

√5th **206.8 Other monocytic leukemia**

Aleukemic: Aleukemic:
   monocytic leukemia   monocytoid leukemia

√5th **206.9 Unspecified monocytic leukemia**

√4th **207 Other specified leukemia**

EXCLUDES   *leukemic reticuloendotheliosis (202.4)*
                plasma cell leukemia (203.1)

The following fifth-digit subclassification is for use with category 207:

   0 without mention of remission
   1 in remission

√5th **207.0 Acute erythremia and erythroleukemia**

Acute erythremic myelosis   Erythremic myelosis
Di Guglielmo's disease

DEF: Erythremia: polycythemia vera.

DEF: Erythroleukemia: a malignant blood dyscrasia (a myeloproliferative disorder).

√5th **207.1 Chronic erythremia**

Heilmeyer-Schöner disease

√5th **207.2 Megakaryocytic leukemia**

Megakaryocytic myelosis   Thrombocytic leukemia

√5th **207.8 Other specified leukemia**

Lymphosarcoma cell leukemia

√4th **208 Leukemia of unspecified cell type**

The following fifth-digit subclassification is for use with category 208:

   0 without mention of remission
   1 in remission

√5th **208.0 Acute**

Acute leukemia NOS   Stem cell leukemia
Blast cell leukemia

EXCLUDES   *acute exacerbation of chronic unspecified leukemia (208.1)*

√5th **208.1 Chronic**

Chronic leukemia NOS

√5th **208.2 Subacute**

Subacute leukemia NOS

√5th **208.8 Other leukemia of unspecified cell type**

√5th **208.9 Unspecified leukemia**

Leukemia NOS

BENIGN NEOPLASMS (210-229)

√4th **210 Benign neoplasm of lip, oral cavity, and pharynx**

EXCLUDES   *cyst (of):*
      jaw (526.0-526.2,526.89)
      oral soft tissue (528.4)
      radicular (522.8)

210.0 Lip

Frenulum labii
Lip (inner aspect) (mucosa) (vermilion border)

EXCLUDES   *labial commissure (210.4)*
             skin of lip (216.0)

210.1 Tongue

Lingual tonsil

210.2 Major salivary glands

Gland: Gland:
   parotid   submandibular
   sublingual

EXCLUDES   *benign neoplasms of minor salivary glands:*
        NOS (210.4)
        buccal mucosa (210.4)
        lips (210.0)
        palate (hard) (soft) (210.4)
        tongue (210.1)
        tonsil, palatine (210.5)

210.3 Floor of mouth

210.4 Other and unspecified parts of mouth

Gingiva   Oral mucosa
Gum (upper) (lower)   Palate (hard) (soft)
Labial commissure   Uvula
Oral cavity NOS

EXCLUDES   *benign odontogenic neoplasms of bone (213.0-213.1)*
        developmental odontogenic cysts (526.0)
        mucosa of lips (210.0)
        nasopharyngeal [posterior] [superior] surface of soft palate (210.7)

210.5 Tonsil

Tonsil (faucial) (palatine)

EXCLUDES   *lingual tonsil (210.1)*
        pharyngeal tonsil (210.7)
        tonsillar:
          fossa (210.6)
          pillars (210.6)

210.6 Other parts of oropharynx

Branchial cleft or vestiges   Tonsillar:
Epiglottis, anterior aspect   fossa
Fauces NOS   pillars
Mesopharynx NOS   Vallecula

EXCLUDES   *epiglottis:*
        NOS(212.1)
        suprahyoid portion (212.1)

210.7 Nasopharynx

Adenoid tissue   Pharyngeal tonsil
Lymphadenoid tissue   Posterior nasal septum

210.8 Hypopharynx

Arytenoid fold   Postcricoidregion
Laryngopharynx   Pyriform fossa

210.9 Pharynx, unspecified

Throat NOS

√4th **211 Benign neoplasm of other parts of digestive system**

211.0 Esophagus

211.1 Stomach

Body ⎫
Cardia ⎬ of stomach
Fundus ⎭

Cardiac orifice
Pylorus

√4th √5th Additional Digit Required   Unspecified Code   Other Specified Code   Manifestation Code   ►◄ Revised Text   ● New Code   ▲ Revised Code Title

211.2 Duodenum, jejunum, and ileum
Small intestine NOS
> EXCLUDES ampulla of Vater (211.5)
> ileocecal valve (211.3)

211.3 Colon
Appendix   Ileocecal valve
Cecum   Large intestine NOS
> EXCLUDES rectosigmoid junction (211.4)

211.4 Rectum and anal canal
Anal canal or sphincter   Rectosigmoid junction
Anus NOS
> EXCLUDES anus:
> margin (216.5)
> skin (216.5)
> perianal skin (216.5)

211.5 Liver and biliary passages
Ampulla of Vater   Gallbladder
Common bile duct   Hepatic duct
Cystic duct   Sphincter of Oddi

211.6 Pancreas, except islets of Langerhans

211.7 Islets of Langerhans
Islet cell tumor
Use additional code to identify any functional
activity

211.8 Retroperitoneum and peritoneum
Mesentery   Omentum
Mesocolon   Retroperitoneal tissue

211.9 Other and unspecified site
Alimentary tract NOS
Digestive system NOS
Gastrointestinal tract NOS
Intestinal tract NOS
Intestine NOS
Spleen, not elsewhere classified

√4ᵗʰ **212 Benign neoplasm of respiratory and intrathoracic organs**

212.0 Nasal cavities, middle ear, and accessory sinuses
Cartilage of nose   Sinus
Eustachian tube   ethomoidal
Nares   frontal
Septum of nose   maxillary
sphenoidal
> EXCLUDES auditory canal (external) (216.2)
> bone of:
> ear (213.0)
> nose [turbinates] (213.0)
> cartilage of ear (215.0)
> ear (external) (skin) (216.2)
> nose NOS (229.8)
> skin (216.3)
> olfactory bulb (225.1)
> polyp of:
> accessory sinus (471.8)
> ear (385.30-385.35)
> nasal cavity (471.0)
> posterior margin of septum and
> choanae (210.7)

212.1 Larynx
Cartilage:
arytenoid
cricoid
cuneiform
thyroid
Epiglottis (suprahyoid portion) NOS
Glottis
Vocal cords (false) (true)
> EXCLUDES epiglottis, anterior aspect (210.6)
> polyp of vocal cord or larynx (478.4)

212.2 Trachea

212.3 Bronchus and lung
Carina   Hilus of lung

212.4 Pleura

212.5 Mediastinum

212.6 Thymus

212.7 Heart
> EXCLUDES great vessels (215.4)

212.8 Other specified sites

212.9 Site unspecified
Respiratory organ NOS
Upper respiratory tract NOS
> EXCLUDES intrathoracic NOS (229.8)
> thoracic NOS (229.8)

√4ᵗʰ **213 Benign neoplasm of bone and articular cartilage**
> INCLUDES cartilage (articular) (joint)
> periosteum
> EXCLUDES cartilage of:
> ear (215.0)
> eyelid (215.0)
> larynx (212.1)
> nose (212.0)
> exostosis NOS (726.91)
> synovia (215.0-215.9)

213.0 Bones of skull and face
> EXCLUDES lower jaw bone (213.1)

213.1 Lower jaw bone

213.2 Vertebral column, excluding sacrum and coccyx

213.3 Ribs, sternum, and clavicle

213.4 Scapula and long bones of upper limb

213.5 Short bones of upper limb

213.6 Pelvic bones, sacrum, and coccyx

213.7 Long bones of lower limb

213.8 Short bones of lower limb

213.9 Bone and articular cartilage, site unspecified

√4ᵗʰ **214 Lipoma**
> INCLUDES angiolipoma
> fibrolipoma
> hibernoma
> lipoma (fetal) (infiltrating) (intramuscular)
> myelolipoma
> myxolipoma

DEF: Benign tumor frequently composed of mature fat cells; may occasionally be composed of fetal fat cells.

214.0 Skin and subcutaneous tissue of face

214.1 Other skin and subcutaneous tissue

214.2 Intrathoracic organs

214.3 Intra-abdominal organs

214.4 Spermatic cord   ♂

214.8 Other specified sites

214.9 Lipoma, unspecified site

√4ᵗʰ **215 Other benign neoplasm of connective and other soft tissue**
> INCLUDES blood vessel
> bursa
> fascia
> ligament
> muscle
> peripheral, sympathetic, and parasympathetic
> nerves and ganglia
> synovia
> tendon (sheath)
> EXCLUDES cartilage:
> articular (213.0-213.9)
> larynx (212.1)
> nose (212.0)
> connective tissue of:
> breast (217)
> internal organ, except lipoma and
> hemangioma—code to benign neoplasm
> of the site
> lipoma (214.0-214.9)

215.0 Head, face, and neck

215.2 Upper limb, including shoulder

215.3 Lower limb, including hip

215.4   Thorax
>   EXCLUDES   *heart (212.7)*
>   *mediastinum (212.5)*
>   *thymus (212.6)*

215.5   Abdomen
>   Abdominal wall   Hypochondrium

215.6   Pelvis
>   Buttock   Inguinal region
>   Groin   Perineum
>   EXCLUDES   *uterine:*
>   *leiomyoma (218.0-218.9)*
>   *ligament, any (221.0)*

215.7   Trunk, unspecified
>   Back NOS   Flank NOS

215.8   Other specified sites

215.9   Site unspecified

✓4ᵗʰ **216 Benign neoplasm of skin**
>   INCLUDES   blue nevus
>   dermatofibroma
>   hydrocystoma
>   pigmented nevus
>   syringoadenoma
>   syringoma
>   EXCLUDES   *skin of genital organs (221.0-222.9)*

216.0   Skin of lip
>   EXCLUDES   *vermilion border of lip (210.0)*

216.1   Eyelid, including canthus
>   EXCLUDES   *cartilage of eyelid (215.0)*

216.2   Ear and external auditory canal
>   Auricle (ear)
>   Auricular canal, external
>   External meatus
>   Pinna
>   EXCLUDES   *cartilage of ear (215.0)*

216.3   Skin of other and unspecified parts of face
>   Cheek, external   Nose, external
>   Eyebrow   Temple

216.4   Scalp and skin of neck

216.5   Skin of trunk, except scrotum
>   Axillary fold   Skin of:
>   Perianal skin   buttock
>   Skin of: chest wall
>   abdominal wall   groin
>   anus   perineum
>   back   Umbilicus
>   breast
>   EXCLUDES   *anal canal (211.4)*
>   *anus NOS (211.4)*
>   *skin of scrotum (222.4)*

216.6   Skin of upper limb, including shoulder

216.7   Skin of lower limb, including hip

216.8   Other specified sites of skin

216.9   Skin, site unspecified

217 Benign neoplasm of breast
>   Breast (male) (female):   Breast (male) (female):
>   connective tissue   soft parts
>   glandular tissue
>   EXCLUDES   *adenofibrosis (610.2)*
>   *benign cyst of breast (610.0)*
>   *fibrocystic disease (610.1)*
>   *skin of breast (216.5)*

✓4ᵗʰ **218 Uterine leiomyoma**
>   INCLUDES   fibroid (bleeding) (uterine)
>   uterine:
>   fibromyoma
>   myoma

DEF: Benign tumor primarily derived from uterine smooth muscle tissue; may contain fibrous, fatty, or epithelial tissue; also called uterine fibroid or myoma.

218.0   Submucous leiomyoma of uterus   ♀

218.1   Intramural leiomyoma of uterus   ♀
>   Interstitial leiomyoma of uterus

218.2   Subserous leiomyoma of uterus   ♀

218.9   Leiomyoma of uterus, unspecified   ♀

✓4ᵗʰ **219 Other benign neoplasm of uterus**

219.0   Cervix uteri   ♀

219.1   Corpus uteri   ♀
>   Endometrium   Myometrium
>   Fundus

219.8   Other specified parts of uterus   ♀

219.9   Uterus, part unspecified   ♀

220 Benign neoplasm of ovary   ♀
>   Use additional code to identify any functional activity (256.0-256.1)
>   EXCLUDES   *cyst:*
>   *corpus albicans (620.2)*
>   *corpus luteum (620.1)*
>   *endometrial (617.1)*
>   *follicular (atretic) (620.0)*
>   *graafian follicle (620.0)*
>   *ovarian NOS (620.2)*
>   *retention (620.2)*

✓4ᵗʰ **221 Benign neoplasm of other female genital organs**
>   INCLUDES   adenomatous polyp
>   benign teratoma
>   EXCLUDES   *cyst:*
>   *epoophoron (752.11)*
>   *fimbrial (752.11)*
>   *Gartner's duct (752.11)*
>   *parovarian (752.11)*

221.0   Fallopian tube and uterine ligaments   ♀
>   Oviduct
>   Parametruim
>   Uterine ligament (broad) (round) (uterosacral)
>   Uterine tube

221.1   Vagina   ♀

221.2   Vulva   ♀
>   Clitoris
>   External female genitalia NOS
>   Greater vestibular [Bartholin's] gland
>   Labia (majora) (minora)
>   Pudendum
>   EXCLUDES   *Bartholin's (duct) (gland) cyst (616.2)*

221.8   Other specified sites of female genital organs   ♀

221.9   Female genital organ, site unspecified   ♀
>   Female genitourinary tract NOS

✓4ᵗʰ **222 Benign neoplasm of male genital organs**

222.0   Testis   ♂
>   Use additional code to identify any functional activity

222.1   Penis   ♂
>   Corpus cavernosum   Prepuce
>   Glans penis

222.2   Prostate   ♂
>   EXCLUDES   *adenomatous hyperplasia of prostate (600.2)*
>   *prostatic:*
>   *adenoma (600.2)*
>   *enlargement (600.0)*
>   *hypertrophy (600.0)*

222.3   Epididymis   ♂

222.4   Scrotum   ♂
>   Skin of scrotum

222.8   Other specified sites of male genital organs   ♂
>   Seminal vesicle
>   Spermatic cord

222.9   Male genital organ, site unspecified   ♂
>   Male genitourinary tract NOS

Neoplasms 215.4–222.9

✓4ᵗʰ ✓5ᵗʰ Additional Digit Required   Unspecified Code   Other Specified Code   Manifestation Code   ►◄ Revised Text   ● New Code   ▲ Revised Code Title

Neoplasms 223–229.9

✓4ᵗʰ **223 Benign neoplasm of kidney and other urinary organs**
     223.0 **Kidney, except pelvis**
         Kidney NOS
         EXCLUDES *renal:*
                 calyces (223.1)
                 pelvis (223.1)
     223.1 **Renal pelvis**
     223.2 **Ureter**
         EXCLUDES *ureteric orifice of bladder (223.3)*
     223.3 **Bladder**
✓5ᵗʰ   223.8 **Other specified sites of urinary organs**
         223.81 **Urethra**
                 EXCLUDES *urethral orifice of bladder*
                             (223.3)
         223.89 **Other**
                 Paraurethral glands
     223.9 **Urinary organ, site unspecified**
         Urinary system NOS
✓4ᵗʰ **224 Benign neoplasm of eye**
         EXCLUDES *cartilage of eyelid (215.0)*
                  eyelid (skin) (216.1)
                  optic nerve (225.1)
                  orbital bone (213.0)
     224.0 **Eyeball, except conjunctiva, cornea, retina, and choroid**
         Ciliary body   Sclera
         Iris   Uveal tract
     224.1 **Orbit**
         EXCLUDES *bone of orbit (213.0)*
     224.2 **Lacrimal gland**
     224.3 **Conjunctiva**
     224.4 **Cornea**
     224.5 **Retina**
         EXCLUDES *hemangioma of retina (228.03)*
     224.6 **Choroid**
     224.7 **Lacrimal duct**
         Lacrimal sac
         Nasolacrimal duct
     224.8 **Other specified parts of eye**
     224.9 **Eye, part unspecified**
✓4ᵗʰ **225 Benign neoplasm of brain and other parts of nervous system**
         EXCLUDES *hemangioma (228.02)*
                  neurofibromatosis (237.7)
                  peripheral, sympathetic, and parasympathetic
                     nerves and ganglia (215.0-215.9)
                  retrobulbar (224.1)
     225.0 **Brain**
     225.1 **Cranial nerves**
     225.2 **Cerebral meninges**
         Meninges NOS   Meningioma (cerebral)
     225.3 **Spinal cord**
         Cauda equina

Eyeball

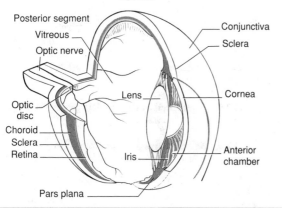

     225.4 **Spinal meninges**
         Spinal meningioma
     225.8 **Other specified sites of nervous system**
     225.9 **Nervous system, part unspecified**
         Nervous system (central) NOS
         EXCLUDES *meninges NOS (225.2)*
226 Benign neoplasm of thyroid glands
         Use additional code to identify any functional activity
✓4ᵗʰ **227 Benign neoplasm of other endocrine glands and related structures**
         Use additional code to identify any functional activity
         EXCLUDES *ovary (220)*
                  pancreas (211.6)
                  testis (222.0)
     227.0 **Adrenal gland**
         Suprarenal gland
     227.1 **Parathyroid gland**
     227.3 **Pituitary gland and craniopharyngeal duct (pouch)**
         Craniobuccal pouch   Rathke's pouch
         Hypophysis   Sella turcica
     227.4 **Pineal gland**
         Pineal body
     227.5 **Carotid body**
     227.6 **Aortic body and other paraganglia**
         Coccygeal body   Para-aortic body
         Glomus jugulare
     227.8 **Other**
     227.9 **Endocrine gland, site unspecified**
✓4ᵗʰ **228 Hemangioma and lymphangioma, any site**
         INCLUDES angioma (benign) (cavernous) (congenital) NOS
                  cavernous nevus
                  glomus tumor
                  hemangioma (benign) (congenital)
         EXCLUDES *benign neoplasm of spleen, except hemangioma*
                  and lymphangioma (211.9)
                  glomus jugulare (227.6)
                  nevus:
                     NOS (216.0-216.9)
                     blue or pigmented (216.0-216.9)
                     vascular (757.32)
✓5ᵗʰ   228.0 **Hemangioma, any site**
         DEF: A common benign tumor usually occurring in infancy; composed of newly formed blood vessels due to malformation of angioblastic tissue.
         228.00 **Of unspecified site**
         228.01 **Of skin and subcutaneous tissue**
         228.02 **Of intracranial structures**
         228.03 **Of retina**
         228.04 **Of intra-abdominal structures**
                 Peritoneum   Retroperitoneal tissue
         228.09 **Of other sites**
                 Systemic angiomatosis
     228.1 **Lymphangioma, any site**
         Congenital lymphangioma
         Lymphatic nevus
✓4ᵗʰ **229 Benign neoplasm of other and unspecified sites**
     229.0 **Lymph nodes**
         EXCLUDES *lymphangioma (228.1)*
     229.8 **Other specified sites**
         Intrathoracic NOS   Thoracic NOS
     229.9 **Site unspecified**

CARCINOMA IN SITU (230-234)

INCLUDES	Bowen's disease
	erythroplasia
	Queyrat's erythroplasia

EXCLUDES	leukoplakia—see Alphabetic Index

DEF: A neoplastic type; with tumor cells confined to epithelium of origin; without further invasion.

✓4ᵗʰ 230 Carcinoma in situ of digestive organs

230.0 Lip, oral cavity, and pharynx

Gingiva	Oropharynx
Hypopharynx	Salivary gland or duct
Mouth [any part]	Tongue
Nasopharynx	

EXCLUDES	aryepiglottic fold or interarytenoid fold,
	laryngeal aspect (231.0)
	epiglottis:
	NOS (231.0)
	suprahyoid portion (231.0)
	skin of lip (232.0)

230.1 Esophagus

230.2 Stomach

Body
Cardia } of stomach
Fundus

Cardiac orifice
Pylorus

230.3 Colon

Appendix	Ileocecal valve
Cecum	Large intestine NOS

EXCLUDES	rectosigmoid junction (230.4)

230.4 Rectum

Rectosigmoid junction

230.5 Anal canal

Anal sphincter

230.6 Anus, unspecified

EXCLUDES	anus:
	margin (232.5)
	skin (232.5)
	perianal skin (232.5)

230.7 Other and unspecified parts of intestine

Duodenum	Jejunum
Ileum	Small intestine NOS

EXCLUDES	ampulla of Vater (230.8)

230.8 Liver and biliary system

Ampulla of Vater	Gallbladder
Common bile duct	Hepatic duct
Cystic duct	Sphincter of Oddi

230.9 Other and unspecified digestive organs

Digestive organ NOS
Gastrointestinal tract NOS
Pancreas
Spleen

✓4ᵗʰ 231 Carcinoma in situ of respiratory system

231.0 Larynx

Cartilage:	Epiglottis:
arytenoid	NOS
cricoid	posterior surface
cuneiform	suprahyoid portion
thyroid	Vocal cords (false) (true)

EXCLUDES	aryepiglottic fold or interarytenoid fold:
	NOS (230.0)
	hypopharyngeal aspect (230.0)
	marginal zone (230.0)

231.1 Trachea

231.2 Bronchus and lung

Carina
Hilus of lung

231.8 Other specified parts of respiratory system

Accessory sinuses	Nasal cavities
Middle ear	Pleura

EXCLUDES	ear (external) (skin) (232.2)
	nose NOS (234.8)
	skin (232.3)

231.9 Respiratory system, part unspecified

Respiratory organ NOS

✓4ᵗʰ 232 Carcinoma in situ of skin

INCLUDES	pigment cells

232.0 Skin of lip

EXCLUDES	vermilion border of lip (230.0)

232.1 Eyelid, including canthus

232.2 Ear and external auditory canal

232.3 Skin of other and unspecified parts of face

232.4 Scalp and skin of neck

232.5 Skin of trunk, except scrotum

Anus, margin	Skin of:
Axillary fold	breast
Perianal skin	buttock
Skin of:	chest wall
abdominal wall	groin
anus	perineum
back	Umbilicus

EXCLUDES	anal canal (230.5)
	anus NOS (230.6)
	skin of genital organs (233.3, 233.5-233.6)

232.6 Skin of upper limb, including shoulder

232.7 Skin of lower limb, including hip

232.8 Other specified sites of skin

232.9 Skin, site unspecified

✓4ᵗʰ 233 Carcinoma in situ of breast and genitourinary system

233.0 Breast

EXCLUDES	Paget's disease (174.0-174.9)
	skin of breast (232.5)

233.1 Cervix uteri   ♀

233.2 Other and unspecified parts of uterus   ♀

233.3 Other and unspecified female genital organs   ♀

233.4 Prostate   ♂

233.5 Penis   ♂

233.6 Other and unspecified male genital organs   ♂

233.7 Bladder

233.9 Other and unspecified urinary organs

✓4ᵗʰ 234 Carcinoma in situ of other and unspecified sites

234.0 Eye

EXCLUDES	cartilage of eyelid (234.8)
	eyelid (skin) (232.1)
	optic nerve (234.8)
	orbital bone (234.8)

234.8 Other specified sites

Endocrine gland [any]

234.9 Site unspecified

Carcinoma in situ NOS

NEOPLASMS OF UNCERTAIN BEHAVIOR (235-238)

Note: Categories 235–238 classify by site certain histomorphologically well-defined neoplasms, the subsequent behavior of which cannot be predicted from the present appearance.

✓4ᵗʰ 235 Neoplasm of uncertain behavior of digestive and respiratory systems

235.0 Major salivary glands

Gland:	Gland:
parotid	submandibular
sublingual	

EXCLUDES	minor salivary glands (235.1)

✓4ᵗʰ Additional Digit Required	Unspecified Code	Other Specified Code	Manifestation Code	▶◀ Revised Text	● New Code	▲ Revised Code Title
✓5ᵗʰ						

2003 ICD•9•CM   **Volume 1 — 41**

Neoplasms 230–235.0

Neoplasms 235.1–238.5

235.1 Lip, oral cavity, and pharynx
Gingiva   Nasopharynx
Hypopharynx   Oropharynx
Minor salivary glands   Tongue
Mouth

> *EXCLUDES*   *aryepiglottic fold or interarytenoid fold,*
> *laryngeal aspect (235.6)*
> *epiglottis:*
>   *NOS (235.6)*
>   *suprahyoid portion (235.6)*
> *skin of lip (238.2)*

235.2 Stomach, intestines, and rectum

235.3 Liver and biliary passages
Ampulla of Vater
Bile ducts [any]
Gallbladder
Liver

235.4 Retroperitoneum and peritoneum

235.5 Other and unspecified digestive organs
Anal:
   canal
   sphincter
Anus NOS
Esophagus
Pancreas
Spleen

> *EXCLUDES*   *anus:*
>   *margin (238.2)*
>   *skin (238.2)*
>   *perianal skin (238.2)*

235.6 Larynx

> *EXCLUDES*   *aryepiglottic fold or interarytenoid fold:*
>   *NOS (235.1)*
>   *hypopharyngeal aspect (235.1)*
>   *marginal zone (235.1)*

235.7 Trachea, bronchus, and lung

235.8 Pleura, thymus, and mediastinum

235.9 Other and unspecified respiratory organs
Accessory sinuses
Middle ear
Nasal cavities
Respiratory organ NOS

> *EXCLUDES*   *ear (external) (skin) (238.2)*
>   *nose (238.8)*
>   *skin (238.2)*

√4th **236 Neoplasm of uncertain behavior of genitourinary organs**

236.0 Uterus ♀

236.1 Placenta ♀
Chorioadenoma (destruens)
Invasive mole
Malignant hydatid(iform) mole

236.2 Ovary ♀
Use additional code to identify any functional
activity

236.3 Other and unspecified female genital organs ♀

236.4 Testis ♂
Use additional code to identify any functional
activity

236.5 Prostate ♂

236.6 Other and unspecified male genital organs ♂

236.7 Bladder

√5th **236.9 Other and unspecified urinary organs**
   236.90 Urinary organ, unspecified
   236.91 Kidney and ureter
   236.99 Other

√4th **237 Neoplasm of uncertain behavior of endocrine glands and nervous system**

237.0 Pituitary gland and craniopharyngeal duct
Use additional code to identify any functional
activity

237.1 Pineal gland

237.2 Adrenal gland
Suprarenal gland
Use additional code to identify any functional
activity

237.3 Paraganglia
Aortic body
Carotid body
Coccygeal body
Glomus jugulare

237.4 Other and unspecified endocrine glands
Parathyroid gland
Thyroid gland

237.5 Brain and spinal cord

237.6 Meninges
Meninges:
   NOS
   cerebral
   spinal

√5th **237.7 Neurofibromatosis**
von Recklinghausen's disease

> DEF: An inherited condition with developmental changes in the
> nervous system, muscles, bones and skin; multiple soft tumors
> (neurofibromas) distributed over the entire body.

237.70 Neurofibromatosis, unspecified

237.71 Neurofibromatosis, type 1 [von Recklinghausen's disease]

237.72 Neurofibromatosis, type 2 [acoustic neurofibromatosis]

> DEF: Inherited condition with cutaneous lesions, benign
> tumors of peripheral nerves and bilateral 8th nerve
> masses.

237.9 Other and unspecified parts of nervous system
Cranial nerves

> *EXCLUDES*   *peripheral, sympathetic, and*
> *parasympathetic nerves and*
> *ganglia (238.1)*

√4th **238 Neoplasm of uncertain behavior of other and unspecified sites and tissues**

238.0 Bone and articular cartilage

> *EXCLUDES*   *cartilage:*
>   *ear (238.1)*
>   *eyelid (238.1)*
>   *larynx (235.6)*
>   *nose (235.9)*
>   *synovia (238.1)*

238.1 Connective and other soft tissue
Peripheral, sympathetic, and parasympathetic
nerves and ganglia

> *EXCLUDES*   *cartilage (of):*
>   *articular (238.0)*
>   *larynx (235.6)*
>   *nose (235.9)*
>   *connective tissue of breast (238.3)*

238.2 Skin

> *EXCLUDES*   *anus NOS (235.5)*
>   *skin of genital organs (236.3, 236.6)*
>   *vermilion border of lip (235.1)*

238.3 Breast

> *EXCLUDES*   *skin of breast (238.2)*

238.4 Polycythemia vera

> DEF: Abnormal proliferation of all bone marrow elements,
> increased red cell mass and total blood volume; unknown etiology,
> frequently associated with splenomegaly, leukocytosis, and
> thrombocythemia.

238.5 Histiocytic and mast cells
Mast cell tumor NOS
Mastocytoma NOS

238.6   **Plasma cells**
Plasmacytoma NOS
Solitary myeloma

238.7   **Other lymphatic and hematopoietic tissues**
Disease:
lymphoproliferative (chronic) NOS
myeloproliferative (chronic) NOS
Idiopathic thrombocythemia
Megakaryocytic myelosclerosis
Myelodysplastic syndrome
Myelosclerosis with myeloid metaplasia
Panmyelosis (acute)

     EXCLUDES   *myelfibrosis (289.8)*
myelosclerosis NOS (289.8)
myelosis:
     NOS (205.9)
       megakaryocytic (207.2)

238.8   **Other specified sites**
Eye
Heart

     EXCLUDES   *eyelid (skin) (238.2)*
cartilage (238.1)

238.9   **Site unspecified**

NEOPLASMS OF UNSPECIFIED NATURE (239)

✓4ᵗʰ **239 Neoplasms of unspecified nature**

Note: Category 239 classifies by site neoplasms of unspecified morphology and behavior. The term "mass," unless otherwise stated, is not to be regarded as a neoplastic growth.

     INCLUDES   "growth" NOS
neoplasm NOS
new growth NOS
tumor NOS

239.0   **Digestive system**

     EXCLUDES   *anus:*
     margin (239.2)
     skin (239.2)
perianal skin (239.2)

239.1   **Respiratory system**

239.2   **Bone, soft tissue, and skin**

     EXCLUDES   *anal canal (239.0)*
anus NOS (239.0)
bone marrow (202.9)
cartilage:
     larynx (239.1)
     nose (239.1)
connective tissue of breast (239.3)
skin of genital organs (239.5)
vermilion border of lip (239.0)

239.3   **Breast**

     EXCLUDES   *skin of breast (239.2)*

239.4   **Bladder**

239.5   **Other genitourinary organs**

239.6   **Brain**

     EXCLUDES   *cerebral meninges (239.7)*
cranial nerves (239.7)

239.7   **Endocrine glands and other parts of nervous system**

     EXCLUDES   *peripheral, sympathetic, and parasympathetic nerves and ganglia (239.2)*

239.8   **Other specified sites**

     EXCLUDES   *eyelid (skin) (239.2)*
cartilage (239.2)
great vessels (239.2)
optic nerve (239.7)

239.9   **Site unspecified**

✓4ᵗʰ / ✓5ᵗʰ Additional Digit Required   Unspecified Code   Other Specified Code   Manifestation Code   ▶◀ Revised Text   ● New Code   ▲ Revised Code Title

2003 ICD•9•CM   **Volume 1 — 43**

Endocrine System

Hypothalamus
Pituitary
(Hypophysis)
gland
Thyroid gland
Thymus gland
Pineal gland
Parathyroid
glands
Adrenal
(Suprarenal)
glands
Ovaries
Pancreas
Testes

3. ENDOCRINE, NUTRITIONAL AND METABOLIC DISEASES, AND IMMUNITY DISORDERS (240-279)

> **EXCLUDES** *endocrine and metabolic disturbances specific to the fetus and newborn (775.0-775.9)*

Note: All neoplasms, whether functionally active or not, are classified in Chapter 2. Codes in Chapter 3 (i.e., 242.8, 246.0, 251-253, 255-259) may be used to identify such functional activity associated with any neoplasm, or by ectopic endocrine tiss256ue.

DISORDERS OF THYROID GLAND (240-246)

✓4th 240 Simple and unspecified goiter

DEF: An enlarged thyroid gland often caused by an inadequate dietary intake of iodine.

240.0 Goiter, specified as simple
Any condition classifiable to 240.9, specified as simple

240.9 Goiter, unspecified
Enlargement of thyroid   Goiter or struma:
Goiter or struma: hyperplastic
   NOS   nontoxic (diffuse)
   diffuse colloid   parenchymatous
   endemic   sporadic
> **EXCLUDES** *congenital (dyshormonogenic) goiter (246.1)*

✓4th 241 Nontoxic nodular goiter
> **EXCLUDES** *adenoma of thyroid (226)*
> *cystadenoma of thyroid (226)*

241.0 Nontoxic uninodular goiter
Thyroid nodule   Uninodular goiter (nontoxic)
DEF: Enlarged thyroid, commonly due to decreased thyroid production, with single nodule; no clinical hypothyroidism.

241.1 Nontoxic multinodular goiter
Multinodular goiter (nontoxic)
DEF: Enlarged thyroid, commonly due to decreased thyroid production with multiple nodules; no clinical hypothyroidism.

241.9 Unspecified nontoxic nodular goiter
Adenomatous goiter
Nodular goiter (nontoxic) NOS
Struma nodosa (simplex)

✓4th 242 Thyrotoxicosis with or without goiter
> **EXCLUDES** *neonatal thyrotoxicosis (775.3)*

The following fifth-digit subclassification is for use with category 242:
   0 without mention of thyrotoxic crisis or storm
   1 with mention of thyrotoxic crisis or storm

DEF: A condition caused by excess quantities of thyroid hormones being introduced into the tissues.

✓5th 242.0 Toxic diffuse goiter
Basedow's disease
Exophthalmic or toxic goiter NOS
Graves' disease
Primary thyroid hyperplasia
DEF: Diffuse thyroid enlargement accompanied by hyperthyroidism, bulging eyes, and dermopathy.

✓5th 242.1 Toxic uninodular goiter
Thyroid nodule   ⎫ toxic or with
Uninodular goiter ⎬ hyperthyroidism

DEF: Symptomatic hyperthyroidism with a single nodule on the enlarged thyroid gland. Abrupt onset of symptoms; including extreme nervousness, insomnia, weight loss, tremors, and psychosis or coma.

✓5th 242.2 Toxic multinodular goiter
Secondary thyroid hyperplasia
DEF: Symptomatic hyperthyroidism with multiple nodules on the enlarged thyroid gland. Abrupt onset of symptoms; including extreme nervousness, insomnia, weight loss, tremors, and psychosis or coma.

✓5th 242.3 Toxic nodular goiter, unspecified
Adenomatous goiter   ⎫
Nodular goiter   ⎬ toxic or with
Struma nodosa   ⎭ hyperthyroidism

Any condition classifiable to 241.9 specified as toxic or with hyperthyroidism

✓5th 242.4 Thyrotoxicosis from ectopic thyroid nodule

✓5th 242.8 Thyrotoxicosis of other specified origin
Overproduction of thyroid-stimulating hormone [TSH]
Thyrotoxicosis:
   factitia from ingestion of excessive thyroid material
Use additional E code to identify cause, if drug-induced

✓5th 242.9 Thyrotoxicosis without mention of goiter or other cause
Hyperthyroidism NOS
Thyrotoxicosis NOS

243 Congenital hypothyroidism
Congenital thyroid insufficiency
Cretinism (athyrotic) (endemic)
Use additional code to identify associated mental retardation
> **EXCLUDES** *congenital (dyshormonogenic) goiter (246.1)*
DEF: Underproduction of thyroid hormone present from birth.

✓4th 244 Acquired hypothyroidism
> **INCLUDES** athyroidism (acquired)
> hypothyroidism (acquired)
> myxedema (adult) (juvenile)
> thyroid (gland) insufficiency (acquired)

244.0 Postsurgical hypothyroidism
DEF: Underproduction of thyroid hormone due to surgical removal of all or part of the thyroid gland.

244.1 Other postablative hypothyroidism
Hypothyroidism following therapy, such as irradiation

244.2 Iodine hypothyroidism
Hypothyroidism resulting from administration or ingestion of iodide
Use additional E code to identify drug

244.3 Other iatrogenic hypothyroidism
Hypothyroidism resulting from:
   P-aminosalicylic acid [PAS]
   Phenylbutazone
   Resorcinol
Iatrogenic hypothyroidism NOS
Use additional E code to identify drug

✓4th
✓5th Additional Digit Required   Unspecified Code   Other Specified Code   Manifestation Code   ►◄ Revised Text   ● New Code   ▲ Revised Code Title

244.8   Other specified acquired hypothyroidism
Secondary hypothyroidism NEC

244.9   Unspecified hypothyroidism

Hypothyroidism
Myxedema   } primary or NOS

√4ᵗʰ **245 Thyroiditis**

245.0   Acute thyroiditis
Abscess of thyroid
Thyroiditis:
    nonsuppurative, acute
    pyogenic
    suppurative
Use additional code to identify organism

DEF: Inflamed thyroid caused by infection, with abscess and liquid puris.

245.1   Subacute thyroiditis
Thyroiditis:
    de Quervain's
    giant cell
    granulomatous
    viral

DEF: Inflammation of the thyroid, characterized by fever and painful enlargement of the thyroid gland, with granulomas in the gland.

245.2   Chronic lymphocytic thyroiditis
Hashimoto's disease
Struma lymphomatosa
Thyroiditis:
    autoimmune
    lymphocytic (chronic)

DEF: Autoimmune disease of thyroid; lymphocytes infiltrate the gland and thyroid antibodies are produced; women more often affected.

245.3   Chronic fibrous thyroiditis
Struma fibrosa
Thyroiditis:
    invasive (fibrous)
    ligneous
    Riedel's

DEF: Persistent fibrosing inflammation of thyroid with adhesions to nearby structures; rare condition.

245.4   Iatrogenic thyroiditis
Use additional code to identify cause

DEF: Thyroiditis resulting from treatment or intervention by physician or in a patient intervention setting.

245.8   Other and unspecified chronic thyroiditis
Chronic thyroiditis:
    NOS
    nonspecific

245.9   Thyroiditis, unspecified
Thyroiditis NOS

√4ᵗʰ **246 Other disorders of thyroid**

246.0   Disorders of thyrocalcitonin secretion
Hypersecretion of calcitonin or thyrocalcitonin

246.1   Dyshormonogenic goiter
Congenital (dyshormonogenic) goiter
Goiter due to enzyme defect in synthesis of thyroid
    hormone
Goitrous cretinism (sporadic)

246.2   Cyst of thyroid
EXCLUDES   cystadenoma of thyroid (226)

246.3   Hemorrhage and infarction of thyroid

246.8   Other specified disorders of thyroid
Abnormality of thyroid-binding globulin
Atrophy of thyroid
Hyper-TBG-nemia
Hypo-TBG-nemia

246.9   Unspecified disorder of thyroid

DISEASES OF OTHER ENDOCRINE GLANDS (250-259)

√4ᵗʰ **250 Diabetes mellitus**
EXCLUDES   gestational diabetes (648.8)
    hyperglycemia NOS (790.6)
    neonatal diabetes mellitus (775.1)
    nonclinical diabetes (790.2)

The following fifth-digit subclassification is for use with category 250:

0   type II [non-insulin dependent type] [NIDDM type] [adult-onset type] or unspecified type, not stated as uncontrolled
Fifth-digit 0 is for use for type II, adult-onset diabetic patients, even if the patient requires insulin

1   type I [insulin dependent type] [IDDM] [juvenile type], not stated as uncontrolled

2   type II [non-insulin dependent type] [NIDDM type] [adult-onset type] or unspecified type, uncontrolled
Fifth-digit 2 is for use for type II, adult-onset diabetic patients, even if the patient requires insulin

3   type I [insulin dependent type] [IDDM] [juvenile type], uncontrolled

DEF: Inability to metabolize carbohydrates, proteins, and fats with insufficient secretion of insulin. Symptoms may be unremarkable, with long-term complications, involving kidneys, nerves, blood vessels, and eyes.

√5ᵗʰ **250.0**   Diabetes mellitus without mention of complication
Diabetes mellitus without mention of complication or manifestation classifiable to 250.1-250.9
Diabetes (mellitus) NOS

√5ᵗʰ **250.1**   Diabetes with ketoacidosis
Diabetic:
    acidosis } without mention
    ketosis   } of coma

DEF: Diabetic hyperglycemic crisis causing ketone presence in body fluids.

√5ᵗʰ **250.2**   Diabetes with hyperosmolarity
Hyperosmolar (nonketotic) coma

√5ᵗʰ **250.3**   Diabetes with other coma
Diabetic coma (with ketoacidosis)
Diabetic hypoglycemic coma
Insulin coma NOS
EXCLUDES   diabetes with hyperosmolar coma (250.2)

DEF: Coma (not hyperosmolar) caused by hyperglycemia or hypoglycemia as complication of diabetes.

√5ᵗʰ **250.4**   Diabetes with renal manifestations
Use additional code to identify manifestation, as:
    diabetic:
       nephropathy NOS (583.81)
       nephrosis (581.81)
       intercapillary glomerulosclerosis (581.81)
       Kimmelstiel-Wilson syndrome (581.81)

√5ᵗʰ **250.5**   Diabetes with ophthalmic manifestations
Use additional code to identify manifestation, as:
    diabetic:
       blindness (369.00-369.9)
       cataract (366.41)
       glaucoma (365.44)
       retinal edema (362.83)
       retinopathy (362.01-362.02)

√5ᵗʰ **250.6**   Diabetes with neurological manifestations
Use additional code to identify manifestation, as:
    diabetic:
       amyotrophy (358.1)
       mononeuropathy (354.0-355.9)
       neurogenic arthropathy (713.5)
       peripheral autonomic neuropathy (337.1)
       polyneuropathy (357.2)

√5ᵗʰ **250.7**   **Diabetes with peripheral circulatory disorders**
Use additional code to identify manifestation, as:
diabetic:
gangrene (785.4)
peripheral angiopathy (443.81)
DEF: Blood vessel damage or disease, usually in the feet, legs, or hands, as a complication of diabetes.

√5ᵗʰ **250.8**   **Diabetes with other specified manifestations**
Diabetic hypoglycemia
Hypoglycemic shock
Use additional code to identify manifestation, as:
any associated ulceration (707.10-707.9)
diabetic bone changes (731.8)
Use additional E code to identify cause, if drug-induced

√5ᵗʰ **250.9**   **Diabetes with unspecified complication**

√4ᵗʰ **251**   **Other disorders of pancreatic internal secretion**

251.0   **Hypoglycemic coma**
Iatrogenic hyperinsulinism
Non-diabetic insulin coma
Use additional E code to identify cause, if drug-induced
   EXCLUDES   *hypoglycemic coma in diabetes mellitus (250.3)*
DEF: Coma induced by low blood sugar in non-diabetic patient.

251.1   **Other specified hypoglycemia**
Hyperinsulinism:
NOS
ectopic
functional
Hyperplasia of pancreatic
islet beta cells NOS
   EXCLUDES   *hypoglycemia:*
in diabetes mellitus (250.8)
in infant of diabetic mother (775.0)
neonatal hypoglycemia (775.6)
hypoglycemic coma (251.0)
Use additional E code to identify cause, if drug-induced.
DEF: Excessive production of insulin by the pancreas; associated with obesity and insulin-producing tumors.

251.2   **Hypoglycemia, unspecified**
Hypoglycemia:
NOS
reactive
spontaneous
   EXCLUDES   *hypoglycemia:*
with coma (251.0)
in diabetes mellitus (250.8)
leucine-induced (270.3)

251.3   **Postsurgical hypoinsulinemia**
Hypoinsulinemia following complete or partial pancreatectomy
Postpancreatectomy hyperglycemia

251.4   **Abnormality of secretion of glucagon**
Hyperplasia of pancreatic islet alpha cells with glucagon excess
DEF: Production malfunction of a pancreatic hormone secreted by cells of the islets of Langerhans

251.5   **Abnormality of secretion of gastrin**
Hyperplasia of pancreatic alpha cells with gastrin excess
Zollinger-Ellison syndrome

251.8   **Other specified disorders of pancreatic internal secretion**

251.9   **Unspecified disorder of pancreatic internal secretion**
Islet cell hyperplasia NOS

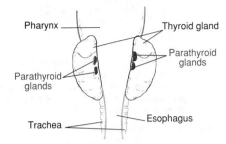

Dorsal View of Parathyroid Glands

Parathyroid glands
↓
Parathyroid hormone (PTH)
↓
Calcium in bones ⟷ Calcium in blood

√4ᵗʰ **252**   **Disorders of parathyroid gland**

252.0   **Hyperparathyroidism**
Hyperplasia of parathyroid
Osteitis fibrosa cystica generalisata
von Recklinghausen's disease of bone
   EXCLUDES   *ectopic hyperparathyroidism (259.3)*
secondary hyperparathyroidism (of renal origin) (588.8)
DEF: Abnormally high secretion of parathyroid hormones causing bone deterioration, reduced renal function, kidney stones.

252.1   **Hypoparathyroidism**
Parathyroiditis (autoimmune)
Tetany:
parathyroid
parathyroprival
   EXCLUDES   *pseudohypoparathyroidism (275.4)*
pseudopseudohypoparathyroidism (275.4)
tetany NOS (781.7)
transitory neonatal hypoparathyroidism (775.4)
DEF: Abnormally low secretion of parathyroid hormones which causes decreased calcium and increased phosphorus in the blood. Resulting in muscle cramps, tetany, urinary frequency and cataracts.

252.8   **Other specified disorders of parathyroid gland**
Cyst
Hemorrhage } of parathyroid gland

252.9   **Unspecified disorder of parathyroid gland**

√4ᵗʰ **253**   **Disorders of the pituitary gland and its hypothalamic control**
   INCLUDES   the listed conditions whether the disorder is in the pituitary or the hypothalamus
   EXCLUDES   *Cushing's syndrome (255.0)*

253.0   **Acromegaly and gigantism**
Overproduction of growth hormone
DEF: Acromegaly: chronic, beginning in middle age; caused by hypersecretion of the pituitary growth hormone; produces enlarged parts of skeleton, especially the nose, ears, jaws, fingers and toes.
DEF: Gigantism: pituitary gigantism caused by excess growth of short flat bones; men may grow 78 to 80 inches tall.

253.1   **Other and unspecified anterior pituitary hyperfunction**
Forbes-Albright syndrome
   EXCLUDES   *overproduction of:*
ACTH (255.3)
thyroid-stimulating hormone [TSH] (242.8)
DEF: Spontaneous galactorrhea-amenorrhea syndrome unrelated to pregnancy; usually related to presence of pituitary tumor.

√4ᵗʰ
√5ᵗʰ   Additional Digit Required   Unspecified Code   Other Specified Code   Manifestation Code   ▶◀ Revised Text   ● New Code   ▲ Revised Code Title

253.2 Panhypopituitarism
Cachexia, pituitary
Necrosis of pituitary (postpartum)
Pituitary insufficiency NOS
Sheehan's syndrome
Simmonds' disease
EXCLUDES   *iatrogenic hypopituitarism (253.7)*

DEF: Damage to or absence of pituitary gland leading to impaired sexual function, weight loss, fatigue, bradycardia, hypotension, pallor, depression, and impaired growth in children; called Simmonds' disease if cachexia is prominent.

253.3 Pituitary dwarfism
Isolated deficiency of (human) growth hormone [HGH]
Lorain-Levi dwarfism

DEF: Dwarfism with infantile physical characteristics due to abnormally low secretion of growth hormone and gonadotropin deficiency.

253.4 Other anterior pituitary disorders
Isolated or partial deficiency of an anterior pituitary hormone, other than growth hormone
Prolactin deficiency

253.5 Diabetes insipidus
Vasopressin deficiency
EXCLUDES   *nephrogenic diabetes insipidus (588.1)*

DEF: Metabolic disorder causing insufficient antidiuretic hormone release; symptoms include frequent urination, thirst, ravenous hunger, loss of weight, fatigue.

253.6 Other disorders of neurohypophysis
Syndrome of inappropriate secretion of antidiuretic hormone [ADH]
EXCLUDES   *ectopic antidiuretic hormone secretion (259.3)*

DEF: Pituitary dysfunction that results from drug therapy, radiation therapy, or surgery, causing mild to severe symptoms.

253.7 Iatrogenic pituitary disorders
Hypopituitarism: Hypopituitarism:
  hormone-induced   postablative
  hypophysectomy-induced   radiotherapy-induced
Use additional E code to identify cause

253.8 Other disorders of the pituitary and other syndromes of diencephalohypophyseal origin
Abscess of pituitary
Adiposogenital dystrophy
Cyst of Rathke's pouch
Fröhlich's syndrome
EXCLUDES   *craniopharyngioma (237.0)*

253.9 Unspecified
Dyspituitarism

✓4ᵗʰ 254 Diseases of thymus gland
EXCLUDES   *aplasia or dysplasia with immunodeficiency (279.2)*
hypoplasia with immunodeficiency (279.2)
myasthenia gravis (358.0)

254.0 Persistent hyperplasia of thymus
Hypertrophy of thymus

DEF: Continued abnormal growth of the twin lymphoid lobes that produce T lymphocytes.

254.1 Abscess of thymus
254.8 Other specified diseases of thymus gland
Atrophy } of thymus
Cyst
EXCLUDES   *thymoma (212.6)*

254.9 Unspecified disease of thymus gland

✓4ᵗʰ 255 Disorders of adrenal glands
INCLUDES   the listed conditions whether the basic disorder is in the adrenals or is pituitary-induced

255.0 Cushing's syndrome
Adrenal hyperplasia due to excess ACTH
Cushing's syndrome:
  NOS
  iatrogenic
  idiopathic
  pituitary-dependent
Ectopic ACTH syndrome
Iatrogenic syndrome of excess cortisol
Overproduction of cortisol
Use additional E code to identify cause, if drug-induced
EXCLUDES   *congenital adrenal hyperplasia (255.2)*

DEF: Due to adrenal cortisol oversecretion or glucocorticoid medications; may cause fatty tissue of the face, neck and body, osteoporosis and curvature of spine, hypertension, diabetes mellitus, female genitourinary problems, male impotence, degeneration of muscle tissues, weakness.

255.1 Hyperaldosteronism
Aldosteronism (primary) (secondary)
Bartter's syndrome
Conn's syndrome

DEF: Oversecretion of aldosterone causing fluid retention, hypertension.

255.2 Adrenogenital disorders
Achard-Thiers syndrome
Adrenogenital syndromes, virilizing or feminizing, whether acquired or associated with congenital adrenal hyperplasia consequent on inborn enzyme defects in hormone synthesis
Congenital adrenal hyperplasia
Female adrenal pseudohermaphroditism
Male:
  macrogenitosomia praecox
  sexual precocity with adrenal hyperplasia
Virilization (female) (suprarenal)
EXCLUDES   *adrenal hyperplasia due to excess ACTH (255.0)*
isosexual virilization (256.4)

255.3 Other corticoadrenal overactivity
Acquired benign adrenal androgenic overactivity
Overproduction of ACTH

255.4 Corticoadrenal insufficiency
Addisonian crisis
Addison's disease NOS
Adrenal:
  atrophy (autoimmune)
  calcification
  crisis
  hemorrhage
  infarction
  insufficiency NOS
EXCLUDES   *tuberculous Addison's disease (017.6)*

DEF: Underproduction of adrenal hormones causing low blood pressure.

255.5 Other adrenal hypofunction
Adrenal medullary insufficiency
EXCLUDES   *Waterhouse-Friderichsen syndrome (meningococcal) (036.3)*

255.6 Medulloadrenal hyperfunction
Catecholamine secretion by pheochromocytoma

255.8 Other specified disorders of adrenal glands
Abnormality of cortisol-binding globulin

255.9 Unspecified disorder of adrenal glands

√4ᵗʰ **256 Ovarian dysfunction**

256.0 Hyperestrogenism   ♀

DEF: Excess secretion of estrogen by the ovaries; characterized by ovaries containing multiple follicular cysts filled with serous fluid .

256.1 Other ovarian hyperfunction   ♀

Hypersecretion of ovarian androgens

256.2 Postablative ovarian failure   ♀

Ovarian failure: Ovarian failure:
    iatrogenic   postsurgical
    postirradiation

▶Use additional code for states associated with artificial menopause (627.4)◀

EXCLUDES *acquired absence of ovary (V45.77)*
asymptomatic age-related (natural) postmenopausal status (V49.81)

DEF: Failed ovarian function after medical or surgical intervention.

√5ᵗʰ **256.3 Other ovarian failure**

Use additional code for states associated with ▶natural menopause (627.2)◀

EXCLUDES *asymptomatic age-related (natural) postmenopausal status (V49.81)*

256.31 Premature menopause   ♀

DEF: Permanent cessation of ovarian function before the age of 40 occuring naturally of unknown cause.

256.39 Other ovarian failure   ♀

Delayed menarche
Ovarian hypofunction
Primary ovarian failure NOS

256.4 Polycystic ovaries   ♀

Isosexual virilization   Stein-Leventhal syndrome

DEF: Multiple serous filled cysts of ovary; symptoms of infertility, hirsutism, oligomenorrhea or amenorrhea.

256.8 Other ovarian dysfunction   ♀

256.9 Unspecified ovarian dysfunction   ♀

√4ᵗʰ **257 Testicular dysfunction**

257.0 Testicular hyperfunction   ♂

Hypersecretion of testicular hormones

257.1 Postablative testicular hypofunction   ♂

Testicular hypofunction: Testicular hypofunction:
    iatrogenic   postsurgical
    postirradiation

257.2 Other testicular hypofunction   ♂

Defective biosynthesis of testicular androgen
Eunuchoidism:
    NOS
    hypogonadotropic
Failure:
    Leydig's cell, adult
    seminiferous tubule, adult
Testicular hypogonadism
EXCLUDES *azoospermia (606.0)*

257.8 Other testicular dysfunction   ♂

Goldberg-Maxwell syndrome
Male pseudohermaphroditism with testicular feminization
Testicular feminization

257.9 Unspecified testicular dysfunction   ♂

√4ᵗʰ **258 Polyglandular dysfunction and related disorders**

258.0 Polyglandular activity in multiple endocrine adenomatosis

Wermer's syndrome

DEF: Wermer's syndrome: A rare hereditary condition characterized by the presence of adenomas or hyperplasia in more than one endocrine gland causing premature aging.

258.1 Other combinations of endocrine dysfunction

Lloyd's syndrome
Schmidt's syndrome

258.8 Other specified polyglandular dysfunction

258.9 Polyglandular dysfunction, unspecified

√4ᵗʰ **259 Other endocrine disorders**

259.0 Delay in sexual development and puberty, not elsewhere classified

Delayed puberty

259.1 Precocious sexual development and puberty, not elsewhere classified   P

Sexual precocity: Sexual precocity:
    NOS   cryptogenic
    constitutional   idiopathic

259.2 Carcinoid syndrome

Hormone secretion by carcinoid tumors

DEF: Presence of carcinoid tumors that spread to liver; characterized by cyanotic flushing of skin, diarrhea, bronchospasm, acquired tricuspid and pulmonary stenosis, sudden drops in blood pressure, edema, ascites.

259.3 Ectopic hormone secretion, not elsewhere classified

Ectopic:
    antidiuretic hormone secretion [ADH]
    hyperparathyroidism
EXCLUDES *ectopic ACTH syndrome (255.0)*

259.4 Dwarfism, not elsewhere classified

Dwarfism:
    NOS
    constitutional
EXCLUDES *dwarfism:*
    achondroplastic (756.4)
    intrauterine (759.7)
    nutritional (263.2)
    pituitary (253.3)
    renal (588.0)
    progeria (259.8)

259.8 Other specified endocrine disorders

Pineal gland dysfunction Werner's syndrome
Progeria

259.9 Unspecified endocrine disorder

Disturbance: Infantilism NOS
    endocrine NOS
    hormone NOS

NUTRITIONAL DEFICIENCIES (260-269)

EXCLUDES *deficiency anemias (280.0-281.9)*

260 Kwashiorkor

Nutritional edema with dyspigmentation of skin and hair

DEF: Syndrome, particularly of children; excessive carbohydrate with inadequate protein intake, inhibited growth potential, anomalies in skin and hair pigmentation, edema and liver disease.

261 Nutritional marasmus

Nutritional atrophy
Severe calorie deficiency
Severe malnutrition NOS

DEF: Protein-calorie malabsorption or malnutrition of children; characterized by tissue wasting, dehydration, and subcutaneous fat depletion; may occur with infectious disease; also called infantile atrophy.

262 Other severe, protein-calorie malnutrition

Nutritional edema without mention of dyspigmentation of skin and hair

√4ᵗʰ **263 Other and unspecified protein-calorie malnutrition**

263.0 Malnutrition of moderate degree

DEF: Malnutrition characterized by biochemical changes in electrolytes, lipids, blood plasma.

263.1 Malnutrition of mild degree

263.2 Arrested development following protein-calorie malnutrition

Nutritional dwarfism
Physical retardation due to malnutrition

263.8 Other protein-calorie malnutrition

263.9 Unspecified protein-calorie malnutrition

Dystrophy due to malnutrition
Malnutrition (calorie) NOS
EXCLUDES *nutritional deficiency NOS (269.9)*

Endocrine, Nutritional and Metabolic, Immunity 256–263.9

√4ᵗʰ
√5ᵗʰ Additional Digit Required   Unspecified Code   Other Specified Code   Manifestation Code   ▶◀ Revised Text   ● New Code   ▲ Revised Code Title

✓4th **264 Vitamin A deficiency**

264.0 With conjunctival xerosis
DEF: Vitamin A deficiency with conjunctival dryness.

264.1 With conjunctival xerosis and Bitot's spot
Bitot's spot in the young child
DEF: Vitamin A deficiency with conjunctival dryness, superficial spots of keratinized epithelium.

264.2 With corneal xerosis
DEF: Vitamin A deficiency with corneal dryness.

264.3 With corneal ulceration and xerosis
DEF: Vitamin A deficiency with corneal dryness, epithelial ulceration.

264.4 With keratomalacia
DEF: Vitamin A deficiency creating corneal dryness; progresses to corneal insensitivity, softness, necrosis; usually bilateral.

264.5 With night blindness
DEF: Vitamin A deficiency causing vision failure in dim light.

264.6 With xerophthalmic scars of cornea
DEF: Vitamin A deficiency with corneal scars from dryness.

264.7 Other ocular manifestations of vitamin A deficiency
Xerophthalmia due to vitamin A deficiency

264.8 Other manifestations of vitamin A deficiency
Follicular keratosis ⎫ due to vitamin A
Xeroderma ⎭ deficiency

264.9 Unspecified vitamin A deficiency
Hypovitaminosis A NOS

✓4th **265 Thiamine and niacin deficiency states**

265.0 Beriberi
DEF: Inadequate vitamin B_1 (thiamine) intake, affects heart and peripheral nerves; individual may become edematous and develop cardiac disease due to the excess fluid; alcoholics and people with a diet of excessive polished rice prone to the disease.

265.1 Other and unspecified manifestations of thiamine deficiency
Other vitamin B_1 deficiency states

265.2 Pellagra
Deficiency: Deficiency:
niacin (-tryptophan)   vitamin PP
nicotinamide   Pellagra (alcoholic)
nicotinic acid
DEF: Niacin deficiency causing dermatitis, inflammation of mucous membranes, diarrhea, and psychic disturbances.

✓4th **266 Deficiency of B-complex components**

266.0 Ariboflavinosis
Riboflavin [vitamin B_2] deficiency
DEF: Vitamin B_2 (riboflavin) deficiency marked by swollen lips and tongue fissures, corneal vascularization, scaling lesions, and anemia.

266.1 Vitamin B_6 deficiency
Deficiency: Deficiency:
pyridoxal   pyridoxine
pyridoxamine   Vitamin B_6 deficiency
syndrome
EXCLUDES *vitamin B_6-responsive sideroblastic anemia (285.0)*
DEF: Vitamin B_6 deficiency causing skin, lip, and tongue disturbances, peripheral neuropathy; and convulsions in infants.

266.2 Other B-complex deficiencies
Deficiency: Deficiency:
cyanocobalamin   vitamin B_{12}
folic acid
EXCLUDES *combined system disease with anemia (281.0-281.1)*
deficiency anemias (281.0-281.9)
subacute degeneration of spinal cord with anemia (281.0-281.1)

266.9 Unspecified vitamin B deficiency

267 Ascorbic acid deficiency
Deficiency of vitamin C
Scurvy
EXCLUDES *scorbutic anemia (281.8)*
DEF: Vitamin C deficiency causing swollen gums, myalgia, weight loss, and weakness.

✓4th **268 Vitamin D deficiency**
EXCLUDES *vitamin D-resistant:*
osteomalacia (275.3)
rickets (275.3)

268.0 Rickets, active
EXCLUDES *celiac rickets (579.0)*
renal rickets (588.0)
DEF: Inadequate vitamin D intake, usually in pediatrics, that affects bones most involved with muscular action; may cause nodules on ends and sides of bones; delayed closure of fontanels in infants; symptoms may include muscle soreness, and profuse sweating.

268.1 Rickets, late effect
Any condition specified as due to rickets and stated to be a late effect or sequela of rickets
Use additional code to identify the nature of late effect
DEF: Distorted or demineralized bones as a result of vitamin D deficiency.

268.2 Osteomalacia, unspecified
DEF: Softening of bones due to decrease in calcium; marked by pain, tenderness, muscular weakness, anorexia, and weight loss.

268.9 Unspecified vitamin D deficiency
Avitaminosis D

✓4th **269 Other nutritional deficiencies**

269.0 Deficiency of vitamin K
EXCLUDES *deficiency of coagulation factor due to vitamin K deficiency (286.7)*
vitamin K deficiency of newborn (776.0)

269.1 Deficiency of other vitamins
Deficiency: Deficiency:
vitamin E   vitamin P

269.2 Unspecified vitamin deficiency
Multiple vitamin deficiency NOS

269.3 Mineral deficiency, not elsewhere classified
Deficiency: Deficiency:
calcium, dietary   iodine
EXCLUDES *deficiency:*
calcium NOS (275.4)
potassium (276.8)
sodium (276.1)

269.8 Other nutritional deficiency
EXCLUDES *adult failure to thrive (783.7)*
failure to thrive in childhood (783.41)
feeding problems (783.3)
newborn (779.3)

269.9 Unspecified nutritional deficiency

OTHER METABOLIC AND IMMUNITY DISORDERS (270-279)

Use additional code to identify any associated mental retardation

✓4th 270 Disorders of amino-acid transport and metabolism

    EXCLUDES   *abnormal findings without manifest disease (790.0-796.9)*
                     disorders of purine and pyrimidine metabolism (277.1-277.2)
                     gout (274.0-274.9)

270.0 Disturbances of amino-acid transport
- Cystinosis
- Cystinuria
- Fanconi (-de Toni) (-Debré) syndrome
- Glycinuria (renal)
- Hartnup disease

270.1 Phenylketonuria [PKU]
- Hyperphenylalaninemia

DEF: Inherited metabolic condition causing excess phenylpyruvic and other acids in urine; results in mental retardation, neurological manifestations, including spasticity and tremors, light pigmentation, eczema, and mousy odor.

270.2 Other disturbances of aromatic amino-acid metabolism
- Albinism
- Alkaptonuria
- Alkaptonuric ochronosis
- Disturbances of metabolism of tyrosine and tryptophan
- Homogentisic acid defects
- Hydroxykynureninuria
- Hypertyrosinemia
- Indicanuria
- Kynureninase defects
- Oasthouse urine disease
- Ochronosis
- Tyrosinosis
- Tyrosinuria
- Waardenburg syndrome

    EXCLUDES   *vitamin B$_6$-deficiency syndrome (266.1)*

270.3 Disturbances of branched-chain amino-acid metabolism
- Disturbances of metabolism of leucine, isoleucine, and valine
- Hypervalinemia
- Intermittent branched-chain ketonuria
- Leucine-induced hypoglycemia
- Leucinosis
- Maple syrup urine disease

270.4 Disturbances of sulphur-bearing amino-acid metabolism
- Cystathioninemia
- Cystathioninuria
- Disturbances of metabolism of methionine, homocystine, and cystathionine
- Homocystinuria
- Hypermethioninemia
- Methioninemia

270.5 Disturbances of histidine metabolism
- Carnosinemia
- Histidinemia
- Hyperhistidinemia
- Imidazole aminoaciduria

270.6 Disorders of urea cycle metabolism
- Argininosuccinic aciduria
- Citrullinemia
- Disorders of metabolism of ornithine, citrulline, argininosuccinic acid, arginine, and ammonia
- Hyperammonemia
- Hyperornithinemia

270.7 Other disturbances of straight-chain amino-acid metabolism
- Glucoglycinuria
- Glycinemia (with methyl-malonic acidemia)
- Hyperglycinemia
- Hyperlysinemia
- Other disturbances of metabolism of glycine, threonine, serine, glutamine, and lysine
- Pipecolic acidemia
- Saccharopinuria

270.8 Other specified disorders of amino-acid metabolism

Alaninemia	Iminoacidopathy
Ethanolaminuria	Prolinemia
Glycoprolinuria	Prolinuria
Hydroxyprolinemia	Sarcosinemia
Hyperprolinemia	

270.9 Unspecified disorder of amino-acid metabolism

✓4th 271 Disorders of carbohydrate transport and metabolism

    EXCLUDES   *abnormality of secretion of glucagon (251.4)*
                     diabetes mellitus (250.0-250.9)
                     hypoglycemia NOS (251.2)
                     mucopolysaccharidosis (277.5)

271.0 Glycogenosis
- Amylopectinosis
- Glucose-6-phosphatase deficiency
- Glycogen storage disease
- McArdle's disease
- Pompe's disease
- von Gierke's disease

DEF: Excess glycogen storage; rare inherited trait affects liver, kidneys; causes various symptoms depending on type, though often weakness, and muscle cramps.

271.1 Galactosemia
- Galactose-1-phosphate uridyl transferase deficiency
- Galactosuria

DEF: Any of three genetic disorders due to defective galactose metabolism; symptoms include failure to thrive in infancy, jaundice, liver and spleen damage, cataracts, and mental retardation.

271.2 Hereditary fructose intolerance
- Essential benign fructosuria   Fructosemia

DEF: Chromosome recessive disorder of carbohydrate metabolism; in infants, occurs after dietary sugar introduced; characterized by enlarged spleen, yellowish cast to skin, and progressive inability to thrive.

271.3 Intestinal disaccharidase deficiencies and disaccharide malabsorption
- Intolerance or malabsorption (congenital) (of):
  - glucose-galactose
  - lactose
  - sucrose-isomaltose

271.4 Renal glycosuria
- Renal diabetes

DEF: Persistent abnormal levels of glucose in urine, with normal blood glucose levels; caused by failure of the renal tubules to reabsorb glucose.

271.8 Other specified disorders of carbohydrate transport and metabolism

Essential benign pentosuria	Mannosidosis
Fucosidosis	Oxalosis
Glycolic aciduria	Xylosuria
Hyperoxaluria (primary)	Xylulosuria

271.9 Unspecified disorder of carbohydrate transport and metabolism

---

✓4th
✓5th Additional Digit Required   Unspecified Code   Other Specified Code   Manifestation Code   ▶◀ Revised Text   ● New Code   ▲ Revised Code Title

2003 ICD•9•CM   **Volume 1 — 51**

Endocrine, Nutritional and Metabolic, Immunity 272–273.9

Lipid Metabolism

✓4th 272 Disorders of lipoid metabolism
EXCLUDES   *localized cerebral lipidoses (330.1)*

272.0 Pure hypercholesterolemia
Familial hypercholesterolemia
Fredrickson Type IIa hyperlipoproteinemia
Hyperbetalipoproteinemia
Hyperlipidemia, Group A
Low-density-lipoid-type [LDL] hyperlipoproteinemia

272.1 Pure hyperglyceridemia
Endogenous hyperglyceridemia
Fredrickson Type IV hyperlipoproteinemia
Hyperlipidemia, Group B
Hyperprebetalipoproteinemia
Hypertriglyceridemia, essential
Very-low-density-lipoid-type [VLDL]
    hyperlipoproteinemia

272.2 Mixed hyperlipidemia
Broad- or floating-betalipoproteinemia
Fredrickson Type IIb or III hyperlipoproteinemia
Hypercholesterolemia with endogenous
    hyperglyceridemia
Hyperbetalipoproteinemia with
    prebetalipoproteinemia
Tubo-eruptive xanthoma
Xanthoma tuberosum
DEF: Elevated levels of lipoprotein, a complex of fats and proteins, in blood due to inherited metabolic disorder.

272.3 Hyperchylomicronemia
Bürger-Grütz syndrome
Fredrickson type I or V hyperlipoproteinemia
Hyperlipidemia, Group D
Mixed hyperglyceridemia

272.4 Other and unspecified hyperlipidemia
Alpha-lipoproteinemia
Combined hyperlipidemia
Hyperlipidemia NOS
Hyperlipoproteinemia NOS
DEF: Hyperlipoproteinemia: elevated levels of transient chylomicrons in the blood which are a form of lipoproteins which transport dietary cholesterol and triglycerides from the small intestine to the blood.

272.5 Lipoprotein deficiencies
Abetalipoproteinemia
Bassen-Kornzweig syndrome
High-density lipoid deficiency (familial)
Hypoalphalipoproteinemia
Hypobetalipoproteinemia
DEF: Abnormally low levels of lipoprotein, a complex of fats and protein, in the blood.

272.6 Lipodystrophy
Barraquer-Simons disease
Progressive lipodystrophy
Use additional E code to identify cause, if iatrogenic
EXCLUDES   *intestinal lipodystrophy (040.2)*
DEF: Disturbance of fat metabolism resulting in loss of fatty tissue in some areas of the body.

272.7 Lipidoses
Chemically-induced lipidosis
Disease:
    Anderson's
    Fabry's
    Gaucher's
    I cell [mucolipidosis I]
    lipoid storage NOS
    Niemann-Pick
    pseudo-Hurler's or mucolipidosis III
    triglyceride storage, Type I or II
    Wolman's or triglyceride storage, Type III
Mucolipidosis II
Primary familial xanthomatosis
EXCLUDES   *cerebral lipidoses (330.1)*
       Tay-Sachs disease (330.1)
DEF: Lysosomal storage diseases marked by an abnormal amount of lipids in reticuloendothelial cells.

272.8 Other disorders of lipoid metabolism
Hoffa's disease or liposynovitis prepatellaris
Launois-Bensaude's lipomatosis
Lipoid dermatoarthritis

272.9 Unspecified disorder of lipoid metabolism

✓4th 273 Disorders of plasma protein metabolism
EXCLUDES   *agammaglobulinemia and*
       hypogammaglobulinemia (279.0-279.2)
    coagulation defects (286.0-286.9)
    hereditary hemolytic anemias (282.0-282.9)

273.0 Polyclonal hypergammaglobulinemia
Hypergammaglobulinemic purpura:
    benign primary
    Waldenström's
DEF: Elevated blood levels of gamma globulins, frequently found in patients with chronic infectious diseases.

273.1 Monoclonal paraproteinemia
Benign monoclonal hypergammaglobulinemia [BMH]
Monoclonal gammopathy:
    NOS
    associated with lymphoplasmacytic dyscrasias
    benign
Paraproteinemia:
    benign (familial)
    secondary to malignant or inflammatory disease
DEF: Elevated blood levels of macroglobulins (plasma globulins of high weight); characterized by malignant neoplasms of bone marrow, spleen, liver, or lymph nodes; symptoms include weakness, fatigue, bleeding disorders, and vision problems.

273.2 Other paraproteinemias
Cryoglobulinemic: Mixed cryoglobulinemia
    purpura
    vasculitis

273.3 Macroglobulinemia
Macroglobulinemia (idiopathic) (primary)
Waldenström's macroglobulinemia

273.8 Other disorders of plasma protein metabolism
Abnormality of transport protein
Bisalbuminemia

273.9 Unspecified disorder of plasma protein metabolism

✓4th **274 Gout**

> EXCLUDES *lead gout (984.0-984.9)*

> DEF: Purine and pyrimidine metabolic disorders; manifested by hyperuricemia and recurrent acute inflammatory arthritis; monosodium urate or monohydrate crystals may be deposited in and around the joints, leading to joint destruction, and severe crippling.

274.0 Gouty arthropathy

✓5th **274.1 Gouty nephropathy**

> **274.10 Gouty nephropathy, unspecified**

> **274.11 Uric acid nephrolithiasis**
>> DEF: Sodium urate stones in the kidney.

> **274.19 Other**

✓5th **274.8 Gout with other specified manifestations**

> **274.81 Gouty tophi of ear**
>> DEF: Chalky sodium urate deposit in the ear due to gout; produces chronic inflammation of external ear.

> **274.82 Gouty tophi of other sites**
>> Gouty tophi of heart

> **274.89 Other**
>> Use additional code to identify manifestations, as:
>> gouty:
>>> iritis (364.11)
>>> neuritis (357.4)

274.9 Gout, unspecified

✓4th **275 Disorders of mineral metabolism**

> EXCLUDES *abnormal findings without manifest disease (790.0-796.9)*

275.0 Disorders of iron metabolism
> Bronzed diabetes
> Hemochromatosis
> Pigmentary cirrhosis (of liver)
>> EXCLUDES *anemia:*
>>> *iron deficiency (280.0-280.9)*
>>> *sideroblastic (285.0)*

275.1 Disorders of copper metabolism
> Hepatolenticular degeneration
> Wilson's disease

275.2 Disorders of magnesium metabolism
> Hypermagnesemia
> Hypomagnesemia

275.3 Disorders of phosphorus metabolism
> Familial hypophosphatemia
> Hypophosphatasia
> Vitamin D-resistant:
>> osteomalacia
>> rickets

✓5th **275.4 Disorders of calcium metabolism**
> EXCLUDES *parathyroid disorders (252.0-252.9)*
> *vitamin D deficiency (268.0-268.9)*

> **275.40 Unspecified disorder of calcium metabolism**

> **275.41 Hypocalcemia**
>> DEF: Abnormally decreased blood calcium level; symptoms include hyperactive deep tendon reflexes, muscle, abdominal cramps, and carpopedal spasm.

> **275.42 Hypercalcemia**
>> DEF: Abnormally increased blood calcium level; symptoms include muscle weakness, fatigue, nausea, depression, and constipation.

> **275.49 Other disorders of calcium metabolism**
>> Nephrocalcinosis
>> Pseudohypoparathyroidism
>> Pseudopseudohypoparathryoidism

>> DEF: Nephrocalcinosis: calcium phosphate deposits in the tubules of the kidney with resultant renal insufficiency.

>> DEF: Pseudohypoparathyroidism: inherited disorder with signs and symptoms of hypoparathyroidism; caused by inadequate response to parathyroid hormone, not hormonal deficiency. Symptoms include muscle cramps, tetany, urinary frequency, blurred vision due to cataracts, and dry scaly skin.

>> DEF: Pseudopseudohypoparathyroidism: clinical manifestations of hypoparathyroidism without affecting blood calcium levels.

275.8 Other specified disorders of mineral metabolism

275.9 Unspecified disorder of mineral metabolism

✓4th **276 Disorders of fluid, electrolyte, and acid-base balance**
> EXCLUDES *diabetes insipidus (253.5)*
> *familial periodic paralysis (359.3)*

276.0 Hyperosmolality and/or hypernatremia
> Sodium [Na] excess   Sodium [Na] overload

276.1 Hyposmolality and/or hyponatremia
> Sodium [Na] deficiency

276.2 Acidosis
> Acidosis: Acidosis:
> NOS   metabolic
> lactic   respiratory
>> EXCLUDES *diabetic acidosis (250.1)*

> DEF: Disorder involves decrease of pH (hydrogen ion) concentration in blood and cellular tissues; caused by increase in acid and decrease in bicarbonate.

276.3 Alkalosis
> Alkalosis: Alkalosis:
> NOS   respiratory
> metabolic

> DEF: Accumulation of base (non-acid part of salt), or loss of acid without relative loss of base in body fluids; caused by increased arterial plasma bicarbonate concentration or loss of carbon dioxide due to hyperventilation.

276.4 Mixed acid-base balance disorder
> Hypercapnia with mixed acid-base disorder

276.5 Volume depletion
> Dehydration
> Depletion of volume of plasma or extracellular fluid
> Hypovolemia
>> EXCLUDES *hypovolemic shock:*
>>> *postoperative (998.0)*
>>> *traumatic (958.4)*

276.6 Fluid overload
> Fluid retention
>> EXCLUDES *ascites (789.5)*
>>> *localized edema (782.3)*

276.7 Hyperpotassemia
> Hyperkalemia   Potassium [K]:
> Potassium [K]:   intoxication
> excess   overload

> DEF: Elevated blood levels of potassium; symptoms include abnormal EKG readings, weakness; related to defective renal excretion.

276.8 Hypopotassemia
> Hypokalemia   Potassium [K] deficiency

> DEF: Decreased blood levels of potassium; symptoms include neuromuscular disorders.

✓4th ✓5th Additional Digit Required   Unspecified Code   Other Specified Code   Manifestation Code   ►◄ Revised Text   ● New Code   ▲ Revised Code Title

2003 ICD•9•CM   **Volume 1 — 53**

276.9 Electrolyte and fluid disorders not elsewhere classified

Electrolyte imbalance Hypochloremia
Hyperchloremia

> **EXCLUDES** electrolyte imbalance:
> associated with hyperemesis
> gravidarum (643.1)
> complicating labor and delivery
> (669.0)
> following abortion and ectopic or
> molar pregnancy (634-638
> with .4, 639.4)

√4th **277 Other and unspecified disorders of metabolism**

√5th **277.0 Cystic fibrosis**

Fibrocystic disease of the pancreas
Mucoviscidosis

DEF: Generalized, genetic disorder of infants, children, and young adults marked by exocrine gland dysfunction; characterized by chronic pulmonary disease with excess mucus production, pancreatic deficiency, high levels of electrolytes in the sweat.

277.00 Without mention of meconium ileus
▶Cystic fibrosis NOS◀

277.01 With meconium ileus   N

Meconium:
ileus (of newborn)
obstruction of intestine in mucoviscidosis

277.02 With pulmonary manifestations

Cystic fibrosis with pulmonary exacerbation
Use additional code to identify any
infectious organism present, such as:
pseudomonas (041.7)

277.03 With gastrointestinal manifestations

> **EXCLUDES** with meconium ileus (277.01)

277.09 With other manifestations

277.1 Disorders of porphyrin metabolism

Hematoporphyria
Hematoporphyrinuria
Hereditary coproporphyria
Porphyria
Porphyrinuria
Protocoproporphyria
Protoporphyria
Pyrroloporphyria

277.2 Other disorders of purine and pyrimidine metabolism

Hypoxanthine-guanine-phosphoribosyltransferase
deficiency [HG-PRT deficiency]
Lesch-Nyhan syndrome
Xanthinuria

> **EXCLUDES** gout (274.0-274.9)
> orotic aciduric anemia (281.4)

277.3 Amyloidosis

Amyloidosis:
NOS
inherited systemic
nephropathic
neuropathic (Portuguese) (Swiss)
secondary
Benign paroxysmal peritonitis
Familial Mediterranean fever
Hereditary cardiac amyloidosis

DEF: Conditions of diverse etiologies characterized by the accumulation of insoluble fibrillar proteins (amyloid) in various organs and tissues of the body, compromising vital functions.

277.4 Disorders of bilirubin excretion

Hyperbilirubinemia:	Syndrome:
congenital	Dubin-Johnson
constitutional	Gilbert's
Syndrome:	Rotor's
Crigler-Najjar	

> **EXCLUDES** hyperbilirubinemias specific to the
> perinatal period (774.0-774.7)

277.5 Mucopolysaccharidosis

Gargoylism	Morquio-Brailsford disease
Hunter's syndrome	Osteochondrodystrophy
Hurler's syndrome	Sanfilippo's syndrome
Lipochondrodystrophy	Scheie's syndrome
Maroteaux-Lamy syndrome	

DEF: Metabolism disorders evidenced by excretion of various mucopolysaccharides in urine and infiltration of these substances into connective tissue, with resulting various defects of bone, cartilage and connective tissue.

277.6 Other deficiencies of circulating enzymes

Alpha 1-antitrypsin deficiency
Hereditary angioedema

277.7 Dysmetabolic syndrome X   A

Use additional code for associated manifestations,
such as:
cardiovascular disease ▶(414.00-414.06)◀
obesity (278.00-278.01)

DEF: A specific group of metabolic disorders that are related to the state of insulin resistance (decreased cellular response to insulin) without elevated blood sugars; often related to elevated cholesterol and triglycerides, obesity, cardiovascular disease, and high blood pressure.

277.8 Other specified disorders of metabolism

Hand-Schüller-Christian disease
Histiocytosis (acute) (chronic)
Histiocytosis X (chronic)

> **EXCLUDES** histiocytosis:
> acute differentiated progressive
> (202.5)
> X, acute (progressive) (202.5)

277.9 Unspecified disorder of metabolism

Enzymopathy NOS

√4th **278 Obesity and other hyperalimentation**

> **EXCLUDES** hyperalimentation NOS (783.6)
> poisoning by vitamins NOS (963.5)
> polyphagia (783.6)

√5th **278.0 Obesity**

> **EXCLUDES** adiposogenital dystrophy (253.8)
> obesity of endocrine origin NOS (259.9)

278.00 Obesity, unspecified
Obesity NOS

278.01 Morbid obesity

DEF: Increased weight beyond limits of skeletal and physical requirements (125 percent or more over ideal body weight), as a result of excess fat in subcutaneous connective tissues.

278.1 Localized adiposity
Fat pad

278.2 Hypervitaminosis A

278.3 Hypercarotinemia

DEF: Elevated blood carotene level due to ingesting excess carotenoids or the inability to convert carotenoids to vitamin A.

278.4 Hypervitaminosis D

DEF: Weakness, fatigue, loss of weight, and other symptoms resulting from ingesting excessive amounts of vitamin D.

278.8 Other hyperalimentation

√4th **279 Disorders involving the immune mechanism**

√5th **279.0 Deficiency of humoral immunity**

DEF: Inadequate immune response to bacterial infections with potential reinfection by viruses due to lack of circulating immunoglobulins (acquired antibodies).

279.00 Hypogammaglobulinemia, unspecified
Agammaglobulinemia NOS

279.01 Selective IgA immunodeficiency

279.02 Selective IgM immunodeficiency

279.03 Other selective immunoglobulin deficiencies

Selective deficiency of IgG

N Newborn Age: 0   P Pediatric Age: 0-17   M Maternity Age: 12-55   A Adult Age: 15-124   MSP Medicare Secondary Payer

279.04 Congenital hypogammaglobulinemia
Agammaglobulinemia:
　　Bruton's type
　　X-linked

279.05 Immunodeficiency with increased IgM
Immunodeficiency with hyper-IgM:
　　autosomal recessive
　　X-linked

279.06 Common variable immunodeficiency
Dysgammaglobulinemia (acquired)
　　(congenital) (primary)
Hypogammaglobulinemia:
　　acquired primary
　　congenital non-sex-linked
　　sporadic

279.09 Other
Transient hypogammaglobulinemia of
　　infancy

√5ᵗʰ 279.1 Deficiency of cell-mediated immunity

279.10 Immunodeficiency with predominant T-cell defect, unspecified

279.11 DiGeorge's syndrome
Pharyngeal pouch syndrome
Thymic hypoplasia

DEF: Congenital disorder due to defective development of the third and fourth pharyngeal pouches; results in hypoplasia or aplasia of the thymus, parathyroid glands; related to congenital heart defects, anomalies of the great vessels, esophageal atresia, and abnormalities of facial structures.

279.12 Wiskott-Aldrich syndrome

DEF: A disease characterized by chronic conditions, such as eczema, suppurative otitis media and anemia; it results from an X-linked recessive gene and is classified as an immune deficiency syndrome.

279.13 Nezelof's syndrome
Cellular immunodeficiency with abnormal immunoglobulin deficiency

DEF: Immune system disorder characterized by a pathological deficiency in cellular immunity and humoral antibodies resulting in inability to fight infectious diseases.

279.19 Other
　　EXCLUDES *ataxia-telangiectasia (334.8)*

279.2 Combined immunity deficiency
Agammaglobulinemia:
　　autosomal recessive
　　Swiss-type
　　x-linked recessive
Severe combined immunodeficiency [SCID]
Thymic:
　　alymphoplasia
　　aplasia or dysplasia with immunodeficiency
　　EXCLUDES *thymic hypoplasia (279.11)*

DEF: Agammaglobulinemia: no immunoglobulins in the blood.

DEF: Thymic alymphoplasia: severe combined immunodeficiency; result of failed lymphoid tissue development.

279.3 Unspecified immunity deficiency

279.4 Autoimmune disease, not elsewhere classified
Autoimmune disease NOS
　　EXCLUDES *transplant failure or rejection (996.80-996.89)*

279.8 Other specified disorders involving the immune mechanism
Single complement [C1-C9] deficiency or dysfunction

279.9 Unspecified disorder of immune mechanism

√4ᵗʰ
√5ᵗʰ Additional Digit Required   Unspecified Code   Other Specified Code   Manifestation Code   ▶◀ Revised Text   ● New Code   ▲ Revised Code Title

4. DISEASES OF THE BLOOD AND BLOOD-FORMING ORGANS (280-289)

> **EXCLUDES**   *anemia complicating pregnancy or the puerperium (648.2)*

✓4ᵗʰ 280 Iron deficiency anemias

> **INCLUDES**   anemia:
> asiderotic
> hypochromic-microcytic
> sideropenic
>
> **EXCLUDES**   *familial microcytic anemia (282.4)*

280.0 Secondary to blood loss (chronic)
Normocytic anemia due to blood loss
> **EXCLUDES**   *acute posthemorrhagic anemia (285.1)*

280.1 Secondary to inadequate dietary iron intake

280.8 Other specified iron deficiency anemias
Paterson-Kelly syndrome
Plummer-Vinson syndrome
Sideropenic dysphagia

280.9 Iron deficiency anemia, unspecified
Anemia:
achlorhydric
chlorotic
idiopathic hypochromic
iron [Fe] deficiency NOS

✓4ᵗʰ 281 Other deficiency anemias

281.0 Pernicious anemia
Anemia:
Addison's
Biermer's
congenital pernicious
Congenital intrinsic factor [Castle's] deficiency
> **EXCLUDES**   *combined system disease without mention of anemia (266.2)*
> *subacute degeneration of spinal cord without mention of anemia (266.2)*

DEF: Chronic progressive anemia due to Vitamin B_{12} malabsorption; caused by lack of a secretion known as intrinsic factor, which is produced by the gastric mucosa of the stomach.

281.1 Other vitamin B_{12} deficiency anemia
Anemia:
vegan's
vitamin B_{12} deficiency (dietary)
due to selective vitamin B_{12} malabsorption with proteinuria
Syndrome:
Imerslund's
Imerslund-Gräsbeck
> **EXCLUDES**   *combined system disease without mention of anemia (266.2)*
> *subacute degeneration of spinal cord without mention of anemia (266.2)*

281.2 Folate-deficiency anemia
Congenital folate malabsorption
Folate or folic acid deficiency anemia:
NOS
dietary
drug-induced
Goat's milk anemia
Nutritional megaloblastic anemia (of infancy)
Use additional E code to identify drug

DEF: Macrocytic anemia resembles pernicious anemia but without absence of hydrochloric acid secretions; responsive to folic acid therapy.

281.3 Other specified megaloblastic anemias not elsewhere classified
Combined B_{12} and folate-deficiency anemia
Refractory megaloblastic anemia

DEF: Megaloblasts predominant in bone marrow with few normoblasts; rare familial type associated with proteinuria and genitourinary tract anomalies.

281.4 Protein-deficiency anemia
Amino-acid-deficiency anemia

281.8 Anemia associated with other specified nutritional deficiency
Scorbutic anemia

281.9 Unspecified deficiency anemia
Anemia:
dimorphic
macrocytic
megaloblastic NOS
nutritional NOS
simple chronic

✓4ᵗʰ 282 Hereditary hemolytic anemias

DEF: Escalated rate of erythrocyte destruction; similar to all anemias, occurs when imbalance exists between blood loss and blood production.

282.0 Hereditary spherocytosis
Acholuric (familial) jaundice
Congenital hemolytic anemia (spherocytic)
Congenital spherocytosis
Minkowski-Chauffard syndrome
Spherocytosis (familial)
> **EXCLUDES**   *hemolytic anemia of newborn (773.0-773.5)*

DEF: Hereditary, chronic illness marked by abnormal red blood cell membrane; symptoms include enlarged spleen, jaundice; and anemia in severe cases.

282.1 Hereditary elliptocytosis
Elliptocytosis (congenital)
Ovalocytosis (congenital) (hereditary)

DEF: Genetic hemolytic anemia characterized by malformed, elliptical erythrocytes; there is increased destruction of red cells with resulting anemia.

282.2 Anemias due to disorders of glutathione metabolism
Anemia:
6-phosphogluconic dehydrogenase deficiency
enzyme deficiency, drug-induced
erythrocytic glutathione deficiency
glucose-6-phosphate dehydrogenase [G-6-PD] deficiency
glutathione-reductase deficiency
hemolytic nonspherocytic (hereditary), type I
Disorder of pentose phosphate pathway
Favism

282.3 Other hemolytic anemias due to enzyme deficiency
Anemia:
hemolytic nonspherocytic (hereditary), type II
hexokinase deficiency
pyruvate kinase [PK] deficiency
triosephosphate isomerase deficiency

 ✓4ᵗʰ ✓5ᵗʰ Additional Digit Required   Unspecified Code   Other Specified Code   Manifestation Code   ▶◀ Revised Text   ● New Code   ▲ Revised Code Title

282.4 Thalassemias
Cooley's anemia
Hereditary leptocytosis
Mediterranean anemia (with other
hemoglobinopathy)
Microdrepanocytosis
Sickle-cell thalassemia
Thalassemia (alpha) (beta) (intermedia) (major)
(minima) (minor) (mixed) (trait) (with other
hemoglobinopathy)
Thalassemia-Hb-S disease

EXCLUDES *sickle-cell:*
anemia (282.60-282.69)
trait (282.5)

DEF: Group of hereditary anemias occurring in the Mediterranean
and Southeast Asia; characterized by impaired hemoglobin
synthesis; homozygous form may cause death in utero; mild red
blood cell anomalies in heterozygous.

282.5 Sickle-cell trait
Hb-AS genotype
Hemoglobin S [Hb-S] trait
Heterozygous:
hemoglobin S
Hb-S

EXCLUDES *that with other hemoglobinopathy*
(282.60-282.69)
that with thalassemia (282.4)

DEF: Heterozygous genetic makeup characterized by one gene for
normal hemoglobin and one for sickle-cell hemoglobin; clinical
disease rarely present.

√5th **282.6 Sickle-cell anemia**
EXCLUDES *sickle-cell thalassemia (282.4)*
sickle-cell trait (282.5)

DEF: Inherited blood disorder; sickle-shaped red blood cells are
hard and pointed, clogging blood flow; anemia characterized by,
periodic episodes of pain, acute abdominal discomfort, skin
ulcerations of the legs, increased infections; occurs primarily in
persons of African descent.

282.60 Sickle-cell anemia, unspecified
282.61 Hb-S disease without mention of crisis
282.62 Hb-S disease with mention of crisis
Sickle-cell crisis NOS
282.63 Sickle-cell/Hb-C disease
Hb-S/Hb-C disease
282.69 Other
Disease: Disease:
Hb-S/Hb-D   sickle-cell/Hb-D
Hb-S/Hb-E   sickle-cell/Hb-E

282.7 Other hemoglobinopathies
Abnormal hemoglobin NOS
Congenital Heinz-body anemia
Disease:
Hb-Bart's
hemoglobin C [Hb-C]
hemoglobin D [Hb-D]
hemoglobin E [Hb-E]
hemoglobin Zurich [Hb-Zurich]
Hemoglobinopathy NOS
Hereditary persistence of fetal hemoglobin [HPFH]
Unstable hemoglobin hemolytic disease

EXCLUDES *familial polycythemia (289.6)*
hemoglobin M [Hb-M] disease (289.7)
high-oxygen-affinity hemoglobin (289.0)

DEF: Any disorder of hemoglobin due to alteration of molecular
structure; may include overt anemia.

282.8 Other specified hereditary hemolytic anemias
Stomatocytosis
282.9 Hereditary hemolytic anemia, unspecified
Hereditary hemolytic anemia NOS

√4th **283 Acquired hemolytic anemias**
DEF: Non-hereditary anemia characterized by premature destruction of red
blood cells; caused by infectious organisms, poisons, and physical agents.

283.0 Autoimmune hemolytic anemias
Autoimmune hemolytic disease (cold type) (warm
type)
Chronic cold hemagglutinin disease
Cold agglutinin disease or hemoglobinuria
Hemolytic anemia:
cold type (secondary) (symptomatic)
drug-induced
warm type (secondary) (symptomatic)
Use additional E code to identify cause, if drug-
induced

EXCLUDES *Evans' syndrome (287.3)*
*hemolytic disease of newborn (773.0-
773.5)*

√5th **283.1 Non-autoimmune hemolytic anemias**
Use additional E code to identify cause

DEF: Hemolytic anemia and thrombocytopenia with acute renal
failure; relatively rare condition; 50 percent of patients require
renal dialysis.

**283.10 Non-autoimmune hemolytic anemia,
unspecified**
283.11 Hemolytic-uremic syndrome
**283.19 Other non-autoimmune hemolytic
anemias**
Hemolytic anemia:
mechanical
microangiopathic
toxic

**283.2 Hemoglobinuria due to hemolysis from external
causes**
Acute intravascular hemolysis
Hemoglobinuria:
from exertion
march
paroxysmal (cold) (nocturnal)
due to other hemolysis
Marchiafava-Micheli syndrome
Use additional E code to identify cause

283.9 Acquired hemolytic anemia, unspecified
Acquired hemolytic anemia NOS
Chronic idiopathic hemolytic anemia

√4th **284 Aplastic anemia**
DEF: Bone marrow failure to produce the normal amount of blood
components; generally non-responsive to usual therapy.

284.0 Constitutional aplastic anemia
Aplasia, (pure) red cell:
congenital
of infants
primary
Blackfan-Diamond syndrome
Familial hypoplastic anemia
Fanconi's anemia
Pancytopenia with malformations

284.8 Other specified aplastic anemias
Aplastic anemia (due to):
chronic systemic disease
drugs
infection
radiation
toxic (paralytic)
Pancytopenia (acquired)
Red cell aplasia (acquired) (adult) (pure) (with
thymoma)
Use additional E code to identify cause

284.9 Aplastic anemia, unspecified
Anemia:
aplastic (idiopathic) NOS
aregenerative
hypoplastic NOS
nonregenerative
refractory
Medullary hypoplasia

✓4ᵗʰ **285 Other and unspecified anemias**

285.0 Sideroblastic anemia
Anemia:
hypochromic with iron loading
sideroachrestic
sideroblastic
acquired
congenital
hereditary
primary
refractory
secondary (drug-induced) (due to disease)
sex-linked hypochromic
vitamin B₆-responsive
Pyridoxine-responsive (hypochromic) anemia
Use additional E code to identify cause, if drug
induced

DEF: Characterized by a disruption of final heme synthesis; results in iron overload of reticuloendothelial tissues.

285.1 Acute posthemorrhagic anemia
Anemia due to acute blood loss
EXCLUDES *anemia due to chronic blood loss (280.0)*
blood loss anemia NOS (280.0)

✓5ᵗʰ **285.2 Anemia in chronic illness**
285.21 Anemia in end-stage renal disease
285.22 Anemia in neoplastic disease
285.29 Anemia of other chronic illness

285.8 Other specified anemias
Anemia:
dyserythropoietic (congenital)
dyshematopoietic (congenital)
leukoerythroblastic
von Jaksch's
Infantile pseudoleukemia

285.9 Anemia, unspecified
Anemia:
NOS
essential
normocytic, not due to blood loss
profound
progressive
secondary
Oligocythemia
EXCLUDES *anemia (due to):*
blood loss:
acute (285.1)
chronic or unspecified (280.0)
iron deficiency (280.0-280.9)

✓4ᵗʰ **286 Coagulation defects**

286.0 Congenital factor VIII disorder
Antihemophilic globulin [AHG] deficiency
Factor VIII (functional) deficiency
Hemophilia:
NOS
A
classical
familial
hereditary
Subhemophilia
EXCLUDES *factor VIII deficiency with vascular defect (286.4)*

DEF: Hereditary, sex-linked, results in missing antihemophilic globulin (AHG) (factor VIII); causes abnormal coagulation characterized by increased tendency to bleeding, large bruises of skin, soft tissue; may also be bleeding in mouth, nose, gastrointestinal tract; after childhood, hemorrhages in joints, resulting in swelling and impaired function.

286.1 Congenital factor IX disorder
Christmas disease
Deficiency:
factor IX (functional)
plasma thromboplastin component [PTC]
Hemophilia B

DEF: Deficiency of plasma thromboplastin component (PTC) (factor IX) and plasma thromboplastin antecedent (PTA); PTC deficiency clinically indistinguishable from classical hemophilia; PTA deficiency found in both sexes.

286.2 Congenital factor XI deficiency
Hemophilia C
Plasma thromboplastin antecedent [PTA] deficiency
Rosenthal's disease

286.3 Congenital deficiency of other clotting factors
Congenital afibrinogenemia
Deficiency:
AC globulin factor:
I [fibrinogen]
II [prothrombin]
V [labile]
VII [stable]
X [Stuart-Prower]
XII [Hageman]
XIII [fibrin stabilizing]
Laki-Lorand factor
proaccelerin
Disease
Owren's
Stuart-Prower
Dysfibrinogenemia (congenital)
Dysprothrombinemia (constitutional)
Hypoproconvertinemia
Hypoprothrmbinemia (hereditary)
Parahemophilia

286.4 von Willebrand's disease
Angiohemophilia (A) (B)
Constitutional thrombopathy
Factor VIII deficiency with vascular defect
Pseudohemophilia type B
Vascular hemophilia
von Willebrand's (-Jürgens') disease
EXCLUDES *factor VIII deficiency:*
NOS (286.0)
with functional defect (286.0)
hereditary capillary fragility (287.8)

DEF: Abnormal blood coagulation caused by deficient blood Factor VII; congenital; symptoms include excess or prolonged bleeding, such as hemorrhage during menstruation, following birthing, or after surgical procedure.

Blood and Blood-Forming Organs 284.9–286.4

✓4ᵗʰ / ✓5ᵗʰ   Additional Digit Required   Unspecified Code   Other Specified Code   Manifestation Code   ▶◀ Revised Text   ● New Code   ▲ Revised Code Title

2003 ICD•9•CM   **Volume 1 — 59**

286.5 Hemorrhagic disorder due to circulating anticoagulants
Antithrombinemia
Antithromboplastinemia
Antithromboplastino-genemia
Hyperheparinemia
Increase in:
anti-VIIIa
anti-IXa
anti-Xa
anti-XIa
antithrombin
Systemic lupus erythematosus [SLE] inhibitor
Use additional E code to identify cause, if drug induced

286.6 Defibrination syndrome
Afibrinogenemia, acquired
Consumption coagulopathy
Diffuse or disseminated intravascular coagulation [DIC syndrome]
Fibrinolytic hemorrhage, acquired
Hemorrhagic fibrinogenolysis
Pathologic fibrinolysis
Purpura:
fibrinolytic
fulminans

EXCLUDES   *that complicating:*
abortion (634-638 with .1, 639.1)
pregnancy or the puerperium (641.3, 666.3)
disseminated intravascular coagulation in newborn (776.2)

DEF: Characterized by destruction of circulating fibrinogen; often precipitated by other conditions, such as injury, causing release of thromboplastic particles in blood stream.

286.7 Acquired coagulation factor deficiency
Deficiency of coagulation factor due to:
liver disease
vitamin K deficiency
Hypoprothrombinemia, acquired
Use additional E code to identify cause, if drug induced

EXCLUDES   *vitamin K deficiency of newborn (776.0)*

286.9 Other and unspecified coagulation defects
Defective coagulation NOS
Deficiency, coagulation factor NOS
Delay, coagulation
Disorder:
coagulation
hemostasis

EXCLUDES   *abnormal coagulation profile (790.92)*
hemorrhagic disease of newborn (776.0)
that complicating:
abortion (634-638 with .1, 639.1)
pregnancy or the puerperium (641.3, 666.3)

✓4ᵗʰ **287 Purpura and other hemorrhagic conditions**
EXCLUDES   *hemorrhagic thrombocythemia (238.7)*
purpura fulminans (286.6)

287.0 Allergic purpura
Peliosis rheumatica   Purpura:
Purpura: rheumatica
anaphylactoid   Schönlein-Henoch
autoimmune   vascular
Henoch's   Vasculitis, allergic
nonthrombocytopenic:
hemorrhagic
idiopathic

EXCLUDES   *hemorrhagic purpura (287.3)*
purpura annularis telangiectodes (709.1)

DEF: Any hemorrhagic condition, thrombocytic or nonthrombocytopenic in origin, caused by a presumed allergic reaction.

287.1 Qualitative platelet defects
Thrombasthenia (hemorrhagic) (hereditary)
Thrombocytasthenia
Thrombocytopathy (dystrophic)
Thrombopathy (Bernard-Soulier)

EXCLUDES   *von Willebrand's disease (286.4)*

287.2 Other nonthrombocytopenic purpuras
Purpura:
NOS
senile
simplex

287.3 Primary thrombocytopenia
Evans' syndrome
Megakaryocytic hypoplasia
Purpura, thrombocytopenic
congenital
hereditary
idiopathic
Throbocytopenia:
congenital
hereditary
primary
Tidal platelet dysgenesis

EXCLUDES   *thrombotic thrombocytopenic purpura (446.6)*
transient thrombocytopenia of newborn (776.1)

DEF: Decrease in number of blood platelets in circulating blood and purpural skin hemorrhages.

287.4 Secondary thrombocytopenia
Posttransfusion purpura
Thrombocytopenia (due to):
dilutional
drugs
extracorporeal circulation of blood
platelet alloimmunization
Use additional E code to identify cause

EXCLUDES   *transient thrombocytopenia of newborn (776.1)*

DEF: Reduced number of platelets in circulating blood as consequence of an underlying disease or condition.

287.5 Thrombocytopenia, unspecified

287.8 Other specified hemorrhagic conditions
Capillary fragility (hereditary)
Vascular pseudohemophilia

287.9 Unspecified hemorrhagic conditions
Hemorrhagic diathesis (familial)

✓4th **288 Diseases of white blood cells**
> **EXCLUDES** *leukemia (204.0-208.9)*

288.0 Agranulocytosis
Infantile genetic agranulocytosis
Kostmann's syndrome
Neutropenia:
 NOS
 cyclic
 drug-induced
 immune
 periodic
 toxic
Neutropenic splenomegaly
Use additional E code to identify drug or other cause
> **EXCLUDES** *transitory neonatal neutropenia (776.7)*

DEF: Sudden, severe condition characterized by reduced number of white blood cells; results in sores in the throat, stomach or skin; symptoms include chills, fever; some drugs can bring on condition.

288.1 Functional disorders of polymorphonuclear neutrophils
Chronic (childhood) granulomatous disease
Congenital dysphagocytosis
Job's syndrome
Lipochrome histiocytosis (familial)
Progressive septic granulomatosis

288.2 Genetic anomalies of leukocytes
Anomaly (granulation) (granulocyte) or syndrome:
 Alder's (-Reilly)
 Chédiak-Steinbrinck (-Higashi)
 Jordan's
 May-Hegglin
 Pelger-Huet
Hereditary:
 hypersegmentation
 hyposegmentation
 leukomelanopathy

288.3 Eosinophilia
Eosinophilia:
 allergic
 hereditary
 idiopathic
 secondary
Eosinophilic leukocytosis
> **EXCLUDES** *Löffler's syndrome (518.3)*
> *pulmonary eosinophilia (518.3)*

DEF: Elevated number of eosinophils in the blood; characteristic of allergic states and various parasitic infections.

288.8 Other specified disease of white blood cells
Leukemoid reaction
 lymphocytic
 monocytic
 myelocytic
Leukocytosis
Lymphocytopenia
Lymphocytosis (symptomatic)
Lymphopenia
Monocytosis (symptomatic)
Plasmacytosis
> **EXCLUDES** *immunity disorders (279.0-279.9)*

288.9 Unspecified disease of white blood cells

✓4th **289 Other diseases of blood and blood-forming organs**

289.0 Polycythemia, secondary
High-oxygen-affinity hemoglobin
Polycythemia:
 acquired
 benign
 due to:
  fall in plasma volume
  high altitude
 emotional
 erythropoietin
 hypoxemic
 nephrogenous
 relative
 spurious
 stress
> **EXCLUDES** *polycythemia:*
> *neonatal (776.4)*
> *primary (238.4)*
> *vera (238.4)*

DEF: Elevated number of red blood cells in circulating blood as result of reduced oxygen supply to the tissues.

289.1 Chronic lymphadenitis
Chronic:
 adenitis } any lymph node, except
 lymphadenitis } mesenteric
> **EXCLUDES** *acute lymphadenitis (683)*
> *mesenteric (289.2)*
> *enlarged glands NOS (785.6)*

DEF: Persistent inflammation of lymph node tissue; origin of infection is usually elsewhere.

289.2 Nonspecific mesenteric lymphadenitis
Mesenteric lymphadenitis (acute) (chronic)

DEF: Inflammation of the lymph nodes in peritoneal fold that encases abdominal organs; disease resembles acute appendicitis; unknown etiology.

289.3 Lymphadenitis, unspecified, except mesenteric

289.4 Hypersplenism
"Big spleen" syndrome   Hypersplenia
Dyssplenism
> **EXCLUDES** *primary splenic neutropenia (288.0)*

DEF: An overactive spleen; it causes a deficiency of the peripheral blood components, an increase in bone marrow cells and sometimes a notable increase in the size of the spleen.

✓5th ### 289.5 Other diseases of spleen
289.50 Disease of spleen, unspecified
289.51 Chronic congestive splenomegaly
289.59 Other
Lien migrans   Splenic:
Perisplenitis   fibrosis
Splenic: infarction
 abscess   rupture, nontraumatic
 atrophy   Splenitis
 cyst   Wandering spleen
> **EXCLUDES** *bilharzial splenic fibrosis*
> *(120.0-120.9)*
> *hepatolienal fibrosis (571.5)*
> *splenomegaly NOS (789.2)*

289.6 Familial polycythemia
Familial:
 benign polycythemia
 erythrocytosis

DEF: Elevated number of red blood cells.

✓4th ✓5th Additional Digit Required   Unspecified Code   Other Specified Code   Manifestation Code   ►◄ Revised Text   ● New Code   ▲ Revised Code Title

2003 ICD•9•CM   **Volume 1 — 61**

Blood and Blood-Forming Organs 288–289.6

289.7 **Methemoglobinemia**

Congenital NADH [DPNH]-methemoglobin-reductase deficiency

Hemoglobin M [Hb-M] disease

Methemoglobinemia:

NOS

acquired (with sulfhemoglobinemia)

hereditary

toxic

Stokvis' disease

Sulfhemoglobinemia

Use additional E code to identify cause

DEF: Presence in the blood of methemoglobin, a chemically altered form of hemoglobin; causes cyanosis, headache, dizziness, ataxia dyspnea, tachycardia, nausea, stupor, coma, and, rarely, death.

289.8 **Other specified diseases of blood and blood-forming organs**

Hypergammaglobulinemia

Myelofibrosis

Pseudocholinesterase deficiency

289.9 **Unspecified diseases of blood and blood-forming organs**

Blood dyscrasia NOS

Erythroid hyperplasia

5. MENTAL DISORDERS (290-319)

In the *International Classification of Diseases, 9th Revision* (ICD-9), the corresponding Chapter V, "Mental Disorders," includes a glossary which defines the contents of each category. The introduction to Chapter V in ICD-9 indicates that the glossary is intended so that psychiatrists can make the diagnosis based on the descriptions provided rather than from the category titles. Lay coders are instructed to code whatever diagnosis the physician records.

Chapter 5, "Mental Disorders," in ICD-9-CM uses the standard classification format with inclusion and exclusion terms, omitting the glossary as part of the main text.

The mental disorders section of ICD-9-CM has been expanded to incorporate additional psychiatric disorders not listed in ICD-9. The glossary from ICD-9 does not contain all these terms. It now appears in Appendix B, which also contains descriptions and definitions for the terms added in ICD-9-CM. Some of these were provided by the American Psychiatric Association's Task Force on Nomenclature and Statistics who are preparing the Diagnostic and Statistical Manual, Third Edition (DSM-III), and others from A Psychiatric Glossary.

The American Psychiatric Association provided invaluable assistance in modifying Chapter 5 of ICD-9-CM to incorporate detail useful to American clinicians and gave permission to use material from the aforementioned sources.

1. Manual of the *International Statistical Classification of Diseases, Injuries, and Causes of Death, 9th Revision,* World Health Organization, Geneva, Switzerland, 1975.

2. American Psychiatric Association, Task Force on Nomenclature and Statistics, Robert L. Spitzer, M.D., Chairman.

3. *A Psychiatric Glossary,* Fourth Edition, American Psychiatric Association, Washington, D.C., 1975.

PSYCHOSES (290-299)

EXCLUDES   *mental retardation (317-319)*

ORGANIC PSYCHOTIC CONDITIONS (290-294)

INCLUDES   psychotic organic brain syndrome

EXCLUDES   *nonpsychotic syndromes of organic etiology (310.0-310.9)*
psychoses classifiable to 295-298 and without impairment of orientation, comprehension, calculation, learning capacity, and judgment, but associated with physical disease, injury, or condition affecting the brain [eg., following childbirth] (295.0-298.8)

✓4th **290 Senile and presenile organic psychotic conditions**
Code first the associated neurological condition

EXCLUDES   *dementia not classified as senile, presenile, or arteriosclerotic (294.10-294.11)*
psychoses classifiable to 295-298 occurring in the senium without dementia or delirium (295.0-298.8)
senility with mental changes of nonpsychotic severity (310.1)
transient organic psychotic conditions (293.0-293.9)

290.0 Senile dementia, uncomplicated   A
Senile dementia:
  NOS
  simple type

EXCLUDES   *mild memory disturbances, not amounting to dementia, associated with senile brain disease (310.1)*
senile dementia with:
  delirium or confusion (290.3)
  delusional [paranoid] features (290.20)
  depressive features (290.21)

✓5th **290.1 Presenile dementia**
Brain syndrome with presenile brain disease

EXCLUDES   *arteriosclerotic dementia (290.40-290.43)*
dementia associated with other cerebral conditions (294.10-294.11)

290.10 Presenile dementia, uncomplicated   A
Presenile dementia:
  NOS
  simple type

290.11 Presenile dementia with delirium   A
Presenile dementia with acute confusional state

290.12 Presenile dementia with delusional features   A
Presenile dementia, paranoid type

290.13 Presenile dementia with depressive features   A
Presenile dementia, depressed type

✓5th **290.2 Senile dementia with delusional or depressive features**

EXCLUDES   *senile dementia:*
  NOS (290.0)
  with delirium and/or confusion (290.3)

290.20 Senile dementia with delusional features   A
Senile dementia, paranoid type
Senile psychosis NOS

290.21 Senile dementia with depressive features   A

290.3 Senile dementia with delirium   A
Senile dementia with acute confusional state

EXCLUDES   *senile:*
  dementia NOS (290.0)
  psychosis NOS (290.20)

✓5th **290.4 Arteriosclerotic dementia**
Multi-infarct dementia or psychosis
Use additional code to identify cerebral atherosclerosis (437.0)

EXCLUDES   *suspected cases with no clear evidence of arteriosclerosis (290.9)*

290.40 Arteriosclerotic dementia, uncomplicated   A
Arteriosclerotic dementia:
  NOS
  simple type

290.41 Arteriosclerotic dementia with delirium   A
Arteriosclerotic dementia with acute confusional state

290.42 Arteriosclerotic dementia with delusional features   A
Arteriosclerotic dementia, paranoid type

290.43 Arteriosclerotic dementia with depressive features   A
Arteriosclerotic dementia, depressed type

290.8 Other specified senile psychotic conditions
Presbyophrenic psychosis

290.9 Unspecified senile psychotic condition   A

✓4th **291 Alcoholic psychoses**

EXCLUDES   *alcoholism without psychosis (303.0-303.9)*

291.0 Alcohol withdrawal delirium
Alcoholic delirium
Delirium tremens

EXCLUDES   *alcohol withdrawal (291.81)*

Mental Disorders 290–291.0

✓4th
✓5th Additional Digit Required   Unspecified Code   Other Specified Code   Manifestation Code   ▶◀ Revised Text   ● New Code   ▲ Revised Code Title

2003 ICD•9•CM   Volume 1 — 63

291.1 Alcohol amnestic syndrome
Alcoholic polyneuritic psychosis
Korsakoff's psychosis, alcoholic
Wernicke-Korsakoff syndrome (alcoholic)
DEF: Prominent and lasting reduced memory span, disordered time appreciation and confabulation, occurring in alcoholics, as sequel to acute alcoholic psychosis.

291.2 Other alcoholic dementia
Alcoholic dementia NOS
Alcoholism associated with dementia NOS
Chronic alcoholic brain syndrome

291.3 Alcohol withdrawal hallucinosis
Alcoholic:
hallucinosis (acute)
psychosis with hallucinosis
EXCLUDES   alcohol withdrawal with delirium
(291.0)
schizophrenia (295.0-295.9) and
paranoid states (297.0-297.9)
taking the form of chronic
hallucinosis with clear
consciousness in an alcoholic
DEF: Psychosis lasting less than six months with slight or no clouding of consciousness in which auditory hallucinations predominate.

291.4 Idiosyncratic alcohol intoxication
Pathologic:
alcohol intoxication
drunkenness
EXCLUDES   acute alcohol intoxication (305.0)
in alcoholism (303.0)
simple drunkenness (305.0)
DEF: Unique behavioral patterns, like belligerence, after intake of relatively small amounts of alcohol; behavior not due to excess consumption.

291.5 Alcoholic jealousy
Alcoholic:
paranoia
psychosis, paranoid type
EXCLUDES   nonalcoholic paranoid states (297.0-
297.9)
schizophrenia, paranoid type (295.3)

✓5ᵗʰ **291.8 Other specified alcoholic psychosis**
291.81 Alcohol withdrawal
Alcohol:
abstinence syndrome or symptoms
withdrawal syndrome or symptoms
EXCLUDES   alcohol withdrawal:
delirium (291.0)
hallucinosis (291.3)
delirium tremens (291.0)

291.89 Other
291.9 Unspecified alcoholic psychosis
Alcoholic:
mania NOS
psychosis NOS
Alcoholism (chronic) with psychosis

✓4ᵗʰ **292 Drug psychoses**
INCLUDES   drug-induced mental disorders
organic brain syndrome associated with
consumption of drugs
Use additional code for any associated drug dependence
(304.0-304.9)
Use additional E code to identify drug
292.0 Drug withdrawal syndrome
Drug:
abstinence syndrome or symptoms
withdrawal syndrome or symptoms

✓5ᵗʰ **292.1 Paranoid and/or hallucinatory states induced by drugs**
292.11 Drug-induced organic delusional syndrome
Paranoid state induced by drugs
292.12 Drug-induced hallucinosis
Hallucinatory state induced by drugs
EXCLUDES   states following LSD or other
hallucinogens, lasting
only a few days or less
["bad trips"] (305.3)

292.2 Pathological drug intoxication
Drug reaction:
NOS
idiosyncratic   resulting in brief psychotic
pathologic   states

EXCLUDES   expected brief psychotic reactions to
hallucinogens ["bad trips"] (305.3)
physiological side-effects of drugs (e.g.,
dystonias)

✓5ᵗʰ **292.8 Other specified drug-induced mental disorders**
292.81 Drug-induced delirium
292.82 Drug-induced dementia
292.83 Drug-induced amnestic syndrome
292.84 Drug-induced organic affective syndrome
Depressive state induced by drugs
292.89 Other
Drug-induced organic personality syndrome
292.9 Unspecified drug-induced mental disorder
Organic psychosis NOS due to or associated with
drugs

✓4ᵗʰ **293 Transient organic psychotic conditions**
INCLUDES   transient organic mental disorders not
associated with alcohol or drugs
Code first the associated physical or neurological condition
EXCLUDES   confusional state or delirium superimposed on
senile dementia (290.3)
dementia due to:
alcohol (291.0-291.9)
arteriosclerosis (290.40-290.43)
drugs (292.82)
senility (290.0)

293.0 Acute delirium
Acute:
confusional state
infective psychosis
organic reaction
posttraumatic organic psychosis
psycho-organic syndrome
Acute psychosis associated with endocrine,
metabolic, or cerebrovascular disorder
Epileptic:
confusional state
twilight state

293.1 Subacute delirium
Subacute:
confusional state
infective psychosis
organic reaction
posttraumatic organic psychosis
psycho-organic syndrome
psychosis associated with endocrine or metabolic
disorder

✓5ᵗʰ **293.8 Other specified transient organic mental disorders**
293.81 Organic delusional syndrome
Transient organic psychotic condition,
paranoid type
293.82 Organic hallucinosis syndrome
Transient organic psychotic condition,
hallucinatory type

N Newborn Age: 0   P Pediatric Age: 0-17   M Maternity Age: 12-55   A Adult Age: 15-124   MSP Medicare Secondary Payer

293.83 Organic affective syndrome
Transient organic psychotic condition,
depressive type

293.84 Organic anxiety syndrome

293.89 Other

293.9 Unspecified transient organic mental disorder
Organic psychosis:
infective NOS
posttraumatic NOS
transient NOS
Psycho-organic syndrome

✓4th 294 Other organic psychotic conditions (chronic)
INCLUDES organic psychotic brain syndromes (chronic),
not elsewhere classified

294.0 Amnestic syndrome
Korsakoff's psychosis or syndrome (nonalcoholic)
EXCLUDES alcoholic:
amnestic syndrome (291.1)
Korsakoff's psychosis (291.1)

✓5th 294.1 Dementia in conditions classified elsewhere
Code first any underlying physical condition, as:
dementia in:
Alzheimer's disease (331.0)
cerebral lipidoses (330.1)
epilepsy (345.0-345.9)
general paresis [syphilis] (094.1)
hepatolenticular degeneration (275.1)
Huntington's chorea (333.4)
Jakob-Creutzfeldt disease (046.1)
multiple sclerosis (340)
Pick's disease of the brain (331.1)
polyarteritis nodosa (446.0)
syphilis (094.1)
EXCLUDES dementia:
arteriosclerotic (290.40-290.43)
presenile (290.10-290.13)
senile (290.0)
epileptic psychosis NOS (294.8)

294.10 Dementia in conditions classified elsewhere without behavioral disturbance
Dementia in conditions classified elsewhere NOS

294.11 Dementia in conditions classified elsewhere with behavioral disturbance
Aggressive behavior   Violent behavior
Combative behavior   Wandering off

294.8 Other specified organic brain syndromes (chronic)
Epileptic psychosis NOS
Mixed paranoid and affective organic psychotic states
Use additional code for associated epilepsy (345.0-345.9)
EXCLUDES mild memory disturbances, not amounting to dementia (310.1)

294.9 Unspecified organic brain syndrome (chronic)
Organic psychosis (chronic)

OTHER PSYCHOSES (295-299)
Use additional code to identify any associated physical disease, injury, or condition affecting the brain with psychoses classifiable to 295-298

✓4th 295 Schizophrenic disorders
INCLUDES schizophrenia of the types described in 295.0-295.9 occurring in children
EXCLUDES childhood type schizophrenia (299.9)
infantile autism (299.0)

The following fifth-digit subclassification is for use with category 295:
0 unspecified
1 subchronic
2 chronic
3 subchronic with acute exacerbation
4 chronic with acute exacerbation
5 in remission

DEF: Group of disorders with disturbances in thought (delusions, hallucinations), mood (blunted, flattened, inappropriate affect), sense of self, relationship to world; also bizarre, purposeless behavior, repetitive activity, or inactivity.

✓5th 295.0 Simple type
Schizophrenia simplex
EXCLUDES latent schizophrenia (295.5)

✓5th 295.1 Disorganized type
Hebephrenia
Hebephrenic type schizophrenia
DEF: Inappropriate behavior; results in extreme incoherence and disorganization of time, place and sense of social appropriateness; withdrawal from routine social interaction may occur.

✓5th 295.2 Catatonic type
Catatonic (schizophrenia):   Schizophrenic:
agitation   catalepsy
excitation   catatonia
excited type   flexibilitas cerea
stupor
withdrawn type
DEF: Extreme changes in motor activity; one extreme is decreased response or reaction to the environment and the other is spontaneous activity.

✓5th 295.3 Paranoid type
Paraphrenic schizophrenia
EXCLUDES involutional paranoid state (297.2)
paranoia (297.1)
paraphrenia (297.2)
DEF: Preoccupied with delusional suspicions and auditory hallucinations related to single theme; usually hostile, grandiose, overly religious, occasionally hypochondriacal.

✓5th 295.4 Acute schizophrenic episode
Oneirophrenia   Schizophreniform:
Schizophreniform: disorder
attack   psychosis, confusional type
EXCLUDES acute forms of schizophrenia of:
catatonic type (295.2)
hebephrenic type (295.1)
paranoid type (295.3)
simple type (295.0)
undifferentiated type (295.8)

✓5th 295.5 Latent schizophrenia
Latent schizophrenic reaction
Schizophrenia:
borderline
incipient
prepsychotic
prodromal
pseudoneurotic
pseudopsychopathic
EXCLUDES schizoid personality (301.20-301.22)

Mental Disorders 293.83–295.5

Mental Disorders 295.6–296.99

§ ✓5ᵗʰ **295.6 Residual schizophrenia**
Chronic undifferentiated schizophrenia
Restzustand (schizophrenic)
Schizophrenic residual state

§ ✓5ᵗʰ **295.7 Schizo-affective type**
Cyclic schizophrenia
Mixed schizophrenic and affective psychosis
Schizo-affective psychosis
Schizophreniform psychosis, affective type

§ ✓5ᵗʰ **295.8 Other specified types of schizophrenia**
Acute (undifferentiated) schizophrenia
Atypical schizophrenia
Cenesthopathic schizophrenia
EXCLUDES *infantile autism (299.0)*

§ ✓5ᵗʰ **295.9 Unspecified schizophrenia**
Schizophrenia:
  NOS
  mixed NOS
  undifferentiated NOS
Schizophrenic reaction NOS
Schizophreniform psychosis NOS

✓4ᵗʰ **296 Affective psychoses**
INCLUDES episodic affective disorders
EXCLUDES *neurotic depression (300.4)*
reactive depressive psychosis (298.0)
reactive excitation (298.1)

The following fifth-digit subclassification is for use with categories 296.0-296.6:
  0 unspecified
  1 mild
  2 moderate
  3 severe, without mention of psychotic behavior
  4 severe, specified as with psychotic behavior
  5 in partial or unspecified remission
  6 in full remission

✓5ᵗʰ **296.0 Manic disorder, single episode**
Hypomania (mild) NOS
Hypomanic psychosis
Mania (monopolar) NOS
Manic-depressive psychosis
  or reaction: } single episode or unspecified
    hypomanic
    manic
EXCLUDES *circular type, if there was a previous attack of depression (296.4)*

DEF: Mood disorder identified by hyperactivity; may show extreme agitation or exaggerated excitability; speech and thought processes may be accelerated.

✓5ᵗʰ **296.1 Manic disorder, recurrent episode**
Any condition classifiable to 296.0, stated to be recurrent
EXCLUDES *circular type, if there was a previous attack of depression (296.4)*

✓5ᵗʰ **296.2 Major depressive disorder, single episode**
Depressive psychosis
Endogenous depression
Involutional melancholia
Manic-depressive psychosis
  or reaction,   } single episode or unspecified
    depressed type
Monopolar depression
Psychotic depression
EXCLUDES *circular type, if previous attack was of manic type (296.5)*
depression NOS (311)
reactive depression (neurotic) (300.4)
psychotic (298.0)

DEF: Mood disorder that produces depression; may exhibit as sadness, low self-esteem, or guilt feelings; other manifestations may be withdrawal from friends and family; interrupted normal sleep.

✓5ᵗʰ **296.3 Major depressive disorder, recurrent episode**
Any condition classifiable to 296.2, stated to be recurrent
EXCLUDES *circular type, if previous attack was of manic type (296.5)*
depression NOS (311)
reactive depression (neurotic) (300.4)
psychotic (298.0)

✓5ᵗʰ **296.4 Bipolar affective disorder, manic**
Bipolar disorder, now manic
Manic-depressive psychosis, circular type but currently manic
EXCLUDES *brief compensatory or rebound mood swings (296.99)*

✓5ᵗʰ **296.5 Bipolar affective disorder, depressed**
Bipolar disorder, now depressed
Manic-depressive psychosis, circular type but currently depressed
EXCLUDES *brief compensatory or rebound mood swings (296.99)*

✓5ᵗʰ **296.6 Bipolar affective disorder, mixed**
Manic-depressive psychosis, circular type, mixed

296.7 Bipolar affective disorder, unspecified
Atypical bipolar affective disorder NOS
Manic-depressive psychosis, circular type, current condition not specified as either manic or depressive

DEF: Manic-depressive disorder referred to as bipolar because of the mood range from manic to depressive.

✓5ᵗʰ **296.8 Manic-depressive psychosis, other and unspecified**
296.80 Manic-depressive psychosis, unspecified
Manic-depressive:
  reaction NOS
  syndrome NOS
296.81 Atypical manic disorder
296.82 Atypical depressive disorder
296.89 Other
Manic-depressive psychosis, mixed type

✓5ᵗʰ **296.9 Other and unspecified affective psychoses**
EXCLUDES *psychogenic affective psychoses (298.0-298.8)*
296.90 Unspecified affective psychosis
Affective psychosis NOS
Melancholia NOS
296.99 Other specified affective psychoses
Mood swings:
  brief compensatory
  rebound

---

§ Requres fifth-digit. See beginning of category 295 for codes and definitions.

✓4ᵗʰ **297 Paranoid states (Delusional disorders)**
     INCLUDES   paranoid disorders
     EXCLUDES   *acute paranoid reaction (298.3)*
                    alcoholic jealousy or paranoid state (291.5)
                    paranoid schizophrenia (295.3)

297.0 Paranoid state, simple

297.1 Paranoia
     Chronic paranoid psychosis
     Sander's disease
     Systematized delusions
     EXCLUDES   *paranoid personality disorder (301.0)*

297.2 Paraphrenia
     Involutional paranoid state   Paraphrenia
                           (involutional)
     Late paraphrenia
     DEF: Paranoid schizophrenic disorder that persists over a
     prolonged period but does not distort personality despite persistent
     delusions.

297.3 Shared paranoid disorder
     Folie à deux
     Induced psychosis or paranoid disorder
     DEF: Mental disorder two people share; first person with the
     delusional disorder convinces second person because of a close
     relationship and shared experiences to accept the delusions.

297.8 Other specified paranoid states
     Paranoia querulans   Sensitiver Beziehungswahn
     EXCLUDES   *acute paranoid reaction or state (298.3)*
                    senile paranoid state (290.20)

297.9 Unspecified paranoid state
     Paranoid:
         disorder NOS
         psychosis NOS
         reaction NOS
         state NOS

✓4ᵗʰ **298 Other nonorganic psychoses**
     INCLUDES   psychotic conditions due to or provoked by:
                    emotional stress
                    environmental factors as major part of
                    etiology

298.0 Depressive type psychosis
     Psychogenic depressive psychosis
     Psychotic reactive depression
     Reactive depressive psychosis
     EXCLUDES   *manic-depressive psychosis, depressed*
                    type (296.2-296.3)
                    neurotic depression (300.4)
                    reactive depression NOS (300.4)

298.1 Excitative type psychosis
     Acute hysterical psychosis   Reactive excitation
     Psychogenic excitation
     EXCLUDES   *manic-depressive psychosis, manic*
                    type (296.0-296.1)
     DEF: Affective disorder similar to manic-depressive psychosis, in
     the manic phase, seemingly brought on by stress.

298.2 Reactive confusion
     Psychogenic confusion
     Psychogenic twilight state
     EXCLUDES   *acute confusional state (293.0)*
     DEF: Confusion, disorientation, cloudiness in consciousness;
     brought on by severe emotional upheaval.

298.3 Acute paranoid reaction
     Acute psychogenic paranoid psychosis
     Bouffée délirante
     EXCLUDES   *paranoid states (297.0-297.9)*

298.4 Psychogenic paranoid psychosis
     Protracted reactive paranoid psychosis

298.8 Other and unspecified reactive psychosis
     Brief reactive psychosis NOS
     Hysterical psychosis
     Psychogenic psychosis NOS
     Psychogenic stupor
     EXCLUDES   *acute hysterical psychosis (298.1)*

298.9 Unspecified psychosis
     Atypical psychosis
     Psychosis NOS

✓4ᵗʰ **299 Psychoses with origin specific to childhood**
     INCLUDES   pervasive developmental disorders
     EXCLUDES   *adult type psychoses occurring in childhood, as:*
                    affective disorders (296.0-296.9)
                    manic-depressive disorders (296.0-296.9)
                    schizophrenia (295.0-295.9)

The following fifth-digit subclassification is for use with
category 299:
         0 current or active state
         1 residual state

✓5ᵗʰ **299.0 Infantile autism**
     Childhood autism
     Infantile psychosis
     Kanner's syndrome
     EXCLUDES   *disintegrative psychosis (299.1)*
                    Heller's syndrome (299.1)
                    schizophrenic syndrome of childhood
                       (299.9)
     DEF: Severe mental disorder of children, results in impaired social
     behavior; abnormal development of communicative skills, appears
     to be unaware of the need for emotional support and offers little
     emotional response to family members.

✓5ᵗʰ **299.1 Disintegrative psychosis**
     Heller's syndrome
     Use additional code to identify any associated
         neurological disorder
     EXCLUDES   *infantile autism (299.0)*
                    schizophrenic syndrome of childhood
                       (299.9)
     DEF: Mental disease of children identified by impaired development
     of reciprocal social skills, verbal and nonverbal communication
     skills, imaginative play.

✓5ᵗʰ **299.8 Other specified early childhood psychoses**
     Atypical childhood psychosis
     Borderline psychosis of childhood
     EXCLUDES   *simple stereotypes without psychotic*
                    disturbance (307.3)

✓5ᵗʰ **299.9 Unspecified**
     Child psychosis NOS
     Schizophrenia, childhood type NOS
     Schizophrenic syndrome of childhood NOS
     EXCLUDES   *schizophrenia of adult type occurring in*
                    childhood (295.0-295.9)

NEUROTIC DISORDERS, PERSONALITY DISORDERS, AND OTHER NONPSYCHOTIC MENTAL DISORDERS (300-316)

✓4ᵗʰ **300 Neurotic disorders**

✓5ᵗʰ **300.0 Anxiety states**
     EXCLUDES   *anxiety in:*
                    acute stress reaction (308.0)
                    transient adjustment reaction
                       (309.24)
                    neurasthenia (300.5)
                    psychophysiological disorders (306.0-
                       306.9)
                    separation anxiety (309.21)
     DEF: Mental disorder characterized by anxiety and avoidance
     behavior not particularly related to any specific situation or
     stimulus; symptoms include emotional instability, apprehension,
     fatigue.

✓4ᵗʰ / ✓5ᵗʰ Additional Digit Required   Unspecified Code   Other Specified Code   Manifestation Code   ►◄ Revised Text   ● New Code   ▲ Revised Code Title

2003 ICD•9•CM   **Volume 1 — 67**

300.00 Anxiety state, unspecified

Anxiety:	Anxiety:
neurosis	state (neurotic)
reaction	Atypical anxiety disorder

300.01 Panic disorder

Panic:

    attack

    state

DEF: Neurotic disorder characterized by recurrent panic or anxiety, apprehension, fear or terror; symptoms include shortness of breath, palpitations, dizziness, faintness or shakiness; fear of dying may persist or fear of other morbid consequences.

300.02 Generalized anxiety disorder

300.09 Other

√5th **300.1 Hysteria**

    EXCLUDES   *adjustment reaction (309.0-309.9)*

        anorexia nervosa (307.1)

        gross stress reaction (308.0-308.9)

        hysterical personality (301.50-301.59)

        psychophysiologic disorders (306.0-306.9)

300.10 Hysteria, unspecified

300.11 Conversion disorder

Astasia-abasia, hysterical

Conversion hysteria or reaction

Hysterical

    blindness

    deafness

    paralysis

DEF: Mental disorder that impairs physical functions with no physiological basis; sensory motor symptoms include seizures, paralysis, temporary blindness; increase in stress or avoidance of unpleasant responsibilities may precipitate.

300.12 Psychogenic amnesia

Hysterical amnesia

300.13 Psychogenic fugue

Hysterical fugue

DEF: Dissociative hysteria; identified by loss of memory, flight from familiar surroundings; conscious activity is not associated with perception of surroundings, no later memory of episode.

300.14 Multiple personality

Dissociative identity disorder

300.15 Dissociative disorder or reaction, unspecified

DEF: Hysterical neurotic episode; sudden but temporary changes in perceived identity, memory, consciousness, segregated memory patterns exist separate from dominant personality.

300.16 Factitious illness with psychological symptoms

Compensation neurosis

Ganser's syndrome, hysterical

DEF: A disorder characterized by the purposeful assumption of mental illness symptoms; the symptoms are not real, possibly representing what the patient imagines mental illness to be like, and are acted out more often when another person is present.

300.19 Other and unspecified factitious illness

Factitious illness (with physical symptoms) NOS

    EXCLUDES   *multiple operations or hospital addiction syndrome (301.51)*

√5th **300.2 Phobic disorders**

    EXCLUDES   *anxiety state not associated with a specific situation or object (300.00-300.09)*

        obsessional phobias (300.3)

300.20 Phobia, unspecified

Anxiety-hysteria NOS

Phobia NOS

300.21 Agoraphobia with panic attacks

Fear of:

    open spaces

    streets   } with panic

    travel   attacks

300.22 Agoraphobia without mention of panic attacks

Any condition classifiable to 300.21 without mention of panic attacks

300.23 Social phobia

Fear of:	Fear of:
eating in public	washing in public
public speaking	

300.29 Other isolated or simple phobias

Acrophobia	Claustrophobia
Animal phobias	Fear of crowds

300.3 Obsessive-compulsive disorders

Anancastic neurosis	Obsessional phobia [any]
Compulsive neurosis	

    EXCLUDES   *obsessive-compulsive symptoms occurring in:*

        endogenous depression (296.2-296.3)

        organic states (eg., encephalitis)

        schizophrenia (295.0-295.9)

300.4 Neurotic depression

Anxiety depression	Dysthymic disorder
Depression with anxiety	Neurotic depressive state
Depressive reaction	Reactive depression

    EXCLUDES   *adjustment reaction with depressive symptoms (309.0-309.1)*

        depression NOS (311)

        manic-depressive psychosis, depressed type (296.2-296.3)

        reactive depressive psychosis (298.0)

DEF: Depression without psychosis; less severe depression related to personal change or unexpected circumstances; also referred to as "reactional depression."

300.5 Neurasthenia

Fatigue neurosis

Nervous debility

Psychogenic:

    asthenia

    general fatigue

Use additional code to identify any associated physical disorder

    EXCLUDES   *anxiety state (300.00-300.09)*

        neurotic depression (300.4)

        psychophysiological disorders (306.0-306.9)

        specific nonpsychotic mental disorders following organic brain damage (310.0-310.9)

DEF: Physical and mental symptoms caused primarily by what is known as mental exhaustion; symptoms include chronic weakness, fatigue.

300.6 Depersonalization syndrome
Depersonalization disorder
Derealization (neurotic)
Neurotic state with depersonalization episode
> EXCLUDES   depersonalization associated with:
>   anxiety (300.00-300.09)
>   depression (300.4)
>   manic-depressive disorder or
>   psychosis (296.0-296.9)
>   schizophrenia (295.0-295.9)

DEF: Dissociative disorder characterized by feelings of strangeness about self or body image; symptoms include dizziness, anxiety, fear of insanity, loss of reality of surroundings.

300.7 Hypochondriasis
Body dysmorphic disorder
> EXCLUDES   hypochondriasis in:
>   hysteria (300.10-300.19)
>   manic-depressive psychosis,
>   depressed type (296.2-296.3)
>   neurasthenia (300.5)
>   obsessional disorder (300.3)
>   schizophrenia (295.0-295.9)

√5ᵗʰ 300.8 Other neurotic disorders

300.81 Somatization disorder
Briquet's disorder
Severe somatoform disorder

300.82 Undifferentiated somatoform disorder
Atypical somatoform disorder
Somatoform disorder NOS

DEF: Disorders in which patients have symptoms that suggest an organic disease but no evidence of physical disorder after repeated testing.

300.89 Other
Occupational neurosis, including writers' cramp
Psychasthenia
Psychasthenic neurosis

300.9 Unspecified neurotic disorder
Neurosis NOS
Psychoneurosis NOS

√4ᵗʰ 301 Personality disorders
> INCLUDES   character neurosis
Use additional code to identify any associated neurosis or psychosis, or physical condition
> EXCLUDES   nonpsychotic personality disorder associated
>   with organic brain syndromes (310.0-
>   310.9)

301.0 Paranoid personality disorder
Fanatic personality
Paranoid personality (disorder)
Paranoid traits
> EXCLUDES   acute paranoid reaction (298.3)
>   alcoholic paranoia (291.5)
>   paranoid schizophrenia (295.3)
>   paranoid states (297.0-297.9)

√5ᵗʰ 301.1 Affective personality disorder
> EXCLUDES   affective psychotic disorders (296.0-
>   296.9)
>   neurasthenia (300.5)
>   neurotic depression (300.4)

301.10 Affective personality disorder, unspecified

301.11 Chronic hypomanic personality disorder
Chronic hypomanic disorder
Hypomanic personality

301.12 Chronic depressive personality disorder
Chronic depressive disorder
Depressive character or personality

301.13 Cyclothymic disorder
Cycloid personality
Cyclothymia
Cyclothymic personality

√5ᵗʰ 301.2 Schizoid personality disorder
> EXCLUDES   schizophrenia (295.0-295.9)

301.20 Schizoid personality disorder, unspecified

301.21 Introverted personality

301.22 Schizotypal personality

301.3 Explosive personality disorder
Aggressive: Emotional instability
   personality   (excessive)
   reaction   Pathological emotionality
Aggressiveness   Quarrelsomeness
> EXCLUDES   dyssocial personality (301.7)
>   hysterical neurosis (300.10-300.19)

301.4 Compulsive personality disorder
Anancastic personality
Obsessional personality
> EXCLUDES   obsessive-compulsive disorder (300.3)
>   phobic state (300.20-300.29)

√5ᵗʰ 301.5 Histrionic personality disorder
> EXCLUDES   hysterical neurosis (300.10-300.19)

DEF: Extreme emotional behavior, often theatrical; often concerned about own appeal; may demand attention, exhibit seductive behavior.

301.50 Histrionic personality disorder, unspecified
Hysterical personality NOS

301.51 Chronic factitious illness with physical symptoms
Hospital addiction syndrome
Multiple operations syndrome
Munchausen syndrome

301.59 Other histrionic personality disorder
Personality: Personality:
   emotionally unstable   psychoinfantile
   labile

301.6 Dependent personality disorder
Asthenic personality   Passive personality
Inadequate personality
> EXCLUDES   neurasthenia (300.5)
>   passive-aggressive personality (301.84)

DEF: Overwhelming feeling of helplessness; fears of abandonment may persist; difficulty in making personal decisions without confirmation by others; low self-esteem due to irrational sensitivity to criticism.

301.7 Antisocial personality disorder
Amoral personality
Asocial personality
Dyssocial personality
Personality disorder with predominantly sociopathic or asocial manifestation
> EXCLUDES   disturbance of conduct without
>   specifiable personality disorder
>   (312.0-312.9)
>   explosive personality (301.3)

DEF: Continuous antisocial behavior that violates rights of others; social traits include extreme aggression, total disregard for traditional social rules.

√5ᵗʰ 301.8 Other personality disorders

301.81 Narcissistic personality
DEF: Grandiose fantasy or behavior, lack of social empathy, hypersensitive to the lack of others' judgment, exploits others; also sense of entitlement to have expectations met, need for continual admiration.

301.82 Avoidant personality
DEF: Personality disorder marked by feelings of social inferiority; sensitivity to criticism, emotionally restrained due to fear of rejection.

√4ᵗʰ √5ᵗʰ   Additional Digit Required   Unspecified Code   Other Specified Code   Manifestation Code   ▶◀ Revised Text   ● New Code   ▲ Revised Code Title

2003 ICD•9•CM   Volume 1 — 69

301.83 Borderline personality

DEF: Personality disorder characterized by unstable moods, self-image, and interpersonal relationships; uncontrolled anger, impulsive and self-destructive acts, fears of abandonment, feelings of emptiness and boredom, recurrent suicide threats or self-mutilation.

301.84 Passive-aggressive personality

DEF: Pattern of procrastination and refusal to meet standards; introduce own obstacles to success and exploit failure.

301.89 Other

Personality:	Personality:
eccentric	masochistic
"haltlose" type	psychoneurotic
immature	

EXCLUDES   *psychoinfantile personality (301.59)*

301.9 Unspecified personality disorder

Pathological personality NOS
Personality disorder NOS
Psychopathic:
    constitutional state
    personality (disorder)

√4th **302 Sexual deviations and disorders**

EXCLUDES   *sexual disorder manifest in:*
    organic brain syndrome (290.0-294.9, 310.0-310.9)
    psychosis (295.0-298.9)

302.0 Ego-dystonic homosexuality

Ego-dystonic lesbianism
Homosexual conflict disorder

EXCLUDES   *homosexual pedophilia (302.2)*

302.1 Zoophilia

Bestiality

DEF: A sociodeviant disorder marked by engaging in sexual intercourse with animals.

302.2 Pedophilia

DEF: A sociodeviant condition of adults characterized by sexual activity with children.

302.3 Transvestism

EXCLUDES   *trans-sexualism (302.5)*

DEF: The desire to dress in clothing of opposite sex.

302.4 Exhibitionism

DEF: Sexual deviant behavior; exposure of genitals to strangers; behavior prompted by intense sexual urges and fantasies.

√5th **302.5 Trans-sexualism**

EXCLUDES   *transvestism (302.3)*

DEF: Gender identity disturbance; overwhelming desire to change anatomic sex, due to belief that individual is a member of the opposite sex.

302.50 With unspecified sexual history
302.51 With asexual history
302.52 With homosexual history
302.53 With heterosexual history

302.6 Disorders of psychosexual identity

Feminism in boys
Gender identity disorder of childhood

EXCLUDES   *gender identity disorder in adult (302.85)*
    homosexuality (302.0)
    trans-sexualism (302.50-302.53)
    transvestism (302.3)

√5th **302.7 Psychosexual dysfunction**

EXCLUDES   *impotence of organic origin (607.84)*
    normal transient symptoms from ruptured hymen
    transient or occasional failures of erection due to fatigue, anxiety, alcohol, or drugs

302.70 Psychosexual dysfunction, unspecified
302.71 With inhibited sexual desire
302.72 With inhibited sexual excitement
    Frigidity   Impotence
302.73 With inhibited female orgasm   ♀
302.74 With inhibited male orgasm   ♂
302.75 With premature ejaculation   ♂
302.76 With functional dyspareunia   ♀
    Dyspareunia, psychogenic

DEF: Difficult or painful sex due to psychosomatic state.

302.79 With other specified psychosexual dysfunctions

√5th **302.8 Other specified psychosexual disorders**

302.81 Fetishism

DEF: Psychosexual disorder noted for intense sexual urges and arousal precipitated by fantasies; use of inanimate objects, such as clothing, to stimulate sexual arousal, orgasm.

302.82 Voyeurism

DEF: Psychosexual disorder characterized by uncontrollable impulse to observe others, without their knowledge, who are nude or engaged in sexual activity.

302.83 Sexual masochism

DEF: Psychosexual disorder noted for need to achieve sexual gratification through humiliating or hurtful acts inflicted on self.

302.84 Sexual sadism

DEF: Psychosexual disorder noted for need to achieve sexual gratification through humiliating or hurtful acts inflicted on someone else.

302.85 Gender identity disorder of adolescent or adult life

302.89 Other

    Nymphomania   Satyriasis

302.9 Unspecified psychosexual disorder

Pathologic sexuality NOS
Sexual deviation NOS

√4th **303 Alcohol dependence syndrome**

Use additional code to identify any associated condition, as:
    alcoholic psychoses (291.0-291.9)
    drug dependence (304.0-304.9)
    physical complications of alcohol, such as:
       cerebral degeneration (331.7)
       cirrhosis of liver (571.2)
       epilepsy (345.0-345.9)
       gastritis (535.3)
       hepatitis (571.1)
       liver damage NOS (571.3)

EXCLUDES   *drunkenness NOS (305.0)*

The following fifth-digit subclassification is for use with category 303:

    0   unspecified
    1   continuous
    2   episodic
    3   in remission

√5th **303.0 Acute alcoholic intoxication**

Acute drunkenness in alcoholism

√5th **303.9 Other and unspecified alcohol dependence**

Chronic alcoholism
Dipsomania

☑4ᵗʰ **304 Drug dependence**

EXCLUDES   *nondependent abuse of drugs (305.1-305.9)*

The following fifth-digit subclassification is for use with category 304:

     0   unspecified
     1   continuous
     2   episodic
     3   in remission

☑5ᵗʰ **304.0 Opioid type dependence**

Heroin	Opium alkaloids and their
Meperidine	derivatives
Methadone	Synthetics with morphine-like
Morphine	effects
Opium	

☑5ᵗʰ **304.1 Barbiturate and similarly acting sedative or hypnotic dependence**

Barbiturates
Nonbarbiturate sedatives and tranquilizers with a
     similar effect:

chlordiazepoxide	meprobamate
diazepam	methaqualone
glutethimide	

☑5ᵗʰ **304.2 Cocaine dependence**

Coca leaves and derivatives

☑5ᵗʰ **304.3 Cannabis dependence**

Hashish	Marihuana
Hemp	

☑5ᵗʰ **304.4 Amphetamine and other psychostimulant dependence**

Methylphenidate	Phenmetrazine

☑5ᵗʰ **304.5 Hallucinogen dependence**

Dimethyltryptamine [DMT]
Lysergic acid diethylamide [LSD] and derivatives
Mescaline
Psilocybin

☑5ᵗʰ **304.6 Other specified drug dependence**

Absinthe addiction   Glue sniffing

EXCLUDES   *tobacco dependence (305.1)*

☑5ᵗʰ **304.7 Combinations of opioid type drug with any other**

☑5ᵗʰ **304.8 Combinations of drug dependence excluding opioid type drug**

☑5ᵗʰ **304.9 Unspecified drug dependence**

Drug addiction NOS   Drug dependence NOS

☑4ᵗʰ **305 Nondependent abuse of drugs**

Note: Includes cases where a person, for whom no other
diagnosis is possible, has come under medical care
because of the maladaptive effect of a drug on which he
is not dependent and that he has taken on his own
initiative to the detriment of his health or social
functioning.

EXCLUDES   *alcohol dependence syndrome (303.0-303.9)*
drug dependence (304.0-304.9)
drug withdrawal syndrome (292.0)
poisoning by drugs or medicinal substances (960.0-979.9)

The following fifth-digit subclassification is for use with codes 305.0, 305.2-305.9:

     0   unspecified
     1   continuous
     2   episodic
     3   in remission

☑5ᵗʰ **305.0 Alcohol abuse**

Drunkenness NOS
Excessive drinking of alcohol NOS
"Hangover" (alcohol)
Inebriety NOS

EXCLUDES   *acute alcohol intoxication in alcoholism (303.0)*
alcoholic psychoses (291.0-291.9)

305.1 Tobacco use disorder

Tobacco dependence

EXCLUDES   *history of tobacco use (V15.82)*

☑5ᵗʰ **305.2 Cannabis abuse**

☑5ᵗʰ **305.3 Hallucinogen abuse**

Acute intoxication from hallucinogens ["bad trips"]
LSD reaction

☑5ᵗʰ **305.4 Barbiturate and similarly acting sedative or hypnotic abuse**

☑5ᵗʰ **305.5 Opioid abuse**

☑5ᵗʰ **305.6 Cocaine abuse**

☑5ᵗʰ **305.7 Amphetamine or related acting sympathomimetic abuse**

☑5ᵗʰ **305.8 Antidepressant type abuse**

☑5ᵗʰ **305.9 Other, mixed, or unspecified drug abuse**

"Laxative habit"
Misuse of drugs NOS
Nonprescribed use of drugs or patent medicinals

☑4ᵗʰ **306 Physiological malfunction arising from mental factors**

INCLUDES   psychogenic:

physical symptoms	} not involving
physiological	} tissue
manifestations	} damage

EXCLUDES   *hysteria (300.11-300.19)*
physical symptoms secondary to a psychiatric disorder classified elsewhere
psychic factors associated with physical conditions involving tissue damage classified elsewhere (316)
specific nonpsychotic mental disorders following organic brain damage (310.0-310.9)

DEF: Functional disturbances or interruptions due to mental or psychological causes; no tissue damage sustained in these conditions.

306.0 Musculoskeletal

Psychogenic paralysis   Psychogenic torticollis

EXCLUDES   *Gilles de la Tourette's syndrome (307.23)*
paralysis as hysterical or conversion reaction (300.11)
tics (307.20-307.22)

306.1 Respiratory

Psychogenic:	Psychogenic:
air hunger	hyperventilation
cough	yawning
hiccough	

EXCLUDES   *psychogenic asthma (316 and 493.9)*

306.2 Cardiovascular

Cardiac neurosis
Cardiovascular neurosis
Neurocirculatory asthenia
Psychogenic cardiovascular disorder

EXCLUDES   *psychogenic paroxysmal tachycardia (316 and 427.2)*

DEF: Neurocirculatory asthenia: functional nervous and circulatory irregularities with palpitations, dyspnea, fatigue, rapid pulse, precordial pain, fear of effort, discomfort during exercise, anxiety; also called DaCosta's syndrome, Effort syndrome, Irritable or Soldier's Heart.

306.3 Skin

Psychogenic pruritus

EXCLUDES   *psychogenic:*
alopecia (316 and 704.00)
dermatitis (316 and 692.9)
eczema (316 and 691.8 or 692.9)
urticaria (316 and 708.0-708.9)

Mental Disorders 304–306.3

☑4ᵗʰ
☑5ᵗʰ
Additional Digit Required   Unspecified Code   Other Specified Code   Manifestation Code   ▶◀ Revised Text   ● New Code   ▲ Revised Code Title

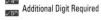 *2003 ICD•9•CM*   Volume 1 — 71

Mental Disorders 306.4–307.48

306.4 Gastrointestinal
Aerophagy
Cyclical vomiting, psychogenic
Diarrhea, psychogenic
Nervous gastritis
Psychogenic dyspepsia

EXCLUDES   cyclical vomiting NOS (536.2)
globus hystericus (300.11)
mucous colitis (316 and 564.9)
psychogenic:
   cardiospasm (316 and 530.0)
   duodenal ulcer (316 and 532.0-
     532.9)
   gastric ulcer (316 and 531.0-531.9)
   peptic ulcer NOS (316 and 533.0-
     533.9)
   vomiting NOS (307.54)

DEF: Aerophagy: excess swallowing of air, usually unconscious; related to anxiety; results in distended abdomen or belching, often interpreted by the patient as a physical disorder.

√5th **306.5 Genitourinary**
EXCLUDES   enuresis, psychogenic (307.6)
frigidity (302.72)
impotence (302.72)
psychogenic dyspareunia (302.76)

306.50 Psychogenic genitourinary malfunction, unspecified

306.51 Psychogenic vaginismus ♀
Functional vaginismus

DEF: Psychogenic response resulting in painful contractions of vaginal canal muscles; can be severe enough to prevent sexual intercourse.

306.52 Psychogenic dysmenorrhea ♀
306.53 Psychogenic dysuria
306.59 Other

306.6 Endocrine
306.7 Organs of special sense
EXCLUDES   hysterical blindness or deafness (300.11)
psychophysical visual disturbances (368.16)

306.8 Other specified psychophysiological malfunction
Bruxism   Teeth grinding

306.9 Unspecified psychophysiological malfunction
Psychophysiologic disorder NOS
Psychosomatic disorder NOS

√4th **307 Special symptoms or syndromes, not elsewhere classified**
Note: This category is intended for use if the psychopathology is manifested by a single specific symptom or group of symptoms which is not part of an organic illness or other mental disorder classifiable elsewhere.

EXCLUDES   those due to mental disorders classified elsewhere
those of organic origin

307.0 Stammering and stuttering
EXCLUDES   dysphasia (784.5)
lisping or lalling (307.9)
retarded development of speech (315.31-315.39)

307.1 Anorexia nervosa
EXCLUDES   eating disturbance NOS (307.50)
feeding problem (783.3)
of nonorganic origin (307.59)
loss of appetite (783.0)
of nonorganic origin (307.59)

√5th **307.2 Tics**
EXCLUDES   nail-biting or thumb-sucking (307.9)
stereotypes occurring in isolation (307.3)
tics of organic origin (333.3)

DEF: Involuntary muscle response usually confined to the face, shoulders.

307.20 Tic disorder, unspecified
307.21 Transient tic disorder of childhood
307.22 Chronic motor tic disorder
307.23 Gilles de la Tourette's disorder
Motor-verbal tic disorder

DEF: Syndrome of facial and vocal tics in childhood; progresses to spontaneous or involuntary jerking, obscene utterances, other uncontrollable actions considered inappropriate.

307.3 Stereotyped repetitive movements
Body-rocking   Spasmus nutans
Head banging   Stereotypes NOS
EXCLUDES   tics (307.20-307.23)
of organic origin (333.3)

√5th **307.4 Specific disorders of sleep of nonorganic origin**
EXCLUDES   narcolepsy (347)
those of unspecified cause (780.50-780.59)

307.40 Nonorganic sleep disorder, unspecified
307.41 Transient disorder of initiating or maintaining sleep

Hyposomnia   } associated with
Insomnia   } intermittent
Sleeplessness } emotional reactions or conflicts

307.42 Persistent disorder of initiating or maintaining sleep
Hyposomnia, insomnia, or sleeplessness associated with:
anxiety
conditioned arousal
depression (major) (minor)
psychosis

307.43 Transient disorder of initiating or maintaining wakefulness
Hypersomnia associated with acute or intermittent emotional reactions or conflicts

307.44 Persistent disorder of initiating or maintaining wakefulness
Hypersomnia associated with depression (major) (minor)

307.45 Phase-shift disruption of 24-hour sleep-wake cycle
Irregular sleep-wake rhythm, nonorganic origin
Jet lag syndrome
Rapid time-zone change
Shifting sleep-work schedule

307.46 Somnambulism or night terrors
DEF: Sleepwalking marked by extreme terror, panic, screaming, confusion; no recall of event upon arousal; term may refer to simply the act of sleepwalking.

307.47 Other dysfunctions of sleep stages or arousal from sleep
Nightmares: Sleep drunkenness
NOS
REM-sleep type

307.48 Repetitive intrusions of sleep
Repetitive intrusion of sleep with:
atypical polysomnographic features
environmental disturbances
repeated REM-sleep interruptions

307.49 Other
"Short-sleeper"
Subjective insomnia complaint

√5th **307.5 Other and unspecified disorders of eating**
EXCLUDES *anorexia:*
nervosa (307-1)
of unspecified cause (783.0)
overeating, of unspecified cause (783.6)
vomiting:
NOS (787.0)
cyclical (536.2)
psychogenic (306.4)

307.50 Eating disorder, unspecified

307.51 Bulimia
Overeating of nonorganic origin
DEF: Mental disorder commonly characterized by binge eating followed by self-induced vomiting; perceptions of being fat; and fear the inability to stop eating voluntarily.

307.52 Pica
Perverted appetite of nonorganic origin
DEF: Compulsive eating disorder characterized by craving for substances, other than food; such as paint chips or dirt.

307.53 Psychogenic rumination
Regurgitation, of nonorganic origin, of food with reswallowing
EXCLUDES *obsessional rumination (300.3)*

307.54 Psychogenic vomiting

307.59 Other
Infantile feeding disturbances } of nonorganic origin
Loss of appetite } origin

307.6 Enuresis
Enuresis (primary) (secondary) of nonorganic origin
EXCLUDES *enuresis of unspecified cause (788.3)*
DEF: Involuntary urination past age of normal control; also called bedwetting; no trace to biological problem; focus on psychological issues.

307.7 Encopresis
Encopresis (continuous) (discontinuous) of nonorganic origin
EXCLUDES *encopresis of unspecified cause (787.6)*
DEF: Inability to control bowel movements; cause traced to psychological, not biological, problems.

√5th **307.8 Psychalgia**
307.80 Psychogenic pain, site unspecified
307.81 Tension headache
EXCLUDES *headache:*
NOS (784.0)
migraine (346.0-346.9)

307.89 Other
Psychogenic backache
EXCLUDES *pains not specifically*
attributable to a
psychological cause (in):
back (724.5)
joint (719.4)
limb (729.5)
lumbago (724.2)
rheumatic (729.0)

307.9 Other and unspecified special symptoms or syndromes, not elsewhere classified
Hair plucking   Masturbation
Lalling   Nail-biting
Lisping   Thumb-sucking

√4th **308 Acute reaction to stress**
INCLUDES catastrophic stress
combat fatigue
gross stress reaction (acute)
transient disorders in response to exceptional physical or mental stress which usually subside within hours or days
EXCLUDES *adjustment reaction or disorder (309.0-309.9)*
chronic stress reaction (309.1-309.9)

308.0 Predominant disturbance of emotions
Anxiety } as acute reaction to
Emotional crisis } exceptional
Panic state } [gross] stress

308.1 Predominant disturbance of consciousness
Fugues as acute reaction to exceptional [gross] stress

308.2 Predominant psychomotor disturbance
Agitation states } as acute reaction to
Stupor } exceptional [gross] stress

308.3 Other acute reactions to stress
Acute situational disturbance
Brief or acute posttraumatic stress disorder
EXCLUDES *prolonged posttraumatic emotional disturbance (309.81)*

308.4 Mixed disorders as reaction to stress

308.9 Unspecified acute reaction to stress

√4th **309 Adjustment reaction**
INCLUDES adjustment disorders
reaction (adjustment) to chronic stress
EXCLUDES *acute reaction to major stress (308.0-308.9)*
neurotic disorders (300.0-300.9)

309.0 Brief depressive reaction
Adjustment disorder with depressed mood
Grief reaction
EXCLUDES *affective psychoses (296.0-296.9)*
neurotic depression (300.4)
prolonged depressive reaction (309.1)
psychogenic depressive psychosis (298.0)

309.1 Prolonged depressive reaction
EXCLUDES *affective psychoses (296.0-296.9)*
brief depressive reaction (309.0)
neurotic depression (300.4)
psychogenic depressive psychosis (298.0)

√5th **309.2 With predominant disturbance of other emotions**
309.21 Separation anxiety disorder
DEF: Abnormal apprehension by a child when physically separated from support environment; byproduct of abnormal symbiotic child-parent relationship.

309.22 Emancipation disorder of adolescence and early adult life
DEF: Adjustment reaction of late adolescence; conflict over independence from parental supervision; symptoms include difficulty in making decisions, increased reliance on parental advice, deliberate adoption of values in opposition of parents.

309.23 Specific academic or work inhibition

309.24 Adjustment reaction with anxious mood

309.28 Adjustment reaction with mixed emotional features
Adjustment reaction with anxiety and depression

309.29 Other
Culture shock

√4th Additional Digit Required
√5th
Unspecified Code   Other Specified Code   Manifestation Code   ▶◀ Revised Text   ● New Code   ▲ Revised Code Title

309.3 With predominant disturbance of conduct

Conduct disturbance ⎫
Destructiveness   ⎬ as adjustment reaction

> EXCLUDES   *destructiveness in child (312.9)*
> *disturbance of conduct NOS (312.9)*
> *dyssocial behavior without manifest psychiatric disorder (V71.01-V71.02)*
> *personality disorder with predominantly sociopathic or asocial manifestations (301.7)*

309.4 With mixed disturbance of emotions and conduct

✓5th **309.8 Other specified adjustment reactions**

309.81 Prolonged posttraumatic stress disorder

Chronic posttraumatic stress disorder
Concentration camp syndrome

> EXCLUDES   *posttraumatic brain syndrome:*
> *nonpsychotic (310.2)*
> *psychotic (293.0-293.9)*

DEF: Preoccupation with traumatic events beyond normal experience; events such as rape, personal assault, combat, natural disasters, accidents, torture precipitate disorder; also recurring flashbacks of trauma; symptoms include difficulty remembering, sleeping, or concentrating, and guilt feelings for surviving.

309.82 Adjustment reaction with physical symptoms

309.83 Adjustment reaction with withdrawal

Elective mutism as adjustment reaction
Hospitalism (in children) NOS

309.89 Other

309.9 Unspecified adjustment reaction

Adaptation reaction NOS
Adjustment reaction NOS

✓4th **310 Specific nonpsychotic mental disorders due to organic brain damage**

> EXCLUDES   *neuroses, personality disorders, or other nonpsychotic conditions occurring in a form similar to that seen with functional disorders but in association with a physical condition (300.0-300.9, 301.0-301.9)*

310.0 Frontal lobe syndrome

Lobotomy syndrome
Postleucotomy syndrome [state]

> EXCLUDES   *postcontusion syndrome (310.2)*

310.1 Organic personality syndrome

Cognitive or personality change of other type, of nonpsychotic severity
Mild memory disturbance
Organic psychosyndrome of nonpsychotic severity
Presbyophrenia NOS
Senility with mental changes of nonpsychotic severity

DEF: Personality disorder caused by organic factors, such as brain lesions, head trauma, or cerebrovascular accident (CVA).

310.2 Postconcussion syndrome

Postcontusion syndrome or encephalopathy
Posttraumatic brain syndrome, nonpsychotic
Status postcommotio cerebri

> EXCLUDES   *frontal lobe syndrome (310.0)*
> *postencephalitic syndrome (310.8)*
> *any organic psychotic conditions following head injury (293.0-294.0)*

DEF: Nonpsychotic disorder due to brain trauma, causes symptoms unrelated to any disease process; symptoms include amnesia, serial headaches, rapid heartbeat, fatigue, disrupted sleep patterns, inability to concentrate.

310.8 Other specified nonpsychotic mental disorders following organic brain damage

Postencephalitic syndrome
Other focal (partial) organic psychosyndromes

310.9 Unspecified nonpsychotic mental disorder following organic brain damage

311 Depressive disorder, not elsewhere classified

Depressive disorder NOS   Depression NOS
Depressive state NOS

> EXCLUDES   *acute reaction to major stress with depressive symptoms (308.0)*
> *affective personality disorder (301.10-301.13)*
> *affective psychoses (296.0-296.9)*
> *brief depressive reaction (309.0)*
> *depressive states associated with stressful events (309.0-309.1)*
> *disturbance of emotions specific to childhood and adolescence, with misery and unhappiness (313.1)*
> *mixed adjustment reaction with depressive symptoms (309.4)*
> *neurotic depression (300.4)*
> *prolonged depressive adjustment reaction (309.1)*
> *psychogenic depressive psychosis (298.0)*

✓4th **312 Disturbance of conduct, not elsewhere classified**

> EXCLUDES   *adjustment reaction with disturbance of conduct (309.3)*
> *drug dependence (304.0-304.9)*
> *dyssocial behavior without manifest psychiatric disorder (V71.01-V71.02)*
> *personality disorder with predominantly sociopathic or asocial manifestations (301.7)*
> *sexual deviations (302.0-302.9)*

The following fifth-digit subclassification is for use with categories 312.0-312.2:

     0   **unspecified**
     1   **mild**
     2   **moderate**
     3   **severe**

✓5th **312.0 Undersocialized conduct disorder, aggressive type**

Aggressive outburst   Unsocialized aggressive
Anger reaction   disorder

DEF: Mental condition identified by behaviors disrespectful of others' rights and of age-appropriate social norms or rules; symptoms include bullying, vandalism, verbal and physical abusiveness, lying, stealing, defiance.

✓5th **312.1 Undersocialized conduct disorder, unaggressive type**

Childhood truancy, unsocialized
Solitary stealing
Tantrums

✓5th **312.2 Socialized conduct disorder**

Childhood truancy, socialized   Group delinquency

> EXCLUDES   *gang activity without manifest psychiatric disorder (V71.01)*

✓5th **312.3 Disorders of impulse control, not elsewhere classified**

312.30 Impulse control disorder, unspecified

312.31 Pathological gambling

312.32 Kleptomania

312.33 Pyromania

312.34 Intermittent explosive disorder

312.35 Isolated explosive disorder

312.39 Other

312.4 Mixed disturbance of conduct and emotions

Neurotic delinquency

> EXCLUDES   *compulsive conduct disorder (312.3)*

N Newborn Age: 0   **P** Pediatric Age: 0-17   **M** Maternity Age: 12-55   **A** Adult Age: 15-124   **MSP** Medicare Secondary Payer

74 — Volume 1   *2003 ICD•9•CM*

✓5ᵗʰ **312.8 Other specified disturbances of conduct, not elsewhere classified**

312.81 Conduct disorder, childhood onset type

312.82 Conduct disorder, adolescent onset type

312.89 Other conduct disorder

312.9 Unspecified disturbance of conduct
Delinquency (juvenile)

✓4ᵗʰ **313 Disturbance of emotions specific to childhood and adolescence**
> **EXCLUDES** *adjustment reaction (309.0-309.9)*
> *emotional disorder of neurotic type (300.0-300.9)*
> *masturbation, nail-biting, thumbsucking, and other isolated symptoms (307.0-307.9)*

313.0 Overanxious disorder
Anxiety and fearfulness ⎫ of childhood and
Overanxious disorder   ⎭ adolescence
> **EXCLUDES** *abnormal separation anxiety (309.21)*
> *anxiety states (300.00-300.09)*
> *hospitalism in children (309.83)*
> *phobic state (300.20-300.29)*

313.1 Misery and unhappiness disorder
> **EXCLUDES** *depressive neurosis (300.4)*

✓5ᵗʰ **313.2 Sensitivity, shyness, and social withdrawal disorder**
> **EXCLUDES** *infantile autism (299.0)*
> *schizoid personality (301.20-301.22)*
> *schizophrenia (295.0-295.9)*

313.21 Shyness disorder of childhood
Sensitivity reaction of childhood or adolescence

313.22 Introverted disorder of childhood
Social withdrawal ⎫ of childhood or
Withdrawal   ⎬ adolescence
reaction   ⎭

313.23 Elective mutism
> **EXCLUDES** *elective mutism as adjustment reaction (309.83)*

313.3 Relationship problems
Sibling jealousy
> **EXCLUDES** *relationship problems associated with aggression, destruction, or other forms of conduct disturbance (312.0-312.9)*

✓5ᵗʰ **313.8 Other or mixed emotional disturbances of childhood or adolescence**

313.81 Oppositional disorder
DEF: Mental disorder of children noted for pervasive opposition, defiance of authority.

313.82 Identity disorder
DEF: Distress of adolescents caused by inability to form acceptable self-identity; uncertainty about career choice, sexual orientation, moral values.

313.83 Academic underachievement disorder

313.89 Other   P

313.9 Unspecified emotional disturbance of childhood or adolescence   P

✓4ᵗʰ **314 Hyperkinetic syndrome of childhood**
> **EXCLUDES** *hyperkinesis as symptom of underlying disorder—code the underlying disorder*

DEF: A behavioral disorder usually diagnosed at an early age; characterized by the inability to focus attention for a normal period of time.

✓5ᵗʰ **314.0 Attention deficit disorder**
Adult   Child

314.00 Without mention of hyperactivity
Predominantly inattentive type

314.01 With hyperactivity
Combined type
Overactivity NOS
Predominantly hyperactive/impulsive type
Simple disturbance of attention with overactivity

314.1 Hyperkinesis with developmental delay
Developmental disorder of hyperkinesis
Use additional code to identify any associated neurological disorder

314.2 Hyperkinetic conduct disorder
Hyperkinetic conduct disorder without developmental delay
> **EXCLUDES** *hyperkinesis with significant delays in specific skills (314.1)*

314.8 Other specified manifestations of hyperkinetic syndrome

314.9 Unspecified hyperkinetic syndrome
Hyperkinetic reaction of childhood or adolescence NOS
Hyperkinetic syndrome NOS

✓4ᵗʰ **315 Specific delays in development**
> **EXCLUDES** *that due to a neurological disorder (320.0-389.9)*

✓5ᵗʰ **315.0 Specific reading disorder**

315.00 Reading disorder, unspecified

315.01 Alexia
DEF: Lack of ability to understand written language; manifestation of aphasia.

315.02 Developmental dyslexia
DEF: Serious impairment of reading skills unexplained in relation to general intelligence and teaching processes; it can be inherited or congenital.

315.09 Other
Specific spelling difficulty

315.1 Specific arithmetical disorder
Dyscalculia

315.2 Other specific learning difficulties
> **EXCLUDES** *specific arithmetical disorder (315.1)*
> *specific reading disorder (315.00-315.09)*

✓5ᵗʰ **315.3 Developmental speech or language disorder**

315.31 Developmental language disorder
Developmental aphasia
Expressive language disorder
Word deafness
> **EXCLUDES** *acquired aphasia (784.3)*
> *elective mutism (309.83, 313.0, 313.23)*

315.32 Receptive language disorder (mixed)
Receptive expressive language disorder

315.39 Other
Developmental articulation disorder
Dyslalia
> **EXCLUDES** *lisping and lalling (307.9)*
> *stammering and stuttering (307.0)*

315.4 Coordination disorder
Clumsiness syndrome   Specific motor development
Dyspraxia syndrome   disorder

315.5 Mixed development disorder

315.8 Other specified delays in development

315.9 Unspecified delay in development
Developmental disorder NOS

✓4ᵗʰ / ✓5ᵗʰ Additional Digit Required   Unspecified Code   Other Specified Code   Manifestation Code   ▶◀ Revised Text   ● New Code   ▲ Revised Code Title

2003 ICD•9•CM   **Volume 1 — 75**

316 Psychic factors associated with diseases classified elsewhere

Psychologic factors in physical conditions classified elsewhere

Use additional code to identify the associated physical condition, as:

psychogenic:
- asthma (493.9)
- dermatitis (692.9)
- duodenal ulcer (532.0-532.9)
- eczema (691.8, 692.9)
- gastric ulcer (531.0-531.9)
- mucous colitis (564.9)
- paroxysmal tachycardia (427.2)
- ulcerative colitis (556)
- urticaria (708.0-708.9)

psychosocial dwarfism (259.4)

EXCLUDES *physical symptoms and physiological malfunctions, not involving tissue damage, of mental origin (306.0-306.9)*

MENTAL RETARDATION (317-319)

Use additional code(s) to identify any associated psychiatric or physical condition(s)

317 Mild mental retardation

High-grade defect

IQ 50-70

Mild mental subnormality

√4ᵗʰ 318 Other specified mental retardation

318.0 Moderate mental retardation

IQ 35-49

Moderate mental subnormality

318.1 Severe mental retardation

IQ 20-34

Severe mental subnormality

318.2 Profound mental retardation

IQ under 20

Profound mental subnormality

319 Unspecified mental retardation

Mental deficiency NOS

Mental subnormality NOS

6. NERVOUS SYSTEM AND SENSE ORGANS (320-389)

INFLAMMATORY DISEASES OF THE CENTRAL NERVOUS SYSTEM
(320-326)

☑4ᵗʰ 320 Bacterial meningitis

INCLUDES	arachnoiditis	
	leptomeningitis	
	meningitis	bacterial
	meningoencephalitis	
	meningomyelitis	
	pachymeningitis	

DEF: Bacterial infection causing inflammation of the lining of the brain and/or spinal cord.

320.0 Hemophilus meningitis
Meningitis due to Hemophilus influenzae [H. influenzae]

320.1 Pneumococcal meningitis

320.2 Streptococcal meningitis

320.3 Staphylococcal meningitis

320.7 *Meningitis in other bacterial diseases classified elsewhere*
Code first underlying disease, as:
actinomycosis (039.8)
listeriosis (027.0)
typhoid fever (002.0)
whooping cough (033.0-033.9)
> EXCLUDES   meningitis (in):
> epidemic (036.0)
> gonococcal (098.82)
> meningococcal (036.0)
> salmonellosis (003.21)
> syphilis:
>   NOS (094.2)
>   congenital (090.42)
>   meningovascular (094.2)
>   secondary (091.81)
> tuberculous (013.0)

☑5ᵗʰ 320.8 Meningitis due to other specified bacteria

320.81 Anaerobic meningitis
Bacteroides (fragilis)
Gram-negative anaerobes

320.82 *Meningitis due to gram-negative bacteria, not elsewhere classified*
Aerobacter aerogenes
Escherichia coli [E. coli]
Friedländer bacillus
Klebsiella pneumoniae
Proteus morganii
Pseudomonas
> EXCLUDES   gram-negative anaerobes (320.81)

320.89 *Meningitis due to other specified bacteria*
Bacillus pyocyaneus

320.9 *Meningitis due to unspecified bacterium*
Meningitis:
bacterial NOS
purulent NOS
pyogenic NOS
suppurative NOS

☑4ᵗʰ 321 Meningitis due to other organisms

INCLUDES	arachnoiditis	
	leptomeningitis	due to organisms
	meningitis	other than
	pachymeningitis	bacteria

DEF: Infection causing inflammation of the lining of the brain and/or spinal cord, due to organisms other than bacteria.

321.0 *Cryptococcal meningitis*
Code first underlying disease (117.5)

321.1 *Meningitis in other fungal diseases*
Code first underlying disease (110.0-118)
> EXCLUDES   meningitis in:
> candidiasis (112.83)
> coccidioidomycosis (114.2)
> histoplasmosis (115.01, 115.11, 115.91)

321.2 *Meningitis due to viruses not elsewhere classified*
Code first underlying disease, as:
meningitis due to arbovirus (060.0-066.9)
> EXCLUDES   meningitis (due to):
> abacterial (047.0-047.9)
> adenovirus (049.1)
> aseptic NOS (047.9)
> Coxsackie (virus)(047.0)
> ECHO virus (047.1)
> enterovirus (047.0-047.9)
> herpes simplex virus (054.72)
> herpes zoster virus (053.0)
> lymphocytic choriomeningitis virus (049.0)
> mumps (072.1)
> viral NOS (047.9)
> meningo-eruptive syndrome (047.1)

321.3 *Meningitis due to trypanosomiasis*
Code first underlying disease (086.0-086.9)

321.4 *Meningitis in sarcoidosis*
Code first underlying disease (135)

321.8 *Meningitis due to other nonbacterial organisms classified elsewhere*
Code first underlying disease
> EXCLUDES   leptospiral meningitis (100.81)

☑4ᵗʰ 322 Meningitis of unspecified cause

INCLUDES	arachnoiditis	
	leptomeningitis	with no organism
	meningitis	specified as
	pachymeningitis	cause

DEF: Infection causing inflammation of the lining of the brain and/or spinal cord, due to unspecified cause.

322.0 Nonpyogenic meningitis
Meningitis with clear cerebrospinal fluid

322.1 Eosinophilic meningitis

322.2 Chronic meningitis

322.9 *Meningitis, unspecified*

☑4ᵗʰ 323 Encephalitis, myelitis, and encephalomyelitis

INCLUDES	acute disseminated encephalomyelitis
	meningoencephalitis, except bacterial
	meningomyelitis, except bacterial
	myelitis (acute):
	ascending
	transverse

> EXCLUDES   bacterial:
> meningoencephalitis (320.0-320.9)
> meningomyelitis (320.0-320.9)

DEF: Encephalitis: inflammation of brain tissues.

DEF: Myelitis: inflammation of the spinal cord.

DEF: Encephalomyelitis: inflammation of brain and spinal cord.

☑4ᵗʰ
☑5ᵗʰ
Additional Digit Required   Unspecified Code   Other Specified Code   Manifestation Code   ▶◀ Revised Text   ● New Code   ▲ Revised Code Title

323.0 Encephalitis in viral diseases classified elsewhere

Code first underlying disease, as:
cat-scratch disease (078.3)
infectious mononucleosis (075)
ornithosis (073.7)

EXCLUDES encephalitis (in):
arthropod-borne viral (062.0-064)
herpes simplex (054.3)
mumps (072.2)
other viral diseases of central
nervous system (049.8-049.9)
poliomyelitis (045.0-045.9)
rubella (056.01)
slow virus infections of central
nervous system (046.0-046.9)
viral NOS (049.9)

323.1 Encephalitis in rickettsial diseases classified elsewhere

Code first underlying disease (080-083.9)

DEF: Inflammation of the brain caused by rickettsial disease carried by louse, tick, or mite.

323.2 Encephalitis in protozoal diseases classified elsewhere

Code first underlying disease, as:
malaria (084.0-084.9)
trypanosomiasis (086.0-086.9)

DEF: Inflammation of the brain caused by protozoal disease carried by mosquitoes and flies.

323.4 Other encephalitis due to infection classified elsewhere

Code first underlying disease

EXCLUDES encephalitis (in):
meningococcal (036.1)
syphilis:
NOS (094.81)
congenital (090.41)
toxoplasmosis (130.0)
tuberculosis (013.6)
meningoencephalitis due to free-living
ameba [Naegleria] (136.2)

323.5 Encephalitis following immunization procedures

Encephalitis
Encephalomyelitis } postimmunization or
postvaccinal

Use additional E code to identify vaccine

323.6 Postinfectious encephalitis

Code first underlying disease

EXCLUDES encephalitis:
postchickenpox (052.0)
postmeasles (055.0)

DEF: Infection, inflammation of brain several weeks following the outbreak of a systemic infection.

323.7 Toxic encephalitis

Code first underlying cause, as:
carbon tetrachloride (982.1)
hydroxyquinoline derivatives (961.3)
lead (984.0-984.9)
mercury (985.0)
thallium (985.8)

323.8 Other causes of encephalitis

323.9 Unspecified cause of encephalitis

√4ᵗʰ **324 Intracranial and intraspinal abscess**

324.0 Intracranial abscess

Abscess (embolic):　　Abscess (embolic) of brain
cerebellar　　　　　　[any part]:
cerebral　　　　　　　epidural
　　　　　　　　　　　extradural
　　　　　　　　　　　otogenic
　　　　　　　　　　　subdural

EXCLUDES tuberculous (013.3)

324.1 Intraspinal abscess

Abscess (embolic) of spinal cord [any part]:
epidural
extradural
subdural

EXCLUDES tuberculous (013.5)

324.9 Of unspecified site

Extradural or subdural abscess NOS

325 Phlebitis and thrombophlebitis of intracranial venous sinuses

Embolism
Endophlebitis
Phlebitis, septic or } of cavernous, lateral, or
suppurative　　　　other intracranial
Thrombophlebitis　　or unspecified
Thrombosis　　　　　intracranial
　　　　　　　　　　venous sinus

EXCLUDES that specified as:
complicating pregnancy, childbirth, or the
puerperium (671.5)
of nonpyogenic origin (437.6)

DEF: Inflammation and formation of blood clot in a vein within the brain or its lining.

326 Late effects of intracranial abscess or pyogenic infection

Note: This category is to be used to indicate conditions whose primary classification is to 320-325 [excluding 320.7, 321.0-321.8, 323.0-323.4, 323.6-323.7] as the cause of late effects, themselves classifiable elsewhere. The "late effects" include conditions specified as such, or as sequelae, which may occur at any time after the resolution of the causal condition.

Use additional code to identify condition, as:
hydrocephalus (331.4)
paralysis (342.0-342.9, 344.0-344.9)

HEREDITARY AND DEGENERATIVE DISEASES OF THE CENTRAL NERVOUS SYSTEM (330-337)

EXCLUDES hepatolenticular degeneration (275.1)
multiple sclerosis (340)
other demyelinating diseases of central nervous
system (341.0-341.9)

√4ᵗʰ **330 Cerebral degenerations usually manifest in childhood**

Use additional code to identify associated mental retardation

330.0 Leukodystrophy

Krabbe's disease　　　Pelizaeus-Merzbacher
Leukodystrophy　　　　disease
NOS　　　　　　　　Sulfatide lipidosis
globoid cell
metachromatic
sudanophilic

DEF: Hereditary disease of arylsulfatase or cerebroside sulfatase; characterized by a diffuse loss of myelin in CNS; infantile form causes blindness, motor disturbances, rigidity, mental deterioration and, occasionally, convulsions.

330.1 Cerebral lipidoses

Amaurotic (familial) idiocy　Disease:
Disease:　　　　　　　　　Spielmeyer-Vogt
Batten　　　　　　　　　　Tay-Sachs
Jansky-Bielschowsky　　　Gangliosidosis
Kufs'

DEF: Genetic disorder causing abnormal lipid accumulation in the reticuloendothelial cells of the brain.

330.2 Cerebral degeneration in generalized lipidoses

Code first underlying disease, as:
Fabry's disease (272.7)
Gaucher's disease (272.7)
Niemann-Pick disease (272.7)
sphingolipidosis (272.7)

N Newborn Age: 0　　　　P Pediatric Age: 0-17　　　　M Maternity Age: 12-55　　　　A Adult Age: 15-124　　　　MSP Medicare Secondary Payer

330.3 Cerebral degeneration of childhood in other diseases classified elsewhere

Code first underlying disease, as:
Hunter's disease (277.5)
mucopolysaccharidosis (277.5)

330.8 Other specified cerebral degenerations in childhood

Alpers' disease or gray-matter degeneration
Infantile necrotizing encephalomyelopathy
Leigh's disease
Subacute necrotizing encephalopathy or encephalomyelopathy

330.9 Unspecified cerebral degeneration in childhood

√4th 331 Other cerebral degenerations

331.0 Alzheimer's disease

DEF: Diffuse atrophy of cerebral cortex; causing a progressive decline in intellectual and physical functions, including memory loss, personality changes and profound dementia.

331.1 Pick's disease

DEF: Rare, progressive degenerative brain disease, similar to Alzheimer's; cortical atrophy affects the frontal and temporal lobes.

331.2 Senile degeneration of brain

EXCLUDES   senility NOS (797)

331.3 Communicating hydrocephalus

EXCLUDES   congenital hydrocephalus (741.0, 742.3)

DEF: Subarachnoid hemorrhage and meningitis causing excess buildup of cerebrospinal fluid in cavities due to nonabsorption of fluid back through fluid pathways.

331.4 Obstructive hydrocephalus

Acquired hydrocephalus NOS

EXCLUDES   congenital hydrocephalus (741.0, 742.3)

DEF: Obstruction of cerebrospinal fluid passage from brain into spinal canal.

331.7 Cerebral degeneration in diseases classified elsewhere

Code first underlying disease, as:
alcoholism (303.0-303.9)
beriberi (265.0)
cerebrovascular disease (430-438)
congenital hydrocephalus (741.0, 742.3)
neoplastic disease (140.0-239.9)
myxedema (244.0-244.9)
vitamin B_{12} deficiency (266.2)

EXCLUDES   cerebral degeneration in:
Jakob-Creutzfeldt disease (046.1)
progressive multifocal leukoencephalopathy (046.3)
subacute spongiform encephalopathy (046.1)

√5th 331.8 Other cerebral degeneration

331.81 Reye's syndrome   P

DEF: Rare childhood illness, often developed after a bout of viral upper respiratory infection; characterized by vomiting, elevated serum transaminase, changes in liver and other viscera; symptoms may be followed by an encephalopathic phase with brain swelling, disturbances of consciousness and seizures; can be fatal.

331.89 Other

Cerebral ataxia

331.9 Cerebral degeneration, unspecified

√4th 332 Parkinson's disease

332.0 Paralysis agitans

Parkinsonism or Parkinson's disease:
NOS
idiopathic
primary

DEF: Form of parkinsonism; progressive, occurs in senior years; characterized by masklike facial expression; condition affects ability to stand erect, walk smoothly; weakened muscles, also tremble and involuntarily movement.

332.1 Secondary Parkinsonism

Parkinsonism due to drugs
Use additional E code to identify drug, if drug-induced

EXCLUDES   Parkinsonism (in):
Huntington's disease (333.4)
progressive supranuclear palsy (333.0)
Shy-Drager syndrome (333.0)
syphilitic (094.82)

√4th 333 Other extrapyramidal disease and abnormal movement disorders

INCLUDES   other forms of extrapyramidal, basal ganglia, or striatopallidal disease

EXCLUDES   abnormal movements of head NOS (781.0)

333.0 Other degenerative diseases of the basal ganglia

Atrophy or degeneration:
olivopontocerebellar [Déjérine-Thomas syndrome]
pigmentary pallidal [Hallervorden-Spatz disease]
striatonigral
Parkinsonian syndrome associated with:
idiopathic orthostatic hypotension
symptomatic orthostatic hypotension
Progressive supranuclear ophthalmoplegia
Shy-Drager syndrome

333.1 Essential and other specified forms of tremor

Benign essential tremor
Familial tremor
Use additional E code to identify drug, if drug-induced

EXCLUDES   tremor NOS (781.0)

333.2 Myoclonus

Familial essential myoclonus
Progressive myoclonic epilepsy
Unverricht-Lundborg disease
Use additional E code to identify drug, if drug-induced

DEF: Spontaneous movements or contractions of muscles.

333.3 Tics of organic origin

Use additional E code to identify drug, if drug-induced

EXCLUDES   Gilles de la Tourette's syndrome (307.23)
habit spasm (307.22)
tic NOS (307.20)

333.4 Huntington's chorea

DEF: Genetic disease; characterized by chronic progressive mental deterioration; dementia and death within 15 years of onset.

333.5 Other choreas

Hemiballism(us)
Paroxysmal choreo-athetosis
Use additional E code to identify drug, if drug-induced

EXCLUDES   Sydenham's or rheumatic chorea (392.0-392.9)

√4th √5th Additional Digit Required   Unspecified Code   Other Specified Code   Manifestation Code   ►◄ Revised Text   ● New Code   ▲ Revised Code Title

2003 ICD•9•CM   **Volume 1 — 79**

Nervous System and Sense Organs 333.6–336.9

333.6 Idiopathic torsion dystonia
Dystonia:
deformans progressiva
musculorum deformans
(Schwalbe-) Ziehen-Oppenheim disease

DEF: Sustained muscular contractions, causing twisting and repetitive movements that result in abnormal postures of trunk and limbs; etiology unknown.

333.7 Symptomatic torsion dystonia
Athetoid cerebral palsy [Vogt's disease]
Double athetosis (syndrome)
Use additional E code to identify drug, if drug-induced

√5ᵗʰ **333.8 Fragments of torsion dystonia**
Use additional E code to identify drug, if drug-induced

     333.81 Blepharospasm
DEF: Uncontrolled winking or blinking due to orbicularis oculi muscle spasm.

     333.82 Orofacial dyskinesia
DEF: Uncontrolled movement of mouth or facial muscles.

     333.83 Spasmodic torticollis
EXCLUDES   torticollis:
NOS (723.5)
hysterical (300.11)
psychogenic (306.0)
DEF: Uncontrolled movement of head due to spasms of neck muscle.

     333.84 Organic writers' cramp
EXCLUDES   pychogenic (300.89)

     333.89 Other

√5ᵗʰ **333.9 Other and unspecified extrapyramidal diseases and abnormal movement disorders**
     333.90 Unspecified extrapyramidal disease and abnormal movement disorder
     333.91 Stiff-man syndrome
     333.92 Neuroleptic malignant syndrome
Use additional E code to identify drug
     333.93 Benign shuddering attacks
     333.99 Other
Restless legs

√4ᵗʰ **334 Spinocerebellar disease**
EXCLUDES   olivopontocerebellar degeneration (333.0)
peroneal muscular atrophy (356.1)

334.0 Friedreich's ataxia
DEF: Genetic recessive disease of children; sclerosis of dorsal, lateral spinal cord columns; characterized by ataxia, speech impairment, swaying and irregular movements, with muscle paralysis, especially of lower limbs.

334.1 Hereditary spastic paraplegia
334.2 Primary cerebellar degeneration
Cerebellar ataxia: Primary cerebellar
   Marie's   degeneration:
   Sanger-Brown   NOS
   Dyssynergia cerebellaris   hereditary
     myoclonica   sporadic

334.3 Other cerebellar ataxia
Cerebellar ataxia NOS
Use additional E code to identify drug, if drug-induced

334.4 Cerebellar ataxia in diseases classified elsewhere
Code first underlying disease, as:
alcoholism (303.0-303.9)
myxedema (244.0-244.9)
neoplastic disease (140.0-239.9)

334.8 Other spinocerebellar diseases
Ataxia-telangiectasia [Louis-Bar syndrome]
Corticostriatal-spinal degeneration

334.9 Spinocerebellar disease, unspecified
√4ᵗʰ **335 Anterior horn cell disease**
335.0 Werdnig-Hoffmann disease
Infantile spinal muscular atrophy
Progressive muscular atrophy of infancy
DEF: Spinal muscle atrophy manifested in prenatal period or shortly after birth; symptoms include hypotonia, atrophy of skeletal muscle; death occurs in infancy.

√5ᵗʰ **335.1 Spinal muscular atrophy**
     335.10 Spinal muscular atrophy, unspecified
     335.11 Kugelberg-Welander disease
Spinal muscular atrophy:
familial
juvenile
DEF: Hereditary; juvenile muscle atrophy; appears during first two decades of life; due to lesions of anterior horns of spinal cord; includes wasting, diminution of lower body muscles and twitching.

     335.19 Other
Adult spinal muscular atrophy

√5ᵗʰ **335.2 Motor neuron disease**
     335.20 Amyotrophic lateral sclerosis   Ⓐ
Motor neuron disease (bulbar) (mixed type)
     335.21 Progressive muscular atrophy
Duchenne-Aran muscular atrophy
Progressive muscular atrophy (pure)
     335.22 Progressive bulbar palsy
     335.23 Pseudobulbar palsy
     335.24 Primary lateral sclerosis
     335.29 Other
335.8 Other anterior horn cell diseases
335.9 Anterior horn cell disease, unspecified

√4ᵗʰ **336 Other diseases of spinal cord**
336.0 Syringomyelia and syringobulbia
336.1 Vascular myelopathies
Acute infarction of spinal cord (embolic) (nonembolic)
Arterial thrombosis of spinal cord
Edema of spinal cord
Hematomyelia
Subacute necrotic myelopathy

336.2 Subacute combined degeneration of spinal cord in diseases classified elsewhere
Code first underlying disease, as:
pernicious anemia (281.0)
other vitamin B_{12} deficiency anemia (281.1)
vitamin B_{12} deficiency (266.2)

336.3 Myelopathy in other diseases classified elsewhere
Code first underlying disease, as:
myelopathy in neoplastic disease (140.0-239.9)
EXCLUDES   myelopathy in:
intervertebral disc disorder (722.70-722.73)
spondylosis (721.1, 721.41-721.42, 721.91)

336.8 Other myelopathy
Myelopathy: Myelopathy:
  drug-induced   radiation-induced
Use additonal E code to identify cause

336.9 Unspecified disease of spinal cord
Cord compression NOS   Myelopathy NOS
EXCLUDES   myelitis (323.0-323.9)
spinal (canal) stenosis (723.0, 724.00-724.09)

✓4th **337　Disorders of the autonomic nervous system**

> INCLUDES　disorders of peripheral autonomic, sympathetic, parasympathetic, or vegetative system
>
> EXCLUDES　*familial dysautonomia [Riley-Day syndrome] (742.8)*

337.0　Idiopathic peripheral autonomic neuropathy
> Carotid sinus syncope or syndrome
> Cervical sympathetic dystrophy or paralysis

337.1　*Peripheral autonomic neuropathy in disorders classified elsewhere*
> *Code first underlying disease, as:*
> amyloidosis (277.3)
> diabetes (250.6)

✓5th **337.2　Reflex sympathetic dystrophy**
> DEF: Disturbance of the sympathetic nervous system evidenced by sweating, pain, pallor and edema following injury to nerves or blood vessels.

　337.20　Reflex sympathetic dystrophy, unspecified

　337.21　Reflex sympathetic dystrophy of the upper limb

　337.22　Reflex sympathetic dystrophy of the lower limb

　337.29　Reflex sympathetic dystrophy of other specified site

337.3　Autonomic dysreflexia
> Use additional code to identify the cause, such as:
> decubitus ulcer (707.0)
> fecal impaction (560.39)
> urinary tract infection (599.0)
>
> DEF: Noxious stimuli evokes paroxysmal hypertension, bradycardia, excess sweating, headache, pilomotor responses, facial flushing, and nasal congestion due to uncontrolled parasympathetic nerve response; usually occurs in patients with spinal cord injury above major sympathetic outflow tract (T_6).

337.9　Unspecified disorder of autonomic nervous system

OTHER DISORDERS OF THE CENTRAL NERVOUS SYSTEM (340-349)

340　Multiple sclerosis　　　　　A
> Disseminated or multiple sclerosis:
> NOS
> brain stem
> cord
> generalized

✓4th **341　Other demyelinating diseases of central nervous system**

341.0　Neuromyelitis optica

341.1　Schilder's disease
> Baló's concentric sclerosis
> Encephalitis periaxialis:
> concentrica [Baló's]
> diffusa [Schilder's]
>
> DEF: Chronic leukoencephalopathy of children and adolescents; symptoms include blindness, deafness, bilateral spasticity and progressive mental deterioration.

341.8　Other demyelinating diseases of central nervous system
> Central demyelination of corpus callosum
> Central pontine myelinosis
> Marchiafava (-Bignami) disease

341.9　Demyelinating disease of central nervous system, unspecified

✓4th **342　Hemiplegia and hemiparesis**
> Note: This category is to be used when hemiplegia (complete) (incomplete) is reported without further specification, or is stated to be old or long-standing but of unspecified cause. The category is also for use in multiple coding to identify these types of hemiplegia resulting from any cause.
>
> EXCLUDES　*congenital (343.1)*
> *hemiplegia due to late effect of cerebrovascular accident (438.20-438.22)*
> *infantile NOS (343.4)*

> The following fifth-digits are for use with codes 342.0-342.9:
> **0　affecting unspecified side**
> **1　affecting dominant side**
> **2　affecting nondominant side**

✓5th **342.0　Flaccid hemiplegia**

✓5th **342.1　Spastic hemiplegia**

✓5th **342.8　Other specified hemiplegia**

✓5th **342.9　Hemiplegia, unspecified**

✓4th **343　Infantile cerebral palsy**
> INCLUDES　cerebral:
> palsy NOS
> spastic infantile paralysis
> congenital spastic paralysis (cerebral)
> Little's disease
> paralysis (spastic) due to birth injury:
> intracranial
> spinal
>
> EXCLUDES　*hereditary cerebral paralysis, such as:*
> *hereditary spastic paraplegia (334.1)*
> *Vogt's disease (333.7)*
> *spastic paralysis specified as noncongenital or noninfantile (344.0-344.9)*

343.0　Diplegic
> Congenital diplegia　　　Congenital paraplegia
> DEF: Paralysis affecting both sides of the body simultaneously.

343.1　Hemiplegic
> Congenital hemiplegia
> EXCLUDES　*infantile hemiplegia NOS (343.4)*

343.2　Quadriplegic
> Tetraplegic

343.3　Monoplegic

343.4　Infantile hemiplegia
> Infantile hemiplegia (postnatal) NOS

343.8　Other specified infantile cerebral palsy

343.9　Infantile cerebral palsy, unspecified
> Cerebral palsy NOS

✓4th **344　Other paralytic syndromes**
> Note: This category is to be used when the listed conditions are reported without further specification or are stated to be old or long-standing but of unspecified cause. The category is also for use in multiple coding to identify these conditions resulting from any cause.
>
> INCLUDES　paralysis (complete) (incomplete), except as classifiable to 342 and 343
>
> EXCLUDES　*congenital or infantile cerebral palsy (343.0-343.9)*
> *hemiplegia (342.0-342.9)*
> *congenital or infantile (343.1, 343.4)*

✓5th **344.0　Quadriplegia and quadriparesis**

　344.00　Quadriplegia unspecified

　344.01　C_1-C_4 complete

　344.02　C_1-C_4 incomplete

　344.03　C_5-C_7 complete

　344.04　C_5-C_7 incomplete

　344.09　Other

344.1　Paraplegia
> Paralysis of both lower limbs
> Paraplegia (lower)

✓4th ✓5th　Additional Digit Required　　　Unspecified Code　　　Other Specified Code　　　Manifestation Code　　　▶◀ Revised Text　　　● New Code　　　▲ Revised Code Title

2003 ICD•9•CM　　　　　**Volume 1 — 81**

344.2 Diplegia of upper limbs
Diplegia (upper)   Paralysis of both upper limbs

√5ᵗʰ **344.3 Monoplegia of lower limb**
Paralysis of lower limb
> **EXCLUDES** *monoplegia of lower limb due to late effect of cerebrovascular accident (438.40-438.42)*

344.30 Affecting unspecified side
344.31 Affecting dominant side
344.32 Affecting nondominant side

√5ᵗʰ **344.4 Monoplegia of upper limb**
Paralysis of upper limb
> **EXCLUDES** *monoplegia of upper limb due to late effect of cerebrovascular accident (438.30-438.32)*

344.40 Affecting unspecified side
344.41 Affecting dominant side
344.42 Affecting nondominant side

344.5 Unspecified monoplegia

√5ᵗʰ **344.6 Cauda equina syndrome**
DEF: Dull pain and paresthesias in sacrum, perineum and bladder due to compression of spinal nerve roots; pain radiates down buttocks, back of thigh, calf of leg and into foot with prickling, burning sensations.

344.60 Without mention of neurogenic bladder
344.61 With neurogenic bladder
Acontractile bladder
Autonomic hyperreflexia of bladder
Cord bladder
Detrusor hyperreflexia

√5ᵗʰ **344.8 Other specified paralytic syndromes**
344.81 Locked-in state
DEF: State of consciousness where patients are paralyzed and unable to respond to environmental stimuli; patients have eye movements, and stimuli can enter the brain but patients cannot respond to stimuli.

344.89 Other specified paralytic syndrome
344.9 Paralysis, unspecified

√4ᵗʰ **345 Epilepsy**
> **EXCLUDES** *progressive myoclonic epilepsy (333.2)*

DEF: Brain disorder characterized by electrical-like disturbances; may include occasional impairment or loss of consciousness, abnormal motor phenomena and psychic or sensory disturbances.

The following fifth-digit subclassification is for use with categories 345.0, .1, .4–.9:
> 0 without mention of intractable epilepsy
> 1 with intractable epilepsy, so stated

√5ᵗʰ **345.0 Generalized nonconvulsive epilepsy**
Absences: Pykno-epilepsy
  atonic   Seizures:
  typical   akinetic
Minor epilepsy   atonic
Petit mal

√5ᵗʰ **345.1 Generalized convulsive epilepsy**
Epileptic seizures: Epileptic seizures:
  clonic   tonic-clonic
  myoclonic   Grand mal
  tonic   Major epilepsy
> **EXCLUDES** *convulsions:*
>   *NOS (780.3)*
>   *infantile (780.3)*
>   *newborn (779.0)*
> *infantile spasms (345.6)*

DEF: Convulsive seizures with tension of limbs (tonic) or rhythmic contractions (clonic).

345.2 Petit mal status
Epileptic absence status
DEF: Minor myoclonic spasms and sudden momentary loss of consciousness in epilepsy.

345.3 Grand mal status
Status epilepticus NOS
> **EXCLUDES** *epilepsia partialis continua (345.7)*
> *status:*
>   *psychomotor (345.7)*
>   *temporal lobe (345.7)*

DEF: Sudden loss of consciousness followed by generalized convulsions in epilepsy.

√5ᵗʰ **345.4 Partial epilepsy, with impairment of consciousness**
Epilepsy:
  limbic system
  partial:
    secondarily generalized
    with memory and ideational disturbances
  psychomotor
  psychosensory
  temporal lobe
Epileptic automatism

√5ᵗʰ **345.5 Partial epilepsy, without mention of impairment of consciousness**
Epilepsy: Epilepsy:
  Bravais-Jacksonian NOS   sensory-induced
  focal (motor) NOS   somatomotor
  Jacksonian NOS   somatosensory
  motor partial   visceral
  partial NOS   visual

√5ᵗʰ **345.6 Infantile spasms**
Hypsarrhythmia   Salaam attacks
Lightning spasms
> **EXCLUDES** *salaam tic (781.0)*

√5ᵗʰ **345.7 Epilepsia partialis continua**
Kojevnikov's epilepsy
DEF: Continuous muscle contractions and relaxation; result of abnormal neural discharge.

√5ᵗʰ **345.8 Other forms of epilepsy**
Epilepsy: Epilepsy:
  cursive [running]   gelastic

√5ᵗʰ **345.9 Epilepsy, unspecified**
Epileptic convulsions, fits, or seizures NOS
> **EXCLUDES** *convulsive seizure or fit NOS (780.3)*

√4ᵗʰ **346 Migraine**
DEF: Benign vascular headache of extreme pain; commonly associated with irritability, nausea, vomiting and often photophobia; premonitory visual hallucination of a crescent in the visual field (scotoma).

The following fifth-digit subclassification is for use with category 346:
> 0 without mention of intractable migraine
> 1 with intractable migraine, so stated

√5ᵗʰ **346.0 Classical migraine**
Migraine preceded or accompanied by transient focal neurological phenomena
Migraine with aura

√5ᵗʰ **346.1 Common migraine**
Atypical migraine   Sick headache

√5ᵗʰ **346.2 Variants of migraine**
Cluster headache   Migraine:
Histamine cephalgia   lower half
Horton's neuralgia   retinal
Migraine: Neuralgia:
  abdominal   ciliary
  basilar   migrainous

√5ᵗʰ **346.8 Other forms of migraine**
Migraine: Migraine:
  hemiplegic   ophthalmoplegic

√5ᵗʰ **346.9 Migraine, unspecified**

347 Cataplexy and narcolepsy

DEF: Cataplexy: sudden onset of muscle weakness with loss of tone and strength; caused by aggressive or spontaneous emotions.

DEF: Narcolepsy: brief, recurrent, uncontrollable episodes of sound sleep.

☑4ᵗʰ **348 Other conditions of brain**

348.0 Cerebral cysts

Arachnoid cyst	Porencephaly, acquired
Porencephalic cyst	Pseudoporencephaly

EXCLUDES   *porencephaly (congenital) (742.4)*

348.1 Anoxic brain damage

EXCLUDES   *that occurring in:*
     abortion (634-638 with .7, 639.8)
     ectopic or molar pregnancy (639.8)
     labor or delivery (668.2, 669.4)
     that of newborn (767.0, 768.0-768.9,
       772.1-772.2)

Use additional E code to identify cause

DEF: Brain injury due to lack of oxygen, other than birth trauma.

348.2 Benign intracranial hypertension

Pseudotumor cerebri

EXCLUDES   *hypertensive encephalopathy (437.2)*

DEF: Elevated pressure in brain due to fluid retention in brain cavities.

348.3 Encephalopathy, unspecified

348.4 Compression of brain

Compression ⎫
Herniation ⎬ brain (stem)
       ⎭

Posterior fossa compression syndrome

DEF: Elevated pressure in brain due to blood clot, tumor, fracture, abscess, other condition.

348.5 Cerebral edema

DEF: Elevated pressure in the brain due to fluid retention in brain tissues.

348.8 Other conditions of brain

Cerebral:	Cerebral:
calcification	fungus

348.9 Unspecified condition of brain

☑4ᵗʰ **349 Other and unspecified disorders of the nervous system**

349.0 Reaction to spinal or lumbar puncture

Headache following lumbar puncture

349.1 Nervous system complications from surgically implanted device

EXCLUDES   *immediate postoperative complications (997.00-997.09)*
     mechanical complications of nervous system device (996.2)

349.2 Disorders of meninges, not elsewhere classified

Adhesions, meningeal (cerebral) (spinal)
Cyst, spinal meninges
Meningocele, acquired
Pseudomeningocele, acquired

☑5ᵗʰ **349.8 Other specified disorders of nervous system**

349.81 Cerebrospinal fluid rhinorrhea

EXCLUDES   *cerebrospinal fluid otorrhea (388.61)*

DEF: Cerebrospinal fluid discharging from the nose; caused by fracture of frontal bone with tearing of dura mater and arachnoid.

349.82 Toxic encephalopathy

Use additional E code, if desired, to identify cause

DEF: Brain tissue degeneration due to toxic substance.

349.89 Other

349.9 Unspecified disorders of nervous system

Disorder of nervous system (central) NOS

DISORDERS OF THE PERIPHERAL NERVOUS SYSTEM (350-359)

EXCLUDES   *diseases of:*
     acoustic [8th] nerve (388.5)
     oculomotor [3rd, 4th, 6th] nerves (378.0-378.9)
     optic [2nd] nerve (377.0-377.9)
     peripheral autonomic nerves (337.0-337.9)
     neuralgia ⎫
     neuritis ⎬ *NOS or "rheumatic"*
     radiculitis ⎭ *(729.2)*

     peripheral neuritis in pregnancy (646.4)

☑4ᵗʰ **350 Trigeminal nerve disorders**

INCLUDES   disorders of 5th cranial nerve

350.1 Trigeminal neuralgia

Tic douloureux	Trigeminal neuralgia NOS
Trifacial neuralgia	

EXCLUDES   *postherpetic (053.12)*

350.2 Atypical face pain

350.8 Other specified trigeminal nerve disorders

350.9 Trigeminal nerve disorder, unspecified

☑4ᵗʰ **351 Facial nerve disorders**

INCLUDES   disorders of 7th cranial nerve

EXCLUDES   *that in newborn (767.5)*

351.0 Bell's palsy

Facial palsy

DEF: Unilateral paralysis of face due to lesion on facial nerve; produces facial distortion.

351.1 Geniculate ganglionitis

Geniculate ganglionitis NOS

EXCLUDES   *herpetic (053.11)*

DEF: Inflammation of tissue at bend in facial nerve.

351.8 Other facial nerve disorders

Facial myokymia
Melkersson's syndrome

351.9 Facial nerve disorder, unspecified

☑4ᵗʰ **352 Disorders of other cranial nerves**

352.0 Disorders of olfactory [1st] nerve

352.1 Glossopharyngeal neuralgia

DEF: Pain between throat and ear along petrosal and jugular ganglia.

352.2 Other disorders of glossopharyngeal [9th] nerve

352.3 Disorders of pneumogastric [10th] nerve

Disorders of vagal nerve

EXCLUDES   *paralysis of vocal cords or larynx (478.30-478.34)*

DEF: Nerve disorder affecting ear, tongue, pharynx, larynx, esophagus, viscera and thorax.

352.4 Disorders of accessory [11th] nerve

DEF: Nerve disorder affecting palate, pharynx, larynx, thoracic viscera, sternocleidomastoid and trapezius muscles.

352.5 Disorders of hypoglossal [12th] nerve

DEF: Nerve disorder affecting tongue muscles.

352.6 Multiple cranial nerve palsies

Collet-Sicard syndrome	Polyneuritis cranialis

352.9 Unspecified disorder of cranial nerves

☑4ᵗʰ **353 Nerve root and plexus disorders**

EXCLUDES   *conditions due to:*
     intervertebral disc disorders (722.0-722.9)
     spondylosis (720.0-721.9)
     vertebrogenic disorders (723.0-724.9)

☑4ᵗʰ
☑5ᵗʰ
Additional Digit Required   Unspecified Code   Other Specified Code   Manifestation Code   ▶◀ Revised Text   ● New Code   ▲ Revised Code Title

2003 ICD•9•CM   Volume 1 — 83

353.0 Brachial plexus lesions
Cervical rib syndrome
Costoclavicular syndrome
Scalenus anticus syndrome
Thoracic outlet syndrome
EXCLUDES brachial neuritis or radiculitis NOS (723.4)
that in newborn (767.6)
DEF: Acquired disorder in tissue along nerves in shoulder; causes corresponding motor and sensory dysfunction.

353.1 Lumbosacral plexus lesions
DEF: Acquired disorder in tissue along nerves in lower back; causes corresponding motor and sensory dysfunction.

353.2 Cervical root lesions, not elsewhere classified
353.3 Thoracic root lesions, not elsewhere classified
353.4 Lumbosacral root lesions, not elsewhere classified
353.5 Neuralgic amyotrophy
Parsonage-Aldren-Turner syndrome
353.6 Phantom limb (syndrome)
DEF: Abnormal tingling or a burning sensation, transient aches, and intermittent or continuous pain perceived as originating in the absent limb.

353.8 Other nerve root and plexus disorders
353.9 Unspecified nerve root and plexus disorder

✓4th 354 Mononeuritis of upper limb and mononeuritis multiplex
DEF: Inflammation of a single nerve; known as mononeuritis multiplex when several nerves in unrelated body areas are affected.

354.0 Carpal tunnel syndrome
Median nerve entrapment   Partial thenar atrophy
DEF: Compression of median nerve by tendons; causes pain, tingling, numbness and burning sensation in hand.

354.1 Other lesion of median nerve
Median nerve neuritis
354.2 Lesion of ulnar nerve
Cubital tunnel syndrome
Tardy ulnar nerve palsy
354.3 Lesion of radial nerve
Acute radial nerve palsy
354.4 Causalgia of upper limb
EXCLUDES causalgia:
NOS (355.9)
lower limb (355.71)
DEF: Peripheral nerve damage, upper limb; usually due to injury; causes burning sensation and trophic skin changes.

354.5 Mononeuritis multiplex
Combinations of single conditions classifiable to 354 or 355
354.8 Other mononeuritis of upper limb
354.9 Mononeuritis of upper limb, unspecified

✓4th 355 Mononeuritis of lower limb
355.0 Lesion of sciatic nerve
EXCLUDES sciatica NOS (724.3)
DEF: Acquired disorder of sciatic nerve; causes motor and sensory dysfunction in back, buttock and leg.

355.1 Meralgia paresthetica
Lateral cutaneous femoral nerve of thigh compression or syndrome
DEF: Inguinal ligament entraps lateral femoral cutaneous nerve; causes tingling, pain and numbness along outer thigh.

355.2 Other lesion of femoral nerve
355.3 Lesion of lateral popliteal nerve
Lesion of common peroneal nerve
355.4 Lesion of medial popliteal nerve
355.5 Tarsal tunnel syndrome
DEF: Compressed, entrapped posterior tibial nerve; causes tingling, pain and numbness in sole of foot.

355.6 Lesion of plantar nerve
Morton's metatarsalgia, neuralgia, or neuroma
✓5th 355.7 Other mononeuritis of lower limb
355.71 Causalgia of lower limb
EXCLUDES causalgia:
NOS (355.9)
upper limb (354.4)
DEF: Dysfunction of lower limb peripheral nerve, usually due to injury; causes burning pain and trophic skin changes.

355.79 Other mononeuritis of lower limb
355.8 Mononeuritis of lower limb, unspecified
355.9 Mononeuritis of unspecified site
Causalgia NOS
EXCLUDES causalgia:
lower limb (355.71)
upper limb (354.4)

✓4th 356 Hereditary and idiopathic peripheral neuropathy
356.0 Hereditary peripheral neuropathy
Déjérine-Sottas disease
356.1 Peroneal muscular atrophy
Charcôt-Marie-Tooth disease
Neuropathic muscular atrophy
DEF: Genetic disorder, in muscles innervated by peroneal nerves; symptoms include muscle wasting in lower limbs and locomotor difficulties.

356.2 Hereditary sensory neuropathy
DEF: Inherited disorder in dorsal root ganglia, optic nerve, and cerebellum, causing sensory losses, shooting pains, and foot ulcers.

356.3 Refsum's disease
Heredopathia atactica polyneuritiformis
DEF: Genetic disorder of lipid metabolism; causes persistent, painful inflammation of nerves and retinitis pigmentosa.

356.4 Idiopathic progressive polyneuropathy
356.8 Other specified idiopathic peripheral neuropathy
Supranuclear paralysis
356.9 Unspecified

✓4th 357 Inflammatory and toxic neuropathy
357.0 Acute infective polyneuritis
Guillain-Barré syndrome Postinfectious polyneuritis
DEF: Guillain-Barré syndrome: acute demyelinatry polyneuropathy preceded by viral illness (i.e., herpes, cytomegalovirus [CMV], Epstein-Barr virus [EBV]) or a bacterial illness; areflexic motor paralysis with mild sensory disturbance and acellular rise in spinal fluid protein.

357.1 Polyneuropathy in collagen vascular disease
Code first underlying disease, as:
disseminated lupus erythematosus (710.0)
polyarteritis nodosa (446.0)
rheumatoid arthritis (714.0)
357.2 Polyneuropathy in diabetes
Code first underlying disease (250.6)
357.3 Polyneuropathy in malignant disease
Code first underlying disease (140.0-208.9)
357.4 Polyneuropathy in other diseases classified elsewhere
Code first underlying disease, as:
amyloidosis (277.3)
beriberi (265.0)
deficiency of B vitamins (266.0-266.9)
diphtheria (032.0-032.9)
hypoglycemia (251.2)
pellagra (265.2)
porphyria (277.1)
sarcoidosis (135)
uremia (585)
EXCLUDES polyneuropathy in:
herpes zoster (053.13)
mumps (072.72)

357.5   **Alcoholic polyneuropathy**

357.6   **Polyneuropathy due to drugs**
Use additional E code to identify drug

357.7   **Polyneuropathy due to other toxic agents**
Use additional E code to identify toxic agent

√5ᵗʰ **357.8**   **Other**

357.81   **Chronic inflammatory demyelinating polyneuritis**

DEF: Chronic inflammatory demyelinating polyneuritis: inflammation of peripheral nerves resulting in destruction of myelin sheath; associated with diabetes mellitus, dysproteinemias, renal failure and malnutrition; symptoms include tingling, numbness, burning pain, diminished tendon reflexes, weakness, and atrophy in lower extremities.

357.82   **Critical illness polyneuropathy**
Acute motor neuropathy

357.89   **Other inflammatory and toxic neuropathy**

357.9   **Unspecified**

√4ᵗʰ **358**   **Myoneural disorders**

358.0   **Myasthenia gravis**

DEF: Autoimmune disorder of acetylcholine at neuromuscular junction; causing fatigue of voluntary muscles.

358.1   *Myasthenic syndromes in diseases classified elsewhere*

Amyotrophy
Eaton-Lambert syndrome   } from stated cause classified elsewhere

Code first underlying disease, as:
    botulism (005.1)
    diabetes mellitus (250.6)
    hypothyroidism (244.0-244.9)
    malignant neoplasm (140.0-208.9)
    pernicious anemia (281.0)
    thyrotoxicosis (242.0-242.9)

358.2   **Toxic myoneural disorders**
Use additional E code to identify toxic agent

358.8   **Other specified myoneural disorders**

358.9   **Myoneural disorders, unspecified**

√4ᵗʰ **359**   **Muscular dystrophies and other myopathies**
EXCLUDES   idiopathic polymyositis (710.4)

359.0   **Congenital hereditary muscular dystrophy**
Benign congenital myopathy
Central core disease
Centronuclear myopathy
Myotubular myopathy
Nemaline body disease
EXCLUDES   arthrogryposis multiplex congenita (754.89)

DEF: Genetic disorder; causing progressive or nonprogressive muscle weakness.

359.1   **Hereditary progressive muscular dystrophy**

Muscular dystrophy: Muscular dystrophy:
    NOS   Gower's
    distal   Landouzy-Déjérine
    Duchenne   limb-girdle
    Erb's   ocular
    fascioscapulohumeral oculopharyngeal

DEF: Genetic degenerative, muscle disease; causes progressive weakness, wasting of muscle with no nerve involvement.

359.2   **Myotonic disorders**

Dystrophia myotonica   Paramyotonia congenita
Eulenburg's disease   Steinert's disease
Myotonia congenita   Thomsen's disease

DEF: Impaired movement due to spasmatic, rigid muscles.

359.3   **Familial periodic paralysis**
Hypokalemic familial periodic paralysis

DEF: Genetic disorder; characterized by rapidly progressive flaccid paralysis; attacks often occur after exercise or exposure to cold or dietary changes.

359.4   **Toxic myopathy**
Use additional E code to identify toxic agent

DEF: Muscle disorder caused by toxic agent.

359.5   *Myopathy in endocrine diseases classified elsewhere*

Code first underlying disease, as:
    Addison's disease (255.4)
    Cushing's syndrome (255.0)
    hypopituitarism (253.2)
    myxedema (244.0-244.9)
    thyrotoxicosis (242.0-242.9)

DEF: Muscle disorder secondary to dysfunction in hormone secretion.

359.6   *Symptomatic inflammatory myopathy in diseases classified elsewhere*

Code first underlying disease, as:
    amyloidosis (277.3)
    disseminated lupus erythematosus (710.0)
    malignant neoplasm (140.0-208.9)
    polyarteritis nodosa (446.0)
    rheumatoid arthritis (714.0)
    sarcoidosis (135)
    scleroderma (710.1)
    Sjögren's disease (710.2)

√5ᵗʰ **359.8**   **Other myopathies**

359.81   **Critical illness myopathy**
Acute necrotizing myopathy
Acute quadriplegic myopathy
Intensive care (ICU) myopathy
Myopathy of critical illness

359.89   **Other myopathies**

359.9   **Myopathy, unspecified**

DISORDERS OF THE EYE AND ADNEXA (360-379)

√4ᵗʰ **360**   **Disorders of the globe**
INCLUDES   disorders affecting multiple structures of eye

√5ᵗʰ **360.0**   **Purulent endophthalmitis**

360.00   **Purulent endophthalmitis, unspecified**

360.01   **Acute endophthalmitis**

360.02   **Panophthalmitis**

360.03   **Chronic endophthalmitis**

360.04   **Vitreous abscess**

√5ᵗʰ **360.1**   **Other endophthalmitis**

360.11   **Sympathetic uveitis**

DEF: Inflammation of vascular layer of uninjured eye; follows injury to other eye.

360.12   **Panuveitis**

DEF: Inflammation of entire vascular layer of eye, including choroid, iris and ciliary body.

360.13   **Parasitic endophthalmitis NOS**

DEF: Parasitic infection causing inflammation of the entire eye.

360.14   **Ophthalmia nodosa**

DEF: Conjunctival inflammation caused by embedded hairs.

360.19   **Other**
Phacoanaphylactic endophthalmitis

√5ᵗʰ **360.2**   **Degenerative disorders of globe**

360.20   **Degenerative disorder of globe, unspecified**

√4ᵗʰ √5ᵗʰ Additional Digit Required   Unspecified Code   Other Specified Code   Manifestation Code   ▶◀ Revised Text   ● New Code   ▲ Revised Code Title

2003 ICD•9•CM   October 2002 • Volume 1 — 85

Nervous System and Sense Organs 357.5–360.20

Nervous System and Sense Organs 360.21–361.19

360.21 Progressive high (degenerative) myopia
Malignant myopia

DEF: Severe, progressive nearsightedness in adults, complicated by serious disease of the choroid; leads to retinal detachment and blindness.

360.23 Siderosis

DEF: Iron pigment deposits within tissue of eyeball; caused by high iron content of blood.

360.24 Other metallosis
Chalcosis

DEF: Metal deposits, other than iron, within eyeball tissues.

360.29 Other
> EXCLUDES   xerophthalmia (264.7)

√5th **360.3 Hypotony of eye**
360.30 Hypotony, unspecified

DEF: Low osmotic pressure causing lack of tone, tension and strength.

360.31 Primary hypotony

360.32 Ocular fistula causing hypotony

DEF: Low intraocular pressure due to leak through abnormal passage.

360.33 Hypotony associated with other ocular disorders

360.34 Flat anterior chamber

DEF: Low pressure behind cornea, causing compression.

√5th **360.4 Degenerated conditions of globe**
360.40 Degenerated globe or eye, unspecified

360.41 Blind hypotensive eye
Atrophy of globe
Phthisis bulbi

DEF: Vision loss due to extremely low intraocular pressure.

360.42 Blind hypertensive eye
Absolute glaucoma

DEF: Vision loss due to painful, high intraocular pressure.

360.43 Hemophthalmos, except current injury
> EXCLUDES   traumatic (871.0-871.9, 921.0-921.9)

DEF: Pool of blood within eyeball, not from current injury.

360.44 Leucocoria

DEF: Whitish mass or reflex in the pupil behind lens; also called cat's eye reflex; often indicative of retinoblastoma.

√5th **360.5 Retained (old) intraocular foreign body, magnetic**
> EXCLUDES   current penetrating injury with magnetic foreign body (871.5)
> retained (old) foreign body of orbit (376.6)

360.50 Foreign body, magnetic, intraocular, unspecified

360.51 Foreign body, magnetic, in anterior chamber

360.52 Foreign body, magnetic, in iris or ciliary body

360.53 Foreign body, magnetic, in lens

360.54 Foreign body, magnetic, in vitreous

360.55 Foreign body, magnetic, in posterior wall

360.59 Foreign body, magnetic, in other or multiple sites

√5th **360.6 Retained (old) intraocular foreign body, nonmagnetic**
Retained (old) foreign body:
NOS
nonmagnetic
> EXCLUDES   current penetrating injury with (nonmagnetic) foreign body (871.6)
> retained (old) foreign body in orbit (376.6)

360.60 Foreign body, intraocular, unspecified

360.61 Foreign body in anterior chamber

360.62 Foreign body in iris or ciliary body

360.63 Foreign body in lens

360.64 Foreign body in vitreous

360.65 Foreign body in posterior wall

360.69 Foreign body in other or multiple sites

√5th **360.8 Other disorders of globe**
360.81 Luxation of globe

DEF: Displacement of eyeball.

360.89 Other

360.9 Unspecified disorder of globe

√4th **361 Retinal detachments and defects**

DEF: Light-sensitive layer at back of eye, separates from blood supply; disrupting vision.

√5th **361.0 Retinal detachment with retinal defect**
Rhegmatogenous retinal detachment
> EXCLUDES   detachment of retinal pigment epithelium (362.42-362.43)
> retinal detachment (serous) (without defect) (361.2)

361.00 Retinal detachment with retinal defect, unspecified

361.01 Recent detachment, partial, with single defect

361.02 Recent detachment, partial, with multiple defects

361.03 Recent detachment, partial, with giant tear

361.04 Recent detachment, partial, with retinal dialysis
Dialysis (juvenile) of retina (with detachment)

361.05 Recent detachment, total or subtotal

361.06 Old detachment, partial
Delimited old retinal detachment

361.07 Old detachment, total or subtotal

√5th **361.1 Retinoschisis and retinal cysts**
> EXCLUDES   juvenile retinoschisis (362.73)
> microcystoid degeneration of retina (362.62)
> parasitic cyst of retina (360.13)

361.10 Retinoschisis, unspecified

DEF: Separation of retina due to degenerative process of aging; should not be confused with acute retinal detachment.

361.11 Flat retinoschisis

DEF: Slow, progressive split of retinal sensory layers.

361.12 Bullous retinoschisis

DEF: Fluid retention between split retinal sensory layers.

361.13 Primary retinal cysts

361.14 Secondary retinal cysts

361.19 Other
Pseudocyst of retina

361.2 Serous retinal detachment
Retinal detachment without retinal defect
> EXCLUDES   *central serous retinopathy (362.41)*
> *retinal pigment epithelium detachment (362.42-362.43)*

√5th **361.3 Retinal defects without detachment**
> EXCLUDES   *chorioretinal scars after surgery for detachment (363.30-363.35)*
> *peripheral retinal degeneration without defect (362.60-362.66)*

     361.30 Retinal defect, unspecified
        Retinal break(s) NOS

     361.31 Round hole of retina without detachment

     361.32 Horseshoe tear of retina without detachment
        Operculum of retina without mention of detachment

     361.33 Multiple defects of retina without detachment

√5th **361.8 Other forms of retinal detachment**
     361.81 Traction detachment of retina
        Traction detachment with vitreoretinal organization

     361.89 Other

361.9 Unspecified retinal detachment

√4th **362 Other retinal disorders**
> EXCLUDES   *chorioretinal scars (363.30-363.35)*
> *chorioretinitis (363.0-363.2)*

√5th **362.0 Diabetic retinopathy**
Code first diabetes (250.5)
DEF: Retinal changes in diabetes of long duration; causes hemorrhages, microaneurysms, waxy deposits and proliferative noninflammatory degenerative disease of retina.

     362.01 *Background diabetic retinopathy*
        Diabetic macular edema
        Diabetic retinal edema
        Diabetic retinal microaneurysms
        Diabetic retinopathy NOS

     362.02 *Proliferative diabetic retinopathy*

√5th **362.1 Other background retinopathy and retinal vascular changes**
     362.10 Background retinopathy, unspecified
     362.11 Hypertensive retinopathy
        DEF: Retinal irregularities caused by systemic hypertension.

     362.12 Exudative retinopathy
        Coats' syndrome

     362.13 Changes in vascular appearance
        Vascular sheathing of retina
        Use additional code for any associated atherosclerosis (440.8)

     362.14 Retinal microaneurysms NOS
        DEF: Microscopic dilation of retinal vessels in nondiabetic.

     362.15 Retinal telangiectasia
        DEF: Dilation of blood vessels of the retina.

     362.16 Retinal neovascularization NOS
        Neovascularization:
          choroidal
          subretinal
        DEF: New and abnormal vascular growth in the retina.

     362.17 Other intraretinal microvascular abnormalities
        Retinal varices

362.18 Retinal vasculitis
     Eales' disease   Retinal:
     Retinal: perivasculitis
       arteritis   phlebitis
       endarteritis
     DEF: Inflammation of retinal blood vessels.

√5th **362.2 Other proliferative retinopathy**
     362.21 Retrolental fibroplasia
        DEF: Fibrous tissue in vitreous, from retina to lens, causing blindness; associated with premature infants requiring high amounts of oxygen.

     362.29 Other nondiabetic proliferative retinopathy

√5th **362.3 Retinal vascular occlusion**
DEF: Obstructed blood flow to and from retina.

     362.30 Retinal vascular occlusion, unspecified
     362.31 Central retinal artery occlusion
     362.32 Arterial branch occlusion
     362.33 Partial arterial occlusion
        Hollenhorst plaque
        Retinal microembolism

     362.34 Transient arterial occlusion
        Amaurosis fugax

     362.35 Central retinal vein occlusion
     362.36 Venous tributary (branch) occlusion
     362.37 Venous engorgement
        Occlusion:
          incipient } of retinal vein
          partial

√5th **362.4 Separation of retinal layers**
> EXCLUDES   *retinal detachment (serous) (361.2)*
> *rhegmatogenous (361.00-361.07)*

     362.40 Retinal layer separation, unspecified
     362.41 Central serous retinopathy
        DEF: Serous-filled blister causing detachment of retina from pigment epithelium.

     362.42 Serous detachment of retinal pigment epithelium
        Exudative detachment of retinal pigment epithelium
        DEF: Blister of fatty fluid causing detachment of retina from pigment epithelium.

     362.43 Hemorrhagic detachment of retinal pigment epithelium
        DEF: Blood-filled blister causing detachment of retina from pigment epithelium.

√5th **362.5 Degeneration of macula and posterior pole**
> EXCLUDES   *degeneration of optic disc (377.21-377.24)*
> *hereditary retinal degeneration [dystrophy] (362.70-362.77)*

     362.50 Macular degeneration (senile), unspecified
     362.51 Nonexudative senile macular degeneration
        Senile macular degeneration:
          atrophic
          dry

     362.52 Exudative senile macular degeneration
        Kuhnt-Junius degeneration
        Senile macular degeneration:
          disciform
          wet
        DEF: Leakage in macular blood vessels with loss of visual acuity.

     362.53 Cystoid macular degeneration
        Cystoid macular edema
        DEF: Retinal swelling and cyst formation in macula.

Nervous System and Sense Organs 361.2–362.53

√4th √5th Additional Digit Required   Unspecified Code   Other Specified Code   Manifestation Code   ▶◀ Revised Text   ● New Code   ▲ Revised Code Title

362.54 Macular cyst, hole, or pseudohole

362.55 Toxic maculopathy

Use additional E code to identify drug, if drug induced

362.56 Macular puckering

Preretinal fibrosis

362.57 Drusen (degenerative)

DEF: White, hyaline deposits on Bruch's membrane (lamina basalis choroideae).

√5th **362.6 Peripheral retinal degenerations**

EXCLUDES   hereditary retinal degeneration [dystrophy] (362.70-362.77)
retinal degeneration with retinal defect (361.00-361.07)

362.60 Peripheral retinal degeneration, unspecified

362.61 Paving stone degeneration

DEF: Degeneration of peripheral retina; causes thinning through which choroid is visible.

362.62 Microcystoid degeneration

Blessig's cysts   Iwanoff's cysts

362.63 Lattice degeneration

Palisade degeneration of retina

DEF: Degeneration of retina; often bilateral, usually benign; characterized by lines intersecting at irregular intervals in peripheral retina; retinal thinning and retinal holes may occur.

362.64 Senile reticular degeneration

DEF: Net-like appearance of retina; sign of degeneration.

362.65 Secondary pigmentary degeneration

Pseudoretinitis pigmentosa

362.66 Secondary vitreoretinal degenerations

√5th **362.7 Hereditary retinal dystrophies**

DEF: Genetically induced progressive changes in retina.

362.70 Hereditary retinal dystrophy, unspecified

362.71 *Retinal dystrophy in systemic or cerebroretinal lipidoses*

Code first underlying disease, as:
cerebroretinal lipidoses (330.1)
systemic lipidoses (272.7)

362.72 *Retinal dystrophy in other systemic disorders and syndromes*

Code first underlying disease, as:
Bassen-Kornzweig syndrome (272.5)
Refsum's disease (356.3)

362.73 Vitreoretinal dystrophies

Juvenile retinoschisis

362.74 Pigmentary retinal dystrophy

Retinal dystrophy, albipunctate
Retinitis pigmentosa

362.75 Other dystrophies primarily involving the sensory retina

Progressive cone(-rod) dystrophy
Stargardt's disease

362.76 Dystrophies primarily involving the retinal pigment epithelium

Fundus flavimaculatus
Vitelliform dystrophy

362.77 Dystrophies primarily involving Bruch's membrane

Dystrophy:
hyaline
pseudoinflammatory foveal
Hereditary drusen

√5th **362.8 Other retinal disorders**

EXCLUDES   chorioretinal inflammations (363.0-363.2)
chorioretinal scars (363.30-363.35)

362.81 Retinal hemorrhage

Hemorrhage:
preretinal
retinal (deep) (superficial)
subretinal

362.82 Retinal exudates and deposits

362.83 Retinal edema

Retinal:
cotton wool spots
edema (localized) (macular) (peripheral)

DEF: Retinal swelling due to fluid accumulation.

362.84 Retinal ischemia

DEF: Reduced retinal blood supply.

362.85 Retinal nerve fiber bundle defects

362.89 Other retinal disorders

362.9 Unspecified retinal disorder

√4th **363 Chorioretinal inflammations, scars, and other disorders of choroid**

√5th **363.0 Focal chorioretinitis and focal retinochoroiditis**

EXCLUDES   focal chorioretinitis or retinochoroiditis in:
histoplasmosis (115.02, 115.12, 115.92)
toxoplasmosis (130.2)
congenital infection (771.2)

363.00 Focal chorioretinitis, unspecified

Focal:
choroiditis or chorioretinitis NOS
retinitis or retinochoroiditis NOS

363.01 Focal choroiditis and chorioretinitis, juxtapapillary

363.03 Focal choroiditis and chorioretinitis of other posterior pole

363.04 Focal choroiditis and chorioretinitis, peripheral

363.05 Focal retinitis and retinochoroiditis, juxtapapillary

Neuroretinitis

363.06 Focal retinitis and retinochoroiditis, macular or paramacular

363.07 Focal retinitis and retinochoroiditis of other posterior pole

363.08 Focal retinitis and retinochoroiditis, peripheral

√5th **363.1 Disseminated chorioretinitis and disseminated retinochoroiditis**

EXCLUDES   disseminated choroiditis or chorioretinitis in secondary syphilis (091.51)
neurosyphilitic disseminated retinitis or retinochoroiditis (094.83)
retinal (peri)vasculitis (362.18)

363.10 Disseminated chorioretinitis, unspecified

Disseminated:
choroiditis or chorioretinitis NOS
retinitis or retinochoroiditis NOS

363.11 Disseminated choroiditis and chorioretinitis, posterior pole

363.12 Disseminated choroiditis and chorioretinitis, peripheral

363.13 *Disseminated choroiditis and chorioretinitis, generalized*

Code first any underlying disease, as:
tuberculosis (017.3)

363.14 **Disseminated retinitis and retinochoroiditis, metastatic**

363.15 **Disseminated retinitis and retinochoroiditis, pigment epitheliopathy**

Acute posterior multifocal placoid pigment epitheliopathy

DEF: Widespread inflammation of retina and choroid; characterized by pigmented epithelium involvement.

√5th 363.2 **Other and unspecified forms of chorioretinitis and retinochoroiditis**

EXCLUDES   panophthalmitis (360.02)
sympathetic uveitis (360.11)
uveitis NOS (364.3)

363.20 Chorioretinitis, unspecified

Choroiditis NOS   Uveitis, posterior NOS
Retinitis NOS

363.21 **Pars planitis**

Posterior cyclitis

DEF: Inflammation of peripheral retina and ciliary body; characterized by bands of white cells.

363.22 **Harada's disease**

DEF: Retinal detachment and bilateral widespread exudative choroiditis; symptoms include headache, vomiting, increased lymphocytes in cerebrospinal fluid; and temporary or permanent deafness may occur.

√5th 363.3 **Chorioretinal scars**

Scar (postinflammatory) (postsurgical) (posttraumatic):
choroid
retina

363.30 Chorioretinal scar, unspecified

363.31 **Solar retinopathy**

DEF: Retinal scarring caused by solar radiation.

363.32 Other macular scars

363.33 Other scars of posterior pole

363.34 **Peripheral scars**

363.35 **Disseminated scars**

√5th 363.4 **Choroidal degenerations**

363.40 Choroidal degeneration, unspecified
Choroidal sclerosis NOS

363.41 **Senile atrophy of choroid**

DEF: Wasting away of choroid; due to aging.

363.42 **Diffuse secondary atrophy of choroid**

DEF: Wasting away of choroid in systemic disease.

363.43 **Angioid streaks of choroid**

DEF: Degeneration of choroid; characterized by dark brown steaks radiating from optic disk; occurs with pseudoxanthoma, elasticum or Paget's disease.

√5th 363.5 **Hereditary choroidal dystrophies**

Hereditary choroidal atrophy:
partial [choriocapillaris]
total [all vessels]

363.50 Hereditary choroidal dystrophy or atrophy, unspecified

363.51 **Circumpapillary dystrophy of choroid, partial**

363.52 **Circumpapillary dystrophy of choroid, total**
Helicoid dystrophy of choroid

363.53 **Central dystrophy of choroid, partial**
Dystrophy, choroidal: Dystrophy, choroidal:
central areolar   circinate

363.54 **Central choroidal atrophy, total**
Dystrophy, choroidal: Dystrophy, choroidal:
central gyrate   serpiginous

363.55 **Choroideremia**

DEF: Hereditary choroid degeneration, occurs in first decade; characterized by constricted visual field and ultimately blindness in males; less debilitating in females.

363.56 Other diffuse or generalized dystrophy, partial
Diffuse choroidal sclerosis

363.57 Other diffuse or generalized dystrophy, total
Generalized gyrate atrophy, choroid

√5th 363.6 **Choroidal hemorrhage and rupture**

363.61 Choroidal hemorrhage, unspecified

363.62 **Expulsive choroidal hemorrhage**

363.63 **Choroidal rupture**

√5th 363.7 **Choroidal detachment**

363.70 Choroidal detachment, unspecified

363.71 **Serous choroidal detachment**

DEF: Detachment of choroid from sclera; due to blister of serous fluid.

363.72 **Hemorrhagic choroidal detachment**

DEF: Detachment of choroid from sclera; due to blood-filled blister.

363.8 Other disorders of choroid

363.9 Unspecified disorder of choroid

√4th 364 **Disorders of iris and ciliary body**

√5th 364.0 **Acute and subacute iridocyclitis**

Anterior uveitis
Cyclitis   acute
Iridocyclitis   subacute
Iritis

EXCLUDES   gonococcal (098.41)
herpes simplex (054.44)
herpes zoster (053.22)

364.00 Acute and subacute iridocyclitis, unspecified

364.01 **Primary iridocyclitis**

364.02 **Recurrent iridocyclitis**

364.03 **Secondary iridocyclitis, infectious**

364.04 **Secondary iridocyclitis, noninfectious**
Aqueous: Aqueous:
cells   flare
fibrin

364.05 **Hypopyon**

DEF: Accumulation of white blood cells between cornea and lens.

√5th 364.1 **Chronic iridocyclitis**

EXCLUDES   posterior cyclitis (363.21)

364.10 Chronic iridocyclitis, unspecified

364.11 *Chronic iridocyclitis in diseases classified elsewhere*
Code first underlying disease, as:
sarcoidosis (135)
tuberculosis (017.3)
EXCLUDES   syphilitic iridocyclitis (091.52)

DEF: Persistent inflammation of iris and ciliary body; due to underlying disease or condition.

√5th 364.2 **Certain types of iridocyclitis**
EXCLUDES   posterior cyclitis (363.21)
sympathetic uveitis (360.11)

364.21 **Fuchs' heterochromic cyclitis**

DEF: Chronic cyclitis characterized by differences in the color of the two irises; the lighter iris appears in the inflamed eye.

Nervous System and Sense Organs 363.14–364.21

√4th √5th Additional Digit Required   Unspecified Code   Other Specified Code   Manifestation Code   ►◄ Revised Text   ● New Code   ▲ Revised Code Title

2003 ICD•9•CM   Volume 1 — 89

Nervous System and Sense Organs 364.22–365.21

364.22 Glaucomatocyclitic crises
DEF: One-sided form of secondary open angle glaucoma; recurrent, uncommon and of short duration; causes high intraocular pressure, rarely damage.

364.23 Lens-induced iridocyclitis
DEF: Inflammation of iris; due to immune reaction to proteins in lens following trauma or other lens abnormality.

364.24 Vogt-Koyanagi syndrome
DEF: Uveomeningitis with exudative iridocyclitis and choroiditis; causes depigmentation of hair and skin; detached retina; tinnitus and loss of hearing may occur.

364.3 Unspecified iridocyclitis
Uveitis NOS

√5ᵗʰ 364.4 Vascular disorders of iris and ciliary body

364.41 Hyphema
Hemorrhage of iris or ciliary body
DEF: Hemorrhage in anterior chamber; also called hyphemia or "blood shot" eyes.

364.42 Rubeosis iridis
Neovascularization of iris or ciliary body
DEF: Blood vessel and connective tissue formation on surface of iris; symptomatic of diabetic retinopathy, central retinal vein occlusion and retinal detachment.

√5ᵗʰ 364.5 Degenerations of iris and ciliary body

364.51 Essential or progressive iris atrophy

364.52 Iridoschisis
DEF: Splitting of iris into two layers.

364.53 Pigmentary iris degeneration
Acquired heterochromia
Pigment dispersion
    syndrome   } of iris
Translucency

364.54 Degeneration of pupillary margin
Atrophy of sphincter
Ectropion of pigment } of iris
    epithelium

364.55 Miotic cysts of pupillary margin
DEF: Serous-filled sacs in pupillary margin of iris.

364.56 Degenerative changes of chamber angle

364.57 Degenerative changes of ciliary body

364.59 Other iris atrophy
Iris atrophy (generalized) (sector shaped)

√5ᵗʰ 364.6 Cysts of iris, ciliary body, and anterior chamber
EXCLUDES   miotic pupillary cyst (364.55)
    parasitic cyst (360.13)

364.60 Idiopathic cysts
DEF: Fluid-filled sacs in iris or ciliary body; unknown etiology.

364.61 Implantation cysts
Epithelial down-growth, anterior chamber
Implantation cysts (surgical) (traumatic)

364.62 Exudative cysts of iris or anterior chamber

364.63 Primary cyst of pars plana
DEF: Fluid-filled sacs of outermost ciliary ring.

364.64 Exudative cyst of pars plana
DEF: Protein, fatty-filled sacs of outermost ciliary ring; due to fluid lead from blood vessels.

√5ᵗʰ 364.7 Adhesions and disruptions of iris and ciliary body
EXCLUDES   flat anterior chamber (360.34)

364.70 Adhesions of iris, unspecified
Synechiae (iris) NOS

364.71 Posterior synechiae
DEF: Adhesion binding iris to lens.

364.72 Anterior synechiae
DEF: Adhesion binding the iris to cornea.

364.73 Goniosynechiae
Peripheral anterior synechiae
DEF: Adhesion binding the iris to cornea at the angle of the anterior chamber.

364.74 Pupillary membranes
Iris bombé   Pupillary:
Pupillary: seclusion
    occlusion
DEF: Membrane traversing the pupil and blocking vision.

364.75 Pupillary abnormalities
Deformed pupil   Rupture of sphincter, pupil
Ectopic pupil

364.76 Iridodialysis
DEF: Separation of the iris from the ciliary body base; due to trauma or surgical accident.

364.77 Recession of chamber angle
DEF: Receding of anterior chamber angle of the eye; restricts vision.

364.8 Other disorders of iris and ciliary body
Prolapse of iris NOS
EXCLUDES   prolapse of iris in recent wound (871.1)

364.9 Unspecified disorder of iris and ciliary body

√4ᵗʰ 365 Glaucoma
EXCLUDES   blind hypertensive eye [absolute glaucoma]
    (360.42)
    congenital glaucoma (743.20-743.22)
DEF: Rise in intraocular pressure which restricts blood flow; multiple causes.

√5ᵗʰ 365.0 Borderline glaucoma [glaucoma suspect]

365.00 Preglaucoma, unspecified

365.01 Open angle with borderline findings
Open angle with:
    borderline intraocular pressure
    cupping of optic discs
DEF: Minor block of aqueous outflow from eye.

365.02 Anatomical narrow angle

365.03 Steroid responders

365.04 Ocular hypertension
DEF: High fluid pressure within eye; no apparent cause.

√5ᵗʰ 365.1 Open-angle glaucoma

365.10 Open-angle glaucoma, unspecified
Wide-angle glaucoma NOS

365.11 Primary open angle glaucoma
Chronic simple glaucoma
DEF: High intraocular pressure, despite free flow of aqueous.

365.12 Low tension glaucoma

365.13 Pigmentary glaucoma
DEF: High intraocular pressure; due to iris pigment granules blocking aqueous flow.

365.14 Glaucoma of childhood
Infantile or juvenile glaucoma

365.15 Residual stage of open angle glaucoma

√5ᵗʰ 365.2 Primary angle-closure glaucoma

365.20 Primary angle-closure glaucoma, unspecified

365.21 Intermittent angle-closure glaucoma
Angle-closure glaucoma:
    interval
    subacute
DEF: Recurring attacks of high intraocular pressure; due to blocked aqueous flow.

N   Newborn Age: 0   P   Pediatric Age: 0-17   M   Maternity Age: 12-55   A   Adult Age: 15-124   MSP   Medicare Secondary Payer

365.22　Acute angle-closure glaucoma

DEF: Sudden, severe rise in intraocular pressure due to blockage in aqueous drainage.

365.23　Chronic angle-closure glaucoma

365.24　Residual stage of angle-closure glaucoma

✓5th **365.3　Corticosteroid-induced glaucoma**

DEF: Elevated intraocular pressure; due to long-term corticosteroid therapy.

365.31　Glaucomatous stage

365.32　Residual stage

✓5th **365.4　Glaucoma associated with congenital anomalies, dystrophies, and systemic syndromes**

365.41　*Glaucoma associated with chamber angle anomalies*

Code first associated disorder, as:
Axenfeld's anomaly (743.44)
Rieger's anomaly or syndrome (743.44)

365.42　*Glaucoma associated with anomalies of iris*

Code first associated disorder, as:
aniridia (743.45)
essential iris atrophy (364.51)

365.43　*Glaucoma associated with other anterior segment anomalies*

Code first associated disorder, as:
microcornea (743.41)

365.44　*Glaucoma associated with systemic syndromes*

Code first associated disease, as
neurofibromatosis (237.7)
Sturge-Weber (-Dimitri) syndrome (759.6)

✓5th **365.5　Glaucoma associated with disorders of the lens**

365.51　Phacolytic glaucoma

Use additional code for associated hypermature cataract (366.18)

DEF: Elevated intraocular pressure; due to lens protein blocking aqueous flow.

365.52　Pseudoexfoliation glaucoma

Use additional code for associated pseudoexfoliation of capsule (366.11)

DEF: Glaucoma characterized by small grayish particles deposited on the lens.

365.59　Glaucoma associated with other lens disorders

Use additional code for associated disorder, as:
dislocation of lens (379.33-379.34)
spherophakia (743.36)

✓5th **365.6　Glaucoma associated with other ocular disorders**

365.60　Glaucoma associated with unspecified ocular disorder

365.61　Glaucoma associated with pupillary block

Use additional code for associated disorder, as:
seclusion of pupil [iris bombé] (364.74)

DEF: Acute, open-angle glaucoma caused by mature cataract; aqueous flow is blocked by lens material and macrophages.

365.62　Glaucoma associated with ocular inflammations

Use additional code for associated disorder, as:
glaucomatocyclitic crises (364.22)
iridocyclitis (364.0-364.3)

365.63　Glaucoma associated with vascular disorders

Use additional code for associated disorder, as:
central retinal vein occlusion (362.35)
hyphema (364.41)

365.64　Glaucoma associated with tumors or cysts

Use additional code for associated disorder, as:
benign neoplasm (224.0-224.9)
epithelial down-growth (364.61)
malignant neoplasm (190.0-190.9)

365.65　Glaucoma associated with ocular trauma

Use additional code for associated condition, as:
contusion of globe (921.3)
recession of chamber angle (364.77)

✓5th **365.8　Other specified forms of glaucoma**

365.81　Hypersecretion glaucoma

365.82　Glaucoma with increased episcleral venous pressure

365.83　Aqueous misdirection

Malignant glaucoma

365.89　Other specified glaucoma

365.9　Unspecified glaucoma

✓4th **366　Cataract**

EXCLUDES　congenital cataract (743.30-743.34)

DEF: A variety of conditions that create a cloudy, or calcified lens that obstructs vision.

✓5th **366.0　Infantile, juvenile, and presenile cataract**

366.00　Nonsenile cataract, unspecified

366.01　Anterior subcapsular polar cataract

DEF: Defect within the front, center lens surface.

366.02　Posterior subcapsular polar cataract

DEF: Defect within the rear, center lens surface.

366.03　Cortical, lamellar, or zonular cataract

DEF: Opacities radiating from center to edge of lens; appear as thin, concentric layers of lens.

366.04　Nuclear cataract

366.09　Other and combined forms of nonsenile cataract

✓5th **366.1　Senile cataract**

366.10　Senile cataract, unspecified　Ⓐ

366.11　Pseudoexfoliation of lens capsule　Ⓐ

366.12　Incipient cataract　Ⓐ

Cataract:　　　Cataract:
coronary　　　punctate
immature NOS　Water clefts

DEF: Minor disorders of lens not affecting vision; due to aging.

366.13　Anterior subcapsular polar senile cataract　Ⓐ

366.14　Posterior subcapsular polar senile cataract　Ⓐ

366.15　Cortical senile cataract　Ⓐ

366.16　Nuclear sclerosis　Ⓐ

Cataracta brunescens
Nuclear cataract

366.17　Total or mature cataract　Ⓐ

366.18　Hypermature cataract　Ⓐ

Morgagni cataract

366.19　Other and combined forms of senile cataract　Ⓐ

✓5th **366.2　Traumatic cataract**

366.20　Traumatic cataract, unspecified

366.21　Localized traumatic opacities

Vossius' ring

366.22　Total traumatic cataract

366.23　Partially resolved traumatic cataract

✓5th **366.3　Cataract secondary to ocular disorders**

366.30　Cataracta complicata, unspecified

✓4th ✓5th　Additional Digit Required　　Unspecified Code　　Other Specified Code　　Manifestation Code　　▶◀ Revised Text　　● New Code　　▲ Revised Code Title

2003 ICD•9•CM　　　　　　　　　　　　　　　　　　　　　October 2002 • Volume 1 — 91

Nervous System and Sense Organs 366.31–368.32

366.31 Glaucomatous flecks (subcapsular)
Code first underlying glaucoma
(365.0-365.9)

366.32 Cataract in inflammatory disorders
Code first underlying condition, as:
chronic choroiditis (363.0-363.2)

366.33 Cataract with neovascularization
Code first underlying condition, as:
chronic iridocyclitis (364.10)

366.34 Cataract in degenerative disorders
Sunflower cataract
Code first underlying condition, as:
chalcosis (360.24)
degenerative myopia (360.21)
pigmentary retinal dystrophy (362.74)

✓5th **366.4 Cataract associated with other disorders**

366.41 Diabetic cataract
Code first diabetes (250.5)

366.42 Tetanic cataract
Code first underlying disease, as:
calcinosis (275.4)
hypoparathyroidism (252.1)

366.43 Myotonic cataract
Code first underlying disorder (359.2)

366.44 Cataract associated with other syndromes
Code first underlying condition, as:
craniofacial dysostosis (756.0)
galactosemia (271.1)

366.45 Toxic cataract
Drug-induced cataract
Use additional E code to identify drug or
other toxic substance

366.46 Cataract associated with radiation and other physical influences
Use additional E code to identify cause

✓5th **366.5 After-cataract**

366.50 After-cataract, unspecified
Secondary cataract NOS

366.51 Soemmering's ring
DEF: A donut-shaped lens remnant and a capsule behind
the pupil as a result of cataract surgery or trauma.

366.52 Other after-cataract, not obscuring vision

366.53 After-cataract, obscuring vision

366.8 Other cataract
Calcification of lens

366.9 Unspecified cataract

✓4th **367 Disorders of refraction and accommodation**

367.0 Hypermetropia
Far-sightedness
Hyperopia
DEF: Refraction error, called also hyperopia, focal point is posterior
to retina; abnormally short anteroposterior diameter or subnormal
refractive power; causes farsightedness.

367.1 Myopia
Near-sightedness
DEF: Refraction error, focal point is anterior to retina; causes near-
sightedness.

✓5th **367.2 Astigmatism**

367.20 Astigmatism, unspecified

367.21 Regular astigmatism

367.22 Irregular astigmatism

✓5th **367.3 Anisometropia and aniseikonia**

367.31 Anisometropia
DEF: Eyes with refractive powers that differ by at least
one diopter.

367.32 Aniseikonia
DEF: Eyes with unequal retinal imaging; usually due to
refractive error.

367.4 Presbyopia
DEF: Loss of crystalline lens elasticity; causes errors of
accommodation; due to aging.

✓5th **367.5 Disorders of accommodation**

367.51 Paresis of accommodation
Cycloplegia
DEF: Partial paralysis of ciliary muscle; causing focus
problems.

367.52 Total or complete internal ophthalmoplegia
DEF: Total paralysis of ciliary muscle; large pupil
incapable of focus.

367.53 Spasm of accommodation
DEF: Abnormal contraction of ciliary muscle; causes
focus problems.

✓5th **367.8 Other disorders of refraction and accommodation**

367.81 Transient refractive change

367.89 Other
Drug-induced } disorders of refraction
Toxic   & accommodation

367.9 Unspecified disorder of refraction and accommodation

✓4th **368 Visual disturbances**
EXCLUDES   electrophysiological disturbances (794.11-
794.14)

✓5th **368.0 Amblyopia ex anopsia**
DEF: Vision impaired due to disuse; esotropia often cause.

368.00 Amblyopia, unspecified

368.01 Strabismic amblyopia
Suppression amblyopia

368.02 Deprivation amblyopia
DEF: Decreased vision associated with suppressed
retinal image of one eye.

368.03 Refractive amblyopia

✓5th **368.1 Subjective visual disturbances**

368.10 Subjective visual disturbance, unspecified

368.11 Sudden visual loss

368.12 Transient visual loss
Concentric fading   Scintillating scotoma

368.13 Visual discomfort
Asthenopia   Photophobia
Eye strain

368.14 Visual distortions of shape and size
Macropsia   Micropsia
Metamorphopsia

368.15 Other visual distortions and entoptic phenomena
Photopsia   Refractive:
Refractive: polyopia
diplopia   Visual halos

368.16 Psychophysical visual disturbances
Visual: Visual:
agnosia   hallucinations
disorientation syndrome

368.2 Diplopia
Double vision

✓5th **368.3 Other disorders of binocular vision**

368.30 Binocular vision disorder, unspecified

368.31 Suppression of binocular vision

368.32 Simultaneous visual perception without fusion

368.33 Fusion with defective stereopsis

DEF: Faulty depth perception though normal ability to focus.

368.34 Abnormal retinal correspondence

√5th **368.4 Visual field defects**

368.40 Visual field defect, unspecified

368.41 Scotoma involving central area

Scotoma: Scotoma:
central   paracentral
centrocecal

DEF: Vision loss (blind spot) in central five degrees of visual field.

368.42 Scotoma of blind spot area

Enlarged: Paracecal scotoma
angioscotoma
blind spot

368.43 Sector or arcuate defects

Scotoma:
arcuate
Bjerrum
Seidel

DEF: Arc-shaped blind spot caused by retinal nerve damage.

368.44 Other localized visual field defect

Scotoma: Visual field defect:
NOS   nasal step
ring   peripheral

368.45 Generalized contraction or constriction

368.46 Homonymous bilateral field defects

Hemianopsia (altitudinal) (homonymous)
Quadrant anopia

DEF: Disorders found in the corresponding vertical halves of the visual fields of both eyes .

368.47 Heteronymous bilateral field defects

Hemianopsia:
binasal
bitemporal

DEF: Disorders in the opposite halves of the visual fields of both eyes.

√5th **368.5 Color vision deficiencies**

Color blindness

368.51 Protan defect

Protanomaly
Protanopia

DEF: Mild difficulty distinguishing green and red hues with shortened spectrum; sex-linked affecting one percent of males.

368.52 Deutan defect

Deuteranomaly
Deuteranopia

DEF: Male-only disorder; difficulty in distinguishing green and red, no shortened spectrum.

368.53 Tritan defect

Tritanomaly
Tritanopia

DEF: Difficulty in distinguishing blue and yellow; occurs often due to drugs, retinal detachment and central nervous system diseases.

368.54 Achromatopsia

Monochromatism (cone) (rod)

DEF: Complete color blindness; caused by disease, injury to retina, optic nerve or pathway.

368.55 Acquired color vision deficiencies

368.59 Other color vision deficiencies

√5th **368.6 Night blindness**

Nyctalopia

DEF: Nyctalopia: disorder of vision in dim light or night blindness.

368.60 Night blindness, unspecified

368.61 Congenital night blindness

Hereditary night blindness
Oguchi's disease

368.62 Acquired night blindness

EXCLUDES   that due to vitamin A deficiency (264.5)

368.63 Abnormal dark adaptation curve

Abnormal threshold
Delayed adaptation } of cones or rods

368.69 Other night blindness

368.8 Other specified visual disturbances

Blurred vision NOS

368.9 Unspecified visual disturbance

√4th **369 Blindness and low vision**

Note: Visual impairment refers to a functional limitation of the eye (e.g., limited visual acuity or visual field). It should be distinguished from visual disability, indicating a limitation of the abilities of the individual (e.g., limited reading skills, vocational skills), and from visual handicap, indicating a limitation of personal and socioeconomic independence (e.g., limited mobility, limited employability).

The levels of impairment defined in the table on page 94 are based on the recommendations of the WHO Study Group on Prevention of Blindness (Geneva, November 6–10, 1972; WHO Technical Report Series 518), and of the International Council of Ophthalmology (1976).

Note that definitions of blindness vary in different settings.

For international reporting WHO defines blindness as profound impairment. This definition can be applied to blindness of one eye (369.1, 369.6) and to blindness of the individual (369.0).

For determination of benefits in the U.S.A., the definition of legal blindness as severe impairment is often used. This definition applies to blindness of the individual only.

EXCLUDES   *correctable impaired vision due to refractive errors (367.0-367.9)*

√5th **369.0 Profound impairment, both eyes**

369.00 Impairment level not further specified

Blindness:
NOS according to WHO definition
both eyes

369.01 Better eye: total impairment; lesser eye: total impairment

369.02 Better eye: near-total impairment; lesser eye: not further specified

369.03 Better eye: near-total impairment; lesser eye: total impairment

369.04 Better eye: near-total impairment; lesser eye: near-total impairment

369.05 Better eye: profound impairment; lesser eye: not further specified

369.06 Better eye: profound impairment; lesser eye: total impairment

369.07 Better eye: profound impairment; lesser eye: near-total impairment

369.08 Better eye: profound impairment; lesser eye: profound impairment

Nervous System and Sense Organs 368.33–369.08

√4th   √5th   Additional Digit Required   Unspecified Code   Other Specified Code   Manifestation Code   ►◄ Revised Text   ● New Code   ▲ Revised Code Title

Nervous System and Sense Organs 369.1–370.07

√5th **369.1 Moderate or severe impairment, better eye, profound impairment lesser eye**

369.10 Impairment level not further specified
Blindness, one eye, low vision other eye

369.11 Better eye: severe impairment; lesser eye: blind, not further specified

369.12 Better eye: severe impairment; lesser eye: total impairment

369.13 Better eye: severe impairment; lesser eye: near-total impairment

369.14 Better eye: severe impairment; lesser eye: profound impairment

369.15 Better eye: moderate impairment; lesser eye: blind, not further specified

369.16 Better eye: moderate impairment; lesser eye: total impairment

369.17 Better eye: moderate impairment; lesser eye: near-total impairment

369.18 Better eye: moderate impairment; lesser eye: profound impairment

√5th **369.2 Moderate or severe impairment, both eyes**

369.20 Impairment level not further specified
Low vision, both eyes NOS

369.21 Better eye: severe impairment; lesser eye: not further specified

369.22 Better eye: severe impairment; lesser eye: severe impairment

369.23 Better eye: moderate impairment; lesser eye: not further specified

369.24 Better eye: moderate impairment; lesser eye: severe impairment

369.25 Better eye: moderate impairment; lesser eye: moderate impairment

369.3 Unqualified visual loss, both eyes
EXCLUDES *blindness NOS:*
legal [U.S.A. definition] (369.4)
WHO definition (369.00)

369.4 Legal blindness, as defined in U.S.A.
Blindness NOS according to U.S.A. definition
EXCLUDES *legal blindness with specification of impairment level (369.01-369.08, 369.11-369.14, 369.21-369.22)*

√5th **369.6 Profound impairment, one eye**

369.60 Impairment level not further specified
Blindness, one eye

369.61 One eye: total impairment; other eye: not specified

369.62 One eye: total impairment; other eye: near-normal vision

369.63 One eye: total impairment; other eye: normal vision

369.64 One eye: near-total impairment; other eye: not specified

369.65 One eye: near-total impairment; other eye: near-normal vision

369.66 One eye: near-total impairment; other eye: normal vision

369.67 One eye: profound impairment; other eye: not specified

369.68 One eye: profound impairment; other eye: near-normal vision

369.69 One eye: profound impairment; other eye: normal vision

√5th **369.7 Moderate or severe impairment, one eye**

369.70 Impairment level not further specified
Low vision, one eye

369.71 One eye: severe impairment; other eye: not specified

369.72 One eye: severe impairment; other eye: near-normal vision

Classification		LEVELS OF VISUAL IMPAIRMENT	Additional descriptors which may be encountered
"legal"	WHO	Visual acuity and/or visual field limitation (whichever is worse)	
	(NEAR-) NORMAL VISION	RANGE OF NORMAL VISION 20/10 20/13 20/16 20/20 20/25 2.0 1.6 1.25 1.0 0.8	
		NEAR-NORMAL VISION 20/30 20/40 20/50 20/60 0.7 0.6 0.5 0.4 0.3	
	LOW VISION	MODERATE VISUAL IMPAIRMENT 20/70 20/80 20/100 20/125 20/160 0.25 0.20 0.16 0.12	Moderate low vision
LEGAL BLINDNESS (U.S.A.) both eyes		SEVERE VISUAL IMPAIRMENT 20/200 20/250 20/320 20/400 0.10 0.08 0.06 0.05 Visual field: 20 degrees or less	Severe low vision, "Legal" blindness
	BLINDNESS (WHO) one or both eyes	PROFOUND VISUAL IMPAIRMENT 20/500 20/630 20/800 20/1000 0.04 0.03 0.025 0.02 Count fingers at: less than 3m (10 ft.) Visual field: 10 degrees or less	Profound low vision, Moderate blindness
		NEAR-TOTAL VISUAL IMPAIRMENT Visual acuity: less than 0.02 (20/1000) Count fingers at: 1m (3 ft.) or less Hand movements: 5m (15 ft.) or less Light projection, light perception Visual field: 5 degrees or less	Severe blindness, Near-total blindness
		TOTAL VISUAL IMPAIRMENT No light perception (NLP)	Total blindness

Visual acuity refers to best achievable acuity with correction.
Non-listed Snellen fractions may be classified by converting to the nearest decimal equivalent, e.g. 10/200 = 0.05, 6/30 = 0.20.
CF (count fingers) without designation of distance, may be classified to profound impairment.
HM (hand motion) without designation of distance, may be classified to near-total impairment.
Visual field measurements refer to the largest field diameter for a 1/100 white test object.

369.73 One eye: severe impairment; other eye: normal vision

369.74 One eye: moderate impairment; other eye: not specified

369.75 One eye: moderate impairment; other eye: near-normal vision

369.76 One eye: moderate impairment; other eye: normal vision

369.8 Unqualified visual loss, one eye

369.9 Unspecified visual loss

√4th **370 Keratitis**

√5th **370.0 Corneal ulcer**
EXCLUDES *that due to vitamin A deficiency (264.3)*

370.00 Corneal ulcer, unspecified

370.01 Marginal corneal ulcer

370.02 Ring corneal ulcer

370.03 Central corneal ulcer

370.04 Hypopyon ulcer
Serpiginous ulcer
DEF: Corneal ulcer with an accumulation of pus in the eye's anterior chamber.

370.05 Mycotic corneal ulcer
DEF: Fungal infection causing corneal tissue loss.

370.06 Perforated corneal ulcer
DEF: Tissue loss through all layers of cornea.

370.07 Mooren's ulcer
DEF: Tissue loss, with chronic inflammation, at junction of cornea and sclera; seen in elderly.

√5th **370.2 Superficial keratitis without conjunctivitis**
  EXCLUDES   dendritic [herpes simplex] keratitis
             (054.42)
  370.20 Superficial keratitis, unspecified
  370.21 Punctate keratitis
    Thygeson's superficial punctate keratitis
    DEF: Formation of cellular and fibrinous deposits (keratic
    precipitates) on posterior surface; deposits develop after
    injury or iridocyclitis.
  370.22 Macular keratitis
    Keratitis: Keratitis:
      areolar   stellate
      nummular   striate
  370.23 Filamentary keratitis
    DEF: Keratitis characterized by twisted filaments of
    mucoid material on the cornea's surface.
  370.24 Photokeratitis
    Snow blindness
    Welders' keratitis
    DEF: Painful, inflamed cornea; due to extended exposure
    to ultraviolet light.

√5th **370.3 Certain types of keratoconjunctivitis**
  370.31 Phlyctenular keratoconjunctivitis
    Phlyctenulosis
    Use additional code for any associated
      tuberculosis (017.3)
    DEF: Miniature blister on conjunctiva or cornea;
    associated with tuberculosis and malnutrition disorders.
  **370.32 Limbar and corneal involvement in vernal
  conjunctivitis**
    Use additional code for vernal conjunctivitis
      (372.13)
    DEF: Corneal itching and inflammation in conjunctivitis;
    often limited to lining of eyelids.
  **370.33 Keratoconjunctivitis sicca, not specified as
  Sjögren's**
    EXCLUDES   Sjögren's syndrome (710.2)
    DEF: Inflammation of conjunctiva and cornea;
    characterized by "horny" looking tissue and excess blood
    in these areas; decreased flow of lacrimal (tear) is a
    contributing factor.
  370.34 Exposure keratoconjunctivitis
    DEF: Incomplete closure of eyelid causing dry, inflamed
    eye.
  370.35 Neurotrophic keratoconjunctivitis

√5th **370.4 Other and unspecified keratoconjunctivitis**
  370.40 Keratoconjunctivitis, unspecified
    Superficial keratitis with conjunctivitis NOS
  **370.44 Keratitis or keratoconjunctivitis in
  exanthema**
    Code first underlying condition (050.0-052.9)
    EXCLUDES   herpes simplex (054.43)
               herpes zoster (053.21)
               measles (055.71)
  370.49 Other
    EXCLUDES   epidemic keratoconjunctivitis
               (077.1)

√5th **370.5 Interstitial and deep keratitis**
  370.50 Interstitial keratitis, unspecified
  370.52 Diffuse interstitial keratitis
    Cogan's syndrome
    DEF: Inflammation of cornea; with deposits in middle
    corneal layers; may obscure vision.
  370.54 Sclerosing keratitis
    DEF: Chronic corneal inflammation leading to opaque
    scarring.

  370.55 Corneal abscess
    DEF: Pocket of pus and inflammation on the cornea.
  370.59 Other
    EXCLUDES   disciform herpes simplex
               keratitis (054.43)
               syphilitic keratitis (090.3)

√5th **370.6 Corneal neovascularization**
  **370.60 Corneal neovascularization,
  unspecified**
  370.61 Localized vascularization of cornea
    DEF: Limited infiltration of cornea by new blood vessels.
  370.62 Pannus (corneal)
    DEF: Buildup of superficial vascularization and
    granulated tissue under epithelium of cornea.
  370.63 Deep vascularization of cornea
    DEF: Deep infiltration of cornea by new blood vessels.
  370.64 Ghost vessels (corneal)
  370.8 Other forms of keratitis
  370.9 Unspecified keratitis

√4th **371 Corneal opacity and other disorders of cornea**
√5th **371.0 Corneal scars and opacities**
    EXCLUDES   that due to vitamin A deficiency (264.6)
  371.00 Corneal opacity, unspecified
    Corneal scar NOS
  371.01 Minor opacity of cornea
    Corneal nebula
  371.02 Peripheral opacity of cornea
    Corneal macula not interfering with central
      vision
  371.03 Central opacity of cornea
    Corneal:
      leucoma ⎫ interfering with central
      macula ⎭   vision
  371.04 Adherent leucoma
    DEF: Dense, opaque corneal growth adhering to the iris;
    also spelled as leukoma.
  371.05 Phthisical cornea
    Code first underlying tuberculosis (017.3)
√5th **371.1 Corneal pigmentations and deposits**
  371.10 Corneal deposit, unspecified
  371.11 Anterior pigmentations
    Stähli's lines
  371.12 Stromal pigmentations
    Hematocornea
  371.13 Posterior pigmentations
    Krukenberg spindle
  371.14 Kayser-Fleischer ring
    DEF: Copper deposits forming ring at outer edge of
    cornea; seen in Wilson's disease and other liver
    disorders.
  **371.15 Other deposits associated with
  metabolic disorders**
  371.16 Argentous deposits
    DEF: Silver deposits in cornea.
√5th **371.2 Corneal edema**
  371.20 Corneal edema, unspecified
  371.21 Idiopathic corneal edema
    DEF: Corneal swelling and fluid retention of unknown
    cause.
  371.22 Secondary corneal edema
    DEF: Corneal swelling and fluid retention caused by an
    underlying disease, injury, or condition.

√4th
√5th Additional Digit Required   Unspecified Code   Other Specified Code   Manifestation Code   ▶◀ Revised Text   ● New Code   ▲ Revised Code Title

Nervous System and Sense Organs 371.23–372.15

371.23 Bullous keratopathy
DEF: Corneal degeneration; characterized by recurring, rupturing epithelial "blisters;" ruptured blebs expose corneal nerves, cause great pain; occurs in glaucoma, iridocyclitis and Fuchs' epithelial dystrophy.

371.24 Corneal edema due to wearing of contact lenses

√5th **371.3 Changes of corneal membranes**
371.30 Corneal membrane change, unspecified
371.31 Folds and rupture of Bowman's membrane
371.32 Folds in Descemet's membrane
371.33 Rupture in Descemet's membrane

√5th **371.4 Corneal degenerations**
371.40 Corneal degeneration, unspecified
371.41 Senile corneal changes
          Arcus senilis   Hassall-Henle bodies
371.42 Recurrent erosion of cornea
          EXCLUDES Mooren's ulcer (370.07)
371.43 Band-shaped keratopathy
          DEF: Horizontal bands of superficial corneal calcium deposits.
371.44 Other calcerous degenerations of cornea
371.45 Keratomalacia NOS
          EXCLUDES that due to vitamin A deficiency (264.4)
          DEF: Destruction of the cornea by keratinization of the epithelium with ulceration and perforation of the cornea; seen in cases of vitamin A deficiency.
371.46 Nodular degeneration of cornea
          Salzmann's nodular dystrophy
371.48 Peripheral degenerations of cornea
          Marginal degeneration of cornea [Terrien's]
371.49 Other
          Discrete colliquative keratopathy

√5th **371.5 Hereditary corneal dystrophies**
DEF: Genetic disorder; leads to opacities, edema or lesions of cornea.

371.50 Corneal dystrophy, unspecified
371.51 Juvenile epithelial corneal dystrophy
371.52 Other anterior corneal dystrophies
          Corneal dystrophy:
            microscopic cystic
            ring-like
371.53 Granular corneal dystrophy
371.54 Lattice corneal dystrophy
371.55 Macular corneal dystrophy
371.56 Other stromal corneal dystrophies
          Crystalline corneal dystrophy
371.57 Endothelial corneal dystrophy
          Combined corneal dystrophy
          Cornea guttata
          Fuchs' endothelial dystrophy
371.58 Other posterior corneal dystrophies
          Polymorphous corneal dystrophy

√5th **371.6 Keratoconus**
DEF: Bilateral bulging protrusion of anterior cornea; often due to noninflammatory thinning.

371.60 Keratoconus, unspecified
371.61 Keratoconus, stable condition
371.62 Keratoconus, acute hydrops

√5th **371.7 Other corneal deformities**
371.70 Corneal deformity, unspecified
371.71 Corneal ectasia
          DEF: Bulging protrusion of thinned, scarred cornea.

371.72 Descemetocele
DEF: Protrusion of Descemet's membrane into cornea.

371.73 Corneal staphyloma
DEF: Protrusion of cornea into adjacent tissue.

√5th **371.8 Other corneal disorders**
371.81 Corneal anesthesia and hypoesthesia
          DEF: Decreased or absent sensitivity of cornea.
371.82 Corneal disorder due to contact lens
          EXCLUDES corneal edema due to contact lens (371.24)
          DEF: Contact lens wear causing cornea disorder, excluding swelling.
371.89 Other

371.9 Unspecified corneal disorder

√4th **372 Disorders of conjunctiva**
          EXCLUDES keratoconjunctivitis (370.3-370.4)

√5th **372.0 Acute conjunctivitis**
372.00 Acute conjunctivitis, unspecified
372.01 Serous conjunctivitis, except viral
          EXCLUDES viral conjunctivitis NOS (077.9)
372.02 Acute follicular conjunctivitis
          Conjunctival folliculosis NOS
          EXCLUDES conjunctivitis:
            adenoviral (acute follicular) (077.3)
            epidemic hemorrhagic (077.4)
            inclusion (077.0)
            Newcastle (077.8)
            epidemic keratoconjunctivitis (077.1)
            pharyngoconjunctival fever (077.2)
          DEF: Severe conjunctival inflammation with dense infiltrations of lymphoid tissues of inner eyelids; may be traced to a viral or chlamydial etiology.
372.03 Other mucopurulent conjunctivitis
          Catarrhal conjunctivitis
          EXCLUDES blennorrhea neonatorum (gonococcal) (098.40)
            neonatal conjunctivitis(771.6)
            ophthalmia neonatorum NOS (771.6)
372.04 Pseudomembranous conjunctivitis
          Membranous conjunctivitis
          EXCLUDES diphtheritic conjunctivitis (032.81)
          DEF: Severe inflammation of conjunctiva; false membrane develops on inner surface of eyelid; membrane can be removed without harming epithelium, due to bacterial infections, toxic and allergic factors, and viral infections.
372.05 Acute atopic conjunctivitis
          DEF: Sudden, severe conjunctivitis due to allergens.

√5th **372.1 Chronic conjunctivitis**
372.10 Chronic conjunctivitis, unspecified
372.11 Simple chronic conjunctivitis
372.12 Chronic follicular conjunctivitis
          DEF: Persistent inflammation of conjunctiva; with infiltration of lymphoid tissue of inner eyelids.
372.13 Vernal conjunctivitis
372.14 Other chronic allergic conjunctivitis
372.15 Parasitic conjunctivitis
          Code first underlying disease, as:
            filariasis (125.0-125.9)
            mucocutaneous leishmaniasis (085.5)

√5th **372.2 Blepharoconjunctivitis**
    372.20 Blepharoconjunctivitis, unspecified
    372.21 Angular blepharoconjunctivitis
        DEF: Inflammation at junction of upper and lower eyelids; may block lacrimal secretions.

    372.22 Contact blepharoconjunctivitis

√5th **372.3 Other and unspecified conjunctivitis**
    372.30 Conjunctivitis, unspecified
    372.31 Rosacea conjunctivitis
        Code first underlying rosacea dermatitis (695.3)

    372.33 Conjunctivitis in mucocutaneous disease
        Code first underlying disease, as:
           erythema multiforme (695.1)
           Reiter's disease (099.3)
        EXCLUDES *ocular pemphigoid (694.61)*

    372.39 Other

√5th **372.4 Pterygium**
    EXCLUDES *pseudopterygium (372.52)*
    DEF: Wedge-shaped, conjunctival thickening that advances from the inner corner of the eye toward the cornea.

    372.40 Pterygium, unspecified
    372.41 Peripheral pterygium, stationary
    372.42 Peripheral pterygium, progressive
    372.43 Central pterygium
    372.44 Double pterygium
    372.45 Recurrent pterygium

√5th **372.5 Conjunctival degenerations and deposits**
    372.50 Conjunctival degeneration, unspecified
    372.51 Pinguecula
        DEF: Proliferative spot on the bulbar conjunctiva located near the sclerocorneal junction, usually on the nasal side; it is seen in elderly people.

    372.52 Pseudopterygium
        DEF: Conjunctival scar joined to the cornea; it looks like a pterygium but is not attached to the tissue.

    372.53 Conjunctival xerosis
        EXCLUDES *conjunctival xerosis due to vitamin A deficiency (264.0, 264.1, 264.7)*
        DEF: Dry conjunctiva due to vitamin A deficiency; related to Bitot's spots; may develop into xerophthalmia and keratomalacia.

    372.54 Conjunctival concretions
        DEF: Calculus or deposit on conjunctiva.

    372.55 Conjunctival pigmentations
        Conjunctival argyrosis
        DEF: Color deposits in conjunctiva.

    372.56 Conjunctival deposits

√5th **372.6 Conjunctival scars**
    372.61 Granuloma of conjunctiva
    372.62 Localized adhesions and strands of conjunctiva
        DEF: Abnormal fibrous connections in conjunctiva.

    372.63 Symblepharon
        Extensive adhesions of conjunctiva
        DEF: Adhesion of the eyelids to the eyeball.

    372.64 Scarring of conjunctiva
        Contraction of eye socket (after enucleation)

√5th **372.7 Conjunctival vascular disorders and cysts**
    372.71 Hyperemia of conjunctiva
        DEF: Conjunctival blood vessel congestion causing eye redness.

    372.72 Conjunctival hemorrhage
        Hyposphagma
        Subconjunctival hemorrhage
    372.73 Conjunctival edema
        Chemosis of conjunctiva
        Subconjunctival edema
        DEF: Fluid retention and swelling in conjunctival tissue.

    372.74 Vascular abnormalities of conjunctiva
        Aneurysm(ata) of conjunctiva
    372.75 Conjunctival cysts
        DEF: Abnormal sacs of fluid in conjunctiva.

√5th **372.8 Other disorders of conjunctiva**
    372.81 Conjunctivochalasis
        DEF: Bilateral condition of redundant conjunctival tissue between globe and lower eyelid margin; may cover lower punctum, interferring with normal tearing.

    372.89 Other disorders of conjunctiva
  372.9 Unspecified disorder of conjunctiva

√4th **373 Inflammation of eyelids**
√5th **373.0 Blepharitis**
    EXCLUDES *blepharoconjunctivitis (372.20-372.22)*
    373.00 Blepharitis, unspecified
    373.01 Ulcerative blepharitis
    373.02 Squamous blepharitis

√5th **373.1 Hordeolum and other deep inflammation of eyelid**
    DEF: Purulent, localized, staphylococcal infection in sebaceous glands of eyelids.

    373.11 Hordeolum externum
        Hordeolum NOS
        Stye
        DEF: Infection of oil gland in eyelash follicles.

    373.12 Hordeolum internum
        Infection of meibomian gland
        DEF: Infection of oil gland of eyelid margin.

    373.13 Abscess of eyelid
        Furuncle of eyelid
        DEF: Inflamed pocket of pus on eyelid.

  373.2 Chalazion
    Meibomian (gland) cyst
    EXCLUDES *infected meibomian gland (373.12)*
    DEF: Chronic inflammation of the meibomian gland, causing an eyelid mass.

√5th **373.3 Noninfectious dermatoses of eyelid**
    373.31 Eczematous dermatitis of eyelid
    373.32 Contact and allergic dermatitis of eyelid
    373.33 Xeroderma of eyelid
    373.34 Discoid lupus erythematosus of eyelid

  373.4 Infective dermatitis of eyelid of types resulting in deformity
    Code first underlying disease, as:
        leprosy (030.0-030.9)
        lupus vulgaris (tuberculous) (017.0)
        yaws (102.0-102.9)

  373.5 Other infective dermatitis of eyelid
    Code first underlying disease, as:
        actinomycosis (039.3)
        impetigo (684)
        mycotic dermatitis (110.0-111.9)
        vaccinia (051.0)
        postvaccination (999.0)
    EXCLUDES *herpes:*
        simplex (054.41)
        zoster (053.20)

Nervous System and Sense Organs 372.2-373.5

√4th √5th Additional Digit Required   Unspecified Code   Other Specified Code   Manifestation Code   ▶◀ Revised Text   ● New Code   ▲ Revised Code Title

Nervous System and Sense Organs 373.6–375.2

373.6 *Parasitic infestation of eyelid*
 Code first underlying disease, as:
  leishmaniasis (085.0-085.9)
  loiasis (125.2)
  onchocerciasis (125.3)
  pediculosis (132.0)

373.8 Other inflammations of eyelids

373.9 Unspecified inflammation of eyelid

✓4ᵗʰ **374** Other disorders of eyelids

✓5ᵗʰ **374.0** Entropion and trichiasis of eyelid
 DEF: Entropion: turning inward of eyelid edge toward eyeball.

 DEF: Trichiasis: ingrowing eyelashes marked by irritation with possible distortion of sight.

 374.00 Entropion, unspecified
 374.01 Senile entropion   A
 374.02 Mechanical entropion
 374.03 Spastic entropion
 374.04 Cicatricial entropion
 374.05 Trichiasis without entropion

✓5ᵗʰ **374.1** Ectropion
 DEF: Turning outward (eversion) of eyelid edge; exposes palpebral conjunctiva; dryness, irritation result.

 374.10 Ectropion, unspecified
 374.11 Senile ectropion   A
 374.12 Mechanical ectropion
 374.13 Spastic ectropion
 374.14 Cicatricial ectropion

✓5ᵗʰ **374.2** Lagophthalmos
 DEF: Incomplete closure of eyes; causes dry eye and other complications.

 374.20 Lagophthalmos, unspecified
 374.21 Paralytic lagophthalmos
 374.22 Mechanical lagophthalmos
 374.23 Cicatricial lagophthalmos

✓5ᵗʰ **374.3** Ptosis of eyelid
 374.30 Ptosis of eyelid, unspecified
 374.31 Paralytic ptosis
  DEF: Drooping of upper eyelid due to nerve disorder.
 374.32 Myogenic ptosis
  DEF: Drooping of upper eyelid due to muscle disorder.
 374.33 Mechanical ptosis
  DEF: Outside force causes drooping of upper eyelid.
 374.34 Blepharochalasis
  Pseudoptosis
  DEF: Loss of elasticity causing skin to hang over eyelid margin; due to intercellular tissue atrophy.

✓5ᵗʰ **374.4** Other disorders affecting eyelid function
 EXCLUDES   blepharoclonus (333.81)
      blepharospasm (333.81)
      facial nerve palsy (351.0)
      third nerve palsy or paralysis (378.51-378.52)
      tic (psychogenic) (307.20-307.23)
      organic (333.3)
 374.41 Lid retraction or lag
 374.43 Abnormal innervation syndrome
  Jaw-blinking
  Paradoxical facial movements
 374.44 Sensory disorders
 374.45 Other sensorimotor disorders
  Deficient blink reflex
 374.46 Blepharophimosis
  Ankyloblepharon
  DEF: Narrowing of palpebral fissure horizontally; caused by laterally displaced inner canthi; either acquired or congenital.

✓5ᵗʰ **374.5** Degenerative disorders of eyelid and periocular area
 374.50 Degenerative disorder of eyelid, unspecified
 374.51 Xanthelasma
  Xanthoma (planum) (tuberosum) of eyelid
  Code first underlying condition (272.0-272.9)
  DEF: Fatty tumors of eyelid linked to high fat content of blood.
 374.52 Hyperpigmentation of eyelid
  Chloasma   Dyspigmentation
  DEF: Excess pigment of eyelid.
 374.53 Hypopigmentation of eyelid
  Vitiligo of eyelid
  DEF: Lack of color pigment of the eyelid.
 374.54 Hypertrichosis of eyelid
  DEF: Excess eyelash growth.
 374.55 Hypotrichosis of eyelid
  Madarosis of eyelid
  DEF: Less than normal, or .absent, eyelashes.
 374.56 Other degenerative disorders of skin affecting eyelid

✓5ᵗʰ **374.8** Other disorders of eyelid
 374.81 Hemorrhage of eyelid
  EXCLUDES   black eye (921.0)
 374.82 Edema of eyelid
  Hyperemia of eyelid
  DEF: Swelling and fluid retention in eyelid.
 374.83 Elephantiasis of eyelid
  DEF: Filarial disease causing dermatitis and enlarged eyelid.
 374.84 Cysts of eyelids
  Sebaceous cyst of eyelid
 374.85 Vascular anomalies of eyelid
 374.86 Retained foreign body of eyelid
 374.87 Dermatochalasis
  DEF: Loss of elasticity causing skin under eye to sag.
 374.89 Other disorders of eyelid

374.9 Unspecified disorder of eyelid

✓4ᵗʰ **375** Disorders of lacrimal system

✓5ᵗʰ **375.0** Dacryoadenitis
 375.00 Dacryoadenitis, unspecified
 375.01 Acute dacryoadenitis
  DEF: Severe, sudden inflammation of lacrimal gland.
 375.02 Chronic dacryoadenitis
  DEF: Persistent inflammation of lacrimal gland.
 375.03 Chronic enlargement of lacrimal gland

✓5ᵗʰ **375.1** Other disorders of lacrimal gland
 375.11 Dacryops
  DEF: Overproduction and constant flow of tears; may cause distended lacrimal duct.
 375.12 Other lacrimal cysts and cystic degeneration
 375.13 Primary lacrimal atrophy
 375.14 Secondary lacrimal atrophy
  DEF: Wasting away of lacrimal gland due to another disease.
 375.15 Tear film insufficiency, unspecified
  Dry eye syndrome
  DEF: Eye dryness and irritation due to insufficient tear production.
 375.16 Dislocation of lacrimal gland

✓5ᵗʰ **375.2** Epiphora
 DEF: Abnormal development of tears due to stricture of lacrimal passages.

N Newborn Age: 0   P Pediatric Age: 0-17   M Maternity Age: 12-55   A Adult Age: 15-124   MSP Medicare Secondary Payer

375.20 Epiphora, unspecified as to cause

375.21 Epiphora due to excess lacrimation
   DEF: Tear overflow due to overproduction.

375.22 Epiphora due to insufficient drainage
   DEF: Tear overflow due to blocked drainage.

√5ᵗʰ 375.3 Acute and unspecified inflammation of lacrimal passages
   EXCLUDES *neonatal dacryocystitis (771.6)*

375.30 Dacryocystitis, unspecified

375.31 Acute canaliculitis, lacrimal

375.32 Acute dacryocystitis
   Acute peridacryocystitis

375.33 Phlegmonous dacryocystitis
   DEF: Infection of tear sac with pockets of pus.

√5ᵗʰ 375.4 Chronic inflammation of lacrimal passages

375.41 Chronic canaliculitis

375.42 Chronic dacryocystitis

375.43 Lacrimal mucocele

√5ᵗʰ 375.5 Stenosis and insufficiency of lacrimal passages

375.51 Eversion of lacrimal punctum
   DEF: Abnormal turning outward of tear duct.

375.52 Stenosis of lacrimal punctum
   DEF: Abnormal narrowing of tear duct.

375.53 Stenosis of lacrimal canaliculi

375.54 Stenosis of lacrimal sac
   DEF: Abnormal narrowing of tear sac.

375.55 Obstruction of nasolacrimal duct, neonatal
   EXCLUDES *congenital anomaly of nasolacrimal duct (743.65)*
   DEF: Acquired, abnormal obstruction of lacrimal system, from eye to nose; in an infant.

375.56 Stenosis of nasolacrimal duct, acquired

375.57 Dacryolith
   DEF: Concretion or stone in lacrimal system.

√5ᵗʰ 375.6 Other changes of lacrimal passages

375.61 Lacrimal fistula
   DEF: Abnormal communication from lacrimal system.

375.69 Other

√5ᵗʰ 375.8 Other disorders of lacrimal system

375.81 Granuloma of lacrimal passages
   DEF: Abnormal nodules within lacrimal system.

375.89 Other

375.9 Unspecified disorder of lacrimal system

√4ᵗʰ 376 Disorders of the orbit

√5ᵗʰ 376.0 Acute inflammation of orbit

376.00 Acute inflammation of orbit, unspecified

376.01 Orbital cellulitis
   Abscess of orbit
   DEF: Infection of tissue between orbital bone and eyeball.

376.02 Orbital periostitis
   DEF: Inflammation of connective tissue covering orbital bone.

376.03 Orbital osteomyelitis
   DEF: Inflammation of orbital bone.

376.04 Tenonitis

√5ᵗʰ 376.1 Chronic inflammatory disorders of orbit

376.10 Chronic inflammation of orbit, unspecified

376.11 Orbital granuloma
   Pseudotumor (inflammatory) of orbit
   DEF: Abnormal nodule between orbital bone and eyeball.

376.12 Orbital myositis
   DEF: Painful inflammation of eye muscles.

376.13 *Parasitic infestation of orbit*
   Code first underlying disease, as:
      hydatid infestation of orbit (122.3, 122.6, 122.9)
      myiasis of orbit (134.0)

√5ᵗʰ 376.2 Endocrine exophthalmos
   Code first underlying thyroid disorder (242.0-242.9)

376.21 *Thyrotoxic exophthalmos*
   DEF: Bulging eyes due to hyperthyroidism.

376.22 *Exophthalmic ophthalmoplegia*
   DEF: Inability to rotate eye due to bulging eyes.

√5ᵗʰ 376.3 Other exophthalmic conditions

376.30 Exophthalmos, unspecified
   DEF: Abnormal protrusion of eyeball.

376.31 Constant exophthalmos
   DEF: Continuous, abnormal protrusion or bulging of eyeball.

376.32 Orbital hemorrhage
   DEF: Bleeding behind the eyeball, causing forward bulge.

376.33 Orbital edema or congestion
   DEF: Fluid retention behind eyeball, causing forward bulge.

376.34 Intermittent exophthalmos

376.35 Pulsating exophthalmos
   DEF: Bulge or protrusion; associated with a carotid-cavernous fistula.

376.36 Lateral displacement of globe
   DEF: Abnormal displacement of the eyeball away from nose, toward temple.

√5ᵗʰ 376.4 Deformity of orbit

376.40 Deformity of orbit, unspecified

376.41 Hypertelorism of orbit
   DEF: Abnormal increase in interorbital distance; associated with congenital facial deformities; may be accompanied by mental deficiency.

376.42 Exostosis of orbit
   DEF: Abnormal bony growth of orbit.

376.43 Local deformities due to bone disease
   DEF: Acquired abnormalities of orbit; due to bone disease.

376.44 Orbital deformities associated with craniofacial deformities

376.45 Atrophy of orbit
   DEF: Wasting away of bone tissue of orbit.

376.46 Enlargement of orbit

376.47 Deformity due to trauma or surgery

√5ᵗʰ 376.5 Enophthalmos
   DEF: Recession of eyeball deep into eye socket.

376.50 Enophthalmos, unspecified as to cause

376.51 Enophthalmos due to atrophy of orbital tissue

376.52 Enophthalmos due to trauma or surgery

376.6 Retained (old) foreign body following penetrating wound of orbit
   Retrobulbar foreign body

√5ᵗʰ 376.8 Other orbital disorders

376.81 Orbital cysts
   Encephalocele of orbit

√4ᵗʰ √5ᵗʰ Additional Digit Required   Unspecified Code   Other Specified Code   Manifestation Code   ►◄ Revised Text   ● New Code   ▲ Revised Code Title

2003 ICD•9•CM   **Volume 1 — 99**

Nervous System and Sense Organs 376.82–378.08

376.82 **Myopathy of extraocular muscles**
DEF: Disease in the muscles that control eyeball movement.

376.89 Other

376.9 Unspecified disorder of orbit

✓4ᵗʰ 377 **Disorders of optic nerve and visual pathways**

✓5ᵗʰ 377.0 **Papilledema**

377.00 Papilledema, unspecified

377.01 **Papilledema associated with increased intracranial pressure**

377.02 **Papilledema associated with decreased ocular pressure**

377.03 **Papilledema associated with retinal disorder**

377.04 **Foster-Kennedy syndrome**
DEF: Retrobulbar optic neuritis, central scotoma and optic atrophy; caused by tumors in frontal lobe of brain that press downward.

✓5ᵗʰ 377.1 **Optic atrophy**

377.10 Optic atrophy, unspecified

377.11 **Primary optic atrophy**
EXCLUDES *neurosyphilitic optic atrophy (094.84)*

377.12 **Postinflammatory optic atrophy**
DEF: Adverse effect of inflammation causing wasting away of eye.

377.13 **Optic atrophy associated with retinal dystrophies**
DEF: Progressive changes in retinal tissue due to metabolic disorder causing wasting away of eye.

377.14 **Glaucomatous atrophy [cupping] of optic disc**

377.15 **Partial optic atrophy**
Temporal pallor of optic disc

377.16 **Hereditary optic atrophy**
Optic atrophy:
dominant hereditary
Leber's

✓5ᵗʰ 377.2 **Other disorders of optic disc**

377.21 **Drusen of optic disc**

377.22 **Crater-like holes of optic disc**

377.23 **Coloboma of optic disc**
DEF: Ocular malformation caused by the failure of fetal fissure of optic stalk to close.

377.24 **Pseudopapilledema**

✓5ᵗʰ 377.3 **Optic neuritis**
EXCLUDES *meningococcal optic neuritis (036.81)*

377.30 Optic neuritis, unspecified

377.31 **Optic papillitis**
DEF: Swelling and inflammation of optic disc.

377.32 **Retrobulbar neuritis (acute)**
EXCLUDES *syphilitic retrobulbar neuritis (094.85)*
DEF: Inflammation of optic nerve immediately behind the eyeball.

377.33 **Nutritional optic neuropathy**
DEF: Malnutrition causing optic nerve disorder.

377.34 **Toxic optic neuropathy**
Toxic amblyopia
DEF: Toxic substance causing optic nerve disorder.

377.39 Other
EXCLUDES *ischemic optic neuropathy (377.41)*

✓5ᵗʰ 377.4 **Other disorders of optic nerve**

377.41 **Ischemic optic neuropathy**
DEF: Decreased blood flow affecting optic nerve.

377.42 **Hemorrhage in optic nerve sheaths**
DEF: Bleeding in meningeal lining of optic nerve.

377.49 Other
Compression of optic nerve

✓5ᵗʰ 377.5 **Disorders of optic chiasm**

377.51 **Associated with pituitary neoplasms and disorders**
DEF: Abnormal pituitary growth causing disruption in nerve chain from retina to brain.

377.52 Associated with other neoplasms
DEF: Abnormal growth, other than pituitary, causing disruption in nerve chain from retina to brain.

377.53 **Associated with vascular disorders**
DEF: Vascular disorder causing disruption in nerve chain from retina to brain.

377.54 **Associated with inflammatory disorders**
DEF: Inflammatory disease causing disruption in nerve chain from retina to brain.

✓5ᵗʰ 377.6 **Disorders of other visual pathways**

377.61 **Associated with neoplasms**

377.62 **Associated with vascular disorders**

377.63 **Associated with inflammatory disorders**

✓5ᵗʰ 377.7 **Disorders of visual cortex**
EXCLUDES *visual:*
agnosia (368.16)
hallucinations (368.16)
halos (368.15)

377.71 **Associated with neoplasms**

377.72 **Associated with vascular disorders**

377.73 **Associated with inflammatory disorders**

377.75 **Cortical blindness**
DEF: Blindness due to brain disorder, rather than eye disorder.

377.9 Unspecified disorder of optic nerve and visual pathways

✓4ᵗʰ 378 **Strabismus and other disorders of binocular eye movements**
EXCLUDES *nystagmus and other irregular eye movements (379.50-379.59)*
DEF: Misalignment of the eyes due to imbalance in extraocular muscles.

✓5ᵗʰ 378.0 **Esotropia**
Convergent concomitant strabismus
EXCLUDES *intermittent esotropia (378.20-378.22)*
DEF: Visual axis deviation created by one eye fixing upon an image and the other eye deviating inward.

378.00 Esotropia, unspecified

378.01 **Monocular esotropia**

378.02 **Monocular esotropia with A pattern**

378.03 **Monocular esotropia with V pattern**

378.04 Monocular esotropia with other noncomitancies
Monocular esotropia with X or Y pattern

378.05 **Alternating esotropia**

378.06 **Alternating esotropia with A pattern**

378.07 **Alternating esotropia with V pattern**

378.08 Alternating esotropia with other noncomitancies
Alternating esotropia with X or Y pattern

N Newborn Age: 0   P Pediatric Age: 0-17   M Maternity Age: 12-55   A Adult Age: 15-124   MSP Medicare Secondary Payer

√5th **378.1 Exotropia**
Divergent concomitant strabismus

> **EXCLUDES** intermittent exotropia (378.20, 378.23-378.24)

DEF: Visual axis deviation created by one eye fixing upon an image and the other eye deviating outward.

378.10 Exotropia, unspecified
378.11 Monocular exotropia
378.12 Monocular exotropia with A pattern
378.13 Monocular exotropia with V pattern
378.14 Monocular exotropia with other noncomitancies
> Monocular exotropia with X or Y pattern

378.15 Alternating exotropia
378.16 Alternating exotropia with A pattern
378.17 Alternating exotropia with V pattern
378.18 Alternating exotropia with other noncomitancies
> Alternating exotropia with X or Y pattern

√5th **378.2 Intermittent heterotropia**

> **EXCLUDES** vertical heterotropia (intermittent) (378.31)

DEF: Deviation of eyes seen only at intervals; it is also called strabismus.

378.20 Intermittent heterotropia, unspecified
> Intermittent:
> esotropia NOS
> exotropia NOS

378.21 Intermittent esotropia, monocular
378.22 Intermittent esotropia, alternating
378.23 Intermittent exotropia, monocular
378.24 Intermittent exotropia, alternating

√5th **378.3 Other and unspecified heterotropia**
378.30 Heterotropia, unspecified
378.31 Hypertropia
> Vertical heterotropia (constant) (intermittent)

378.32 Hypotropia
378.33 Cyclotropia
378.34 Monofixation syndrome
> Microtropia

378.35 Accommodative component in esotropia

√5th **378.4 Heterophoria**

DEF: Deviation occurring only when the other eye is covered.

378.40 Heterophoria, unspecified
378.41 Esophoria
378.42 Exophoria
378.43 Vertical heterophoria
378.44 Cyclophoria
378.45 Alternating hyperphoria

√5th **378.5 Paralytic strabismus**

DEF: Deviation of the eye due to nerve paralysis affecting muscle.

378.50 Paralytic strabismus, unspecified
378.51 Third or oculomotor nerve palsy, partial
378.52 Third or oculomotor nerve palsy, total
378.53 Fourth or trochlear nerve palsy
378.54 Sixth or abducens nerve palsy
378.55 External ophthalmoplegia
378.56 Total ophthalmoplegia

√5th **378.6 Mechanical strabismus**

DEF: Deviation of the eye due to an outside force on extraocular muscle.

378.60 Mechanical strabismus, unspecified

378.61 Brown's (tendon) sheath syndrome
> DEF: Congenital or acquired shortening of the anterior sheath of the superior oblique muscle; the eye is unable to move upward and inward; it is usually unilateral.

378.62 Mechanical strabismus from other musculofascial disorders
378.63 Limited duction associated with other conditions

√5th **378.7 Other specified strabismus**
378.71 Duane's syndrome
> DEF: Congenital, affects one eye; due to abnormal fibrous bands attached to rectus muscle; inability to abduct affected eye with retraction of globe.

378.72 Progressive external ophthalmoplegia
> DEF: Paralysis progressing from one eye muscle to another.

378.73 Strabismus in other neuromuscular disorders

√5th **378.8 Other disorders of binocular eye movements**

> **EXCLUDES** nystagmus (379.50-379.56)

378.81 Palsy of conjugate gaze
> DEF: Muscle dysfunction impairing parallel movement of the eye.

378.82 Spasm of conjugate gaze
> DEF: Muscle contractions impairing parallel movement of eye.

378.83 Convergence insufficiency or palsy
378.84 Convergence excess or spasm
378.85 Anomalies of divergence
378.86 Internuclear ophthalmoplegia
> DEF: Eye movement anomaly due to brainstem lesion.

378.87 Other dissociated deviation of eye movements
> Skew deviation

378.9 **Unspecified disorder of eye movements**
> Ophthalmoplegia NOS Strabismus NOS

√4th **379 Other disorders of eye**

√5th **379.0 Scleritis and episcleritis**

> **EXCLUDES** syphilitic episcleritis (095.0)

379.00 Scleritis, unspecified
> Episcleritis NOS

379.01 Episcleritis periodica fugax
> DEF: Hyperemia (engorgement) of the sclera and overlying conjunctiva characterized by a sudden onset and short duration.

379.02 Nodular episcleritis
> DEF: Inflammation of the outermost layer of the sclera, with formation of nodules.

379.03 Anterior scleritis
379.04 Scleromalacia perforans
> DEF: Scleral thinning, softening and degeneration; seen with rheumatoid arthritis.

379.05 Scleritis with corneal involvement
> Scleroperikeratitis

379.06 Brawny scleritis
> DEF: Severe inflammation of the sclera; with thickened corneal margins.

379.07 Posterior scleritis
> Sclerotenonitis

379.09 Other
> Scleral abscess

√5th **379.1 Other disorders of sclera**

> **EXCLUDES** blue sclera (743.47)

√4th
√5th Additional Digit Required   Unspecified Code   Other Specified Code   Manifestation Code   ▶◀ Revised Text   ● New Code   ▲ Revised Code Title

379.11 Scleral ectasia
Scleral staphyloma NOS
DEF: Protrusion of the contents of the eyeball where the sclera has thinned.

379.12 Staphyloma posticum
DEF: Ring-shaped protrusion or bulging of sclera and uveal tissue at posterior pole of eye.

379.13 Equatorial staphyloma
DEF: Ring-shaped protrusion or bulging of sclera and uveal tissue midway between front and back of eye.

379.14 Anterior staphyloma, localized

379.15 Ring staphyloma

379.16 Other degenerative disorders of sclera

379.19 Other

√5th **379.2 Disorders of vitreous body**
DEF: Disorder of clear gel that fills space between retina and lens.

379.21 Vitreous degeneration
Vitreous: Vitreous:
  cavitation   liquefaction
  detachment

379.22 Crystalline deposits in vitreous
Asteroid hyalitis
Synchysis scintillans

379.23 Vitreous hemorrhage

379.24 Other vitreous opacities
Vitreous floaters

379.25 Vitreous membranes and strands

379.26 Vitreous prolapse
DEF: Slipping of vitreous from normal position.

379.29 Other disorders of vitreous
EXCLUDES   vitreous abscess (360.04)

√5th **379.3 Aphakia and other disorders of lens**
EXCLUDES   after-cataract (366.50-366.53)

379.31 Aphakia
EXCLUDES   cataract extraction status (V45.61)
DEF: Absence of eye's crystalline lens.

379.32 Subluxation of lens

379.33 Anterior dislocation of lens
DEF: Lens displaced toward iris.

379.34 Posterior dislocation of lens
DEF: Lens displaced backward toward vitreous.

379.39 Other disorders of lens

√5th **379.4 Anomalies of pupillary function**

379.40 Abnormal pupillary function, unspecified

379.41 Anisocoria
DEF: Unequal pupil diameter.

379.42 Miosis (persistent), not due to miotics
DEF: Abnormal contraction of pupil less than 2 millimeters.

379.43 Mydriasis (persistent), not due to mydriatics
DEF: Morbid dilation of pupil.

379.45 Argyll Robertson pupil, atypical
Argyll Robertson phenomenon or pupil, nonsyphilitic
EXCLUDES   Argyll Robertson pupil (syphilitic) (094.89)
DEF: Failure of pupil to respond to light; affects both eyes; may be caused by diseases such as syphilis of the central nervous system or miosis.

379.46 Tonic pupillary reaction
Adie's pupil or syndrome

379.49 Other
Hippus
Pupillary paralysis

√5th **379.5 Nystagmus and other irregular eye movements**

379.50 Nystagmus, unspecified
DEF: Involuntary, rapid, rhythmic movement of eyeball; vertical, horizontal, rotatory or mixed; cause may be congenital, acquired, physiological, neurological, myopathic, or due to ocular diseases.

379.51 Congenital nystagmus

379.52 Latent nystagmus

379.53 Visual deprivation nystagmus

379.54 Nystagmus associated with disorders of the vestibular system

379.55 Dissociated nystagmus

379.56 Other forms of nystagmus

379.57 Deficiencies of saccadic eye movements
Abnormal optokinetic response
DEF: Saccadic eye movements; small, rapid, involuntary movements by both eyes simultaneously, due to changing point of fixation on visualized object.

379.58 Deficiencies of smooth pursuit movements

379.59 Other irregularities of eye movements
Opsoclonus

379.8 Other specified disorders of eye and adnexa

√5th **379.9 Unspecified disorder of eye and adnexa**

379.90 Disorder of eye, unspecified

379.91 Pain in or around eye

379.92 Swelling or mass of eye

379.93 Redness or discharge of eye

379.99 Other ill-defined disorders of eye
EXCLUDES   blurred vision NOS (368.8)

DISEASES OF THE EAR AND MASTOID PROCESS (380-389)

√4th **380 Disorders of external ear**

√5th **380.0 Perichondritis of pinna**
Perichondritis of auricle

380.00 Perichondritis of pinna, unspecified

380.01 Acute perichondritis of pinna

380.02 Chronic perichondritis of pinna

√5th **380.1 Infective otitis externa**

380.10 Infective otitis externa, unspecified
Otitis externa (acute):   Otitis externa (acute):
  NOS   hemorrhagica
  circumscribed   infective NOS
  diffuse

380.11 Acute infection of pinna
EXCLUDES   furuncular otitis externa (680.0)

380.12 Acute swimmers' ear
Beach ear   Tank ear
DEF: Otitis externa due to swimming.

380.13 *Other acute infections of external ear*
Code first underlying disease, as:
  erysipelas (035)
  impetigo (684)
  seborrheic dermatitis (690.10-690.18)
EXCLUDES   herpes simplex (054.73)
                     herpes zoster (053.71)

380.14 Malignant otitis externa
DEF: Severe necrotic otitis externa; due to bacteria.

380.15 *Chronic mycotic otitis externa*
Code first underlying disease, as:
  aspergillosis (117.3)
  otomycosis NOS (111.9)
EXCLUDES   candidal otitis externa (112.82)

380.16 **Other chronic infective otitis externa**
Chronic infective otitis externa NOS

√5th 380.2 **Other otitis externa**

380.21 **Cholesteatoma of external ear**
Keratosis obturans of external ear (canal)

EXCLUDES *cholesteatoma NOS (385.30-385.35)*
postmastoidectomy (383.32)

DEF: Cystlike mass filled with debris, including cholesterol; rare, congenital condition.

380.22 **Other acute otitis externa**

Acute otitis externa: Acute otitis externa:
actinic   eczematoid
chemical   reactive
contact

380.23 **Other chronic otitis externa**
Chronic otitis externa NOS

√5th 380.3 **Noninfectious disorders of pinna**

380.30 **Disorder of pinna, unspecified**

380.31 **Hematoma of auricle or pinna**

380.32 **Acquired deformities of auricle or pinna**

EXCLUDES *cauliflower ear (738.7)*

380.39 **Other**

EXCLUDES *gouty tophi of ear (274.81)*

380.4 **Impacted cerumen**
Wax in ear

√5th 380.5 **Acquired stenosis of external ear canal**
Collapse of external ear canal

380.50 **Acquired stenosis of external ear canal, unspecified as to cause**

380.51 **Secondary to trauma**

DEF: Narrowing of external ear canal; due to trauma.

380.52 **Secondary to surgery**

DEF: Postsurgical narrowing of external ear canal.

380.53 **Secondary to inflammation**

DEF: Narrowing, external ear canal; due to chronic inflammation.

√5th 380.8 **Other disorders of external ear**

380.81 **Exostosis of external ear canal**

380.89 **Other**

380.9 **Unspecified disorder of external ear**

√4th 381 **Nonsuppurative otitis media and Eustachian tube disorders**

√5th 381.0 **Acute nonsuppurative otitis media**
Acute tubotympanic catarrh
Otitis media, acute or subacute:
catarrhal
exudative
transudative
with effusion

EXCLUDES *otitic barotrauma (993.0)*

381.00 **Acute nonsuppurative otitis media, unspecified**

381.01 **Acute serous otitis media**
Acute or subacute secretory otitis media

DEF: Sudden, severe infection of middle ear.

381.02 **Acute mucoid otitis media**
Acute or subacute seromucinous otitis media
Blue drum syndrome

DEF: Sudden, severe infection of middle ear, with mucous.

381.03 **Acute sanguinous otitis media**

DEF: Sudden, severe infection of middle ear, with blood.

381.04 **Acute allergic serous otitis media**

381.05 **Acute allergic mucoid otitis media**

381.06 **Acute allergic sanguinous otitis media**

√5th 381.1 **Chronic serous otitis media**
Chronic tubotympanic catarrh

381.10 **Chronic serous otitis media, simple or unspecified**

DEF: Persistent infection of middle ear, without pus.

381.19 **Other**
Serosanguinous chronic otitis media

√5th 381.2 **Chronic mucoid otitis media**
Glue ear

EXCLUDES *adhesive middle ear disease (385.10-385.19)*

DEF: Chronic condition; characterized by viscous fluid in middle ear; due to obstructed Eustachian tube.

381.20 **Chronic mucoid otitis media, simple or unspecified**

381.29 **Other**
Mucosanguinous chronic otitis media

381.3 **Other and unspecified chronic nonsuppurative otitis media**

Otitis media, chronic: Otitis media, chronic:
allergic   seromucinous
exudative   transudative
secretory   with effusion

381.4 **Nonsuppurative otitis media, not specified as acute or chronic**

Otitis media: Otitis media:
allergic   seromucinous
catarrhal   serous
exudative   transudative
mucoid   with effusion
secretory

√5th 381.5 **Eustachian salpingitis**

381.50 **Eustachian salpingitis, unspecified**

381.51 **Acute Eustachian salpingitis**

DEF: Sudden, severe inflammation of Eustachian tube.

381.52 **Chronic Eustachian salpingitis**

DEF: Persistent inflammation of Eustachian tube.

√5th 381.6 **Obstruction of Eustachian tube**

Stenosis ⎫
Stricture ⎬ of Eustachian tube

381.60 **Obstruction of Eustachian tube, unspecified**

381.61 **Osseous obstruction of Eustachian tube**
Obstruction of Eustachian tube from cholesteatoma, polyp, or other osseous lesion

381.62 **Intrinsic cartilagenous obstruction of Eustachian tube**

DEF: Blockage of Eustachian tube; due to cartilage overgrowth.

381.63 **Extrinsic cartilagenous obstruction of Eustachian tube**
Compression of Eustachian tube

381.7 **Patulous Eustachian tube**

DEF: Distended, oversized Eustachian tube.

√5th 381.8 **Other disorders of Eustachian tube**

381.81 **Dysfunction of Eustachian tube**

381.89 **Other**

381.9 **Unspecified Eustachian tube disorder**

√4th 382 **Suppurative and unspecified otitis media**

√5th 382.0 **Acute suppurative otitis media**

Otitis media, acute: Otitis media, acute:
necrotizing NOS   purulent

382.00 **Acute suppurative otitis media without spontaneous rupture of ear drum**

DEF: Sudden, severe inflammation of middle ear, with pus.

Nervous System and Sense Organs 382.01–385.02

382.01 Acute suppurative otitis media with spontaneous rupture of ear drum
DEF: Sudden, severe inflammation of middle ear, with pressure tearing ear drum tissue.

382.02 Acute suppurative otitis media in diseases classified elsewhere
Code first underlying disease, as:
  influenza (487.8)
  scarlet fever (034.1)
EXCLUDES   postmeasles otitis (055.2)

382.1 Chronic tubotympanic suppurative otitis media
Benign chronic suppurative otitis media
Chronic tubotympanic disease
} (with anterior perforation of ear drum)

DEF: Inflammation of tympanic cavity and auditory tube; with pus formation.

382.2 Chronic atticoantral suppurative otitis media
Chronic atticoantral disease
Persistent mucosal disease
} (with posterior or superior marginal perforation of ear drum)

DEF: Inflammation of upper tympanic membrane and mastoid antrum; with pus formation.

382.3 Unspecified chronic suppurative otitis media
Chronic purulent otitis media
EXCLUDES   tuberculous otitis media (017.4)

382.4 Unspecified suppurative otitis media
Purulent otitis media NOS

382.9 Unspecified otitis media
Otitis media: Otitis media:
  NOS   chronic NOS
  acute NOS

√4th **383 Mastoiditis and related conditions**
√5th **383.0 Acute mastoiditis**
Abscess of mastoid   Empyema of mastoid
383.00 Acute mastoiditis without complications
DEF: Sudden, severe inflammation of mastoid air cells.

383.01 Subperiosteal abscess of mastoid
DEF: Pocket of pus within mastoid bone.

383.02 Acute mastoiditis with other complications
Gradenigo's syndrome

383.1 Chronic mastoiditis
Caries of mastoid
Fistula of mastoid
EXCLUDES   tuberculous mastoiditis (015.6)
DEF: Persistent inflammation of mastoid air cells.

√5th **383.2 Petrositis**
Coalescing osteitis
Inflammation
Osteomyelitis
} of petrous bone

383.20 Petrositis, unspecified
383.21 Acute petrositis
DEF: Sudden, severe inflammation of dense bone behind ear.

383.22 Chronic petrositis
DEF: Persistent inflammation of dense bone behind ear.

√5th **383.3 Complications following mastoidectomy**
383.30 Postmastoidectomy complication, unspecified
383.31 Mucosal cyst of postmastoidectomy cavity
DEF: Mucous-lined cyst cavity following removal of mastoid bone.

383.32 Recurrent cholesteatoma of postmastoidectomy cavity
DEF: Cystlike mass of cell debris in cavity following removal of mastoid bone.

383.33 Granulations of postmastoidectomy cavity
Chronic inflammation of postmastoidectomy cavity
DEF: Granular tissue in cavity following removal of mastoid bone.

√5th **383.8 Other disorders of mastoid**
383.81 Postauricular fistula
DEF: Abnormal passage behind mastoid cavity.

383.89 Other
383.9 Unspecified mastoiditis
√4th **384 Other disorders of tympanic membrane**
√5th **384.0 Acute myringitis without mention of otitis media**
384.00 Acute myringitis, unspecified
Acute tympanitis NOS
DEF: Sudden, severe inflammation of ear drum.

384.01 Bullous myringitis
Myringitis bullosa hemorrhagica
DEF: Type of viral otitis media characterized by the appearance of serous or hemorrhagic blebs on the tympanic membrane.

384.09 Other
384.1 Chronic myringitis without mention of otitis media
Chronic tympanitis
DEF: Persistent inflammation of ear drum; with no evidence of middle ear infection.

√5th **384.2 Perforation of tympanic membrane**
Perforation of ear drum: Perforation of ear drum:
  NOS   postinflammatory
  persistent posttraumatic
EXCLUDES   otitis media with perforation of tympanic membrane (382.00-382.9)
                 traumatic perforation [current injury] (872.61)

384.20 Perforation of tympanic membrane, unspecified
384.21 Central perforation of tympanic membrane
384.22 Attic perforation of tympanic membrane
Pars flaccida
384.23 Other marginal perforation of tympanic membrane
384.24 Multiple perforations of tympanic membrane
384.25 Total perforation of tympanic membrane
√5th **384.8 Other specified disorders of tympanic membrane**
384.81 Atrophic flaccid tympanic membrane
Healed perforation of ear drum
384.82 Atrophic nonflaccid tympanic membrane
384.9 Unspecified disorder of tympanic membrane
√4th **385 Other disorders of middle ear and mastoid**
EXCLUDES   mastoiditis (383.0-383.9)
√5th **385.0 Tympanosclerosis**
385.00 Tympanosclerosis, unspecified as to involvement
385.01 Tympanosclerosis involving tympanic membrane only
DEF: Tough, fibrous tissue impeding functions of ear drum.

385.02 Tympanosclerosis involving tympanic membrane and ear ossicles
DEF: Tough, fibrous tissue impeding functions of middle ear bones (stapes, malleus, incus).

385.03 Tympanosclerosis involving tympanic membrane, ear ossicles, and middle ear
DEF: Tough, fibrous tissue impeding functions of ear drum, middle ear bones and middle ear canal.

385.09 Tympanosclerosis involving other combination of structures

√5th **385.1 Adhesive middle ear disease**
Adhesive otitis   Otitis media:
Otitis media: fibrotic
chronic adhesive
EXCLUDES   glue ear (381.20-381.29)
DEF: Adhesions of middle ear structures.

385.10 Adhesive middle ear disease, unspecified as to involvement
385.11 Adhesions of drum head to incus
385.12 Adhesions of drum head to stapes
385.13 Adhesions of drum head to promontorium
385.19 Other adhesions and combinations

√5th **385.2 Other acquired abnormality of ear ossicles**
385.21 Impaired mobility of malleus
Ankylosis of malleus
385.22 Impaired mobility of other ear ossicles
Ankylosis of ear ossicles, except malleus
385.23 Discontinuity or dislocation of ear ossicles
DEF: Disruption in auditory chain; created by malleus, incus and stapes.
385.24 Partial loss or necrosis of ear ossicles
DEF: Tissue loss in malleus, incus and stapes.

√5th **385.3 Cholesteatoma of middle ear and mastoid**
Cholesterosis
Epidermosis
Keratosis   } of (middle) ear
Polyp

EXCLUDES   cholesteatoma:
external ear canal (380.21)
recurrent of postmastoidectomy cavity (383.32)

DEF: Cystlike mass of middle ear and mastoid antrum filled with debris, including cholesterol.

385.30 Cholesteatoma, unspecified
385.31 Cholesteatoma of attic
385.32 Cholesteatoma of middle ear
385.33 Cholesteatoma of middle ear and mastoid
DEF: Cystlike mass of cell debris in middle ear and mastoid air cells behind ear.

385.35 Diffuse cholesteatosis

√5th **385.8 Other disorders of middle ear and mastoid**
385.82 Cholesterin granuloma
DEF: Granuloma formed of fibrotic tissue; contains cholesterol crystals surrounded by foreign-body cells; found in the middle ear and mastoid area.

385.83 Retained foreign body of middle ear
385.89 Other
385.9 Unspecified disorder of middle ear and mastoid

√4th **386 Vertiginous syndromes and other disorders of vestibular system**
EXCLUDES   vertigo NOS (780.4)

√5th **386.0 Ménière's disease**
Endolymphatic hydrops
Lermoyez's syndrome
Ménière's syndrome or vertigo
DEF: Distended membranous labyrinth of middle ear from endolymphatic hydrops; causes ischemia, failure of nerve function; hearing and balance dysfunction; symptoms include fluctuating deafness, ringing in ears and dizziness.

386.00 Ménière's disease, unspecified
Ménière's disease (active)
386.01 Active Ménière's disease, cochleovestibular
386.02 Active Ménière's disease, cochlear
386.03 Active Ménière's disease, vestibular
386.04 Inactive Ménière's disease
Ménière's disease in remission

√5th **386.1 Other and unspecified peripheral vertigo**
EXCLUDES   epidemic vertigo (078.81)
386.10 Peripheral vertigo, unspecified
386.11 Benign paroxysmal positional vertigo
Benign paroxysmal positional nystagmus
386.12 Vestibular neuronitis
Acute (and recurrent) peripheral vestibulopathy
DEF: Transient benign vertigo, unknown cause; characterized by response to caloric stimulation on one side, nystagmus with rhythmic movement of eyes; normal auditory function present; occurs in young adults.

386.19 Other
Aural vertigo
Otogenic vertigo

386.2 Vertigo of central origin
Central positional nystagmus
Malignant positional vertigo

√5th **386.3 Labyrinthitis**
386.30 Labyrinthitis, unspecified
386.31 Serous labyrinthitis
Diffuse labyrinthitis
DEF: Inflammation of labyrinth; with fluid buildup.
386.32 Circumscribed labyrinthitis
Focal labyrinthitis
386.33 Suppurative labyrinthitis
Purulent labyrinthitis
DEF: Inflammation of labyrinth; with pus.
386.34 Toxic labyrinthitis
DEF: Inflammation of labyrinth; due to toxic reaction.
386.35 Viral labyrinthitis

√5th **386.4 Labyrinthine fistula**
386.40 Labyrinthine fistula, unspecified
386.41 Round window fistula
386.42 Oval window fistula
386.43 Semicircular canal fistula
386.48 Labyrinthine fistula of combined sites

√5th **386.5 Labyrinthine dysfunction**
386.50 Labyrinthine dysfunction, unspecified
386.51 Hyperactive labyrinth, unilateral
DEF: Oversensitivity of labyrinth to auditory signals; affecting one ear.
386.52 Hyperactive labyrinth, bilateral
DEF: Oversensitivity of labyrinth to auditory signals; affecting both ears.
386.53 Hypoactive labyrinth, unilateral
DEF: Reduced sensitivity of labyrinth to auditory signals; affecting one ear.
386.54 Hypoactive labyrinth, bilateral
DEF: Reduced sensitivity of labyrinth to auditory signals; affecting both ears.
386.55 Loss of labyrinthine reactivity, unilateral
DEF: Reduced reaction of labyrinth to auditory signals, affecting one ear.

√4th√5th Additional Digit Required   Unspecified Code   Other Specified Code   Manifestation Code   ▶◀ Revised Text   ● New Code   ▲ Revised Code Title

Nervous System and Sense Organs 386.56–389.9

386.56 Loss of labyrinthine reactivity, bilateral
DEF: Reduced reaction of labyrinth to auditory signals; affecting both ears.

386.58 Other forms and combinations

386.8 Other disorders of labyrinth

386.9 Unspecified vertiginous syndromes and labyrinthine disorders

√4th **387 Otosclerosis**
INCLUDES   otospongiosis

DEF: Synonym for otospongiosis, spongy bone formation in the labyrinth bones of the ear; it causes progressive hearing impairment.

387.0 Otosclerosis involving oval window, nonobliterative
DEF: Tough, fibrous tissue impeding functions of oval window.

387.1 Otosclerosis involving oval window, obliterative
DEF: Tough, fibrous tissue blocking oval window.

387.2 Cochlear otosclerosis
Otosclerosis involving: Otosclerosis involving:
   otic capsule   round window
DEF: Tough, fibrous tissue impeding functions of cochlea.

387.8 Other otosclerosis

387.9 Otosclerosis, unspecified

√4th **388 Other disorders of ear**

√5th **388.0 Degenerative and vascular disorders of ear**

388.00 Degenerative and vascular disorders, unspecified

388.01 Presbyacusis
DEF: Progressive, bilateral perceptive hearing loss caused by advancing age; it is also known as presbycusis.

388.02 Transient ischemic deafness
DEF: Restricted blood flow to auditory organs causing temporary hearing loss.

√5th **388.1 Noise effects on inner ear**

388.10 Noise effects on inner ear, unspecified

388.11 Acoustic trauma (explosive) to ear
Otitic blast injury

388.12 Noise-induced hearing loss

388.2 Sudden hearing loss, unspecified

√5th **388.3 Tinnitus**
DEF: Abnormal noises in ear; may be heard by others beside the affected individual; noises include ringing, clicking, roaring and buzzing.

388.30 Tinnitus, unspecified

388.31 Subjective tinnitus

388.32 Objective tinnitus

√5th **388.4 Other abnormal auditory perception**

388.40 Abnormal auditory perception, unspecified

388.41 Diplacusis
DEF: Perception of a single auditory sound as two sounds at two different levels of intensity.

388.42 Hyperacusis
DEF: Exceptionally acute sense of hearing caused by such conditions as Bell's palsy; this term may also refer to painful sensitivity to sounds.

388.43 Impairment of auditory discrimination
DEF: Impaired ability to distinguish tone of sound.

388.44 Recruitment
DEF: Perception of abnormally increased loudness caused by a slight increase in sound intensity; it is a term used in audiology.

388.5 Disorders of acoustic nerve
Acoustic neuritis
Degeneration } of acoustic or eighth nerve
Disorder
EXCLUDES   acoustic neuroma (225.1)
        syphilitic acoustic neuritis (094.86)

√5th **388.6 Otorrhea**

388.60 Otorrhea, unspecified
Discharging ear NOS

388.61 Cerebrospinal fluid otorrhea
EXCLUDES   cerebrospinal fluid rhinorrhea (349.81)
DEF: Spinal fluid leakage from ear.

388.69 Other
Otorrhagia

√5th **388.7 Otalgia**

388.70 Otalgia, unspecified
Earache NOS

388.71 Otogenic pain

388.72 Referred pain

388.8 Other disorders of ear

388.9 Unspecified disorder of ear

√4th **389 Hearing loss**

√5th **389.0 Conductive hearing loss**
Conductive deafness

DEF: Dysfunction in sound-conducting structures of external or middle ear causing hearing loss.

389.00 Conductive hearing loss, unspecified

389.01 Conductive hearing loss, external ear

389.02 Conductive hearing loss, tympanic membrane

389.03 Conductive hearing loss, middle ear

389.04 Conductive hearing loss, inner ear

389.08 Conductive hearing loss of combined types

√5th **389.1 Sensorineural hearing loss**
Perceptive hearing loss or deafness
EXCLUDES   abnormal auditory perception (388.40-388.44)
        psychogenic deafness (306.7)

DEF: Nerve conduction causing hearing loss.

389.10 Sensorineural hearing loss, unspecified

389.11 Sensory hearing loss

389.12 Neural hearing loss

389.14 Central hearing loss

389.18 Sensorineural hearing loss of combined types

389.2 Mixed conductive and sensorineural hearing loss
Deafness or hearing loss of type classifiable to 389.0 with type classifiable to 389.1

389.7 Deaf mutism, not elsewhere classifiable
Deaf, nonspeaking

389.8 Other specified forms of hearing loss

389.9 Unspecified hearing loss
Deafness NOS

7. DISEASES OF THE CIRCULATORY SYSTEM (390-459)

ACUTE RHEUMATIC FEVER (390-392)

DEF: Febrile disease occurs mainly in children or young adults following throat infection by group A streptococci; symptoms include fever, joint pain, lesions of heart, blood vessels and joint connective tissue, abdominal pain, skin changes, and chorea.

390 Rheumatic fever without mention of heart involvement
Arthritis, rheumatic, acute or subacute
Rheumatic fever (active) (acute)
Rheumatism, articular, acute or subacute
EXCLUDES *that with heart involvement (391.0-391.9)*

√4ᵗʰ 391 Rheumatic fever with heart involvement
EXCLUDES *chronic heart diseases of rheumatic origin (393.0-398.9) unless rheumatic fever is also present or there is evidence of recrudescence or activity of the rheumatic process*

391.0 Acute rheumatic pericarditis
Rheumatic:
fever (active) (acute) with pericarditis
pericarditis (acute)
Any condition classifiable to 390 with pericarditis
EXCLUDES *that not specified as rheumatic (420.0-420.9)*
DEF: Sudden, severe inflammation of heart lining due to rheumatic fever.

391.1 Acute rheumatic endocarditis
Rheumatic:
endocarditis, acute
fever (active) (acute) with endocarditis or valvulitis
valvulitis acute
Any condition classifiable to 390 with endocarditis or valvulitis
DEF: Sudden, severe inflammation of heart cavities due to rheumatic fever.

391.2 Acute rheumatic myocarditis
Rheumatic fever (active) (acute) with myocarditis
Any condition classifiable to 390 with myocarditis
DEF: Sudden, severe inflammation of heart muscles due to rheumatic fever.

391.8 Other acute rheumatic heart disease
Rheumatic:
fever (active) (acute) with other or multiple types of heart involvement
pancarditis, acute
Any condition classifiable to 390 with other or multiple types of heart involvement

391.9 Acute rheumatic heart disease, unspecified
Rheumatic:
carditis, acute
fever (active) (acute) with unspecified type of heart involvement
heart disease, active or acute
Any condition classifiable to 390 with unspecified type of heart involvement

√4ᵗʰ 392 Rheumatic chorea
INCLUDES Sydenham's chorea
EXCLUDES *chorea:*
NOS (333.5)
Huntington's (333.4)
DEF: Childhood disease linked with rheumatic fever and streptococcal infections; symptoms include spasmodic, involuntary movements of limbs or facial muscles, psychic symptoms, and irritability.

392.0 With heart involvement
Rheumatic chorea with heart involvement of any type classifiable to 391

392.9 Without mention of heart involvement

CHRONIC RHEUMATIC HEART DISEASE (393-398)

393 Chronic rheumatic pericarditis
Adherent pericardium, rheumatic
Chronic rheumatic:
mediastinopericarditis
myopericarditis
EXCLUDES *pericarditis NOS or not specified as rheumatic (423.0-423.9)*
DEF: Persistent inflammation of heart lining due to rheumatic heart disease.

√4ᵗʰ 394 Diseases of mitral valve
EXCLUDES *that with aortic valve involvement (396.0-396.9)*

394.0 Mitral stenosis
Mitral (valve):
obstruction (rheumatic)
stenosis NOS
DEF: Narrowing, of mitral valve between left atrium and left ventricle due to rheumatic heart disease.

394.1 Rheumatic mitral insufficiency
Rheumatic mitral: Rheumatic mitral:
incompetence   regurgitation
EXCLUDES *that not specified as rheumatic (424.0)*
DEF: Malfunction of mitral valve between left atrium and left ventricle due to rheumatic heart disease.

394.2 Mitral stenosis with insufficiency
Mitral stenosis with incompetence or regurgitation
DEF: A narrowing or stricture of the mitral valve situated between the left atrium and left ventricle. The stenosis interferes with blood flow from the atrium into the ventricle. If the valve does not completely close, it becomes insufficient (inadequate) and cannot prevent regurgitation (abnormal backward flow) into the atrium when the left ventricle contracts. This abnormal function is also called incompetence.

394.9 Other and unspecified mitral valve diseases
Mitral (valve):   Mitral (valve):
disease (chronic)   failure

√4ᵗʰ 395 Diseases of aortic valve
EXCLUDES *that not specified as rheumatic (424.1)*
that with mitral valve involvement (396.0-396.9)

395.0 Rheumatic aortic stenosis
Rheumatic aortic (valve) obstruction
DEF: Narrowing of the aortic valve; results in backflow into ventricle due to rheumatic heart disease.

395.1 Rheumatic aortic insufficiency
Rheumatic aortic: Rheumatic aortic:
incompetence   regurgitation
DEF: Malfunction of the aortic valve; results in backflow into left ventricle due to rheumatic heart disease.

395.2 Rheumatic aortic stenosis with insufficiency
Rheumatic aortic stenosis with incompetence or regurgitation
DEF: Malfunction and narrowing, of the aortic valve; results in backflow into left ventricle due to rheumatic heart disease.

395.9 Other and unspecified rheumatic aortic diseases
Rheumatic aortic (valve) disease

√4ᵗʰ 396 Diseases of mitral and aortic valves
INCLUDES involvement of both mitral and aortic valves, whether specified as rheumatic or not

396.0 Mitral valve stenosis and aortic valve stenosis
Atypical aortic (valve) stenosis
Mitral and aortic (valve) obstruction (rheumatic)

396.1 Mitral valve stenosis and aortic valve insufficiency

396.2 Mitral valve insufficiency and aortic valve stenosis

396.3 Mitral valve insufficiency and aortic valve insufficiency
Mitral and aortic (valve):   Mitral and aortic (valve):
incompetence   regurgitation

Circulatory System 390–396.3

396.8　Multiple involvement of mitral and aortic valves

Stenosis and insufficiency of mitral or aortic valve
with stenosis or insufficiency, or both, of the
other valve

396.9　Mitral and aortic valve diseases, unspecified

√4ᵗʰ **397　Diseases of other endocardial structures**

397.0　Diseases of tricuspid valve

Tricuspid (valve) (rheumatic):
　disease
　insufficiency
　obstruction
　regurgitation
　stenosis

DEF: Malfunction of the valve between right atrium and right
ventricle due to rheumatic heart disease.

397.1　Rheumatic diseases of pulmonary valve

EXCLUDES　　*that not specified as rheumatic (424.3)*

**397.9　Rheumatic diseases of endocardium, valve
unspecified**

Rheumatic:
　endocarditis (chronic)
　valvulitis (chronic)

EXCLUDES　　*that not specified as rheumatic
(424.90-424.99)*

√4ᵗʰ **398　Other rheumatic heart disease**

398.0　Rheumatic myocarditis

Rheumatic degeneration of myocardium

EXCLUDES　　*myocarditis not specified as rheumatic
(429.0)*

DEF: Chronic inflammation of heart muscle due to rheumatic heart
disease.

√5ᵗʰ **398.9　Other and unspecified rheumatic heart diseases**

398.90　Rheumatic heart disease, unspecified

Rheumatic:　　　Rheumatic:
　carditis　　　　　heart disease NOS

EXCLUDES　　*carditis not specified as
rheumatic (429.89)*
*heart disease NOS not
specified as rheumatic
(429.9)*

398.91　Rheumatic heart failure (congestive)

Rheumatic left ventricular failure

DEF: Decreased cardiac output, edema and hypertension
due to rheumatic heart disease.

398.99　Other

HYPERTENSIVE DISEASE (401-405)

EXCLUDES　　*that complicating pregnancy, childbirth, or the
puerperium (642.0-642.9)*
that involving coronary vessels (410.00-414.9)

√4ᵗʰ **401　Essential hypertension**

INCLUDES
　high blood pressure
　hyperpiesia
　hyperpiesis
　hypertension (arterial) (essential) (primary)
　　(systemic)
　hypertensive vascular:
　　degeneration
　　disease

EXCLUDES　　*elevated blood pressure without diagnosis of
hypertension (796.2)*
pulmonary hypertension (416.0-416.9)
that involving vessels of:
　brain (430-438)
　eye (362.11)

DEF: Hypertension that occurs without apparent organic cause; idiopathic.

401.0　Malignant

DEF: Severe high arterial blood pressure; results in necrosis in
kidney, retina, etc.; hemorrhages occur and death commonly due to
uremia or rupture of cerebral vessel.

401.1　Benign

DEF: Mildly elevated arterial blood pressure.

401.9　Unspecified

√4ᵗʰ **402　Hypertensive heart disease**

▶Use additional code to specify type of heart failure (428.0,
428.20-428.23, 428.30-428.33, 428.40-428.43)◀

INCLUDES　　hypertensive:
　cardiomegaly
　cardiopathy
　cardiovascular disease
　heart (disease) (failure)
any condition classifiable to 428, 429.0-429.3,
　429.8, 429.9 due to hypertension

√5ᵗʰ **402.0　Malignant**

▲　　**402.00　Without heart failure**
▲　　**402.01　With heart failure**

√5ᵗʰ **402.1　Benign**

▲　　**402.10　Without heart failure**
▲　　**402.11　With heart failure**

√5ᵗʰ **402.9　Unspecified**

▲　　**402.90　Without heart failure**
▲　　**402.91　With heart failure**

√4ᵗʰ **403　Hypertensive renal disease**

INCLUDES　　arteriolar nephritis
arteriosclerosis of:
　kidney
　renal arterioles
arteriosclerotic nephritis (chronic) (interstitial)
hypertensive:
　nephropathy
　renal failure
　uremia (chronic)
nephrosclerosis
renal sclerosis with hypertension
any condition classifiable to 585, 586, or 587
　with any condition classifiable to 401

EXCLUDES　　*acute renal failure (584.5-584.9)*
renal disease stated as not due to hypertension
*renovascular hypertension (405.0-405.9 with
fifth-digit 1)*

The following fifth-digit subclassification is for use with
category 403:
　　0　without mention of renal failure
　　1　with renal failure

√5ᵗʰ **403.0　Malignant**

√5ᵗʰ **403.1　Benign**

√5ᵗʰ **403.9　Unspecified**

√4ᵗʰ **404　Hypertensive heart and renal disease**

▶Use additional code to specify type of heart failure (428.0,
428.20-428.23, 428.30-428.33, 428.40-428.43)◀

INCLUDES　　disease:
　cardiorenal
　cardiovascular renal
any condition classifiable to 402 with any
　condition classifiable to 403

The following fifth-digit subclassification is for use with
category 404:
▲　　**0　without mention of heart failure or renal
failure**
▲　　**1　with heart failure**
▲　　**2　with renal failure**
▲　　**3　with heart failure and renal failure**

√5ᵗʰ **404.0　Malignant**

✓5th **404.1** Benign
✓5th **404.9** Unspecified

✓4th **405 Secondary hypertension**
DEF: High arterial blood pressure due to or with a variety of primary diseases, such as renal disorders, CNS disorders, endocrine, and vascular diseases.

✓5th **405.0** Malignant
405.01 Renovascular
405.09 Other

✓5th **405.1** Benign
405.11 Renovascular
405.19 Other

✓5th **405.9** Unspecified
405.91 Renovascular
405.99 Other

ISCHEMIC HEART DISEASE (410-414)

INCLUDES that with mention of hypertension
Use additional code to identify presence of hypertension (401.0-405.9)

✓4th **410 Acute myocardial infarction**
INCLUDES cardiac infarction
coronary (artery):
embolism
occlusion
rupture
thrombosis
infarction of heart, myocardium, or ventricle
rupture of heart, myocardium, or ventricle
any condition classifiable to 414.1-414.9
specified as acute or with a stated
duration of 8 weeks or less

DEF: A sudden insufficiency of blood supply to an area of the heart muscle; usually due to a coronary artery occlusion.

The following fifth-digit subclassification is for use with category 410:

0 episode of care unspecified
Use when the source document does not contain sufficient information for the assignment of fifth digit 1 or 2.

1 initial episode of care
Use fifth-digit 1 to designate the first episode of care (regardless of facility site) for a newly diagnosed myocardial infarction. The fifth-digit 1 is assigned regardless of the number of times a patient may be transferred during the initial episode of care.

2 subsequent episode of care
Use fifth-digit 2 to designate an episode of care following the initial episode when the patient is admitted for further observation, evaluation or treatment for a myocardial infarction that has received initial treatment, but is still less than 8 weeks old.

✓5th **410.0** Of anterolateral wall A

✓5th **410.1** Of other anterior wall A
Infarction:
anterior (wall)
NOS
anteroapical   (with contiguous portion of
anteroseptal   intraventricular septum)

✓5th **410.2** Of inferolateral wall A

✓5th **410.3** Of inferoposterior wall A

✓5th **410.4** Of other inferior wall A
Infarction:
diaphragmatic   (with contiguous portion
wall NOS   of intraventricular
inferior (wall) NOS septum)

✓5th **410.5** Of other lateral wall A
Infarction: Infarction:
apical-lateral   high lateral
basal-lateral   posterolateral

✓5th **410.6** True posterior wall infarction A
Infarction: Infarction:
posterobasal   strictly posterior

✓5th **410.7** Subendocardial infarction A
Nontransmural infarction

✓5th **410.8** Of other specified sites A
Infarction of: Infarction of:
atrium   septum alone
papillary muscle

✓5th **410.9** Unspecified site A
Acute myocardial infarction NOS
Coronary occlusion NOS

✓4th **411 Other acute and subacute forms of ischemic heart disease**
411.0 Postmyocardial infarction syndrome A
Dressler's syndrome
DEF: Complication developing several days/weeks after myocardial infarction; symptoms include fever, leukocytosis, chest pain, evidence of pericarditis, pleurisy, and pneumonitis; tendency to recur.

411.1 Intermediate coronary syndrome A
Impending infarction   Preinfarction syndrome
Preinfarction angina   Unstable angina
EXCLUDES angina (pectoris) (413.9)
decubitus (413.0)

DEF: A condition representing an intermediate stage between angina of effort and acute myocardial infarction. It is often documented by the physician as "unstable angina."

Sections of Heart Muscle

Pericardial layers:
Pleural
Fibrous
Parietal
Epicardium
Serous (fluid)
Pericardial cavity
Endocardium
Myocardium (muscular)
Endocardial cavity
Septum:
Membranous
Muscular
Sectional Schematic
Pericardial sac
Pericardial reflection (layers fused)
Pericardial sinus

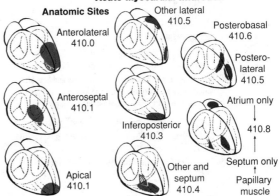

Acute Myocardial Infarction

Anatomic Sites
Anterolateral 410.0
Other lateral 410.5
Posterobasal 410.6
Postero-lateral 410.5
Anteroseptal 410.1
Atrium only 410.8
Inferoposterior 410.3
Septum only
Apical 410.1
Other and septum 410.4
Papillary muscle

✓4th
✓5th Additional Digit Required   Unspecified Code   Other Specified Code   Manifestation Code   ►◄ Revised Text   ● New Code   ▲ Revised Code Title

Circulatory System 404.1–411.1

Circulatory System 411.8–415.0

√5ᵗʰ **411.8 Other**

411.81 Acute coronary occlusion without myocardial infarction   A

Acute coronary (artery):

embolism   ⎫ without or not
obstruction   ⎬ resulting in
occlusion   ⎭ myocardial
thrombosis   infarction

EXCLUDES   *obstruction without infarction due to atherosclerosis* ▶*(414.00-414.06)*◀
occlusion without infarction due to atherosclerosis ▶*(414.00-414.06)*◀

DEF: Interrupted blood flow to a portion of the heart; without tissue death.

411.89 Other   A

Coronary insufficiency (acute)
Subendocardial ischemia

412 Old myocardial infarction   A

Healed myocardial infarction
Past myocardial infarction diagnosed on ECG [EKG] or other special investigation, but currently presenting no symptoms

√4ᵗʰ **413 Angina pectoris**

DEF: Severe constricting pain in the chest, often radiating from the precordium to the left shoulder and down the arm, due to ischemia of the heart muscle; usually caused by coronary disease; pain is often precipitated by effort or excitement.

413.0 Angina decubitus   A

Nocturnal angina

DEF: Angina occurring only in the recumbent position.

413.1 Prinzmetal angina   A

Variant angina pectoris

DEF: Angina occurring when patient is recumbent; associated with ST-segment elevations.

413.9 Other and unspecified angina pectoris   A

Angina: Anginal syndrome
  NOS   Status anginosus
  cardiac   Stenocardia
  of effort   Syncope anginosa

EXCLUDES   *preinfarction angina (411.1)*

√4ᵗʰ **414 Other forms of chronic ischemic heart disease**

EXCLUDES   *arteriosclerotic cardiovascular disease [ASCVD] (429.2)*
cardiovascular:
  arteriosclerosis or sclerosis (429.2)
  degeneration or disease (429.2)

√5ᵗʰ **414.0 Coronary atherosclerosis**

Arteriosclerotic heart disease [ASHD]
Atherosclerotic heart disease
Coronary (artery):
  arteriosclerosis
  arteritis or endarteritis
  atheroma
  sclerosis
  stricture

EXCLUDES   *embolism of graft (996.72)*
occlusion NOS of graft (996.72)
thrombus of graft (996.72)

DEF: A chronic condition marked by thickening and loss of elasticity of the coronary artery; caused by deposits of plaque containing cholesterol, lipoid material and lipophages.

414.00 Of unspecified type of vessel, native or graft   A

414.01 Of native coronary artery   A

DEF: Plaque deposits in natural heart vessels.

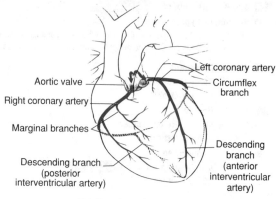

Arteries of the Heart

Aortic valve
Right coronary artery
Marginal branches
Descending branch (posterior interventricular artery)
Left coronary artery
Circumflex branch
Descending branch (anterior interventricular artery)

414.02 Of autologous vein bypass graft   A

DEF: Plaque deposit in grafted vein originating within patient.

414.03 Of nonautologous biological bypass graft   A

DEF: Plaque deposits in grafted vessel originating outside patient.

414.04 Of artery bypass graft   A

Internal mammary artery

DEF: Plaque deposits in grafted artery originating within patient.

414.05 Of unspecified type of bypass graft   A

Bypass graft NOS

● **414.06 Of coronary artery of transplanted heart**

▲ √5ᵗʰ **414.1 Aneurysm and dissection of heart**

▲ **414.10 Aneurysm of heart (wall)**

Aneurysm (arteriovenous):
  mural
  ventricular

▲ **414.11 Aneurysm of coronary vessels**

Aneurysm (arteriovenous) of coronary vessels

● **414.12 Dissection of coronary artery**

▲ **414.19 Other aneurysm of heart**

Arteriovenous fistula, acquired, of heart

414.8 Other specified forms of chronic ischemic heart disease

Chronic coronary insufficiency
Ischemia, myocardial (chronic)
Any condition classifiable to 410 specified as chronic, or presenting with symptoms after 8 weeks from date of infarction

EXCLUDES   *coronary insufficiency (acute) (411.89)*

414.9 Chronic ischemic heart disease, unspecified

Ischemic heart disease NOS

DISEASES OF PULMONARY CIRCULATION (415-417)

√4ᵗʰ **415 Acute pulmonary heart disease**

415.0 Acute cor pulmonale

EXCLUDES   *cor pulmonale NOS (416.9)*

DEF: A heart-lung disease marked by dilation and failure of the right side of heart; due to pulmonary embolism; ventilatory function is impaired and pulmonary hypertension results within hours.

N Newborn Age: 0   P Pediatric Age: 0-17   M Maternity Age: 12-55   A Adult Age: 15-124   MSP Medicare Secondary Payer

√5ᵗʰ **415.1 Pulmonary embolism and infarction**
Pulmonary (artery) (vein):
    apoplexy
    embolism
    infarction (hemorrhagic)
    thrombosis

EXCLUDES   *that complicating:*
    abortion (634-638 with .6, 639.6)
    ectopic or molar pregnancy (639.6)
    pregnancy, childbirth, or the
        puerperium (673.0-673.8)

DEF: Embolism: closure of the pulmonary artery or branch; due to
thrombosis (blood clot).

DEF: Infarction: necrosis of lung tissue; due to obstructed arterial
blood supply, most often by pulmonary embolism.

**415.11 Iatrogenic pulmonary embolism and
infarction**

415.19 Other

√4ᵗʰ **416 Chronic pulmonary heart disease**

416.0 Primary pulmonary hypertension
Idiopathic pulmonary arteriosclerosis
Pulmonary hypertension (essential) (idiopathic)
    (primary)

DEF: A rare increase in pulmonary circulation, often resulting in
right ventricular failure or fatal syncope.

416.1 Kyphoscoliotic heart disease
DEF: High blood pressure within the lungs as a result of curvature
of the spine.

416.8 Other chronic pulmonary heart diseases
Pulmonary hypertension, secondary

416.9 Chronic pulmonary heart disease, unspecified
Chronic cardiopulmonary disease
Cor pulmonale (chronic) NOS

√4ᵗʰ **417 Other diseases of pulmonary circulation**

417.0 Arteriovenous fistula of pulmonary vessels
EXCLUDES   *congenital arteriovenous fistula (747.3)*
DEF: Abnormal communication between blood vessels within lung.

417.1 Aneurysm of pulmonary artery
EXCLUDES   *congenital aneurysm (747.3)*

**417.8 Other specified diseases of pulmonary
circulation**

Pulmonary:	Pulmonary:
arteritis	endarteritis
Rupture	of pulmonary vessel
Stricture	

417.9 Unspecified disease of pulmonary circulation

OTHER FORMS OF HEART DISEASE (420-429)

√4ᵗʰ **420 Acute pericarditis**
INCLUDES   acute:
    mediastinopericarditis
    myopericarditis
    pericardial effusion
    pleuropericarditis
    pneumopericarditis

EXCLUDES   *acute rheumatic pericarditis (391.0)*
    postmyocardial infarction syndrome [Dressler's]
        (411.0)

DEF: Inflammation of the pericardium (heart sac); pericardial friction rub
results from this inflammation and is heard as a scratchy or leathery sound.

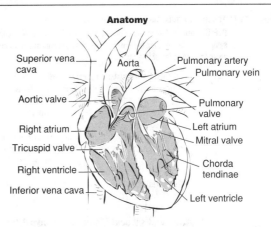

Anatomy

Superior vena cava • Aorta • Pulmonary artery • Pulmonary vein • Aortic valve • Pulmonary valve • Right atrium • Left atrium • Mitral valve • Tricuspid valve • Chorda tendinae • Right ventricle • Inferior vena cava • Left ventricle

Blood Flow

**420.0 Acute pericarditis in diseases classified
elsewhere**
Code first underlying disease, as:
    actinomycosis (039.8)
    amebiasis (006.8)
    nocardiosis (039.8)
    tuberculosis (017.9)
    uremia (585)

EXCLUDES   *pericarditis (acute) (in):*
    Coxsackie (virus) (074.21)
    gonococcal (098.83)
    histoplasmosis (115.0-115.9 with
        fifth-digit 3)
    meningococcal infection (036.41)
    syphilitic (093.81)

√5ᵗʰ **420.9 Other and unspecified acute pericarditis**

420.90 Acute pericarditis, unspecified
Pericarditis (acute):	Pericarditis (acute):
NOS	sicca
infective NOS	

420.91 Acute idiopathic pericarditis
Pericarditis, acute:	Pericarditis, acute:
benign	viral
nonspecific	

420.99 Other
Pericarditis (acute):
    pneumococcal
    purulent
    staphylococcal
    streptococcal
    suppurative
Pneumopyopericardium
Pyopericardium

EXCLUDES   *pericarditis in diseases*
    classified elsewhere
    (420.0)

Circulatory System 415.1–420.99

 Additional Digit Required   Unspecified Code   Other Specified Code   Manifestation Code   ►◄ Revised Text   ● New Code   ▲ Revised Code Title

2003 ICD•9•CM   **Volume 1 — 111**

Circulatory System 421–424.1

✓4th **421 Acute and subacute endocarditis**

DEF: Bacterial inflammation of the endocardium (intracardiac area); major symptoms include fever, fatigue, heart murmurs, splenomegaly, embolic episodes and areas of infarction.

421.0 Acute and subacute bacterial endocarditis

Endocarditis (acute) (chronic) (subacute):
bacterial
infective NOS
lenta
malignant
purulent
septic

Endocarditis (acute) (chronic) (subacute):
ulcerative
vegetative
Infective aneurysm
Subacute bacterial endocarditis [SBE]

Use additional code to identify infectious organism [e.g., Streptococcus 041.0, Staphylococcus 041.1]

421.1 Acute and subacute infective endocarditis in diseases classified elsewhere

Code first underlying disease, as:
blastomycosis (116.0)
Q fever (083.0)
typhoid (fever) (002.0)

EXCLUDES endocarditis (in):
Coxsackie (virus) (074.22)
gonococcal (098.84)
histoplasmosis (115.0-115.9 with fifth-digit 4)
meningococcal infection (036.42)
monilial (112.81)

421.9 Acute endocarditis, unspecified

Endocarditis
Myoendocarditis } acute or subacute
Periendocarditis

EXCLUDES acute rheumatic endocarditis (391.1)

✓4th **422 Acute myocarditis**

EXCLUDES acute rheumatic myocarditis (391.2)

DEF: Acute inflammation of the muscular walls of the heart (myocardium).

422.0 Acute myocarditis in diseases classified elsewhere

Code first underlying disease, as:
myocarditis (acute):
influenzal (487.8)
tuberculous (017.9)

EXCLUDES myocarditis (acute) (due to):
aseptic, of newborn (074.23)
Coxsackie (virus) (074.23)
diphtheritic (032.82)
meningococcal infection (036.43)
syphilitic (093.82)
toxoplasmosis (130.3)

✓5th **422.9 Other and unspecified acute myocarditis**

422.90 Acute myocarditis, unspecified

Acute or subacute (interstitial) myocarditis

422.91 Idiopathic myocarditis

Myocarditis (acute or subacute):
Fiedler's
giant cell
isolated (diffuse) (granulomatous)
nonspecific granulomatous

422.92 Septic myocarditis

Myocarditis, acute or subacute:
pneumococcal
staphylococcal

Use additional code to identify infectious organism [e.g., Staphylococcus 041.1]

EXCLUDES myocarditis, acute or subacute:
in bacterial diseases classified elsewhere (422.0)
streptococcal (391.2)

422.93 Toxic myocarditis

DEF: Inflammation of the heart muscle due to an adverse reaction to certain drugs or chemicals reaching the heart through the bloodstream.

422.99 Other

✓4th **423 Other diseases of pericardium**

EXCLUDES that specified as rheumatic (393)

423.0 Hemopericardium

DEF: Blood in the pericardial sac (pericardium).

423.1 Adhesive pericarditis

Adherent pericardium
Fibrosis of pericardium
Milk spots
Pericarditis:
adhesive
obliterative
Soldiers' patches

DEF: Two layers of serous pericardium adhere to each other by fibrous adhesions.

423.2 Constrictive pericarditis

Concato's disease
Pick's disease of heart (and liver)

DEF: Inflammation identified by a rigid, thickened and sometimes calcified pericardium; ventricles of the heart cannot be adequately filled and congestive heart failure may result.

423.8 Other specified diseases of pericardium

Calcification
Fistula } of pericardium

423.9 Unspecified disease of pericardium

✓4th **424 Other diseases of endocardium**

EXCLUDES bacterial endocarditis (421.0-421.9)
rheumatic endocarditis (391.1, 394.0-397.9)
syphilitic endocarditis (093.20-093.24)

424.0 Mitral valve disorders

Mitral (valve):
incompetence
insufficiency } NOS of specified cause, except rheumatic
regurgitation

EXCLUDES mitral (valve):
disease (394.9)
failure (394.9)
stenosis (394.0)
the listed conditions:
specified as rheumatic (394.1)
unspecified as to cause but with mention of:
diseases of aortic valve (396.0-396.9)
mitral stenosis or obstruction (394.2)

424.1 Aortic valve disorders

Aortic (valve):
incompetence
insufficiency
regurgitation } NOS of specified cause, except rheumatic
stenosis

EXCLUDES hypertrophic subaortic stenosis (425.1)
that specified as rheumatic (395.0-395.9)
that of unspecified cause but with mention of diseases of mitral valve (396.0-396.9)

424.2 Tricuspid valve disorders, specified as nonrheumatic

Tricuspid valve:
incompetence
insufficiency   } of specified cause,
regurgitation   except
stenosis   rheumatic

> **EXCLUDES** *rheumatic or of unspecified cause (397.0)*

424.3 Pulmonary valve disorders

Pulmonic: Pulmonic:
incompetence NOS   regurgitation NOS
insufficiency NOS   stenosis NOS

> **EXCLUDES** *that specified as rheumatic (397.1)*

✓5th **424.9 Endocarditis, valve unspecified**

424.90 Endocarditis, valve unspecified, unspecified cause

Endocarditis (chronic):
NOS
nonbacterial thrombotic
Valvular:
incompetence
insufficiency   } of unspecified
regurgitation   valve,
stenosis   unspecified
Valvulitis (chronic) } cause

424.91 *Endocarditis in diseases classified elsewhere*

Code first underlying disease as:
atypical verrucous endocarditis [Libman-Sacks] (710.0)
disseminated lupus erythematosus (710.0)
tuberculosis (017.9)

> **EXCLUDES** *syphilitic (093.20-093.24)*

Normal Heart Valve Function

Heart Valve Disorders

424.99 Other

Any condition classifiable to 424.90 with specified cause, except rheumatic

> **EXCLUDES** *endocardial fibroelastosis (425.3)*
> *that specified as rheumatic (397.9)*

✓4th **425 Cardiomyopathy**

> **INCLUDES** myocardiopathy

425.0 Endomyocardial fibrosis

425.1 Hypertrophic obstructive cardiomyopathy

Hypertrophic subaortic stenosis (idiopathic)

DEF: Cardiomyopathy marked by left ventricle hypertrophy, enlarged septum; results in obstructed blood flow.

425.2 Obscure cardiomyopathy of Africa

Becker's disease
Idiopathic mural endomyocardial disease

425.3 Endocardial fibroelastosis

Elastomyofibrosis

DEF: A condition marked by left ventricle hypertrophy and conversion of the endocardium into a thick fibroelastic coat; capacity of the ventricle may be reduced, but is often increased.

425.4 Other primary cardiomyopathies

Cardiomyopathy: Cardiomyopathy:
NOS   idiopathic
congestive   nonobstructive
constrictive   obstructive
familial   restrictive
hypertrophic   Cardiovascular collagenosis

425.5 Alcoholic cardiomyopathy

DEF: Heart disease as result of excess alcohol consumption.

425.7 *Nutritional and metabolic cardiomyopathy*

Code first underlying disease, as:
amyloidosis (277.3)
beriberi (265.0)
cardiac glycogenosis (271.0)
mucopolysaccharidosis (277.5)
thyrotoxicosis (242.0-242.9)

> **EXCLUDES** *gouty tophi of heart (274.82)*

425.8 *Cardiomyopathy in other diseases classified elsewhere*

Code first underlying disease, as:
Friedreich's ataxia (334.0)
myotonia atrophica (359.2)
progressive muscular dystrophy (359.1)
sarcoidosis (135)

> **EXCLUDES** *cardiomyopathy in Chagas' disease (086.0)*

425.9 Secondary cardiomyopathy, unspecified

Nerve Conduction of the Heart

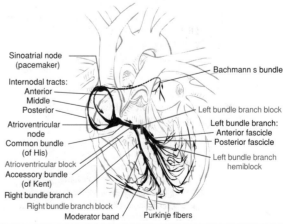

✓4th ✓5th **Additional Digit Required**   Unspecified Code   Other Specified Code   Manifestation Code   ▶◀ Revised Text   ● New Code   ▲ Revised Code Title

2003 ICD•9•CM   **Volume 1 — 113**

Circulatory System 424.2–425.9

Circulatory System 426–427.81

√4ᵗʰ **426 Conduction disorders**
DEF: Disruption or disturbance in the electrical impulses that regulate heartbeats.

426.0 Atrioventricular block, complete
Third degree atrioventricular block

√5ᵗʰ **426.1 Atrioventricular block, other and unspecified**
426.10 Atrioventricular block, unspecified
Atrioventricular [AV] block (incomplete) (partial)
426.11 First degree atrioventricular block
Incomplete atrioventricular block, first degree
Prolonged P-R interval NOS
426.12 Mobitz (type) II atrioventricular block
Incomplete atrioventricular block:
Mobitz (type) II
second degree, Mobitz (type) II
DEF: Impaired conduction of excitatory impulse from cardiac atrium to ventricle through AV node.
426.13 Other second degree atrioventricular block
Incomplete atrioventricular block:
Mobitz (type) I [Wenckebach's]
second degree:
NOS
Mobitz (type) I
with 2:1 atrioventricular response [block]
Wenckebach's phenomenon
DEF: Wenckebach's phenomenon: impulses generated at constant rate to sinus node, P-R interval lengthens; results in cycle of ventricular inadequacy and shortened P-R interval; second-degree A-V block commonly called "Mobitz type 1."

426.2 Left bundle branch hemiblock
Block:
left anterior fascicular
left posterior fascicular
426.3 Other left bundle branch block
Left bundle branch block:
NOS
anterior fascicular with posterior fascicular
complete
main stem
426.4 Right bundle branch block
√5ᵗʰ **426.5 Bundle branch block, other and unspecified**
426.50 Bundle branch block, unspecified
426.51 Right bundle branch block and left posterior fascicular block
426.52 Right bundle branch block and left anterior fascicular block
426.53 Other bilateral bundle branch block
Bifascicular block NOS
Bilateral bundle branch block NOS
Right bundle branch with left bundle branch block (incomplete) (main stem)
426.54 Trifascicular block
426.6 Other heart block
Intraventricular block: Sinoatrial block
NOS   Sinoauricular block
diffuse
myofibrillar
426.7 Anomalous atrioventricular excitation
Atrioventricular conduction:
accelerated
accessory
pre-excitation
Ventricular pre-excitation
Wolff-Parkinson-White syndrome
DEF: Wolff-Parkinson-White: normal conduction pathway is bypassed; results in short P-R interval on EKG; tendency to supraventricular tachycardia.

√5ᵗʰ **426.8 Other specified conduction disorders**
426.81 Lown-Ganong-Levine syndrome
Syndrome of short P-R interval, normal QRS complexes, and supraventricular tachycardias
426.89 Other
Dissociation:
atrioventricular [AV]
interference
isorhythmic
Nonparoxysmal AV nodal tachycardia
426.9 Conduction disorder, unspecified
Heart block NOS
Stokes-Adams syndrome

√4ᵗʰ **427 Cardiac dysrhythmias**
EXCLUDES   that complicating:
abortion (634-638 with .7, 639.8)
ectopic or molar pregnancy (639.8)
labor or delivery (668.1, 669.4)
DEF: Disruption or disturbance in the rhythm of heartbeats.

427.0 Paroxysmal supraventricular tachycardia
Paroxysmal tachycardia: Paroxysmal tachycardia:
atrial [PAT]   junctional
atrioventricular [AV]   nodal
DEF: Rapid atrial rhythm.
427.1 Paroxysmal ventricular tachycardia
Ventricular tachycardia (paroxysmal)
DEF: Rapid ventricular rhythm.
427.2 Paroxysmal tachycardia, unspecified
Bouveret-Hoffmann syndrome
Paroxysmal tachycardia:
NOS
essential
√5ᵗʰ **427.3 Atrial fibrillation and flutter**
427.31 Atrial fibrillation
DEF: Irregular, rapid atrial contractions.
427.32 Atrial flutter
DEF: Regular, rapid atrial contractions.
√5ᵗʰ **427.4 Ventricular fibrillation and flutter**
427.41 Ventricular fibrillation
DEF: Irregular, rapid ventricular contractions.
427.42 Ventricular flutter
DEF: Regular, rapid, ventricular contractions.
427.5 Cardiac arrest
Cardiorespiratory arrest
√5ᵗʰ **427.6 Premature beats**
427.60 Premature beats, unspecified
Ectopic beats   Premature contractions
Extrasystoles   or systoles NOS
Extrasystolic arrhythmia
427.61 Supraventricular premature beats
Atrial premature beats, contractions, or systoles
427.69 Other
Ventricular premature beats, contractions, or systoles
√5ᵗʰ **427.8 Other specified cardiac dysrhythmias**
427.81 Sinoatrial node dysfunction
Sinus bradycardia:
persistent
severe
Syndrome:
sick sinus
tachycardia-bradycardia
EXCLUDES   sinus bradycardia NOS (427.89)
DEF: Complex cardiac arrhythmia; appears as severe sinus bradycardia, sinus bradycardia with tachycardia, or sinus bradycardia with atrioventricular block.

427.89 Other

Rhythm disorder: Rhythm disorder:
   coronary sinus   nodal
   ectopic   Wandering (atrial)
       pacemaker

EXCLUDES   *carotid sinus syncope (337.0)*
▶*neonatal bradycardia*
  (779.81)◀
▶*neonatal tachycardia*
  (779.82)◀
reflex bradycardia (337.0)
tachycardia NOS (785.0)

427.9 Cardiac dysrhythmia, unspecified
Arrhythmia (cardiac) NOS

✓4th 428 Heart failure

EXCLUDES   *following cardiac surgery (429.4)*
rheumatic (398.91)
that complicating:
  abortion (634-638 with .7, 639.8)
  ectopic or molar pregnancy (639.8)
  labor or delivery (668.1, 669.4)
▶Code, if applicable, heart failure due to hypertension first (402.0-402.9, with fifth-digit 1 or 404.0-404.9 with fifth-digit 1 or 3)◀

▲ **428.0 Congestive heart failure, unspecified**
Congestive heart disease
Right heart failure (secondary to left heart failure)
EXCLUDES ▶*fluid overload NOS (276.6)*◀

DEF: Mechanical inadequacy; caused by inability of heart to pump and circulate blood; results in fluid collection in lungs, hypertension, congestion and edema of tissue.

428.1 Left heart failure
Acute edema of lung ⎫
Acute pulmonary   ⎬ with heart disease NOS
   edema   ⎭ or heart failure

Cardiac asthma
Left ventricular failure

DEF: Mechanical inadequacy of left ventricle; causing fluid in lungs.

● **✓5th 428.2 Systolic heart failure**
EXCLUDES   *combined systolic and diastolic heart failure (428.40-428.43)*

●   **428.20 Unspecified**
●   **428.21 Acute**
●   **428.22 Chronic**
●   **428.23 Acute on chronic**
● **✓5th 428.3 Diastolic heart failure**
EXCLUDES   *combined systolic and diastolic heart failure (428.40-428.43)*

●   **428.30 Unspecified**
●   **428.31 Acute**
●   **428.32 Chronic**
●   **428.33 Acute on chronic**
● **✓5th 428.4 Combined systolic and diastolic heart failure**
●   **428.40 Unspecified**
●   **428.41 Acute**
●   **428.42 Chronic**
●   **428.43 Acute on chronic**
   428.9 Heart failure, unspecified
Cardiac failure NOS   Myocardial failure NOS
Heart failure NOS   Weak heart

✓4th 429 Ill-defined descriptions and complications of heart disease

429.0 Myocarditis, unspecified
Myocarditis: ⎫
  NOS   ⎪
  chronic (interstitial) ⎬ (with mention of
  fibroid   ⎪   arteriosclerosis)
  senile   ⎭

Use additional code to identify presence of arteriosclerosis
EXCLUDES   *acute or subacute (422.0-422.9)*
rheumatic (398.0)
  acute (391.2)
that due to hypertension (402.0-402.9)

429.1 Myocardial degeneration
Degeneration of heart or ⎫
  myocardium: ⎪
  fatty   ⎪
  mural   ⎬ (with mention of
  muscular   ⎪   arteriosclerosis)
Myocardial: ⎪
  degeneration   ⎪
  disease   ⎭

Use additional code to identify presence of arteriosclerosis
EXCLUDES   *that due to hypertension (402.0-402.9)*

429.2 Cardiovascular disease, unspecified
Arteriosclerotic cardiovascular disease [ASCVD]
Cardiovascular arteriosclerosis
Cardiovascular: ⎫
  degeneration   ⎬ (with mention of
  disease   ⎪   arteriosclerosis)
  sclerosis   ⎭

Use additional code to identify presence of arteriosclerosis
EXCLUDES   *that due to hypertension (402.0-402.9)*

429.3 Cardiomegaly
Cardiac: Ventricular dilatation
  dilatation
  hypertrophy
EXCLUDES   *that due to hypertension (402.0-402.9)*

429.4 Functional disturbances following cardiac surgery
Cardiac insufficiency ⎫ following cardiac surgery
Heart failure   ⎬   or due to prosthesis

Postcardiotomy syndrome
Postvalvulotomy syndrome
EXCLUDES   *cardiac failure in the immediate postoperative period (997.1)*

429.5 Rupture of chordae tendineae
DEF: Torn tissue, between heart valves and papillary muscles.

429.6 Rupture of papillary muscle
DEF: Torn muscle, between chordae tendineae and heart wall.

✓5th 429.7 Certain sequelae of myocardial infarction, not elsewhere classified
Use additional code to identify the associated myocardial infarction:
   with onset of 8 weeks or less (410.00-410.92)
   with onset of more than 8 weeks (414.8)
EXCLUDES   *congenital defects of heart (745, 746)*
coronary aneurysm (414.11)
disorders of papillary muscle (429.6, 429.81)
postmyocardial infarction syndrome (411.0)
rupture of chordae tendineae (429.5)

429.71 Acquired cardiac septal defect
EXCLUDES   *acute septal infarction (410.00-410.92)*

DEF: Abnormal communication, between opposite heart chambers; due to defect of septum; not present at birth.

✓4th / **✓5th** Additional Digit Required   Unspecified Code   Other Specified Code   Manifestation Code   ▶◀ Revised Text   ● New Code   ▲ Revised Code Title

Circulatory System 429.79–435.1

429.79 Other
Mural thrombus (atrial) (ventricular), acquired, following myocardial infarction

✓5ᵗʰ 429.8 Other ill-defined heart diseases

429.81 Other disorders of papillary muscle
Papillary muscle: Papillary muscle:
   atrophy   incompetence
   degeneration   incoordination
   dysfunction   scarring

429.82 Hyperkinetic heart disease
DEF: Condition of unknown origin in young adults; marked by increased cardiac output at rest, increased rate of ventricular ejection; may lead to heart failure.

429.89 Other
Carditis
> **EXCLUDES**   *that due to hypertension (402.0-402.9)*

429.9 Heart disease, unspecified
Heart disease (organic) NOS   Morbus cordis NOS
> **EXCLUDES**   *that due to hypertension (402.0-402.9)*

CEREBROVASCULAR DISEASE (430-438)
> **INCLUDES**   with mention of hypertension (conditions classifiable to 401-405)

Use additional code to identify presence of hypertension
> **EXCLUDES**   *any condition classifiable to 430-434, 436, 437 occurring during pregnancy, childbirth, or the puerperium, or specified as puerperal (674.0)*
> ▶*iatrogenic cerebrovascular infarction or hemorrhage (997.02)*◀

430 Subarachnoid hemorrhage
Meningeal hemorrhage
Ruptured:
   berry aneurysm
   (congenital) cerebral aneurysm NOS
> **EXCLUDES**   *syphilitic ruptured cerebral aneurysm (094.87)*

DEF: Bleeding in space between brain and lining.

431 Intracerebral hemorrhage
Hemorrhage (of):   Hemorrhage (of):
   basilar   internal capsule
   bulbar   intrapontine
   cerebellar   pontine
   cerebral   subcortical
   cerebromeningeal   ventricular
   cortical   Rupture of blood vessel in brain

DEF: Bleeding within the brain.

✓4ᵗʰ 432 Other and unspecified intracranial hemorrhage

432.0 Nontraumatic extradural hemorrhage
Nontraumatic epidural hemorrhage
DEF: Bleeding, nontraumatic, between skull and brain lining.

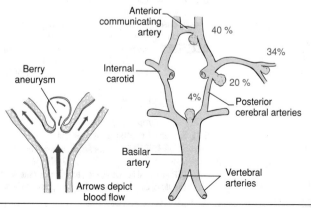

Berry Aneurysm

Anterior communicating artery — 40 %

34%

Internal carotid — 20 %

4%

Berry aneurysm

Posterior cerebral arteries

Basilar artery

Vertebral arteries

Arrows depict blood flow

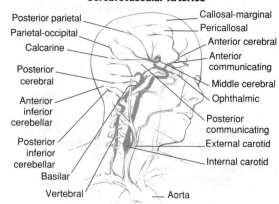

Cerebrovascular Arteries

Posterior parietal
Parietal-occipital
Calcarine
Posterior cerebral
Anterior inferior cerebellar
Posterior inferior cerebellar
Basilar
Vertebral

Callosal-marginal
Pericallosal
Anterior cerebral
Anterior communicating
Middle cerebral
Ophthalmic
Posterior communicating
External carotid
Internal carotid
Aorta

432.1 Subdural hemorrhage
Subdural hematoma, nontraumatic
DEF: Bleeding, between outermost and other layers of brain lining.

432.9 Unspecified intracranial hemorrhage
Intracranial hemorrhage NOS

✓4ᵗʰ 433 Occlusion and stenosis of precerebral arteries
> **INCLUDES**   embolism
> narrowing   } of basilar, carotid, and
> obstruction   vertebral arteries
> thrombosis

> **EXCLUDES**   *insufficiency NOS of precerebral arteries (435.0-435.9)*

DEF: Blockage, stricture, arteries branching into brain.

The following fifth-digit subclassification is for use with category 433:
   0   without mention of cerebral infarction
   1   with cerebral infarction

✓5ᵗʰ	**433.0**	**Basilar artery**
✓5ᵗʰ	**433.1**	**Carotid artery**
✓5ᵗʰ	**433.2**	**Vertebral artery**
✓5ᵗʰ	**433.3**	**Multiple and bilateral**
✓5ᵗʰ	**433.8**	**Other specified precerebral artery**
✓5ᵗʰ	**433.9**	**Unspecified precerebral artery**

Precerebral artery NOS

✓4ᵗʰ 434 Occlusion of cerebral arteries
The following fifth-digit subclassification is for use with category 434:
   0   without mention of cerebral infarction
   1   with cerebral infarction

✓5ᵗʰ	**434.0**	**Cerebral thrombosis**	A
		Thrombosis of cerebral arteries	
✓5ᵗʰ	**434.1**	**Cerebral embolism**	A
✓5ᵗʰ	**434.9**	**Cerebral artery occlusion, unspecified**	A

✓4ᵗʰ 435 Transient cerebral ischemia
> **INCLUDES**   cerebrovascular insufficiency (acute) with transient focal neurological signs and symptoms
> insufficiency of basilar, carotid, and vertebral arteries
> spasm of cerebral arteries

> **EXCLUDES**   *acute cerebrovascular insufficiency NOS (437.1)*
> *that due to any condition classifiable to 433 (433.0-433.9)*

DEF: Temporary restriction of blood flow, to arteries branching into brain.

435.0 Basilar artery syndrome
435.1 Vertebral artery syndrome

N	Newborn Age: 0	P	Pediatric Age: 0-17	M	Maternity Age: 12-55	A	Adult Age: 15-124	MSP	Medicare Secondary Payer

435.2 Subclavian steal syndrome

DEF: Cerebrovascular insufficiency, due to occluded subclavian artery; symptoms include pain in mastoid and posterior head regions, flaccid paralysis of arm and diminished or absent radical pulse on affected side.

435.3 Vertebrobasilar artery syndrome

DEF: Transient ischemic attack; due to brainstem dysfunction; symptoms include confusion, vertigo, binocular blindness, diplopia, unilateral or bilateral weakness and paresthesis of extremities.

435.8 Other specified transient cerebral ischemias   A

435.9 Unspecified transient cerebral ischemia   A

    Impending cerebrovascular accident
    Intermittent cerebral ischemia
    Transient ischemic attack [TIA]

436 Acute, but ill-defined, cerebrovascular disease   A

    Apoplexy, apoplectic: Cerebral seizure
        NOS   Cerebrovascular accident
        attack   [CVA] NOS
        cerebral   Stroke
        seizure

        EXCLUDES   *any condition classifiable to categories 430-435*
               ▶*postoperative cerebrovascular accident*
                   (997.02)◀

√4ᵗʰ **437 Other and ill-defined cerebrovascular disease**

437.0 Cerebral atherosclerosis   A

    Atheroma of cerebral arteries
    Cerebral arteriosclerosis

437.1 Other generalized ischemic cerebrovascular disease

    Acute cerebrovascular insufficiency NOS
    Cerebral ischemia (chronic)

437.2 Hypertensive encephalopathy

DEF: Cerebral manifestations (such as visual disturbances and headache) due to high blood pressure.

437.3 Cerebral aneurysm, nonruptured

    Internal carotid artery, intracranial portion
    Internal carotid artery NOS

        EXCLUDES   *congenital cerebral aneurysm,*
                   nonruptured (747.81)
                internal carotid artery, extracranial
                   portion (442.81)

437.4 Cerebral arteritis

DEF: Inflammation of a cerebral artery or arteries.

437.5 Moyamoya disease

DEF: Cerebrovascular ischemia; vessels occlude and rupture causing tiny hemorrhages at base of brain; predominantly affects Japanese.

437.6 Nonpyogenic thrombosis of intracranial venous sinus

        EXCLUDES   *pyogenic (325)*

437.7 Transient global amnesia

DEF: Episode of short-term memory loss, not often recurrent; pathogenesis unknown; with no signs or symptoms of neurological disorder.

437.8 Other

437.9 Unspecified

    Cerebrovascular disease or lesion NOS

√4ᵗʰ **438 Late effects of cerebrovascular disease**

    Note: This category is to be used to indicate conditions in 430-437 as the cause of late effects. The "late effects" include conditions specified as such, as sequelae, which may occur at any time after the onset of the causal condition.

438.0 Cognitive deficits

√5ᵗʰ **438.1 Speech and language deficits**

    438.10 Speech and language deficit, unspecified

438.11 Aphasia

DEF: Impairment or absence of the ability to communicate by speech, writing or signs or to comprehend the spoken or written language due to disease or injury to the brain. Total aphasia is the loss of function of both sensory and motor areas of the brain.

438.12 Dysphasia

DEF: Impaired speech; marked by inability to sequence language.

438.19 Other speech and language deficits

√5ᵗʰ **438.2 Hemiplegia/hemiparesis**

DEF: Paralysis of one side of the body.

    438.20 Hemiplegia affecting unspecified side
    438.21 Hemiplegia affecting dominant side
    438.22 Hemiplegia affecting nondominant side

√5ᵗʰ **438.3 Monoplegia of upper limb**

DEF: Paralysis of one limb or one muscle group.

    438.30 Monoplegia of upper limb affecting unspecified side
    438.31 Monoplegia of upper limb affecting dominant side
    438.32 Monoplegia of upper limb affecing nondominant side

√5ᵗʰ **438.4 Monoplegia of lower limb**

    438.40 Monoplegia of lower limb affecting unspecified side
    438.41 Monoplegia of lower limb affecting dominant side
    438.42 Monoplegia of lower limb affecting nondominant side

√5ᵗʰ **438.5 Other paralytic syndrome**

    Use additional code to identify type of paralytic syndrome, such as:
        locked-in state (344.81)
        quadriplegia (344.00-344.09)

        EXCLUDES   *late effects of cerebrovascular accident*
                   with:
                hemiplegia/hemiparesis (438.20-
                   438.22)
                monoplegia of lower limb (438.40-
                   438.42)
                monoplegia of upper limb (438.30-
                   438.32)

    438.50 Other paralytic syndrome affecting unspecified side
    438.51 Other paralytic syndrome affecting dominant side
    438.52 Other paralytic syndrome affecting nondominant side
    438.53 Other paralytic syndrome, bilateral

● **438.6 Alterations of sensations**

    Use additional code to identify the altered sensation

● **438.7 Disturbances of vision**

    Use additional code to identify the visual disturbance

√5ᵗʰ **438.8 Other late effects of cerebrovascular disease**

438.81 Apraxia

DEF: Inability to activate learned movements; no known sensory or motor impairment.

438.82 Dysphagia

DEF: Inability or difficulty in swallowing.

● **438.83 Facial weakness**

    Facial droop

● **438.84 Ataxia**

● **438.85 Vertigo**

√4ᵗʰ
√5ᵗʰ Additional Digit Required   Unspecified Code   Other Specified Code   Manifestation Code   ▶◀ Revised Text   ● New Code   ▲ Revised Code Title

Map of Major Arteries

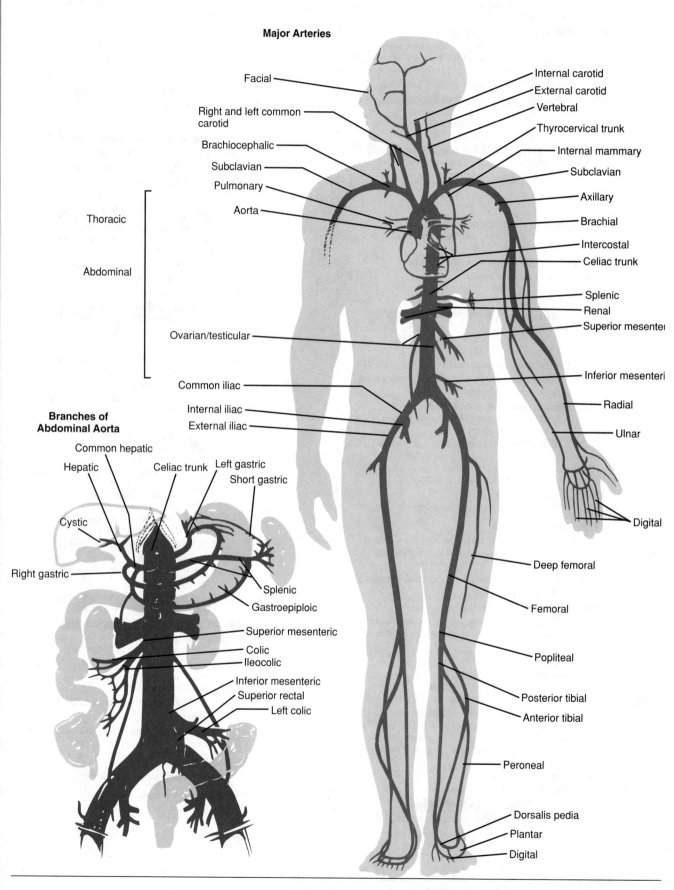

Major Arteries

Facial

Internal carotid

External carotid

Vertebral

Right and left common carotid

Thyrocervical trunk

Brachiocephalic

Internal mammary

Subclavian

Subclavian

Pulmonary

Axillary

Aorta

Brachial

Thoracic

Intercostal

Celiac trunk

Abdominal

Splenic

Renal

Superior mesenter

Ovarian/testicular

Inferior mesenteri

Common iliac

Radial

Branches of Abdominal Aorta

Internal iliac

External iliac

Ulnar

Common hepatic

Hepatic

Celiac trunk

Left gastric

Short gastric

Digital

Cystic

Right gastric

Splenic

Gastroepiploic

Deep femoral

Superior mesenteric

Femoral

Colic

Ileocolic

Popliteal

Inferior mesenteric

Superior rectal

Left colic

Posterior tibial

Anterior tibial

Peroneal

Dorsalis pedia

Plantar

Digital

Circulatory System

N Newborn Age: 0   P Pediatric Age: 0-17   M Maternity Age: 12-55   A Adult Age: 15-124   MSP Medicare Secondary Payer

438.89 Other late effects of cerebrovascular disease

Use additional code to identify the late effect

438.9 Unspecified late effects of cerebrovascular disease

DISEASES OF ARTERIES, ARTERIOLES, AND CAPILLARIES (440-448)

√4ᵗʰ **440** Atherosclerosis

INCLUDES arteriolosclerosis
arteriosclerosis (obliterans) (senile)
arteriosclerotic vascular disease
atheroma
degeneration:
  arterial
  arteriovascular
  vascular
endarteritis deformans or obliterans
senile:
  arteritis
  endarteritis

EXCLUDES ►atheroembolism (445.01-445.89)◄
atherosclerosis of bypass graft of the extremities (403.30-403.32)

DEF: Stricture and reduced elasticity of an artery; due to plaque deposits.

440.0 Of aorta ⒜

440.1 Of renal artery ⒜

EXCLUDES atherosclerosis of renal arterioles (403.00-403.91)

√5ᵗʰ **440.2** Of native arteries of the extremities

EXCLUDES atherosclerosis of bypass graft of the extremities (440.30-440.32)

440.20 Atherosclerosis of the extremities, unspecified ⒜

440.21 Atherosclerosis of the extremities with intermittent claudication ⒜

DEF: Atherosclerosis; marked by pain, tension and weakness after walking; no symptoms while at rest.

440.22 Atherosclerosis of the extremities with rest pain ⒜

INCLUDES any condition classifiable to 440.21

DEF: Atherosclerosis, marked by pain, tension and weakness while at rest.

440.23 Atherosclerosis of the extremities with ulceration ⒜

Use additional code for any associated ulceration (707.10-707.9)

INCLUDES any condition classifiable to 440.21 and 440.22

440.24 Atherosclerosis of the extremities with gangrene ⒜

INCLUDES any condition classifiable to 440.21, 440.22, and 440.23 with ischemic gangrene 785.4

EXCLUDES gas gangrene (040.0)

440.29 Other ⒜

√5ᵗʰ **440.3** Of bypass graft of extremities

EXCLUDES atherosclerosis of native arteries of the extremities (440.21-440.24)
embolism [occlusion NOS] [thrombus] of graft (996.74)

440.30 Of unspecified graft ⒜

440.31 Of autologous vein bypass graft ⒜

440.32 Of nonautologous biological bypass graft ⒜

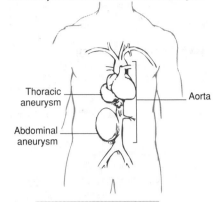

Thoracic, Abdominal and Aortic Aneurysm

Thoracic aneurysm

Aorta

Abdominal aneurysm

440.8 Of other specified arteries ⒜

EXCLUDES basilar (433.0)
carotid (433.1)
cerebral (437.0)
coronary ►(414.00-414.06)◄
mesenteric (557.1)
precerebral (433.0-433.9)
pulmonary (416.0)
vertebral (433.2)

440.9 Generalized and unspecified atherosclerosis ⒜

Arteriosclerotic vascular disease NOS

EXCLUDES arteriosclerotic cardiovascular disease [ASCVD] (429.2)

√4ᵗʰ **441** Aortic aneurysm and dissection

EXCLUDES syphilitic aortic aneurysm (093.0)
traumatic aortic aneurysm (901.0, 902.0)

√5ᵗʰ **441.0** Dissection of aorta

DEF: Dissection or splitting of wall of the aorta; due to blood entering through intimal tear or interstitial hemorrhage.

441.00 Unspecified site ⒜

441.01 Thoracic ⒜

441.02 Abdominal ⒜

441.03 Thoracoabdominal ⒜

441.1 Thoracic aneurysm, ruptured ⒜

441.2 Thoracic aneurysm without mention of rupture ⒜

441.3 Abdominal aneurysm, ruptured ⒜

441.4 Abdominal aneurysm without mention of rupture ⒜

441.5 Aortic aneurysm of unspecified site, ruptured ⒜

Rupture of aorta NOS

441.6 Thoracoabdominal aneurysm, ruptured ⒜

441.7 Thoracoabdominal aneurysm, without mention of rupture ⒜

441.9 Aortic aneurysm of unspecified site without mention of rupture ⒜

Aneurysm
Dilatation   } of aorta
Hyaline necrosis

√4ᵗʰ **442** Other aneurysm

INCLUDES aneurysm (ruptured) (cirsoid) (false) (varicose) aneurysmal varix

EXCLUDES arteriovenous aneurysm or fistula:
acquired (447.0)
congenital (747.60-747.69)
traumatic (900.0-904.9)

DEF: Dissection or splitting of arterial wall; due to blood entering through intimal tear or interstitial hemorrhage.

442.0 Of artery of upper extremity ⒜

442.1 Of renal artery ⒜

442.2 Of iliac artery ⒜

√4ᵗʰ
√5ᵗʰ Additional Digit Required   Unspecified Code   Other Specified Code   Manifestation Code   ►◄ Revised Text   ● New Code   ▲ Revised Code Title

2003 ICD•9•CM

October 2002 • Volume 1 — 119

Circulatory System 438.89–442.2

Circulatory System 442.3–444.9

442.3   Of artery of lower extremity   A

Aneurysm:

femoral
popliteal }   artery

✓5ᵗʰ   **442.8   Of other specified artery**

442.81   Artery of neck   A

Aneurysm of carotid artery (common)
(external) (internal, extracranial
portion)

EXCLUDES   *internal carotid artery,
intracranial portion
(437.3)*

442.82   Subclavian artery   A

442.83   Splenic artery   A

442.84   Other visceral artery   A

Aneurysm:

celiac
gastroduodenal
gastroepiploic
hepatic }   artery
pancreaticoduodenal
superior mesenteric

442.89   Other   A

Aneurysm:

mediastinal
spinal }   artery

EXCLUDES   *cerebral (nonruptured) (437.3)
congenital (747.81)
ruptured (430)
coronary (414.11)
heart (414.10)
pulmonary (417.1)*

442.9   Of unspecified site   A

✓4ᵗʰ   **443   Other peripheral vascular disease**

443.0   Raynaud's syndrome

Raynaud's:

disease
phenomenon (secondary)

Use additional code to identify gangrene (785.4)

DEF: Constriction of the arteries, due to cold or stress; bilateral
ischemic attacks of fingers, toes, nose or ears; symptoms include
pallor, paresthesia and pain; more common in females.

443.1   Thromboangiitis obliterans [Buerger's disease]

Presenile gangrene

DEF: Inflammatory disease of extremity blood vessels, mainly the
lower; occurs primarily in young men and leads to tissue ischemia
and gangrene.

●   ✓5ᵗʰ   **443.2   Other arterial dissection**

EXCLUDES   *dissection of aorta (441.00-441.03)
dissection of coronary arteries (414.12)*

●   **443.21   Dissection of carotid artery**

●   **443.22   Dissection of iliac artery**

●   **443.23   Dissection of renal artery**

●   **443.24   Dissection of vertebral artery**

●   **443.29   Dissection of other artery**

✓5ᵗʰ   **443.8   Other specified peripheral vascular diseases**

**443.81   *Peripheral angiopathy in diseases
classified elsewhere***

Code first underlying disease, as:
diabetes mellitus (250.7)

443.89   Other

Acrocyanosis   Erythrocyanosis
Acroparesthesia: Erythromelalgia
   simple [Schultze's type]
   vasomotor [Nothnagel's type]

EXCLUDES   *chilblains (991.5)
frostbite (991.0-991.3)
immersion foot (991.4)*

Arterial Diseases and Disorders

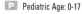

443.9   **Peripheral vascular disease, unspecified**

Intermittent claudication NOS
Peripheral:
   angiopathy NOS
   vascular disease NOS
Spasm of artery

EXCLUDES   *atherosclerosis of the arteries of the
extremities (440.20-440.22)
spasm of cerebral artery (435.0-435.9)*

✓4ᵗʰ   **444   Arterial embolism and thrombosis**

INCLUDES   infarction:
   embolic
   thrombotic
   occlusion

EXCLUDES   ▶*atheroembolism (445.01-445.89)*◀
*that complicating:
   abortion (634-638 with .6, 639.6)
   ectopic or molar pregnancy (639.6)
   pregnancy, childbirth, or the pueperium
     (673.0-673.8)*

444.0   Of abdominal aorta

Aortic bifurcation syndrome
Aortoiliac obstruction
Leriche's syndrome
Saddle embolus

444.1   Of thoracic aorta

Embolism or thrombosis of aorta (thoracic)

✓5ᵗʰ   **444.2   Of arteries of the extremities**

444.21   Upper extremity

444.22   Lower extremity

Arterial embolism or thrombosis:
   femoral
   peripheral NOS
   popliteal

EXCLUDES   *iliofemoral (444.81)*

✓5ᵗʰ   **444.8   Of other specified artery**

444.81   Iliac artery

444.89   Other

EXCLUDES   *basilar (433.0)
carotid (433.1)
cerebral (434.0-434.9)
coronary (410.00-410.92)
mesenteric (557.0)
ophthalmic (362.30-362.34)
precerebral (433.0-433.9)
pulmonary (415.19)
renal (593.81)
retinal (362.30-362.34)
vertebral (433.2)*

444.9   Of unspecified artery

| N | Newborn Age: 0 | P | Pediatric Age: 0-17 | M | Maternity Age: 12-55 | A | Adult Age: 15-124 | MSP | Medicare Secondary Payer |

● ✓4ᵗʰ **445 Atheroembolism**

       INCLUDES   atherothrombotic microembolism
                      cholesterol embolism

●   ✓5ᵗʰ **445.0   Of extremities**

●   **445.01 Upper extremity**

●   **445.02 Lower extremity**

●   ✓5ᵗʰ **445.8   Of other sites**

●   **445.81 Kidney**

                Use additional code for any associated
                kidney failure (584, 585)

●   **445.89 Other site**

✓4ᵗʰ **446 Polyarteritis nodosa and allied conditions**

       446.0   Polyarteritis nodosa

            Disseminated necrotizing periarteritis
            Necrotizing angiitis
            Panarteritis (nodosa)
            Periarteritis (nodosa)

            DEF: Inflammation of small and mid-size arteries; symptoms related to involved arteries in kidneys, muscles, gastrointestinal tract and heart; results in tissue death.

       446.1   Acute febrile mucocutaneous lymph node syndrome [MCLS]

            Kawasaki disease

            DEF: Acute febrile disease of children; marked by erythema of conjunctiva and mucous membranes of upper respiratory tract, skin eruptions and edema.

   ✓5ᵗʰ **446.2   Hypersensitivity angiitis**

            EXCLUDES   *antiglomerular basement membrane disease without pulmonary hemorrhage (583.89)*

       446.20 Hypersensitivity angiitis, unspecified

       446.21 Goodpasture's syndrome

            Antiglomerular basement membrane antibody-mediated nephritis with pulmonary hemorrhage
            Use additional code to identify renal disease (583.81)

            DEF: Glomerulonephritis associated with hematuria, progresses rapidly; results in death from renal failure.

       446.29 Other specified hypersensitivity angiitis

       446.3   Lethal midline granuloma

            Malignant granuloma of face

            DEF: Granulomatous lesion; in nose or paranasal sinuses; often fatal; occurs chiefly in males.

       446.4   Wegener's granulomatosis

            Necrotizing respiratory granulomatosis
            Wegener's syndrome

            DEF: A disease occurring mainly in men; marked by necrotizing granulomas and ulceration of the upper respiratory tract; underlying condition is a vasculitis affecting small vessels and is possibly due to an immune disorder.

       446.5   Giant cell arteritis

            Cranial arteritis   Temporal arteritis
            Horton's disease

            DEF: Inflammation of arteries; due to giant cells affecting carotid artery branches, resulting in occlusion; symptoms include fever, headache and neurological problems; occurs in elderly.

       446.6   Thrombotic microangiopathy

            Moschcowitz's syndrome
            Thrombotic thrombocytopenic purpura

            DEF: Blockage of small blood vessels; due to hyaline deposits; symptoms include purpura, CNS disorders; results in protracted disease or rapid death.

       446.7   Takayasu's disease

            Aortic arch arteritis
            Pulseless disease

            DEF: Progressive obliterative arteritis of brachiocephalic trunk, left subclavian, and left common carotid arteries above aortic arch; results in ischemia in brain, heart and arm; pulses impalpable in head, neck and arms; more common in young adult females.

✓4ᵗʰ **447 Other disorders of arteries and arterioles**

       447.0   Arteriovenous fistula, acquired

            Arteriovenous aneurysm, acquired

            EXCLUDES   *cerebrovascular (437.3)*
                          coronary (414.19)
                          pulmonary (417.0)
                          surgically created arteriovenous shunt or fistula:
                             complication (996.1, 996.61-996.62)
                             status or presence (V45.1)
                          traumatic (900.0-904.9)

            DEF: Communication between an artery and vein caused by error in healing.

       447.1   Stricture of artery

       447.2   Rupture of artery

            Erosion
            Fistula, except arteriovenous   } of artery
            Ulcer

            EXCLUDES   *traumatic rupture of artery (900.0-904.9)*

       447.3   Hyperplasia of renal artery

            Fibromuscular hyperplasia of renal artery

            DEF: Overgrowth of cells in muscular lining of renal artery.

       447.4   Celiac artery compression syndrome

            Celiac axis syndrome
            Marable's syndrome

       447.5   Necrosis of artery

       447.6   Arteritis, unspecified

            Aortitis NOS   Endarteritis NOS

            EXCLUDES   *arteritis, endarteritis:*
                          aortic arch (446.7)
                          cerebral (437.4)
                          coronary ▶(414.00-414.06)◀
                          deformans (440.0-440.9)
                          obliterans (440.0-440.9)
                          pulmonary (417.8)
                          senile (440.0-440.9)
                          polyarteritis NOS (446.0)
                          syphilitic aortitis (093.1)

       447.8   Other specified disorders of arteries and arterioles

            Fibromuscular hyperplasia of arteries, except renal

       447.9   Unspecified disorders of arteries and arterioles

✓4ᵗʰ **448 Disease of capillaries**

       448.0   Hereditary hemorrhagic telangiectasia

            Rendu-Osler-Weber disease

            DEF: Genetic disease with onset after puberty; results in multiple telangiectases, dilated venules on skin and mucous membranes; recurrent bleeding may occur.

       448.1   Nevus, non-neoplastic

            Nevus: Nevus:
               araneus   spider
               senile   stellar

            EXCLUDES   *neoplastic (216.0-216.9)*
                          port wine (757.32)
                          strawberry (757.32)

            DEF: Enlarged or malformed blood vessels of skin; results in reddish swelling, skin patch, or birthmark.

Circulatory System 445–448.1

✓4ᵗʰ / ✓5ᵗʰ   Additional Digit Required   Unspecified Code   Other Specified Code   Manifestation Code   ▶◄ Revised Text   ● New Code   ▲ Revised Code Title

Map of Major Veins

2003 ICD•9•CM

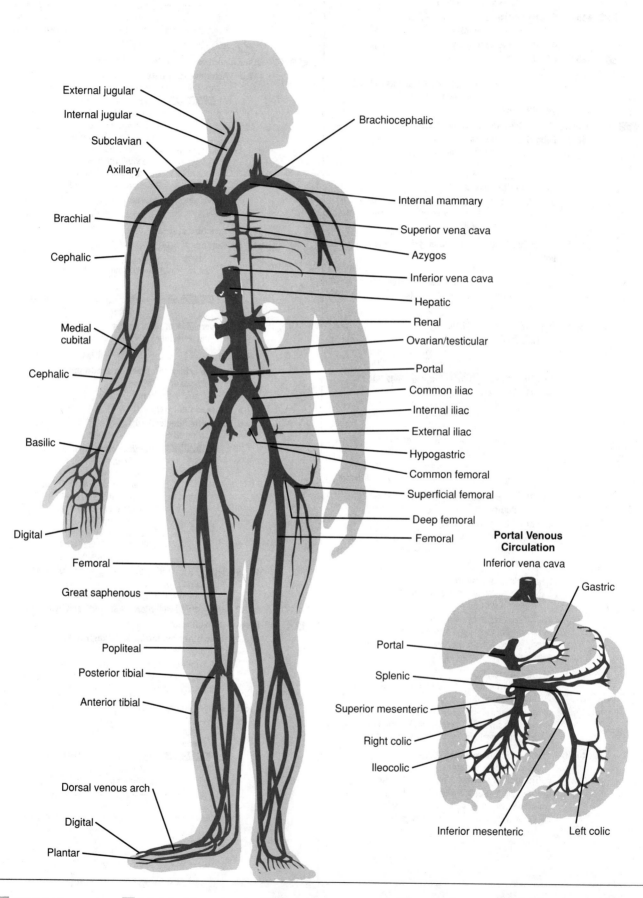

Portal Venous Circulation

Circulatory System

448.9 Other and unspecified capillary diseases
Capillary: Capillary:
hemorrhage   thrombosis
hyperpermeability
EXCLUDES capillary fragility (hereditary) (287.8)

DISEASES OF VEINS AND LYMPHATICS, AND OTHER DISEASES OF CIRCULATORY SYSTEM (451-459)

√4th **451 Phlebitis and thrombophlebitis**
INCLUDES endophlebitis
inflammation, vein
periphlebitis
suppurative phlebitis
Use additional E code to identify drug, if drug-induced
EXCLUDES that complicating:
abortion (634-638 with .7, 639.8)
ectopic or molar pregnancy (639.8)
pregnancy, childbirth, or the puerperium
(671.0-671.9)
that due to or following:
implant or catheter device (996.61-996.62)
infusion, perfusion, or transfusion (999.2)

DEF: Inflammation of a vein (phlebitis) with formation of a thrombus (thrombophlebitis).

451.0 Of superficial vessels of lower extremities
Saphenous vein (greater) (lesser)
√5th **451.1 Of deep vessels of lower extremities**
451.11 Femoral vein (deep) (superficial)
451.19 Other
Femoropopliteal vein   Tibial vein
Popliteal vein
451.2 Of lower extremities, unspecified
√5th **451.8 Of other sites**
EXCLUDES intracranial venous sinus (325)
nonpyogenic (437.6)
portal (vein) (572.1)
451.81 Iliac vein
451.82 Of superficial veins of upper extremities
Antecubital vein   Cephalic vein
Basilic vein
451.83 Of deep veins of upper extremities
Brachial vein   Ulnar vein
Radial vein
451.84 Of upper extremities, unspecified
451.89 Other
Axillary vein   Thrombophlebitis of
Jugular vein   breast (Mondor's
Subclavian vein   disease)
451.9 Of unspecified site
452 Portal vein thrombosis
Portal (vein) obstruction
EXCLUDES hepatic vein thrombosis (453.0)
phlebitis of portal vein (572.1)
DEF: Formation of a blood clot in main vein of liver.

√4th **453 Other venous embolism and thrombosis**
EXCLUDES that complicating:
abortion (634-638 with .7, 639.8)
ectopic or molar pregnancy (639.8)
pregnancy, childbirth, or the puerperium
(671.0-671.9)
that with inflammation, phlebitis, and
thrombophlebitis (451.0-451.9)
453.0 Budd-Chiari syndrome
Hepatic vein thrombosis
DEF: Thrombosis or other obstruction of hepatic vein; symptoms include enlarged liver, extensive collateral vessels, intractable ascites and severe portal hypertension.

453.1 Thrombophlebitis migrans
DEF: Slow, advancing thrombophlebitis; appearing first in one vein then another.
453.2 Of vena cava
453.3 Of renal vein
453.8 Of other specified veins
EXCLUDES cerebral (434.0-434.9)
coronary (410.00-410.92)
intracranial venous sinus (325)
nonpyogenic (437.6)
mesenteric (557.0)
portal (452)
precerebral (433.0-433.9)
pulmonary (415.19)
453.9 Of unspecified site
Embolism of vein   Thrombosis (vein)
√4th **454 Varicose veins of lower extremities**
EXCLUDES that complicating pregnancy, childbirth, or the puerperium (671.0)
DEF: Dilated leg veins; due to incompetent vein valves that allow reversed blood flow and cause tissue erosion or weakness of wall; may be painful.

454.0 With ulcer   A
Varicose ulcer (lower extremity, any part)
Varicose veins with ulcer of lower extremity [any part] or of unspecified site
Any condition classifiable to 454.9 with ulcer or specified as ulcerated
454.1 With inflammation   A
Stasis dermatitis
Varicose veins with inflammation of lower extremity [any part] or of unspecified site
Any condition classifiable to 454.9 with inflammation or specified as inflamed
454.2 With ulcer and inflammation   A
Varicose veins with ulcer and inflammation of lower extremity [any part] or of unspecified site
Any condition classifiable to 454.9 with ulcer and inflammation
● **454.8 With other complications**
Edema
Pain
Swelling
▲ **454.9 Asymptomatic varicose veins**   A
Phlebectasia ⎫ of lower extremity [any part]
Varicose veins ⎬ or of unspecified site
Varix   ⎭
►Varicose veins NOS◄
√4th **455 Hemorrhoids**
INCLUDES hemorrhoids (anus) (rectum)
piles
varicose veins, anus or rectum
EXCLUDES that complicating pregnancy, childbirth, or the puerperium (671.8)
DEF: Varicose condition of external hemorrhoidal veins causing painful swellings at the anus.

455.0 Internal hemorrhoids without mention of complication
455.1 Internal thrombosed hemorrhoids
455.2 Internal hemorrhoids with other complication
Internal hemorrhoids: Internal hemorrhoids:
bleeding   strangulated
prolapsed   ulcerated
455.3 External hemorrhoids without mention of complication
455.4 External thrombosed hemorrhoids
455.5 External hemorrhoids with other complication
External hemorrhoids: External hemorrhoids:
bleeding   strangulated
prolapsed   ulcerated

Circulatory System 455.6–459.3

455.6 **Unspecified hemorrhoids without mention of complication**
Hemorrhoids NOS

455.7 **Unspecified thrombosed hemorrhoids**
Thrombosed hemorrhoids, unspecified whether internal or external

455.8 **Unspecified hemorrhoids with other complication**
Hemorrhoids, unspecified whether internal or external:
bleeding
prolapsed
strangulated
ulcerated

455.9 **Residual hemorrhoidal skin tags**
Skin tags, anus or rectum

✓4ᵗʰ **456** **Varicose veins of other sites**

456.0 **Esophageal varices with bleeding**
DEF: Distended, tortuous, veins of lower esophagus, usually due to portal hypertension.

456.1 **Esophageal varices without mention of bleeding**

✓5ᵗʰ **456.2** **Esophageal varices in diseases classified elsewhere**
Code first underlying disease, as:
cirrhosis of liver (571.0-571.9)
portal hypertension (572.3)

456.20 **With bleeding**

456.21 **Without mention of bleeding**

456.3 **Sublingual varices**
DEF: Distended, tortuous veins beneath tongue.

456.4 **Scrotal varices** ♂
Varicocele

456.5 **Pelvic varices**
Varices of broad ligament

456.6 **Vulval varices** ♀
Varices of perineum
EXCLUDES   that complicating pregnancy, childbirth, or the puerperium (671.1)

456.8 **Varices of other sites**
Varicose veins of nasal septum (with ulcer)
EXCLUDES   placental varices (656.7)
retinal varices (362.17)
varicose ulcer of unspecified site (454.0)
varicose veins of unspecified site (454.9)

✓4ᵗʰ **457** **Noninfectious disorders of lymphatic channels**

457.0 **Postmastectomy lymphedema syndrome** [A]
Elephantiasis
Obliteration of lymphatic vessel } due to mastectomy
DEF: Reduced lymphatic circulation following mastectomy; symptoms include swelling of the arm on the operative side.

457.1 **Other lymphedema**
Elephantiasis (nonfilarial) NOS
Lymphangiectasis
Lymphedema: acquired (chronic)
Lymphedema: praecox
secondary
Obliteration, lymphatic vessel
EXCLUDES   elephantiasis (nonfilarial):
congenital (757.0)
eyelid (374.83)
vulva (624.8)
DEF: Fluid retention due to reduced lymphatic circulation; due to other than mastectomy.

457.2 **Lymphangitis**
Lymphangitis: Lymphangitis:
NOS   subacute
chronic
EXCLUDES   acute lymphangitis (682.0-682.9)

457.8 **Other noninfectious disorders of lymphatic channels**
Chylocele (nonfilarial)   Lymph node or vessel:
Chylous: fistula
ascites   infarction
cyst   rupture
EXCLUDES   chylocele:
filarial (125.0-125.9)
tunica vaginalis (nonfilarial) (608.84)

457.9 **Unspecified noninfectious disorder of lymphatic channels**

✓4ᵗʰ **458** **Hypotension**
INCLUDES   hypopiesis
EXCLUDES   cardiovascular collapse (785.50)
maternal hypotension syndrome (669.2)
shock (785.50-785.59)
Shy-Drager syndrome (333.0)

458.0 **Orthostatic hypotension**
Hypotension: Hypotension:
orthostatic (chronic)   postural
DEF: Low blood pressure; occurs when standing.

458.1 **Chronic hypotension**
Permanent idiopathic hypotension
DEF: Persistent low blood pressure.

458.2 **Iatrogenic hypotension**
Postoperative hypotension
DEF: Abnormally low blood pressure; due to medical treatment.

458.8 **Other specified hypotension**

458.9 **Hypotension, unspecified**
Hypotension (arterial) NOS

✓4ᵗʰ **459** **Other disorders of circulatory system**

459.0 **Hemorrhage, unspecified**
Rupture of blood vessel NOS
Spontaneous hemorrhage NEC
EXCLUDES   hemorrhage:
gastrointestinal NOS (578.9)
in newborn NOS (772.9)
secondary or recurrent following trauma (958.2)
traumatic rupture of blood vessel (900.0-904.9)

✓5ᵗʰ **459.1** **Postphlebitic syndrome**
►Chronic venous hypertension due to deep vein thrombosis◄
EXCLUDES   ►chronic venous hypertension without deep vein thrombosis (459.30-459.39)◄
DEF: Various conditions following deep vein thrombosis; including edema, pain, stasis dermatitis, cellulitis, varicose veins and ulceration of the lower leg.

● **459.10** **Postphlebitic syndrome without complications**
Asymptomatic postphlebitic syndrome
Postphlebitic syndrome NOS

● **459.11** **Postphlebitic syndrome with ulcer**
● **459.12** **Postphlebitic syndrome with inflammation**
● **459.13** **Postphlebitic syndrome with ulcer and inflammation**

● **459.19** **Postphlebitic syndrome with other complication**

459.2 **Compression of vein**
Stricture of vein
Vena cava syndrome (inferior) (superior)

● ✓5ᵗʰ **459.3** **Chronic venous hypertension (idiopathic)**
Stasis edema
EXCLUDES   chronic venous hypertension due to deep vein thrombosis (459.10-459.19)
varicose veins (454.0-454.9)

[N] Newborn Age: 0   [P] Pediatric Age: 0-17   [M] Maternity Age: 12-55   [A] Adult Age: 15-124   [MSP] Medicare Secondary Payer

124 — Volume 1 • October 2002   2003 ICD•9•CM

- 459.30 **Chronic venous hypertension without complications**
  Asymptomatic chronic venous hypertension
  Chronic venous hypertension NOS
- 459.31 **Chronic venous hypertension with ulcer**
- 459.32 **Chronic venous hypertension with inflammation**
- 459.33 **Chronic venous hypertension with ulcer and inflammation**
- 459.39 **Chronic venous hypertension with other complication**

√5th 459.8 **Other specified disorders of circulatory system**

459.81 **Venous (peripheral) insufficiency, unspecified**
  Chronic venous insufficiency NOS
  Use additional code for any associated ulceration (707.10-707.9)

  DEF: Insufficient drainage, venous blood, any part of body, results in edema or dermatosis.

459.89 **Other**
  Collateral circulation (venous), any site
  Phlebosclerosis
  Venofibrosis

459.9 **Unspecified circulatory system disorder**

Circulatory System 459.30–459.9

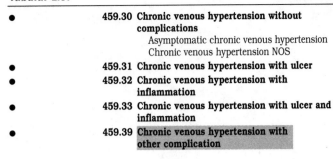
Additional Digit Required   Unspecified Code   Other Specified Code   Manifestation Code   ►◄ Revised Text   ● New Code   ▲ Revised Code Title

2003 ICD•9•CM   October 2002 • Volume 1 — 125

8. DISEASES OF THE RESPIRATORY SYSTEM (460-519)

Use additional code to identify infectious organism

ACUTE RESPIRATORY INFECTIONS (460-466)

> `EXCLUDES` *pneumonia and influenza (480.0-487.8)*

460 Acute nasopharyngitis [common cold]

Coryza (acute)
Nasal catarrh, acute
Nasopharyngitis:
   NOS
   acute

Nasopharyngitis:
   infective NOS
Rhinitis:
   acute
   infective

> `EXCLUDES` *nasopharyngitis, chronic (472.2)*
> *pharyngitis:*
>   *acute or unspecified (462)*
>   *chronic (472.1)*
> *rhinitis:*
>   *allergic (477.0-477.9)*
>   *chronic or unspecified (472.0)*
> *sore throat:*
>   *acute or unspecified (462)*
>   *chronic (472.1)*

DEF: Acute inflammation of mucous membranes; extends from nares to pharynx.

√4ᵗʰ 461 Acute sinusitis

> `INCLUDES` abscess
> empyema
> infection   acute, of sinus (accessory)
> inflammation   (nasal)
> suppuration

> `EXCLUDES` *chronic or unspecified sinusitis (473.0-473.9)*

461.0 Maxillary
   Acute antritis

461.1 Frontal

461.2 Ethmoidal

461.3 Sphenoidal

461.8 Other acute sinusitis
   Acute pansinusitis

461.9 Acute sinusitis, unspecified
   Acute sinusitis NOS

462 Acute pharyngitis

Acute sore throat NOS
Pharyngitis (acute):
   NOS
   gangrenous
   infective
   phlegmonous
   pneumococcal

Pharyngitis (acute):
   staphylococcal
   suppurative
   ulcerative
Sore throat (viral) NOS
Viral pharyngitis

> `EXCLUDES` *abscess:*
>   *peritonsillar [quinsy] (475)*
>   *pharyngeal NOS (478.29)*
>   *retropharyngeal (478.24)*
> *chronic pharyngitis (472.1)*
> *infectious mononucleosis (075)*
> *that specified as (due to):*
>   *Coxsackie (virus) (074.0)*
>   *gonococcus (098.6)*
>   *herpes simplex (054.79)*
>   *influenza (487.1)*
>   *septic (034.0)*
>   *streptococcal (034.0)*

463 Acute tonsillitis

Tonsillitis (acute):
   NOS
   follicular
   gangrenous
   infective
   pneumococcal

Tonsillitis (acute):
   septic
   staphylococcal
   suppurative
   ulcerative
   viral

> `EXCLUDES` *chronic tonsillitis (474.0)*
> *hypertrophy of tonsils (474.1)*
> *peritonsillar abscess [quinsy] (475)*
> *sore throat:*
>   *acute or NOS (462)*
>   *septic (034.0)*
> *streptococcal tonsillitis (034.0)*

√4ᵗʰ 464 Acute laryngitis and tracheitis

> `EXCLUDES` *that associated with influenza (487.1)*
> *that due to Streptococcus (034.0)*

√5ᵗʰ 464.0 Acute laryngitis

Laryngitis (acute):
   NOS
   edematous
   Hemophilus influenzae [H. influenzae]
   pneumococcal
   septic
   suppurative
   ulcerative

> `EXCLUDES` *chronic laryngitis (476.0-476.1)*
> *influenzal laryngitis (487.1)*

464.00 Without mention of obstruction

464.01 With obstruction

√5ᵗʰ 464.1 Acute tracheitis

Tracheitis (acute):
   NOS
   catarrhal

Tracheitis (acute):
   viral

> `EXCLUDES` *chronic tracheitis (491.8)*

464.10 Without mention of obstruction

464.11 With obstruction

√5ᵗʰ 464.2 Acute laryngotracheitis

Laryngotracheitis (acute)
Tracheitis (acute) with laryngitis (acute)

> `EXCLUDES` *chronic laryngotracheitis (476.1)*

464.20 Without mention of obstruction

464.21 With obstruction

√5ᵗʰ 464.3 Acute epiglottitis

Viral epiglottitis

> `EXCLUDES` *epiglottitis, chronic (476.1)*

464.30 Without mention of obstruction

464.31 With obstruction

464.4 Croup

Croup syndrome

DEF: Acute laryngeal obstruction due to allergy, foreign body or infection; symptoms include barking cough, hoarseness and harsh, persistent high-pitched respiratory sound.

√5ᵗʰ 464.5 Supraglottitis, unspecified

DEF: ▶ A rapidly advancing generalized upper respiratory infection of the lingual tonsillar area, epiglottic folds, false vocal cords, and the epiglottis; seen most commonly in children, but can affect people of any age. ◀

464.50 Without mention of obstruction

464.51 With obstruction

√4ᵗʰ 465 Acute upper respiratory infections of multiple or unspecified sites

> `EXCLUDES` *upper respiratory infection due to:*
>   *influenza (487.1)*
>   *Streptococcus (034.0)*

465.0 Acute laryngopharyngitis

DEF: Acute infection of the vocal cords and pharynx.

√4ᵗʰ / √5ᵗʰ   Additional Digit Required   Unspecified Code   Other Specified Code   Manifestation Code   ▶◀ Revised Text   ● New Code   ▲ Revised Code Title

Respiratory System 465.8–473.9

Respiratory System

Upper Respiratory System

465.8   **Other multiple sites**
Multiple URI

465.9   **Unspecified site**
Acute URI NOS
Upper respiratory infection (acute)

✓4th **466**   **Acute bronchitis and bronchiolitis**

INCLUDES   that with:
     bronchospasm
     obstruction

466.0   **Acute bronchitis**

Bronchitis, acute or subacute:	Bronchitis, acute or subacute:
fibrinous	viral
membranous	with tracheitis
pneumococcal	Croupous bronchitis
purulent	Tracheobronchitis, acute
septic	

EXCLUDES   acute bronchitis with:
     bronchiectasis (494.1)
     chronic obstructive pulmonary disease
     (491.21)

DEF: Acute inflammation of main branches of bronchial tree due to infectious or irritant agents; symptoms include cough with a varied production of sputum, fever, substernal soreness, and lung rales.

✓5th **466.1**   **Acute bronchiolitis**
Bronchiolitis (acute)   Capillary pneumonia

DEF: Acute inflammation of finer subdivisions of bronchial tree due to infectious or irritant agents; symptoms include cough with a varied production of sputum, fever, substernal soreness, and lung rales.

     466.11   **Acute bronchiolitis due to respiratory syncytial virus (RSV)**

     466.19   **Acute bronchiolitis due to other infectious organisms**
         Use additional code to identify organism

OTHER DISEASES OF THE UPPER RESPIRATORY TRACT (470-478)

470   **Deviated nasal septum**
Deflected septum (nasal) (acquired)
EXCLUDES   congenital (754.0)

✓4th **471**   **Nasal polyps**
EXCLUDES   adenomatous polyps (212.0)

471.0   **Polyp of nasal cavity**

Polyp:	Polyp:
choanal	nasopharyngeal

471.1   **Polypoid sinus degeneration**
Woakes' syndrome or ethmoiditis

471.8   **Other polyp of sinus**

Polyp of sinus:	Polyp of sinus:
accessory	maxillary
ethmoidal	sphenoidal

471.9   **Unspecified nasal polyp**
Nasal polyp NOS

✓4th **472**   **Chronic pharyngitis and nasopharyngitis**

472.0   **Chronic rhinitis**

Ozena	Rhinitis:
Rhinitis:	hypertrophic
NOS	obstructive
atrophic	purulent
granulomatous	ulcerative

EXCLUDES   allergic rhinitis (477.0-477.9)

DEF: Persistent inflammation of mucous membranes of nose.

472.1   **Chronic pharyngitis**

Chronic sore throat	Pharyngitis:
Pharyngitis:	granular (chronic)
atrophic	hypertrophic

472.2   **Chronic nasopharyngitis**
EXCLUDES   acute or unspecified nasopharyngitis (460)

DEF: Persistent inflammation of mucous membranes extending from nares to pharynx.

✓4th **473**   **Chronic sinusitis**

INCLUDES   abscess
     empyema   (chronic) of sinus
     infection   (accessory) (nasal)
     suppuration

EXCLUDES   acute sinusitis (461.0-461.9)

473.0   **Maxillary**
Antritis (chronic)

473.1   **Frontal**

473.2   **Ethmoidal**
EXCLUDES   Woakes' ethmoiditis (471.1)

473.3   **Sphenoidal**

473.8   **Other chronic sinusitis**
Pansinusitis (chronic)

473.9   **Unspecified sinusitis (chronic)**
Sinusitis (chronic) NOS

Paranasal Sinuses

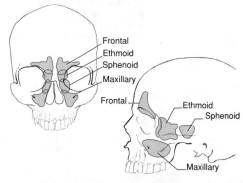

✓4ᵗʰ **474 Chronic disease of tonsils and adenoids**

    ✓5ᵗʰ **474.0 Chronic tonsillitis and adenoiditis**

         EXCLUDES *acute or unspecified tonsillitis (463)*

         474.00 Chronic tonsillitis

         474.01 Chronic adenoiditis

         474.02 Chronic tonsillitis and adenoiditis

    ✓5ᵗʰ **474.1 Hypertrophy of tonsils and adenoids**

         Enlargement
         Hyperplasia   } of tonsils or adenoids
         Hypertrophy

         EXCLUDES *that with:*
             adenoiditis (474.01)
             adenoiditis and tonsillitis (474.02)
             tonsillitis (474.00)

         474.10 Tonsils with adenoids

         474.11 Tonsils alone

         474.12 Adenoids alone

     474.2 Adenoid vegetations

         DEF: Fungus-like growth of lymph tissue between the nares and pharynx.

     474.8 Other chronic disease of tonsils and adenoids

         Amygdalolith   Tonsillar tag
         Calculus, tonsil   Ulcer, tonsil
         Cicatrix of tonsil (and adenoid)

     474.9 Unspecified chronic disease of tonsils and adenoids

         Disease (chronic) of tonsils (and adenoids)

    475 Peritonsillar abscess

         Abscess of tonsil   Quinsy
         Peritonsillar cellulitis

         EXCLUDES *tonsillitis:*
             acute or NOS (463)
             chronic (474.0)

✓4ᵗʰ **476 Chronic laryngitis and laryngotracheitis**

     476.0 Chronic laryngitis

         Laryngitis: Laryngitis:
           catarrhal   sicca
           hypertrophic

     476.1 Chronic laryngotracheitis

         Laryngitis, chronic, with tracheitis (chronic)
         Tracheitis, chronic, with laryngitis

         EXCLUDES *chronic tracheitis (491.8)*
             laryngitis and tracheitis, acute or
             unspecified (464.00-464.51)

✓4ᵗʰ **477 Allergic rhinitis**

     INCLUDES allergic rhinitis (nonseasonal) (seasonal)
         hay fever
         spasmodic rhinorrhea

     EXCLUDES *allergic rhinitis with asthma (bronchial) (493.0)*

     DEF: True immunoglobulin E (IgE)-mediated allergic reaction of nasal mucosa; seasonal (typical hay fever) or perennial (year-round allergens: dust, food, dander).

     477.0 Due to pollen
         Pollinosis

     477.1 Due to food

     477.8 Due to other allergen

     477.9 Cause unspecified

✓4ᵗʰ **478 Other diseases of upper respiratory tract**

     478.0 Hypertrophy of nasal turbinates

         DEF: Overgrowth, enlargement of shell-shaped bones, in nasal cavity.

     478.1 Other diseases of nasal cavity and sinuses

         Abscess
         Necrosis } of nose (septum)
         Ulcer

         Cyst or mucocele of sinus (nasal)
         Rhinolith

         EXCLUDES *varicose ulcer of nasal septum (456.8)*

    ✓5ᵗʰ **478.2 Other diseases of pharynx, not elsewhere classified**

         478.20 Unspecified disease of pharynx

         478.21 Cellulitis of pharynx or nasopharynx

         478.22 Parapharyngeal abscess

         478.24 Retropharyngeal abscess

            DEF: Purulent infection, behind pharynx and front of precerebral fascia.

         478.25 Edema of pharynx or nasopharynx

         478.26 Cyst of pharynx or nasopharynx

         478.29 Other

            Abscess of pharynx or nasopharynx

            EXCLUDES *ulcerative pharyngitis (462)*

    ✓5ᵗʰ **478.3 Paralysis of vocal cords or larynx**

         DEF: Loss of motor ability of vocal cords or larynx; due to nerve or muscle damage.

         478.30 Paralysis, unspecified
            Laryngoplegia   Paralysis of glottis

         478.31 Unilateral, partial

         478.32 Unilateral, complete

         478.33 Bilateral, partial

         478.34 Bilateral, complete

     478.4 Polyp of vocal cord or larynx

         EXCLUDES *adenomatous polyps (212.1)*

     478.5 Other diseases of vocal cords

         Abscess
         Cellulitis
         Granuloma   } of vocal cords
         Leukoplakia

         Chorditis (fibrinous) (nodosa) (tuberosa)
         Singers' nodes

     478.6 Edema of larynx

         Edema (of):   Edema (of):
           glottis   supraglottic
           subglottic

    ✓5ᵗʰ **478.7 Other diseases of larynx, not elsewhere classified**

         478.70 Unspecified disease of larynx

         478.71 Cellulitis and perichondritis of larynx

            DEF: Inflammation of deep soft tissues or lining of bone of the larynx.

         478.74 Stenosis of larynx

         478.75 Laryngeal spasm
            Laryngismus (stridulus)

            DEF: Involuntary muscle contraction of the larynx.

         478.79 Other

            Abscess
            Necrosis
            Obstruction } of larynx
            Pachyderma
            Ulcer

            EXCLUDES *ulcerative laryngitis (464.00-464.01)*

     478.8 Upper respiratory tract hypersensitivity reaction, site unspecified

         EXCLUDES *hypersensitivity reaction of lower respiratory tract, as:*
            extrinsic allergic alveolitis (495.0-495.9)
            pneumoconiosis (500-505)

     478.9 Other and unspecified diseases of upper respiratory tract

         Abscess
         Cicatrix } of trachea

✓4ᵗʰ **Additional Digit Required**   **Unspecified Code**   **Other Specified Code**   **Manifestation Code**   ►◄ Revised Text   ● New Code   ▲ Revised Code Title

2002 ICD•9•CM   **Volume 1 — 129**

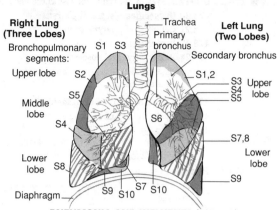

Lungs

PNEUMONIA AND INFLUENZA (480-487)

EXCLUDES   pneumonia:
    allergic or eosinophilic (518.3)
    aspiration:
        NOS (507.0)
        newborn (770.1)
        solids and liquids (507.0-507.8)
    congenital (770.0)
    lipoid (507.1)
    passive (514)
    rheumatic (390)

√4ᵗʰ 480 Viral pneumonia
    480.0   Pneumonia due to adenovirus
    480.1   Pneumonia due to respiratory syncytial virus
    480.2   Pneumonia due to parainfluenza virus
    480.8   Pneumonia due to other virus not elsewhere classified
             EXCLUDES   congenital rubella pneumonitis (771.0)
                 influenza with pneumonia, any form (487.0)
                 pneumonia complicating viral diseases classified elsewhere (484.1-484.8)
    480.9   Viral pneumonia, unspecified
    481 Pneumococcal pneumonia [Streptococcus pneumoniae pneumonia]
             Lobar pneumonia, organism unspecified
√4ᵗʰ 482 Other bacterial pneumonia
    482.0   Pneumonia due to Klebsiella pneumoniae
    482.1   Pneumonia due to Pseudomonas
    482.2   Pneumonia due to Hemophilus influenzae [H. influenzae]
    √5ᵗʰ 482.3   Pneumonia due to Streptococcus
             EXCLUDES   Streptococcus pneumoniae (481)
        482.30 Streptococcus, unspecified
        482.31 Group A
        482.32 Group B
        482.39 Other Streptococcus
    √5ᵗʰ 482.4   Pneumonia due to Staphylococcus
        482.40 Pneumonia due to Staphylococcus, unspecified
        482.41 Pneumonia due to Staphylococcus aureus
        482.49 Other Staphylococcus pneumonia
    √5ᵗʰ 482.8   Pneumonia due to other specified bacteria
             EXCLUDES   pneumonia, complicating infectious disease classified elsewhere (484.1-484.8)
        482.81 Anaerobes
             Bacteroides (melaninogenicus)
             Gram-negative anaerobes
        482.82 Escherichia coli [E. coli]

    482.83 Other gram-negative bacteria
             Gram-negative pneumonia NOS
             Proteus
             Serratia marcescens
             EXCLUDES   gram-negative anaerobes (482.81)
                 Legionnaires' disease (482.84)
    482.84 Legionnaires' disease
             DEF: Severe and often fatal infection by *Legionella pneumophilia*; symptoms include high fever, gastrointestinal pain, headache, myalgia, dry cough, and pneumonia; transmitted airborne via air conditioning systems, humidifiers, water faucets, shower heads; not person-to-person contact.
    482.89 Other specified bacteria
    482.9   Bacterial pneumonia unspecified
√4ᵗʰ 483 Pneumonia due to other specified organism
    483.0   Mycoplasma pneumoniae
             Eaton's agent
             Pleuropneumonia-like organism [PPLO]
    483.1   Chlamydia
    483.8   Other specified organism
√4ᵗʰ 484 Pneumonia in infectious diseases classified elsewhere
             EXCLUDES   influenza with pneumonia, any form (487.0)
    484.1   Pneumonia in cytomegalic inclusion disease
             Code first underlying disease, as (078.5)
    484.3   Pneumonia in whooping cough
             Code first underlying disease, as (033.0-033.9)
    484.5   Pneumonia in anthrax
             Code first underlying disease (022.1)
    484.6   Pneumonia in aspergillosis
             Code first underlying disease (117.3)
    484.7   Pneumonia in other systemic mycoses
             Code first underlying disease
             EXCLUDES   pneumonia in:
                 candidiasis (112.4)
                 coccidioidomycosis (114.0)
                 histoplasmosis (115.0-115.9 with fifth-digit 5)
    484.8   Pneumonia in other infectious diseases classified elsewhere
             Code first underlying disease, as:
                 Q fever (083.0)
                 typhoid fever (002.0)
             EXCLUDES   pneumonia in:
                 actinomycosis (039.1)
                 measles (055.1)
                 nocardiosis (039.1)
                 ornithosis (073.0)
                 Pneumocystis carinii (136.3)
                 salmonellosis (003.22)
                 toxoplasmosis (130.4)
                 tuberculosis (011.6)
                 tularemia (021.2)
                 varicella (052.1)
    485 Bronchopneumonia, organism unspecified
             Bronchopneumonia: Pneumonia:
                 hemorrhagic   lobular
                 terminal   segmental
             Pleurobronchopneumonia
             EXCLUDES   bronchiolitis (acute) (466.11-466.19)
                 chronic (491.8)
                 lipoid pneumonia (507.1)
    486 Pneumonia, organism unspecified
             EXCLUDES   hypostatic or passive pneumonia (514)
                 influenza with pneumonia, any form (487.0)
                 inhalation or aspiration pneumonia due to foreign materials (507.0-507.8)
                 pneumonitis due to fumes and vapors (506.0)

N Newborn Age: 0   P Pediatric Age: 0-17   M Maternity Age: 12-55   A Adult Age: 15-124   MSP Medicare Secondary Payer

☑4ᵗʰ **487 Influenza**

> **EXCLUDES** *Hemophilus influenzae [H. influenzae]:*
> *infection NOS (041.5)*
> *laryngitis (464.00-464.01)*
> *meningitis (320.0)*
> *pneumonia (482.2)*

487.0 With pneumonia
Influenza with pneumonia, any form
Influenzal:
bronchopneumonia
pneumonia

487.1 With other respiratory manifestations
Influenza NOS
Influenzal:
laryngitis
pharyngitis
respiratory infection (upper) (acute)

487.8 With other manifestations
Encephalopathy due to influenza
Influenza with involvement of gastrointestinal tract

> **EXCLUDES** *"intestinal flu" [viral gastroenteritis]*
> *(008.8)*

CHRONIC OBSTRUCTIVE PULMONARY DISEASE AND ALLIED CONDITIONS (490-496)

490 Bronchitis, not specified as acute or chronic
Bronchitis NOS:
catarrhal
with tracheitis NOS
Tracheobronchitis NOS

> **EXCLUDES** *bronchitis:*
> *allergic NOS (493.9)*
> *asthmatic NOS (493.9)*
> *due to fumes and vapors (506.0)*

☑4ᵗʰ **491 Chronic bronchitis**

> **EXCLUDES** *chronic obstructive asthma (493.2)*

491.0 Simple chronic bronchitis
Catarrhal bronchitis, chronic
Smokers' cough

491.1 Mucopurulent chronic bronchitis
Bronchitis (chronic) (recurrent):
fetid
mucopurulent
purulent

DEF: Chronic bronchial infection characterized by both mucus and pus secretions in the bronchial tree; recurs after asymptomatic periods; signs are coughing, expectoration and secondary changes in the lung.

Bronchioli and Alveoli

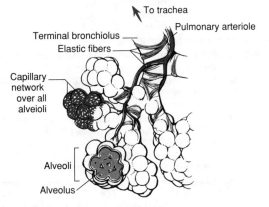

To trachea
Pulmonary arteriole
Terminal bronchiolus
Elastic fibers
Capillary network over all alveioli
Alveoli
Alveolus

☑5ᵗʰ **491.2 Obstructive chronic bronchitis**
Bronchitis:
emphysematous
obstructive (chronic) (diffuse)
Bronchitis with:
chronic airway obstruction
emphysema

> **EXCLUDES** *asthmatic bronchitis (acute) NOS*
> *(493.9)*
> *chronic obstructive asthma (493.2)*

491.20 Without mention of acute exacerbation
Emphysema with chronic bronchitis

491.21 With acute exacerbation
Acute bronchitis with chronic obstructive pulmonary disease [COPD]
Acute and chronic obstructive bronchitis
Acute exacerbation of chronic obstructive pulmonary disease [COPD]
Emphysema with both acute and chronic bronchitis

> **EXCLUDES** *chronic obstructive asthma*
> *with acute exacerbation*
> *(493.22)*

491.8 Other chronic bronchitis

Chronic:	Chronic:
tracheitis	tracheobronchitis

491.9 Unspecified chronic bronchitis

☑4ᵗʰ **492 Emphysema**

492.0 Emphysematous bleb
Giant bullous emphysema
Ruptured emphysematous bleb
Tension pneumatocele
Vanishing lung

DEF: Formation of vesicle or bulla in emphysematous lung, more than one millimeter; contains serum or blood.

492.8 Other emphysema

Emphysema (lung or pulmonary):	Emphysema (lung or pulmonary):
NOS	unilateral
centriacinar	vesicular
centrilobular	MacLeod's syndrome
obstructive	Swyer-James syndrome
panacinar	Unilateral hyperlucent lung
panlobular	

> **EXCLUDES** *emphysema:*
> *with both acute and chronic*
> *bronchitis (491.21)*
> *with chronic bronchitis (491.2)*
> *compensatory (518.2)*
> *due to fumes and vapors (506.4)*
> *interstitial (518.1)*
> *newborn (770.2)*
> *mediastinal (518.1)*
> *surgical (subcutaneous) (998.81)*
> *traumatic (958.7)*

☑4ᵗʰ **493 Asthma**

> **EXCLUDES** *wheezing NOS (786.07)*

The following fifth-digit subclassification is for use with category 493:
> **0** **without mention of status asthmaticus or acute exacerbation or unspecified**
> **1** **with status asthmaticus**
> **2** **with acute exacerbation**

DEF: Status asthmaticus: Severe, intractable episode of asthma unresponsive to normal therapeutic measures.

Respiratory System 487–493

☑4ᵗʰ / ☑5ᵗʰ Additional Digit Required   Unspecified Code   Other Specified Code   Manifestation Code   ▶◀ Revised Text   ● New Code   ▲ Revised Code Title

2003 ICD•9•CM   **Volume 1 — 131**

Respiratory System 493.0–506.3

√5ᵗʰ **493.0 Extrinsic asthma**

Asthma: Asthma:
allergic with   hay
    stated cause   platinum
atopic   Hay fever with asthma
childhood

EXCLUDES   asthma:
           allergic NOS (493.9)
           detergent (507.8)
           miners' (500)
           wood (495.8)

DEF: Transient stricture of airway diameters of bronchi; due to environmental factor; also called allergic (bronchial) asthma.

√5ᵗʰ **493.1 Intrinsic asthma**

Late-onset asthma

DEF: Transient stricture, of airway diameters of bronchi; due to pathophysiological disturbances.

√5ᵗʰ **493.2 Chronic obstructive asthma**

Asthma with chronic obstructive pulmonary disease [COPD]

►Chronic asthmatic bronchitis◄

EXCLUDES   acute bronchitis (466.0)
           chronic obstructive bronchitis (491.2)

DEF: Persistent narrowing of airway diameters in the bronchial tree, restricting airflow and causing constant labored breathing.

√5ᵗʰ **493.9 Asthma, unspecified**

Asthma (bronchial) (allergic NOS)
Bronchitis:
allergic
asthmatic

√4ᵗʰ **494 Bronchiectasis**

Bronchiectasis (fusiform) (postinfectious) (recurrent)
Bronchiolectasis

EXCLUDES   congenital (748.61)
           tuberculous bronchiectasis (current disease) (011.5)

DEF: Dilation of bronchi; due to infection or chronic conditions; causes decreased lung capacity and recurrent infections of lungs.

494.0 Bronchiectasis without acute exacerbation

494.1 Bronchiectasis with acute exacerbation

Acute bronchitis with bronchiectasis

√4ᵗʰ **495 Extrinsic allergic alveolitis**

INCLUDES   allergic alveolitis and pneumonitis due to inhaled organic dust particles of fungal, thermophilic actinomycete, or other origin

DEF: Pneumonitis due to particles inhaled into lung, often at workplace; symptoms include cough, chills, fever, increased heart and respiratory rates; develops within hours of exposure.

495.0 Farmers' lung

495.1 Bagassosis

495.2 Bird-fanciers' lung

Budgerigar-fanciers' disease or lung
Pigeon-fanciers' disease or lung

495.3 Suberosis

Cork-handlers' disease or lung

495.4 Malt workers' lung

Alveolitis due to Aspergillus clavatus

495.5 Mushroom workers' lung

495.6 Maple bark-strippers' lung

Alveolitis due to Cryptostroma corticale

495.7 "Ventilation" pneumonitis

Allergic alveolitis due to fungal, thermophilic actinomycete, and other organisms growing in ventilation [air conditioning] systems

495.8 Other specified allergic alveolitis and pneumonitis

Cheese-washers' lung
Coffee workers' lung
Fish-meal workers' lung
Furriers' lung
Grain-handlers' disease or lung
Pituitary snuff-takers' disease
Sequoiosis or red-cedar asthma
Wood asthma

495.9 Unspecified allergic alveolitis and pneumonitis

Alveolitis, allergic (extrinsic)
Hypersensitivity pneumonitis

496 Chronic airway obstruction, not elsewhere classified   A

Note: This code is not to be used with any code from categories 491-493
Chronic:
nonspecific lung disease
obstructive lung disease
obstructive pulmonary disease [COPD] NOS

EXCLUDES   chronic obstructive lung disease [COPD]
           specified (as) (with):
           allergic alveolitis (495.0-495.9)
           asthma (493.2)
           bronchiectasis (494.0-494.1)
           bronchitis (491.20-491.21)
             with emphysema (491.20-491.21)
           emphysema (492.0-492.8)

PNEUMOCONIOSES AND OTHER LUNG DISEASES DUE TO EXTERNAL AGENTS (500-508)

DEF: Permanent deposits of particulate matter, within lungs; due to occupational or environmental exposure; results in chronic induration and fibrosis. (See specific listings in 500-508 code range)

500 Coal workers' pneumoconiosis   A

Anthracosilicosis   Coal workers' lung
Anthracosis   Miner's asthma
Black lung disease

501 Asbestosis   A

502 Pneumoconiosis due to other silica or silicates

Pneumoconiosis due to talc
Silicotic fibrosis (massive) of lung
Silicosis (simple) (complicated)

503 Pneumoconiosis due to other inorganic dust

Aluminosis (of lung)   Graphite fibrosis (of lung)
Bauxite fibrosis (of lung)   Siderosis
Berylliosis   Stannosis

504 Pneumonopathy due to inhalation of other dust

Byssinosis   Flax-dressers' disease
Cannabinosis

EXCLUDES   allergic alveolitis (495.0-495.9)
           asbestosis (501)
           bagassosis (495.1)
           farmers' lung (495.0)

505 Pneumoconiosis, unspecified

√4ᵗʰ **506 Respiratory conditions due to chemical fumes and vapors**

Use additional E code to identify cause

506.0 Bronchitis and pneumonitis due to fumes and vapors

Chemical bronchitis (acute)

506.1 Acute pulmonary edema due to fumes and vapors

Chemical pulmonary edema (acute)

EXCLUDES   acute pulmonary edema NOS (518.4)
           chronic or unspecified pulmonary edema (514)

506.2 Upper respiratory inflammation due to fumes and vapors

506.3 Other acute and subacute respiratory conditions due to fumes and vapors

506.4 Chronic respiratory conditions due to fumes and vapors

Emphysema (diffuse) (chronic)   ⎫
Obliterative bronchiolitis (chronic) (subacute)   ⎬ due to inhalation of chemical fumes and vapors
Pulmonary fibrosis (chronic)   ⎭

506.9 Unspecified respiratory conditions due to fumes and vapors

Silo-fillers' disease

✓4ᵗʰ 507 Pneumonitis due to solids and liquids

EXCLUDES   *fetal aspiration pneumonitis (770.1)*

507.0 Due to inhalation of food or vomitus

Aspiration pneumonia (due to):
   NOS
   food (regurgitated)
   gastric secretions

Aspiration pneumonia (due to):
   milk
   saliva
   vomitus

507.1 Due to inhalation of oils and essences

Lipoid pneumonia (exogenous)

EXCLUDES   *endogenous lipoid pneumonia (516.8)*

507.8 Due to other solids and liquids

Detergent asthma

✓4ᵗʰ 508 Respiratory conditions due to other and unspecified external agents

Use additional E code to identify cause

508.0 Acute pulmonary manifestations due to radiation

Radiation pneumonitis

508.1 Chronic and other pulmonary manifestations due to radiation

Fibrosis of lung following radiation

508.8 Respiratory conditions due to other specified external agents

508.9 Respiratory conditions due to unspecified external agent

OTHER DISEASES OF RESPIRATORY SYSTEM (510-519)

✓4ᵗʰ 510 Empyema

Use additional code to identify infectious organism (041.0-041.9)

EXCLUDES   *abscess of lung (513.0)*

DEF: Purulent infection, within pleural space.

510.0 With fistula

Fistula:
   bronchocutaneous
   bronchopleural
   hepatopleural

Fistula:
   mediastinal
   pleural
   thoracic

Any condition classifiable to 510.9 with fistula

DEF: Purulent infection of respiratory cavity; with communication from cavity to another structure.

510.9 Without mention of fistula

Abscess:
   pleura
   thorax
Empyema (chest) (lung) (pleura)
Fibrinopurulent pleurisy
Pleurisy:
   purulent

Pleurisy:
   septic
   seropurulent
   suppurative
Pyopneumothorax
Pyothorax

✓4ᵗʰ 511 Pleurisy

EXCLUDES   *malignant pleural effusion (197.2)*
pleurisy with mention of tuberculosis, current disease (012.0)

DEF: Inflammation of serous membrane of lungs and lining of thoracic cavity; causes exudation in cavity or membrane surface.

511.0 Without mention of effusion or current tuberculosis

Adhesion, lung or pleura
Calcification of pleura
Pleurisy (acute) (sterile):
   diaphragmatic
   fibrinous
   interlobar

Pleurisy:
   NOS
   pneumococcal
   staphylococcal
   streptococcal
Thickening of pleura

511.1 With effusion, with mention of a bacterial cause other than tuberculosis

Pleurisy with effusion (exudative) (serous):
   pneumococcal
   staphylococcal
   streptococcal
   other specified nontuberculous bacterial cause

511.8 Other specified forms of effusion, except tuberculous

Encysted pleurisy
Hemopneumothorax
Hemothorax

Hydropneumothorax
Hydrothorax

EXCLUDES   *traumatic (860.2-860.5, 862.29, 862.39)*

511.9 Unspecified pleural effusion

Pleural effusion NOS
Pleurisy:
   exudative
   serofibrinous

Pleurisy:
   serous
   with effusion NOS

✓4ᵗʰ 512 Pneumothorax

DEF: Collapsed lung; due to gas or air in pleural space.

512.0 Spontaneous tension pneumothorax

DEF: Leaking air from lung into lining causing collapse.

512.1 Iatrogenic pneumothorax

Postoperative pneumothorax

DEF: Air trapped in the lining of the lung following surgery.

512.8 Other spontaneous pneumothorax

Pneumothorax:
   NOS
   acute

Pneumothorax:
   chronic

EXCLUDES   *pneumothorax:*
congenital (770.2)
traumatic (860.0-860.1, 860.4-860.5)
tuberculous, current disease (011.7)

✓4ᵗʰ 513 Abscess of lung and mediastinum

513.0 Abscess of lung

Abscess (multiple) of lung
Gangrenous or necrotic pneumonia
Pulmonary gangrene or necrosis

513.1 Abscess of mediastinum

514 Pulmonary congestion and hypostasis

Hypostatic:
   bronchopneumonia
   pneumonia
Passive pneumonia
Pulmonary congestion (chronic) (passive)

Pulmonary edema:
   NOS
   chronic

EXCLUDES   *acute pulmonary edema:*
NOS (518.4)
with mention of heart disease or failure (428.1)

DEF: Excessive retention of interstitial fluid in the lungs and pulmonary vessels; due to poor circulation.

515 Postinflammatory pulmonary fibrosis

Cirrhosis of lung   ⎫
Fibrosis of lung (atrophic) (confluent) (massive) (perialveolar) (peribronchial)   ⎬ chronic or unspecified
Induration of lung   ⎭

DEF: Fibrosis and scarring of the lungs due to inflammatory reaction.

✓4ᵗʰ / ✓5ᵗʰ   Additional Digit Required   Unspecified Code   Other Specified Code   Manifestation Code   ►◄ Revised Text   ● New Code   ▲ Revised Code Title

☑4ᵗʰ **516 Other alveolar and parietoalveolar pneumonopathy**

516.0 Pulmonary alveolar proteinosis

DEF: Reduced ventilation; due to proteinaceous deposits on alveoli; symptoms include dyspnea, cough, chest pain, weakness, weight loss, and hemoptysis.

516.1 Idiopathic pulmonary hemosiderosis

Essential brown induration of lung
Code first underlying disease (275.0)

DEF: Fibrosis of alveolar walls; marked by abnormal amounts hemosiderin in lungs; primarily affects children; symptoms include anemia, fluid in lungs, and blood in sputum; etiology unknown.

516.2 Pulmonary alveolar microlithiasis

DEF: Small calculi in pulmonary alveoli resembling sand-like particles on x-ray.

516.3 Idiopathic fibrosing alveolitis

Alveolar capillary block
Diffuse (idiopathic) (interstitial) pulmonary fibrosis
Hamman-Rich syndrome

516.8 Other specified alveolar and parietoalveolar pneumonopathies

Endogenous lipoid pneumonia
Interstitial pneumonia (desquamative) (lymphoid)

EXCLUDES *lipoid pneumonia, exogenous or unspecified (507.1)*

516.9 Unspecified alveolar and parietoalveolar pneumonopathy

☑4ᵗʰ **517 Lung involvement in conditions classified elsewhere**

EXCLUDES *rheumatoid lung (714.81)*

517.1 Rheumatic pneumonia

Code first underlying disease (390)

517.2 Lung involvement in systemic sclerosis

Code first underlying disease (710.1)

517.8 Lung involvement in other diseases classified elsewhere

Code first underlying disease, as:
amyloidosis (277.3)
polymyositis (710.4)
sarcoidosis (135)
Sjögren's disease (710.2)
systemic lupus erythematosus (710.0)

EXCLUDES *syphilis (095.1)*

☑4ᵗʰ **518 Other diseases of lung**

518.0 Pulmonary collapse

Atelectasis   Middle lobe syndrome
Collapse of lung

EXCLUDES *atelectasis:*
congenital (partial) (770.5)
primary (770.4)
tuberculous, current disease (011.8)

518.1 Interstitial emphysema

Mediastinal emphysema

EXCLUDES *surgical (subcutaneous) emphysema (998.81)*
that in fetus or newborn (770.2)
traumatic emphysema (958.7)

DEF: Escaped air from the alveoli trapped in the interstices of the lung; trauma or cough may cause the disease.

518.2 Compensatory emphysema

DEF: Distention of all or part of the lung caused by disease processes or surgical intervention that decreased volume in another part of the lung; overcompensation reaction to the loss of capacity in another part of the lung.

518.3 Pulmonary eosinophilia

Eosinophilic asthma   Pneumonia:
Löffler's syndrome   eosinophilic
Pneumonia: Tropical eosinophilia
   allergic

DEF: Infiltration, into pulmonary parenchyma of eosinophilia; results in cough, fever, and dyspnea.

518.4 Acute edema of lung, unspecified

Acute pulmonary edema NOS
Pulmonary edema, postoperative

EXCLUDES *pulmonary edema:*
acute, with mention of heart disease or failure (428.1)
chronic or unspecified (514)
due to external agents (506.0-508.9)

DEF: Severe, sudden fluid retention within lung tissues.

518.5 Pulmonary insufficiency following trauma and surgery

Adult respiratory distress syndrome
Pulmonary insufficiency following:
   shock
   surgery
   trauma
Shock lung

EXCLUDES *adult respiratory distress syndrome associated with other conditions (518.82)*
pneumonia:
aspiration (507.0)
hypostatic (514)
respiratory failure in other conditions (518.81, 518.83-518.84)

518.6 Allergic bronchopulmonary aspegillosis

DEF: Noninvasive hypersensitive reaction; due to allergic reaction to *Aspergillus fumigatus* (mold).

☑5ᵗʰ **518.8 Other diseases of lung**

518.81 Acute respiratory failure

Respiratory failure NOS

EXCLUDES *acute and chronic respiratory failure (518.84)*
acute respiratory distress (518.82)
chronic respiratory failure (518.83)
respiratory arrest (799.1)
respiratory failure, newborn ▶(770.84)◀

518.82 Other pulmonary insufficiency, not elsewhere classified

Acute respiratory distress
Acute respiratory insufficiency
Adult respiratory distress syndrome NEC

EXCLUDES *adult respiratory distress syndrome associated with trauma and surgery (518.5)*
pulmonary insufficiency following trauma and surgery (518.5)
respiratory distress:
NOS (786.09)
newborn ▶(770.89)◀
syndrome, newborn (769)
shock lung (518.5)

518.83 Chronic respiratory failure

518.84 Acute and chronic respiratory failure

Acute on chronic respiratory failure

518.89 Other diseases of lung, not elsewhere classified

Broncholithiasis   Lung disease NOS
Calcification of lung   Pulmolithiasis

DEF: Broncholithiasis: calculi in lumen of transbronchial tree.

DEF: Pulmolithiasis: calculi in lung.

☑4ᵗʰ **519 Other diseases of respiratory system**

☑5ᵗʰ **519.0 Tracheostomy complications**

519.00 Tracheostomy complication, unspecified

519.01 Infection of tracheostomy
Use additional code to identify type of infection, such as:
abscess or cellulitis of neck (682.1)
septicemia (038.0-038.9)
Use additional code to identify organism (041.00-041.9)

519.02 Mechanical complication of tracheostomy
Tracheal stenosis due to tracheostomy

519.09 Other tracheostomy complications
Hemorrhage due to tracheostomy
Tracheoesophageal fistula due to tracheostomy

519.1 Other diseases of trachea and bronchus, not elsewhere classified
Calcification ⎫
Stenosis ⎬ of bronchus or trachea
Ulcer ⎭

519.2 Mediastinitis
DEF: Inflammation of tissue between organs behind sternum.

519.3 Other diseases of mediastinum, not elsewhere classified
Fibrosis ⎫
Hernia ⎬ of mediastinum
Retraction ⎭

519.4 Disorders of diaphragm
Diaphragmitis   Relaxation of diaphragm
Paralysis of diaphragm
EXCLUDES *congenital defect of diaphragm (756.6)*
diaphragmatic hernia (551-553 with .3)
congenital (756.6)

519.8 Other diseases of respiratory system, not elsewhere classified

519.9 Unspecified disease of respiratory system
Respiratory disease (chronic) NOS

9. DISEASES OF THE DIGESTIVE SYSTEM (520-579)

DISEASES OF ORAL CAVITY, SALIVARY GLANDS, AND JAWS
(520-529)

√4ᵗʰ 520 Disorders of tooth development and eruption

520.0 Anodontia
Absence of teeth (complete) (congenital) (partial)
Hypodontia
Oligodontia
> **EXCLUDES** *acquired absence of teeth (525.10-525.19)*

520.1 Supernumerary teeth
Distomolar   Paramolar
Fourth molar   Supplemental teeth
Mesiodens
> **EXCLUDES** *supernumerary roots (520.2)*

520.2 Abnormalities of size and form
Concrescence
Fusion   } of teeth
Gemination

Dens evaginatus   Microdontia
Dens in dente   Peg-shaped [conical] teeth
Dens invaginatus   Supernumerary roots
Enamel pearls   Taurodontism
Macrodontia   Tuberculum paramolare
> **EXCLUDES** *that due to congenital syphilis (090.5)*
> *tuberculum Carabelli, which is regarded as a normal variation*

520.3 Mottled teeth
Dental fluorosis
Mottling of enamel
Nonfluoride enamel opacities

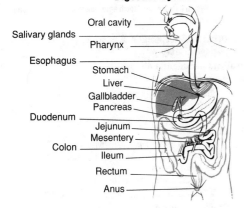

Digestive System

Salivary glands
Oral cavity
Pharynx
Esophagus
Stomach
Liver
Gallbladder
Pancreas
Duodenum
Jejunum
Mesentery
Colon
Ileum
Rectum
Anus

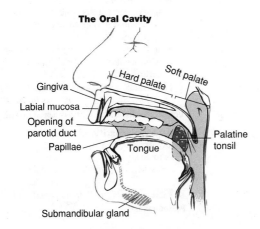

The Oral Cavity

Gingiva
Hard palate
Soft palate
Labial mucosa
Opening of parotid duct
Papillae
Tongue
Palatine tonsil
Submandibular gland

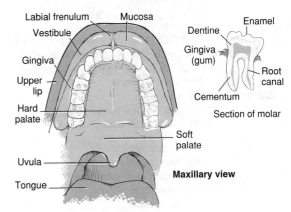

Teeth

Labial frenulum
Mucosa
Vestibule
Gingiva
Upper lip
Hard palate
Uvula
Tongue
Soft palate

Dentine
Enamel
Gingiva (gum)
Root canal
Cementum
Section of molar

Maxillary view

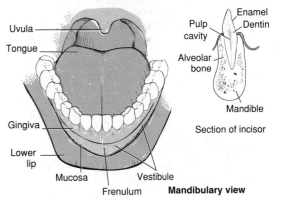

Uvula
Tongue
Gingiva
Lower lip
Mucosa
Vestibule
Frenulum

Enamel
Dentin
Pulp cavity
Alveolar bone
Mandible

Section of incisor

Mandibulary view

520.4 Disturbances of tooth formation
Aplasia and hypoplasia of cementum
Dilaceration of tooth
Enamel hypoplasia (neonatal) (postnatal) (prenatal)
Horner's teeth
Hypocalcification of teeth
Regional odontodysplasia
Turner's tooth
> **EXCLUDES** *Hutchinson's teeth and mulberry molars in congenital syphilis (090.5)*
> *mottled teeth (520.3)*

520.5 Hereditary disturbances in tooth structure, not elsewhere classified
Amelogenesis
Dentinogenesis } imperfecta
Odontogenesis

Dentinal dysplasia   Shell teeth

520.6 Disturbances in tooth eruption
Teeth: Tooth eruption:
  embedded   late
  impacted   obstructed
  natal   premature
  neonatal
  primary [deciduous]:
    persistent
    shedding, premature
> **EXCLUDES** *exfoliation of teeth (attributable to disease of surrounding tissues) (525.0-525.19)*
> *impacted or embedded teeth with abnormal position of such teeth or adjacent teeth (524.3)*

520.7 Teething syndrome

√4ᵗʰ √5ᵗʰ Additional Digit Required   **Unspecified Code**   **Other Specified Code**   **Manifestation Code**   ►◄ Revised Text   ● New Code   ▲ Revised Code Title

2003 ICD•9•CM   **Volume 1 — 137**

Digestive System 520.8–523.5

520.8   Other specified disorders of tooth development and eruption
Color changes during tooth formation
Pre-eruptive color changes
> EXCLUDES   *posteruptive color changes (521.7)*

520.9   Unspecified disorder of tooth development and eruption

√4th **521 Diseases of hard tissues of teeth**

√5th **521.0 Dental caries**

521.00 Dental caries, unspecified

521.01 Dental caries limited to enamel
Initial caries
White spot lesion

521.02 Dental caries extending into dentine

521.03 Dental caries extending into pulp

521.04 Arrested dental caries

521.05 Odontoclasia
Infantile melanodontia
Melanodontoclasia
> EXCLUDES   *internal and external resorption of teeth (521.4)*

DEF:▶ A pathological dental condition described as stained areas, loss of tooth substance, and hypoplasia linked to nutritional deficiencies during tooth development and to cariogenic oral conditions; synonyms are melanodontoclasia and infantile melanodontia.◀

521.09 Other dental caries

521.1 Excessive attrition
Approximal wear   Occlusal wear

521.2 Abrasion
Abrasion:
  dentifrice
  habitual
  occupational   } of teeth
  ritual
  traditional
Wedge defect NOS

521.3 Erosion
Erosion of teeth:
  NOS
  due to:
    medicine
    persistent vomiting
  idiopathic
  occupational

521.4 Pathological resorption
Internal granuloma of pulp
Resorption of tooth or root (external) (internal)
DEF: Loss of dentin and cementum due to disease process.

521.5 Hypercementosis
Cementation hyperplasia
DEF: Excess deposits of cementum, on tooth root.

521.6 Ankylosis of teeth
DEF: Adhesion of tooth to surrounding bone.

521.7 Posteruptive color changes
Staining [discoloration] of teeth:
  NOS
  due to:
    drugs
    metals
    pulpal bleeding
> EXCLUDES   *accretions [deposits] on teeth (523.6)*
> *pre-eruptive color changes (520.8)*

521.8 Other specified diseases of hard tissues of teeth
Irradiated enamel
Sensitive dentin

521.9 Unspecified disease of hard tissues of teeth

√4th **522 Diseases of pulp and periapical tissues**

522.0 Pulpitis
Pulpal:
  abscess
  polyp
Pulpitis:
  acute
  chronic (hyperplastic) (ulcerative)
  suppurative

522.1 Necrosis of the pulp
Pulp gangrene
DEF: Death of pulp tissue.

522.2 Pulp degeneration
Denticles   Pulp stones
Pulp calcifications

522.3 Abnormal hard tissue formation in pulp
Secondary or irregular dentin

522.4 Acute apical periodontitis of pulpal origin
DEF: Severe inflammation of periodontal ligament due to pulpal inflammation or necrosis.

522.5 Periapical abscess without sinus
Abscess: Abscess:
  dental   dentoalveolar
> EXCLUDES   *periapical abscess with sinus (522.7)*

522.6 Chronic apical periodontitis
Apical or periapical granuloma
Apical periodontitis NOS

522.7 Periapical abscess with sinus
Fistula: Fistula:
  alveolar process   dental

522.8 Radicular cyst
Cyst: Cyst:
  apical (periodontal)   radiculodental
  periapical   residual radicular
> EXCLUDES   *lateral developmental or lateral periodontal cyst (526.0)*
DEF: Cyst in tissue around tooth apex due to chronic infection of granuloma around root.

522.9 Other and unspecified diseases of pulp and periapical tissues

√4th **523 Gingival and periodontal diseases**

523.0 Acute gingivitis
> EXCLUDES   *acute necrotizing ulcerative gingivitis (101)*
> *herpetic gingivostomatitis (054.2)*

523.1 Chronic gingivitis
Gingivitis (chronic):   Gingivitis (chronic):
  NOS   simple marginal
  desquamative   ulcerative
  hyperplastic   Gingivostomatitis
> EXCLUDES   *herpetic gingivostomatitis (054.2)*

523.2 Gingival recession
Gingival recession (generalized) (localized) (postinfective) (postoperative)

523.3 Acute periodontitis
Acute: Paradontal abscess
  pericementitis   Periodontal abscess
  pericoronitis
> EXCLUDES   *acute apical periodontitis (522.4)*
> *periapical abscess (522.5, 522.7)*
DEF: Severe inflammation, of tissues supporting teeth.

523.4 Chronic periodontitis
Alveolar pyorrhea   Periodontitis:
Chronic pericoronitis   NOS
Pericementitis (chronic)   complex
     simplex
> EXCLUDES   *chronic apical periodontitis (522.6)*

523.5 Periodontosis

523.6 Accretions on teeth

Dental calculus:
  subgingival
  supragingival

Deposits on teeth:
  materia alba
  soft

Deposits on teeth:
  betel

  tartar
  tobacco

DEF: Foreign material on tooth surface, usually plaque or calculus.

523.8 Other specified periodontal diseases

Giant cell:
  epulis
  peripheral granuloma
Gingival:
  cysts
  enlargement NOS
  fibromatosis
Gingival polyp
Periodontal lesions due to traumatic occlusion
Peripheral giant cell granuloma

EXCLUDES   *leukoplakia of gingiva (528.6)*

523.9 Unspecified gingival and periodontal disease

✓4th 524 Dentofacial anomalies, including malocclusion

✓5th 524.0 Major anomalies of jaw size

EXCLUDES   *hemifacial atrophy or hypertrophy (754.0)*
unilateral condylar hyperplasia or hypoplasia of mandible (526.89)

524.00 Unspecified anomaly

DEF: Unspecified deformity of jaw size.

524.01 Maxillary hyperplasia

DEF: Overgrowth or overdevelopment of upper jaw bone.

524.02 Mandibular hyperplasia

DEF: Overgrowth or overdevelopment of lower jaw bone.

524.03 Maxillary hypoplasia

DEF: Incomplete or underdeveloped, upper jaw bone.

524.04 Mandibular hypoplasia

DEF: Incomplete or underdeveloped, lower jaw bone.

524.05 Macrogenia

DEF: Enlarged, jaw, especially chin; affects bone, soft tissue, or both.

524.06 Microgenia

DEF: Underdeveloped mandible, characterized by an extremely small chin.

524.09 Other specified anomaly

✓5th 524.1 Anomalies of relationship of jaw to cranial base

524.10 Unspecified anomaly

  Prognathism   Retrognathism

DEF: Prognathism: protrusion of lower jaw.

DEF: Retrognathism: jaw is located posteriorly to a normally positioned jaw; backward position of mandible.

524.11 Maxillary asymmetry

DEF: Absence of symmetry of maxilla.

524.12 Other jaw asymmetry

524.19 Other specified anomaly

524.2 Anomalies of dental arch relationship

Crossbite (anterior) (posterior)
Disto-occlusion
Mesio-occlusion
Midline deviation
Open bite (anterior) (posterior)
Overbite (excessive):
  deep
  horizontal
  vertical
Overjet
Posterior lingual occlusion of mandibular teeth
Soft tissue impingement

EXCLUDES   *hemifacial atrophy or hypertrophy (754.0)*
unilateral condylar hyperplasia or hypoplasia of mandible (526.89)

524.3 Anomalies of tooth position

Crowding
Diastema
Displacement   } of tooth, teeth
Rotation
Spacing, abnormal
Transposition

Impacted or embedded teeth with abnormal position of such teeth or adjacent teeth

524.4 Malocclusion, unspecified

DEF: Malposition of top and bottom teeth; interferes with chewing.

524.5 Dentofacial functional abnormalities

Abnormal jaw closure
Malocclusion due to:
  abnormal swallowing
  mouth breathing
  tongue, lip, or finger habits

✓5th 524.6 Temporomandibular joint disorders

EXCLUDES   *current temporomandibular joint:*
dislocation (830.0-830.1)
strain (848.1)

524.60 Temporomandibular joint disorders, unspecified

Temporomandibular joint-pain-dysfunction syndrome [TMJ]

524.61 Adhesions and ankylosis (bony or fibrous)

DEF: Stiffening or union of temporomandibular joint due to bony or fibrous union across joint.

524.62 Arthralgia of temporomandibular joint

DEF: Pain in temporomandibular joint; not inflammatory in nature.

524.63 Articular disc disorder (reducing or non-reducing)

524.69 Other specified temporomandibular joint disorders

✓5th 524.7 Dental alveolar anomalies

524.70 Unspecified alveolar anomaly

524.71 Alveolar maxillary hyperplasia

DEF: Excessive tissue formation in the dental alveoli of upper jaw.

524.72 Alveolar mandibular hyperplasia

DEF: Excessive tissue formation in the dental alveoli of lower jaw.

524.73 Alveolar maxillary hypoplasia

DEF: Incomplete or underdeveloped, alveolar tissue of upper jaw.

524.74 Alveolar mandibular hypoplasia

DEF: Incomplete or underdeveloped, alveolar tissue of lower jaw.

524.79 Other specified alveolar anomaly

✓4th
✓5th   Additional Digit Required   Unspecified Code   Other Specified Code   Manifestation Code   ▶◀ Revised Text   ● New Code   ▲ Revised Code Title

2003 ICD•9•CM   **Volume 1 — 139**

Digestive System 524.8–528.1

524.8 Other specified dentofacial anomalies

524.9 Unspecified dentofacial anomalies

√4ᵗʰ **525 Other diseases and conditions of the teeth and supporting structures**

     525.0 Exfoliation of teeth due to systemic causes

         DEF: Deterioration of teeth and surrounding structures due to systemic disease.

     √5ᵗʰ **525.1 Loss of teeth due to trauma, extraction, or periodontal disease**

         525.10 Acquired absence of teeth, unspecified
            Edentulism
            Tooth extraction status, NOS

         525.11 Loss of teeth due to trauma

         525.12 Loss of teeth due to periodontal disease

         525.13 Loss of teeth due to caries

         525.19 Other loss of teeth

     525.2 Atrophy of edentulous alveolar ridge

     525.3 Retained dental root

     525.8 Other specified disorders of the teeth and supporting structures
         Enlargement of alveolar ridge NOS
         Irregular alveolar process

     525.9 Unspecified disorder of the teeth and supporting structures

√4ᵗʰ **526 Diseases of the jaws**

     526.0 Developmental odontogenic cysts
         Cyst: Cyst:
         dentigerous   lateral periodontal
         eruption   primordial
         follicular   Keratocyst
         lateral developmental
         EXCLUDES   radicular cyst (522.8)

     526.1 Fissural cysts of jaw
         Cyst:
         globulomaxillary
         incisor canal
         median anterior maxillary
         median palatal
         nasopalatine
         palatine of papilla
         EXCLUDES   cysts of oral soft tissues (528.4)

     526.2 Other cysts of jaws
         Cyst of jaw: Cyst of jaw:
         NOS   hemorrhagic
         aneurysmal   traumatic

     526.3 Central giant cell (reparative) granuloma
         EXCLUDES   peripheral giant cell granuloma (523.8)

     526.4 Inflammatory conditions
         Abscess
         Osteitis
         Osteomyelitis   } of jaw (acute) (chronic)
         (neonatal)   (suppurative)
         Periostitis

         Sequestrum of jaw bone
         EXCLUDES   alveolar osteitis (526.5)

     526.5 Alveolitis of jaw
         Alveolar osteitis
         Dry socket
         DEF: Inflammation, of alveoli or tooth socket.

     √5ᵗʰ **526.8 Other specified diseases of the jaws**
         526.81 Exostosis of jaw
            Torus mandibularis
            Torus palatinus
            DEF: Spur or bony outgrowth on the jaw.

         526.89 Other
            Cherubism
            Fibrous dysplasia   } of jaw(s)
            Latent bone cyst
            Osteoradionecrosis

         Unilateral condylar hyperplasia or hypoplasia of mandible

     526.9 Unspecified disease of the jaws

√4ᵗʰ **527 Diseases of the salivary glands**

     527.0 Atrophy
         DEF: Wasting away, necrosis of salivary gland tissue.

     527.1 Hypertrophy
         DEF: Overgrowth or overdeveloped salivary gland tissue.

     527.2 Sialoadenitis
         Parotitis: Sialoangitis
         NOS   Sialodochitis
         allergic
         toxic
         EXCLUDES   epidemic or infectious parotitis (072.0-072.9)
            uveoparotid fever (135)
         DEF: Inflammation of salivary gland.

     527.3 Abscess

     527.4 Fistula
         EXCLUDES   congenital fistula of salivary gland (750.24)

     527.5 Sialolithiasis
         Calculus   } of salivary gland or duct
         Stone
         Sialodocholithiasis

     527.6 Mucocele
         Mucous:
         extravasation cyst of salivary gland
         retention cyst of salivary gland
         Ranula
         DEF: Dilated salivary gland cavity filled with mucous.

     527.7 Disturbance of salivary secretion
         Hyposecretion   Sialorrhea
         Ptyalism   Xerostomia

     527.8 Other specified diseases of the salivary glands
         Benign lymphoepithelial lesion of salivary gland
         Sialectasia
         Sialosis
         Stenosis   } of salivary duct
         Stricture

     527.9 Unspecified disease of the salivary glands

√4ᵗʰ **528 Diseases of the oral soft tissues, excluding lesions specific for gingiva and tongue**

     528.0 Stomatitis
         Stomatitis: Vesicular stomatitis
         NOS
         ulcerative
         EXCLUDES   stomatitis:
            acute necrotizing ulcerative (101)
            aphthous (528.2)
            gangrenous (528.1)
            herpetic (054.2)
            Vincent's (101)
         DEF: Inflammation of oral mucosa; labial and buccal mucosa, tongue, plate, floor of the mouth, and gingivae.

     528.1 Cancrum oris
         Gangrenous stomatitis
         Noma
         DEF: A severely gangrenous lesion of mouth due to fusospirochetal infection; destroys buccal, labial and facial tissues; can be fatal; found primarily in debilitated and malnourished children.

528.2 Oral aphthae
Aphthous stomatitis
Canker sore
Periadenitis mucosa necrotica recurrens
Recurrent aphthous ulcer
Stomatitis herpetiformis
EXCLUDES *herpetic stomatitis (054.2)*

DEF: Small oval or round ulcers of the mouth marked by a grayish exudate and a red halo effect.

528.3 Cellulitis and abscess
Cellulitis of mouth (floor) Oral fistula
Ludwig's angina
EXCLUDES *abscess of tongue (529.0)*
cellulitis or abscess of lip (528.5)
fistula (of):
dental (522.7)
lip (528.5)
gingivitis (523.0-523.1)

528.4 Cysts
Dermoid cyst
Epidermoid cyst
Epstein's pearl   } of mouth
Lymphoepithelial cyst
Nasoalveolar cyst
Nasolabial cyst
EXCLUDES *cyst:*
gingiva (523.8)
tongue (529.8)

528.5 Diseases of lips
Abscess
Cellulitis   } of lip(s)
Fistula
Hypertrophy

Cheilitis: Cheilodynia
NOS   Cheilosis
angular
EXCLUDES *actinic cheilitis (692.79)*
congenital fistula of lip (750.25)
leukoplakia of lips (528.6)

528.6 Leukoplakia of oral mucosa, including tongue
Leukokeratosis of   Leukoplakia of:
oral mucosa   lips
Leukoplakia of: tongue
gingiva
EXCLUDES *carcinoma in situ (230.0, 232.0)*
leukokeratosis nicotina palati (528.7)

DEF: Thickened white patches of epithelium on mucous membranes of mouth.

528.7 Other disturbances of oral epithelium, including tongue

Erythroplakia
Focal epithelial hyperplasia } of mouth or tongue
Leukoedema

Leukokeratosis nicotina palati
EXCLUDES *carcinoma in situ (230.0, 232.0)*
leukokeratosis NOS (702)

528.8 Oral submucosal fibrosis, including of tongue
528.9 Other and unspecified diseases of the oral soft tissues
Cheek and lip biting
Denture sore mouth
Denture stomatitis
Melanoplakia
Papillary hyperplasia of palate
Eosinophilic granuloma
Irritative hyperplasia   } of oral mucosa
Pyogenic granuloma
Ulcer (traumatic)

√4th **529 Diseases and other conditions of the tongue**
529.0 Glossitis
Abscess   }
Ulceration (traumatic) } of tongue
EXCLUDES *glossitis:*
benign migratory (529.1)
Hunter's (529.4)
median rhomboid (529.2)
Moeller's (529.4)

529.1 Geographic tongue
Benign migratory glossitis
Glossitis areata exfoliativa

DEF: Chronic glossitis; marked by filiform papillae atrophy and inflammation; no known etiology.

529.2 Median rhomboid glossitis

DEF: A noninflammatory, congenital disease characterized by rhomboid-like lesions at the middle third of the tongue's dorsal surface.

529.3 Hypertrophy of tongue papillae
Black hairy tongue   Hypertrophy of foliate papillae
Coated tongue   Lingua villosa nigra

529.4 Atrophy of tongue papillae
Bald tongue   Glossitis:
Glazed tongue   Moeller's
Glossitis: Glossodynia exfoliativa
Hunter's   Smooth atrophic tongue

529.5 Plicated tongue
Fissured   }
Furrowed   } tongue
Scrotal   }
EXCLUDES *fissure of tongue, congenital (750.13)*

DEF: Cracks, fissures or furrows, on dorsal surface of tongue.

529.6 Glossodynia
Glossopyrosis   Painful tongue
EXCLUDES *glossodynia exfoliativa (529.4)*

529.8 Other specified conditions of the tongue

Atrophy
Crenated   }
Enlargement } (of) tongue
Hypertrophy }

Glossocele
Glossoptosis
EXCLUDES *erythroplasia of tongue (528.7)*
leukoplakia of tongue (528.6)
macroglossia (congenital) (750.15)
microglossia (congenital) (750.16)
oral submucosal fibrosis (528.8)

529.9 Unspecified condition of the tongue

DISEASES OF ESOPHAGUS, STOMACH, AND DUODENUM (530-537)

√4th **530 Diseases of esophagus**
EXCLUDES *esophageal varices (456.0-456.2)*

530.0 Achalasia and cardiospasm
Achalasia (of cardia) Megaesophagus
Aperistalsis of esophagus
EXCLUDES *congenital cardiospasm (750.7)*

DEF: Failure of smooth muscle fibers to relax, at gastrointestinal junctures; such as esophagogastric sphincter when swallowing.

√5th **530.1 Esophagitis**
Abscess of esophagus Esophagitis:
Esophagitis: peptic
NOS   postoperative
chemical   regurgitant
Use additional E code to identify cause, if induced
by chemical
EXCLUDES *tuberculous esophagitis (017.8)*

530.10 Esophagitis, unspecified

√4th √5th Additional Digit Required   Unspecified Code   Other Specified Code   Manifestation Code   ▶◀ Revised Text   ● New Code   ▲ Revised Code Title

530.11 Reflux esophagitis

DEF: Inflammation of lower esophagus; due to regurgitated gastric acid from malfunctioning lower esophageal sphincter; causes heartburn and substernal pain.

530.12 Acute esophagitis

DEF: ▶ An acute inflammation of the mucous lining or submucosal coat of the esophagus ◀

530.19 Other esophagitis

530.2 Ulcer of esophagus

Ulcer of esophagus
    fungal
    peptic
Ulcer of esophagus due to ingestion of:
    aspirin
    chemicals
    medicines
Use additional E code to identify cause, if induced by chemical or drug

530.3 Stricture and stenosis of esophagus

Compression of esophagus
Obstruction of esophagus

EXCLUDES   *congenital stricture of esophagus (750.3)*

530.4 Perforation of esophagus

Rupture of esophagus

EXCLUDES   *traumatic perforation of esophagus (862.22, 862.32, 874.4-874.5)*

530.5 Dyskinesia of esophagus

Corkscrew esophagus   Esophagospasm
Curling esophagus   Spasm of esophagus

EXCLUDES   *cardiospasm (530.0)*

DEF: Difficulty performing voluntary esophageal movements.

530.6 Diverticulum of esophagus, acquired

Diverticulum, acquired:
    epiphrenic
    pharyngoesophageal
    pulsion
    subdiaphragmatic
    traction
    Zenker's (hypopharyngeal)
Esophageal pouch, acquired
Esophagocele, acquired

EXCLUDES   *congenital diverticulum of esophagus (750.4)*

530.7 Gastroesophageal laceration-hemorrhage syndrome

Mallory-Weiss syndrome

DEF: Laceration of distal esophagus and proximal stomach due to vomiting, hiccups or other sustained activity.

✓5th 530.8 Other specified disorders of esophagus

530.81 Esophageal reflux

Gastroesophageal reflux

EXCLUDES   *reflux esophagitis (530.11)*

DEF: Regurgitation of the gastric contents into esophagus and possibly pharynx; where aspiration may occur between the vocal cords and down into the trachea.

Esophagus

Pharyngeal constrictors
Front view
Epiglottis
Cricoid cartilage
Trachea
C6
Pharyngoesophageal sphincter
Gastroesophageal sphincter
Diaphragm
Side view
Stomach

530.82 Esophageal hemorrhage

EXCLUDES   *hemorrhage due to esophageal varices (456.0-456.2)*

530.83 Esophageal leukoplakia

530.84 Tracheoesophageal fistula

EXCLUDES   *congenital tracheoesophageal fistula (750.3)*

530.89 Other

EXCLUDES   *Paterson-Kelly syndrome (280.8)*

530.9 Unspecified disorder of esophagus

✓4th 531 Gastric ulcer

INCLUDES   ulcer (peptic):
                prepyloric
                pylorus
                stomach

Use additional E code to identify drug, if drug-induced

EXCLUDES   *peptic ulcer NOS (533.0-533.9)*

The following fifth-digit subclassification is for use with category 531:

    0 without mention of obstruction
    1 with obstruction

DEF: Destruction of tissue in lumen of stomach due to action of gastric acid and pepsin on gastric mucosa decreasing resistance to ulcers.

✓5th 531.0 Acute with hemorrhage

✓5th 531.1 Acute with perforation

✓5th 531.2 Acute with hemorrhage and perforation

✓5th 531.3 Acute without mention of hemorrhage or perforation

✓5th 531.4 Chronic or unspecified with hemorrhage

✓5th 531.5 Chronic or unspecified with perforation

✓5th 531.6 Chronic or unspecified with hemorrhage and perforation

✓5th 531.7 Chronic without mention of hemorrhage or perforation

✓5th 531.9 Unspecified as acute or chronic, without mention of hemorrhage or perforation

✓4th 532 Duodenal ulcer

INCLUDES   erosion (acute) of duodenum
                ulcer (peptic):
                    duodenum
                    postpyloric

Use additional E code to identify drug, if drug-induced

EXCLUDES   *peptic ulcer NOS (533.0-533.9)*

The following fifth-digit subclassification is for use with category 532:

    0 without mention of obstruction
    1 with obstruction

DEF: Ulcers in duodenum due to action of gastric acid and pepsin on mucosa decreasing resistance to ulcers.

Stomach

Esophagus
Diaphragm
Cardiac portion
Stomach
Fundus
Pylorus
Greater curvature
Pancreas
Sphincter of Oddi
Pancreatic duct
Common bile duct
Proximal duodenum

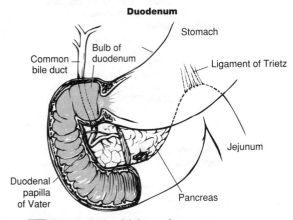

Duodenum

Stomach

Common bile duct

Bulb of duodenum

Ligament of Trietz

Jejunum

Duodenal papilla of Vater

Pancreas

✓5ᵗʰ	**532.0**	**Acute with hemorrhage**
✓5ᵗʰ	**532.1**	**Acute with perforation**
✓5ᵗʰ	**532.2**	**Acute with hemorrhage and perforation**
✓5ᵗʰ	**532.3**	**Acute without mention of hemorrhage or perforation**
✓5ᵗʰ	**532.4**	**Chronic or unspecified with hemorrhage**
✓5ᵗʰ	**532.5**	**Chronic or unspecified with perforation**
✓5ᵗʰ	**532.6**	**Chronic or unspecified with hemorrhage and perforation**
✓5ᵗʰ	**532.7**	**Chronic without mention of hemorrhage or perforation**
✓5ᵗʰ	**532.9**	**Unspecified as acute or chronic, without mention of hemorrhage or perforation**

✓4ᵗʰ **533 Peptic ulcer, site unspecified**

     INCLUDES   gastroduodenal ulcer NOS
                      peptic ulcer NOS
                      stress ulcer NOS

     Use additional E code to identify drug, if drug-induced

     EXCLUDES   *peptic ulcer:*
                  duodenal (532.0-532.9)
                  gastric (531.0-531.9)

The following fifth-digit subclassification is for use with category 533:
        0 without mention of obstruction
        1 with obstruction

✓5ᵗʰ	**533.0**	**Acute with hemorrhage**
✓5ᵗʰ	**533.1**	**Acute with perforation**
✓5ᵗʰ	**533.2**	**Acute with hemorrhage and perforation**
✓5ᵗʰ	**533.3**	**Acute without mention of hemorrhage and perforation**
✓5ᵗʰ	**533.4**	**Chronic or unspecified with hemorrhage**
✓5ᵗʰ	**533.5**	**Chronic or unspecified with perforation**
✓5ᵗʰ	**533.6**	**Chronic or unspecified with hemorrhage and perforation**
✓5ᵗʰ	**533.7**	**Chronic without mention of hemorrhage or perforation**
✓5ᵗʰ	**533.9**	**Unspecified as acute or chronic, without mention of hemorrhage or perforation**

✓4ᵗʰ **534 Gastrojejunal ulcer**

     INCLUDES   ulcer (peptic) or erosion:
                       anastomotic
                       gastrocolic
                       gastrointestinal
                       gastrojejunal
                       jejunal
                       marginal
                       stomal

     EXCLUDES   *primary ulcer of small intestine (569.82)*

The following fifth-digit subclassification is for use with category 534:
        0 without mention of obstruction
        1 with obstruction

✓5ᵗʰ	**534.0**	**Acute with hemorrhage**
✓5ᵗʰ	**534.1**	**Acute with perforation**
✓5ᵗʰ	**534.2**	**Acute with hemorrhage and perforation**
✓5ᵗʰ	**534.3**	**Acute without mention of hemorrhage or perforation**
✓5ᵗʰ	**534.4**	**Chronic or unspecified with hemorrhage**
✓5ᵗʰ	**534.5**	**Chronic or unspecified with perforation**
✓5ᵗʰ	**534.6**	**Chronic or unspecified with hemorrhage and perforation**
✓5ᵗʰ	**534.7**	**Chronic without mention of hemorrhage or perforation**
✓5ᵗʰ	**534.9**	**Unspecified as acute or chronic, without mention of hemorrhage or perforation**

✓4ᵗʰ **535 Gastritis and duodenitis**

The following fifth-digit subclassification is for use with category 535:
        0 without mention of hemorrhage
        1 with hemorrhage

✓5ᵗʰ	**535.0**	**Acute gastritis**
✓5ᵗʰ	**535.1**	**Atrophic gastritis**

        Gastritis: Gastritis:
          atrophic-hyperplastic   chronic (atrophic)

        DEF: Inflammation of stomach, with mucous membrane atrophy and peptic gland destruction.

✓5ᵗʰ	**535.2**	**Gastric mucosal hypertrophy**

        Hypertrophic gastritis

✓5ᵗʰ	**535.3**	**Alcoholic gastritis**
✓5ᵗʰ	**535.4**	**Other specified gastritis**

        Gastritis:
          allergic
          bile induced
          irritant
          superficial
          toxic

✓5ᵗʰ	**535.5**	**Unspecified gastritis and gastroduodenitis**
✓5ᵗʰ	**535.6**	**Duodenitis**

        DEF: Inflammation of intestine, between pylorus and jejunum.

✓4ᵗʰ **536 Disorders of function of stomach**

     EXCLUDES   *functional disorders of stomach specified as psychogenic (306.4)*

        536.0 Achlorhydria

        DEF: Absence of gastric acid due to gastric mucosa atrophy; unresponsive to histamines; also known as gastric anacidity.

        536.1 Acute dilatation of stomach

          Acute distention of stomach

        536.2 Persistent vomiting

          Habit vomiting
          Persistent vomiting [not of pregnancy]
          Uncontrollable vomiting

        EXCLUDES   *excessive vomiting in pregnancy (643.0-643.9)*
                       vomiting NOS (787.0)

Digestive System 532.0–536.2

✓4ᵗʰ / ✓5ᵗʰ   Additional Digit Required   Unspecified Code   Other Specified Code   Manifestation Code   ▶◀ Revised Text   ● New Code   ▲ Revised Code Title

2003 ICD•9•CM   **Volume 1 — 143**

Digestive System 536.3–543.9

536.3 Gastroparesis

DEF: Slight degree of paralysis within muscular coat of stomach.

√5th **536.4 Gastrostomy complications**

536.40 Gastrostomy complication, unspecified

536.41 Infection of gastrostomy

Use additional code to specify type of infection, such as:
abscess or cellulitis of abdomen (682.2)
septicemia (038.0-038.9)
Use additional code to identify organism (041.00-041.9)

536.42 Mechanical complication of gastrostomy

536.49 Other gastrostomy complications

536.8 Dyspepsia and other specified disorders of function of stomach

Achylia gastrica   Hyperchlorhydria
Hourglass contraction   Hypochlorhydria
    of stomach   Indigestion
Hyperacidity

EXCLUDES   achlorhydria (536.0)
            heartburn (787.1)

536.9 Unspecified functional disorder of stomach

Functional gastrointestinal:
disorder
disturbance
irritation

√4th **537 Other disorders of stomach and duodenum**

537.0 Acquired hypertrophic pyloric stenosis

Constriction ⎫
Obstruction ⎬ of pylorus, acquired or
Stricture ⎭   adult

EXCLUDES   congenital or infantile pyloric stenosis (750.5)

537.1 Gastric diverticulum

EXCLUDES   congenital diverticulum of stomach (750.7)

DEF: Herniated sac or pouch, within stomach or duodenum.

537.2 Chronic duodenal ileus

DEF: Persistent obstruction between pylorus and jejunum.

537.3 Other obstruction of duodenum

Cicatrix ⎫
Stenosis ⎬
Stricture ⎬ of duodenum
Volvulus ⎭

EXCLUDES   congenital obstruction of duodenum (751.1)

537.4 Fistula of stomach or duodenum

Gastrocolic fistula   Gastrojejunocolic fistula

537.5 Gastroptosis

DEF: Downward displacement of stomach.

537.6 Hourglass stricture or stenosis of stomach

Cascade stomach

EXCLUDES   congenital hourglass stomach (750.7)
            hourglass contraction of stomach (536.8)

√5th **537.8 Other specified disorders of stomach and duodenum**

537.81 Pylorospasm

EXCLUDES   congenital pylorospasm (750.5)

DEF: Spasm of the pyloric sphincter.

537.82 Angiodysplasia of stomach and duodenum (without mention of hemorrhage)

537.83 Angiodysplasia of stomach and duodenum with hemorrhage

DEF: Bleeding of stomach and duodenum due to vascular abnormalities.

● **537.84 Dieulafoy lesion (hemorrhagic) of stomach and duodenum**

537.89 Other

Gastric or duodenal:
prolapse
rupture
Intestinal metaplasia of gastric mucosa
Passive congestion of stomach

EXCLUDES   diverticula of duodenum (562.00-562.01)
            gastrointestinal hemorrhage (578.0-578.9)

537.9 Unspecified disorder of stomach and duodenum

APPENDICITIS (540-543)

√4th **540 Acute appendicitis**

DEF: Inflammation of vermiform appendix due to fecal obstruction, neoplasm or foreign body of appendiceal lumen; causes infection, edema and infarction of appendiceal wall; may result in mural necrosis, and perforation.

540.0 With generalized peritonitis

Appendicitis (acute): ⎫
fulminating   ⎬ with:
gangrenous   ⎬   perforation
obstructive   ⎬   peritonitis
Cecitis (acute)   ⎭   (generalized)
                 rupture

Rupture of appendix

EXCLUDES   acute appendicitis with peritoneal abscess (540.1)

540.1 With peritoneal abscess

With generalized peritonitis
Abscess of appendix

540.9 Without mention of peritonitis

Acute:
appendicitis: ⎫
fulminating   ⎬ without mention of
gangrenous   ⎬   perforation,
inflamed   ⎬   peritonitis, or rupture
obstructive   ⎬
cecitis   ⎭

541 Appendicitis, unqualified

542 Other appendicitis

Appendicitis: Appendicitis:
chronic   relapsing
recurrent   subacute

EXCLUDES   hyperplasia (lymphoid) of appendix (543.0)

√4th **543 Other diseases of appendix**

543.0 Hyperplasia of appendix (lymphoid)

DEF: Proliferation of cells in appendix tissue.

543.9 Other and unspecified diseases of appendix

Appendicular or appendiceal:
colic
concretion
fistula
Diverticulum ⎫
Fecalith   ⎬
Intussusception ⎬ of appendix
Mucocele   ⎬
Stercolith   ⎭

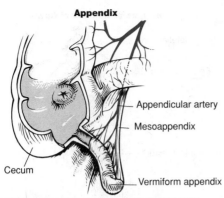

Appendix

Appendicular artery

Mesoappendix

Cecum

Vermiform appendix

HERNIA OF ABDOMINAL CAVITY (550-553)

INCLUDES   hernia:
acquired
congenital, except diaphragmatic or hiatal

✓4ᵗʰ **550 Inguinal hernia**

INCLUDES   bubonocele
inguinal hernia (direct) (double) (indirect)
(oblique) (sliding)
scrotal hernia

The following fifth-digit subclassification is for use with
category 550:

   **0 unilateral or unspecified (not specified as
       recurrent)**
       Unilateral NOS
   1 unilateral or unspecified, recurrent
   2 bilateral (not specified as recurrent)
       Bilateral NOS
   3 bilateral, recurrent

DEF: Hernia: protrusion of an abdominal organ or tissue through inguinal
canal.

DEF: Indirect inguinal hernia: (external or oblique) leaves abdomen through
deep inguinal ring, passes through inguinal canal lateral to the inferior
epigastric artery.

DEF: Direct inguinal hernia: (internal) emerges between inferior epigastric
artery and rectus muscle edge.

Inguinal Hernia

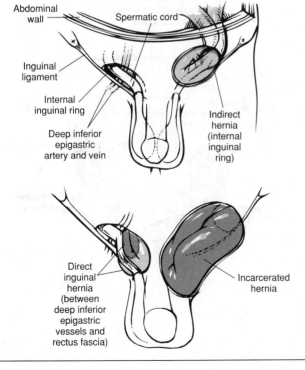

Abdominal
wall

Spermatic cord

Inguinal
ligament

Internal
inguinal ring

Indirect
hernia
(internal
inguinal
ring)

Deep inferior
epigastric
artery and vein

Direct
inguinal
hernia
(between
deep inferior
epigastric
vessels and
rectus fascia)

Incarcerated
hernia

✓5ᵗʰ **550.0 Inguinal hernia, with gangrene**
        Inguinal hernia with gangrene (and obstruction)

✓5ᵗʰ **550.1 Inguinal hernia, with obstruction, without mention
        of gangrene**
        Inguinal hernia with mention of incarceration,
        irreducibility, or strangulation

✓5ᵗʰ **550.9 Inguinal hernia, without mention of obstruction or
        gangrene**
        Inguinal hernia NOS

✓4ᵗʰ **551 Other hernia of abdominal cavity, with gangrene**
        INCLUDES   that with gangrene (and obstruction)

✓5ᵗʰ **551.0 Femoral hernia with gangrene**

        **551.00 Unilateral or unspecified (not specified as
                recurrent)**
                Femoral hernia NOS with gangrene

        551.01 Unilateral or unspecified, recurrent

        551.02 Bilateral (not specified as recurrent)

        551.03 Bilateral, recurrent

        551.1 Umbilical hernia with gangrene
                Parumbilical hernia specified as gangrenous

✓5ᵗʰ **551.2 Ventral hernia with gangrene**

        551.20 Ventral, unspecified, with gangrene

        551.21 Incisional, with gangrene
                Hernia:
                postoperative   } specified as
                recurrent, ventral } gangrenous

        551.29 Other
                Epigastric hernia specified as gangrenous

        551.3 Diaphragmatic hernia with gangrene
                Hernia:
                hiatal (esophageal) }
                (sliding)   } specified as
                paraesophageal   } gangrenous
                Thoracic stomach   }

                EXCLUDES   congenital diaphragmatic hernia
                            (756.6)

        551.8 Hernia of other specified sites, with gangrene
                Any condition classifiable to 553.8 if specified as
                gangrenous

        551.9 Hernia of unspecified site, with gangrene
                Any condition classifiable to 553.9 if specified as
                gangrenous

✓4ᵗʰ **552 Other hernia of abdominal cavity, with obstruction, but
        without mention of gangrene**
        EXCLUDES   that with mention of gangrene (551.0-551.9)

✓5ᵗʰ **552.0 Femoral hernia with obstruction**
                Femoral hernia specified as incarcerated,
                irreducible, strangulated, or causing
                obstruction

        **552.00 Unilateral or unspecified (not specified as
                recurrent)**

        552.01 Unilateral or unspecified, recurrent

        552.02 Bilateral (not specified as recurrent)

        552.03 Bilateral, recurrent

        552.1 Umbilical hernia with obstruction
                Parumbilical hernia specified as incarcerated,
                irreducible, strangulated, or causing
                obstruction

✓5ᵗʰ **552.2 Ventral hernia with obstruction**
                Ventral hernia specified as incarcerated, irreducible,
                strangulated, or causing obstruction

        552.20 Ventral, unspecified, with obstruction

✓4ᵗʰ
✓5ᵗʰ Additional Digit Required   Unspecified Code   Other Specified Code   Manifestation Code   ►◄ Revised Text   ● New Code   ▲ Revised Code Title

2003 ICD•9•CM   Volume 1 — 145

552.21 Incisional, with obstruction
Hernia:
postoperative
recurrent,   } specified as
ventral   incarcerated,
                    irreducible,
                    strangulated, or
                    causing
                    obstruction

552.29 Other
Epigastric hernia specified as incarcerated,
irreducible, strangulated, or causing
obstruction

552.3 Diaphragmatic hernia with obstruction
Hernia:
hiatal (esophageal)
(sliding)   } specified as incarcerated,
paraesophageal   irreducible,
Thoracic stomach   strangulated, or
                    causing obstruction

EXCLUDES *congenital diaphragmatic hernia
(756.6)*

**552.8 Hernia of other specified sites, with
obstruction**
Any condition classifiable to 553.8 if specified as
incarcerated, irreducible, strangulated, or
causing obstruction

552.9 Hernia of unspecified site, with obstruction
Any condition classifiable to 553.9 if specified as
incarcerated, irreducible, strangulated, or
causing obstruction

✓4ᵗʰ **553 Other hernia of abdominal cavity without mention of
obstruction or gangrene**
EXCLUDES *the listed conditions with mention of:
gangrene (and obstruction) (551.0-551.9)
obstruction (552.0-552.9)*

✓5ᵗʰ **553.0 Femoral hernia**
**553.00 Unilateral or unspecified (not specified as
recurrent)**
Femoral hernia NOS
553.01 Unilateral or unspecified, recurrent
553.02 Bilateral (not specified as recurrent)
553.03 Bilateral, recurrent
553.1 Umbilical hernia
Parumbilical hernia
✓5ᵗʰ **553.2 Ventral hernia**
553.20 Ventral, unspecified
553.21 Incisional
Hernia:
postoperative
recurrent, ventral
553.29 Other
Hernia:
epigastric
spigelian

Hernias of Abdominal Cavity

Hiatal hernia
Diaphragm
Epigastric hernia
Incisional hernia
Umbilical hernia
Inguinal hernia

553.3 Diaphragmatic hernia
Hernia:
hiatal (esophageal) (sliding)
paraesophageal
Thoracic stomach
EXCLUDES *congenital:
diaphragmatic hernia (756.6)
hiatal hernia (750.6)
esophagocele (530.6)*

553.8 Hernia of other specified sites
Hernia:
ischiatic
ischiorectal
lumbar
obturator
pudendal
retroperitoneal
sciatic
Other abdominal hernia of specified site
EXCLUDES *vaginal enterocele (618.6)*

553.9 Hernia of unspecified site
Enterocele
Epiplocele
Hernia:
NOS
interstitial
intestinal
intra-abdominal
Rupture (nontraumatic)
Sarcoepiplocele

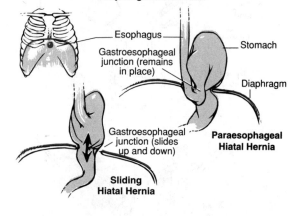

Diaphragmatic Hernia

Esophagus
Gastroesophageal
junction (remains
in place)
Stomach
Diaphragm
Gastroesophageal
junction (slides
up and down)
**Paraesophageal
Hiatal Hernia**
**Sliding
Hiatal Hernia**

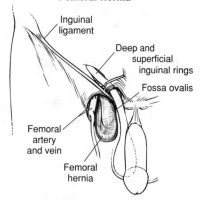

Femoral Hernia

Inguinal
ligament
Deep and
superficial
inguinal rings
Fossa ovalis
Femoral
artery
and vein
Femoral
hernia

NONINFECTIOUS ENTERITIS AND COLITIS (555-558)

☑4ᵗʰ **555 Regional enteritis**

> INCLUDES   Crohn's disease
>   Granulomatous enteritis
>   EXCLUDES   *ulcerative colitis (556)*

DEF: Inflammation of intestine; classified to site.

555.0 Small intestine

Ileitis:	Regional enteritis or
regional	Crohn's disease of:
segmental	duodenum
terminal	ileum
	jejunum

555.1 Large intestine

Colitis:	Regional enteritis or
granulmatous	Crohn's disease of:
regional	colon
transmural	large bowel
	rectum

555.2 Small intestine with large intestine
Regional ileocolitis

555.9 Unspecified site
Crohn's disease NOS
Regional enteritis NOS

☑4ᵗʰ **556 Ulcerative colitis**

DEF: Chronic inflammation of mucosal lining of intestinal tract; may be single area or entire colon.

556.0 Ulcerative (chronic) enterocolitis
556.1 Ulcerative (chronic) ileocolitis
556.2 Ulcerative (chronic) proctitis
556.3 Ulcerative (chronic) proctosigmoiditis
556.4 Pseudopolyposis of colon
556.5 Left-sided ulcerative (chronic) colitis
556.6 Universal ulcerative (chronic) colitis
Pancolitis
556.8 Other ulcerative colitis
556.9 Ulcerative colitis, unspecified
Ulcerative enteritis NOS

☑4ᵗʰ **557 Vascular insufficiency of intestine**

> EXCLUDES   *necrotizing enterocolitis of the newborn (777.5)*

DEF: Inadequacy of intestinal vessels.

557.0 Acute vascular insufficiency of intestine
Acute:
  hemorrhagic enterocolitis
  ischemic colitis, enteritis, or enterocolitis
  massive necrosis of intestine
Bowel infarction
Embolism of mesenteric artery
Fulminant enterocolitis
Hemorrhagic necrosis of intestine
Infarction of appendices epiploicae
Intestinal gangrene
Intestinal infarction (acute) (agnogenic)
  (hemorrhagic) (nonocclusive)
Mesenteric infarction (embolic) (thrombotic)
Necrosis of intestine
Terminal hemorrhagic enteropathy
Thrombosis of mesenteric artery

557.1 Chronic vascular insufficiency of intestine
Angina, abdominal
Chronic ischemic colitis, enteritis, or enterocolitis
Ischemic stricture of intestine
Mesenteric:
  angina
  artery syndrome (superior)
  vascular insufficiency

557.9 Unspecified vascular insufficiency of intestine
Alimentary pain due to vascular insufficiency
Ischemic colitis, enteritis, or enterocolitis NOS

☑4ᵗʰ **558 Other and unspecified noninfectious gastroenteritis and colitis**

> EXCLUDES   *infectious:*
>   *colitis, enteritis, or gastroenteritis (009.0-*
>   *009.1)*
>   *diarrhea (009.2-009.3)*

558.1 Gastroenteritis and colitis due to radiation
Radiation enterocolitis

558.2 Toxic gastroenteritis and colitis
Use additional E code, if desired, to identify cause

558.3 Allergic gastroenteritis and colitis
DEF: True immunoglobulin E (IgE)-mediated allergic reaction of the lining of the stomach, intestines, or colon to food proteins; causes nausea, vomiting, diarrhea, and abdominal cramping.

558.9 Other and unspecified noninfectious gastroenteritis and colitis

Colitis	
Enteritis	
Gastroenteritis	NOS, dietetic, or
Ileitis	noninfectious
Jejunitis	
Sigmoiditis	

OTHER DISEASES OF INTESTINES AND PERITONEUM (560-569)

☑4ᵗʰ **560 Intestinal obstruction without mention of hernia**

> EXCLUDES   *duodenum (537.2-537.3)*
>   *inguinal hernia with obstruction (550.1)*
>   *intestinal obstruction complicating hernia*
>   *(552.0-552.9)*
>   *mesenteric:*
>   *embolism (557.0)*
>   *infarction (557.0)*
>   *thrombosis (557.0)*
>   *neonatal intestinal obstruction (277.01, 777.1-*
>   *777.2, 777.4)*

560.0 Intussusception
Intussusception (colon) (intestine) (rectum)
Invagination of intestine or colon

> EXCLUDES   *intussusception of appendix (543.9)*

DEF: Prolapse of a bowel section into adjacent section; occurs primarily in children; symptoms include paroxysmal pain, vomiting, presence of lower abdominal tumor and blood, and mucous passage from rectum.

560.1 Paralytic ileus
Adynamic ileus
Ileus (of intestine) (of bowel) (of colon)
Paralysis of intestine or colon

> EXCLUDES   *gallstone ileus (560.31)*

DEF: Obstruction of ileus due to inhibited bowel motility.

560.2 Volvulus

Knotting	
Strangulation	of intestine, bowel, or
Torsion	colon
Twist	

DEF: Entanglement of bowel; causes obstruction; may compromise bowel circulation.

Large Intestine

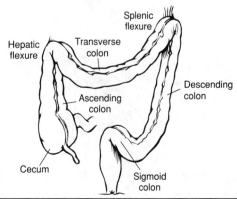

☑4ᵗʰ   Additional Digit Required   Unspecified Code   Other Specified Code   Manifestation Code   ▶◀ Revised Text   ● New Code   ▲ Revised Code Title

2003 ICD•9•CM   **Volume 1 — 147**

Digestive System 560.3–564.6

☑5ᵗʰ **560.3　Impaction of intestine**
　560.30　Impaction of intestine, unspecified
　　　Impaction of colon
　560.31　Gallstone ileus
　　　Obstruction of intestine by gallstone
　560.39　Other
　　　Concretion of intestine
　　　Enterolith
　　　Fecal impaction

☑5ᵗʰ **560.8　Other specified intestinal obstruction**
　560.81　Intestinal or peritoneal adhesions with obstruction (postoperative) (postinfection)
　　　EXCLUDES　*adhesions without obstruction (568.0)*
　　　DEF: Obstruction of peritoneum or intestine due to abnormal union of tissues.
　560.89　Other
　　　Mural thickening causing obstruction
　　　EXCLUDES　*ischemic stricture of intestine (557.1)*

　560.9　Unspecified intestinal obstruction
　　　Enterostenosis
　　　Obstruction
　　　Occlusion　　　⎫
　　　Stenosis　　　⎬　of intestine or colon
　　　Stricture　　　⎭
　　　EXCLUDES　*congenital stricture or stenosis of intestine (751.1-751.2)*

☑4ᵗʰ **562　Diverticula of intestine**
　　Use additional code to identify any associated:
　　peritonitis (567.0-567.9)
　　EXCLUDES　*congenital diverticulum of colon (751.5)*
　　　　　　　diverticulum of appendix (543.9)
　　　　　　　Meckel's diverticulum (751.0)

☑5ᵗʰ **562.0　Small intestine**
　562.00　Diverticulosis of small intestine (without mention of hemorrhage)
　　　Diverticulosis:　　　⎫
　　　　duodenum　　　⎬　without mention of
　　　　ileum　　　　　⎬　　diverticulitis
　　　　jejunum　　　 ⎭
　　　DEF: Saclike herniations of mucous lining of small intestine.

　562.01　Diverticulitis of small intestine (without mention of hemorrhage)
　　　Diverticulitis (with diverticulosis):
　　　　duodenum
　　　　ileum
　　　　jejunum
　　　　small intestine
　　　DEF: Inflamed saclike herniations of mucous lining of small intestine.

Volvulus, Diverticulitis

Knotted intestine (volvulus)

Diverticulum

　562.02　Diverticulosis of small intestine with hemorrhage
　562.03　Diverticulitis of small intestine with hemorrhage

☑5ᵗʰ **562.1　Colon**
　562.10　Diverticulosis of colon (without mention of hemorrhage)
　　　Diverticulosis:　　　⎫
　　　　NOS　　　　　　　⎬　without mention
　　　　intestine (large)　⎬　　of
　　　Diverticular disease ⎬　　diverticulitis
　　　　(colon)　　　　　 ⎭
　　　DEF: Saclike herniations of mucous lining of large intestine

　562.11　Diverticulitis of colon (without mention of hemorrhage)
　　　Diverticulitis (with diverticulosis):
　　　　NOS　　　　　intestine (large)
　　　　colon
　　　DEF: Inflamed saclike herniations of mucosal lining of large intestine.

　562.12　Diverticulosis of colon with hemorrhage
　562.13　Diverticulitis of colon with hemorrhage

☑4ᵗʰ **564　Functional digestive disorders, not elsewhere classified**
　　EXCLUDES　*functional disorders of stomach (536.0-536.9)*
　　　　　　　those specified as psychogenic (306.4)

☑5ᵗʰ **564.0　Constipation**
　564.00　Constipation, unspecified
　564.01　Slow transit constipation
　　　DEF: ▶ Delay in the transit of fecal material through the colon secondary to smooth muscle dysfunction or decreased peristaltic contractions along the colon: also called colonic inertia or delayed transit. ◀
　564.02　Outlet dysfunction constipation
　　　DEF: ▶Failure to relax the paradoxical contractions of the striated pelvic floor muscles during the attempted defecation.◀
　564.09　Other constipation
　564.1　Irritable bowel syndrome
　　　Irritable colon
　　　Spastic colon
　　　DEF: Functional gastrointestinal disorder (FGID); symptoms following meals include diarrhea, constipation, abdominal pain; other symptoms include bloating, gas, distended abdomen, nausea, vomiting, appetite loss, emotional distress, and depression.

　564.2　Postgastric surgery syndromes
　　　Dumping syndrome　　Postgastrectomy syndrome
　　　Jejunal syndrome　　　Postvagotomy syndrome
　　　EXCLUDES　*malnutrition following gastrointestinal surgery (579.3)*
　　　　　　　postgastrojejunostomy ulcer (534.0-534.9)

　564.3　Vomiting following gastrointestinal surgery
　　　Vomiting (bilious) following gastrointestinal surgery
　564.4　Other postoperative functional disorders
　　　Diarrhea following gastrointestinal surgery
　　　EXCLUDES　*colostomy and enterostomy complications (569.60-569.69)*

　564.5　Functional diarrhea
　　　EXCLUDES　*diarrhea:*
　　　　　　　NOS (787.91)
　　　　　　　psychogenic (306.4)
　　　DEF: Diarrhea with no detectable organic cause.

　564.6　Anal spasm
　　　Proctalgia fugax

N Newborn Age: 0　　　　P Pediatric Age: 0-17　　　　M Maternity Age: 12-55　　　　A Adult Age: 15-124　　　　MSP Medicare Secondary Payer

564.7 Megacolon, other than Hirschsprung's
Dilatation of colon

> EXCLUDES megacolon:
> congenital [Hirschsprung's] (751.3)
> toxic (556)

DEF: Enlarged colon; congenital or acquired; can occur acutely or become chronic.

✓5th **564.8 Other specified functional disorders of intestine**
> EXCLUDES malabsorption (579.0-579.9)

564.81 Neurogenic bowel
DEF: Disorder of bowel due to spinal cord lesion above conus medullaris; symptoms include precipitous micturition, nocturia, catheter intolerance, headache, sweating, nasal obstruction and spastic contractions.

564.89 Other functional disorders of intestine
Atony of colon
DEF: Absence of normal bowel tone or strength.

564.9 Unspecified functional disorder of intestine

✓4th **565 Anal fissure and fistula**

565.0 Anal fissure
Tear of anus, nontraumatic
> EXCLUDES traumatic (863.89, 863.99)

DEF: Ulceration of cleft at anal mucosa; causes pain, itching, bleeding, infection, and sphincter spasm; may occur with hemorrhoids.

565.1 Anal fistula
Fistula:
anorectal
rectal
rectum to skin
> EXCLUDES fistula of rectum to internal organs—
> see Alphabetic Index
> ischiorectal fistula (566)
> rectovaginal fistula (619.1)

DEF: Abnormal opening on cutaneous surface near anus; may lack connection with rectum.

566 Abscess of anal and rectal regions
Abscess:
ischiorectal
perianal
perirectal
Cellulitis:
anal
perirectal
rectal
Ischiorectal fistula

✓4th **567 Peritonitis**
> EXCLUDES peritonitis:
> benign paroxysmal (277.3)
> pelvic, female (614.5, 614.7)
> periodic familial (277.3)
> puerperal (670)
> with or following:
> abortion (634-638 with .0, 639.0)
> appendicitis (540.0-540.1)
> ectopic or molar pregnancy (639.0)

DEF: Inflammation of the peritoneal cavity.

567.0 *Peritonitis in infectious diseases classified elsewhere*
Code first underlying disease
> EXCLUDES peritonitis:
> gonococcal (098.86)
> syphilitic (095.2)
> tuberculous (014.0)

567.1 Pneumococcal peritonitis

567.2 Other suppurative peritonitis
Abscess (of):	Abscess (of):
abdominopelvic	subhepatic
mesenteric	subphrenic
omentum	Peritonitis (acute):
peritoneum	general
retrocecal	pelvic, male
retroperitoneal	subphrenic
subdiaphragmatic	suppurative

567.8 Other specified peritonitis
Chronic proliferative peritonitis	Peritonitis due to:
	bile
Fat necrosis of peritoneum	urine
Mesenteric saponification	

567.9 Unspecified peritonitis
Peritonitis:	Peritonitis:
NOS	of unspecified cause

✓4th **568 Other disorders of peritoneum**

568.0 Peritoneal adhesions (postoperative) (postinfection)
Adhesions (of):	Adhesions (of):
abdominal (wall)	mesenteric
diaphragm	omentum
intestine	stomach
male pelvis	Adhesive bands
> EXCLUDES adhesions:
> pelvic, female (614.6)
> with obstruction:
> duodenum (537.3)
> intestine (560.81)

DEF: Abnormal union of tissues in peritoneum.

✓5th **568.8 Other specified disorders of peritoneum**
568.81 Hemoperitoneum (nontraumatic)
568.82 Peritoneal effusion (chronic)
> EXCLUDES ascites NOS (789.5)

DEF: Persistent leakage of fluid within peritoneal cavity.

Anal Fistula and Abscess

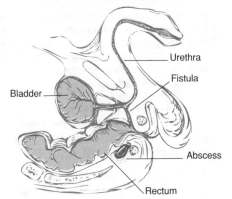

Urethra
Fistula
Bladder
Abscess
Rectum

Rectum and Anus

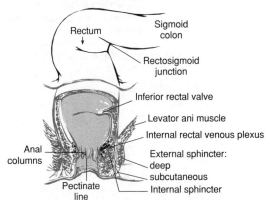

Rectum
Sigmoid colon
Rectosigmoid junction
Inferior rectal valve
Levator ani muscle
Internal rectal venous plexus
External sphincter:
deep
subcutaneous
Internal sphincter
Anal columns
Pectinate line

✓4th ✓5th Additional Digit Required Unspecified Code Other Specified Code Manifestation Code ▶◀ Revised Text ● New Code ▲ Revised Code Title

2003 ICD•9•CM Volume 1 — 149

568.89 Other
Peritoneal:
cyst
granuloma

568.9 Unspecified disorder of peritoneum

√4th **569 Other disorders of intestine**

569.0 Anal and rectal polyp
Anal and rectal polyp NOS
EXCLUDES adenomatous anal and rectal polyp (211.4)

569.1 Rectal prolapse
Procidentia:
anus (sphincter)
rectum (sphincter)
Proctoptosis
Prolapse:
anal canal
rectal mucosa
EXCLUDES prolapsed hemorrhoids (455.2, 455.5)

569.2 Stenosis of rectum and anus
Stricture of anus (sphincter)

569.3 Hemorrhage of rectum and anus
EXCLUDES gastrointestinal bleeding NOS (578.9)
melena (578.1)

√5th **569.4 Other specified disorders of rectum and anus**

569.41 Ulcer of anus and rectum
Solitary ulcer } of anus (sphincter) or
Stercoral ulcer } rectum (sphincter)

569.42 Anal or rectal pain

569.49 Other
Granuloma } of rectum (sphincter)
Rupture }

Hypertrophy of anal papillae
Proctitis NOS
EXCLUDES fistula of rectum to:
internal organs—see
Alphabetic Index
skin (565.1)
hemorrhoids (455.0-455.9)
incontinence of sphincter ani
(787.6)

569.5 Abscess of intestine
EXCLUDES appendiceal abscess (540.1)

√5th **569.6 Colostomy and enterostomy complications**
DEF: Complication in a surgically created opening, from intestine to surface skin.

569.60 Colostomy and enterostomy complication, unspecified

569.61 Infection of colostomy or enterostomy
Use additional code to identify organism (041.00-041.9)
Use additional code to specify type of infection, such as:
abscess or cellulitis of abdomen (682.2)
septicemia (038.0-038.9)

569.62 Mechanical complication of colostomy and enterostomy
Malfunction of colostomy and enterostomy

569.69 Other complication
Fistula
Hernia
Prolapse

√5th **569.8 Other specified disorder of intestine**

569.81 Fistula of intestine, excluding rectum and anus
Fistula: Fistula:
abdominal wall   enteroenteric
enterocolic   ileorectal
EXCLUDES fistula of intestine to internal organs—see Alphabetic Index
persistent postoperative fistula (998.6)

569.82 Ulceration of intestine
Primary ulcer of intestine
Ulceration of colon
EXCLUDES that with perforation (569.83)

569.83 Perforation of intestine

569.84 Angiodysplasia of intestine (without mention of hemorrhage)
DEF: Small vascular abnormalities of the intestinal tract without bleeding problems.

569.85 Angiodysplasia of intestine with hemorrhage
DEF: Small vascular abnormalities of the intestinal tract with bleeding problems.

569.86 Dieulafoy lesion (hemorrhagic) of intestine

569.89 Other
Enteroptosis
Granuloma } of intestine
Prolapse }

Pericolitis
Perisigmoiditis
Visceroptosis
EXCLUDES gangrene of intestine, mesentery, or omentum (557.0)
hemorrhage of intestine NOS (578.9)
obstruction of intestine (560.0-560.9)

569.9 Unspecified disorder of intestine

OTHER DISEASES OF DIGESTIVE SYSTEM (570-579)

570 Acute and subacute necrosis of liver
Acute hepatic failure
Acute or subacute hepatitis, not specified as infective
Necrosis of liver (acute) (diffuse) (massive) (subacute)
Parenchymatous degeneration of liver
Yellow atrophy (liver) (acute) (subacute)
EXCLUDES icterus gravis of newborn (773.0-773.2)
serum hepatitis (070.2-070.3)
that with:
abortion (634-638 with .7, 639.8)
ectopic or molar pregnancy (639.8)
pregnancy, childbirth, or the puerperium (646.7)
viral hepatitis (070.0-070.9)

√4th **571 Chronic liver disease and cirrhosis**

571.0 Alcoholic fatty liver   A

571.1 Acute alcoholic hepatitis   A
Acute alcoholic liver disease

571.2 Alcoholic cirrhosis of liver   A
Florid cirrhosis
Laennec's cirrhosis (alcoholic)
DEF: Fibrosis and dysfunction, of liver; due to alcoholic liver disease.

571.3 Alcoholic liver damage, unspecified   A

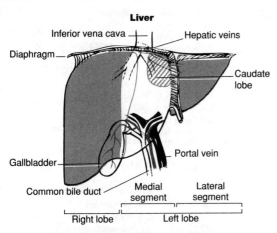

Liver

☑5ᵗʰ **571.4 Chronic hepatitis**
> EXCLUDES *viral hepatitis (acute) (chronic) (070.0-070.9)*

571.40 Chronic hepatitis, unspecified

571.41 Chronic persistent hepatitis

571.49 Other
Chronic hepatitis:
active
aggressive
Recurrent hepatitis

571.5 Cirrhosis of liver without mention of alcohol
Cirrhosis of liver: Cirrhosis of liver:
NOS   postnecrotic
cryptogenic   Healed yellow atrophy
macronodular   (liver)
micronodular   Portal cirrhosis
posthepatitic
DEF: Fibrosis and dysfunction of liver; not alcohol related.

571.6 Biliary cirrhosis
Chronic nonsuppurative destructive cholangitis
Cirrhosis:
cholangitic
cholestatic

571.8 Other chronic nonalcoholic liver disease
Chronic yellow atrophy (liver)
Fatty liver, without mention of alcohol

571.9 Unspecified chronic liver disease without mention of alcohol

☑4ᵗʰ **572 Liver abscess and sequelae of chronic liver disease**

572.0 Abscess of liver
> EXCLUDES *amebic liver abscess (006.3)*

572.1 Portal pyemia
Phlebitis of portal vein   Pylephlebitis
Portal thrombophlebitis   Pylethrombophlebitis
DEF: Inflammation of portal vein or branches; may be due to intestinal disease; symptoms include fever, chills, jaundice, sweating, and abscess in various body parts.

572.2 Hepatic coma
Hepatic encephalopathy
Hepatocerebral intoxication
Portal-systemic encephalopathy

572.3 Portal hypertension
DEF: Abnormally high blood pressure in the portal vein.

572.4 Hepatorenal syndrome
> EXCLUDES *that following delivery (674.8)*
DEF: Hepatic and renal failure characterized by cirrhosis with ascites or obstructive jaundice, oliguria, and low sodium concentration.

572.8 Other sequelae of chronic liver disease

☑4ᵗʰ **573 Other disorders of liver**
> EXCLUDES *amyloid or lardaceous degeneration of liver (277.3)*
> *congenital cystic disease of liver (751.62)*
> *glycogen infiltration of liver (271.0)*
> *hepatomegaly NOS (789.1)*
> *portal vein obstruction (452)*

573.0 Chronic passive congestion of liver
DEF: Blood accumulation in liver tissue.

573.1 Hepatitis in viral diseases classified elsewhere
Code first underlying disease as:
Coxsackie virus disease (074.8)
cytomegalic inclusion virus disease (078.5)
infectious mononucleosis (075)
> EXCLUDES *hepatitis (in):*
> *mumps (072.71)*
> *viral (070.0-070.9)*
> *yellow fever (060.0-060.9)*

573.2 Hepatitis in other infectious diseases classified elsewhere
Code first underlying disease, as:
malaria (084.9)
> EXCLUDES *hepatitis in:*
> *late syphilis (095.3)*
> *secondary syphilis (091.62)*
> *toxoplasmosis (130.5)*

573.3 Hepatitis, unspecified
Toxic (noninfectious) hepatitis
Use additional E code to identify cause

573.4 Hepatic infarction

573.8 Other specified disorders of liver
Hepatoptosis

573.9 Unspecified disorder of liver

☑4ᵗʰ **574 Cholelithiasis**
The following fifth-digit subclassification is for use with category 574:
   0 without mention of obstruction
   1 with obstruction

☑5ᵗʰ **574.0 Calculus of gallbladder with acute cholecystitis** ▲
Biliary calculus
Calculus of cystic duct } with acute cholecystitis
Cholelithiasis
Any condition classifiable to 574.2 with acute cholecystitis

☑5ᵗʰ **574.1 Calculus of gallbladder with other cholecystitis** ▲
Biliary calculus
Calculus of cystic duct } with cholecystitis
Cholelithiasis
Cholecystitis with cholelithiasis NOS
Any condition classifiable to 574.2 with cholecystitis (chronic)

Gallbladder and Bile Ducts

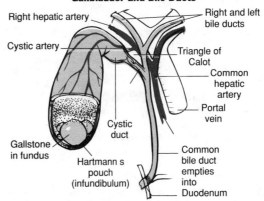

☑4ᵗʰ / ☑5ᵗʰ Additional Digit Required   Unspecified Code   Other Specified Code   Manifestation Code   ▶◀ Revised Text   ● New Code   ▲ Revised Code Title

2003 ICD•9•CM   **Volume 1 — 151**

Digestive System 574.2–576.9

§ ✓5ᵗʰ **574.2 Calculus of gallbladder without mention of cholecystitis**   A

    Biliary: Cholelithiasis NOS
        calculus NOS   Colic (recurrent) of
        colic NOS   gallbladder
    Calculus of cystic duct   Gallstone (impacted)

§ ✓5ᵗʰ **574.3 Calculus of bile duct with acute cholecystitis**   A

    Calculus of bile
       duct [any]   } with acute cholecystitis
    Choledocholithiasis

    Any condition classifiable to 574.5 with acute
       cholecystitis

§ ✓5ᵗʰ **574.4 Calculus of bile duct with other cholecystitis**   A

    Calculus of bile duct
       [any]   } with cholecystitis
    Choledocholithiasis   (chronic)

    Any condition classifiable to 574.5 with cholecystitis
       (chronic)

§ ✓5ᵗʰ **574.5 Calculus of bile duct without mention of cholecystitis**   A

    Calculus of: Choledocholithiasis
       bile duct [any]   Hepatic:
       common duct   colic (recurrent)
       hepatic duct   lithiasis

§ ✓5ᵗʰ **574.6 Calculus of gallbladder and bile duct with acute cholecystitis**   A

    Any condition classifiable to 574.0 and 574.3

§ ✓5ᵗʰ **574.7 Calculus of gallbladder and bile duct with other cholecystitis**   A

    Any condition classifiable to 574.1 and 574.4

§ ✓5ᵗʰ **574.8 Calculus of gallbladder and bile duct with acute and chronic cholecystitis**   A

    Any condition classifiable to 574.6 and 574.7

§ ✓5ᵗʰ **574.9 Calculus of gallbladder and bile duct without cholecystitis**   A

    Any condition classifiable to 574.2 and 574.5

✓4ᵗʰ **575 Other disorders of gallbladder**

    575.0 Acute cholecystitis   A

       Abscess of gallbladder
       Angiocholecystitis
       Cholecystitis:
          emphysematous (acute)   } without mention
          gangrenous   of calculus
          suppurative
       Empyema of gallbladder
       Gangrene of gallbladder

       EXCLUDES   *that with:*
            acute and chronic cholecystitis
              (575.12)
            choledocholithiasis (574.3)
            choledocholithiasis and
              cholelithiasis (574.6)
            cholelithiasis (574.0)

    ✓5ᵗʰ **575.1 Other cholecystitis**   A

       Cholecystitis:
          NOS   } without mention of calculus
          chronic

       EXCLUDES   *that with:*
            choledocholithiasis (574.4)
            choledocholithiasis and
              cholelithiasis (574.8)
            cholelithiasis (574.1)

    575.10 Cholecystitis, unspecified
       Cholecystitis NOS

    575.11 Chronic cholecystitis

    575.12 Acute and chronic cholecystitis

    575.2 Obstruction of gallbladder   A

       Occlusion
       Stenosis   } of cystic duct or gallbladder without
       Stricture   mention of calculus

       EXCLUDES   *that with calculus (574.0-574.2 with*
                  fifth-digit 1)

    575.3 Hydrops of gallbladder   A
       Mucocele of gallbladder
       DEF: Serous fluid accumulation in bladder.

    575.4 Perforation of gallbladder
       Rupture of cystic duct or gallbladder

    575.5 Fistula of gallbladder
       Fistula: Fistula:
         cholecystoduodenal   cholecystoenteric

    575.6 Cholesterolosis of gallbladder
       Strawberry gallbladder
       DEF: Cholesterol deposits in gallbladder tissue.

    575.8 Other specified disorders of gallbladder

       Adhesions
       Atrophy
       Cyst
       Hypertrophy   } (of) cystic duct or gallbladder
       Nonfunctioning
       Ulcer

       Biliary dyskinesia
       EXCLUDES   *Hartmann's pouch of intestine (V44.3)*
                  nonvisualization of gallbladder (793.3)

    575.9 Unspecified disorder of gallbladder

✓4ᵗʰ **576 Other disorders of biliary tract**
       EXCLUDES   *that involving the:*
            cystic duct (575.0-575.9)
            gallbladder (575.0-575.9)

    576.0 Postcholecystectomy syndrome   A
       DEF: Jaundice or abdominal pain following cholecystectomy.

    576.1 Cholangitis
       Cholangitis: Cholangitis:
         NOS   recurrent
         acute   sclerosing
         ascending   secondary
         chronic   stenosing
         primary   suppurative

    576.2 Obstruction of bile duct
       Occlusion   } of bile duct, except cystic
       Stenosis   duct, without mention
       Stricture   of calculus

       EXCLUDES   *congenital (751.61)*
            that with calculus (574.3-574.5 with
                fifth-digit 1)

    576.3 Perforation of bile duct
       Rupture of bile duct, except cystic duct

    576.4 Fistula of bile duct
       Choledochoduodenal fistula

    576.5 Spasm of sphincter of Oddi

    576.8 Other specified disorders of biliary tract

       Adhesions
       Atrophy
       Cyst
       Hypertrophy   } of bile duct [any]
       Stasis
       Ulcer

       EXCLUDES   *congenital choledochal cyst (751.69)*

    576.9 Unspecified disorder of biliary tract

---

§ Requires fifth-digit. See beginning of category 574 for codes and definitions.

N Newborn Age: 0   P Pediatric Age: 0-17   M Maternity Age: 12-55   A Adult Age: 15-124   MSP Medicare Secondary Payer

Pancreas

Head   Neck   Body   Tail

Common bile duct

Accesory pancreatic duct

Spleen

Pancreatic duct (of Wirsung)

Uncinate process

Duodenum

Superior mesenteric artery and vein

✓4ᵗʰ 577 Diseases of pancreas

577.0 Acute pancreatitis

Abscess of pancreas   Pancreatitis:
Necrosis of pancreas: acute (recurrent)
   acute   apoplectic
   infective   hemorrhagic
Pancreatitis: subacute
   NOS   suppurative

     EXCLUDES   *mumps pancreatitis (072.3)*

A

577.1 Chronic pancreatitis

Chronic pancreatitis: Pancreatitis:
   NOS   painless
   infectious   recurrent
   interstitial   relapsing

577.2 Cyst and pseudocyst of pancreas

577.8 Other specified diseases of pancreas

Atrophy
Calculus
Cirrhosis   } of pancreas
Fibrosis

Pancreatic: Pancreatic:
   infantilism   necrosis:
   necrosis: fat
     NOS   Pancreatolithiasis
     aseptic

     EXCLUDES   *fibrocystic disease of pancreas*
                 ▶*(277.00-277.09)*◀
                 islet cell tumor of pancreas (211.7)
                 pancreatic steatorrhea (579.4)

577.9 Unspecified disease of pancreas

✓4ᵗʰ 578 Gastrointestinal hemorrhage

     EXCLUDES   *that with mention of:*
         angiodysplasia of stomach and duodenum
            (537.83)
         angiodysplasia of intestine (569.85)
         diverticulitis, intestine:
            large (562.13)
            small (562.03)
         diverticulosis, intestine:
            large (562.12)
            small (562.02)
         gastritis and duodenitis (535.0-535.6)
         ulcer:
            duodenal, gastric, gastrojejuunal or peptic
            (531.00-534.91)

578.0 Hematemesis
     Vomiting of blood

578.1 Blood in stool
     Melena

     EXCLUDES   *melena of the newborn (772.4, 777.3)*
                 occult blood (792.1)

578.9 Hemorrhage of gastrointestinal tract, unspecified
     Gastric hemorrhage
     Intestinal hemorrhage

✓4ᵗʰ 579 Intestinal malabsorption

579.0 Celiac disease

Celiac: Gee (-Herter) disease
   crisis   Gluten enteropathy
   infantilism   Idiopathic steatorrhea
   rickets   Nontropical sprue

DEF: Malabsorption syndrome due to gluten consumption; symptoms include fetid, bulky, frothy, oily stools; distended abdomen, gas, weight loss, asthenia, electrolyte depletion and vitamin B, D and K deficiency.

579.1 Tropical sprue

Sprue: Tropical steatorrhea
   NOS
   tropical

DEF: Diarrhea, occurs in tropics; may be due to enteric infection and malnutrition.

579.2 Blind loop syndrome
     Postoperative blind loop syndrome

DEF: Obstruction or impaired passage in small intestine due to alterations, from strictures or surgery; causes stasis, abnormal bacterial flora, diarrhea, weight loss, multiple vitamin deficiency, and megaloblastic anemia.

579.3 Other and unspecified postsurgical nonabsorption

Hypoglycemia   } following gastrointestinal
Malnutrition   surgery

579.4 Pancreatic steatorrhea

DEF: Excess fat in feces due to absence of pancreatic juice in intestine.

579.8 Other specified intestinal malabsorption

Enteropathy: Steatorrhea (chronic)
   exudative
   protein-losing

579.9 Unspecified intestinal malabsorption
     Malabsorption syndrome NOS

✓4ᵗʰ / ✓5ᵗʰ Additional Digit Required   Unspecified Code   Other Specified Code   Manifestation Code   ▶◀ Revised Text   ● New Code   ▲ Revised Code Title

2003 ICD•9•CM   **October 2002 • Volume 1 — 153**

Kidney

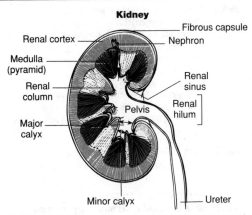

- Renal cortex
- Fibrous capsule
- Nephron
- Medulla (pyramid)
- Renal column
- Renal sinus
- Renal hilum
- Pelvis
- Major calyx
- Minor calyx
- Ureter

10. DISEASES OF THE GENITOURINARY SYSTEM (580-629)

NEPHRITIS, NEPHROTIC SYNDROME, AND NEPHROSIS (580-589)

EXCLUDES *hypertensive renal disease (403.00-403.91)*

√4th 580 Acute glomerulonephritis

INCLUDES acute nephritis

DEF: Acute, severe inflammation in tuft of capillaries that filter the kidneys.

580.0 With lesion of proliferative glomerulonephritis
Acute (diffuse) proliferative glomerulonephritis
Acute poststreptococcal glomerulonephritis

580.4 With lesion of rapidly progressive glomerulonephritis
Acute nephritis with lesion of necrotizing glomerulitis

DEF: Acute glomerulonephritis; progresses to ESRD with diffuse epithelial proliferation.

√5th 580.8 With other specified pathological lesion in kidney

580.81 Acute glomerulonephritis in diseases classified elsewhere
Code first underlying disease, as:
infectious hepatitis (070.0-070.9)
mumps (072.79)
subacute bacterial endocarditis (421.0)
typhoid fever (002.0)

580.89 Other
Glomerulonephritis, acute, with lesion of:
exudative nephritis
interstitial (diffuse) (focal) nephritis

580.9 Acute glomerulonephritis with unspecified pathological lesion in kidney

Glomerulonephritis:
NOS
hemorrhagic
Nephritis
Nephropathy
    } specified as acute

Nephron

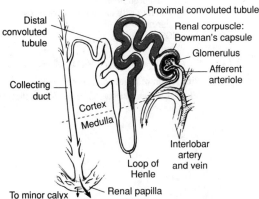

- Distal convoluted tubule
- Proximal convoluted tubule
- Renal corpuscle: Bowman's capsule
- Glomerulus
- Afferent arteriole
- Collecting duct
- Cortex
- Medulla
- Interlobar artery and vein
- Loop of Henle
- Renal papilla
- To minor calyx

√4th 581 Nephrotic syndrome

DEF: Disease process marked by symptoms such as; extensive edema, notable proteinuria, hypoalbuminemia, and susceptibility to intercurrent infections.

581.0 With lesion of proliferative glomerulonephritis

581.1 With lesion of membranous glomerulonephritis
Epimembranous nephritis
Idiopathic membranous glomerular disease
Nephrotic syndrome with lesion of:
focal glomerulosclerosis
sclerosing membranous glomerulonephritis
segmental hyalinosis

581.2 With lesion of membranoproliferative glomerulonephritis
Nephrotic syndrome with lesion (of):
endothelial
hypocomplementemic persistent
lobular
mesangiocapillary
mixed membranous and proliferative
    } glomerulonephritis

DEF: Glomerulonephritis combined with clinical features of nephrotic syndrome; characterized by uneven thickening of glomerular capillary walls and mesangial cell increase; slowly progresses to ESRD.

581.3 With lesion of minimal change glomerulonephritis
Foot process disease
Lipoid nephrosis
Minimal change: glomerular disease
Minimal change:
glomerulitis
nephrotic syndrome

√5th 581.8 With other specified pathological lesion in kidney

581.81 Nephrotic syndrome in diseases classified elsewhere
Code first underlying disease, as:
amyloidosis (277.3)
diabetes mellitus (250.4)
malaria (084.9)
polyarteritis (446.0)
systemic lupus erythematosus (710.0)
EXCLUDES *nephrosis in epidemic hemorrhagic fever (078.6)*

581.89 Other
Glomerulonephritis with edema and lesion of:
exudative nephritis
interstitial (diffuse) (focal) nephritis

581.9 Nephrotic syndrome with unspecified pathological lesion in kidney
Glomerulonephritis with edema NOS
Nephritis:
nephrotic NOS
with edema NOS
Nephrosis NOS
Renal disease with edema NOS

√4th 582 Chronic glomerulonephritis

INCLUDES chronic nephritis

DEF: Slow progressive type of nephritis characterized by inflammation of the capillary loops in the glomeruli of the kidney, which leads to renal failure.

582.0 With lesion of proliferative glomerulonephritis
Chronic (diffuse) proliferative glomerulonephritis

582.1 With lesion of membranous glomerulonephritis
Chronic glomerulonephritis:
membranous
sclerosing
Focal glomerulosclerosis
Segmental hyalinosis

√4th √5th Additional Digit Required   Unspecified Code   Other Specified Code   Manifestation Code   ►◄ Revised Text   ● New Code   ▲ Revised Code Title

2003 ICD•9•CM   **Volume 1 — 155**

582.2   With lesion of membranoproliferative glomerulonephritis
Chronic glomerulonephritis:
endothelial
hypocomplementemic persistent
lobular
membranoproliferative
mesangiocapillary
mixed membranous and proliferative
DEF: Chronic glomerulonephritis with mesangial cell proliferation.

582.4   With lesion of rapidly progressive glomerulonephritis
Chronic nephritis with lesion of necrotizing glomerulitis
DEF: Chronic glomerulonephritisrapidly progresses to ESRD; marked by diffuse epithelial proliferation.

√5th **582.8   With other specified pathological lesion in kidney**
582.81   Chronic glomerulonephritis in diseases classified elsewhere
Code first underlying disease, as:
amyloidosis (277.3)
systemic lupus erythematosus (710.0)
582.89   Other
Chronic glomerulonephritis with lesion of:
exudative nephritis
interstitial (diffuse) (focal) nephritis

582.9   Chronic glomerulonephritis with unspecified pathological lesion in kidney
Glomerulonephritis:
NOS
hemorrhagic   } specified as chronic
Nephritis
Nephropathy

√4th **583   Nephritis and nephropathy, not specified as acute or chronic**
INCLUDES   "renal disease" so stated, not specified as acute or chronic but with stated pathology or cause

583.0   With lesion of proliferative glomerulonephritis
Proliferative: Proliferative:
glomerulonephritis   nephritis NOS
(diffuse) NOS   nephropathy NOS

583.1   With lesion of membranous glomerulonephritis
Membranous:
glomerulonephritis NOS
nephritis NOS
Membranous nephropathy:
NOS
DEF: Kidney inflammation or dysfunction with deposits on glomerular capillary basement membranes.

583.2   With lesion of membranoproliferative glomerulonephritis
Membranoproliferative:
glomerulonephritis NOS
nephritis NOS
nephropathy NOS
Nephritis NOS, with lesion of:
hypocomplementemic
persistent
lobular
mesangiocapillary   } glomerulonephritis
mixed membranous
and proliferative
DEF: Kidney inflammation or dysfunction with mesangial cell proliferation.

583.4   With lesion of rapidly progressive glomerulonephritis
Necrotizing or rapidly progressive:
glomerulitis NOS
glomerulonephritis NOS
nephritis NOS
nephropathy NOS
Nephritis, unspecified, with lesion of necrotizing glomerulitis
DEF: Kidney inflammation or dysfunction; rapidly progresses to ESRD marked by diffuse epithelial proliferation.

583.6   With lesion of renal cortical necrosis
Nephritis NOS   } with (renal) cortical
Nephropathy NOS   }   necrosis
Renal cortical necrosis NOS

583.7   With lesion of renal medullary necrosis
Nephritis NOS   } with (renal) medullary
Nephropathy NOS   } [papillary] necrosis

√5th **583.8   With other specified pathological lesion in kidney**
583.81   Nephritis and nephropathy, not specified as acute or chronic, in diseases classified elsewhere
Code first underlying disease, as:
amyloidosis (277.3)
diabetes mellitus (250.4)
gonococcal infection (098.19)
Goodpasture's syndrome (446.21)
systemic lupus erythematosus (710.0)
tuberculosis (016.0)
EXCLUDES   *gouty nephropathy (274.10)*
syphilitic nephritis (095.4)
583.89   Other
Glomerulitis   } with lesion of:
Glomerulonephritis } exudative
Nephritis   } nephritis
Nephropathy   } interstitial
Renal disease   } nephritis

583.9   With unspecified pathological lesion in kidney
Glomerulitis NOS   Nephritis NOS
Glomerulonephritis NOS   Nephropathy NOS
EXCLUDES   *nephropathy complicating pregnancy, labor, or the puerperium (642.0-642.9, 646.2)*
renal disease NOS with no stated cause (593.9)

√4th **584   Acute renal failure**
EXCLUDES   *following labor and delivery (669.3)*
posttraumatic (958.5)
that complicating:
abortion (634-638 with .3, 639.3)
ectopic or molar pregnancy (639.3)
DEF: State resulting from increasing urea and related substances from the blood (azotemia), often with urine output of less than 500 ml per day.

584.5   With lesion of tubular necrosis
Lower nephron nephrosis
Renal failure with (acute) tubular necrosis
Tubular necrosis:
NOS
acute
DEF: Acute decline in kidney efficiency with destruction of tubules.

584.6   With lesion of renal cortical necrosis
DEF: Acute decline in kidney efficiency with destruction of renal tissues that filter blood.

N Newborn Age: 0   P Pediatric Age: 0-17   M Maternity Age: 12-55   A Adult Age: 15-124   MSP Medicare Secondary Payer

584.7 With lesion of renal medullary [papillary] necrosis
Necrotizing renal papillitis
DEF: Acute decline in kidney efficiency with destruction of renal tissues that collect urine.

584.8 With other specified pathological lesion in kidney

584.9 Acute renal failure, unspecified

585 Chronic renal failure
Chronic uremia
Use additional code to identify manifestation as:
uremic:
neuropathy (357.4)
pericarditis (420.0)
EXCLUDES   *that with any condition classifiable to 401*
(403.0-403.9 with fifth-digit 1)

586 Renal failure, unspecified
Uremia NOS
EXCLUDES   *following labor and delivery (669.3)*
posttraumatic renal failure (958.5)
that complicating:
abortion (634-638 with .3, 639.3)
ectopic or molar pregnancy (639.3)
uremia:
extrarenal (788.9)
prerenal (788.9)
with any condition classifiable to 401 (403.0-
403.9 with fifth-digit 1)

DEF: Renal failure: kidney functions cease; malfunction may be due to inability to excrete metabolized substances or retain level of electrolytes.

DEF: Uremia: excess urea, creatinine and other nitrogenous products of protein and amino acid metabolism in blood due to reduced excretory function in bilateral kidney disease; also called azotemia.

587 Renal sclerosis, unspecified
Atrophy of kidney
Contracted kidney
Renal:
cirrhosis
fibrosis
EXCLUDES   *nephrosclerosis (arteriolar) (arteriosclerotic)*
(403.00-403.92)
with hypertension (403.00-403.91)

✓4th 588 Disorders resulting from impaired renal function
588.0 Renal osteodystrophy
Azotemic osteodystrophy
Phosphate-losing tubular disorders
Renal:
dwarfism
infantilism
rickets

DEF: Bone disorder that results in various bone diseases such as osteomalacia, osteoporosis or osteosclerosis; caused by impaired renal function, an abnormal level of phosphorus in the blood and impaired stimulation of the parathyroid.

588.1 Nephrogenic diabetes insipidus
EXCLUDES   *diabetes insipidus NOS (253.5)*

DEF: Type of diabetes due to renal tubules inability to reabsorb water; not responsive to vasopressin; may develop into chronic renal insufficiency.

588.8 Other specified disorders resulting from impaired renal function
Hypokalemic nephropathy
Secondary hyperparathyroidism (of renal origin)
EXCLUDES   *secondary hypertension (405.0-405.9)*

588.9 Unspecified disorder resulting from impaired renal function

✓4th 589 Small kidney of unknown cause
589.0 Unilateral small kidney
589.1 Bilateral small kidneys
589.9 Small kidney, unspecified

Genitourinary System

Inferior vena cava — Aorta — Left kidney — Right kidney — Ureter — Anterior division of internal iliac artery — Ovarian or testicular artery and vein — Superior and Inferior vesicular arteries — Urinary bladder — Ureteral orifice — Urethra — Urogenital diaphragm

OTHER DISEASES OF URINARY SYSTEM (590-599)

✓4th 590 Infections of kidney
Use additional code to identify organism, such as Escherichia coli [E. coli] (041.4)

✓5th 590.0 Chronic pyelonephritis
Chronic pyelitis
Chronic pyonephrosis
►Code, if applicable, any causal condition first◄

590.00 Without lesion of renal medullary necrosis

590.01 With lesion of renal medullary necrosis

✓5th 590.1 Acute pyelonephritis
Acute pyelitis   Acute pyonephrosis

590.10 Without lesion of renal medullary necrosis

590.11 With lesion of renal medullary necrosis

590.2 Renal and perinephric abscess
Abscess: Abscess:
kidney   perirenal
nephritic   Carbuncle of kidney

590.3 Pyeloureteritis cystica
Infection of renal pelvis and ureter
Ureteritis cystica

DEF: Inflammation and formation of submucosal cysts in the kidney, pelvis, and ureter.

✓5th 590.8 Other pyelonephritis or pyonephrosis, not specified as acute or chronic

590.80 Pyelonephritis, unspecified
Pyelitis NOS
Pyelonephritis NOS

590.81 *Pyelitis or pyelonephritis in diseases classified elsewhere*
Code first underlying disease, as:
tuberculosis (016.0)

590.9 Infection of kidney, unspecified
EXCLUDES   *urinary tract infection NOS (599.0)*

591 Hydronephrosis
Hydrocalycosis   Hydroureteronephrosis
Hydronephrosis
EXCLUDES   *congenital hydronephrosis (753.29)*
hydroureter (593.5)

DEF: Distention of kidney and pelvis, with urine build-up due to ureteral obstruction; pyonephrosis may result.

✓4th 592 Calculus of kidney and ureter
EXCLUDES   *nephrocalcinosis (275.4)*

592.0 Calculus of kidney
Nephrolithiasis NOS   Staghorn calculus
Renal calculus or stone   Stone in kidney
EXCLUDES   *uric acid nephrolithiasis (274.11)*

592.1 Calculus of ureter
Ureteric stone   Ureterolithiasis

592.9 Urinary calculus, unspecified

✓4th ✓5th Additional Digit Required   Unspecified Code   Other Specified Code   Manifestation Code   ►◄ Revised Text   ● New Code   ▲ Revised Code Title

2003 ICD•9•CM   **October 2002 • Volume 1 — 157**

✓4th **593 Other disorders of kidney and ureter**

593.0 Nephroptosis
     Floating kidney   Mobile kidney

593.1 Hypertrophy of kidney

593.2 Cyst of kidney, acquired
     Cyst (multiple) (solitary) of kidney, not congenital
     Peripelvic (lymphatic) cyst
     EXCLUDES   *calyceal or pyelogenic cyst of kidney*
                    (591)
                    congenital cyst of kidney (753.1)
                    polycystic (disease of) kidney (753.1)
     DEF: Abnormal, fluid-filled sac in the kidney, not present at birth.

593.3 Stricture or kinking of ureter
     Angulation   } of ureter (post-operative)
     Constriction
     Stricture of pelviureteric junction
     DEF: Stricture or knot in tube connecting kidney to bladder.

593.4 Other ureteric obstruction
     Idiopathic retroperitoneal fibrosis
     Occlusion NOS of ureter
     EXCLUDES   *that due to calculus (592.1)*

593.5 Hydroureter
     EXCLUDES   *congenital hydroureter (753.22)*
                    hydroureteronephrosis (591)

593.6 Postural proteinuria
     Benign postural proteinuria
     Orthostatic proteinuria
     EXCLUDES   *proteinuria NOS (791.0)*
     DEF: Excessive amounts of serum protein in the urine caused by the body position, e.g., orthostatic and lordotic.

✓5th **593.7 Vesicoureteral reflux**
     DEF: Backflow of urine, from bladder into ureter due to obstructed bladder neck.

     593.70 Unspecified or without reflux nephropathy

     593.71 With reflux nephropathy, unilateral

     593.72 With reflux nephropathy, bilateral

     593.73 With reflux nephropathy NOS

✓5th **593.8 Other specified disorders of kidney and ureter**

     593.81 Vascular disorders of kidney
         Renal (artery):   Renal (artery):
           embolism   thrombosis
           hemorrhage   Renal infarction

     593.82 Ureteral fistula
         Intestinoureteral fistula
         EXCLUDES   *fistula between ureter and*
                        female genital tract
                        (619.0)
         DEF: Abnormal communication, between tube connecting kidney to bladder and another structure.

     593.89 Other
         Adhesions, kidney   Polyp of ureter
           or ureter   Pyelectasia
         Periureteritis   Ureterocele
         EXCLUDES   *tuberculosis of ureter (016.2)*
                        ureteritis cystica (590.3)

593.9 Unspecified disorder of kidney and ureter
     Renal disease NOS
     Salt-losing nephritis or syndrome
     EXCLUDES   *cystic kidney disease (753.1)*
                    nephropathy, so stated (583.0-583.9)
                    renal disease:
                       acute (580.0-580.9)
                       arising in pregnancy or the
                           puerperium (642.1-642.2,
                           642.4-642.7, 646.2)
                       chronic (582.0-582.9)
                       not specified as acute or chronic, but
                         with stated pathology or cause
                         (583.0-583.9)

✓4th **594 Calculus of lower urinary tract**

594.0 Calculus in diverticulum of bladder
     DEF: Stone or mineral deposit in abnormal sac on the bladder wall.

594.1 Other calculus in bladder
     Urinary bladder stone
     EXCLUDES   *staghorn calculus (592.0)*
     DEF: Stone or mineral deposit in bladder.

594.2 Calculus in urethra
     DEF: Stone or mineral deposit in tube that empties urine from bladder.

594.8 Other lower urinary tract calculus

594.9 Calculus of lower urinary tract, unspecified
     EXCLUDES   *calculus of urinary tract NOS (592.9)*

✓4th **595 Cystitis**
     EXCLUDES   *prostatocystitis (601.3)*
     Use additional code to identify organism, such as Escherichia coli [E. coli] (041.4)

595.0 Acute cystitis
     EXCLUDES   *trigonitis (595.3)*
     DEF: Acute inflammation of bladder.

595.1 Chronic interstitial cystitis
     Hunner's ulcer   Submucous cystitis
     Panmural fibrosis of bladder
     DEF: Inflamed lesion affecting bladder wall; symptoms include urinary frequency, pain on bladder filling, nocturia, and distended bladder.

595.2 Other chronic cystitis
     Chronic cystitis NOS   Subacute cystitis
     EXCLUDES   *trigonitis (595.3)*
     DEF: Persistent inflammation of bladder.

595.3 Trigonitis
     Follicular cystitis   Urethrotrigonitis
     Trigonitis (acute) (chronic)
     DEF: Inflammation of the triangular area of the bladder called the trigonum vesicae.

595.4 Cystitis in diseases classified elsewhere
     Code first underlying disease, as:
         actinomycosis (039.8)
         amebiasis (006.8)
         bilharziasis (120.0-120.9)
         Echinococcus infestation (122.3, 122.6)
     EXCLUDES   *cystitis:*
                  diphtheritic (032.84)
                  gonococcal (098.11, 098.31)
                  monilial (112.2)
                  trichomonal (131.09)
                  tuberculous (016.1)

N Newborn Age: 0   **P** Pediatric Age: 0-17   **M** Maternity Age: 12-55   **A** Adult Age: 15-124   **MSP** Medicare Secondary Payer

158 — Volume 1   *2003 ICD•9•CM*

√5th **595.8　Other specified types of cystitis**

595.81　Cystitis cystica

DEF: Inflammation of the bladder characterized by formation of multiple cysts.

595.82　Irradiation cystitis

Use additional E code to identify cause

DEF: Inflammation of the bladder due to effects of radiation.

595.89　Other

Abscess of bladder　　　　Cystitis:
Cystitis:　　　　　　　　　　emphysematous
　bullous　　　　　　　　　　glandularis

595.9　Cystitis, unspecified

√4th **596　Other disorders of bladder**

Use additional code to identify urinary incontinence (625.6, 788.30-788.39)

596.0　Bladder neck obstruction

Contracture (acquired)　}　of bladder neck or
Obstruction (acquired)　}　vesicourethral
Stenosis (acquired)　　 }　orifice

EXCLUDES　*congenital (753.6)*

DEF: Bladder outlet and vesicourethral obstruction; occurs more often in males as a consequence of benign prostatic hypertrophy or prostatic cancer; may also occur in either sex due to strictures, following radiation, cystoscopy, catheterization, injury, infection, blood clots, bladder cancer, impaction or disease compressing bladder neck.

596.1　Intestinovesical fistula

Fistula:　　　　　　　　　Fistula:
　enterovesical　　　　　　　vesicoenteric
　vesicocolic　　　　　　　　vesicorectal

DEF: Abnormal communication, between intestine and bladder.

596.2　Vesical fistula, not elsewhere classified

Fistula:　　　　　　　　　Fistula:
　bladder NOS　　　　　　　vesicocutaneous
　urethrovesical　　　　　　vesicoperineal

EXCLUDES　*fistula between bladder and female genital tract (619.0)*

DEF: Abnormal communication between bladder and another structure.

596.3　Diverticulum of bladder

Diverticulitis　　　　　　 }　of bladder
Diverticulum (acquired) (false)

EXCLUDES　*that with calculus in diverticulum of bladder (594.0)*

DEF: Abnormal pouch in bladder wall.

596.4　Atony of bladder

High compliance bladder
Hypotonicity　}　of bladder
Inertia　　　　}

EXCLUDES　*neurogenic bladder (596.54)*

DEF: Distended, bladder with loss of expulsive force; linked to CNS disease.

√5th **596.5　Other functional disorders of bladder**

EXCLUDES　*cauda equina syndrome with neurogenic bladder (344.61)*

596.51　Hypertonicity of bladder

Hyperactivity
Overactive bladder

DEF: Abnormal tension of muscular wall of bladder; may appear after surgery of voluntary nerve.

596.52　Low bladder compliance

DEF: Low bladder capacity; causes increased pressure and frequent urination.

596.53　Paralysis of bladder

DEF: Impaired bladder motor function due to nerve or muscle damage.

596.54　Neurogenic bladder NOS

DEF: Unspecified dysfunctional bladder due to lesion of central, peripheral nervous system; may result in incontinence, residual urine retention, urinary infection, stones and renal failure.

596.55　Detrusor sphincter dyssynergia

DEF: Instability of the urinary bladder sphincter muscle associated with urinary incontinence.

596.59　Other functional disorder of bladder

Detrusor instability

DEF: Detrusor instability: instability of bladder; marked by uninhibited contractions often leading to incontinence.

596.6　Rupture of bladder, nontraumatic

596.7　Hemorrhage into bladder wall

Hyperemia of bladder

EXCLUDES　*acute hemorrhagic cystitis (595.0)*

596.8　Other specified disorders of bladder

Bladder:　　　　　　　　　Bladder:
　calcified　　　　　　　　　hemorrhage
　contracted　　　　　　　　hypertrophy

EXCLUDES　*cystocele, female (618.0, 618.2-618.4)*
hernia or prolapse of bladder, female (618.0, 618.2-618.4)

596.9　Unspecified disorder of bladder

Bladder

Anterior View

Fundus

Right ureter

Left ureter

Lateral wall

Ureteral orifice

Trigone

Uvula of bladder

Urethra

Lateral View

Urachus

Left ureter

Peritoneum

Pubic bone

Urogenital diaphragm

√4th √5th Additional Digit Required　　Unspecified Code　　Other Specified Code　　Manifestation Code　　►◄ Revised Text　　● New Code　　▲ Revised Code Title

2003 ICD•9•CM　　　　　　　　　　　　　　　　　　　　　　　　　　　　　　　　**Volume 1 — 159**

Genitourinary System 597–600.1

✓4ᵗʰ 597 Urethritis, not sexually transmitted, and urethral syndrome
> **EXCLUDES** *nonspecific urethritis, so stated (099.4)*

597.0 Urethral abscess
> Abscess:　　　　　　　　Abscess of:
>   periurethral　　　　　　Cowper's gland
>   urethral (gland)　　　　Littré's gland
> Abscess of:　　　　　　Periurethral cellulitis
>   bulbourethral gland
>
> **EXCLUDES** *urethral caruncle (599.3)*
>
> DEF: Pocket of pus in tube that empties urine from the bladder.

✓5ᵗʰ 597.8 Other urethritis
597.80 Urethritis, unspecified
597.81 Urethral syndrome NOS
597.89 Other
> Adenitis, Skene's glands
> Cowperitis
> Meatitis, urethral
> Ulcer, urethra (meatus)
> Verumontanitis
> **EXCLUDES** *trichomonal (131.02)*

✓4ᵗʰ 598 Urethral stricture
> Use additional code to identify urinary incontinence (625.6, 788.30-788.39)
>
> **INCLUDES** pinhole meatus
>   stricture of urinary meatus
>
> **EXCLUDES** *congenital stricture of urethra and urinary meatus (753.6)*
>
> DEF: Narrowing of tube that empties urine from bladder.

✓5ᵗʰ 598.0 Urethral stricture due to infection
598.00 Due to unspecified infection
598.01 Due to infective diseases classified elsewhere
> *Code first underlying disease, as:*
>   gonococcal infection (098.2)
>   schistosomiasis (120.0-120.9)
>   syphilis (095.8)

598.1 Traumatic urethral stricture
> Stricture of urethra:　　Stricture of urethra:
>   late effect of injury　　postobstetric
> **EXCLUDES** *postoperative following surgery on genitourinary tract (598.2)*

598.2 Postoperative urethral stricture
> Postcatheterization stricture of urethra

598.8 Other specified causes of urethral stricture
598.9 Urethral stricture, unspecified

✓4ᵗʰ 599 Other disorders of urethra and urinary tract
599.0 Urinary tract infection, site not specified
> **EXCLUDES** *candidiasis of urinary tract (112.2)*
>   ▶*urinary tract infection of newborn (771.82)*◀
> Use additional code to identify organism, such as Escherichia coli [E. coli] (041.4)

599.1 Urethral fistula
> Fistula:　　　　　　　Urinary fistula NOS
>   urethroperineal
>   urethrorectal
> **EXCLUDES** *fistula:*
>   *urethroscrotal (608.89)*
>   *urethrovaginal (619.0)*
>   *urethrovesicovaginal (619.0)*

599.2 Urethral diverticulum
> DEF: Abnormal pouch in urethral wall.

599.3 Urethral caruncle
> Polyp of urethra

599.4 Urethral false passage
> DEF: Abnormal opening in urethra due to surgery, trauma or disease.

599.5 Prolapsed urethral mucosa
> Prolapse of urethra　　Urethrocele
> **EXCLUDES** *urethrocele, female (618.0, 618.2-618.4)*

599.6 Urinary obstruction, unspecified
> Obstructive uropathy NOS
> Urinary (tract) obstruction NOS
> Use additional code to identify urinary incontinence (625.6, 788.30-788.39)
> **EXCLUDES** *obstructive nephropathy NOS (593.89)*

599.7 Hematuria
> Hematuria (benign) (essential)
> **EXCLUDES** *hemoglobinuria (791.2)*
>
> DEF: Blood in urine.

✓5ᵗʰ 599.8 Other specified disorders of urethra and urinary tract
> Use additional code to identify urinary incontinence (625.6, 788.30-788.39)
> **EXCLUDES** *symptoms and other conditions classifiable to 788.0-788.2, 788.4-788.9, 791.0-791.9*

599.81 Urethral hypermobility
> DEF: Hyperactive urethra.

599.82 Intrinsic (urethral) spincter deficiency [ISD]
> DEF: Malfunctioning urethral sphincter.

599.83 Urethral instability
> DEF: Inconsistent functioning of urethra.

599.84 Other specified disorders of urethra
> Rupture of urethra (nontraumatic)
> Urethral:
>   cyst
>   granuloma
>
> DEF: Rupture of urethra; due to herniation or breaking down of tissue; not due to trauma.
>
> DEF: Urethral cyst: abnormal sac in urethra; usually fluid filled.
>
> DEF: Granuloma: inflammatory cells forming small nodules in urethra.

599.89 Other specified disorders of urinary tract

599.9 Unspecified disorder of urethra and urinary tract

DISEASES OF MALE GENITAL ORGANS (600-608)

✓4ᵗʰ 600 Hyperplasia of prostate
> Use additional code to identify urinary incontinence (788.30-788.39)
>
> DEF: Fibrostromal proliferation in periurethral glands, causes blood in urine; etiology unknown.

600.0 Hypertrophy (benign) of prostate　　　Ａ♂
> Benign prostatic hypertrophy
> Enlargement of prostate
> Smooth enlarged prostate
> Soft enlarged prostate

600.1 Nodular prostate　　　Ａ♂
> Hard, firm prostate　　Multinodular prostate
> **EXCLUDES** *malignant neoplasm of prostate (185)*
>
> DEF: Hard, firm nodule in prostate.

Ⓝ Newborn Age: 0　　Ⓟ Pediatric Age: 0-17　　Ⓜ Maternity Age: 12-55　　Ⓐ Adult Age: 15-124　　ᴹˢᴾ Medicare Secondary Payer

Male Pelvic Organs

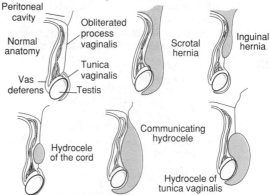

Common Inguinal Canal Anomalies

600.2 Benign localized hyperplasia of prostate A ♂
Adenofibromatous hypertrophy of prostate
Adenoma of prostate
Fibroadenoma of prostate
Fibroma of prostate
Myoma of prostate
Polyp of prostate
> EXCLUDES   benign neoplasms of prostate (222.2)
> hypertrophy of prostate (600.0)
> malignant neoplasm of prostate (185)

DEF: Benign localized hyperplasia is a clearly defined epithelial tumor. Other terms used for this condition are adenofibromatous hypertrophy of prostate, adenoma of prostate, fibroadenoma of prostate, fibroma of prostate, myoma of prostate, and polyp of prostate.

600.3 Cyst of prostate A ♂
DEF: Sacs of fluid, which differentiate this from either nodular or adenomatous tumors.

600.9 Hyperplasia of prostate, unspecified A ♂
Median bar
Prostatic obstruction NOS

√4th 601 Inflammatory diseases of prostate
Use additional code to identify organism, such as Staphylococcus (041.1), or Streptococcus (041.0)

601.0 Acute prostatitis A ♂
601.1 Chronic prostatitis A ♂
601.2 Abscess of prostate A ♂
601.3 Prostatocystitis A ♂
601.4 Prostatitis in diseases classified elsewhere A ♂
Code first underlying disease, as:
actinomycosis (039.8)
blastomycosis (116.0)
syphilis (095.8)
tuberculosis (016.5)
> EXCLUDES   prostatitis:
> gonococcal (098.12, 098.32)
> monilial (112.2)
> trichomonal (131.03)

601.8 Other specified inflammatory diseases of prostate A ♂
Prostatitis: Prostatitis:
cavitary   granulomatous
diverticular

601.9 Prostatitis, unspecified A ♂
Prostatitis NOS

√4th 602 Other disorders of prostate
602.0 Calculus of prostate A ♂
Prostatic stone
DEF: Stone or mineral deposit in prostate.

602.1 Congestion or hemorrhage of prostate A ♂
DEF: Bleeding or fluid collection in prostate.

602.2 Atrophy of prostate A ♂
602.3 Dysplasia of prostate A ♂
Prostatic intraepithelial ▶neoplasia◀ I (PIN I)
Prostatic intraepithelial ▶neoplasia◀ II (PIN II)
> EXCLUDES   prostatic intraepithelial ▶neoplasia◀ III (PIN III) (233.4)

DEF: Abnormality of shape and size of the intraepithelial tissues of the prostate; pre-malignant condition characterized by stalks and absence of a basilar cell layer; synonyms are intraductal dysplasia, large acinar atypical hyperplasia, atypical primary hyperplasia, hyperplasia with malignant changes, marked atypia, or duct-acinar dysplasia.

602.8 Other specified disorders of prostate A ♂
Fistula
Infarction } of prostate
Stricture
Periprostatic adhesions

602.9 Unspecified disorder of prostate A ♂

√4th 603 Hydrocele
> INCLUDES   hydrocele of spermatic cord, testis, or tunica vaginalis
> EXCLUDES   congenital (778.6)

DEF: Circumscribed collection of fluid in tunica vaginalis, spermatic cord or testis.

603.0 Encysted hydrocele
603.1 Infected hydrocele
Use additional code to identify organism
603.8 Other specified types of hydrocele
603.9 Hydrocele, unspecified

√4th 604 Orchitis and epididymitis
Use additional code to identify organism, such as Escherichia coli [E. coli] (041.4), Staphylococcus (041.1), or Streptococcus (041.0)

604.0 Orchitis, epididymitis, and epididymo-orchitis, with abscess ♂
Abscess of epididymis or testis

√5th 604.9 Other orchitis, epididymitis, and epididymo-orchitis, without mention of abscess
604.90 Orchitis and epididymitis, unspecified ♂
604.91 Orchitis and epididymitis in diseases classified elsewhere ♂
Code first underlying disease, as:
diphtheria (032.89)
filariasis (125.0-125.9)
syphilis (095.8)
> EXCLUDES   orchitis:
> gonococcal (098.13, 098.33)
> mumps (072.0)
> tuberculous (016.5)
> tuberculous epididymitis (016.4)

604.99 Other ♂

Genitourinary System 600.2–604.99

Genitourinary System 605–608.83

605 Redundant prepuce and phimosis ♂
  Adherent prepuce   Phimosis (congenital)
  Paraphimosis   Tight foreskin

  DEF: Constriction of preputial orifice causing inability of the prepuce to be drawn back over the glans; it may be congenital or caused by infection.

√4ᵗʰ 606 Infertility, male
  606.0 Azoospermia [A] ♂
    Absolute infertility
    Infertility due to:
      germinal (cell) aplasia
      spermatogenic arrest (complete)

    DEF: Absence of spermatozoa in the semen or inability to produce spermatozoa.

  606.1 Oligospermia ♂ [A]
    Infertility due to:
      germinal cell desquamation
      hypospermatogenesis
      incomplete spermatogenic arrest

    DEF: Insufficient number of sperm in semen.

  606.8 Infertility due to extratesticular causes [A] ♂
    Infertility due to: Infertility due to:
      drug therapy   radiation
      infection   systemic disease
      obstruction of efferent
        ducts

  606.9 Male infertility, unspecified [A] ♂

√4ᵗʰ 607 Disorders of penis
  EXCLUDES   phimosis (605)

  607.0 Leukoplakia of penis ♂
    Kraurosis of penis
    EXCLUDES   carcinoma in situ of penis (233.5)
                erythroplasia of Queyrat (233.5)

    DEF: White, thickened patches on glans penis.

  607.1 Balanoposthitis ♂
    Balanitis
    Use additional code to identify organism
    DEF: Inflammation of glans penis and prepuce.

  607.2 Other inflammatory disorders of penis ♂
    Abscess   ⎫
    Boil   ⎬ of corpus cavernosum or penis
    Carbuncle ⎪
    Cellulitis ⎭

    Cavernitis (penis)
    Use additional code to identify organism
    EXCLUDES   herpetic infection (054.13)

  607.3 Priapism ♂
    Painful erection
    DEF: Prolonged penile erection without sexual stimulation.

  √5ᵗʰ 607.8 Other specified disorders of penis
    607.81 Balanitis xerotica obliterans ♂
      Induratio penis plastica
      DEF: Inflammation of the glans penis, caused by stricture of the opening of the prepuce.

    607.82 Vascular disorders of penis ♂
      Embolism   ⎫
      Hematoma   ⎪ of corpus
        (nontraumatic) ⎬ cavernosum
      Hemorrhage ⎪ or penis
      Thrombosis ⎭

    607.83 Edema of penis ♂
      DEF: Fluid retention within penile tissues.

    607.84 Impotence of organic origin [A] ♂
      EXCLUDES   nonorganic or unspecified (302.72)
      DEF: Physiological cause interfering with erection.

Torsion of Testes

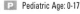

Torsion of testis   Testes after correction showing bilateral fixation

  607.89 Other ♂
    Atrophy   ⎫
    Fibrosis   ⎬ of corpus cavernosum
    Hypertrophy ⎪ or penis
    Ulcer (chronic) ⎭

  607.9 Unspecified disorder of penis ♂

√4ᵗʰ 608 Other disorders of male genital organs
  608.0 Seminal vesiculitis ♂
    Abscess   ⎫
    Cellulitis ⎬ of seminal vesicle

    Vesiculitis (seminal)
    Use additional code to identify organism
    EXCLUDES   gonococcal infection (098.14, 098.34)

    DEF: Inflammation of seminal vesicle.

  608.1 Spermatocele ♂
    DEF: Cystic enlargement of the epididymis or the testis; the cysts contain spermatozoa.

  608.2 Torsion of testis ♂
    Torsion of: Torsion of:
      epididymis   testicle
      spermatic cord

    DEF: Twisted or rotated testis; may compromise blood flow.

  608.3 Atrophy of testis ♂

  608.4 Other inflammatory disorders of male genital organs ♂
    Abscess   ⎫
    Boil   ⎪ of scrotum, spermatic cord, testis
    Carbuncle ⎬ [except abscess], tunica
    Cellulitis ⎭ vaginalis, or vas deferens

    Vasitis
    Use additional code to identify organism
    EXCLUDES   abscess of testis (604.0)

  √5ᵗʰ 608.8 Other specified disorders of male genital organs
    608.81 Disorders of male genital organs in diseases classified elsewhere ♂
      Code first underlying disease, as:
        filariasis (125.0-125.9)
        tuberculosis (016.5)

    608.82 Hematospermia ♂
      DEF: ▶Presence of blood in the ejaculate; relatively common, affecting men of any age after puberty; cause is often difficult to determine since the semen originates in several organs, often the result of a viral bacterial infection and inflammation.◄

    608.83 Vascular disorders ♂
      Hematoma   ⎫
        (non-   ⎪ of seminal vesicle,
        traumatic) ⎬ spermatic cord,
      Hemorrhage ⎪ testis, scrotum,
      Thrombosis ⎭ tunica vaginalis,
                     or vas deferens

      Hematocele NOS, male

[N] Newborn Age: 0   [P] Pediatric Age: 0-17   [M] Maternity Age: 12-55   [A] Adult Age: 15-124   [MSP] Medicare Secondary Payer

608.84 Chylocele of tunica vaginalis ♂

DEF: Chylous effusion into tunica vaginalis; due to infusion of lymphatic fluids.

608.85 Stricture ♂

Stricture of: Stricture of:
   spermatic cord   vas deferens
   tunica vaginalis

608.86 Edema ♂

608.87 Retrograde ejaculation ♂

DEF: ▶Condition where the semen travels to the bladder rather than out through the urethra due to damaged nerves causing the bladder neck to remain open during ejaculation.◀

608.89 Other ♂

Atrophy   } of seminal vesicle,
Fibrosis   } spermatic cord,
Hypertrophy   } testis, scrotum,
Ulcer   } tunica vaginalis, or
            } vas deferens

> EXCLUDES   atrophy of testis (608.3)

608.9 Unspecified disorder of male genital organs ♂

DISORDERS OF BREAST (610-611)

✓4ᵗʰ **610 Benign mammary dysplasias**

610.0 Solitary cyst of breast
Cyst (solitary) of breast

610.1 Diffuse cystic mastopathy A
Chronic cystic mastitis   Fibrocystic disease of
Cystic breast   breast

DEF: Extensive formation of nodular cysts in breast tissue; symptoms include tenderness, change in size and hyperplasia of ductal epithelium.

610.2 Fibroadenosis of breast
Fibroadenosis of breast: Fibroadenosis of breast:
   NOS   diffuse
   chronic   periodic
   cystic   segmental

DEF: Non-neoplastic nodular condition of breast.

610.3 Fibrosclerosis of breast

DEF: Fibrous tissue in breast.

610.4 Mammary duct ectasia
Comedomastitis   Mastitis:
Duct ectasia   periductal
               plasma cell

DEF: Atrophy of duct epithelium; causes distended collecting ducts of mammary gland; drying up of breast secretion, intraductal inflammation and periductal and interstitial chronic inflammatory reaction.

610.8 Other specified benign mammary dysplasias
Mazoplasia   Sebaceous cyst of breast

610.9 Benign mammary dysplasia, unspecified

✓4ᵗʰ **611 Other disorders of breast**

> EXCLUDES   that associated with lactation or the puerperium (675.0-676.9)

611.0 Inflammatory disease of breast
Abscess (acute) (chronic)   Mastitis (acute) (subacute)
   (nonpuerperal) of: (nonpuerperal):
     areola   NOS
     breast   infective
     Mammillary fistula   retromammary
                   submammary

> EXCLUDES   carbuncle of breast (680.2)
> chronic cystic mastitis (610.1)
> neonatal infective mastitis (771.5)
> thrombophlebitis of breast [Mondor's disease] (451.89)

611.1 Hypertrophy of breast
Gynecomastia
Hypertrophy of breast:
   NOS
   massive pubertal

611.2 Fissure of nipple

611.3 Fat necrosis of breast
Fat necrosis (segmental) of breast

DEF: Splitting of neutral fats in adipose tissue cells as a result of trauma; a firm circumscribed mass is then formed in the breast.

611.4 Atrophy of breast

611.5 Galactocele

DEF: Milk-filled cyst in breast; due to blocked duct.

611.6 Galactorrhea not associated with childbirth

DEF: Flow of milk not associated with childbirth or pregnancy.

✓5ᵗʰ **611.7 Signs and symptoms in breast**

611.71 Mastodynia
Pain in breast

611.72 Lump or mass in breast

611.79 Other
Induration of breast   Nipple discharge
Inversion of nipple   Retraction of nipple

611.8 Other specified disorders of breast
Hematoma (nontraumatic) } of breast
Infarction   }

Occlusion of breast duct
Subinvolution of breast (postlactational) (postpartum)

611.9 Unspecified breast disorder

INFLAMMATORY DISEASE OF FEMALE PELVIC ORGANS (614-616)

Use additional code to identify organism, such as Staphylococcus (041.1), or Streptococcus (041.0)

> EXCLUDES   that associated with pregnancy, abortion, childbirth, or the puerperium (630-676.9)

✓4ᵗʰ **614 Inflammatory disease of ovary, fallopian tube, pelvic cellular tissue, and peritoneum**

> EXCLUDES   endometritis (615.0-615.9)
> major infection following delivery (670)
> that complicating:
>   abortion (634-638 with .0, 639.0)
>   ectopic or molar pregnancy (639.0)
>   pregnancy or labor (646.6)

614.0 Acute salpingitis and oophoritis ♀
Any condition classifiable to 614.2, specified as acute or subacute

DEF: Acute inflammation, of ovary and fallopian tube.

614.1 Chronic salpingitis and oophoritis ♀
Hydrosalpinx
Salpingitis:
   follicularis
   isthmica nodosa
Any condition classifiable to 614.2, specified as chronic

DEF: Persistent inflammation of ovary and fallopian tube.

614.2 Salpingitis and oophoritis not specified as acute, subacute, or chronic ♀
Abscess (of):   Pyosalpinx
   fallopian tube   Perisalpingitis
   ovary   Salpingitis
   tubo-ovarian   Salpingo-oophoritis
Oophoritis   Tubo-ovarian inflammatory
Perioophoritis   disease

> EXCLUDES   gonococcal infection (chronic) (098.37)
> acute (098.17)
> tuberculous (016.6)

✓4ᵗʰ / ✓5ᵗʰ Additional Digit Required   Unspecified Code   Other Specified Code   Manifestation Code   ▶◀ Revised Text   ● New Code   ▲ Revised Code Title

2003 ICD•9•CM   **January 2002 • Volume 1 — 163**

614.3 Acute parametritis and pelvic cellulitis ♀
Acute inflammatory pelvic disease
Any condition classifiable to 614.4, specified as acute

DEF: Parametritis: inflammation of the parametrium; pelvic cellulitis is a synonym for parametritis.

614.4 Chronic or unspecified parametritis and pelvic cellulitis ♀
Abscess (of):
broad ligament
parametrium
pelvis, female   } chronic or NOS
pouch of Douglas

Chronic inflammatory pelvic disease
Pelvic cellulitis, female
EXCLUDES   tuberculous (016.7)

614.5 Acute or unspecified pelvic peritonitis, female ♀
614.6 Pelvic peritoneal adhesions, female (postoperative) (postinfection) ♀
Adhesions:
peritubal
tubo-ovarian
Use additional code to identify any associated infertility (628.2)

DEF: Fibrous scarring abnormally joining structures within abdomen.

614.7 Other chronic pelvic peritonitis, female ♀
EXCLUDES   tuberculous (016.7)

614.8 Other specified inflammatory disease of female pelvic organs and tissues ♀

614.9 Unspecified inflammatory disease of female pelvic organs and tissues ♀
Pelvic infection or inflammation, female NOS
Pelvic inflammatory disease [PID]

√4ᵗʰ **615 Inflammatory diseases of uterus, except cervix**
EXCLUDES   following delivery (670)
hyperplastic endometritis (621.3)
that complicating:
abortion (634-638 with .0, 639.0)
ectopic or molar pregnancy (639.0)
pregnancy or labor (646.6)

615.0 Acute ♀
Any condition classifiable to 615.9, specified as acute or subacute

615.1 Chronic ♀
Any condition classifiable to 615.9, specified as chronic

615.9 Unspecified inflammatory disease of uterus ♀
Endometritis   Perimetritis
Endomyometritis   Pyometra
Metritis   Uterine abscess
Myometritis

√4ᵗʰ **616 Inflammatory disease of cervix, vagina, and vulva**
EXCLUDES   that complicating:
abortion (634-638 with .0, 639.0)
ectopic or molar pregnancy (639.0)
pregnancy, childbirth, or the puerperium (646.6)

616.0 Cervicitis and endocervicitis ♀
Cervicitis   } with or without mention of
Endocervicitis   } erosion or ectropion

Nabothian (gland) cyst or follicle
EXCLUDES   erosion or ectropion without mention of cervicitis (622.0)

√5ᵗʰ **616.1 Vaginitis and vulvovaginitis**
DEF: Inflammation or infection of vagina or external female genitalia.

616.10 Vaginitis and vulvovaginitis, unspecified ♀
Vaginitis:
NOS
postirradiation
Vulvitis NOS
Vulvovaginitis NOS
Use additional code to identify organism, such as Escherichia coli [E. coli] (041.4), Staphylococcus (041.1), or Streptococcus (041.0)
EXCLUDES   noninfective leukorrhea (623.5)
postmenopausal or senile vaginitis (627.3)

616.11 Vaginitis and vulvovaginitis in diseases classified elsewhere ♀
Code first underlying disease, as:
pinworm vaginitis (127.4)
EXCLUDES   herpetic vulvovaginitis (054.11)
monilial vulvotaginitis (112.1)
trichomonal vaginitis or vulvovaginitis (131.01)

616.2 Cyst of Bartholin's gland ♀
Bartholin's duct cyst
DEF: Fluid-filled sac within gland of vaginal orifice.

616.3 Abscess of Bartholin's gland ♀
Vulvovaginal gland abscess

616.4 Other abscess of vulva ♀
Abscess
Carbuncle   } of vulva
Furuncle

√5ᵗʰ **616.5 Ulceration of vulva**
616.50 Ulceration of vulva, unspecified ♀
Ulcer NOS of vulva

616.51 Ulceration of vulva in diseases classified elsewhere ♀
Code first underlying disease, as:
Behçet's syndrome (136.1)
tuberculosis (016.7)
EXCLUDES   vulvar ulcer (in):
gonococcal (098.0)
herpes simplex (054.12)
syphilitic (091.0)

Female Genitourinary System

Uterine (fallopian) tube
Ovary
Rectouterine pouch (of Douglas)
Uterus (fundus)
Cervix
Bladder
Rectum
Pubic bone
Clitoris
Urogenital diaphragm
Anus
Urethral orifice (meatus)
Labia minora
Labia majora
Vaginal canal

N Newborn Age: 0   **P** Pediatric Age: 0-17   **M** Maternity Age: 12-55   **A** Adult Age: 15-124   **MSP** Medicare Secondary Payer

164 — Volume 1   *2003 ICD•9•CM*

Common Sites of Endometriosis

Common sites of
endometriosis, in
descending order
of frequency:
(1) ovary
(2) cul de sac
(3) utersacral ligaments
(4) broad ligaments
(5) fallopian tube
(6) uterovesical fold
(7) round ligament
(8) vermiform appedix
(9) vagina
(10) rectovaginal septum

**616.8   Other specified inflammatory diseases of
cervix, vagina, and vulva**   ♀
> Caruncle, vagina or labium
> Ulcer, vagina
>> **EXCLUDES**   *noninflammatory disorders of:*
>>   *cervix (622.0-622.9)*
>>   *vagina (623.0-623.9)*
>>   *vulva (624.0-624.9)*

**616.9   Unspecified inflammatory disease of cervix,
vagina and vulva**   ♀

OTHER DISORDERS OF FEMALE GENITAL TRACT (617-629)

✓4ᵗʰ **617 Endometriosis**
> **DEF:** What resembles uterine mucosa (endometrial tissue) is found in the
> pelvic cavity.

617.0   Endometriosis of uterus   ♀
> Adenomyosis   Endometriosis:
> Endometriosis: internal
>   cervix   myometrium
>> **EXCLUDES**   *stromal endometriosis (236.0)*
> **DEF:** Aberrant uterine mucosal tissue; creating products of menses
> and inflamed uterine tissues.

617.1   Endometriosis of ovary   ♀
> Chocolate cyst of ovary
> Endometrial cystoma of ovary
> **DEF:** Aberrant uterine tissue; creating products of menses and
> inflamed ovarian tissues.

617.2   Endometriosis of fallopian tube   ♀
> **DEF:** Aberrant uterine tissue; creating products of menses and
> inflamed tissues of fallopian tubes.

617.3   Endometriosis of pelvic peritoneum   ♀
> Endometriosis: Endometriosis:
>   broad ligament   parametrium
>   cul-de-sac (Douglas')   round ligament
> **DEF:** Aberrant uterine tissue; creating products of menses and
> inflamed peritoneum tissues.

**617.4   Endometriosis of rectovaginal septum and
vagina**   ♀
> **DEF:** Aberrant uterine tissue; creating products of menses and
> inflamed tissues in and behind vagina.

617.5   Endometriosis of intestine   ♀
> Endometriosis: Endometriosis:
>   appendix   rectum
>   colon
> **DEF:** Aberrant uterine tissue; creating products of menses and
> inflamed intestinal tissues.

617.6   Endometriosis in scar of skin   ♀

617.8   Endometriosis of other specified sites   ♀
> Endometriosis: Endometriosis:
>   bladder   umbilicus
>   lung   vulva

617.9   Endometriosis, site unspecified   ♀

✓4ᵗʰ **618 Genital prolapse**
> Use additional code to identify urinary incontinence (625.6,
> 788.31, 788.33-788.39)
>> **EXCLUDES**   *that complicating pregnancy, labor, or delivery*
>>   *(654.4)*

**618.0   Prolapse of vaginal walls without mention of
uterine prolapse**   ♀
> Cystocele
> Cystourethrocele
> Proctocele, female   ⎫
> Rectocele   ⎬ without mention of uterine
> Urethrocele, female   ⎪   prolapse
> Vaginal prolapse   ⎭
>> **EXCLUDES**   *that with uterine prolapse (618.2-*
>>   *618.4)*
>>   *enterocele (618.6)*
>>   *vaginal vault prolapse following*
>>   *hysterectomy (618.5)*

**618.1   Uterine prolapse without mention of vaginal
wall prolapse**   ♀
> Descensus uteri   Uterine prolapse:
> Uterine prolapse: first degree
>   NOS   second degree
>   complete   third degree
>> **EXCLUDES**   *that with mention of cystocele,*
>>   *urethrocele, or rectocele (618.2-*
>>   *618.4)*

618.2   Uterovaginal prolapse, incomplete   ♀
> **DEF:** Downward displacement of uterus downward into vagina.

618.3   Uterovaginal prolapse, complete   ♀
> **DEF:** Downward displacement of uterus exposed within external
> genitalia.

618.4   Uterovaginal prolapse, unspecified   ♀
618.5   Prolapse of vaginal vault after hysterectomy   ♀
618.6   Vaginal enterocele, congenital or acquired   ♀
> Pelvic enterocele, congenital or acquired
> **DEF:** Vaginal vault hernia formed by the loop of the small intestine
> protruding into the rectal vaginal pouch; can also accompany
> uterine prolapse or follow hysterectomy.

618.7   Old laceration of muscles of pelvic floor   ♀
618.8   Other specified genital prolapse   ♀
> Incompetence or weakening of pelvic fundus
> Relaxation of vaginal outlet or pelvis

618.9   Unspecified genital prolapse   ♀

Types of Vaginal Hernias

2003 ICD•9•CM

✓4ᵗʰ
✓5ᵗʰ Additional Digit Required | Unspecified Code | Other Specified Code | Manifestation Code | ▶◀ Revised Text | ● New Code | ▲ Revised Code Title

Volume 1 — 165

√4ᵗʰ **619 Fistula involving female genital tract**
> EXCLUDES *vesicorectal and intestinovesical fistula (596.1)*

619.0 Urinary-genital tract fistula, female ♀
Fistula: Fistula:
  cervicovesical uteroureteric
  ureterovaginal uterovesical
  urethrovaginal vesicocervicovaginal
  urethrovesicovaginal vesicovaginal

619.1 Digestive-genital tract fistula, female ♀
Fistula: Fistula:
  intestinouterine rectovulval
  intestinovaginal sigmoidovaginal
  rectovaginal uterorectal

619.2 Genital tract-skin fistula, female ♀
Fistula:
  uterus to abdominal wall
  vaginoperineal

619.8 Other specified fistulas involving female genital tract ♀
Fistula: Fistula:
  cervix uterus
  cul-de-sac (Douglas') vagina
DEF: Abnormal communication between female reproductive tract and skin.

619.9 Unspecified fistula involving female genital tract ♀

√4ᵗʰ **620 Noninflammatory disorders of ovary, fallopian tube, and broad ligament**
> EXCLUDES *hydrosalpinx (614.1)*

620.0 Follicular cyst of ovary ♀
Cyst of graafian follicle
DEF: Fluid-filled, encapsulated cyst due to occluded follicle duct that secretes hormones into ovaries.

620.1 Corpus luteum cyst or hematoma ♀
Corpus luteum hemorrhage or rupture
Lutein cyst
DEF: Fluid-filled cyst due to serous developing from corpus luteum or clotted blood.

620.2 Other and unspecified ovarian cyst ♀
Cyst:
  NOS
  corpus albicans
  retention NOS } of ovary
  serous
  theca-lutein

Simple cystoma of ovary
> EXCLUDES *cystadenoma (benign) (serous) (220)*
> *developmental cysts (752.0)*
> *neoplastic cysts (220)*
> *polycystic ovaries (256.4)*
> *Stein-Leventhal syndrome (256.4)*

620.3 Acquired atrophy of ovary and fallopian tube ♀
Senile involution of ovary

620.4 Prolapse or hernia of ovary and fallopian tube ♀
Displacement of ovary and fallopian tube
Salpingocele

620.5 Torsion of ovary, ovarian pedicle, or fallopian tube ♀
Torsion: Torsion:
  accessory tube hydatid of Morgagni

620.6 Broad ligament laceration syndrome ♀
Masters-Allen syndrome

620.7 Hematoma of broad ligament ♀
Hematocele, broad ligament
DEF: Blood within peritoneal fold that supports uterus.

Uterus and Ovaries

620.8 Other noninflammatory disorders of ovary, fallopian tube, and broad ligament ♀
Cyst
Polyp } of broad ligament or fallopian tube

Infarction
Rupture } of ovary or fallopian tube

Hematosalpinx
> EXCLUDES *hematosalpinx in ectopic pregnancy (639.2)*
> *peritubal adhesions (614.6)*
> *torsion of ovary, ovarian pedicle, or fallopian tube (620.5)*

620.9 Unspecified noninflammatory disorder of ovary, fallopian tube, and broad ligament ♀

√4ᵗʰ **621 Disorders of uterus, not elsewhere classified**

621.0 Polyp of corpus uteri ♀
Polyp: Polyp:
  endometrium uterus NOS
> EXCLUDES *cervical polyp NOS (622.7)*

621.1 Chronic subinvolution of uterus ♀
> EXCLUDES *puerperal (674.8)*
DEF: Abnormal size of uterus after delivery; the uterus does not return to its normal size after the birth of a child.

621.2 Hypertrophy of uterus ♀
Bulky or enlarged uterus
> EXCLUDES *puerperal (674.8)*

621.3 Endometrial cystic hyperplasia ♀
Hyperplasia (adenomatous) (cystic) (glandular) of endometrium
Hyperplastic endometritis
DEF: Abnormal cystic overgrowth of endometrial tissue.

621.4 Hematometra ♀
Hemometra
> EXCLUDES *that in congenital anomaly (752.2-752.3)*
DEF: Accumulated blood in uterus.

621.5 Intrauterine synechiae ♀
Adhesions of uterus
Band(s) of uterus

621.6 Malposition of uterus ♀
Anteversion
Retroflexion } of uterus
Retroversion
> EXCLUDES *malposition complicating pregnancy, labor, or delivery (654.3-654.4)*
> *prolapse of uterus (618.1-618.4)*

N Newborn Age: 0   **P** Pediatric Age: 0-17   **M** Maternity Age: 12-55   **A** Adult Age: 15-124   **MSP** Medicare Secondary Payer

621.7 Chronic inversion of uterus ♀
> EXCLUDES   *current obstetrical trauma (665.2)*
> *prolapse of uterus (618.1-618.4)*

621.8 Other specified disorders of uterus, not elsewhere classified ♀

Atrophy, acquired
Cyst
Fibrosis NOS   } of uterus
Old laceration (postpartum)
Ulcer

> EXCLUDES   *bilharzial fibrosis (120.0-120.9)*
> *endometriosis (617.0)*
> *fistulas (619.0-619.8)*
> *inflammatory diseases (615.0-615.9)*

621.9 Unspecified disorder of uterus ♀

✓4ᵗʰ 622 Noninflammatory disorders of cervix
> EXCLUDES   *abnormality of cervix complicating pregnancy, labor, or delivery (654.5-654.6)*
> *fistula (619.0-619.8)*

622.0 Erosion and ectropion of cervix ♀

Eversion } of cervix
Ulcer

> EXCLUDES   *that in chronic cervicitis (616.0)*

DEF: Ulceration or turning outward of uterine cervix.

622.1 Dysplasia of cervix (uteri) ♀
Anaplasia of cervix
Cervical atypism
▶Cervical intraepithelial neoplasia I (CIN I)
Cervical intraepithelial neoplasia II (CIN II)
High grade squamous intraepithelial dysplasia (HGSIL)
Low grade squamous intraepithelial dysplasia (LGSIL)◀
> EXCLUDES   *carcinoma in situ of cervix (233.1)*
> *cervical intraepithelial neoplasia III [CIN III] (233.1)*

622.2 Leukoplakia of cervix (uteri) ♀
DEF: Abnormal cell structures in portal between uterus and vagina.

> EXCLUDES   *carcinoma in situ of cervix (233.1)*

DEF: Thickened, white patches on portal between uterus and vagina.

622.3 Old laceration of cervix ♀
Adhesions
Band(s) } of cervix
Cicatrix (postpartum)
> EXCLUDES   *current obstetrical trauma (665.3)*

DEF: Scarring or other evidence of old wound on cervix.

622.4 Stricture and stenosis of cervix ♀
Atresia (acquired)
Contracture } of cervix
Occlusion

Pinpoint os uteri
> EXCLUDES   *congenital (752.49)*
> *that complicating labor (654.6)*

622.5 Incompetence of cervix ♀
> EXCLUDES   *complicating pregnancy (654.5)*
> *that affecting fetus or newborn (761.0)*

DEF: Inadequate functioning of cervix; marked by abnormal widening during pregnancy; causing miscarriage.

622.6 Hypertrophic elongation of cervix ♀
DEF: Overgrowth of cervix tissues extending down into vagina.

622.7 Mucous polyp of cervix ♀
Polyp NOS of cervix
> EXCLUDES   *adenomatous polyp of cervix (219.0)*

622.8 Other specified noninflammatory disorders of cervix ♀

Atrophy (senile)
Cyst
Fibrosis } of cervix
Hemorrhage

> EXCLUDES   *endometriosis (617.0)*
> *fistula (619.0-619.8)*
> *inflammatory diseases (616.0)*

622.9 Unspecified noninflammatory disorder of cervix ♀

✓4ᵗʰ 623 Noninflammatory disorders of vagina
> EXCLUDES   *abnormality of vagina complicating pregnancy, labor, or delivery (654.7)*
> *congenital absence of vagina (752.49)*
> *congenital diaphragm or bands (752.49)*
> *fistulas involving vagina (619.0-619.8)*

623.0 Dysplasia of vagina ♀
> EXCLUDES   *carcinoma in situ of vagina (233.3)*

623.1 Leukoplakia of vagina ♀
DEF: Thickened white patches on vaginal canal.

623.2 Stricture or atresia of vagina ♀
Adhesions (postoperative) (postradiation) of vagina
Occlusion of vagina
Stenosis, vagina
Use additional E code to identify any external cause
> EXCLUDES   *congenital atresia or stricture (752.49)*

623.3 Tight hymenal ring ♀
Rigid hymen
Tight hymenal ring } acquired or congenital
Tight introitus
> EXCLUDES   *imperforate hymen (752.42)*

623.4 Old vaginal laceration ♀
> EXCLUDES   *old laceration involving muscles of pelvic floor (618.7)*

DEF: Scarring or other evidence of old wound on vagina.

623.5 Leukorrhea, not specified as infective ♀
Leukorrhea NOS of vagina
Vaginal discharge NOS
> EXCLUDES   *trichomonal (131.00)*

DEF: Viscid whitish discharge, from vagina.

623.6 Vaginal hematoma ♀
> EXCLUDES   *current obstetrical trauma (665.7)*

623.7 Polyp of vagina ♀

623.8 Other specified noninflammatory disorders of vagina ♀

Cyst
Hemorrhage } of vagina

623.9 Unspecified noninflammatory disorder of vagina ♀

✓4ᵗʰ 624 Noninflammatory disorders of vulva and perineum
> EXCLUDES   *abnormality of vulva and perineum complicating pregnancy, labor, or delivery (654.8)*
> *condyloma acuminatum (078.1)*
> *fistulas involving:*
> *perineum — see Alphabetic Index*
> *vulva (619.0-619.8)*
> *vulval varices (456.6)*
> *vulvar involvement in skin conditions (690-709.9)*

624.0 Dystrophy of vulva ♀
Kraurosis
Leukoplakia } of vulva

> EXCLUDES   *carcinoma in situ of vulva (233.3)*

624.1 Atrophy of vulva ♀

✓4ᵗʰ
✓5ᵗʰ Additional Digit Required   Unspecified Code   Other Specified Code   Manifestation Code   ▶◀ Revised Text   ● New Code   ▲ Revised Code Title

2003 ICD•9•CM   **October 2002 • Volume 1 — 167**

624.2 Hypertrophy of clitoris ♀
> EXCLUDES   *that in endocrine disorders (255.2, 256.1)*

624.3 Hypertrophy of labia ♀
Hypertrophy of vulva NOS
DEF: Overgrowth of fleshy folds on either side of vagina.

624.4 Old laceration or scarring of vulva ♀
DEF: Scarring or other evidence of old wound on external female genitalia.

624.5 Hematoma of vulva ♀
> EXCLUDES   *that complicating delivery (664.5)*

DEF: Blood in tissue of external genitalia.

624.6 Polyp of labia and vulva ♀

624.8 Other specified noninflammatory disorders of vulva and perineum ♀

Cyst ⎫
Edema ⎬ of vulva
Stricture ⎭

624.9 Unspecified noninflammatory disorder of vulva and perineum ♀

✓4th **625 Pain and other symptoms associated with female genital organs**

625.0 Dyspareunia ♀
> EXCLUDES   *psychogenic dyspareunia (302.76)*

DEF: Difficult or painful sexual intercourse.

625.1 Vaginismus ♀
Colpospasm   Vulvismus
> EXCLUDES   *psychogenic vaginismus (306.51)*

DEF: Vaginal spasms; due to involuntary contraction of musculature; prevents intercourse.

625.2 Mittelschmerz ♀
Intermenstrual pain   Ovulation pain
DEF: Pain occurring between menstrual periods.

625.3 Dysmenorrhea ♀
Painful menstruation
> EXCLUDES   *psychogenic dysmenorrhea (306.52)*

625.4 Premenstrual tension syndromes ♀
Menstrual:
    migraine
    molimen
Premenstual syndrome
Premenstrual tension NOS

625.5 Pelvic congestion syndrome ♀
Congestion-fibrosis syndrome   Taylor's syndrome
DEF: Excessive accumulated of blood in vessels of pelvis; may occur after orgasm; causes abnormal menstruation, lower back pain and vaginal discharge.

625.6 Stress incontinence, female ♀
> EXCLUDES   *mixed incontinence (788.33)*
> *stress incontinence, male (788.32)*

DEF: Involuntary leakage of urine due to insufficient sphincter control; occurs upon sneezing, laughing, coughing, sudden movement or lifting.

625.8 Other specified symptoms associated with female genital organs ♀

625.9 Unspecified symptom associated with female genital organs ♀

✓4th **626 Disorders of menstruation and other abnormal bleeding from female genital tract**
> EXCLUDES   *menopausal and premenopausal bleeding (627.0)*
> *pain and other symptoms associated with menstrual cycle (625.2-625.4)*
> *postmenopausal bleeding (627.1)*

626.0 Absence of menstruation ♀
Amenorrhea (primary) (secondary)

626.1 Scanty or infrequent menstruation ♀
Hypomenorrhea   Oligomenorrhea

626.2 Excessive or frequent menstruation ♀
Heavy periods   Menorrhagia
Menometrorrhagia   Plymenorrhea
> EXCLUDES   *premenopausal(627.0)*
> *that in puberty (626.3)*

626.3 Puberty bleeding ♀
Excessive bleeding associated with onset of menstrual periods
Pubertal menorrhagia

626.4 Irregular menstrual cycle ♀
Irregular: Irregular:
  bleeding NOS   periods
  menstruation

626.5 Ovulation bleeding ♀
Regular intermenstrual bleeding

626.6 Metrorrhagia ♀
Bleeding unrelated to menstrual cycle
Irregular intermenstrual bleeding

626.7 Postcoital bleeding ♀
DEF: Bleeding from vagina after sexual intercourse.

626.8 Other ♀
Dysfunctional or functional uterine hemorrhage NOS
Menstruation:
  retained
  suppression of

626.9 Unspecified ♀

✓4th **627 Menopausal and postmenopausal disorders**
> EXCLUDES   *asymptomatic age-related (natural) postmenopausal status (V49.81)*

627.0 Premenopausal menorrhagia ♀
Excessive bleeding associated with onset of menopause
Menorrhagia:
  climacteric
  menopausal
  preclimacteric

627.1 Postmenopausal bleeding ♀

▲ **627.2 Symptomatic menopausal or female climacteric states** ♀
Symptoms, such as flushing, sleeplessness, headache, lack of concentration, associated with the menopause

627.3 Postmenopausal atrophic vaginitis ♀
Senile (atrophic) vaginitis

▲ **627.4 Symptomatic states associated with artificial menopause** ♀
Postartificial menopause syndromes
Any condition classifiable to 627.1, 627.2, or 627.3 which follows induced menopause
DEF: Conditions arising after hysterectomy.

627.8 Other specified menopausal and postmenopausal disorders ♀
> EXCLUDES   *premature menopause NOS (256.31)*

627.9 Unspecified menopausal and postmenopausal disorder ♀

✓4ᵗʰ **628 Infertility, female**

INCLUDES   primary and secondary sterility

DEF: Infertility: inability to conceive for at least one year with regular intercourse.

DEF: Primary infertility: occurring in patients who have never conceived.

DEF: Secondary infertility; occurring in patients who have previously conceived.

628.0   Associated with anovulation   ♀
Anovulatory cycle
Use additional code for any associated Stein-Leventhal syndrome (256.4)

628.1   *Of pituitary-hypothalamic origin*   ♀
Code first underlying cause, as:
adiposogenital dystrophy (253.8)
anterior pituitary disorder (253.0-253.4)

628.2   Of tubal origin   ♀
Infertility associated with congenital anomaly of tube
Tubal:
block
occlusion
stenosis
Use additional code for any associated peritubal adhesions (614.6)

628.3   Of uterine origin   ♀
Infertility associated with congenital anomaly of uterus
Nonimplantation
Use additional code for any associated tuberculous endometritis (016.7)

628.4   Of cervical or vaginal origin   ♀
Infertility associated with:
anomaly of cervical mucus
congenital structural anomaly
dysmucorrhea

628.8   Of other specified origin   ♀

628.9   Of unspecified origin   ♀

✓4ᵗʰ **629 Other disorders of female genital organs**

629.0   Hematocele, female, not elsewhere classified   ♀
EXCLUDES   *hematocele or hematoma:*
broad ligament (620.7)
fallopian tube (620.8)
*that associated with ectopic
pregnancy* ▶*(633.00-633.91)*◀
uterus (621.4)
vagina (623.6)
vulva (624.5)

629.1   Hydrocele, canal of Nuck   ♀
Cyst of canal of Nuck (acquired)
EXCLUDES   *congenital (752.41)*

629.8   Other specified disorders of female genital organs   ♀

629.9   Unspecified disorder of female genital organs   ♀
Habitual aborter without current pregnancy

✓4ᵗʰ
✓5ᵗʰ   Additional Digit Required   Unspecified Code   Other Specified Code   Manifestation Code   ▶◀ Revised Text   ● New Code   ▲ Revised Code Title

2003 ICD•9•CM   October 2002 • Volume 1 — 169

11. COMPLICATIONS OF PREGNANCY, CHILDBIRTH, AND THE PUERPERIUM (630-677)

ECTOPIC AND MOLAR PREGNANCY (630-633)

Use additional code from category 639 to identify any complications

630 Hydatidiform mole 　Ⓜ♀

Trophoblastic disease NOS
Vesicularmole

> **EXCLUDES** chorioadenoma (destruens) (236.1)
> chorionepithelioma (181)
> malignant hydatidiform mole (236.1)

DEF: Abnormal product of pregnancy; marked by mass of cysts resembling bunch of grapes due to chorionic villi proliferation, and dissolution; must be surgically removed.

631 Other abnormal product of conception 　Ⓜ♀

Blighted ovum
Mole:
　NOS
　carneous
　fleshy
　stone

632 Missed abortion 　Ⓜ♀

Early fetal death before completion of 22 weeks' gestation with retention of dead fetus
Retained products of conception, not following spontaneous or induced abortion or delivery

> **EXCLUDES** failed induced abortion (638.0-638.9)
> fetal death (intrauterine) (late) (656.4)
> missed delivery (656.4)
> that with abnormal product of conception (630, 631)

√4th **633 Ectopic pregnancy**

> **INCLUDES** ruptured ectopic pregnancy

DEF: Fertilized egg develops outside uterus.

√5th **633.0 Abdominal pregnancy**
Intraperitoneal pregnancy

- **633.00 Abdominal pregnancy without intrauterine pregnancy** 　Ⓜ♀
- **633.01 Abdominal pregnancy with intrauterine pregnancy** 　Ⓜ♀

√5th **633.1 Tubal pregnancy**
Fallopian pregnancy
Rupture of (fallopian) tube due to pregnancy
Tubal abortion

- **633.10 Tubal pregnancy without intrauterine pregnancy** 　Ⓜ♀
- **633.11 Tubal pregnancy with intrauterine pregnancy** 　Ⓜ♀

√5th **633.2 Ovarian pregnancy**

- **633.20 Ovarian pregnancy without intrauterine pregnancy** 　Ⓜ♀
- **633.21 Ovarian pregnancy with intrauterine pregnancy** 　Ⓜ♀

√5th **633.8 Other ectopic pregnancy**

Pregnancy: 　　Pregnancy:
　cervical 　　intraligamentous
　combined 　　mesometric
　cornual 　　mural

- **633.80 Other ectopic pregnancy without intrauterine pregnancy** 　Ⓜ♀
- **633.81 Other ectopic pregnancy with intrauterine pregnancy** 　Ⓜ♀

√5th **633.9 Unspecified ectopic pregnancy**

- **633.90 Unspecified ectopic pregnancy without intrauterine pregnancy** 　Ⓜ♀
- **633.91 Unspecified ectopic pregnancy with intrauterine pregnancy** 　Ⓜ♀

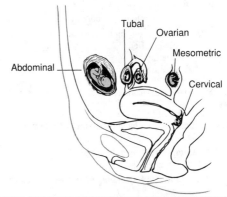

Ectopic Pregnancy Sites

Tubal
Ovarian
Mesometric
Abdominal
Cervical

OTHER PREGNANCY WITH ABORTIVE OUTCOME (634-639)

The following fourth-digit subdivisions are for use with categories 634-638:

.0 Complicated by genital tract and pelvic infection
Endometritis
Salpingo-oophoritis
Sepsis NOS
Septicemia NOS
Any condition classifiable to 639.0, with condition classifiable to 634-638

> **EXCLUDES** urinary tract infection (634-638 with .7)

.1 Complicated by delayed or excessive hemorrhage
Afibrinogenemia
Defibrination syndrome
Intravascular hemolysis
Any condition classifiable to 639.1, with condition classifiable to 634-638

.2 Complicated by damage to pelvic organs and tissues
Laceration, perforation, or tear of:
　bladder
　uterus
Any condition classifiable to 639.2, with condition classifiable to 634-638

.3 Complicated by renal failure
Oliguria
Uremia
Any condition classifiable to 639.3, with condition classifiable to 634-638

.4 Complicated by metabolic disorder
Electrolyte imbalance with conditions classifiable to 634-638

.5 Complicated by shock
Circulatory collapse
Shock (postoperative) (septic)
Any condition classifiable to 639.5, with condition classifiable to 634-638

.6 Complicated by embolism
Embolism:
　NOS
　amniotic fluid
　pulmonary
Any condition classifiable to 639.6, with condition classifiable to 634-638

.7 With other specified complications
Cardiac arrest or failure
Urinary tract infection
Any condition classifiable to 639.8, with condition classifiable to 634-638

.8 With unspecified complication
.9 Without mention of complication

Complications of Pregnancy, Childbirth, & Puerperium 630–633.91

√4th / √5th Additional Digit Required　　Unspecified Code　　Other Specified Code　　Manifestation Code　　▶◀ Revised Text　　● New Code　　▲ Revised Code Title

Complications of Pregnancy, Childbirth, & Puerperium 634–639

§ ✓4ᵗʰ **634 Spontaneous abortion**

> INCLUDES   miscarriage
>   spontaneous abortion
>
> Requires fifth-digit to identify stage:
>   **0 unspecified**
>   **1 incomplete**
>   **2 complete**

DEF: Spontaneous premature expulsion of the products of conception from the uterus.

✓5ᵗʰ **634.0 Complicated by genital tract and pelvic infection**   Ⓜ♀

✓5ᵗʰ **634.1 Complicated by delayed or excessive hemorrhage**   Ⓜ♀

✓5ᵗʰ **634.2 Complicated by damage to pelvic organs or tissues**   Ⓜ♀

✓5ᵗʰ **634.3 Complicated by renal failure**   Ⓜ♀

✓5ᵗʰ **634.4 Complicated by metabolic disorder**   Ⓜ♀

✓5ᵗʰ **634.5 Complicated by shock**   Ⓜ♀

✓5ᵗʰ **634.6 Complicated by embolism**   Ⓜ♀

✓5ᵗʰ **634.7 With other specified complications**   Ⓜ♀

✓5ᵗʰ **634.8 With unspecified complication**   Ⓜ♀

✓5ᵗʰ **634.9 Without mention of complication**   Ⓜ♀

§ ✓4ᵗʰ **635 Legally induced abortion**

> INCLUDES   abortion or termination of pregnancy:
>   elective
>   legal
>   therapeutic
>
> EXCLUDES   *menstrual extraction or regulation (V25.3)*
>
> Requires fifth-digit to identify stage:
>   **0 unspecified**
>   **1 incomplete**
>   **2 complete**

DEF: Intentional expulsion of products of conception from uterus performed by medical professionals inside boundaries of law.

✓5ᵗʰ **635.0 Complicated by genital tract and pelvic infection**   Ⓜ♀

✓5ᵗʰ **635.1 Complicated by delayed or excessive hemorrhage**   Ⓜ♀

✓5ᵗʰ **635.2 Complicated by damage to pelvic organs or tissues**   Ⓜ♀

✓5ᵗʰ **635.3 Complicated by renal failure**   Ⓜ♀

✓5ᵗʰ **635.4 Complicated by metabolic disorder**   Ⓜ♀

✓5ᵗʰ **635.5 Complicated by shock**   Ⓜ♀

✓5ᵗʰ **635.6 Complicated by embolism**   Ⓜ♀

✓5ᵗʰ **635.7 With other specified complications**   Ⓜ♀

✓5ᵗʰ **635.8 With unspecified complication**   Ⓜ♀

✓5ᵗʰ **635.9 Without mention of complication**   Ⓜ♀

§ ✓4ᵗʰ **636 Illegally induced abortion**

> INCLUDES   abortion:
>   criminal
>   illegal
>   self-induced
>
> Requires fifth-digit to identify stage:
>   **0 unspecified**
>   **1 incomplete**
>   **2 complete**

DEF: Intentional expulsion of products of conception from uterus; outside boundaries of law.

✓5ᵗʰ **636.0 Complicated by genital tract and pelvic infection**   Ⓜ♀

✓5ᵗʰ **636.1 Complicated by delayed or excessive hemorrhage**   Ⓜ♀

✓5ᵗʰ **636.2 Complicated by damage to pelvic organs or tissues**   Ⓜ♀

✓5ᵗʰ **636.3 Complicated by renal failure**   Ⓜ♀

✓5ᵗʰ **636.4 Complicated by metabolic disorder**   Ⓜ♀

✓5ᵗʰ **636.5 Complicated by shock**   Ⓜ♀

✓5ᵗʰ **636.6 Complicated by embolism**   Ⓜ♀

✓5ᵗʰ **636.7 With other specified complications**   Ⓜ♀

✓5ᵗʰ **636.8 With unspecified complication**   Ⓜ♀

✓5ᵗʰ **636.9 Without mention of complication**   Ⓜ♀

§ ✓4ᵗʰ **637 Unspecified abortion**

> INCLUDES   abortion NOS
>   retained products of conception following abortion, not classifiable elsewhere
>
> Requires fifth-digit to identify stage:
>   **0 unspecified**
>   **1 incomplete**
>   **2 complete**

✓5ᵗʰ **637.0 Complicated by genital tract and pelvic infection**   Ⓜ♀

✓5ᵗʰ **637.1 Complicated by delayed or excessive hemorrhage**   Ⓜ♀

✓5ᵗʰ **637.2 Complicated by damage to pelvic organs or tissues**   Ⓜ♀

✓5ᵗʰ **637.3 Complicated by renal failure**   Ⓜ♀

✓5ᵗʰ **637.4 Complicated by metabolic disorder**   Ⓜ♀

✓5ᵗʰ **637.5 Complicated by shock**   Ⓜ♀

✓5ᵗʰ **637.6 Complicated by embolism**   Ⓜ♀

✓5ᵗʰ **637.7 With other specified complications**   Ⓜ♀

✓5ᵗʰ **637.8 With unspecified complication**   Ⓜ♀

✓5ᵗʰ **637.9 Without mention of complication**   Ⓜ♀

§ ✓4ᵗʰ **638 Failed attempted abortion**

> INCLUDES   failure of attempted induction of (legal) abortion
>
> EXCLUDES   *incomplete abortion (634.0-637.9)*

DEF: Continued pregnancy despite an attempted legal abortion.

638.0 Complicated by genital tract and pelvic infection   Ⓜ♀

638.1 Complicated by delayed or excessive hemorrhage   Ⓜ♀

638.2 Complicated by damage to pelvic organs or tissues   Ⓜ♀

638.3 Complicated by renal failure   Ⓜ♀

638.4 Complicated by metabolic disorder   Ⓜ♀

638.5 Complicated by shock   Ⓜ♀

638.6 Complicated by embolism   Ⓜ♀

638.7 With other specified complications   Ⓜ♀

638.8 With unspecified complication   Ⓜ♀

638.9 Without mention of complication   Ⓜ♀

✓4ᵗʰ **639 Complications following abortion and ectopic and molar pregnancies**

Note: This category is provided for use when it is required to classify separately the complications classifiable to the fourth-digit level in categories 634-638; for example:

a) when the complication itself was responsible for an episode of medical care, the abortion, ectopic or molar pregnancy itself having been dealt with at a previous episode

b) when these conditions are immediate complications of ectopic or molar pregnancies classifiable to 630-633 where they cannot be identified at fourth-digit level.

§ See beginning of section 634–639 for fourth-digit definitions.

639.0 Genital tract and pelvic infection Ⓜ ♀

Endometritis
Parametritis
Pelvic peritonitis
Salpingitis — following conditions classifiable to 630-638
Salpingo-oophoritis
Sepsis NOS
Septicemia NOS

EXCLUDES *urinary tract infection (639.8)*

639.1 Delayed or excessive hemorrhage Ⓜ ♀

Afibrinogenemia
Defibrination syndrome — following conditions classifiable to 630-638
Intravascular hemolysis

639.2 Damage to pelvic organs and tissues Ⓜ ♀

Laceration, perforation, or tear of:
bladder
bowel
broad ligament — following conditions classifiable to 630-638
cervix
periurethral tissue
uterus
vagina

639.3 Renal failure Ⓜ ♀

Oliguria
Renal:
failure (acute)
shutdown — following conditions classifiable to 630-638
tubular necrosis
Uremia

639.4 Metabolic disorders Ⓜ ♀

Electrolyte imbalance following conditions classifiable to 630-638

639.5 Shock Ⓜ ♀

Circulatory collapse
Shock (postoperative) — following conditions classifiable to 630-638
(septic)

639.6 Embolism Ⓜ ♀

Embolism:
NOS
air
amniotic fluid
blood-clot
fat — following conditions classifiable to 630-638
pulmonary
pyemic
septic
soap

639.8 Other specified complications following abortion or ectopic and molar pregnancy Ⓜ ♀

Acute yellow atrophy or necrosis of liver
Cardiac arrest or failure — following conditions classifiable to 630-638
Cerebral anoxia
Urinary tract infection

639.9 Unspecified complication following abortion or ectopic and molar pregnancy Ⓜ ♀

Complication(s) not further specified following conditions classifiable to 630-638

COMPLICATIONS MAINLY RELATED TO PREGNANCY (640-648)

INCLUDES the listed conditions even if they arose or were present during labor, delivery, or the puerperium

The following fifth-digit subclassification is for use with categories 640-648 to denote the current episode of care. Valid fifth-digits are in [brackets] under each code.

0 unspecified as to episode of care or not applicable

1 delivered, with or without mention of antepartum condition
Antepartum condition with delivery
Delivery NOS (with mention of antepartum complication during current episode of care)
Intrapartum obstetric condition (with mention of antepartum complication during current episode of care)
Pregnancy, delivered (with mention of antepartum complication during current episode of care)

2 delivered, with mention of postpartum complication
Delivery with mention of puerperal complication during current episode of care

3 antepartum condition or complication
Antepartum obstetric condition, not delivered during the current episode of care

4 postpartum condition or complication
Postpartum or puerperal obstetric condition or complication following delivery that occurred:
during previous episode of care
outside hospital, with subsequent admission for observation or care

✓4th **640 Hemorrhage in early pregnancy**

INCLUDES hemorrhage before completion of 22 weeks' gestation

§ ✓5th **640.0 Threatened abortion** Ⓜ ♀
[0,1,3] DEF: Bloody discharge during pregnancy; cervix may be dilated and pregnancy is threatened, but the pregnancy is not terminated.

§ ✓5th **640.8 Other specified hemorrhage in early pregnancy** Ⓜ ♀
[0,1,3]

§ ✓5th **640.9 Unspecified hemorrhage in early pregnancy** Ⓜ ♀
[0,1,3]

✓4th **641 Antepartum hemorrhage, abruptio placentae, and placenta previa**

§ ✓5th **641.0 Placenta previa without hemorrhage** Ⓜ ♀
[0,1,3]
Low implantation of placenta
Placenta previa noted: — without hemorrhage
during pregnancy
before labor (and delivered by cesarean delivery)

DEF: Placenta implanted in lower segment of uterus; commonly causes hemorrhage in the last trimester of pregnancy.

§ ✓5th **641.1 Hemorrhage from placenta previa** Ⓜ ♀
[0,1,3]
Low-lying placenta
Placenta previa: — NOS or with hemorrhage (intrapartum)
incomplete
marginal
partial
total

EXCLUDES *hemorrhage from vasa previa (663.5)*

§ Requires fifth digit. Valid digits are in [brackets] under each code. See beginning of section 640–648 for codes and definitions.

Complications of Pregnancy, Childbirth, & Puerperium 639.0–641.1

✓4th ✓5th **Additional Digit Required** | **Unspecified Code** | **Other Specified Code** | **Manifestation Code** | ▶◀ Revised Text | ● New Code | ▲ Revised Code Title

2003 ICD•9•CM | **Volume 1 — 173**

Complications of Pregnancy, Childbirth, & Puerperium 641.2–643

Placenta Previa

| Low (marginal) implantation | Partial placenta previa | Total placenta previa |

§ ✓5ᵗʰ **641.2 Premature separation of placenta** Ⓜ ♀
[0,1,3]
  Ablatio placentae
  Abruptio placentae
  Accidental antepartum hemorrhage
  Couvelaire uterus
  Detachment of placenta (premature)
  Premature separation of normally implanted
    placenta

DEF: Abruptio placentae: premature detachment of the placenta, characterized by shock, oliguria and decreased fibrinogen.

§ ✓5ᵗʰ **641.3 Antepartum hemorrhage associated with** Ⓜ ♀
[0,1,3] **coagulation defects**
  Antepartum or intrapartum hemorrhage associated
    with:
    afibrinogenemia
    hyperfibrinolysis
    hypofibrinogenemia

DEF: Uterine hemorrhage prior to delivery.

§ ✓5ᵗʰ **641.8 Other antepartum hemorrhage** Ⓜ ♀
[0,1,3]
  Antepartum or intrapartum hemorrhage associated
    with:
    trauma
    uterine leiomyoma

§ ✓5ᵗʰ **641.9 Unspecified antepartum hemorrhage** Ⓜ ♀
[0,1,3]
  Hemorrhage: Hemorrhage:
    antepartum NOS   of pregnancy NOS
    intrapartum NOS

✓4ᵗʰ **642 Hypertension complicating pregnancy, childbirth, and the puerperium**

Abruptio Placentae

| Partial separation (concealed bleeding) | Partial separation (apparent hemorrhage) | Complete separation (concealed hemorrhage) |

§ ✓5ᵗʰ **642.0 Benign essential hypertension complicating** Ⓜ ♀
[0-4] **pregnancy, childbirth, and the puerperium**
  Hypertension: specified as complicating,
    benign essential   or as a reason for
    chronic NOS   obstetric care during
    essential   pregnancy,
    pre-existing NOS   childbirth, or the
                            puerperium

§ ✓5ᵗʰ **642.1 Hypertension secondary to renal disease,** Ⓜ ♀
[0-4] **complicating pregnancy, childbirth, and the**
  puerperium
  Hypertension secondary to renal disease, specified
    as complicating, or as a reason for obstetric
    care during pregnancy, childbirth, or the
    puerperium

§ ✓5ᵗʰ **642.2 Other pre-existing hypertension complicating** Ⓜ ♀
[0-4] **pregnancy, childbirth, and the puerperium**
  Hypertensive: specified as complicating,
    heart and renal   or as a reason for
      disease   obstetric care
    heart disease   during pregnancy,
    renal disease   childbirth, or the
  Malignant   puerperium
    hypertension

§ ✓5ᵗʰ **642.3 Transient hypertension of pregnancy** Ⓜ ♀
[0-4]
  Gestational hypertension
  Transient hypertension, so described, in pregnancy,
    childbirth, or the puerperium

§ ✓5ᵗʰ **642.4 Mild or unspecified pre-eclampsia** Ⓜ ♀
[0-4]
  Hypertension in pregnancy, childbirth, or the
    puerperium, not specified as pre-existing, with
    either albuminuria or edema, or both; mild or
    unspecified
  Pre-eclampsia: Toxemia (pre-eclamptic):
    NOS   NOS
    mild   mild
  EXCLUDES *albuminuria in pregnancy, without*
    mention of hypertension (646.2)
    edema in pregnancy, without mention
    of hypertension (646.1)

§ ✓5ᵗʰ **642.5 Severe pre-eclampsia** Ⓜ ♀
[0-4]
  Hypertension in pregnancy, childbirth, or the
    puerperium, not specified as pre-existing, with
    either albuminuria or edema, or both; specified
    as severe
  Pre-eclampsia, severe
  Toxemia (pre-eclamptic), severe

§ ✓5ᵗʰ **642.6 Eclampsia** Ⓜ ♀
[0-4]
  Toxemia:
    eclamptic
    with convulsions

§ ✓5ᵗʰ **642.7 Pre-eclampsia or eclampsia superimposed on** Ⓜ ♀
[0-4] **pre existing hypertension**
  Conditions classifiable to 642.4-642.6, with
    conditions classifiable to 642.0-642.2

§ ✓5ᵗʰ **642.9 Unspecified hypertension complicating** Ⓜ ♀
[0-4] **pregnancy, childbirth, or the puerperium**
  Hypertension NOS, without mention of albuminuria
    or edema, complicating pregnancy, childbirth,
    or the puerperium

✓4ᵗʰ **643 Excessive vomiting in pregnancy**
  INCLUDES hyperemesis
    vomiting: arising during pregnancy
      persistent
      vicious

  hyperemesis gravidarum

§ Requires fifth digit. Valid digits are in [brackets] under each code. See beginning of section 640–648 for codes and definitions.

Ⓝ Newborn Age: 0   Ⓟ Pediatric Age: 0-17   Ⓜ Maternity Age: 12-55   Ⓐ Adult Age: 15-124   **MSP** Medicare Secondary Payer

§ ✓5ᵗʰ **643.0 Mild hyperemesis gravidarum** M ♀
[0,1,3]   Hyperemesis gravidarum, mild or unspecified, starting before the end of the 22nd week of gestation

      DEF: Detrimental vomiting and nausea.

§ ✓5ᵗʰ **643.1 Hyperemesis gravidarum with metabolic** M ♀
[0,1,3] **disturbance**
     Hyperemesis gravidarum, starting before the end of the 22nd week of gestation, with metabolic disturbance, such as:
      carbohydrate depletion
      dehydration
      electrolyte imbalance

§ ✓5ᵗʰ **643.2 Late vomiting of pregnancy** M ♀
[0,1,3]   Excessive vomiting starting after 22 completed weeks of gestation

§ ✓5ᵗʰ **643.8 Other vomiting complicating pregnancy** M ♀
[0,1,3]   Vomiting due to organic disease or other cause, specified as complicating pregnancy, or as a reason for obstetric care during pregnancy
     Use additional code to specify cause

§ ✓5ᵗʰ **643.9 Unspecified vomiting of pregnancy** M ♀
[0,1,3]   Vomiting as a reason for care during pregnancy, length of gestation unspecified

✓4ᵗʰ **644 Early or threatened labor**

§ ✓5ᵗʰ **644.0 Threatened premature labor** M ♀
[0,3]   Premature labor after 22 weeks, but before 37 completed weeks of gestation without delivery
      EXCLUDES *that occurring before 22 completed weeks of gestation (640.0)*

§ ✓5ᵗʰ **644.1 Other threatened labor** M ♀
[0,3]   False labor:
      NOS
      after 37 completed weeks of gestation } without delivery
      Threatened labor NOS

§ ✓5ᵗʰ **644.2 Early onset of delivery** M ♀
[0,1]   Onset (spontaneous) of delivery } before 37 completed weeks of gestation
      Premature labor with onset of delivery

✓4ᵗʰ **645 Late pregnancy**

§ ✓5ᵗʰ **645.1 Post term pregnancy** M ♀
[0,1,3]   Pregnancy over 40 completed weeks to 42 completed weeks gestation

§ ✓5ᵗʰ **645.2 Prolonged pregnancy** M ♀
[0,1,3]   Pregnancy which has advanced beyond 42 completed weeks of gestation

✓4ᵗʰ **646 Other complications of pregnancy, not elsewhere classified**
     Use additional code(s) to further specify complication

§ ✓5ᵗʰ **646.0 Papyraceous fetus** M ♀
[0,1,3]   DEF: Fetus retained in the uterus beyond natural term, exhibits parchment-like skin.

§ ✓5ᵗʰ **646.1 Edema or excessive weight gain in pregnancy,** M ♀
[0-4] **without mention of hypertension**
     Gestational edema   Maternal obesity syndrome
      EXCLUDES *that with mention of hypertension (642.0-642.)*

§ ✓5ᵗʰ **646.2 Unspecified renal disease in pregnancy,** M ♀
[0-4] **without mention of hypertension**
     Albuminuria
     Nephropathy NOS   } in pregnancy or the
     Renal disease NOS   puerperium,
     Uremia   without mention of hypertension

     Gestational proteinuria
      EXCLUDES *that with mention of hypertension (642.0-642.9)*

§ ✓5ᵗʰ **646.3 Habitual aborter** M ♀
[0,1,3]   EXCLUDES *with current abortion (634.0-634.9)*
                    without current pregnancy (629.9)

     DEF: Three or more consecutive spontaneous abortions.

§ ✓5ᵗʰ **646.4 Peripheral neuritis in pregnancy** M ♀
[0-4]

§ ✓5ᵗʰ **646.5 Asymptomatic bacteriuria in pregnancy** M ♀
[0-4]

§ ✓5ᵗʰ **646.6 Infections of genitourinary tract in pregnancy** M ♀
[0-4]   Conditions classifiable to 590, 595, 597, 599.0, 616 complicating pregnancy, childbirth, or the puerperium
     Conditions classifiable to ▶(614.0-614.5, 614.7-614.9, 615)◀ complicating pregnancy or labor
      EXCLUDES *major puerperal infection (670)*

§ ✓5ᵗʰ **646.7 Liver disorders in pregnancy** M ♀
[0,1,3]   Acute yellow atrophy of liver (obstetric) (true)
     Icterus gravis   } of pregnancy
     Necrosis of liver

      EXCLUDES *hepatorenal syndrome following delivery (674.8)*
                   viral hepatitis (647.6)

§ ✓5ᵗʰ **646.8 Other specified complications of pregnancy** M ♀
[0-4]   Fatigue during pregnancy
     Herpes gestationis
     Insufficient weight gain of pregnancy
     Uterine size-date discrepancy

§ ✓5ᵗʰ **646.9 Unspecified complication of pregnancy** M ♀
[0,1,3]

✓4ᵗʰ **647 Infectious and parasitic conditions in the mother classifiable elsewhere, but complicating pregnancy, childbirth, or the puerperium**
      INCLUDES the listed conditions when complicating the pregnant state, aggravated by the pregnancy, or when a main reason for obstetric care
      EXCLUDES *those conditions in the mother known or suspected to have affected the fetus (655.0-655.9)*
     Use additional code(s) to further specify complication

§ ✓5ᵗʰ **647.0 Syphilis** M ♀
[0-4]   Conditions classifiable to 090-097

§ ✓5ᵗʰ **647.1 Gonorrhea** M ♀
[0-4]   Conditions classifiable to 098

§ ✓5ᵗʰ **647.2 Other venereal diseases** M ♀
[0-4]   Conditions classifiable to 099

§ ✓5ᵗʰ **647.3 Tuberculosis** M ♀
[0-4]   Conditions classifiable to 010-018

§ ✓5ᵗʰ **647.4 Malaria** M ♀
[0-4]   Conditions classifiable to 084

§ ✓5ᵗʰ **647.5 Rubella** M ♀
[0-4]   Conditions classifiable to 056

---

§ Requires fifth digit. Valid digits are in [brackets] under each code. See beginning of section 640–648 for codes and definitions.

 Additional Digit Required   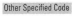 Unspecified Code   Other Specified Code   Manifestation Code   ▶◀ Revised Text   ● New Code   ▲ Revised Code Title

§ ☑5ᵗʰ **647.6 Other viral diseases** Ⓜ♀
[0-4]   Conditions classifiable to 042 and 050-079, except 056

§ ☑5ᵗʰ **647.8 Other specified infectious and parasitic** Ⓜ♀
[0-4]   **diseases**

§ ☑5ᵗʰ **647.9 Unspecified infection or infestation** Ⓜ♀
[0-4]

☑4ᵗʰ **648 Other current conditions in the mother classifiable elsewhere, but complicating pregnancy, childbirth, or the puerperium**

> **INCLUDES** the listed conditions when complicating the pregnant state, aggravated by the pregnancy, or when a main reason for obstetric care
>
> **EXCLUDES** *those conditions in the mother known or suspected to have affected the fetus (655.0-665.9)*

Use additional code(s) to identify the condition

§ ☑5ᵗʰ **648.0 Diabetes mellitus** Ⓜ♀
[0-4]   Conditions classifiable to 250
> **EXCLUDES** *gestational diabetes (648.8)*

§ ☑5ᵗʰ **648.1 Thyroid dysfunction** Ⓜ♀
[0-4]   Conditions classifiable to 240-246

§ ☑5ᵗʰ **648.2 Anemia** Ⓜ♀
[0-4]   Conditions classifiable to 280-285

§ ☑5ᵗʰ **648.3 Drug dependence** Ⓜ♀
[0-4]   Conditions classifiable to 304

§ ☑5ᵗʰ **648.4 Mental disorders** Ⓜ♀
[0-4]   Conditions classifiable to 290-303, 305-316, 317-319

§ ☑5ᵗʰ **648.5 Congenital cardiovascular disorders** Ⓜ♀
[0-4]   Conditions classifiable to 745-747

§ ☑5ᵗʰ **648.6 Other cardiovascular diseases** Ⓜ♀
[0-4]   Conditions classifiable to 390-398, 410-429
> **EXCLUDES** *cerebrovascular disorders in the puerperium (674.0)*
> *venous complications (671.0-671.9)*

§ ☑5ᵗʰ **648.7 Bone and joint disorders of back, pelvis, and** Ⓜ♀
[0-4]   **lower limbs**
Conditions classifiable to 720-724, and those classifiable to 711-719 or 725-738, specified as affecting the lower limbs

§ ☑5ᵗʰ **648.8 Abnormal glucose tolerance** Ⓜ♀
[0-4]   Conditions classifiable to 790.2
Gestational diabetes
> **DEF:** Glucose intolerance arising in pregnancy, resolving at end of pregnancy.

§ ☑5ᵗʰ **648.9 Other current conditions classifiable** Ⓜ♀
[0-4]   **elsewhere**
Conditions classifiable to 440-459
Nutritional deficiencies [conditions classifiable to 260-269]

NORMAL DELIVERY, AND OTHER INDICATIONS FOR CARE IN PREGNANCY, LABOR, AND DELIVERY (650-659)

The following fifth-digit subclassification is for use with categories 651-659 to denote the current episode of care. Valid fifth-digits are in [brackets] under each code.

    0 unspecified as to episode of care or not applicable
    1 delivered, with or without mention of antepartum condition
    2 delivered, with mention of postpartum complication
    3 antepartum condition or complication
    4 postpartum condition or complication

650 Normal delivery Ⓜ♀
Delivery requiring minimal or no assistance, with or without episiotomy, without fetal manipulation [e.g., rotation version] or instrumentation [forceps] of spontaneous, cephalic, vaginal, full-term, single, live-born infant. This code is for use as a single diagnosis code and is not to be used with any other code in the range 630-676.
> **EXCLUDES** *breech delivery (assisted) (spontaneous) NOS (652.2)*
> *delivery by vacuum extractor, forceps, cesarean section, or breech extraction, without specified complication (669.5-669.7)*

Use additional code to indicate outcome of delivery (V27.0)

☑4ᵗʰ **651 Multiple gestation**

§ ☑5ᵗʰ **651.0 Twin pregnancy** Ⓜ♀
[0,1,3]

§ ☑5ᵗʰ **651.1 Triplet pregnancy** Ⓜ♀
[0,1,3]

§ ☑5ᵗʰ **651.2 Quadruplet pregnancy** Ⓜ♀
[0,1,3]

§ ☑5ᵗʰ **651.3 Twin pregnancy with fetal loss and retention** Ⓜ♀
[0,1,3]   **of one fetus**
Vanishing twin syndrome (651.33)

§ ☑5ᵗʰ **651.4 Triplet pregnancy with fetal loss and** Ⓜ♀
[0,1,3]   **retention of one or more fetus(es)**

§ ☑5ᵗʰ **651.5 Quadruplet pregnancy with fetal loss and** Ⓜ♀
[0,1,3]   **retention of one or more fetus(es)**

§ ☑5ᵗʰ **651.6 Other multiple pregnancy with fetal loss and** Ⓜ♀
[0,1,3]   **retention of one or more fetus(es)**

§ ☑5ᵗʰ **651.8 Other specified multiple gestation** Ⓜ♀
[0,1,3]

§ ☑5ᵗʰ **651.9 Unspecified multiple gestation** Ⓜ♀
[0,1,3]

☑4ᵗʰ **652 Malposition and malpresentation of fetus**
Code first any associated obstructed labor (660.0)

§ ☑5ᵗʰ **652.0 Unstable lie** Ⓜ♀
[0,1,3]   **DEF:** Changing fetal position.

§ ☑5ᵗʰ **652.1 Breech or other malpresentation successfully** Ⓜ♀
[0,1,3]   **converted to cephalic presentation**
Cephalic version NOS

§ ☑5ᵗʰ **652.2 Breech presentation without mention of** Ⓜ♀
[0,1,3]   **version**
Breech delivery (assisted) (spontaneous) NOS
Buttocks presentation
Complete breech
Frank breech
> **EXCLUDES** *footling presentation (652.8)*
> *incomplete breech (652.8)*

DEF: Fetal presentation of buttocks or feet at birth canal.

---

§ Requires fifth digit. Valid digits are in [brackets] under each code. See beginning of section 640–648 for codes and definitions.

Ⓝ Newborn Age: 0   Ⓟ Pediatric Age: 0-17   Ⓜ Maternity Age: 12-55   Ⓐ Adult Age: 15-124   **MSP** Medicare Secondary Payer

Malposition and Malpresentation

Breech

Mother's pelvis

Shoulder (arm prolapse)

Face (mentum)

Compound (extremity together with head)

Oblique

Cephalopelvic Disproportion

Pubic symphysis

Cephalopelvic disproportion due to: Contraction of pelvic inlet, or large fetus, or hydrocephalus

Ischial tuberosity

Contraction of pelvic outlet (from below)

Pubic symphysis

Pelvic inlet from above

§ ✓5ᵗʰ **652.3 Transverse or oblique presentation**   Ⓜ♀
   [0,1,3]
     Oblique lie   Transverse lie
     EXCLUDES *transverse arrest of fetal head (660.3)*
     DEF: Delivery of fetus, shoulder first.

§ ✓5ᵗʰ **652.4 Face or brow presentation**   Ⓜ♀
   [0,1,3]
     Mentum presentation

§ ✓5ᵗʰ **652.5 High head at term**   Ⓜ♀
   [0,1,3]
     Failure of head to enter pelvic brim

§ ✓5ᵗʰ **652.6 Multiple gestation with malpresentation**   Ⓜ♀
   [0,1,3] **of one fetus or more**

§ ✓5ᵗʰ **652.7 Prolapsed arm**   Ⓜ♀
   [0,1,3]

§ ✓5ᵗʰ **652.8 Other specified malposition or**   Ⓜ♀
   [0,1,3] **malpresentation**
     Compound presentation

§ ✓5ᵗʰ **652.9 Unspecified malposition or malpresentation**   Ⓜ♀
   [0,1,3]

✓4ᵗʰ **653 Disproportion**
     Code first any associated obstructed labor (660.1)

§ ✓5ᵗʰ **653.0 Major abnormality of bony pelvis, not further**   Ⓜ♀
   [0,1,3] **specified**
     Pelvic deformity NOS

§ ✓5ᵗʰ **653.1 Generally contracted pelvis**   Ⓜ♀
   [0,1,3]
     Contracted pelvis NOS

§ ✓5ᵗʰ **653.2 Inlet contraction of pelvis**   Ⓜ♀
   [0,1,3]
     Inlet contraction (pelvis)

§ ✓5ᵗʰ **653.3 Outlet contraction of pelvis**   Ⓜ♀
   [0,1,3]
     Outlet contraction (pelvis)

§ ✓5ᵗʰ **653.4 Fetopelvic disproportion**   Ⓜ♀
   [0,1,3]
     Cephalopelvic disproportion NOS
     Disproportion of mixed maternal and fetal origin,
       with normally formed fetus

§ ✓5ᵗʰ **653.5 Unusually large fetus causing disproportion**   Ⓜ♀
   [0,1,3]
     Disproportion of fetal origin with normally formed
       fetus
     Fetal disproportion NOS
     EXCLUDES *that when the reason for medical care*
       was concern for the fetus (656.6)

§ ✓5ᵗʰ **653.6 Hydrocephalic fetus causing disproportion**   Ⓜ♀
   [0,1,3] **EXCLUDES** *that when the reason for medical care*
       was concern for the fetus (655.0)

§ ✓5ᵗʰ **653.7 Other fetal abnormality causing disproportion**   Ⓜ♀
   [0,1,3]
     Conjoined twins   Fetal:
     Fetal: myelomeningocele
       ascites   sacral teratoma
       hydrops   tumor

§ ✓5ᵗʰ **653.8 Disproportion of other origin**   Ⓜ♀
   [0,1,3] **EXCLUDES** *shoulder (girdle) dystocia (660.4)*

§ ✓5ᵗʰ **653.9 Unspecified disproportion**   Ⓜ♀
   [0,1,3]

✓4ᵗʰ **654 Abnormality of organs and soft tissues of pelvis**
     INCLUDES the listed conditions during pregnancy,
       childbirth, or the puerperium
     Code first any associated obstructed labor (660.2)

§ ✓5ᵗʰ **654.0 Congenital abnormalities of uterus**   Ⓜ♀
   [0-4]
     Double uterus   Uterus bicornis

§ ✓5ᵗʰ **654.1 Tumors of body of uterus**   Ⓜ♀
   [0-4]
     Uterine fibroids

§ ✓5ᵗʰ **654.2 Previous cesarean delivery**   Ⓜ♀
   [0,1,3]
     Uterine scar from previous cesarean delivery

§ ✓5ᵗʰ **654.3 Retroverted and incarcerated gravid uterus**   Ⓜ♀
   [0-4]
     DEF: Retroverted: tilted back uterus; no change in angle of
     longitudinal axis.
     DEF: Incarcerated: immobile, fixed uterus.

§ ✓5ᵗʰ **654.4 Other abnormalities in shape or position of**   Ⓜ♀
   [0-4] **gravid uterus and of neighboring structures**
     Cystocele   Prolapse of gravid uterus
     Pelvic floor repair   Rectocele
     Pendulous abdomen Rigid pelvic floor

§ ✓5ᵗʰ **654.5 Cervical incompetence**   Ⓜ♀
   [0-4]
     Presence of Shirodkar suture with or without
       mention of cervical incompetence
     DEF: Abnormal cervix; tendency to dilate in second trimester;
     causes premature fetal expulsion.
     DEF: Shirodkar suture: purse-string suture used to artificially close
     incompetent cervix.

§ ✓5ᵗʰ **654.6 Other congenital or acquired abnormality of**   Ⓜ♀
   [0-4] **cervix**
     Cicatricial cervix   Rigid cervix (uteri)
     Polyp of cervix   Stenosis or stricture of cervix
     Previous surgery to cervix Tumor of cervix

§ ✓5ᵗʰ **654.7 Congenital or acquired abnormality of vagina**   Ⓜ♀
   [0-4]
     Previous surgery to vagina Stricture of vagina
     Septate vagina   Tumor of vagina
     Stenosis of vagina (acquired) (congenital)

§ ✓5ᵗʰ **654.8 Congenital or acquired abnormality of vulva**   Ⓜ♀
   [0-4]
     Fibrosis of perineum Rigid perineum
     Persistent hymen   Tumor of vulva
     Previous surgery to
       perineum or vulva
     EXCLUDES *varicose veins of vulva (671.1)*

§ ✓5ᵗʰ **654.9 Other and unspecified**   Ⓜ♀
   [0-4]
     Uterine scar NEC

§ Requires fifth digit. Valid digits are in [brackets] under each code. See beginning of section 640–648 for codes and definitions.

✓4ᵗʰ **655 Known or suspected fetal abnormality affecting management of mother**

> INCLUDES   the listed conditions in the fetus as a reason for observation or obstetrical care of the mother, or for termination of pregnancy

§ ✓5ᵗʰ **655.0 Central nervous system malformation in fetus** Ⓜ ♀
[0,1,3]
> Fetal or suspected fetal:
> anencephaly
> hydrocephalus
> spina bifida (with myelomeningocele)

§ ✓5ᵗʰ **655.1 Chromosomal abnormality in fetus** Ⓜ ♀
[0,1,3]

§ ✓5ᵗʰ **655.2 Hereditary disease in family possibly affecting fetus** Ⓜ ♀
[0,1,3]

§ ✓5ᵗʰ **655.3 Suspected damage to fetus from viral disease in the mother** Ⓜ ♀
[0,1,3]
> Suspected damage to fetus from maternal rubella

§ ✓5ᵗʰ **655.4 Suspected damage to fetus from other disease in the mother** Ⓜ ♀
[0,1,3]
> Suspected damage to fetus from maternal:
> alcohol addiction
> listeriosis
> toxoplasmosis

§ ✓5ᵗʰ **655.5 Suspected damage to fetus from drugs** Ⓜ ♀
[0,1,3]

§ ✓5ᵗʰ **655.6 Suspected damage to fetus from radiation** Ⓜ ♀
[0,1,3]

§ ✓5ᵗʰ **655.7 Decreased fetal movements** Ⓜ ♀
[0,1,3]

§ ✓5ᵗʰ **655.8 Other known or suspected fetal abnormality, not elsewhere classified** Ⓜ ♀
[0,1,3]
> Suspected damage to fetus from:
> environmental toxins
> intrauterine contraceptive device

§ ✓5ᵗʰ **655.9 Unspecified** Ⓜ ♀
[0,1,3]

✓4ᵗʰ **656 Other fetal and placental problems affecting management of mother**

§ ✓5ᵗʰ **656.0 Fetal-maternal hemorrhage** Ⓜ ♀
[0,1,3]
> Leakage (microscopic) of fetal blood into maternal circulation

§ ✓5ᵗʰ **656.1 Rhesus isoimmunization** Ⓜ ♀
[0,1,3]
> Anti-D [Rh] antibodies
> Rh incompatibility
> DEF: Antibodies developing against Rh factor; mother with Rh negative develops antibodies against Rh positive fetus.

§ ✓5ᵗʰ **656.2 Isoimmunization from other and unspecified blood-group incompatibility** Ⓜ ♀
[0,1,3]
> ABO isoimmunization

§ ✓5ᵗʰ **656.3 Fetal distress** Ⓜ ♀
[0,1,3]
> Fetal metabolic acidemia
> EXCLUDES   abnormal fetal acid-base balance (656.8)
> abnormality in fetal heart rate or rhythm (659.7)
> fetal bradycardia (659.7)
> fetal tachycardia (659.7)
> meconium in liquor (656.8)
> DEF: Life-threatening disorder; fetal anoxia, hemolytic disease and other miscellaneous diseases cause fetal distress.

§ ✓5ᵗʰ **656.4 Intrauterine death** Ⓜ ♀
[0,1,3]
> Fetal death:
> NOS
> after completion of 22 weeks' gestation
> late
> Missed delivery
> EXCLUDES   missed abortion (632)

§ ✓5ᵗʰ **656.5 Poor fetal growth** Ⓜ ♀
[0,1,3]
> "Light-for-dates"   "Small-for-dates"
> "Placental insufficiency"

§ ✓5ᵗʰ **656.6 Excessive fetal growth** Ⓜ ♀
[0,1,3]
> "Large-for-dates"

§ ✓5ᵗʰ **656.7 Other placental conditions** Ⓜ ♀
[0,1,3]
> Abnormal placenta   Placental infarct
> EXCLUDES   placental polyp (674.4)
> placentitis (658.4)

§ ✓5ᵗʰ **656.8 Other specified fetal and placental problems** Ⓜ ♀
[0,1,3]
> Abnormal acid-base balance
> Intrauterine acidosis
> Lithopedian
> Meconium in liquor
> DEF: Lithopedion: Calcified fetus; not expelled by mother.

§ ✓5ᵗʰ **656.9 Unspecified fetal and placental problem** Ⓜ ♀
[0,1,3]

✓4ᵗʰ **657 Polyhydramnios** Ⓜ ♀
[0,1,3]
§ ✓5ᵗʰ   Use 0 as fourth-digit for this category
> Hydramnios
> DEF: Excess amniotic fluid.

✓4ᵗʰ **658 Other problems associated with amniotic cavity and membranes**
> EXCLUDES   amniotic fluid embolism (673.1)

§ ✓5ᵗʰ **658.0 Oligohydramnios** Ⓜ ♀
[0,1,3]
> Oligohydramnios without mention of rupture of membranes
> DEF: Deficient amount of amniotic fluid.

§ ✓5ᵗʰ **658.1 Premature rupture of membranes** Ⓜ ♀
[0,1,3]
> Rupture of amniotic sac less than 24 hours prior to the onset of labor

§ ✓5ᵗʰ **658.2 Delayed delivery after spontaneous or unspecified rupture of membranes** Ⓜ ♀
[0,1,3]
> Prolonged rupture of membranes NOS
> Rupture of amniotic sac 24 hours or more prior to the onset of labor

§ ✓5ᵗʰ **658.3 Delayed delivery after artificial rupture of membranes** Ⓜ ♀
[0,1,3]

§ ✓5ᵗʰ **658.4 Infection of amniotic cavity** Ⓜ ♀
[0,1,3]
> Amnionitis   Membranitis
> Chorioamnionitis   Placentitis

§ ✓5ᵗʰ **658.8 Other** Ⓜ ♀
[0,1,3]
> Amnion nodosum   Amniotic cyst

§ ✓5ᵗʰ **658.9 Unspecified** Ⓜ ♀
[0,1,3]

✓4ᵗʰ **659 Other indications for care or intervention related to labor and delivery, not elsewhere classified**

§ ✓5ᵗʰ **659.0 Failed mechanical induction** Ⓜ ♀
[0,1,3]
> Failure of induction of labor by surgical or other instrumental methods

§ ✓5ᵗʰ **659.1 Failed medical or unspecified induction** Ⓜ ♀
[0,1,3]
> Failed induction NOS
> Failure of induction of labor by medical methods, such as oxytocic drugs

§ ✓5ᵗʰ **659.2 Maternal pyrexia during labor, unspecified** Ⓜ ♀
[0,1,3]
> DEF: Fever during labor.

---

§ Requires fifth digit. Valid digits are in [brackets] under each code. See beginning of section 640–648 for codes and definitions.

Ⓝ Newborn Age: 0   Ⓟ Pediatric Age: 0-17   Ⓜ Maternity Age: 12-55   Ⓐ Adult Age: 15-124   MSP Medicare Secondary Payer

§ ✓5ᵗʰ **659.3 Generalized infection during labor**   Ⓜ♀
[0,1,3]   Septicemia during labor

§ ✓5ᵗʰ **659.4 Grand multiparity**   Ⓜ♀
[0,1,3]   **EXCLUDES** *supervision only, in pregnancy (V23.3)*
           without current pregnancy (V61.5)
   DEF: Having borne six or more children previously.

§ ✓5ᵗʰ **659.5 Elderly primigravida**   Ⓜ♀
[0,1,3]   First pregnancy in a woman who will be 35 years of
       age or older at expected date of delivery
     EXCLUDES *supervision only, in pregnancy (V23.81)*

§ ✓5ᵗʰ **659.6 Elderly multigravida**   Ⓜ♀
[0,1,3]   Second or more pregnancy in a woman who will be
       35 years of age or older at expected date of
       delivery
     EXCLUDES *elderly primigravida 659.5*
            supervision only, in pregnancy (V23.82)

§ ✓5ᵗʰ **659.7 Abnormality in fetal heart rate or rhythm**   Ⓜ♀
[0,1,3]   Depressed fetal heart tones
     Fetal:
       bradycardia
       tachycardia
     Fetal heart rate decelerations
     Non-reassuring fetal heart rate or rhythm

§ ✓5ᵗʰ **659.8 Other specified indications for care or**   Ⓜ♀
[0,1,3] **intervention related to labor and delivery**
     Pregnancy in a female less than 16 years old at
       expected date of delivery
     Very young maternal age

§ ✓5ᵗʰ **659.9 Unspecified indication for care or**   Ⓜ♀
[0,1,3] **intervention related to labor and delivery**

COMPLICATIONS OCCURRING MAINLY IN THE COURSE OF LABOR AND DELIVERY (660-669)

The following fifth-digit subclassification is for use with
categories 660-669 to denote the current episode of care.
Valid fifth-digits are in [brackets] under each code.
     0 unspecified as to episode of care or not
       applicable
     1 delivered, with or without mention of
       antepartum condition
     2 delivered, with mention of postpartum
       complication
     3 antepartum condition or complication
     4 postpartum condition or complication

✓4ᵗʰ **660 Obstructed labor**

§ ✓5ᵗʰ **660.0 Obstruction caused by malposition of fetus**   Ⓜ♀
[0,1,3] **at onset of labor**
     Any condition classifiable to 652, causing
       obstruction during labor
     Use additional code from 652.0-652.9 to identify
       condition

§ ✓5ᵗʰ **660.1 Obstruction by bony pelvis**   Ⓜ♀
[0,1,3]   Any condition classifiable to 653, causing
       obstruction during labor
     Use additional code from 653.0-653.9 to identify
       condition

§ ✓5ᵗʰ **660.2 Obstruction by abnormal pelvic soft tissues**   Ⓜ♀
[0,1,3]   Prolapse of anterior lip of cervix
     Any condition classifiable to 654, causing
       obstruction during labor
     Use additional code from 654.0-654.9 to identify
       condition

§ ✓5ᵗʰ **660.3 Deep transverse arrest and persistent**   Ⓜ♀
[0,1,3] **occipitoposterior position**

§ ✓5ᵗʰ **660.4 Shoulder (girdle) dystocia**   Ⓜ♀
[0,1,3]   Impacted shoulders
   DEF: Obstructed labor due to impacted fetal shoulders.

§ ✓5ᵗʰ **660.5 Locked twins**   Ⓜ♀
[0,1,3]

§ ✓5ᵗʰ **660.6 Failed trial of labor, unspecified**   Ⓜ♀
[0,1,3]   Failed trial of labor, without mention of condition or
       suspected condition

§ ✓5ᵗʰ **660.7 Failed forceps or vacuum extractor,**   Ⓜ♀
[0,1,3] **unspecified**
     Application of ventouse or forceps, without mention
       of condition

§ ✓5ᵗʰ **660.8 Other causes of obstructed labor**   Ⓜ♀
[0,1,3]

§ ✓5ᵗʰ **660.9 Unspecified obstructed labor**   Ⓜ♀
[0,1,3]   Dystocia: Dystocia:
       NOS   maternal NOS
       fetal NOS

✓4ᵗʰ **661 Abnormality of forces of labor**

§ ✓5ᵗʰ **661.0 Primary uterine inertia**   Ⓜ♀
[0,1,3]   Failure of cervical dilation
     Hypotonic uterine dysfunction, primary
     Prolonged latent phase of labor
   DEF: Lack of efficient contractions during labor causing prolonged
   labor.

§ ✓5ᵗʰ **661.1 Secondary uterine inertia**   Ⓜ♀
[0,1,3]   Arrested active phase of labor
     Hypotonic uterine dysfunction, secondary

§ ✓5ᵗʰ **661.2 Other and unspecified uterine inertia**   Ⓜ♀
[0,1,3]   Desultory labor   Poor contractions
     Irregular labor   Slow slope active phase
                         of labor

§ ✓5ᵗʰ **661.3 Precipitate labor**   Ⓜ♀
[0,1,3]   **DEF: Rapid labor and delivery.**

§ ✓5ᵗʰ **661.4 Hypertonic, incoordinate, or prolonged**   Ⓜ♀
[0,1,3] **uterine contractions**
     Cervical spasm
     Contraction ring (dystocia)
     Dyscoordinate labor
     Hourglass contraction of uterus
     Hypertonic uterine dysfunction
     Incoordinate uterine action
     Retraction ring (Bandl's) (pathological)
     Tetanic contractions
     Uterine dystocia NOS
     Uterine spasm

§ ✓5ᵗʰ **661.9 Unspecified abnormality of labor**   Ⓜ♀
[0,1,3]

✓4ᵗʰ **662 Long labor**

§ ✓5ᵗʰ **662.0 Prolonged first stage**   Ⓜ♀
[0,1,3]

§ ✓5ᵗʰ **662.1 Prolonged labor, unspecified**   Ⓜ♀
[0,1,3]

§ ✓5ᵗʰ **662.2 Prolonged second stage**   Ⓜ♀
[0,1,3]

§ ✓5ᵗʰ **662.3 Delayed delivery of second twin, triplet, etc.**   Ⓜ♀
[0,1,3]

✓4ᵗʰ **663 Umbilical cord complications**

§ ✓5ᵗʰ **663.0 Prolapse of cord**   Ⓜ♀
[0,1,3]   Presentation of cord
   DEF: Abnormal presentation of fetus; marked by protruding
   umbilical cord during labor; can cause fetal death.

---

§ Requires fifth digit. Valid digits are in [brackets] under each code. See beginning of section 640–648 for codes and definitions.

  Additional Digit Required   Unspecified Code   Other Specified Code   Manifestation Code   ►◄ Revised Text   ● New Code   ▲ Revised Code Title

2003 ICD•9•CM   **Volume 1 — 179**

§ ✓5ᵗʰ **663.1 Cord around neck, with compression**   M ♀
[0,1,3]   Cord tightly around neck

§ ✓5ᵗʰ **663.2 Other and unspecified cord entanglement, with compression**   M ♀
[0,1,3]   Entanglement of cords of twins in mono-amniotic sac
   Knot in cord (with compression)

§ ✓5ᵗʰ **663.3 Other and unspecified cord entanglement, without mention of compression**   M ♀
[0,1,3]

§ ✓5ᵗʰ **663.4 Short cord**   M ♀
[0,1,3]

§ ✓5ᵗʰ **663.5 Vasa previa**   M ♀
[0,1,3]   **DEF:** Abnormal presentation of fetus marked by blood vessels of umbilical cord in front of fetal head.

§ ✓5ᵗʰ **663.6 Vascular lesions of cord**   M ♀
[0,1,3]   Bruising of cord   Thrombosis of vessels of
   Hematoma of cord   cord

§ ✓5ᵗʰ **663.8 Other umbilical cord complications**   M ♀
[0,1,3]   Velamentous insertion of umbilical cord

§ ✓5ᵗʰ **663.9 Unspecified umbilical cord complication**   M ♀
[0,1,3]

✓4ᵗʰ **664 Trauma to perineum and vulva during delivery**
    INCLUDES   damage from instruments
               that from extension of episiotomy

§ ✓5ᵗʰ **664.0 First-degree perineal laceration**   M ♀
[0,1,4]   Perineal laceration, rupture, or tear involving:
     fourchette   skin
     hymen   vagina
     labia   vulva

§ ✓5ᵗʰ **664.1 Second-degree perineal laceration**   M ♀
[0,1,4]   Perineal laceration, rupture, or tear (following episiotomy) involving:
     pelvic floor
     perineal muscles
     vaginal muscles
      EXCLUDES   *that involving anal sphincter (664.2)*

§ ✓5ᵗʰ **664.2 Third-degree perineal laceration**   M ♀
[0,1,4]   Perineal laceration, rupture, or tear (following episiotomy) involving:
     anal sphincter
     rectovaginal septum
     sphincter NOS
      EXCLUDES   *that with anal or rectal mucosal laceration (664.3)*

§ ✓5ᵗʰ **664.3 Fourth-degree perineal laceration**   M ♀
[0,1,4]   Perineal laceration, rupture, or tear as classifiable to 664.2 and involving also:
     anal mucosa
     rectal mucosa

Perineal Lacerations

First degree
Anus
Second degree
Third degree
Fourth degree

§ ✓5ᵗʰ **664.4 Unspecified perineal laceration**   M ♀
[0,1,4]   Central laceration

§ ✓5ᵗʰ **664.5 Vulval and perineal hematoma**   M ♀
[0,1,4]

§ ✓5ᵗʰ **664.8 Other specified trauma to perineum and vulva**   M ♀
[0,1,4]

§ ✓5ᵗʰ **664.9 Unspecified trauma to perineum and vulva**   M ♀
[0,1,4]

✓4ᵗʰ **665 Other obstetrical trauma**
    INCLUDES   damage from instruments

§ ✓5ᵗʰ **665.0 Rupture of uterus before onset of labor**   M ♀
[0,1,3]

§ ✓5ᵗʰ **665.1 Rupture of uterus during labor**   M ♀
[0,1]   Rupture of uterus NOS

§ ✓5ᵗʰ **665.2 Inversion of uterus**   M ♀
[0,2,4]

§ ✓5ᵗʰ **665.3 Laceration of cervix**   M ♀
[0,1,4]

§ ✓5ᵗʰ **665.4 High vaginal laceration**   M ♀
[0,1,4]   Laceration of vaginal wall or sulcus without mention of perineal laceration

§ ✓5ᵗʰ **665.5 Other injury to pelvic organs**   M ♀
[0,1,4]   Injury to:
     bladder
     urethra

§ ✓5ᵗʰ **665.6 Damage to pelvic joints and ligaments**   M ♀
[0,1,4]   Avulsion of inner symphyseal cartilage
   Damage to coccyx
   Separation of symphysis (pubis)

§ ✓5ᵗʰ **665.7 Pelvic hematoma**   M ♀
[0,1,2,4]   Hematoma of vagina

§ ✓5ᵗʰ **665.8 Other specified obstetrical trauma**   M ♀
[0-4]

§ ✓5ᵗʰ **665.9 Unspecified obstetrical trauma**   M ♀
[0-4]

✓4ᵗʰ **666 Postpartum hemorrhage**

§ ✓5ᵗʰ **666.0 Third-stage hemorrhage**   M ♀
[0,2,4]   Hemorrhage associated with retained, trapped, or adherent placenta
   Retained placenta NOS

§ ✓5ᵗʰ **666.1 Other immediate postpartum hemorrhage**   M ♀
[0,2,4]   Atony of uterus
   Hemorrhage within the first 24 hours following delivery of placenta
   Postpartum hemorrhage (atonic) NOS

§ ✓5ᵗʰ **666.2 Delayed and secondary postpartum hemorrhage**   M ♀
[0,2,4]   Hemorrhage:
     after the first 24 hours following delivery
     associated with retained portions of placenta or membranes
   Postpartum hemorrhage specified as delayed or secondary
   Retained products of conception NOS, following delivery

§ ✓5ᵗʰ **666.3 Postpartum coagulation defects**   M ♀
[0,2,4]   Postpartum: Postpartum:
     afibrinogenemia   fibrinolysis

✓4ᵗʰ **667 Retained placenta or membranes, without hemorrhage**
    Requires fifth-digit; valid digits are in [brackets] under each code. See beginning of section 660-669 for definitions.
    DEF: Postpartum condition resulting from failure to expel placental membrane tissues due to failed contractions of uterine wall.

---

§ Requires fifth digit. Valid digits are in [brackets] under each code. See beginning of section 640–648 for codes and definitions.

N Newborn Age: 0   P Pediatric Age: 0-17   M Maternity Age: 12-55   A Adult Age: 15-124   MSP Medicare Secondary Payer

§ ✓5th **667.0**   **Retained placenta without hemorrhage**   Ⓜ♀
[0,2,4]

Placenta accreta
Retained placenta: } without hemorrhage
NOS
total

§ ✓5th **667.1**   **Retained portions of placenta or membranes,**   Ⓜ♀
[0,2,4]   **without hemorrhage**

Retained products of conception following delivery,
without hemorrhage

✓4th **668**   **Complications of the administration of anesthetic or other sedation in labor and delivery**

INCLUDES   complications arising from the administration of a general or local anesthetic, analgesic, or other sedation in labor and delivery

EXCLUDES   *reaction to spinal or lumbar puncture (349.0)*
spinal headache (349.0)

Use additional code(s) to further specify complication

§ ✓5th **668.0**   **Pulmonary complications**   Ⓜ♀
[0-4]

Inhalation [aspiration] of   following anesthesia
  stomach contents   or other
  or secretions   } sedation in
Mendelson's syndrome   labor or
Pressure collapse of lung   delivery

§ ✓5th **668.1**   **Cardiac complications**   Ⓜ♀
[0-4]
Cardiac arrest or failure following anesthesia or other sedation in labor and delivery

§ ✓5th **668.2**   **Central nervous system complications**   Ⓜ♀
[0-4]
Cerebral anoxia following anesthesia or other sedation in labor and delivery

§ ✓5th **668.8**   **Other complications of anesthesia or other sedation in labor and delivery**   Ⓜ♀
[0-4]

§ ✓5th **668.9**   **Unspecified complication of anesthesia and other sedation**   Ⓜ♀
[0-4]

✓4th **669**   **Other complications of labor and delivery, not elsewhere classified**

§ ✓5th **669.0**   **Maternal distress**   Ⓜ♀
[0-4]
Metabolic disturbance in labor and delivery

§ ✓5th **669.1**   **Shock during or following labor and delivery**   Ⓜ♀
[0-4]
Obstetric shock

§ ✓5th **669.2**   **Maternal hypotension syndrome**   Ⓜ♀
[0-4]
DEF: Low arterial blood pressure, in mother, during labor and delivery.

§ ✓5th **669.3**   **Acute renal failure following labor and delivery** Ⓜ♀
[0,2,4]

§ ✓5th **669.4**   **Other complications of obstetrical surgery and procedures**   Ⓜ♀
[0-4]

Cardiac: following cesarean or other
  arrest   obstetrical surgery or
  failure   } procedure, including
Cerebral anoxia   delivery NOS

EXCLUDES   *complications of obstetrical surgical wounds (674.1-674.3)*

§ ✓5th **669.5**   **Forceps or vacuum extractor delivery**   Ⓜ♀
[0,1]   **without mention of indication**
Delivery by ventouse, without mention of indication

§ ✓5th **669.6**   **Breech extraction, without mention of**   Ⓜ♀
[0,1]   **indication**
EXCLUDES   *breech delivery NOS (652.2)*

§ ✓5th **669.7**   **Cesarean delivery, without mention of**   Ⓜ♀
[0,1]   **indication**

§ ✓5th **669.8**   **Other complications of labor and delivery**   Ⓜ♀
[0-4]

§ ✓5th **669.9**   **Unspecified complication of labor and delivery** Ⓜ♀
[0-4]

COMPLICATIONS OF THE PUERPERIUM (670-677)

Note: Categories 671 and 673-676 include the listed conditions even if they occur during pregnancy or childbirth.

The following fifth-digit subclassification is for use with categories 670-676 to denote the current episode of care. Valid fifth-digits are in [brackets] under each code.
  0   **unspecified as to episode of care or not applicable**
  1   **delivered, with or without mention of antepartum condition**
  2   **delivered, with mention of postpartum complication**
  3   **antepartum condition or complication**
  4   **postpartum condition or complication**

✓4th **670**   **Major puerperal infection**
[0,2,4]

§ ✓5th   Use 0 as fourth-digit for this category
Puerperal:
  endometritis
  fever (septic)
  pelvic:
    cellulitis
    sepsis
  peritonitis
  pyemia
  salpingitis
  septicemia

EXCLUDES   *infection following abortion (639.0)*
minor genital tract infection following delivery (646.6)
puerperal pyrexia NOS (672)
puerperal fever NOS (672)
puerperal pyrexia of unknown origin (672)
urinary tract infection following delivery (646.6)

DEF: Infection and inflammation, following childbirth.

✓4th **671**   **Venous complications in pregnancy and the puerperium**

§ ✓5th **671.0**   **Varicose veins of legs**   Ⓜ♀
[0-4]   Varicose veins NOS
DEF: Distended, tortuous veins on legs associated with pregnancy.

§ ✓5th **671.1**   **Varicose veins of vulva and perineum**   Ⓜ♀
[0-4]   DEF: Distended, tortuous veins on external female genitalia associated with pregnancy.

§ ✓5th **671.2**   **Superficial thrombophlebitis**   Ⓜ♀
[0-4]   Thrombophlebitis (superficial)

§ ✓5th **671.3**   **Deep phlebothrombosis, antepartum**   Ⓜ♀
[0,1,3]   Deep-vein thrombosis, antepartum

§ ✓5th **671.4**   **Deep phlebothrombosis, postpartum**   Ⓜ♀
[0,2,4]   Deep-vein thrombosis, postpartum
Pelvic thrombophlebitis, postpartum
Phlegmasia alba dolens (puerperal)

§ ✓5th **671.5**   **Other phlebitis and thrombosis**   Ⓜ♀
[0-4]   Cerebral venous thrombosis
Thrombosis of intracranial venous sinus

§ ✓5th **671.8**   **Other venous complications**   Ⓜ♀
[0-4]   Hemorrhoids

§ ✓5th **671.9**   **Unspecified venous complication**   Ⓜ♀
[0-4]   Phlebitis NOS   Thrombosis NOS

✓4th **672**   **Pyrexia of unknown origin during the puerperium**
[0,2,4]

§ ✓5th   Use 0 as fourth-digit for this category
Postpartum fever NOS
Puerperal fever NOS
Puerperal pyrexia NOS
DEF: Fever of unknown origin experienced by the mother after childbirth.

§ Requires fifth digit. Valid digits are in [brackets] under each code. See beginning of section 640–648 for codes and definitions.

✓4th / ✓5th Additional Digit Required   Unspecified Code   Other Specified Code   Manifestation Code   ►◄ Revised Text   ● New Code   ▲ Revised Code Title

Complications of Pregnancy, Childbirth, & Puerperium 667.0–672

√4th **673 Obstetrical pulmonary embolism**

Requires fifth-digit; valid digits are in [brackets] under each code. See beginning of section 670-676 for definitions.

INCLUDES pulmonary emboli in pregnancy, childbirth, or the puerperium, or specified as puerperal

EXCLUDES embolism following abortion (639.6)

§ √5th **673.0 Obstetrical air embolism** M ♀
[0-4]
DEF: Sudden blocking of pulmonary artery with air or nitrogen bubbles during puerperium..

§ √5th **673.1 Amniotic fluid embolism** M ♀
[0-4]
DEF: Sudden onset of pulmonary artery blockage from amniotic fluid entering the mother's circulation near the end of pregnancy due to strong uterine contractions.

§ √5th **673.2 Obstetrical blood-clot embolism** M ♀
[0-4]
Puerperal pulmonary embolism NOS
DEF: Blood clot blocking artery in the lung; associated with pregnancy.

§ √5th **673.3 Obstetrical pyemic and septic embolism** M ♀
[0-4]

§ √5th **673.8 Other pulmonary emboli** M ♀
[0-4]
Fat embolism

√4th **674 Other and unspecified complications of the puerperium, not elsewhere classified**

§ √5th **674.0 Cerebrovascular disorders in the puerperium** M ♀
[0-4]
Any condition classifiable to 430-434, 436-437 occurring during pregnancy, childbirth, or the puerperium, or specified as puerperal
EXCLUDES intracranial venous sinus thrombosis (671.5)

§ √5th **674.1 Disruption of cesarean wound** M ♀
[0,2,4]
Dehiscence or disruption of uterine wound
EXCLUDES ▶uterine rupture before onset of labor (665.0)
uterine rupture during labor (665.1)◀

§ √5th **674.2 Disruption of perineal wound** M ♀
[0,2,4]
Breakdown of perineum   Disruption of wound of:
Disruption of wound of: perineal laceration
episiotomy   Secondary perineal tear

§ √5th **674.3 Other complications of obstetrical surgical wounds** M ♀
[0,2,4]

Hematoma
Hemorrhage } of cesarean section or perineal
Infection   wound

EXCLUDES damage from instruments in delivery (664.0-665.9)

§ √5th **674.4 Placental polyp** M ♀
[0,2,4]

§ √5th **674.8 Other** M ♀
[0,2,4]
Hepatorenal syndrome, following delivery
Postpartum:
cardiomyopathy
subinvolution of uterus
uterine hypertrophy

§ √5th **674.9 Unspecified** M ♀
[0,2,4]
Sudden death of unknown cause during the puerperium

√4th **675 Infections of the breast and nipple associated with childbirth**
INCLUDES the listed conditions during pregnancy, childbirth, or the puerperium

§ √5th **675.0 Infections of nipple** M ♀
[0-4]
Abscess of nipple

§ √5th **675.1 Abscess of breast** M ♀
[0-4]
Abscess: Mastitis:
mammary   purulent
subareolar   retromammary
submammary   submammary

§ √5th **675.2 Nonpurulent mastitis** M ♀
[0-4]
Lymphangitis of breast   Mastitis:
Mastitis: interstitial
NOS   parenchymatous

§ √5th **675.8 Other specified infections of the breast and nipple** M ♀
[0-4]

§ √5th **675.9 Unspecified infection of the breast and nipple** M ♀
[0-4]

√4th **676 Other disorders of the breast associated with childbirth and disorders of lactation**
INCLUDES the listed conditions during pregnancy, the puerperium, or lactation

§ √5th **676.0 Retracted nipple** M ♀
[0-4]

§ √5th **676.1 Cracked nipple** M ♀
[0-4]
Fissure of nipple

§ √5th **676.2 Engorgement of breasts** M ♀
[0-4]
DEF: Abnormal accumulation of milk in ducts of breast.

§ √5th **676.3 Other and unspecified disorder of breast** M ♀
[0-4]

§ √5th **676.4 Failure of lactation** M ♀
[0-4]
Agalactia
DEF: Abrupt ceasing of milk secretion by breast.

§ √5th **676.5 Suppressed lactation** M ♀
[0-4]

§ √5th **676.6 Galactorrhea** M ♀
[0-4]
EXCLUDES galactorrhea not associated with childbirth (611.6)
DEF: Excessive or persistent milk secretion by breast; may be in absence of nursing.

§ √5th **676.8 Other disorders of lactation** M ♀
[0-4]
Galactocele
DEF: Galactocele: obstructed mammary gland, creating retention cyst, results in milk-filled cysts enlarging mammary gland.

§ √5th **676.9 Unspecified disorder of lactation** M ♀
[0-4]

677 Late effect of complication of pregnancy, childbirth, and the puerperium M ♀
Note: This category is to be used to indicate conditions in 632-648.9 and 651-676.9 as the cause of the late effect, themselves classifiable elsewhere. The "late effects" include conditions specified as such, or as sequelae, which may occur at any time after puerperium.
Code first any sequelae

§ Requires fifth digit. Valid digits are in [brackets] under each code. See beginning of section 670–676 for codes and definitions.

12. DISEASES OF THE SKIN AND SUBCUTANEOUS TISSUE (680-709)

INFECTIONS OF SKIN AND SUBCUTANEOUS TISSUE (680-686)

> **EXCLUDES** *certain infections of skin classified under "Infectious and Parasitic Diseases," such as:*
> *erysipelas (035)*
> *erysipeloid of Rosenbach (027.1)*
> *herpes:*
> *simplex (054.0-054.9)*
> *zoster (053.0-053.9)*
> *molluscum contagiosum (078.0)*
> *viral warts (078.1)*

✓4th 680 Carbuncle and furuncle

> **INCLUDES** boil
> furunculosis

DEF: Carbuncle: necrotic boils in skin and subcutaneous tissue of neck or back mainly due to staphylococcal infection.

DEF: Furuncle: Circumscribed inflammation of corium and subcutaneous tissue due to staphylococcal infection.

680.0 Face
Ear [any part]   Nose (septum)
Face [any part, except eye] Temple (region)
> **EXCLUDES** *eyelid (373.13)*
> *lacrimal apparatus (375.31)*
> *orbit (376.01)*

680.1 Neck

680.2 Trunk
Abdominal wall   Flank
Back [any part, except   Groin
   buttocks]   Pectoral region
Breast   Perineum
Chest wall   Umbilicus
> **EXCLUDES** *buttocks (680.5)*
> *external genital organs:*
> *female (616.4)*
> *male (607.2, 608.4)*

680.3 Upper arm and forearm
Arm [any part, except hand]
Axilla
Shoulder

680.4 Hand
Finger [any]   Wrist
Thumb

680.5 Buttock
Anus   Gluteal region

680.6 Leg, except foot
Ankle   Knee
Hip   Thigh

680.7 Foot
Heel
Toe

680.8 Other specified sites
Head [any part, except face]
Scalp
> **EXCLUDES** *external genital organs:*
> *female (616.4)*
> *male (607.2, 608.4)*

680.9 Unspecified site
Boil NOS   Furuncle NOS
Carbuncle NOS

✓4th 681 Cellulitis and abscess of finger and toe

> **INCLUDES** that with lymphangitis

Use additional code to identify organism, such as Staphylococcus (041.1)

DEF: Acute suppurative inflammation and edema in subcutaneous tissue or muscle of finger or toe.

✓5th 681.0 Finger

681.00 Cellulitis and abscess, unspecified

681.01 Felon
Pulp abscess   Whitlow
> **EXCLUDES** *herpetic whitlow (054.6)*

DEF: Painful abscess of fingertips caused by infection in the closed space of terminal phalanx.

681.02 Onychia and paronychia of finger
Panaritium ⎫
Perionychia ⎭ of finger

DEF: Onychia: inflammation of nail matrix; causes nail loss.

DEF: Paronychia: inflammation of tissue folds around nail.

✓5th 681.1 Toe

681.10 Cellulitis and abscess, unspecified

681.11 Onychia and paronychia of toe
Panaritium ⎫
Perionychia ⎭ of toe

681.9 Cellulitis and abscess of unspecified digit
Infection of nail NOS

✓4th 682 Other cellulitis and abscess

> **INCLUDES** abscess (acute)   ⎫ (with lymphangitis)
> cellulitis (diffuse)   ⎬ except of finger
> lymphangitis, acute   ⎭ or toe

Use additional code to identify organism, such as Staphylococcus (041.1)
> **EXCLUDES** *lymphangitis (chronic) (subacute) (457.2)*

DEF: Cellulitis: Acute suppurative inflammation of deep subcutaneous tissue and sometimes muscle due to infection of wound, burn or other lesion.

682.0 Face
Cheek, external   Nose, external
Chin   Submandibular
Forehead   Temple (region)
> **EXCLUDES** *ear [any part] (380.10-380.16)*
> *eyelid (373.13)*
> *lacrimal apparatus (375.31)*
> *lip (528.5)*
> *mouth (528.3)*
> *nose (internal) (478.1)*
> *orbit (376.01)*

682.1 Neck

Skin and Subcutaneous Layer

Hair follicle
Epidermis
Dermis
Hypodermis (subcutaneous layer)
Bulb
Sebaceous gland
Arrector pili muscle
Thick-skin epidermis
Hair shaft
Pacinian corpuscle
Hair matrix
Sweat (eccrine gland)
Sensory nerve
Blood vessels

Additional Digit Required   Unspecified Code   Other Specified Code   Manifestation Code   ►◄ Revised Text   ● New Code   ▲ Revised Code Title

682.2   Trunk

Abdominal wall	Groin
Back [any part, except buttock]	Pectoral region
	Perineum
Chest wall	Umbilicus, except newborn
Flank	

EXCLUDES   anal and rectal regions (566)
   breast:
      NOS (611.0)
      puerperal (675.1)
   external genital organs:
      female (616.3-616.4)
      male (604.0, 607.2, 608.4)
   umbilicus, newborn (771.4)

682.3   Upper arm and forearm
   Arm [any part, except hand]
   Axilla
   Shoulder
      EXCLUDES   hand (682.4)

682.4   Hand, except fingers and thumb
   Wrist
      EXCLUDES   finger and thumb (681.00-681.02)

682.5   Buttock
   Gluteal region
      EXCLUDES   anal and rectal regions (566)

682.6   Leg, except foot

Ankle	Knee
Hip	Thigh

682.7   Foot, except toes
   Heel
      EXCLUDES   toe (681.10-681.11)

682.8   Other specified sites
   Head [except face]
   Scalp
      EXCLUDES   face (682.0)

682.9   Unspecified site

Abscess NOS	Lymphangitis, acute NOS
Cellulitis NOS	

      EXCLUDES   lymphangitis NOS (457.2)

683 Acute lymphadenitis
   Abscess (acute)
   Adenitis, acute   } lymph gland or node,
   Lymphadenitis, acute   except mesenteric

   Use additional code to identify organism, such as
      Staphylococcus (041.1)
      EXCLUDES   enlarged glands NOS (785.6)
         lymphadenitis:
            chronic or subacute, except mesenteric
               (289.1)
            mesenteric (acute) (chronic) (subacute) (289.2)
            unspecified (289.3)

DEF: Acute inflammation of lymph nodes due to primary infection located elsewhere in the body.

▶ Lymphatic System of Head and Neck◀

Schematic of lymph node

Lymphatic drainage of the head, neck, and face

Stages of Pilonidal Disease

Normal follicle
Stretched follicle
Infected follicle
Acute abscess
Chronic abscess
Epithelial tube

684 Impetigo
   Impetiginization of other dermatoses
   Impetigo (contagiosa) [any site] [any organism]:

bullous	neonatorum
circinate	simplex

   Pemphigus neonatorum
      EXCLUDES   impetigo herpetiformis (694.3)

DEF: Infectious skin disease commonly occurring in children; caused by group A streptococci or *Staphylococcus aureus*; skin lesions usually appear on the face and consist of subcorneal vesicles and bullae that burst and form yellow crusts.

√4ᵗʰ 685 Pilonidal cyst
      INCLUDES   fistula } coccygeal or pilonidal
                  sinus

DEF: Hair-containing cyst or sinus in the tissues of the sacrococcygeal area; often drains through opening at the postanal dimple.

685.0   With abscess
685.1   Without mention of abscess

√4ᵗʰ 686 Other local infections of skin and subcutaneous tissue
      Use additional code to identify any infectious organism
         (041.0-041.8)

√5ᵗʰ 686.0   Pyoderma

Dermatitis:	Dermatitis:
purulent	suppurative
septic	

DEF: Nonspecific purulent skin disease related most to furuncles, pustules, or possibly carbuncles.

686.00   Pyoderma, unspecified
686.01   Pyoderma gangrenosum
      DEF: Persistent debilitating skin disease, characterized by irregular, boggy, blue-red ulcerations, with central healing and undermined edges.

686.09   Other pyoderma

686.1   Pyogenic granuloma

Granuloma:	Granuloma:
septic	telangiectaticum
suppurative	

      EXCLUDES   pyogenic granuloma of oral mucosa
                  (528.9)

DEF: Solitary polypoid capillary hemangioma often associated with local irritation, trauma, and superimposed inflammation; located on the skin and gingival or oral mucosa.

686.8   Other specified local infections of skin and subcutaneous tissue

Bacterid (pustular)	Ecthyma
Dermatitis vegetans	Perlèche

      EXCLUDES   dermatitis infectiosa eczematoides
                  (690.8)
         panniculitis (729.30-729.39)

686.9 **Unspecified local infection of skin and subcutaneous tissue**
　　　Fistula of skin NOS
　　　Skin infection NOS
　　　　EXCLUDES　*fistula to skin from internal organs — see Alphabetic Index*

OTHER INFLAMMATORY CONDITIONS OF SKIN AND SUBCUTANEOUS TISSUE (690-698)

　　　EXCLUDES　*panniculitis (729.30-729.39)*

✓4th **690** **Erythematosquamous dermatosis**
　　　EXCLUDES　*eczematous dermatitis of eyelid (373.31)*
　　　　　parakeratosis variegata (696.2)
　　　　　psoriasis (696.0-696.1)
　　　　　seborrheic keratosis (702.11-702.19)

　　　DEF: Dry material desquamated from the scalp, associated with disease.

✓5th **690.1** **Seborrheic dermatitis**

　　690.10 **Seborrheic dermatitis, unspecified**
　　　　Seborrheic dermatitis NOS

　　690.11 **Seborrhea capitis**　　P
　　　　Cradle cap

　　690.12 **Seborrheic infantile dermatitis**　　P

　　690.18 **Other seborrheic dermatitis**

　690.8 **Other erythematosquamous dermatosis**

✓4th **691** **Atopic dermatitis and related conditions**
　　DEF: Atopic dermatitis: chronic, pruritic, inflammatory skin disorder found on the face and antecubital and popliteal fossae; noted in persons with a hereditary predisposition to pruritus, and often accompanied by allergic rhinitis, hay fever, asthma, and extreme itching; also called allergic dermatitis, allergic or atopic eczema, or disseminated neurodermatitis.

　691.0 **Diaper or napkin rash**
　　　Ammonia dermatitis　　Diaper or napkin:
　　　Diaper or napkin:　　　rash
　　　　dermatitis　　　Psoriasiform napkin eruption
　　　　erythema

　691.8 **Other atopic dermatitis and related conditions**
　　　Atopic dermatitis　　Neurodermatitis:
　　　Besnier's prurigo　　　atopic
　　　Eczema:　　　　diffuse (of Brocq)
　　　　atopic
　　　　flexural
　　　　intrinsic (allergic)

✓4th **692** **Contact dermatitis and other eczema**
　　　INCLUDES　dermatitis:
　　　　　NOS
　　　　　contact
　　　　　occupational
　　　　　venenata
　　　　eczema (acute) (chronic):
　　　　　NOS
　　　　　allergic
　　　　　erythematous
　　　　　occupational
　　　EXCLUDES　*allergy NOS (995.3)*
　　　　　contact dermatitis of eyelids (373.32)
　　　　　dermatitis due to substances taken internally (693.0-693.9)
　　　　　eczema of external ear (380.22)
　　　　　perioral dermatitis (695.3)
　　　　　urticarial reactions (708.0-708.9, 995.1)

　　DEF: Contact dermatitis: acute or chronic dermatitis caused by initial irritant effect of a substance, or by prior sensitization to a substance coming once again in contact with skin.

　692.0 **Due to detergents**
　692.1 **Due to oils and greases**

692.2 **Due to solvents**
　　　Dermatitis due to solvents of:
　　　　chlorocompound ⎤
　　　　cyclohexane ⎥
　　　　ester ⎥
　　　　glycol ⎥ group
　　　　hydrocarbon ⎥
　　　　ketone ⎦

692.3 **Due to drugs and medicines in contact with skin**
　　Dermatitis (allergic)　　Dermatitis (allergic)
　　　(contact) due to:　　　(contact) due to:
　　　arnica　　　　neomycin
　　　fungicides　　　pediculocides
　　　iodine　　　　phenols
　　　keratolytics　　　scabicides
　　　mercurials　　　any drug applied to skin
　　Dermatitis medicamentosa due to drug applied to skin
　　Use additional E code to identify drug
　　　EXCLUDES　*allergy NOS due to drugs (995.2)*
　　　　　dermatitis due to ingested drugs (693.0)
　　　　　dermatitis medicamentosa NOS (693.0)

692.4 **Due to other chemical products**
　　Dermatitis due to:　　Dermatitis due to:
　　　acids　　　　insecticide
　　　adhesive plaster　　nylon
　　　alkalis　　　　plastic
　　　caustics　　　rubber
　　　dichromate

692.5 **Due to food in contact with skin**
　　Dermatitis, contact,　　Dermatitis, contact,
　　　due to:　　　　due to:
　　　cereals　　　　fruit
　　　fish　　　　meat
　　　flour　　　　milk
　　　EXCLUDES　*dermatitis due to:*
　　　　　dyes (692.89)
　　　　　ingested foods (693.1)
　　　　　preservatives (692.89)

692.6 **Due to plants [except food]**
　　Dermatitis due to:
　　　lacquer tree [Rhus verniciflua]
　　　poison:
　　　　ivy [Rhus toxicodendron]
　　　　oak [Rhus diversiloba]
　　　　sumac [Rhus venenata]
　　　　vine [Rhus radicans]
　　　primrose [Primula]
　　　ragweed [Senecio jacobae]
　　　other plants in contact with the skin
　　　EXCLUDES　*allergy NOS due to pollen (477.0)*
　　　　　nettle rash (708.8)

✓5th **692.7** **Due to solar radiation**
　　　EXCLUDES　*sunburn due to other ultraviolet radiation exposure (692.82)*

　　692.70 **Unspecified dermatitis due to sun**
　　692.71 **Sunburn**
　　　　First degree sunburn
　　　　Sunburn NOS

 Additional Digit Required　　**Unspecified Code**　　Other Specified Code　　Manifestation Code　　►◄ Revised Text　　● New Code　　▲ Revised Code Title

2003 ICD•9•CM　　　　　**Volume 1 — 185**

692.72 Acute dermatitis due to solar radiation
Acute solar skin damage NOS
Berlogue dermatitis
Photoallergic response
Phototoxic response
Polymorphus light eruption
> EXCLUDES *sunburn (692.71, 692.76-692.77)*

Use additional E code to identify drug, if drug induced

DEF: Berloque dermatitis: phytophotodermatitis due to sun exposure after use of a product containing bergamot oil; causes red patches, which may turn brown.

DEF: Photoallergic response: dermatitis due to hypersensitivity to the sun; causes papulovesicular, eczematous or exudative eruptions.

DEF: Phototoxic response: chemically induced sensitivity to sun causes burn-like reaction, occasionally vesiculation and subsequent hyperpigmentation.

DEF: Polymorphous light eruption: inflammatory skin eruptions due to sunlight exposure; eruptions differ in size and shape.

DEF: Acute solar skin damage (NOS): rapid, unspecified injury to skin from sun.

692.73 Actinic reticuloid and actinic granuloma

DEF: Actinic reticuloid: dermatosis aggravated by light, causes chronic eczema-like eruption on exposed skin which extends to other unexposed surfaces; occurs in the eldery.

DEF: Actinic granuloma: inflammatory response of skin to sun causing small nodule of microphages.

692.74 Other chronic dermatitis due to solar radiation
Solar elastosis
Chronic solar skin damage NOS
> EXCLUDES *actinic [solar] keratosis (702.0)*

DEF: Solar elastosis: premature aging of skin of light-skinned people; causes inelasticity, thinning or thickening, wrinkling, dryness, scaling and hyperpigmentation.

DEF: Chronic solar skin damage (NOS): chronic skin impairment due to exposure to the sun, not otherwise specified.

692.75 Disseminated superficial actinic porokeratosis (DSAP)

DEF: Autosomal dominant skin condition occurring in skin that has been overexposed to the sun. Primarily affects women over the age of 16; characterized by numerous superficial annular, keratotic, brownish-red spots or thickenings with depressed centers and sharp, ridged borders. High risk that condition will evolve into squamous cell carcinoma.

692.76 Sunburn of second degree
692.77 Sunburn of third degree
692.79 Other dermatitis due to solar radiation
Hydroa aestivale
Photodermatitis   } (due to sun)
Photosensitiveness

Solar skin damage NOS

692.8 Due to other specified agents
692.81 Dermatitis due to cosmetics
692.82 Dermatitis due to other radiation
Infrared rays   Tanning bed
Light   Ultraviolet rays
Radiation NOS   X-rays
> EXCLUDES *solar radiation (692.70-692.79)*

692.83 Dermatitis due to metals
Jewelry
692.89 Other
Dermatitis due to:
cold weather
dyes
furs
hot weather
preservatives
ultraviolet rays, except from sun
> EXCLUDES *allergy NOS due to animal hair, dander (animal), or dust (477.8)*
> *sunburn (692.71, 692.76-692.77)*

692.9 Unspecified cause
Dermatitis: Dermatitis:
NOS   venenata NOS
contact NOS   Eczema NOS

693 Dermatitis due to substances taken internally
> EXCLUDES *adverse effect NOS of drugs and medicines (995.2)*
> *allergy NOS (995.3)*
> *contact dermatitis (692.0-692.9)*
> *urticarial reactions (708.0-708.9, 995.1)*

DEF: Inflammation of skin due to ingested substance.

693.0 Due to drugs and medicines
Dermatitis medicamentosa NOS
Use additional E code to identify drug
> EXCLUDES *that due to drugs in contact with skin (692.3)*

693.1 Due to food
693.8 Due to other specified substances taken internally
693.9 Due to unspecified substance taken internally
> EXCLUDES *dermatitis NOS (692.9)*

694 Bullous dermatoses
694.0 Dermatitis herpetiformis
Dermatosis herpetiformis Hydroa herpetiformis
Duhring's disease
> EXCLUDES *herpes gestationis (646.8)*
> *dermatitis herpetiformis:*
> *juvenile (694.2)*
> *senile (694.5)*

DEF: Chronic, relapsing multisystem disease manifested most in the cutaneous system; seen as an extremely pruritic eruption of various combinations of lesions that frequently heal leaving hyperpigmentation or hypopigmentation and occasionally scarring; usually associated with an asymptomatic gluten-sensitive enteropathy, and immunogenic factors are believed to play a role in its origin.

694.1 Subcorneal pustular dermatosis
Sneddon-Wilkinson disease or syndrome

DEF: Chronic relapses of sterile pustular blebs beneath the horny skin layer of the trunk and skin folds; resembles dermatitis herpetiformis.

694.2 Juvenile dermatitis herpetiformis
Juvenile pemphigoid
694.3 Impetigo herpetiformis

DEF: Rare dermatosis associated with pregnancy; marked by itching pustules in third trimester, hypocalcemia, tetany, fever and lethargy; may result in maternal or fetal death.

N Newborn Age: 0   P Pediatric Age: 0-17   M Maternity Age: 12-55   A Adult Age: 15-124   MSP Medicare Secondary Payer

694.4 Pemphigus

Pemphigus: Pemphigus:
NOS   malignant
erythematosus   vegetans
foliaceus   vulgaris

EXCLUDES   *pemphigus neonatorum (684)*

DEF: Chronic, relapsing, sometimes fatal skin diseases; causes vesicles, bullae; autoantibodies against intracellular connections cause acantholysis.

694.5 Pemphigoid

Benign pemphigus NOS
Bullous pemphigoid
Herpes circinatus bullosus
Senile dermatitis herpetiformis

✓5th **694.6 Benign mucous membrane pemphigoid**

Cicatricial pemphigoid
Mucosynechial atrophic bullous dermatitis

694.60 Without mention of ocular involvement

694.61 With ocular involvement

Ocular pemphigus

694.8 Other specified bullous dermatoses

EXCLUDES   *herpes gestationis (646.8)*

694.9 Unspecified bullous dermatoses

✓4th **695 Erythematous conditions**

695.0 Toxic erythema

Erythema venenatum

695.1 Erythema multiforme

Erythema iris   Scalded skin syndrome
Herpes iris   Stevens-Johnson syndrome
Lyell's syndrome   Toxic epidermal necrolysis

DEF: Symptom complex with a varied skin eruption pattern of macular, bullous, papular, nodose, or vesicular lesions on the neck, face, and legs; gastritis and rheumatic pains are also noticeable, first-seen symptoms; complex is secondary to a number of factors, including infections, ingestants, physical agents, malignancy and pregnancy.

695.2 Erythema nodosum

EXCLUDES   *tuberculous erythema nodosum (017.1)*

DEF: Panniculitis (an inflammatory reaction of the subcutaneous fat) of women, usually seen as a hypersensitivity reaction to various infections, drugs, sarcoidosis, and specific enteropathies; the acute stage is often associated with other symptoms, including fever, malaise, and arthralgia; the lesions are pink to blue in color, appear in crops as tender nodules and are found on the front of the legs below the knees.

695.3 Rosacea

Acne: Perioral dermatitis
erythematosa   Rhinophyma
rosacea

DEF: Chronic skin disease, usually of the face, characterized by persistent erythema and sometimes by telangiectasis with acute episodes of edema, engorgement papules, and pustules.

695.4 Lupus erythematosus

Lupus:
erythematodes (discoid)
erythematosus (discoid), not disseminated

EXCLUDES   *lupus (vulgaris) NOS (017.0)*
                systemic [disseminated] lupus
                   erythematosus (710.0)

DEF: Group of connective tissue disorders occurring as various cutaneous diseases of unknown origin; it primarily affects women between the ages of 20 and 40.

✓5th **695.8 Other specified erythematous conditions**

695.81 Ritter's disease

Dermatitis exfoliativa neonatorum

DEF: Infectious skin disease of infants and young children marked by eruptions ranging from a localized bullous type to widespread development of easily ruptured fine vesicles and bullae; results in exfoliation of large planes of skin and leaves raw areas; also called staphylococcal scalded skin syndrome.

695.89 Other

Erythema intertrigo
Intertrigo
Pityriasis rubra (Hebra)

EXCLUDES   *mycotic intertrigo (111.0-*
                 111.9)

695.9 Unspecified erythematous condition

Erythema NOS   Erythroderma (secondary)

✓4th **696 Psoriasis and similar disorders**

696.0 Psoriatic arthropathy

DEF: Psoriasis associated with inflammatory arthritis; often involves interphalangeal joints.

696.1 Other psoriasis

Acrodermatitis continua
Dermatitis repens
Psoriasis:
NOS
any type, except arthropathic

EXCLUDES   *psoriatic arthropathy (696.0)*

696.2 Parapsoriasis

Parakeratosis variegata
Parapsoriasis lichenoides chronica
Pityriasis lichenoides et varioliformis

DEF: Erythrodermas similar to lichen, planus and psoriasis; symptoms include redness and itching; resistant to treatment.

696.3 Pityriasis rosea

Pityriasis circinata (et maculata)

DEF: Common, self-limited rash of unknown etiology marked by a solitary erythematous, salmon or fawn-colored herald plaque on the trunk, arms or thighs; followed by development of papular or macular lesions that tend to peel and form a scaly collarette.

696.4 Pityriasis rubra pilaris

Devergie's disease   Lichen ruber acuminatus

EXCLUDES   *pityriasis rubra (Hebra) (695.89)*

DEF: Inflammatory disease of hair follicles; marked by firm, red lesions topped by horny plugs; may form patches; occurs on fingers elbows, knees.

696.5 Other and unspecified pityriasis

Pityriasis: Pityriasis:
NOS   streptogenes
alba

EXCLUDES   *pityriasis:*
                simplex (690.18)
                versicolor (111.0)

696.8 Other

✓4th **697 Lichen**

EXCLUDES   *lichen:*
           obtusus corneus (698.3)
           pilaris (congenital) (757.39)
           ruber acuminatus (696.4)
           sclerosus et atrophicus (701.0)
           scrofulosus (017.0)
           simplex chronicus (698.3)
           spinulosus (congenital) (757.39)
           urticatus (698.2)

Skin and Subcutaneous Tissue 694.4–697

✓4th ✓5th Additional Digit Required   Unspecified Code   Other Specified Code   Manifestation Code   ▶◀ Revised Text   ● New Code   ▲ Revised Code Title

2003 ICD•9•CM   **Volume 1 — 187**

697.0　Lichen planus
Lichen:　　　　　　Lichen:
　planopilaris　　　　　ruber planus
DEF: Inflammatory, pruritic skin disease; marked by angular, flat-top, violet-colored papules; may be acute and widespread or chronic and localized.

697.1　Lichen nitidus
Pinkus' disease
DEF: Chronic, inflammatory, usually asymptomatic skin disorder, characterized by numerous glistening, flat-topped, discrete, smooth, skin-colored micropapules most often on penis, lower abdomen, inner thighs, wrists, forearms, breasts and buttocks.

697.8　Other lichen, not elsewhere classified
Lichen:　　　　　　Lichen:
　ruber moniliforme　　　striata

697.9　Lichen, unspecified

✓4ᵗʰ 698　Pruritus and related conditions
EXCLUDES　pruritus specified as psychogenic (306.3)
DEF: Pruritus: Intense, persistent itching due to irritation of sensory nerve endings from organic or psychogenic causes.

698.0　Pruritus ani
Perianal itch

698.1　Pruritus of genital organs

698.2　Prurigo
Lichen urticatus　　　Prurigo:
Prurigo:　　　　　　　mitis
　NOS　　　　　　　　simplex
　Hebra's　　　　　Urticaria papulosa (Hebra)
EXCLUDES　prurigo nodularis (698.3)

698.3　Lichenification and lichen simplex chronicus
Hyde's disease
Neurodermatitis (circumscripta) (local)
Prurigo nodularis
EXCLUDES　neurodermatitis, diffuse (of Brocq) (691.8)

DEF: Lichenification: thickening of skin due to prolonged rubbing or scratching.

DEF: Lichen simplex chronicus: eczematous dermatitis, of face, neck, extremities, scrotum, vulva, and perianal region due to repeated itching, rubbing and scratching; spontaneous or evolves with other dermatoses.

698.4　Dermatitis factitia [artefacta]
Dermatitis ficta
Neurotic excoriation
Use additional code to identify any associated mental disorder
DEF: Various types of self-inflicted skin lesions characterized in appearance as an erythema to a gangrene.

698.8　Other specified pruritic conditions
Pruritus:　　　　Winter itch
　hiemalis
　senilis

698.9　Unspecified pruritic disorder
Itch NOS
Pruritus NOS

OTHER DISEASES OF SKIN AND SUBCUTANEOUS TISSUE (700-709)
EXCLUDES　conditions confined to eyelids (373.0-374.9)
　　　　congenital conditions of skin, hair, and nails (757.0-757.9)

700　Corns and callosities
Callus
Clavus
DEF: Corns: conical or horny thickening of skin on toes, due to friction, pressure from shoes and hosiery; pain and inflammation may develop.

DEF: Callosities: localized overgrowth (hyperplasia) of the horny epidermal layer due to pressure or friction.

✓4ᵗʰ 701　Other hypertrophic and atrophic conditions of skin
EXCLUDES　dermatomyositis (710.3)
　　　　hereditary edema of legs (757.0)
　　　　scleroderma (generalized) (710.1)

701.0　Circumscribed scleroderma
Addison's keloid
Dermatosclerosis, localized
Lichen sclerosus et atrophicus
Morphea
Scleroderma, circumscribed or localized
DEF: Thickened, hardened, skin and subcutaneous tissue; may involve musculoskeletal system.

701.1　Keratoderma, acquired
Acquired:
　ichthyosis
　keratoderma palmaris et plantaris
Elastosis perforans serpiginosa
Hyperkeratosis:
　NOS
　follicularis in cutem penetrans
　palmoplantaris climacterica
Keratoderma:
　climactericum
　tylodes, progressive
Keratosis (blennorrhagica)
EXCLUDES　Darier's disease [keratosis follicularis] (congenital) (757.39)
　　　　keratosis:
　　　　　arsenical (692.4)
　　　　　gonococcal (098.81)

701.2　Acquired acanthosis nigricans
Keratosis nigricans
DEF: Diffuse velvety hyperplasia of the spinous skin layer of the axilla and other body folds marked by gray, brown, or black pigmentation; in adult form it is often associated with an internal carcinoma (malignant acanthosis nigricans) in a benign, nevoid form it is relatively generalized; benign juvenile form with obesity is sometimes caused by an endocrine disturbance.

701.3　Striae atrophicae
Atrophic spots of skin
Atrophoderma maculatum
Atrophy blanche (of Milian)
Degenerative colloid atrophy
Senile degenerative atrophy
Striae distensae
DEF: Bands of atrophic, depressed, wrinkled skin associated with stretching of skin from pregnancy, obesity, or rapid growth during puberty.

701.4　Keloid scar
Cheloid　　　　　　Keloid
Hypertrophic scar
DEF: Overgrowth of scar tissue due to excess amounts of collagen during connective tissue repair; occurs mainly on upper trunk, face.

701.5　Other abnormal granulation tissue
Excessive granulation

701.8　Other specified hypertrophic and atrophic conditions of skin
Acrodermatitis atrophicans chronica
Atrophia cutis senilis
Atrophoderma neuriticum
Confluent and reticulate papillomatosis
Cutis laxa senilis
Elastosis senilis
Folliculitis ulerythematosa reticulata
Gougerot-Carteaud syndrome or disease

701.9　Unspecified hypertrophic and atrophic conditions of skin
Atrophoderma

☑4ᵗʰ **702 Other dermatoses**
> EXCLUDES   *carcinoma in situ (232.0-232.9)*

702.0   Actinic keratosis
> DEF: Wart-like growth, red or skin-colored; may form a cutaneous horn.

☑5ᵗʰ **702.1   Seborrheic keratosis**
> DEF: Common, benign, lightly pigmented, warty growth composed of basaloid cells.

    702.11   Inflamed seborrheic keratosis
    702.19   Other seborrheic keratosis
        Seborrheic keratosis NOS

702.8   Other specified dermatoses

☑4ᵗʰ **703 Diseases of nail**
> EXCLUDES   *congenital anomalies (757.5)*
> *onychia and paronychia (681.02, 681.11)*

703.0   Ingrowing nail
    Ingrowing nail with infection   Unguis incarnatus
> EXCLUDES   *infection, nail NOS (681.9)*

703.8   Other specified diseases of nail
    Dystrophia unguium   Onychauxis
    Hypertrophy of nail   Onychogryposis
    Koilonychia   Onycholysis
    Leukonychia (punctata) (striata)

703.9   Unspecified disease of nail

☑4ᵗʰ **704 Diseases of hair and hair follicles**
> EXCLUDES   *congenital anomalies (757.4)*

☑5ᵗʰ **704.0   Alopecia**
> EXCLUDES   *madarosis (374.55)*
> *syphilitic alopecia (091.82)*

> DEF: Lack of hair, especially on scalp; often called baldness; may be partial or total; occurs at any age.

    704.00   Alopecia, unspecified
        Baldness   Loss of hair

    704.01   Alopecia areata
        Ophiasis
> DEF: Alopecia areata: usually reversible, inflammatory, patchy hair loss found in beard or scalp.

> DEF: Ophiasis: alopecia areata of children; marked by band around temporal and occipital scalp margins.

    704.02   Telogen effluvium
> DEF: Shedding of hair from premature telogen development in follicles due to stress, including shock, childbirth, surgery, drugs or weight loss.

    704.09   Other
        Folliculitis decalvans
        Hypotrichosis:
            NOS
            postinfectional NOS
        Pseudopelade

704.1   Hirsutism
    Hypertrichosis: Polytrichia
        NOS
        lanuginosa, acquired
> EXCLUDES   *hypertrichosis of eyelid (374.54)*

> DEF: Excess hair growth; often in unexpected places and amounts.

704.2   Abnormalities of the hair
    Atrophic hair   Trichiasis:
    Clastothrix   NOS
    Fragilitas crinium   cicatrical
            Trichorrhexis (nodosa)
> EXCLUDES   *trichiasis of eyelid (374.05)*

704.3   Variations in hair color
    Canities (premature)
    Grayness, hair (premature)
    Heterochromia of hair
    Poliosis:
        NOS
        circumscripta, acquired

704.8   Other specified diseases of hair and hair follicles
    Folliculitis: Sycosis:
        NOS   NOS
        abscedens et suffodiens   barbae [not parasitic]
        pustular   lupoid
    Perifolliculitis: vulgaris
        NOS
        capitis abscedens et suffodiens
        scalp

704.9   Unspecified disease of hair and hair follicles

☑4ᵗʰ **705 Disorders of sweat glands**

705.0   Anhidrosis
    Hypohidrosis   Oligohidrosis
> DEF: Lack or deficiency of ability to sweat.

705.1   Prickly heat
    Heat rash   Sudamina
    Miliaria rubra (tropicalis)

☑5ᵗʰ **705.8   Other specified disorders of sweat glands**

    705.81   Dyshidrosis
        Cheiropompholyx   Pompholyx
> DEF: Vesicular eruption, on hands, feet causing itching and burning.

    705.82   Fox-Fordyce disease
> DEF: Chronic, usually pruritic disease chiefly of women evidenced by small follicular papular eruptions, especially in the axillary and pubic areas; develops from the closure and rupture of the affected apocrine glands' intraepidermal portion of the ducts.

    705.83   Hidradenitis
        Hidradenitis suppurativa
> DEF: Inflamed sweat glands.

    705.89   Other
        Bromhidrosis   Granulosis rubra nasi
        Chromhidrosis   Urhidrosis
> EXCLUDES   *hidrocystoma (216.0-216.9)*
> *hyperhidrosis (780.8)*

> DEF: Bromhidrosis: foul-smelling axillary sweat due to decomposed bacteria.

> DEF: Chromhidrosis: secretion of colored sweat.

> DEF: Granulosis ubra nasi: ideopathic condition of children; causes redness, sweating around nose, face and chin; tends to end by puberty.

> DEF: Urhidrosis: urinous substance, such as uric acid, in sweat; occurs in uremia.

705.9   Unspecified disorder of sweat glands
    Disorder of sweat glands NOS

☑4ᵗʰ **706 Diseases of sebaceous glands**

706.0   Acne varioliformis
    Acne: Acne:
        frontalis   necrotica
> DEF: Rare form of acne characterized by persistent brown papulopustules usually on the brow and temporoparietal part of the scalp.

706.1   Other acne
    Acne: Acne:
        NOS   vulgaris
        conglobata   Blackhead
        cystic   Comedo
        pustular
> EXCLUDES   *acne rosacea (695.3)*

Skin and Subcutaneous Tissue 702–706.1

☑4ᵗʰ / ☑5ᵗʰ Additional Digit Required   Unspecified Code   Other Specified Code   Manifestation Code   ▶◀ Revised Text   ● New Code   ▲ Revised Code Title

2003 ICD•9•CM   **Volume 1 — 189**

Skin and Subcutaneous Tissue 706.2–709.2

706.2   Sebaceous cyst
Atheroma, skin   Wen
Keratin cyst
DEF: Benign epidermal cyst, contains sebum and keratin; presents as firm, circumscribed nodule.

706.3   Seborrhea
EXCLUDES   seborrhea:
    capitis (690.11)
    sicca (690.18)
   seborrheic:
    dermatitis (690.10)
    keratosis (702.11-702.19)
DEF: Seborrheic dermatitis marked by excessive secretion of sebum; the sebum forms an oily coating, crusts, or scales on the skin; it is also called hypersteatosis.

706.8   Other specified diseases of sebaceous glands
Asteatosis (cutis)   Xerosis cutis

706.9   Unspecified disease of sebaceous glands

√4ᵗʰ 707   Chronic ulcer of skin
INCLUDES   non-infected sinus of skin
non-healing ulcer
EXCLUDES   specific infections classified under "Infectious and Parasitic Diseases" (001.0-136.9)
varicose ulcer (454.0, 454.2)

707.0   Decubitus ulcer
Bed sore   Plaster ulcer
Decubitus ulcer [any site]   Pressure ulcer

√5ᵗʰ 707.1   Ulcer of lower limbs, except decubitus
Ulcer, chronic:
   neurogenic } of lower limb
   trophic
►Code, if applicable, any casual condition first:◄
atherosclerosis of the extremities with ulceration (440.23)
►chronic venous hypertension with ulcer (459.31)
chronic venous hypertension with ulcer and inflammation (459.33)◄
diabetes mellitus (250.80-250.83)
►postphlebitic syndrome with ulcer (459.11)
postphlebitic syndrome with ulcer and inflammation (459.13)◄

707.10   Ulcer of lower limb, unspecified
707.11   Ulcer of thigh
707.12   Ulcer of calf
707.13   Ulcer of ankle
707.14   Ulcer of heel and midfoot
Plantar surface of midfoot
707.15   Ulcer of other part of foot
Toes
707.19   Ulcer of other part of lower limb

707.8   Chronic ulcer of other specified sites
Ulcer, chronic:
   neurogenic } of other specified sites
   trophic

707.9   Chronic ulcer of unspecified site
Chronic ulcer NOS   Tropical ulcer NOS
Trophic ulcer NOS   Ulcer of skin NOS

√4ᵗʰ 708   Urticaria
EXCLUDES   edema:
    angioneurotic (995.1)
    Quincke's (995.1)
   hereditary angioedema (277.6)
   urticaria:
    giant (995.1)
    papulosa (Hebra) (698.2)
    pigmentosa (juvenile) (congenital) (757.33)
DEF: Skin disorder marked by raised edematous patches of skin or mucous membrane with intense itching; also called hives.

708.0   Allergic urticaria
708.1   Idiopathic urticaria
708.2   Urticaria due to cold and heat
Thermal urticaria
708.3   Dermatographic urticaria
Dermatographia   Factitial urticaria
708.4   Vibratory urticaria
708.5   Cholinergic urticaria
708.8   Other specified urticaria
Nettle rash   Urticaria:
Urticaria: recurrent periodic
   chronic
708.9   Urticaria, unspecified
Hives NOS

√4ᵗʰ 709   Other disorders of skin and subcutaneous tissue
√5ᵗʰ 709.0   Dyschromia
EXCLUDES   albinism (270.2)
   pigmented nevus (216.0-216.9)
   that of eyelid (374.52-374.53)
DEF: Pigment disorder of skin or hair.

709.00   Dyschromia, unspecified
709.01   Vitiligo
DEF: Persistent, progressive development of nonpigmented white patches on otherwise normal skin.

709.09   Other
709.1   Vascular disorders of skin
Angioma serpiginosum
Purpura (primary)annularis telangiectodes
709.2   Scar conditions and fibrosis of skin
Adherent scar (skin)   Fibrosis, skin NOS
Cicatrix   Scar NOS
Disfigurement (due to scar)
EXCLUDES   keloid scar (701.4)

Six Stages of Decubitus Ulcers

First Stage — Skin is warm, firm, or stretched

Second Stage — Bacteria enter

Third Stage — Fat layer exposed

Fourth Stage — Muscle necrosis

Fifth Stage — Advanced muscle necrosis

Sixth Stage — Bone necrosis

Cutaneous Lesions
Surface Lesions

Fissure   Polyp growth   Ulcer

Solid Lesions
Flat macule   Slightly elevated wheal   Solid papule

Sac Lesions

Cyst   Clear fluid vesicle   Pustule

N Newborn Age: 0   P Pediatric Age: 0-17   M Maternity Age: 12-55   A Adult Age: 15-124   MSP Medicare Secondary Payer

709.3 **Degenerative skin disorders**

Calcinosis: Degeneration, skin
  circumscripta Deposits, skin
  cutis Senile dermatosis NOS
Colloid milium Subcutaneous calcification

709.4 **Foreign body granuloma of skin and subcutaneous tissue**

> EXCLUDES *residual foreign body without*
> *granuloma of skin and*
> *subcutaneous tissue (729.6)*
> *that of muscle (728.82)*

709.8 **Other specified disorders of skin**

Epithelial hyperplasia Vesicular eruption
Menstrual dermatosis

DEF: Epithelial hyperplasia: increased number of epitheleal cells.

DEF: Vesicular eruption: liquid-filled structures appearing through skin.

709.9 **Unspecified disorder of skin and subcutaneous tissue**

Dermatosis NOS

✓4ᵗʰ
✓5ᵗʰ Additional Digit Required   Unspecified Code   Other Specified Code   Manifestation Code   ▶◀ Revised Text   ● New Code   ▲ Revised Code Title

2003 ICD•9•CM   Volume 1 — 191

13. DISEASES OF THE MUSCULOSKELETAL SYSTEM AND CONNECTIVE TISSUE (710-739)

The following fifth-digit subclassification is for use with categories 711-712, 715-716, 718-719, and 730:

0 site unspecified

1 shoulder region
　　Acromioclavicular joint(s)
　　Clavicle
　　Glenohumeral joint(s)
　　Scapula
　　Sternoclavicular joint(s)

2 upper arm
　　Elbow joint　　　　　Humerus

3 forearm
　　Radius　　　　　　　Wrist joint
　　Ulna

4 hand
　　Carpus　　　　　　　Phalanges [fingers]
　　Metacarpus

5 pelvic region and thigh
　　Buttock　　　　　　　Hip (joint)
　　Femur

6 lower leg
　　Fibula　　　　　　　Patella
　　Knee joint　　　　　Tibia

7 ankle and foot
　　Ankle joint　　　　　Phalanges, foot
　　Digits [toes]　　　　Tarsus
　　Metatarsus　　　　　Other joints in foot

8 other specified sites
　　Head　　　　　　　　Skull
　　Neck　　　　　　　　Trunk
　　Ribs　　　　　　　　Vertebral column

9 multiple sites

ARTHROPATHIES AND RELATED DISORDERS (710-719)

　EXCLUDES　*disorders of spine (720.0-724.9)*

✓4ᵗʰ **710 Diffuse diseases of connective tissue**

　INCLUDES　all collagen diseases whose effects are not mainly confined to a single system

　EXCLUDES　*those affecting mainly the cardiovascular system, i.e., polyarteritis nodosa and allied conditions (446.0-446.7)*

710.0 Systemic lupus erythematosus
　Disseminated lupus erythematosus
　Libman-Sacks disease
　Use additional code to identify manifestation, as:
　　endocarditis (424.91)
　　nephritis (583.81)
　　　chronic (582.81)
　　nephrotic syndrome (581.81)
　　EXCLUDES　*lupus erythematosus (discoid) NOS (695.4)*

DEF: A chronic multisystemic inflammatory disease affecting connective tissue; marked by anemia, leukopenia, muscle and joint pains, fever, rash of a butterfly pattern around cheeks and forehead area; of unknown etiology.

710.1 Systemic sclerosis
　Acrosclerosis　　　　Progressive systemic sclerosis
　CRST syndrome　　　Scleroderma
　　EXCLUDES　*circumscribed scleroderma (701.0)*
　▶Use additional code to identify manifestation, as:
　　lung involvement (517.8)
　　myopathy (359.6)◀

DEF: Systemic disease, involving excess fibrotic collagen build-up; symptoms include thickened skin; fibrotic degenerative changes in various organs; and vascular abnomalities; condition occurs more often in females.

Joint Structures

710.2 Sicca syndrome
　Keratoconjunctivitis sicca
　Sjögren's disease

DEF: Autoimmune disease; associated with keratoconjunctivitis, laryngopharyngitis, rhinitis, dry mouth, enlarged parotid gland, and chronic polyarthritis.

710.3 Dermatomyositis
　Poikilodermatomyositis
　Polymyositis with skin involvement

DEF: Polymyositis associated with flat-top purple papules on knuckles; marked by upper eyelid rash, edema of eyelids and orbit area, red rash on forehead, neck, shoulders, trunk and arms; symptoms include fever, weight loss aching muscles; visceral cancer (in individuals older than 40).

710.4 Polymyositis

DEF: Chronic, progressive, inflammatory skeletal muscle disease; causes weakness of limb girdles, neck, pharynx; may precede or follow scleroderma, Sjogren's disease, systemic lupus erythematosus, arthritis, or malignancy.

710.5 Eosinophilia myalgia syndrome
　Toxic oil syndrome
　Use additional E code to identify drug, if drug induced

DEF: Eosinophilia myalgia syndrome (EMS): inflammatory, multisystem fibrosis; associated with ingesting elemetary L-tryptophan; symptoms include myalgia, weak limbs and bulbar muscles, distal sensory loss, areflexia, arthralgia, cough, fever, fatigue, skin rashes, myopathy, and eosinophil counts greater than 1000/microliter.

DEF: Toxic oil syndrome: syndrome silimar to EMS due to ingesting contaminated cooking oil.

710.8 Other specified diffuse diseases of connective tissue
　Multifocal fibrosclerosis (idiopathic) NEC
　Systemic fibrosclerosing syndrome

710.9 Unspecified diffuse connective tissue disease
　Collagen disease NOS

✓4ᵗʰ ✓5ᵗʰ Additional Digit Required　　Unspecified Code　　Other Specified Code　　Manifestation Code　　▶◀ Revised Text　　● New Code　　▲ Revised Code Title

2003 ICD•9•CM　　　　　　　　　　　　　　　　　　　　　　**October 2002 • Volume 1 — 193**

✓4ᵗʰ **711 Arthropathy associated with infections**

INCLUDES	arthritis	}	associated with
	arthropathy		conditions
	polyarthritis		classifiable
	polyarthropathy		below

     EXCLUDES   rheumatic fever (390)

The following fifth-digit subclassification is for use with category 711; valid digits are in [brackets] under each code.

     0   site unspecified
     1   shoulder region
     2   upper arm
     3   forearm
     4   hand
     5   pelvic region and thigh
     6   lower leg
     7   ankle and foot
     8   other specified sites
     9   multiple sites

§ ✓5ᵗʰ **711.0 Pyogenic arthritis**
[0-9]   Arthritis or polyarthritis (due to):
     coliform [Escherichia coli]
     Hemophilus influenzae [H. influenzae]
     pneumococcal
     Pseudomonas
     staphylococcal
     streptococcal
     Pyarthrosis
     Use additional code to identify infectious organism (041.0-041.8)

DEF: Infectious arthritis caused by various bacteria; marked by inflamed synovial membranes, and purulent effusion in joints.

§ ✓5ᵗʰ **711.1 Arthropathy associated with Reiter's disease and nonspecific urethritis**
[0-9]   *Code first underlying disease as:*
     nonspecific urethritis (099.4)
     Reiter's disease (099.3)

DEF: Reiter's disease: joint disease marked by diarrhea, urethritis, conjunctivitis, keratosis and arthritis; of unknown etiology; affects young males.

DEF: Urethritis: inflamed urethra.

§ ✓5ᵗʰ **711.2 Arthropathy in Behçet's syndrome**
[0-9]   *Code first underlying disease (136.1)*

DEF: Behçet's syndrome: chronic inflammatory disorder, of unknown etiology; affects small blood vessels; causes ulcers of oral and pharyngeal mucous membranes and genitalia, skin lesions, retinal vasculitis, optic atrophy and severe uveitis.

§ ✓5ᵗʰ **711.3 Postdysenteric arthropathy**
[0-9]   *Code first underlying disease as:*
     dysentery (009.0)
     enteritis, infectious (008.0-009.3)
     paratyphoid fever (002.1-002.9)
     typhoid fever (002.0)
     EXCLUDES   salmonella arthritis (003.23)

§ ✓5ᵗʰ **711.4 Arthropathy associated with other bacterial diseases**
[0-9]   *Code first underlying disease as:*
     diseases classifiable to 010-040, 090-099, except as in 711.1, 711.3, and 713.5
     leprosy (030.0-030.9)
     tuberculosis (015.0-015.9)
     EXCLUDES   gonococcal arthritis (098.50)
            meningococcal arthritis (036.82)

§ ✓5ᵗʰ **711.5 Arthropathy associated with other viral diseases**
[0-9]   *Code first underlying disease as:*
     diseases classifiable to 045-049, 050-079, 480, 487
     O'nyong nyong (066.3)
     EXCLUDES   that due to rubella (056.71)

§ ✓5ᵗʰ **711.6 Arthropathy associated with mycoses**
[0-9]   *Code first underlying disease (110.0-118)*

§ ✓5ᵗʰ **711.7 Arthropathy associated with helminthiasis**
[0-9]   *Code first underlying disease as:*
     filariasis (125.0-125.9)

§ ✓5ᵗʰ **711.8 Arthropathy associated with other infectious and parasitic diseases**
[0-9]   *Code first underlying disease as:*
     diseases classifiable to 080-088, 100-104, 130-136
     EXCLUDES   arthropathy associated with sarcoidosis (713.7)

§ ✓5ᵗʰ **711.9 Unspecified infective arthritis**
[0-9]   Infective arthritis or polyarthritis (acute) (chronic) (subacute) NOS

✓4ᵗʰ **712 Crystal arthropathies**

     INCLUDES   crystal-induced arthritis andsynovitis
     EXCLUDES   gouty arthropathy (274.0)

DEF: Joint disease due to urate crystal deposit in joints or synovial membranes.

The following fifth-digit subclassification is for use with category 712; valid digits are in [brackets] under each code. See definitions prior to category 710.

     0   site unspecified
     1   shoulder region
     2   upper arm
     3   forearm
     4   hand
     5   pelvic region and thigh
     6   lower leg
     7   ankle and foot
     8   other specified sites
     9   multiple sites

§ ✓5ᵗʰ **712.1 Chondrocalcinosis due to dicalcium phosphate crystals**
[0-9]   Chondrocalcinosis due to dicalcium phosphate crystals (with other crystals)
     Code first underlying disease (275.4)

§ ✓5ᵗʰ **712.2 Chondrocalcinosis due to pyrophosphate crystals**
[0-9]   *Code first underlying disease (275.4)*

§ ✓5ᵗʰ **712.3 Chondrocalcinosis, unspecified**
[0-9]   *Code first underlying disease (275.4)*

§ ✓5ᵗʰ **712.8 Other specified crystal arthropathies**
[0-9]

§ ✓5ᵗʰ **712.9 Unspecified crystal arthropathy**
[0-9]

✓4ᵗʰ **713 Arthropathy associated with other disorders classified elsewhere**

INCLUDES	arthritis	}	associated with
	arthropathy		conditions
	polyarthritis		classifiable below
	polyarthropathy		

---

§ Requires fifth digit. Valid digits are in [brackets] under each code. See beginning of section 710–739 for codes and definitions.

N Newborn Age: 0   P Pediatric Age: 0-17   M Maternity Age: 12-55   A Adult Age: 15-124   MSP Medicare Secondary Payer

713.0   *Arthropathy associated with other endocrine and metabolic disorders*

Code first underlying disease as:
acromegaly (253.0)
hemochromatosis (275.0)
hyperparathyroidism (252.0)
hypogammaglobulinemia (279.00-279.09)
hypothyroidism (243-244.9)
lipoid metabolism disorder (272.0-272.9)
ochronosis (270.2)

   EXCLUDES   *arthropathy associated with:*
amyloidosis (713.7)
crystal deposition disorders, except gout (712.1-712.9)
diabetic neuropathy (713.5)
gouty arthropathy (274.0)

713.1   *Arthropathy associated with gastrointestinal conditions other than infections*

Code first underlying disease as:
regional enteritis (555.0-555.9)
ulcerative colitis (556)

713.2   *Arthropathy associated with hematological disorders*

Code first underlying disease as:
hemoglobinopathy (282.4-282.7)
hemophilia (286.0-286.2)
leukemia (204.0-208.9)
malignant reticulosis (202.3)
multiple myelomatosis (203.0)

   EXCLUDES   *arthropathy associated with Henoch-Schönlein purpura (713.6)*

713.3   *Arthropathy associated with dermatological disorders*

Code first underlying disease as:
erythema multiforme (695.1)
erythema nodosum (695.2)

   EXCLUDES   *psoriatic arthropathy (696.0)*

713.4   *Arthropathy associated with respiratory disorders*

Code first underlying disease as:
diseases classifiable to 490-519

   EXCLUDES   *arthropathy associated with respiratory infections (711.0, 711.4-711.8)*

713.5   *Arthropathy associated with neurological disorders*

Charcôt's arthropathy
Neuropathic arthritis
    } associated with diseases classifiable elsewhere

Code first underlying disease as:
neuropathic joint disease [Charcôt's joints]:
NOS (094.0)
diabetic (250.6)
syringomyelic (336.0)
tabetic [syphilitic] (094.0)

713.6   *Arthropathy associated with hypersensitivity reaction*

Code first underlying disease as:
Henoch (-Schönlein) purpura (287.0)
serum sickness (999.5)

   EXCLUDES   *allergic arthritis NOS (716.2)*

713.7   *Other general diseases with articular involvement*

Code first underlying disease as:
amyloidosis (277.3)
familial Mediterranean fever (277.3)
sarcoidosis (135)

713.8   *Arthropathy associated with other conditions classifiable elsewhere*

Code first underlying disease as:
conditions classifiable elsewhere except as in 711.1-711.8, 712, and 713.0-713.7

✓4ᵗʰ 714 Rheumatoid arthritis and other inflammatory polyarthropathies

   EXCLUDES   *rheumatic fever (390)*
rheumatoid arthritis of spine NOS (720.0)

714.0   **Rheumatoid arthritis**

Arthritis or polyarthritis:
atrophic
rheumatic (chronic)
Use additional code to identify manifestation, as:
myopathy (359.6)
polyneuropathy (357.1)

   EXCLUDES   *juvenile rheumatoid arthritis NOS (714.30)*

DEF: Chronic systemic disease principally of joints, manifested by inflammatory changes in articular structures and synovial membranes, atrophy, and loss in bone density.

714.1   **Felty's syndrome**

Rheumatoid arthritis with splenoadenomegaly and leukopenia

DEF: Syndrome marked by rheumatoid arthritis, splenomegaly, leukopenia, pigmented spots on lower extremity skin, anemia, and thrombocytopenia.

714.2   **Other rheumatoid arthritis with visceral or systemic involvement**

Rheumatoid carditis

✓5ᵗʰ 714.3   **Juvenile chronic polyarthritis**

DEF: Rheumatoid arthritis of more than one joint; lasts longer than six weeks in age 17 or younger; symptoms include fever, erythematous rash, weight loss, lymphadenopathy, hepatosplenomegaly and pericarditis.

    714.30   **Polyarticular juvenile rheumatoid arthritis, chronic or unspecified**
Juvenile rheumatoid arthritis NOS
Still's disease

    714.31   **Polyarticular juvenile rheumatoid arthritis, acute**

    714.32   **Pauciarticular juvenile rheumatoid arthritis**

    714.33   **Monoarticular juvenile rheumatoid arthritis**

714.4   **Chronic postrheumatic arthropathy**
Chronic rheumatoid nodular fibrositis
Jaccoud's syndrome

DEF: Persistent joint disorder; follows previous rheumatic infection.

✓5ᵗʰ 714.8   **Other specified inflammatory polyarthropathies**

    714.81   **Rheumatoid lung**
Caplan's syndrome
Diffuse interstitial rheumatoid disease of lung
Fibrosing alveolitis, rheumatoid

DEF: Lung disorders associated with rheumatoid arthritis.

    714.89   **Other**

714.9   **Unspecified inflammatory polyarthropathy**
Inflammatory polyarthropathy or polyarthritis NOS

   EXCLUDES   *polyarthropathy NOS (716.5)*

✓4ᵗʰ / ✓5ᵗʰ Additional Digit Required   Unspecified Code   Other Specified Code   Manifestation Code   ▶◀ Revised Text   ● New Code   ▲ Revised Code Title

2003 ICD•9•CM   **Volume 1 — 195**

Musculoskeletal System and Connective Tissue 715–717.49

√4ᵗʰ 715 Osteoarthrosis and allied disorders

Note: Localized, in the subcategories below, includes bilateral involvement of the same site.

INCLUDES   arthritis or polyarthritis:
     degenerative
     hypertrophic
     degenerative joint disease
     osteoarthritis

EXCLUDES   *Marie-Strümpell spondylitis (720.0)*
osteoarthrosis [osteoarthritis] of spine (721.0-721.9)

The following fifth-digit subclassification is for use with category 715; valid digits are in [brackets] under each code. See definitions prior to category 710.

  0   site unspecified
  1   shoulder region
  2   upper arm
  3   forearm
  4   hand
  5   pelvic region and thigh
  6   lower leg
  7   ankle and foot
  8   other specified sites
  9   multiple sites

§ √5ᵗʰ 715.0 Osteoarthrosis, generalized
[0,4,9]   Degenerative joint disease, involving multiple joints
     Primary generalized hypertrophic osteoarthrosis

DEF: Chronic noninflammatory arthritis; marked by degenerated articular cartilage and enlarged bone; symptoms include pain and stiffness with activity; occurs among elderly.

§ √5ᵗʰ 715.1 Osteoarthrosis, localized, primary
[0-8]   Localized osteoarthropathy, idiopathic

§ √5ᵗʰ 715.2 Osteoarthrosis, localized, secondary
[0-8]   Coxae malum senilis

§ √5ᵗʰ 715.3 Osteoarthrosis, localized, not specified whether primary or secondary
[0-8]   Otto's pelvis

§ √5ᵗʰ 715.8 Osteoarthrosis involving, or with mention of more than one site, but not specified as generalized
[0,9]

§ √5ᵗʰ 715.9 Osteoarthrosis, unspecified whether generalized or localized
[0-8]

√4ᵗʰ 716 Other and unspecified arthropathies

EXCLUDES   *cricoarytenoid arthropathy (478.79)*

The following fifth-digit subclassification is for use with category 716; valid digits are in [brackets] under each code. See definitions prior to category 710.

  0   site unspecified
  1   shoulder region
  2   upper arm
  3   forearm
  4   hand
  5   pelvic region and thigh
  6   lower leg
  7   ankle and foot
  8   other specified sites
  9   multiple sites

§ √5ᵗʰ 716.0 Kaschin-Beck disease
[0-9]   Endemic polyarthritis

DEF: Chronic degenerative disease of spine and peripheral joints; occurs in eastern Siberian, northern Chinese, and Korean youth; may a mycotoxicosis caused by eating cereals infected with fungus.

§ √5ᵗʰ 716.1 Traumatic arthropathy
[0-9]

§ √5ᵗʰ 716.2 Allergic arthritis
[0-9]   EXCLUDES   *arthritis associated with Henoch-Schönlein purpura or serum sickness (713.6)*

§ √5ᵗʰ 716.3 Climacteric arthritis   ♀
[0-9]   Menopausal arthritis

DEF: Ovarian hormone deficiency; causes pain in small joints, shoulders, elbows or knees; affects females at menopause; also called arthropathia ovaripriva.

§ √5ᵗʰ 716.4 Transient arthropathy
[0-9]   EXCLUDES   *palindromic rheumatism (719.3)*

§ √5ᵗʰ 716.5 Unspecified polyarthropathy or polyarthritis
[0-9]

§ √5ᵗʰ 716.6 Unspecified monoarthritis
[0-8]   Coxitis

§ √5ᵗʰ 716.8 Other specified arthropathy
[0-9]

§ √5ᵗʰ 716.9 Arthropathy, unspecified
[0-9]

Arthritis
Arthropathy } (acute) (chronic) (subacute)

Articular rheumatism (chronic)
Inflammation of joint NOS

√4ᵗʰ 717 Internal derangement of knee

INCLUDES   degeneration
     rupture, old } of articular cartilage or meniscus of knee
     tear, old

EXCLUDES   *acute derangement of knee (836.0-836.6)*
ankylosis (718.5)
contracture (718.4)
current injury (836.0-836.6)
deformity (736.4-736.6)
recurrent dislocation (718.3)

717.0 Old bucket handle tear of medial meniscus
     Old bucket handle tear of unspecified cartilage

717.1 Derangement of anterior horn of medial meniscus

717.2 Derangement of posterior horn of medial meniscus

717.3 Other and unspecified derangement of medial meniscus
     Degeneration of internal semilunar cartilage

√5ᵗʰ 717.4 Derangement of lateral meniscus

     717.40 Derangement of lateral meniscus, unspecified

     717.41 Bucket handle tear of lateral meniscus

     717.42 Derangement of anterior horn of lateral meniscus

     717.43 Derangement of posterior horn of lateral meniscus

     717.49 Other

Disruption and Tears of Meniscus

Disruptions and Tears of Meniscus

Bucket-handle

Flap-type

Peripheral   Radial

Horizontal   Vertical   Congenital discoid

---

§ Requires fifth digit. Valid digits are in [brackets] under each code. See beginning of section 710–739 for codes and definitions.

Internal Derangements of Knee

Disruptions of Cruciate Ligament

Chondromalacia of Patella

Anterior

Posterior

"Kissing" lesion of femur

717.5 Derangement of meniscus, not elsewhere classified
Congenital discoid meniscus
Cyst of semilunar cartilage
Derangement of semilunar cartilage NOS

717.6 Loose body in knee
Joint mice, knee
Rice bodies, knee (joint)
DEF: The presence in the joint synovial area of a small, frequently calcified, loose body created from synovial membrane, organized fibrin fragments of articular cartilage or arthritis osteophytes.

717.7 Chondromalacia of patella
Chondromalacia patellae
Degeneration [softening] of articular cartilage of patella
DEF: Softened patella cartilage.

√5th **717.8 Other internal derangement of knee**
717.81 Old disruption of lateral collateral ligament
717.82 Old disruption of medial collateral ligament
717.83 Old disruption of anterior cruciate ligament
717.84 Old disruption of posterior cruciate ligament
717.85 Old disruption of other ligaments of knee
Capsular ligament of knee
717.89 Other
Old disruption of ligaments of knee NOS

717.9 Unspecified internal derangement of knee
Derangement NOS of knee

√4th **718 Other derangement of joint**
EXCLUDES current injury (830.0-848.9)
jaw (524.6)

The following fifth-digit subclassification is for use with category 718; valid digits are in [brackets] under each code. See definitions prior to category 710.
  0 site unspecified
  1 shoulder region
  2 upper arm
  3 forearm
  4 hand
  5 pelvic region and thigh
  6 lower leg
  7 ankle and foot
  8 other specified sites
  9 multiple sites

§ √5th **718.0 Articular cartilage disorder**
[0-5,7-9] Meniscus: Meniscus:
disorder   tear, old
rupture, old   Old rupture of ligament(s) of joint NOS
EXCLUDES articular cartilage disorder:
in ochronosis (270.2)
knee (717.0-717.9)
chondrocalcinosis (275.4)
metastatic calcification (275.4)

§ √5th **718.1 Loose body in joint**
[0-5,7-9] Joint mice
EXCLUDES knee (717.6)
DEF: Calcified loose bodies in synovial fluid; due to arthritic osteophytes.

§ √5th **718.2 Pathological dislocation**
[0-9] Dislocation or displacement of joint, not recurrent and not current injury
Spontaneous dislocation (joint)

§ √5th **718.3 Recurrent dislocation of joint**
[0-9]

§ √5th **718.4 Contracture of joint**
[0-9]

§ √5th **718.5 Ankylosis of joint**
[0-9] Ankylosis of joint (fibrous) (osseous)
EXCLUDES spine (724.9)
stiffness of joint without mention of ankylosis (719.5)
DEF: Immobility and solidification, of joint; due to disease, injury or surgical procedure.

§ √5th **718.6 Unspecified intrapelvic protrusion of acetabulum**
[0,5] Protrusio acetabuli, unspecified
DEF: Sinking of the floor of acetabulum; causing femoral head to protrude, limits hip movement; of unknown etiology.

§ √5th **718.7 Developmental dislocation of joint**
[0-9] EXCLUDES ▶congenital dislocation of joint (754.0-755.8)
traumatic dislocation of joint (830-839)◀

§ √5th **718.8 Other joint derangement, not elsewhere classified**
[0-9] Flail joint (paralytic)
Instability of joint
EXCLUDES deformities classifiable to 736 (736.0-736.9)

§ √5th **718.9 Unspecified derangement of joint**
[0-5,7-9] EXCLUDES knee (717.9)

√4th **719 Other and unspecified disorders of joint**
EXCLUDES jaw (524.6)

The following fifth-digit subclassification is for use with category 719; valid digits are in [brackets] under each code. See definitions prior to category 710.
  0 site unspecified
  1 shoulder region
  2 upper arm
  3 forearm
  4 hand
  5 pelvic region and thigh
  6 lower leg
  7 ankle and foot
  8 other specified sites
  9 multiple sites

Musculoskeletal System and Connective Tissue 717.5–719

§ Requires fifth digit. Valid digits are in [brackets] under each code. See beginning of section 710–739 for codes and definitions.

√4th √5th Additional Digit Required   Unspecified Code   Other Specified Code   Manifestation Code   ▶◀ Revised Text   ● New Code   ▲ Revised Code Title

Joint Derangements and Disorders

Loose body in joint

Dislocation of joint

Joint contracture | Ankylosis of joint | Synovial effusion (fluid) | Hemarthrosis (blood)

§ ✓5ᵗʰ **719.0 Effusion of joint**
[0-9]
Hydrarthrosis
Swelling of joint, with or without pain
EXCLUDES intermittent hydrarthrosis (719.3)

§ ✓5ᵗʰ **719.1 Hemarthrosis**
[0-9]
EXCLUDES current injury (840.0-848.9)

§ ✓5ᵗʰ **719.2 Villonodular synovitis**
[0-9]
DEF: Overgrowth of synovial tissue, especially at knee joint; due to macrophage infiltration of giant cells in synovial villi and fibrous nodules.

§ ✓5ᵗʰ **719.3 Palindromic rheumatism**
[0-9]
Hench-Rosenberg syndrome
Intermittent hydrarthrosis

DEF: Recurrent episodes of afebrile arthritis and periarthritis marked by their complete disappearance after a few days or hours; causes swelling, redness, and disability usually affecting only one joint; no known cause; affects adults of either sex.

§ ✓5ᵗʰ **719.4 Pain in joint**
[0-9]
Arthralgia

§ ✓5ᵗʰ **719.5 Stiffness of joint, not elsewhere classified**
[0-9]

§ ✓5ᵗʰ **719.6 Other symptoms referable to joint**
[0-9]
Joint crepitus   Snapping hip

§ ✓5ᵗʰ **719.7 Difficulty in walking**
[0,5-9]
EXCLUDES abnormality of gait (781.2)

§ ✓5ᵗʰ **719.8 Other specified disorders of joint**
[0-9]
Calcification of joint   Fistula of joint
EXCLUDES temporomandibular joint-pain-dysfunction syndrome [Costen's syndrome] (524.6)

§ ✓5ᵗʰ **719.9 Unspecified disorder of joint**
[0-9]

DORSOPATHIES (720-724)
EXCLUDES curvature of spine (737.0-737.9)
osteochondrosis of spine (juvenile) (732.0)
adult (732.8)

✓4ᵗʰ **720 Ankylosing spondylitis and other inflammatory spondylopathies**

720.0 Ankylosing spondylitis
Rheumatoid arthritis of spine NOS
Spondylitis:
Marie-Strümpell
rheumatoid

DEF: Rheumatoid arthritis of spine and sacroiliac joints; fusion and deformity in spine follows; affects mainly males; cause unknown.

720.1 Spinal enthesopathy
Disorder of peripheral ligamentous or muscular attachments of spine
Romanus lesion
DEF: Tendinous or muscular vertebral bone attachment abnormality.

720.2 Sacroiliitis, not elsewhere classified
Inflammation of sacroiliac joint NOS
DEF: Pain due to inflammation in joint, at juncture of sacrum and hip.

✓5ᵗʰ **720.8 Other inflammatory spondylopathies**

720.81 Inflammatory spondylopathies in diseases classified elsewhere
Code first underlying disease as:
tuberculosis (015.0)

720.89 Other

720.9 Unspecified inflammatory spondylopathy
Spondylitis NOS

✓4ᵗʰ **721 Spondylosis and allied disorders**
DEF: Degenerative changes in spinal joint.

721.0 Cervical spondylosis without myelopathy
Cervical or cervicodorsal: Cervical or cervicodorsal:
arthritis   spondylarthritis
osteoarthritis

721.1 Cervical spondylosis with myelopathy
Anterior spinal artery compression syndrome
Spondylogenic compression of cervical spinal cord
Vertebral artery compression syndrome

721.2 Thoracic spondylosis without myelopathy
Thoracic: Thoracic:
arthritis   spondylarthritis
osteoarthritis

721.3 Lumbosacral spondylosis without myelopathy
Lumbar or lumbosacral: Lumbar or lumbosacral:
arthritis   spondylarthritis
osteoarthritis

✓5ᵗʰ **721.4 Thoracic or lumbar spondylosis with myelopathy**

721.41 Thoracic region
Spondylogenic compression of thoracic spinal cord

721.42 Lumbar region
Spondylogenic compression of lumbar spinal cord

721.5 Kissing spine
Baastrup's syndrome
DEF: Compression of spinous processes of adjacent vertebrae; due to mutual contact.

721.6 Ankylosing vertebral hyperostosis

721.7 Traumatic spondylopathy
Kümmell's disease or spondylitis

721.8 Other allied disorders of spine

Normal Anatomy of Vertebral Disc

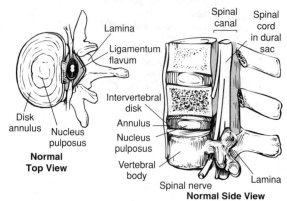

Lamina
Ligamentum flavum
Spinal canal
Spinal cord in dural sac
Intervertebral disk
Annulus
Nucleus pulposus
Disk annulus
Nucleus pulposus
Vertebral body
Spinal nerve
Lamina
Normal Top View
Normal Side View

§ Requires fifth digit. Valid digits are in [brackets] under each code. See beginning of section 710–739 for codes and definitions.

√5th **721.9 Spondylosis of unspecified site**
 721.90 **Without mention of myelopathy**
  Spinal:
   arthritis (deformans) (degenerative)
    (hypertrophic)
  osteoarthritis NOS
  Spondylarthrosis NOS
 721.91 **With myelopathy**
  Spondylogenic compression of spinal cord
   NOS

√4th **722 Intervertebral disc disorders**
 722.0 **Displacement of cervical intervertebral disc** A
  without myelopathy
  Neuritis (brachial) or radiculitis due to displacement
   or rupture of cervical intervertebral disc
  Any condition classifiable to 722.2 of the cervical or
   cervicothoracic intervertebral disc

√5th 722.1 **Displacement of thoracic or lumbar intervertebral**
  disc without myelopathy
  722.10 **Lumbar intervertebral disc without** A
   myelopathy
   Lumbago or sciatica due to displacement of
    intervertebral disc
   Neuritis or radiculitis due to displacement
    or rupture of lumbar intervertebral
    disc
   Any condition classifiable to 722.2 of the
    lumbar or lumbosacral intervertebral
    disc
  722.11 **Thoracic intervertebral disc without** A
   myelopathy
   Any condition classifiable to 722.2 of
    thoracic intervertebral disc

 722.2 **Displacement of intervertebral disc, site** A
  unspecified, without myelopathy
  Discogenic syndrome NOS
  Herniation of nucleus pulposus NOS
  Intervertebral disc NOS:
   extrusion
   prolapse
   protrusion
   rupture
  Neuritis or radiculitis due to displacement or
   rupture of intervertebral disc

√5th 722.3 **Schmorl's nodes**
  DEF: Irregular bone defect in the margin of the vertebral body;
  causes herniation into end plate of vertebral body.

  722.30 **Unspecified region** A
  722.31 **Thoracic region** A
  722.32 **Lumbar region** A
  722.39 **Other** A
 722.4 **Degeneration of cervical intervertebral disc** A
  Degeneration of cervicothoracic intervertebral disc

√5th 722.5 **Degeneration of thoracic or lumbar intervertebral**
  disc
  722.51 **Thoracic or thoracolumbar** A
   intervertebral disc
  722.52 **Lumbar or lumbosacral intervertebral** A
   disc
 722.6 **Degeneration of intervertebral disc, site** A
  unspecified
  Degenerative disc disease NOS
  Narrowing of intervertebral disc or space NOS

√5th 722.7 **Intervertebral disc disorder with myelopathy**
  722.70 **Unspecified region** A
  722.71 **Cervical region** A
  722.72 **Thoracic region** A
  722.73 **Lumbar region** A
√5th 722.8 **Postlaminectomy syndrome**
  DEF: Spinal disorder due to spinal laminectomy surgery.

  722.80 **Unspecified region** A
  722.81 **Cervical region** A
  722.82 **Thoracic region** A
  722.83 **Lumbar region** A
√5th 722.9 **Other and unspecified disc disorder**
  Calcification of intervertebral cartilage or disc
  Discitis
  722.90 **Unspecified region** A
  722.91 **Cervical region** A
  722.92 **Thoracic region** A
  722.93 **Lumbar region** A

√4th **723 Other disorders of cervical region**
  EXCLUDES conditions due to:
    intervertebral disc disorders (722.0-722.9)
    spondylosis (721.0-721.9)
 723.0 **Spinal stenosis in cervical region**
 723.1 **Cervicalgia**
  Pain in neck
  DEF: Pain in cervical spine or neck region.

 723.2 **Cervicocranial syndrome**
  Barré-Liéou syndrome
  Posterior cervical sympathetic syndrome
  DEF: Neurologic disorder of upper cervical spine and nerve roots.

 723.3 **Cervicobrachial syndrome (diffuse)**
  DEF: Complex of symptoms due to scalenus anterior muscle
  compressing the brachial plexus; pain radiates from shoulder to
  arm or back of neck.

 723.4 **Brachial neuritis or radiculitis NOS**
  Cervical radiculitis
  Radicular syndrome of upper limbs

Derangement of Vertebral Disc

Spinal Stenosis in Cervical Region

√4th
√5th Additional Digit Required   Unspecified Code   Other Specified Code   Manifestation Code   ▶◀ Revised Text   ● New Code   ▲ Revised Code Title

Musculoskeletal System and Connective Tissue 721.9–723.4

723.5 Torticollis, unspecified
Contracture of neck
EXCLUDES congenital (754.1)
due to birth injury (767.8)
hysterical (300.11)
►ocular torticollis (781.93)◄
psychogenic (306.0)
spasmodic (333.83)
traumatic, current (847.0)

DEF: Abnormally positioned neck relative to head; due to cervical muscle or fascia contractions; also called wryneck.

723.6 Panniculitis specified as affecting neck
DEF: Inflammation of the panniculus adiposus (subcutaneous fat) in the neck.

723.7 Ossification of posterior longitudinal ligament in cervical region

723.8 Other syndromes affecting cervical region
Cervical syndrome NEC
Klippel's disease
Occipital neuralgia

723.9 Unspecified musculoskeletal disorders and symptoms referable to neck
Cervical (region) disorder NOS

√4th 724 Other and unspecified disorders of back
EXCLUDES collapsed vertebra (code to cause, e.g., osteoporosis, 733.00-733.09)
conditions due to:
intervertebral disc disorders (722.0-722.9)
spondylosis (721.0-721.9)

√5th 724.0 Spinal stenosis, other than cervical
724.00 Spinal stenosis, unspecified region [A]
724.01 Thoracic region [A]
724.02 Lumbar region [A]
724.09 Other [A]

724.1 Pain in thoracic spine

724.2 Lumbago
Low back pain   Lumbalgia
Low back syndrome

724.3 Sciatica
Neuralgia or neuritis of sciatic nerve
EXCLUDES specified lesion of sciatic nerve (355.0)

724.4 Thoracic or lumbosacral neuritis or radiculitis, unspecified
Radicular syndrome of lower limbs

724.5 Backache, unspecified
Vertebrogenic (pain) syndrome NOS

724.6 Disorders of sacrum
Ankylosis
Instability } lumbosacral or sacroiliac (joint)

√5th 724.7 Disorders of coccyx
724.70 Unspecified disorder of coccyx
724.71 Hypermobility of coccyx
724.79 Other
Coccygodynia

724.8 Other symptoms referable to back
Ossification of posterior longitudinal ligament NOS
Panniculitis specified as sacral or affecting back

724.9 Other unspecified back disorders
Ankylosis of spine NOS
Compression of spinal nerve root NEC
Spinal disorder NOS
EXCLUDES sacroiliitis (720.2)

RHEUMATISM, EXCLUDING THE BACK (725-729)
INCLUDES disorders of muscles and tendons and their attachments, and of other soft tissues

725 Polymyalgia rheumatica
DEF: Joint and muscle pain, pelvis, and shoulder girdle stiffness, high sedimentation rate and temporal arteritis; occurs in elderly.

√4th 726 Peripheral enthesopathies and allied syndromes
Note: Enthesopathies are disorders of peripheral ligamentous or muscular attachments.
EXCLUDES spinal enthesopathy (720.1)

726.0 Adhesive capsulitis of shoulder

√5th 726.1 Rotator cuff syndrome of shoulder and allied disorders
726.10 Disorders of bursae and tendons in shoulder region, unspecified
Rotator cuff syndrome NOS
Supraspinatus syndrome NOS
726.11 Calcifying tendinitis of shoulder
726.12 Bicipital tenosynovitis
726.19 Other specified disorders
EXCLUDES complete rupture of rotator cuff, nontraumatic (727.61)

726.2 Other affections of shoulder region, not elsewhere classified
Periarthritis of shoulder   Scapulohumeral fibrositis

√5th 726.3 Enthesopathy of elbow region
726.30 Enthesopathy of elbow, unspecified
726.31 Medial epicondylitis
726.32 Lateral epicondylitis
Epicondylitis NOS   Tennis elbow
Golfers' elbow
726.33 Olecranon bursitis
Bursitis of elbow
726.39 Other

726.4 Enthesopathy of wrist and carpus
Bursitis of hand or wrist
Periarthritis of wrist

726.5 Enthesopathy of hip region
Bursitis of hip   Psoas tendinitis
Gluteal tendinitis   Trochanteric tendinitis
Iliac crest spur

√5th 726.6 Enthesopathy of knee
726.60 Enthesopathy of knee, unspecified
Bursitis of knee NOS
726.61 Pes anserinus tendinitis or bursitis
DEF: Inflamed tendons of sartorius, gracilis and semitendinosus muscles of medial aspect of knee.
726.62 Tibial collateral ligament bursitis
Pellegrini-Stieda syndrome
726.63 Fibular collateral ligament bursitis
726.64 Patellar tendinitis
726.65 Prepatellar bursitis
726.69 Other
Bursitis:
infrapatellar
subpatellar

√5th 726.7 Enthesopathy of ankle and tarsus
726.70 Enthesopathy of ankle and tarsus, unspecified
Metatarsalgia NOS
EXCLUDES Morton's metatarsalgia (355.6)
726.71 Achilles bursitis or tendinitis
726.72 Tibialis tendinitis
Tibialis (anterior) (posterior) tendinitis
726.73 Calcaneal spur
DEF: Overgrowth of calcaneal bone; causes pain on walking; due to chronic avulsion injury of plantar fascia from calcaneus.
726.79 Other
Peroneal tendinitis

726.8 Other peripheral enthesopathies

N Newborn Age: 0   P Pediatric Age: 0-17   M Maternity Age: 12-55   A Adult Age: 15-124   MSP Medicare Secondary Payer

Bunion

Normal metatarsophalangeal joint

Exostosis

Ganglia

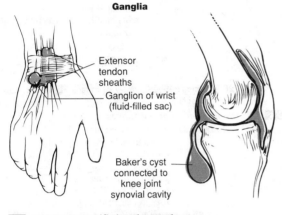

Extensor tendon sheaths

Ganglion of wrist (fluid-filled sac)

Baker's cyst connected to knee joint synovial cavity

√5th **726.9 Unspecified enthesopathy**

    726.90 Enthesopathy of unspecified site
        Capsulitis NOS
        Periarthritis NOS
        Tendinitis NOS

    726.91 Exostosis of unspecified site
        Bone spur NOS

√4th **727 Other disorders of synovium, tendon, and bursa**

  √5th **727.0 Synovitis and tenosynovitis**

    727.00 Synovitis and tenosynovitis, unspecified
        Synovitis NOS
        Tenosynovitis NOS

    727.01 *Synovitis and tenosynovitis in diseases classified elsewhere*
        Code first underlying disease as:
        tuberculosis (015.0-015.9)
        EXCLUDES *crystal-induced (275.4)*
                gonococcal (098.51)
                gouty (274.0)
                syphilitic (095.7)

    727.02 Giant cell tumor of tendon sheath

    727.03 Trigger finger (acquired)
        DEF: Stenosing tenosynovitis or nodule in flexor tendon; cessation of flexion or extension movement in finger, followed by snapping into place.

    727.04 Radial styloid tenosynovitis
        de Quervain's disease

    727.05 Other tenosynovitis of hand and wrist

    727.06 Tenosynovitis of foot and ankle

    727.09 Other

  727.1 Bunion
    DEF: Enlarged first metatarsal head due to inflamed bursa; results in laterally displaced great toe.

727.2 Specific bursitides often of occupational origin
    Beat: Miners':
      elbow   elbow
      hand   knee
      knee
    Chronic crepitant synovitis of wrist

727.3 Other bursitis
    Bursitis NOS
    EXCLUDES *bursitis:*
        gonococcal (098.52)
        subacromial (726.19)
        subcoracoid (726.19)
        subdeltoid (726.19)
        syphilitic (095.7)
        "frozen shoulder" (726.0)

√5th **727.4 Ganglion and cyst of synovium, tendon, and bursa**

    727.40 Synovial cyst, unspecified
        EXCLUDES *that of popliteal space (727.51)*

    727.41 Ganglion of joint

    727.42 Ganglion of tendon sheath

    727.43 Ganglion, unspecified

    727.49 Other
        Cyst of bursa

√5th **727.5 Rupture of synovium**

    727.50 Rupture of synovium, unspecified

    727.51 Synovial cyst of popliteal space
        Baker's cyst (knee)

    727.59 Other

√5th **727.6 Rupture of tendon, nontraumatic**

    727.60 Nontraumatic rupture of unspecified tendon

    727.61 Complete rupture of rotator cuff

    727.62 Tendons of biceps (long head)

    727.63 Extensor tendons of hand and wrist

    727.64 Flexor tendons of hand and wrist

    727.65 Quadriceps tendon

    727.66 Patellar tendon

    727.67 Achilles tendon

    727.68 Other tendons of foot and ankle

    727.69 Other

√5th **727.8 Other disorders of synovium, tendon, and bursa**

    727.81 Contracture of tendon (sheath)
        Short Achilles tendon (acquired)

    727.82 Calcium deposits in tendon and bursa
        Calcification of tendon NOS
        Calcific tendinitis NOS
        EXCLUDES *peripheral ligamentous or muscular attachments (726.0-726.9)*

    727.83 Plica syndrome
        Plica knee
        DEF: A fold in the synovial tissue that begins to form before birth, creating a septum between two pockets of synovial tissue; two most common plicae are the medial patellar plica and the suprapatellar plica. Plica syndrome, or plica knee, refers to symptomatic plica. Experienced by females more commonly than males.

    727.89 Other
        Abscess of bursa or tendon
        EXCLUDES *xanthomatosis localized to tendons (272.7)*

  727.9 Unspecified disorder of synovium, tendon, and bursa

√4th **728 Disorders of muscle, ligament, and fascia**
    EXCLUDES *enthesopathies (726.0-726.9)*
        muscular dystrophies (359.0-359.1)
        myoneural disorders (358.0-358.9)
        myopathies (359.2-359.9)
        old disruption of ligaments of knee (717.81-717.89)

√4th
√5th Additional Digit Required   Unspecified Code   Other Specified Code   Manifestation Code   ►◄ Revised Text   ● New Code   ▲ Revised Code Title

728.0 Infective myositis
Myositis:
   purulent
   suppurative
> **EXCLUDES**   myositis:
>   epidemic (074.1)
>   interstitial (728.81)
>   syphilitic (095.6)
>   tropical (040.81)

DEF: Inflamed connective septal tissue of muscle.

✓5ᵗʰ 728.1 Muscular calcification and ossification

728.10 Calcification and ossification, unspecified
Massive calcification (paraplegic)

728.11 Progressive myositis ossificans
DEF: Progressive myositic disease; marked by bony tissue formed by voluntary muscle; occurs among very young.

728.12 Traumatic myositis ossificans
Myositis ossificans (circumscripta)

728.13 Postoperative heterotopic calcification
DEF: Abnormal formation of calcium deposits in muscular tissue after surgery, marked by a corresponding loss of muscle tone and tension.

728.19 Other
Polymyositis ossificans

728.2 Muscular wasting and disuse atrophy, not elsewhere classified
Amyotrophia NOS
Myofibrosis
> **EXCLUDES**   neuralgic amyotrophy (353.5)
>   progressive muscular atrophy (335.0-335.9)

728.3 Other specific muscle disorders
Arthrogryposis
Immobility syndrome (paraplegic)
> **EXCLUDES**   arthrogryposis multiplex congenita (754.89)
>   stiff-man syndrome (333.91)

728.4 Laxity of ligament

728.5 Hypermobility syndrome

728.6 Contracture of palmar fascia   **A**
Dupuytren's contracture
DEF: Dupuytren's contracture: flexion deformity of finger, due to shortened, thickened fibrosing of palmar fascia; cause unknown; associated with long-standing epilepsy; occurs more often in males.

✓5ᵗʰ 728.7 Other fibromatoses

728.71 Plantar fascial fibromatosis
Contracture of plantar fascia
Plantar fasciitis (traumatic)
DEF: Plantar fascia fibromatosis; causes nodular swelling and pain; not associated with contractures.

728.79 Other
Garrod's or knuckle pads
Nodular fasciitis
Pseudosarcomatous fibromatosis (proliferative) (subcutaneous)
DEF: Knuckle pads: pea-size nodules on dorsal surface of interphalangeal joints; new growth of fibrous tissue with thickened dermis and epidermis.

✓5ᵗʰ 728.8 Other disorders of muscle, ligament, and fascia

728.81 Interstitial myositis
DEF: Inflammation of septal connective parts of muscle tissue.

728.82 Foreign body granuloma of muscle
Talc granuloma of muscle

728.83 Rupture of muscle, nontraumatic

728.84 Diastasis of muscle
Diastasis recti (abdomen)
> **EXCLUDES**   diastasis recti complicating pregnancy, labor, and delivery (665.8)

DEF: Muscle separation, such as recti abdominis after repeated pregnancies.

728.85 Spasm of muscle

728.86 Necrotizing fasciitis
Use additional code to identify:
   infectious organism (041.00-041.89)
   gangrene (785.4), if applicable
DEF: Fulminating infection begins with extensive cellulitis, spreads to superficial and deep fascia; causes thrombosis of subcutaneous vessels, and gangrene of underlying tissue.

728.89 Other
Eosinophilic fasciitis
Use additional E code to identify drug, if drug induced
DEF: Eosinophilic fasciitis: inflammation of fascia of extremities associated with eosinophilia, edema, and swelling; occurs alone or as part of myalgia syndrome.

728.9 Unspecified disorder of muscle, ligament, and fascia

✓4ᵗʰ 729 Other disorders of soft tissues
> **EXCLUDES**   acroparesthesia (443.89)
>   carpal tunnel syndrome (354.0)
>   disorders of the back (720.0-724.9)
>   entrapment syndromes (354.0-355.9)
>   palindromic rheumatism (719.3)
>   periarthritis (726.0-726.9)
>   psychogenic rheumatism (306.0)

729.0 Rheumatism, unspecified and fibrositis
DEF: General term describes diseases of muscle, tendon, nerve, joint, or bone; symptoms include pain and stiffness.

729.1 Myalgia and myositis, unspecified
Fibromyositis NOS
DEF: Myalgia: muscle pain.

DEF: Myositis: inflamed voluntary muscle.

DEF: Fibromyositis: inflamed fibromuscular tissue.

729.2 Neuralgia, neuritis, and radiculitis, unspecified
> **EXCLUDES**   brachial radiculitis (723.4)
>   cervical radiculitis (723.4)
>   lumbosacral radiculitis (724.4)
>   mononeuritis (354.0-355.9)
>   radiculitis due to intervertebral disc involvement (722.0-722.2, 722.7)
>   sciatica (724.3)

DEF: Neuralgia: [aroxysmal pain along nerve symptoms include brief pain and tenderness at point nerve exits.

DEF: Neuritis: inflamed nerve, symptoms include paresthesia, paralysis and loss of reflexes at nerve site.

DEF: Radiculitis: inflamed nerve root.

✓5ᵗʰ 729.3 Panniculitis, unspecified
DEF: Inflammatory reaction of subcutaneous fat; causes nodules; often develops in abdominal region.

729.30 Panniculitis, unspecified site
Weber-Christian disease
DEF: Febrile, nodular, nonsuppurative, relapsing inflammation of subcutaneous fat.

729.31 Hypertrophy of fat pad, knee
Hypertrophy of infrapatellar fat pad

N Newborn Age: 0   **P** Pediatric Age: 0-17   **M** Maternity Age: 12-55   **A** Adult Age: 15-124   **MSP** Medicare Secondary Payer

202 — Volume 1   *2003 ICD•9•CM*

729.39 Other site

    EXCLUDES *panniculitis specified as*
        (affecting):
        back (724.8)
        neck (723.6)
        sacral (724.8)

729.4 Fasciitis, unspecified

    EXCLUDES *necrotizing fasciitis (728.86)*
        nodular fasciitis (728.79)

729.5 Pain in limb

729.6 Residual foreign body in soft tissue

    EXCLUDES *foreign body granuloma:*
        muscle (728.82)
        skin and subcutaneous tissue
          (709.4)

✓5ᵗʰ 729.8 Other musculoskeletal symptoms referable to limbs

    729.81 Swelling of limb

    729.82 Cramp

    729.89 Other

       EXCLUDES *abnormality of gait (781.2)*
           tetany (781.7)
           transient paralysis of limb
             (781.4)

729.9 Other and unspecified disorders of soft tissue
    Polyalgia

OSTEOPATHIES, CHONDROPATHIES, AND ACQUIRED MUSCULOSKELETAL DEFORMITIES (730-739)

✓4ᵗʰ 730 Osteomyelitis, periostitis, and other infections involving bone

    EXCLUDES *jaw (526.4-526.5)*
          petrous bone (383.2)

Use additional code to identify organism, such as Staphylococcus (041.1)

DEF: Osteomyelitis: bacterial inflammation of bone tissue and marrow.

DEF: Periostitis: inflammation of specialized connective tissue; causes swelling of bone and aching pain.

The following fifth-digit subclassification is for use with category 730; valid digits are in [brackets] under each code. See definitions prior to category 710.

    0 site unspecified
    1 shoulder region
    2 upper arm
    3 forearm
    4 hand
    5 pelvic region and thigh
    6 lower leg
    7 ankle and foot
    8 other specified sites
    9 multiple sites

§ ✓5ᵗʰ 730.0 Acute osteomyelitis
    [0-9]
       Abscess of any bone except accessory sinus, jaw, or mastoid
       Acute or subacute osteomyelitis, with or without mention of periostitis

§ ✓5ᵗʰ 730.1 Chronic osteomyelitis
    [0-9]
       Brodie's abscess
       Chronic or old osteomyelitis, with or without mention of periostitis
       Sequestrum of bone
       Sclerosing osteomyelitis of Garré

       EXCLUDES *aseptic necrosis of bone (733.40-733.49)*

§ ✓5ᵗʰ 730.2 Unspecified osteomyelitis
    [0-9]
       Osteitis or osteomyelitis NOS, with or without mention of periostitis

§ ✓5ᵗʰ 730.3 Periostitis without mention of osteomyelitis
    [0-9]
       Abscess of periosteum } without mention of
       Periostosis   osteomyelitis

       EXCLUDES *that in secondary syphilis (091.61)*

§ ✓5ᵗʰ 730.7 *Osteopathy resulting from poliomyelitis*
    [0-9]
       Code first underlying disease (045.0-045.9)

§ ✓5ᵗʰ 730.8 *Other infections involving bone in diseases classified elsewhere*
    [0-9]
       Code first underlying disease as:
         tuberculosis (015.0-015.9)
         typhoid fever (002.0)

       EXCLUDES *syphilis of bone NOS (095.5)*

§ ✓5ᵗʰ 730.9 Unspecified infection of bone
    [0-9]

✓4ᵗʰ 731 Osteitis deformans and osteopathies associated with other disorders classified elsewhere

DEF: Osteitis deformans: Bone disease marked by episodes of increased bone loss, excessive repair attempts follow; causes weakened, deformed bones with increased mass, bowed long bones, deformed flat bones, pain and pathological fractures; may be fatal if associated with congestive heart failure, giant cell tumors or bone sarcoma; also called Paget's disease.

731.0 Osteitis deformans without mention of bone tumor
    Paget's disease of bone

731.1 *Osteitis deformans in diseases classified elsewhere*
    Code first underlying disease as:
       malignant neoplasm of bone (170.0-170.9)

731.2 Hypertrophic pulmonary osteoarthropathy
    Bamberger-Marie disease

DEF: Clubbing, of fingers and toes; related to enlarged ends of long bones; due to chronic lung and heart disease.

731.8 *Other bone involvement in diseases classified elsewhere*
    Code first underlying disease as:
       diabetes mellitus (250.8)
    Use additional code to specify bone condition, such as:
       acute osteomyelitis (730.00-730.09)

✓4ᵗʰ 732 Osteochondropathies

DEF: Conditions related to both bone and cartilage, or conditions in which cartilage is converted to bone (enchondral ossification).

732.0 Juvenile osteochondrosis of spine
    Juvenile osteochondrosis (of):
       marginal or vertebral epiphysis (of Scheuermann)
       spine NOS
    Vertebral epiphysitis

    EXCLUDES *adolescent postural kyphosis (737.0)*

732.1 Juvenile osteochondrosis of hip and pelvis
    Coxa plana
    Ischiopubic synchondrosis (of van Neck)
    Osteochondrosis (juvenile) of:
       acetabulum
       head of femur (of Legg-Calvé-Perthes)
       iliac crest (of Buchanan)
       symphysis pubis (of Pierson)
    Pseudocoxalgia

732.2 Nontraumatic slipped upper femoral epiphysis
    Slipped upper femoral epiphysis NOS

Musculoskeletal System and Connective Tissue 729.39-732.2

§ Requires fifth digit. Valid digits are in [brackets] under each code. See beginning of section 710–739 for codes and definitions.

✓4ᵗʰ / ✓5ᵗʰ Additional Digit Required   Unspecified Code   Other Specified Code   Manifestation Code   ►◄ Revised Text   ● New Code   ▲ Revised Code Title

732.3   Juvenile osteochondrosis of upper extremity
Osteochondrosis (juvenile) of:
   capitulum of humerus (of Panner)
   carpal lunate (of Kienbock)
   hand NOS
   head of humerus (of Haas)
   heads of metacarpals (of Mauclaire)
   lower ulna (of Burns)
   radial head (of Brailsford)
   upper extremity NOS

732.4   Juvenile osteochondrosis of lower extremity, excluding foot
Osteochondrosis (juvenile) of:
   lower extremity NOS
   primary patellar center (of Köhler)
   proximal tibia (of Blount)
   secondary patellar center (of Sinding-Larsen)
   tibial tubercle (of Osgood-Schlatter)
Tibia vara

732.5   Juvenile osteochondrosis of foot
Calcaneal apophysitis
Epiphysitis, os calcis
Osteochondrosis (juvenile) of:
   astragalus (of Diaz)
   calcaneum (of Sever)
   foot NOS
   metatarsal:
      second (of Freiberg)
      fifth (of Iselin)
   os tibiale externum (of Haglund)
   tarsal navicular (of Köhler)

732.6   Other juvenile osteochondrosis
Apophysitis ⎫
Epiphysitis ⎬ specified as juvenile, of other
Osteochondritis ⎪   site, or site NOS
Osteochondrosis ⎭

732.7   Osteochondritis dissecans

732.8   Other specified forms of osteochondropathy
Adult osteochondrosis of spine

732.9   Unspecified osteochondropathy
Apophysitis ⎫
Epiphysitis ⎬ NOS
Osteochondritis ⎪ not specified as adult or juve-
Osteochondrosis ⎭   nile, of unspecified site

✓4th 733   Other disorders of bone and cartilage
   EXCLUDES   bone spur (726.91)
                cartilage of, or loose body in, joint (717.0-717.9, 718.0-718.9)
                giant cell granuloma of jaw (526.3)
                osteitis fibrosa cystica generalisata (252.0)
                osteomalacia (268.2)
                polyostotic fibrous dysplasia of bone (756.54)
                prognathism, retrognathism (524.1)
                xanthomatosis localized to bone (272.7)

✓5th 733.0   Osteoporosis
DEF: Bone mass reduction that ultimately results in fractures after minimal trauma; dorsal kyphosis or loss of height often occur.

733.00   Osteoporosis, unspecified
Wedging of vertebra NOS

733.01   Senile osteoporosis
Postmenopausal osteoporosis

733.02   Idiopathic osteoporosis

733.03   Disuse osteoporosis

733.09   Other
Drug-induced osteoporosis
Use additional E code to identify drug

✓5th 733.1   Pathologic fracture
Spontaneous fracture
   EXCLUDES   stress fracture (733.93-733.95)
                traumatic fracture (800-829)

DEF: Fracture due to bone structure weakening by pathological processes (e.g., osteoporosis, neoplasms and osteomalacia).

733.10   Pathologic fracture, unspecified site

733.11   Pathologic fracture of humerus

733.12   Pathologic fracture of distal radius and ulna
Wrist NOS

733.13   Pathologic fracture of vertebrae
Collapse of vertebra NOS

733.14   Pathologic fracture of neck of femur
Femur NOS   Hip NOS

733.15   Pathologic fracture of other specified part of femur

733.16   Pathologic fracture of tibia or fibula
Ankle NOS

733.19   Pathologic fracture of other specified site

✓5th 733.2   Cyst of bone

733.20   Cyst of bone (localized), unspecified

733.21   Solitary bone cyst
Unicameral bone cyst

733.22   Aneurysmal bone cyst
DEF: Solitary bone lesion, bulges into periosteum; marked by calcified rim.

733.29   Other
Fibrous dysplasia (monostotic)
   EXCLUDES   cyst of jaw (526.0-526.2, 526.89)
                osteitis fibrosa cystica (252.0)
                polyostotic fibrousdyplasia of bone (756.54)

733.3   Hyperostosis of skull
Hyperostosis interna frontalis
Leontiasis ossium
DEF: Abnormal bone growth on inner aspect of cranial bones.

✓5th 733.4   Aseptic necrosis of bone
   EXCLUDES   osteochondropathies (732.0-732.9)
DEF: Infraction of bone tissue due to a nonfectious etiology, such as a fracture, ischemic disorder or administration of immunosuppressive drugs; leads to degenerative joint disease or nonunion of fractures.

733.40   Aseptic necrosis of bone, site unspecified

733.41   Head of humerus

733.42   Head and neck of femur
Femur NOS
   EXCLUDES   Legg-Calvé-Perthes disease (732.1)

733.43   Medial femoral condyle

733.44   Talus

733.49   Other

733.5   Osteitis condensans
Piriform sclerosis of ilium
DEF: Idiopathic condition marked by low back pain; associated with oval or triangular sclerotic, opaque bone next to sacroiliac joints in the ileum.

733.6   Tietze's disease
Costochondral junction syndrome
Costochondritis
DEF: Painful, idiopathic, nonsuppurative, swollen costal cartilage sometimes confused with cardiac symptoms because the anterior chest pain resembles that of coronary artery disease.

Acquired Deformities of Toe

733.7 Algoneurodystrophy
Disuse atrophy of bone
Sudeck's atrophy
DEF: Painful, idiopathic.

√5ᵗʰ **733.8 Malunion and nonunion of fracture**
    733.81 Malunion of fracture
    733.82 Nonunion of fracture
        Pseudoarthrosis (bone)

√5ᵗʰ **733.9 Other and unspecified disorders of bone and cartilage**
    733.90 Disorder of bone and cartilage, unspecified
    733.91 Arrest of bone development or growth
        Epiphyseal arrest
    733.92 Chondromalacia
        Chondromalacia:
          NOS
          localized, except patella
          systemic
          tibial plateau
        EXCLUDES   *chondromalacia of patella (717.7)*
        DEF: Articular cartilage softening.
    733.93 Stress fracture of tibia or fibula
        Stress reaction of tibia or fibula
    733.94 Stress fracture of the metatarsals
        Stress reaction of metatarsals
    733.95 Stress fracture of other bone
        Stress reaction of other bone
    733.99 Other
        Diaphysitis
        Hypertrophy of bone
        Relapsing polychondritis

734 Flat foot
    Pes planus (acquired)
    Talipes planus (acquired)
    EXCLUDES   *congenital (754.61)*
                rigid flat foot (754.61)
                spastic (everted) flat foot (754.61)

√4ᵗʰ **735 Acquired deformities of toe**
    EXCLUDES   *congenital (754.60-754.69, 755.65-755.66)*
    735.0 Hallux valgus (acquired)
        DEF: Angled displacement of the great toe, causing it to ride over or under other toes.
    735.1 Hallux varus (acquired)
        DEF: Angled displacement of the great toe toward the body midline, away from the other toes.
    735.2 Hallux rigidus
        DEF: Limited flexion movement at metatarsophalangeal joint of great toe; due to degenerative joint disease.

Acquired Deformities of Forearm

    735.3 Hallux malleus
        DEF: Extended proximal phalanx, flexed distal phalanges, of great toe; foot resembles claw or hammer.
    735.4 Other hammer toe (acquired)
    735.5 Claw toe (acquired)
        DEF: Hyperextended proximal phalanges, flexed middle and distal phalanges.
    735.8 Other acquired deformities of toe
    735.9 Unspecified acquired deformity of toe

√4ᵗʰ **736 Other acquired deformities of limbs**
    EXCLUDES   *congenital (754.3-755.9)*
√5ᵗʰ **736.0 Acquired deformities of forearm, excluding fingers**
    736.00 Unspecified deformity
        Deformity of elbow, forearm, hand, or wrist (acquired) NOS
    736.01 Cubitus valgus (acquired)
        DEF: Deviation of the elbow away from the body midline upon extension; it occurs when the palm is turning outward.
    736.02 Cubitus varus (acquired)
        DEF: Elbow joint displacement angled laterally; when the forearm is extended, it is deviated toward the midline of the body; also called "gun stock" deformity.
    736.03 Valgus deformity of wrist (acquired)
        DEF: Abnormal angulation away from the body midline.
    736.04 Varus deformity of wrist (acquired)
        DEF: Abnormal angulation toward the body midline.
    736.05 Wrist drop (acquired)
        DEF: Inability to extend the hand at the wrist due to extensor muscle paralysis.
    736.06 Claw hand (acquired)
        DEF: Flexion and atrophy of the hand and fingers; found in ulnar nerve lesions, syringomyelia, and leprosy.
    736.07 Club hand, acquired
        DEF: Twisting of the hand out of shape or position; caused by the congenital absence of the ulna or radius.
    736.09 Other
    736.1 Mallet finger
        DEF: Permanently flexed distal phalanx.
√5ᵗʰ **736.2 Other acquired deformities of finger**
    736.20 Unspecified deformity
        Deformity of finger (acquired) NOS
    736.21 Boutonniere deformity
        DEF: A complete or partial protrusion of a joint finger through a defect in the extensor aponeurosis; also called buttonhole deformity.

√4ᵗʰ √5ᵗʰ Additional Digit Required   Unspecified Code   Other Specified Code   Manifestation Code   ►◄ Revised Text   ● New Code   ▲ Revised Code Title

736.22 Swan-neck deformity

DEF: Flexed distal and hyperextended proximal interphalangeal joint.

736.29 Other

EXCLUDES   trigger finger (727.03)

✓5th **736.3 Acquired deformities of hip**

736.30 Unspecified deformity

Deformity of hip (acquired) NOS

736.31 Coxa valga (acquired)

DEF: Increase of at least 140 degrees in the angle formed by the axis of the head and the neck of the femur, and the axis of its shaft.

736.32 Coxa vara (acquired)

DEF: The bending downward of the neck of the femur: causing difficulty in movement; a right angle or less may be formed by the axis of the head and neck of the femur, and the axis of its shaft.

736.39 Other

✓5th **736.4 Genu valgum or varum (acquired)**

736.41 Genu valgum (acquired)

DEF: Abnormally close together and an abnormally large space between the ankles; also called "knock-knees."

736.42 Genu varum (acquired)

DEF: Abnormally separated knees and the inward bowing of the legs; it is also called "bowlegs."

736.5 Genu recurvatum (acquired)

DEF: Hyperextended knees; also called "backknee."

736.6 Other acquired deformities of knee

Deformity of knee (acquired) NOS

✓5th **736.7 Other acquired deformities of ankle and foot**

EXCLUDES   deformities of toe (acquired) (735.0-735.9)
pes planus (acquired) (734)

Acquired Deformities of Hip

Genu valga (knock-knee)   Normal angle   Coxa valga   Coxa vara   Genu vara (bowleg)

Acquired Deformities of Lower Limb

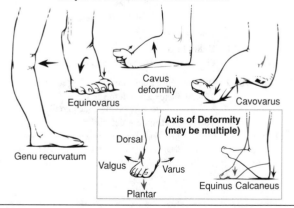

Equinovarus   Cavus deformity   Cavovarus

Genu recurvatum

Axis of Deformity (may be multiple)
Dorsal
Valgus   Varus
Plantar   Equinus   Calcaneus

736.70 Unspecified deformity of ankle and foot, acquired

736.71 Acquired equinovarus deformity

Clubfoot, acquired

EXCLUDES   clubfoot not specified as acquired (754.5-754.7)

736.72 Equinus deformity of foot, acquired

DEF: A plantar flexion deformity that forces people to walk on their toes.

736.73 Cavus deformity of foot

EXCLUDES   that with claw foot (736.74)

DEF: Abnormally high longitudinal arch of the foot.

736.74 Claw foot, acquired

DEF: High foot arch with hyperextended toes at metatarsophalangeal joint and flexed toes at distal joints; also called "main en griffe."

736.75 Cavovarus deformity of foot, acquired

DEF: Inward turning of the heel from the midline of the leg and an abnormally high longitudinal arch.

736.76 Other calcaneus deformity

736.79 Other

Acquired:

pes
talipes   } not elsewhere classified

✓5th **736.8 Acquired deformities of other parts of limbs**

736.81 Unequal leg length (acquired)

736.89 Other

Deformity (acquired):
arm or leg, not elsewhere classified
shoulder

736.9 Acquired deformity of limb, site unspecified

✓4th **737 Curvature of spine**

EXCLUDES   congenital (754.2)

737.0 Adolescent postural kyphosis

EXCLUDES   osteochondrosis of spine (juvenile) (732.0)
adult (732.8)

✓5th **737.1 Kyphosis (acquired)**

737.10 Kyphosis (acquired) (postural)

737.11 Kyphosis due to radiation

737.12 Kyphosis, postlaminectomy

737.19 Other

EXCLUDES   that associated with conditions classifiable elsewhere (737.41)

Kyphosis and Lordosis

Kyphosis (hump)

Lordosis (concave)

Scoliosis and Kyphoscoliosis

Scoliosis

Kyphoscoliosis

√5ᵗʰ **737.2 Lordosis (acquired)**

DEF: Swayback appearance created by an abnormally increased spinal curvature; it is also referred to as "hollow back" or "saddle back."

737.20 Lordosis (acquired) (postural)
737.21 Lordosis, postlaminectomy
737.22 Other postsurgical lordosis
737.29 Other

> EXCLUDES *that associated with conditions classifiable elsewhere (737.42)*

√5ᵗʰ **737.3 Kyphoscoliosis and scoliosis**

DEF: Kyphoscoliosis: backward and lateral curvature of the spinal column; it is found in vertebral osteochondrosis.

DEF: Scoliosis: an abnormal deviation of the spine to the left or right of the midline

737.30 Scoliosis [and kyphoscoliosis], idiopathic
737.31 Resolving infantile idiopathic scoliosis
737.32 Progressive infantile idiopathic scoliosis
737.33 Scoliosis due to radiation
737.34 Thoracogenic scoliosis
737.39 Other

> EXCLUDES *that associated with conditions classifiable elsewhere (737.43)*
> *that in kyphoscoliotic heart disease (416.1)*

√5ᵗʰ **737.4 Curvature of spine associated with other conditions**

Code first associated condition as:
  Charcôt-Marie-Tooth disease (356.1)
  mucopolysaccharidosis (277.5)
  neurofibromatosis (237.7)
  osteitis deformans (731.0)
  osteitis fibrosa cystica (252.0)
  osteoporosis (733.00-733.09)
  poliomyelitis (138)
  tuberculosis [Pott's curvature] (015.0)

737.40 *Curvature of spine, unspecified*
737.41 *Kyphosis*
737.42 *Lordosis*
737.43 *Scoliosis*

737.8 Other curvatures of spine
737.9 Unspecified curvature of spine

Curvature of spine (acquired) (idiopathic) NOS
Hunchback, acquired

> EXCLUDES *deformity of spine NOS (738.5)*

√4ᵗʰ **738 Other acquired deformity**

> EXCLUDES *congenital (754.0-756.9, 758.0-759.9)*
> *dentofacial anomalies (524.0-524.9)*

738.0 Acquired deformity of nose

Deformity of nose (acquired)
Overdevelopment of nasal bones

> EXCLUDES *deflected or deviated nasal septum (470)*

√5ᵗʰ **738.1 Other acquired deformity of head**

738.10 Unspecified deformity
738.11 Zygomatic hyperplasia

DEF: Abnormal enlargement of the zygoma (processus zygomaticus temporalis).

738.12 Zygomatic hypoplasia

DEF: Underdevelopment of the zygoma (processus zygomaticus temporalis).

738.19 Other specified deformity

738.2 Acquired deformity of neck
738.3 Acquired deformity of chest and rib

Deformity:	Pectus:
chest (acquired)	carinatum, acquired
rib (acquired)	excavatum, acquired

738.4 Acquired spondylolisthesis

Degenerative spondylolisthesis
Spondylolysis, acquired

> EXCLUDES *congenital (756.12)*

DEF: Vertebra displaced forward over another; due to bilateral defect in vertebral arch, eroded articular surface of posterior facts and elongated pedicle between fifth lumbar vertebra and sacrum.

738.5 Other acquired deformity of back or spine

Deformity of spine NOS

> EXCLUDES *curvature of spine (737.0-737.9)*

738.6 Acquired deformity of pelvis

Pelvic obliquity

> EXCLUDES *intrapelvic protrusion of acetabulum (718.6)*
> *that in relation to labor and delivery (653.0-653.4, 653.8-653.9)*

DEF: Pelvic obliquity: slanting or inclination of the pelvis at an angle between 55 and 60 degrees between the plane of the pelvis and the horizontal plane.

738.7 Cauliflower ear

DEF: Abnormal external ear; due to injury, subsequent perichondritis.

738.8 Acquired deformity of other specified site

Deformity of clavicle

738.9 Acquired deformity of unspecified site

√4ᵗʰ **739 Nonallopathic lesions, not elsewhere classified**

> INCLUDES segmental dysfunction
> somatic dysfunction

DEF: Disability, loss of function or abnormality of a body part that is neither classifiable to a particular system nor brought about therapeutically to counteract another disease.

739.0 Head region
  Occipitocervical region
739.1 Cervical region
  Cervicothoracic region
739.2 Thoracic region
  Thoracolumbar region
739.3 Lumbar region
  Lumbosacral region
739.4 Sacral region
  Sacrococcygeal region Sacroiliac region
739.5 Pelvic region
  Hip region
  Pubic region

Musculoskeletal System and Connective Tissue 737.2–739.5

739.6   **Lower extremities**

739.7   **Upper extremities**
     Acromioclavicular region
     Sternoclavicular region

739.8   **Rib cage**
     Costochondral region   Sternochondral region
     Costovertebral region

739.9   **Abdomen and other**

N Newborn Age: 0   P Pediatric Age: 0-17   M Maternity Age: 12-55   A Adult Age: 15-124   MSP Medicare Secondary Payer

14. CONGENITAL ANOMALIES (740-759)

✓4th 740 Anencephalus and similar anomalies

740.0 Anencephalus

Acrania   Hemicephaly
Amyelencephalus   Hemianencephaly

DEF: Fetus without cerebrum, cerebellum and flat bones of skull.

740.1 Craniorachischisis

DEF: Congenital slit in cranium and vertebral column.

740.2 Iniencephaly

DEF: Spinal cord passes through enlarged occipital bone (foramen magnum); absent vertebral bone layer and spinal processes; resulting in both reduction in number and proper fusion of the vertebrae.

✓4th 741 Spina bifida

> **EXCLUDES**   spina bifida occulta (756.17)

DEF: Lack of closure of spinal cord's bony encasement; marked by cord protrusion into lumbosacral area; evident by elevated alpha-fetoprotein of amniotic fluid.

> The following fifth-digit subclassification is for use with category 741:
> 0 unspecified region
> 1 cervical region
> 2 dorsal [thoracic] region
> 3 lumbar region

✓5th 741.0 With hydrocephalus

Arnold-Chiari syndrome, type II
Any condition classifiable to 741.9 with any condition classifiable to 742.3
Chiari malformation, type II

✓5th 741.9 Without mention of hydrocephalus

Hydromeningocele (spinal)   Myelocystocele
Hydromyelocele   Rachischisis
Meningocele (spinal)   Spina bifida (aperta)
Meningomyelocele   Syringomyelocele
Myelocele

✓4th 742 Other congenital anomalies of nervous system

742.0 Encephalocele

Encephalocystocele   Hydromeningocele, cranial
Encephalomyelocele   Meningocele, cerebral
Hydroencephalocele   Meningoencephalocele

DEF: Brain tissue protrudes through skull defect.

742.1 Microcephalus

Hydromicrocephaly
Micrencephaly

DEF: Extremely small head or brain.

742.2 Reduction deformities of brain

Absence
Agenesis ⎫
Aplasia ⎬ of part of brain
Hypoplasia ⎭

Agyria   Holoprosencephaly
Arhinencephaly   Microgyria

742.3 Congenital hydrocephalus

Aqueduct of Sylvius:
 anomaly
 obstruction, congenital
 stenosis
Atresia of foramina of Magendie and Luschka
Hydrocephalus in newborn

> **EXCLUDES**   hydrocephalus:
> acquired (331.3-331.4)
> due to congenital toxoplasmosis (771.2)
> with any condition classifiable to 741.9 (741.0)

DEF: Fluid accumulation within the skull; involves subarachnoid (external) or ventricular (internal) brain spaces.

742.4 Other specified anomalies of brain

Congenital cerebral cyst   Multiple anomalies of brain
Macroencephaly   NOS
Macrogyria   Porencephaly
Megalencephaly   Ulegyria

✓5th 742.5 Other specified anomalies of spinal cord

742.51 Diastematomyelia

DEF: Congenital anomaly often associated with spina bifida; the spinal cord is separated into halves by a bony tissue resembling a "spike" (a spicule), each half surrounded by a dural sac.

742.53 Hydromyelia

Hydrorhachis

DEF: Dilated central spinal cord canal; characterized by increased fluid accumulation.

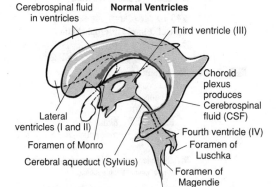

Normal Ventricles and Hydrocephalus

Normal Ventricles

Cerebrospinal fluid in ventricles
Third ventricle (III)
Choroid plexus produces Cerebrospinal fluid (CSF)
Lateral ventricles (I and II)
Fourth ventricle (IV)
Foramen of Monro
Foramen of Luschka
Cerebral aqueduct (Sylvius)
Foramen of Magendie

Spina Bifida

Normal spinal cord
Skin
Cerebrospinal fluid space

Spinal cord (placode) in section
Cerebrospinal fluid
Skin
Unfused posterior vertebral bone

Hydrocephalus

Blockage of any CSF passage increases pressure in skull, which may push tissue through the Incisura tentorii or through the Foramen magnum

Enlarged ventricles

✓4th ✓5th Additional Digit Required   Unspecified Code   Other Specified Code   Manifestation Code   ▶◀ Revised Text   ● New Code   ▲ Revised Code Title

2003 ICD•9•CM   **Volume 1 — 209**

742.59 Other
Amyelia
Atelomyelia
Congenital anomaly of spinal meninges
Defective development of cauda equina
Hypoplasia of spinal cord
Myelatelia
Myelodysplasia

742.8 Other specified anomalies of nervous system
Agenesis of nerve
Displacement of brachial plexus
Familial dysautonomia
Jaw-winking syndrome
Marcus-Gunn syndrome
Riley-Day syndrome
EXCLUDES *neurofibromatosis (237.7)*

742.9 Unspecified anomaly of brain, spinal cord, and nervous system

Anomaly
Congenital:
   disease } of: brain
   lesion } nervous system
Deformity } spinal cord

✓4ᵗʰ **743 Congenital anomalies of eye**

✓5ᵗʰ **743.0 Anophthalmos**
DEF: Complete absence of the eyes or the presence of vestigial eyes.

743.00 Clinical anophthalmos, unspecified
Agenesis }
Congenital absence } of eye

Anophthalmos NOS

743.03 Cystic eyeball, congenital

743.06 Cryptophthalmos
DEF: Eyelids continue over eyeball, results in apparent absence of eyelids.

✓5ᵗʰ **743.1 Microphthalmos**
Dysplasia }
Hypoplasia } of eye

Rudimentary eye

DEF: Abnormally small eyeballs, may be opacities of cornea and lens, scarring of choroid and retina.

743.10 Microphthalmos, unspecified

743.11 Simple microphthalmos

743.12 Microphthalmos associated with other anomalies of eye and adnexa

✓5ᵗʰ **743.2 Buphthalmos**
Glaucoma: Hydrophthalmos
  congenital
  newborn
EXCLUDES *glaucoma of childhood (365.14)*
traumatic glaucoma due to birth injury (767.8)

DEF: Distended, enlarged fibrous coats of eye; due to intraocular pressure of congenital glaucoma.

743.20 Buphthalmos, unspecified

743.21 Simple buphthalmos

743.22 Buphthalmos associated with other ocular anomalies

Keratoglobus, }
  congenital } associated with
Megalocornea } buphthalmos

✓5ᵗʰ **743.3 Congenital cataract and lens anomalies**
EXCLUDES *infantile cataract (366.00-366.09)*
DEF: Opaque eye lens.

743.30 Congenital cataract, unspecified

743.31 Capsular and subcapsular cataract

743.32 Cortical and zonular cataract

743.33 Nuclear cataract

743.34 Total and subtotal cataract, congenital

743.35 Congenital aphakia
Congenital absence of lens

743.36 Anomalies of lens shape
Microphakia   Spherophakia

743.37 Congenital ectopic lens

743.39 Other

✓5ᵗʰ **743.4 Coloboma and other anomalies of anterior segment**
DEF: Coloboma: ocular tissue defect associated with defect of ocular fetal intraocular fissure; may cause small pit on optic disk, major defects of iris, ciliary body, choroid, and retina.

743.41 Anomalies of corneal size and shape
Microcornea
EXCLUDES *that associated with buphthalmos (743.22)*

743.42 Corneal opacities, interfering with vision, congenital

743.43 Other corneal opacities, congenital

743.44 Specified anomalies of anterior chamber, chamber angle, and related structures
Anomaly: Anomaly:
  Axenfeld's   Rieger's
  Peters'

743.45 Aniridia
DEF: Incompletely formed or absent iris; affects both eyes; dominant trait; also called congenital hyperplasia of iris.

743.46 Other specified anomalies of iris and ciliary body
Anisocoria, congenital   Coloboma of iris
Atresia of pupil   Corectopia

743.47 Specified anomalies of sclera

743.48 Multiple and combined anomalies of anterior segment

743.49 Other

✓5ᵗʰ **743.5 Congenital anomalies of posterior segment**

743.51 Vitreous anomalies
Congenital vitreous opacity

743.52 Fundus coloboma
DEF: Absent retinal and choroidal tissue; occurs in lower fundus; a bright white ectatic zone of exposed sclera extends into and changes the optic disk.

743.53 Chorioretinal degeneration, congenital

743.54 Congenital folds and cysts of posterior segment

743.55 Congenital macular changes

743.56 Other retinal changes, congenital

743.57 Specified anomalies of optic disc
Coloboma of optic disc (congenital)

743.58 Vascular anomalies
Congenital retinal aneurysm

743.59 Other

✓5ᵗʰ **743.6 Congenital anomalies of eyelids, lacrimal system, and orbit**

743.61 Congenital ptosis
DEF: Drooping of eyelid.

743.62 Congenital deformities of eyelids
Ablepharon   Congenital:
Absence of eyelid   ectropion
Accessory eyelid   entropion

743.63 Other specified congenital anomalies of eyelid
Absence, agenesis, of cilia

743.64 Specified congenital anomalies of lacrimal gland

743.65 Specified congenital anomalies of lacrimal passages
  Absence, agenesis of:
    lacrimal apparatus
    punctum lacrimale
    Accessory lacrimal canal

743.66 Specified congenital anomalies of orbit

743.69 Other
  Accessory eye muscles

743.8 Other specified anomalies of eye
  EXCLUDES   *congenital nystagmus (379.51)*
  ocular albinism (270.2)
  retinitis pigmentosa (362.74)

743.9 Unspecified anomaly of eye
  Congenital:
    anomaly NOS   } of eye [any part]
    deformity NOS }

✓4th **744 Congenital anomalies of ear, face, and neck**
  EXCLUDES   *anomaly of:*
  cervical spine (754.2, 756.10-756.19)
  larynx (748.2-748.3)
  nose (748.0-748.1)
  parathyroid gland (759.2)
  thyroid gland (759.2)
  cleft lip (749.10-749.25)

✓5th **744.0 Anomalies of ear causing impairment of hearing**
  EXCLUDES   *congenital deafness without mention of cause (389.0-389.9)*

  744.00 Unspecified anomaly of ear with impairment of hearing

  744.01 Absence of external ear
    Absence of:
      auditory canal (external)
      auricle (ear) (with stenosis or atresia of auditory canal)

  744.02 Other anomalies of external ear with impairment of hearing
    Atresia or stricture of auditory canal (external)

  744.03 Anomaly of middle ear, except ossicles
    Atresia or stricture of osseous meatus (ear)

  744.04 Anomalies of ear ossicles
    Fusion of ear ossicles

  744.05 Anomalies of inner ear
    Congenital anomaly of:
      membranous labyrinth
      organ of Corti

  744.09 Other
    Absence of ear, congenital

744.1 Accessory auricle
  Accessory tragus   Supernumerary:
  Polyotia   ear
  Preauricular appendage   lobule
  DEF: Redundant tissue or structures of ear.

✓5th **744.2 Other specified anomalies of ear**
  EXCLUDES   *that with impairment of hearing (744.00-744.09)*

  744.21 Absence of ear lobe, congenital

  744.22 Macrotia
    DEF: Abnormally large pinna of ear.

  744.23 Microtia
    DEF: Hypoplasia of pinna; associated with absent or closed auditory canal.

  744.24 Specified anomalies of Eustachian tube
    Absence of Eustachian tube

  744.29 Other
    Bat ear   Prominence of auricle
    Darwin's tubercle   Ridge ear
    Pointed ear
    EXCLUDES   *preauricular sinus (744.46)*

744.3 Unspecified anomaly of ear
  Congenital:
    anomaly NOS   } of ear, not elsewhere
    deformity NOS }   classified

✓5th **744.4 Branchial cleft cyst or fistula; preauricular sinus**
  DEF: Coloboma: malclosure of the intraocular fissure in embryo resulting in defects to optic disk, iris, ciliary body, choroid, or retina.

  744.41 Branchial cleft sinus or fistula
    Branchial:
      sinus (external) (internal)
      vestige
    DEF: Cyst due to failed closure of embryonic branchial cleft.

  744.42 Branchial cleft cyst

  744.43 Cervical auricle

  744.46 Preauricular sinus or fistula

  744.47 Preauricular cyst

  744.49 Other
    Fistula (of):   Fistula (of):
      auricle, congenital   cervicoaural

744.5 Webbing of neck
  Pterygium colli
  DEF: Thick, triangular skinfold, stretches from lateral side of neck across shoulder; associated with Turner's and Noonan's syndromes.

✓5th **744.8 Other specified anomalies of face and neck**

  744.81 Macrocheilia
    Hypertrophy of lip, congenital
    DEF: Abnormally large lips.

  744.82 Microcheilia
    DEF: Abnormally small lips.

  744.83 Macrostomia
    DEF: Bilateral or unilateral anomaly, of mouth due to malformed maxillary and mandibular processes; results in mouth extending toward ear.

  744.84 Microstomia
    DEF: Abnormally small mouth.

  744.89 Other
    EXCLUDES   *congenital fistula of lip (750.25)*
    musculoskeletal anomalies (754.0-754.1, 756.0)

744.9 Unspecified anomalies of face and neck
  Congenital:
    anomaly NOS   } of face [any part] or
    deformity NOS }   neck [any part]

✓4th **745 Bulbus cordis anomalies and anomalies of cardiac septal closure**

  745.0 Common truncus
    Absent septum   }
    Communication   } between aorta and
    (abnormal)   } pulmonary artery

    Aortic septal defect
    Common aortopulmonary trunk
    Persistent truncus arteriosus

✓5th **745.1 Transposition of great vessels**

  745.10 Complete transposition of great vessels
    Transposition of great vessels:
      NOS
      classical

✓4th
✓5th
Additional Digit Required   Unspecified Code   Other Specified Code   Manifestation Code   ►◄ Revised Text   ● New Code   ▲ Revised Code Title

2003 ICD•9•CM   **Volume 1 — 211**

Heart Defects

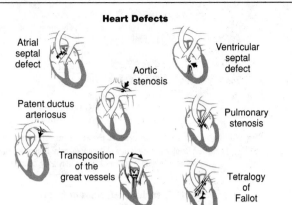

Atrial septal defect

Ventricular septal defect

Aortic stenosis

Patent ductus arteriosus

Pulmonary stenosis

Transposition of the great vessels

Tetralogy of Fallot

745.11 Double outlet right ventricle
Dextratransposition of aorta
Incomplete transposition of great vessels
Origin of both great vessels from right ventricle
Taussig-Bing syndrome or defect

745.12 Corrected transposition of great vessels

745.19 Other

745.2 Tetralogy of Fallot
Fallot's pentalogy
Ventricular septal defect with pulmonary stenosis or atresia, dextraposition of aorta, and hypertrophy of right ventricle
> **EXCLUDES** *Fallot's triad (746.09)*

DEF: Obstructed cardiac outflow causes pulmonary stenosis, interventricular septal defect and right ventricular hypertrophy.

745.3 Common ventricle
Cor triloculare biatriatum
Single ventricle

745.4 Ventricular septal defect
Eisenmenger's defect or complex
Gerbo dedefect
Interventricular septal defect
Left ventricular-right atrial communication
Roger's disease
> **EXCLUDES** *common atrioventricular canal type (745.69)*
> *single ventricle (745.3)*

745.5 Ostium secundum type atrial septal defect
Defect: Patent or persistent:
   atrium secundum   foramen ovale
   fossa ovalis   ostium secundum
Lutembacher's syndrome

DEF: Opening in atrial septum due to failure of the septum secondum and the endocardial cushions to fuse; there is a rim of septum surrounding the defect.

√5th 745.6 Endocardial cushion defects

DEF: Atrial and/or ventricular septa defects causing abnormal fusion of cushions in atrioventricular canal.

745.60 Endocardial cushion defect, unspecified type

DEF: Septal defect due to imperfect fusion of endocardial cushions.

745.61 Ostium primum defect
Persistent ostium primum

DEF: Opening in low, posterior septum primum; causes cleft in basal portion of atrial septum; associated with cleft mitral valve.

745.69 Other
Absence of atrial septum
Atrioventricular canal type ventricular septal defect
Common atrioventricular canal
Common atrium

745.7 Cor biloculare
Absence of atrial and ventricular septa

DEF: Atrial and ventricular septal defect; marked by heart with two cardiac chambers (one atrium, one ventricle), and one atrioventricular valve.

745.8 Other

745.9 Unspecified defect of septal closure
Septal defect NOS

√4th 746 Other congenital anomalies of heart
> **EXCLUDES** *endocardial fibroelastosis (425.3)*

√5th 746.0 Anomalies of pulmonary valve
> **EXCLUDES** *infundibular or subvalvular pulmonic stenosis (746.83)*
> *tetralogy of Fallot (745.2)*

746.00 Pulmonary valve anomaly, unspecified

746.01 Atresia, congenital
Congenital absence of pulmonary valve

746.02 Stenosis, congenital

DEF: Stenosis of opening between pulmonary artery and right ventricle; causes obstructed blood outflow from right ventricle.

746.09 Other
Congenital insufficiency of pulmonary valve
Fallot's triad or trilogy

746.1 Tricuspid atresia and stenosis, congenital
Absence of tricuspid valve

746.2 Ebstein's anomaly

DEF: Malformation of the tricuspid valve characterized by septal and posterior leaflets attaching to the wall of the right ventricle; causing the right ventricle to fuse with the atrium producing a large right atrium and a small ventricle; causes a malfunction of the right ventricle with accompanying complications such as heart failure and abnormal cardiac rhythm.

746.3 Congenital stenosis of aortic valve
Congenital aortic stenosis
> **EXCLUDES** *congenital:*
> *subaortic stenosis (746.81)*
> *supravalvular aortic stenosis (747.22)*

DEF: Stenosis of orifice of aortic valve; obstructs blood outflow from left ventricle.

746.4 Congenital insufficiency of aortic valve
Bicuspid aortic valve
Congenital aortic insufficiency

DEF: Impaired functioning of aortic valve due to incomplete closure; causes backflow (regurgitation) of blood from aorta to left ventricle.

746.5 Congenital mitral stenosis
Fused commissure ⎫
Parachute deformity ⎬ of mitral valve
Supernumerary cusps ⎭

DEF: Stenosis of left atrioventricular orifice.

746.6 Congenital mitral insufficiency

DEF: Impaired functioning of mitral valve due to incomplete closure; causes backflow of blood from left ventricle to left atrium.

746.7 Hypoplastic left heart syndrome
Atresia, or marked hypoplasia, of aortic orifice or valve, with hypoplasia of ascending aorta and defective development of left ventricle (with mitral valve atresia)

√5ᵗʰ **746.8 Other specified anomalies of heart**

746.81 Subaortic stenosis

DEF: Stenosis, of left ventricular outflow tract due to fibrous tissue ring or septal hypertrophy below aortic valve.

746.82 Cor triatriatum

DEF: Transverse septum divides left atrium due to failed resorption of embryonic common pulmonary vein; results in three atrial chambers.

746.83 Infundibular pulmonic stenosis

Subvalvular pulmonic stenosis

DEF: Stenosis of right ventricle outflow tract within infundibulum due to fibrous diaphragm below valve or long, narrow fibromuscular channel.

746.84 Obstructive anomalies of heart, not elsewhere classified

Uhl's disease

746.85 Coronary artery anomaly

Anomalous origin or communication of coronary artery
Arteriovenous malformation of coronary artery
Coronary artery:
  absence
  arising from aorta or pulmonary trunk
  single

746.86 Congenital heart block

Complete or incomplete atrioventricular [AV] block

DEF: Impaired conduction of electrical impulses; due to maldeveloped junctional tissue.

746.87 Malposition of heart and cardiac apex

Abdominal heart   Levocardia (isolated)
Dextrocardia   Mesocardia
Ectopia cordis

> **EXCLUDES**   *dextrocardia with complete transposition of viscera (759.3)*

746.89 Other

Atresia   } of cardiac vein
Hypoplasia

Congenital:
  cardiomegaly
  diverticulum, left ventricle
  pericardial defect

746.9 Unspecified anomaly of heart

Congenital:
  anomaly of heart NOS
  heart disease NOS

√4ᵗʰ **747 Other congenital anomalies of circulatory system**

747.0 Patent ductus arteriosus

Patent ductus Botalli   Persistent ductus arteriosus

DEF: Open lumen in ductus arteriosus causes arterial blood recirculation in lungs; inhibits blood supply to aorta; symptoms such as shortness of breath more noticeable upon activity.

√5ᵗʰ **747.1 Coarctation of aorta**

DEF: Localized deformity of aortic media seen as a severe constriction of the vessel lumen; major symptom is high blood pressure in the arms and low pressure in the legs; a CVA, rupture of the aorta, bacterial endocarditis or congestive heart failure can follow if left untreated.

747.10 Coarctation of aorta (preductal) (postductal)

Hypoplasia of aortic arch

747.11 Interruption of aortic arch

√5ᵗʰ **747.2 Other anomalies of aorta**

747.20 Anomaly of aorta, unspecified

747.21 Anomalies of aortic arch

Anomalous origin, right subclavian artery
Dextraposition of aorta
Double aortic arch
Kommerell's diverticulum
Overriding aorta
Persistent:
  convolutions, aortic arch
  right aortic arch
Vascular ring

> **EXCLUDES**   *hypoplasia of aortic arch (747.10)*

747.22 Atresia and stenosis of aorta

Absence   }
Aplasia   } of aorta
Hypoplasia   }
Stricture   }

Supra (valvular)-aortic stenosis

> **EXCLUDES**   *congenital aortic (valvular) stenosis or stricture, so stated (746.3)*
> *hypoplasia of aorta in hypoplastic left heart syndrome (746.7)*

747.29 Other

Aneurysm of sinus of Valsalva
Congenital:
  aneurysm } of aorta
  dilation   }

747.3 Anomalies of pulmonary artery

Agenesis   }
Anomaly   }
Atresia   } of pulmonary artery
Coarctation }
Hypoplasia   }
Stenosis   }

Pulmonary arteriovenous aneurysm

√5ᵗʰ **747.4 Anomalies of great veins**

747.40 Anomaly of great veins, unspecified

Anomaly NOS of:
  pulmonary veins
  vena cava

747.41 Total anomalous pulmonary venous connection

Total anomalous pulmonary venous return [TAPVR]:
  subdiaphragmatic
  supradiaphragmatic

747.42 Partial anomalous pulmonary venous connection

Partial anomalous pulmonary venous return

747.49 Other anomalies of great veins

Absence   } of vena cava (inferior)
Congenital   } (superior)
  stenosis   }

Persistent:
  left posterior cardinal vein
  left superior vena cava
Scimitar syndrome
Transposition of pulmonary veins NOS

747.5 Absence or hypoplasia of umbilical artery

Single umbilical artery

√4ᵗʰ
√5ᵗʰ   Additional Digit Required   Unspecified Code   Other Specified Code   Manifestation Code   ▶◀ Revised Text   ● New Code   ▲ Revised Code Title

2003 ICD•9•CM   **Volume 1 — 213**

√5th **747.6 Other anomalies of peripheral vascular system**

Absence ⎱
Anomaly ⎬ of artery or vein, not elsewhere
Atresia ⎰   classified

Arteriovenous aneurysm   Congenital:
   (peripheral)   phlebectasia
Arteriovenous malformation   stricture, artery
   of the peripheral   varix
   vascular system   Multiple renal arteries
Congenital:
   aneurysm (peripheral)

> EXCLUDES   anomalies of:
>   cerebral vessels (747.81)
>   pulmonary artery (747.3)
>   congenital retinal aneurysm (743.58)
>   hemangioma (228.00-228.09)
>   lymphangioma (228.1)

747.60 Anomaly of the peripheral vascular system, unspecified site

747.61 Gastrointestinal vessel anomaly

747.62 Renal vessel anomaly

747.63 Upper limb vessel anomaly

747.64 Lower limb vessel anomaly

747.69 Anomalies of other specified sites of peripheral vascular system

√5th **747.8 Other specified anomalies of circulatory system**

747.81 Anomalies of cerebrovascular system

Arteriovenous malformation of brain
Cerebral arteriovenous aneurysm, congenital
Congenital anomalies of cerebral vessels

> EXCLUDES   ruptured cerebral
>   (arteriovenous)
>   aneurysm (430)

747.82 Spinal vessel anomaly

Arteriovenous malformation of spinal vessel

747.83 Persistent fetal circulation

Persistent pulmonary hypertension
Primary pulmonary hypertension of newborn

747.89 Other

Aneurysm, congenital, specified site not elsewhere classified

> EXCLUDES   congenital aneurysm:
>   coronary (746.85)
>   peripheral (747.6)
>   pulmonary (747.3)
>   retinal (743.58)

747.9 Unspecified anomaly of circulatory system

√4th **748 Congenital anomalies of respiratory system**

> EXCLUDES   congenital defect of diaphragm (756.6)

748.0 Choanal atresia

Atresia ⎱ of nares (anterior)
Congenital stenosis ⎰   (posterior)

DEF: Occluded posterior nares (choana), bony or membranous due to failure of embryonic bucconasal membrane to rupture.

748.1 Other anomalies of nose

Absent nose   Congenital:
Accessory nose   notching of tip of nose
Cleft nose   perforation of wall of
Congenital: nasal sinus
   deformity of nose   Deformity of wall of nasal
             sinus

> EXCLUDES   congenital deviation of nasal septum
>   (754.0)

748.2 Web of larynx

Web of larynx: Web of larynx:
   NOS   subglottic
   glottic

DEF: Malformed larynx; marked by thin, translucent, or thick, fibrotic spread between vocal folds; affects speech.

748.3 Other anomalies of larynx, trachea, and bronchus

Absence or agenesis of: Congenital:
   bronchus   dilation, trachea
   larynx   stenosis:
   trachea   larynx
Anomaly(of):   trachea
   cricoid cartilage   tracheocele
   epiglottis   Diverticulum:
   thyroid cartilage   bronchus
   tracheal cartilage   trachea
Atresia (of):   Fissure of epiglottis
   epiglottis   Laryngocele
   glottis   Posterior cleft of cricoid
   larynx   cartilage (congenital)
   trachea   Rudimentary tracheal
Cleft thyroid, cartilage,   bronchus
   congenital   Stridor, laryngeal,
             congenital

748.4 Congenital cystic lung

Disease, lung: Honeycomb lung, congenital
   cystic, congenital
   polycystic, congenital

> EXCLUDES   acquired or unspecified cystic lung
>   (518.89)

DEF: Enlarged air spaces of lung parenchyma.

748.5 Agenesis, hypoplasia, and dysplasia of lung

Absence of lung (fissures) (lobe)
Aplasia of lung
Hypoplasia of lung (lobe)
Sequestration of lung

√5th **748.6 Other anomalies of lung**

748.60 Anomaly of lung, unspecified

748.61 Congenital bronchiectasis

748.69 Other

Accessory lung (lobe)
Azygos lobe (fissure), lung

748.8 Other specified anomalies of respiratory system

Abnormal communication between pericardial and pleural sacs
Anomaly, pleural folds
Atresia of nasopharynx
Congenital cyst of mediastinum

748.9 Unspecified anomaly of respiratory system

Anomaly of respiratory system NOS

√4th **749 Cleft palate and cleft lip**

√5th **749.0 Cleft palate**

749.00 Cleft palate, unspecified

749.01 Unilateral, complete

749.02 Unilateral, incomplete

Cleft uvula

749.03 Bilateral, complete

749.04 Bilateral, incomplete

√5th **749.1 Cleft lip**

Cheiloschisis   Harelip
Congenital fissure of lip   Labium leporinum

749.10 Cleft lip, unspecified

749.11 Unilateral, complete

749.12 Unilateral, incomplete

749.13 Bilateral, complete

749.14 Bilateral, incomplete

Cleft Lip and Palate

Unilateral cleft lip — No cleft palate

Cleft lip with cleft alveolar ridge — No cleft palate

Unilateral cleft lip and cleft palate — Alveolar ridge — Cleft palate

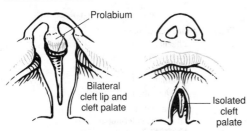

Prolabium — Bilateral cleft lip and cleft palate

Isolated cleft palate

✓5th **749.2 Cleft palate with cleft lip**
Cheilopalatoschisis

749.20 Cleft palate with cleft lip, unspecified

749.21 Unilateral, complete

749.22 Unilateral, incomplete

749.23 Bilateral, complete

749.24 Bilateral, incomplete

749.25 Other combinations

✓4th **750 Other congenital anomalies of upper alimentary tract**
> EXCLUDES   *dentofacial anomalies (524.0-524.9)*

750.0 Tongue tie
Ankyloglossia

DEF: Restricted tongue movement due to lingual frenum extending toward tip of tongue. Tongue may be fused to mouth floor affecting speech.

✓5th **750.1 Other anomalies of tongue**

750.10 Anomaly of tongue, unspecified

750.11 Aglossia

DEF: Absence of tongue.

750.12 Congenital adhesions of tongue

750.13 Fissure of tongue
Bifid tongue   Double tongue

750.15 Macroglossia
Congenital hypertrophy of tongue

750.16 Microglossia
Hypoplasia of tongue

750.19 Other

✓5th **750.2 Other specified anomalies of mouth and pharynx**

750.21 Absence of salivary gland

750.22 Accessory salivary gland

750.23 Atresia, salivary duct
Imperforate salivary duct

750.24 Congenital fistula of salivary gland

750.25 Congenital fistula of lip
Congenital (mucus) lip pits

750.26 Other specified anomalies of mouth
Absence of uvula

750.27 Diverticulum of pharynx
Pharyngeal pouch

750.29 Other specified anomalies of pharynx
Imperforate pharynx

750.3 Tracheoesophageal fistula, esophageal atresia and stenosis

Absent esophagus
Atresia of esophagus
Congenital:
    esophageal ring
    stenosis of esophagus
    stricture of esophagus

Congenital fistula:
    esophagobronchial
    esophagotracheal
Imperforate esophagus
Webbed esophagus

750.4 Other specified anomalies of esophagus

Dilatation, congenital
Displacement, congenital
Diverticulum   } (of) esophagus
Duplication
Giant

Esophageal pouch
> EXCLUDES   *congenital hiatus hernia (750.6)*

750.5 Congenital hypertrophic pyloric stenosis
Congenital or infantile:
    constriction
    hypertrophy
    spasm   } of pylorus
    stenosis
    stricture

DEF: Obstructed pylorus due to overgrowth of pyloric muscle.

750.6 Congenital hiatus hernia
Displacement of cardia through esophageal hiatus
> EXCLUDES   *congenital diaphragmatic hernia (756.6)*

750.7 Other specified anomalies of stomach
Congenital:
    cardiospasm
    hourglass stomach
Displacement of stomach
Diverticulum of stomach, congenital
Duplication of stomach
Megalogastria
Microgastria
Transposition of stomach

750.8 Other specified anomalies of upper alimentary tract

750.9 Unspecified anomaly of upper alimentary tract
Congenital:
    anomaly NOS   } of upper alimentary tract
    deformity NOS   [any part, except tongue]

✓4th **751 Other congenital anomalies of digestive system**

751.0 Meckel's diverticulum
Meckel's diverticulum (displaced) (hypertrophic)
Persistent:
    omphalomesenteric duct
    vitelline duct

DEF: Malformed sacs or appendages of ileum of small intestine; can cause strangulation, volvulus and intussusception.

751.1 Atresia and stenosis of small intestine   P
Atresia of: Atresia of:
    duodenum   intestine NOS
    ileum
Congenital:
    absence
    obstruction   } of small intestine or
    stenosis   intestine NOS
    stricture

Imperforate jejunum

✓4th / ✓5th Additional Digit Required   Unspecified Code   Other Specified Code   Manifestation Code   ▶◀ Revised Text   ● New Code   ▲ Revised Code Title

2003 ICD•9•CM   **Volume 1 — 215**

Congenital Anomalies 751.2–752.2

751.2 **Atresia and stenosis of large intestine, rectum, and anal canal** P
Absence:
anus (congenital)
appendix, congenital
large intestine, congenital
rectum
Atresia of:
anus
colon
rectum
Congenital or infantile:
obstruction of large intestine
occlusion of anus
stricture of anus
Imperforate:
anus
rectum
Stricture of rectum, congenital

751.3 **Hirschsprung's disease and other congenital functional disorders of colon**
Aganglionosis
Congenital dilation of colon
Congenital megacolon
Macrocolon

DEF: Hirschsprung's disease: enlarged or dilated colon (megacolon), with absence of ganglion cells in the narrowed wall distally; causes inability to defecate.

751.4 **Anomalies of intestinal fixation**
Congenital adhesions: Rotation of cecum or colon:
omental, anomalous   failure of
peritoneal   incomplete
Jackson's membrane   insufficient
Malrotation of colon   Universal mesentery

751.5 **Other anomalies of intestine**
Congenital diverticulum, colon
Dolichocolon
Duplication of:
anus
appendix
cecum
intestine
Ectopic anus
Megaloappendix
Megaloduodenum
Microcolon
Persistent cloaca
Transposition of:
appendix
colon
intestine

✓5ᵗʰ **751.6** **Anomalies of gallbladder, bile ducts, and liver**

751.60 **Unspecified anomaly of gallbladder, bile ducts, and liver**

751.61 **Biliary atresia** P
Congenital:
absence
hypoplasia   } of bile duct (common)
obstruction   or passage
stricture

751.62 **Congenital cystic disease of liver**
Congenital polycystic disease of liver
Fibrocystic disease of liver

751.69 **Other anomalies of gallbladder, bile ducts, and liver**
Absence of:
gallbladder, congenital
liver (lobe)
Accessory:
hepatic ducts
liver
Congenital:
choledochal cyst
hepatomegaly
Duplication of:
biliary duct
cystic duct
gallbladder
liver
Floating:
gallbladder
liver
Intrahepatic gallbladder

751.7 **Anomalies of pancreas**
Absence
Accessory
Agenesis   } (of) pancreas
Annular
Hypoplasia

Ectopic pancreatic tissue
Pancreatic heterotopia
EXCLUDES   *diabetes mellitus:*
congenital (250.0-250.9)
neonatal (775.1)
fibrocystic disease of pancreas
▶*(277.00-277.09)*◀

751.8 **Other specified anomalies of digestive system**
Absence (complete) (partial) of alimentary tract NOS
Duplication   } of digestive organs NOS
Malposition, congenital
EXCLUDES   *congenital diaphragmatic hernia*
(756.6)
congenital hiatus hernia (750.6)

751.9 **Unspecified anomaly of digestive system**
Congenital:
anomaly NOS   } of digestive system NOS
deformity NOS

✓4ᵗʰ **752 Congenital anomalies of genital organs**
EXCLUDES   *syndromes associated with anomalies in the*
number and form of chromosomes (758.0-
758.9)
testicular feminization syndrome (257.8)

752.0 **Anomalies of ovaries** ♀
Absence, congenital
Accessory
Ectopic   } (of) ovary
Streak

✓5ᵗʰ **752.1** **Anomalies of fallopian tubes and broad ligaments**
752.10 **Unspecified anomaly of fallopian tubes and broad ligaments** ♀

752.11 **Embryonic cyst of fallopian tubes and broad ligaments** ♀
Cyst: Cyst:
epoophoron   Gartner's duct
fimbrial   parovarian

752.19 **Other** ♀
Absence
Accessory   } (of) fallopian tube or
Atresia   broad ligament

752.2 **Doubling of uterus** ♀
Didelphic uterus
Doubling of uterus [any degree] (associated with doubling of cervix and vagina)

 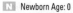

752.3   **Other anomalies of uterus**   ♀

Absence, congenital ⎫
Agenesis   ⎬ (of) uterus
Aplasia   ⎪
Bicornuate   ⎭

Uterus unicornis
Uterus with only one functioning horn

√5th **752.4**   **Anomalies of cervix, vagina, and external female genitalia**

752.40 Unspecified anomaly of cervix, vagina, and external female genitalia   ♀

752.41 Embryonic cyst of cervix, vagina, and external female genitalia   ♀

Cyst of:
canal of Nuck, congenital
vagina, embryonal
vulva, congenital

DEF: Embryonic fluid-filled cysts, of cervix, vagina or external female genitalia.

752.42 Imperforate hymen   ♀

DEF: Complete closure of membranous fold around external opening of vagina.

752.49 Other anomalies of cervix, vagina, and external female genitalia   ♀

Absence   ⎫ of cervix, clitoris,
Agenesis   ⎬   vagina, or vulva

Congenital stenosis or stricture of:
cervical canal
vagina

EXCLUDES   double vagina associated with total duplication (752.2)

√5th **752.5**   **Undescended and retractile testicle**

752.51 Undescended testis   ♂
Cryptorchism
Ectopic testis

752.52 Retractile testis   ♂

√5th **752.6**   **Hypospadias and epispadias and other penile anomalies**

752.61 Hypospadias   ♂

DEF: Hypospadias: abnormal opening of urethra on the ventral surface of the penis or perineum; also a rare defect of vagina.

752.62 Epispadias   ♂
Anaspadias

DEF: Epispadias: urethra opening on dorsal surface of penis; in females appears as a slit in the upper wall of urethra.

752.63 Congenital chordee   ♂

DEF: Ventral bowing of penis due to fibrous band along corpus spongiosum; occurs with hypospadias.

752.64 Micropenis   ♂

752.65 Hidden penis   ♂

752.69 Other penile anomalies   ♂

752.7   **Indeterminate sex and pseudohermaphroditism**

Gynandrism   Pseudohermaphroditism
Hermaphroditism   (male) (female)
Ovotestis   Pure gonadal dysgenesis

EXCLUDES   pseudohermaphroditism:
female, with adrenocortical disorder (255.2)
male, with gonadal disorder (257.8)
with specified chromosomal anomaly (758.0-758.9)
testicular feminization syndrome (257.8)

DEF: Pseudohermaphroditism: presence of gonads of one sex and external genitalia of other sex.

▶ **Hypospadias and Epispadias** ◀

Hypospadias   **Epispadias**
(ventral view)   **(dorsal view)**

752.8   **Other specified anomalies of genital organs**

Absence of: Atresia of:
prostate   ejaculatory duct
spermatic cord   vas deferens
vas deferens   Fusion of testes
Anorchism   Hypoplasia of testis
Aplasia (congenital) of: Monorchism
prostate   Polyorchism
round ligament
testicle

EXCLUDES   congenital hydrocele (778.6)
penile anomalies (752.61-752.69)
phimosis or paraphimosis (605)

752.9   **Unspecified anomaly of genital organs**

Congenital:
anomaly NOS   ⎫ of genital organ, not
deformity NOS   ⎬   elsewhere classified

√4th **753**   **Congenital anomalies of urinary system**

753.0   **Renal agenesis and dysgenesis**

Atrophy of kidney:
congenital
infantile
Congenital absence of kidney(s)
Hypoplasia of kidney(s)

√5th **753.1**   **Cystic kidney disease**

EXCLUDES   acquired cyst of kidney (593.2)

753.10 Cystic kidney disease, unspecified

753.11 Congenital single renal cyst

753.12 Polycystic kidney, unspecified type

753.13 Polycystic kidney, autosomal dominant

DEF: Slow progressive disease characterized by bilateral cysts causing increased kidney size and impaired function.

753.14 Polycystic kidney, autosomal recessive

DEF: Rare disease characterized by multiple cysts involving kidneys and liver, producing renal and hepatic failure in childhood or adolescence.

753.15 Renal dysplasia

753.16 Medullary cystic kidney
Nephronopthisis

DEF: Diffuse kidney disease results in uremia onset prior to age 20.

753.17 Medullary sponge kidney

DEF: Dilated collecting tubules; usually asymptomatic but calcinosis in tubules may cause renal insufficiency.

753.19 Other specified cystic kidney disease
Multicystic kidney

√5th **753.2**   **Obstructive defects of renal pelvis and ureter**

753.20 Unspecified obstructive defect of renal pelvis and ureter

753.21 Congenital obstruction of ureteropelvic junction

DEF: Stricture at junction of ureter and renal pelvis.

√4th
√5th Additional Digit Required   Unspecified Code   Other Specified Code   Manifestation Code   ▶◀ Revised Text   ● New Code   ▲ Revised Code Title

753.22 Congenital obstruction of ureterovesical junction
    Adynamic ureter
    Congenital hydroureter
    DEF: Stricture at junction of ureter and bladder.

753.23 Congenital ureterocele

753.29 Other

753.3 Other specified anomalies of kidney
    Accessory kidney   Fusion of kidneys
    Congenital: Giant kidney
      calculus of kidney   Horseshoe kidney
      displaced kidney   Hyperplasia of kidney
    Discoid kidney   Lobulation of kidney
    Double kidney with   Malrotation of kidney
      double pelvis   Trifid kidney (pelvis)
    Ectopic kidney

753.4 Other specified anomalies of ureter
    Absent ureter   Double ureter
    Accessory ureter   Ectopic ureter
    Deviation of ureter   Implantation, anomalous
    Displaced ureteric orifice   of ureter

753.5 Exstrophy of urinary bladder
    Ectopia vesicae
    Extroversion of bladder
    DEF: Absence of lower abdominal and anterior bladder walls with posterior bladder wall protrusion.

753.6 Atresia and stenosis of urethra and bladder neck
    Congenital obstruction:
      bladder neck
      urethra
    Congenital stricture of:
      urethra (valvular)
      urinary meatus
      vesicourethral orifice
    Imperforate urinary meatus
    Impervious urethra
    Urethral valve formation

753.7 Anomalies of urachus
    Cyst
    Fistula   } (of) urachussinus
    Patent

    Persistent umbilical sinus

753.8 Other specified anomalies of bladder and urethra
    Absence, congenital of: Congenital urethrorectal
      bladder   fistula
      urethra   Congenital prolapse of:
    Accessory: bladder (mucosa)
      bladder   urethra
      urethra   Double:
    Congenital: urethra
      diverticulum of bladder   urinary meatus
      hernia of bladder

753.9 Unspecified anomaly of urinary system
    Congenital:
      anomaly NOS   } of urinary system [any part,
      deformity NOS   except urachus]

√4ᵗʰ 754 Certain congenital musculoskeletal deformities
    INCLUDES   nonteratogenic deformities which are considered to be due to intrauterine malposition and pressure

754.0 Of skull, face, and jaw
    Asymmetry of face   Dolichocephaly
    Compression facies   Plagiocephaly
    Depressions in skull   Potter's facies
    Deviation of nasal   Squashed or bent nose,
      septum, congenital   congenital
    EXCLUDES   dentofacial anomalies (524.0-524.9)
       syphilitic saddle nose (090.5)

754.1 Of sternocleidomastoid muscle
    Congenital sternomastoid torticollis
    Congenital wryneck
    Contracture of sternocleidomastoid (muscle)
    Sternomastoid tumor

754.2 Of spine
    Congenital postural:
      lordosis
      scoliosis

√5ᵗʰ 754.3 Congenital dislocation of hip
    754.30 Congenital dislocation of hip, unilateral
      Congenital dislocation of hip NOS
    754.31 Congenital dislocation of hip, bilateral
    754.32 Congenital subluxation of hip, unilateral
      Congenital flexion deformity, hip or thigh
      Predislocation status of hip at birth
      Preluxation of hip, congenital
    754.33 Congenital subluxation of hip, bilateral
    754.35 Congenital dislocation of one hip with subluxation of other hip

√5ᵗʰ 754.4 Congenital genu recurvatum and bowing of long bones of leg
    754.40 Genu recurvatum
      DEF: Backward curving of knee joint.
    754.41 Congenital dislocation of knee (with genu recurvatum)
      DEF: Elevated, outward rotation of heel; also called clubfoot.
    754.42 Congenital bowing of femur
    754.43 Congenital bowing of tibia and fibula
    754.44 Congenital bowing of unspecified long bones of leg

√5ᵗʰ 754.5 Varus deformities of feet
    EXCLUDES   acquired (736.71, 736.75, 736.79)
    754.50 Talipes varus
      Congenital varus deformity of foot, unspecified
      Pes varus
      DEF: Inverted foot marked by outer sole resting on ground.
    754.51 Talipes equinovarus
      Equinovarus (congenital)
    754.52 Metatarsus primus varus
      DEF: Malformed first metatarsal bone, with bone angled toward body.
    754.53 Metatarsus varus
      DEF: Osseous adhesion of radius and ulna.
    754.59 Other
      Talipes calcaneovarus

√5ᵗʰ 754.6 Valgus deformities of feet
    EXCLUDES   valgus deformity of foot (acquired) (736.79)
    754.60 Talipes valgus
      Congenital valgus deformity of foot, unspecified
    754.61 Congenital pes planus
      Congenital rocker bottom flat foot
      Flat foot, congenital
      EXCLUDES   pes planus (acquired) (734)
    754.62 Talipes calcaneovalgus
    754.69 Other
      Talipes: Talipes:
        equinovalgus   planovalgus

√5ᵗʰ 754.7 Other deformities of feet
    EXCLUDES   acquired (736.70-736.79)
    754.70 Talipes, unspecified
      Congenital deformity of foot NOS
    754.71 Talipes cavus
      Cavus foot (congenital)

754.79 Other
     Asymmetric talipes   Talipes:
     Talipes: equinus
         calcaneus

√5ᵗʰ 754.8 Other specified nonteratogenic anomalies
   754.81 Pectus excavatum
     Congenital funnel chest
   754.82 Pectus carinatum
     Congenital pigeon chest [breast]
   754.89 Other
     Club hand (congenital)
     Congenital:
       deformity of chest wall
       dislocation of elbow
     Generalized flexion contractures of lower
       limb joints, congenital
     Spade-like hand (congenital)

√4ᵗʰ 755 Other congenital anomalies of limbs
   EXCLUDES *those deformities classifiable to 754.0-754.8*

√5ᵗʰ 755.0 Polydactyly
   755.00 Polydactyly, unspecified digits
     Supernumerary digits
   755.01 Of fingers
     Accessory fingers
   755.02 Of toes
     Accessory toes

√5ᵗʰ 755.1 Syndactyly
     Symphalangy   Webbing of digits
   755.10 Of multiple and unspecified sites
   755.11 Of fingers without fusion of bone
   755.12 Of fingers with fusion of bone
   755.13 Of toes without fusion of bone
   755.14 Of toes with fusion of bone

√5ᵗʰ 755.2 Reduction deformities of upper limb
   755.20 Unspecified reduction deformity of upper limb
     Ectromelia NOS ⎫
     Hemimelia NOS ⎬ of upper limb
     Shortening of arm, congenital
   755.21 Transverse deficiency of upper limb
     Amelia of upper limb
     Congenital absence of:
       fingers, all (complete or partial)
       forearm, including hand and fingers
       upper limb, complete
     Congenital amputation of upper limb
     Transverse hemimelia of upper limb
   755.22 Longitudinal deficiency of upper limb, not elsewhere classified
     Phocomelia NOS of upper limb
     Rudimentary arm
   755.23 Longitudinal deficiency, combined, involving humerus, radius, and ulna (complete or incomplete)
     Congenital absence of arm and forearm
       (complete or incomplete) with or
       without metacarpal deficiency and/or
       phalangeal deficiency, incomplete
     Phocomelia, complete, of upper limb
   755.24 Longitudinal deficiency, humeral, complete or partial (with or without distal deficiencies, incomplete)
     Congenital absence of humerus (with or
       without absence of some [but not all]
       distal elements)
     Proximal phocomelia of upper limb

755.25 Longitudinal deficiency, radioulnar, complete or partial (with or without distal deficiencies, incomplete)
     Congenital absence of radius and ulna (with
       or without absence of some [but not
       all] distal elements)
     Distal phocomelia of upper limb
755.26 Longitudinal deficiency, radial, complete or partial (with or without distal deficiencies, incomplete)
     Agenesis of radius
     Congenital absence of radius (with or
       without absence of some [but not all]
       distal elements)
755.27 Longitudinal deficiency, ulnar, complete or partial (with or without distal deficiencies, incomplete)
     Agenesis of ulna
     Congenital absence of ulna (with or without
       absence of some [but not all] distal
       elements)
755.28 Longitudinal deficiency, carpals or metacarpals, complete or partial (with or without incomplete phalangeal deficiency)
755.29 Longitudinal deficiency, phalanges, complete or partial
     Absence of finger, congenital
     Aphalangia of upper limb, terminal,
       complete or partial
   EXCLUDES *terminal deficiency of all five*
                   digits (755.21)
                  transverse deficiency of
                     phalanges (755.21)

√5ᵗʰ 755.3 Reduction deformities of lower limb
   755.30 Unspecified reduction deformity of lower limb
     Ectromelia NOS ⎫
     Hemimelia NOS ⎬ of lower limb
     Shortening of leg, congenital
   755.31 Transverse deficiency of lower limb
     Amelia of lower limb
     Congenital absence of:
       foot
       leg, including foot and toes
       lower limb, complete
       toes, all, complete
     Transverse hemimelia of lower limb
   755.32 Longitudinal deficiency of lower limb, not elsewhere classified
     Phocomelia NOS of lower limb
   755.33 Longitudinal deficiency, combined, involving femur, tibia, and fibula (complete or incomplete)
     Congenital absence of thigh and (lower) leg
       (complete or incomplete) with or
       without metacarpal deficiency and/or
       phalangeal deficiency, incomplete
     Phocomelia, complete, of lower limb
   755.34 Longitudinal deficiency, femoral, complete or partial (with or without distal deficiencies, incomplete)
     Congenital absence of femur (with or
       without absence of some [but not all]
       distal elements)
     Proximal phocomelia of lower limb
   755.35 Longitudinal deficiency, tibiofibular, complete or partial (with or without distal deficiencies, incomplete)
     Congenital absence of tibia and fibula (with
       or without absence of some [but not
       all] distal elements)
     Distal phocomelia of lower limb

√4ᵗʰ
√5ᵗʰ Additional Digit Required   Unspecified Code   Other Specified Code   Manifestation Code   ▶◀ Revised Text   ● New Code   ▲ Revised Code Title

2003 ICD•9•CM   **Volume 1 — 219**

Congenital Anomalies 755.36–756.11

755.36 Longitudinal deficiency, tibia, complete or partial (with or without distal deficiencies, incomplete)
Agenesis of tibia
Congenital absence of tibia (with or without absence of some [but not all] distal elements)

755.37 Longitudinal deficiency, fibular, complete or partial (with or without distal deficiencies, incomplete)
Agenesis of fibula
Congenital absence of fibula (with or without absence of some [but not all] distal elements)

755.38 Longitudinal deficiency, tarsals or metatarsals, complete or partial (with or without incomplete phalangeal deficiency)

755.39 Longitudinal deficiency, phalanges, complete or partial
Absence of toe, congenital
Aphalangia of lower limb, terminal, complete or partial
EXCLUDES   *terminal deficiency of all five digits (755.31)*
transverse deficiency of phalanges (755.31)

755.4 Reduction deformities, unspecified limb
Absence, congenital (complete or partial) of limb NOS
Amelia
Ectromelia   } of unspecified limb
Hemimelia
Phocomelia

√5th **755.5 Other anomalies of upper limb, including shoulder girdle**

755.50 Unspecified anomaly of upper limb

755.51 Congenital deformity of clavicle

755.52 Congenital elevation of scapula
Sprengel's deformity

755.53 Radioulnar synostosis

755.54 Madelung's deformity
DEF: Distal ulnar overgrowth or radial shortening; also called carpus curvus.

755.55 Acrocephalosyndactyly
Apert's syndrome
DEF: Premature cranial suture fusion (craniostenosis); marked by cone-shaped or pointed (acrocephaly) head and webbing of the fingers (syndactyly); it is very similar to craniofacial dysostosis.

755.56 Accessory carpal bones

755.57 Macrodactylia (fingers)
DEF: Abnormally large fingers, toes.

755.58 Cleft hand, congenital
Lobster-claw hand
DEF: Extended separation between fingers into metacarpus; also may refer to large fingers and absent middle fingers of hand.

755.59 Other
Cleidocranial dysostosis
Cubitus:
valgus, congenital
varus, congenital
EXCLUDES   *club hand (congenital) (754.89)*
congenital dislocation of elbow (754.89)

√5th **755.6 Other anomalies of lower limb, including pelvic girdle**

755.60 Unspecified anomaly of lower limb

755.61 Coxa valga, congenital
DEF: Abnormally wide angle between the neck and shaft of the femur.

755.62 Coxa vara, congenital
DEF: Diminished angle between neck and shaft of femur.

755.63 Other congenital deformity of hip (joint)
Congenital anteversion of femur (neck)
EXCLUDES   *congenital dislocation of hip (754.30-754.35)*

755.64 Congenital deformity of knee (joint)
Congenital:
absence of patella
genu valgum [knock-knee]
genu varum [bowleg]
Rudimentary patella

755.65 Macrodactylia of toes
DEF: Abnormally large toes.

755.66 Other anomalies of toes
Congenital: Congenital:
hallux valgus   hammer toe
hallux varus

755.67 Anomalies of foot, not elsewhere classified
Astragaloscaphoid synostosis
Calcaneonavicular bar
Coalition of calcaneus
Talonavicular synostosis
Tarsal coalitions

755.69 Other
Congenital:
angulation of tibia
deformity (of):
ankle (joint)
sacroiliac (joint)
fusion of sacroiliac joint

755.8 Other specified anomalies of unspecified limb

755.9 Unspecified anomaly of unspecified limb
Congenital:
anomaly NOS   } of unspecified limb
deformity NOS
EXCLUDES   *reduction deformity of unspecified limb (755.4)*

√4th **756 Other congenital musculoskeletal anomalies**
EXCLUDES   *those deformities classifiable to 754.0-754.8*

756.0 Anomalies of skull and face bones
Absence of skull bones   Imperfect fusion of skull
Acrocephaly   Oxycephaly
Congenital deformity   Platybasia
of forehead   Premature closure of
Craniosynostosis   cranial sutures
Crouzon's disease   Tower skull
Hypertelorism   Trigonocephaly
EXCLUDES   *acrocephalosyndactyly [Apert's syndrome] (755.55)*
dentofacial anomalies (524.0-524.9)
skull defects associated with brain anomalies, such as:
anencephalus (740.0)
encephalocele (742.0)
hydrocephalus (742.3)
microcephalus (742.1)

√5th **756.1 Anomalies of spine**

756.10 Anomaly of spine, unspecified

756.11 Spondylolysis, lumbosacral region
Prespondylolisthesis (lumbosacral)
DEF: Bilateral or unilateral defect through the pars interarticularis of a vertebra causes spondylolisthesis.

N Newborn Age: 0   **P** Pediatric Age: 0-17   **M** Maternity Age: 12-55   **A** Adult Age: 15-124   **MSP** Medicare Secondary Payer

756.12 Spondylolisthesis

DEF: Downward slipping of lumbar vertebra over next vertebra; usually related to pelvic deformity.

756.13 Absence of vertebra, congenital

756.14 Hemivertebra

DEF: Incomplete development of one side of a vertebra.

756.15 Fusion of spine [vertebra], congenital

756.16 Klippel-Feil syndrome

DEF: Short, wide neck; limits range of motion due to abnormal number of cervical vertebra or fused hemivertebrae.

756.17 Spina bifida occulta

EXCLUDES　spina bifida (aperta) (741.0-741.9)

DEF: Spina bifida marked by a bony spinal canal defect without a protrusion of the cord or meninges; it is diagnosed by radiography and has no symptoms.

756.19 Other

Platyspondylia
Supernumerary vertebra

756.2 Cervical rib

Supernumerary rib in the cervical region

DEF: Costa cervicalis: extra rib attached to cervical vertebra.

756.3 Other anomalies of ribs and sternum

Congenital absence of: Congenital:
　rib　　　　　　　fissure of sternum
　sternum　　　　　fusion of ribs
　　　　　　　　　　Sternum bifidum

EXCLUDES　nonteratogenic deformity of chest wall (754.81-754.89)

756.4 Chondrodystrophy

Achondroplasia　　　　　Enchondromatosis
Chondrodystrophia (fetalis)　Ollier's disease
Dyschondroplasia

EXCLUDES　lipochondrodystrophy [Hurler's syndrome] (277.5)
　　　　　　　Morquio's disease (277.5)

DEF: Abnormal development of cartilage.

√5ᵗʰ 756.5 Osteodystrophies

756.50 Osteodystrophy, unspecified

756.51 Osteogenesis imperfecta

Fragilitas ossium
Osteopsathyrosis

DEF: A collagen disorder commonly characterized by brittle, osteoporotic, easily fractured bones, hypermobility of joints, blue sclerae, and a tendency to hemorrhage.

756.52 Osteopetrosis

DEF: Abnormally dense bone, optic atrophy, hepatosplenomegaly, deafness; sclerosing depletes bone marrow and nerve foramina of skull; often fatal.

756.53 Osteopoikilosis

DEF: Multiple sclerotic foci on ends of long bones, stippling in round, flat bones; identified by x-ray.

756.54 Polyostotic fibrous dysplasia of bone

DEF: Fibrous tissue displaces bone results in segmented ragged-edge café-au-lait spots; occurs in girls of early puberty.

756.55 Chondroectodermal dysplasia

Ellis-van Creveld syndrome

DEF: Inadequate enchondral bone formation; impaired development of hair and teeth, polydactyly, and cardiac septum defects.

756.56 Multiple epiphyseal dysplasia

756.59 Other

Albright (-McCune)-Sternberg syndrome

756.6 Anomalies of diaphragm

Absence of diaphragm　　Congenital hernia:
Congenital hernia:　　　　foramen of Morgagni
　diaphragmatic　　　　Eventration of diaphragm

EXCLUDES　congenital hiatus hernia (750.6)

√5ᵗʰ 756.7 Anomalies of abdominal wall

756.70 Anomaly of abdominal wall, unspecified

756.71 Prune belly syndrome

Eagle-Barrett syndrome
Prolapse of bladder mucosa

DEF: Prune belly syndrome: absence of lower rectus abdominis muscle and lower and medial oblique muscles; results in dilated bladder and ureters, dysplastic kidneys and hydronephrosis; more common in male infants with undescended testicles.

756.79 Other congenital anomalies of abdominal wall

Exomphalos
Gastroschisis
Omphalocele

EXCLUDES　umbilical hernia (551-553 with .1)

DEF: Exomphalos: umbilical hernia prominent navel.

DEF: Gastroschisis: fissure of abdominal wall, results in protruding small or large intestine.

DEF: Omphalocele: hernia of umbilicus due to impaired abdominal wall; results in membrane-covered intestine protruding through peritoneum and amnion.

√5ᵗʰ 756.8 Other specified anomalies of muscle, tendon, fascia, and connective tissue

756.81 Absence of muscle and tendon

Absence of muscle (pectoral)

756.82 Accessory muscle

756.83 Ehlers-Danlos syndrome

DEF: Danlos syndrome: connective tissue disorder causes hyperextended skin and joints; results in fragile blood vessels with bleeding, poor wound healing and subcutaneous pseudotumors.

756.89 Other

Amyotrophia congenita
Congenital shortening of tendon

756.9 Other and unspecified anomalies of musculoskeletal system

Congenital:
anomaly NOS　} of musculoskeletal system,
deformity NOS　} not elsewhere classified

√4ᵗʰ 757 Congenital anomalies of the integument

INCLUDES　anomalies of skin, subcutaneous tissue, hair, nails, and breast

EXCLUDES　hemangioma (228.00-228.09)
　　　　　　　pigmented nevus (216.0-216.9)

757.0 Hereditary edema of legs

Congenital lymphedema
Hereditary trophedema
Milroy's disease

757.1 Ichthyosis congenita

Congenital ichthyosis
Harlequin fetus
Ichthyosiform erythroderma

DEF: Overproduction of skin cells causes scaling of skin; may result in stillborn fetus or death soon after birth.

757.2 Dermatoglyphic anomalies

Abnormal palmar creases

DEF: Abnormal skin-line patterns of fingers, palms, toes and soles; initial finding of possible chromosomal abnormalities.

Congenital Anomalies 756.12–757.2

√4ᵗʰ / **√5ᵗʰ** Additional Digit Required　　Unspecified Code　　Other Specified Code　　Manifestation Code　　▶◀ Revised Text　　● New Code　　▲ Revised Code Title

2003 ICD•9•CM　　　　　　　　　　　　　　　　　　　　　　　　　　Volume 1 — 221

Congenital Anomalies 757.3–759.4

✓5th **757.3 Other specified anomalies of skin**

757.31 Congenital ectodermal dysplasia

DEF: Tissues and structures originate in embryonic ectoderm; includes anhidrotic and hidrotic ectodermal dysplasia and EEC syndrome.

757.32 Vascular hamartomas

Birthmarks   Strawberry nevus
Port-wine stain

DEF: Benign tumor of blood vessels; due to malformed angioblastic tissues.

757.33 Congenital pigmentary anomalies of skin

Congenital poikiloderma
Urticaria pigmentosa
Xeroderma pigmentosum
EXCLUDES   albinism (270.2)

757.39 Other

Accessory skin tags, congenital
Congenital scar
Epidermolysis bullosa
Keratoderma (congenital)
EXCLUDES   pilonidal cyst (685.0-685.1)

757.4 Specified anomalies of hair

Congenital: Congenital:
alopecia   hypertrichosis
atrichosis   monilethrix
beaded hair   Persistent lanugo

757.5 Specified anomalies of nails

Anonychia   Congenital:
Congenital: leukonychia
clubnail   onychauxis
koilonychia   pachyonychia

757.6 Specified anomalies of breast

Absent
Accessory } breast or nipple
Supernumerary

Hypoplasia of breast
EXCLUDES   absence of pectoral muscle (756.81)

757.8 Other specified anomalies of the integument

757.9 Unspecified anomaly of the integument

Congenital:
anomaly NOS } of integument
deformity NOS

✓4th **758 Chromosomal anomalies**

INCLUDES   syndromes associated with anomalies in the number and form of chromosomes

758.0 Down's syndrome

Mongolism   Trisomy:
Translocation Down's   21 or 22
syndrome   G

758.1 Patau's syndrome

Trisomy: Trisomy:
13   D_1

DEF: Trisomy of 13th chromosome; characteristic failure to thrive, severe mental impairment, seizures, abnormal eyes, low-set ears and sloped forehead.

758.2 Edwards' syndrome

Trisomy: Trisomy:
18   E_3

DEF: Trisomy of 18th chromosome; characteristic mental and physical impairments; mainly affects females.

758.3 Autosomal deletion syndromes

Antimongolism syndrome
Cri-du-chat syndrome

DEF: Antimongolism syndrome: Deletions in 21st chromosome; characteristic oblique palpebral fissures, hypertonia, micrognathia, microcephaly, high-arched palate and impaired mental and physical growth.

DEF: Cri-du-chat syndrome: Abnormally large distance between two organs or parts, abnormally small brain and severe mental impairment; characteristic of abnormal 5th chromosome.

758.4 Balanced autosomal translocation in normal individual

758.5 Other conditions due to autosomal anomalies

Accessory autosomes NEC

758.6 Gonadal dysgenesis

Ovarian dysgenesis   XO syndrome
Turner's syndrome
EXCLUDES   pure gonadal dysgenesis (752.7)

DEF: Impaired embryonic development of seminiferous tubes; results in small testes, azoospermia, infertility and enlarged mammary glands.

758.7 Klinefelter's syndrome   ♂

XXY syndrome

✓5th **758.8 Other conditions due to chromosome anomalies**

758.81 Other conditions due to sex chromosome anomalies

758.89 Other

758.9 Conditions due to anomaly of unspecified chromosome

✓4th **759 Other and unspecified congenital anomalies**

759.0 Anomalies of spleen

Aberrant
Absent } spleen
Accessory

Congenital splenomegaly
Ectopic spleen
Lobulation of spleen

759.1 Anomalies of adrenal gland

Aberrant
Absent } adrenal gland
Accessory

EXCLUDES   adrenogenital disorders (255.2)
congenital disorders of steroid metabolism (255.2)

759.2 Anomalies of other endocrine glands

Absent parathyroid gland
Accessory thyroid gland
Persistent thyroglossal or thyrolingual duct
Thyroglossal (duct) cyst
EXCLUDES   congenital:
goiter (246.1)
hypothyroidism (243)

759.3 Situs inversus

Situs inversus or transversus:
abdominalis
thoracis
Transposition of viscera:
abdominal
thoracic
EXCLUDES   dextrocardia without mention of complete transposition (746.87)

DEF: Laterally transposed thoracic and abdominal viscera.

759.4 Conjoined twins

Craniopagus   Thoracopagus
Dicephalus   Xiphopagus
Pygopagus

N Newborn Age: 0   **P** Pediatric Age: 0-17   **M** Maternity Age: 12-55   **A** Adult Age: 15-124   **MSP** Medicare Secondary Payer

222 — Volume 1   *2003 ICD•9•CM*

759.5 Tuberous sclerosis

Bourneville's disease   Epiloia

DEF: Hamartomas of brain, retina and viscera, impaired mental ability, seizures and adenoma sebaceum.

759.6 Other hamartoses, not elsewhere classified

Syndrome:	Syndrome:
Peutz-Jeghers	von Hippel-Lindau
Sturge-Weber (-Dimitri)	

EXCLUDES *neurofibromatosis (237.7)*

DEF: Peutz-Jeghers: hereditary syndrome characterized by hamartomas of small intestine

DEF: Sturge-Weber: congenital syndrome characterized by unilateral port-wine stain over trigeminal nerve, underlying meninges and cerebral cortex.

DEF: von Hipple-Lindau: hereditary syndrome of congenital angiomatosis of the retina and cerebellum.

759.7 Multiple congenital anomalies, so described

Congenital:
    anomaly, multiple NOS
    deformity, multiple NOS

√5ᵗʰ **759.8 Other specified anomalies**

  759.81 Prader-Willi syndrome

  759.82 Marfan syndrome

  759.83 Fragile X syndrome

  759.89 Other

    Congenital malformation syndromes affecting multiple systems, not elsewhere classified

    Laurence-Moon-Biedl syndrome

759.9 Congenital anomaly, unspecified

√4ᵗʰ √5ᵗʰ Additional Digit Required   Unspecified Code   Other Specified Code   Manifestation Code   ▶◀ Revised Text   ● New Code   ▲ Revised Code Title

2003 ICD•9•CM   **Volume 1 — 223**

15. CERTAIN CONDITIONS ORIGINATING IN THE PERINATAL PERIOD (760-779)

> **INCLUDES**   conditions which have their origin in the perinatal period even though death or morbidity occurs later
>
> Use additional code(s) to further specify condition

MATERNAL CAUSES OF PERINATAL MORBIDITY AND MORTALITY (760-763)

√4th 760 Fetus or newborn affected by maternal conditions which may be unrelated to present pregnancy

> **INCLUDES**   the listed maternal conditions only when specified as a cause of mortality or morbidity of the fetus or newborn
>
> **EXCLUDES**   *maternal endocrine and metabolic disorders affecting fetus or newborn (775.0-775.9)*

760.0 Maternal hypertensive disorders
Fetus or newborn affected by maternal conditions classifiable to 642

760.1 Maternal renal and urinary tract diseases
Fetus or newborn affected by maternal conditions classifiable to 580-599

760.2 Maternal infections
Fetus or newborn affected by maternal infectious disease classifiable to 001-136 and 487, but fetus or newborn not manifesting that disease

> **EXCLUDES**   *congenital infectious diseases (771.0-771.8)*
> *maternal genital tract and other localized infections (760.8)*

760.3 Other chronic maternal circulatory and respiratory diseases
Fetus or newborn affected by chronic maternal conditions classifiable to 390-459, 490-519, 745-748

760.4 Maternal nutritional disorders
Fetus or newborn affected by:
maternal disorders classifiable to 260-269
maternal malnutrition NOS

> **EXCLUDES**   *fetal malnutrition (764.10-764.29)*

760.5 Maternal injury
Fetus or newborn affected by maternal conditions classifiable to 800-995

760.6 Surgical operation on mother

> **EXCLUDES**   *cesarean section for present delivery (763.4)*
> *damage to placenta from amniocentesis, cesarean section, or surgical induction (762.1)*
> *previous surgery to uterus or pelvic organs (763.89)*

√5th 760.7 Noxious influences affecting fetus via placenta or breast milk
Fetus or newborn affected by noxious substance transmitted via placenta or breast milk

> **EXCLUDES**   *anesthetic and analgesic drugs administered during labor and delivery (763.5)*
> *drug withdrawal syndrome in newborn (779.5)*

760.70 Unspecified noxious substance
Fetus or newborn affected by:
Drug NEC

760.71 Alcohol
Fetal alcohol syndrome

760.72 Narcotics

760.73 Hallucinogenic agents

760.74 Anti-infectives
Antibiotics

760.75 Cocaine

760.76 Diethylstilbestrol [DES]

760.79 Other
Fetus or newborn affected by:
immune sera	transmitted via
medicinal agents	placenta
NEC	or breast
toxic substance NEC	milk

760.8 Other specified maternal conditions affecting fetus or newborn
Maternal genital tract and other localized infection affecting fetus or newborn, but fetus or newborn not manifesting that disease

> **EXCLUDES**   *maternal urinary tract infection affecting fetus or newborn (760.1)*

760.9 Unspecified maternal condition affecting fetus or newborn

√4th 761 Fetus or newborn affected by maternal complications of pregnancy

> **INCLUDES**   the listed maternal conditions only when specified as a cause of mortality or morbidity of the fetus or newborn

761.0 Incompetent cervix

DEF: Inadequate functioning of uterine cervix.

761.1 Premature rupture of membranes

761.2 Oligohydramnios

> **EXCLUDES**   *that due to premature rupture of membranes (761.1).*

DEF: Deficient amniotic fluid.

761.3 Polyhydramnios
Hydramnios (acute) (chronic)

DEF: Excess amniotic fluid.

761.4 Ectopic pregnancy
Pregnancy:	Pregnancy:
abdominal	tubal
intraperitoneal	

761.5 Multiple pregnancy
Triplet (pregnancy)   Twin (pregnancy)

761.6 Maternal death

761.7 Malpresentation before labor
Breech presentation	
External version	
Oblique lie	before labor
Transverse lie	
Unstable lie	

761.8 Other specified maternal complications of pregnancy affecting fetus or newborn
Spontaneous abortion, fetus

761.9 Unspecified maternal complication of pregnancy affecting fetus or newborn

√4th 762 Fetus or newborn affected by complications of placenta, cord, and membranes

> **INCLUDES**   the listed maternal conditions only when specified as a cause of mortality or morbidity in the fetus or newborn

762.0 Placenta previa   N

DEF: Placenta developed in lower segment of uterus; causes hemorrhaging in last trimester.

762.1 Other forms of placental separation and hemorrhage   N
Abruptio placentae
Antepartum hemorrhage
Damage to placenta from amniocentesis, cesarean section, or surgical induction
Maternal blood loss
Premature separation of placenta
Rupture of marginal sinus

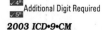

√4th Additional Digit Required   Unspecified Code   Other Specified Code   Manifestation Code   ►◄ Revised Text   ● New Code   ▲ Revised Code Title
√5th

2003 ICD•9•CM   **Volume 1 — 225**

Conditions in the Perinatal Period 760–762.1

762.2 Other and unspecified morphological and functional abnormalities of placenta   N
Placental: Placental:
    dysfunction   insufficiency
    infarction

762.3 Placental transfusion syndromes   N
Placental and cord abnormality resulting in twin-to-twin or other transplacental transfusion
Use additional code to indicate resultant condition in fetus or newborn:
    fetal blood loss (772.0)
    polycythemia neonatorum (776.4)

762.4 Prolapsed cord   N
Cord presentation

762.5 Other compression of umbilical cord   N
Cord around neck   Knot in cord
Entanglement of cord   Torsion of cord

762.6 Other and unspecified conditions of umbilical cord   N
Short cord
Thrombosis
Varices   } of umbilical cord
Velamentous insertion
Vasa previa
    EXCLUDES   *infection of umbilical cord (771.4)*
            single umbilical artery (747.5)

762.7 Chorioamnionitis   N
Amnionitis   Placentitis
Membranitis
DEF: Inflamed fetal membrane.

762.8 Other specified abnormalities of chorion and amnion   N

762.9 Unspecified abnormality of chorion and amnion   N

√4ᵗʰ **763 Fetus or newborn affected by other complications of labor and delivery**
    INCLUDES   the listed conditions only when specified as a cause of mortality or morbidity in the fetus or newborn

763.0 Breech delivery and extraction   N

763.1 Other malpresentation, malposition, and disproportion during labor and delivery   N
Fetus or newborn affected by:
    abnormality of bony pelvis
    contracted pelvis
    persistent occipitoposterior position
    shoulder presentation
    transverse lie
    conditions classifiable to 652, 653, and 660

763.2 Forceps delivery   N
Fetus or newborn affected by forceps extraction

763.3 Delivery by vacuum extractor   N

763.4 Cesarean delivery   N
    EXCLUDES   *placental separation or hemorrhage from cesarean section (762.1)*

763.5 Maternal anesthesia and analgesia   N
Reactions and intoxications from maternal opiates and tranquilizers during labor and delivery
    EXCLUDES   *drug withdrawal syndrome in newborn (779.5)*

763.6 Precipitate delivery   N
Rapid second stage

763.7 Abnormal uterine contractions   N
Fetus or newborn affected by:
    contraction ring
    hypertonic labor
    hypotonic uterine dysfunction
    uterine inertia or dysfunction
    conditions classifiable to 661, except 661.3

√5ᵗʰ **763.8 Other specified complications of labor and delivery affecting fetus or newborn**

763.81 Abnormality in fetal heart rate or rhythm before the onset of labor   N

763.82 Abnormality in fetal heart rate or rhythm during labor   N

763.83 Abnormality in fetal heart rate or rhythm, unspecified as to time of onset   N

763.89 Other specified complications of labor and delivery affecting fetus or newborn   N
Fetus or newborn affected by:
    abnormality of maternal soft tissues
    destructive operation on live fetus to facilitate delivery
    induction of labor (medical)
    previous surgery to uterus or pelvic organs
    other conditions classifiable to 650-669
    other procedures used in labor and delivery

763.9 Unspecified complication of labor and delivery affecting fetus or newborn   N

OTHER CONDITIONS ORIGINATING IN THE PERINATAL PERIOD (764-779)

The following fifth-digit subclassification is for use with ▶category 764 and codes 765.0 and 765.1◀ to denote birthweight:
    0   unspecified [weight]
    1   less than 500 grams
    2   500-749 grams
    3   750-999 grams
    4   1,000-1,249 grams
    5   1,250-1,499 grams
    6   1,500-1,749 grams
    7   1,750-1,999 grams
    8   2,000-2,499 grams
    9   2,500 grams and over

√4ᵗʰ **764 Slow fetal growth and fetal malnutrition**

√5ᵗʰ **764.0 "Light-for-dates" without mention of fetal malnutrition**   N
Infants underweight for gestational age
"Small-for-dates"

√5ᵗʰ **764.1 "Light-for-dates" with signs of fetal malnutrition**   N
Infants "light-for-dates" classifiable to 764.0, who in addition show signs of fetal malnutrition, such as dry peeling skin and loss of subcutaneous tissue

√5ᵗʰ **764.2 Fetal malnutrition without mention of "light-for-dates"**   N
Infants, not underweight for gestational age, showing signs of fetal malnutrition, such as dry peeling skin and loss of subcutaneous tissue
Intrauterine malnutrition

√5ᵗʰ **764.9 Fetal growth retardation, unspecified**   N
Intrauterine growth retardation

√4ᵗʰ **765 Disorders relating to short gestation and low birthweight**
    INCLUDES   the listed conditions, without further specification, as causes of mortality, morbidity, or additional care, in fetus or newborn

√5ᵗʰ **765.0 Extreme immaturity**   N
Note: Usually implies a birthweight of less than 1000 grams.
▶Use additional code for weeks of gestation (765.20-765.29)◀

√5ᵗʰ **765.1 Other preterm infants**   N

Note: Usually implies a birthweight of 1000-2499 grams.

Prematurity NOS

Prematurity or small size, not classifiable to 765.0 or as "light-for-dates" in 764

▶Use additional code for weeks of gestation (765.20-765.29)◀

√5ᵗʰ **765.2 Weeks of gestation**

765.20 Unspecified weeks of gestation   N

765.21 Less than 24 completed weeks of gestation   N

765.22 24 completed weeks of gestation   N

765.23 25-26 completed weeks of gestation   N

765.24 27-28 completed weeks of gestation   N

765.25 29-30 completed weeks of gestation   N

765.26 31-32 completed weeks of gestation   N

765.27 33-34 completed weeks of gestation   N

765.28 35-36 completed weeks of gestation   N

765.29 37 or more completed weeks of gestation   N

√4ᵗʰ **766 Disorders relating to long gestation and high birthweight**

INCLUDES the listed conditions, without further specification, as causes of mortality, morbidity, or additional care, in fetus or newborn

766.0 Exceptionally large baby   N

Note: Usually implies a birthweight of 4500 grams or more.

766.1 Other "heavy-for-dates" infants   N

Other fetus or infant "heavy-" or "large-for-dates" regardless of period of gestation

766.2 Post-term infant, not "heavy-for-dates"   N

Fetus or infant with gestation period of 294 days or more [42 or more completed weeks], not "heavy-" or "large-for-dates"

Postmaturity NOS

√4ᵗʰ **767 Birth trauma**

767.0 Subdural and cerebral hemorrhage   N

Subdural and cerebral hemorrhage, whether described as due to birth trauma or to intrapartum anoxia or hypoxia

Subdural hematoma (localized)

Tentorial tear

Use additional code to identify cause

EXCLUDES intraventricular hemorrhage (772.10-772.14)

subarachnoid hemorrhage (772.2)

767.1 Injuries to scalp   N

Caput succedaneum

Cephalhematoma

Chignon (from vacuum extraction)

Massive epicranial subaponeurotic hemorrhage

767.2 Fracture of clavicle   N

767.3 Other injuries to skeleton   N

Fracture of: Fracture of:

long bones   skull

EXCLUDES congenital dislocation of hip (754.30-754.35)

fracture of spine, congenital (767.4)

767.4 Injury to spine and spinal cord   N

Dislocation ⎫

Fracture   ⎬ of spine or spinal cord

Laceration   ⎪ due to birth trauma

Rupture   ⎭

767.5 Facial nerve injury   N

Facial palsy

767.6 Injury to brachial plexus   N

Palsy or paralysis: Palsy or paralysis:

brachial   Klumpke (-Déjérine)

Erb (-Duchenne)

767.7 Other cranial and peripheral nerve injuries   N

Phrenic nerve paralysis

767.8 Other specified birth trauma   N

Eye damage   Rupture of:

Hematoma of: liver

liver (subcapsular)   spleen

testes   Scalpel wound

vulva   Traumatic glaucoma

EXCLUDES *hemorrhage classifiable to 772.0-772.9*

767.9 Birth trauma, unspecified   N

Birth injury NOS

√4ᵗʰ **768 Intrauterine hypoxia and birth asphyxia**

Use only when associated with newborn morbidity classifiable elsewhere

DEF: Oxygen intake insufficiency due to interrupted placental circulation or premature separation of placenta.

768.0 Fetal death from asphyxia or anoxia before onset of labor or at unspecified time   N

768.1 Fetal death from asphyxia or anoxia during labor   N

768.2 Fetal distress before onset of labor, in liveborn infant   N

Fetal metabolic acidemia before onset of labor, in liveborn infant

768.3 Fetal distress first noted during labor, in liveborn infant   N

Fetal metabolic acidemia first noted during labor, in liveborn infant

768.4 Fetal distress, unspecified as to time of onset, in liveborn infant   N

Fetal metabolic acidemia unspecified as to time of onset, in liveborn infant

768.5 Severe birth asphyxia   N

Birth asphyxia with neurologic involvement

768.6 Mild or moderate birth asphyxia   N

Other specified birth asphyxia (without mention of neurologic involvement)

768.9 Unspecified birth asphyxia in liveborn infant   N

Anoxia ⎫

Asphyxia ⎬ NOS, in liveborn infant

Hypoxia ⎭

769 Respiratory distress syndrome   N

Cardiorespiratory distress syndrome of newborn

Hyaline membrane disease (pulmonary)

Idiopathic respiratory distress syndrome [IRDS or RDS] of newborn

Pulmonary hypoperfusion syndrome

EXCLUDES *transient tachypnea of newborn (770.6)*

DEF: Severe chest contractions upon air intake and expiratory grunting; infant appears blue due to oxygen deficiency and has rapid respiratory rate; formerly called hyaline membrane disease.

√4ᵗʰ **770 Other respiratory conditions of fetus and newborn**

770.0 Congenital pneumonia   N

Infective pneumonia acquired prenatally

EXCLUDES *pneumonia from infection acquired after birth (480.0-486)*

770.1 Meconium aspiration syndrome   N

Aspiration of contents of birth canal NOS

Meconium aspiration below vocal cords

Pneumonitis:

fetal aspiration

meconium

DEF: Aspiration of meconium by the newborn infant prior to delivery. Presence of meconium in the trachea or chest x-ray indicating patchy infiltrates in conjunction with chest hyperextension establishes this diagnosis.

√4ᵗʰ / √5ᵗʰ Additional Digit Required   Unspecified Code   Other Specified Code   Manifestation Code   ▶◀ Revised Text   ● New Code   ▲ Revised Code Title

Conditions in the Perinatal Period 770.2–772.6

770.2 **Interstitial emphysema and related conditions** [N]

Pneumomediastinum ⎫
Pneumopericardium ⎬ originating in the
Pneumothorax ⎭ perinatal period

770.3 **Pulmonary hemorrhage** [N]

Hemorrhage:
    alveolar (lung) ⎫
    intra-alveolar (lung) ⎬ originating in the
    massive pulmonary ⎭ perinatal period

770.4 **Primary atelectasis** [N]

Pulmonary immaturity NOS

DEF: Alveoli fail to expand causing insufficient air intake by newborn.

770.5 **Other and unspecified atelectasis** [N]

Atelectasis: ⎫
    NOS ⎪
    partial ⎬ originating in the
    secondary ⎪ perinatal period
Pulmonary collapse ⎭

770.6 **Transitory tachypnea of newborn** [N]

Idiopathic tachypnea of newborn
Wet lung syndrome

EXCLUDES   respiratory distress syndrome (769)

DEF: Quick, shallow breathing of newborn; short-term problem.

770.7 **Chronic respiratory disease arising in the perinatal period** [N]

Bronchopulmonary dysplasia
Interstitial pulmonary fibrosis of prematurity
Wilson-Mikity syndrome

√5th **770.8** **Other respiratory problems after birth**

●   **770.81** **Primary apnea of newborn** [N]

Apneic spells of newborn NOS
Essential apnea of newborn
Sleep apnea of newborn

●   **770.82** **Other apnea of newborn** [N]

Obstructive apnea of newborn

●   **770.83** **Cyanotic attacks of newborn** [N]

●   **770.84** **Respiratory failure of newborn** [N]

EXCLUDES   respiratory distress syndrome (769)

●   **770.89** **Other respiratory problems after birth** [N]

770.9 **Unspecified respiratory condition of fetus and newborn** [N]

√4th **771** **Infections specific to the perinatal period**

INCLUDES   infections acquired before or during birth or via the umbilicus

EXCLUDES   congenital pneumonia (770.0)
     congenital syphilis (090.0-090.9)
     maternal infectious disease as a cause of mortality or morbidity in fetus or newborn, but fetus or newborn not manifesting the disease (760.2)
     ophthalmia neonatorum due to gonococcus (098.40)
     other infections not specifically classified to this category

771.0 **Congenital rubella** [N]

Congenital rubella pneumonitis

771.1 **Congenital cytomegalovirus infection** [N]

Congenital cytomegalic inclusion disease

771.2 **Other congenital infections** [N]

Congenital: Congenital:
  herpes simplex   toxoplasmosis
  listeriosis   tuberculosis
  malaria

771.3 **Tetanus neonatorum** [N]

Tetanus omphalitis

EXCLUDES   hypocalcemic tetany (775.4)

DEF: Severe infection of central nervous system; due to exotoxin of tetanus bacillus from navel infection prompted by nonsterile technique during umbilical ligation.

771.4 **Omphalitis of the newborn** [N]

Infection:
  navel cord
  umbilical stump

EXCLUDES   tetanus omphalitis (771.3)

DEF: Inflamed umbilicus.

771.5 **Neonatal infective mastitis** [N]

EXCLUDES   noninfective neonatal mastitis (778.7)

771.6 **Neonatal conjunctivitis and dacryocystitis** [N]

Ophthalmia neonatorum NOS

EXCLUDES   ophthalmia neonatorum due to gonococcus (098.40)

771.7 **Neonatal Candida infection** [N]

Neonatal moniliasis   Thrush in newborn

√5th **771.8** **Other infection specific to the perinatal period**

▶Use additional code to identify organism◀

●   **771.81** **Septicemia [sepsis] of newborn** [N]

●   **771.82** **Urinary tract infection of newborn** [N]

●   **771.83** **Bacteremia of newborn** [N]

●   **771.89** **Other infections specific to the perinatal period** [N]

Intra-amniotic infection of fetus NOS
Infection of newborn NOS

√4th **772** **Fetal and neonatal hemorrhage**

EXCLUDES   hematological disorders of fetus and newborn (776.0-776.9)

772.0 **Fetal blood loss** [N]

Fetal blood loss from:
  cut end of co-twin's cord
  placenta
  ruptured cord
  vasa previa
Fetal exsanguination
Fetal hemorrhage into:
  co-twin
  mother's circulation

√5th **772.1** **Intraventricular hemorrhage** [N]

Intraventricular hemorrhage from any perinatal cause

772.10 **Unspecified grade**

772.11 **Grade I**

Bleeding into germinal matrix

772.12 **Grade II**

Bleeding into ventricle

772.13 **Grade III**

Bleeding with enlargement of ventricle

772.14 **Grade IV**

Bleeding into cerebral cortex

772.2 **Subarachnoid hemorrhage** [N]

Subarachnoid hemorrhage from any perinatal cause

EXCLUDES   subdural and cerebral hemorrhage (767.0)

772.3 **Umbilical hemorrhage after birth** [N]

Slipped umbilical ligature

772.4 **Gastrointestinal hemorrhage** [N]

EXCLUDES   swallowed maternal blood (777.3)

772.5 **Adrenal hemorrhage** [N]

772.6 **Cutaneous hemorrhage** [N]

Bruising ⎫
Ecchymoses ⎬
Petechiae ⎬ in fetus or newborn
Superficial hematoma ⎭

[N] Newborn Age: 0   [P] Pediatric Age: 0-17   [M] Maternity Age: 12-55   [A] Adult Age: 15-124   [MSP] Medicare Secondary Payer

228 — Volume 1 • October 2002   *2003 ICD•9•CM*

772.8   Other specified hemorrhage of fetus or newborn N

> EXCLUDES   *hemorrhagic disease of newborn (776.0)*
> *pulmonary hemorrhage (770.3)*

772.9   Unspecified hemorrhage of newborn N

√4th **773   Hemolytic disease of fetus or newborn, due to isoimmunization**

DEF: Hemolytic anemia of fetus or newborn due to maternal antibody formation against fetal erythrocytes; infant blood contains nonmaternal antigen.

773.0   Hemolytic disease due to Rh isoimmunization N

Anemia	
Erythroblastosis (fetalis)	due to RH:
Hemolytic disease (fetus) (newborn)	antibodies
	isoimmunization
	maternal/fetal
Jaundice	incompatibility

Rh hemolytic disease
Rh isoimmunization

773.1   Hemolytic disease due to ABO isoimmunization N

ABO hemolytic disease
ABO isoimmunization

Anemia	
Erythroblastosis (fetalis)	due to ABO:
	antibodies
Hemolytic disease (fetus) (newborn)	isoimmunization
	maternal/fetal
Jaundice	incompatibility

DEF: Incompatible Rh fetal-maternal blood grouping; prematurely destroys red blood cells; detected by Coombs test.

773.2   Hemolytic disease due to other and unspecified isoimmunization N

Eythroblastosis (fetalis) (neonatorum) NOS
Hemolytic disease (fetus) (newborn) NOS
Jaundice or anemia due to other and unspecified blood-group incompatibility

773.3   Hydrops fetalis due to isoimmunization N

Use additional code to identify type of isoimmunization (773.0-773.2)

DEF: Massive edema of entire body and severe anemia; may result in fetal death or stillbirth.

773.4   Kernicterus due to isoimmunization N

Use additional code to identify type of isoimmunization (773.0-773.2)

DEF: Complication of erythroblastosis fetalis associated with severe neural symptoms, high blood bilirubin levels and nerve cell destruction; results in bilirubin-pigmented gray matter of central nervous system.

773.5   Late anemia due to isoimmunization

√4th **774   Other perinatal jaundice**

774.0   *Perinatal jaundice from hereditary hemolytic anemias* N

Code first underlying disease (282.0-282.9)

774.1   Perinatal jaundice from other excessive hemolysis N

Fetal or neonatal jaundice from:
  bruising
  drugs or toxins transmitted from mother
  infection
  polycythemia
  swallowed maternal blood
Use additional code to identify cause

> EXCLUDES   *jaundice due to isoimmunization (773.0-773.2)*

774.2   Neonatal jaundice associated with preterm delivery N

Hyperbilirubinemia of prematurity
Jaundice due to delayed conjugation associated with preterm delivery

√5th **774.3   Neonatal jaundice due to delayed conjugation from other causes**

774.30   Neonatal jaundice due to delayed conjugation, cause unspecified N

DEF: Jaundice of newborn with abnormal bilirubin metabolism; causes excess accumulated unconjugated bilirubin in blood.

774.31   *Neonatal jaundice due to delayed conjugation in diseases classified elsewhere* N

Code first underlying diseases as:
  congenital hypothyroidism (243)
  Crigler-Najjar syndrome (277.4)
  Gilbert's syndrome (277.4)

774.39   Other N

Jaundice due to delayed conjugation from causes, such as:
  breast milk inhibitors
  delayed development of conjugating system

774.4   Perinatal jaundice due to hepatocellular damage N

Fetal or neonatal hepatitis
Giant cell hepatitis
Inspissated bile syndrome

774.5   *Perinatal jaundice from other causes* N

Code first underlying cause as:
  congenital obstruction of bile duct (751.61)
  galactosemia (271.1)
  Mucoviscidosis ▶(277.00-277.09)◀

774.6   Unspecified fetal and neonatal jaundice N

Icterus neonatorum
Neonatal hyperbilirubinemia (transient)
Physiologic jaundice NOS in newborn

> EXCLUDES   *that in preterm infants (774.2)*

774.7   Kernicterus not due to isoimmunization N

Bilirubin encephalopathy
Kernicterus of newborn NOS

> EXCLUDES   *kernicterus due to isoimmunization (773.4)*

√4th **775   Endocrine and metabolic disturbances specific to the fetus and newborn**

> INCLUDES   transitory endocrine and metabolic disturbances caused by the infant's response to maternal endocrine and metabolic factors, its removal from them, or its adjustment to extrauterine existence

775.0   Syndrome of "infant of a diabetic mother" N

Maternal diabetes mellitus affecting fetus or newborn (with hypoglycemia)

775.1   Neonatal diabetes mellitus N

Diabetes mellitus syndrome in newborn infant

775.2   Neonatal myasthenia gravis N

775.3   Neonatal thyrotoxicosis N

Neonatal hyperthyroidism (transient)

775.4   Hypocalcemia and hypomagnesemia of newborn N

Cow's milk hypocalcemia
Hypocalcemic tetany, neonatal
Neonatal hypoparathyroidism
Phosphate-loading hypocalcemia

775.5   Other transitory neonatal electrolyte disturbances N

Dehydration, neonatal

775.6   Neonatal hypoglycemia N

> EXCLUDES   *infant of mother with diabetes mellitus (775.0)*

775.7   Late metabolic acidosis of newborn N

775.8   Other transitory neonatal endocrine and metabolic disturbances N

Amino-acid metabolic disorders described as transitory

√4th
√5th Additional Digit Required   Unspecified Code   Other Specified Code   Manifestation Code   ▶◀ Revised Text   ● New Code   ▲ Revised Code Title

775.9 Unspecified endocrine and metabolic disturbances specific to the fetus and newborn N

✓4th 776 Hematological disorders of fetus and newborn
INCLUDES disorders specific to the fetus or newborn

776.0 Hemorrhagic disease of newborn N
Hemorrhagic diathesis of newborn
Vitamin K deficiency of newborn
EXCLUDES fetal or neonatal hemorrhage (772.0-772.9)

776.1 Transient neonatal thrombocytopenia N
Neonatal thrombocytopenia due to:
exchange transfusion
idiopathic maternal thrombocytopenia
isoimmunization
DEF: Temporary decrease in blood platelets of newborn.

776.2 Disseminated intravascular coagulation in newborn N
DEF: Disseminated intravascular coagulation of newborn: clotting disorder due to excess thromboplastic agents in blood as a result of disease or trauma; causes blood clotting within vessels and reduces available elements necessary for blood coagulation.

776.3 Other transient neonatal disorders of coagulation N
Transient coagulation defect, newborn

776.4 Polycythemia neonatorum N
Plethora of newborn   Polycythemia due to:
Polycythemia due to: maternal-fetal transfusion
donor twin transfusion
DEF: Abnormal increase of total red blood cells of newborn.

776.5 Congenital anemia N
Anemia following fetal blood loss
EXCLUDES anemia due to isoimmunization (773.0-773.2, 773.5)
hereditary hemolytic anemias (282.0-282.9)

776.6 Anemia of prematurity N

776.7 Transient neonatal neutropenia N
Isoimmune neutropenia
Maternal transfer neutropenia
EXCLUDES congenital neutropenia (nontransient) (288.0)
DEF: Decreased neutrophilic leukocytes in blood of newborn.

776.8 Other specified transient hematological disorders N

776.9 Unspecified hematological disorder specific to fetus or newborn N

✓4th 777 Perinatal disorders of digestive system
INCLUDES disorders specific to the fetus and newborn
EXCLUDES intestinal obstruction classifiable to 560.0-560.9

777.1 Meconium obstruction N
Congenital fecaliths
Delayed passage of meconium
Meconium ileus NOS
Meconium plug syndrome
EXCLUDES meconium ileus in cystic fibrosis (277.01)
DEF: Meconium blocked digestive tract of newborn.

777.2 Intestinal obstruction due to inspissated milk N

777.3 Hematemesis and melena due to swallowed maternal blood N
Swallowed blood syndrome in newborn
EXCLUDES that not due to swallowed maternal blood (772.4)

777.4 Transitory ileus of newborn N
EXCLUDES Hirschsprung's disease (751.3)

777.5 Necrotizing enterocolitis in fetus or newborn N
Pseudomembranous enterocolitis in newborn
DEF: Acute inflammation of small intestine due to pseudomembranous plaque over ulceration; may be due to aggressive antibiotic therapy.

777.6 Perinatal intestinal perforation N
Meconium peritonitis

777.8 Other specified perinatal disorders of digestive system N

777.9 Unspecified perinatal disorder of digestive system N

✓4th 778 Conditions involving the integument and temperature regulation of fetus and newborn

778.0 Hydrops fetalis not due to isoimmunization N
Idiopathic hydrops
EXCLUDES hydrops fetalis due to isoimmunization (773.3)
DEF: Edema of entire body, unrelated to immune response.

778.1 Sclerema neonatorum N
Subcutaneous fat necrosis
DEF: Diffuse, rapidly progressing white, waxy, nonpitting hardening of tissue, usually of legs and feet, life-threatening; found in preterm or debilitated infants; unknown etiology.

778.2 Cold injury syndrome of newborn N
778.3 Other hypothermia of newborn N
778.4 Other disturbances of temperature regulation of newborn N
Dehydration fever in newborn
Environmentally-induced pyrexia
Hyperthermia in newborn
Transitory fever of newborn

778.5 Other and unspecified edema of newborn N
Edema neonatorum

778.6 Congenital hydrocele N
Congenital hydrocele of tunica vaginalis

778.7 Breast engorgement in newborn N
Noninfective mastitis of newborn
EXCLUDES infective mastitis of newborn (771.5)

778.8 Other specified conditions involving the integument of fetus and newborn N
Urticaria neonatorum
EXCLUDES impetigo neonatorum (684)
pemphigus neonatorum (684)

778.9 Unspecified condition involving the integument and temperature regulation of fetus and newborn N

✓4th 779 Other and ill-defined conditions originating in the perinatal period

779.0 Convulsions in newborn N
Fits
Seizures } in newborn

779.1 Other and unspecified cerebral irritability in newborn N

779.2 Cerebral depression, coma, and other abnormal cerebral signs N
CNS dysfunction in newborn NOS

779.3 Feeding problems in newborn N
Regurgitation of food
Slow feeding } in newborn
Vomiting

779.4 Drug reactions and intoxications specific to newborn N
Gray syndrome from chloramphenicol administration in newborn
EXCLUDES fetal alcohol syndrome (760.71)
reactions and intoxications from maternal opiates and tranquilizers (763.5)

779.5   **Drug withdrawal syndrome in newborn**   N

Drug withdrawal syndrome in infant of dependent mother

> EXCLUDES   *fetal alcohol syndrome (760.71)*

779.6   **Termination of pregnancy (fetus)**   N

Fetal death due to:
    induced abortion
    termination of pregnancy

> EXCLUDES   *spontaneous abortion (fetus) (761.8)*

779.7   **Periventricular leukomalacia**

DEF: Necrosis of white matter adjacent to lateral ventricles with the formation of cysts; cause of PVL has not been firmly established, but thought to be related to inadequate blood flow in certain areas of the brain.

√5ᵗʰ **779.8**   **Other specified conditions originating in the perinatal period**

     779.81   **Neonatal bradycardia**   N

> EXCLUDES   *abnormality in fetal heart rate or rhythm complicating labor and delivery (763.81-763.83)*
> *bradycardia due to birth asphyxia (768.5-768.9)*

     779.82   **Neonatal tachycardia**   N

> EXCLUDES   *abnormality in fetal heart rate or rhythm complicating labor and delivery (763.81-763.83)*

     779.89   **Other specified conditions originating in the perinatal period**   N

779.9   **Unspecified condition originating in the perinatal period**   N

Congenital debility NOS
Stillbirth NEC

√4ᵗʰ
√5ᵗʰ   Additional Digit Required   Unspecified Code   Other Specified Code   Manifestation Code   ▶◀ Revised Text   ● New Code   ▲ Revised Code Title

2003 ICD•9•CM   October 2002 • Volume 1 — 231

16. SYMPTOMS, SIGNS, AND ILL-DEFINED CONDITIONS (780-799)

This section includes symptoms, signs, abnormal results of laboratory or other investigative procedures, and ill-defined conditions regarding which no diagnosis classifiable elsewhere is recorded.

Signs and symptoms that point rather definitely to a given diagnosis are assigned to some category in the preceding part of the classification. In general, categories 780-796 include the more ill-defined conditions and symptoms that point with perhaps equal suspicion to two or more diseases or to two or more systems of the body, and without the necessary study of the case to make a final diagnosis. Practically all categories in this group could be designated as "not otherwise specified," or as "unknown etiology," or as "transient." The Alphabetic Index should be consulted to determine which symptoms and signs are to be allocated here and which to more specific sections of the classification; the residual subcategories numbered .9 are provided for other relevant symptoms which cannot be allocated elsewhere in the classification.

The conditions and signs or symptoms included in categories 780-796 consist of: (a) cases for which no more specific diagnosis can be made even after all facts bearing on the case have been investigated; (b) signs or symptoms existing at the time of initial encounter that proved to be transient and whose causes could not be determined; (c) provisional diagnoses in a patient who failed to return for further investigation or care; (d) cases referred elsewhere for investigation or treatment before the diagnosis was made; (e) cases in which a more precise diagnosis was not available for any other reason; (f) certain symptoms which represent important problems in medical care and which it might be desired to classify in addition to a known cause.

SYMPTOMS (780-789)

✓4ᵗʰ **780 General symptoms**

✓5ᵗʰ **780.0 Alteration of consciousness**

> **EXCLUDES** coma:
> diabetic (250.2-250.3)
> hepatic (572.2)
> originating in the perinatal period (779.2)

780.01 Coma
DEF: State of unconsciousness from which the patient cannot be awakened.

780.02 Transient alteration of awareness
DEF: Temporary, recurring spells of reduced consciousness.

780.03 Persistent vegetative state
DEF: Persistent wakefulness without consciousness due to nonfunctioning cerebral cortex.

780.09 Other
Drowsiness　　　　Stupor
Semicoma　　　　Unconsciousness
Somnolence

780.1 Hallucinations
Hallucinations:　　　　Hallucinations:
NOS　　　　olfactory
auditory　　　　tactile
gustatory

> **EXCLUDES** those associated with mental disorders, as functional psychoses (295.0-298.9)
> organic brain syndromes (290.0-294.9, 310.0-310.9)
> visual hallucinations (368.16)

DEF: Perception of external stimulus in absence of stimulus; inability to distinguish between real and imagined.

780.2 Syncope and collapse
Blackout　　　　(Near) (Pre) syncope
Fainting　　　　Vasovagal attack

> **EXCLUDES** carotid sinus syncope (337.0)
> heat syncope (992.1)
> neurocirculatory asthenia (306.2)
> orthostatic hypotension (458.0)
> shock NOS (785.50)

DEF: Sudden unconsciousness due to reduced blood flow to brain.

✓5ᵗʰ **780.3 Convulsions**

> **EXCLUDES** convulsions:
> epileptic (345.10-345.91)
> in newborn (779.0)

DEF: Sudden, involuntary contractions of the muscles.

780.31 Febrile convulsions
Febrile seizure

780.39 Other convulsions
Convulsive disorder NOS
Fit NOS
Seizure NOS

780.4 Dizziness and giddiness
Light-headedness　　　　Vertigo NOS

> **EXCLUDES** Ménière's disease and other specified vertiginous syndromes (386.0-386.9)

DEF: Whirling sensations in head with feeling of falling.

✓5ᵗʰ **780.5 Sleep disturbances**

> **EXCLUDES** that of nonorganic origin (307.40-307.49)

780.50 Sleep disturbance, unspecified

780.51 Insomnia with sleep apnea
DEF: Transient cessation of breathing disturbing sleep.

780.52 Other insomnia
Insomnia NOS
DEF: Inability to maintain adequate sleep cycle.

780.53 Hypersomnia with sleep apnea
DEF: Autonomic response inhibited during sleep; causes insufficient oxygen intake, acidosis and pulmonary hypertension.

780.54 Other hypersomnia
Hypersomnia NOS
DEF: Prolonged sleep cycle.

780.55 Disruptions of 24-hour sleep-wake cycle
Inversion of sleep rhythm
Irregular sleep-wake rhythm NOS
Non-24-hour sleep-wake rhythm

780.56 Dysfunctions associated with sleep stages or arousal from sleep

780.57 Other and unspecified sleep apnea

780.59 Other

780.6 Fever
Chills with fever
Fever NOS
Fever of unknown origin (FUO)
Hyperpyrexia NOS
Pyrexia
Pyrexia of unknown origin

> **EXCLUDES** pyrexia of unknown origin (during):
> in newborn (778.4)
> labor (659.2)
> the puerperium (672)

DEF: Elevated body temperature; no known cause.

✓4ᵗʰ
✓5ᵗʰ Additional Digit Required　　　Unspecified Code　　　Other Specified Code　　　Manifestation Code　　　▶◀ Revised Text　　　● New Code　　　▲ Revised Code Title

Symptoms, Signs, and Ill-Defined Conditions 780.7–782.0

✓5th **780.7 Malaise and fatigue**

EXCLUDES debility, unspecified (799.3)
fatigue (during):
combat (308.0-308.9)
heat (992.6)
pregnancy (646.8)
neurasthenia (300.5)
senile asthenia (797)

DEF: Indefinite feeling of debility or lack of good health.

780.71 Chronic fatigue syndrome

DEF: Persistent fatigue, symptoms include weak muscles, sore throat, lymphadenitis, headache, depression and mild fever; no known cause; also called chronic mononucleosis, benign myalgic encephalomyelitis, Iceland disease and neurosthenia.

780.79 Other malaise and fatigue
Asthenia NOS
Lethargy
Postviral (asthenic) syndrome
Tiredness

DEF: Asthenia: any weakness, lack of strength or loss of energy, especially neuromuscular.

DEF: Lethargy: listlessness, drowsiness, stupor and apathy.

DEF: Postviral (asthenia) syndrome: listlessness, drowsiness, stupor and apathy; follows acute viral infection.

DEF: Tiredness: general exhaustion or fatigue.

780.8 Hyperhidrosis
Diaphoresis
Excessive sweating

DEF: Excessive sweating, appears as droplets on skin; general or localized.

✓5th **780.9 Other general symptoms**

EXCLUDES hypothermia:
NOS (accidental) (991.6)
due to anesthesia (995.89)
of newborn (778.2-778.3)
memory disturbance as part of a
pattern of mental disorder

● **780.91 Fussy infant (baby)**
● **780.92 Excessive crying of infant (baby)**
● **780.99 Other general symptoms**
Amnesia (retrograde)
Chill(s) NOS
Generalized pain
Hypothermia, not associated with low
environmental temperature

✓4th **781 Symptoms involving nervous and musculoskeletal systems**

EXCLUDES depression NOS (311)
disorders specifically relating to:
back (724.0-724.9)
hearing (388.0-389.9)
joint (718.0-719.9)
limb (729.0-729.9)
neck (723.0-723.9)
vision (368.0-369.9)
pain in limb (729.5)

781.0 Abnormal involuntary movements
Abnormal head movements Spasms NOS
Fasciculation Tremor NOS

EXCLUDES abnormal reflex (796.1)
chorea NOS (333.5)
infantile spasms (345.60-345.61)
spastic paralysis (342.1, 343.0-344.9)
specified movement disorders
classifiable to 333 (333.0-333.9)
that of nonorganic origin (307.2-307.3)

781.1 Disturbances of sensation of smell and taste
Anosmia Parosmia
Parageusia

DEF: Anosmia: loss of sense of smell due to organic factors, including loss of olfactory nerve conductivity, cerebral disease, nasal fossae formation and peripheral olfactory nerve diseases; can also be psychological disorder.

DEF: Parageusia: distorted sense of taste, or bad taste in mouth.

DEF: Parosmia: distorted sense of smell.

781.2 Abnormality of gait
Gait: Gait:
ataxic spastic
paralytic staggering

EXCLUDES ataxia:
NOS (781.3)
locomotor (progressive) (094.0)
difficulty in walking (719.7)

DEF: Abnormal, asymmetric gait.

781.3 Lack of coordination
Ataxia NOS Muscular incoordination

EXCLUDES ataxic gait (781.2)
cerebellar ataxia (334.0-334.9)
difficulty in walking (719.7)
vertigo NOS (780.4)

781.4 Transient paralysis of limb
Monoplegia, transient NOS

EXCLUDES paralysis (342.0-344.9)

781.5 Clubbing of fingers

DEF: Enlarged soft tissue of distal fingers.

781.6 Meningismus
Dupré's syndrome Meningism

DEF: Condition with signs and symptoms that resemble meningeal irritation; it is associated with febrile illness and dehydration with no evidence of infection.

781.7 Tetany
Carpopedal spasm

EXCLUDES tetanus neonatorum (771.3)
tetany:
hysterical (300.11)
newborn (hypocalcemic) (775.4)
parathyroid (252.1)
psychogenic (306.0)

DEF: Nerve and muscle hyperexcitability; symptoms include muscle spasms, twitching, cramps, laryngospasm with inspiratory stridor, hyperreflexia and choreiform movements.

781.8 Neurologic neglect syndrome
Asomatognosia Left-sided neglect
Hemi-akinesia Sensory extinction
Hemi-inattention Sensory neglect
Hemispatial neglect Visuospatial neglect

✓5th **781.9 Other symptoms involving nervous and musculoskeletal systems**

781.91 Loss of height

EXCLUDES osteoporosis (733.00-733.09)

781.92 Abnormal posture
● **781.93 Ocular torticollis**
781.99 Other symptoms involving nervous and musculoskeletal systems

✓4th **782 Symptoms involving skin and other integumentary tissue**

EXCLUDES symptoms relating to breast (611.71-611.79)

782.0 Disturbance of skin sensation
Anesthesia of skin
Burning or prickling sensation
Hyperesthesia
Hypoesthesia
Numbness
Paresthesia
Tingling

782.1 Rash and other nonspecific skin eruption
Exanthem
EXCLUDES *vesicular eruption (709.8)*

782.2 Localized superficial swelling, mass, or lump
Subcutaneous nodules
EXCLUDES *localized adiposity (278.1)*

782.3 Edema
Anasarca   Localized edema NOS
Dropsy
EXCLUDES *ascites (789.5)*
edema of:
newborn NOS (778.5)
pregnancy (642.0-642.9, 646.1)
fluid retention (276.6)
hydrops fetalis (773.3, 778.0)
hydrothorax (511.8)
nutritional edema (260, 262)

DEF: Edema: excess fluid in intercellular body tissue.

DEF: Anasarca: massive edema in all body tissues.

DEF: Dropsy: serous fluid accumulated in body cavity or cellular tissue.

DEF: Localized edema: edema in specific body areas.

782.4 Jaundice, unspecified, not of newborn
Cholemia NOS   Icterus NOS
EXCLUDES *jaundice in newborn (774.0-774.7)*
due to isoimmunization (773.0-773.2, 773.4)

DEF: Bilirubin deposits of skin, causing yellow cast.

782.5 Cyanosis
EXCLUDES *newborn ▶(770.83)◀*

DEF: Deficient oxygen of blood; causes blue cast to skin.

✓5ᵗʰ **782.6 Pallor and flushing**
782.61 Pallor
782.62 Flushing
Excessive blushing

782.7 Spontaneous ecchymoses
Petechiae
EXCLUDES *ecchymosis in fetus or newborn (772.6)*
purpura (287.0-287.9)

DEF: Hemorrhagic spots of skin; resemble freckles.

782.8 Changes in skin texture
Induration ⎫
Thickening ⎭ of skin

782.9 Other symptoms involving skin and integumentary tissues

✓4ᵗʰ **783 Symptoms concerning nutrition, metabolism, and development**
783.0 Anorexia
Loss of appetite
EXCLUDES *anorexia nervosa (307.1)*
loss of appetite of nonorganic origin (307.59)

783.1 Abnormal weight gain
EXCLUDES *excessive weight gain in pregnancy (646.1)*
obesity (278.00)
morbid (278.01)

✓5ᵗʰ **783.2 Abnormal loss of weight and underweight**
783.21 Loss of weight
783.22 Underweight

783.3 Feeding difficulties and mismanagement
Feeding problem (elderly) (infant)
EXCLUDES *feeding disturbance or problems:*
in newborn (779.3)
of nonorganic origin (307.50-307.59)

✓5ᵗʰ **783.4 Lack of expected normal physiological development in childhood**
EXCLUDES *delay in sexual development and puberty (259.0)*
gonadal dysgenesis (758.6)
pituitary dwarfism (253.3)
slow fetal growth and fetal malnutrition (764.00-764.99)
specific delays in mental development (315.0-315.9)

783.40 Lack of normal physiological development, unspecified
Inadequate development
Lack of development

783.41 Failure to thrive
Failure to gain weight

DEF: Organic failure to thrive: acute or chronic illness that interferes with nutritional intake, absorption, metabolism excretion and energy requirements. Nonorganic FTT is symptom of neglect or abuse.

783.42 Delayed milestones
Late talker
Late walker

783.43 Short stature
Growth failure
Growth retardation
Lack of growth
Physical retardation

DEF: Constitutional short stature: stature inconsistent with chronological age. Genetic short stature is when skeletal maturation matches chronological age.

783.5 Polydipsia
Excessive thirst

783.6 Polyphagia
Excessive eating   Hyperalimentation NOS
EXCLUDES *disorders of eating of nonorganic origin (307.50-307.59)*

783.7 Adult failure to thrive

783.9 Other symptoms concerning nutrition, metabolism, and development
Hypometabolism
EXCLUDES *abnormal basal metabolic rate (794.7)*
dehydration (276.5)
other disorders of fluid, electrolyte, and acid-base balance (276.0-276.9)

✓4ᵗʰ **784 Symptoms involving head and neck**
EXCLUDES *encephalopathy NOS (348.3)*
specific symptoms involving neck classifiable to 723 (723.0-723.9)

784.0 Headache
Facial pain   Pain in head NOS
EXCLUDES *atypical face pain (350.2)*
migraine (346.0-346.9)
tension headache (307.81)

784.1 Throat pain
EXCLUDES *dysphagia (787.2)*
neck pain (723.1)
sore throat (462)
chronic (472.1)

784.2 Swelling, mass, or lump in head and neck
Space-occupying lesion, intracranial NOS

784.3 Aphasia
EXCLUDES *developmental aphasia (315.31)*

DEF: Inability to communicate through speech, written word, or sign language.

✓5ᵗʰ **784.4 Voice disturbance**
784.40 Voice disturbance, unspecified
784.41 Aphonia
Loss of voice

✓4ᵗʰ ✓5ᵗʰ Additional Digit Required   Unspecified Code   Other Specified Code   Manifestation Code   ▶◄ Revised Text   ● New Code   ▲ Revised Code Title

2003 ICD•9•CM   **October 2002 • Volume 1 — 235**

784.49 Other

Change in voice	Hypernasality
Dysphonia	Hyponasality
Hoarseness	

784.5 Other speech disturbance

Dysarthria	Slurred speech
Dysphasia	

> EXCLUDES   stammering and stuttering (307.0)
> that of nonorganic origin (307.0, 307.9)

√5th **784.6 Other symbolic dysfunction**

> EXCLUDES   developmental learning delays (315.0-315.9)

784.60 Symbolic dysfunction, unspecified

784.61 Alexia and dyslexia

Alexia (with agraphia)

DEF: Alexia: Inability to understand written word due to central brain lesion.

DEF: Dyslexia: Ability to recognize letters but inability to read, spell, and write words; genetic.

784.69 Other

Acalculia	Agraphia NOS
Agnosia	Apraxia

784.7 Epistaxis

Hemorrhage from nose
Nosebleed

784.8 Hemorrhage from throat

> EXCLUDES   hemoptysis (786.3)

784.9 Other symptoms involving head and neck

Choking sensation	Mouth breathing
Halitosis	Sneezing

√4th **785 Symptoms involving cardiovascular system**

> EXCLUDES   heart failure NOS (428.9)

785.0 Tachycardia, unspecified

Rapid heart beat

> EXCLUDES   ▶neonatal tachycardia (779.82)◀
> paroxysmal tachycardia (427.0-427.2)

DEF: Excessively rapid heart rate.

785.1 Palpitations

Awareness of heart beat

> EXCLUDES   specified dysrhythmias (427.0-427.9)

DEF: Shock syndrome: associated with myocardial infarction, cardiac tamponade and massive pulmonary embolism; symptoms include mental torpor, reduced blood pressure, tachycardia, pallor and cold, clammy skin.

785.2 Undiagnosed cardiac murmurs

Heart murmurs NOS

785.3 Other abnormal heart sounds

Cardiac dullness, increased or decreased
Friction fremitus, cardiac
Precordial friction

785.4 Gangrene

Gangrene:
  NOS
  spreading cutaneous
Gangrenous cellulitis
Phagedena
Code first any associated underlying condition

> EXCLUDES   gangrene of certain sites — see
> Alphabetic Index
> gangrene with atherosclerosis of the
> extremities (440.24)
> gas gangrene (040.0)

DEF: Gangrene: necrosis of skin tissue due to bacterial infection, diabetes, embolus and vascular supply loss.

DEF: Gangrenous cellulitis: group A streptococcal infection; begins with severe cellulitis, spreads to superficial and deep fascia; produces gangrene of underlying tissues.

√5th **785.5 Shock without mention of trauma**

785.50 Shock, unspecified

Failure of peripheral circulation

785.51 Cardiogenic shock

DEF: Peripheral circulatory failure due to heart insufficiencies.

785.59 Other

Shock:	Shock:
endotoxic	hypovolemic
gram-negative	septic

> EXCLUDES   shock (due to):
> anesthetic (995.4)
> anaphylactic (995.0)
> due to serum (999.4)
> electric (994.8)
> following abortion (639.5)
> lightning (994.0)
> obstetrical (669.1)
> postoperative (998.0)
> traumatic (958.4)

785.6 Enlargement of lymph nodes

Lymphadenopathy	"Swollen glands"

> EXCLUDES   lymphadenitis (chronic) (289.1-289.3)
> acute (683)

785.9 Other symptoms involving cardiovascular system

Bruit (arterial)	Weak pulse

√4th **786 Symptoms involving respiratory system and other chest symptoms**

√5th **786.0 Dyspnea and respiratory abnormalities**

786.00 Respiratory abnormality, unspecified

786.01 Hyperventilation

> EXCLUDES   hyperventilation, psychogenic (306.1)

DEF: Rapid breathing causes carbon dioxide loss from blood.

786.02 Orthopnea

DEF: Difficulty breathing except in upright position.

786.03 Apnea

> EXCLUDES   ▶apnea of newborn (770.81, 770.82)◀
> sleep apnea (780.51, 780.53, 780.57)

DEF: Cessation of breathing.

786.04 Cheyne-Stokes respiration

DEF: Rhythmic increase of depth and frequency of breathing with apnea; occurs in frontal lobe and diencephalic dysfunction.

786.05 Shortness of breath

DEF: Inability to take in sufficient oxygen.

786.06 Tachypnea

> EXCLUDES   transitory tachypnea of newborn (770.6)

DEF: Abnormal rapid respiratory rate; called hyperventilation.

786.07 Wheezing

> EXCLUDES   asthma (493.00-493.92)

DEF: Stenosis of respiratory passageway; causes whistling sound; due to asthma, coryza, croup, emphysema, hay fever, edema, and pleural effusion.

N Newborn Age: 0   **P** Pediatric Age: 0-17   **M** Maternity Age: 12-55   **A** Adult Age: 15-124   **MSP** Medicare Secondary Payer

236 — Volume 1 • October 2002   *2003 ICD•9•CM*

786.09 Other

> EXCLUDES   *respiratory distress:*
> *following trauma and*
> *surgery (518.5)*
> *newborn ▶(770.89)◀*
> *syndrome (newborn) (769)*
> *adult (518.5)*
> *respiratory failure (518.81,*
> *518.83-518.84)*
> *newborn ▶(770.84)◀*

786.1 Stridor

> EXCLUDES   *congenital laryngeal stridor (748.3)*

DEF: Obstructed airway causes harsh sound.

786.2 Cough

> EXCLUDES   *cough:*
> *psychogenic (306.1)*
> *smokers' (491.0)*
> *with hemorrhage (786.3)*

786.3 Hemoptysis

Cough with hemorrhage
Pulmonary hemorrhage NOS

> EXCLUDES   *pulmonary hemorrhage of newborn*
> *(770.3)*

DEF: Coughing up blood or blood-stained sputum.

786.4 Abnormal sputum

Abnormal:
amount
color   ⎫
odor   ⎬ (of) sputum
Excessive ⎭

√5ᵗʰ 786.5 Chest pain

786.50 Chest pain, unspecified

786.51 Precordial pain

DEF: Chest pain over heart and lower thorax.

786.52 Painful respiration

Pain: Pleurodynia
anterior chest wall
pleuritic

> EXCLUDES   *epidemic pleurodynia (074.1)*

786.59 Other

Discomfort ⎫
Pressure   ⎬ in chest
Tightness ⎭

> EXCLUDES   *pain in breast (611.71)*

786.6 Swelling, mass, or lump in chest

> EXCLUDES   *lump in breast (611.72)*

786.7 Abnormal chest sounds

Abnormal percussion, chest   Rales
Friction sounds, chest   Tympany, chest

> EXCLUDES   *wheezing (786.07)*

786.8 Hiccough

> EXCLUDES   *psychogenic hiccough (306.1)*

786.9 Other symptoms involving respiratory system and chest

Breath-holding spell

√4ᵗʰ 787 Symptoms involving digestive system

> EXCLUDES   *constipation (564.00-564.09)*
> *pylorospasm (537.81)*
> *congenital (750.5)*

√5ᵗʰ 787.0 Nausea and vomiting

Emesis

> EXCLUDES   *hematemesis NOS (578.0)*
> *vomiting:*
> *bilious, following gastrointestinal*
> *surgery (564.3)*
> *cyclical (536.2)*
> *psychogenic (306.4)*
> *excessive, in pregnancy (643.0-*
> *643.9)*
> *habit (536.2)*
> *of newborn (779.3)*
> *psychogenic NOS (307.54)*

787.01 Nausea with vomiting

787.02 Nausea alone

787.03 Vomiting alone

787.1 Heartburn

Pyrosis   Waterbrash

> EXCLUDES   *dyspepsia or indigestion (536.8)*

787.2 Dysphagia

Difficulty in swallowing

787.3 Flatulence, eructation, and gas pain

Abdominal distention (gaseous)
Bloating
Tympanites (abdominal) (intestinal)

> EXCLUDES   *aerophagy (306.4)*

DEF: Flatulence: excess air or gas in intestine or stomach.

DEF: Eructation: belching, expelling gas through mouth.

DEF: Gas pain: gaseous pressure affecting gastrointestinal system.

787.4 Visible peristalsis

Hyperperistalsis

DEF: Increase in involuntary movements of intestines.

787.5 Abnormal bowel sounds

Absent bowel sounds
Hyperactive bowel sounds

787.6 Incontinence of feces

Encopresis NOS
Incontinence of sphincter ani

> EXCLUDES   *that of nonorganic origin (307.7)*

787.7 Abnormal feces

Bulky stools

> EXCLUDES   *abnormal stool content (792.1)*
> *melena:*
> *NOS (578.1)*
> *newborn (772.4, 777.3)*

√5ᵗʰ 787.9 Other symptoms involving digestive system

> EXCLUDES   *gastrointestinal hemorrhage (578.0-*
> *578.9)*
> *intestinal obstruction (560.0-560.9)*
> *specific functional digestive disorders:*
> *esophagus (530.0-530.9)*
> *stomach and duodenum (536.0-*
> *536.9)*
> *those not elsewhere classified*
> *(564.00-564.9)*

787.91 Diarrhea

Diarrhea NOS

787.99 Other

Change in bowel habits
Tenesmus (rectal)

DEF: Tenesmus: painful, ineffective straining at the rectum with limited passage of fecal matter.

√4ᵗʰ √5ᵗʰ Additional Digit Required   Unspecified Code   Other Specified Code   Manifestation Code   ▶◀ Revised Text   ● New Code   ▲ Revised Code Title

2003 ICD•9•CM   **October 2002 • Volume 1 — 237**

✓4ᵗʰ 788 Symptoms involving urinary system

> **EXCLUDES** *hematuria (599.7)*
> *nonspecific findings on examination of the urine (791.0-791.9)*
> *small kidney of unknown cause (589.0-589.9)*
> *uremia NOS (586)*

788.0 Renal colic
Colic (recurrent) of: Colic (recurrent) of:
  kidney   ureter
DEF: Kidney pain.

788.1 Dysuria
Painful urination   Strangury

✓5ᵗʰ 788.2 Retention of urine
DEF: Inability to void.

788.20 Retention of urine, unspecified
788.21 Incomplete bladder emptying
788.29 Other specified retention of urine

✓5ᵗʰ 788.3 Incontinence of urine
▶Code, if applicable, any causal condition first, such as:◀
congenital ureterocele (753.23)
genital prolapse (618.0-618.9)
> **EXCLUDES** *that of nonorganic origin (307.6)*

788.30 Urinary incontinence, unspecified
Enuresis NOS

788.31 Urge incontinence
DEF: Inability to control urination, upon urge to urinate.

788.32 Stress incontinence, male   ♂
> **EXCLUDES** *stress incontinence, female (625.6)*
DEF: Inability to control urination associated with weak sphincter in males.

788.33 Mixed incontinence, (male) (female)
Urge and stress
DEF: Urge, stress incontinence: involuntary discharge of urine due to anatomic displacement.

788.34 Incontinence without sensory awareness
DEF: Involuntary discharge of urine without sensory warning.

788.35 Post-void dribbling
DEF: Involuntary discharge of residual urine after voiding.

788.36 Nocturnal enuresis
DEF: Involuntary discharge of urine during the night.

788.37 Continuous leakage
DEF: Continuous, involuntary urine seepage.

788.39 Other urinary incontinence

✓5ᵗʰ 788.4 Frequency of urination and polyuria
788.41 Urinary frequency
Frequency of micturition
788.42 Polyuria
DEF: Excessive urination.

788.43 Nocturia
DEF: Urination affecting sleep patterns.

788.5 Oliguria and anuria
Deficient secretion of urine
Suppression of urinary secretion
> **EXCLUDES** *that complicating:*
> *abortion (634-638 with .3, 639.3)*
> *ectopic or molar pregnancy (639.3)*
> *pregnancy, childbirth, or the puerperium (642.0-642.9, 646.2)*

DEF: Oliguria: diminished urinary secretion related to fluid intake.

DEF: Anuria: lack of urinary secretion due to renal failure or obstructed urinary tract.

✓5ᵗʰ 788.6 Other abnormality of urination
788.61 Splitting of urinary stream
Intermittent urinary stream
788.62 Slowing of urinary stream
Weak stream
788.69 Other

788.7 Urethral discharge
Penile discharge   Urethrorrhea

788.8 Extravasation of urine
DEF: Leaking or infiltration of urine into tissues.

788.9 Other symptoms involving urinary system
Extrarenal uremia   Vesical:
Vesical: tenesmus
  pain

✓4ᵗʰ 789 Other symptoms involving abdomen and pelvis
> **EXCLUDES** *symptoms referable to genital organs:*
> *female (625.0-625.9)*
> *male (607.0-608.9)*
> *psychogenic (302.70-302.79)*

The following fifth-digit subclassification is to be used for codes 789.0, 789.3, 789.4, 789.6:

  0 **unspecified site**
  1 **right upper quadrant**
  2 **left upper quadrant**
  3 **right lower quadrant**
  4 **left lower quadrant**
  5 **periumbilic**
  6 **epigastric**
  7 **generalized**
  9 **other specified site**
      Multiple sites

✓5ᵗʰ 789.0 Abdominal pain
Colic:
  NOS
  infantile
Cramps, abdominal
> **EXCLUDES** *renal colic (788.0)*

789.1 Hepatomegaly
Enlargement of liver

789.2 Splenomegaly
Enlargement of spleen

✓5ᵗʰ 789.3 Abdominal or pelvic swelling, mass, or lump
Diffuse or generalized swelling or mass:
  abdominal NOS
  umbilical
> **EXCLUDES** *abdominal distention (gaseous) (787.3)*
> *ascites (789.5)*

✓5ᵗʰ 789.4 Abdominal rigidity

789.5 Ascites
Fluid in peritoneal cavity
DEF: Serous fluid effusion and accumulation in abdominal cavity.

✓5ᵗʰ 789.6 Abdominal tenderness
Rebound tenderness

789.9 Other symptoms involving abdomen and pelvis
Umbilical: Umbilical:
  bleeding   discharge

NONSPECIFIC ABNORMAL FINDINGS (790-796)

√4ᵗʰ 790 Nonspecific findings on examination of blood

　　EXCLUDES　*abnormality of:*
　　　　platelets (287.0-287.9)
　　　　thrombocytes (287.0-287.9)
　　　　white blood cells (288.0-288.9)

√5ᵗʰ 790.0　Abnormality of red blood cells

　　EXCLUDES　*anemia:*
　　　　congenital (776.5)
　　　　newborn, due to isoimmunization
　　　　　(773.0-773.2, 773.5)
　　　　of premature infant (776.6)
　　　　other specified types (280.0-285.9)
　　　hemoglobin disorders (282.5-282.7)
　　　polycythemia:
　　　　familial (289.6)
　　　　neonatorum (776.4)
　　　　secondary (289.0)
　　　　vera (238.4)

790.01　Precipitous drop in hematocrit
　　　Drop in hematocrit

790.09　Other abnormality of red blood cells
　　　Abnormal red cell morphology NOS
　　　Abnormal red cell volume NOS
　　　Anisocytosis
　　　Poikilocytosis

790.1　Elevated sedimentation rate

790.2　Abnormal glucose tolerance test
　　EXCLUDES　*that complicating pregnancy, childbirth,*
　　　　or the puerperium (648.8)

790.3　Excessive blood level of alcohol
　　　Elevated blood-alcohol

790.4　Nonspecific elevation of levels of transaminase or lactic acid dehydrogenase [LDH]

790.5　Other nonspecific abnormal serum enzyme levels
　　　Abnormal serum level of:
　　　　acid phosphatase
　　　　alkaline phosphatase
　　　　amylase
　　　　lipase
　　EXCLUDES　*deficiency of circulating enzymes (277.6)*

790.6　Other abnormal blood chemistry
　　　Abnormal blood level of:　Abnormal blood level of:
　　　　cobalt　　　　　　　　magnesium
　　　　copper　　　　　　　 mineral
　　　　iron　　　　　　　　 zinc
　　　　lithium
　　EXCLUDES　*abnormality of electrolyte or acid-base balance (276.0-276.9)*
　　　　hypoglycemia NOS (251.2)
　　　　specific finding indicating abnormality of:
　　　　　amino-acid transport and metabolism (270.0-270.9)
　　　　　carbohydrate transport and metabolism (271.0-271.9)
　　　　　lipid metabolism (272.0-272.9)
　　　　uremia NOS (586)

790.7　Bacteremia
　　EXCLUDES　▶*bacteremia of newborn (771.83)*◀
　　　　septicemia (038)
　　　Use additional code to identify organism (041)
　　DEF: Bacterial infection of blood with no signs of infection.

790.8　Viremia, unspecified
　　DEF: Presence of a virus in the blood stream.

√5ᵗʰ 790.9　Other nonspecific findings on examination of blood

790.91　Abnormal arterial blood gases

790.92　Abnormal coagulation profile
　　　Abnormal or prolonged:
　　　　bleeding time
　　　　coagulation time
　　　　partial thromboplastin time [PTT]
　　　　prothrombin time [PT]
　　EXCLUDES　*coagulation (hemorrhagic) disorders (286.0-286.9)*

790.93　Elevated prostate specific antigen, (PSA) A ♂

790.94　Euthyroid sick syndrome
　　DEF: Transient alteration of thyroid hormone metabolism due to nonthyroid illness or stress.

790.99　Other

√4ᵗʰ 791 Nonspecific findings on examination of urine
　　EXCLUDES　*hematuria NOS (599.7)*
　　　specific findings indicating abnormality of:
　　　　amino-acid transport and metabolism (270.0-270.9)
　　　　carbohydrate transport and metabolism (271.0-271.9)

791.0　Proteinuria
　　　Albuminuria　　　　Bence-Jones proteinuria
　　EXCLUDES　*postural proteinuria (593.6)*
　　　　that arising during pregnancy or the puerperium (642.0-642.9, 646.2)
　　DEF: Excess protein in urine.

791.1　Chyluria
　　EXCLUDES　*filarial (125.0-125.9)*
　　DEF: Excess chyle in urine.

791.2　Hemoglobinuria
　　DEF: Free hemoglobin in blood due to rapid hemolysis of red blood cells.

791.3　Myoglobinuria
　　DEF: Myoglobin (oxygen-transporting pigment) in urine.

791.4　Biliuria
　　DEF: Bile pigments in urine.

791.5　Glycosuria
　　EXCLUDES　*renal glycosuria (271.4)*
　　DEF: Sugar in urine.

791.6　Acetonuria
　　　Ketonuria
　　DEF: Excess acetone in urine.

791.7　Other cells and casts in urine

791.9　Other nonspecific findings on examination of urine
　　　Crystalluria　　　　　　Elevated urine levels of:
　　　Elevated urine levels of:　　vanillylmandelic
　　　　17-ketosteroids　　　　　 acid [VMA]
　　　　catecholamines　　　　Melanuria
　　　　indolacetic acid

√4ᵗʰ 792 Nonspecific abnormal findings in other body substances
　　EXCLUDES　*that in chromosomal analysis (795.2)*

792.0　Cerebrospinal fluid

792.1　Stool contents
　　　Abnormal stool color　Occult stool
　　　Fat in stool　　　　　Pus in stool
　　　Mucus in stool
　　EXCLUDES　*blood in stool [melena] (578.1)*
　　　　newborn (772.4, 777.3)

792.2　Semen　♂
　　　Abnormal spermatozoa
　　EXCLUDES　*azoospermia (606.0)*
　　　　oligospermia (606.1)

792.3　Amniotic fluid　M ♀
　　DEF: Nonspecific abnormal findings in amniotic fluid.

792.4　Saliva
　　EXCLUDES　*that in chromosomal analysis (795.2)*

Symptoms, Signs, and Ill-Defined Conditions 790–792.4

√4ᵗʰ / √5ᵗʰ　Additional Digit Required　　Unspecified Code　　Other Specified Code　　Manifestation Code　　▶◀ Revised Text　　● New Code　　▲ Revised Code Title

2003 ICD•9•CM　　　　　　　　　　　　　　　　　　　　October 2002 • Volume 1 — 239

Symptoms, Signs, and III-Defined Conditions 792.5–795.09

792.5 Cloudy (hemodialysis) (peritoneal) dialysis effluent

792.9 Other nonspecific abnormal findings in body substances

Peritoneal fluid   Synovial fluid
Pleural fluid   Vaginal fluids

✓4ᵗʰ **793** Nonspecific abnormal findings on radiological and other examination of body structure

INCLUDES   nonspecific abnormal findings of:
thermography
ultrasound examination [echogram]
x-ray examination

EXCLUDES   *abnormal results of function studies and radioisotope scans (794.0-794.9)*

793.0 Skull and head

EXCLUDES   *nonspecific abnormal echoencephalogram (794.01)*

793.1 Lung field

Coin lesion
Shadow } (of) lung

DEF: Coin lesion of lung: coin-shaped, solitary pulmonary nodule; diagnosis includes tuberculoma, histoplasmoma, blastomycoma, coccidioidomycoma, primary carcinoma of the lung, metastatic carcinoma and benign pulmonary tumor.

793.2 Other intrathoracic organ

Abnormal: Abnormal:
echocardiogram   ultrasound cardiogram
heart shadow   Mediastinal shift

793.3 Biliary tract

Nonvisualization of gallbladder

793.4 Gastrointestinal tract

793.5 Genitourinary organs

Filling defect: Filling defect:
bladder   ureter
kidney

793.6 Abdominal area, including retroperitoneum

793.7 Musculoskeletal system

✓5ᵗʰ **793.8** Breast

793.80 Abnormal mammogram, unspecified

793.81 Mammographic microcalcification

DEF: Calcium and cellular debris deposits in the breast that cannot be felt but can be detected on a mammogram; can be a sign of cancer, benign conditions, or changes in the breast tissue as a result of inflammation, injury, or obstructed duct.

793.89 Other abnormal findings on radiological examination of breast

793.9 Other

Abnormal:
placental finding by x-ray or ultrasound method
radiological findings in skin and subcutaneous tissue

EXCLUDES   *abnormal finding by radioisotope localization of placenta (794.9)*

✓4ᵗʰ **794** Nonspecific abnormal results of function studies

INCLUDES   radioisotope:
scans
uptake studies
scintiphotography

✓5ᵗʰ **794.0** Brain and central nervous system

794.00 Abnormal function study, unspecified

794.01 Abnormal echoencephalogram

794.02 Abnormal electroencephalogram [EEG]

794.09 Other

Abnormal brain scan

✓5ᵗʰ **794.1** Peripheral nervous system and special senses

794.10 Abnormal response to nerve stimulation, unspecified

794.11 Abnormal retinal function studies

Abnormal electroretinogram [ERG]

794.12 Abnormal electro-oculogram [EOG]

794.13 Abnormal visually evoked potential

794.14 Abnormal oculomotor studies

794.15 Abnormal auditory function studies

794.16 Abnormal vestibular function studies

794.17 Abnormal electromyogram [EMG]

EXCLUDES   *that of eye (794.14)*

794.19 Other

794.2 Pulmonary

Abnormal lung scan   Reduced:
Reduced: vital capacity
ventilatory capacity

✓5ᵗʰ **794.3** Cardiovascular

794.30 Abnormal function study, unspecified

794.31 Abnormal electrocardiogram [ECG] [EKG]

794.39 Other

Abnormal: Abnormal:
ballistocardiogram   vectorcardiogram
phonocardiogram

794.4 Kidney

Abnormal renal function test

794.5 Thyroid

Abnormal thyroid: Abnormal thyroid:
scan   uptake

794.6 Other endocrine function study

794.7 Basal metabolism

Abnormal basal metabolic rate [BMR]

794.8 Liver

Abnormal liver scan

794.9 Other

Bladder   Placenta
Pancreas   Spleen

✓4ᵗʰ **795** Nonspecific abnormal histological and immunological findings

EXCLUDES   *nonspecific abnormalities of red blood cells (790.01-790.09)*

✓5ᵗʰ **795.0** Nonspecific abnormal Papanicolaou smear of cervix

EXCLUDES   ▸*carcinoma in-situ of cervix (233.1)*
cervical intraepithelial neoplasia I (CIN I) (622.1)
cervical intraepithelial neoplasia II (CIN II) (622.1)
cervical intraepithelial neoplasia III (CIN III) (233.1)
dyplasia of cervix (uteri) (622.1)
high grade squamous intraepithelial dysplasia (HGSIL) (622.1)
low grade squamous intraepithelial dysplasia (LGSIL) (622.1)◄

● **795.00** Nonspecific abnormal Papanicolaou smear of cervix, unspecified ♀

● **795.01** Atypical squamous cell changes of undetermined significance favor benign (ASCUS favor benign) ♀

Atypical glandular cell changes of undetermined significance favor benign (AGCUS favor benign)

● **795.02** Atypical squamous cell changes of undetermined significance favor dysplasia (ASCUS favor dysplasia) ♀

Atypical glandular cell changes of undetermined significance favor dysplasia (AGCUS favor dysplasia)

● **795.09** Other nonspecific abnormal Papanicolaou smear of cervix ♀

Benign cellular changes
Unsatisfactory smear

795.1 Nonspecific abnormal Papanicolaou smear of other site

795.2 Nonspecific abnormal findings on chromosomal analysis
  Abnormal karyotype

√5th **795.3 Nonspecific positive culture findings**
  Positive culture findings in:
    nose
    sputum
    throat
    wound
    EXCLUDES *that of:*
      blood (790.7-790.8)
      urine (791.9)

● **795.31 Nonspecific positive findings for anthrax**
    Positive findings by nasal swab

● **795.39 Other nonspecific positive culture findings**

795.4 Other nonspecific abnormal histological findings

795.5 Nonspecific reaction to tuberculin skin test without active tuberculosis
  Abnormal result of Mantoux test
  PPD positive
  Tuberculin (skin test):
    positive
    reactor

795.6 False positive serological test for syphilis
  False positive Wassermann reaction

√5th **795.7 Other nonspecific immunological findings**
    EXCLUDES *isoimmunization, in pregnancy (656.1-656.2)*
      affecting fetus or newborn (773.0-773.2)

795.71 Nonspecific serologic evidence of human immunodeficiency virus [HIV]
    Inclusive human immunodeficiency [HIV] test (adult) (infant)
    Note: This code is ONLY to be used when a test finding is reported as nonspecific. Asymptomatic positive findings are coded to V08. If any HIV infection symptom or condition is present, see code 042. Negative findings are not coded.
    EXCLUDES *acquired immunodeficiency syndrome [AIDS] (042)*
      asymptomatic human immunodeficiency virus, [HIV] infection status (V08)
      HIV infection, symptomatic (042)
      human immunodeficiency virus [HIV] disease (042)
      positive (status) NOS (V08)

795.79 Other and unspecified nonspecific immunological findings
    Raised antibody titer
    Raised level of immunoglobulins

√4th **796 Other nonspecific abnormal findings**

796.0 Nonspecific abnormal toxicological findings
    Abnormal levels of heavy metals or drugs in blood, urine, or other tissue
    EXCLUDES *excessive blood level of alcohol (790.3)*

796.1 Abnormal reflex

796.2 Elevated blood pressure reading without diagnosis of hypertension
    Note: This category is to be used to record an episode of elevated blood pressure in a patient in whom no formal diagnosis of hypertension has been made, or as an incidental finding.

796.3 Nonspecific low blood pressure reading

796.4 Other abnormal clinical findings

796.5 Abnormal finding on antenatal screening M♀

796.9 Other

ILL-DEFINED AND UNKNOWN CAUSES OF MORBIDITY AND MORTALITY (797-799)

797 Senility without mention of psychosis
  Old age   Senile:
  Senescence   debility
  Senile asthenia   exhaustion
    EXCLUDES *senile psychoses (290.0-290.9)*

√4th **798 Sudden death, cause unknown**

798.0 Sudden infant death syndrome P
    Cot death   Sudden death of nonspecific
    Crib death   cause in infancy
    DEF: Sudden Infant Death Syndrome (SIDS): death of infant under age one due to nonspecific cause.

798.1 Instantaneous death

798.2 Death occurring in less than 24 hours from onset of symptoms, not otherwise explained
    Death known not to be violent or instantaneous, for which no cause could be discovered
    Died without sign of disease

798.9 Unattended death
    Death in circumstances where the body of the deceased was found and no cause could be discovered
    Found dead

√4th **799 Other ill-defined and unknown causes of morbidity and mortality**
  DEF: Weakened organ functions due to complex chronic medical conditions.

799.0 Asphyxia
    EXCLUDES *asphyxia (due to):*
      carbon monoxide (986)
      inhalation of food or foreign body (932-934.9)
      newborn (768.0-768.9)
      traumatic (994.7)
    DEF: Lack of oxygen.

799.1 Respiratory arrest
    Cardiorespiratory failure
    EXCLUDES *cardiac arrest (427.5)*
      failure of peripheral circulation (785.50)
      respiratory distress:
        NOS (786.09)
        acute (518.82)
        following trauma and surgery (518.5)
        newborn ▶(770.89)◀
        syndrome (newborn) (769)
          adult (following trauma and surgery) (518.5)
        other (518.82)
      respiratory failure (518.81, 518.83-518.84)
        newborn ▶(770.84)◀
      respiratory insufficiency (786.09)
        acute (518.82)

799.2 Nervousness
    "Nerves"

799.3 Debility, unspecified
    EXCLUDES *asthenia (780.79)*
      nervous debility (300.5)
      neurasthenia (300.5)
      senile asthenia (797)

799.4 Cachexia
    Wasting disease
    EXCLUDES *nutritional marasmus (261)*

√4th √5th Additional Digit Required   Unspecified Code   Other Specified Code   Manifestation Code   ▶◀ Revised Text   ● New Code   ▲ Revised Code Title

799.8   **Other ill-defined conditions**

DEF: General ill health and poor nutrition.

799.9   **Other unknown and unspecified cause**

Undiagnosed disease, not specified as to site or system involved

Unknown cause of morbidity or mortality

17. INJURY AND POISONING (800-999)

Use E code(s) to identify the cause and intent of the injury or poisoning (E800-E999)

Note:

1. The principle of multiple coding of injuries should be followed wherever possible. Combination categories for multiple injuries are provided for use when there is insufficient detail as to the nature of the individual conditions, or for primary tabulation purposes when it is more convenient to record a single code; otherwise, the component injuries should be coded separately.

   Where multiple sites of injury are specified in the titles, the word "with" indicates involvement of both sites, and the word "and" indicates involvement of either or both sites. The word "finger" thumb.

2. Categories for "late effect" of injuries are to be found at 905-909.

FRACTURES (800-829)

EXCLUDES   *malunion (733.81)*
nonunion (733.82)
pathological or spontaneous fracture (733.10-733.19)
stress fractures (733.93-733.95)

The terms "condyle," "coronoid process," "ramus," and "symphysis" indicate the portion of the bone fractured, not the name of the bone involved.

The descriptions "closed" and "open" used in the fourth-digit subdivisions include the following terms:

closed (with or without delayed healing):

comminuted	impacted
depressed	linear
elevated	simple
fissured	slipped epiphysis
fracture NOS	spiral
greenstick	

open (with or without delayed healing):

compound	puncture
infected	with foreign body
missile	

A fracture not indicated as closed or open should be classified as closed.

FRACTURE OF SKULL (800-804)

The following fifth-digit subclassification is for use with the appropriate codes in categories 800, 801, 803, and 804:

0   unspecified state of consciousness
1   with no loss of consciousness
2   with brief [less than one hour] loss of consciousness
3   with moderate [1-24 hours] loss of consciousness
4   with prolonged [more than 24 hours] loss of consciousness and return to pre-existing conscious level
5   with prolonged [more than 24 hours] loss of consciousness, without return to pre-existing conscious level
     Use fifth-digit 5 to designate when a patient is unconscious and dies before regaining consciousness, regardless of the duration of the loss of consciousness
6   with loss of consciousness of unspecified duration
9   with concussion, unspecified

Fractures

Fracture-dislocation   Impacted
Avulsion
Open (skin broken)
Oblique
Epiphyseal
March
Closed spiral
Linear (fissured)
Greenstick
Depressed
Comminuted

✓4th 800 Fracture of vault of skull
     INCLUDES   frontal bone
                    parietal bone
     DEF: Fracture of bone that forms skull dome and protects brain.

§ ✓5th   **800.0**   Closed without mention of intracranial injury   **MSP**
§ ✓5th   **800.1**   Closed with cerebral laceration and contusion   **MSP**
§ ✓5th   **800.2**   Closed with subarachnoid, subdural, and extradural hemorrhage   **MSP**
§ ✓5th   **800.3**   Closed with other and unspecified intracranial hemorrhage   **MSP**
§ ✓5th   **800.4**   Closed with intracranial injury of other and unspecified nature   **MSP**
§ ✓5th   **800.5**   Open without mention of intracranial injury   **MSP**
§ ✓5th   **800.6**   Open with cerebral laceration and contusion   **MSP**
§ ✓5th   **800.7**   Open with subarachnoid, subdural, and extradural hemorrhage   **MSP**
§ ✓5th   **800.8**   Open with other and unspecified intracranial hemorrhage   **MSP**
§ ✓5th   **800.9**   Open with intracranial injury of other and unspecified nature   **MSP**

✓4th 801 Fracture of base of skull
     INCLUDES   fossa:
                     anterior
                     middle
                     posterior
                occiput bone
                orbital roof
                sinus:
                     ethmoid
                     frontal
                sphenoid bone
                temporal bone
     DEF: Fracture of bone that forms skull floor.

§ ✓5th   **801.0**   Closed without mention of intracranial injury   **MSP**
§ ✓5th   **801.1**   Closed with cerebral laceration and contusion   **MSP**
§ ✓5th   **801.2**   Closed with subarachnoid, subdural, and extradural hemorrhage   **MSP**
§ ✓5th   **801.3**   Closed with other and unspecified intracranial hemorrhage   **MSP**
§ ✓5th   **801.4**   Closed with intracranial injury of other and unspecified nature   **MSP**
§ ✓5th   **801.5**   Open without mention of intracranial injury   **MSP**
§ ✓5th   **801.6**   Open with cerebral laceration and contusion   **MSP**
§ ✓5th   **801.7**   Open with subarachnoid, subdural, and extradural hemorrhage   **MSP**
§ ✓5th   **801.8**   Open with other and unspecified intracranial hemorrhage   **MSP**

§ Requires fifth-digit. See beginning of section 800–804 for codes and definitions.

✓4th / ✓5th Additional Digit Required   Unspecified Code   Other Specified Code   Manifestation Code   ▶◀ Revised Text   ● New Code   ▲ Revised Code Title

Injury and Poisoning 800–801.8

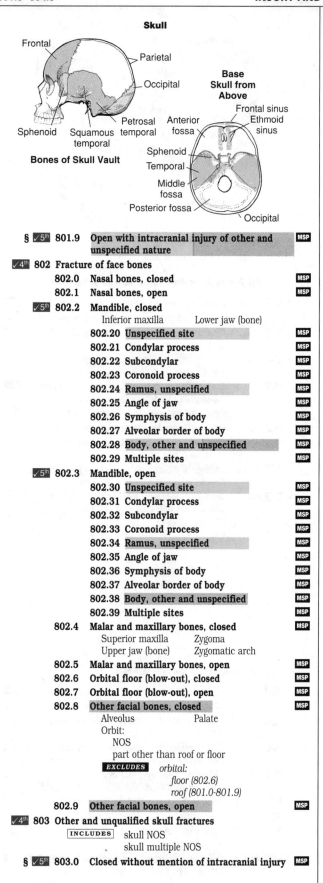

Skull

Frontal
Parietal
Occipital

Base Skull from Above

Sphenoid
Petrosal temporal
Squamous temporal

Frontal sinus
Ethmoid sinus
Anterior fossa
Sphenoid
Temporal
Middle fossa
Posterior fossa
Occipital

Bones of Skull Vault

Facial Fractures

Frontal bone
Nasal bone
Type III
Type II
Type I
Maxilla

LeFort Fracture Types

Orbital floor
Zygomatic bone (malar) and arch
Subcondylar
Body
Angle
Symphysis
Parasymphysis

Common Fracture Sites of Mandible

§ ✓5th **801.9** Open with intracranial injury of other and unspecified nature `MSP`

✓4th **802 Fracture of face bones**

802.0 Nasal bones, closed `MSP`

802.1 Nasal bones, open `MSP`

✓5th **802.2** Mandible, closed
Inferior maxilla   Lower jaw (bone)

802.20 Unspecified site `MSP`
802.21 Condylar process `MSP`
802.22 Subcondylar `MSP`
802.23 Coronoid process `MSP`
802.24 Ramus, unspecified `MSP`
802.25 Angle of jaw `MSP`
802.26 Symphysis of body `MSP`
802.27 Alveolar border of body `MSP`
802.28 Body, other and unspecified `MSP`
802.29 Multiple sites `MSP`

✓5th **802.3** Mandible, open

802.30 Unspecified site `MSP`
802.31 Condylar process `MSP`
802.32 Subcondylar `MSP`
802.33 Coronoid process `MSP`
802.34 Ramus, unspecified `MSP`
802.35 Angle of jaw `MSP`
802.36 Symphysis of body `MSP`
802.37 Alveolar border of body `MSP`
802.38 Body, other and unspecified `MSP`
802.39 Multiple sites `MSP`

802.4 Malar and maxillary bones, closed `MSP`
Superior maxilla   Zygoma
Upper jaw (bone)   Zygomatic arch

802.5 Malar and maxillary bones, open `MSP`

802.6 Orbital floor (blow-out), closed `MSP`

802.7 Orbital floor (blow-out), open `MSP`

802.8 Other facial bones, closed `MSP`
Alveolus   Palate
Orbit:
    NOS
    part other than roof or floor
    `EXCLUDES` orbital:
        floor (802.6)
        roof (801.0-801.9)

802.9 Other facial bones, open `MSP`

✓4th **803 Other and unqualified skull fractures**
`INCLUDES` skull NOS
skull multiple NOS

§ ✓5th **803.0** Closed without mention of intracranial injury `MSP`

§ ✓5th **803.1** Closed with cerebral laceration and contusion `MSP`

§ ✓5th **803.2** Closed with subarachnoid, subdural, and extradural hemorrhage `MSP`

§ ✓5th **803.3** Closed with other and unspecified intracranial hemorrhage `MSP`

§ ✓5th **803.4** Closed with intracranial injury of other and unspecified nature `MSP`

§ ✓5th **803.5** Open without mention of intracranial injury `MSP`

§ ✓5th **803.6** Open with cerebral laceration and contusion `MSP`

§ ✓5th **803.7** Open with subarachnoid, subdural, and extradural hemorrhage `MSP`

§ ✓5th **803.8** Open with other and unspecified intracranial hemorrhage `MSP`

§ ✓5th **803.9** Open with intracranial injury of other and unspecified nature `MSP`

✓4th **804 Multiple fractures involving skull or face with other bones**

§ ✓5th **804.0** Closed without mention of intracranial injury `MSP`

§ ✓5th **804.1** Closed with cerebral laceration and contusion `MSP`

§ ✓5th **804.2** Closed with subarachnoid, subdural, and extradural hemorrhage `MSP`

§ ✓5th **804.3** Closed with other and unspecified intracranial hemorrhage `MSP`

§ ✓5th **804.4** Closed with intracranial injury of other and unspecified nature `MSP`

§ ✓5th **804.5** Open without mention of intracranial injury `MSP`

§ ✓5th **804.6** Open with cerebral laceration and contusion `MSP`

§ ✓5th **804.7** Open with subarachnoid, subdural, and extradural hemorrage `MSP`

§ ✓5th **804.8** Open with other and unspecified intracranial hemorrhage `MSP`

§ ✓5th **804.9** Open with intracranial injury of other and unspecified nature `MSP`

§ Requires fifth-digit. See beginning of section 800–804 for codes and definitions.

`N` Newborn Age: 0   `P` Pediatric Age: 0-17   `M` Maternity Age: 12-55   `A` Adult Age: 15-124   `MSP` Medicare Secondary Payer

FRACTURE OF NECK AND TRUNK (805-809)

√4ᵗʰ **805 Fracture of vertebral column without mention of spinal cord injury**

> INCLUDES   neural arch
> spine
> spinous process
> transverse process
> vertebra

The following fifth-digit subclassification is for use with codes 805.0-805.1:

0 cervical vertebra, unspecified level
1 first cervical vertebra
2 second cervical vertebra
3 third cervical vertebra
4 fourth cervical vertebra
5 fifth cervical vertebra
6 sixth cervical vertebra
7 seventh cervical vertebra
8 multiple cervical vertebrae

√5ᵗʰ **805.0 Cervical, closed** `MSP`
    Atlas
    Axis

√5ᵗʰ **805.1 Cervical, open** `MSP`
805.2 Dorsal [thoracic], closed `MSP`
805.3 Dorsal [thoracic], open `MSP`
805.4 Lumbar, closed `MSP`
805.5 Lumbar, open `MSP`
805.6 Sacrum and coccyx, closed `MSP`
805.7 Sacrum and coccyx, open `MSP`
805.8 Unspecified, closed `MSP`
805.9 Unspecified, open `MSP`

√4ᵗʰ **806 Fracture of vertebral column with spinal cord injury**

> INCLUDES   any condition classifiable to 805 with:
> complete or incomplete transverse lesion (of cord)
> hematomyelia
> injury to:
>   cauda equina
>   nerve
> paralysis
> paraplegia
> quadriplegia
> spinal concussion

√5ᵗʰ **806.0 Cervical, closed**

806.00 C_1-C_4 level with unspecified spinal cord injury `MSP`
    Cervical region NOS with spinal cord injury NOS

806.01 C_1-C_4 level with complete lesion of cord `MSP`

806.02 C_1-C_4 level with anterior cord syndrome `MSP`

806.03 C_1-C_4 level with central cord syndrome `MSP`

806.04 C_1-C_4 level with other specified spinal cord injury `MSP`
    C_1-C_4 level with:
      incomplete spinal cord lesion NOS
      posterior cord syndrome

806.05 C_5-C_7 level with unspecified spinal cord injury `MSP`

806.06 C_5-C_7 level with complete lesion of cord `MSP`

806.07 C_5-C_7 level with anterior cord syndrome `MSP`

806.08 C_5-C_7 level with central cord syndrome `MSP`

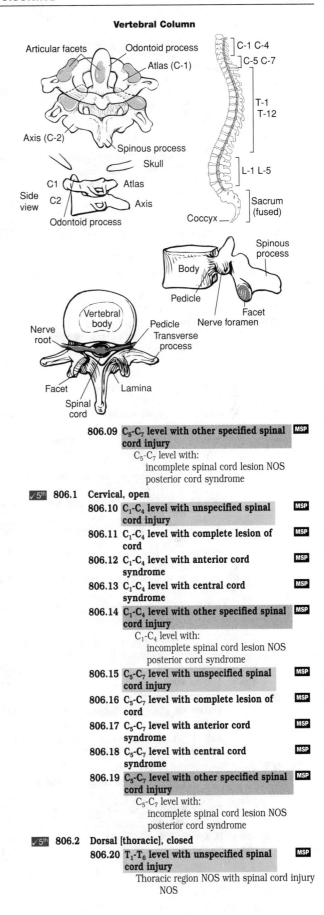

Vertebral Column

Articular facets — Odontoid process — Atlas (C-1) — Axis (C-2) — Spinous process — Skull — Side view — C1 — C2 — Atlas — Axis — Odontoid process — C-1 C-4 — C-5 C-7 — T-1 T-12 — L-1 L-5 — Sacrum (fused) — Coccyx — Spinous process — Body — Pedicle — Facet — Nerve root — Vertebral body — Pedicle — Nerve foramen — Transverse process — Facet — Lamina — Spinal cord

806.09 C_5-C_7 level with other specified spinal cord injury `MSP`
    C_5-C_7 level with:
      incomplete spinal cord lesion NOS
      posterior cord syndrome

√5ᵗʰ **806.1 Cervical, open**

806.10 C_1-C_4 level with unspecified spinal cord injury `MSP`

806.11 C_1-C_4 level with complete lesion of cord `MSP`

806.12 C_1-C_4 level with anterior cord syndrome `MSP`

806.13 C_1-C_4 level with central cord syndrome `MSP`

806.14 C_1-C_4 level with other specified spinal cord injury `MSP`
    C_1-C_4 level with:
      incomplete spinal cord lesion NOS
      posterior cord syndrome

806.15 C_5-C_7 level with unspecified spinal cord injury `MSP`

806.16 C_5-C_7 level with complete lesion of cord `MSP`

806.17 C_5-C_7 level with anterior cord syndrome `MSP`

806.18 C_5-C_7 level with central cord syndrome `MSP`

806.19 C_5-C_7 level with other specified spinal cord injury `MSP`
    C_5-C_7 level with:
      incomplete spinal cord lesion NOS
      posterior cord syndrome

√5ᵗʰ **806.2 Dorsal [thoracic], closed**

806.20 T_1-T_6 level with unspecified spinal cord injury `MSP`
    Thoracic region NOS with spinal cord injury NOS

√4ᵗʰ / √5ᵗʰ Additional Digit Required   Unspecified Code   Other Specified Code   Manifestation Code   ►◄ Revised Text   ● New Code   ▲ Revised Code Title

Injury and Poisoning 806.21–808.9

806.21 T_1-T_6 level with complete lesion of cord   `MSP`

806.22 T_1-T_6 level with anterior cord syndrome   `MSP`

806.23 T_1-T_6 level with central cord syndrome   `MSP`

806.24 T_1-T_6 level with other specified spinal cord injury   `MSP`
    T_1-T_6 level with:
      incomplete spinal cord lesion NOS
      posterior cord syndrome

806.25 T_7-T_{12} level with unspecified spinal cord injury   `MSP`

806.26 T_7-T_{12} level with complete lesion of cord   `MSP`

806.27 T_7-T_{12} level with anterior cord syndrome   `MSP`

806.28 T_7-T_{12} level with central cord syndrome   `MSP`

806.29 T_7-T_{12} level with other specified spinal cord injury   `MSP`
    T_7-T_{12} level with:
      incomplete spinal cord lesion NOS
      posterior cord syndrome

✓5th **806.3** Dorsal [thoracic], open

806.30 T_1-T_6 level with unspecified spinal cord injury   `MSP`

806.31 T_1-T_6 level with complete lesion of cord   `MSP`

806.32 T_1-T_6 level with anterior cord syndrome   `MSP`

806.33 T_1-T_6 level with central cord syndrome   `MSP`

806.34 T_1-T_6 level with other specified spinal cord injury   `MSP`
    T_1-T_6 level with:
      incomplete spinal cord lesion NOS
      posterior cord syndrome

806.35 T_7-T_{12} level with unspecified spinal cord injury   `MSP`

806.36 T_7-T_{12} level with complete lesion of cord   `MSP`

806.37 T_7-T_{12} level with anterior cord syndrome   `MSP`

806.38 T_7-T_{12} level with central cord syndrome   `MSP`

806.39 T_7-T_{12} level with other specified spinal cord injury   `MSP`
    T_7-T_{12} level with:
      incomplete spinal cord lesion NOS
      posterior cord syndrome

806.4 Lumbar, closed   `MSP`

806.5 Lumbar, open   `MSP`

✓5th **806.6** Sacrum and coccyx, closed

806.60 With unspecified spinal cord injury   `MSP`

806.61 With complete cauda equina lesion   `MSP`

806.62 With other cauda equina injury   `MSP`

806.69 With other spinal cord injury   `MSP`

✓5th **806.7** Sacrum and coccyx, open

806.70 With unspecified spinal cord injury   `MSP`

806.71 With complete cauda equina lesion   `MSP`

806.72 With other cauda equina injury   `MSP`

806.79 With other spinal cord injury   `MSP`

806.8 Unspecified, closed   `MSP`

806.9 Unspecified, open   `MSP`

✓4th **807** Fracture of rib(s), sternum, larynx, and trachea

The following fifth-digit subclassification is for use with codes 807.0-807.1:

    0   rib(s), unspecified
    1   one rib
    2   two ribs
    3   three ribs
    4   four ribs
    5   five ribs
    6   six ribs
    7   seven ribs
    8   eight or more ribs
    9   multiple ribs, unspecified

✓5th **807.0** Rib(s), closed   `MSP`

✓5th **807.1** Rib(s), open   `MSP`

807.2 Sternum, closed   `MSP`
    DEF: Break in flat bone (breast bone) in anterior thorax.

807.3 Sternum, open   `MSP`
    DEF: Break, with open wound, in flat bone in mid anterior thorax.

807.4 Flail chest   `MSP`

807.5 Larynx and trachea, closed   `MSP`
    Hyoid bone   Trachea
    Thyroid cartilage

807.6 Larynx and trachea, open   `MSP`

✓4th **808** Fracture of pelvis

808.0 Acetabulum, closed

808.1 Acetabulum, open

808.2 Pubis, closed

808.3 Pubis, open

✓5th **808.4** Other specified part, closed

808.41 Ilium

808.42 Ischium

808.43 Multiple pelvic fractures with disruption of pelvic circle

808.49 Other
    Innominate bone   Pelvic rim

✓5th **808.5** Other specified part, open

808.51 Ilium

808.52 Ischium

808.53 Multiple pelvic fractures with disruption of pelvic circle

808.59 Other

808.8 Unspecified, closed

808.9 Unspecified, open

Pelvis and Pelvic Fractures

Fractures Disrupting Pelvic Circle — Pelvic circle — Stable — Unstable (two-place fracture)

Iliac crest — Ilium — L5 — Anterior superior iliac spine — Ischial spine — Acetabulum — Femur — Ischial tuberosity

Pelvic Bones — Sacrum — Coccyx — Pubis — Pubic symphysis

Acetabular Fractures — Posterior pillar — Transverse

 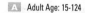

✓4th **809 Ill-defined fractures of bones of trunk**

> INCLUDES   bones of trunk with other bones except those of skull and face
> multiple bones of trunk
>
> EXCLUDES   *multiple fractures of:*
> *pelvic bones alone (808.0-808.9)*
> *ribs alone (807.0-807.1, 807.4)*
> *ribs or sternum with limb bones (819.0-819.1, 828.0-828.1)*
> *skull or face with other bones (804.0-804.9)*

809.0   Fracture of bones of trunk, closed

809.1   Fracture of bones of trunk, open

FRACTURE OF UPPER LIMB (810-819)

✓4th **810 Fracture of clavicle**

> INCLUDES   collar bone
> interligamentous part of clavicle

The following fifth-digit subclassification is for use with category 810:

0   unspecified part
   Clavicle NOS
1   sternal end of clavicle
2   shaft of clavicle
3   acromial end of clavicle

✓5th **810.0   Closed**   MSP
✓5th **810.1   Open**   MSP

✓4th **811 Fracture of scapula**

> INCLUDES   shoulder blade

The following fifth-digit subclassification is for use with category 811:

0   unspecified part
1   acromial process
   Acromion (process)
2   coracoid process
3   glenoid cavity and neck of scapula
9   other

✓5th **811.0   Closed**   MSP
✓5th **811.1   Open**   MSP

✓4th **812 Fracture of humerus**

✓5th **812.0   Upper end, closed**
   812.00   Upper end, unspecified part
      Proximal end   Shoulder
   812.01   Surgical neck
      Neck of humerus NOS
   812.02   Anatomical neck
   812.03   Greater tuberosity
   812.09   Other
      Head   Upper epiphysis

✓5th **812.1   Upper end, open**
   812.10   Upper end, unspecified part
   812.11   Surgical neck

Right Clavicle and Scapula, Anterior View

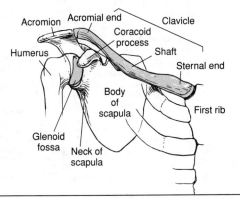

✓4th **810 Fracture of clavicle**

Right Humerus, Anterior View

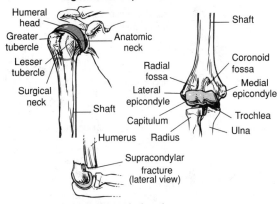

   812.12   Anatomical neck
   812.13   Greater tuberosity
   812.19   Other

✓5th **812.2   Shaft or unspecified part, closed**
   812.20   Unspecified part of humerus
      Humerus NOS   Upper arm NOS
   812.21   Shaft of humerus

✓5th **812.3   Shaft or unspecified part, open**
   812.30   Unspecified part of humerus
   812.31   Shaft of humerus

✓5th **812.4   Lower end, closed**
   Distal end of humerus
   Elbow
   812.40   Lower end, unspecified part
   812.41   Supracondylar fracture of humerus
   812.42   Lateral condyle
      External condyle
   812.43   Medial condyle
      Internal epicondyle
   812.44   Condyle(s), unspecified
      Articular process NOS
      Lower epiphysis NOS
   812.49   Other
      Multiple fractures of lower end
      Trochlea

✓5th **812.5   Lower end, open**
   812.50   Lower end, unspecified part
   812.51   Supracondylar fracture of humerus
   812.52   Lateral condyle
   812.53   Medial condyle
   812.54   Condyle(s), unspecified
   812.59   Other

✓4th **813 Fracture of radius and ulna**

✓5th **813.0   Upper end, closed**
   Proximal end
   813.00   Upper end of forearm, unspecified
   813.01   Olecranon process of ulna
   813.02   Coronoid process of ulna
   813.03   Monteggia's fracture

   > DEF: Fracture near the head of the ulnar shaft, causing dislocation of the radial head.

   813.04   Other and unspecified fractures of proximal end of ulna (alone)
      Multiple fractures of ulna, upper end
   813.05   Head of radius
   813.06   Neck of radius
   813.07   Other and unspecified fractures of proximal end of radius (alone)
      Multiple fractures of radius, upper end
   813.08   Radius with ulna, upper end [any part]

✓4th
✓5th   Additional Digit Required   Unspecified Code   Other Specified Code   Manifestation Code   ►◄ Revised Text   ● New Code   ▲ Revised Code Title

2003 ICD•9•CM   Volume 1 — 247

Right Radius and Ulna, Anterior View

Labels: Olecranon process, Coronoid process, Radius, Ulna, Colles fracture, Radius, Shafts, Humerus (lateral view), Radius dislocated, Radial styloid process, Ulnar styloid process, Monteggia's fracture-dislocation

√5th **813.1 Upper end, open**
813.10 Upper end of forearm, unspecified
813.11 Olecranon process of ulna
813.12 Coronoid process of ulna
813.13 Monteggia's fracture
813.14 Other and unspecified fractures of proximal end of ulna (alone)
813.15 Head of radius
813.16 Neck of radius
813.17 Other and unspecified fractures of proximal end of radius (alone)
813.18 Radius with ulna, upper end [any part]

√5th **813.2 Shaft, closed**
813.20 Shaft, unspecified
813.21 Radius (alone)
813.22 Ulna (alone)
813.23 Radius with ulna

√5th **813.3 Shaft, open**
813.30 Shaft, unspecified
813.31 Radius (alone)
813.32 Ulna (alone)
813.33 Radius with ulna

√5th **813.4 Lower end, closed**
Distal end
813.40 Lower end of forearm, unspecified
813.41 Colles' fracture
Smith's fracture
DEF: Break of lower end of radius; associated with backward movement of the radius lower section.
813.42 Other fractures of distal end of radius (alone)
Dupuytren's fracture, radius
Radius, lower end
DEF: Dupuytren's fracture: fracture and dislocation of the forearm; the fracture is of the radius above the wrist, and the dislocation is of the ulna at the lower end.
813.43 Distal end of ulna (alone)
Ulna: Ulna:
  head   lower epiphysis
  lower end   styloid process
813.44 Radius with ulna, lower end
813.45 Torus fracture of radius

√5th **813.5 Lower end, open**
813.50 Lower end of forearm, unspecified
813.51 Colles' fracture
813.52 Other fractures of distal end of radius (alone)
813.53 Distal end of ulna (alone)
813.54 Radius with ulna, lower end

√5th **813.8 Unspecified part, closed**
813.80 Forearm, unspecified
813.81 Radius (alone)
813.82 Ulna (alone)
813.83 Radius with ulna

√5th **813.9 Unspecified part, open**
813.90 Forearm, unspecified
813.91 Radius (alone)
813.92 Ulna (alone)
813.93 Radius with ulna

√4th **814 Fracture of carpal bone(s)**

The following fifth-digit subclassification is for use with category 814:
0 carpal bone, unspecified
    Wrist NOS
1 navicular [scaphoid] of wrist
2 lunate [semilunar] bone of wrist
3 triquetral [cuneiform] bone of wrist
4 pisiform
5 trapezium bone [larger multangular]
6 trapezoid bone [smaller multangular]
7 capitate bone [os magnum]
8 hamate [unciform] bone
9 other

√5th 814.0 Closed
√5th 814.1 Open

√4th **815 Fracture of metacarpal bone(s)**
INCLUDES   hand [except finger]
           metacarpus

The following fifth-digit subclassification is for use with category 815:
0 metacarpal bone(s), site unspecified
1 base of thumb [first] metacarpal
    Bennett's fracture
2 base of other metacarpal bone(s)
3 shaft of metacarpal bone(s)
4 neck of metacarpal bone(s)
9 multiple sites of metacarpus

√5th 815.0 Closed
√5th 815.1 Open

√4th **816 Fracture of one or more phalanges of hand**
INCLUDES   finger(s) thumb

The following fifth-digit subclassification is for use with category 816:
0 phalanx or phalanges, unspecified
1 middle or proximal phalanx or phalanges
2 distal phalanx or phalanges
3 multiple sites

Hand Fractures

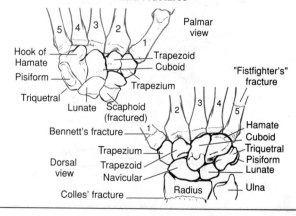

Labels: Palmar view, Hook of Hamate, Pisiform, Triquetral, Lunate, Scaphoid (fractured), Bennett's fracture, Trapezium, Trapezoid, Navicular, Colles' fracture, Trapezoid, Cuboid, Trapezium, Dorsal view, "Fistfighter's" fracture, Hamate, Cuboid, Triquetral, Pisiform, Lunate, Radius, Ulna

---

N Newborn Age: 0   P Pediatric Age: 0-17   M Maternity Age: 12-55   A Adult Age: 15-124   MSP Medicare Secondary Payer

☑5th **816.0 Closed**

☑5th **816.1 Open**

☑4th **817 Multiple fractures of hand bones**

> INCLUDES   metacarpal bone(s) with phalanx or phalanges of same hand

    817.0 Closed

    817.1 Open

☑4th **818 Ill-defined fractures of upper limb**

> INCLUDES   arm NOS
> multiple bones of same upper limb
>
> EXCLUDES   *multiple fractures of:*
>   *metacarpal bone(s) with phalanx or*
>   *phalanges (817.0-817.1)*
>   *phalanges of hand alone (816.0-816.1)*
>   *radius with ulna (813.0-813.9)*

    818.0 Closed

    818.1 Open

☑4th **819 Multiple fractures involving both upper limbs, and upper limb with rib(s) and sternum**

> INCLUDES   arm(s) with rib(s) or sternum
> both arms [any bones]

    819.0 Closed

    819.1 Open

FRACTURE OF LOWER LIMB (820-829)

☑4th **820 Fracture of neck of femur**

☑5th **820.0 Transcervical fracture, closed**

    820.00 Intracapsular section, unspecified

    820.01 Epiphysis (separation) (upper)
      Transepiphyseal

    820.02 Midcervical section
      Transcervical NOS

    820.03 Base of neck
      Cervicotrochanteric section

    820.09 Other
      Head of femur   Subcapital

☑5th **820.1 Transcervical fracture, open**

    820.10 Intracapsular section, unspecified

    820.11 Epiphysis (separation) (upper)

    820.12 Midcervical section

    820.13 Base of neck

    820.19 Other

☑5th **820.2 Pertrochanteric fracture, closed**

    820.20 Trochanteric section, unspecified
      Trochanter: Trochanter:
      NOS   lesser
      greater

    820.21 Intertrochanteric section

    820.22 Subtrochanteric section

☑5th **820.3 Pertrochanteric fracture, open**

    820.30 Trochanteric section, unspecified

    820.31 Intertrochanteric section

    820.32 Subtrochanteric section

    820.8 Unspecified part of neck of femur, closed
      Hip NOS   Neck of femur NOS

    820.9 Unspecified part of neck of femur, open

☑4th **821 Fracture of other and unspecified parts of femur**

☑5th **821.0 Shaft or unspecified part, closed**

    821.00 Unspecified part of femur
      Thigh   Upper leg

> EXCLUDES   *hip NOS (820.8)*

    821.01 Shaft

☑5th **821.1 Shaft or unspecified part, open**

    821.10 Unspecified part of femur

    821.11 Shaft

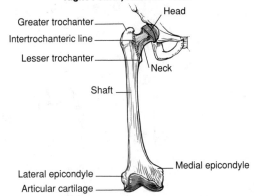

Right Femur, Anterior View

Head — Greater trochanter — Intertrochanteric line — Lesser trochanter — Neck — Shaft — Medial epicondyle — Lateral epicondyle — Articular cartilage

☑5th **821.2 Lower end, closed**
    Distal end

    821.20 Lower end, unspecified part

    821.21 Condyle, femoral

    821.22 Epiphysis, lower (separation)

    821.23 Supracondylar fracture of femur
      Multiple fractures of lower end

    821.29 Other
      Multiple fractures of lower end

☑5th **821.3 Lower end, open**

    821.30 Lower end, unspecified part

    821.31 Condyle, femoral

    821.32 Epiphysis, lower (separation)

    821.33 Supracondylar fracture of femur

    821.39 Other

☑4th **822 Fracture of patella**

    822.0 Closed

    822.1 Open

☑4th **823 Fracture of tibia and fibula**

> EXCLUDES   *Dupuytren's fracture (824.4-824.5)*
>   *ankle (824.4-824.5)*
>   *radius (813.42, 813.52)*
>   *Pott's fracture (824.4-824.5)*
>   *that involving ankle (824.0-824.9)*

> The following fifth-digit subclassification is for use with category 823:
>
>   0   tibia alone
>   1   fibula alone
>   2   fibula with tibia

☑5th **823.0 Upper end, closed**
    Head   Tibia:
    Proximal end   condyles
                     tuberosity

☑5th **823.1 Upper end, open**

☑5th **823.2 Shaft, closed**

☑5th **823.3 Shaft, open**

● ☑5th **823.4 Torus fracture**

☑5th **823.8 Unspecified part, closed**
    Lower leg NOS

☑5th **823.9 Unspecified part, open**

☑4th **824 Fracture of ankle**

    824.0 Medial malleolus, closed
      Tibia involving: Tibia involving:
      ankle   malleolus

    824.1 Medial malleolus, open

    824.2 Lateral malleolus, closed
      Fibula involving: Fibula involving:
      ankle   malleolus

    824.3 Lateral malleolus, open

☑4th / ☑5th **Additional Digit Required**   Unspecified Code   Other Specified Code   Manifestation Code   ▶◀ Revised Text   ● New Code   ▲ Revised Code Title

Injury and Poisoning 824.4–830.1

Right Tibula and Fibula, Anterior View

Right Foot, Dorsal

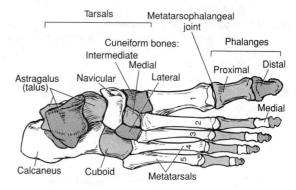

824.4 Bimalleolar, closed
Dupuytren's fracture, fibula   Pott's fracture

DEF: Bimalleolar, closed: Breaking of both nodules (malleoli) on either side of ankle joint, without an open wound.

DEF: Dupuytren's fracture (Pott's fracture): The breaking of the farthest end of the lower leg bone (fibula), with injury to the farthest end joint of the other lower leg bone (tibia).

824.5 Bimalleolar, open

824.6 Trimalleolar, closed
Lateral and medial malleolus with anterior or posterior lip of tibia

824.7 Trimalleolar, open

824.8 Unspecified, closed
Ankle NOS

824.9 Unspecified, open

√4ᵗʰ **825 Fracture of one or more tarsal and metatarsal bones**

825.0 Fracture of calcaneus, closed
Heel bone   Os calcis

825.1 Fracture of calcaneus, open

√5ᵗʰ **825.2 Fracture of other tarsal and metatarsal bones, closed**

825.20 Unspecified bone(s) of foot [except toes]
Instep

825.21 Astragalus
Talus

825.22 Navicular [scaphoid], foot

825.23 Cuboid

825.24 Cuneiform, foot

825.25 Metatarsal bone(s)

825.29 Other
Tarsal with metatarsal bone(s) only
EXCLUDES calcaneus (825.0)

√5ᵗʰ **825.3 Fracture of other tarsal and metatarsal bones, open**

825.30 Unspecified bone(s) of foot [except toes]

825.31 Astragalus

825.32 Navicular [scaphoid], foot

825.33 Cuboid

825.34 Cuneiform, foot

825.35 Metatarsal bone(s)

825.39 Other

√4ᵗʰ **826 Fracture of one or more phalanges of foot**
INCLUDES toe(s)

826.0 Closed

826.1 Open

√4ᵗʰ **827 Other, multiple, and ill-defined fractures of lower limb**
INCLUDES leg NOS
multiple bones of same lower limb
EXCLUDES multiple fractures of:
ankle bones alone (824.4-824.9)
phalanges of foot alone (826.0-826.1)
tarsal with metatarsal bones (825.29, 825.39)
tibia with fibula (823.0-823.9 with fifth-digit 2)

827.0 Closed

827.1 Open

√4ᵗʰ **828 Multiple fractures involving both lower limbs, lower with upper limb, and lower limb(s) with rib(s) and sternum**
INCLUDES arm(s) with leg(s) [any bones]
both legs [any bones]
leg(s) with rib(s) or sternum

828.0 Closed   MSP

828.1 Open   MSP

√4ᵗʰ **829 Fracture of unspecified bones**

829.0 Unspecified bone, closed

829.1 Unspecified bone, open

DISLOCATION (830-839)
INCLUDES displacement
subluxation
EXCLUDES congenital dislocation (754.0-755.8)
pathological dislocation (718.2)
recurrent dislocation (718.3)

The descriptions "closed" and "open," used in the fourth-digit subdivisions, include the following terms:

closed: open:
complete   compound
dislocation NOS   infected
partial   with foreign body
simple
uncomplicated

A dislocation not indicated as closed or open should be classified as closed.

√4ᵗʰ **830 Dislocation of jaw**
INCLUDES jaw (cartilage) (meniscus)
mandible
maxilla (inferior)
temporomandibular (joint)

830.0 Closed dislocation

830.1 Open dislocation

831 Dislocation of shoulder ✓4th

    EXCLUDES   *sternoclavicular joint (839.61, 839.71)*
                     sternum (839.61, 839.71)

The following fifth-digit subclassification is for use with category 831:

  0 shoulder, unspecified
      Humerus NOS
  1 anterior dislocation of humerus
  2 posterior dislocation of humerus
  3 inferior dislocation of humerus
  4 acromioclavicular (joint)
      Clavicle
  9 other
      Scapula

✓5th **831.0 Closed dislocation**
✓5th **831.1 Open dislocation**

832 Dislocation of elbow ✓4th

The following fifth-digit subclassification is for use with category 832:

  0 elbow unspecified
  1 anterior dislocation of elbow
  2 posterior dislocation of elbow
  3 medial dislocation of elbow
  4 lateral dislocation of elbow
  9 other

✓5th **832.0 Closed dislocation**
✓5th **832.1 Open dislocation**

833 Dislocation of wrist ✓4th

The following fifth-digit subclassification is for use with category 833:

  0 wrist, unspecified part
      Carpal (bone)
      Radius, distal end
  1 radioulnar (joint), distal
  2 radiocarpal (joint)
  3 midcarpal (joint)
  4 carpometacarpal (joint)
  5 metacarpal (bone), proximal end
  9 other
      Ulna, distal end

✓5th **833.0 Closed dislocation**
✓5th **833.1 Open dislocation**

834 Dislocation of finger ✓4th

    INCLUDES   finger(s)
                     phalanx of hand
                     thumb

The following fifth-digit subclassification is for use with category 834:

  0 finger, unspecified part
  1 metacarpophalangeal (joint)
      Metacarpal (bone), distal end
  2 interphalangeal (joint), hand

✓5th **834.0 Closed dislocation**
✓5th **834.1 Open dislocation**

835 Dislocation of hip ✓4th

The following fifth-digit subclassification is for use with category 835:

  0 dislocation of hip, unspecified
  1 posterior dislocation
  2 obturator dislocation
  3 other anterior dislocation

✓5th **835.0 Closed dislocation**
✓5th **835.1 Open dislocation**

836 Dislocation of knee ✓4th

    EXCLUDES   *dislocation of knee:*
                   old or pathological (718.2)
                   recurrent (718.3)
            internal derangement of knee joint (717.0-717.5,
                   717.8-717.9)
            old tear of cartilage or meniscus of knee (717.0-
                   717.5, 717.8-717.9)

836.0 Tear of medial cartilage or meniscus of knee, current

    Bucket handle tear:
      NOS   } current injury
      medial meniscus

836.1 Tear of lateral cartilage or meniscus of knee, current

836.2 Other tear of cartilage or meniscus of knee, current

    Tear of:
      cartilage   } current injury, not
        (semilunar)   specified as
      meniscus   } medial or lateral

836.3 Dislocation of patella, closed
836.4 Dislocation of patella, open

✓5th **836.5 Other dislocation of knee, closed**
  836.50 Dislocation of knee, unspecified
  836.51 Anterior dislocation of tibia, proximal end
      Posterior dislocation of femur, distal end
  836.52 Posterior dislocation of tibia, proximal end
      Anterior dislocation of femur, distal end
  836.53 Medial dislocation of tibia, proximal end
  836.54 Lateral dislocation of tibia, proximal end
  836.59 Other

✓5th **836.6 Other dislocation of knee, open**
  836.60 Dislocation of knee, unspecified
  836.61 Anterior dislocation of tibia, proximal end
  836.62 Posterior dislocation of tibia, proximal end
  836.63 Medial dislocation of tibia, proximal end
  836.64 Lateral dislocation of tibia, proximal end
  836.69 Other

837 Dislocation of ankle ✓4th

    INCLUDES   astragalus
                     fibula, distal end
                     navicular, foot
                     scaphoid, foot
                     tibia, distal end

837.0 Closed dislocation
837.1 Open dislocation

838 Dislocation of foot ✓4th

The following fifth-digit subclassification is for use with category 838:

  0 foot, unspecified
  1 tarsal (bone), joint unspecified
  2 midtarsal (joint)
  3 tarsometatarsal (joint)
  4 metatarsal (bone), joint unspecified
  5 metatarsophalangeal (joint)
  6 interphalangeal (joint), foot
  9 other
      Phalanx of foot
      Toe(s)

✓5th **838.0 Closed dislocation**
✓5th **838.1 Open dislocation**

839 Other, multiple, and ill-defined dislocations ✓4th

✓5th **839.0 Cervical vertebra, closed**
    Cervical spine   Neck
  839.00 Cervical vertebra, unspecified   **MSP**
  839.01 First cervical vertebra   **MSP**

Injury and Poisoning 831–839.01

✓4th / ✓5th   Additional Digit Required   Unspecified Code   Other Specified Code   Manifestation Code   ►◄ Revised Text   ● New Code   ▲ Revised Code Title

2003 ICD•9•CM   **Volume 1 — 251**

839.02   Second cervical vertebra   MSP
839.03   Third cervical vertebra   MSP
839.04   Fourth cervical vertebra   MSP
839.05   Fifth cervical vertebra   MSP
839.06   Sixth cervical vertebra   MSP
839.07   Seventh cervical vertebra   MSP
839.08   Multiple cervical vertebrae   MSP

√5th 839.1   **Cervical vertebra, open**
839.10   Cervical vertebra, unspecified   MSP
839.11   First cervical vertebra   MSP
839.12   Second cervical vertebra   MSP
839.13   Third cervical vertebra   MSP
839.14   Fourth cervical vertebra   MSP
839.15   Fifth cervical vertebra   MSP
839.16   Sixth cervical vertebra   MSP
839.17   Seventh cervical vertebra   MSP
839.18   Multiple cervical vertebrae   MSP

√5th 839.2   **Thoracic and lumbar vertebra, closed**
839.20   Lumbar vertebra   MSP
839.21   Thoracic vertebra   MSP
     Dorsal [thoracic] vertebra

√5th 839.3   **Thoracic and lumbar vertebra, open**
839.30   Lumbar vertebra   MSP
839.31   Thoracic vertebra   MSP

√5th 839.4   **Other vertebra, closed**
839.40   Vertebra, unspecified site
     Spine NOS
839.41   Coccyx
839.42   Sacrum
     Sacroiliac (joint)
839.49   Other

√5th 839.5   **Other vertebra, open**
839.50   Vertebra, unspecified site
839.51   Coccyx
839.52   Sacrum
839.59   Other

√5th 839.6   **Other location, closed**
839.61   Sternum
     Sternoclavicular joint
839.69   Other
     Pelvis

√5th 839.7   **Other location, open**
839.71   Sternum   MSP
839.79   Other   MSP

839.8   **Multiple and ill-defined, closed**   MSP
     Arm
     Back
     Hand
     Multiple locations, except fingers or toes alone
     Other ill-defined locations
     Unspecified location

839.9   **Multiple and ill-defined, open**   MSP

SPRAINS AND STRAINS OF JOINTS AND ADJACENT MUSCLES
(840-848)

INCLUDES   avulsion
     hemarthrosis
     laceration   of:
     rupture   joint capsule
     sprain   ligament
     strain   muscle
     tear   tendon

EXCLUDES   *laceration of tendon in open wounds (880-884 and 890-894 with .2)*

√4th 840   **Sprains and strains of shoulder and upper arm**
840.0   Acromioclavicular (joint) (ligament)
840.1   Coracoclavicular (ligament)
840.2   Coracohumeral (ligament)
840.3   Infraspinatus (muscle) (tendon)
840.4   Rotator cuff (capsule)
     EXCLUDES   *complete rupture of rotator cuff, nontraumatic (727.61)*
840.5   Subscapularis (muscle)
840.6   Supraspinatus (muscle) (tendon)
840.7   Superior glenoid labrum lesion
     SLAP lesion
     DEF: ▶ Detachment injury of the superior aspect of the glenoid labrum which is the ring of fibrocartilage attached to the rim of the glenoid cavity of the scapula.◀
840.8   Other specified sites of shoulder and upper arm
840.9   Unspecified site of shoulder and upper arm
     Arm NOS
     Shoulder NOS

√4th 841   **Sprains and strains of elbow and forearm**
841.0   Radial collateral ligament
841.1   Ulnar collateral ligament
841.2   Radiohumeral (joint)
841.3   Ulnohumeral (joint)
841.8   Other specified sites of elbow and forearm
841.9   Unspecified site of elbow and forearm
     Elbow NOS

√4th 842   **Sprains and strains of wrist and hand**
√5th 842.0   **Wrist**
842.00   Unspecified site
842.01   Carpal (joint)
842.02   Radiocarpal (joint) (ligament)
842.09   Other
     Radioulnar joint, distal
√5th 842.1   **Hand**
842.10   Unspecified site
842.11   Carpometacarpal (joint)
842.12   Metacarpophalangeal (joint)
842.13   Interphalangeal (joint)
842.19   Other
     Midcarpal (joint)

√4th 843   **Sprains and strains of hip and thigh**
843.0   Iliofemoral (ligament)
843.1   Ischiocapsular (ligament)
843.8   Other specified sites of hip and thigh
843.9   Unspecified site of hip and thigh
     Hip NOS
     Thigh NOS

√4th 844   **Sprains and strains of knee and leg**
844.0   Lateral collateral ligament of knee
844.1   Medial collateral ligament of knee
844.2   Cruciate ligament of knee
844.3   Tibiofibular (joint) (ligament), superior
844.8   Other specified sites of knee and leg
844.9   Unspecified site of knee and leg
     Knee NOS   Leg NOS

√4th 845   **Sprains and strains of ankle and foot**
√5th 845.0   **Ankle**
845.00   Unspecified site
845.01   Deltoid (ligament), ankle
     Internal collateral (ligament), ankle
845.02   Calcaneofibular (ligament)
845.03   Tibiofibular (ligament), distal
845.09   Other
     Achilles tendon

✓5ᵗʰ **845.1 Foot**
     845.10 Unspecified site
     845.11 Tarsometatarsal (joint) (ligament)
     845.12 Metatarsophalangeal (joint)
     845.13 Interphalangeal (joint), toe
     845.19 Other

✓4ᵗʰ **846 Sprains and strains of sacroiliac region**
     846.0 Lumbosacral (joint) (ligament)
     846.1 Sacroiliac ligament
     846.2 Sacrospinatus (ligament)
     846.3 Sacrotuberous (ligament)
     846.8 Other specified sites of sacroiliac region
     846.9 Unspecified site of sacroiliac region

✓4ᵗʰ **847 Sprains and strains of other and unspecified parts of back**
     EXCLUDES *lumbosacral (846.0)*
     847.0 Neck   [MSP]
         Anterior longitudinal (ligament), cervical
         Atlanto-axial (joints)
         Atlanto-occipital (joints)
         Whiplash injury
         EXCLUDES *neck injury NOS (959.0)*
                   thyroid region (848.2)
     847.1 Thoracic
     847.2 Lumbar
     847.3 Sacrum
         Sacrococcygeal (ligament)
     847.4 Coccyx
     847.9 Unspecified site of back
         Back NOS

✓4ᵗʰ **848 Other and ill-defined sprains and strains**
     848.0 Septal cartilage of nose
     848.1 Jaw
         Temporomandibular (joint) (ligament)
     848.2 Thyroid region
         Cricoarytenoid (joint) (ligament)
         Cricothyroid (joint) (ligament)
         Thyroid cartilage
     848.3 Ribs
         Chondrocostal
           (joint)   } without mention of injury to
         Costal cartilage }   sternum

✓5ᵗʰ **848.4 Sternum**
     848.40 Unspecified site
     848.41 Sternoclavicular (joint) (ligament)
     848.42 Chondrosternal (joint)
     848.49 Other
         Xiphoid cartilage
     848.5 Pelvis
         Symphysis pubis
         EXCLUDES *that in childbirth (665.6)*
     848.8 Other specified sites of sprains and strains
     848.9 Unspecified site of sprain and strain

INTRACRANIAL INJURY, EXCLUDING THOSE WITH SKULL FRACTURE (850-854)

     EXCLUDES *intracranial injury with skull fracture (800-801 and 803-804, except .0 and .5)*
                   open wound of head without intracranial injury (870.0-873.9)
                   skull fracture alone (800-801 and 803-804 with .0, .5)

The description "with open intracranial wound," used in the fourth-digit subdivisions, those specified as open or with mention of infection or foreign body.

The following fifth-digit subclassification is for use with categories 851-854:

   0   unspecified state of consciousness
   1   with no loss of consciousness
   2   with brief [less than one hour] loss of consciousness
   3   with moderate [1-24 hours] loss of consciousness
   4   with prolonged [more than 24 hours] loss of consciousness and return to pre-existing conscious level
   5   with prolonged [more than 24 hours] loss of consciousness, without return to pre-existing conscious level
        Use fifth-digit 5 to designate when a patient is unconscious and dies before regaining consciousness, regardless of the duration of the loss of consciousness
   6   with loss of consciousness of unspecified duration
   9   with concussion, unspecified

✓4ᵗʰ **850 Concussion**
     INCLUDES commotio cerebri
     EXCLUDES *concussion with:*
                cerebral laceration or contusion (851.0-851.9)
                cerebral hemorrhage (852-853)
         head injury NOS (959.01)

     850.0 With no loss of consciousness   [MSP]
         Concussion with mental confusion or disorientation, without loss of consciousness
     850.1 With brief loss of consciousness   [MSP]
         Loss of consciousness for less than one hour
     850.2 With moderate loss of consciousness   [MSP]
         Loss of consciousness for 1-24 hours
     850.3 With prolonged loss of consciousness and return to pre-existing conscious level   [MSP]
         Loss of consciousness for more than 24 hours with complete recovery
     850.4 With prolonged loss of consciousness, without return to pre-existing conscious level   [MSP]
     850.5 With loss of consciousness of unspecified duration   [MSP]
     850.9 Concussion, unspecified   [MSP]

✓4ᵗʰ **851 Cerebral laceration and contusion**
   § ✓5ᵗʰ **851.0** Cortex (cerebral) contusion without mention of open intracranial wound   [MSP]
   § ✓5ᵗʰ **851.1** Cortex (cerebral) contusion with open intracranial wound   [MSP]
   § ✓5ᵗʰ **851.2** Cortex (cerebral) laceration without mention of open intracranial wound   [MSP]
   § ✓5ᵗʰ **851.3** Cortex (cerebral) laceration with open intracranial wound   [MSP]
   § ✓5ᵗʰ **851.4** Cerebellar or brain stem contusion without mention of open intracranial wound   [MSP]
   § ✓5ᵗʰ **851.5** Cerebellar or brain stem contusion with open intracranial wound   [MSP]

§ Requires fifth-digit. See beginning of section 850-854 for codes and definitions.

Injury and Poisoning 845.1–851.5

 Additional Digit Required   Unspecified Code   Other Specified Code   Manifestation Code   ►◄ Revised Text   ● New Code   ▲ Revised Code Title

2003 ICD•9•CM   **Volume 1 — 253**

§ ✓5ᵗʰ **851.6**   **Cerebellar or brain stem laceration without mention of open intracranial wound**   `MSP`

§ ✓5ᵗʰ **851.7**   **Cerebellar or brain stem laceration with open intracranial wound**   `MSP`

§ ✓5ᵗʰ **851.8**   **Other and unspecified cerebral laceration and contusion, without mention of open intracranial wound**   `MSP`
     Brain (membrane) NOS

§ ✓5ᵗʰ **851.9**   **Other and unspecified cerebral laceration and contusion, with open intracranial wound**   `MSP`

✓4ᵗʰ **852**   **Subarachnoid, subdural, and extradural hemorrhage, following injury**

   `EXCLUDES`   *Cerebral contusion or laceration (with hemorrhage) (851.0-851.9)*

   DEF: Bleeding from lining of brain; due to injury.

§ ✓5ᵗʰ **852.0**   **Subarachnoid hemorrhage following injury without mention of open intracranial wound**   `MSP`
     Middle meningeal hemorrhage following injury

§ ✓5ᵗʰ **852.1**   **Subarachnoid hemorrhage following injury with open intracranial wound**   `MSP`

§ ✓5ᵗʰ **852.2**   **Subdural hemorrhage following injury without mention of open intracranialwound**   `MSP`

§ ✓5ᵗʰ **852.3**   **Subdural hemorrhage following injury with open intracranial wound**   `MSP`

§ ✓5ᵗʰ **852.4**   **Extradural hemorrhage following injury without mention of open intracranial wound**   `MSP`
     Epidural hematoma following injury

§ ✓5ᵗʰ **852.5**   **Extradural hemorrhage following injury with open intracranial wound**   `MSP`

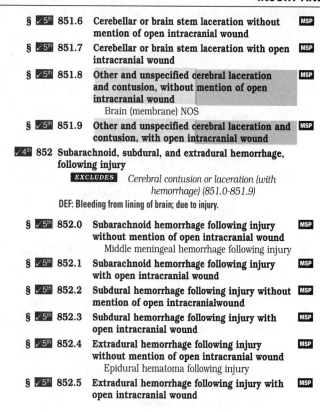

Brain

Corpus callosum
Cerebrum
Hypothalamus
Interventricular foramen
Fornix
Third ventricle
Pineal body
Optic chiasm
Hypophysis
Pons
Mamillary body
Peduncle
Medulla oblangata
Corpora quadrigemina
Cerebral aqueduct
Vermis
Fourth ventricle
Median aperture
Spinal cord

Precentral gyrus (motor)
Anterior horn of lateral ventricle
Intraventricular foramen
Third ventricle
Lateral sulcus
Central sulcus
Postcentral gyrus (sensory)
Body and posterior horn of lateral ventricle
Inferior horn of lateral ventricle
Cerebral aqueduct
Lateral aperture
Fourth ventricle
Median aperture

✓4ᵗʰ **853**   **Other and unspecified intracranial hemorrhage following injury**

§ ✓5ᵗʰ **853.0**   **Without mention of open intracranial wound**   `MSP`
     Cerebral compression due to injury
     Intracranial hematoma following injury
     Traumatic cerebral hemorrhage

§ ✓5ᵗʰ **853.1**   **With open intracranial wound**   `MSP`

✓4ᵗʰ **854**   **Intracranial injury of other and unspecified nature**

   `INCLUDES`   brain injury NOS
                cavernous sinus
                intracranial injury

   `EXCLUDES`   *any condition classifiable to 850-853*
                head injury NOS (959.01)

§ ✓5ᵗʰ **854.0**   **Without mention of open intracranial wound**   `MSP`

§ ✓5ᵗʰ **854.1**   **With open intracranial wound**   `MSP`

INTERNAL INJURY OF THORAX, ABDOMEN, AND PELVIS (860-869)

   `INCLUDES`   blast injuries
                blunt trauma
                bruise
                concussion injuries
                    (except cerebral)
                crushing   of internal
                hematoma   organs
                laceration
                puncture
                tear
                traumatic rupture

   `EXCLUDES`   *concussion NOS (850.0-850.9)*
                flail chest (807.4)
                foreign body entering through orifice (930.0-939.9)
                injury to blood vessels (901.0-902.9)

The description "with open wound," used in the fourth-digit subdivisions, those with mention of infection or foreign body.

✓4ᵗʰ **860**   **Traumatic pneumothorax and hemothorax**

   DEF: Traumatic pneumothorax: air or gas leaking into pleural space of lung due to trauma.

   DEF: Traumatic hemothorax: blood buildup in pleural space of lung due to trauma.

   860.0   **Pneumothorax without mention of open wound into thorax**   `MSP`

   860.1   **Pneumothorax with open wound into thorax**   `MSP`

   860.2   **Hemothorax without mention of open wound into thorax**   `MSP`

   860.3   **Hemothorax with open wound into thorax**   `MSP`

   860.4   **Pneumohemothorax without mention of open wound into thorax**   `MSP`

   860.5   **Pneumohemothorax with open wound into thorax**   `MSP`

✓4ᵗʰ **861**   **Injury to heart and lung**

   `EXCLUDES`   *injury to blood vessels of thorax (901.0-901.9)*

✓5ᵗʰ **861.0**   **Heart, without mention of open wound into thorax**

   861.00   **Unspecified injury**   `MSP`

   861.01   **Contusion**   `MSP`
       Cardiac contusion
       Myocardial contusion

       DEF: Bruising within the pericardium with no mention of open wound.

   861.02   **Laceration without penetration of heart chambers**   `MSP`

       DEF: Tearing injury of heart tissue, without penetration of chambers; no open wound.

---

§ Requires fifth-digit. See beginning of section 850–854 for codes and definitions.

`N` Newborn Age: 0   `P` Pediatric Age: 0-17   `M` Maternity Age: 12-55   `A` Adult Age: 15-124   `MSP` Medicare Secondary Payer

861.03 Laceration with penetration of heart chambers **MSP**

✓5ᵗʰ 861.1 **Heart, with open wound into thorax**
861.10 Unspecified injury **MSP**
861.11 Contusion **MSP**
861.12 Laceration without penetration of heart chambers **MSP**
861.13 Laceration with penetration of heart chambers **MSP**

✓5ᵗʰ 861.2 **Lung, without mention of open wound into thorax**
861.20 Unspecified injury **MSP**
861.21 Contusion **MSP**
>>> DEF: Bruising of lung without mention of open wound.
861.22 Laceration **MSP**

✓5ᵗʰ 861.3 **Lung, with open wound into thorax**
861.30 Unspecified injury **MSP**
861.31 Contusion **MSP**
861.32 Laceration **MSP**

✓4ᵗʰ 862 **Injury to other and unspecified intrathoracic organs**
>>> **EXCLUDES** *injury to blood vessels of thorax (901.0-901.9)*
862.0 **Diaphragm, without mention of open wound into cavity**
862.1 **Diaphragm, with open wound into cavity**
✓5ᵗʰ 862.2 **Other specified intrathoracic organs, without mention of open wound into cavity**
862.21 Bronchus
862.22 Esophagus
862.29 Other
>>> Pleura Thymus gland
✓5ᵗʰ 862.3 **Other specified intrathoracic organs, with open wound into cavity**
862.31 Bronchus
862.32 Esophagus
862.39 Other
862.8 **Multiple and unspecified intrathoracic organs, without mention of open wound into cavity** **MSP**
>>> Crushed chest
>>> Multiple intrathoracic organs
862.9 **Multiple and unspecified intrathoracic organs, with open wound into cavity**

✓4ᵗʰ 863 **Injury to gastrointestinal tract**
>>> **EXCLUDES** *anal sphincter laceration during delivery (664.2)*
>>> *bile duct (868.0-868.1 with fifth-digit 2)*
>>> *gallbladder (868.0-868.1 with fifth-digit 2)*
863.0 **Stomach, without mention of open wound into cavity** **MSP**
863.1 **Stomach, with open wound into cavity** **MSP**
✓5ᵗʰ 863.2 **Small intestine, without mention of open wound into cavity**
863.20 Small intestine, unspecified site **MSP**
863.21 Duodenum **MSP**
863.29 Other **MSP**
✓5ᵗʰ 863.3 **Small intestine, with open wound into cavity**
863.30 Small intestine, unspecified site **MSP**
863.31 Duodenum **MSP**
863.39 Other **MSP**
✓5ᵗʰ 863.4 **Colon or rectum, without mention of open wound into cavity**
863.40 Colon, unspecified site **MSP**
863.41 Ascending [right] colon **MSP**
863.42 Transverse colon **MSP**
863.43 Descending [left] colon **MSP**
863.44 Sigmoid colon **MSP**
863.45 Rectum **MSP**
863.46 Multiple sites in colon and rectum **MSP**
863.49 Other **MSP**

✓5ᵗʰ 863.5 **Colon or rectum, with open wound into cavity**
863.50 Colon, unspecified site **MSP**
863.51 Ascending [right] colon **MSP**
863.52 Transverse colon **MSP**
863.53 Descending [left] colon **MSP**
863.54 Sigmoid colon **MSP**
863.55 Rectum **MSP**
863.56 Multiple sites in colon and rectum **MSP**
863.59 Other **MSP**

✓5ᵗʰ 863.8 **Other and unspecified gastrointestinal sites, without mention of open wound into cavity** **MSP**
863.80 Gastrointestinal tract, unspecified site **MSP**
863.81 Pancreas, head **MSP**
863.82 Pancreas, body **MSP**
863.83 Pancreas, tail **MSP**
863.84 Pancreas, multiple and unspecified sites **MSP**
863.85 Appendix **MSP**
863.89 Other **MSP**
>>> Intestine NOS

✓5ᵗʰ 863.9 **Other and unspecified gastrointestinal sites, with open wound into cavity**
863.90 Gastrointestinal tract, unspecified site **MSP**
863.91 Pancreas, head **MSP**
863.92 Pancreas, body **MSP**
863.93 Pancreas, tail **MSP**
863.94 Pancreas, multiple and unspecified sites **MSP**
863.95 Appendix **MSP**
863.99 Other **MSP**

✓4ᵗʰ 864 **Injury to liver**
>>> The following fifth-digit subclassification is for use with category 864:
>>> 0 unspecified injury
>>> 1 hematoma and contusion
>>> 2 laceration, minor
>>> >>> Laceration involving capsule only, or without significant involvement of hepatic parenchyma [i.e., less than 1 cm deep]
>>> 3 laceration, moderate
>>> >>> Laceration involving parenchyma but without major disruption of parenchyma [i.e., less than 10 cm long and less than 3 cm deep]
>>> 4 laceration, major
>>> >>> Laceration with significant disruption of hepatic parenchyma [i.e., 10 cm long and 3 cm deep]
>>> >>> Multiple moderate lacerations, with or without hematoma
>>> >>> Stellate lacerations of liver
>>> 5 laceration, unspecified
>>> 9 other

✓5ᵗʰ 864.0 **Without mention of open wound into cavity** **MSP**
✓5ᵗʰ 864.1 **With open wound into cavity** **MSP**

✓4ᵗʰ 865 **Injury to spleen**
>>> The following fifth-digit subclassification is for use with category 865:
>>> 0 unspecified injury
>>> 1 hematoma without rupture of capsule
>>> 2 capsular tears, without major disruption of parenchyma
>>> 3 laceration extending into parenchyma
>>> 4 massive parenchymal disruption
>>> 9 other

✓5ᵗʰ 865.0 **Without mention of open wound into cavity** **MSP**
✓5ᵗʰ 865.1 **With open wound into cavity** **MSP**

✓4ᵗʰ / ✓5ᵗʰ **Additional Digit Required** Unspecified Code Other Specified Code Manifestation Code ▶◀ Revised Text ● New Code ▲ Revised Code Title

2003 ICD•9•CM Volume 1 — 255

Injury and Poisoning 861.03–865.1

Injury and Poisoning 866–872.02

✓4ᵗʰ **866 Injury to kidney**

The following fifth-digit subclassification is for use with category 866:

     0   unspecified injury
     1   hematoma without rupture of capsule
     2   laceration
     3   complete disruption of kidney parenchyma

✓5ᵗʰ **866.0 Without mention of open wound into cavity**   MSP

✓5ᵗʰ **866.1 With open wound into cavity**   MSP

✓4ᵗʰ **867 Injury to pelvic organs**

     EXCLUDES   *injury during delivery (664.0-665.9)*

     867.0 Bladder and urethra, without mention of open wound into cavity   MSP

     867.1 Bladder and urethra, with open wound into cavity   MSP

     867.2 Ureter, without mention of open wound into cavity   MSP

     867.3 Ureter, with open wound into cavity   MSP

     867.4 Uterus, without mention of open wound into cavity   ♀ MSP

     867.5 Uterus, with open wound into cavity   ♀ MSP

     867.6 Other specified pelvic organs, without mention of open wound into cavity   MSP

        Fallopian tube   Seminal vesicle
        Ovary   Vas deferens
        Prostate

     867.7 Other specified pelvic organs, with open wound into cavity   MSP

     867.8 Unspecified pelvic organ, without mention of open wound into cavity   MSP

     867.9 Unspecified pelvic organ, with open wound into cavity   MSP

✓4ᵗʰ **868 Injury to other intra-abdominal organs**

The following fifth-digit subclassification is for use with category 868:

     0   unspecified intra-abdominal organ
     1   adrenal gland
     2   bile duct and gallbladder
     3   peritoneum
     4   retroperitoneum
     9   other and multiple intra-abdominal organs

✓5ᵗʰ **868.0 Without mention of open wound into cavity**   MSP

✓5ᵗʰ **868.1 With open wound into cavity**   MSP

✓4ᵗʰ **869 Internal injury to unspecified or ill-defined organs**

     INCLUDES   internal injury NOS
                  multiple internal injury NOS

     869.0 Without mention of open wound into cavity   MSP

     869.1 With open wound into cavity   MSP

OPEN WOUND (870-897)

     INCLUDES   animal bite
                  avulsion
                  cut
                  laceration
                  puncture wound
                  traumatic amputation

     EXCLUDES   *burn (940.0-949.5)*
                  crushing (925-929.9)
                  puncture of internal organs (860.0-869.1)
                  superficial injury (910.0-919.9)
                  that incidental to:
                     dislocation (830.0-839.9)
                     fracture (800.0-829.1)
                     internal injury (860.0-869.1)
                     intracranial injury (851.0-854.1)

The description "complicated" used in the fourth-digit subdivisions includes those with mention of delayed healing, delayed treatment, foreign body, or infection.

Use additional code to identify infection

OPEN WOUND OF HEAD, NECK, AND TRUNK (870-879)

✓4ᵗʰ **870 Open wound of ocular adnexa**

     870.0 Laceration of skin of eyelid and periocular area

     870.1 Laceration of eyelid, full-thickness, not involving lacrimal passages

     870.2 Laceration of eyelid involving lacrimal passages

     870.3 Penetrating wound of orbit, without mention of foreign body

     870.4 Penetrating wound of orbit with foreign body

        EXCLUDES   *retained (old) foreign body in orbit (376.6)*

     870.8 Other specified open wounds of ocular adnexa

     870.9 Unspecified open wound of ocular adnexa

✓4ᵗʰ **871 Open wound of eyeball**

     EXCLUDES   *2nd cranial nerve [optic] injury (950.0-950.9)*
                  3rd cranial nerve [oculomotor] injury (951.0)

     871.0 Ocular laceration without prolapse of intraocular tissue

        DEF: Tear in ocular tissue without displacing structures.

     871.1 Ocular laceration with prolapse or exposure of intraocular tissue

     871.2 Rupture of eye with partial loss of intraocular tissue

        DEF: Forcible tearing of eyeball, with tissue loss.

     871.3 Avulsion of eye

        Traumatic enucleation

        DEF: Traumatic extraction of eyeball from socket.

     871.4 Unspecified laceration of eye

     871.5 Penetration of eyeball with magnetic foreign body

        EXCLUDES   *retained (old) magnetic foreign body in globe (360.50-360.59)*

     871.6 Penetration of eyeball with (nonmagnetic) foreign body

        EXCLUDES   *retained (old) (nonmagnetic) foreign body in globe (360.60-360.69)*

     871.7 Unspecified ocular penetration

     871.9 Unspecified open wound of eyeball

✓4ᵗʰ **872 Open wound of ear**

✓5ᵗʰ **872.0 External ear, without mention of complication**

     872.00 External ear, unspecified site

     872.01 Auricle, ear

        Pinna

        DEF: Open wound of fleshy, outer ear.

     872.02 Auditory canal

        DEF: Open wound of passage from external ear to eardrum.

N Newborn Age: 0   P Pediatric Age: 0-17   M Maternity Age: 12-55   A Adult Age: 15-124   MSP Medicare Secondary Payer

✓5th **872.1** **External ear, complicated**
    872.10 External ear, unspecified site
    872.11 Auricle, ear
    872.12 Auditory canal

✓5th **872.6** **Other specified parts of ear, without mention of complication**
    872.61 Ear drum
        Drumhead   Tympanic membrane
    872.62 Ossicles
    872.63 Eustachian tube
        DEF: Open wound of channel between nasopharynx and tympanic cavity.
    872.64 Cochlea
        DEF: Open wound of snail shell shaped tube of inner ear.
    872.69 Other and multiple sites

✓5th **872.7** **Other specified parts of ear, complicated**
    872.71 Ear drum
    872.72 Ossicles
    872.73 Eustachian tube
    872.74 Cochlea
    872.79 Other and multiple sites

872.8 **Ear, part unspecified, without mention of complication**
    Ear NOS

872.9 **Ear, part unspecified, complicated**

✓4th **873 Other open wound of head**
  873.0 **Scalp, without mention of complication**
  873.1 **Scalp, complicated**

✓5th **873.2** **Nose, without mention of complication**
    873.20 Nose, unspecified site
    873.21 Nasal septum
        DEF: Open wound between nasal passages.
    873.22 Nasal cavity
        DEF: Open wound of nostrils.
    873.23 Nasal sinus
        DEF: Open wound of mucous-lined respiratory cavities.
    873.29 Multiple sites

✓5th **873.3** **Nose, complicated**
    873.30 Nose, unspecified site
    873.31 Nasal septum
    873.32 Nasal cavity
    873.33 Nasal sinus
    873.39 Multiple sites

✓5th **873.4** **Face, without mention of complication**
    873.40 Face, unspecified site
    873.41 Cheek
    873.42 Forehead
        Eyebrow
    873.43 Lip
    873.44 Jaw
    873.49 Other and multiple sites

✓5th **873.5** **Face, complicated**
    873.50 Face, unspecified site
    873.51 Cheek
    873.52 Forehead
    873.53 Lip
    873.54 Jaw
    873.59 Other and multiple sites

✓5th **873.6** **Internal structures of mouth, without mention of complication**
    873.60 Mouth, unspecified site
    873.61 Buccal mucosa
        DEF: Open wound of inside of cheek.

    873.62 Gum (alveolar process)
    873.63 Tooth (broken)
    873.64 Tongue and floor of mouth
    873.65 Palate
        DEF: Open wound of roof of mouth.
    873.69 Other and multiple sites

✓5th **873.7** **Internal structures of mouth, complicated**
    873.70 Mouth, unspecified site
    873.71 Buccal mucosa
    873.72 Gum (alveolar process)
    873.73 Tooth (broken)
    873.74 Tongue and floor of mouth
    873.75 Palate
    873.79 Other and multiple sites

  873.8 **Other and unspecified open wound of head without mention of complication**
    Head NOS

  873.9 **Other and unspecified open wound of head, complicated**

✓4th **874 Open wound of neck**

✓5th **874.0** **Larynx and trachea, without mention of complication**
    874.00 Larynx with trachea
    874.01 Larynx
    874.02 Trachea

✓5th **874.1** **Larynx and trachea, complicated**
    874.10 Larynx with trachea
    874.11 Larynx
    874.12 Trachea

  874.2 **Thyroid gland, without mention of complication**
  874.3 **Thyroid gland, complicated**
  874.4 **Pharynx, without mention of complication**
    Cervical esophagus
  874.5 **Pharynx, complicated**
  874.8 **Other and unspecified parts, without mention of complication**
    Nape of neck   Throat NOS
    Supraclavicular region
  874.9 **Other and unspecified parts, complicated**

✓4th **875 Open wound of chest (wall)**
    EXCLUDES   open wound into thoracic cavity (860.0-862.9)
                traumatic pneumothorax and hemothorax (860.1, 860.3, 860.5)
  875.0 **Without mention of complication**
  875.1 **Complicated**

✓4th **876 Open wound of back**
    INCLUDES   loin
                lumbar region
    EXCLUDES   open wound into thoracic cavity (860.0-862.9)
                traumatic pneumothorax and hemothorax (860.1, 860.3, 860.5)
  876.0 **Without mention of complication**
  876.1 **Complicated**

✓4th **877 Open wound of buttock**
    INCLUDES   sacroiliac region
  877.0 **Without mention of complication**
  877.1 **Complicated**

✓4th **878 Open wound of genital organs (external), including traumatic amputation**
    EXCLUDES   injury during delivery (664.0-665.9)
                internal genital organs (867.0-867.9)
  878.0 **Penis, without mention of complication**   ♂
  878.1 **Penis, complicated**   ♂
  878.2 **Scrotum and testes, without mention of complication**   ♂
  878.3 **Scrotum and testes, complicated**   ♂

✓4th / ✓5th Additional Digit Required   Unspecified Code   Other Specified Code   Manifestation Code   ►◄ Revised Text   ● New Code   ▲ Revised Code Title

Injury and Poisoning 878.4–895.1

878.4   **Vulva, without mention of complication**   ♀
Labium (majus) (minus)

878.5   **Vulva, complicated**   ♀

878.6   **Vagina, without mention of complication**   ♀

878.7   **Vagina, complicated**   ♀

878.8   **Other and unspecified parts, without mention of complication**

878.9   **Other and unspecified parts, complicated**

✓4ᵗʰ **879 Open wound of other and unspecified sites, except limbs**

879.0   **Breast, without mention of complication**

879.1   **Breast, complicated**

879.2   **Abdominal wall, anterior, without mention of complication**
Abdominal wall NOS   Pubic region
Epigastric region   Umbilical region
Hypogastric region

879.3   **Abdominal wall, anterior, complicated**

879.4   **Abdominal wall, lateral, without mention of complication**
Flank   Iliac (region)
Groin   Inguinal region
Hypochondrium

879.5   **Abdominal wall, lateral, complicated**

879.6   **Other and unspecified parts of trunk, without mention of complication**
Pelvic region   Trunk NOS
Perineum

879.7   **Other and unspecified parts of trunk, complicated**

879.8   **Open wound(s) (multiple) of unspecified site(s) without mention of complication**
Multiple open wounds NOS   Open wound NOS

879.9   **Open wound(s) (multiple) of unspecified site(s), complicated**

OPEN WOUND OF UPPER LIMB (880-887)

✓4ᵗʰ **880 Open wound of shoulder and upper arm**

The following fifth-digit subclassification is for use with category 880:
     0   shoulder region
     1   scapular region
     2   axillary region
     3   upper arm
     9   multiple sites

✓5ᵗʰ 880.0   **Without mention of complication**

✓5ᵗʰ 880.1   **Complicated**

✓5ᵗʰ 880.2   **With tendon involvement**

✓4ᵗʰ **881 Open wound of elbow, forearm, and wrist**

The following fifth-digit subclassification is for use with category 881:
     0   forearm
     1   elbow
     2   wrist

✓5ᵗʰ 881.0   **Without mention of complication**

✓5ᵗʰ 881.1   **Complicated**

✓5ᵗʰ 881.2   **With tendon involvement**

✓4ᵗʰ **882 Open wound of hand except finger(s) alone**

882.0   **Without mention of complication**

882.1   **Complicated**

882.2   **With tendon involvement**

✓4ᵗʰ **883 Open wound of finger(s)**
INCLUDES   fingernail
thumb (nail)

883.0   **Without mention of complication**

883.1   **Complicated**

883.2   **With tendon involvement**

✓4ᵗʰ **884 Multiple and unspecified open wound of upper limb**
INCLUDES   arm NOS
multiple sites of one upper limb
upper limb NOS

884.0   **Without mention of complication**

884.1   **Complicated**

884.2   **With tendon involvement**

✓4ᵗʰ **885 Traumatic amputation of thumb (complete) (partial)**
INCLUDES   thumb(s) (with finger(s) of either hand)

885.0   **Without mention of complication**

885.1   **Complicated**

✓4ᵗʰ **886 Traumatic amputation of other finger(s) (complete) (partial)**
INCLUDES   finger(s) of one or both hands, without mention of thumb(s)

886.0   **Without mention of complication**

886.1   **Complicated**

✓4ᵗʰ **887 Traumatic amputation of arm and hand (complete) (partial)**

887.0   **Unilateral, below elbow, without mention of complication**   MSP

887.1   **Unilateral, below elbow, complicated**   MSP

887.2   **Unilateral, at or above elbow, without mention of complication**   MSP

887.3   **Unilateral, at or above elbow, complicated**   MSP

887.4   **Unilateral, level not specified, without mention of complication**   MSP

887.5   **Unilateral, level not specified, complicated**   MSP

887.6   **Bilateral [any level], without mention of complication**   MSP
One hand and other arm

887.7   **Bilateral [any level], complicated**   MSP

OPEN WOUND OF LOWER LIMB (890-897)

✓4ᵗʰ **890 Open wound of hip and thigh**

890.0   **Without mention of complication**

890.1   **Complicated**

890.2   **With tendon involvement**

✓4ᵗʰ **891 Open wound of knee, leg [except thigh], and ankle**
INCLUDES   leg NOS
multiple sites of leg, except thigh
EXCLUDES   *that of thigh (890.0-890.2)*
with multiple sites of lower limb (894.0-894.2)

891.0   **Without mention of complication**

891.1   **Complicated**

891.2   **With tendon involvement**

✓4ᵗʰ **892 Open wound of foot except toe(s) alone**
INCLUDES   heel

892.0   **Without mention of complication**

892.1   **Complicated**

892.2   **With tendon involvement**

✓4ᵗʰ **893 Open wound of toe(s)**
INCLUDES   toenail

893.0   **Without mention of complication**

893.1   **Complicated**

893.2   **With tendon involvement**

✓4ᵗʰ **894 Multiple and unspecified open wound of lower limb**
INCLUDES   lower limb NOS
multiple sites of one lower limb, with thigh

894.0   **Without mention of complication**

894.1   **Complicated**

894.2   **With tendon involvement**

✓4ᵗʰ **895 Traumatic amputation of toe(s) (complete) (partial)**
INCLUDES   toe(s) of one or both feet

895.0   **Without mention of complication**

895.1   **Complicated**

N Newborn Age: 0   P Pediatric Age: 0-17   M Maternity Age: 12-55   A Adult Age: 15-124   MSP Medicare Secondary Payer

√4th **896 Traumatic amputation of foot (complete) (partial)**

     896.0 Unilateral, without mention of complication   `MSP`

     • 896.1 Unilateral, complicated   `MSP`

     896.2 Bilateral, without mention of complication   `MSP`

         EXCLUDES   *one foot and other leg (897.6-897.7)*

     896.3 Bilateral, complicated   `MSP`

√4th **897 Traumatic amputation of leg(s) (complete) (partial)**

     897.0 Unilateral, below knee, without mention of complication   `MSP`

     897.1 Unilateral, below knee, complicated   `MSP`

     897.2 Unilateral, at or above knee, without mention of complication   `MSP`

     897.3 Unilateral, at or above knee, complicated   `MSP`

     897.4 Unilateral, level not specified, without mention of complication   `MSP`

     897.5 Unilateral, level not specified, complicated   `MSP`

     897.6 Bilateral [any level], without mention of complication   `MSP`

         One foot and other leg

     897.7 Bilateral [any level], complicated   `MSP`

INJURY TO BLOOD VESSELS (900-904)

`INCLUDES`

arterial hematoma
avulsion
cut
laceration
rupture
traumatic aneurysm
or fistula
(arteriovenous)

} of blood vessel, secondary to other injuries e.g., fracture or open wound

`EXCLUDES`   *accidental puncture or laceration during medical procedure (998.2)*
intracranial hemorrhage following injury (851.0-854.1)

√4th **900 Injury to blood vessels of head and neck**

   √5th 900.0 Carotid artery

     900.00 Carotid artery, unspecified   `MSP`

     900.01 Common carotid artery   `MSP`

     900.02 External carotid artery   `MSP`

     900.03 Internal carotid artery   `MSP`

     900.1 Internal jugular vein   `MSP`

   √5th 900.8 Other specified blood vessels of head and neck

     900.81 External jugular vein   `MSP`

         Jugular vein NOS

     900.82 Multiple blood vessels of head and neck   `MSP`

     900.89 Other   `MSP`

     900.9 Unspecified blood vessel of head and neck   `MSP`

√4th **901 Injury to blood vessels of thorax**

         `EXCLUDES`   *traumatic hemothorax (860.2-860.5)*

     901.0 Thoracic aorta

     901.1 Innominate and subclavian arteries

     901.2 Superior vena cava

     901.3 Innominate and subclavian veins

   √5th 901.4 Pulmonary blood vessels

     901.40 Pulmonary vessel(s), unspecified

     901.41 Pulmonary artery

     901.42 Pulmonary vein

   √5th 901.8 Other specified blood vessels of thorax

     901.81 Intercostal artery or vein

     901.82 Internal mammary artery or vein

     901.83 Multiple blood vessels of thorax

     901.89 Other

         Azygos vein
         Hemiazygos vein

     901.9 Unspecified blood vessel of thorax

√4th **902 Injury to blood vessels of abdomen and pelvis**

     902.0 Abdominal aorta

   √5th 902.1 Inferior vena cava

     902.10 Inferior vena cava, unspecified

     902.11 Hepatic veins

     902.19 Other

   √5th 902.2 Celiac and mesenteric arteries

     902.20 Celiac and mesenteric arteries, unspecified

     902.21 Gastric artery

     902.22 Hepatic artery

     902.23 Splenic artery

     902.24 Other specified branches of celiac axis

     902.25 Superior mesenteric artery (trunk)

     902.26 Primary branches of superior mesenteric artery

         Ileocolic artery

     902.27 Inferior mesenteric artery

     902.29 Other

   √5th 902.3 Portal and splenic veins

     902.31 Superior mesenteric vein and primary subdivisions

         Ileocolic vein

     902.32 Inferior mesenteric vein

     902.33 Portal vein

     902.34 Splenic vein

     902.39 Other

         Cystic vein   Gastric vein

   √5th 902.4 Renal blood vessels

     902.40 Renal vessel(s), unspecified

     902.41 Renal artery

     902.42 Renal vein

     902.49 Other

         Suprarenal arteries

   √5th 902.5 Iliac blood vessels

     902.50 Iliac vessel(s), unspecified

     902.51 Hypogastric artery

     902.52 Hypogastric vein

     902.53 Iliac artery

     902.54 Iliac vein

     902.55 Uterine artery   ♀

     902.56 Uterine vein   ♀

     902.59 Other

   √5th 902.8 Other specified blood vessels of abdomen and pelvis

     902.81 Ovarian artery   ♀

     902.82 Ovarian vein   ♀

     902.87 Multiple blood vessels of abdomen and pelvis

     902.89 Other

     902.9 Unspecified blood vessel of abdomen and pelvis

√4th **903 Injury to blood vessels of upper extremity**

   √5th 903.0 Axillary blood vessels

     903.00 Axillary vessel(s), unspecified

     903.01 Axillary artery

     903.02 Axillary vein

     903.1 Brachial blood vessels

     903.2 Radial blood vessels

     903.3 Ulnar blood vessels

     903.4 Palmar artery

     903.5 Digital blood vessels

     903.8 Other specified blood vessels of upper extremity

         Multiple blood vessels of upper extremity

     903.9 Unspecified blood vessel of upper extremity

√4th / √5th Additional Digit Required   Unspecified Code   Other Specified Code   Manifestation Code   ▶◀ Revised Text   ● New Code   ▲ Revised Code Title

✓4ᵗʰ **904 Injury to blood vessels of lower extremity and unspecified sites**

    904.0 **Common femoral artery**
        Femoral artery above profunda origin

    904.1 **Superficial femoral artery**

    904.2 **Femoral veins**

    904.3 **Saphenous veins**
        Saphenous vein (greater) (lesser)

  ✓5ᵗʰ 904.4 **Popliteal blood vessels**
        904.40 Popliteal vessel(s), unspecified
        904.41 **Popliteal artery**
        904.42 **Popliteal vein**

  ✓5ᵗʰ 904.5 **Tibial blood vessels**
        904.50 Tibial vessel(s), unspecified
        904.51 **Anterior tibial artery**
        904.52 **Anterior tibial vein**
        904.53 **Posterior tibial artery**
        904.54 **Posterior tibial vein**

    904.6 **Deep plantar blood vessels**

    904.7 **Other specified blood vessels of lower extremity**
        Multiple blood vessels of lower extremity

    904.8 **Unspecified blood vessel of lower extremity**

    904.9 **Unspecified site**
        Injury to blood vessel NOS

LATE EFFECTS OF INJURIES, POISONINGS, TOXIC EFFECTS, AND OTHER EXTERNAL CAUSES (905-909)

Note: These categories are to be used to indicate conditions classifiable to 800-999 as the cause of late effects, which are themselves classified elsewhere. The "late effects" include those specified as such, or as sequelae, which may occur at any time after the acute injury.

✓4ᵗʰ **905 Late effects of musculoskeletal and connective tissue injuries**

    905.0 **Late effect of fracture of skull and face bones**
        Late effect of injury classifiable to 800-804

    905.1 **Late effect of fracture of spine and trunk without mention of spinal cord lesion**
        Late effect of injury classifiable to 805, 807-809

    905.2 **Late effect of fracture of upper extremities**
        Late effect of injury classifiable to 810-819

    905.3 **Late effect of fracture of neck of femur**
        Late effect of injury classifiable to 820

    905.4 **Late effect of fracture of lower extremities**
        Late effect of injury classifiable to 821-827

    905.5 **Late effect of fracture of multiple and unspecified bones**
        Late effect of injury classifiable to 828-829

    905.6 **Late effect of dislocation**
        Late effect of injury classifiable to 830-839

    905.7 **Late effect of sprain and strain without mention of tendon injury**
        Late effect of injury classifiable to 840-848, except tendon injury

    905.8 **Late effect of tendon injury**
        Late effect of tendon injury due to:
          open wound [injury classifiable to 880-884 with .2, 890-894 with .2]
          sprain and strain [injury classifiable to 840-848]

    905.9 **Late effect of traumatic amputation**
        Late effect of injury classifiable to 885-887, 895-897
        EXCLUDES *late amputation stump complication (997.60-997.69)*

✓4ᵗʰ **906 Late effects of injuries to skin and subcutaneous tissues**

    906.0 **Late effect of open wound of head, neck, and trunk**
        Late effect of injury classifiable to 870-879

    906.1 **Late effect of open wound of extremities without mention of tendon injury**
        Late effect of injury classifiable to 880-884, 890-894 except .2

    906.2 **Late effect of superficial injury**
        Late effect of injury classifiable to 910-919

    906.3 **Late effect of contusion**
        Late effect of injury classifiable to 920-924

    906.4 **Late effect of crushing**
        Late effect of injury classifiable to 925-929

    906.5 **Late effect of burn of eye, face, head, and neck**
        Late effect of injury classifiable to 940-941

    906.6 **Late effect of burn of wrist and hand**
        Late effect of injury classifiable to 944

    906.7 **Late effect of burn of other extremities**
        Late effect of injury classifiable to 943 or 945

    906.8 **Late effect of burns of other specified sites**
        Late effect of injury classifiable to 942, 946-947

    906.9 **Late effect of burn of unspecified site**
        Late effect of injury classifiable to 948-949

✓4ᵗʰ **907 Late effects of injuries to the nervous system**

    907.0 **Late effect of intracranial injury without mention of skull fracture**
        Late effect of injury classifiable to 850-854

    907.1 **Late effect of injury to cranial nerve**
        Late effect of injury classifiable to 950-951

    907.2 **Late effect of spinal cord injury**
        Late effect of injury classifiable to 806, 952

    907.3 **Late effect of injury to nerve root(s), spinal plexus(es), and other nerves of trunk**
        Late effect of injury classifiable to 953-954

    907.4 **Late effect of injury to peripheral nerve of shoulder girdle and upper limb**
        Late effect of injury classifiable to 955

    907.5 **Late effect of injury to peripheral nerve of pelvic girdle and lower limb**
        Late effect of injury classifiable to 956

    907.9 **Late effect of injury to other and unspecified nerve**
        Late effect of injury classifiable to 957

✓4ᵗʰ **908 Late effects of other and unspecified injuries**

    908.0 **Late effect of internal injury to chest**
        Late effect of injury classifiable to 860-862

    908.1 **Late effect of internal injury to intra-abdominal organs**
        Late effect of injury classifiable to 863-866, 868

    908.2 **Late effect of internal injury to other internal organs**
        Late effect of injury classifiable to 867 or 869

    908.3 **Late effect of injury to blood vessel of head, neck, and extremities**
        Late effect of injury classifiable to 900, 903-904

    908.4 **Late effect of injury to blood vessel of thorax, abdomen, and pelvis**
        Late effect of injury classifiable to 901-902

    908.5 **Late effect of foreign body in orifice**
        Late effect of injury classifiable to 930-939

    908.6 **Late effect of certain complications of trauma**
        Late effect of complications classifiable to 958

    908.9 **Late effect of unspecified injury**
        Late effect of injury classifiable to 959

Ⓝ Newborn Age: 0   Ⓟ Pediatric Age: 0-17   Ⓜ Maternity Age: 12-55   Ⓐ Adult Age: 15-124   MSP Medicare Secondary Payer

✓4ᵗʰ **909 Late effects of other and unspecified external causes**

909.0 Late effect of poisoning due to drug, medicinal or biological substance

Late effect of conditions classifiable to 960-979

EXCLUDES   *late effect of adverse effect of drug, medicinal or biological substance (909.5)*

909.1 Late effect of toxic effects of nonmedical substances

Late effect of conditions classifiable to 980-989

909.2 Late effect of radiation

Late effect of conditions classifiable to 990

909.3 Late effect of complications of surgical and medical care

Late effect of conditions classifiable to 996-999

909.4 Late effect of certain other external causes

Late effect of conditions classifiable to 991-994

909.5 Late effect of adverse effect of drug, medical or biological substance

EXCLUDES   *late effect of poisoning due to drug, medical or biological substance (909.0)*

909.9 Late effect of other and unspecified external causes

SUPERFICIAL INJURY (910-919)

EXCLUDES   *burn (blisters) (940.0-949.5)*
contusion (920-924.9)
foreign body:
     granuloma (728.82)
     inadvertently left in operative wound (998.4)
     residual in soft tissue (729.6)
insect bite, venomous (989.5)
open wound with incidental foreign body (870.0-897.7)

✓4ᵗʰ **910 Superficial injury of face, neck, and scalp except eye**

INCLUDES   cheek
        ear
        gum
        lip
        nose
        throat

EXCLUDES   *eye and adnexa (918.0-918.9)*

910.0 Abrasion or friction burn without mention of infection

910.1 Abrasion or friction burn, infected

910.2 Blister without mention of infection

910.3 Blister, infected

910.4 Insect bite, nonvenomous, without mention of infection

910.5 Insect bite, nonvenomous, infected

910.6 Superficial foreign body (splinter) without major open wound and without mention of infection

910.7 Superficial foreign body (splinter) without major open wound, infected

910.8 Other and unspecified superficial injury of face, neck, and scalp without mention of infection

910.9 Other and unspecified superficial injury of face, neck, and scalp, infected

✓4ᵗʰ **911 Superficial injury of trunk**

INCLUDES   abdominal wall
        anus
        back
        breast
        buttock
        mchest wall
        flank
        groin
        interscapular region
        labium (majus) (minus)
        penis
        perineum
        scrotum
        testis
        vagina
        vulva

EXCLUDES   *hip (916.0-916.9)*
scapular region (912.0-912.9)

911.0 Abrasion or friction burn without mention of infection

911.1 Abrasion or friction burn, infected

911.2 Blister without mention of infection

911.3 Blister, infected

911.4 Insect bite, nonvenomous, without mention of infection

911.5 Insect bite, nonvenomous, infected

911.6 Superficial foreign body (splinter) without major open wound and without mention of infection

911.7 Superficial foreign body (splinter) without major open wound, infected

911.8 Other and unspecified superficial injury of trunk, without mention of infection

911.9 Other and unspecified superficial injury of trunk, infected

✓4ᵗʰ **912 Superficial injury of shoulder and upper arm**

INCLUDES   axilla
        scapular region

912.0 Abrasion or friction burn without mention of infection

912.1 Abrasion or friction burn, infected

912.2 Blister without mention of infection

912.3 Blister, infected

912.4 Insect bite, nonvenomous, without mention of infection

912.5 Insect bite, nonvenomous, infected

912.6 Superficial foreign body (splinter) without major open wound and without mention of infection

912.7 Superficial foreign body (splinter) without major open wound, infected

912.8 Other and unspecified superficial injury of shoulder and upper arm without mention of infection

912.9 Other and unspecified superficial injury of shoulder and upper arm, infected

✓4ᵗʰ **913 Superficial injury of elbow, forearm, and wrist**

913.0 Abrasion or friction burn without mention of infection

913.1 Abrasion or friction burn, infected

913.2 Blister without mention of infection

913.3 Blister, infected

913.4 Insect bite, nonvenomous, without mention of infection

913.5 Insect bite, nonvenomous, infected

913.6 Superficial foreign body (splinter) without major open wound and without mention of infection

913.7 Superficial foreign body (splinter) without major open wound, infected

---

✓4ᵗʰ
✓5ᵗʰ   Additional Digit Required   Unspecified Code   Other Specified Code   Manifestation Code   ▶◀ Revised Text   ● New Code   ▲ Revised Code Title

2003 ICD•9•CM   **Volume 1 — 261**

Injury and Poisoning 913.8–921.9

913.8 Other and unspecified superficial injury of elbow, forearm, and wrist without mention of infection

913.9 Other and unspecified superficial injury of elbow, forearm, and wrist, infected

✓4th **914** Superficial injury of hand(s) except finger(s) alone

914.0 Abrasion or friction burn without mention of infection

914.1 Abrasion or friction burn, infected

914.2 Blister without mention of infection

914.3 Blister, infected

914.4 Insect bite, nonvenomous, without mention of infection

914.5 Insect bite, nonvenomous, infected

914.6 Superficial foreign body (splinter) without major open wound and without mention of infection

914.7 Superficial foreign body (splinter) without major open wound, infected

914.8 Other and unspecified superficial injury of hand without mention of infection

914.9 Other and unspecified superficial injury of hand, infected

✓4th **915** Superficial injury of finger(s)

     INCLUDES   fingernail
                      thumb (nail)

915.0 Abrasion or friction burn without mention of infection

915.1 Abrasion or friction burn, infected

915.2 Blister without mention of infection

915.3 Blister, infected

915.4 Insect bite, nonvenomous, without mention of infection

915.5 Insect bite, nonvenomous, infected

915.6 Superficial foreign body (splinter) without major open wound and without mention of infection

915.7 Superficial foreign body (splinter) without major open wound, infected

915.8 Other and unspecified superficial injury of fingers without mention of infection

915.9 Other and unspecified superficial injury of fingers, infected

✓4th **916** Superficial injury of hip, thigh, leg, and ankle

916.0 Abrasion or friction burn without mention of infection

916.1 Abrasion or friction burn, infected

916.2 Blister without mention of infection

916.3 Blister, infected

916.4 Insect bite, nonvenomous, without mention of infection

916.5 Insect bite, nonvenomous, infected

916.6 Superficial foreign body (splinter) without major open wound and without mention of infection

916.7 Superficial foreign body (splinter) without major open wound, infected

916.8 Other and unspecified superficial injury of hip, thigh, leg, and ankle without mention of infection

916.9 Other and unspecified superficial injury of hip, thigh, leg, and ankle, infected

✓4th **917** Superficial injury of foot and toe(s)

     INCLUDES   heel
                      toenail

917.0 Abrasion or friction burn without mention of infection

917.1 Abrasion or friction burn, infected

917.2 Blister without mention of infection

917.3 Blister, infected

917.4 Insect bite, nonvenomous, without mention of infection

917.5 Insect bite, nonvenomous, infected

917.6 Superficial foreign body (splinter) without major open wound and without mention of infection

917.7 Superficial foreign body (splinter) without major open wound, infected

917.8 Other and unspecified superficial injury of foot and toes without mention of infection

917.9 Other and unspecified superficial injury of foot and toes, infected

✓4th **918** Superficial injury of eye and adnexa

     EXCLUDES   burn (940.0-940.9)
                      foreign body on external eye (930.0-930.9)

918.0 Eyelids and periocular area

Abrasion   Superficial foreign body
Insect bite   (splinter)

918.1 Cornea

Corneal abrasion   Superficial laceration

     EXCLUDES   corneal injury due to contact lens (371.82)

918.2 Conjunctiva

918.9 Other and unspecified superficial injuries of eye

Eye (ball) NOS

✓4th **919** Superficial injury of other, multiple, and unspecified sites

     EXCLUDES   multiple sites classifiable to the same three-digit category (910.0-918.9)

919.0 Abrasion or friction burn without mention of infection

919.1 Abrasion or friction burn, infected

919.2 Blister without mention of infection

919.3 Blister, infected

919.4 Insect bite, nonvenomous, without mention of infection

919.5 Insect bite, nonvenomous, infected

919.6 Superficial foreign body (splinter) without major open wound and without mention of infection

919.7 Superficial foreign body (splinter) without major open wound, infected

919.8 Other and unspecified superficial injury without mention of infection

919.9 Other and unspecified superficial injury, infected

CONTUSION WITH INTACT SKIN SURFACE (920-924)

     INCLUDES   bruise } without fracture or open
                   hematoma }   wound

     EXCLUDES   concussion (850.0-850.9)
                   hemarthrosis (840.0-848.9)
                   internal organs (860.0-869.1)
                   that incidental to:
                      crushing injury (925-929.9)
                      dislocation (830.0-839.9)
                      fracture (800.0-829.1)
                      internal injury (860.0-869.1)
                      intracranial injury (850.0-854.1)
                      nerve injury (950.0-957.9)
                      open wound (870.0-897.7)

920 Contusion of face, scalp, and neck except eye(s)

Cheek   Mandibular joint area
Ear (auricle)   Nose
Gum   Throat
Lip

✓4th **921** Contusion of eye and adnexa

921.0 Black eye, not otherwise specified

921.1 Contusion of eyelids and periocular area

921.2 Contusion of orbital tissues

921.3 Contusion of eyeball

921.9 Unspecified contusion of eye

Injury of eye NOS

☑4ᵗʰ **922 Contusion of trunk**

     922.0 **Breast**

     922.1 **Chest wall**

     922.2 **Abdominal wall**

         Flank   Groin

☑5ᵗʰ 922.3 **Back**

         922.31 **Back**

             EXCLUDES   *interscapular region (922.33)*

         922.32 **Buttock**

         922.33 **Interscapular region**

     922.4 **Genital organs**

         Labium (majus) (minus)   Vulva

         Penis   Vagina

         Perineum   Testis

         Scrotum

     922.8 **Multiple sites of trunk**

     922.9 **Unspecified part**

         Trunk NOS

☑4ᵗʰ **923 Contusion of upper limb**

☑5ᵗʰ 923.0 **Shoulder and upper arm**

         923.00 **Shoulder region**

         923.01 **Scapular region**

         923.02 **Axillary region**

         923.03 **Upper arm**

         923.09 **Multiple sites**

☑5ᵗʰ 923.1 **Elbow and forearm**

         923.10 **Forearm**

         923.11 **Elbow**

☑5ᵗʰ 923.2 **Wrist and hand(s), except finger(s) alone**

         923.20 **Hand(s)**

         923.21 **Wrist**

     923.3 **Finger**

         Fingernail   Thumb (nail)

     923.8 **Multiple sites of upper limb**

     923.9 **Unspecified part of upper limb**

         Arm NOS

☑4ᵗʰ **924 Contusion of lower limb and of other and unspecified sites**

☑5ᵗʰ 924.0 **Hip and thigh**

         924.00 **Thigh**

         924.01 **Hip**

☑5ᵗʰ 924.1 **Knee and lower leg**

         924.10 **Lower leg**

         924.11 **Knee**

☑5ᵗʰ 924.2 **Ankle and foot, excluding toe(s)**

         924.20 **Foot**

            Heel

         924.21 **Ankle**

     924.3 **Toe**

         Toenail

     924.4 **Multiple sites of lower limb**

     924.5 **Unspecified part of lower limb**

         Leg NOS

     924.8 **Multiple sites, not elsewhere classified**

     924.9 **Unspecified site**

CRUSHING INJURY (925-929)

     EXCLUDES   *concussion (850.0-850.9)*

         fractures (800-829)

         internal organs (860.0-869.1)

         that incidental to:

            internal injury (860.0-869.1)

            intracranial injury (850.0-854.1)

☑4ᵗʰ **Crushing injury of face, scalp, and neck**

     Cheek   Pharynx

     Ear   Throat

     Larynx

     925.1 **Crushing injury of face and scalp**   MSP

         Cheek   Ear

     925.2 **Crushing injury of neck**   MSP

         Larynx   Throat

         Pharynx

☑4ᵗʰ **Crushing injury of trunk**

     EXCLUDES   *crush injury of internal organs (860.0-869.1)*

     926.0 **External genitalia**

         Labium (majus) (minus)   Testis

         Penis   Vulva

         Scrotum

☑5ᵗʰ 926.1 **Other specified sites**

         926.11 **Back**

         926.12 **Buttock**

         926.19 **Other**

            Breast

            EXCLUDES   *crushing of chest (860.0-862.9)*

     926.8 **Multiple sites of trunk**   MSP

     926.9 **Unspecified site**

         Trunk NOS

☑4ᵗʰ **Crushing injury of upper limb**

☑5ᵗʰ 927.0 **Shoulder and upper arm**

         927.00 **Shoulder region**

         927.01 **Scapular region**

         927.02 **Axillary region**

         927.03 **Upper arm**

         927.09 **Multiple sites**

☑5ᵗʰ 927.1 **Elbow and forearm**

         927.10 **Forearm**

         927.11 **Elbow**

☑5ᵗʰ 927.2 **Wrist and hand(s), except finger(s) alone**

         927.20 **Hand(s)**

         927.21 **Wrist**

     927.3 **Finger(s)**

     927.8 **Multiple sites of upper limb**

     927.9 **Unspecified site**

         Arm NOS

☑4ᵗʰ **928 Crushing injury of lower limb**

☑5ᵗʰ 928.0 **Hip and thigh**

         928.00 **Thigh**

         928.01 **Hip**

☑5ᵗʰ 928.1 **Knee and lower leg**

         928.10 **Lower leg**

         928.11 **Knee**

☑5ᵗʰ 928.2 **Ankle and foot, excluding toe(s) alone**

         928.20 **Foot**

            Heel

         928.21 **Ankle**

     928.3 **Toe(s)**

     928.8 **Multiple sites of lower limb**

     928.9 **Unspecified site**

         Leg NOS

☑4ᵗʰ **929 Crushing injury of multiple and unspecified sites**

     EXCLUDES   *multiple internal injury NOS (869.0-869.1)*

     929.0 **Multiple sites, not elsewhere classified**   MSP

     929.9 **Unspecified site**   MSP

Injury and Poisoning 922–929.9

☑4ᵗʰ ☑5ᵗʰ Additional Digit Required   Unspecified Code   Other Specified Code   Manifestation Code   ▶◀ Revised Text   ● New Code   ▲ Revised Code Title

2003 ICD•9•CM   **Volume 1 — 263**

EFFECTS OF FOREIGN BODY ENTERING THROUGH ORIFICE (930-939)

> **EXCLUDES**   *foreign body:*
> *granuloma (728.82)*
> *inadvertently left in operative wound (998.4, 998.7)*
> *in open wound (800-839, 851-897)*
> *residual in soft tissues (729.6)*
> *superficial without major open wound (910-919 with .6 or .7)*

✓4th **930 Foreign body on external eye**

> **EXCLUDES**   *foreign body in penetrating wound of:*
> *eyeball (871.5-871.6)*
> *retained (old) (360.5-360.6)*
> *ocular adnexa (870.4)*
> *retained (old) (376.6)*

930.0   **Corneal foreign body**
930.1   **Foreign body in conjunctival sac**
930.2   **Foreign body in lacrimal punctum**
930.8   **Other and combined sites**
930.9   **Unspecified site**
    External eye NOS

931 **Foreign body in ear**
    Auditory canal   Auricle

932 **Foreign body in nose**
    Nasal sinus   Nostril

✓4th **933 Foreign body in pharynx and larynx**

933.0   **Pharynx**
    Nasopharynx   Throat NOS

933.1   **Larynx**
    Asphyxia due to foreign body
    Choking due to:
        food (regurgitated)
        phlegm

✓4th **934 Foreign body in trachea, bronchus, and lung**

934.0   **Trachea**
934.1   **Main bronchus**
934.8   **Other specified parts**
    Bronchioles   Lung
934.9   **Respiratory tree, unspecified**
    Inhalation of liquid or vomitus, lower respiratory tract NOS

✓4th **935 Foreign body in mouth, esophagus, and stomach**

935.0   **Mouth**
935.1   **Esophagus**
935.2   **Stomach**

936 **Foreign body in intestine and colon**

937 **Foreign body in anus and rectum**
    Rectosigmoid (junction)

938 **Foreign body in digestive system, unspecified**
    Alimentary tract NOS
    Swallowed foreign body

✓4th **939 Foreign body in genitourinary tract**

939.0   **Bladder and urethra**
939.1   **Uterus, any part**   ♀

> **EXCLUDES**   *intrauterine contraceptive device:*
> *complications from (996.32, 996.65)*
> *presence of (V45.51)*

939.2   **Vulva and vagina**   ♀
939.3   **Penis**   ♂
939.9   **Unspecified site**

Burns

Degrees of Burns

BURNS (940-949)

> **INCLUDES**   burns from:
> electrical heating appliance
> electricity
> flame
> hot object
> lightning
> radiation
> chemical burns (external) (internal)
> scalds

> **EXCLUDES**   *friction burns (910-919 with .0, .1)*
> *sunburn (692.71, 692.76-692.77)*

✓4th **940 Burn confined to eye and adnexa**

940.0   **Chemical burn of eyelids and periocular area**
940.1   **Other burns of eyelids and periocular area**
940.2   **Alkaline chemical burn of cornea and conjunctival sac**
940.3   **Acid chemical burn of cornea and conjunctival sac**
940.4   **Other burn of cornea and conjunctival sac**
940.5   **Burn with resulting rupture and destruction of eyeball**
940.9   **Unspecified burn of eye and adnexa**

✓4th **941 Burn of face, head, and neck**

> **EXCLUDES**   *mouth (947.0)*

The following fifth-digit subclassification is for use with category 941:

0   **face and head, unspecified site**
1   **ear [any part]**
2   **eye (with other parts of face, head, and neck)**
3   **lip(s)**
4   **chin**
5   **nose (septum)**
6   **scalp [any part]**
        Temple (region)
7   **forehead and cheek**
8   **neck**
9   **multiple sites [except with eye] of face, head, and neck**

✓5th 941.0   **Unspecified degree**
✓5th 941.1   **Erythema [first degree]**
✓5th 941.2   **Blisters, epidermal loss [second degree]**
✓5th 941.3   **Full-thickness skin loss [third degree NOS]**
✓5th 941.4   **Deep necrosis of underlying tissues [deep third degree] without mention of loss of a body part**
✓5th 941.5   **Deep necrosis of underlying tissues [deep third degree] with loss of a body part**

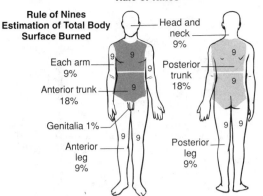

Rule of Nines

Rule of Nines
Estimation of Total Body
Surface Burned

Head and neck 9%

Each arm 9%

Posterior trunk 18%

Anterior trunk 18%

Genitalia 1%

Anterior leg 9%

Posterior leg 9%

✓4ᵗʰ **942 Burn of trunk**

EXCLUDES *scapular region (943.0-943.5 with fifth-digit 6)*

The following fifth-digit subclassification is for use with category 942:

   0   trunk, unspecified site
   1   breast
   2   chest wall, excluding breast and nipple
   3   abdominal wall
      Flank   Groin
   4   back [any part]
      Buttock   Interscapular region
   5   genitalia
      Labium (majus) (minus)   Scrotum
      Penis   Testis
      Perineum   Vulva
   9   other and multiple sites of trunk

✓5ᵗʰ   **942.0**   Unspecified degree
✓5ᵗʰ   **942.1**   Erythema [first degree]
✓5ᵗʰ   **942.2**   Blisters, epidermal loss [second degree]
✓5ᵗʰ   **942.3**   Full-thickness skin loss [third degree NOS]
✓5ᵗʰ   **942.4**   Deep necrosis of underlying tissues [deep third degree] without mention of loss of a body part
✓5ᵗʰ   **942.5**   Deep necrosis of underlying tissues [deep third degree] with loss of a body part

✓4ᵗʰ **943 Burn of upper limb, except wrist and hand**

The following fifth-digit subclassification is for use with category 943:

   0   upper limb, unspecified site
   1   forearm
   2   elbow
   3   upper arm
   4   axilla
   5   shoulder
   6   scapular region
   9   multiple sites of upper limb, except wrist and hand

✓5ᵗʰ   **943.0**   Unspecified degree
✓5ᵗʰ   **943.1**   Erythema [first degree]
✓5ᵗʰ   **943.2**   Blisters, epidermal loss [second degree]
✓5ᵗʰ   **943.3**   Full-thickness skin loss [third degree NOS]
✓5ᵗʰ   **943.4**   Deep necrosis of underlying tissues [deep third degree] without mention of loss of a body part
✓5ᵗʰ   **943.5**   Deep necrosis of underlying tissues [deep third degree] with loss of a body part

✓4ᵗʰ **944 Burn of wrist(s) and hand(s)**

The following fifth-digit subclassification is for use with category 944:

   0   hand, unspecified site
   1   single digit [finger (nail)] other than thumb
   2   thumb (nail)
   3   two or more digits, not including thumb
   4   two or more digits including thumb
   5   palm
   6   back of hand
   7   wrist
   8   multiple sites of wrist(s) and hand(s)

✓5ᵗʰ   **944.0**   Unspecified degree
✓5ᵗʰ   **944.1**   Erythema [first degree]
✓5ᵗʰ   **944.2**   Blisters, epidermal loss [second degree]
✓5ᵗʰ   **944.3**   Full-thickness skin loss [third degree NOS]
✓5ᵗʰ   **944.4**   Deep necrosis of underlying tissues [deep third degree] without mention of loss of a body part
✓5ᵗʰ   **944.5**   Deep necrosis of underlying tissues [deep third degree] with loss of a body part

✓4ᵗʰ **945 Burn of lower limb(s)**

The following fifth-digit subclassification is for use with category 945:

   0   lower limb [leg], unspecified site
   1   toe(s) (nail)
   2   foot
   3   ankle
   4   lower leg
   5   knee
   6   thigh [any part]
   9   multiple sites of lower limb(s)

✓5ᵗʰ   **945.0**   Unspecified degree
✓5ᵗʰ   **945.1**   Erythema [first degree]
✓5ᵗʰ   **945.2**   Blisters, epidermal loss [second degree]
✓5ᵗʰ   **945.3**   Full-thickness skin loss [third degree NOS]
✓5ᵗʰ   **945.4**   Deep necrosis of underlying tissues [deep third degree] without mention of loss of a body part
✓5ᵗʰ   **945.5**   Deep necrosis of underlying tissues [deep third degree] with loss of a body part

✓4ᵗʰ **946 Burns of multiple specified sites**

INCLUDES   burns of sites classifiable to more than one three-digit category in 940-945

EXCLUDES   *multiple burns NOS (949.0-949.5)*

   946.0   Unspecified degree
   946.1   Erythema [first degree]
   946.2   Blisters, epidermal loss [second degree]
   946.3   Full-thickness skin loss [third degree NOS]
   946.4   Deep necrosis of underlying tissues [deep third degree] without mention of loss of a body part
   946.5   Deep necrosis of underlying tissues [deep third degree] with loss of a body part

✓4ᵗʰ **947 Burn of internal organs**

INCLUDES   burns from chemical agents (ingested)

   947.0   **Mouth and pharynx**
           Gum   Tongue
   947.1   **Larynx, trachea, and lung**
   947.2   **Esophagus**
   947.3   **Gastrointestinal tract**
           Colon   Small intestine
           Rectum   Stomach
   947.4   **Vagina and uterus**   ♀
   947.8   **Other specified sites**
   947.9   **Unspecified site**

Injury and Poisoning 942–947.9

✓4ᵗʰ / ✓5ᵗʰ   Additional Digit Required   Unspecified Code   Other Specified Code   Manifestation Code   ▶◀ Revised Text   ● New Code   ▲ Revised Code Title

2003 ICD•9•CM   **Volume 1 — 265**

✓4ᵗʰ **948 Burns classified according to extent of body surface involved**

Note: This category is to be used when the site of the burn is unspecified, or with categories 940-947 when the site is specified.

EXCLUDES *sunburn (692.71, 692.76-692.77)*

The following fifth-digit subclassification is for use with category 948 to indicate the percent of body surface with third degree burn; valid digits are in [brackets] under each code:

0   less than 10 percent or unspecified
1   10-19%
2   20-29%
3   30-39%
4   40-49%
5   50-59%
6   60-69%
7   70-79%
8   80-89%
9   90% or more of body surface

✓5ᵗʰ **948.0** Burn [any degree] involving less than 10 percent of
[0]   body surface

✓5ᵗʰ **948.1** 10-19 percent of body surface
[0-1]

✓5ᵗʰ **948.2** 20-29 percent of body surface
[0-2]

✓5ᵗʰ **948.3** 30-39 percent of body surface
[0-3]

✓5ᵗʰ **948.4** 40-49 percent of body surface
[0-4]

✓5ᵗʰ **948.5** 50-59 percent of body surface
[0-5]

✓5ᵗʰ **948.6** 60-69 percent of body surface
[0-6]

✓5ᵗʰ **948.7** 70-79 percent of body surface
[0-7]

✓5ᵗʰ **948.8** 80-89 percent of body surface
[0-8]

✓5ᵗʰ **948.9** 90 percent or more of body surface
[0-9]

✓4ᵗʰ **949 Burn, unspecified**

INCLUDES   burn NOS multiple burns NOS

EXCLUDES   *burn of unspecified site but with statement of the extent of body surface involved (948.0-948.9)*

949.0   **Unspecified degree**
949.1   **Erythema [first degree]**
949.2   **Blisters, epidermal loss [second degree]**
949.3   **Full-thickness skin loss [third degree NOS]**
949.4   **Deep necrosis of underlying tissues [deep third degree] without mention of loss of a body part**
949.5   **Deep necrosis of underlying tissues [deep third degree] with loss of a body part**

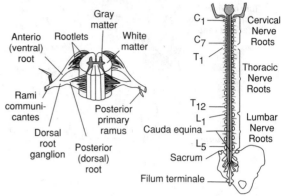

Spinal Nerve Roots

INJURY TO NERVES AND SPINAL CORD (950-957)

INCLUDES   division of nerve
lesion in continuity
traumatic neuroma   } (with open wound)
traumatic transient paralysis

EXCLUDES   *accidental puncture or laceration during medical procedure (998.2)*

✓4ᵗʰ **950 Injury to optic nerve and pathways**

950.0   **Optic nerve injury**
Second cranial nerve

950.1   **Injury to optic chiasm**

950.2   **Injury to optic pathways**

950.3   **Injury to visual cortex**

950.9   **Unspecified**
Traumatic blindness NOS

✓4ᵗʰ **951 Injury to other cranial nerve(s)**

951.0   **Injury to oculomotor nerve**
Third cranial nerve

951.1   **Injury to trochlear nerve**
Fourth cranial nerve

951.2   **Injury to trigeminal nerve**
Fifth cranial nerve

951.3   **Injury to abducens nerve**
Sixth cranial nerve

951.4   **Injury to facial nerve**
Seventh cranial nerve

951.5   **Injury to acoustic nerve**
Auditory nerve   Traumatic deafness NOS
Eighth cranial nerve

951.6   **Injury to accessory nerve**
Eleventh cranial nerve

951.7   **Injury to hypoglossal nerve**
Twelfth cranial nerve

951.8   **Injury to other specified cranial nerves**
Glossopharyngeal [9th cranial] nerve
Olfactory [1st cranial] nerve
Pneumogastric [10th cranial] nerve
Traumatic anosmia NOS
Vagus [10th cranial] nerve

951.9   **Injury to unspecified cranial nerve**

✓4ᵗʰ **952 Spinal cord injury without evidence of spinal bone injury**

✓5ᵗʰ **952.0**   **Cervical**

952.00   **C_1-C_4 level with unspecified spinal cord injury**
Spinal cord injury, cervical region NOS

952.01   **C_1-C_4 level with complete lesion of spinal cord**

952.02   **C_1-C_4 level with anterior cord syndrome**

952.03   **C_1-C_4 level with central cord syndrome**

N Newborn Age: 0   P Pediatric Age: 0-17   M Maternity Age: 12-55   A Adult Age: 15-124   MSP Medicare Secondary Payer

952.04 C_1-C_4 level with other specified spinal cord injury
     Incomplete spinal cord lesion at C_1-C_4 level:
        NOS
        with posterior cord syndrome

952.05 C_5-C_7 level with unspecified spinal cord injury

952.06 C_5-C_7 level with complete lesion of spinal cord

952.07 C_5-C_7 level with anterior cord syndrome

952.08 C_5-C_7 level with central cord syndrome

952.09 C_5-C_7 level with other specified spinal cord injury
     Incomplete spinal cord lesion at C_5-C_7 level:
        NOS
        with posterior cord syndrome

√5th   **952.1**   **Dorsal [thoracic]**

952.10 T_1-T_6 level with unspecified spinal cord injury
     Spinal cord injury, thoracic region NOS

952.11 T_1-T_6 level with complete lesion of spinal cord

952.12 T_1-T_6 level with anterior cord syndrome

952.13 T_1-T_6 level with central cord syndrome

952.14 T_1-T_6 level with other specified spinal cord injury
     Incomplete spinal cord lesion at T_1-T_6 level:
        NOS
        with posterior cord syndrome

952.15 T_7-T_{12} level with unspecified spinal cord injury

952.16 T_7-T_{12} level with complete lesion of spinal cord

952.17 T_7-T_{12} level with anterior cord syndrome

952.18 T_7-T_{12} level with central cord syndrome

952.19 T_7-T_{12} level with other specified spinal cord injury
     Incomplete spinal cord lesion at T_7-T_{12} level:
        NOS
        with posterior cord syndrome

952.2   **Lumbar**

952.3   **Sacral**

952.4   **Cauda equina**

952.8   **Multiple sites of spinal cord**

952.9   **Unspecified site of spinal cord**

√4th   **953**   **Injury to nerve roots and spinal plexus**

953.0   **Cervical root**

953.1   **Dorsal root**

953.2   **Lumbar root**

953.3   **Sacral root**

953.4   **Brachial plexus**

953.5   **Lumbosacral plexus**

953.8   **Multiple sites**

953.9   **Unspecified site**

√4th   **954**   **Injury to other nerve(s) of trunk, excluding shoulder and pelvic girdles**

954.0   **Cervical sympathetic**

954.1   **Other sympathetic**
     Celiac ganglion or plexus   Splanchnic nerve(s)
     Inferior mesenteric plexus   Stellate ganglion

954.8   **Other specified nerve(s) of trunk**

954.9   **Unspecified nerve of trunk**

√4th   **955**   **Injury to peripheral nerve(s) of shoulder girdle and upper limb**

955.0   **Axillary nerve**

955.1   **Median nerve**

955.2   **Ulnar nerve**

955.3   **Radial nerve**

955.4   **Musculocutaneous nerve**

955.5   **Cutaneous sensory nerve, upper limb**

955.6   **Digital nerve**

955.7   **Other specified nerve(s) of shoulder girdle and upper limb**

955.8   **Multiple nerves of shoulder girdle and upper limb**

955.9   **Unspecified nerve of shoulder girdle and upper limb**

√4th   **956**   **Injury to peripheral nerve(s) of pelvic girdle and lower limb**

956.0   **Sciatic nerve**

956.1   **Femoral nerve**

956.2   **Posterior tibial nerve**

956.3   **Peroneal nerve**

956.4   **Cutaneous sensory nerve, lower limb**

956.5   **Other specified nerve(s) of pelvic girdle and lower limb**

956.8   **Multiple nerves of pelvic girdle and lower limb**

956.9   **Unspecified nerve of pelvic girdle and lower limb**

√4th   **957**   **Injury to other and unspecified nerves**

957.0   **Superficial nerves of head and neck**

957.1   **Other specified nerve(s)**

957.8   **Multiple nerves in several parts**
     Multiple nerve injury NOS

957.9   **Unspecified site**
     Nerve injury NOS

CERTAIN TRAUMATIC COMPLICATIONS AND UNSPECIFIED INJURIES (958-959)

√4th   **958**   **Certain early complications of trauma**
     EXCLUDES   *adult respiratory distress syndrome (518.5)*
         flail chest (807.4)
         shock lung (518.5)
         that occurring during or following medical procedures (996.0-999.9)

958.0   **Air embolism**
     Pneumathemia
     EXCLUDES   *that complicating:*
         abortion (634-638 with .6, 639.6)
         ectopic or molar pregnancy (639.6)
         pregnancy, childbirth, or the puerperium (673.0)

     DEF: Arterial obstruction due to introduction of air bubbles into the veins following surgery or trauma.

958.1   **Fat embolism**
     EXCLUDES   *that complicating:*
         abortion (634-638 with .6, 639.6)
         pregnancy, childbirth, or the puerperium (673.8)

     DEF: Arterial blockage due to the entrance of fat in circulatory system, after fracture of large bones or administration of corticosteroids.

958.2   **Secondary and recurrent hemorrhage**

958.3   **Posttraumatic wound infection, not elsewhere classified**
     EXCLUDES   *infected open wounds — code to complicated open wound of site*

√4th
√5th
Additional Digit Required   Unspecified Code   Other Specified Code   Manifestation Code   ►◄ Revised Text   ● New Code   ▲ Revised Code Title

2003 ICD•9•CM   Volume 1 — 267

958.4 Traumatic shock `MSP`

Shock (immediate) (delayed) following injury

> `EXCLUDES` shock:
>> anaphylactic (995.0)
>>> due to serum (999.4)
>> anesthetic (995.4)
>> electric (994.8)
>> following abortion (639.5)
>> lightning (994.0)
>> nontraumatic NOS (785.50)
>> obstetric (669.1)
>> postoperative (998.0)

DEF: Shock, immediate or delayed following injury.

958.5 Traumatic anuria `MSP`

Crush syndrome

Renal failure following crushing

> `EXCLUDES` that due to a medical procedure (997.5)

DEF: Complete suppression of urinary secretion by kidneys due to trauma.

958.6 Volkmann's ischemic contracture

Posttraumatic muscle contracture

DEF: Muscle deterioration due to loss of blood supply from injury or tourniquet; causes muscle contraction and results in inability to extend the muscles fully.

958.7 Traumatic subcutaneous emphysema

> `EXCLUDES` subcutaneous emphysema resulting from a procedure (998.81)

958.8 Other early complications of trauma

DEF: Compartmental syndrome is abnormal pressure in confined anatomical space, as in swollen muscle restricted by fascia.

√4ᵗʰ **959 Injury, other and unspecified**

> `INCLUDES` injury NOS
> `EXCLUDES` injury NOS of:
>> blood vessels (900.0-904.9)
>> eye (921.0-921.9)
>> internal organs (860.0-869.1)
>> intracranial sites (854.0-854.1)
>> nerves (950.0-951.9, 953.0-957.9)
>> spinal cord (952.0-952.9)

√5ᵗʰ **959.0 Head, face and neck**

959.01 Head injury, unspecified `MSP`

> `EXCLUDES` concussion (850.1-850.9)
>> with head injury NOS (850.0-850.9)
>> ►head injury NOS with loss of consciousness (850.1-850.5)◄
>> specified injuries (850.0-854.1)

959.09 Injury of face and neck `MSP`

Cheek	Mouth
Ear	Nose
Eyebrow	Throat
Lip	

959.1 Trunk

Abdominal wall	External genital organs
Back	Flank
Breast	Groin
Buttock	Interscapular region
Chest wall	Perineum

> `EXCLUDES` scapular region (959.2)

959.2 Shoulder and upper arm

Axilla	Scapular region

959.3 Elbow, forearm, and wrist

959.4 Hand, except finger

959.5 Finger

Fingernail	Thumb (nail)

959.6 Hip and thigh

Upper leg

959.7 Knee, leg, ankle, and foot

959.8 Other specified sites, including multiple

> `EXCLUDES` multiple sites classifiable to the same four-digit category (959.0-959.7)

959.9 Unspecified site

POISONING BY DRUGS, MEDICINAL AND BIOLOGICAL SUBSTANCES (960-979)

> `INCLUDES` overdose of these substances
>> wrong substance given or taken in error
> `EXCLUDES` adverse effects ["hypersensitivity," "reaction," etc.] of correct substance properly administered. Such cases are to be classified according to the nature of the adverse effect, such as:
>> adverse effect NOS (995.2)
>> allergic lymphadenitis (289.3)
>> aspirin gastritis (535.4)
>> blood disorders (280.0-289.9)
>> dermatitis:
>>> contact (692.0-692.9)
>>> due to ingestion (693.0-693.9)
>> nephropathy (583.9)
>> [The drug giving rise to the adverse effect may be identified by use of categories E930-E949.]
>> drug dependence (304.0-304.9)
>> drug reaction and poisoning affecting the newborn (760.0-779.9)
>> nondependent abuse of drugs (305.0-305.9)
>> pathological drug intoxication (292.2)

Use additional code to specify the effects of the poisoning

√4ᵗʰ **960 Poisoning by antibiotics**

> `EXCLUDES` antibiotics:
>> ear, nose, and throat (976.6)
>> eye (976.5)
>> local (976.0)

960.0 Penicillins

Ampicillin	Cloxacillin
Carbenicillin	Penicillin G

960.1 Antifungal antibiotics

Amphotericin B	Nystatin
Griseofulvin	Trichomycin

> `EXCLUDES` preparations intended for topical use (976.0-976.9)

960.2 Chloramphenicol group

Chloramphenicol	Thiamphenicol

960.3 Erythromycin and other macrolides

Oleandomycin	Spiramycin

960.4 Tetracycline group

Doxycycline	Oxytetracycline
Minocycline	

960.5 Cephalosporin group

Cephalexin	Cephaloridine
Cephaloglycin	Cephalothin

960.6 Antimycobacterial antibiotics

Cycloserine	Rifampin
Kanamycin	Streptomycin

960.7 Antineoplastic antibiotics

Actinomycin such as:
- Bleomycin
- Cactinomycin
- Dactinomycin
- Daunorubicin
- Mitomycin

960.8 Other specified antibiotics

960.9 Unspecified antibiotic

`N` Newborn Age: 0   `P` Pediatric Age: 0-17   `M` Maternity Age: 12-55   `A` Adult Age: 15-124   `MSP` Medicare Secondary Payer

268 — Volume 1 • October 2002   2003 ICD•9•CM

✓4ᵗʰ **961 Poisoning by other anti-infectives**

    EXCLUDES *anti-infectives:*
        ear, nose, and throat (976.6)
        eye (976.5)
        local (976.0)

961.0 Sulfonamides
    Sulfadiazine   Sulfamethoxazole
    Sulfafurazole

961.1 Arsenical anti-infectives

961.2 Heavy metal anti-infectives
    Compounds of: Compounds of:
      antimony   lead
      bismuth   mercury
    EXCLUDES *mercurial diuretics (974.0)*

961.3 Quinoline and hydroxyquinoline derivatives
    Chiniofon   Diiodohydroxyquin
    EXCLUDES *antimalarial drugs (961.4)*

961.4 Antimalarials and drugs acting on other blood protozoa
    Chloroquine   Proguanil [chloroguanide]
    Cycloguanil   Pyrimethamine
    Primaquine   Quinine

961.5 Other antiprotozoal drugs
    Emetine

961.6 Anthelmintics
    Hexylresorcinol   Thiabendazole
    Piperazine

961.7 Antiviral drugs
    Methisazone
    EXCLUDES *amantadine (966.4)*
        cytarabine (963.1)
        idoxuridine (976.5)

961.8 Other antimycobacterial drugs
    Ethambutol   Para-aminosalicylic acid
    Ethionamide   derivatives
    Isoniazid   Sulfones

961.9 Other and unspecified anti-infectives
    Flucytosine   Nitrofuran derivatives

✓4ᵗʰ **962 Poisoning by hormones and synthetic substitutes**
    EXCLUDES *oxytocic hormones (975.0)*

962.0 Adrenal cortical steroids
    Cortisone derivatives
    Desoxycorticosterone derivatives
    Fluorinated corticosteroids

962.1 Androgens and anabolic congeners
    Methandriol   Oxymetholone
    Nandrolone   Testosterone

962.2 Ovarian hormones and synthetic substitutes
    Contraceptives, oral
    Estrogens
    Estrogens and progestogens, combined
    Progestogens

962.3 Insulins and antidiabetic agents
    Acetohexamide
    Biguanide derivatives, oral
    Chlorpropamide
    Glucagon
    Insulin
    Phenformin
    Sulfonylurea derivatives, oral
    Tolbutamide

962.4 Anterior pituitary hormones
    Corticotropin   Somatotropin [growth
    Gonadotropin   hormone]

962.5 Posterior pituitary hormones
    Vasopressin
    EXCLUDES *oxytocic hormones (975.0)*

962.6 Parathyroid and parathyroid derivatives

962.7 Thyroid and thyroid derivatives
    Dextrothyroxin   Liothyronine
    Levothyroxine sodium   Thyroglobulin

962.8 Antithyroid agents
    Iodides   Thiourea
    Thiouracil

962.9 Other and unspecified hormones and synthetic substitutes

✓4ᵗʰ **963 Poisoning by primarily systemic agents**

963.0 Antiallergic and antiemetic drugs
    Antihistamines   Diphenylpyraline
    Chlorpheniramine   Thonzylamine
    Diphenhydramine   Tripelennamine
    EXCLUDES *phenothiazine-based tranquilizers (969.1)*

963.1 Antineoplastic and immunosuppressive drugs
    Azathioprine   Cytarabine
    Busulfan   Fluorouracil
    Chlorambucil   Mercaptopurine
    Cyclophosphamide   thio-TEPA
    EXCLUDES *antineoplastic antibiotics (960.7)*

963.2 Acidifying agents

963.3 Alkalizing agents

963.4 Enzymes, not elsewhere classified
    Penicillinase

963.5 Vitamins, not elsewhere classified
    Vitamin A   Vitamin D
    EXCLUDES *nicotinic acid (972.2)*
        vitamin K (964.3)

963.8 Other specified systemic agents
    Heavy metal antagonists

963.9 Unspecified systemic agent

✓4ᵗʰ **964 Poisoning by agents primarily affecting blood constituents**

964.0 Iron and its compounds
    Ferric salts
    Ferrous sulfate and other ferrous salts

964.1 Liver preparations and other antianemic agents
    Folic acid

964.2 Anticoagulants
    Coumarin   Phenindione
    Heparin   Warfarin sodium

964.3 Vitamin K [phytonadione]

964.4 Fibrinolysis-affecting drugs
    Aminocaproic acid   Streptokinase
    Streptodornase   Urokinase

964.5 Anticoagulant antagonists and other coagulants
    Hexadimethrine   Protamine sulfate

964.6 Gamma globulin

964.7 Natural blood and blood products
    Blood plasma   Packed red cells
    Human fibrinogen   Whole blood
    EXCLUDES *transfusion reactions (999.4-999.8)*

964.8 Other specified agents affecting blood constituents
    Macromolecular blood substitutes
    Plasma expanders

964.9 Unspecified agent affecting blood constituents

✓4ᵗʰ **965 Poisoning by analgesics, antipyretics, and antirheumatics**
    EXCLUDES *drug dependence (304.0-304.9)*
        nondependent abuse (305.0-305.9)

✓5ᵗʰ **965.0 Opiates and related narcotics**

    965.00 Opium (alkaloids), unspecified

    965.01 Heroin
        Diacetylmorphine

    965.02 Methadone

    965.09 Other
        Codeine [methylmorphine]
        Meperidine [pethidine]
        Morphine

965.1 Salicylates
    Acetylsalicylic acid [aspirin]   Salicylic acid salts

✓4ᵗʰ / ✓5ᵗʰ Additional Digit Required   Unspecified Code   Other Specified Code   Manifestation Code   ▶◀ Revised Text   ● New Code   ▲ Revised Code Title

965.4 Aromatic analgesics, not elsewhere classified
Acetanilid   Phenacetin [acetophenetidin]
Paracetamol [acetaminophen]

965.5 Pyrazole derivatives
Aminophenazone [aminopyrine]
Phenylbutazone

✓5th **965.6 Antirheumatics [antiphlogistics]**
> EXCLUDES   salicylates (965.1)
>   steroids (962.0-962.9)

965.61 Propionic acid derivatives
Fenoprofen
Flurbiprofen
Ibuprofen
Ketoprofen
Naproxen
Oxaprozin

965.69 Other antirheumatics
Gold salts
Indomethacin

965.7 Other non-narcotic analgesics
Pyrabital

965.8 Other specified analgesics and antipyretics
Pentazocine

965.9 Unspecified analgesic and antipyretic

✓4th **966 Poisoning by anticonvulsants and anti-Parkinsonism drugs**

966.0 Oxazolidine derivatives
Paramethadione   Trimethadione

966.1 Hydantoin derivatives
Phenytoin

966.2 Succinimides
Ethosuximide   Phensuximide

966.3 Other and unspecified anticonvulsants
Primidone
> EXCLUDES   barbiturates (967.0)
>   sulfonamides (961.0)

966.4 Anti-Parkinsonism drugs
Amantadine
Ethopropazine [profenamine]
Levodopa [L-dopa]

✓4th **967 Poisoning by sedatives and hypnotics**
> EXCLUDES   drug dependence (304.0-304.9)
>   nondependent abuse (305.0-305.9)

967.0 Barbiturates
Amobarbital [amylobarbitone]
Barbital [barbitone]
Butabarbital [butabarbitone]
Pentobarbital [pentobarbitone]
Phenobarbital [phenobarbitone]
Secobarbital [quinalbarbitone]
> EXCLUDES   thiobarbiturate anesthetics (968.3)

967.1 Chloral hydrate group

967.2 Paraldehyde

967.3 Bromine compounds
Bromide   Carbromal (derivatives)

967.4 Methaqualone compounds

967.5 Glutethimide group

967.6 Mixed sedatives, not elsewhere classified

967.8 Other sedatives and hypnotics

967.9 Unspecified sedative or hypnotic
Sleeping:
   drug
   pill   } NOS
   tablet

✓4th **968 Poisoning by other central nervous system depressants and anesthetics**
> EXCLUDES   drug dependence (304.0-304.9)
>   nondependent abuse (305.0-305.9)

968.0 Central nervous system muscle-tone depressants
Chlorphenesin (carbamate)   Methocarbamol
Mephenesin

968.1 Halothane

968.2 Other gaseous anesthetics
Ether
Halogenated hydrocarbon derivatives, except
   halothane
Nitrous oxide

968.3 Intravenous anesthetics
Ketamine
Methohexital [methohexitone]
Thiobarbiturates, such as thiopental sodium

968.4 Other and unspecified general anesthetics

968.5 Surface [topical] and infiltration anesthetics
Cocaine   Procaine
Lidocaine [lignocaine] Tetracaine

968.6 Peripheral nerve- and plexus-blocking anesthetics

968.7 Spinal anesthetics

968.9 Other and unspecified local anesthetics

✓4th **969 Poisoning by psychotropic agents**
> EXCLUDES   drug dependence (304.0-304.9)
>   nondependent abuse (305.0-305.9)

969.0 Antidepressants
Amitriptyline
Imipramine
Monoamine oxidase [MAO] inhibitors

969.1 Phenothiazine-based tranquilizers
Chlorpromazine   Prochlorperazine
Fluphenazine   Promazine

969.2 Butyrophenone-based tranquilizers
Haloperidol   Trifluperidol
Spiperone

969.3 Other antipsychotics, neuroleptics, and major tranquilizers

969.4 Benzodiazepine-based tranquilizers
Chlordiazepoxide   Lorazepam
Diazepam   Medazepam
Flurazepam   Nitrazepam

969.5 Other tranquilizers
Hydroxyzine   Meprobamate

969.6 Psychodysleptics [hallucinogens]
Cannabis (derivatives)   Mescaline
Lysergide [LSD]   Psilocin
Marihuana (derivatives) Psilocybin

969.7 Psychostimulants
Amphetamine   Caffeine
> EXCLUDES   central appetite depressants (977.0)

969.8 Other specified psychotropic agents

969.9 Unspecified psychotropic agent

✓4th **970 Poisoning by central nervous system stimulants**

970.0 Analeptics
Lobeline
Nikethamide

970.1 Opiate antagonists
Levallorphan
Nalorphine
Naloxone

970.8 Other specified central nervous system stimulants

970.9 Unspecified central nervous system stimulant

✓4th **971 Poisoning by drugs primarily affecting the autonomic nervous system**

971.0 Parasympathomimetics [cholinergics]
Acetylcholine   Pilocarpine
Anticholinesterase:
   organophosphorus
   reversible

971.1 Parasympatholytics [anticholinergics and antimuscarinics] and spasmolytics
Atropine   Quaternary ammonium
Homatropine   derivatives
Hyoscine [scopolamine]
> EXCLUDES   papaverine (972.5)

971.2 **Sympathomimetics [adrenergics]**
Epinephrine [adrenalin]   Levarterenol [noradrenalin]

971.3 **Sympatholytics [antiadrenergics]**
Phenoxybenzamine   Tolazolinehydrochloride

971.9 **Unspecified drug primarily affecting autonomic nervous system**

✓4th 972 **Poisoning by agents primarily affecting the cardiovascular system**

972.0 **Cardiac rhythm regulators**
Practolol   Propranolol
Procainamide   Quinidine
EXCLUDES lidocaine (968.5)

972.1 **Cardiotonic glycosides and drugs of similar action**
Digitalis glycosides   Strophanthins
Digoxin

972.2 **Antilipemic and antiarteriosclerotic drugs**
Clofibrate   Nicotinic acid derivatives

972.3 **Ganglion-blocking agents**
Pentamethonium bromide

972.4 **Coronary vasodilators**
Dipyridamole   Nitrites
Nitrates [nitroglycerin]

972.5 **Other vasodilators**
Cyclandelate   Papaverine
Diazoxide
EXCLUDES nicotinic acid (972.2)

972.6 **Other antihypertensive agents**
Clonidine   Rauwolfia alkaloids
Guanethidine   Reserpine

972.7 **Antivaricose drugs, including sclerosing agents**
Sodium morrhuate   Zinc salts

972.8 **Capillary-active drugs**
Adrenochrome derivatives   Metaraminol

972.9 **Other and unspecified agents primarily affecting the cardiovascular system**

✓4th 973 **Poisoning by agents primarily affecting the gastrointestinal system**

973.0 **Antacids and antigastric secretion drugs**
Aluminum hydroxide   Magnesium trisilicate

973.1 **Irritant cathartics**
Bisacodyl   Phenolphthalein
Castor oil

973.2 **Emollient cathartics**
Dioctyl sulfosuccinates

973.3 **Other cathartics, including intestinal atonia drugs**
Magnesium sulfate

973.4 **Digestants**
Pancreatin   Pepsin
Papain

973.5 **Antidiarrheal drugs**
Kaolin   Pectin
EXCLUDES anti-infectives (960.0-961.9)

973.6 **Emetics**

973.8 **Other specified agents primarily affecting the gastrointestinal system**

973.9 **Unspecified agent primarily affecting the gastrointestinal system**

✓4th 974 **Poisoning by water, mineral, and uric acid metabolism drugs**

974.0 **Mercurial diuretics**
Chlormerodrin   Mersalyl
Mercaptomerin

974.1 **Purine derivative diuretics**
Theobromine   Theophylline
EXCLUDES aminophylline [theophylline ethylenediamine] (975.7)
caffeine (969.7)

974.2 **Carbonic acid anhydrase inhibitors**
Acetazolamide

974.3 **Saluretics**
Benzothiadiazides   Chlorothiazide group

974.4 **Other diuretics**
Ethacrynic acid   Furosemide

974.5 **Electrolytic, caloric, and water-balance agents**

974.6 **Other mineral salts, not elsewhere classified**

974.7 **Uric acid metabolism drugs**
Allopurinol   Probenecid
Colchicine

✓4th 975 **Poisoning by agents primarily acting on the smooth and skeletal muscles and respiratory system**

975.0 **Oxytocic agents**
Ergot alkaloids   Prostaglandins
Oxytocin

975.1 **Smooth muscle relaxants**
Adiphenine   Metaproterenol [orciprenaline]
EXCLUDES papaverine (972.5)

975.2 **Skeletal muscle relaxants**

975.3 **Other and unspecified drugs acting on muscles**

975.4 **Antitussives**
Dextromethorphan   Pipazethate

975.5 **Expectorants**
Acetylcysteine   Terpin hydrate
Guaifenesin

975.6 **Anti-common cold drugs**

975.7 **Antiasthmatics**
Aminophylline [theophylline ethylenediamine]

975.8 **Other and unspecified respiratory drugs**

✓4th 976 **Poisoning by agents primarily affecting skin and mucous membrane, ophthalmological, otorhinolaryngological, and dental drugs**

976.0 **Local anti-infectives and anti-inflammatory drugs**

976.1 **Antipruritics**

976.2 **Local astringents and local detergents**

976.3 **Emollients, demulcents, and protectants**

976.4 **Keratolytics, keratoplastics, other hair treatment drugs and preparations**

976.5 **Eye anti-infectives and other eye drugs**
Idoxuridine

976.6 **Anti-infectives and other drugs and preparations for ear, nose, and throat**

976.7 **Dental drugs topically applied**
EXCLUDES anti-infectives (976.0)
local anesthetics (968.5)

976.8 **Other agents primarily affecting skin and mucous membrane**
Spermicides [vaginal contraceptives]

976.9 **Unspecified agent primarily affecting skin and mucous membrane**

✓4th 977 **Poisoning by other and unspecified drugs and medicinal substances**

977.0 **Dietetics**
Central appetite depressants

977.1 **Lipotropic drugs**

977.2 **Antidotes and chelating agents, not elsewhere classified**

977.3 **Alcohol deterrents**

977.4 **Pharmaceutical excipients**
Pharmaceutical adjuncts

977.8 **Other specified drugs and medicinal substances**
Contrast media used for diagnostic x-ray procedures
Diagnostic agents and kits

977.9 **Unspecified drug or medicinal substance**

✓4th 978 **Poisoning by bacterial vaccines**

978.0 **BCG**

978.1 **Typhoid and paratyphoid**

978.2 **Cholera**

978.3 **Plague**

978.4 **Tetanus**

978.5 **Diphtheria**

✓4th ✓5th Additional Digit Required   Unspecified Code   Other Specified Code   Manifestation Code   ▶◀ Revised Text   ● New Code   ▲ Revised Code Title

2003 ICD•9•CM   Volume 1 — 271

Injury and Poisoning 978.6–988.9

978.6   Pertussis vaccine, including combinations with a pertussis component

978.8   Other and unspecified bacterial vaccines

978.9   Mixed bacterial vaccines, except combinations with a pertussis component

✓4ᵗʰ **979 Poisoning by other vaccines and biological substances**

EXCLUDES   *gamma globulin (964.6)*

979.0   Smallpox vaccine

979.1   Rabies vaccine

979.2   Typhus vaccine

979.3   Yellow fever vaccine

979.4   Measles vaccine

979.5   Poliomyelitis vaccine

979.6   Other and unspecified viral and rickettsial vaccines

     Mumps vaccine

979.7   Mixed viral-rickettsial and bacterial vaccines, except combinations with a pertussis component

EXCLUDES   *combinations with a pertussis component (978.6)*

979.9   Other and unspecified vaccines and biological substances

TOXIC EFFECTS OF SUBSTANCES CHIEFLY NONMEDICINAL AS TO SOURCE (980-989)

EXCLUDES   *burns from chemical agents (ingested) (947.0-947.9)*
localized toxic effects indexed elsewhere (001.0-799.9)
respiratory conditions due to external agents (506.0-508.9)

Use additional code to specify the nature of the toxic effect

✓4ᵗʰ **980 Toxic effect of alcohol**

980.0   Ethyl alcohol

     Denatured alcohol   Grain alcohol
     Ethanol
     Use additional code to identify any associated:
       acute alcohol intoxication (305.0)
         in alcoholism (303.0)
       drunkenness (simple) (305.0)
       pathological (291.4)

980.1   Methyl alcohol

     Methanol   Wood alcohol

980.2   Isopropyl alcohol

     Dimethyl carbinol   Rubbing alcohol
     Isopropanol

980.3   Fusel oil

     Alcohol: Alcohol:
       amyl   propyl
       butyl

980.8   Other specified alcohols

980.9   Unspecified alcohol

981 Toxic effect of petroleum products

     Benzine   Petroleum:
     Gasoline   ether
     Kerosene   naphtha
     Paraffin wax   spirit

✓4ᵗʰ **982 Toxic effect of solvents other than petroleum-based**

982.0   Benzene and homologues

982.1   Carbon tetrachloride

982.2   Carbon disulfide

     Carbon bisulfide

982.3   Other chlorinated hydrocarbon solvents

     Tetrachloroethylene   Trichloroethylene

EXCLUDES   *chlorinated hydrocarbon preparations other than solvents (989.2)*

982.4   Nitroglycol

982.8   Other nonpetroleum-based solvents

     Acetone

✓4ᵗʰ **983 Toxic effect of corrosive aromatics, acids, and caustic alkalis**

983.0   Corrosive aromatics

     Carbolic acid or phenol   Cresol

983.1   Acids

     Acid: Acid:
       hydrochloric   sulfuric
       nitric

983.2   Caustic alkalis

     Lye   Sodium hydroxide
     Potassium hydroxide

983.9   Caustic, unspecified

✓4ᵗʰ **984 Toxic effect of lead and its compounds (including fumes)**

INCLUDES   that from all sources except medicinal substances

984.0   Inorganic lead compounds

     Lead dioxide   Lead salts

984.1   Organic lead compounds

     Lead acetate   Tetraethyl lead

984.8   Other lead compounds

984.9   Unspecified lead compound

✓4ᵗʰ **985 Toxic effect of other metals**

INCLUDES   that from all sources except medicinal substances

985.0   Mercury and its compounds

     Minamata disease

985.1   Arsenic and its compounds

985.2   Manganese and its compounds

985.3   Beryllium and its compounds

985.4   Antimony and its compounds

985.5   Cadmium and its compounds

985.6   Chromium

985.8   Other specified metals

     Brass fumes   Iron compounds
     Copper salts   Nickel compounds

985.9   Unspecified metal

986 Toxic effect of carbon monoxide

     Carbon monoxide from any source

✓4ᵗʰ **987 Toxic effect of other gases, fumes, or vapors**

987.0   Liquefied petroleum gases

     Butane   Propane

987.1   Other hydrocarbon gas

987.2   Nitrogen oxides

     Nitrogen dioxide   Nitrous fumes

987.3   Sulfur dioxide

987.4   Freon

     Dichloromonofluoromethane

987.5   Lacrimogenic gas

     Bromobenzyl cyanide   Ethyliodoacetate
     Chloroacetophenone

987.6   Chlorine gas

987.7   Hydrocyanic acid gas

987.8   Other specified gases, fumes, or vapors

     Phosgene   Polyester fumes

987.9   Unspecified gas, fume, or vapor

✓4ᵗʰ **988 Toxic effect of noxious substances eaten as food**

EXCLUDES   *allergic reaction to food, such as:*
       gastroenteritis (558.3)
       rash (692.5, 693.1)
     food poisoning (bacterial) (005.0-005.9)
     toxic effects of food contaminants, such as:
       aflatoxin and other mycotoxin (989.7)
       mercury (985.0)

988.0   Fish and shellfish

988.1   Mushrooms

988.2   Berries and other plants

988.8   Other specified noxious substances eaten as food

988.9   Unspecified noxious substance eaten as food

N Newborn Age: 0   P Pediatric Age: 0-17   M Maternity Age: 12-55   A Adult Age: 15-124   MSP Medicare Secondary Payer

☑4ᵗʰ **989 Toxic effect of other substances, chiefly nonmedicinal as to source**

    989.0 Hydrocyanic acid and cyanides
         Potassium cyanide   Sodium cyanide
         EXCLUDES   *gas and fumes (987.7)*

    989.1 Strychnine and salts

    989.2 Chlorinated hydrocarbons
         Aldrin   DDT
         Chlordane   Dieldrin
         EXCLUDES   *chlorinated hydrocarbon solvents (982.0-982.3)*

    989.3 Organophosphate and carbamate
         Carbaryl   Parathion
         Dichlorvos   Phorate
         Malathion   Phosdrin

    989.4 Other pesticides, not elsewhere classified
         Mixtures of insecticides

    989.5 Venom
         Bites of venomous snakes, lizards, and spiders
         Tick paralysis

    989.6 Soaps and detergents

    989.7 Aflatoxin and other mycotoxin [food contaminants]

☑5ᵗʰ   **989.8 Other substances, chiefly nonmedicinal as to source**
        989.81 Asbestos
             EXCLUDES   *asbestosis (501)*
                             exposure to asbestos (V15.84)

        989.82 Latex
        989.83 Silicone
             EXCLUDES   *silicone used in medical devices, implants and grafts (996.00-996.79)*

        989.84 Tobacco
        989.89 Other

    989.9 Unspecified substance, chiefly nonmedicinal as to source

OTHER AND UNSPECIFIED EFFECTS OF EXTERNAL CAUSES (990-995)

990 Effects of radiation, unspecified
     Complication of:
         phototherapy
         radiation therapy
     Radiation sickness
     EXCLUDES   *specified adverse effects of radiation. Such conditions are to be classified according to the nature of the adverse effect, as:*
                burns (940.0-949.5)
                dermatitis (692.7-692.8)
                leukemia (204.0-208.9)
                pneumonia (508.0)
                sunburn (692.71, 692.76-692.77)
                [The type of radiation giving rise to the adverse effect may be identified by use of the E codes.]

☑4ᵗʰ **991 Effects of reduced temperature**
    991.0 Frostbite of face
    991.1 Frostbite of hand
    991.2 Frostbite of foot
    991.3 Frostbite of other and unspecified sites
    991.4 Immersion foot
         Trench foot
     DEF: Paresthesia, edema, blotchy cyanosis of foot, the skin is soft (macerated), pale and wrinkled, and the sole is swollen with surface ridging and following sustained immersion in water.

    991.5 Chilblains
         Erythema pernio   Perniosis
     DEF: Red, swollen, itchy skin; follows damp cold exposure; also associated with pruritus and a burning feeling, in hands, feet, ears, and face in children, legs and toes in women, and hands and fingers in men.

    991.6 Hypothermia
         Hypothermia (accidental)
         EXCLUDES   *hypothermia following anesthesia (995.89)*
                        hypothermia not associated with low environmental temperature ▶(780.99)◀
     DEF: Reduced body temperature due to low environmental temperatures.

    991.8 Other specified effects of reduced temperature
    991.9 Unspecified effect of reduced temperature
         Effects of freezing or excessive cold NOS

☑4ᵗʰ **992 Effects of heat and light**
     EXCLUDES   *burns (940.0-949.5)*
                diseases of sweat glands due to heat (705.0-705.9)
                malignant hyperpyrexia following anesthesia (995.86)
                sunburn (692.71, 692.76-692.77)

    992.0 Heat stroke and sunstroke
         Heat apoplexy   Siriasis
         Heat pyrexia   Thermoplegia
         Ictus solaris
     DEF: Headache, vertigo, cramps and elevated body temperature due to high environmental temperatures.

    992.1 Heat syncope
         Heat collapse

    992.2 Heat cramps

    992.3 Heat exhaustion, anhydrotic
         Heat prostration due to water depletion
         EXCLUDES   *that associated with salt depletion (992.4)*

    992.4 Heat exhaustion due to salt depletion
         Heat prostration due to salt (and water) depletion

    992.5 Heat exhaustion, unspecified
         Heat prostration NOS

    992.6 Heat fatigue, transient

    992.7 Heat edema
     DEF: Fluid retention due to high environmental temperatures.

    992.8 Other specified heat effects
    992.9 Unspecified

☑4ᵗʰ **993 Effects of air pressure**
    993.0 Barotrauma, otitic
         Aero-otitis media
         Effects of high altitude on ears
     DEF: Ringing ears, deafness, pain and vertigo due to air pressure changes.

    993.1 Barotrauma, sinus
         Aerosinusitis
         Effects of high altitude on sinuses

    993.2 Other and unspecified effects of high altitude
         Alpine sickness   Hypobaropathy
         Andes disease   Mountain sickness
         Anoxia due to high altitude

    993.3 Caisson disease
         Bends   Decompression sickness
         Compressed-air disease   Divers' palsy or paralysis
     DEF: Rapid reduction in air pressure while breathing compressed air; symptoms include skin lesions, joint pains, respiratory and neurological problems.

    993.4 Effects of air pressure caused by explosion
    993.8 Other specified effects of air pressure
    993.9 Unspecified effect of air pressure

☑4ᵗʰ
☑5ᵗʰ
Additional Digit Required   Unspecified Code   Other Specified Code   Manifestation Code   ▶◀ Revised Text   ● New Code   ▲ Revised Code Title

2003 ICD•9•CM   **October 2002 • Volume 1 — 273**

Injury and Poisoning 994–995.69

✓4ᵗʰ **994 Effects of other external causes**

> EXCLUDES   *certain adverse effects not elsewhere classified (995.0-995.8)*

994.0 Effects of lightning
Shock from lightning   Struck by lightning NOS
> EXCLUDES   *burns (940.0-949.5)*

994.1 Drowning and nonfatal submersion
Bathing cramp   Immersion

994.2 Effects of hunger
Deprivation of food   Starvation

994.3 Effects of thirst
Deprivation of water

994.4 Exhaustion due to exposure

994.5 Exhaustion due to excessive exertion
Overexertion

994.6 Motion sickness
Air sickness   Travel sickness
Seasickness

994.7 Asphyxiation and strangulation
Suffocation (by):   Suffocation (by):
    bedclothes   plastic bag
    cave-in   pressure
    constriction   strangulation
    mechanical
> EXCLUDES   *asphyxia from:*
>   *carbon monoxide (986)*
>   *inhalation of food or foreign body (932-934.9)*
>   *other gases, fumes, and vapors (987.0-987.9)*

994.8 Electrocution and nonfatal effects of electric current
Shock from electric current
> EXCLUDES   *electric burns (940.0-949.5)*

994.9 Other effects of external causes
Effects of:
    abnormal gravitational [G] forces or states
    weightlessness

✓4ᵗʰ **995 Certain adverse effects not elsewhere classified**

> EXCLUDES   *complications of surgical and medical care (996.0-999.9)*

995.0 Other anaphylactic shock
Allergic shock   NOS or due to adverse effect of
Anaphylactic   correct medicinal
   reaction   substance properly
Anaphylaxis   administered
Use additional E code to identify external cause, such as:
    adverse effects of correct medicinal substance properly administered [E930-E949]
> EXCLUDES   *anaphylactic reaction to serum (999.4)*
>   *anaphylactic shock due to adverse food reaction (995.60-995.69)*

DEF: Immediate sensitivity response after exposure to specific antigen; results in life-threatening respiratory distress; usually followed by vascular collapse, shock , urticaria, angioedema and pruritus.

995.1 Angioneurotic edema
Giant urticaria
> EXCLUDES   *urticaria:*
>   *due to serum (999.5)*
>   *other specified (698.2, 708.0-708.9, 757.33)*

DEF: Circulatory response of deep dermis, subcutaneous or submucosal tissues; causes localized edema and wheals.

995.2 Unspecified adverse effect of drug, medicinal and biological substance
Adverse effect   ⎫
Allergic reaction   ⎬ (due) to correct medicinal
Hypersensitivity   ⎪   substance properly
Idiosyncrasy   ⎭   administered

Drug: Drug:
  hypersensitivity NOS   reaction NOS
> EXCLUDES   *pathological drug intoxication (292.2)*

995.3 Allergy, unspecified
Allergic reaction NOS   Idiosyncrasy NOS
Hypersensitivity NOS
> EXCLUDES   *allergic reaction NOS to correct medicinal substance properly administered (995.2)*
>   *specific types of allergic reaction, such as:*
>   *allergic diarrhea (558.3)*
>   *dermatitis (691.0-693.9)*
>   *hayfever (477.0-477.9)*

995.4 Shock due to anesthesia
Shock due to anesthesia in which the correct substance was properly administered
> EXCLUDES   *complications of anesthesia in labor or delivery (668.0-668.9)*
>   *overdose or wrong substance given (968.0-969.9)*
>   *postoperative shock NOS (998.0)*
>   *specified adverse effects of anesthesia classified elsewhere, such as:*
>   *anoxic brain damage (348.1)*
>   *hepatitis (070.0-070.9), etc.*
>   *unspecified adverse effect of anesthesia (995.2)*

✓5ᵗʰ **995.5 Child maltreatment syndrome**
Use additional code(s), if applicable, to identify any associated injuries
Use additional E code to identify:
    nature of abuse (E960-E968)
    perpetrator (E967.0-E967.9)

995.50 Child abuse, unspecified   P

995.51 Child emotional/psychological abuse   P

995.52 Child neglect (nutritional)   P

995.53 Child sexual abuse   P

995.54 Child physical abuse   P
Battered baby or child syndrome
> EXCLUDES   *shaken infant syndrome (995.55)*

995.55 Shaken infant syndrome   P
Use additional code(s) to identify any associated injuries

995.59 Other child abuse and neglect   P
Multiple forms of abuse

✓5ᵗʰ **995.6 Anaphylactic shock due to adverse food reaction**
Anaphylactic shock due to nonpoisonous foods

995.60 Due to unspecified food

995.61 Due to peanuts

995.62 Due to crustaceans

995.63 Due to fruits and vegetables

995.64 Due to tree nuts and seeds

995.65 Due to fish

995.66 Due to food additives

995.67 Due to milk products

995.68 Due to eggs

995.69 Due to other specified food

995.7 **Other adverse food reactions, not elsewhere classified**

Use additional code to identify the type of reaction, such as:

hives (708.0)

wheezing (786.07)

EXCLUDES *anaphylactic shock due to adverse food reaction (995.60-995.69)*

asthma (493.0, 493.9)

dermatitis due to food (693.1)

in contact with the skin (692.5)

gastroenteritis and colitis due to food (558.3)

rhinitis due to food (477.1)

√5ᵗʰ **995.8** **Other specified adverse effects, not elsewhere classified**

995.80 **Adult maltreatment, unspecified** [A]

Abused person NOS

Use additional code to identify:

any associated injury

perpetrator (E967.0-E967.9)

995.81 **Adult physical abuse** [A]

Battered:

person syndrome NEC

man

spouse

woman

Use additional code to identify:

any association injury

nature of abuse (E960-E968)

perpetrator (E967.0-E967.9)

995.82 **Adult emotional/psychological abuse** [A]

Use additional E code to identify perpetrator (E967.0-E967.9)

995.83 **Adult sexual abuse** [A]

Use additional code to identify:

any associated injury

perpetrator (E967.0-E967.9)

995.84 **Adult neglect (nutritional)** [A]

Use addition code to identify:

intent of neglect (E904.0, E968.4)

perpetrator (E967.0-E967.9)

995.85 **Other adult abuse and neglect** [A]

Multiple forms of abuse and neglect

Use additional code to identify:

any associated injury

intent of neglect (E904.0, E968.4)

nature of abuse (E960-E968)

perpetrator (E967.0-E967.9)

995.86 **Malignant hyperthermia**

Malignant hyperpyrexia due to anesthesia

995.89 **Other**

Hypothermia due to anesthesia

● √5ᵗʰ **995.9** **Systemic inflammatory response syndrome (SIRS)**

● **995.90** **Systemic inflammatory response syndrome, unspecified**

SIRS NOS

● **995.91** **Systemic inflammatory response syndrome due to infectious process without organ dysfunction**

● **995.92** **Systemic inflammatory response syndrome due to infectious process with organ dysfunction**

Severe sepsis

Use additional code to specify organ dysfunction, such as:

encephalopathy (348.3)

heart failure (428.0-428.9)

kidney failure (584.5-584.9, 585, 586)

● **995.93** **Systemic inflammatory response syndrome due to noninfectious process without organ dysfunction**

● **995.94** **Systemic inflammatory response syndrome due to noninfectious process with organ dysfunction**

Use additional code to specify organ dysfunction, such as:

encephalopathy (348.3)

heart failure (428.0-428.9)

kidney failure (584.5-584.9, 585, 586)

COMPLICATIONS OF SURGICAL AND MEDICAL CARE, NOT ELSEWHERE CLASSIFIED (996-999)

EXCLUDES *adverse effects of medicinal agents (001.0-799.9, 995.0-995.8)*

burns from local applications and irradiation (940.0-949.5)

complications of:

conditions for which the procedure was performed

surgical procedures during abortion, labor, and delivery (630-676.9)

poisoning and toxic effects of drugs and chemicals (960.0-989.9)

postoperative conditions in which no complications are present, such as:

artificial opening status (V44.0-V44.9)

closure of external stoma (V55.0-V55.9)

fitting of prosthetic device (V52.0-V52.9)

specified complications classified elsewhere

anesthetic shock (995.4)

electrolyte imbalance (276.0-276.9)

postlaminectomy syndrome (722.80-722.83)

postmastectomy lymphedema syndrome (457.0)

postoperative psychosis (293.0-293.9)

any other condition classified elsewhere in the Alphabetic Index when described as due to a procedure

√4ᵗʰ **996** **Complications peculiar to certain specified procedures**

INCLUDES complications, not elsewhere classified, in the use of artificial substitutes [e.g., Dacron, metal, Silastic, Teflon] or natural sources [e.g., bone] involving:

anastomosis (internal)

graft (bypass) (patch)

implant

internal device:

catheter

electronic

fixation

prosthetic

reimplant

transplant

EXCLUDES *accidental puncture or laceration during procedure (998.2)*

complications of internal anastomosis of:

gastrointestinal tract (997.4)

urinary tract (997.5)

other specified complications classified elsewhere, such as:

hemolytic anemia (283.1)

functional cardiac disturbances (429.4)

serum hepatitis (070.2-070.3)

√5ᵗʰ **996.0** **Mechanical complication of cardiac device, implant, and graft**

Breakdown (mechanical)

Displacement

Leakage

Obstruction, mechanical

Perforation

Protrusion

996.00 **Unspecified device, implant, and graft** [MSP]

996.01 **Due to cardiac pacemaker (electrode)** [MSP]

√4ᵗʰ
√5ᵗʰ Additional Digit Required   Unspecified Code   Other Specified Code   Manifestation Code   ▶◀ Revised Text   ● New Code   ▲ Revised Code Title

996.02 Due to heart valve prosthesis `MSP`

996.03 Due to coronary bypass graft `MSP`

> EXCLUDES   *atherosclerosis of graft (414.02, 414.03)*
> *embolism [occlusion NOS] [thrombus] of graft (996.72)*

996.04 Due to automatic implantable cardiac defibrillator

996.09 Other `MSP`

996.1 Mechanical complication of other vascular device, implant, and graft `MSP`

femoral-popliteal bypass graft
Mechanical complications involving:
aortic (bifurcation) graft (replacement)
arteriovenous:
dialysis catheter
fistula   } surgically created
shunt

balloon (counterpulsation) device, intra-aortic
carotid artery bypass graft
umbrella device, vena cava

> EXCLUDES   *atherosclerosis of biological graft (440.30-440.32)*
> *embolism [occlusion NOS] [thrombus] of (biological) (synthetic) graft (996.74)*
> *peritoneal dialysis catheter (996.56)*

996.2 Mechanical complication of nervous system device, implant, and graft `MSP`

Mechanical complications involving:
dorsal column stimulator
electrodes implanted in brain [brain "pacemaker"]
peripheral nerve graft
ventricular (communicating) shunt

√5ᵗʰ **996.3 Mechanical complication of genitourinary device, implant, and graft**

996.30 Unspecified device, implant, and graft `MSP`

996.31 Due to urethral [indwelling] catheter `MSP`

996.32 Due to intrauterine contraceptive device ♀ `MSP`

996.39 Other `MSP`

Cystostomy catheter
Prosthetic reconstruction of vas deferens
Repair (graft) of ureter without mention of resection

> EXCLUDES   *complications due to:*
> *external stoma of urinary tract (997.5)*
> *internal anastomosis of urinary tract (997.5)*

996.4 Mechanical complication of internal orthopedic device, implant, and graft `MSP`

Mechanical complications involving:
external (fixation) device utilizing internal screw(s), pin(s) or other methods of fixation
grafts of bone, cartilage, muscle, or tendon
internal (fixation) device such as nail, plate, rod, etc.

> EXCLUDES   *complications of external orthopedic device, such as:*
> *pressure ulcer due to cast (707.0)*

√5ᵗʰ **996.5 Mechanical complications of other specified prosthetic device, implant, and graft**

Mechanical complications involving:
prosthetic implant in: prosthetic implant in:
bile duct   chin
breast   orbit of eye
nonabsorbable surgical material NOS
other graft, implant, and internal device, not elsewhere classified

996.51 Due to corneal graft

996.52 Due to graft of other tissue, not elsewhere classified

Skin graft failure or rejection

> EXCLUDES   *failure of artificial skin graft (996.55)*
> *failure of decellularized allodermis (996.55)*
> *sloughing of temporary skin allografts or xenografts (pigskin)—omit code*

996.53 Due to ocular lens prosthesis

> EXCLUDES   *contact lenses—code to condition*

996.54 Due to breast prosthesis

Breast capsule (prosthesis)
Mammary implant

996.55 Due to artificial skin graft and decellularized allodermis

Dislodgement
Displacement
Failure
Non-adherence
Poor incorporation
Shearing

996.56 Due to peritoneal dialysis catheter

> EXCLUDES   *mechanical complication of arteriovenous dialysis catheter (996.1)*

996.59 Due to other implant and internal device, not elsewhere classified

Nonabsorbable surgical material NOS
Prosthetic implant in:
bile duct
chin
orbit of eye

√5ᵗʰ **996.6 Infection and inflammatory reaction due to internal prosthetic device, implant, and graft**

Infection (causing obstruction)   } due to (presence of) any device, implant, and graft classifiable to 996.0-996.5
Inflammation

Use additional code to identify specified infections

996.60 Due to unspecified device, implant, and graft

996.61 Due to cardiac device, implant, and graft

Cardiac pacemaker or defibrillator:
electrode(s), lead(s)
pulse generator
subcutaneous pocket
Coronary artery bypass graft
Heart valve prosthesis

996.62 Due to other vascular device, implant, and graft

Arterial graft
Arteriovenous fistula or shunt
Infusion pump
Vascular catheter (arterial) (dialysis) (venous)

996.63 Due to nervous system device, implant, and graft

Electrodes implanted in brain
Peripheral nerve graft
Spinal canal catheter
Ventricular (communicating) shunt (catheter)

996.64 Due to indwelling urinary catheter

Use additional code to identify specified infections, such as:
Cystitis (595.0-595.9)
Sepsis (038.0-038.9)

`N` Newborn Age: 0   `P` Pediatric Age: 0-17   `M` Maternity Age: 12-55   `A` Adult Age: 15-124   `MSP` Medicare Secondary Payer

276 — Volume 1   2003 ICD•9•CM

996.65 Due to other genitourinary device, implant, and graft
Intrauterine contraceptive device

996.66 Due to internal joint prosthesis

996.67 Due to other internal orthopedic device, implant, and graft
Bone growth stimulator (electrode)
Internal fixation device (pin) (rod) (screw)

996.68 Due to peritoneal dialysis catheter
Exit-site infection or inflammation

996.69 Due to other internal prosthetic device, implant, and graft
Breast prosthesis
Ocular lens prosthesis
Prosthetic orbital implant

√5th **996.7 Other complications of internal (biological) (synthetic) prosthetic device, implant, and graft**

Complication NOS ⎫
occlusion NOS ⎪
Embolism ⎪ due to (presence of) any
Fibrosis ⎬ device, implant, and
Hemorrhage ⎪ graft classifiable to
Pain ⎪ 996.0-996.5
Stenosis ⎪
Thrombus ⎭

> **EXCLUDES** *transplant rejection (996.8)*

996.70 Due to unspecified device, implant, and graft

996.71 Due to heart valve prosthesis

996.72 Due to other cardiac device, implant, and graft
Cardiac pacemaker or defibrillator:
electrode(s), lead(s)
subcutaneous pocket
Coronary artery bypass (graft)
> **EXCLUDES** *occlusion due to atherosclerosis*
> ►*(414.02-414.06)*◄

996.73 Due to renal dialysis device, implant, and graft

996.74 Due to other vascular device, implant, and graft
> **EXCLUDES** *occlusion of biological graft due to atherosclerosis (440.30-440.32)*

996.75 Due to nervous system device, implant, and graft

996.76 Due to genitourinary device, implant, and graft

996.77 Due to internal joint prosthesis

996.78 Due to other internal orthopedic device, implant, and graft

996.79 Due to other internal prosthetic device, implant, and graft

√5th **996.8 Complications of transplanted organ**
Transplant failure or rejection
Use additional code to identify nature of complication, such as:
Cytomegalovirus (CMV) infection (078.5)

996.80 Transplanted organ, unspecified

996.81 Kidney

996.82 Liver

996.83 Heart

996.84 Lung

996.85 Bone marrow
Graft-versus-host disease (acute) (chronic)

996.86 Pancreas

996.87 Intestine

996.89 Other specified transplanted organ

√5th **996.9 Complications of reattached extremity or body part**

996.90 Unspecified extremity

996.91 Forearm

996.92 Hand

996.93 Finger(s)

996.94 Upper extremity, other and unspecified

996.95 Foot and toe(s)

996.96 Lower extremity, other and unspecified

996.99 Other specified body part

√4th **997 Complications affecting specified body system, not elsewhere classified**
Use additional code to identify complications
> **EXCLUDES** *the listed conditions when specified as:*
> *causing shock (998.0)*
> *complications of:*
> *anesthesia:*
> *adverse effect (001.0-799.9, 995.0-995.8)*
> *in labor or delivery (668.0-668.9)*
> *poisoning (968.0-969.9)*
> *implanted device or graft (996.0-996.9)*
> *obstetrical procedures (669.0-669.4)*
> *reattached extremity (996.90-996.96)*
> *transplanted organ (996.80-996.89)*

√5th **997.0 Nervous system complications**

997.00 Nervous system complication, unspecified

997.01 Central nervous system complication
Anoxic brain damage
Cerebral hypoxia
> **EXCLUDES** *cerebrovascular hemorrhage or infarction (997.02)*

997.02 Iatrogenic cerbrovascular infarction or hemorrhage
Postoperative stroke

997.09 Other nervous system complications

997.1 Cardiac complications
Cardiac: ⎫
arrest ⎪ during or resulting
insufficiency ⎬ from a
Cardiorespiratory failure ⎪ procedure
Heart failure ⎭
> **EXCLUDES** *the listed conditions as long-term effects of cardiac surgery or due to the presence of cardiac prosthetic device (429.4)*

997.2 Peripheral vascular complications
Phlebitis or thrombophlebitis during or resulting from a procedure
> **EXCLUDES** *the listed conditions due to:*
> *implant or catheter device (996.62)*
> *infusion, perfusion, or transfusion (999.2)*
> *complications affecting blood vessels (997.71-997.79)*

√4th
√5th Additional Digit Required   Unspecified Code   Other Specified Code   Manifestation Code   ►◄ Revised Text   ● New Code   ▲ Revised Code Title

2003 ICD•9•CM   **October 2002 • Volume 1 — 277**

997.3   **Respiratory complications**

Mendelson's syndrome ⎤
Pneumonia (aspiration) ⎦ resulting from a procedure

> **EXCLUDES**   *iatrogenic [postoperative] pneumothorax (512.1)*
> *iatrogenic pulmonary embolism (415.11)*
> *Mendelson's syndrome in labor and delivery (668.0)*
> *specified complications classified elsewhere, such as:*
>   *adult respiratory distress syndrome (518.5)*
>   *pulmonary edema, postoperative (518.4)*
>   *respiratory insufficiency, acute, postoperative (518.5)*
>   *shock lung (518.5)*
>   *tracheostomy complications (519.00-519.09)*

DEF: Mendelson's syndrome: acid pneumonitis due to aspiration of gastric acids, may occur after anesthesia or sedation.

997.4   **Digestive system complications**

Complications of:
    intestinal (internal) anastomosis and bypass, not elsewhere classified, except that involving urinary tract

Hepatic failure ⎤
Hepatorenal syndrome ⎬ specified as due to a procedure
Intestinal obstruction NOS ⎦

> **EXCLUDES**   *gastrostomy complications (536.40-536.49)*
> *specified gastrointestinal complications classified elsewhere, such as:*
> *blind loop syndrome (579.2)*
> *colostomy and enterostomy complications (569.60-569.69)*
> *gastrojejunal ulcer (534.0-534.9)*
> *infection of external stoma (569.61)*
> *pelvic peritoneal adhesions, female (614.6)*
> *peritoneal adhesions (568.0)*
> *peritoneal adhesions with obstruction (560.81)*
> *postcholecystectomy syndrome (576.0)*
> *postgastric surgery syndromes (564.2)*

997.5   **Urinary complications**

Complications of:
    external stoma of urinary tract
    internal anastomosis and bypass of urinary tract, including that involving intestinal tract

Oliguria or anuria ⎤
Renal: ⎥
    failure (acute) ⎬ specified as due to procedure
    insufficiency (acute) ⎥
Tubular necrosis (acute) ⎦

> **EXCLUDES**   *specified complications classified elsewhere, such as:*
> *postoperative stricture of:*
>   *ureter (593.3)*
>   *urethra (598.2)*

✓5ᵗʰ **997.6**   **Amputation stump complication**

> **EXCLUDES**   *admission for treatment for a current traumatic amputation — code to complicated traumatic amputation*
> *phantom limb (syndrome) (353.6)*

997.60   **Unspecified complication**

997.61   **Neuroma of amputation stump**

DEF: Hyperplasia generated nerve cell mass following amputation.

997.62   **Infection (chronic)**

Use additional code to identify organism

997.69   **Other**

✓5ᵗʰ **997.7**   **Vascular complications of other vessels**

> **EXCLUDES**   *peripheral vascular complications (997.2)*

997.71   **Vascular complications of mesenteric artery**

997.72   **Vascular complications of renal artery**

997.79   **Vascular complications of other vessels**

✓5ᵗʰ **997.9**   **Complications affecting other specified body systems, not elsewhere classified**

> **EXCLUDES**   *specified complications classified elsewhere, such as:*
> *broad ligament laceration syndrome (620.6)*
> *postartificial menopause syndrome (627.4)*
> *postoperative stricture of vagina (623.2)*

997.91   **Hypertension**

> **EXCLUDES**   *essential hypertension (401.0-401.9)*

997.99   **Other**

Vitreous touch syndrome

DEF: Vitreous protruding through pupil and attaches to corneal epithelium; causes aqueous fluid in vitreous body; marked by corneal edema, loss of lucidity; complication of cataract surgery.

✓4ᵗʰ **998**   **Other complications of procedures, not elsewhere classified**

998.0   **Postoperative shock**

Collapse NOS ⎤
Shock (endotoxic) ⎬ during or resulting from a surgical procedure
    (hypovolemic) (septic) ⎦

> **EXCLUDES**   *shock:*
> *anaphylactic due to serum (999.4)*
> *anesthetic (995.4)*
> *electric (994.8)*
> *following abortion (639.5)*
> *obstetric (669.1)*
> *traumatic (958.4)*

✓5ᵗʰ **998.1**   **Hemorrhage or hematoma or seroma complicating a procedure**

> **EXCLUDES**   *hemorrhage, hematoma, or seroma:*
> *complicating cesarean section or puerperal perineal wound (674.3)*

998.11   **Hemorrhage complicating a procedure**

998.12   **Hematoma complicating a procedure**

998.13   **Seroma complicating a procedure**

998.2 Accidental puncture or laceration during a procedure

Accidental perforation by catheter or other instrument during a procedure on:
- blood vessel
- nerve
- organ

EXCLUDES   *iatrogenic [postoperative] pneumothorax (512.1)*
puncture or laceration caused by implanted device intentionally left in operation wound (996.0-996.5)
specified complications classified elsewhere, such as:
broad ligament laceration syndrome (620.6)
trauma from instruments during delivery (664.0-665.9)

√5ᵗʰ **998.3 Disruption of operation wound**

Dehiscence ⎫
Rupture   ⎬ of operation wound

EXCLUDES   *disruption of:*
cesarean wound (674.1)
perineal wound, puerperal (674.2)

● **998.31 Disruption of internal operation wound**

● **998.32 Disruption of external operation wound**
Disruption of operation wound NOS

998.4 Foreign body accidentally left during a procedure

Adhesions   ⎫ due to foreign body accidentally
Obstruction ⎬ left in operative wound or
Perforation ⎭ body cavity during a procedure

EXCLUDES   *obstruction or perforation caused by implanted device intentionally left in body (996.0-996.5)*

√5ᵗʰ **998.5 Postoperative infection**

EXCLUDES   *infection due to:*
implanted device (996.60-996.69)
infusion, perfusion, or transfusion (999.3)
postoperative obstetrical wound infection (674.3)

998.51 Infected postoperative seroma
Use additional code to identify organism

998.59 Other postoperative infection

Abscess:
- intra-abdominal
- stitch ⎫
- subphrenic ⎬ postoperative
- wound
Septicemia ⎭

Use additional code to identify infection

998.6 Persistent postoperative fistula

998.7 Acute reaction to foreign substance accidentally left during a procedure

Peritonitis: Peritonitis:
aseptic   chemical

√5ᵗʰ **998.8 Other specified complications of procedures, not elsewhere classified**

998.81 Emphysema (subcutaneous) (surgical) resulting from a procedure

998.82 Cataract fragments in eye following cataract surgery

998.83 Non-healing surgical wound

998.89 Other specified complications

998.9 Unspecified complication of procedure, not elsewhere classified

Postoperative complication NOS

EXCLUDES   *complication NOS of obstetrical, surgery or procedure (669.4)*

√4ᵗʰ **999 Complications of medical care, not elsewhere classified**

INCLUDES   complications, not elsewhere classified, of:
- dialysis (hemodialysis) (peritoneal) (renal)
- extracorporeal circulation
- hyperalimentation therapy
- immunization
- infusion
- inhalation therapy
- injection
- inoculation
- perfusion
- transfusion
- vaccination
- ventilation therapy

EXCLUDES   *specified complications classified elsewhere such as:*
complications of implanted device (996.0-996.9)
contact dermatitis due to drugs (692.3)
dementia dialysis (294.8)
transient (293.9)
dialysis disequilibrium syndrome (276.0-276.9)
poisoning and toxic effects of drugs and chemicals (960.0-989.9)
postvaccinal encephalitis (323.5)
water and electrolyte imbalance (276.0-276.9)

999.0 Generalized vaccinia

DEF: Skin eruption, self-limiting; follows vaccination; due to transient viremia with virus localized in skin.

999.1 Air embolism

Air embolism to any site following infusion, perfusion, or transfusion

EXCLUDES   *embolism specified as:*
complicating:
abortion (634-638 with .6, 639.6)
ectopic or molar pregnancy (639.6)
pregnancy, childbirth, or the puerperium (673.0)
due to implanted device (996.7)
traumatic (958.0)

999.2 Other vascular complications

Phlebitis   ⎫ following infusion,
Thromboembolism ⎬ perfusion, or
Thrombophlebitis ⎭ transfusion

EXCLUDES   *the listed conditions when specified as:*
due to implanted device (996.61-996.62. 996.72-996.74)
postoperative NOS (997.2, 997.71-997.79)

999.3 Other infection

Infection ⎫ following infusion, injection,
Sepsis   ⎬ transfusion, or
Septicemia ⎭ vaccination

EXCLUDES   *the listed conditions when specified as:*
due to implanted device (996.60-996.69)
postoperative NOS (998.51-998.59)

999.4 Anaphylactic shock due to serum

EXCLUDES   *shock:*
allergic NOS (995.0)
anaphylactic:
NOS (995.0)
due to drugs and chemicals (995.0)

DEF: Life-threatening hypersensitivity to foreign serum; causes respiratory distress, vascular collapse, and shock.

√4ᵗʰ / √5ᵗʰ Additional Digit Required   Unspecified Code   Other Specified Code   Manifestation Code   ▶◀ Revised Text   ● New Code   ▲ Revised Code Title

999.5   **Other serum reaction**

Intoxication by serum   Serum sickness
Protein sickness   Urticaria due to serum
Serum rash

> **EXCLUDES**   *serum hepatitis (070.2-070.3)*

DEF: Serum sickness: Hypersensitivity to foreign serum; causes fever, hives, swelling, and lymphadenopathy.

999.6   **ABO incompatibility reaction**

Incompatible blood transfusion
Reaction to blood group incompatibility in infusion or transfusion

999.7   **Rh incompatibility reaction**

Reactions due to Rh factor in infusion or transfusion

999.8   **Other transfusion reaction**

Septic shock due to transfusion
Transfusion reaction NOS

> **EXCLUDES**   *postoperative shock (998.0)*

999.9   **Other and unspecified complications of medical care, not elsewhere classified**

Complications, not elsewhere classified, of:

electroshock ⎫
inhalation   ⎬ therapy
ultrasound   ⎭
ventilation

Unspecified misadventure of medical care

> **EXCLUDES**   *unspecified complication of:*
>   *phototherapy (990)*
>   *radiation therapy (990)*

N Newborn Age: 0   **P** Pediatric Age: 0-17   **M** Maternity Age: 12-55   **A** Adult Age: 15-124   **MSP** Medicare Secondary Payer

280 — Volume 1   *2003 ICD•9•CM*

Injury and Poisoning 999.5–999.9

SUPPLEMENTARY CLASSIFICATION OF FACTORS INFLUENCING HEALTH STATUS AND CONTACT WITH HEALTH SERVICES (V01-V83)

This classification is provided to deal with occasions when circumstances other than a disease or injury classifiable to categories 001-999 (the main part of ICD) are recorded as "diagnoses" or "problems." This can arise mainly in three ways:

a) When a person who is not currently sick encounters the health services for some specific purpose, such as to act as a donor of an organ or tissue, to receive prophylactic vaccination, or to discuss a problem which is in itself not a disease or injury. This will be a fairly rare occurrence among hospital inpatients, but will be relatively more common among hospital outpatients and patients of family practitioners, health clinics, etc.

b) When a person with a known disease or injury, whether it is current or resolving, encounters the health care system for a specific treatment of that disease or injury (e.g., dialysis for renal disease; chemotherapy for malignancy; cast change).

c) When some circumstance or problem is present which influences the person's health status but is not in itself a current illness or injury. Such factors may be elicited during population surveys, when the person may or may not be currently sick, or be recorded as an additional factor to be borne in mind when the person is receiving care for some current illness or injury classifiable to categories 001-999.

In the latter circumstances the V code should be used only as a supplementary code and should not be the one selected for use in primary, single cause tabulations. Examples of these circumstances are a personal history of certain diseases, or a person with an artificial heart valve in situ.

PERSONS WITH POTENTIAL HEALTH HAZARDS RELATED TO COMMUNICABLE DISEASES (V01-V06)

> **EXCLUDES**   *family history of infectious and parasitic diseases (V18.8)*
> *personal history of infectious and parasitic diseases (V12.0)*

✓4th **V01 Contact with or exposure to communicable diseases**

V01.0 **Cholera**
Conditions classifiable to 001

V01.1 **Tuberculosis**
Conditions classifiable to 010-018

V01.2 **Poliomyelitis**
Conditions classifiable to 045

V01.3 **Smallpox**
Conditions classifiable to 050

V01.4 **Rubella**
Conditions classifiable to 056

V01.5 **Rabies**
Conditions classifiable to 071

V01.6 **Venereal diseases**
Conditions classifiable to 090-099

V01.7 **Other viral diseases**
Conditions classifiable to 042-078 and V08, except as above

✓5th V01.8 **Other communicable diseases**
Conditions classifiable to 001-136, except as above

● V01.81 **Anthrax**

● V01.89 **Other communicable diseases**

V01.9 **Unspecified communicable disease**

✓4th **V02 Carrier or suspected carrier of infectious diseases**

V02.0 **Cholera**

V02.1 **Typhoid**

V02.2 **Amebiasis**

V02.3 **Other gastrointestinal pathogens**

V02.4 **Diphtheria**

✓5th V02.5 **Other specified bacterial diseases**

V02.51 **Group B streptococcus**

V02.52 **Other streptococcus**

V02.59 **Other specified bacterial disease**
Meningococcal
Staphylococcal

✓5th V02.6 **Viral hepatitis**
Hepatitis Australian-antigen [HAA] [SH] carrier
Serum hepatitis carrier

V02.60 **Viral hepatitis carrier, unspecified**

V02.61 **Hepatitis B carrier**

V02.62 **Hepatitis C carrier**

V02.69 **Other viral hepatitis carrier**

V02.7 **Gonorrhea**

V02.8 **Other venereal diseases**

V02.9 **Other specified infectious organism**

✓4th **V03 Need for prophylactic vaccination and inoculation against bacterial diseases**

> **EXCLUDES**   *vaccination not carried out because of contraindication (V64.0)*
> *vaccines against combinations of diseases (V06.0-V06.9)*

V03.0 **Cholera alone**

V03.1 **Typhoid-paratyphoid alone [TAB]**

V03.2 **Tuberculosis [BCG]**

V03.3 **Plague**

V03.4 **Tularemia**

V03.5 **Diphtheria alone**

V03.6 **Pertussis alone**

V03.7 **Tetanus toxoid alone**

✓5th V03.8 **Other specified vaccinations against single bacterial diseases**

V03.81 **Hemophilus influenza, type B [Hib]**

V03.82 **Streptococcus pneumoniae [pneumococcus]**

V03.89 **Other specified vaccination**

V03.9 **Unspecified single bacterial disease**

✓4th **V04 Need for prophylactic vaccination and inoculation against certain viral diseases**

> **EXCLUDES**   *vaccines against combinations of diseases (V06.0-V06.9)*

V04.0 **Poliomyelitis**

V04.1 **Smallpox**

V04.2 **Measles alone**

V04.3 **Rubella alone**

V04.4 **Yellow fever**

V04.5 **Rabies**

V04.6 **Mumps alone**

V04.7 **Common cold**

V04.8 **Influenza**

✓4th **V05 Need for other prophylactic vaccination and inoculation against single diseases**

> **EXCLUDES**   *vaccines against combinations of diseases (V06.0-V06.9)*

V05.0 **Arthropod-borne viral encephalitis**

V05.1 **Other arthropod-borne viral diseases**

V05.2 **Leishmaniasis**

V05.3 **Viral hepatitis**

V05.4 **Varicella**
Chickenpox

V05.8 **Other specified disease**

V05.9 **Unspecified single disease**

✓4th **V06 Need for prophylactic vaccination and inoculation against combinations of diseases**

Note: Use additional single vaccination codes from categories V03-V05 to identify any vaccinations not included in a combination code.

V06.0 **Cholera with typhoid-paratyphoid [cholera+TAB]**

V06.1 **Diphtheria-tetanus-pertussis, combined [DTP]**

V06.2 **Diphtheria-tetanus-pertussis with typhoid-paratyphoid [DTP+TAB]**

✓4th ✓5th   Additional Digit Required   Unspecified Code   Other Specified Code   Manifestation Code   ►◄ Revised Text   ● New Code   ▲ Revised Code Title

2003 ICD•9•CM   October 2002 • Volume 1 — 281

V Codes V06.3–V10.48

V06.3 Diphtheria-tetanus-pertussis with poliomyelitis [DTP+polio]

V06.4 Measles-mumps-rubella [MMR]

V06.5 Tetanus-diphtheria [Td]

V06.6 Streptococcus pneumoniae [pneumococcus] and influenza

V06.8 Other combinations

> EXCLUDES *multiple single vaccination codes (V03.0-V05.9)*

V06.9 Unspecified combined vaccine

PERSONS WITH NEED FOR ISOLATION, OTHER POTENTIAL HEALTH HAZARDS AND PROPHYLACTIC MEASURES (V07-V09)

√4th **V07** Need for isolation and other prophylactic measures

> EXCLUDES *prophylactic organ removal (V50.41-V50.49)*

V07.0 Isolation

Admission to protect the individual from his surroundings or for isolation of individual after contact with infectious diseases

V07.1 Desensitization to allergens

V07.2 Prophylactic immunotherapy

Administration of:
antivenin
immune sera [gamma globulin]
RhoGAM
tetanus antitoxin

√5th **V07.3** Other prophylactic chemotherapy

V07.31 Prophylactic fluoride administration

V07.39 Other prophylactic chemotherapy

> EXCLUDES *maintenance chemotherapy following disease (V58.1)*

V07.4 Postmenopausal hormone replacement therapy ♀

V07.8 Other specified prophylactic measure

V07.9 Unspecified prophylactic measure

V08 Asymptomatic human immunodeficiency virus [HIV] infection status

HIV positive NOS

Note: This code is ONLY to be used when NO HIV infection symptoms or conditions are present. If any HIV infection symptoms or conditions are present, see code 042.

> EXCLUDES *AIDS (042)*
> *human immunodeficiency virus [HIV] disease (042)*
> *exposure to HIV (V01.7)*
> *nonspecific serologic evidence of HIV (795.71)*
> *symptomatic human immunodeficiency virus [HIV] infection (042)*

√4th **V09** Infection with drug-resistant microorganisms

Note: This category is intended for use as an additional code for infectious conditions classified elsewhere to indicate the presence of drug-resistance of the infectious organism.

V09.0 Infection with microorganisms resistant to penicillins `SDx`

V09.1 Infection with microorganisms resistant to cephalosporins and other B-lactam antibiotics `SDx`

V09.2 Infection with microorganisms resistant to macrolides `SDx`

V09.3 Infection with microorganisms resistant to tetracyclines `SDx`

V09.4 Infection with microorganisms resistant to aminoglycosides `SDx`

√5th **V09.5** Infection with microorganisms resistant to quinolones and fluoroquinolones

V09.50 Without mention of resistance to multiple quinolones and fluoroquinoles `SDx`

V09.51 With resistance to multiple quinolones and fluoroquinoles `SDx`

V09.6 Infection with microorganisms resistant to sulfonamides `SDx`

√5th **V09.7** Infection with microorganisms resistant to other specified antimycobacterial agents

> EXCLUDES *Amikacin (V09.4)*
> *Kanamycin (V09.4)*
> *Streptomycin [SM] (V09.4)*

V09.70 Without mention of resistance to multiple antimycobacterial agents `SDx`

V09.71 With resistance to multiple antimycobacterial agents `SDx`

√5th **V09.8** Infection with microorganisms resistant to other specified drugs

V09.80 Without mention of resistance to multiple drugs `SDx`

V09.81 With resistance to multiple drugs `SDx`

√5th **V09.9** Infection with drug-resistant microorganisms, unspecified

Drug resistance, NOS

V09.90 Without mention of multiple drug resistance `SDx`

V09.91 With multiple drug resistance `SDx`

Multiple drug resistance NOS

PERSONS WITH POTENTIAL HEALTH HAZARDS RELATED TO PERSONAL AND FAMILY HISTORY

> EXCLUDES *obstetric patients where the possibility that the fetus might be affected is the reason for observation or management during pregnancy (655.0-655.9)*

√4th **V10** Personal history of malignant neoplasm

√5th **V10.0** Gastrointestinal tract

History of conditions classifiable to 140-159

V10.00 Gastrointestinal tract, unspecified

V10.01 Tongue

V10.02 Other and unspecified oral cavity and pharynx

V10.03 Esophagus

V10.04 Stomach

V10.05 Large intestine

V10.06 Rectum, rectosigmoid junction, and anus

V10.07 Liver

V10.09 Other

√5th **V10.1** Trachea, bronchus, and lung

History of conditions classifiable to 162

V10.11 Bronchus and lung

V10.12 Trachea

√5th **V10.2** Other respiratory and intrathoracic organs

History of conditions classifiable to 160, 161, 163-165

V10.20 Respiratory organ, unspecified

V10.21 Larynx

V10.22 Nasal cavities, middle ear, and accessory sinuses

V10.29 Other

V10.3 Breast

History of conditions classifiable to 174 and 175

√5th **V10.4** Genital organs

History of conditions classifiable to 179-187

V10.40 Female genital organ, unspecified ♀

V10.41 Cervix uteri ♀

V10.42 Other parts of uterus ♀

V10.43 Ovary ♀

V10.44 Other female genital organs ♀

V10.45 Male genital organ, unspecified ♂

V10.46 Prostate ♂

V10.47 Testis ♂

V10.48 Epididymis ♂

N Newborn Age: 0   P Pediatric Age: 0-17   M Maternity Age: 12-55   A Adult Age: 15-124   MSP Medicare Secondary Payer

V10.49 Other male genital organs ♂

✓5th **V10.5 Urinary organs**
History of conditions classifiable to 188 and 189
V10.50 Urinary organ, unspecified
V10.51 Bladder
V10.52 Kidney
EXCLUDES *renal pelvis (V10.53)*
V10.53 Renal pelvis
V10.59 Other

✓5th **V10.6 Leukemia**
Conditions classifiable to 204-208
EXCLUDES *leukemia in remission (204-208)*
V10.60 Leukemia, unspecified
V10.61 Lymphoid leukemia
V10.62 Myeloid leukemia
V10.63 Monocytic leukemia
V10.69 Other

✓5th **V10.7 Other lymphatic and hematopoietic neoplasms**
Conditions classifiable to 200-203
EXCLUDES *listed conditions in 200-203 in remission*
V10.71 Lymphosarcoma and reticulosarcoma
V10.72 Hodgkin's disease
V10.79 Other

✓5th **V10.8 Personal history of malignant neoplasm of other sites**
History of conditions classifiable to 170-173, 190-195
V10.81 Bone
V10.82 Malignant melanoma of skin
V10.83 Other malignant neoplasm of skin
V10.84 Eye
V10.85 Brain
V10.86 Other parts of nervous system
EXCLUDES *peripheral sympathetic, and parasympathetic nerves (V10.89)*
V10.87 Thyroid
V10.88 Other endocrine glands and related structures
V10.89 Other

V10.9 Unspecified personal history of malignant neoplasm

✓4th **V11 Personal history of mental disorder**
V11.0 Schizophrenia SDx
EXCLUDES *that in remission (295.0-295.9 with fifth-digit 5)*

V11.1 Affective disorders SDx
Personal history of manic-depressive psychosis
EXCLUDES *that in remission (296.0-296.6 with fifth-digit 5, 6)*

V11.2 Neurosis SDx
V11.3 Alcoholism SDx
V11.8 Other mental disorders SDx
V11.9 Unspecified mental disorder SDx

✓4th **V12 Personal history of certain other diseases**
✓5th **V12.0 Infectious and parasitic diseases**
V12.00 Unspecified infectious and parasitic disease SDx
V12.01 Tuberculosis SDx
V12.02 Poliomyelitis SDx
V12.03 Malaria SDx
V12.09 Other SDx
V12.1 Nutritional deficiency SDx
V12.2 Endocrine, metabolic, and immunity disorders SDx
EXCLUDES *history of allergy (V14.0-V14.9, V15.01-V15.09)*

V12.3 Diseases of blood and blood-forming organs SDx

✓5th **V12.4 Disorders of nervous system and sense organs**
V12.40 Unspecified disorder of nervous system and sense organs SDx
V12.41 Benign neoplasm of the brain SDx
V12.49 Other disorders of nervous system and sense organs SDx

✓5th **V12.5 Diseases of circulatory system**
EXCLUDES *old myocardial infarction (412) postmyocardial infarction syndrome (411.0)*
V12.50 Unspecified circulatory disease SDx
V12.51 Venous thrombosis and embolism SDx
Pulmonary embolism
V12.52 Thrombophlebitis SDx
V12.59 Other SDx
V12.6 Diseases of respiratory system SDx

✓5th **V12.7 Diseases of digestive system**
V12.70 Unspecified digestive disease SDx
V12.71 Peptic ulcer disease SDx
V12.72 Colonic polyps SDx
V12.79 Other SDx

✓4th **V13 Personal history of other diseases**
✓5th **V13.0 Disorders of urinary system**
V13.00 Unspecified urinary disorder SDx
V13.01 Urinary calculi SDx
V13.09 Other SDx
V13.1 Trophoblastic disease SDx ♀
EXCLUDES *supervision during a current pregnancy (V23.1)*

✓5th **V13.2 Other genital system and obstetric disorders**
EXCLUDES *supervision during a current pregnancy of a woman with poor obstetric history (V23.0-V23.9) habitual aborter (646.3) without current pregnancy (629.9)*
● V13.21 Personal history of pre-term labor SDx
EXCLUDES *current pregnancy with history of pre-term labor (V23.41)*
● V13.29 Other genital system and obstetric disorders SDx
V13.3 Diseases of skin and subcutaneous tissue SDx
V13.4 Arthritis SDx
V13.5 Other musculoskeletal disorders SDx

✓5th **V13.6 Congenital malformations**
V13.61 Hypospadias SDx ♂
V13.69 Other congenital malformations SDx
V13.7 Perinatal problems SDx
EXCLUDES *low birth weight status (V21.30-V21.35)*
V13.8 Other specified diseases SDx
V13.9 Unspecified disease SDx

✓4th **V14 Personal history of allergy to medicinal agents**
V14.0 Penicillin SDx
V14.1 Other antibiotic agent SDx
V14.2 Sulfonamides SDx
V14.3 Other anti-infective agent SDx
V14.4 Anesthetic agent SDx
V14.5 Narcotic agent SDx
V14.6 Analgesic agent SDx
V14.7 Serum or vaccine SDx
V14.8 Other specified medicinal agents SDx
V14.9 Unspecified medicinal agent SDx

✓4th ✓5th Additional Digit Required   Unspecified Code   Other Specified Code   Manifestation Code   ►◄ Revised Text   ● New Code   ▲ Revised Code Title

☑4ᵗʰ V15 Other personal history presenting hazards to health

    ☑5ᵗʰ **V15.0 Allergy, other than to medicinal agents**

          EXCLUDES *allergy to food substance used as base for medicinal agent (V14.0-V14.9)*

        V15.01 Allergy to peanuts `SDx`

        V15.02 Allergy to milk products `SDx`

          EXCLUDES *lactose intolerance (271.3)*

        V15.03 Allergy to eggs `SDx`

        V15.04 Allergy to seafood `SDx`
            Seafood (octopus) (squid) ink
            Shellfish

        V15.05 Allergy to other foods `SDx`
            Food additives
            Nuts other than peanuts

        V15.06 Allergy to insects `SDx`
            Bugs
            Insect bites and stings
            Spiders

        V15.07 Allergy to latex `SDx`
            Latex sensitivity

        V15.08 Allergy to radiographic dye `SDx`
            Contrast media used for diagnostic x-ray procedures

        V15.09 Other allergy, other than to medicinal agents `SDx`

    V15.1 Surgery to heart and great vessels `SDx`

        EXCLUDES *replacement by transplant or other means (V42.1-V42.2, V43.2-V43.4)*

    V15.2 Surgery to other major organs `SDx`

        EXCLUDES *replacement by transplant or other means (V42.0-V43.8)*

    V15.3 Irradiation `SDx`
        Previous exposure to therapeutic or other ionizing radiation

    ☑5ᵗʰ **V15.4 Psychological trauma**

        EXCLUDES *history of condition classifiable to 290-316 (V11.0-V11.9)*

        V15.41 History of physical abuse `SDx`
            Rape

        V15.42 History of emotional abuse `SDx`
            Neglect

        V15.49 Other `SDx`

    V15.5 Injury `SDx`

    V15.6 Poisoning `SDx`

    V15.7 Contraception `SDx`

        EXCLUDES *current contraceptive management (V25.0-V25.4)*
               presence of intrauterine contraceptive device as incidental finding (V45.5)

    ☑5ᵗʰ **V15.8 Other specified personal history presenting hazards to health**

        V15.81 Noncompliance with medical treatment `SDx`

        V15.82 History of tobacco use `SDx`
            EXCLUDES *tobacco dependence (305.1)*

        V15.84 Exposure to asbestos `SDx`

        V15.85 Exposure to potentially hazardous body fluids `SDx`

        V15.86 Exposure to lead `SDx`

        V15.89 Other `SDx`

    V15.9 Unspecified personal history presenting hazards to health `SDx`

☑4ᵗʰ V16 Family history of malignant neoplasm

    V16.0 Gastrointestinal tract
        Family history of condition classifiable to 140-159

    V16.1 Trachea, bronchus, and lung
        Family history of condition classifiable to 162

    V16.2 Other respiratory and intrathoracic organs
        Family history of condition classifiable to 160-161, 163-165

    V16.3 Breast
        Family history of condition classifiable to 174

    ☑5ᵗʰ **V16.4 Genital organs**
        Family history of condition classifiable to 179-187

        V16.40 Genital organ, unspecified

        V16.41 Ovary

        V16.42 Prostate

        V16.43 Testis

        V16.49 Other

    ☑5ᵗʰ **V16.5 Urinary organs**
        Family history of condition classifiable to 189

        V16.51 Kidney

        V16.59 Other

    V16.6 Leukemia
        Family history of condition classifiable to 204-208

    V16.7 Other lymphatic and hematopoietic neoplasms
        Family history of condition classifiable to 200-203

    V16.8 Other specified malignant neoplasm
        Family history of other condition classifiable to 140-199

    V16.9 Unspecified malignant neoplasm

☑4ᵗʰ V17 Family history of certain chronic disabling diseases

    V17.0 Psychiatric condition

        EXCLUDES *family history of mental retardation (V18.4)*

    V17.1 Stroke (cerebrovascular)

    V17.2 Other neurological diseases
        Epilepsy
        Huntington's chorea

    V17.3 Ischemic heart disease

    V17.4 Other cardiovascular diseases

    V17.5 Asthma

    V17.6 Other chronic respiratory conditions

    V17.7 Arthritis

    V17.8 Other musculoskeletal diseases

☑4ᵗʰ V18 Family history of certain other specific conditions

    V18.0 Diabetes mellitus

    V18.1 Other endocrine and metabolic diseases

    V18.2 Anemia

    V18.3 Other blood disorders

    V18.4 Mental retardation

    V18.5 Digestive disorders

    ☑5ᵗʰ **V18.6 Kidney diseases**

        V18.61 Polycystic kidney

        V18.69 Other kidney diseases

    V18.7 Other genitourinary diseases

    V18.8 Infectious and parasitic diseases

☑4ᵗʰ V19 Family history of other conditions

    V19.0 Blindness or visual loss

    V19.1 Other eye disorders

    V19.2 Deafness or hearing loss

    V19.3 Other ear disorders

    V19.4 Skin conditions

    V19.5 Congenital anomalies

    V19.6 Allergic disorders

    V19.7 Consanguinity

    V19.8 Other condition

N Newborn Age: 0   **P** Pediatric Age: 0-17   **M** Maternity Age: 12-55   **A** Adult Age: 15-124   **MSP** Medicare Secondary Payer

284 — Volume 1   `SDx` Secondary Diagnosis   `PDx` Primary Diagnosis   *2003 ICD•9•CM*

PERSONS ENCOUNTERING HEALTH SERVICES IN CIRCUMSTANCES RELATED TO REPRODUCTION AND DEVELOPMENT (V20-V28)

√4ᵗʰ **V20 Health supervision of infant or child**

V20.0 Foundling `PDx` `P`

V20.1 Other healthy infant or child receiving care `PDx` `P`
> Medical or nursing care supervision of healthy infant in cases of:
> maternal illness, physical or psychiatric
> socioeconomic adverse condition at home
> too many children at home preventing or interfering with normal care

V20.2 Routine infant or child health check `PDx` `P`
> Developmental testing of infant or child
> Immunizations appropriate for age
> Routine vision and hearing testing
> Use additional code(s) to identify:
> special screening examination(s) performed (V73.0-V82.9)
>> *EXCLUDES*   *special screening for developmental handicaps (V79.3)*

√4ᵗʰ **V21 Constitutional states in development**

V21.0 Period of rapid growth in childhood `SDx`

V21.1 Puberty `SDx`

V21.2 Other adolescence `SDx`

√5ᵗʰ **V21.3 Low birth weight status**
>> *EXCLUDES*   *history of perinatal problems (V13.7)*

V21.30 Low birth weight status, unspecified `SDx`

V21.31 Low birth weight status, less than 500 grams `SDx`

V21.32 Low birth weight status, 500-999 grams `SDx`

V21.33 Low birth weight status, 1000-1499 grams `SDx`

V21.34 Low birth weight status, 1500-1999 grams `SDx`

V21.35 Low birth weight status, 2000-2500 grams `SDx`

V21.8 Other specified constitutional states in development `SDx`

V21.9 Unspecified constitutional state in development `SDx`

√4ᵗʰ **V22 Normal pregnancy**
>> *EXCLUDES*   *pregnancy examination or test, pregnancy unconfirmed (V72.4)*

V22.0 Supervision of normal first pregnancy `PDx` ♀

V22.1 Supervision of other normal pregnancy `PDx` ♀

V22.2 Pregnant state, incidental `SDx` ♀
> Pregnant state NOS

√4ᵗʰ **V23 Supervision of high-risk pregnancy**

V23.0 Pregnancy with history of infertility `M` ♀

V23.1 Pregnancy with history of trophoblastic disease `M` ♀
> Pregnancy with history of:
> hydatidiform mole
> vesicular mole
>> *EXCLUDES*   *that without current pregnancy (V13.1)*

V23.2 Pregnancy with history of abortion `SDx` `M` ♀
> Pregnancy with history of conditions classifiable to 634-638
>> *EXCLUDES*   *habitual aborter:*
>> *care during pregnancy (646.3)*
>> *that without current pregnancy (629.9)*

V23.3 Grand multiparity `M` ♀
>> *EXCLUDES*   *care in relation to labor and delivery (659.4)*
>> *that without current pregnancy (V61.5)*

√5ᵗʰ **V23.4 Pregnancy with other poor obstetric history**
> Pregnancy with history of other conditions classifiable to 630-676

● **V23.41 Pregnancy with history of pre-term labor** `M` ♀

● **V23.49 Pregnancy with other poor obstetric history** `M` ♀

V23.5 Pregnancy with other poor reproductive history `M` ♀
> Pregnancy with history of stillbirth or neonatal death

V23.7 Insufficient prenatal care `M` ♀
> History of little or no prenatal care

√5ᵗʰ **V23.8 Other high-risk pregnancy**

V23.81 Elderly primigravida `M` ♀
> First pregnancy in a woman who will be 35 years of age or older at expected date of delivery
>> *EXCLUDES*   *elderly primigravida complicating pregnancy (659.5)*

V23.82 Elderly multigravida `M` ♀
> Second or more pregnancy in a woman who will be 35 years of age or older at expected date of delivery
>> *EXCLUDES*   *elderly multigravida complicating pregnancy (659.6)*

V23.83 Young primigravida `M` ♀
> First pregnancy in a female less than 16 years old at expected date of delivery
>> *EXCLUDES*   *young primigravida complicating pregnancy (659.8)*

V23.84 Young multigravida `M` ♀
> Second or more pregnancy in a female less than 16 years old at expected date of delivery
>> *EXCLUDES*   *young multigravida complicating pregnancy (659.8)*

V23.89 Other high-risk pregnancy `M` ♀

V23.9 Unspecified high-risk pregnancy `M` ♀

√4ᵗʰ **V24 Postpartum care and examination**

V24.0 Immediately after delivery `PDx` `M` ♀
> Care and observation in uncomplicated cases

V24.1 Lactating mother `PDx` ♀
> Supervision of lactation

V24.2 Routine postpartum follow-up `PDx` ♀

√4ᵗʰ **V25 Encounter for contraceptive management**

√5ᵗʰ **V25.0 General counseling and advice**

V25.01 Prescription of oral contraceptives ♀

V25.02 Initiation of other contraceptive measures ♀
> Fitting of diaphragm
> Prescription of foams, creams, or other agents

V25.09 Other
> Family planning advice

V25.1 Insertion of intrauterine contraceptive device ♀

V25.2 Sterilization
> Admission for interruption of fallopian tubes or vas deferens

V25.3 Menstrual extraction ♀
> Menstrual regulation

√4ᵗʰ / √5ᵗʰ Additional Digit Required   Unspecified Code   Other Specified Code   Manifestation Code   ►◄ Revised Text   ● New Code   ▲ Revised Code Title

V Codes V25.4–V40.9

✓5th **V25.4 Surveillance of previously prescribed contraceptive methods**

Checking, reinsertion, or removal of contraceptive device

Repeat prescription for contraceptive method

Routine examination in connection with contraceptive maintenance

> EXCLUDES   *presence of intrauterine contraceptive device as incidental finding (V45.5)*

V25.40 Contraceptive surveillance, unspecified

V25.41 Contraceptive pill ♀

V25.42 Intrauterine contraceptive device ♀

Checking, reinsertion, or removal of intrauterine device

V25.43 Implantable subdermal contraceptive ♀

V25.49 Other contraceptive method

V25.5 Insertion of implantable subdermal contraceptive ♀

V25.8 Other specified contraceptive management

Postvasectomy sperm count

> EXCLUDES   *sperm count following sterilization reversal (V26.22)*
> *sperm count for fertility testing (V26.21)*

V25.9 Unspecified contraceptive management

✓4th **V26 Procreative management**

V26.0 Tuboplasty or vasoplasty after previous sterilization

V26.1 Artificial insemination ♀

✓5th **V26.2 Investigation and testing**

> EXCLUDES   *postvasectomy sperm count (V25.8)*

V26.21 Fertility testing

Fallopian insufflation

Sperm count for fertility testing

> EXCLUDES   *Genetic counseling and testing (V26.3)*

V26.22 Aftercare following sterilization reversal

Fallopian insufflation following sterilization reversal

Sperm count following sterilization reversal

V26.29 Other investigation and testing

V26.3 Genetic counseling and testing

> EXCLUDES   *fertility testing (V26.21)*

V26.4 General counseling and advice

✓5th **V26.5 Sterilization status**

V26.51 Tubal ligation status SDx ♀

> EXCLUDES   *infertility not due to previous tubal ligation (628.0-628.9)*

V26.52 Vasectomy status SDx ♂

V26.8 Other specified procreative management

V26.9 Unspecified procreative management

✓4th **V27 Outcome of delivery**

Note: This category is intended for the coding of the outcome of delivery on the mother's record.

V27.0 Single liveborn M SDx ♀

V27.1 Single stillborn M SDx ♀

V27.2 Twins, both liveborn M SDx ♀

V27.3 Twins, one liveborn and one stillborn M SDx ♀

V27.4 Twins, both stillborn M SDx ♀

V27.5 Other multiple birth, all liveborn M SDx ♀

V27.6 Other multiple birth, some liveborn M SDx ♀

V27.7 Other multiple birth, all stillborn M SDx ♀

V27.9 Unspecified outcome of delivery M SDx ♀

Single birth } outcome to infant

Multiple birth } unspecified

✓4th **V28 Antenatal screening**

> EXCLUDES   *abnormal findings on screening — code to findings*
> *routine prenatal care (V22.0-V23.9)*

V28.0 Screening for chromosomal anomalies by amniocentesis M ♀

V28.1 Screening for raised alpha-fetoprotein levels in amniotic fluid M ♀

V28.2 Other screening based on amniocentesis M ♀

V28.3 Screening for malformation using ultrasonics

V28.4 Screening for fetal growth retardation using ultrasonics

V28.5 Screening for isoimmunization

V28.6 Screening for Streptococcus B M ♀

V28.8 Other specified antenatal screening

V28.9 Unspecified antenatal screening

✓4th **V29 Observation and evaluation of newborns and infants for suspected condition not found**

Note: This category is to be used for newborns, within the neonatal period, (the first 28 days of life) who are suspected of having an abnormal condition resulting from exposure from the mother or the birth process, but without signs or symptoms, and, which after examination and observation, is found not to exist.

V29.0 Observation for suspected infectious condition N PDx

V29.1 Observation for suspected neurological condition N PDx

V29.2 Observation for suspected respiratory condition N PDx

V29.3 Observation for suspected genetic or metabolic condition N PDx

V29.8 Observation for other specified suspected condition PDx

V29.9 Observation for unspecified suspected condition PDx

LIVEBORN INFANTS ACCORDING TO TYPE OF BIRTH (V30-V39)

Note: These categories are intended for the coding of liveborn infants who are consuming health care [e.g., crib or bassinet occupancy].

The following fourth-digit subdivisions are for use with categories V30-V39:

✓5th   0 Born in hospital N

     1 Born before admission to hospital N

     2 Born outside hospital and not hospitalized

The following two fifth-digits are for use with the fourth-digit .0, Born in hospital:

     0 delivered without mention of cesarean delivery

     1 delivered by cesarean delivery

✓4th **V30 Single liveborn** PDx

✓4th **V31 Twin, mate liveborn** PDx

✓4th **V32 Twin, mate stillborn** PDx

✓4th **V33 Twin, unspecified** PDx

✓4th **V34 Other multiple, mates all liveborn** PDx

✓4th **V35 Other multiple, mates all stillborn** PDx

✓4th **V36 Other multiple, mates live- and stillborn** PDx

✓4th **V37 Other multiple, unspecified** PDx

✓4th **V39 Unspecified** PDx

PERSONS WITH A CONDITION INFLUENCING THEIR HEALTH STATUS (V40-V49)

Note: These categories are intended for use when these conditions are recorded as "diagnoses" or "problems."

✓4th **V40 Mental and behavioral problems**

V40.0 Problems with learning SDx

V40.1 Problems with communication [including speech] SDx

V40.2 Other mental problems SDx

V40.3 Other behavioral problems SDx

V40.9 Unspecified mental or behavioral problem SDx

✓4ᵗʰ **V41 Problems with special senses and other special functions**

    V41.0 Problems with sight `SDx`

    V41.1 Other eye problems `SDx`

    V41.2 Problems with hearing `SDx`

    V41.3 Other ear problems `SDx`

    V41.4 Problems with voice production `SDx`

    V41.5 Problems with smell and taste `SDx`

    V41.6 Problems with swallowing and mastication `SDx`

    V41.7 Problems with sexual function `SDx`

        `EXCLUDES` *marital problems (V61.10)*
                psychosexual disorders (302.0-302.9)

    V41.8 Other problems with special functions `SDx`

    V41.9 Unspecified problem with special functions `SDx`

✓4ᵗʰ **V42 Organ or tissue replaced by transplant**

    `INCLUDES` homologous or heterologous (animal) (human) transplant organ status

    V42.0 Kidney `SDx`

    V42.1 Heart `SDx`

    V42.2 Heart valve `SDx`

    V42.3 Skin `SDx`

    V42.4 Bone `SDx`

    V42.5 Cornea `SDx`

    V42.6 Lung `SDx`

    V42.7 Liver `SDx`

  ✓5ᵗʰ **V42.8** Other specified organ or tissue

        V42.81 Bone marrow `SDx`

        V42.82 Peripheral stem cells `SDx`

        V42.83 Pancreas `SDx`

        V42.84 Intestines `SDx`

        V42.89 Other `SDx`

    V42.9 Unspecified organ or tissue `SDx`

✓4ᵗʰ **V43 Organ or tissue replaced by other means**

    `INCLUDES` replacement of organ by:
                artificial device
                mechanical device
                prosthesis

    `EXCLUDES` *cardiac pacemaker in situ (V45.01)*
             fitting and adjustment of prosthetic device
               (V52.0-V52.9)
             renal dialysis status (V45.1)

    V43.0 Eye globe `SDx`

    V43.1 Lens `SDx`

        Pseudophakos

    V43.2 Heart `SDx`

    V43.3 Heart valve `SDx`

    V43.4 Blood vessel `SDx`

    V43.5 Bladder `SDx`

  ✓5ᵗʰ **V43.6** Joint

        V43.60 Unspecified joint `SDx`

        V43.61 Shoulder `SDx`

        V43.62 Elbow `SDx`

        V43.63 Wrist `SDx`

        V43.64 Hip `SDx`

        V43.65 Knee `SDx`

        V43.66 Ankle `SDx`

        V43.69 Other `SDx`

    V43.7 Limb `SDx`

  ✓5ᵗʰ **V43.8** Other organ or tissue

        V43.81 Larynx `SDx`

        V43.82 Breast `SDx`

        V43.83 Artificial skin `SDx`

        V43.89 Other `SDx`

✓4ᵗʰ **V44 Artificial opening status**

    `EXCLUDES` *artificial openings requiring attention or*
             management (V55.0-V55.9)

    V44.0 Tracheostomy `SDx`

    V44.1 Gastrostomy `SDx`

    V44.2 Ileostomy `SDx`

    V44.3 Colostomy `SDx`

    V44.4 Other artificial opening of gastrointestinal tract `SDx`

  ✓5ᵗʰ **V44.5** Cystostomy

        V44.50 Cystostomy, unspecified `SDx`

        V44.51 Cutaneous-vesicostomy `SDx`

        V44.52 Appendico-vesicostomy `SDx`

        V44.59 Other cystostomy `SDx`

    V44.6 Other artificial opening of urinary tract `SDx`

        Nephrostomy   Urethrostomy
        Ureterostomy

    V44.7 Artificial vagina `SDx`

    V44.8 Other artificial opening status `SDx`

    V44.9 Unspecified artificial opening status `SDx`

✓4ᵗʰ **V45 Other postsurgical states**

    `EXCLUDES` *aftercare management (V51-V58.9)*
             malfunction or other complication — code to
               condition

  ✓5ᵗʰ **V45.0** Cardiac device in situ

        V45.00 Unspecified cardiac device `SDx`

        V45.01 Cardiac pacemaker `SDx`

        V45.02 Automatic implantable cardiac defibrillator `SDx`

        V45.09 Other specified cardiac device `SDx`

            Carotid sinus pacemaker in situ

    V45.1 Renal dialysis status `SDx`

        Patient requiring intermittent renal dialysis

        Presence of arterial-venous shunt (for dialysis)

        `EXCLUDES` *admission for dialysis treatment or*
                 session (V56.0)

    V45.2 Presence of cerebrospinal fluid drainage device `SDx`

        Cerebral ventricle (communicating) shunt, valve, or device in situ

        `EXCLUDES` *malfunction (996.2)*

    V45.3 Intestinal bypass or anastomosis status `SDx`

    V45.4 Arthrodesis status `SDx`

  ✓5ᵗʰ **V45.5** Presence of contraceptive device

        `EXCLUDES` *checking, reinsertion, or removal of*
                 device (V25.42)
                 complication from device (996.32)
                 insertion of device (V25.1)

        V45.51 Intrauterine contraceptive device `SDx` ♀

        V45.52 Subdermal contraceptive implant `SDx`

        V45.59 Other `SDx`

  ✓5ᵗʰ **V45.6** States following surgery of eye and adnexa

        Cataract extraction   ⎫
        Filtering bleb   ⎬ state following eye surgery
        Surgical eyelid adhesion ⎭

        `EXCLUDES` *aphakia (379.31)*
                 artificial eye globe (V43.0)

        V45.61 Cataract extraction status `SDx`

            Use additional code for associated artificial lens status (V43.1)

        V45.69 Other states following surgery of eye and adnexa `SDx`

  ✓5ᵗʰ **V45.7** Acquired absence of organ

        V45.71 Acquired absence of breast

        V45.72 Acquired absence of intestine (large) (small)

        V45.73 Acquired absence of kidney

        V45.74 Other parts of urinary tract

            Bladder

        V45.75 Stomach

        V45.76 Lung

        V45.77 Genital organs

        V45.78 Eye

        V45.79 Other acquired absence of organ

✓4ᵗʰ Additional Digit Required   `Unspecified Code`   `Other Specified Code`   `Manifestation Code`   ►◄ Revised Text   ● New Code   ▲ Revised Code Title

V Codes V45.8–V50.9

√5ᵗʰ **V45.8 Other postsurgical status**
      V45.81 Aortocoronary bypass status `SDx`
      V45.82 Percutaneous transluminal coronary `SDx`
            angioplasty status
      V45.83 Breast implant removal status `SDx`
      V45.84 Dental restoration status `SDx`
            Dental crowns status
            Dental fillings status
      V45.89 Other `SDx`
            Presence of neuropacemaker or other
            electronic device
            EXCLUDES *artificial heart valve in situ*
                             (V43.3)
                         vascular prosthesis in situ
                             (V43.4)

√4ᵗʰ **V46 Other dependence on machines**
    V46.0 Aspirator `SDx`
    V46.1 Respirator `SDx`
            Iron lung
●   **V46.2 Supplemental oxygen** `SDx`
            Long-term oxygen therapy
    V46.8 Other enabling machines `SDx`
            Hyperbaric chamber
            Possum [Patient-Operated-Selector-Mechanism]
            EXCLUDES *cardiac pacemaker (V45.0)*
                          kidney dialysis machine (V45.1)
    V46.9 Unspecified machine dependence `SDx`

√4ᵗʰ **V47 Other problems with internal organs**
    V47.0 Deficiencies of internal organs `SDx`
    V47.1 Mechanical and motor problems with internal `SDx`
            organs
    V47.2 Other cardiorespiratory problems `SDx`
            Cardiovascular exercise intolerance with pain (with):
               at rest
               less than ordinary activity
               ordinary activity
    V47.3 Other digestive problems `SDx`
    V47.4 Other urinary problems `SDx`
    V47.5 Other genital problems `SDx`
    V47.9 Unspecified `SDx`

√4ᵗʰ **V48 Problems with head, neck, and trunk**
    V48.0 Deficiencies of head `SDx`
            EXCLUDES *deficiencies of ears, eyelids, and nose*
                            (V48.8)
    V48.1 Deficiencies of neck and trunk `SDx`
    V48.2 Mechanical and motor problems with head `SDx`
    V48.3 Mechanical and motor problems with neck `SDx`
            and trunk
    V48.4 Sensory problem with head `SDx`
    V48.5 Sensory problem with neck and trunk `SDx`
    V48.6 Disfigurements of head `SDx`
    V48.7 Disfigurements of neck and trunk `SDx`
    V48.8 Other problems with head, neck, and trunk `SDx`
    V48.9 Unspecified problem with head, neck, or `SDx`
            trunk

√4ᵗʰ **V49 Other conditions influencing health status**
    V49.0 Deficiencies of limbs
    V49.1 Mechanical problems with limbs
    V49.2 Motor problems with limbs
    V49.3 Sensory problems with limbs
    V49.4 Disfigurements of limbs
    V49.5 Other problems of limbs
√5ᵗʰ **V49.6 Upper limb amputation status**
      V49.60 Unspecified level `SDx`
      V49.61 Thumb `SDx`
      V49.62 Other finger(s) `SDx`
      V49.63 Hand `SDx`

      V49.64 Wrist `SDx`
            Disarticulation of wrist
      V49.65 Below elbow `SDx`
      V49.66 Above elbow `SDx`
            Disarticulation of elbow
      V49.67 Shoulder `SDx`
            Disarticulation of shoulder
√5ᵗʰ **V49.7 Lower limb amputation status**
      V49.70 Unspecified level `SDx`
      V49.71 Great toe `SDx`
      V49.72 Other toe(s) `SDx`
      V49.73 Foot `SDx`
      V49.74 Ankle `SDx`
            Disarticulation of ankle
      V49.75 Below knee `SDx`
      V49.76 Above knee `SDx`
            Disarticulation of knee
      V49.77 Hip `SDx`
            Disarticulation of hip
√5ᵗʰ **V49.8 Other specified conditions influencing health status**
      V49.81 Asymptomatic postmenopausal `A` ♂
            status (age-related) (natural)
            EXCLUDES *menopausal and*
                           premenopausal
                           disorders (627.0-627.9)
                         postsurgical menopause
                           (256.2)
                         premature menopause
                           (256.31)
                         symptomatic menopause
                           (627.0-627.9)
      V49.82 Dental sealant status `SDx`
      V49.89 Other specified conditions influencing `SDx`
            health status
    V49.9 Unspecified `SDx`

PERSONS ENCOUNTERING HEALTH SERVICES FOR SPECIFIC PROCEDURES AND AFTERCARE (V50-V59)

    Note: Categories V51-V58 are intended for use to indicate a reason for care in patients who may have already been treated for some disease or injury not now present, or who are receiving care to consolidate the treatment, to deal with residual states, or to prevent recurrence.
    EXCLUDES *follow-up examination for medical surveillance following treatment (V67.0-V67.9)*

√4ᵗʰ **V50 Elective surgery for purposes other than remedying health states**
    V50.0 Hair transplant
    V50.1 Other plastic surgery for unacceptable cosmetic appearance
            Breast augmentation or reduction
            Face-lift
            EXCLUDES *plastic surgery following healed injury or operation (V51)*
    V50.2 Routine or ritual circumcision ♂
            Circumcision in the absence of significant medical indication
    V50.3 Ear piercing
√5ᵗʰ **V50.4 Prophylactic organ removal**
            EXCLUDES *organ donations (V59.0-V59.9)*
                        therapeutic organ removal — code to condition
      V50.41 Breast
      V50.42 Ovary ♀
      V50.49 Other
    V50.8 Other
    V50.9 Unspecified

V51 Aftercare involving the use of plastic surgery
Plastic surgery following healed injury or operation
> EXCLUDES   *cosmetic plastic surgery (V50.1)*
> *plastic surgery as treatment for current injury — code to condition*
> *repair of scarred tissue — code to scar*

√4ᵗʰ V52 Fitting and adjustment of prosthetic device and implant
> INCLUDES   removal of device
> EXCLUDES   *malfunction or complication of prosthetic device (996.0-996.7)*
> *status only, without need for care (V43.0-V43.8)*

- **V52.0 Artificial arm (complete) (partial)**
- **V52.1 Artificial leg (complete) (partial)**
- **V52.2 Artificial eye**
- **V52.3 Dental prosthetic device**
- **V52.4 Breast prosthesis and implant** ♀
  > EXCLUDES   *admission for implant insertion (V50.1)*
- **V52.8 Other specified prosthetic device**
- **V52.9 Unspecified prosthetic device**

√4ᵗʰ V53 Fitting and adjustment of other device
> INCLUDES   removal of device
> replacement of device
> EXCLUDES   *status only, without need for care (V45.0-V45.8)*

- **√5ᵗʰ V53.0 Devices related to nervous system and special senses**
  - **V53.01 Fitting and adjustment of cerebral ventricular (communicating) shunt**
  - **V53.02 Neuropacemaker (brain) (peripheral nerve) (spinal cord)**
  - **V53.09 Fitting and adjustment of other devices related to nervous system and special senses**
    - Auditory substitution device
    - Visual substitution device
- **V53.1 Spectacles and contact lenses**
- **V53.2 Hearing aid**
- **√5ᵗʰ V53.3 Cardiac device**
  - Reprogramming
  - **V53.31 Cardiac pacemaker**
    > EXCLUDES   *mechanical complication of cardiac pacemaker (996.01)*
  - **V53.32 Automatic implantable cardiac defibrillator**
  - **V53.39 Other cardiac device**
- **V53.4 Orthodontic devices**
- **V53.5 Other intestinal appliance**
  > EXCLUDES   *colostomy (V55.3)*
  > *ileostomy (V55.2)*
  > *other artificial opening of digestive tract (V55.4)*
- **V53.6 Urinary devices**
  - Urinary catheter
  > EXCLUDES   *cystostomy (V55.5)*
  > *nephrostomy (V55.6)*
  > *ureterostomy (V55.6)*
  > *urethrostomy (V55.6)*
- **V53.7 Orthopedic devices**
  - Orthopedic:
    - brace
    - cast
    - corset
    - shoes
  > EXCLUDES   *other orthopedic aftercare (V54)*
- **V53.8 Wheelchair**
- **V53.9 Other and unspecified device**

√4ᵗʰ V54 Other orthopedic aftercare
- **V54.0 Aftercare involving removal of fracture plate or other internal fixation device**
  - Removal of:
    - pins
    - plates
    - rods
    - screws
  > EXCLUDES   *malfunction of internal orthopedic device (996.4)*
  > *other complication of nonmechanical nature (996.60-996.79)*
  > *removal of external fixation device ▶(V54.89)◀*

- **√5ᵗʰ V54.1 Aftercare for healing traumatic fracture**
  - **V54.10 Aftercare for healing traumatic fracture of arm, unspecified**
  - **V54.11 Aftercare for healing traumatic fracture of upper arm**
  - **V54.12 Aftercare for healing traumatic fracture of lower arm**
  - **V54.13 Aftercare for healing traumatic fracture of hip**
  - **V54.14 Aftercare for healing traumatic fracture of leg, unspecified**
  - **V54.15 Aftercare for healing traumatic fracture of upper leg**
    > EXCLUDES   *aftercare for healing traumatic fracture of hip (V54.13)*
  - **V54.16 Aftercare for healing traumatic fracture of lower leg**
  - **V54.17 Aftercare for healing traumatic fracture of vertebrae**
  - **V54.19 Aftercare for healing traumatic fracture of other bone**
- **√5ᵗʰ V54.2 Aftercare for healing pathologic fracture**
  - **V54.20 Aftercare for healing pathologic fracture of arm, unspecified**
  - **V54.21 Aftercare for healing pathologic fracture of upper arm**
  - **V54.22 Aftercare for healing pathologic fracture of lower arm**
  - **V54.23 Aftercare for healing pathologic fracture of hip**
  - **V54.24 Aftercare for healing pathologic fracture of leg, unspecified**
  - **V54.25 Aftercare for healing pathologic fracture of upper leg**
    > EXCLUDES   *aftercare for healing pathologic fracture of hip (V54.23)*
  - **V54.26 Aftercare for healing pathologic fracture of lower leg**
  - **V54.27 Aftercare for healing pathologic fracture of vertebrae**
  - **V54.29 Aftercare for healing pathologic fracture of other bone**
- **√5ᵗʰ V54.8 Other orthopedic aftercare**
  - **V54.81 Aftercare following joint replacement**
    - Use additional code to identify joint replacement site (V43.60-V43.69)
  - **V54.89 Other orthopedic aftercare**
    - Aftercare for healing fracture NOS
- **V54.9 Unspecified orthopedic aftercare**

√4ᵗʰ / √5ᵗʰ Additional Digit Required   Unspecified Code   Other Specified Code   Manifestation Code   ▶◀ Revised Text   ● New Code   ▲ Revised Code Title

2003 ICD•9•CM   October 2002 • Volume 1 — 289

V Codes V51–V54.9

✓4ᵗʰ V55 Attention to artificial openings

> INCLUDES   adjustment or repositioning of catheter
> closure
> passage of sounds or bougies
> reforming
> removal or replacement of catheter
> toilet or cleansing
>
> EXCLUDES   *complications of external stoma (519.00-519.09,*
> *569.60-569.69, 997.4, 997.5)*
> *status only, without need for care (V44.0-V44.9)*

V55.0 Tracheostomy

V55.1 Gastrostomy

V55.2 Ileostomy

V55.3 Colostomy

V55.4 Other artificial opening of digestive tract

V55.5 Cystostomy

V55.6 Other artificial opening of urinary tract
> Nephrostomy   Urethrostomy
> Ureterostomy

V55.7 Artificial vagina

V55.8 Other specified artificial opening

V55.9 Unspecified artificial opening

✓4ᵗʰ V56 Encounter for dialysis and dialysis catheter care

> Use additional code to identify the associated condition
>
> EXCLUDES   *dialysis preparation — code to condition*

V56.0 Extracorporeal dialysis
> Dialysis (renal) NOS
>
> EXCLUDES   *dialysis status (V45.1)*

V56.1 Fitting and adjustment of extracorporeal dialysis catheter
> Removal or replacement of catheter
> Toilet or cleansing
> Use additional code for any concurrent
> extracorporeal dialysis (V56.0)

V56.2 Fitting and adjustment of peritoneal dialysis catheter
> Use additional code for any concurrent peritoneal
> dialysis (V56.8)

✓5ᵗʰ V56.3 Encounter for adequacy testing for dialysis

> **V56.31 Encounter for adequacy testing for hemodialysis**
>
> **V56.32 Encounter for adequacy testing for peritoneal dialysis**
> > Peritoneal equilibration test

V56.8 Other dialysis
> Peritoneal dialysis

✓4ᵗʰ V57 Care involving use of rehabilitation procedures
> Use additional code to identify underlying condition

V57.0 Breathing exercises

V57.1 Other physical therapy
> Therapeutic and remedial exercises, except
> breathing

✓5ᵗʰ V57.2 Occupational therapy and vocational rehabilitation

> **V57.21 Encounter for occupational therapy**
>
> **V57.22 Encounter for vocational therapy**

V57.3 Speech therapy

V57.4 Orthoptic training

✓5ᵗʰ V57.8 Other specified rehabilitation procedure

> **V57.81 Orthotic training**
> > Gait training in the use of artificial limbs
>
> **V57.89 Other**
> > Multiple training or therapy

V57.9 Unspecified rehabilitation procedure

✓4ᵗʰ V58 Encounter for other and unspecified procedures and aftercare

> EXCLUDES   *convalescence and palliative care (V66)*

V58.0 Radiotherapy
> Encounter or admission for radiotherapy
>
> EXCLUDES   *encounter for radioactive implant —*
> *code to condition*
> *radioactive iodine therapy — code to*
> *condition*

V58.1 Chemotherapy
> Encounter or admission for chemotherapy
>
> EXCLUDES   *prophylactic chemotherapy against*
> *disease which has never been*
> *present (V03.0-V07.9)*

V58.2 Blood transfusion, without reported diagnosis

V58.3 Attention to surgical dressings and sutures
> Change of dressings
> Removal of sutures

✓5ᵗʰ V58.4 Other aftercare following surgery

> EXCLUDES   *aftercare following sterilization reversal*
> *surgery (V26.22)*
> *attention to artificial openings (V55.0-*
> *V55.9)*
> *orthopedic aftercare (V54.0-V54.9)*
>
> ▶Note: Codes from this subcategory should be used in
> conjunction with other aftercare codes to fully
> identify the reason for the aftercare encounter◄

> **V58.41 Encounter for planned postoperative wound closure**
>
> > EXCLUDES   *disruption of operative wound*
> > *(998.3)*
>
> • **V58.42 Aftercare following surgery for neoplasm**
> > Conditions classifiable to 140-239
>
> • **V58.43 Aftercare following surgery for injury and trauma**
> > Conditions classifiable to 800-999
> >
> > EXCLUDES   *aftercare for healing traumatic*
> > *fracture (V54.10-V54.19)*
>
> **V58.49 Other specified aftercare following surgery**

V58.5 Orthodontics
> EXCLUDES   *fitting and adjustment of orthodontic*
> *device (V53.4)*

✓5ᵗʰ V58.6 Long-term (current) drug use
> EXCLUDES   *drub abuse (305.00-305.93)*
> *drug dependence (304.00-304.93)*

> **V58.61 Long-term (current) use of anticoagulants**
>
> **V58.62 Long-term (current) use of antibiotics**
>
> **V58.69 Long-term (current) use of other medications**
> > High-risk medications

• ✓5ᵗʰ V58.7 Aftercare following surgery to specified body systems, not elsewhere classified

> Note: Codes from this subcategory should be used
> in conjunction with other aftercare codes to
> fully identify the reason for the aftercare
> encounter

> • **V58.71 Aftercare following surgery of the sense organs, NEC**
> > Conditions classifiable to 360-379, 380-389
>
> • **V58.72 Aftercare following surgery of the nervous system, NEC**
> > Conditions classifiable to 320-359
> >
> > EXCLUDES   *aftercare following surgery of*
> > *the sense organs, NEC*
> > *(V58.71)*
>
> • **V58.73 Aftercare following surgery of the circulatory system, NEC**
> > Conditions classifiable to 390-459
>
> • **V58.74 Aftercare following surgery of the respiratory system, NEC**
> > Conditions classifiable to 460-519

●   **V58.75 Aftercare following surgery of the teeth, oral cavity and digestive system, NEC**
Conditions classifiable to 520-579

●   **V58.76 Aftercare following surgery of the genitourinary system, NEC**
Conditions classifiable to 580-629
> **EXCLUDES**   *aftercare following sterilization reversal (V26.22)*

●   **V58.77 Aftercare following surgery of the skin and subcutaneous tissue, NEC**
Conditions classifiable to 680-709

●   **V58.78 Aftercare following surgery of the musculoskeletal system, NEC**
Conditions classifiable to 710-739

√5ᵗʰ **V58.8 Other specified procedures and aftercare**

   V58.81 Fitting and adjustment of vascular catheter
Removal or replacement of catheter
Toilet or cleansing
> **EXCLUDES**   *complication of renal dialysis (996.73)*
> *complication of vascular catheter (996.74)*
> *dialysis preparation — code to condition*
> *encounter for dialysis (V56.0-V56.8)*
> *fitting and adjustment of dialysis catheter (V56.1)*

   V58.82 Fitting and adjustment of nonvascular catheter, NEC
Removal or replacement of catheter
Toilet or cleansing
> **EXCLUDES**   *fitting and adjustment of peritoneal dialysis catheter (V56.2)*
> *fitting and adjustment of urinary catheter (V53.6)*

   V58.83 Encounter for therapeutic drug monitoring
> **EXCLUDES**   *blood-drug testing for medicolegal reasons (V70.4)*
> ▶Use additional code for any associated long-term (current) drug use (V58.61-V58.69)◀

   V58.89 Other specified aftercare

   V58.9 Unspecified aftercare   `SDx`

√4ᵗʰ **V59 Donors**
> **EXCLUDES**   *examination of potential donor (V70.8)*
> *self-donation of organ or tissue — code to condition*

√5ᵗʰ **V59.0 Blood**
   V59.01 Whole blood   `PDx`
   V59.02 Stem cells   `PDx`
   V59.09 Other   `PDx`
   V59.1 Skin   `PDx`
   V59.2 Bone   `PDx`
   V59.3 Bone marrow   `PDx`
   V59.4 Kidney   `PDx`
   V59.5 Cornea   `PDx`
   V59.6 Liver   `PDx`
   V59.8 Other specified organ or tissue   `PDx`
   V59.9 Unspecified organ or tissue   `PDx`

PERSONS ENCOUNTERING HEALTH SERVICES IN OTHER CIRCUMSTANCES (V60-V68)

√4ᵗʰ **V60 Housing, household, and economic circumstances**

   V60.0 Lack of housing   `SDx`
Hobos   Transients
Social migrants   Vagabonds
Tramps

   V60.1 Inadequate housing   `SDx`
Lack of heating
Restriction of space
Technical defects in home preventing adequate care

   V60.2 Inadequate material resources   `SDx`
Economic problem   Poverty NOS

   V60.3 Person living alone   `SDx`

   V60.4 No other household member able to render care   `SDx`
Person requiring care (has) (is):
family member too handicapped, ill, or otherwise unsuited to render care
partner temporarily away from home
temporarily away from usual place of abode
> **EXCLUDES**   *holiday relief care (V60.5)*

   V60.5 Holiday relief care   `SDx`
Provision of health care facilities to a person normally cared for at home, to enable relatives to take a vacation

   V60.6 Person living in residential institution   `SDx`
Boarding school resident

   V60.8 Other specified housing or economic circumstances   `SDx`

   V60.9 Unspecified housing or economic circumstance   `SDx`

√4ᵗʰ **V61 Other family circumstances**
> **INCLUDES**   when these circumstances or fear of them, affecting the person directly involved or others, are mentioned as the reason, justified or not, for seeking or receiving medical advice or care

   V61.0 Family disruption
Divorce   Estrangement

√5ᵗʰ **V61.1 Counseling for marital and partner problems**
> **EXCLUDES**   *problems related to:*
> *psychosexual disorders (302.0-302.9)*
> *sexual function (V41.7)*

   V61.10 Counseling for marital and partner problems, unspecified
Marital conflict
Partner conflict

   V61.11 Counseling for victim of spousal and partner abuse
> **EXCLUDES**   *encounter for treatment of current injuries due to abuse (995.80-995.85)*

   V61.12 Counseling for perpetrator of spousal and partner abuse

√5ᵗʰ **V61.2 Parent-child problems**

   V61.20 Counseling for parent-child problem, unspecified
Concern about behavior of child
Parent-child conflict

   V61.21 Counseling for victim of child abuse
Child battering   Child neglect
> **EXCLUDES**   *current injuries due to abuse (995.50-995.59)*

   V61.22 Counseling for perpetrator of parent child abuse
> **EXCLUDES**   *counseling for non-parental abuser (V62.83)*

√4ᵗʰ / √5ᵗʰ **Additional Digit Required**   **Unspecified Code**   **Other Specified Code**   **Manifestation Code**   ▶◀ **Revised Text**   ● **New Code**   ▲ **Revised Code Title**

V61.29 Other
         Problem concerning adopted or foster child

V61.3 Problems with aged parents or in-laws

✓5th **V61.4 Health problems within family**

V61.41 Alcoholism in family

V61.49 Other

Care of	}	sick or handicapped
Presence		person in family or
of		household

V61.5 Multiparity

V61.6 Illegitimacy or illegitimate pregnancy M ♀

V61.7 Other unwanted pregnancy M ♀

V61.8 Other specified family circumstances
         Problems with family members NEC

V61.9 Unspecified family circumstance

✓4th **V62 Other psychosocial circumstances**

> INCLUDES   those circumstances or fear of them, affecting the person directly involved or others, mentioned as the reason, justified or not, for seeking or receiving medical advice or care

> EXCLUDES   previous psychological trauma (V15.41-V15.49)

V62.0 Unemployment SDx

> EXCLUDES   circumstances when main problem is economic inadequacy or poverty (V60.2)

V62.1 Adverse effects of work environment SDx

V62.2 Other occupational circumstances or maladjustment SDx
         Career choice problem
         Dissatisfaction with employment

V62.3 Educational circumstances SDx
         Dissatisfaction with school environment
         Educational handicap

V62.4 Social maladjustment SDx
         Cultural deprivation
         Political, religious, or sex discrimination
         Social:
             isolation
             persecution

V62.5 Legal circumstances SDx
         Imprisonment
         Legal investigation
         Litigation
         Prosecution

V62.6 Refusal of treatment for reasons of religion or conscience SDx

✓5th **V62.8 Other psychological or physical stress, not elsewhere classified**

V62.81 Interpersonal problems, not elsewhere classified SDx

V62.82 Bereavement, uncomplicated SDx

> EXCLUDES   bereavement as adjustment reaction (309.0)

V62.83 Counseling for perpetrator of physical/sexual abuse SDx

> EXCLUDES   counseling for perpetrator of parental child abuse (V61.22)
> counseling for perpetrator of spousal and partner abuse (V61.12)

V62.89 Other SDx
         Life circumstance problems
         Phase of life problems

V62.9 Unspecified psychosocial circumstance SDx

✓4th **V63 Unavailability of other medical facilities for care**

V63.0 Residence remote from hospital or other health care facility

V63.1 Medical services in home not available

> EXCLUDES   no other household member able to render care (V60.4)

V63.2 Person awaiting admission to adequate facility elsewhere

V63.8 Other specified reasons for unavailability of medical facilities
         Person on waiting list undergoing social agency investigation

V63.9 Unspecified reason for unavailability of medical facilities

✓4th **V64 Persons encountering health services for specific procedures, not carried out**

V64.0 Vaccination not carried out because of contraindication SDx

V64.1 Surgical or other procedure not carried out because of contraindication SDx

V64.2 Surgical or other procedure not carried out because of patient's decision SDx

V64.3 Procedure not carried out for other reasons SDx

V64.4 Laparoscopic surgical procedure converted to open procedure SDx

✓4th **V65 Other persons seeking consultation without complaint or sickness**

V65.0 Healthy person accompanying sick person
         Boarder

V65.1 Person consulting on behalf of another person
         Advice or treatment for nonattending third party

> EXCLUDES   concern (normal) about sick person in family (V61.41-V61.49)

V65.2 Person feigning illness
         Malingerer
         Peregrinating patient

V65.3 Dietary surveillance and counseling
         Dietary surveillance and counseling (in):
             NOS
             colitis
             diabetes mellitus
             food allergies or intolerance
             gastritis
             hypercholesterolemia
             hypoglycemia
             obesity

✓5th **V65.4 Other counseling, not elsewhere classified**
         Health:
             advice
             education
             instruction

> EXCLUDES   counseling (for):
> contraception (V25.40-V25.49)
> genetic (V26.3)
> on behalf of third party (V65.1)
> procreative management (V26.4)

V65.40 Counseling NOS

V65.41 Exercise counseling

V65.42 Counseling on substance use and abuse

V65.43 Counseling on injury prevention

V65.44 Human immunodeficiency virus [HIV] counseling

V65.45 Counseling on other sexually transmitted diseases

V65.49 Other specified counseling

V65.5 Person with feared complaint in whom no diagnosis was made
         Feared condition not demonstrated
         Problem was normal state
         "Worried well"

V65.8 Other reasons for seeking consultation

> EXCLUDES   specified symptoms

V65.9 Unspecified reason for consultation

√4ᵗʰ **V66 Convalescence and palliative care**
    V66.0 Following surgery `PDx`
    V66.1 Following radiotherapy `PDx`
    V66.2 Following chemotherapy `PDx`
    V66.3 Following psychotherapy and other treatment `PDx`
        for mental disorder
    V66.4 Following treatment of fracture `PDx`
    V66.5 Following other treatment `PDx`
    V66.6 Following combined treatment `PDx`
    V66.7 Encounter for palliative care `SDx`
        End-of-life care
        Hospice care
        Terminal care
        Code first underlying disease
    V66.9 Unspecified convalescence `PDx`

√4ᵗʰ **V67 Follow-up examination**
    `INCLUDES` surveillance only following completed treatment
    `EXCLUDES` surveillance of contraception (V25.40-V25.49)
  √5ᵗʰ **V67.0 Following surgery**
    V67.00 Following surgery, unspecified
    V67.01 Follow-up vaginal pap smear ♀
        Vaginal pap-smear, status-post hysterectomy for malignant condition
        Use additional code to identify:
          acquired absence of uterus (V45.77)
          personal history of malignant neoplasm (V10.40-V10.44)
        `EXCLUDES` *vaginal pap smear status-post hysterectomy for non-malignant condition (V76.47)*
    V67.09 Following other surgery
        `EXCLUDES` *sperm count following sterilization reversal (V26.22)*
                  sperm count for fertility testing (V26.21)
    V67.1 Following radiotherapy
    V67.2 Following chemotherapy
        Cancer chemotherapy follow-up
    V67.3 Following psychotherapy and other treatment for mental disorder
    V67.4 Following treatment of healed fracture
        `EXCLUDES` *current (healing) fracture aftercare (V54.0-V54.9)*
  √5ᵗʰ **V67.5 Following other treatment**
    V67.51 Following completed treatment with high-risk medications, not elsewhere classified
        `EXCLUDES` *long-term (current) drug use (V58.61-V58.69)*
    V67.59 Other
    V67.6 Following combined treatment
    V67.9 Unspecified follow-up examination

√4ᵗʰ **V68 Encounters for administrative purposes**
    V68.0 Issue of medical certificates `PDx`
        Issue of medical certificate of:
          cause of death
          fitness
          incapacity
        `EXCLUDES` *encounter for general medical examination (V70.0-V70.9)*
    V68.1 Issue of repeat prescriptions `PDx`
        Issue of repeat prescription for:
          appliance
          glasses
          medications
        `EXCLUDES` *repeat prescription for contraceptives (V25.41-V25.49)*

    V68.2 Request for expert evidence `PDx`
  √5ᵗʰ **V68.8 Other specified administrative purpose**
    V68.81 Referral of patient without `PDx`
        examination or treatment
    V68.89 Other `PDx`
    V68.9 Unspecified administrative purpose `PDx`

√4ᵗʰ **V69 Problems related to lifestyle**
    V69.0 Lack of physical exercise
    V69.1 Inappropriate diet and eating habits
        `EXCLUDES` *anorexia nervosa (307.1)*
                  bulimia (783.6)
                  malnutrition and other nutritional deficiencies (260-269.9)
                  other and unspecified eating disorders (307.50-307.59)
    V69.2 High-risk sexual behavior
    V69.3 Gambling and betting
        `EXCLUDES` *pathological gambling (312.31)*
    V69.8 Other problems related to lifestyle
        Self-damaging behavior
    V69.9 Problem related to lifestyle, unspecified

PERSONS WITHOUT REPORTED DIAGNOSIS ENCOUNTERED DURING EXAMINATION AND INVESTIGATION OF INDIVIDUALS AND POPULATIONS (V70-V83)

Note: Nonspecific abnormal findings disclosed at the time of these examinations are classifiable to categories 790-796.

√4ᵗʰ **V70 General medical examination**
    Use additional code(s) to identify any special screening examination(s) performed (V73.0-V82.9)
    V70.0 Routine general medical examination at a `PDx`
        health care facility
        Health checkup
        `EXCLUDES` *health checkup of infant or child (V20.2)*
    V70.1 General psychiatric examination, requested `PDx`
        by the authority
    V70.2 General psychiatric examination, other and unspecified `PDx`
    V70.3 Other medical examination for administrative purposes `PDx`
        General medical examination for:
          admission to old age home
          adoption
          camp
          driving license
          immigration and naturalization
          insurance certification
          marriage
          prison
          school admission
          sports competition
        `EXCLUDES` *attendance for issue of medical certificates (V68.0)*
                  pre-employment screening (V70.5)
    V70.4 Examination for medicolegal reasons `PDx`
        Blood-alcohol tests
        Blood-drug tests
        Paternity testing
        `EXCLUDES` *examination and observation following:*
                  accidents (V71.3, V71.4)
                  assault (V71.6)
                  rape (V71.5)
    V70.5 Health examination of defined subpopulations `PDx`

Armed forces personnel	Prisoners
Inhabitants of institutions	Prostitutes
Occupational health	Refugees
examinations	School children
Pre-employment screening	Students
Preschool children	

√4ᵗʰ √5ᵗʰ Additional Digit Required   Unspecified Code   Other Specified Code   Manifestation Code   ►◄ Revised Text   ● New Code   ▲ Revised Code Title

2003 ICD•9•CM   **Volume 1 — 293**

V Codes V66–V70.5

V Codes V70.6–V74.6

V70.6 Health examination in population surveys `PDx`
  EXCLUDES special screening (V73.0-V82.9)

V70.7 Examination of participant in clinical trial
  Examination of participant or control in clinical research

V70.8 Other specified general medical examinations `PDx`
  Examination of potential donor of organ or tissue

V70.9 Unspecified general medical examination `PDx`

✓4th **V71 Observation and evaluation for suspected conditions not found**
  INCLUDES This category is to be used when persons without a diagnosis are suspected of having an abnormal condition, without signs or symptoms, which requires study, but after examination and observation, is found not to exist. This category is also for use for administrative and legal observation status.

✓5th **V71.0 Observation for suspected mental condition**
  V71.01 Adult antisocial behavior `A` `PDx`
    Dyssocial behavior or gang activity in adult without manifest psychiatric disorder
  V71.02 Childhood or adolescent antisocial behavior `PDx`
    Dyssocial behavior or gang activity in child or adolescent without manifest psychiatric disorder
  V71.09 Other suspected mental condition `PDx`

V71.1 Observation for suspected malignant neoplasm `PDx`

V71.2 Observation for suspected tuberculosis `PDx`

V71.3 Observation following accident at work `PDx`

V71.4 Observation following other accident `PDx`
  Examination of individual involved in motor vehicle traffic accident

V71.5 Observation following alleged rape or seduction `PDx`
  Examination of victim or culprit

V71.6 Observation following other inflicted injury `PDx`
  Examination of victim or culprit

V71.7 Observation for suspected cardiovascular disease `PDx`

✓5th **V71.8 Observation and evaluation for other specified suspected conditions**
  V71.81 Abuse and neglect `PDx`
    EXCLUDES adult abuse and neglect (995.80-995.85)
      child abuse and neglect (995.50-995.59)
  V71.82 Observation and evaluation for suspected exposure to anthrax
  V71.83 Observation and evaluation for suspected exposure to other biological agent
  V71.89 Other specified suspected conditions `PDx`

V71.9 Observation for unspecified suspected condition `PDx`

✓4th **V72 Special investigations and examinations**
  INCLUDES routine examination of specific system
  EXCLUDES general medical examination (V70.0-V70.4)
    general screening examination of defined population groups (V70.5, V70.6, V70.7)
    routine examination of infant or child (V20.2)
  Use additional code(s) to identify any special screening examination(s) performed (V73.0-V82.9)

V72.0 Examination of eyes and vision `PDx`
V72.1 Examination of ears and hearing `PDx`
V72.2 Dental examination `PDx`

V72.3 Gynecological examination `PDx` ♀
  Papanicolaou cervical smear as part of general gynecological examination
  Pelvic examination (annual) (periodic)
  Use additional code to identify routine vaginal Papanicolaou smear (V76.47)
  EXCLUDES cervical Papanicolaou smear without general gynecological examination (V76.2)
    routine examination in contraceptive management (V25.40-V25.49)

V72.4 Pregnancy examination or test, pregnancy unconfirmed `PDx` ♀
  Possible pregnancy, not (yet) confirmed
  EXCLUDES pregnancy examination with immediate confirmation (V22.0-V22.1)

V72.5 Radiological examination, not elsewhere classified `SDx`
  Routine chest x-ray
  EXCLUDES examination for suspected tuberculosis (V71.2)

V72.6 Laboratory examination `SDx`
  EXCLUDES that for suspected disorder (V71.0-V71.9)

V72.7 Diagnostic skin and sensitization tests `PDx`
  Allergy tests   Skin tests for hypersensitivity
  EXCLUDES diagnostic skin tests for bacterial diseases (V74.0-V74.9)

✓5th **V72.8 Other specified examinations**
  V72.81 Pre-operative cardiovascular examination `PDx`
  V72.82 Pre-operative respiratory examination `PDx`
  V72.83 Other specified pre-operative examination `PDx`
  V72.84 Pre-operative examination, unspecified `PDx`
  V72.85 Other specified examination `PDx`

V72.9 Unspecified examination `PDx`

✓4th **V73 Special screening examination for viral and chlamydial diseases**
  V73.0 Poliomyelitis
  V73.1 Smallpox
  V73.2 Measles
  V73.3 Rubella
  V73.4 Yellow fever
  V73.5 Other arthropod-borne viral diseases
    Dengue fever   Viral encephalitis:
    Hemorrhagic fever   mosquito-borne
         tick-borne
  V73.6 Trachoma
  ✓5th **V73.8 Other specified viral and chlamydial diseases**
    V73.88 Other specified chlamydial diseases
    V73.89 Other specified viral diseases
  ✓5th **V73.9 Unspecified viral and chlamydial disease**
    V73.98 Unspecified chlamydial disease
    V73.99 Unspecified viral disease

✓4th **V74 Special screening examination for bacterial and spirochetal diseases**
  INCLUDES diagnostic skin tests for these diseases
  V74.0 Cholera
  V74.1 Pulmonary tuberculosis
  V74.2 Leprosy [Hansen's disease]
  V74.3 Diphtheria
  V74.4 Bacterial conjunctivitis
  V74.5 Venereal disease
  V74.6 Yaws

V74.8 **Other specified bacterial and spirochetal diseases**
- Brucellosis   Tetanus
- Leptospirosis   Whooping cough
- Plague

V74.9 **Unspecified bacterial and spirochetal disease**

√4ᵗʰ V75 **Special screening examination for other infectious diseases**

V75.0 **Rickettsial diseases**

V75.1 **Malaria**

V75.2 **Leishmaniasis**

V75.3 **Trypanosomiasis**
- Chagas' disease
- Sleeping sickness

V75.4 **Mycotic infections**

V75.5 **Schistosomiasis**

V75.6 **Filariasis**

V75.7 **Intestinal helminthiasis**

V75.8 **Other specified parasitic infections**

V75.9 **Unspecified infectious disease**

√4ᵗʰ V76 **Special screening for malignant neoplasms**

V76.0 **Respiratory organs**

√5ᵗʰ V76.1 **Breast**

V76.10 **Breast screening, unspecified**

V76.11 **Screening mammogram for high-risk patient** ♀

V76.12 **Other screening mammogram**

V76.19 **Other screening breast examination**

V76.2 **Cervix** ♀
- Routine cervical Papanicolaou smear
- **EXCLUDES** *that as part of a general gynecological examination (V72.3)*

V76.3 **Bladder**

√5ᵗʰ V76.4 **Other sites**

V76.41 **Rectum**

V76.42 **Oral cavity**

V76.43 **Skin**

V76.44 **Prostate** ♂

V76.45 **Testis** ♂

V76.46 **Ovary**

V76.47 **Vagina**
- Vaginal pap smear status-post hysterectomy for non-malignant condition
- Use additional code to identify acquired absence of uterus (V45.77)
- **EXCLUDES** *vaginal pap smear status-post hysterectomy for malignant condition (V67.01)*

V76.49 **Other sites**

√5ᵗʰ V76.5 **Intestine**

V76.50 **Intestine, unspecified**

V76.51 **Colon**
- **EXCLUDES** *rectum (V76.41)*

V76.52 **Small intestine**

√5ᵗʰ V76.8 **Other neoplasm**

V76.81 **Nervous system**

V76.89 **Other neoplasm**

V76.9 **Unspecified**

√4ᵗʰ V77 **Special screening for endocrine, nutritional, metabolic, and immunity disorders**

V77.0 **Thyroid disorders**

V77.1 **Diabetes mellitus**

V77.2 **Malnutrition**

V77.3 **Phenylketonuria [PKU]**

V77.4 **Galactosemia**

V77.5 **Gout**

V77.6 **Cystic fibrosis**
- Screening for mucoviscidosis

V77.7 **Other inborn errors of metabolism**

V77.8 **Obesity**

√5ᵗʰ V77.9 **Other and unspecified endocrine, nutritional, metabolic, and immunity disorders**

V77.91 **Screening for lipoid disorders**
- Screening cholesterol level
- Screening for hypercholesterolemia
- Screening for hyperlipidemia

V77.99 **Other and unspecified endocrine, nutritional, metabolic, and immunity disorders**

√4ᵗʰ V78 **Special screening for disorders of blood and blood-forming organs**

V78.0 **Iron deficiency anemia**

V78.1 **Other and unspecified deficiency anemia**

V78.2 **Sickle cell disease or trait**

V78.3 **Other hemoglobinopathies**

V78.8 **Other disorders of blood and blood-forming organs**

V78.9 **Unspecified disorder of blood and blood-forming organs**

√4ᵗʰ V79 **Special screening for mental disorders and developmental handicaps**

V79.0 **Depression**

V79.1 **Alcoholism**

V79.2 **Mental retardation**

V79.3 **Developmental handicaps in early childhood**

V79.8 **Other specified mental disorders and developmental handicaps**

V79.9 **Unspecified mental disorder and developmental handicap**

√4ᵗʰ V80 **Special screening for neurological, eye, and ear diseases**

V80.0 **Neurological conditions**

V80.1 **Glaucoma**

V80.2 **Other eye conditions**
- Screening for:
  - cataract
  - congenital anomaly of eye
  - senile macular lesions
- **EXCLUDES** *general vision examination (V72.0)*

V80.3 **Ear diseases**
- **EXCLUDES** *general hearing examination (V72.1)*

√4ᵗʰ V81 **Special screening for cardiovascular, respiratory, and genitourinary diseases**

V81.0 **Ischemic heart disease**

V81.1 **Hypertension**

V81.2 **Other and unspecified cardiovascular conditions**

V81.3 **Chronic bronchitis and emphysema**

V81.4 **Other and unspecified respiratory conditions**
- **EXCLUDES** *screening for:*
  - *lung neoplasm (V76.0)*
  - *pulmonary tuberculosis (V74.1)*

V81.5 **Nephropathy**
- Screening for asymptomatic bacteriuria

V81.6 **Other and unspecified genitourinary conditions**

√4ᵗʰ V82 **Special screening for other conditions**

V82.0 **Skin conditions**

V82.1 **Rheumatoid arthritis**

V82.2 **Other rheumatic disorders**

V82.3 **Congenital dislocation of hip**

V82.4 **Maternal postnatal screening for chromosomal anomalies** ♀
- **EXCLUDES** *antenatal screening by amniocentesis (V28.0)*

V Codes V74.8–V82.4

√4ᵗʰ / √5ᵗʰ Additional Digit Required   Unspecified Code   Other Specified Code   Manifestation Code   ►◄ Revised Text   ● New Code   ▲ Revised Code Title

2002 ICD•9•CM   **Volume 1 — 295**

V82.5   Chemical poisoning and other contamination
         Screening for:
            heavy metal poisoning
            ingestion of radioactive substance
            poisoning from contaminated water supply
            radiation exposure

V82.6   **Multiphasic screening**

✓5th **V82.8**   **Other specified conditions**

     V82.81 Osteoporosis
         Use additional code to identify:
            postmenopausal hormone replacement
              therapy status (V07.4)
            postmenopausal (natural) status (V49.81)

     V82.89 Other specified conditions

V82.9   **Unspecified condition**

✓4th **V83**   **Genetic carrier status**

    ✓5th **V83.0**   **Hemophilia A carrier**

     V83.01 Asymptomatic hemophilia A carrier
     V83.02 Symptomatic hemophilia A carrier

●   ✓5th **V83.8**   **Other genetic carrier status**

●   **V83.81 Cystic fibrosis gene carrier**

●   **V83.89 Other genetic carrier status**

SUPPLEMENTARY CLASSIFICATION OF EXTERNAL CAUSES OF INJURY AND POISONING (E800-E999)

This section is provided to permit the classification of environmental events, circumstances, and conditions as the cause of injury, poisoning, and other adverse effects. Where a code from this section is applicable, it is intended that it shall be used in addition to a code from one of the main chapters of ICD-9-CM, indicating the nature of the condition. Certain other conditions which may be stated to be due to external causes are classified in Chapters 1 to 16 of ICD-9-CM. For these, the "E" code classification should be used as an additional code for more detailed analysis.

Machinery accidents [other than those connected with transport] are classifiable to category E919, in which the fourth-digit allows a broad classification of the type of machinery involved. If a more detailed classification of type of machinery is required, it is suggested that the "Classification of Industrial Accidents according to Agency," prepared by the International Labor Office, be used in addition. This is reproduced in Appendix D for optional use.

Categories for "late effects" of accidents and other external causes are to be found at E929, E959, E969, E977, E989, and E999.

DEFINITIONS AND EXAMPLES RELATED TO TRANSPORT ACCIDENTS

(a) A **transport accident** (E800-E848) is any accident involving a device designed primarily for, or being used at the time primarily for, conveying persons or goods from one place to another.

INCLUDES accidents involving:
aircraft and spacecraft (E840-E845)
watercraft (E830-E838)
motor vehicle (E810-E825)
railway (E800-E807)
other road vehicles (E826-E829)

In classifying accidents which involve more than one kind of transport, the above order of precedence of transport accidents should be used.

Accidents involving agricultural and construction machines, such as tractors, cranes, and bulldozers, are regarded as transport accidents only when these vehicles are under their own power on a highway [otherwise the vehicles are regarded as machinery]. Vehicles which can travel on land or water, such as hovercraft and other amphibious vehicles, are regarded as watercraft when on the water, as motor vehicles when on the highway, and as off-road motor vehicles when on land, but off the highway.

EXCLUDES accidents:
in sports which involve the use of transport but where the transport vehicle itself was not involved in the accident
involving vehicles which are part of industrial equipment used entirely on industrial premises
occurring during transportation but unrelated to the hazards associated with the means of transportation [e.g., injuries received in a fight on board ship; transport vehicle involved in a cataclysm such as an earthquake]
to persons engaged in the maintenance or repair of transport equipment or vehicle not in motion, unless injured by another vehicle in motion

(b) A **railway accident** is a transport accident involving a railway train or other railway vehicle operated on rails, whether in motion or not.

EXCLUDES accidents:
in repair shops
in roundhouse or on turntable
on railway premises but not involving a train or other railway vehicle

(c) A **railway train** or **railway vehicle** is any device with or without cars coupled to it, desiged for traffic on a railway.

INCLUDES interurban:
electric car ⎫ (operated chiefly on its
streetcar ⎬ own right-of-way,
⎭ not open to other traffic)
railway train, any power [diesel] [electric] [steam]
funicular
monorail or two-rail
subterranean or elevated
other vehicle designed to run on a railway track

EXCLUDES interurban electric cars [streetcars] specified to be operating on a right-of-way that forms part of the public street or highway [definition (n)]

(d) A **railway** or **railroad** is a right-of-way designed for traffic on rails, which is used by carriages or wagons transporting passengers or freight, and by other rolling stock, and which is not open to other public vehicular traffic.

(e) A **motor vehicle accident** is a transport accident involving a motor vehicle. It is defined as a motor vehicle traffic accident or as a motor vehicle nontraffic accident according to whether the accident occurs on a public highway or elsewhere.

EXCLUDES injury or damage due to cataclysm
injury or damage while a motor vehicle, not under its own power, is being loaded on, or unloaded from, another conveyance

(f) A **motor vehicle traffic accident** is any motor vehicle accident occurring on a public highway [i.e., originating, terminating, or involving a vehicle partially on the highway]. A motor vehicle accident is assumed to have occurred on the highway unless another place is specified, except in the case of accidents involving only off-road motor vehicles which are classified as nontraffic accidents unless the contrary is stated.

(g) A **motor vehicle nontraffic accident** is any motor vehicle accident which occurs entirely in any place other than a public highway.

(h) A **public highway [trafficway]** or **street** is the entire width between property lines [or other boundary lines] of every way or place, of which any part is open to the use of the public for purposes of vehicular traffic as a matter of right or custom. A **roadway** is that part of the public highway designed, improved, and ordinarily used, for vehicular travel.

INCLUDES approaches (public) to:
docks
public building
station

EXCLUDES driveway (private)
parking lot
ramp
roads in:
airfield
farm
industrial premises
mine
private grounds
quarry

E Codes

(i) A **motor vehicle** is any mechanically or electrically powered device, not operated on rails, upon which any person or property may be transported or drawn upon a highway. Any object such as a trailer, coaster, sled, or wagon being towed by a motor vehicle is considerd a part of the motor vehicle.

> INCLUDES   automobile [any type]
> bus
> construction machinery, farm and industrial machinery, steam roller, tractor, army tank, highway grader, or similar vehicle on wheels or treads, while in transport under own power
> fire engine (motorized)
> motorcycle
> motorized bicycle [moped] or scooter
> trolley bus not operating on rails
> truck
> van
>
> EXCLUDES   *devices used solely to move persons or materials within the confines of a building and its premises, such as:*
> *building elevator*
> *coal car in mine*
> *electric baggage or mail truck used solely within a railroad station*
> *electric truck used solely within an industrial plant*
> *moving overhead crane*

(j) A **motorcycle** is a two-wheeled motor vehicle having one or two riding saddles and sometimes having a third wheel for the support of a sidecar. The sidecar is considered part of the motorcycle.

> INCLUDES   motorized:
> bicycle [moped]
> scooter
> tricycle

(k) An **off-road motor vehicle** is a motor vehicle of special design, to enable it to negotiate rough or soft terrain or snow. Examples of special design are high construction, special wheels and tires, driven by treads, or support on a cushion of air.

> INCLUDES   all terrain vehicle [ATV]
> army tank
> hovercraft, on land or swamp
> snowmobile

(l) A **driver** of a motor vehicle is the occupant of the motor vehicle operating it or intending to operate it. A **motorcyclist** is the driver of a motorcycle. Other authorized occupants of a motor vehicle are **passengers**.

(m) An **other road vehicle** is any device, except a motor vehicle, in, on, or by which any person or property may be transported on a highway.

> INCLUDES   animal carrying a person or goods
> animal-drawn vehicles
> animal harnessed to conveyance
> bicycle [pedal cycle]
> streetcar
> tricycle (pedal)
>
> EXCLUDES   *pedestrian conveyance [definition (q)]*

(n) A **streetcar** is a device designed and used primarily for transporting persons within a municipality, running on rails, usually subject to normal traffic control signals, and operated principally on a right-of-way that forms part of the traffic way. A trailer being towed by a streetcar is considered a part of the streetcar.

> INCLUDES   interurban or intraurban electric or streetcar, when specified to be operating on a street or public highway
> tram (car)
> trolley (car)

(o) A **pedal cycle** is any road transport vehicle operated solely by pedals.

> INCLUDES   bicycle
> pedal cycle
> tricycle
>
> EXCLUDES   *motorized bicycle [definition (i)]*

(p) A **pedal cyclist** is any person riding on a pedal cycle or in a sidecar attached to such a vehicle.

(q) A **pedestrian conveyance** is any human powered device by which a pedestrian may move other than by walking or by which a walking person may move another pedestrian.

> INCLUDES   baby carriage
> coaster wagon
> ice skates
> perambulator
> pushcart
> pushchair
> roller skates
> scooter
> skateboard
> skis
> sled
> wheelchair

(r) A **pedestrian** is any person involved in an accident who was not at the time of the accident riding in or on a motor vehicle, railroad train, streetcar, animal-drawn or other vehicle, or on a bicycle or animal.

> INCLUDES   person:
> changing tire of vehicle
> in or operating a pedestrian conveyance
> making adjustment to motor of vehicle
> on foot

(s) A **watercraft** is any device for transporting passengers or goods on the water.

(t) A **small boat** is any watercraft propelled by paddle, oars, or small motor, with a passenger capacity of less than ten.

> INCLUDES   boat NOS
> canoe
> coble
> dinghy
> punt
> raft
> rowboat
> rowing shell
> scull
> skiff
> small motorboat
>
> EXCLUDES   *barge*
> *lifeboat (used after abandoning ship)*
> *raft (anchored) being used as a diving platform*
> *yacht*

(u) An **aircraft** is any device for transporting passengers or goods in the air.

> INCLUDES   airplane [any type]
> balloon
> bomber
> dirigible
> glider (hang)
> military aircraft
> parachute

(v) A **commercial transport aircraft** is any device for collective passenger or freight transportation by air, whether run on commercial lines for profit or by government authorities, with the exception of military craft.

▨◁▷ Fourth-digit Required   ▶◀ Revised Text   ● New Code   ▲ Revised Code Title

RAILWAY ACCIDENTS (E800-E807)

Note: For definitions of railway accident and related terms see definitions (a) to (d).

EXCLUDES *accidents involving railway train and:*
aircraft (E840.0-E845.9)
motor vehicle (E810.0-E825.9)
watercraft (E830.0-E838.9)

The following fourth-digit subdivisions are for use with categories E800-E807 to identify the injured person:

.0 Railway employee
Any person who by virtue of his employment in connection with a railway, whether by the railway company or not, is at increased risk of involvement in a railway accident, such as:
catering staff of train
driver
guard
porter
postal staff on train
railway fireman
shunter
sleeping car attendant

.1 Passenger on railway
Any authorized person traveling on a train, except a railway employee.

    EXCLUDES *intending passenger waiting at station (.8)*
unauthorized rider on railway vehicle (.8)

.2 Pedestrian
See definition (r)

.3 Pedal cyclist
See definition (p)

.8 Other specified person
Intending passenger or bystander waiting at station
Unauthorized rider on railway vehicle

.9 Unspecified person

§ ✓4ᵗʰ **E800 Railway accident involving collision with rolling stock**

    INCLUDES collision between railway trains or railway vehicles, any kind
collision NOS on railway
derailment with antecedent collision with rolling stock or NOS

§ ✓4ᵗʰ **E801 Railway accident involving collision with other object**

    INCLUDES collision of railway train with:
buffers
fallen tree on railway
gates
platform
rock on railway
streetcar
other nonmotor vehicle
other object

    EXCLUDES *collision with:*
aircraft (E840.0-E842.9)
motor vehicle (E810.0-E810.9, E820.0-E822.9)

§ ✓4ᵗʰ **E802 Railway accident involving derailment without antecedent collision**

§ ✓4ᵗʰ **E803 Railway accident involving explosion, fire, or burning**

    EXCLUDES *explosion or fire, with antecedent derailment (E802.0-E802.9)*
explosion or fire, with mention of antecedent collision (E800.0-E801.9)

§ ✓4ᵗʰ **E804 Fall in, on, or from railway train**

    INCLUDES fall while alighting from or boarding railway train

    EXCLUDES *fall related to collision, derailment, or explosion of railway train (E800.0-E803.9)*

§ ✓4ᵗʰ **E805 Hit by rolling stock**

    INCLUDES crushed
injured
killed
knocked down
run over
} by railway train or part

    EXCLUDES *pedestrian hit by object set in motion by railway train (E806.0-E806.9)*

§ ✓4ᵗʰ **E806 Other specified railway accident**

    INCLUDES hit by object falling in railway train
injured by door or window on railway train
nonmotor road vehicle or pedestrian hit by object set in motion by railway train
railway train hit by falling:
earth NOS
rock
tree
other object

    EXCLUDES *railway accident due to cataclysm (E908-E909)*

§ ✓4ᵗʰ **E807 Railway accident of unspecified nature**

    INCLUDES found dead
injured
} on railway right-of-way NOS

railway accident NOS

MOTOR VEHICLE TRAFFIC ACCIDENTS (E810-E819)

Note: For definitions of motor vehicle traffic accident, and related terms, see definitions (e) to (k).

EXCLUDES *accidents involving motor vehicle and aircraft (E840.0-E845.9)*

The following fourth-digit subdivisions are for use with categories E810-E819 to identify the injured person:

.0 Driver of motor vehicle other than motorcycle
See definition (1)

.1 Passenger in motor vehicle other than motorcycle
See definition (1)

.2 Motorcyclist
See definition (1)

.3 Passenger on motorcycle
See definition (1)

.4 Occupant of streetcar

.5 Rider of animal; occupant of animal-drawn vehicle

.6 Pedal cyclist
See definition (p)

.7 Pedestrian
See definition (r)

.8 Other specified person
Occupant of vehicle other than above
Person in railway train involved in accident
Unauthorized rider of motor vehicle

.9 Unspecified person

§§ ✓4ᵗʰ **E810 Motor vehicle traffic accident involving collision with train**

    EXCLUDES *motor vehicle collision with object set in motion by railway train (E815.0-E815.9)*
railway train hit by object set in motion by motor vehicle (E818.0-E818.9)

---

§ Requires fourth-digit. See beginning of section E800-E807 for codes and definitions.
§§ Requires fourth-digit. See beginning of section E810-E819 for codes and definitions.

✓4ᵗʰ Fourth-digit Required   ▶◀ Revised Text   ● New Code   ▲ Revised Code Title

§ ☑4ᵗʰ **E811 Motor vehicle traffic accident involving re-entrant collision with another motor vehicle**

INCLUDES   collision between motor vehicle which accidentally leaves the roadway then re-enters the same roadway, or the opposite roadway on a divided highway, and another motor vehicle

EXCLUDES   *collision on the same roadway when none of the motor vehicles involved have left and re-entered the highway (E812.0-E812.9)*

§ ☑4ᵗʰ **E812 Other motor vehicle traffic accident involving collision with motor vehicle**

INCLUDES   collision with another motor vehicle parked, stopped, stalled, disabled, or abandoned on the highway

          motor vehicle collision NOS

EXCLUDES   *collision with object set in motion by another motor vehicle (E815.0-E815.9)*

          re-entrant collision with another motor vehicle (E811.0-E811.9)

§ ☑4ᵗʰ **E813 Motor vehicle traffic accident involving collision with other vehicle**

INCLUDES   collision between motor vehicle, any kind, and:

          other road (nonmotor transport) vehicle, such as:

             animal carrying a person

             animal-drawn vehicle

             pedal cycle

             streetcar

EXCLUDES   *collision with:*

          object set in motion by nonmotor road vehicle (E815.0-E815.9)

          pedestrian (E814.0-E814.9)

          nonmotor road vehicle hit by object set in motion by motor vehicle (E818.0-E818.9)

§ ☑4ᵗʰ **E814 Motor vehicle traffic accident involving collision with pedestrian**

INCLUDES   collision between motor vehicle, any kind, and pedestrian

          pedestrian dragged, hit, or run over by motor vehicle, any kind

EXCLUDES   *pedestrian hit by object set in motion by motor vehicle (E818.0-E818.9)*

§ ☑4ᵗʰ **E815 Other motor vehicle traffic accident involving collision on the highway**

INCLUDES   collision (due to loss of control) (on highway) between motor vehicle, any kind, and:

          abutment (bridge) (overpass)

          animal (herded) (unattended)

          fallen stone, traffic sign, tree, utility pole

          guard rail or boundary fence

          interhighway divider

          landslide (not moving)

          object set in motion by railway train or road vehicle (motor) (nonmotor)

          object thrown in front of motor vehicle

          other object, fixed, movable, or moving

          safety island

          temporary traffic sign or marker

          wall of cut made for road

EXCLUDES   *collision with:*

          any object off the highway (resulting from loss of control) (E816.0-E816.9)

          any object which normally would have been off the highway and is not stated to have been on it (E816.0-E816.9)

          motor vehicle parked, stopped, stalled, disabled, or abandoned on highway (E812.0-E812.9)

          moving landslide (E909)

       motor vehicle hit by object:

          set in motion by railway train or road vehicle (motor) (nonmotor) (E818.0-E818.9)

          thrown into or on vehicle (E818.0-E818.9)

§ ☑4ᵗʰ **E816 Motor vehicle traffic accident due to loss of control, without collision on the highway**

INCLUDES   motor vehicle:

          failing to make

             curve   and:

          going out of control   coliding with

             (due to):   object

             blowout   off the

             burst tire   highway

             driver falling   overturning

                asleep   stopping

             driver inattention   abruptly

             excessive speed   off the

             failure of   highway

                mechanical

                part

EXCLUDES   *collision on highway following loss of control (E810.0-E815.9)*

          loss of control of motor vehicle following collision on the highway (E810.0-E815.9)

§ ☑4ᵗʰ **E817 Noncollision motor vehicle traffic accident while boarding or alighting**

INCLUDES   fall down stairs of motor bus

          fall from car in street

          injured by moving part of the vehicle   while boarding or alighting

          trapped by door of motor bus

---

§   Requires fourth-digit. See beginning of section E810-E819 for codes and definitions.

            ☑4ᵗʰ Fourth-digit Required   ▶◀ Revised Text   ● New Code   ▲ Revised Code Title

§§ ✓4ᵗʰ **E818 Other noncollision motor vehicle traffic accident**

INCLUDES   accidental poisoning
                          from exhaust gas
                          generated by
                 breakage of any part of
                 explosion of any part of
                 fall, jump, or being   ⎫
                          accidentally pushed   ⎪   motor
                          from   ⎬   vehicle
                 fire starting in   ⎪   while
                 hit by object thrown into   ⎪   in
                          or on   ⎪   motion
                 injured by being thrown   ⎪
                          against some part   ⎪
                          of, or object in   ⎭
                 injury from moving part
                          of
                 object falling in or on
                 object thrown on

           collision of railway train or road vehicle except
                          motor vehicle, with object set in motion
                          by motor vehicle
           motor vehicle hit by object set in motion by
                          railway train or road vehicle (motor)
                          (nonmotor)
           pedestrian, railway train, or road vehicle
                          (motor) (nonmotor) hit by object set in
                          motion by motor vehicle

EXCLUDES   *collision between motor vehicle and:*
                     object set in motion by railway train or road
                          vehicle (motor) (nonmotor) (E815.0-
                          E815.9)
                     object thrown towards the motor vehicle
                          (E815.0-E815.9)
                     person overcome by carbon monoxide generated
                          by stationary motor vehicle off the
                          roadway with motor running (E868.2)

§§ ✓4ᵗʰ **E819 Motor vehicle traffic accident of unspecified nature**

INCLUDES   motor vehicle traffic accident NOS
                 traffic accident NOS

MOTOR VEHICLE NONTRAFFIC ACCIDENTS (E820-E825)

           Note: For definitions of motor vehicle nontraffic accident and
                     related terms see definition (a) to (k).

INCLUDES   accidents involving motor vehicles being used
                          in recreational or sporting activities off
                          the highway
                 collision and noncollision motor vehicle
                          accidents occurring entirely off the
                          highway

EXCLUDES   *accidents involving motor vehicle and:*
                     aircraft (E840.0-E845.9)
                     watercraft (E830.0-E838.9)
                 accidents, not on the public highway, involving
                     agricultural and construction machinery
                     but not involving another motor vehicle
                     (E919.0, E919.2, E919.7)

The following fourth-digit subdivisions are for use with
categories E820-E825 to identify the injured person:

   .0 Driver of motor vehicle other than motorcycle
          See definition (l)
   **.1 Passenger in motor vehicle other than
        motorcycle**
          See definition (l)
   .2 Motorcyclist
          See definition (l)
   .3 Passenger on motorcycle
          See definition (l)
   .4 Occupant of streetcar
   **.5 Rider of animal; occupant of animal-drawn
        vehicle**
   .6 Pedal cyclist
          See definition (p)
   .7 Pedestrian
          See definition (r)
   .8 Other specified person
          Occupant of vehicle other than above
          Person on railway train involved in accident
          Unauthorized rider of motor vehicle
   .9 Unspecified person

§ ✓4ᵗʰ **E820 Nontraffic accident involving motor-driven snow vehicle**

INCLUDES   breakage of part of   ⎫ motor-driven
                 fall from   ⎪ snow
                 hit by   ⎬ vehicle (not
                 overturning of   ⎪ on public
                 run over or dragged by ⎭ highway)

           collision of motor-driven snow vehicle with:
                 animal (being ridden) (-drawn vehicle)
                 another off-road motor vehicle
                 other motor vehicle, not on public highway
                 railway train
                 other object, fixed or movable
           injury caused by rough landing of motor-
                 driven snow vehicle (after leaving ground
                 on rough terrain)

EXCLUDES   *accident on the public highway involving motor*
                 driven snow vehicle (E810.0-E819.9)

§ ✓4ᵗʰ **E821 Nontraffic accident involving other off-road motor vehicle**

INCLUDES   breakage of part of   ⎫ off-road motor
                 fall from   ⎪ vehicle,
                 hit by   ⎪ except
                 overturning of   ⎬ snow
                 run over or dragged by ⎪ vehicle (not
                 thrown against some   ⎪ on public
                          part of or object in ⎭ highway)

           collision with:
                 animal (being ridden) (-drawn vehicle)
                 another off-road motor vehicle, except snow
                          vehicle
                 other motor vehicle, not on public highway
                 other object, fixed or movable

EXCLUDES   *accident on public highway involving off-road*
                     motor vehicle (E810.0-E819.9)
                 collision between motor driven snow vehicle and
                     other off-road motor vehicle (E820.0-
                     E820.9)
                 hovercraft accident on water (E830.0-E838.9)

---

§ Requires fourth-digit. See beginning of section E820-E825 for codes and definitions.
§§ Requires fourth-digit. See beginning of section E810-E819 for codes and definitions

✓4ᵗʰ Fourth-digit Required   ▶◀ Revised Text   ● New Code   ▲ Revised Code Title

§§ ✓4ᵗʰ **E822 Other motor vehicle nontraffic accident involving collision with moving object**

     INCLUDES   collision, not on public highway, between motor vehicle, except off-road motor vehicle and:
         animal
         nonmotor vehicle
         other motor vehicle, except off-road motor vehicle
         pedestrian
         railway train
         other moving object

     EXCLUDES   *collision with:*
         motor-driven snow vehicle (E820.0-E820.9)
         other off-road motor vehicle (E821.0-E821.9)

§§ ✓4ᵗʰ **E823 Other motor vehicle nontraffic accident involving collision with stationary object**

     INCLUDES   collision, not on public highway, between motor vehicle, except off-road motor vehicle, and any object, fixed or movable, but not in motion

§§ ✓4ᵗʰ **E824 Other motor vehicle nontraffic accident while boarding and alighting**

     INCLUDES   fall
         injury from
             moving part of motor vehicle
         trapped by door of motor vehicle
             } while boarding or alighting from motor vehicle, except off-road motor vehicle, not on public highway

§§ ✓4ᵗʰ **E825 Other motor vehicle nontraffic accident of other and unspecified nature**

     INCLUDES   accidental poisoning from carbon monoxide generated by
         breakage of any part of
         explosion of any part of
         fall, jump, or being accidentally pushed from
         fire starting in
         hit by object thrown into, towards, or on
         injured by being thrown against some part of, or object in
         injury from moving part of
         object falling in or on
         } motor vehicle while in motion, not on public highway

         motor vehicle nontraffic accident NOS

     EXCLUDES   *fall from or in stationary motor vehicle (E884.9, E885.9)*
         overcome by carbon monoxide or exhaust gas generated by stationary motor vehicle off the roadway with motor running (E868.2)
         struck by falling object from or in stationary motor vehicle (E916)

OTHER ROAD VEHICLE ACCIDENTS (E826-E829)

Note: Other road vehicle accidents are transport accidents involving road vehicles other than motor vehicles. For definitions of other road vehicle and related terms see definitions (m) to (o).

     INCLUDES   accidents involving other road vehicles being used in recreational or sporting activities

     EXCLUDES   *collision of other road vehicle [any] with:*
         aircraft (E840.0-E845.9)
         motor vehicle (E813.0-E813.9, E820.0-E822.9)
         railway train (E801.0-E801.9)

The following fourth-digit subdivisions are for use with categories E826-E829 to identify the injured person.
   .0 Pedestrian
      See definition (r)
   .1 Pedal cyclist
      See definition (p)
   .2 Rider of animal
   .3 Occupant of animal-drawn vehicle
   .4 Occupant of streetcar
   .8 Other specified person
   .9 Unspecified person

§ ✓4ᵗʰ **E826 Pedal cycle accident**
[0-9]

     INCLUDES   breakage of any part of pedal cycle
         collision between pedal cycle and:
            animal (being ridden) (herded) (unattended)
            another pedal cycle
            any pedestrian
            nonmotor road vehicle
            other object, fixed, movable, or moving, not set in motion by motor vehicle, railway train, or aircraft
         entanglement in wheel of pedal cycle
         fall from pedal cycle
         hit by object falling or thrown on the pedal cycle
         pedal cycle accident NOS
         pedal cycle overturned

§ ✓4ᵗʰ **E827 Animal-drawn vehicle accident**
[0,2-4,8,9]

     INCLUDES   breakage of any part of vehicle
         collision between animal-drawn vehicle and:
            animal (being ridden) (herded) (unattended)
            nonmotor road vehicle, except pedal cycle
            pedestrian, pedestrian conveyance, or pedestrian vehicle
            other object, fixed, movable, or moving, not set in motion by motor vehicle, railway train, or aircraft
         fall from
         knocked down by
         overturning of
         run over by
         thrown from
         } animal-drawn vehicle

     EXCLUDES   *collision of animal-drawn vehicle with pedal cycle (E826.0-E826.9)*

---

§ Requires fourth-digit. Valid digits are in [brackets] under each code. See beginning of section E826-E829 for codes and definitions.
§§ Requires fourth-digit. See beginning of section E820-E825 for codes and definitions.

✓4ᵗʰ Fourth-digit Required   ►◄ Revised Text   ● New Code   ▲ Revised Code Title

§§ ☑4ᵗʰ **E828 Accident involving animal being ridden**

[0,2,4,8,9]   `INCLUDES`   collision between animal being ridden and:
      another animal
      nonmotor road vehicle, except pedal cycle,
          and animal-drawn vehicle
      pedestrian, pedestrian conveyance, or
          pedestrian vehicle
      other object, fixed, movable, or moving, not
          set in motion by motor vehicle, railway
          train, or aircraft

      fall from
      knocked down by   } animal being
      thrown from   ridden
      trampled by

      ridden animal stumbled and fell

      `EXCLUDES`   *collision of animal being ridden with:*
         animal-drawn vehicle (E827.0-E827.9)
         pedal cycle (E826.0-E826.9)

§§ ☑4ᵗʰ **E829 Other road vehicle accidents**

[0,4,8,9]   `INCLUDES`   accident while
        boarding or
        alighting from   streetcar
    blow from object in   nonmotor road
    breakage of any part of   vehicle not
    caught in door of-   classifiable
    derailment of   to E826-
    fall in, on, or from   E828
    fire in

    collision between streetcar or nonmotor road
      vehicle, except as in E826-E828, and:
      animal (not being ridden)
      another nonmotor road vehicle not
        classifiable to E826-E828
      pedestrian
      other object, fixed, movable, or moving, not
        set in motion by motor vehicle, railway
        train, or aircraft
    nonmotor road vehicle accident NOS
    streetcar accident NOS

      `EXCLUDES`   *collision with:*
         animal being ridden (E828.0-E828.9)
         animal-drawn vehicle (E827.0-E827.9)
         pedal cycle (E826.0-E826.9)

WATER TRANSPORT ACCIDENTS (E830-E838)

    Note: For definitions of water transport accident and related
      terms see definitions (a), (s), and (t).

    `INCLUDES`   watercraft accidents in the course of
       recreational activities

    `EXCLUDES`   *accidents involving both aircraft, including*
       objects set in motion by aircraft, and
       watercraft (E840.0-E845.9)

The following fourth-digit subdivisions are for use with
categories E830-E838 to identify the injured person:

.0 Occupant of small boat, unpowered

.1 Occupant of small boat, powered
    See definition (t)
    `EXCLUDES`   *water skier (.4)*

.2 Occupant of other watercraft — crew
    Persons:
      engaged in operation of watercraft
      providing passenger services [cabin
        attendants, ship's physician, catering
        personnel]
      working on ship during voyage in other
        capacity [musician in band, operators
        of shops and beauty parlors]

**.3 Occupant of other watercraft — other than
crew**
    Passenger
    Occupant of lifeboat, other than crew, after
      abandoning ship

.4 Water skier

.5 Swimmer

.6 Dockers, stevedores
    Longshoreman employed on the dock in
      loading and unloading ships

.8 Other specified person
    Immigration and custom officials on board
      ship
    Person:
      accompanying passenger or member of crew
        visiting boat
    Pilot (guiding ship into port)

.9 Unspecified person

§ ☑4ᵗʰ **E830 Accident to watercraft causing submersion**

    `INCLUDES`   submersion and drowning due to:
      boat overturning
      boat submerging
      falling or jumping from burning ship
      falling or jumping from crushed watercraft
      ship sinking
      other accident to watercraft

§ ☑4ᵗʰ **E831 Accident to watercraft causing other injury**

    `INCLUDES`   any injury, except submersion and drowning,
       as a result of an accident to watercraft
      burned while ship on fire
      crushed between ships in collision
      crushed by lifeboat after abandoning ship
      fall due to collision or other accident to
       watercraft
      hit by falling object due to accident to
       watercraft
      injured in watercraft accident involving
       collision
      struck by boat or part thereof after fall or jump
       from damaged boat

    `EXCLUDES`   *burns from localized fire or explosion on board*
       ship (E837.0-E837.9)

§ ☑4ᵗʰ **E832 Other accidental submersion or drowning in water transport
accident**

    `INCLUDES`   submersion or drowning as a result of an
       accident other than accident to the
       watercraft, such as:
      fall:
        from gangplank
        from ship
        overboard
      thrown overboard by motion of ship
      washed overboard

    `EXCLUDES`   *submersion or drowning of swimmer or diver*
       who voluntarily jumps from boat not
       involved in an accident (E910.0-E910.9)

---

§   Requires fourth-digit. See beginning of section E830-E838 for codes and definitions.
§§ Requires fourth-digit. Valid digits are in [brackets] under each code. See beginning of section E826-E829 for codes and definitions.

☑4ᵗʰ Fourth-digit Required   ►◄ Revised Text   ● New Code   ▲ Revised Code Title

§§ ☑4ᵗʰ **E833 Fall on stairs or ladders in water transport**

> EXCLUDES   *fall due to accident to watercraft (E831.0-E831.9)*

§§ ☑4ᵗʰ **E834 Other fall from one level to another in water transport**

> EXCLUDES   *fall due to accident to watercraft (E831.0-E831.9)*

§§ ☑4ᵗʰ **E835 Other and unspecified fall in water transport**

> EXCLUDES   *fall due to accident to watercraft (E831.0-E831.9)*

§§ ☑4ᵗʰ **E836 Machinery accident in water transport**

> INCLUDES   injuries in water transport caused by:
>
> deck
> engine room
> galley   ⎫ machinery
> laundry
> loading

§§ ☑4ᵗʰ **E837 Explosion, fire, or burning in watercraft**

> INCLUDES   explosion of boiler on steamship
> localized fire on ship
>
> EXCLUDES   *burning ship (due to collision or explosion) resulting in:*
>   *submersion or drowning (E830.0-E830.9)*
>   *other injury (E831.0-E831.9)*

§§ ☑4ᵗʰ **E838 Other and unspecified water transport accident**

> INCLUDES   accidental poisoning by gases or fumes on ship
> atomic power plant malfunction in watercraft
> crushed between ship and stationary object [wharf]
> crushed between ships without accident to watercraft
> crushed by falling object on ship or while loading or unloading
> hit by boat while water skiing
> struck by boat or part thereof (after fall from boat)
> watercraft accident NOS

AIR AND SPACE TRANSPORT ACCIDENTS (E840-E845)

Note: For definition of aircraft and related terms see definitions (u) and (v).

The following fourth-digit subdivisions are for use with categories E840-E845 to identify the injured person. Valid fourth digits are in [brackets] under codes E842-E845.

.0 Occupant of spacecraft

.1 Occupant of military aircraft, any

Crew in military aircraft [air force] [army] [national guard] [navy]
Passenger (civilian) (military) in military aircraft [air force] [army] [national guard] [navy]
Troops in military aircraft [air force] [army] [national guard] [navy]

> EXCLUDES   *occupants of aircraft operated under jurisdiction of police departments (.5)*
> *parachutist (.7)*

.2 Crew of commercial aircraft (powered) in surface to surface transport

.3 Other occupant of commercial aircraft (powered) in surface to surface transport

Flight personnel:
   not part of crew
   on familiarization flight
Passenger on aircraft (powered) NOS

.4 Occupant of commercial aircraft (powered) in surface to air transport

Occupant [crew] [passenger] of aircraft (powered) engaged in activities, such as:
   aerial spraying (crops) (fire retardants)
   air drops of emergency supplies
   air drops of parachutists, except from military craft
   crop dusting
   lowering of construction material [bridge or telephone pole]
   sky writing

.5 Occupant of other powered aircraft

Occupant [crew][passenger] of aircraft [powered] engaged in activities, such as:
   aerobatic flying
   aircraft racing
   rescue operation
   storm surveillance
   traffic surveillance
Occupant of private plane NOS

.6 Occupant of unpowered aircraft, except parachutist

Occupant of aircraft classifiable to E842

.7 Parachutist (military) (other)

Person making voluntary descent

> EXCLUDES   *person making descent after accident to aircraft (.1-.6)*

.8 Ground crew, airline employee

Persons employed at airfields (civil) (military) or launching pads, not occupants of aircraft

.9 Other person

§ ☑4ᵗʰ **E840 Accident to powered aircraft at takeoff or landing**

> INCLUDES   collision of aircraft
>   with any object, fixed, movable, or moving   ⎫
> crash   ⎬ while taking off or landing
> explosion on aircraft
> fire on aircraft
> forced landing   ⎭

§ ☑4ᵗʰ **E841 Accident to powered aircraft, other and unspecified**

> INCLUDES   aircraft accident NOS
> aircraft crash or wreck NOS
> any accident to powered aircraft while in transit or when not specified whether in transit, taking off, or landing
> collision of aircraft with another aircraft, bird, or any object, while in transit
> explosion on aircraft while in transit
> fire on aircraft while in transit

§ ☑4ᵗʰ **E842 Accident to unpowered aircraft**

[6-9]

> INCLUDES   any accident, except collision with powered aircraft, to:
>   balloon
>   glider
>   hang glider
>   kite carrying a person
> hit by object falling from unpowered aircraft

§ ☑4ᵗʰ **E843 Fall in, on, or from aircraft**

[0-9]

> INCLUDES   accident in boarding or alighting from aircraft, any kind
> fall in, on, or from aircraft [any kind], while in transit, taking off, or landing, except when as a result of an accident to aircraft

---

§   Requires fourth-digit. See beginning of section E840-E845 for codes and definitions.
§§ Requires fourth-digit. See beginning of section E830-E838 for codes and definitions.

☑4ᵗʰ Fourth-digit Required   ▶◀ Revised Text   ● New Code   ▲ Revised Code Title

§ ✓4ᵗʰ **E844 Other specified air transport accidents**

[0-9] ⬛INCLUDES hit by:
  aircraft
  object falling from
    aircraft
  injury by or from:
    machinery on
      aircraft ⎫
    rotating propeller ⎬ without
    voluntary parachute ⎪ accident
      descent ⎭ to aircraft
  poisoning by carbon
    monoxide from
    aircraft while in
    transit
  sucked into jet

any accident involving other transport vehicle
  (motor) (nonmotor) due to being hit by
  object set in motion by aircraft (powered)

⬛EXCLUDES air sickness (E903)
  effects of:
    high altitude (E902.0-E902.1)
    pressure change (E902.0-E902.1)
  injury in parachute descent due to accident to
    aircraft (E840.0-E842.9)

§ ✓4ᵗʰ **E845 Accident involving spacecraft**

[0,8,9] ⬛INCLUDES launching pad accident
⬛EXCLUDES effects of weightlessness in spacecraft (E928.0)

VEHICLE ACCIDENTS NOT ELSEWHERE CLASSIFIABLE (E846-E848)

E846 Accidents involving powered vehicles used solely within the buildings and premises of industrial or commercial establishment

Accident to, on, or involving:
  battery powered airport passenger vehicle
  battery powered trucks (baggage) (mail)
  coal car in mine
  logging car
  self propelled truck, industrial
  station baggage truck (powered)
  tram, truck, or tub (powered) in mine or quarry
Collision with:
  pedestrian
  other vehicle or object within premises
Explosion of ⎫
Fall from ⎬ powered vehicle, industrial
Overturning of ⎪ or commercial
Struck by ⎭

⬛EXCLUDES accidental poisoning by exhaust gas from
  vehicle not elsewhere classifiable (E868.2)
  injury by crane, lift (fork), or elevator (E919.2)

E847 Accidents involving cable cars not running on rails

Accident to, on, or involving:
  cable car, not on rails
  ski chair-lift
  ski-lift with gondola
  téléférique
Breakage of cable
Caught or dragged by ⎫
Fall or jump from ⎬ cable car, not on rails
Object thrown from or in ⎭

E848 Accidents involving other vehicles, not elsewhere classifiable

Accident to, on, or involving:
  ice yacht
  land yacht
  nonmotor, nonroad vehicle NOS

✓4ᵗʰ **E849 Place of occurrence**

The following category is for use to denote the place where
the injury or poisoning occurred.

E849.0 Home

Apartment | Private:
Boarding house | garage
Farm house | garden
Home premises | home
House (residential) | walk
Noninstitutional | Swimming pool in private
  place of residence | house or garden
Private: | Yard of home
  driveway |

⬛EXCLUDES home under construction but not yet
  occupied (E849.3)
  institutional place of residence (E849.7)

E849.1 Farm

Farm:
  buildings
  land under cultivation

⬛EXCLUDES farm house and home premises of farm
  (E849.0)

E849.2 Mine and quarry

Gravel pit | Tunnel under
Sand pit | construction

E849.3 Industrial place and premises

Building under | Industrial yard
  construction | Loading platform (factory)
Dockyard | (store)
Dry dock | Plant, industrial
Factory | Railway yard
  building | Shop (place of work)
  premises | Warehouse
Garage (place of work) | Workhouse

E849.4 Place for recreation and sport

Amusement park | Public park
Baseball field | Racecourse
Basketball court | Resort NOS
Beach resort | Riding school
Cricket ground | Rifle range
Fives court | Seashore resort
Football field | Skating rink
Golf course | Sports palace
Gymnasium | Stadium
Hockey field | Swimming pool, public
Holiday camp | Tennis court
Ice palace | Vacation resort
Lake resort |
Mountain resort |
Playground, including school playground

⬛EXCLUDES that in private house or garden
  (E849.0)

E849.5 Street and highway

E849.6 Public building

Building (including adjacent grounds) used by the
  general public or by a particular group of the
  public, such as:

airport | music hall
bank | nightclub
café | office
casino | office building
church | opera house
cinema | post office
clubhouse | public hall
courthouse | radio broadcasting station
dance hall | restaurant
garage building (for | school (state) (public)
  car storage) | (private)
hotel | shop, commercial
market (grocery or | station (bus) (railway)
  other | store
  commodity) | theater
movie house |

⬛EXCLUDES home garage (E849.0)
  industrial building or workplace
  (E849.3)

§ Requires fourth-digit. See beginning of section E840-E845 for codes and definitions.

✓4ᵗʰ Fourth-digit Required ▶◀ Revised Text ● New Code ▲ Revised Code Title

E849.7 Residential institution

Children's home	Old people's home
Dormitory	Orphanage
Hospital	Prison
Jail	Reform school

E849.8 Other specified places

Beach NOS	Pond or pool (natural)
Canal	Prairie
Caravan site NOS	Public place NOS
Derelict house	Railway line
Desert	Reservoir
Dock	River
Forest	Sea
Harbor	Seashore NOS
Hill	Stream
Lake NOS	Swamp
Mountain	Trailer court
Parking lot	Woods
Parking place	

E849.9 Unspecified place

ACCIDENTAL POISONING BY DRUGS, MEDICINAL SUBSTANCES, AND BIOLOGICALS (E850-E858)

INCLUDES accidental overdose of drug, wrong drug given or taken in error, and drug taken inadvertently

accidents in the use of drugs and biologicals in medical and surgical procedures

EXCLUDES administration with suicidal or homicidal intent or intent to harm, or in circumstances classifiable to E980-E989 (E950.0-E950.5, E962.0, E980.0-E980.5)

correct drug properly administered in therapeutic or prophylactic dosage, as the cause of adverse effect (E930.0-E949.9)

See Alphabetic Index for more complete list of specific drugs to be classified under the fourth-digit subdivisions. The American Hospital Formulary numbers can be used to classify new drugs listed by the American Hospital Formulary Service (AHFS). See Appendix C.

✓4ᵗʰ E850 Accidental poisoning by analgesics, antipyretics, and antirheumatics

E850.0 Heroin
Diacetylmorphine

E850.1 Methadone

E850.2 Other opiates and related narcotics

Codeine [methylmorphine]	Morphine
Meperidine [pethidine]	Opium (alkaloids)

E850.3 Salicylates
Acetylsalicylic acid [aspirin]
Amino derivatives of salicylic acid
Salicylic acid salts

E850.4 Aromatic analgesics, not elsewhere classified
Acetanilid
Paracetamol [acetaminophen]
Phenacetin [acetophenetidin]

E850.5 Pyrazole derivatives
Aminophenazone [amidopyrine]
Phenylbutazone

E850.6 Antirheumatics [antiphlogistics]
Gold salts
Indomethacin

EXCLUDES salicylates (E850.3)
steroids (E858.0)

E850.7 Other non-narcotic analgesics
Pyrabital

E850.8 Other specified analgesics and antipyretics
Pentazocine

E850.9 Unspecified analgesic or antipyretic

E851 Accidental poisoning by barbiturates
Amobarbital [amylobarbitone]
Barbital [barbitone]
Butabarbital [butabarbitone]
Pentobarbital [pentobarbitone]
Phenobarbital [phenobarbitone]
Secobarbital [quinalbarbitone]

EXCLUDES thiobarbiturates (E855.1)

✓4ᵗʰ E852 Accidental poisoning by other sedatives and hypnotics

E852.0 Chloral hydrate group

E852.1 Paraldehyde

E852.2 Bromine compounds
Bromides
Carbromal (derivatives)

E852.3 Methaqualone compounds

E852.4 Glutethimide group

E852.5 Mixed sedatives, not elsewhere classified

E852.8 Other specified sedatives and hypnotics

E852.9 Unspecified sedative or hypnotic
Sleeping:
  drug
  pill   } NOS
  tablet

✓4ᵗʰ E853 Accidental poisoning by tranquilizers

E853.0 Phenothiazine-based tranquilizers

Chlorpromazine	Prochlorperazine
Fluphenazine	Promazine

E853.1 Butyrophenone-based tranquilizers

Haloperidol	Trifluperidol
Spiperone	

E853.2 Benzodiazepine-based tranquilizers

Chlordiazepoxide	Lorazepam
Diazepam	Medazepam
Flurazepam	Nitrazepam

E853.8 Other specified tranquilizers

Hydroxyzine	Meprobamate

E853.9 Unspecified tranquilizer

✓4ᵗʰ E854 Accidental poisoning by other psychotropic agents

E854.0 Antidepressants
Amitriptyline
Imipramine
Monoamine oxidase [MAO] inhibitors

E854.1 Psychodysleptics [hallucinogens]

Cannabis derivatives	Mescaline
Lysergide [LSD]	Psilocin
Marihuana (derivatives)	Psilocybin

E854.2 Psychostimulants

Amphetamine	Caffeine

EXCLUDES central appetite depressants (E858.8)

E854.3 Central nervous system stimulants

Analeptics	Opiate antagonists

E854.8 Other psychotropic agents

✓4ᵗʰ E855 Accidental poisoning by other drugs acting on central and autonomic nervous system

E855.0 Anticonvulsant and anti-Parkinsonism drugs
Amantadine
Hydantoin derivatives
Levodopa [L-dopa]
Oxazolidine derivatives [paramethadione] [trimethadione]
Succinimides

E855.1 Other central nervous system depressants
Ether
Gaseous anesthetics
Halogenated hydrocarbon derivatives
Intravenous anesthetics
Thiobarbiturates, such as thiopental sodium

E855.2 Local anesthetics

Cocaine	Procaine
Lidocaine [lignocaine]	Tetracaine

E855.3 Parasympathomimetics [cholinergics]
- Acetylcholine   Pilocarpine
- Anticholinesterase:
  - organophosphorus
  - reversible

E855.4 Parasympatholytics [anticholinergics and antimuscarinics] and spasmolytics
- Atropine
- Homatropine
- Hyoscine [scopolamine]
- Quaternary ammonium derivatives

E855.5 Sympathomimetics [adrenergics]
- Epinephrine [adrenalin]
- Levarterenol [noradrenalin]

E855.6 Sympatholytics [antiadrenergics]
- Phenoxybenzamine
- Tolazoline hydrochloride

E855.8 Other specified drugs acting on central and autonomic nervous systems

E855.9 Unspecified drug acting on central and autonomic nervous systems

E856 Accidental poisoning by antibiotics

E857 Accidental poisoning by other anti-infectives

✓4th E858 Accidental poisoning by other drugs

E858.0 Hormones and synthetic substitutes

E858.1 Primarily systemic agents

E858.2 Agents primarily affecting blood constituents

E858.3 Agents primarily affecting cardiovascular system

E858.4 Agents primarily affecting gastrointestinal system

E858.5 Water, mineral, and uric acid metabolism drugs

E858.6 Agents primarily acting on the smooth and skeletal muscles and respiratory system

E858.7 Agents primarily affecting skin and mucous membrane, ophthalmological, otorhinolaryngological, and dental drugs

E858.8 Other specified drugs
- Central appetite depressants

E858.9 Unspecified drug

ACCIDENTAL POISONING BY OTHER SOLID AND LIQUID SUBSTANCES, GASES, AND VAPORS (E860-E869)

Note: Categories in this section are intended primarily to indicate the external cause of poisoning states classifiable to 980-989. They may also be used to indicate external causes of localized effects classifiable to 001-799.

✓4th E860 Accidental poisoning by alcohol, not elsewhere classified

E860.0 Alcoholic beverages
- Alcohol in preparations intended for consumption

E860.1 Other and unspecified ethyl alcohol and its products
- Denatured alcohol   Grain alcohol NOS
- Ethanol NOS   Methylated spirit

E860.2 Methyl alcohol
- Methanol   Wood alcohol

E860.3 Isopropyl alcohol
- Dimethyl carbinol   Rubbing alcohol subsitute
- Isopropanol   Secondary propyl alcohol

E860.4 Fusel oil
- Alcohol: Alcohol:
  - amyl   propyl
  - butyl

E860.8 Other specified alcohols

E860.9 Unspecified alcohol

✓4th E861 Accidental poisoning by cleansing and polishing agents, disinfectants, paints, and varnishes

E861.0 Synthetic detergents and shampoos

E861.1 Soap products

E861.2 Polishes

E861.3 Other cleansing and polishing agents
- Scouring powders

E861.4 Disinfectants
- Household and other disinfectants not ordinarily used on the person
- **EXCLUDES** *carbolic acid or phenol (E864.0)*

E861.5 Lead paints

E861.6 Other paints and varnishes
- Lacquers   Paints, other than lead
- Oil colors   White washes

E861.9 Unspecified

✓4th E862 Accidental poisoning by petroleum products, other solvents and their vapors, not elsewhere classified

E862.0 Petroleum solvents
- Petroleum: Petroleum:
  - ether   naphtha
  - benzine

E862.1 Petroleum fuels and cleaners
- Antiknock additives to petroleum fuels
- Gas oils
- Gasoline or petrol
- Kerosene
- **EXCLUDES** *kerosene insecticides (E863.4)*

E862.2 Lubricating oils

E862.3 Petroleum solids
- Paraffin wax

E862.4 Other specified solvents
- Benzene

E862.9 Unspecified solvent

✓4th E863 Accidental poisoning by agricultural and horticultural chemical and pharmaceutical preparations other than plant foods and fertilizers
- **EXCLUDES** *plant foods and fertilizers (E866.5)*

E863.0 Insecticides of organochlorine compounds
- Benzene hexachloride   Dieldrin
- Chlordane   Endrine
- DDT   Toxaphene

E863.1 Insecticides of organophosphorus compounds
- Demeton   Parathion
- Diazinon   Phenylsulphthion
- Dichlorvos   Phorate
- Malathion   Phosdrin
- Methyl parathion

E863.2 Carbamates
- Aldicarb   Propoxur
- Carbaryl

E863.3 Mixtures of insecticides

E863.4 Other and unspecified insecticides
- Kerosene insecticides

E863.5 Herbicides
- 2, 4-Dichlorophenoxyacetic acid [2, 4-D]
- 2, 4, 5-Trichlorophenoxyacetic acid [2, 4, 5-T]
- Chlorates
- Diquat
- Mixtures of plant foods and fertilizers with herbicides
- Paraquat

E863.6 Fungicides
- Organic mercurials (used in seed dressing)
- Pentachlorophenols

E863.7 Rodenticides
- Fluoroacetates   Warfarin
- Squill and derivatives   Zinc phosphide
- Thallium

E863.8 Fumigants
- Cyanides   Phosphine
- Methyl bromide

E863.9 Other and unspecified

E Codes E855.3–E863.9

✓4ᵗʰ **E864 Accidental poisoning by corrosives and caustics, not elsewhere classified**

> EXCLUDES   *those as components of disinfectants (E861.4)*

E864.0 Corrosive aromatics
> Carbolic acid or phenol

E864.1 Acids
> Acid:
>> hydrochloric
>> nitric
>> sulfuric

E864.2 Caustic alkalis
> Lye

E864.3 Other specified corrosives and caustics

E864.4 Unspecified corrosives and caustics

✓4ᵗʰ **E865 Accidental poisoning from poisonous foodstuffs and poisonous plants**

> INCLUDES   any meat, fish, or shellfish
> plants, berries, and fungi eaten as, or in mistake for, food, or by a child

> EXCLUDES   *anaphylactic shock due to adverse food reaction (995.60-995.69)*
> *food poisoning (bacterial) (005.0-005.9)*
> *poisoning and toxic reactions to venomous plants (E905.6-E905.7)*

E865.0 Meat

E865.1 Shellfish

E865.2 Other fish

E865.3 Berries and seeds

E865.4 Other specified plants

E865.5 Mushrooms and other fungi

E865.8 Other specified foods

E865.9 Unspecified foodstuff or poisonous plant

✓4ᵗʰ **E866 Accidental poisoning by other and unspecified solid and liquid substances**

> EXCLUDES   *these substances as a component of:*
> *medicines (E850.0-E858.9)*
> *paints (E861.5-E861.6)*
> *pesticides (E863.0-E863.9)*
> *petroleum fuels (E862.1)*

E866.0 Lead and its compounds and fumes

E866.1 Mercury and its compounds and fumes

E866.2 Antimony and its compounds and fumes

E866.3 Arsenic and its compounds and fumes

E866.4 Other metals and their compounds and fumes
> Beryllium (compounds)   Iron (compounds)
> Brass fumes   Manganese (compounds)
> Cadmium (compounds)   Nickel (compounds)
> Copper salts   Thallium (compounds)

E866.5 Plant foods and fertilizers
> EXCLUDES   *mixtures with herbicides (E863.5)*

E866.6 Glues and adhesives

E866.7 Cosmetics

E866.8 Other specified solid or liquid substances

E866.9 Unspecified solid or liquid substance

E867 Accidental poisoning by gas distributed by pipeline
> Carbon monoxide from incomplete combustion of piped gas
> Coal gas NOS
> Liquefied petroleum gas distributed through pipes (pure or mixed with air)
> Piped gas (natural) (manufactured)

✓4ᵗʰ **E868 Accidental poisoning by other utility gas and other carbon monoxide**

E868.0 Liquefied petroleum gas distributed in mobile containers
> Butane
> Liquefied
>> hydrocarbon
>> gas NOS
> Propane
> } or carbon monoxide from incomplete combustion of these gases

E868.1 Other and unspecified utility gas
> Acetylene
> Gas NOS used for lighting, heating, or cooking
> Water gas
> } or carbon monoxide from incomplete combustion of these gases

E868.2 Motor vehicle exhaust gas
> Exhaust gas from:
>> farm tractor, not in transit
>> gas engine
>> motor pump
>> motor vehicle, not in transit
>> any type of combustion engine not in watercraft

> EXCLUDES   *poisoning by carbon monoxide from:*
> *aircraft while in transit (E844.0-E844.9)*
> *motor vehicle while in transit (E818.0-E818.9)*
> *watercraft whether or not in transit (E838.0-E838.9)*

E868.3 Carbon monoxide from incomplete combustion of other domestic fuels
> Carbon monoxide from incomplete combustion of:
>> coal
>> coke
>> kerosene
>> wood
>> } in domestic stove or fireplace

> EXCLUDES   *carbon monoxide from smoke and fumes due to conflagration (E890.0-E893.9)*

E868.8 Carbon monoxide from other sources
> Carbon monoxide from:
>> blast furnace gas
>> incomplete combustion of fuels in industrial use
>> kiln vapor

E868.9 Unspecified carbon monoxide

✓4ᵗʰ **E869 Accidental poisoning by other gases and vapors**
> EXCLUDES   *effects of gases used as anesthetics (E855.1, E938.2)*
> *fumes from heavy metals (E866.0-E866.4)*
> *smoke and fumes due to conflagration or explosion (E890.0-E899)*

E869.0 Nitrogen oxides

E869.1 Sulfur dioxide

E869.2 Freon

E869.3 Lacrimogenic gas [tear gas]
> Bromobenzyl cyanide   Ethyliodoacetate
> Chloroacetophenone

E869.4 Second-hand tobacco smoke

E869.8 Other specified gases and vapors
> Chlorine   Hydrocyanic acid gas

E869.9 Unspecified gases and vapors

MISADVENTURES TO PATIENTS DURING SURGICAL AND MEDICAL CARE (E870-E876)

> EXCLUDES   *accidental overdose of drug and wrong drug given in error (E850.0-E858.9)*
> *surgical and medical procedures as the cause of abnormal reaction by the patient, without mention of misadventure at the time of procedure (E878.0-E879.9)*

✓4ᵗʰ **E870 Accidental cut, puncture, perforation, or hemorrhage during medical care**

E870.0 Surgical operation

E870.1 Infusion or transfusion

E870.2 Kidney dialysis or other perfusion

E870.3 Injection or vaccination

E870.4 Endoscopic examination

✓4ᵗʰ Fourth-digit Required   ▶◀ Revised Text   ● New Code   ▲ Revised Code Title

E870.5 **Aspiration of fluid or tissue, puncture, and
  catheterization**
  Abdominal paracentesis Lumbar puncture
  Aspirating needle biopsy Thoracentesis
  Blood sampling
  EXCLUDES *heart catheterization (E870.6)*

E870.6 **Heart catheterization**

E870.7 **Administration of enema**

E870.8 **Other specified medical care**

E870.9 **Unspecified medical care**

√4th E871 **Foreign object left in body during procedure**

E871.0 **Surgical operation**

E871.1 **Infusion or transfusion**

E871.2 **Kidney dialysis or other perfusion**

E871.3 **Injection or vaccination**

E871.4 **Endoscopic examination**

E871.5 **Aspiration of fluid or tissue, puncture, and
  catheterization**
  Abdominal paracentesis Lumbar puncture
  Aspiration needle biopsy Thoracentesis
  Blood sampling
  EXCLUDES *heart catheterization (E871.6)*

E871.6 **Heart catheterization**

E871.7 **Removal of catheter or packing**

E871.8 **Other specified procedures**

E871.9 **Unspecified procedure**

√4th E872 **Failure of sterile precautions during procedure**

E872.0 **Surgical operation**

E872.1 **Infusion or transfusion**

E872.2 **Kidney dialysis and other perfusion**

E872.3 **Injection or vaccination**

E872.4 **Endoscopic examination**

E872.5 **Aspiration of fluid or tissue, puncture, and
  catheterization**
  Abdominal paracentesis Lumbar puncture
  Aspiration needle biopsy Thoracentesis
  Blood sampling
  EXCLUDES *heart catheterization (E872.6)*

E872.6 **Heart catheterization**

E872.8 **Other specified procedures**

E872.9 **Unspecified procedure**

√4th E873 **Failure in dosage**
  EXCLUDES *accidental overdose of drug, medicinal or
    biological substance (E850.0-E858.9)*

E873.0 **Excessive amount of blood or other fluid during
  transfusion or infusion**

E873.1 **Incorrect dilution of fluid during infusion**

E873.2 **Overdose of radiation in therapy**

E873.3 **Inadvertent exposure of patient to radiation during
  medical care**

E873.4 **Failure in dosage in electroshock or insulin-shock
  therapy**

E873.5 **Inappropriate [too hot or too cold] temperature in
  local application and packing**

E873.6 **Nonadministration of necessary drug or medicinal
  substance**

E873.8 **Other specified failure in dosage**

E873.9 **Unspecified failure in dosage**

√4th E874 **Mechanical failure of instrument or apparatus during
  procedure**

E874.0 **Surgical operation**

E874.1 **Infusion and transfusion**
  Air in system

E874.2 **Kidney dialysis and other perfusion**

E874.3 **Endoscopic examination**

E874.4 **Aspiration of fluid or tissue, puncture, and
  catheterization**
  Abdominal paracentesis Lumbar puncture
  Aspiration needle biopsy Thoracentesis
  Blood sampling
  EXCLUDES *heart catheterization (E874.5)*

E874.5 **Heart catheterization**

E874.8 **Other specified procedures**

E874.9 **Unspecified procedure**

√4th E875 **Contaminated or infected blood, other fluid, drug, or
  biological substance**
  INCLUDES presence of:
    bacterial pyrogens
    endotoxin-producing bacteria
    serum hepatitis-producing agent

E875.0 **Contaminated substance transfused or infused**

E875.1 **Contaminated substance injected or used for
  vaccination**

E875.2 **Contaminated drug or biological substance
  administered by other means**

E875.8 **Other**

E875.9 **Unspecified**

√4th E876 **Other and unspecified misadventures during medical care**

E876.0 **Mismatched blood in transfusion**

E876.1 **Wrong fluid in infusion**

E876.2 **Failure in suture and ligature during surgical
  operation**

E876.3 **Endotracheal tube wrongly placed during anesthetic
  procedure**

E876.4 **Failure to introduce or to remove other tube or
  instrument**
  EXCLUDES *foreign object left in body during
    procedure (E871.0-E871.9)*

E876.5 **Performance of inappropriate operation**

E876.8 **Other specified misadventures during medical care**
  Performance of inappropriate treatment NEC

E876.9 **Unspecified misadventure during medical care**

SURGICAL AND MEDICAL PROCEDURES AS THE CAUSE OF ABNORMAL REACTION OF PATIENT OR LATER COMPLICATION, WITHOUT MENTION OF MISADVENTURE AT THE TIME OF PROCEDURE (E878-E879)

INCLUDES procedures as the cause of abnormal reaction,
    such as:
    displacement or malfunction of prosthetic
      device
    hepatorenal failure, postoperative
    malfunction of external stoma
    postoperative intestinal obstruction
    rejection of transplanted organ

EXCLUDES *anesthetic management properly carried out as
    the cause of adverse effect (E937.0-
    E938.9)*
  *infusion and transfusion, without mention of
    misadventure in the technique of
    procedure (E930.0-E949.9)*

√4th E878 **Surgical operation and other surgical procedures as the
  cause of abnormal reaction of patient, or of later
  complication, without mention of misadventure at the time
  of operation**

E878.0 **Surgical operation with transplant of whole organ**
  Transplantation of: Transplantation of:
    heart   liver
    kidney

E878.1 **Surgical operation with implant of artificial internal
  device**
  Cardiac pacemaker Heart valve prosthesis
  Electrodes implanted in Internal orthopedic
    brain   device

√4th Fourth-digit Required ►◄ Revised Text ● New Code ▲ Revised Code Title

E Codes E878.2–E888.9

E878.2 **Surgical operation with anastomosis, bypass, or graft, with natural or artificial tissues used as implant**

Anastomosis: Graft of blood vessel,
   arteriovenous   tendon, or skin
   gastrojejunal

EXCLUDES   *external stoma (E878.3)*

E878.3 **Surgical operation with formation of external stoma**

Colostomy   Gastrostomy
Cystostomy   Ureterostomy
Duodenostomy

E878.4 **Other restorative surgery**

E878.5 **Amputation of limb(s)**

E878.6 **Removal of other organ (partial) (total)**

E878.8 **Other specified surgical operations and procedures**

E878.9 **Unspecified surgical operations and procedures**

√4ᵗʰ E879 **Other procedures, without mention of misadventure at the time of procedure, as the cause of abnormal reaction of patient, or of later complication**

E879.0 **Cardiac catheterization**

E879.1 **Kidney dialysis**

E879.2 **Radiological procedure and radiotherapy**

EXCLUDES   *radio-opaque dyes for diagnostic x-ray procedures (E947.8)*

E879.3 **Shock therapy**

Electroshock therapy
Insulin-shock therapy

E879.4 **Aspiration of fluid**

Lumbar puncture
Thoracentesis

E879.5 **Insertion of gastric or duodenal sound**

E879.6 **Urinary catheterization**

E879.7 **Blood sampling**

E879.8 **Other specified procedures**

Blood transfusion

E879.9 **Unspecified procedure**

ACCIDENTAL FALLS (E880-E888)

EXCLUDES   *falls (in or from):*
   burning building (E890.8, E891.8)
   into fire (E890.0-E899)
   into water (with submersion or drowning) (E910.0-E910.9)
   machinery (in operation) (E919.0-E919.9)
   on edged, pointed, or sharp object (E920.0-E920.9)
   transport vehicle (E800.0-E845.9)
   vehicle not elsewhere classifiable (E846-E848)

√4ᵗʰ E880 **Fall on or from stairs or steps**

E880.0 **Escalator**

E880.1 **Fall on or from sidewalk curb**

EXCLUDES   *fall from moving sidewalk (E885.9)*

E880.9 **Other stairs or steps**

√4ᵗʰ E881 **Fall on or from ladders or scaffolding**

E881.0 **Fall from ladder**

E881.1 **Fall from scaffolding**

E882 **Fall from or out of building or other structure**

Fall from: Fall from:
   balcony   turret
   bridge   viaduct
   building   wall
   flagpole   window
   tower   Fall through roof

EXCLUDES   *collapse of a building or structure (E916)*
   fall or jump from burning building (E890.8, E891.8)

√4ᵗʰ E883 **Fall into hole or other opening in surface**

INCLUDES   fall into: fall into:
   cavity   shaft
   dock   swimming pool
   hole   tank
   pit   well
   quarry

EXCLUDES   *fall into water NOS (E910.9)*
   that resulting in drowning or submersion without mention of injury (E910.0-E910.9)

E883.0 **Accident from diving or jumping into water [swimming pool]**

Strike or hit:
   against bottom when jumping or diving into water
   wall or board of swimming pool
   water surface

EXCLUDES   *diving with insufficient air supply (E913.2)*
   effects of air pressure from diving (E902.2)

E883.1 **Accidental fall into well**

E883.2 **Accidental fall into storm drain or manhole**

E883.9 **Fall into other hole or other opening in surface**

√4ᵗʰ E884 **Other fall from one level to another**

E884.0 **Fall from playground equipment**

EXCLUDES   *recreational machinery (E919.8)*

E884.1 **Fall from cliff**

E884.2 **Fall from chair**

E884.3 **Fall from wheelchair**

E884.4 **Fall from bed**

E884.5 **Fall from other furniture**

E884.6 **Fall from commode**

Toilet

E884.9 **Other fall from one level to another**

Fall from:
   embankment
   haystack
   stationary vehicle
   tree

√4ᵗʰ E885 **Fall on same level from slipping, tripping, or stumbling**

● E885.0 **Fall from (nonmotorized) scooter**

E885.1 **Fall from roller skates**

In-line skates

E885.2 **Fall from skateboard**

E885.3 **Fall from skis**

E885.4 **Fall from snowboard**

E885.9 **Fall from other slipping, tripping, or stumbling**

Fall on moving sidewalk

√4ᵗʰ E886 **Fall on same level from collision, pushing, or shoving, by or with other person**

EXCLUDES   *crushed or pushed by a crowd or human stampede (E917.1, E917.6)*

E886.0 **In sports**

Tackles in sports

EXCLUDES   *kicked, stepped on, struck by object, in sports (E917.0, E917.5)*

E886.9 **Other and unspecified**

Fall from collision of pedestrian (conveyance) with another pedestrian (conveyance)

E887 **Fracture, cause unspecified**

√4ᵗʰ E888 **Other and unspecified fall**

Accidental fall NOS
Fall on same level NOS

E888.0 **Fall resulting in striking against sharp object**

Use additional external cause code to identify object (E920)

E888.1 **Fall resulting in striking against other object**

E888.8 **Other fall**

E888.9 **Unspecified fall**

Fall NOS

√4ᵗʰ Fourth-digit Required   ▶◀ Revised Text   ● New Code   ▲ Revised Code Title

ACCIDENTS CAUSED BY FIRE AND FLAMES (E890-E899)

> INCLUDES   asphyxia or poisoning due to conflagration or
>   ignition
>   burning by fire
>   secondary fires resulting from explosion
>
> EXCLUDES   *arson (E968.0)*
>   *fire in or on:*
>   *machinery (in operation) (E919.0-E919.9)*
>   *transport vehicle other than stationary*
>   *vehicle (E800.0-E845.9)*
>   *vehicle not elsewhere classifiable (E846-*
>   *E848)*

✓4ᵗʰ E890 Conflagration in private dwelling

> INCLUDES   conflagration in: conflagration in:
>   apartment   lodging house
>   boarding house   mobile home
>   camping place   private garage
>   caravan   rooming house
>   farmhouse   tenement
>   house
>   conflagration originating from sources
>   classifiable to E893-E898 in the above
>   buildings

E890.0 **Explosion caused by conflagration**

E890.1 **Fumes from combustion of polyvinylchloride [PVC]
and similar material in conflagration**

E890.2 **Other smoke and fumes from conflagration**

Carbon monoxide ⎫ from conflagration in
Fumes NOS   ⎬ private building
Smoke NOS   ⎭

E890.3 **Burning caused by conflagration**

E890.8 **Other accident resulting from conflagration**

Collapse of   ⎫
Fall from   ⎬ burning private
Hit by object falling from ⎬ building
Jump from   ⎭

E890.9 **Unspecified accident resulting from conflagration in
private dwelling**

✓4ᵗʰ E891 Conflagration in other and unspecified building or structure

Conflagration in: Conflagration in:
barn   farm outbuildings
church   hospital
convalescent and other   hotel
    residential home   school
dormitory of educational   store
    institution   theater
factory
Conflagration originating from sources classifiable to E893-
    E898, in the above buildings

E891.0 **Explosion caused by conflagration**

E891.1 **Fumes from combustion of polyvinylchloride [PVC]
and similar material in conflagration**

E891.2 **Other smoke and fumes from conflagration**

Carbon monoxide ⎫ from conflagration in
Fumes NOS   ⎬ building or
Smoke NOS   ⎭ structure

E891.3 **Burning caused by conflagration**

E891.8 **Other accident resulting from conflagration**

Collapse of   ⎫
Fall from   ⎬ burning building or
Hit by object falling from ⎬ structure
Jump from   ⎭

E891.9 **Unspecified accident resulting from conflagration of
other and unspecified building or structure**

E892 Conflagration not in building or structure

Fire (uncontrolled) (in) (of):   Fire (uncontrolled) (in) (of):
forest   prairie
grass   transport vehicle [any],
hay   except while in
lumber   transit
mine   tunnel

✓4ᵗʰ E893 Accident caused by ignition of clothing

> EXCLUDES   *ignition of clothing:*
>   *from highly inflammable material (E894)*
>   *with conflagration (E890.0-E892)*

E893.0 **From controlled fire in private dwelling**

Ignition of clothing from:
normal fire (charcoal) ⎫
    (coal) (electric)   ⎬
    (gas) (wood) in: ⎬ in private dwelling
brazier   ⎬ (as listed in
fireplace   ⎬ E890)
furnace   ⎬
stove   ⎭

E893.1 **From controlled fire in other building or structure**

Ignition of clothing from:
normal fire (charcoal) ⎫
    (coal) (electric)   ⎬
    (gas) (wood) in: ⎬ in other building or
brazier   ⎬ structure (as
fireplace   ⎬ listed in E81)
furnace   ⎬
stove   ⎭

E893.2 **From controlled fire not in building or structure**

Ignition of clothing from:
bonfire (controlled)
brazier fire (controlled), not in building or
    structure
trash fire (controlled)

> EXCLUDES   *conflagration not in building (E892)*
>   *trash fire out of control (E892)*

E893.8 **From other specified sources**

Ignition of clothing from:
blowlamp
blowtorch
burning bedspread
candle
cigar
cigarette
lighter
matches
pipe
welding torch

E893.9 **Unspecified source**

Ignition of clothing (from controlled fire NOS) (in
    building NOS) NOS

E894 Ignition of highly inflammable material

Ignition of:
benzine   ⎫
gasoline ⎬
fat   ⎬
kerosene ⎬ (with ignition of clothing)
paraffin ⎬
petrol   ⎭

> EXCLUDES   *ignition of highly inflammable material with:*
>   *conflagration (E890.0-E892)*
>   *explosion (E923.0-E923.9)*

◤4ᵗʰ Fourth-digit Required   ▶◀ Revised Text   ● New Code   ▲ Revised Code Title

E895 Accident caused by controlled fire in private dwelling

Burning by (flame of)
normal fire (charcoal)
(coal) (electric) (gas)
(wood) in:
brazier
fireplace
furnace
stove
} in private dwelling (as listed in E890)

EXCLUDES burning by hot objects not producing fire or flames (E924.0-E924.9)
ignition of clothing from these sources (E893.0)
poisoning by carbon monoxide from incomplete combustion of fuel (E867-E868.9)
that with conflagration (E890.0-E890.9)

E896 Accident caused by controlled fire in other and unspecified building or structure

Burning by (flame of) normal fire (charcoal) (coal) (electric) (gas) (wood) in:
brazier
fireplace
furnace
stove
} in other building or structure (as listed in E891)

EXCLUDES burning by hot objects not producing fire or flames (E924.0-E924.9)
ignition of clothing from these sources (E893.1)
poisoning by carbon monoxide from incomplete combustion of fuel (E867-E868.9)
that with conflagration (E891.0-E891.9)

E897 Accident caused by controlled fire not in building or structure

Burns from flame of:
bonfire
brazier fire, not in building or structure
trash fire
} controlled

EXCLUDES ignition of clothing from these sources (E893.2)
trash fire out of control (E892)
that with conflagration (E892)

✓4ᵗʰ E898 Accident caused by other specified fire and flames

EXCLUDES conflagration (E890.0-E892)
that with ignition of:
clothing (E893.0-E893.9)
highly inflammable material (E894)

E898.0 Burning bedclothes
Bed set on fire NOS

E898.1 Other
Burning by:
blowlamp
blowtorch
candle
cigar
cigarette
fire in room NOS

Burning by:
lamp
lighter
matches
pipe
welding torch

E899 Accident caused by unspecified fire
Burning NOS

ACCIDENTS DUE TO NATURAL AND ENVIRONMENTAL FACTORS (E900-E909)

✓4ᵗʰ E900 Excessive heat

E900.0 Due to weather conditions
Excessive heat as the external cause of:
ictus solaris
siriasis
sunstroke

E900.1 Of man-made origin
Heat (in):
boiler room
drying room
factory
furnace room

Heat (in):
generated in transport vehicle
kitchen

E900.9 Of unspecified origin

✓4ᵗʰ E901 Excessive cold

E901.0 Due to weather conditions
Excessive cold as the cause of:
chilblains NOS
immersion foot

E901.1 Of man-made origin
Contact with or inhalation of:
dry ice
liquid air
liquid hydrogen
liquid nitrogen
Prolonged exposure in:
deep freeze unit
refrigerator

E901.8 Other specified origin

E901.9 Of unspecified origin

✓4ᵗʰ E902 High and low air pressure and changes in air pressure

E902.0 Residence or prolonged visit at high altitude
Residence or prolonged visit at high altitude as the cause of:
Acosta syndrome
Alpine sickness
altitude sickness
Andes disease
anoxia, hypoxia
barotitis, barodontalgia, barosinusitis, otitic barotrauma
hypobarism, hypobaropathy
mountain sickness
range disease

E902.1 In aircraft
Sudden change in air pressure in aircraft during ascent or descent as the cause of:
aeroneurosis
aviators' disease

E902.2 Due to diving
High air pressure from rapid descent in water
Reduction in atmospheric pressure while surfacing from deep water diving
} as the cause of:
caisson disease
divers' disease
divers' palsy or paralysis

E902.8 Due to other specified causes
Reduction in atmospheric pressure while surfacing from underground

E902.9 Unspecified cause

E903 Travel and motion

✓4ᵗʰ E904 Hunger, thirst, exposure, and neglect

EXCLUDES any condition resulting from homicidal intent (E968.0-E968.9)
hunger, thirst, and exposure resulting from accidents connected with transport (E800.0-E848)

E904.0 Abandonment or neglect of infants and helpless persons
Exposure to weather conditions
Hunger or thirst
} resulting from abandonment or neglect

Desertion of newborn
Inattention at or after birth
Lack of care (helpless person) (infant)
EXCLUDES criminal [purposeful] neglect (E968.4)

E904.1 Lack of food
Lack of food as the cause of:
inanition
insufficient nourishment
starvation
EXCLUDES hunger resulting from abandonment or neglect (E904.0)

✓4ᵗʰ Fourth-digit Required   ►◄ Revised Text   ● New Code   ▲ Revised Code Title

E904.2 **Lack of water**
  Lack of water as the cause of:
    dehydration
    inanition
    EXCLUDES   *dehydration due to acute fluid loss (276.5)*

E904.3 **Exposure (to weather conditions), not elsewhere classifiable**
  Exposure NOS
  Humidity
  Struck by hailstones
    EXCLUDES   *struck by lightning (E907)*

E904.9 **Privation, unqualified**
  Destitution

✓4ᵗʰ E905 **Venomous animals and plants as the cause of poisoning and toxic reactions**
    INCLUDES   chemical released by animal
               insects
               release of venom through fangs, hairs, spines, tentacles, and other venom apparatus
    EXCLUDES   *eating of poisonous animals or plants (E865.0-E865.9)*

E905.0 **Venomous snakes and lizards**
  Cobra   Mamba
  Copperhead snake   Rattlesnake
  Coral snake   Sea snake
  Fer de lance   Snake (venomous)
  Gila monster   Viper
  Krait   Water moccasin
    EXCLUDES   *bites of snakes and lizards known to be nonvenomous (E906.2)*

E905.1 **Venomous spiders**
  Black widow spider   Tarantula (venomous)
  Brown spider

E905.2 **Scorpion**

E905.3 **Hornets, wasps, and bees**
  Yellow jacket

E905.4 **Centipede and venomous millipede (tropical)**

E905.5 **Other venomous arthropods**
  Sting of:
    ant
    caterpillar

E905.6 **Venomous marine animals and plants**
  Puncture by sea urchin spine
  Sting of:
    coral
    jelly fish
    nematocysts
    sea anemone
    sea cucumber
    other marine animal or plant
    EXCLUDES   *bites and other injuries caused by nonvenomous marine animal (E906.2-E906.8)*
               bite of sea snake (venomous) (E905.0)

E905.7 **Poisoning and toxic reactions caused by other plants**
  Injection of poisons or toxins into or through skin by plant thorns, spines, or other mechanisms
    EXCLUDES   *puncture wound NOS by plant thorns or spines (E920.8)*

E905.8 **Other specified**

E905.9 **Unspecified**
  Sting NOS
  Venomous bite NOS

✓4ᵗʰ E906 **Other injury caused by animals**
    EXCLUDES   *poisoning and toxic reactions caused by venomous animals and insects (E905.0-E905.9)*
               road vehicle accident involving animals (E827.0-E828.9)
               tripping or falling over an animal (E885.9)

E906.0 **Dog bite**

E906.1 **Rat bite**

E906.2 **Bite of nonvenomous snakes and lizards**

E906.3 **Bite of other animal except arthropod**
  Cats   Rodents, except rats
  Moray eel   Shark

E906.4 **Bite of nonvenomous arthropod**
  Insect bite NOS

E906.5 **Bite by unspecified animal**
  Animal bite NOS

E906.8 **Other specified injury caused by animal**
  Butted by animal
  Fallen on by horse or other animal, not being ridden
  Gored by animal
  Implantation of quills of porcupine
  Pecked by bird
  Run over by animal, not being ridden
  Stepped on by animal, not being ridden
    EXCLUDES   *injury by animal being ridden (E828.0-E828.9)*

E906.9 **Unspecified injury caused by animal**

E907 **Lightning**
    EXCLUDES   *injury from:*
               fall of tree or other object caused by lightning (E916)
               fire caused by lightning (E890.0-E892)

✓4ᵗʰ E908 **Cataclysmic storms, and floods resulting from storms**
    EXCLUDES   *collapse of dam or man-made structure causing flood (E909.3)*

E908.0 **Hurricane**
  Storm surge
  "Tidal wave" caused by storm action
  Typhoon

E908.1 **Tornado**
  Cyclone
  Twisters

E908.2 **Floods**
  Torrential rainfall
  Flash flood
    EXCLUDES   *collapse of dam or man-made structure causing flood (E909.3)*

E908.3 **Blizzard (snow) (ice)**

E908.4 **Dust storm**

E908.8 **Other cataclysmic storms**

E908.9 **Unspecified cataclysmic storms, and floods resulting from storms**
  Storm NOS

✓4ᵗʰ E909 **Cataclysmic earth surface movements and eruptions**

E909.0 **Earthquakes**

E909.1 **Volcanic eruptions**
  Burns from lava
  Ash inhalation

E909.2 **Avalanche, landslide, or mudslide**

E909.3 **Collapse of dam or man-made structure**

E909.4 **Tidalwave caused by earthquake**
  Tidalwave NOS
  Tsunami
    EXCLUDES   *tidalwave caused by tropical storm (E908.0)*

E909.8 **Other cataclysmic earth surface movements and eruptions**

E909.9 **Unspecified cataclysmic earth surface movements and eruptions**

✓4ᵗʰ Fourth-digit Required   ▶◀ Revised Text   ● New Code   ▲ Revised Code Title

ACCIDENTS CAUSED BY SUBMERSION, SUFFOCATION, AND FOREIGN BODIES (E910-E915)

☑4ᵗʰ **E910 Accidental drowning and submersion**

    INCLUDES   immersion
                    swimmers' cramp

    EXCLUDES   *diving accident (NOS) (resulting in injury except*
                    drowning) (E883.0)
                  diving with insufficient air supply (E913.2)
                  drowning and submersion due to:
                    cataclysm (E908-E909)
                    machinery accident (E919.0-E919.9)
                    transport accident (E800.0-E845.9)
                  effect of high and low air pressure (E902.2)
                  injury from striking against objects while in
                    running water (E917.2)

E910.0 While water-skiing
      Fall from water skis with submersion or drowning

       EXCLUDES   *accident to water-skier involving a*
                    watercraft and resulting in
                    submersion or other injury
                    (E830.4, E831.4)

E910.1 While engaged in other sport or recreational activity with diving equipment
      Scuba diving NOS   Underwater spear
      Skin diving NOS   fishing NOS

E910.2 While engaged in other sport or recreational activity without diving equipment
      Fishing or hunting, except from boat or with diving
          equipment
      Ice skating
      Playing in water
      Surfboarding
      Swimming NOS
      Voluntarily jumping from boat, not involved in
          accident, for swim NOS
      Wading in water

       EXCLUDES   *jumping into water to rescue another*
                    person (E910.3)

E910.3 While swimming or diving for purposes other than recreation or sport
      Marine salvage
      Pearl diving
      Placement of fishing nets
      Rescue (attempt) of   (with diving
          another person   equipment)
      Underwater construction
          or repairs

E910.4 In bathtub

E910.8 Other accidental drowning or submersion
      Drowning in: Drowning in:
         quenching tank   swimming pool

E910.9 Unspecified accidental drowning or submersion
      Accidental fall into water NOS
      Drowning NOS

E911 Inhalation and ingestion of food causing obstruction of respiratory tract or suffocation
      Aspiration and inhalation of food [any] (into respiratory tract)
         NOS

      Asphyxia by
      Choked on   }   food [including bone, seed in
      Suffocation by   food, regurgitated food]

      Compression of trachea
      Interruption of respiration   }   by food lodged in
      Obstruction of respiration   esophagus

      Obstruction of pharynx by food (bolus)

       EXCLUDES   *injury, except asphyxia and obstruction of*
                    respiratory passage, caused by food
                    (E915)
                  obstruction of esophagus by food without
                    mention of asphyxia or obstruction of
                    respiratory passage (E915)

E912 Inhalation and ingestion of other object causing obstruction of respiratory tract or suffocation
      Aspiration and inhalation of foreign body except food (into
         respiratory tract) NOS
      Foreign object [bean] [marble] in nose
      Obstruction of pharynx by foreign body

      Compression
      Interruption of respiration   }   by foreign body in
      Obstruction of respiration   esophagus

       EXCLUDES   *injury, except asphyxia and obstruction of*
                    respiratory passage, caused by foreign
                    body (E915)
                  obstruction of esophagus by foreign body
                    without mention of asphyxia or
                    obstruction in respiratory passage (E915)

☑4ᵗʰ **E913 Accidental mechanical suffocation**

       EXCLUDES   *mechanical suffocation from or by:*
                    accidental inhalation or ingestion of:
                    food (E911)
                    foreign object (E912)
                    cataclysm (E908-E909)
                    explosion (E921.0-E921.9, E923.0-E923.9)
                    machinery accident (E919.0-E919.9)

E913.0 In bed or cradle
       EXCLUDES   *suffocation by plastic bag (E913.1)*

E913.1 By plastic bag

E913.2 Due to lack of air (in closed place)
      Accidentally closed up in refrigerator or other
         airtight enclosed space
      Diving with insufficient air supply
       EXCLUDES   *suffocation by plastic bag (E913.1)*

E913.3 By falling earth or other substance
      Cave-in NOS
       EXCLUDES   *cave-in caused by cataclysmic earth*
                    surface movements and eruptions
                    (E909)
                  struck by cave-in without asphyxiation
                    or suffocation (E916)

E913.8 Other specified means
      Accidental hanging, except in bed or cradle

E913.9 Unspecified means
      Asphyxia, mechanical NOS   Suffocation NOS
      Strangulation NOS

E914 Foreign body accidentally entering eye and adnexa
       EXCLUDES   *corrosive liquid (E924.1)*

E915 Foreign body accidentally entering other orifice
       EXCLUDES   *aspiration and inhalation of foreign body, any,*
                    (into respiratory tract) NOS (E911-E912)

OTHER ACCIDENTS (E916-E928)

E916 Struck accidentally by falling object
      Collapse of building, except on fire
      Falling:
         rock
         snowslide NOS
         stone
         tree
      Object falling from:
         machine, not in operation
         stationary vehicle
      Code first:
         collapse of building on fire (E890.0-E891.9)
         falling object in:
            cataclysm (E908-E909)
            machinery accidents (E919.0-E919.9)
            transport accidents (E800.0-E845.9)
            vehicle accidents not elsewhere classifiable (E846-
              E848)
         object set in motion by:
            explosion (E921.0-E921.9, E923.0-E923.9)
            firearm (E922.0-E922.9)
            projected object (E917.0-E917.9)

☑4ᵗʰ **E917 Striking against or struck accidentally by objects or persons**

| INCLUDES | bumping into or against
colliding with
kicking against
stepping on
struck by | } object (moving)
(projected)
(stationary)
pedestrian conveyance
person |

| EXCLUDES | *fall from:*
collision with another person, except when
caused by a crowd (E886.0-E886.9)
stumbling over object (E885.9)
fall resulting in striking against object (E888.0,
E888.1)
injury caused by:
assault (E960.0-E960.1, E967.0-E967.9)
cutting or piercing instrument (E920.0-
E920.9)
explosion (E921.0-E921.9, E923.0-E923.9)
firearm (E922.0-E922.9)
machinery (E919.0-E919.9)
transport vehicle (E800.0-E845.9)
vehicle not elsewhere classifiable (E846-
E848) |

E917.0 In sports without subsequent fall
Kicked or stepped on during game (football) (rugby)
Struck by hit or thrown ball
Struck by hockey stick or puck

E917.1 Caused by a crowd, by collective fear or panic without subsequent fall
Crushed
Pushed   } by crowd or human stampede
Stepped on

E917.2 In running water without subsequent fall
| EXCLUDES | *drowning or submersion (E910.0-*
E910.9)
that in sports (E917.0, E917.5) |

E917.3 Furniture without subsequent fall
| EXCLUDES | *fall from furniture (E884.2, E884.4-*
E884.5) |

E917.4 Other stationary object without subsequent fall
Bath tub
Fence
Lamp-post

E917.5 Object in sports with subsequent fall
Knocked down while boxing

E917.6 Caused by a crowd, by collective fear or panic with subsequent fall

E917.7 Furniture with subsequent fall
| EXCLUDES | *fall from furniture (E884.2, E884.4-*
E884.5) |

E917.8 Other stationary object with subsequent fall
Bath tub
Fence
Lamp-post

E917.9 Other striking against with or without subsequent fall

E918 Caught accidentally in or between objects
Caught, crushed, jammed, or pinched in or between moving or stationary objects, such as:
escalator
folding object
hand tools, appliances, or implements
sliding door and door frame
under packing crate
washing machine wringer
| EXCLUDES | *injury caused by:*
cutting or piercing instrument (E920.0-
E920.9)
machinery (E919.0-E919.9)
transport vehicle (E800.0-E845.9)
vehicle not elsewhere classifiable (E846-
E848)
struck accidentally by:
falling object (E916)
object (moving) (projected) (E917.0-E917.9) |

☑4ᵗʰ **E919 Accidents caused by machinery**

| INCLUDES | burned by
caught in (moving
    parts of)
collapse of
crushed by
cut or pierced by
drowning or
    submersion
    caused by
explosion of, on, in
fall from or into
    moving part of
fire starting in or on
mechanical
    suffocation
    caused by
object falling from, on,
    in motion by
overturning of
pinned under
run over by
struck by
thrown from | } machinery
(accident) |

caught between machinery and other object
machinery accident NOS
| EXCLUDES | *accidents involving machinery, not in operation*
(E884.9, E916-E918)
injury caused by:
electric current in connection with machinery
(E925.0-E925.9)
escalator (E880.0, E918)
explosion of pressure vessel in connection
with machinery (E921.0-E921.9)
moving sidewalk (E885.9)
powered hand tools, appliances, and
implements (E916-E918, E920.0-
E921.9, E923.0-E926.9)
transport vehicle accidents involving
machinery (E800.0-E848.9)
poisoning by carbon monoxide generated by
machine (E868.8) |

☑4ᵗʰ Fourth-digit Required   ▶◀ Revised Text   ● New Code   ▲ Revised Code Title

E919.0 Agricultural machines
  Animal-powered agricultural machine
  Combine
  Derrick, hay
  Farm machinery NOS
  Farm tractor
  Harvester
  Hay mower or rake
  Reaper
  Thresher
  EXCLUDES *that in transport under own power on the highway (E810.0-E819.9)*
              that being towed by another vehicle on the highway (E810.0-E819.9, E827.0-E827.9, E829.0-E829.9)
              that involved in accident classifiable to E820-E829 (E820.0-E829.9)

E919.1 Mining and earth-drilling machinery
  Bore or drill (land) (seabed)   Shaft lift
  Shaft hoist   Under-cutter
  EXCLUDES *coal car, tram, truck, and tub in mine (E846)*

E919.2 Lifting machines and appliances
  Chain hoist
  Crane
  Derrick
  Elevator (building) (grain)   except in agricultural or mining operations
  Forklift truck
  Lift
  Pulley block
  Winch
  EXCLUDES *that being towed by another vehicle on the highway (E810.0-E819.9, E827.0-E827.9, E829.0-829.9)*
              that in transport under own power on the highway (E810.0-E819.9)
              that involved in accident classifiable to E820-E829 (E820.0-E829.9)

E919.3 Metalworking machines
  Abrasive wheel   Metal:
  Forging machine   drilling machine
  Lathe   milling machine
  Mechanical shears   power press
                        rolling-mill
                        sawing machine

E919.4 Woodworking and forming machines
  Band saw   Overhead plane
  Bench saw   Powered saw
  Circular saw   Radial saw
  Molding machine Sander
  EXCLUDES *hand saw (E920.1)*

E919.5 Prime movers, except electrical motors
  Gas turbine
  Internal combustion engine
  Steam engine
  Water driven turbine
  EXCLUDES *that being towed by other vehicle on the highway (E810.0-E819.9, E827.0-E827.9, E829.0-E829.9)*
              that in transport under own power on the highway (E810.0-E819.9)

E919.6 Transmission machinery
  Transmission: Transmission:
    belt   pinion
    cable   pulley
    chain   shaft
    gear

E919.7 Earth moving, scraping, and other excavating machines
  Bulldozer   Steam shovel
  Road scraper
  EXCLUDES *that being towed by other vehicle on the highway (E810.0-E819.9, E827.0-E827.9, E829.0-E829.9)*
              that in transport under own power on the highway (E810.0-E819.9)

E919.8 Other specified machinery
  Machines for manufacture of:
    clothing
    foodstuffs and beverages
    paper
  Printing machine
  Recreational machinery
  Spinning, weaving, and textile machines

E919.9 Unspecified machinery

√4th **E920 Accidents caused by cutting and piercing instruments or objects**
  INCLUDES accidental injury (by) } object:
                                      edged
                                      pointed
                                      sharp

E920.0 Powered lawn mower
E920.1 Other powered hand tools
  Any powered hand tool [compressed air] [electric] [explosive cartridge] [hydraulic power], such as:
    drill
    hand saw
    hedge clipper
    rivet gun
    snow blower
    staple gun
  EXCLUDES *band saw (E919.4)*
              bench saw (E919.4)

E920.2 Powered household appliances and implements
  Blender
  Electric:
    beater or mixer
    can opener
    fan
    knife
    sewing machine
  Garbage disposal appliance

E920.3 Knives, swords, and daggers
E920.4 Other hand tools and implements
  Axe   Paper cutter
  Can opener NOS   Pitchfork
  Chisel   Rake
  Fork   Scissors
  Hand saw   Screwdriver
  Hoe   Sewing machine, not powered
  Ice pick   Shovel
  Needle (sewing)

E920.5 Hypodermic needle
  Contaminated needle
  Needle stick

E920.8 Other specified cutting and piercing instruments or objects
  Arrow   Nail
  Broken glass   Plant thorn
  Dart   Splinter
  Edge of stiff paper Tin can lid
  Lathe turnings
  EXCLUDES *animal spines or quills (E906.8)*
              flying glass due to explosion (E921.0-E923.9)

E920.9 Unspecified cutting and piercing instrument or object

▨4ᵗʰ Fourth-digit Required   ▶◀ Revised Text   ● New Code   ▲ Revised Code Title

✓4ᵗʰ **E921 Accident caused by explosion of pressure vessel**

> INCLUDES accidental explosion of pressure vessels, whether or not part of machinery
>
> EXCLUDES *explosion of pressure vessel on transport vehicle (E800.0-E845.9)*

E921.0 Boilers

E921.1 Gas cylinders
> Air tank
> Pressure gas tank

E921.8 Other specified pressure vessels
> Aerosol can   Pressure cooker
> Automobile tire

E921.9 Unspecified pressure vessel

✓4ᵗʰ **E922 Accident caused by firearm, and air gun missile**

E922.0 Handgun
> Pistol   Revolver
>
> EXCLUDES *Verey pistol (E922.8)*

E922.1 Shotgun (automatic)

E922.2 Hunting rifle

E922.3 Military firearms
> Army rifle   Machine gun

E922.4 Air gun
> BB gun
> Pellet gun

● **E922.5 Paintball gun**

E922.8 Other specified firearm missile
> Verey pistol [flare]

E922.9 Unspecified firearm missile
> Gunshot wound NOS
> Shot NOS

✓4ᵗʰ **E923 Accident caused by explosive material**

> INCLUDES flash burns and other injuries resulting from explosion of explosive material
> ignition of highly explosive material with explosion
>
> EXCLUDES *explosion:*
> *in or on machinery (E919.0-E919.9)*
> *on any transport vehicle, except stationary motor vehicle (E800.0-E848)*
> *with conflagration (E890.0, E891.0,E892)*
> *secondary fires resulting from explosion (E890.0-E899)*

E923.0 Fireworks

E923.1 Blasting materials
> Blasting cap
> Detonator
> Dynamite
> Explosive [any] used in blasting operations

E923.2 Explosive gases
> Acetylene   Fire damp
> Butane   Gasoline fumes
> Coal gas   Methane
> Explosion in mine NOS Propane

E923.8 Other explosive materials
> Bomb   Torpedo
> Explosive missile Explosion in munitions:
> Grenade   dump
> Mine   factory
> Shell

E923.9 Unspecified explosive material
> Explosion NOS

✓4ᵗʰ **E924 Accident caused by hot substance or object, caustic or corrosive material, and steam**

> EXCLUDES *burning NOS (E899)*
> *chemical burn resulting from swallowing a corrosive substance (E860.0-E864.4)*
> *fire caused by these substances and objects (E890.0-E894)*
> *radiation burns (E926.0-E926.9)*
> *therapeutic misadventures (E870.0-E876.9)*

E924.0 Hot liquids and vapors, including steam
> Burning or scalding by:
> boiling water
> hot or boiling liquids not primarily caustic or corrosive
> liquid metal
> steam
> other hot vapor
>
> EXCLUDES *hot (boiling) tap water (E924.2)*

E924.1 Caustic and corrosive substances
> Burning by: Burning by:
> acid [any kind]   corrosive substance
> ammonia   lye
> caustic oven cleaner vitriol
>   or other substance

E924.2 Hot (boiling) tap water

E924.8 Other
> Burning by:
> heat from electric heating appliance
> hot object NOS
> light bulb
> steam pipe

E924.9 Unspecified

✓4ᵗʰ **E925 Accident caused by electric current**

> INCLUDES electric current from exposed wire, faulty appliance, high voltage cable, live rail, or open electric socket as the cause of:
> burn
> cardiac fibrillation
> convulsion
> electric shock
> electrocution
> puncture wound
> respiratory paralysis
>
> EXCLUDES *burn by heat from electrical appliance (E924.8)*
> *lightning (E907)*

E925.0 Domestic wiring and appliances

E925.1 Electric power generating plants, distribution stations, transmission lines
> Broken power line

E925.2 Industrial wiring, appliances, and electrical machinery
> Conductors
> Control apparatus
> Electrical equipment and machinery
> Transformers

E925.8 Other electric current
> Wiring and appliances in or on:
> farm [not farmhouse]
> outdoors
> public building
> residential institutions
> schools

E925.9 Unspecified electric current
> Burns or other injury from electric current NOS
> Electric shock NOS
> Electrocution NOS

✓4ᵗʰ **E926 Exposure to radiation**

> EXCLUDES *abnormal reaction to or complication of treatment without mention of misadventure (E879.2)*
> *atomic power plant malfunction in water transport (E838.0-E838.9)*
> *misadventure to patient in surgical and medical procedures (E873.2-E873.3)*
> *use of radiation in war operations (E996-E997.9)*

E Codes E921–E926

E926.0 Radiofrequency radiation

Overexposure to: from:
    microwave   high-powered radio and
      radiation   television
    radar radiation   transmitters
    radiofrequency   industrial
    radiofrequency   radiofrequency
      radiation   induction heaters
    [any]   radar installations

E926.1 Infrared heaters and lamps

Exposure to infrared radiation from heaters and
  lamps as the cause of:
    blistering
    burning
    charring
    inflammatory change

    EXCLUDES *physical contact with heater or lamp*
              (E924.8)

E926.2 Visible and ultraviolet light sources

Arc lamps   Oxygas welding torch
Black light sources   Sun rays
Electrical welding arc   Tanning bed

    EXCLUDES *excessive heat from these sources*
              (E900.1-E900.9)

E926.3 X-rays and other electromagnetic ionizing radiation

Gamma rays
X-rays (hard) (soft)

E926.4 Lasers

E926.5 Radioactive isotopes

Radiobiologicals
Radiopharmaceuticals

E926.8 Other specified radiation

Artificially accelerated beams of ionized particles
  generated by:
    betatrons
    synchrotrons

E926.9 Unspecified radiation

Radiation NOS

E927 Overexertion and strenuous movements

Excessive physical exercise   Strenuous movements in:
Overexertion (from):   recreational activities
  lifting   other activities
  pulling
  pushing

✓4ᵗʰ E928 Other and unspecified environmental and accidental causes

E928.0 Prolonged stay in weightless environment

Weightlessness in spacecraft (simulator)

E928.1 Exposure to noise

Noise (pollution)   Supersonic waves
Sound waves

E928.2 Vibration

E928.3 Human bite

E928.8 Other

E928.9 Unspecified accident

Accident NOS
Blow NOS
Casualty (not due   } stated as accidentally
  to war)   inflicted
Decapitation

Knocked down
Killed
Injury [any part of   } stated as accidentally
  body, or   inflicted, but not
  unspecified]   otherwise specified
Mangled
Wound

    EXCLUDES *fracture, cause unspecified (E887)*
              injuries undetermined whether
              accidentally or purposely inflicted
              (E980.0-E989)

LATE EFFECTS OF ACCIDENTAL INJURY (E929)

Note: This category is to be used to indicate accidental injury
as the cause of death or disability from late effects,
which are themselves classifiable elsewhere. The "late
effects" include conditions reported as such, or as
sequelae which may occur at any time after the
attempted suicide or self-inflicted injury.

✓4ᵗʰ E929 Late effects of accidental injury

    EXCLUDES *late effects of:*
            surgical and medical procedures (E870.0-
              E879.9)
            therapeutic use of drugs and medicines
              (E930.0-E949.9)

E929.0 Late effects of motor vehicle accident

Late effects of accidents classifiable to E810-E825

E929.1 Late effects of other transport accident

Late effects of accidents classifiable to E800-E807,
  E826-E838, E840-E848

E929.2 Late effects of accidental poisoning

Late effects of accidents classifiable to E850-E858,
  E860-E869

E929.3 Late effects of accidental fall

Late effects of accidents classifiable to E880-E888

E929.4 Late effects of accident caused by fire

Late effects of accidents classifiable to E890-E899

**E929.5 Late effects of accident due to natural and
environmental factors**

Late effects of accidents classifiable to E900-E909

E929.8 Late effects of other accidents

Late effects of accidents classifiable to E910-E928.8

E929.9 Late effects of unspecified accident

Late effects of accidents classifiable to E928.9

DRUGS, MEDICINAL AND BIOLOGICAL SUBSTANCES CAUSING ADVERSE EFFECTS IN THERAPEUTIC USE (E930-E949)

    INCLUDES correct drug properly administered in
            therapeutic or prophylactic dosage, as
            the cause of any adverse effect including
            allergic or hypersensitivity reactions

    EXCLUDES *accidental overdose of drug and wrong drug*
            given or taken in error (E850.0-E858.9)
            accidents in the technique of administration of
            drug or biological substance, such as
            accidental puncture during injection, or
            contamination of drug (E870.0-E876.9)
            administration with suicidal or homicidal intent
            or intent to harm, or in circumstances
            classifiable to E980-E989 (E950.0-E950.5,
            E962.0, E980.0-E980.5)

See Alphabetic Index for more complete list of specific
drugs to be classified under the fourth-digit subdivisions.
The American Hospital Formulary numbers can be used to
classify new drugs listed by the American Hospital
Formulary Service (AHFS). See Appendix C.

✓4ᵗʰ E930 Antibiotics

    EXCLUDES *that used as eye, ear, nose, and throat [ENT],*
            and local anti-infectives (E946.0-E946.9)

E930.0 Penicillins

Natural   Semisynthetic, such as:
Synthetic   nafcillin
Semisynthetic, such as: oxacillin
  ampicillin
  cloxacillin

E930.1 Antifungal antibiotics

Amphotericin B   Hachimycin [trichomycin]
Griseofulvin   Nystatin

E930.2 Chloramphenicol group

Chloramphenicol   Thiamphenicol

E930.3 Erythromycin and other macrolides

Oleandomycin   Spiramycin

    ✓4ᵗʰ Fourth-digit Required   ▶◀ Revised Text   ● New Code   ▲ Revised Code Title

E930.4 Tetracycline group
Doxycycline   Oxytetracycline
Minocycline

E930.5 Cephalosporin group
Cephalexin   Cephaloridine
Cephaloglycin   Cephalothin

E930.6 Antimycobacterial antibiotics
Cycloserine   Rifampin
Kanamycin   Streptomycin

E930.7 Antineoplastic antibiotics
Actinomycins, such as: Actinomycins, such as:
Bleomycin   Daunorubicin
Cactinomycin   Mitomycin
Dactinomycin
EXCLUDES *other antineoplastic drugs (E933.1)*

E930.8 Other specified antibiotics

E930.9 Unspecified antibiotic

✓4th **E931 Other anti-infectives**
EXCLUDES *ENT, and local anti-infectives (E946.0-E946.9)*

E931.0 Sulfonamides
Sulfadiazine   Sulfamethoxazole
Sulfafurazole

E931.1 Arsenical anti-infectives

E931.2 Heavy metal anti-infectives
Compounds of: Compounds of:
antimony   lead
bismuth   mercury
EXCLUDES *mercurial diuretics (E944.0)*

E931.3 Quinoline and hydroxyquinoline derivatives
Chiniofon   Diiodohydroxyquin
EXCLUDES *antimalarial drugs (E931.4)*

E931.4 Antimalarials and drugs acting on other blood protozoa
Chloroquine phosphate   Proguanil [chloroguanide]
Cycloguanil   Pyrimethamine
Primaquine   Quinine (sulphate)

E931.5 Other antiprotozoal drugs
Emetine

E931.6 Anthelmintics
Hexylresorcinol   Piperazine
Male fern oleoresin   Thiabendazole

E931.7 Antiviral drugs
Methisazone
EXCLUDES *amantadine (E936.4)*
cytarabine (E933.1)
idoxuridine (E946.5)

E931.8 Other antimycobacterial drugs
Ethambutol   Para-aminosalicylic
Ethionamide   acid derivatives
Isoniazid   Sulfones

E931.9 Other and unspecified anti-infectives
Flucytosine   Nitrofuranderivatives

✓4th **E932 Hormones and synthetic substitutes**

E932.0 Adrenal cortical steroids
Cortisone derivatives
Desoxycorticosterone derivatives
Fluorinated corticosteroid

E932.1 Androgens and anabolic congeners
Nandrolone phenpropionate
Oxymetholone
Testosterone and preparations

E932.2 Ovarian hormones and synthetic substitutes
Contraceptives, oral
Estrogens
Estrogens and progestogens combined
Progestogens

E932.3 Insulins and antidiabetic agents
Acetohexamide   Phenformin
Biguanide derivatives, oral Sulfonylurea
Chlorpropamide   derivatives,
Glucagon   oral
Insulin   Tolbutamide
EXCLUDES *adverse effect of insulin administered for shock therapy (E879.3)*

E932.4 Anterior pituitary hormones
Corticotropin
Gonadotropin
Somatotropin [growth hormone]

E932.5 Posterior pituitary hormones
Vasopressin
EXCLUDES *oxytocic agents (E945.0)*

E932.6 Parathyroid and parathyroid derivatives

E932.7 Thyroid and thyroid derivatives
Dextrothyroxine   Liothyronine
Levothyroxine sodium Thyroglobulin

E932.8 Antithyroid agents
Iodides   Thiourea
Thiouracil

E932.9 Other and unspecified hormones and synthetic substitutes

✓4th **E933 Primarily systemic agents**

E933.0 Antiallergic and antiemetic drugs
Antihistamines   Diphenylpyraline
Chlorpheniramine   Thonzylamine
Diphenhydramine   Tripelennamine
EXCLUDES *phenothiazine-based tranquilizers (E939.1)*

E933.1 Antineoplastic and immunosuppressive drugs
Azathioprine
Busulfan
Chlorambucil
Cyclophosphamide
Cytarabine
Fluorouracil
Mechlorethamine hydrochloride
Mercaptopurine
Triethylenethiophosphoramide [thio-TEPA]
EXCLUDES *antineoplastic antibiotics (E930.7)*

E933.2 Acidifying agents

E933.3 Alkalizing agents

E933.4 Enzymes, not elsewhere classified
Penicillinase

E933.5 Vitamins, not elsewhere classified
Vitamin A   Vitamin D
EXCLUDES *nicotinic acid (E942.2)*
vitamin K (E934.3)

E933.8 Other systemic agents, not elsewhere classified
Heavy metal antagonists

E933.9 Unspecified systemic agent

✓4th **E934 Agents primarily affecting blood constituents**

E934.0 Iron and its compounds
Ferric salts
Ferrous sulphate and other ferrous salts

E934.1 Liver preparations and other antianemic agents
Folic acid

E934.2 Anticoagulants
Coumarin
Heparin
Phenindione
Prothrombin synthesis inhibitor
Warfarin sodium

E934.3 Vitamin K [phytonadione]

E934.4 Fibrinolysis-affecting drugs
Aminocaproic acid   Streptokinase
Streptodornase   Urokinase

E Codes E930.4–E934.4

✓4th Fourth-digit Required   ▶◀ Revised Text   ● New Code   ▲ Revised Code Title

E Codes E934.5–E941.0

E934.5 Anticoagulant antagonists and other coagulants
Hexadimethrine bromide
Protamine sulfate

E934.6 Gamma globulin

E934.7 Natural blood and blood products
Blood plasma   Packed red cells
Human fibrinogen   Whole blood

E934.8 Other agents affecting blood constituents
Macromolecular blood substitutes

E934.9 Unspecified agent affecting blood constituents

✓4ᵗʰ **E935 Analgesics, antipyretics, and antirheumatics**

E935.0 Heroin
Diacetylmorphine

E935.1 Methadone

E935.2 Other opiates and related narcotics
Codeine [methylmorphine]   Morphine
Meperidine [pethidine]   Opium (alkaloids)

E935.3 Salicylates
Acetylsalicylic acid [aspirin]
Amino derivatives of salicylic acid
Salicylic acid salts

E935.4 Aromatic analgesics, not elsewhere classified
Acetanilid
Paracetamol [acetaminophen]
Phenacetin [acetophenetidin]

E935.5 Pyrazole derivatives
Aminophenazone [aminopyrine]
Phenylbutazone

E935.6 Antirheumatics [antiphlogistics]
Gold salts   Indomethacin
EXCLUDES   salicylates (E935.3)
             steroids (E932.0)

E935.7 Other non-narcotic analgesics
Pyrabital

E935.8 Other specified analgesics and antipyretics
Pentazocine

E935.9 Unspecified analgesic and antipyretic

✓4ᵗʰ **E936 Anticonvulsants and anti-Parkinsonism drugs**

E936.0 Oxazolidine derivatives
Paramethadione
Trimethadione

E936.1 Hydantoin derivatives
Phenytoin

E936.2 Succinimides
Ethosuximide
Phensuximide

E936.3 Other and unspecified anticonvulsants
Beclamide
Primidone

E936.4 Anti-Parkinsonism drugs
Amantadine
Ethopropazine [profenamine]
Levodopa [L-dopa]

✓4ᵗʰ **E937 Sedatives and hypnotics**

E937.0 Barbiturates
Amobarbital [amylobarbitone]
Barbital [barbitone]
Butabarbital [butabarbitone]
Pentobarbital [pentobarbitone]
Phenobarbital [phenobarbitone]
Secobarbital [quinalbarbitone]
EXCLUDES   thiobarbiturates (E938.3)

E937.1 Chloral hydrate group

E937.2 Paraldehyde

E937.3 Bromine compounds
Bromide
Carbromal (derivatives)

E937.4 Methaqualone compounds

E937.5 Glutethimide group

E937.6 Mixed sedatives, not elsewhere classified

E937.8 Other sedatives and hypnotics

E937.9 Unspecified
Sleeping:
   drug
   pill   } NOS
   tablet

✓4ᵗʰ **E938 Other central nervous system depressants and anesthetics**

E938.0 Central nervous system muscle-tone depressants
Chlorphenesin (carbamate)
Mephenesin
Methocarbamol

E938.1 Halothane

E938.2 Other gaseous anesthetics
Ether
Halogenated hydrocarbon derivatives, except
   halothane
Nitrous oxide

E938.3 Intravenous anesthetics
Ketamine
Methohexital [methohexitone]
Thiobarbiturates, such as thiopental sodium

E938.4 Other and unspecified general anesthetics

E938.5 Surface and infiltration anesthetics
Cocaine   Procaine
Lidocaine [lignocaine]   Tetracaine

E938.6 Peripheral nerve- and plexus-blocking anesthetics

E938.7 Spinal anesthetics

E938.9 Other and unspecified local anesthetics

✓4ᵗʰ **E939 Psychotropic agents**

E939.0 Antidepressants
Amitriptyline
Imipramine
Monoamine oxidase [MAO] inhibitors

E939.1 Phenothiazine-based tranquilizers
Chlorpromazine   Prochlorperazine
Fluphenazine   Promazine
Phenothiazine

E939.2 Butyrophenone-based tranquilizers
Haloperidol   Trifluperidol
Spiperone

E939.3 Other antipsychotics, neuroleptics, and major tranquilizers

E939.4 Benzodiazepine-based tranquilizers
Chlordiazepoxide   Lorazepam
Diazepam   Medazepam
Flurazepam   Nitrazepam

E939.5 Other tranquilizers
Hydroxyzine   Meprobamate

E939.6 Psychodysleptics [hallucinogens]
Cannabis (derivatives)   Mescaline
Lysergide [LSD]   Psilocin
Marihuana (derivatives)   Psilocybin

E939.7 Psychostimulants
Amphetamine   Caffeine
EXCLUDES   central appetite depressants (E947.0)

E939.8 Other psychotropic agents

E939.9 Unspecified psychotropic agent

✓4ᵗʰ **E940 Central nervous system stimulants**

E940.0 Analeptics
Lobeline   Nikethamide

E940.1 Opiate antagonists
Levallorphan   Naloxone
Nalorphine

E940.8 Other specified central nervous system stimulants

E940.9 Unspecified central nervous system stimulant

✓4ᵗʰ **E941 Drugs primarily affecting the autonomic nervous system**

E941.0 Parasympathomimetics [cholinergics]
Acetylcholine
Anticholinesterase:
   organophosphorus
   reversible
Pilocarpine

✓4ᵗʰ Fourth-digit Required   ►◄ Revised Text   ● New Code   ▲ Revised Code Title

E941.1 Parasympatholytics [anticholinergics and antimuscarinics] and spasmolytics

Atropine	Hyoscine [scopolamine]
Homatropine	Quaternary ammonium derivatives

> **EXCLUDES** *papaverine (E942.5)*

E941.2 Sympathomimetics [adrenergics]

Epinephrine [adrenalin] Levarterenol [noradrenalin]

E941.3 Sympatholytics [antiadrenergics]

Phenoxybenzamine
Tolazolinehydrochloride

E941.9 Unspecified drug primarily affecting the autonomic nervous system

✓4ᵗʰ **E942 Agents primarily affecting the cardiovascular system**

E942.0 Cardiac rhythm regulators

Practolol	Propranolol
Procainamide	Quinidine

E942.1 Cardiotonic glycosides and drugs of similar action

Digitalis glycosides	Strophanthins
Digoxin	

E942.2 Antilipemic and antiarteriosclerotic drugs

Cholestyramine	Nicotinic acid derivatives
Clofibrate	Sitosterols

> **EXCLUDES** *dextrothyroxine (E932.7)*

E942.3 Ganglion-blocking agents

Pentamethonium bromide

E942.4 Coronary vasodilators

Dipyridamole	Nitrites
Nitrates [nitroglycerin]	Prenylamine

E942.5 Other vasodilators

Cyclandelate	Hydralazine
Diazoxide	Papaverine

E942.6 Other antihypertensive agents

Clonidine	Rauwolfia alkaloids
Guanethidine	Reserpine

E942.7 Antivaricose drugs, including sclerosing agents

Monoethanolamine Zinc salts

E942.8 Capillary-active drugs

Adrenochrome derivatives
Bioflavonoids
Metaraminol

E942.9 Other and unspecified agents primarily affecting the cardiovascular system

✓4ᵗʰ **E943 Agents primarily affecting gastrointestinal system**

E943.0 Antacids and antigastric secretion drugs

Aluminum hydroxide
Magnesium trisilicate

E943.1 Irritant cathartics

Bisacodyl	Phenolphthalein
Castor oil	

E943.2 Emollient cathartics

Sodium dioctyl sulfosuccinate

E943.3 Other cathartics, including intestinal atonia drugs

Magnesium sulfate

E943.4 Digestants

Pancreatin	Pepsin
Papain	

E943.5 Antidiarrheal drugs

Bismuth subcarbonate Pectin
Kaolin

> **EXCLUDES** *anti-infectives (E930.0-E931.9)*

E943.6 Emetics

E943.8 Other specified agents primarily affecting the gastrointestinal system

E943.9 Unspecified agent primarily affecting the gastrointestinal system

✓4ᵗʰ **E944 Water, mineral, and uric acid metabolism drugs**

E944.0 Mercurial diuretics

Chlormerodrin	Mercurophylline
Mercaptomerin	Mersalyl

E944.1 Purine derivative diuretics

Theobromine Theophylline

> **EXCLUDES** *aminophylline [theophylline ethylenediamine] (E945.7)*

E944.2 Carbonic acid anhydrase inhibitors

Acetazolamide

E944.3 Saluretics

Benzothiadiazides Chlorothiazide group

E944.4 Other diuretics

Ethacrynic acid Furosemide

E944.5 Electrolytic, caloric, and water-balance agents

E944.6 Other mineral salts, not elsewhere classified

E944.7 Uric acid metabolism drugs

Cinchophen and congeners	Phenoquin
Colchicine	Probenecid

✓4ᵗʰ **E945 Agents primarily acting on the smooth and skeletal muscles and respiratory system**

E945.0 Oxytocic agents

Ergot alkaloids
Prostaglandins

E945.1 Smooth muscle relaxants

Adiphenine
Metaproterenol [orciprenaline]

> **EXCLUDES** *papaverine (E942.5)*

E945.2 Skeletal muscle relaxants

Alcuronium chloride
Suxamethonium chloride

E945.3 Other and unspecified drugs acting on muscles

E945.4 Antitussives

Dextromethorphan
Pipazethate hydrochloride

E945.5 Expectorants

Acetylcysteine	Ipecacuanha
Cocillana	Terpin hydrate
Guaifenesin [glyceryl guaiacolate]	

E945.6 Anti-common cold drugs

E945.7 Antiasthmatics

Aminophylline [theophylline ethylenediamine]

E945.8 Other and unspecified respiratory drugs

✓4ᵗʰ **E946 Agents primarily affecting skin and mucous membrane, ophthalmological, otorhinolaryngological, and dental drugs**

E946.0 Local anti-infectives and anti-inflammatory drugs

E946.1 Antipruritics

E946.2 Local astringents and local detergents

E946.3 Emollients, demulcents, and protectants

E946.4 Keratolytics, kerstoplastics, other hair treatment drugs and preparations

E946.5 Eye anti-infectives and other eye drugs

Idoxuridine

E946.6 Anti-infectives and other drugs and preparations for ear, nose, and throat

E946.7 Dental drugs topically applied

E946.8 Other agents primarily affecting skin and mucous membrane

Spermicides

E946.9 Unspecified agent primarily affecting skin and mucous membrane

✓4ᵗʰ **E947 Other and unspecified drugs and medicinal substances**

E947.0 Dietetics

E947.1 Lipotropic drugs

E947.2 Antidotes and chelating agents, not elsewhere classified

E947.3 Alcohol deterrents

E947.4 Pharmaceutical excipients

E947.8 Other drugs and medicinal substances

Contrast media used for diagnostic x-ray procedures
Diagnostic agents and kits

E947.9 Unspecified drug or medicinal substance

✓4ᵗʰ Fourth-digit Required ▶◀ Revised Text ● New Code ▲ Revised Code Title

√4ᵗʰ **E948 Bacterial vaccines**

     E948.0   BCG vaccine

     E948.1   Typhoid and paratyphoid

     E948.2   Cholera

     E948.3   Plague

     E948.4   Tetanus

     E948.5   Diphtheria

     E948.6   Pertussis vaccine, including combinations with a pertussis component

     E948.8   Other and unspecified bacterial vaccines

     E948.9   Mixed bacterial vaccines, except combinations with a pertussis component

√4ᵗʰ **E949 Other vaccines and biological substances**

        EXCLUDES   *gamma globulin (E934.6)*

     E949.0   Smallpox vaccine

     E949.1   Rabies vaccine

     E949.2   Typhus vaccine

     E949.3   Yellow fever vaccine

     E949.4   Measles vaccine

     E949.5   Poliomyelitis vaccine

     E949.6   Other and unspecified viral and rickettsial vaccines
            Mumps vaccine

     E949.7   Mixed viral-rickettsial and bacterial vaccines, except combinations with a pertussis component
         EXCLUDES   *combinations with a pertussis component (E948.6)*

     E949.9   Other and unspecified vaccines and biological substances

SUICIDE AND SELF-INFLICTED INJURY (E950-E959)

     INCLUDES   injuries in suicide and attempted suicide
                     self-inflicted injuries specified as intentional

√4ᵗʰ **E950 Suicide and self-inflicted poisoning by solid or liquid substances**

     E950.0   Analgesics, antipyretics, and antirheumatics

     E950.1   Barbiturates

     E950.2   Other sedatives and hypnotics

     E950.3   Tranquilizers and other psychotropic agents

     E950.4   Other specified drugs and medicinal substances

     E950.5   Unspecified drug or medicinal substance

     E950.6   Agricultural and horticultural chemical and pharmaceutical preparations other than plant foods and fertilizers

     E950.7   Corrosive and caustic substances
            Suicide and self-inflicted poisoning by substances classifiable to E864

     E950.8   Arsenic and its compounds

     E950.9   Other and unspecified solid and liquid substances

√4ᵗʰ **E951 Suicide and self-inflicted poisoning by gases in domestic use**

     E951.0   Gas distributed by pipeline

     E951.1   Liquefied petroleum gas distributed in mobile containers

     E951.8   Other utility gas

√4ᵗʰ **E952 Suicide and self-inflicted poisoning by other gases and vapors**

     E952.0   Motor vehicle exhaust gas

     E952.1   Other carbon monoxide

     E952.8   Other specified gases and vapors

     E952.9   Unspecified gases and vapors

√4ᵗʰ **E953 Suicide and self-inflicted injury by hanging, strangulation, and suffocation**

     E953.0   Hanging

     E953.1   Suffocation by plastic bag

     E953.8   Other specified means

     E953.9   Unspecified means

E954 Suicide and self-inflicted injury by submersion [drowning]

√4ᵗʰ **E955 Suicide and self-inflicted injury by firearms, air guns and explosives**

     E955.0   Handgun

     E955.1   Shotgun

     E955.2   Hunting rifle

     E955.3   Military firearms

     E955.4   Other and unspecified firearm
            Gunshot NOS   Shot NOS

     E955.5   Explosives

     E955.6   Air gun
            BB gun
            Pellet gun

●   E955.7   Paintball gun

     E955.9   Unspecified

E956 Suicide and self-inflicted injury by cutting and piercing instrument

√4ᵗʰ **E957 Suicide and self-inflicted injuries by jumping from high place**

     E957.0   Residential premises

     E957.1   Other man-made structures

     E957.2   Natural sites

     E957.9   Unspecified

√4ᵗʰ **E958 Suicide and self-inflicted injury by other and unspecified means**

     E958.0   Jumping or lying before moving object

     E958.1   Burns, fire

     E958.2   Scald

     E958.3   Extremes of cold

     E958.4   Electrocution

     E958.5   Crashing of motor vehicle

     E958.6   Crashing of aircraft

     E958.7   Caustic substances, except poisoning
         EXCLUDES   *poisoning by caustic substance (E950.7)*

     E958.8   Other specified means

     E958.9   Unspecified means

E959 Late effects of self-inflicted injury

     Note: This category is to be used to indicate circumstances classifiable to E950-E958 as the cause of death or disability from late effects, which are themselves classifiable elsewhere. The "late effects" include conditions reported as such, or as sequelae which may occur at any time after the attempted suicide or self-inflicted injury.

HOMICIDE AND INJURY PURPOSELY INFLICTED BY OTHER PERSONS (E960-E969)

     INCLUDES   injuries inflicted by another person with intent to injure or kill, by any means

     EXCLUDES   *injuries due to:*
            legal intervention (E970-E978)
            operations of war (E990-E999)
            ►*terrorism (E979)*◄

√4ᵗʰ **E960 Fight, brawl, rape**

     E960.0   Unarmed fight or brawl
            Beatings NOS
            Brawl or fight with hands, fists, feet
            Injured or killed in fight NOS
         EXCLUDES   *homicidal:*
            injury by weapons (E965.0-E966, E969)
            strangulation (E963)
            submersion (E964)

     E960.1   Rape

√4ᵗʰ Fourth-digit Required   ►◄ Revised Text   ● New Code   ▲ Revised Code Title

E961 Assault by corrosive or caustic substance, except poisoning
  Injury or death purposely caused by corrosive or caustic substance, such as:
  acid [any]
  corrosive substance
  vitriol
  EXCLUDES *burns from hot liquid (E968.3)*
  chemical burns from swallowing a corrosive substance (E962.0-E962.9)

✓4ᵗʰ **E962 Assault by poisoning**
  E962.0 Drugs and medicinal substances
    Homicidal poisoning by any drug or medicinal substance
  E962.1 Other solid and liquid substances
  E962.2 Other gases and vapors
  E962.9 Unspecified poisoning

E963 Assault by hanging and strangulation
  Homicidal (attempt):   Homicidal (attempt):
  garrotting or ligature   strangulation
  hanging   suffocation

E964 Assault by submersion [drowning]

✓4ᵗʰ **E965 Assault by firearms and explosives**
  E965.0 Handgun
    Pistol   Revolver
  E965.1 Shotgun
  E965.2 Hunting rifle
  E965.3 Military firearms
  E965.4 Other and unspecified firearm
  E965.5 Antipersonnel bomb
  E965.6 Gasoline bomb
  E965.7 Letter bomb
  E965.8 Other specified explosive
    Bomb NOS (placed in):   Dynamite
      car
      house
  E965.9 Unspecified explosive

E966 Assault by cutting and piercing instrument
  Assassination (attempt), homicide (attempt) by any instrument classifiable under E920
  Homicidal:
  cut
  puncture } any part of body
  stab
  Stabbed

✓4ᵗʰ **E967 Perpetrator of child and adult abuse**
  Note: Selection of the correct perpetrator code is based on the relationship between the perpetrator and the victim
  E967.0 By father, stepfather, or boyfriend
    Male partner of child's parent or guardian
  E967.1 By other specified person
  E967.2 By mother, stepmother, or girlfriend
    Female partner of child's parent or guardian
  E967.3 By spouse or partner
    Abuse of spouse or partner by ex-spouse or ex-partner
  E967.4 By child
  E967.5 By sibling
  E967.6 By grandparent
  E967.7 By other relative
  E967.8 By non-related caregiver
  E967.9 By unspecified person

✓4ᵗʰ **E968 Assault by other and unspecified means**
  E968.0 Fire
    Arson
    Homicidal burns NOS
    EXCLUDES *burns from hot liquid (E968.3)*
  E968.1 Pushing from a high place
  E968.2 Striking by blunt or thrown object

E968.3 Hot liquid
  Homicidal burns by scalding
E968.4 Criminal neglect
  Abandonment of child, infant, or other helpless person with intent to injure or kill
E968.5 Transport vehicle
  Being struck by other vehicle or run down with intent to injure
  Pushed in front of, thrown from, or dragged by moving vehicle with intent to injure
E968.6 Air gun
  BB gun
  Pellet gun
E968.7 Human bite
E968.8 Other specified means
E968.9 Unspecified means
  Assassination (attempt) NOS
  Homicidal (attempt):
    injury NOS
    wound NOS
  Manslaughter (nonaccidental)
  Murder (attempt) NOS
  Violence, non-accidental

E969 Late effects of injury purposely inflicted by other person
  Note: This category is to be used to indicate circumstances classifiable to E960-E968 as the cause of death or disability from late effects, which are themselves classifiable elsewhere. The "late effects" include conditions reported as such, or as sequelae which may occur at any time after injury purposely inflicted by another person.

LEGAL INTERVENTION (E970-E978)
  INCLUDES injuries inflicted by the police or other law-enforcing agents, including military on duty, in the course of arresting or attempting to arrest lawbreakers, suppressing disturbances, maintaining order, and other legal action
  legal execution
  EXCLUDES *injuries caused by civil insurrections (E990.0-E999)*

E970 Injury due to legal intervention by firearms
  Gunshot wound   Injury by:
  Injury by: rifle pellet or
    machine gun   rubber bullet
    revolver   shot NOS
E971 Injury due to legal intervention by explosives
  Injury by: Injury by:
    dynamite   grenade
    explosive shell   mortar bomb
E972 Injury due to legal intervention by gas
  Asphyxiation by gas   Poisoning by gas
  Injury by tear gas
E973 Injury due to legal intervention by blunt object
  Hit, struck by: Hit, struck by:
    baton (nightstick)   stave
    blunt object
E974 Injury due to legal intervention by cutting and piercing instrument
  Cut   Injured by bayonet
  Incised wound   Stab wound
E975 Injury due to legal intervention by other specified means
  Blow   Manhandling
E976 Injury due to legal intervention by unspecified means
E977 Late effects of injuries due to legal intervention
  Note: This category is to be used to indicate circumstances classifiable to E970-E976 as the cause of death or disability from late effects, which are themselves classifiable elsewhere. The "late effects" include conditions reported as such, or as sequelae, which may occur at any time after the injury due to legal intervention.

✓4ᵗʰ Fourth-digit Required   ▶◀ Revised Text   ● New Code   ▲ Revised Code Title

E978 Legal execution

All executions performed at the behest of the judiciary or ruling authority [whether permanent or temporary] as:
asphyxiation by gas
beheading, decapitation (by guillotine)
capital punishment
electrocution
hanging
poisoning
shooting
other specified means

TERRORISM (E979)

● ✓4ᵗʰ **E979 Terrorism**

Injuries resulting from the unlawful use of force or violence against persons or property to intimidate or coerce a Government, the civilian population, or any segment thereof, in furtherance of political or social objective

● **E979.0 Terrorism involving explosion of marine weapons**
Depth-charge
Marine mine
Mine NOS, at sea or in harbour
Sea-based artillery shell
Torpedo
Underwater blast

● **E979.1 Terrorism involving destruction of aircraft**
Aircraft used as a weapon
Aircraft:
burned
exploded
shot down
Crushed by falling aircraft

● **E979.2 Terrorism involving other explosions and fragments**
Antipersonnel bomb (fragments)
Blast NOS
Explosion (of):
artillery shell
breech-block
cannon block
mortar bomb
munitions being used in terrorism
NOS
Fragments from:
artillery shell
bomb
grenade
guided missile
land-mine
rocket
shell
shrapnel
Mine NOS

● **E979.3 Terrorism involving fires, conflagraton and hot substances**
Burning building or structure:
collapse of
fall from
hit by falling object in
jump from
Conflagraton NOS
Fire (causing):
Asphyxia
Burns
NOS
Other injury
Melting of fittings and furniture in burning
Petrol bomb
Smouldering building or structure

● **E979.4 Terrorism involving firearms**
Bullet:
carbine
machine gun
pistol
rifle
rubber (rifle)
Pellets (shotgun)

● **E979.5 Terrorism involving nuclear weapons**
Blast effects
Exposure to ionizing radiation from nuclear weapon
Fireball effects
Heat from nuclear weapon
Other direct and secondary effects of nuclear weapons

● **E979.6 Terrorism involving biological weapons**
Anthrax
Cholera
Smallpox

● **E979.7 Terrorism involving chemical weapons**
Gases, fumes, chemicals
Hydrogen cyanide
Phosgene
Sarin

● **E979.8 Terrorism involving other means**
Drowning and submersion
Lasers
Piercing or stabbing instruments
Terrorism NOS

● **E979.9 Terrorism, secondary effects**
Note: This code is for use to identify conditions occurring subsequent to a terrorist attack not those that are due to the initial terrorist act
EXCLUDES *late effect of terrorist attack (E999.1)*

INJURY UNDETERMINED WHETHER ACCIDENTALLY OR PURPOSELY INFLICTED (E980-E989)

Note: Categories E980-E989 are for use when it is unspecified or it cannot be determined whether the injuries are accidental (unintentional), suicide (attempted), or assault.

✓4ᵗʰ **E980 Poisoning by solid or liquid substances, undetermined whether accidentally or purposely inflicted**
E980.0 Analgesics, antipyretics, and antirheumatics
E980.1 Barbiturates
E980.2 Other sedatives and hypnotics
E980.3 Tranquilizers and other psychotropic agents
E980.4 Other specified drugs and medicinal substances
E980.5 Unspecified drug or medicinal substance
E980.6 Corrosive and caustic substances
Poisoning, undetermined whether accidental or purposeful, by substances classifiable to E864
E980.7 Agricultural and horticultural chemical and pharmaceutical preparations other than plant foods and fertilizers
E980.8 Arsenic and its compounds
E980.9 Other and unspecified solid and liquid substances

✓4ᵗʰ **E981 Poisoning by gases in domestic use, undetermined whether accidentally or purposely inflicted**
E981.0 Gas distributed by pipeline
E981.1 Liquefied petroleum gas distributed in mobile containers
E981.8 Other utility gas

✓4ᵗʰ **E982 Poisoning by other gases, undetermined whether accidentally or purposely inflicted**
E982.0 Motor vehicle exhaust gas
E982.1 Other carbon monoxide
E982.8 Other specified gases and vapors
E982.9 Unspecified gases and vapors

✓4ᵗʰ **E983 Hanging, strangulation, or suffocation, undetermined whether accidentally or purposely inflicted**
E983.0 Hanging
E983.1 Suffocation by plastic bag
E983.8 Other specified means
E983.9 Unspecified means

✓4ᵗʰ Fourth-digit Required   ▶◀ Revised Text   ● New Code   ▲ Revised Code Title

E984 Submersion [drowning], undetermined whether accidentally or purposely inflicted

✓4ᵗʰ E985 Injury by firearms, air guns and explosives, undetermined whether accidentally or purposely inflicted

   E985.0 Handgun

   E985.1 Shotgun

   E985.2 Hunting rifle

   E985.3 Military firearms

   E985.4 Other and unspecified firearm

   E985.5 Explosives

   E985.6 Air gun
      BB gun
      Pellet gun

●   E985.7 Paintball gun

E986 Injury by cutting and piercing instruments, undetermined whether accidentallyor purposely inflicted

✓4ᵗʰ E987 Falling from high place, undetermined whether accidentally or purposely inflicted

   E987.0 Residential premises

   E987.1 Other man-made structures

   E987.2 Natural sites

   E987.9 Unspecified site

✓4ᵗʰ E988 Injury by other and unspecified means, undetermined whether accidentally or purposely inflicted

   E988.0 Jumping or lying before moving object

   E988.1 Burns, fire

   E988.2 Scald

   E988.3 Extremes of cold

   E988.4 Electrocution

   E988.5 Crashing of motor vehicle

   E988.6 Crashing of aircraft

   E988.7 Caustic substances, except poisoning

   E988.8 Other specified means

   E988.9 Unspecified means

E989 Late effects of injury, undetermined whether accidentally or purposely inflicted

   Note: This category is to be used to indicate circumstances classifiable to E980-E988 as the cause of death or disability from late effects, which are themselves classifiable elsewhere. The "late effects" include conditions reported as such, or as sequelae, which may occur at any time after injury, undetermined whether accidentally or purposely inflicted.

INJURY RESULTING FROM OPERATIONS OF WAR (E990-E999)

   INCLUDES   injuries to military personnel and civilians caused by war and civil insurrections and occurring during the time of war and insurrection

   EXCLUDES   *accidents during training of military personnel manufacture of war material and transport, unless attributable to enemy action*

✓4ᵗʰ E990 Injury due to war operations by fires and conflagrations

   INCLUDES   asphyxia, burns, or other injury originating from fire caused by a fire-producing device or indirectly by any conventional weapon

   E990.0 From gasoline bomb

   E990.9 From other and unspecified source

✓4ᵗʰ E991 Injury due to war operations by bullets and fragments

   E991.0 Rubber bullets (rifle)

   E991.1 Pellets (rifle)

   E991.2 Other bullets
      Bullet [any, except rubber bullets and pellets]
       carbine
       machine gun
       pistol
       rifle
       shotgun

   E991.3 Antipersonnel bomb (fragments)

   E991.9 Other and unspecified fragments
     Fragments from: Fragments from:
      artillery shell   land mine
      bombs, except   rockets
       anti-personnel shell
      grenade   Shrapnel
      guided missile

E992 Injury due to war operations by explosion of marine weapons
   Depth charge   Sea-based artillery shell
   Marine mines   Torpedo
   Mine NOS, at sea or in harbor Underwater blast

E993 Injury due to war operations by other explosion
   Accidental explosion of   Explosion of:
    munitions being used   artillery shell
    in war   breech block
   Accidental explosion of own cannon block
    weapons   mortar bomb
   Air blast NOS   Injury by weapon burst
   Blast NOS
   Explosion NOS

E994 Injury due to war operations by destruction of aircraft
   Airplane: Airplane:
    burned   shot down
    exploded   Crushed by falling
               airplane

E995 Injury due to war operations by other and unspecified forms of conventional warfare
   Battle wounds
   Bayonet injury
   Drowned in war operations

E996 Injury due to war operations by nuclear weapons
   Blast effects
   Exposure to ionizing radiation from nuclear weapons
   Fireball effects
   Heat
   Other direct and secondary effects of nuclear weapons

✓4ᵗʰ E997 Injury due to war operations by other forms of unconventional warfare

   E997.0 Lasers

   E997.1 Biological warfare

   E997.2 Gases, fumes, and chemicals

   E997.8 Other specified forms of unconventional warfare

   E997.9 Unspecified form of unconventional warfare

E998 Injury due to war operations but occurring after cessation of hostilities
   Injuries due to operations of war but occurring after cessation of hostilities by any means classifiable under E990-E997
   Injuries by explosion of bombs or mines placed in the course of operations of war, if the explosion occurred after cessation of hostilities

▲✓4ᵗʰ E999 Late effect of injury due to war operations and terrorism

   Note: This category is to be used to indicate circumstances classifiable to ▶E979,◀ E990-E998 as the cause of death or disability from late effects, which are themselves classifiable elsewhere. The "late effects" include conditions reported as such, or as sequelae, which may occur at any time after the injury, resulting from operations of war ▶or terrorism◀.

●   E999.0 Late effect of injury due to war operations

●   E999.1 Late effect of injury due to terrorism

   ✓4ᵗʰ Fourth-digit Required   ▶◀ Revised Text   ● New Code   ▲ Revised Code Title

Official ICD•9•CM Government Appendixes

MORPHOLOGY OF NEOPLASMS

The World Health Organization has published an adaptation of the International Classification of Diseases for oncology (ICD-O). It contains a coded nomenclature for the morphology of neoplasms, which is reproduced here for those who wish to use it in conjunction with Chapter 2 of the International Classification of Diseases, 9th Revision, Clinical Modification.

The morphology code numbers consist of five digits; the first four identify the histological type of the neoplasm and the fifth indicates its behavior. The one-digit behavior code is as follows:

- /0 Benign
- /1 Uncertain whether benign or malignant
  Borderline malignancy
- /2 Carcinoma in situ
  Intraepithelial
  Noninfiltrating
  Noninvasive
- /3 Malignant, primary site
- /6 Malignant, metastatic site
  Secondary site
- /9 Malignant, uncertain whether primary or metastatic site

In the nomenclature below, the morphology code numbers include the behavior code appropriate to the histological type of neoplasm, but this behavior code should be changed if other reported information makes this necessary. For example, "chordoma (M9370/3)" is assumed to be malignant; the term "benign chordoma" should be coded M9370/0. Similarly, "superficial spreading adenocarcinoma (M8143/3)" described as "noninvasive" should be coded M8143/2 and "melanoma (M8720/3)" described as "secondary" should be coded M8720/6.

The following table shows the correspondence between the morphology code and the different sections of Chapter 2:

Morphology Code Histology/Behavior			ICD-9-CM Chapter 2
Any	0	210-229	Benign neoplasms
M8000- M8004	1	239	Neoplasms of unspecified nature
M8010+	1	235-238	Neoplasms of uncertain behavior
Any	2	230-234	Carcinoma in situ
Any	3	140-195	Malignant neoplasms, stated or presumed
		200-208	to be primary
Any	6	196-198	Malignant neoplasms, stated or presumed to be secondary

The ICD-O behavior digit /9 is inapplicable in an ICD context, since all malignant neoplasms are presumed to be primary (/3) or secondary (/6) according to other information on the medical record.

Only the first-listed term of the full ICD-O morphology nomenclature appears against each code number in the list below. The ICD-9-CM Alphabetical Index (Volume 2), however, includes all the ICD-O synonyms as well as a number of other morphological names still likely to be encountered on medical records but omitted from ICD-O as outdated or otherwise undesirable.

A coding difficulty sometimes arises where a morphological diagnosis contains two qualifying adjectives that have different code numbers. An example is "transitional cell epidermoid carcinoma." "Transitional cell carcinoma NOS" is M8120/3 and "epidermoid carcinoma NOS" is M8070/3. In such circumstances, the higher number (M8120/3 in this example) should be used, as it is usually more specific.

CODED NOMENCLATURE FOR MORPHOLOGY OF NEOPLASMS

M800	**Neoplasms NOS**
M8000/0	Neoplasm, benign
M8000/1	Neoplasm, uncertain whether benign or malignant
M8000/3	Neoplasm, malignant
M8000/6	Neoplasm, metastatic
M8000/9	Neoplasm, malignant, uncertain whether primary or metastatic
M8001/0	Tumor cells, benign
M8001/1	Tumor cells, uncertain whether benign or malignant
M8001/3	Tumor cells, malignant
M8002/3	Malignant tumor, small cell type
M8003/3	Malignant tumor, giant cell type
M8004/3	Malignant tumor, fusiform cell type
M801-M804	**Epithelial neoplasms NOS**
M8010/0	Epithelial tumor, benign
M8010/2	Carcinoma in situ NOS
M8010/3	Carcinoma NOS
M8010/6	Carcinoma, metastatic NOS
M8010/9	Carcinomatosis
M8011/0	Epithelioma, benign
M8011/3	Epithelioma, malignant
M8012/3	Large cell carcinoma NOS
M8020/3	Carcinoma, undifferentiated type NOS
M8021/3	Carcinoma, anaplastic type NOS
M8022/3	Pleomorphic carcinoma
M8030/3	Giant cell and spindle cell carcinoma
M8031/3	Giant cell carcinoma
M8032/3	Spindle cell carcinoma
M8033/3	Pseudosarcomatous carcinoma
M8034/3	Polygonal cell carcinoma
M8035/3	Spheroidal cell carcinoma
M8040/1	Tumorlet
M8041/3	Small cell carcinoma NOS
M8042/3	Oat cell carcinoma
M8043/3	Small cell carcinoma, fusiform cell type
M805-M808	**Papillary and squamous cell neoplasms**
M8050/0	Papilloma NOS (except Papilloma of urinary bladder M8120/1)
M8050/2	Papillary carcinoma in situ
M8050/3	Papillary carcinoma NOS
M8051/0	Verrucous papilloma
M8051/3	Verrucous carcinoma NOS
M8052/0	Squamous cell papilloma
M8052/3	Papillary squamous cell carcinoma
M8053/0	Inverted papilloma
M8060/0	Papillomatosis NOS
M8070/2	Squamous cell carcinoma in situ NOS
M8070/3	Squamous cell carcinoma NOS
M8070/6	Squamous cell carcinoma, metastatic NOS
M8071/3	Squamous cell carcinoma, keratinizing type NOS
M8072/3	Squamous cell carcinoma, large cell, nonkeratinizing type
M8073/3	Squamous cell carcinoma, small cell, nonkeratinizing type
M8074/3	Squamous cell carcinoma, spindle cell type
M8075/3	Adenoid squamous cell carcinoma
M8076/2	Squamous cell carcinoma in situ with questionable stromal invasion
M8076/3	Squamous cell carcinoma, microinvasive
M8080/2	Queyrat's erythroplasia
M8081/2	Bowen's disease
M8082/3	Lymphoepithelial carcinoma
M809-M811	**Basal cell neoplasms**
M8090/1	Basal cell tumor
M8090/3	Basal cell carcinoma NOS
M8091/3	Multicentric basal cell carcinoma
M8092/3	Basal cell carcinoma, morphea type
M8093/3	Basal cell carcinoma, fibroepithelial type
M8094/3	Basosquamous carcinoma
M8095/3	Metatypical carcinoma
M8096/0	Intraepidermal epithelioma of Jadassohn
M8100/0	Trichoepithelioma
M8101/0	Trichofolliculoma
M8102/0	Tricholemmoma
M8110/0	Pilomatrixoma
M812-M813	**Transitional cell papillomas and carcinomas**
M8120/0	Transitional cell papilloma NOS
M8120/1	Urothelial papilloma
M8120/2	Transitional cell carcinoma in situ
M8120/3	Transitional cell carcinoma NOS
M8121/0	Schneiderian papilloma
M8121/1	Transitional cell papilloma, inverted type
M8121/3	Schneiderian carcinoma
M8122/3	Transitional cell carcinoma, spindle cell type

M8123/3	Basaloid carcinoma
M8124/3	Cloacogenic carcinoma
M8130/3	Papillary transitional cell carcinoma

M814-M838 Adenomas and adenocarcinomas

M8140/0	Adenoma NOS
M8140/1	Bronchial adenoma NOS
M8140/2	Adenocarcinoma in situ
M8140/3	Adenocarcinoma NOS
M8140/6	Adenocarcinoma, metastatic NOS
M8141/3	Scirrhous adenocarcinoma
M8142/3	Linitis plastica
M8143/3	Superficial spreading adenocarcinoma
M8144/3	Adenocarcinoma, intestinal type
M8145/3	Carcinoma, diffuse type
M8146/0	Monomorphic adenoma
M8147/0	Basal cell adenoma
M8150/0	Islet cell adenoma
M8150/3	Islet cell carcinoma
M8151/0	Insulinoma NOS
M8151/3	Insulinoma, malignant
M8152/0	Glucagonoma NOS
M8152/3	Glucagonoma, malignant
M8153/1	Gastrinoma NOS
M8153/3	Gastrinoma, malignant
M8154/3	Mixed islet cell and exocrine adenocarcinoma
M8160/0	Bile duct adenoma
M8160/3	Cholangiocarcinoma
M8161/0	Bile duct cystadenoma
M8161/3	Bile duct cystadenocarcinoma
M8170/0	Liver cell adenoma
M8170/3	Hepatocellular carcinoma NOS
M8180/0	Hepatocholangioma, benign
M8180/3	Combined hepatocellular carcinoma and cholangiocarcinoma
M8190/0	Trabecular adenoma
M8190/3	Trabecular adenocarcinoma
M8191/0	Embryonal adenoma
M8200/0	Eccrine dermal cylindroma
M8200/3	Adenoid cystic carcinoma
M8201/3	Cribriform carcinoma
M8210/0	Adenomatous polyp NOS
M8210/3	Adenocarcinoma in adenomatous polyp
M8211/0	Tubular adenoma NOS
M8211/3	Tubular adenocarcinoma
M8220/0	Adenomatous polyposis coli
M8220/3	Adenocarcinoma in adenomatous polyposis coli
M8221/0	Multiple adenomatous polyps
M8230/3	Solid carcinoma NOS
M8231/3	Carcinoma simplex
M8240/1	Carcinoid tumor NOS
M8240/3	Carcinoid tumor, malignant
M8241/1	Carcinoid tumor, argentaffin NOS
M8241/3	Carcinoid tumor, argentaffin, malignant
M8242/1	Carcinoid tumor, nonargentaffin NOS
M8242/3	Carcinoid tumor, nonargentaffin, malignant
M8243/3	Mucocarcinoid tumor, malignant
M8244/3	Composite carcinoid
M8250/1	Pulmonary adenomatosis
M8250/3	Bronchiolo-alveolar adenocarcinoma
M8251/0	Alveolar adenoma
M8251/3	Alveolar adenocarcinoma
M8260/0	Papillary adenoma NOS
M8260/3	Papillary adenocarcinoma NOS
M8261/1	Villous adenoma NOS

M8261/3	Adenocarcinoma in villous adenoma
M8262/3	Villous adenocarcinoma
M8263/0	Tubulovillous adenoma
M8270/0	Chromophobe adenoma
M8270/3	Chromophobe carcinoma
M8280/0	Acidophil adenoma
M8280/3	Acidophil carcinoma
M8281/0	Mixed acidophil-basophil adenoma
M8281/3	Mixed acidophil-basophil carcinoma
M8290/0	Oxyphilic adenoma
M8290/3	Oxyphilic adenocarcinoma
M8300/0	Basophil adenoma
M8300/3	Basophil carcinoma
M8310/0	Clear cell adenoma
M8310/3	Clear cell adenocarcinoma NOS
M8311/1	Hypernephroid tumor
M8312/3	Renal cell carcinoma
M8313/0	Clear cell adenofibroma
M8320/3	Granular cell carcinoma
M8321/0	Chief cell adenoma
M8322/0	Water-clear cell adenoma
M8322/3	Water-clear cell adenocarcinoma
M8323/0	Mixed cell adenoma
M8323/3	Mixed cell adenocarcinoma
M8324/0	Lipoadenoma
M8330/0	Follicular adenoma
M8330/3	Follicular adenocarcinoma NOS
M8331/3	Follicular adenocarcinoma, well differentiated type
M8332/3	Follicular adenocarcinoma, trabecular type
M8333/0	Microfollicular adenoma
M8334/0	Macrofollicular adenoma
M8340/3	Papillary and follicular adenocarcinoma
M8350/3	Nonencapsulated sclerosing carcinoma
M8360/1	Multiple endocrine adenomas
M8361/1	Juxtaglomerular tumor
M8370/0	Adrenal cortical adenoma NOS
M8370/3	Adrenal cortical carcinoma
M8371/0	Adrenal cortical adenoma, compact cell type
M8372/0	Adrenal cortical adenoma, heavily pigmented variant
M8373/0	Adrenal cortical adenoma, clear cell type
M8374/0	Adrenal cortical adenoma, glomerulosa cell type
M8375/0	Adrenal cortical adenoma, mixed cell type
M8380/0	Endometrioid adenoma NOS
M8380/1	Endometrioid adenoma, borderline malignancy
M8380/3	Endometrioid carcinoma
M8381/0	Endometrioid adenofibroma NOS
M8381/1	Endometrioid adenofibroma, borderline malignancy
M8381/3	Endometrioid adenofibroma, malignant

M839-M842 Adnexal and skin appendage neoplasms

M8390/0	Skin appendage adenoma
M8390/3	Skin appendage carcinoma
M8400/0	Sweat gland adenoma
M8400/1	Sweat gland tumor NOS
M8400/3	Sweat gland adenocarcinoma
M8401/0	Apocrine adenoma
M8401/3	Apocrine adenocarcinoma
M8402/0	Eccrine acrospiroma
M8403/0	Eccrine spiradenoma
M8404/0	Hidrocystoma
M8405/0	Papillary hydradenoma

M8406/0	Papillary syringadenoma
M8407/0	Syringoma NOS
M8410/0	Sebaceous adenoma
M8410/3	Sebaceous adenocarcinoma
M8420/0	Ceruminous adenoma
M8420/3	Ceruminous adenocarcinoma

M843 Mucoepidermoid neoplasms

M8430/1	Mucoepidermoid tumor
M8430/3	Mucoepidermoid carcinoma

M844-M849 Cystic, mucinous, and serous neoplasms

M8440/0	Cystadenoma NOS
M8440/3	Cystadenocarcinoma NOS
M8441/0	Serous cystadenoma NOS
M8441/1	Serous cystadenoma, borderline malignancy
M8441/3	Serous cystadenocarcinoma NOS
M8450/0	Papillary cystadenoma NOS
M8450/1	Papillary cystadenoma, borderline malignancy
M8450/3	Papillary cystadenocarcinoma NOS
M8460/0	Papillary serous cystadenoma NOS
M8460/1	Papillary serous cystadenoma, borderline malignancy
M8460/3	Papillary serous cystadenocarcinoma
M8461/0	Serous surface papilloma NOS
M8461/1	Serous surface papilloma, borderline malignancy
M8461/3	Serous surface papillary carcinoma
M8470/0	Mucinous cystadenoma NOS
M8470/1	Mucinous cystadenoma, borderline malignancy
M8470/3	Mucinous cystadenocarcinoma NOS
M8471/0	Papillary mucinous cystadenoma NOS
M8471/1	Papillary mucinous cystadenoma, borderline malignancy
M8471/3	Papillary mucinous cystadenocarcinoma
M8480/0	Mucinous adenoma
M8480/3	Mucinous adenocarcinoma
M8480/6	Pseudomyxoma peritonei
M8481/3	Mucin-producing adenocarcinoma
M8490/3	Signet ring cell carcinoma
M8490/6	Metastatic signet ring cell carcinoma

M850-M854 Ductal, lobular, and medullary neoplasms

M8500/2	Intraductal carcinoma, noninfiltrating NOS
M8500/3	Infiltrating duct carcinoma
M8501/2	Comedocarcinoma, noninfiltrating
M8501/3	Comedocarcinoma NOS
M8502/3	Juvenile carcinoma of the breast
M8503/0	Intraductal papilloma
M8503/2	Noninfiltrating intraductal papillary adenocarcinoma
M8504/0	Intracystic papillary adenoma
M8504/2	Noninfiltrating intracystic carcinoma
M8505/0	Intraductal papillomatosis NOS
M8506/0	Subareolar duct papillomatosis
M8510/3	Medullary carcinoma NOS
M8511/3	Medullary carcinoma with amyloid stroma
M8512/3	Medullary carcinoma with lymphoid stroma
M8520/2	Lobular carcinoma in situ
M8520/3	Lobular carcinoma NOS

M8521/3	Infiltrating ductular carcinoma	M8730/0	Nonpigmented nevus	M8860/0	Angiomyolipoma
M8530/3	Inflammatory carcinoma	M8730/3	Amelanotic melanoma	M8860/3	Angiomyoliposarcoma
M8540/3	Paget's disease, mammary	M8740/0	Junctional nevus	M8861/0	Angiolipoma NOS
M8541/3	Paget's disease and infiltrating duct carcinoma of breast	M8740/3	Malignant melanoma in junctional nevus	M8861/1	Angiolipoma, infiltrating
M8542/3	Paget's disease, extramammary (except Paget's disease of bone)	M8741/2	Precancerous melanosis NOS	M8870/0	Myelolipoma
		M8741/3	Malignant melanoma in precancerous melanosis	M8880/0	Hibernoma
				M8881/0	Lipoblastomatosis

M855   **Acinar cell neoplasms**

M8550/0	Acinar cell adenoma	M8742/2	Hutchinson's melanotic freckle		
M8550/1	Acinar cell tumor	M8742/3	Malignant melanoma in Hutchinson's melanotic freckle		
M8550/3	Acinar cell carcinoma				

M889-M892   **Myomatous neoplasms**

				M8890/0	Leiomyoma NOS
				M8890/1	Intravascular leiomyomatosis
				M8890/3	Leiomyosarcoma NOS

M856-M858   **Complex epithelial neoplasms**

M8560/3	Adenosquamous carcinoma	M8743/3	Superficial spreading melanoma	M8891/1	Epithelioid leiomyoma
M8561/0	Adenolymphoma	M8750/0	Intradermal nevus	M8891/3	Epithelioid leiomyosarcoma
M8570/3	Adenocarcinoma with squamous metaplasia	M8760/0	Compound nevus	M8892/1	Cellular leiomyoma
M8571/3	Adenocarcinoma with cartilaginous and osseous metaplasia	M8761/1	Giant pigmented nevus	M8893/0	Bizarre leiomyoma
		M8761/3	Malignant melanoma in giant pigmented nevus	M8894/0	Angiomyoma
M8572/3	Adenocarcinoma with spindle cell metaplasia	M8770/0	Epithelioid and spindle cell nevus	M8894/3	Angiomyosarcoma
M8573/3	Adenocarcinoma with apocrine metaplasia	M8771/3	Epithelioid cell melanoma	M8895/0	Myoma
		M8772/3	Spindle cell melanoma NOS	M8895/3	Myosarcoma
M8580/0	Thymoma, benign	M8773/3	Spindle cell melanoma, type A	M8900/0	Rhabdomyoma NOS
M8580/3	Thymoma, malignant	M8774/3	Spindle cell melanoma, type B	M8900/3	Rhabdomyosarcoma NOS
		M8775/3	Mixed epithelioid and spindle cell melanoma	M8901/3	Pleomorphic rhabdomyosarcoma

M859-M867   **Specialized gonadal neoplasms**

				M8902/3	Mixed type rhabdomyosarcoma
M8590/1	Sex cord-stromal tumor	M8780/0	Blue nevus NOS	M8903/0	Fetal rhabdomyoma
M8600/0	Thecoma NOS	M8780/3	Blue nevus, malignant	M8904/0	Adult rhabdomyoma
M8600/3	Theca cell carcinoma	M8790/0	Cellular blue nevus	M8910/3	Embryonal rhabdomyosarcoma

M8610/0	Luteoma NOS			M8920/3	Alveolar rhabdomyosarcoma

M880   **Soft tissue tumors and sarcomas NOS**

M893-M899   **Complex mixed and stromal neoplasms**

M8620/1	Granulosa cell tumor NOS	M8800/0	Soft tissue tumor, benign		
M8620/3	Granulosa cell tumor, malignant	M8800/3	Sarcoma NOS	M8930/3	Endometrial stromal sarcoma
M8621/1	Granulosa cell-theca cell tumor	M8800/9	Sarcomatosis NOS	M8931/1	Endolymphatic stromal myosis
M8630/0	Androblastoma, benign	M8801/3	Spindle cell sarcoma	M8932/0	Adenomyoma
M8630/1	Androblastoma NOS	M8802/3	Giant cell sarcoma (except of bone M9250/3)	M8940/0	Pleomorphic adenoma
M8630/3	Androblastoma, malignant	M8803/3	Small cell sarcoma	M8940/3	Mixed tumor, malignant NOS
M8631/0	Sertoli-Leydig cell tumor	M8804/3	Epithelioid cell sarcoma	M8950/3	Mullerian mixed tumor
M8632/1	Gynandroblastoma			M8951/3	Mesodermal mixed tumor

M881-M883   **Fibromatous neoplasms**

M8640/0	Tubular androblastoma NOS	M8810/0	Fibroma NOS	M8960/1	Mesoblastic nephroma
M8640/3	Sertoli cell carcinoma	M8810/3	Fibrosarcoma NOS	M8960/3	Nephroblastoma NOS
M8641/0	Tubular androblastoma with lipid storage	M8811/0	Fibromyxoma	M8961/3	Epithelial nephroblastoma
		M8811/3	Fibromyxosarcoma	M8962/3	Mesenchymal nephroblastoma
M8650/0	Leydig cell tumor, benign	M8812/0	Periosteal fibroma	M8970/3	Hepatoblastoma
M8650/1	Leydig cell tumor NOS	M8812/3	Periosteal fibrosarcoma	M8980/3	Carcinosarcoma NOS
M8650/3	Leydig cell tumor, malignant	M8813/0	Fascial fibroma	M8981/3	Carcinosarcoma, embryonal type
M8660/0	Hilar cell tumor	M8813/3	Fascial fibrosarcoma		
M8670/0	Lipid cell tumor of ovary	M8814/3	Infantile fibrosarcoma	M8982/0	Myoepithelioma
M8671/0	Adrenal rest tumor	M8820/0	Elastofibroma	M8990/0	Mesenchymoma, benign

M868-M871   **Paragangliomas and glomus tumors**

		M8821/1	Aggressive fibromatosis	M8990/1	Mesenchymoma NOS
		M8822/1	Abdominal fibromatosis	M8990/3	Mesenchymoma, malignant
M8680/1	Paraganglioma NOS	M8823/1	Desmoplastic fibroma	M8991/3	Embryonal sarcoma
M8680/3	Paraganglioma, malignant	M8830/0	Fibrous histiocytoma NOS		

M900-M903   **Fibroepithelial neoplasms**

M8681/1	Sympathetic paraganglioma	M8830/1	Atypical fibrous histiocytoma	M9000/0	Brenner tumor NOS
M8682/1	Parasympathetic paraganglioma	M8830/3	Fibrous histiocytoma, malignant	M9000/1	Brenner tumor, borderline malignancy
M8690/1	Glomus jugulare tumor	M8831/0	Fibroxanthoma NOS		
M8691/1	Aortic body tumor	M8831/1	Atypical fibroxanthoma	M9000/3	Brenner tumor, malignant
M8692/1	Carotid body tumor	M8831/3	Fibroxanthoma, malignant	M9010/0	Fibroadenoma NOS
M8693/1	Extra-adrenal paraganglioma NOS	M8832/0	Dermatofibroma NOS	M9011/0	Intracanalicular fibroadenoma NOS
		M8832/1	Dermatofibroma protuberans		
M8693/3	Extra-adrenal paraganglioma, malignant	M8832/3	Dermatofibrosarcoma NOS	M9012/0	Pericanalicular fibroadenoma

M884   **Myxomatous neoplasms**

				M9013/0	Adenofibroma NOS
M8700/0	Pheochromocytoma NOS	M8840/0	Myxoma NOS	M9014/0	Serous adenofibroma
M8700/3	Pheochromocytoma, malignant	M8840/3	Myxosarcoma	M9015/0	Mucinous adenofibroma

M885-M888   **Lipomatous neoplasms**

M8710/3	Glomangiosarcoma			M9020/0	Cellular intracanalicular fibroadenoma
M8711/0	Glomus tumor	M8850/0	Lipoma NOS		
M8712/0	Glomangioma	M8850/3	Liposarcoma NOS	M9020/1	Cystosarcoma phyllodes NOS

M872-M879   **Nevi and melanomas**

		M8851/0	Fibrolipoma	M9020/3	Cystosarcoma phyllodes, malignant
M8720/0	Pigmented nevus NOS	M8851/3	Liposarcoma, well differentiated type		
M8720/3	Malignant melanoma NOS			M9030/0	Juvenile fibroadenoma
M8721/3	Nodular melanoma	M8852/0	Fibromyxolipoma		

M904   **Synovial neoplasms**

M8722/0	Balloon cell nevus	M8852/3	Myxoid liposarcoma	M9040/0	Synovioma, benign
M8722/3	Balloon cell melanoma	M8853/3	Round cell liposarcoma	M9040/3	Synovial sarcoma NOS
M8723/3	Halo nevus	M8854/3	Pleomorphic liposarcoma	M9041/3	Synovial sarcoma, spindle cell type
M8724/0	Fibrous papule of the nose	M8855/3	Mixed type liposarcoma		
M8725/0	Neuronevus	M8856/0	Intramuscular lipoma	M9042/3	Synovial sarcoma, epithelioid cell type
M8726/0	Magnocellular nevus	M8857/0	Spindle cell lipoma		
				M9043/3	Synovial sarcoma, biphasic type
				M9044/3	Clear cell sarcoma of tendons and aponeuroses

Appendix A: Morphology of Neoplasms

M905 — **Mesothelial neoplasms**
M9050/0 — *Mesothelioma, benign*
M9050/3 — *Mesothelioma, malignant*
M9051/0 — *Fibrous mesothelioma, benign*
M9051/3 — *Fibrous mesothelioma, malignant*
M9052/0 — *Epithelioid mesothelioma, benign*
M9052/3 — *Epithelioid mesothelioma, malignant*
M9053/0 — *Mesothelioma, biphasic type, benign*
M9053/3 — *Mesothelioma, biphasic type, malignant*
M9054/0 — *Adenomatoid tumor NOS*

M906-M909 — **Germ cell neoplasms**
M9060/0 — *Dysgerminoma*
M9061/3 — *Seminoma NOS*
M9062/3 — *Seminoma, anaplastic type*
M9063/3 — *Spermatocytic seminoma*
M9064/3 — *Germinoma*
M9070/3 — *Embryonal carcinoma NOS*
M9071/3 — *Endodermal sinus tumor*
M9072/3 — *Polyembryoma*
M9073/1 — *Gonadoblastoma*
M9080/0 — *Teratoma, benign*
M9080/1 — *Teratoma NOS*
M9080/3 — *Teratoma, malignant NOS*
M9081/3 — *Teratocarcinoma*
M9082/3 — *Malignant teratoma, undifferentiated type*
M9083/3 — *Malignant teratoma, intermediate type*
M9084/0 — *Dermoid cyst*
M9084/3 — *Dermoid cyst with malignant transformation*
M9090/0 — *Struma ovarii NOS*
M9090/3 — *Struma ovarii, malignant*
M9091/1 — *Strumal carcinoid*

M910 — **Trophoblastic neoplasms**
M9100/0 — *Hydatidiform mole NOS*
M9100/1 — *Invasive hydatidiform mole*
M9100/3 — *Choriocarcinoma*
M9101/3 — *Choriocarcinoma combined with teratoma*
M9102/3 — *Malignant teratoma, trophoblastic*

M911 — **Mesonephromas**
M9110/0 — *Mesonephroma, benign*
M9110/1 — *Mesonephric tumor*
M9110/3 — *Mesonephroma, malignant*
M9111/1 — *Endosalpingioma*

M912-M916 — **Blood vessel tumors**
M9120/0 — *Hemangioma NOS*
M9120/3 — *Hemangiosarcoma*
M9121/0 — *Cavernous hemangioma*
M9122/0 — *Venous hemangioma*
M9123/0 — *Racemose hemangioma*
M9124/3 — *Kupffer cell sarcoma*
M9130/0 — *Hemangioendothelioma, benign*
M9130/1 — *Hemangioendothelioma NOS*
M9130/3 — *Hemangioendothelioma, malignant*
M9131/0 — *Capillary hemangioma*
M9132/0 — *Intramuscular hemangioma*
M9140/3 — *Kaposi's sarcoma*
M9141/0 — *Angiokeratoma*
M9142/0 — *Verrucous keratotic hemangioma*
M9150/0 — *Hemangiopericytoma, benign*
M9150/1 — *Hemangiopericytoma NOS*
M9150/3 — *Hemangiopericytoma, malignant*
M9160/0 — *Angiofibroma NOS*
M9161/1 — *Hemangioblastoma*

M917 — **Lymphatic vessel tumors**
M9170/0 — *Lymphangioma NOS*
M9170/3 — *Lymphangiosarcoma*
M9171/0 — *Capillary lymphangioma*
M9172/0 — *Cavernous lymphangioma*
M9173/0 — *Cystic lymphangioma*
M9174/0 — *Lymphangiomyoma*
M9174/1 — *Lymphangiomyomatosis*
M9175/0 — *Hemolymphangioma*

M918-M920 — **Osteomas and osteosarcomas**
M9180/0 — *Osteoma NOS*
M9180/3 — *Osteosarcoma NOS*
M9181/3 — *Chondroblastic osteosarcoma*
M9182/3 — *Fibroblastic osteosarcoma*
M9183/3 — *Telangiectatic osteosarcoma*
M9184/3 — *Osteosarcoma in Paget's disease of bone*
M9190/3 — *Juxtacortical osteosarcoma*
M9191/0 — *Osteoid osteoma NOS*
M9200/0 — *Osteoblastoma*

M921-M924 — **Chondromatous neoplasms**
M9210/0 — *Osteochondroma*
M9210/1 — *Osteochondromatosis NOS*
M9220/0 — *Chondroma NOS*
M9220/1 — *Chondromatosis NOS*
M9220/3 — *Chondrosarcoma NOS*
M9221/0 — *Juxtacortical chondroma*
M9221/3 — *Juxtacortical chondrosarcoma*
M9230/0 — *Chondroblastoma NOS*
M9230/3 — *Chondroblastoma, malignant*
M9240/3 — *Mesenchymal chondrosarcoma*
M9241/0 — *Chondromyxoid fibroma*

M925 — **Giant cell tumors**
M9250/1 — *Giant cell tumor of bone NOS*
M9250/3 — *Giant cell tumor of bone, malignant*
M9251/1 — *Giant cell tumor of soft parts NOS*
M9251/3 — *Malignant giant cell tumor of soft parts*

M926 — **Miscellaneous bone tumors**
M9260/3 — *Ewing's sarcoma*
M9261/3 — *Adamantinoma of long bones*
M9262/0 — *Ossifying fibroma*

M927-M934 — **Odontogenic tumors**
M9270/0 — *Odontogenic tumor, benign*
M9270/1 — *Odontogenic tumor NOS*
M9270/3 — *Odontogenic tumor, malignant*
M9271/0 — *Dentinoma*
M9272/0 — *Cementoma NOS*
M9273/0 — *Cementoblastoma, benign*
M9274/0 — *Cementifying fibroma*
M9275/0 — *Gigantiform cementoma*
M9280/0 — *Odontoma NOS*
M9281/0 — *Compound odontoma*
M9282/0 — *Complex odontoma*
M9290/0 — *Ameloblastic fibro-odontoma*
M9290/3 — *Ameloblastic odontosarcoma*
M9300/0 — *Adenomatoid odontogenic tumor*
M9301/0 — *Calcifying odontogenic cyst*
M9310/0 — *Ameloblastoma NOS*
M9310/3 — *Ameloblastoma, malignant*
M9311/0 — *Odontoameloblastoma*
M9312/0 — *Squamous odontogenic tumor*
M9320/0 — *Odontogenic myxoma*
M9321/0 — *Odontogenic fibroma NOS*
M9330/0 — *Ameloblastic fibroma*
M9330/3 — *Ameloblastic fibrosarcoma*
M9340/0 — *Calcifying epithelial odontogenic tumor*

M935-M937 — **Miscellaneous tumors**
M9350/1 — *Craniopharyngioma*
M9360/1 — *Pinealoma*
M9361/1 — *Pineocytoma*
M9362/3 — *Pineoblastoma*
M9363/0 — *Melanotic neuroectodermal tumor*
M9370/3 — *Chordoma*

M938-M948 — **Gliomas**
M9380/3 — *Glioma, malignant*
M9381/3 — *Gliomatosis cerebri*
M9382/3 — *Mixed glioma*
M9383/1 — *Subependymal glioma*
M9384/1 — *Subependymal giant cell astrocytoma*
M9390/0 — *Choroid plexus papilloma NOS*
M9390/3 — *Choroid plexus papilloma, malignant*
M9391/3 — *Ependymoma NOS*
M9392/3 — *Ependymoma, anaplastic type*
M9393/1 — *Papillary ependymoma*
M9394/1 — *Myxopapillary ependymoma*
M9400/3 — *Astrocytoma NOS*
M9401/3 — *Astrocytoma, anaplastic type*
M9410/3 — *Protoplasmic astrocytoma*
M9411/3 — *Gemistocytic astrocytoma*
M9420/3 — *Fibrillary astrocytoma*
M9421/3 — *Pilocytic astrocytoma*
M9422/3 — *Spongioblastoma NOS*
M9423/3 — *Spongioblastoma polare*
M9430/3 — *Astroblastoma*
M9440/3 — *Glioblastoma NOS*
M9441/3 — *Giant cell glioblastoma*
M9442/3 — *Glioblastoma with sarcomatous component*
M9443/3 — *Primitive polar spongioblastoma*
M9450/3 — *Oligodendroglioma NOS*
M9451/3 — *Oligodendroglioma, anaplastic type*
M9460/3 — *Oligodendroblastoma*
M9470/3 — *Medulloblastoma NOS*
M9471/3 — *Desmoplastic medulloblastoma*
M9472/3 — *Medullomyoblastoma*
M9480/3 — *Cerebellar sarcoma NOS*
M9481/3 — *Monstrocellular sarcoma*

M949-M952 — **Neuroepitheliomatous neoplasms**
M9490/0 — *Ganglioneuroma*
M9490/3 — *Ganglioneuroblastoma*
M9491/0 — *Ganglioneuromatosis*
M9500/3 — *Neuroblastoma NOS*
M9501/3 — *Medulloepithelioma NOS*
M9502/3 — *Teratoid medulloepithelioma*
M9503/3 — *Neuroepithelioma NOS*
M9504/3 — *Spongioneuroblastoma*
M9505/1 — *Ganglioglioma*
M9506/0 — *Neurocytoma*
M9507/0 — *Pacinian tumor*
M9510/3 — *Retinoblastoma NOS*
M9511/3 — *Retinoblastoma, differentiated type*
M9512/3 — *Retinoblastoma, undifferentiated type*
M9520/3 — *Olfactory neurogenic tumor*
M9521/3 — *Esthesioneurocytoma*
M9522/3 — *Esthesioneuroblastoma*
M9523/3 — *Esthesioneuroepithelioma*

M953 — **Meningiomas**
M9530/0 — *Meningioma NOS*
M9530/1 — *Meningiomatosis NOS*
M9530/3 — *Meningioma, malignant*
M9531/0 — *Meningotheliomatous meningioma*
M9532/0 — *Fibrous meningioma*
M9533/0 — *Psammomatous meningioma*
M9534/0 — *Angiomatous meningioma*
M9535/0 — *Hemangioblastic meningioma*
M9536/0 — *Hemangiopericytic meningioma*
M9537/0 — *Transitional meningioma*
M9538/1 — *Papillary meningioma*
M9539/3 — *Meningeal sarcomatosis*

M954-M957 — **Nerve sheath tumor**
M9540/0 — *Neurofibroma NOS*
M9540/1 — *Neurofibromatosis NOS*
M9540/3 — *Neurofibrosarcoma*
M9541/0 — *Melanotic neurofibroma*
M9550/0 — *Plexiform neurofibroma*
M9560/0 — *Neurilemmoma NOS*

M9560/1	*Neurinomatosis*
M9560/3	*Neurilemmoma, malignant*
M9570/0	*Neuroma NOS*
M958	**Granular cell tumors and alveolar soft part sarcoma**
M9580/0	*Granular cell tumor NOS*
M9580/3	*Granular cell tumor, malignant*
M9581/3	*Alveolar soft part sarcoma*
M959-M963	**Lymphomas, NOS or diffuse**
M9590/0	*Lymphomatous tumor, benign*
M9590/3	*Malignant lymphoma NOS*
M9591/3	*Malignant lymphoma, non Hodgkin's type*
M9600/3	*Malignant lymphoma, undifferentiated cell type NOS*
M9601/3	*Malignant lymphoma, stem cell type*
M9602/3	*Malignant lymphoma, convoluted cell type NOS*
M9610/3	*Lymphosarcoma NOS*
M9611/3	*Malignant lymphoma, lymphoplasmacytoid type*
M9612/3	*Malignant lymphoma, immunoblastic type*
M9613/3	*Malignant lymphoma, mixed lymphocytic-histiocytic NOS*
M9614/3	*Malignant lymphoma, centroblastic-centrocytic, diffuse*
M9615/3	*Malignant lymphoma, follicular center cell NOS*
M9620/3	*Malignant lymphoma, lymphocytic, well differentiated NOS*
M9621/3	*Malignant lymphoma, lymphocytic, intermediate differentiation NOS*
M9622/3	*Malignant lymphoma, centrocytic*
M9623/3	*Malignant lymphoma, follicular center cell, cleaved NOS*
M9630/3	*Malignant lymphoma, lymphocytic, poorly differentiated NOS*
M9631/3	*Prolymphocytic lymphosarcoma*
M9632/3	*Malignant lymphoma, centroblastic type NOS*
M9633/3	*Malignant lymphoma, follicular center cell, noncleaved NOS*
M964	***Reticulosarcomas***
M9640/3	*Reticulosarcoma NOS*
M9641/3	*Reticulosarcoma, pleomorphic cell type*
M9642/3	*Reticulosarcoma, nodular*
M965-M966	***Hodgkin's disease***
M9650/3	*Hodgkin's disease NOS*
M9651/3	*Hodgkin's disease, lymphocytic predominance*
M9652/3	*Hodgkin's disease, mixed cellularity*
M9653/3	*Hodgkin's disease, lymphocytic depletion NOS*

M9654/3	*Hodgkin's disease, lymphocytic depletion, diffuse fibrosis*
M9655/3	*Hodgkin's disease, lymphocytic depletion, reticular type*
M9656/3	*Hodgkin's disease, nodular sclerosis NOS*
M9657/3	*Hodgkin's disease, nodular sclerosis, cellular phase*
M9660/3	*Hodgkin's paragranuloma*
M9661/3	*Hodgkin's granuloma*
M9662/3	*Hodgkin's sarcoma*
M969	**Lymphomas, nodular or follicular**
M9690/3	*Malignant lymphoma, nodular NOS*
M9691/3	*Malignant lymphoma, mixed lymphocytic-histiocytic, nodular*
M9692/3	*Malignant lymphoma, centroblastic-centrocytic, follicular*
M9693/3	*Malignant lymphoma, lymphocytic, well differentiated, nodular*
M9694/3	*Malignant lymphoma, lymphocytic, intermediate differentiation, nodular*
M9695/3	*Malignant lymphoma, follicular center cell, cleaved, follicular*
M9696/3	*Malignant lymphoma, lymphocytic, poorly differentiated, nodular*
M9697/3	*Malignant lymphoma, centroblastic type, follicular*
M9698/3	*Malignant lymphoma, follicular center cell, noncleaved, follicular*
M970	**Mycosis fungoides**
M9700/3	*Mycosis fungoides*
M9701/3	*Sezary's disease*
M971-M972	**Miscellaneous reticuloendothelial neoplasms**
M9710/3	*Microglioma*
M9720/3	*Malignant histiocytosis*
M9721/3	*Histiocytic medullary reticulosis*
M 722/3	*Letterer-Siwe's disease*
M973	**Plasma cell tumors**
M9730/3	*Plasma cell myeloma*
M9731/0	*Plasma cell tumor, benign*
M9731/1	*Plasmacytoma NOS*
M9731/3	*Plasma cell tumor, malignant*
M974	**Mast cell tumors**
M9740/1	*Mastocytoma NOS*
M9740/3	*Mast cell sarcoma*
M9741/3	*Malignant mastocytosis*
M975	**Burkitt's tumor**
M9750/3	*Burkitt's tumor*
M980-M994	**Leukemias**
M980	**Leukemias NOS**
M9800/3	*Leukemia NOS*
M9801/3	*Acute leukemia NOS*

M9802/3	*Subacute leukemia NOS*
M9803/3	*Chronic leukemia NOS*
M9804/3	*Aleukemic leukemia NOS*
M981	**Compound leukemias**
M9810/3	*Compound leukemia*
M982	**Lymphoid leukemias**
M9820/3	*Lymphoid leukemia NOS*
M9821/3	*Acute lymphoid leukemia*
M9822/3	*Subacute lymphoid leukemia*
M9823/3	*Chronic lymphoid leukemia*
M9824/3	*Aleukemic lymphoid leukemia*
M9825/3	*Prolymphocytic leukemia*
M983	**Plasma cell leukemias**
M9830/3	*Plasma cell leukemia*
M984	**Erythroleukemias**
M9840/3	*Erythroleukemia*
M9841/3	*Acute erythremia*
M9842/3	*Chronic erythremia*
M985	**Lymphosarcoma cell leukemias**
M9850/3	*Lymphosarcoma cell leukemia*
M986	**Myeloid leukemias**
M9860/3	*Myeloid leukemia NOS*
M9861/3	*Acute myeloid leukemia*
M9862/3	*Subacute myeloid leukemia*
M9863/3	*Chronic myeloid leukemia*
M9864/3	*Aleukemic myeloid leukemia*
M9865/3	*Neutrophilic leukemia*
M9866/3	*Acute promyelocytic leukemia*
M987	**Basophilic leukemias**
M9870/3	*Basophilic leukemia*
M988	**Eosinophilic leukemias**
M9880/3	*Eosinophilic leukemia*
M989	**Monocytic leukemias**
M9890/3	*Monocytic leukemia NOS*
M9891/3	*Acute monocytic leukemia*
M9892/3	*Subacute monocytic leukemia*
M9893/3	*Chronic monocytic leukemia*
M9894/3	*Aleukemic monocytic leukemia*
M990-M994	**Miscellaneous leukemias**
M9900/3	*Mast cell leukemia*
M9910/3	*Megakaryocytic leukemia*
M9920/3	*Megakaryocytic myelosis*
M9930/3	*Myeloid sarcoma*
M9940/3	*Hairy cell leukemia*
M995-M997	**Miscellaneous myeloproliferative and lymphoproliferative disorders**
M9950/1	*Polycythemia vera*
M9951/1	*Acute panmyelosis*
M9960/1	*Chronic myeloproliferative disease*
M9961/1	*Myelosclerosis with myeloid metaplasia*
M9962/1	*Idiopathic thrombocythemia*
M9970/1	*Chronic lymphoproliferative disease*

Glossary of Mental Disorders

The psychiatric terms which appear in Chapter 5, "Mental Disorders," are listed here in alphabetic sequence. Many of the glossary descriptions originally appeared in the section on Mental Disorders in the *International Classification of Diseases, 9th Revision*,[1] and others are included to define the psychiatric conditions added to *ICD-9-CM*. The additional definitions are based on material furnished by the *American Psychiatric Association's Task Force on Nomenclature and Statistics*[2] and from *A Psychiatric Glossary*.[3] In a few instances definitions were obtained from *Dorland's Illustrated Medical Dictionary*[4] and from *Stedman's Medical Dictionary, Illustrated*.[5]

1. *Manual of the International Classification of Diseases, Injuries, and Causes of Death*, 9th Revision. World Health Organization, Geneva, Switzerland, 1975.
2. American Psychiatric Association, Task Force on Nomenclature and Statistics, Robert L. Spitzer, Chairman.
3. *A Psychiatric Glossary*, Fourth Edition, American Psychiatric Association, Washington, D.C., 1975.
4. *Dorland's Illustrated Medical Dictionary*, Twenty-fifth Edition, W.B. Saunders Company, Philadelphia, 1974.
5. *Stedman's Medical Dictionary*, Illustrated, Twenty-third Edition, the Williams and Wilkins Company, Baltimore, 1976.

Academic underachievement disorder – Failure to achieve in most school tasks despite adequate intellectual capacity, a supportive and encouraging social environment, and apparent effort. The failure occurs in the absence of a demonstrable specific learning disability and is caused by emotional conflict not clearly associated with any other mental disorder.[2]

Adaptation reaction — *see* Adjustment reaction

Adjustment reaction or disorder – Mild or transient disorders lasting longer than acute stress reactions which occur in individuals of any age without any apparent pre-existing mental disorder. Such disorders are often relatively circumscribed or situation-specific, are generally reversible, and usually last only a few months. They are usually closely related in time and content to stresses such as bereavement, migration, or other experiences. Reactions to major stress that last longer than a few days are also included. In children such disorders are associated with no significant distortion of development.[1]

  conduct disturbance – Mild or transient disorders in which the main disturbance predominantly involves a disturbance of conduct (e.g., an adolescent grief reaction resulting in aggressive or antisocial disorder).[1]

  depressive reaction – States of depression, not specifiable as manic-depressive, psychotic, or neurotic.[1]

    brief – Generally transient, in which the depressive symptoms are usually closely related in time and content to some stressful event.[1]

    prolonged – Generally long-lasting, usually developing in association with prolonged exposure to a stressful situation.[1]

  emotional disturbance – An adjustment disorder in which the main symptoms are emotional in type (e.g., anxiety, fear, worry) but not specifically depressive.[1]

  mixed conduct and emotional disturbance – An adjustment reaction in which both emotional disturbance and disturbance of conduct are prominent features.[1]

Affective psychoses – Mental disorders, usually recurrent, in which there is a severe disturbance of mood (mostly compounded of depression and anxiety but also manifested as elation, and excitement) which is accompanied by one or more of the following – delusions, perplexity, disturbed attitude to self, disorder of perception and behavior; these are all in keeping with the individual's prevailing mood (as are hallucinations when they occur). There is a strong tendency to suicide. For practical reasons, mild disorders of mood may also be included here if the symptoms match closely the descriptions given; this applies particularly to mild hypomania.[1]

  bipolar – A manic-depressive psychosis which has appeared in both the depressive and manic form, either alternating or separated by an interval of normality.[1]

    atypical – An episode of affective psychosis with some, but not all, of the features of the one form of the disorder in individuals who have had a previous episode of the other form of the disorder.[2]

    depressed – A manic-depressive psychosis, circular type, in which the depressive form is currently present.[1]

    manic – A manic-depressive psychosis, circular type, in which the manic form is currently present.[1]

    mixed – A manic-depressive psychosis, circular type, in which both manic and depressive symptoms are present at the same time.[1]

  depressed type – A manic-depressive psychosis in which there is a widespread depressed mood of gloom and wretchedness with some degree of anxiety. There is often reduced activity but there may be restlessness and agitation. There is marked tendency to recurrence; in a few cases this may be at regular intervals.[1]

    atypical – An affective depressive disorder that cannot be classified as a manic-depressive psychosis, depressed type, or chronic depressive personality disorder, or as an adjustment disorder.[2]

  manic type – A manic-depressive psychosis characterized by states of elation or excitement out of keeping with the individual's circumstances and varying from enhanced liveliness (hypomania) to violent, almost uncontrollable, excitement. Aggression and anger, flight of ideas, distractibility, impaired judgment, and grandiose ideas are common.[1]

    mixed type – Manic-depressive psychosis syndromes corresponding to both the manic and depressed types, but which for other reasons cannot be classified more specifically.[1]

Aggressive personality — *see* Personality disorder, explosive type

Agoraphobia — *see* agoraphobia under Phobia

Alcohol dependence syndrome – A state, psychic and usually also physical, resulting from taking alcohol, characterized by behavioral and other responses that always include a compulsion to take alcohol on a continuous or periodic basis in order to experience its psychic effects, and sometimes to avoid the discomfort of its absence; tolerance may or may not be present. A person may be dependent on alcohol and other drugs; if so, also record the diagnosis of drug dependence to identify the agent. If alcohol dependence is associated with alcoholic psychosis or with physical complications, *both* diagnoses should be recorded.[1]

Alcohol intoxication

  acute – A psychic and physical state resulting from alcohol ingestion characterized by slurred speech, unsteady gait, poor coordination, flushed facies, nystagmus, sluggish reflexes, fetor alcoholica, loud speech, emotional instability (e.g., jollity followed by lugubriousness), excessive conviviality, loquacity, and poorly inhibited sexual and aggressive behavior.[2]

  idiosyncratic – Acute psychotic episodes induced by relatively small amounts of alcohol. These are regarded as individual idiosyncratic reactions to alcohol, not due to excessive consumption and without conspicuous neurological signs of intoxication.[1]

  pathological – *see* Alcohol intoxication, idiosyncratic

Alcoholic psychoses – Organic psychotic states due mainly to excessive consumption of alcohol; defects of nutrition are thought to play an important role.[1]

  alcohol abstinence syndrome — *see* alcohol withdrawal syndrome below

  alcohol amnestic syndrome – A syndrome of prominent and lasting reduction of memory span, including striking loss of recent memory, disordered time appreciation and confabulation, occurring in alcoholics as the sequel to an acute alcoholic psychosis (especially delirium tremens) or, more rarely, in the course of chronic alcoholism. It is usually accompanied by peripheral neuritis and may be associated with Wernicke's encephalopathy.[1]

  alcohol withdrawal delirium [delirium tremens] – Acute or subacute organic psychotic states in alcoholics, characterized by clouded consciousness, disorientation, fear, illusions, delusions, hallucinations of any kind, notably visual and tactile, and restlessness, tremor and sometimes fever.[1]

  alcohol withdrawal hallucinosis – A psychosis usually of less than six months' duration, with slight or no clouding of consciousness and much

Appendix B: Glossary of Mental Disorders

anxious restlessness in which auditory hallucinations, mostly of voices uttering insults and threats, predominate.[1]

alcohol withdrawal syndrome – Tremor of hands, tongue, and eyelids following cessation of prolonged heavy drinking of alcohol. Nausea and vomiting, dry mouth, headache, heavy perspiration, fitful sleep, acute anxiety attacks, mood depression, feelings of guilt and remorse, and irritability are associated features.[2]

alcohol delirium — *see* alcohol withdrawal delirium above

alcoholic dementia – Nonhallucinatory dementias occurring in association with alcoholism, but not characterized by the features of either alcohol withdrawal delirium [delirium tremens] or alcohol amnestic syndrome [Korsakoff's alcoholic psychosis].[1]

alcoholic hallucinosis — *see* alcohol withdrawal hallucinosis above

alcoholic jealousy – Chronic paranoid psychosis characterized by delusional jealousy and associated with alcoholism.[1]

alcoholic paranoia — *see* Alcoholic jealousy

alcoholic polyneuritic psychosis — *see* alcohol amnestic syndrome above

Alcoholism

acute — *see* Alcohol intoxication, acute

chronic — *see* Alcohol dependence syndrome

Alexia – Loss of a previously possessed reading facility that cannot be explained by defective visual acuity.[3]

Amnesia, psychogenic – A form of dissociative hysteria in which there is a temporary disturbance in the ability to recall important personal information which has already been registered and stored in memory. The sudden onset of this disturbance in the absence of an underlying organic mental disorder, and the extent of the disturbance being too great to be explained by ordinary forgetfulness, are the essential features.[2]

Amnestic syndrome – A syndrome of prominent and lasting reduction of memory span, including striking loss of recent memory, disordered time appreciation, and confabulation. The commonest causes are chronic alcoholism [alcohol amnestic syndrome; Korsakoff's alcoholic psychosis], chronic barbiturate dependence, and malnutrition. An amnestic syndrome may be the predominating disturbance in the early states of presenile and senile dementia, arteriosclerotic dementia, and in encephalitis and other inflammatory and degenerative diseases in which there is particular bilateral involvement of the temporal lobes, and certain temporal lobe tumors.[2]

alcoholic — *see* alcohol amnestic syndrome under Alcoholic psychoses

Amoral personality — *see* Personality disorder, antisocial type

Anancastic [anankastic] neurosis — *see* Neurotic disorder, obsessive-compulsive

Anancastic [anankastic] personality — *see* Personality disorder, compulsive type

Anorexia nervosa – A disorder in which the main features are persistent active refusal to eat and marked loss of weight.

The level of activity and alertness is characteristically high in relation to the degree of emaciation. Typically the disorder begins in teenage girls but it may sometimes begin before puberty and rarely it occurs in males. Amenorrhea is usual and there may be a variety of other physiological changes including slow pulse and respiration, low body temperature, and dependent edema. Unusual eating habits and attitudes toward food are typical and sometimes starvation follows or alternates with periods of overeating. The accompanying psychiatric symptoms are diverse.[1]

Anxiety hysteria — *see* phobia under Neurotic disorders

Anxiety state (neurotic) – Apprehension, tension, or uneasiness that stems from the anticipation of danger, the source of which is largely unknown or unrecognized.[3]

atypical – An anxiety disorder that does not fulfill the criteria of generalized or panic attack anxiety. An example might be an individual with a single morbid fear.[2]

generalized – A disorder of at least six months' duration in which the predominant feature is limited to diffuse and persistent anxiety without the specific symptoms that characterize phobic disorders, panic disorder, or obsessive-compulsive disorder.[2]

panic attack – An episodic and often chronic, recurrent disorder in which the predominant features are anxiety attacks and nervousness. The anxiety attacks are manifested by discrete periods of sudden onset of intense apprehension, fearfulness, or terror often associated with feelings of impending doom.[2]

Aphasia, developmental – A delay in the production of spoken language. Rarely, there is also a developmental delay in the comprehension of speech sounds.[1]

Arteriosclerotic dementia – Dementia attributable, because of physical signs (on examination of the central nervous system), to degenerative arterial disease of the brain. Symptoms suggesting a focal lesion in the brain are common. There may be a fluctuating or patchy intellectual defect with insight, and an intermittent course is common. Clinical differentiation from senile or presenile dementia, which may coexist with it, may be very difficult or impossible. The diagnosis of cerebral atherosclerosis should also be recorded.[1]

Asocial personality — *see* Personality disorder, antisocial type

Astasia-abasia, hysterical – A form of conversion hysteria in which the individual is unable to stand or walk although the legs are otherwise under control.[4]

Asthenia, psychogenic — *see* neurasthenia under Neurotic disorders

Asthenic personality — *see* Personality disorder, dependent type

Attention deficit disorder — *see* Attention deficit disorder under Hyperkinetic syndrome of childhood.

Autism, infantile – A syndrome present from birth or beginning almost invariably in the first 30 months. Responses to

auditory and sometimes to visual stimuli are abnormal, and there are usually severe problems in the understanding of spoken language. Speech is delayed and, if it develops, is characterized by echolalia, the reversal of pronouns, immature grammatical structure, and inability to use abstract terms. There is generally an impairment in the social use of both verbal and gestural language. Problems in social relationships are most severe before the age of five years and include an impairment in the development of eye-to-eye gaze, social attachments, and cooperative play. Ritualistic behavior is usual and may include abnormal routines, resistance to change, attachment to odd objects, and stereotyped patterns of play. The capacity for abstract or symbolic thought and for imaginative play is diminished. Intelligence ranges from severely subnormal to normal or above. Performance is usually better on tasks involving rote memory or visuospatial skills than on those requiring symbolic or linguistic skills.[1]

Avoidant personality — *see* Personality disorder, avoidant type

"Bad trips" – Acute intoxication from hallucinogen abuse, manifested by hallucinatory states lasting only a few days or less.[1]

Barbiturate abuse – Cases where an individual has taken the drug to the detriment of his health or social functioning, in doses above or for periods beyond those normally regarded as therapeutic.[1]

Bestiality — *see* Zoophilia

Bipolar disorder — *see* Affective psychosis, bipolar

atypical — *see* Affective psychosis, bipolar, atypical

Body-rocking — *see* Stereotyped repetitive movements

Borderline personality — *see* Personality disorder, borderline type

Borderline psychosis of childhood — *see* Psychosis, atypical childhood

Borderline schizophrenia — *see* Schizophrenia, latent

Bouffée délirante — *see* Paranoid reaction, acute

Briquet's disorder — *see* Somatization disorder under Neurotic disorders

Bulimia – An episodic pattern of overeating [binge eating] accompanied by an awareness of the disordered eating pattern with a fear of not being able to stop eating voluntarily. Depressive moods and self-deprecating thoughts follow the episodes of binge eating.[2]

Catalepsy schizophrenia — *see* Schizophrenia, catatonic type

Catastrophic stress — *see* Gross stress reaction

Catatonia (schizophrenic) — *see* Schizophrenia, catatonic type

Character neurosis — *see* Personality disorders

Childhood autism — *see* Autism, infantile

Childhood type schizophrenia — *see* Psychosis, child

Chronic alcoholic brain syndrome — *see* Alcoholic dementia under Alcoholic psychoses

Clay-eating — *see* Pica

Clumsiness syndrome — *see* Coordination disorder under Developmental delay disorders, specific

Combat fatigue — *see* Posttraumatic disorder, acute

Compensation neurosis — *see* Compensation neurosis under Neurotic disorders

Compulsive conduct disorder — *see* Impulse control disorders under Conduct disorders

Compulsive neurosis — *see* Neurotic disorder, obsessive-compulsive

Compulsive personality — *see* Personality disorder, compulsive type

Concentration camp syndrome — *see* Posttraumatic stress disorder, prolonged

Conduct disorders – Disorders mainly involving aggressive and destructive behavior and disorders involving delinquency. It should be used for abnormal behavior, in individuals of any age, which gives rise to social disapproval but which is not part of any other psychiatric condition. Minor emotional disturbances may also be present. To be included, the behavior, as judged by its frequency, severity, and type of associations with other symptoms, must be abnormal in its context. Disturbances of conduct are distinguished from an adjustment reaction by a longer duration and by a lack of close relationship in time and content to some stress. They differ from a personality disorder by the absence of deeply ingrained maladaptive patterns of behavior present from adolescence or earlier.[1]

impulse control disorders – A failure to resist an impulse, drive, or temptation to perform some action which is harmful to the individual or to others. The impulse may or may not be consciously resisted, and the act may or may not be premeditated or planned. Prior to committing the act, there is an increasing sense of tension, and at the time of committing the act, there is an experience of either pleasure, gratification, or release. Immediately following the act, there may or may not be genuine regret, self-reproach, or guilt.[2] *See also* Intermittent explosive disorder, Isolated explosive disorder, Kleptomania, Pathological gambling, and Pyromania.

mixed disturbance of conduct and emotions – A disorder characterized by features of undersocialized and socialized disturbance of conduct, but in which there is also considerable emotional disturbance as shown, for example, by anxiety, misery, or obsessive manifestations.[1]

socialized conduct disorder – Conduct disorders in individuals who have acquired the values or behavior of a delinquent peer group to whom they are loyal and with whom they characteristically steal, play truant, and stay out late at night. There may also be sexual promiscuity.[1]

undersocialized conduct disturbance
aggressive type – A disorder characterized by a persistent pattern of disrespect for the feelings and well-being of others (bullying, physical aggression, cruel behavior, hostility, verbal abusiveness, impudence, defiance, negativism), aggressive antisocial behavior (destructiveness, stealing, persistent lying, frequent truancy, and vandalism), and failure to develop close and stable relationships with others.[2]

unaggressive type – A disorder in which there is a lack of concern for the rights and feelings of others to a degree which indicates a failure to establish a normal degree of affection, empathy, or bond with others. There are two patterns of behavior found. In one, the child is fearful and timid, lacking self-assertiveness, resorts to self-protective and manipulative lying, indulges in whining demandingness and temper tantrums, feels rejected and unfairly treated, and is mistrustful of others. In the other pattern of the disorder, the child approaches others strictly for his own gains and acts exclusively because of exploitative and extractive goals. The child lies brazenly and steals, appearing to feel no guilt, and forms no social bonds to other individuals.[2]

Confusion, psychogenic — *see* Psychosis, reactive confusion

Confusion, reactive — *see* Psychosis, reactive confusion

Confusional state
acute — *see* Delirium, acute
epileptic — *see* Delirium, acute
subacute — *see* Delirium, subacute

Conversion hysteria — *see* Hysteria, conversion type under Neurotic disorders

Coordination disorder — *see* Coordination disorder under Developmental delay disorders, specific

Culture shock – A form of stress reaction associated with an individual's assimilation into a new culture which is vastly different from that in which he was raised.[5]

Cyclic schizophrenia — *see* Schizophrenia, schizo-affective type

Cyclothymic personality or disorder — *see* Personality disorder, cyclothymic type

Delirium – Transient organic psychotic conditions with a short course in which there is a rapidly developing onset of disorganization of higher mental processes manifested by some degree of impairment of information processing, impaired or abnormal attention, perception, memory, and thinking. Clouded consciousness, confusion, disorientation, delusions, illusions, and often vivid hallucinations predominate in the clinical picture.[1, 2]

acute – short-lived states, lasting hours or days, of the above type.[1]

subacute – states of the above type in which the symptoms, usually less florid, last for several weeks or longer, during which they may show marked fluctuations in intensity.[1]

Delirium tremens — *see* Alcohol withdrawal delirium under Alcoholic psychoses

Delusions, systematized — *see* Paranoia

Dementia – A decrement in intellectual functioning of sufficient severity to interfere with occupational or social performance, or both. There is impairment of memory and abstract thinking, the ability to learn new skills, problem solving, and judgment. There is often also personality change or impairment in impulse control. Dementia in organic psychoses may be of a chronic or progressive nature, which if untreated are usually irreversible and terminal.[1, 2]

alcoholic — *see* Alcoholic dementia under Alcoholic psychoses

arteriosclerotic — *see* Arteriosclerotic dementia

multi-infarct — *see* Arteriosclerotic dementia

presenile — *see* Presenile dementia

repeated infarct — *see* Arteriosclerotic dementia

senile — *see* Senile dementia

Depersonalization syndrome — *see* Depersonalization syndrome under Neurotic disorders

Depression – States of depression, usually of moderate but occasionally of marked intensity, which have no specifically manic-depressive or other psychotic depressive features, and which do not appear to be associated with stressful events or other features specified under neurotic depression.[1]

anxiety — *see* Depression under Neurotic disorders

endogenous — *see* Affective psychosis, depressed type

monopolar — *see* Affective psychosis, depressed type

neurotic — *see* Depression under Neurotic disorders

psychotic — *see* Affective psychosis, depressed type

psychotic reactive — *see* Psychosis, depressive

reactive — *see* Depression under Neurotic disorders

reactive psychotic — *see* Psychosis, depressive

Depressive personality or character — *see* Personality disorder, chronic depressive type

Depressive reaction — *see* Depressive reaction under Adjustment reaction

Depressive psychosis — *see* Affective psychosis, depressed type

Derealization (neurotic) — *see* Depersonalization syndrome under Neurotic disorders

Developmental delay disorders, specific – A group of disorders in which a specific delay in development is the main feature. For many the delay is not explicable in terms of general intellectual retardation or of inadequate schooling. In each case development is related to biological maturation, but it is also influenced by nonbiological factors. A diagnosis of a specific developmental delay carries no etiological implications. A diagnosis of specific delay in development should not be made if it is due to a known neurological disorder.[1]

arithmetical disorder – Disorders in which the main feature is a serious impairment in the development of arithmetical skills.[1]

articulation disorder – A delay in the development of normal word-sound production resulting in defects of articulation. Omissions or substitutions of consonants are most frequent.[1]

coordination disorder – Disorders in which the main feature is a serious impairment in the development of motor coordination which is not explicable in terms of general intellectual retardation. The clumsiness is commonly associated with perceptual difficulties.[1]

mixed development disorder – A delay in the development of one specific skill (e.g., reading, arithmetic, speech, or coordination) is frequently associated with lesser delays in other skills. When this occurs, the diagnosis should be made according to the skill most seriously impaired. The mixed category should be used only where the mixture of delayed skills is such that no one skill is preponderantly affected.[1]

motor retardation — *see* Coordination disorder above

reading disorder or retardation – Disorders in which the main feature is a serious impairment in the development of reading or spelling skills which is not explicable in terms of general intellectual retardation or of inadequate schooling. Speech or language difficulties, impaired right-left differentiation, perceptuo-motor problems, and coding difficulties are frequently associated. Similar problems are often present in other members of the family. Adverse psychosocial factors may be present.[1]

speech or language disorder – Disorders in which the main feature is a serious impairment in the development of speech or language (syntax or semantic) which is not explicable in terms of general intellectual retardation. Most commonly there is a delay in the development of normal word-sound production resulting in defects of articulation. Omissions or substitutions of consonants are most frequent. There may also be a delay in the production of spoken language. Rarely, there is also a developmental delay in the comprehension of sounds. Includes cases in which delay is largely due to environmental privation.[1]

Dipsomania — *see* Alcohol dependence syndrome

Disorganized schizophrenia — *see* Schizophrenia, disorganized type

Dissociative hysteria — *see* Hysteria, dissociative type under Neurotic disorders

Drug abuse – Includes cases where an individual, for whom no other diagnosis is possible, has come under medical care because of the maladaptive effect of a drug on which he is not dependent (*see* Drug dependence) and that he has taken on his own initiative to the detriment of his health or social functioning. When drug abuse is secondary to a psychiatric disorder, record the disorder as an additional diagnosis.[1]

Drug dependence – A state, psychic and sometimes also physical dependence, resulting from taking a drug, characterized by behavioral and other responses that always include a compulsion to take a drug on a continuous or periodic basis in order to experience its psychic effects, and sometimes to avoid the discomfort of its absence. Tolerance may or may not be present. A person may be dependent on more than one drug.[1]

Drug psychoses – Organic mental syndromes which are due to consumption of drugs (notably amphetamines, barbiturates, and opiate and LSD groups) and solvents. Some of the syndromes in this group are not as severe as most conditions labeled "psychotic," but they are included here for practical reasons. The drug should be identified, and also a diagnosis of drug dependence should be recorded, if present.[1]

drug-induced hallucinosis – Hallucinatory states of more than a few days, but not more than a few months' duration, associated with large or prolonged intake of drugs, notably of the amphetamine and LSD groups. Auditory hallucinations usually predominate and there may be anxiety or restlessness. States following LSD or other hallucinogens lasting only a few days or less ["bad trips"] are not included.[1]

drug-induced organic delusional syndrome – Paranoid states of more than a few days, but not more than a few months' duration, associated with large or prolonged intake of drugs, notably of the amphetamine and LSD groups.[1]

drug withdrawal syndrome – States associated with drug withdrawal ranging from severe, as specified for alcohol withdrawal delirium [delirium tremens], to less severe states characterized by one or more symptoms such as convulsions, tremor, anxiety, restlessness, gastrointestinal and muscular complaints, and mild disorientation and memory disturbance.[1]

Drunkenness

acute — *see* Alcohol intoxication, acute

pathologic — *see* Alcohol intoxication, idiosyncratic

simple – A state of inebriation due to alcohol consumption without conspicuous neurological signs of intoxication.[2]

sleep – An inability to fully arouse from the sleep state characterized by failure to attain full consciousness after arousal.[2]

Dyscalculia — *see* Arithmetical disorder under Developmental delay disorders, specific

Dyslalia — *see* Articulation disorder under Developmental delay disorders, specific

Dyslexia, developmental – A disorder in which the main feature is a serious impairment of reading skills which is not explicable in terms of general intellectual retardation or of inadequate schooling. Word-blindness and strephosymbolia (tendency to reverse letters and words in reading) are included.[1,3]

Dysmenorrhea, psychogenic – Painful menstruation due to disturbance of psychic control.[4]

Dyspareunia, functional — *see* Functional dyspareunia under Psychosexual dysfunctions

Dyspraxia syndrome — *see* Coordination disorder under Developmental delay disorders, specific

Dyssocial personality — *see* Personality disorder, antisocial type

Dysuria, psychogenic – Difficulty in passing urine due to psychic factors.[4]

Eating disorders – A group of disorders characterized by a conspicuous disturbance in eating behavior.[2] *See also* Bulimia, Pica, and Rumination, psychogenic.

Eccentric personality — *see* Personality disorder, eccentric type

Elective mutism – A pervasive and persistent refusal to speak in situations not attributable to a mental disorder. In some cases the behavior may manifest a form of withdrawal reaction to a specific stressful situation, or as a predominant feature in children exhibiting shyness or social withdrawal disorders.[2]

Emancipation disorder – An adjustment reaction in adolescents or young adults in which there is symptomatic expression (e.g., difficulty in making independent decisions, increased dependence on parental advice, adoption of values deliberately oppositional to parents) of a conflict over independence following the recent assumption of a status in which the individual is more independent of parental control or supervision.[2]

Emotional disturbances specific to childhood and adolescence – Less well-differentiated emotional disorders characteristic of the childhood period. When the emotional disorder takes the form of a neurosis, the appropriate diagnosis should be made. These disorders differ from adjustment reactions in terms of longer duration and by the lack of close relationship in time and content to some stress.[1] *See also* Academic underachievement disorder, Elective mutism, Identity disorder, Introverted disorder of childhood, Misery and unhappiness disorder, Oppositional disorder, Overanxious disorder, and Shyness disorder of childhood.

Encopresis – A disorder in which the main manifestation is the persistent voluntary or involuntary passage of formed stools of normal or near-normal consistency into places not intended for that purpose in the individual's own sociocultural setting. Sometimes the child has failed to gain bowel control, and sometimes he has gained control but then later again became encopretic. There may be a variety of associated psychiatric symptoms and there may be smearing of feces. The condition would not usually be diagnosed under the age of four years.[1]

Endogenous depression — *see* Affective psychosis, depressed type

Enuresis – A disorder in which the main manifestation is a persistent involuntary voiding of urine by day or night which is considered abnormal for the age of the individual. Sometimes the child will have failed to gain bladder control and in other cases he will have gained control and then lost it. Episodic or fluctuating enuresis should be included. The disorder would not usually be diagnosed under the age of four years.[1]

Epileptic confusional or twilight state — *see* Delirium, acute

Excitation

catatonic — *see* Schizophrenia, catatonic type

psychogenic — *see* Psychosis, excitative type

reactive — *see* Psychosis, excitative type

Exhaustion delirium — *see* Stress reaction, acute

Exhibitionism – Sexual deviation in which the main sexual pleasure and gratification is derived from exposure of the genitals to a person of the opposite sex.[1]

Explosive personality disorder — *see* Personality disorder, explosive type

Factitious illness – A form of hysterical neurosis in which there are physical or psychological symptoms that are not real, genuine, or natural, which are produced by the individual and are under his voluntary control.[2]

> **physical symptom type** – The presentation of physical symptoms that may be total fabrication, self-inflicted, an exaggeration or exacerbation of a pre-existing physical condition, or any combination or variation of these.[2]

> **psychological symptom type** – The voluntary production of symptoms suggestive of a mental disorder. Behavior may mimic psychosis or, rather, the individual's idea of psychosis.[2]

Fanatic personality — *see* Personality disorder, paranoid type

Fatigue neurosis — *see* Neurasthenia under Neurotic disorders

Feeble-minded — *see* Mental retardation, mild

Fetishism – A sexual deviation in which nonliving objects are utilized as a preferred or exclusive method of stimulating erotic arousal.[2]

Finger-flicking — *see* Stereotyped repetitive movements

Folie à deux — *see* Shared paranoid disorder

Frigidity – A psychosexual dysfunction in which there is partial or complete failure to attain or maintain the lubrication-swelling response of sexual excitement until completion of the sexual act.[2]

Frontal lobe syndrome – Changes in behavior following damage to the frontal areas of the brain or following interference with the connections of those areas. There is a general diminution of self-control, foresight, creativity, and spontaneity, which may be manifest as increased irritability, selfishness, restlessness, and lack of concern for others. Conscientiousness and powers of concentration are often diminished, but measurable deterioration of intellect or memory is not necessarily present. The overall picture is often one of emotional dullness, lack of drive, and slowness; but, particularly in persons previously with energetic, restless, or aggressive characteristics, there may be a change towards impulsiveness, boastfulness, temper outbursts, silly fatuous humor, and the development of unrealistic ambitions; the direction of change usually depends upon the previous personality. A considerable degree of recovery is possible and may continue over the course of several years.[1]

Fugue, psychogenic – A form of dissociative hysteria characterized by an episode of wandering with inability to recall one's prior identity. Both onset and recovery are rapid. Following recovery there is no recollection of events which took place during the fugue state.[2]

Ganser's syndrome (hysterical) – A form of factitious illness in which the patient voluntarily produces symptoms suggestive of a mental disorder.[2]

Gender identity disorder — *see* Gender identity disorder under Psychosexual identity disorders

Gilles de la Tourette's disorder or syndrome — *see* Gilles de la Tourette's disorder under Tics

Grief reaction — *see* Depressive reaction, brief under Adjustment reaction

Gross stress reaction — *see* Stress reaction, acute

Group delinquency — *see* Socialized conduct disorder under Conduct disorders

Habit spasm — *see* Chronic motor tic disorder under Tics

Hangover (alcohol) — *see* Drunkenness, simple

Head-banging — *see* Stereotyped repetitive movements

Hebephrenia — *see* Schizophrenia, disorganized type

Heller's syndrome — *see* Psychosis, disintegrative

High grade defect — *see* Mental retardation, mild

Homosexuality – Exclusive or predominant sexual attraction for persons of the same sex with or without physical relationship. Record homosexuality as a diagnosis whether or not it is considered as a mental disorder.[1]

Hospital addiction syndrome — *see* Munchausen syndrome

Hospital hoboes — *see* Munchausen syndrome

Hospitalism – A mild or transient adjustment reaction characterized by withdrawal seen in hospitalized patients. In young children this may be manifested by elective mutism.[1]

Hyperkinetic syndrome of childhood – Disorders in which the essential features are short attention span and distractibility. In early childhood the most striking symptom is disinhibited, poorly organized and poorly regulated extreme overactivity but in adolescence this may be replaced by underactivity. Impulsiveness, marked mood fluctuations, and aggression are also common symptoms. Delays in the development of specific skills are often present and disturbed, poor relationships are common. If the hyperkinesis is symptomatic of an underlying disorder, the diagnosis of the underlying disorder is recorded instead.[1]

> **attention deficit disorder** – Cases of hyperkinetic syndrome in which short attention span, distractibility, and overactivity are the main manifestations without significant disturbance of conduct or delay in specific skills.[1]

> **hyperkinesis with developmental delay** – Cases in which the hyperkinetic syndrome is associated with speech delay, clumsiness, reading difficulties, or other delays of specific skills.[1]

> **hyperkinetic conduct disorder** – Cases in which the hyperkinetic syndrome is associated with marked conduct disturbance but not developmental delay.[1]

Hypersomnia – A disorder of initiating arousal from sleep or maintaining wakefulness.[2]

> **persistent** – Chronic difficulty in initiating arousal from sleep or maintaining wakefulness associated with major or minor depressive mental disorders.[2]

> **transient** – Episodes of difficulty in arousal from sleep or maintaining wakefulness associated with acute or intermittent emotional reactions or conflicts.[2]

Hypochondriasis — *see* Hypochondriasis under Neurotic disorders

Hypomania — *see* Affective psychosis, manic type

Hypomanic personality — *see* Personality disorder, chronic hypomanic type

Hyposomnia — *see* Insomnia

Hysteria — *see* Hysteria under Neurotic disorders

> **anxiety** — *see* Phobia under Neurotic disorders

> **psychosis** — *see* Psychosis, reactive

> **acute** — *see* Psychosis, excitative type

Hysterical personality — *see* Personality disorder, histrionic type

Identity disorder – An emotional disorder caused by distress over the inability to reconcile aspects of the self into a relatively coherent and acceptable sense of self, not secondary to another mental disorder. The disturbance is manifested by intense subjective distress regarding uncertainty about a variety of issues relating to identity, including long-term goals, career choice, friendship patterns, values, and loyalties.[2]

Idiocy — *see* Mental retardation, profound

Imbecile — *see* Mental retardation, moderate

Impotence – A psychosexual dysfunction in which there is partial or complete failure to attain or maintain erection until completion of the sexual act.[2]

Impulse control disorder — *see* Impulse control disorders under Conduct disorders

Inadequate personality — *see* Personality disorder, dependent type

Induced paranoid disorder — *see* Shared paranoid disorder

Inebriety — *see* Drunkenness, simple

Infantile autism — *see* Autism, infantile

Insomnia – A disorder of initiating or maintaining sleep.[2]

> **persistent** – A chronic state of sleeplessness associated with chronic anxiety, major or minor depressive disorders, or psychoses.[2]

> **transient** – Episodes of sleeplessness associated with acute or intermittent emotional reactions or conflicts.[2]

Intermittent explosive disorder – Recurrent episodes of sudden and significant loss of control of aggressive impulses, not accounted for by any other mental disorder, which results in serious assault or destruction of property. The magnitude of the behavior during an episode is grossly out of proportion to any psychosocial stressors which may have played a role in eliciting the episode of lack of control. Following each episode there is genuine regret or self-reproach at the consequences of the action and the inability to control the aggressive impulse.[2]

Introverted disorder of childhood – An emotional disturbance in children chiefly manifested by a lack of interest in social relationships and indifference to social praise or criticism.[2]

Introverted personality — *see* Personality disorder, introverted type

Involutional melancholia — *see* Affective psychosis, depressed type

Involutional paranoid state — *see* Paraphrenia

Isolated explosive disorder – A disorder of impulse control in which there is a single discrete episode characterized by failure to resist an impulse which leads to a single, violent externally-directed act, which has a catastrophic impact on others, and for which the available information does not justify the diagnosis of another mental disorder.[2]

Isolated phobia — *see* Simple phobia under Phobia

Jet lag syndrome – A phase-shift disruption of the 24-hour sleep-wake cycle due to rapid time-zone changes experienced in long-distance travel.[2]

Kanner's syndrome — *see* Autism, infantile

Kleptomania – A disorder of impulse control characterized by a recurrent failure to resist impulses to steal objects not for immediate use or their monetary value. An increasing sense of tension is experienced prior to committing the act, with an intense experience of gratification at the time of committing the theft.[2]

Korsakoff's psychosis
  alcoholic — *see* Alcohol amnestic syndrome under Alcoholic psychoses
  nonalcoholic — *see* Amnestic syndrome

Latent schizophrenia — *see* Schizophrenia, latent

Lesbianism — *see* Homosexuality

Lobotomy syndrome — *see* Frontal lobe syndrome

LSD reaction – Acute intoxication from hallucinogen abuse, manifested by hallucinatory states lasting only a few days or less.[1]

Major depressive disorder — *see* Affective psychosis, depressed type

Malingering – A clinical picture in which the predominant feature is the presentation of fake or grossly exaggerated physical or psychiatric illness apparently under voluntary control. In contrast to factitious illness, the symptoms produced in malingering are in pursuit of a goal which, when known, is recognizable and obviously understandable in light of knowledge of the individual's circumstances. Examples of understandable goals include, but are not limited to, becoming a "patient" in order to avoid conscription or military duty, avoid work, obtain financial compensation, evade criminal prosecution, and obtain drugs.[2]

Mania (monopolar) — *see* Affective psychosis, manic type

Manic-depressive psychosis
  circular type — *see* Affective psychosis, bipolar

depressed type — *see* Affective psychosis, depressed type

manic type — *see* Affective psychosis, manic type

mixed type — *see* Affective psychosis, mixed type

Manic disorder — *see* Affective psychosis, manic type
  atypical — *see* Affective psychosis, manic type, atypical

Masochistic personality — *see* Personality disorder, masochistic type

Melancholia — *see* Affective psychoses
  involutional — *see* Affective psychosis, depressed type

Mental retardation – A condition of arrested or incomplete development of mind which is especially characterized by subnormality of intelligence. The coding should be made on the individual's *current* level of functioning *without regard to its nature* or causation, such as psychosis, cultural deprivation, Down's syndrome, etc. Where there is a specific cognitive handicap — such as in speech — the diagnosis of mental retardation should be based on assessments of cognition *outside the area of specific handicap*. The assessment of intellectual level should be based on whatever information is available, including clinical evidence, adaptive behavior, and psychometric findings. The IQ levels given are based on a test with a mean of 100 and a standard deviation of 15, such as the Wechsler scales. They are provided only as a guide and should not be applied rigidly. Mental retardation often involves psychiatric disturbances and may often develop as a result of some physical disease or injury. In these cases, an additional diagnosis should be recorded to identify any associated condition, psychiatric or physical.[1]

mild mental retardation – IQ criteria 50–70. Individuals with this level of retardation are usually educable. During the preschool period they can develop social and communication skills, have minimal retardation in sensorimotor areas, and often are not distinguished from normal children until a later age. During the school age period they can learn academic skills up to approximately the sixth-grade level. During the adult years, they can usually achieve social and vocational skills adequate for minimum self-support, but may need guidance and assistance when under social or economic stress.[1]

moderate mental retardation – IQ criteria 35–49. Individuals with this level of retardation are usually trainable. During the preschool period they can talk or learn to communicate. They have poor social awareness and fair motor development. During the school age period they can profit from training in social and occupational skills, but are unlikely to progress beyond the second-grade level in academic subjects. During their adult years they may achieve self-maintenance in unskilled or semi-skilled work under sheltered conditions. They need supervision and guidance when under mild social or economic stress.[2]

severe mental retardation – IQ criteria 20–34. Individuals with this level of retardation evidence poor motor development, minimal speech, and are generally unable to profit from training and self-help during the preschool period. During the school age period they can talk or learn to communicate, can be trained in elementary health habits, and may profit from systematic habit training. During the adult years they may contribute partially to self-maintenance under complete supervision.[2]

profound mental retardation – IQ criteria under 20. Individuals with this level of retardation evidence minimal capacity for sensorimotor functioning and need nursing care during the preschool period. During the school age period some further motor development may occur, and they may respond to minimal or limited training in self-help. During the adult years some motor and speech development may occur, and they may achieve very limited self-care and need nursing care.[2]

Merycism — *see* Rumination, psychogenic

Minimal brain dysfunction [MBD] — *see* Hyperkinetic syndrome of childhood

Misery and unhappiness disorder – An emotional disorder characteristic of childhood in which the main symptoms involve misery and unhappiness. There may also be eating and sleep disturbances.

Mood swings (brief compensatory) (rebound) – Mild disorders of mood (depression and anxiety or elation and excitement, occurring alternatingly or episodically) seen in affective psychosis.[1]

Motor tic disorders — *see* Tics

Motor-verbal tic disorder — *see* Gilles de la Tourette's disorder under Tics

Multi-infarct dementia or psychosis — *see* Arteriosclerotic dementia

Multiple operations syndrome — *see* Munchausen syndrome

Multiple personality – A form of dissociative hysteria in which there is the domination of the individual at any one time by one of two or more distinct personalities. Each personality is a fully-integrated and complex unit with memories, behavior patterns, and social friendships which determine the nature of the individual's acts when uppermost in consciousness.[2]

Munchausen syndrome – A chronic form of factitious illness in which the individual demonstrates a plausible presentation of voluntarily produced physical symptomatology of such a degree that he is able to obtain and sustain multiple hospitalizations.[2]

Narcissistic personality — *see* Personality disorder, narcissistic type

Nervous debility — *see* Neurasthenia under Neurotic disorders

Neurasthenia — *see* Neurasthenia under Neurotic disorders

Neurotic delinquency — *see* Mixed disturbance of conduct and emotions under Conduct disorders

Neurotic disorders – Neurotic disorders are mental disorders without any demonstrable organic basis in which the individual may have considerable insight and has unimpaired reality testing, in that he usually does not confuse his morbid subjective experiences and fantasies with external reality. Behavior may be greatly affected although usually remaining within socially acceptable limits, but personality is not disorganized. The principal manifestations include excessive anxiety, hysterical symptoms, phobias, obsessional and compulsive symptoms, and depression.[1]

anxiety states – Various combinations of physical and mental manifestations of anxiety, not attributable to real danger and occurring either in attacks [*see* Anxiety state, panic attacks] or as a persisting state [*see* Anxiety state, generalized]. The anxiety is usually diffuse and may extend to panic. Other neurotic features such as obsessional or hysterical symptoms may be present but do not dominate the clinical picture.[1]

compensation neurosis – Certain unconscious neurotic reactions in which features of secondary gain, such as a situational or financial advantage, are prominent.[3]

depersonalization – A neurotic disorder with an unpleasant state of disturbed perception in which external objects or parts of one's own body are experienced as changed in their quality, unreal, remote, or automatized. The patient is aware of the subjective nature of the change he experiences. If depersonalization occurs as a feature of anxiety, schizophrenia, or other mental disorder, the condition is classified according to the major psychiatric disorder.[1]

depression – A neurotic disorder characterized by disproportionate depression which has usually recognizably ensued on a distressing experience; it does not include among its features delusions or hallucinations, and there is often preoccupation with the psychic trauma which preceded the illness, e.g., loss of a cherished person or possession. Anxiety is also frequently present and mixed states of anxiety and depression should be included here. The distinction between depressive neurosis and psychosis should be made not only upon the degree of depression but also on the presence or absence of other neurotic and psychotic characteristics, and upon the degree of disturbance of the individual's behavior.[1]

hypochondriasis – A neurotic disorder in which the conspicuous features are excessive concern with one's health in general or the integrity and functioning of some part of one's body, or less frequently, one's mind. It is usually associated with anxiety and depression. It may occur as a feature of some other severe mental disorder (e.g., manic-depressive psychosis, depressed type, schizophrenia, hysteria) and in that case should be classified according to the corresponding major disorder.[1]

hysteria – A neurotic mental disorder in which motives, of which the patient seems unaware, produce either a restriction of the field of consciousness or disturbances of motor or sensory function which may seem to have psychological advantage or symbolic value.[1] There are three subtypes –

conversion type – The chief or only symptoms of the hysterical neurosis consist of psychogenic disturbance of function in some part of the body, e.g., paralysis, tremor, blindness, deafness, seizures.[1]

dissociative type – The most prominent feature of the hysterical neurosis is a narrowing of the field of consciousness which seems to serve an unconscious purpose and is commonly accompanied or followed by a selective amnesia. There may be dramatic but essentially superficial changes of personality [multiple personality], or sometimes the patient enters into a wandering state [fugue].[1]

factitious illness – Physical or psychological symptoms that are not real, genuine, or natural, which are produced by the individual and are under his voluntary control.[2]

neurasthenia – A neurotic disorder characterized by fatigue, irritability, headache, depression, insomnia, difficulty in concentration, and lack of capacity for enjoyment [anhedonia]. It may follow or accompany an infection or exhaustion, or arise from continued emotional stress. If neurasthenia is associated with a physical disorder, the latter should also be recorded as a diagnosis.[1]

obsessive-compulsive – States in which the outstanding symptom is a feeling of subjective compulsion, which must be resisted, to carry out some action, to dwell on an idea, to recall an experience, or to ruminate on an abstract topic. Unwanted thoughts which intrude, the insistency of words or ideas, ruminations or trains of thought are perceived by the individual to be inappropriate or nonsensical. The obsessional urge or idea is recognized as alien to the personality but as coming from within the self. Obsessional actions may be quasi-ritual performances designed to relieve anxiety, e.g., washing the hands to cope with contamination. Attempts to dispel the unwelcome thoughts or urges may lead to a severe inner struggle, with intense anxiety.[1]

occupational – A neurosis characterized by a functional disorder of a group of muscles used chiefly in one's occupation, marked by the occurrence of spasm, paresis, or incoordination on attempt to repeat the habitual movements (e.g., writer's cramp).[5]

phobic disorders – Neurotic states with abnormally intense dread of certain objects or specific situations which would not normally have that effect. If the anxiety tends to spread from a specified situation or object to a wider range of circumstances, it becomes

akin to or identical with anxiety state and should be classified as such.[1] *See also* Phobia.

somatization disorder – A chronic, but fluctuating, neurotic disorder which begins early in life and is characterized by recurrent and multiple somatic complaints for which medical attention is sought but which are not apparently due to any physical illness. Complaints are presented in a dramatic, vague, or exaggerated way, or are part of a complicated medical history in which often many specific diagnoses have allegedly been made by other physicians. Complaints invariably refer to many organ systems (headache, fatigue, palpitations, fainting, nausea and vomiting, abdominal pains, bowel trouble, allergies, menstrual and sexual difficulties), and the individual frequently receives medical care from a number of physicians, sometimes simultaneously.[2]

Neurosis — *see* Neurotic disorders

Nightmares – Anxiety attacks occurring in dreams during REM sleep.[2]

Night terrors – A pathology of arousal from stage 4 sleep in which the individual experiences excessive terror and extreme panic (screaming, verbalizations), symptoms of autonomic activity, confusion, and poor recall for event.[2]

Nymphomania – Abnormal and excessive need or desire in the woman for sexual intercourse.[3]

Obsessional personality — *see* Personality disorder, compulsive type

Occupational neurosis — *see* Neurotic disorder, occupational

Oneirophrenia — *see* Schizophrenia, acute episode

Oppositional disorder of childhood or adolescence – A disorder characterized by pervasive opposition to all in authority regardless of self-interest, a continuous argumentativeness, and an unwillingness to respond to reasonable persuasion, not accounted for by a conduct disorder, adjustment disorder, or a psychosis of childhood. The oppositional behavior in this disorder is evoked by any demand, rule, suggestion, request, or admonishment placed on the individual.[2]

Organic affective syndrome – A clinical picture in which the predominating symptoms closely resemble those seen in either the depressive or manic affective disorders, occurring in the presence of evidence or history of a specific organic factor which is etiologically related to the disturbance, such as head trauma, endocranial tumors, and exocranial tumors secreting neurotoxic diatheses (e.g., pancreatic carcinoma). Excessive use of steroids, Cushing's syndrome, and other endocrine disorders may lead to an organic affective syndrome.[2]

Organic personality syndrome – Chronic, mild states of memory disturbance and intellectual deterioration, of nonpsychotic nature, often accompanied by increased irritability, querulousness, lassitude, and complaints of physical weakness. These states are often associated with old age, and may precede more severe states due to brain damage classifiable under senile or presenile dementia, dementia associated with other chronic organic psychotic brain syndromes, or delirium, delusions, hallucinosis, and depression in transient organic psychotic conditions.[1]

Organic psychosyndrome, focal (partial) – A nonpsychotic organic mental disorder resembling the postconcussion syndrome associated with localized diseases of the brain or surrounding tissues.[1]

Organic psychotic conditions – Syndromes in which there is impairment of orientation, memory, comprehension, calculation, learning capacity, and judgment. These are the essential features but there may also be shallowness or lability of affect, or a more persistent disturbance of mood, lowering of ethical standards and exaggeration or emergence of personality traits, and diminished capacity for independent decision.[1] See also Alcohol psychoses, Arteriosclerotic dementia, Drug psychoses, Presenile dementia, and Senile dementia.

mixed paranoid and affective – Organic psychosis in which depressive and paranoid symptoms are the main features.[1]

transient – States characterized by clouded consciousness, confusion, disorientation, illusions, and often vivid hallucinations. They are usually due to some intra- or extracerebral toxic, infectious, metabolic or other systemic disturbance and are generally reversible. Depressive and paranoid symptoms may also be present but are not the main feature. The diagnosis of the associated physical or neurological condition should also be recorded.[1]

acute delirium – Short-lived states, lasting hours or days, of the above type.[1]

subacute delirium – States of the above type in which the symptoms, usually less florid, last for several weeks or longer during which they may show marked fluctuations in intensity.[1]

Organic reaction — see Organic psychotic conditions, transient

Overanxious disorder – An ill-defined emotional disorder characteristic of childhood in which the main symptoms involve anxiety and fearfulness.[1]

Panic disorder — see Panic attack under Anxiety state

Paranoia – A rare chronic psychosis in which logically constructed systematized delusions have developed gradually without concomitant hallucinations or the schizophrenic type of disordered thinking. The delusions are mostly of grandeur (the paranoiac prophet or inventor), persecution, or somatic abnormality.[1]

alcoholic — see Alcoholic jealousy under Alcoholic psychoses

querulans – A paranoid state which, though in many ways akin to schizophrenic or affective states, differs from other paranoid states and psychogenic paranoid psychosis.[1]

senile — see Paraphrenia

Paranoid personality — see Personality disorder, paranoid type

Paranoid reaction, acute – Paranoid states apparently provoked by some emotional stress. The stress is often misconstrued as an attack or threat. Such states are particularly prone to occur in prisoners or as acute reactions to a strange and threatening environment, e.g., in immigrants.[1]

Paranoid schizophrenia — see Schizophrenia, paranoid type

Paranoid state

involutional — see Paraphrenia

senile — see Paraphrenia

simple – A psychosis, acute or chronic, not classifiable as schizophrenia or affective psychosis, in which delusions, especially of being influenced, persecuted, or treated in some special way, are the main symptoms. The delusions are of a fairly fixed, elaborate, and systematized kind.[1]

Paranoid traits — see Personality disorder, paranoid type

Paraphilia — see Sexual deviations

Paraphrenia – Paranoid psychosis in which there are conspicuous hallucinations, often in several modalities. Affective symptoms and disordered thinking, if present, do not dominate the clinical picture, and the personality is well preserved.[1]

Paraphrenic schizophrenia — see Schizophrenia, paranoid type

Passive-aggressive personality — see Personality disorder, passive-aggressive type

Passive personality — see Personality disorder, dependent type

Pathological

alcohol intoxication — see Alcohol intoxication, idiosyncratic

drug intoxication – Individual idiosyncratic reactions to comparatively small quantities of a drug, which take the form of acute, brief psychotic states of any type.[1]

drunkenness — see Alcohol intoxication, idiosyncratic

gambling – A disorder of impulse control characterized by a chronic and progressive preoccupation with gambling and urge to gamble, with subsequent gambling behavior that compromises, disrupts, or damages personal, family, and vocational pursuits.[2]

personality — see Personality disorder

Pedophilia – Sexual deviations in which an adult engages in sexual activity with a child of the same or opposite sex.[1]

Peregrinating patient — see Malingering

Personality disorders – Deeply ingrained maladaptive patterns of behavior generally recognizable by the time of adolescence or earlier and continuing throughout most of adult life, although often becoming less obvious in middle or old age. The personality is abnormal either in the balance of its components, their quality and expression, or in its total aspect. Because of this deviation or psychopathy the patient suffers or others have to suffer, and there is an adverse effect upon the individual or on society. It includes what is sometimes called psychopathic personality, but if this is determined primarily by malfunctioning of the brain, it should be classified as one of the nonpsychotic organic brain syndromes. When the patient exhibits an anomaly of personali-

ty directly related to his neurosis or psychosis, e.g., schizoid personality and schizophrenia or anancastic personality and obsessive compulsive neurosis, the relevant neurosis or psychosis which is in evidence should be diagnosed in addition.[1]

affective type – A chronic personality disorder characterized by lifelong predominance of a pronounced mood. The illness does not have a clear onset, and there may be intermittent periods of disturbed mood separated by periods of normal mood.[1]

anancastic [anankastic] type — see Personality disorder, compulsive type

antisocial type – A personality disorder characterized by disregard for social obligations, lack of feeling for others, and impetuous violence or callous unconcern. There is a gross disparity between behavior and the prevailing social norms. Behavior is not readily modifiable by experience, including punishment. People with this personality are often affectively cold, and may be abnormally aggressive or irresponsible. Their tolerance to frustration is low; they blame others or offer plausible rationalizations for the behavior which brings them into conflict with society.[1]

asthenic type — see Personality disorder, dependent type

avoidant type – Individuals with this disorder exhibit excessive social inhibitions and shyness, a tendency to withdraw from opportunities for developing close relationships, and a fearful expectation that they will be belittled and humiliated. Desires for affection and acceptance are strong, but they are unwilling to enter relationships unless given unusually strong guarantees that they will be uncritically accepted. Therefore, they have few close relationships and suffer from feelings of loneliness and isolation.[2]

borderline type – Individuals with this disorder are characterized by instability in a variety of areas, including interpersonal relationships, behavior, mood, and self image. Interpersonal relationships are often intense and unstable with marked shifts of attitude over time. Frequently there is impulsive and unpredictable behavior which is potentially physically self-damaging. There may be problems tolerating being alone, and chronic feelings of emptiness or boredom.[2]

chronic depressive type – An affective personality disorder characterized by lifelong predominance of a chronic nonpsychotic disturbance involving either intermittent or sustained periods of depressed mood (marked by worry, pessimism, low output of energy, and a sense of futility).[2]

chronic hypomanic type – An affective personality disorder characterized by lifelong predominance of a chronic nonpsychotic disturbance involving either intermittent or sustained periods of abnormally elevated mood (unshakable optimism and an enhanced zest for life and activity).[2]

compulsive type – A personality disorder characterized by feelings of personal insecurity, doubt, and incompleteness leading to excessive conscientiousness, checking, stubbornness, and caution. There may be insistent and unwelcome thoughts or impulses which do not attain the severity of an obsessional neurosis. There is perfectionism and meticulous accuracy and a need to check repeatedly in an attempt to ensure this. Rigidity and excessive doubt may be conspicuous.[1]

cyclothymic type – A chronic nonpsychotic disturbance involving depressed and elevated mood, lasting at least two years, separated by periods of normal mood.[2]

dependent type – A personality disorder characterized by passive compliance with the wishes of elders and others and a weak inadequate response to the demands of daily life. Lack of vigor may show itself in the intellectual or emotional spheres; there is little capacity for enjoyment.[1]

eccentric type – A personality disorder characterized by oddities of behavior which do not conform to the clinical syndromes of personality disorders described elsewhere.[2]

explosive type – A personality disorder characterized by instability of mood with liability to intemperate outbursts of anger, hate, violence, or affection. Aggression may be expressed in words or in physical violence. The outbursts cannot readily be controlled by the affected persons, who are not otherwise prone to antisocial behavior.[1]

histrionic type – A personality disorder characterized by shallow, labile affectivity, dependence on others, craving for appreciation and attention, suggestibility, and theatricality. There is often sexual immaturity, e.g., frigidity and over-responsiveness to stimuli. Under stress hysterical symptoms [neurosis] may develop.[1]

hysterical type — *see* Personality disorder, histrionic type

inadequate type — *see* Personality disorder, dependent type

introverted type – A form of schizoid personality in which the essential features are a profound defect in the ability to form social relationships and to respond to the usual forms of social reinforcements. Such patients are characteristically "loners" who do not appear distressed by their social distance and are not interested in greater social involvement.[2]

masochistic type – A personality disorder in which the individual appears to arrange life situations so as to be defeated and humiliated.[2]

narcissistic type – A personality disorder in which interpersonal difficulties are caused by an inflated sense of self-worth, and indifference to the welfare of others. Achievement deficits and social irresponsibilities are justified and sustained by a boastful arrogance, expansive fantasies, facile rationalization, and frank prevarication.[2]

paranoid type – A personality disorder in which there is excessive sensitiveness to setbacks or to what are taken to be humiliations and rebuffs, a tendency to distort experience by misconstruing the neutral or friendly actions of others as hostile or contemptuous, and a combative and tenacious sense of personal rights. There may be a proneness to jealousy or excessive self-importance. Such persons may feel helplessly humiliated and put upon; others, likewise excessively sensitive, are aggressive and insistent. In all cases there is excessive self-reference.[1]

passive-aggressive type – A personality disorder characterized by aggressive behavior manifested in passive ways, such as obstructionism, pouting, procrastination, intentional inefficiency, or stubbornness. The *aggression* often arises from resentment at failing to find gratification in a relationship with an individual or institution upon which the individual is overdependent.[3]

passive type — *see* Personality disorder, dependent type

schizoid type – A personality disorder in which there is withdrawal from affectional, social, and other contacts with autistic preference for fantasy and introspective reserve. Behavior may be slightly eccentric or indicate avoidance of competitive situations. Apparent coolness and detachment may mask an incapacity to express feeling.[1]

schizotypal type – A form of schizoid personality in which individuals with this disorder manifest various oddities of thinking, perception, communication, and behavior. The disturbance in thinking may be expressed as magical thinking, ideas of reference, or paranoid ideation. Perceptual disturbances may include recurrent illusions and derealization [depersonalization]. Frequently, but not invariably, the behavioral manifestations include social isolation and constricted or inappropriate affect which interferes with rapport in face-to-face interaction without any of the frank psychotic features which characterize schizophrenia.[2]

Phobia – Neurotic states with abnormally intense dread of certain objects or specific situations which would not normally have that effect. If the anxiety tends to spread from a specified situation or object to a wider range of circumstances, it becomes akin to or identical with anxiety state, and should be classified as such.[1]

acrophobia – Fear of heights[3]

agoraphobia – Fear of leaving the familiar setting of the home, and is almost always preceded by a phase during which there are recurrent panic attacks. Because of the anticipatory fear of helplessness when having a panic attack, the patient is reluctant or refuses to be alone, travel or walk alone, or to be in situations where there is no ready access to help, such as in crowds, closed or open spaces, or crowded stores.[2]

ailurophobia – Fear of cats[3]

algophobia – Fear of pain[3]

claustrophobia – Fear of closed spaces[3]

isolated phobia — *see* Simple phobia below

mysophobia – Fear of dirt or germs[3]

obsessional — *see* Neurotic disorder, obsessive-compulsive

panphobia – Fear of everything[3]

simple phobia – Fear of a discrete object or situation which is neither fear of leaving the familiar setting of the home [agoraphobia], or of being observed by others in certain situations [social phobia]. Examples of simple phobia are fear of animals, acrophobia, and claustrophobia.[2]

social phobia – Fear of situations in which the subject is exposed to possible scrutiny by others, and the possibility exists that he may act in a fashion that will be considered shameful. The most common social phobias are fears of public speaking, blushing, eating in public, writing in front of others, or using public lavatories.[2]

xenophobia – Fear of strangers[3]

Pica – Perverted appetite of nonorganic origin in which there is persistent eating of non-nutritional substances. Typically, infants ingest paint, plaster, string, hair, or cloth. Older children may have access to animal droppings, sand, bugs, leaves, or pebbles. In the adult, eating of starch or clay-earth has been observed.[2]

Postconcussion syndrome – States occurring after generalized contusion of the brain, in which the symptom picture may resemble that of the frontal lobe syndrome or that of any of the neurotic disorders, but in which in addition, headache, giddiness, fatigue, insomnia, and a subjective feeling of impaired intellectual ability are usually prominent. Mood may fluctuate, and quite ordinary stress may produce exaggerated fear and apprehension. There may be marked intolerance of mental and physical exertion, undue sensitivity to noise, and hypochondriacal preoccupation. The symptoms are more common in persons who have previously suffered from neurotic or personality disorders, or when there is a possibility of compensation. This syndrome is particularly associated with the closed type of head injury when signs of localized brain damage are slight or absent, but it may also occur in other conditions.[1]

Postcontusion syndrome or encephalopathy — *see* Postconcussion syndrome

Postencephalitic syndrome – A nonpsychotic organic mental disorder resembling the postconcussion syndrome associated with central nervous system infections.[1]

Postleucotomy syndrome — *see* Frontal lobe syndrome

Posttraumatic brain syndrome, nonpsychotic — *see* Postconcussion syndrome

Posttraumatic organic psychosis — *see* Organic psychotic conditions, transient

Posttraumatic stress disorder – The development of characteristic symptoms (re-experiencing the traumatic event, numbing of responsiveness to or involvement with the external world, and a variety of other autonomic, dysphoric, or cognitive symptoms) after experiencing a psychologically traumatic event or events outside the normal range of human experience (e.g., rape or assault, military combat, natural catastrophes such as flood or earthquake, or other disaster, such as airplane crash, fires, bombings).[2]

acute – Brief, episodic, or recurrent disorders lasting less than six months' duration after the onset of trauma.[2]

prolonged – Chronic disorders of the above type lasting six months or more following the trauma.[2]

Premature ejaculation — *see* Premature ejaculation under Psychosexual dysfunctions

Prepsychotic schizophrenia — *see* Schizophrenia, latent

Presbyophrenia — *see* Organic personality syndrome

Presenile dementia – Dementia occurring usually before the age of 65 in patients with the relatively rare forms of diffuse or lobar cerebral atrophy. The associated neurological condition (e.g., Alzheimer's disease, Pick's disease, Jakob-Creutzfeldt disease) should also be recorded as a diagnosis.[1]

Prodromal schizophrenia — *see* Schizophrenia, latent

Pseudoneurotic schizophrenia — *see* Schizophrenia, latent

Psychalgia – Pains of mental origin, e.g., headache or backache, for which a more precise medical or psychiatric diagnosis cannot be made.[1]

Psychasthenia – A functioning neurosis marked by stages of pathological fear or anxiety, obsessions, fixed ideas, tics, feelings of inadequacy, self-accusation, and pecular feelings of strangeness, unreality, and depersonalization.[4]

Psychic shock – A sudden disturbance of mental equilibrium produced by strong emotion in response to physical or mental stress.[4]

Psychic factors associated with physical diseases – Mental disturbances or psychic factors of any type thought to have played a major part in the etiology of physical conditions, usually involving tissue damage, classified elsewhere. The mental disturbance is usually mild and nonspecific, and the psychic factors (worry, fear, conflict, etc.) may be present without any overt psychiatric disorder. Examples of these conditions are asthma, dermatitis, eczema, duodenal ulcer, ulcerative colitis, and urticaria, specified as due to psychogenic factors. Use an additional diagnosis to identify the physical condition. In the rare instance that an overt psychiatric disorder is thought to have caused the physical condition, the psychiatric diagnosis should be recorded in addition.[1]

Psychoneurosis — *see* Neurotic disorders

Psycho-organic syndrome — *see* Organic psychotic conditions, transient

Psychopathic constitutional state — *see* Personality disorders

Psychopathic personality — *see* Personality disorders

Psychophysiological disorders – A variety of physical symptoms or types of physiological malfunctions of mental origin, not involving tissue damage, and usually mediated through the autonomic nervous system. The disorders are classified according to the body system involved. If the physical symptom is secondary to a psychiatric disorder classifiable elsewhere, the physical symptom is not classified as a psychophysiological disorder. If tissue damage is involved, then the diagnosis is classified as a *Psychic factor associated with diseases classified elsewhere.*[1]

Psychosexual dysfunctions – A group of disorders in which there is recurrent and persistent dysfunction encountered during sexual activity. The dysfunction may be lifelong or acquired, generalized or situational, and total or partial.[2]

functional dyspareunia – Recurrent and persistent genital pain associated with coitus.[2]

functional vaginismus – A history of recurrent and persistent involuntary spasm of the musculature of the outer one-third of the vagina that interferes with sexual activity.[2]

inhibited female orgasm – Recurrent and persistent inhibition of the female orgasm as manifested by a delay or absence of orgasm following a normal sexual excitement phase during sexual activity.[2]

inhibited male orgasm – Recurrent and persistent inhibition of the male orgasm as manifested by a delay or absence of either the emission or ejaculation phases, or more usually, both following an adequate phase of sexual excitement.[2]

inhibited sexual desire – Persistent inhibition of desire for engaging in a particular form of sexual activity.[2]

inhibited sexual excitement – Recurrent and persistent inhibition of sexual excitement during sexual activity, manifested either by partial or complete failure to attain or maintain erection until completion of the sexual act [impotence], or partial or complete failure to attain or maintain the lubrication-swelling response of sexual excitement until completion of the sexual act [frigidity].[2]

premature ejaculation – Ejaculation occurs before the individual wishes it, because of recurrent and persistent absence of reasonable voluntary control of ejaculation and orgasm during sexual activity.[2]

Psychosexual gender identity disorders – Behavior occurring in preadolescents of immature psychosexuality, or in adults, in which there is an incongruence between the individual's anatomic sex and gender identity.[2]

gender identity disorder – In children or in adults a condition in which the individual would prefer to be of the other sex, and strongly prefers the clothes, toys, activities, and companionship of the other sex. Cross-dressing is intermittent, although it may be frequent. In children the commonest form is feminism in boys.[2]

trans-sexualism – A psychosexual identity disorder centered around fixed beliefs that the overt bodily sex is wrong. The resulting behavior is directed towards either changing the sexual organs by operation, or completely concealing the bodily sex by adopting both the dress and behavior of the opposite sex.[1]

Psychosomatic disorders — *see* Psychophysiological disorders

Psychosis – Mental disorders in which impairment of mental function has developed to a degree that interferes grossly with insight, ability to meet some ordinary demands of life or to maintain adequate contact with reality. It is not an exact or well defined term. Mental retardation is excluded.[1]

affective — *see* Affective psychoses

alcoholic — *see* Alcoholic psychoses

atypical childhood – A variety of atypical infantile psychoses which may show some, but not all, of the features of infantile autism. Symptoms may include stereotyped repetitive movements, hyperkinesis, self-injury, retarded speech development, echolalia, and impaired social relationships. Such disorders may occur in children of any level of intelligence but are particularly common in those with mental retardation.[1]

borderline, of childhood — *see* Psychosis, atypical childhood

child – A group of disorders in children, characterized by distortions in the timing, rate, and sequence of many psychological functions involving language development and social relations in which the severe qualitative abnormalities are not normal for any stage of development.[2] *See also* Autism, infantile, Psychosis, disintegrative, Psychosis, atypical childhood.

depressive — *see* Affective psychosis, depressed type

depressive type – A depressive psychosis which can be similar in its symptoms to manic-depressive psychosis, depressed type but is apparently provoked by saddening stress such as a bereavement, or a severe disappointment or frustration. There may be less diurnal variation of symptoms than in manic-depressive psychosis, depressed type, and the delusions are more often understandable in the context of the life experiences. There is usually a serious disturbance of behavior, e.g., major suicidal attempt.[1]

disintegrative – A disorder in which normal or near-normal development for the first few years is followed by a loss of social skills and of speech, together with a severe disorder of emotions, behavior, and relationships. Usually this loss of speech and of social competence takes place over a period of a few months and is accompanied by the emergence of overactivity and of stereotypies. In most cases there is intellectual impairment, but this is not a necessary part of the disorder. The condition may follow overt brain disease, such as measles encephalitis, but it may also occur in the absence of any known organic brain disease or damage. Any associated neurological disorder should also be recorded.[1]

epileptic – An organic psychotic condition associated with epilepsy.[1]

excitative type – An affective psychosis similar in its symptoms to manic-depressive psychosis, manic type, but apparently provoked by emotional stress.[1]

hypomanic — *see* Affective psychosis, manic type

hysterical — *see* Psychosis, reactive
   acute — *see* Psychosis, excitative type

induced — *see* Shared paranoid disorder

infantile — *see* Autism, infantile

infective — *see* Organic psychotic conditions, transient

Korsakoff's
   alcoholic — *see* alcohol amnestic syndrome under Alcoholic psychoses
   nonalcoholic — *see* Amnestic syndrome

manic-depressive — *see* Affective psychoses

multi-infarct — *see* Arteriosclerotic dementia

paranoid
   chronic — *see* Paranoia
   protracted reactive — *see* Psychosis, paranoid, psychogenic
   psychogenic – Psychogenic or reactive paranoid psychosis of any type which is more protracted than the reactions described under Paranoid reaction, acute.[1]
     acute — *see* Paranoid reaction, acute

postpartum — *see* Psychosis, puerperal

psychogenic — *see* Psychosis, reactive
   depressive — *see* Psychosis, depressive type

puerperal – Any psychosis occurring within a fixed period (approximately 90 days) after childbirth.[3] The diagnosis should be classified according to the predominant symptoms or characteristics, such as schizophrenia, affective psychosis, paranoid states, or other specified psychosis.

reactive – A psychotic condition which is largely or entirely attributable to a recent life experience. This diagnosis is not used for the wider range of psychoses in which environmental factors play some, but not the *major*, part in etiology.[1]
   brief – A florid psychosis of at least a few hours' duration but lasting no more than two weeks, with sudden onset immediately following a severe environmental stress and eventually terminating in complete recovery to the pre-psychotic state.[2]
   confusion – Mental disorders with clouded consciousness, disorientation (though less marked than in organic confusion), and diminished accessibility often accompanied by excessive activity and apparently provoked by emotional stress.[1]
   depressive — *see* Psychosis, depressive type
   schizo-affective — *see* Schizophrenia, schizo-affective type

schizophrenic — *see* Schizophrenia

schizophreniform — *see* Schizophrenia
   affective type — *see* Schizophrenia, schizo-affective type
   confusional type — *see* Schizophrenia, acute episode
   senile — *see* Senile dementia, delusional type

Pyromania – A disorder of impulse control characterized by a recurrent failure to resist impulses to set fires without regard for the consequences, or with deliberate destructive intent. Invariably there is intense fascination with the setting of fires, seeing fires burn, and a satisfaction with the resultant destruction.[2]

Relationship problems of childhood – Emotional disorders characteristic of childhood in which the main symptoms involve relationship problems.[1]

Repeated infarct dementia — *see* Arteriosclerotic dementia

Residual schizophrenia — *see* Schizophrenia, residual type

Restzustand (schizophrenia) — *see* Schizophrenia, residual type

Rumination
   obsessional – The constant preoccupation with certain thoughts, with inability to dismiss them from the mind.[4] *See* Neurotic disorder, obsessive-compulsive.
   psychogenic – In children the regurgitation of food, with failure to thrive or weight loss developing after a period of normal functioning. Food is brought up without nausea, retching, or disgust. The food is then ejected from the mouth, or chewed and reswallowed.[2]

Sander's disease — *see* Paranoia

Satyriasis – Pathologic or exaggerated sexual desire or excitement in the man.[3]

Schizoid personality disorder — *see* Personality disorder, schizoid type

Schizophrenia – A group of psychoses in which there is a fundamental disturbance of personality, a characteristic distortion of thinking, often a sense of being controlled by alien forces, delusions which may be bizarre, disturbed perception, abnormal affect out of keeping with the real situation, and autism. Nevertheless, clear consciousness and intellectual capacity are usually maintained. The disturbance of personality involves its most basic functions which give the normal person his feeling of individuality, uniqueness, and self-direction. The most intimate thoughts, feelings, and acts are often felt to be known to or shared by others and explanatory delusions may develop, to the effect that natural or supernatural forces are at work to influence the schizophrenic person's thoughts and actions in ways that are often bizarre. He may see himself as the pivot of all that happens. Hallucinations, especially of hearing, are common and may comment on the patient or address him. Perception is frequently disturbed in other ways; there may be perplexity, irrelevant features may become all-important and accompanied by passivity feelings, may lead the patient to believe that everyday objects and situations possess a special, usually sinister, meaning intended for him. In the characteristic schizophrenic disturbance of thinking, peripheral and irrelevant features of a total concept, which are inhibited in normal directed mental activity, are brought to the forefront and utilized in place of the elements relevant and appropriate to the situation. Thus, thinking becomes vague, elliptical and obscure, and its expression in speech sometimes incomprehensible. Breaks and interpolations in the flow of consecutive thought are frequent, and the patient may be convinced that his thoughts are being withdrawn by some outside agency. Mood may be shallow, capricious, or incongruous. Ambivalence and disturbance of volition may appear as inertia, negativism, or stupor. Catatonia may be present. The diagnosis "schizophrenia" should not be made unless there is, or has been evident during the same illness, characteristic disturbance of thought, perception, mood, conduct, or personality — preferably in at least two of these areas. The diagnosis should not be restricted to conditions running a protracted, deteriorating, or chronic course. In addition to making the diagnosis on the criteria just given, effort should be made to specify one of the following subtypes of schizophrenia, according to the predominant symptoms.[1]

   acute (undifferentiated) – Schizophrenia of florid nature which cannot be classified as simple, catatonic, hebephrenic, paranoid, or any other types.[1]

   acute episode – Schizophrenic disorders, other than simple, hebephrenic, catatonic, and paranoid, in which there is a dream-like state with slight clouding of consciousness and perplexity. External things, people, and events may become charged with personal significance for the patient. There may be ideas of reference and emotional turmoil. In many such cases remission occurs within a few weeks or months, even without treatment.[1]

   atypical — *see* Schizophrenia, acute (undifferentiated)

   borderline — *see* Schizophrenia, latent

   catatonic type – Includes as an essential feature prominent psychomotor disturbances often alternating between extremes such as hyperkinesis and stupor, or automatic obedience and negativism. Constrained attitudes may be maintained for long periods – if the patient's limbs are put in some unnatural position, they may be held there for some time after the external force has been removed. Severe excitement may be a striking feature of the condition. Depressive or hypomanic concomitants may be present.[1]

   cenesthopathic — *see* Schizophrenia, acute (undifferentiated)

   childhood type — *see* Psychosis, child

   chronic undifferentiated — *see* Schizophrenia, residual

   cyclic — *see* Schizophrenia, schizo-affective type

   disorganized type – A form of schizophrenia in which affective changes are prominent, delusions and hallucinations fleeting and fragmentary, behavior irresponsible and unpredictable, and mannerisms common. The mood is shallow and inappropriate, accompanied by giggling or self-satisfied, self-absorbed smiling, or by a lofty manner, grimaces, mannerisms, pranks, hypochondriacal complaints, and reiterated phrases. Thought is disorganized. There is a tendency to remain solitary, and behavior seems empty of purpose and feeling. This form of schizophrenia usually starts between the ages of 15 and 25 years.[1]

hebephrenic type — *see* Schizophrenia, disorganized type

latent – It has not been possible to produce a generally acceptable description for this condition. It is not recommended for general use, but a description is provided for those who believe it to be useful – a condition of eccentric or inconsequent behavior and anomalies of affect which give the impression of schizophrenia though no definite and characteristic schizophrenic anomalies, present or past, have been manifest.[1]

paranoid type – The form of schizophrenia in which relatively stable delusions, which may be accompanied by hallucinations, dominate the clinical picture. The delusions are frequently of persecution, but may take other forms (for example, of jealousy, exalted birth, Messianic mission, or bodily change). Hallucinations and erratic behavior may occur; in some cases conduct is seriously disturbed from the outset, thought disorder may be gross, and affective flattening with fragmentary delusions and hallucinations may develop.[1]

prepsychotic — *see* Schizophrenia, latent

prodromal — *see* Schizophrenia, latent

pseudoneurotic — *see* Schizophrenia, latent

pseudopsychopathic — *see* Schizophrenia, latent

residual – A chronic form of schizophrenia in which the symptoms that persist from the acute phase have mostly lost their sharpness. Emotional response is blunted and thought disorder, even when gross, does not prevent the accomplishment of routine work.[1]

schizo-affective type – A psychosis in which pronounced manic or depressive features are intermingled with schizophrenic features and which tends towards remission without permanent defect, but which is prone to recur. The diagnosis should be made only when both the affective and schizophrenic symptoms are pronounced.[1]

simple type – A psychosis in which there is insidious development of oddities of conduct, inability to meet the demands of society, and decline in total performance. Delusions and hallucinations are not in evidence and the condition is less obviously psychotic than are the hebephrenic, catatonic, and paranoid types of schizophrenia. With increasing social impoverishment vagrancy may ensue and the patient becomes self-absorbed, idle, and aim-

less. Because the schizophrenic symptoms are not clear-cut, diagnosis of this form should be made sparingly, if at all.[1]

simplex — *see* Schizophrenia, simple type

Schizophrenic syndrome of childhood — *see* Psychosis, child

Schizophreniform

attack — *see* Schizophrenia, acute episode

disorder — *see* Schizophrenia, acute episode

psychosis — *see* Schizophrenia

affective type — *see* Schizophrenia, schizo-affective type

confusional type — *see* Schizophrenia, acute episode

Schizotypal personality — *see* Personality disorder, schizotypal type

Senile dementia – Dementia occurring usually after the age of 65 in which any cerebral pathology other than that of senile atrophic change can be reasonably excluded.[1]

delirium – Senile dementia with a superimposed reversible episode of acute confusional state.[1]

delusional type – A type of senile dementia characterized by development in advanced old age, progressive in nature, in which delusions, varying from simple poorly formed paranoid delusions to highly formed paranoid delusional states, and hallucinations are also present.[1, 2]

depressed type – A type of senile dementia characterized by development in advanced old age, progressive in nature, in which depressive features, ranging from mild to severe forms of manic-depressive affective psychosis, are also present. Disturbance of the sleep-waking cycle and preoccupation with dead people are often particularly prominent.[1, 2]

paranoid type — *see* Senile dementia, delusional type

simple type — *see* Senile dementia

Sensitiver Beziehungswahn – A paranoid state which, though in many ways akin to schizophrenic or affective states, differs from paranoia, simple paranoid state, shared paranoid disorder, or psychogenic psychosis.[1]

Sensitivity reaction of childhood or adolescence — *see* Shyness disorder of childhood

Separation anxiety disorder – A clinical disorder in children in which the predominant disturbance is exaggerated distress at separation from parents, home, or other familial surroundings. When separation is instituted, the child may experience anxiety to the point of panic. In adults a similar disorder is seen in agoraphobic reactions.[2]

Sexual deviations – Abnormal sexual inclinations or behavior which are part of a referral problem. The limits and features of normal sexual behavior have not been stated absolutely in different societies and cultures, but are broadly such as serve approved social and biological purposes. The sexual activity of affected persons is directed primarily either towards people not of the opposite sex, or

towards sexual acts not associated with coitus normally, or towards coitus performed under abnormal circumstances. If the anomalous behavior becomes manifest only during psychosis or other mental illness the condition should be classified under the major illness. It is common for more than one anomaly to occur together in the same individual; in that case the predominant deviation is classified. It is preferable not to diagnose sexual deviation in individuals who perform deviant sexual acts when normal sexual outlets are not available to them.[1] *See also* Exhibitionism, Fetishism, Homosexuality, Nymphomania, Pedophilia, Satyriasis, Sexual masochism, Sexual sadism, Transvestism, Voyeurism, and Zoophilia. Gender identity disorder and trans-sexualism are considered to be psychosexual gender identity disorders and are not included here.

Sexual masochism – A sexual deviation in which sexual arousal and pleasure is produced in an individual by his own physical or psychological suffering, and in which there are insistent and persistent fantasies wherein sexual excitement is produced as a result of suffering.[2]

Sexual sadism – A sexual deviation in which physical or psychological suffering inflicted on another person is utilized as a method of stimulating erotic excitement and orgasm, and in which there are insistent and persistent fantasies wherein sexual excitement is produced as a result of suffering inflicted on the partner.[2]

Shared paranoid disorder – Mainly delusional psychosis, usually chronic and often without florid features, which appears to have developed as a result of a close, if not dependent, relationship with another person who already has an established similar psychosis. The delusions are at least partly shared. The rare cases in which several persons are affected should also be included here.[1]

Shifting sleep-work schedule – A sleep disorder in which the phase-shift disruption of the 24-hour sleep-wake cycle occurs due to rapid changes in the individual's work schedule.[2]

Short sleeper – Individuals who typically need only 4–6 hours of sleep within the 24-hour cycle.[2]

Shyness disorder of childhood – A persistent and excessive shrinking from familiarity or contact with all strangers of sufficient severity as to interfere with peer functioning, yet there are warm and satisfying relationships with family members. A critical feature of this disorder is that the avoidant behavior with strangers persists even after prolonged exposure or contact.[2]

Sibling jealousy or rivalry – An emotional disorder related to competition between siblings for the love of a parent or for other recognition or gain.[3]

Simple phobia — *see* Simple phobia under Phobia

Situational disturbance, acute — *see* Stress reaction, acute

Social phobia — *see* Social phobia under Phobia

Social withdrawal of childhood — *see* Introverted disorder of childhood

Socialized conduct disorder — *see* Socialized conduct disorder under Conduct disorders

Somatization disorder — *see* Somatization disorder under Neurotic disorders

Somatoform disorder, atypical — *see* Hypochondriasis under Neurotic disorders

Spasmus nutans — *see* Stereotyped repetitive movements

Specific academic or work inhibition – An adjustment reaction in which a specific academic or work inhibition occurs in an individual whose intellectual capacity, skills, and previous academic or work performance have been at least adequate, and in which the inhibition occurs despite apparent effort and is not due to any other mental disorder.[2]

Stammering — *see* Stuttering

Starch-eating — *see* Pica

Status postcommotio cerebri — *see* Postconcussion syndrome

Stereotyped repetitive movements – Disorders in which voluntary repetitive stereotyped movements, which are not due to any psychiatric or neurological condition, constitute the main feature. Includes head-banging, spasmus nutans, rocking, twirling, finger-flicking mannerisms, and eye poking. Such movements are particularly common in cases of mental retardation with sensory impairment or with environmental monotony.[1]

Stereotypies — *see* Stereotyped repetitive movements

Stress reaction
    acute – Acute transient disorders of any severity and nature of emotions, consciousness, and psychomotor states (singly or in combination) which occur in individuals, without any apparent pre-existing mental disorder, in response to exceptional physical or mental stress, such as natural catastrophe or battle, and which usually subside within hours or days.[1]
    chronic — *see* Adjustment reaction

Stupor
    catatonic — *see* Schizophrenia, catatonic type
    psychogenic — *see* Psychosis, reactive

Stuttering – Disorders in the rhythm of speech, in which the individual knows precisely what he wishes to say, but at the time is unable to say it because of an involuntary, repetitive prolongation or cessation of a sound.[1]

Subjective insomnia complaint – A complaint of insomnia made by the individual, which has not been investigated or proven.[2]

Tension headache – Headache of mental origin for which a more precise medical or psychiatric diagnosis cannot be made.[1]

Systematized delusions — *see* Paranoia

Tics – Disorders of no known organic origin in which the outstanding feature consists of quick, involuntary, apparently purposeless, and frequently repeated movements which are not due to any neurological condition. Any part of the body may be involved but the face is most frequently affected. Only one form of tic may be present, or there may be a combination of tics which are carried out simultaneously, alternatively, or consecutively.[1]
    chronic motor tic disorder – A tic disorder starting in childhood and persisting into adult life. The tic is limited to no more than three motor areas, and rarely has a verbal component.[2]
    Gilles de la Tourette's disorder [motor-verbal tic disorder] – A rare disorder occurring in individuals of any level of intelligence in which facial tics and tic-like throat noises become more marked and more generalized, and in which later whole words or short sentences (often with obscene content) are ejaculated spasmodically and involuntarily. There is some overlap with other varieties of tic.[1]
    transient tic disorder of childhood – Facial or other tics beginning in childhood, but limited to one year in duration.[2]

Tobacco use disorder – Cases in which tobacco is used to the detriment of a person's health or social functioning or in which there is tobacco dependence. Dependence is included here rather than under drug dependence because tobacco differs from other drugs of dependence in its psychotoxic effects.[1]

Tranquilizer abuse – Cases where an individual has taken the drug to the detriment of his health or social functioning, in doses above or for periods beyond those normally regarded as therapeutic.[1]

Transient organic psychotic condition — *see* Organic psychotic conditions, transient

Trans-sexualism — *see* Trans-sexualism under Psychosexual identity disorders

Transvestism – Sexual deviation in which there is recurrent and persistent dressing in clothes of the opposite sex, and initially in the early stage of the illness, for the purpose of sexual arousal.[2]

Twilight state
    confusional — *see* Delirium, acute
    psychogenic — *see* Psychosis, reactive confusion

Undersocialized conduct disorder — *see* Undersocialized conduct disorder under Conduct disorders

Unsocialized aggressive disorder — *see* Undersocialized conduct disorder, aggressive type under Conduct disorders

Vaginismus, functional — *see* Functional vaginismus under Psychosexual dysfunctions

Vorbeireden – The symptom of the approximate answer or talking past the point, seen in the Ganser syndrome, a form of factitious illness.[2]

Voyeurism – A sexual deviation in which the individual repetitively seeks out situations in which he engages in looking at unsuspecting women who are either naked, in the act of disrobing, or engaging in sexual activity. The act of looking is accompanied by sexual excitement, frequently with orgasm. In its severe form, the act of peeping constitutes the preferred to exclusive sexual activity of the individual.[2]

Wernicke-Korsakoff syndrome — *see* Alcohol amnestic syndrome under Alcoholic psychoses

Withdrawal reaction of childhood or adolescence — *see* Introverted disorder of childhood

Word-deafness – A developmental delay in the comprehension of speech sounds.[1]

Zoophilia – Sexual or anal intercourse with animals.[1]

CLASSIFICATION OF DRUGS BY AMERICAN HOSPITAL FORMULARY SERVICE LIST NUMBER AND THEIR ICD-9-CM EQUIVALENTS

The coding of adverse effects of drugs is keyed to the continually revised Hospital Formulary of the American Hospital Formulary Service (AHFS) published under the direction of the American Society of Hospital Pharmacists.

The following section gives the ICD-9-CM diagnosis code for each AHFS list.

AHFS* List	ICD-9-CM Diagnosis Code
4:00 ANTIHISTAMINE DRUGS	963.0
8:00 ANTI-INFECTIVE AGENTS	
8:04 Amebacides	961.5
hydroxyquinoline derivatives	961.3
arsenical anti-infectives	961.1
8:08 Anthelmintics	961.6
quinoline derivatives	961.3
8:12.04 Antifungal Antibiotics	960.1
nonantibiotics	961.9
8:12.06 Cephalosporins	960.5
8:12.08 Chloramphenicol	960.2
8:12.12 The Erythromycins	960.3
8:12.16 The Penicillins	960.0
8:12.20 The Streptomycins	960.6
8:12.24 The Tetracyclines	960.4
8:12.28 Other Antibiotics	960.8
antimycobacterial antibiotics	960.6
macrolides	960.3
8:16 Antituberculars	961.8
antibiotics	960.6
8:18 Antivirals	961.7
8:20 Plasmodicides (antimalarials)	961.4
8:24 Sulfonamides	961.0
8:26 The Sulfones	961.8
8:28 Treponemicides	961.2
8:32 Trichomonacides	961.5
hydroxyquinoline derivatives	961.3
nitrofuran derivatives	961.9
8:36 Urinary Germicides	961.9
quinoline derivatives	961.3
8:40 Other Anti-Infectives	961.9
10:00 ANTINEOPLASTIC AGENTS	963.1
antibiotics	960.7
progestogens	962.2
12:00 AUTONOMIC DRUGS	
12:04 Parasympathomimetic (Cholinergic) Agents	971.0
12:08 Parasympatholytic (Cholinergic Blocking) Agents	971.1
12:12 Sympathomimetic (Adrenergic) Agents	971.2
12:16 Sympatholytic (Adrenergic Blocking) Agents	971.3
12:20 Skeletal Muscle Relaxants	975.2
central nervous system muscle-tone depressants	968.0
16:00 BLOOD DERIVATIVES	964.7
20:00 BLOOD FORMATION AND COAGULATION	
20:04 Antianemia Drugs	964.1
20:04.04 Iron Preparations	964.0
20:04.08 Liver and Stomach Preparations	964.1
20:12.04 Anticoagulants	964.2
20:12.08 Antiheparin Agents	964.5
20:12.12 Coagulants	964.5
20:12.16 Hemostatics	964.5
capillary-active drugs	972.8
fibrinolysis-affecting agents	964.4
natural products	964.7
24:00 CARDIOVASCULAR DRUGS	
24:04 Cardiac Drugs	972.9
cardiotonic agents	972.1
rhythm regulators	972.0
24:06 Antilipemic Agents	972.2
thyroid derivatives	962.7
24:08 Hypotensive Agents	972.6
adrenergic blocking agents	971.3
ganglion-blocking agents	972.3
vasodilators	972.5

AHFS* List	ICD-9-CM Diagnosis Code
24:12 Vasodilating Agents	972.5
coronary	972.4
nicotinic acid derivatives	972.2
24:16 Sclerosing Agents	972.7
28:00 CENTRAL NERVOUS SYSTEM DRUGS	
28:04 General Anesthetics	968.4
gaseous anesthetics	968.2
halothane	968.1
intravenous anesthetics	968.3
28:08 Analgesics and Antipyretics	965.9
antirheumatics	965.6
aromatic analgesics	965.4
non-narcotics NEC	965.7
opium alkaloids	965.00
heroin	965.01
methadone	965.02
specified type NEC	965.09
pyrazole derivatives	965.5
salicylates	965.1
specified type NEC	965.8
28:10 Narcotic Antagonists	970.1
28:12 Anticonvulsants	966.3
barbiturates	967.0
benzodiazepine-based tranquilizers	969.4
bromides	967.3
hydantoin derivatives	966.1
oxazolidine derivative	966.0
succinimides	966.2
28:16.04 Antidepressants	969.0
28:16.08 Tranquilizers	969.5
benzodiazepine-based	969.4
butyrophenone-based	969.2
major NEC	969.3
phenothiazine-based	969.1
28:16.12 Other Psychotherapeutic Agents	969.8
28:20 Respiratory and Cerebral Stimulants	970.9
analeptics	970.0
anorexigenic agents	977.0
psychostimulants	969.7
specified type NEC	970.8
28:24 Sedatives and Hypnotics	967.9
barbiturates	967.0
benzodiazepine-based tranquilizers	969.4
chloral hydrate group	967.1
glutethamide group	967.5
intravenous anesthetics	968.3
methaqualone	967.4
paraldehyde	967.2
phenothiazine-based tranquilizers	969.1
specified type NEC	967.8
thiobarbiturates	968.3
tranquilizer NEC	969.5
36:00 DIAGNOSTIC AGENTS	977.8
40:00 ELECTROLYTE, CALORIC, AND WATER BALANCE AGENTS NEC	974.5
40:04 Acidifying Agents	963.2
40:08 Alkalinizing Agents	963.3
40:10 Ammonia Detoxicants	974.5
40:12 Replacement Solutions NEC	974.5
plasma volume expanders	964.8
40:16 Sodium-Removing Resins	974.5
40:18 Potassium-Removing Resins	974.5
40:20 Caloric Agents	974.5
40:24 Salt and Sugar Substitutes	974.5
40:28 Diuretics NEC	974.4
carbonic acid anhydrase inhibitors	974.2
mercurials	974.0
purine derivatives	974.1
saluretics	974.3
40:36 Irrigating Solutions	974.5
40:40 Uricosuric Agents	974.7
44:00 ENZYMES NEC	963.4
fibrinolysis-affecting agents	964.4
gastric agents	973.4

Appendix C: Classification of Drugs by AHFS List

AHFS* List		ICD-9-CM Diagnosis Code
48:00	EXPECTORANTS AND COUGH PREPARATIONS	
	antihistamine agents	963.0
	antitussives	975.4
	codeine derivatives	965.09
	expectorants	975.5
	narcotic agents NEC	965.09
52:00	EYE, EAR, NOSE, AND THROAT PREPARATIONS	
52:04	Anti-Infectives	
	ENT	976.6
	ophthalmic	976.5
52:04.04	Antibiotics	
	ENT	976.6
	ophthalmic	976.5
52:04.06	Antivirals	
	ENT	976.6
	ophthalmic	976.5
52:04.08	Sulfonamides	
	ENT	976.6
	ophthalmic	976.5
52:04.12	Miscellaneous Anti-Infectives	
	ENT	976.6
	ophthalmic	976.5
52:08	Anti-Inflammatory Agents	
	ENT	976.6
	ophthalmic	976.5
52:10	Carbonic Anhydrase Inhibitors	974.2
52:12	Contact Lens Solutions	976.5
52:16	Local Anesthetics	968.5
52:20	Miotics	971.0
52:24	Mydriatics	
	adrenergics	971.2
	anticholinergics	971.1
	antimuscarinics	971.1
	parasympatholytics	971.1
	spasmolytics	971.1
	sympathomimetics	971.2
52:28	Mouth Washes and Gargles	976.6
52:32	Vasoconstrictors	971.2
52:36	Unclassified Agents	
	ENT	976.6
	ophthalmic	976.5
56:00	GASTROINTESTINAL DRUGS	
56:04	Antacids and Absorbents	973.0
56:08	Anti-Diarrhea Agents	973.5
56:10	Antiflatulents	973.8
56:12	Cathartics NEC	973.3
	emollients	973.2
	irritants	973.1
56:16	Digestants	973.4
56:20	Emetics and Antiemetics	
	antiemetics	963.0
	emetics	973.6
56:24	Lipotropic Agents	977.1
60:00	GOLD COMPOUNDS	965.6
64:00	HEAVY METAL ANTAGONISTS	963.8
68:00	HORMONES AND SYNTHETIC SUBSTITUTES	
68:04	Adrenals	962.0
68:08	Androgens	962.1
68:12	Contraceptives	962.2
68:16	Estrogens	962.2
68:18	Gonadotropins	962.4
68:20	Insulins and Antidiabetic Agents	962.3
68:20.08	Insulins	962.3
68:24	Parathyroid	962.6
68:28	Pituitary	
	anterior	962.4
	posterior	962.5
68:32	Progestogens	962.2
68:34	Other Corpus Luteum Hormones	962.2
68:36	Thyroid and Antithyroid	
	antithyroid	962.8
	thyroid	962.7

AHFS* List		ICD-9-CM Diagnosis Code
72:00	LOCAL ANESTHETICS NEC	968.9
	topical (surface) agents	968.5
	infiltrating agents (intradermal) (subcutaneous) (submucosal)	968.5
	nerve blocking agents (peripheral) (plexus) (regional)	968.6
	spinal	968.7
76:00	OXYTOCICS	975.0
78:00	RADIOACTIVE AGENTS	990
80:00	SERUMS, TOXOIDS, AND VACCINES	
80:04	Serums	979.9
	immune globulin (gamma) (human)	964.6
80:08	Toxoids NEC	978.8
	diphtheria	978.5
	and tetanus	978.9
	with pertussis component	978.6
	tetanus	978.4
	and diphtheria	978.9
	with pertussis component	978.6
80:12	Vaccines NEC	979.9
	bacterial NEC	978.8
	with	
	other bacterial component	978.9
	pertussis component	978.6
	viral and rickettsial component	979.7
	rickettsial NEC	979.6
	with	
	bacterial component	979.7
	pertussis component	978.6
	viral component	979.7
	viral NEC	979.6
	with	
	bacterial component	979.7
	pertussis component	978.6
	rickettsial component	979.7
84:00	SKIN AND MUCOUS MEMBRANE PREPARATIONS	
84:04	Anti-Infectives	976.0
84:04.04	Antibiotics	976.0
84:04.08	Fungicides	976.0
84:04.12	Scabicides and Pediculicides	976.0
84:04.16	Miscellaneous Local Anti-Infectives	976.0
84:06	Anti-Inflammatory Agents	976.0
84:08	Antipruritics and Local Anesthetics	
	antipruritics	976.1
	local anesthetics	968.5
84:12	Astringents	976.2
84:16	Cell Stimulants and Proliferants	976.8
84:20	Detergents	976.2
84:24	Emollients, Demulcents, and Protectants	976.3
84:28	Keratolytic Agents	976.4
84:32	Keratoplastic Agents	976.4
84:36	Miscellaneous Agents	976.8
86:00	SPASMOLYTIC AGENTS	975.1
	antiasthmatics	975.7
	papaverine	972.5
	theophyllin	974.1
88:00	VITAMINS	
88:04	Vitamin A	963.5
88:08	Vitamin B Complex	963.5
	hematopoietic vitamin	964.1
	nicotinic acid derivatives	972.2
88:12	Vitamin C	963.5
88:16	Vitamin D	963.5
88:20	Vitamin E	963.5
88:24	Vitamin K Activity	964.3
88:28	Multivitamin Preparations	963.5
92:00	UNCLASSIFIED THERAPEUTIC AGENTS	977.8

* American Hospital Formulary Service

CLASSIFICATION OF INDUSTRIAL ACCIDENTS ACCORDING TO AGENCY

Annex B to the Resolution concerning Statistics of Employment Injuries adopted by the Tenth International Conference of Labor Statisticians on 12 October 1962

1 MACHINES

11   **Prime-Movers, except Electrical Motors**
111   *Steam engines*
112   *Internal combustion engines*
119   *Others*
12   **Transmission Machinery**
121   *Transmission shafts*
122   *Transmission belts, cables, pulleys, pinions, chains, gears*
129   *Others*
13   **Metalworking Machines**
131   *Power presses*
132   *Lathes*
133   *Milling machines*
134   *Abrasive wheels*
135   *Mechanical shears*
136   *Forging machines*
137   *Rolling-mills*
139   *Others*
14   **Wood and Assimilated Machines**
141   *Circular saws*
142   *Other saws*
143   *Molding machines*
144   *Overhand planes*
149   *Others*
15   **Agricultural Machines**
151   *Reapers (including combine reapers)*
152   *Threshers*
159   *Others*
16   **Mining Machinery**
161   *Under-cutters*
169   *Others*
19   **Other Machines Not Elsewhere Classified**
191   *Earth-moving machines, excavating and scraping machines, except means of transport*
192   *Spinning, weaving and other textile machines*
193   *Machines for the manufacture of foodstuffs and beverages*
194   *Machines for the manufacture of paper*
195   *Printing machines*
199   *Others*

2 MEANS OF TRANSPORT AND LIFTING EQUIPMENT

21   **Lifting Machines and Appliances**
211   *Cranes*
212   *Lifts and elevators*
213   *Winches*
214   *Pulley blocks*
219   *Others*
22   **Means of Rail Transport**
221   *Inter-urban railways*
222   *Rail transport in mines, tunnels, quarries, industrial establishments, docks, etc.*
229   *Others*
23   **Other Wheeled Means of Transport, Excluding Rail Transport**
231   *Tractors*
232   *Lorries*
233   *Trucks*
234   *Motor vehicles, not elsewhere classified*
235   *Animal-drawn vehicles*
236   *Hand-drawn vehicles*
239   *Others*
24   **Means of Air Transport**
25   **Means of Water Transport**
251   *Motorized means of water transport*
252   *Non-motorized means of water transport*
26   **Other Means of Transport**
261   *Cable-cars*
262   *Mechanical conveyors, except cable-cars*
269   *Others*

3 OTHER EQUIPMENT

31   **Pressure Vessels**
311   *Boilers*
312   *Pressurized containers*
313   *Pressurized piping and accessories*
314   *Gas cylinders*
315   *Caissons, diving equipment*
319   *Others*
32   **Furnaces, Ovens, Kilns**
321   *Blast furnaces*
322   *Refining furnaces*
323   *Other furnaces*
324   *Kilns*
325   *Ovens*
33   **Refrigerating Plants**
34   **Electrical Installations, Including Electric Motors, but Excluding Electric Hand Tools**
341   *Rotating machines*
342   *Conductors*
343   *Transformers*
344   *Control apparatus*
349   *Others*
35   **Electric Hand Tools**
36   **Tools, Implements, and Appliances, Except Electric Hand Tools**
361   *Power-driven hand tools, except electric hand tools*
362   *Hand tools, not power-driven*
369   *Others*
37   **Ladders, Mobile Ramps**
38   **Scaffolding**
39   **Other Equipment, Not Elsewhere Classified**

4 MATERIALS, SUBSTANCES AND RADIATIONS

41   **Explosives**
42   **Dusts, Gases, Liquids and Chemicals, Excluding Explosives**
421   *Dusts*
422   *Gases, vapors, fumes*
423   *Liquids, not elsewhere classified*
424   *Chemicals, not elsewhere classified*
43   **Flying Fragments**
44   **Radiations**
441   *Ionizing radiations*
449   *Others*
49   **Other Materials and Substances Not Elsewhere Classified**

5 WORKING ENVIRONMENT

51   **Outdoor**
511   *Weather*
512   *Traffic and working surfaces*
513   *Water*
519   *Others*
52   **Indoor**
521   *Floors*
522   *Confined quarters*
523   *Stairs*
524   *Other traffic and working surfaces*
525   *Floor openings and wall openings*
526   *Environmental factors (lighting, ventilation, temperature, noise, etc.)*
529   *Others*
53   **Underground**
531   *Roofs and faces of mine roads and tunnels, etc.*
532   *Floors of mine roads and tunnels, etc.*
533   *Working-faces of mines, tunnels, etc.*
534   *Mine shafts*
535   *Fire*
536   *Water*
539   *Others*

6 OTHER AGENCIES, NOT ELSEWHERE CLASSIFIED

61   **Animals**
611   *Live animals*
612   *Animal products*
69   **Other Agencies, Not Elsewhere Classified**

7 AGENCIES NOT CLASSIFIED FOR LACK OF SUFFICIENT DATA

LIST OF THREE-DIGIT CATEGORIES

1. INFECTIOUS AND PARASITIC DISEASES

Intestinal infectious diseases (001-009)
001 Cholera
002 Typhoid and paratyphoid fevers
003 Other salmonella infections
004 Shigellosis
005 Other food poisoning (bacterial)
006 Amebiasis
007 Other protozoal intestinal diseases
008 Intestinal infections due to other organisms
009 Ill-defined intestinal infections

Tuberculosis (010-018)
010 Primary tuberculous infection
011 Pulmonary tuberculosis
012 Other respiratory tuberculosis
013 Tuberculosis of meninges and central nervous system
014 Tuberculosis of intestines, peritoneum, and mesenteric glands
015 Tuberculosis of bones and joints
016 Tuberculosis of genitourinary system
017 Tuberculosis of other organs
018 Miliary tuberculosis

Zoonotic bacterial diseases (020-027)
020 Plague
021 Tularemia
022 Anthrax
023 Brucellosis
024 Glanders
025 Melioidosis
026 Rat-bite fever
027 Other zoonotic bacterial diseases

Other bacterial diseases (030-042)
030 Leprosy
031 Diseases due to other mycobacteria
032 Diphtheria
033 Whooping cough
034 Streptococcal sore throat and scarlatina
035 Erysipelas
036 Meningococcal infection
037 Tetanus
038 Septicemia
039 Actinomycotic infections
040 Other bacterial diseases
041 Bacterial infection in conditions classified elsewhere and of unspecified site

Human immunodeficiency virus (042)
042 Human immunodeficiency virus [HIV] disease

Poliomyelitis and other non-arthropod-borne viral diseases of central nervous system (045-049)
045 Acute poliomyelitis
046 Slow virus infection of central nervous system
047 Meningitis due to enterovirus
048 Other enterovirus diseases of central nervous system
049 Other non-arthropod-borne viral diseases of central nervous system

Viral diseases accompanied by exanthem (050-057)
050 Smallpox
051 Cowpox and paravaccinia
052 Chickenpox
053 Herpes zoster
054 Herpes simplex
055 Measles
056 Rubella
057 Other viral exanthemata

Arthropod-borne viral diseases (060-066)
060 Yellow fever
061 Dengue
062 Mosquito-borne viral encephalitis
063 Tick-borne viral encephalitis
064 Viral encephalitis transmitted by other and unspecified arthropods
065 Arthropod-borne hemorrhagic fever
066 Other arthropod-borne viral diseases

Other diseases due to viruses and Chlamydiae (070-079)
070 Viral hepatitis
071 Rabies
072 Mumps
073 Ornithosis
074 Specific diseases due to Coxsackievirus
075 Infectious mononucleosis
076 Trachoma
077 Other diseases of conjunctiva due to viruses and Chlamydiae
078 Other diseases due to viruses and Chlamydiae
079 Viral infection in conditions classified elsewhere and of unspecified site

Rickettsioses and other arthropod-borne diseases (080-088)
080 Louse-borne [epidemic] typhus
081 Other typhus
082 Tick-borne rickettsioses
083 Other rickettsioses
084 Malaria
085 Leishmaniasis
086 Trypanosomiasis
087 Relapsing fever
088 Other arthropod-borne diseases

Syphilis and other venereal diseases (090-099)
090 Congenital syphilis
091 Early syphilis, symptomatic
092 Early syphilis, latent
093 Cardiovascular syphilis
094 Neurosyphilis
095 Other forms of late syphilis, with symptoms
096 Late syphilis, latent
097 Other and unspecified syphilis
098 Gonococcal infections
099 Other venereal diseases

Other spirochetal diseases (100-104)
100 Leptospirosis
101 Vincent's angina
102 Yaws
103 Pinta
104 Other spirochetal infection

Mycoses (110-118)
110 Dermatophytosis
111 Dermatomycosis, other and unspecified
112 Candidiasis
114 Coccidioidomycosis
115 Histoplasmosis
116 Blastomycotic infection
117 Other mycoses
118 Opportunistic mycoses

Helminthiases (120-129)
120 Schistosomiasis [bilharziasis]
121 Other trematode infections
122 Echinococcosis
123 Other cestode infection
124 Trichinosis
125 Filarial infection and dracontiasis
126 Ancylostomiasis and necatoriasis
127 Other intestinal helminthiases
128 Other and unspecified helminthiases
129 Intestinal parasitism, unspecified

Other infectious and parasitic diseases (130-136)
130 Toxoplasmosis
131 Trichomoniasis
132 Pediculosis and phthirus infestation
133 Acariasis
134 Other infestation
135 Sarcoidosis
136 Other and unspecified infectious and parasitic diseases

Late effects of infectious and parasitic diseases (137-139)
137 Late effects of tuberculosis
138 Late effects of acute poliomyelitis
139 Late effects of other infectious and parasitic diseases

2. NEOPLASMS

Malignant neoplasm of lip, oral cavity, and pharynx (140-149)
140 Malignant neoplasm of lip
141 Malignant neoplasm of tongue
142 Malignant neoplasm of major salivary glands
143 Malignant neoplasm of gum
144 Malignant neoplasm of floor of mouth
145 Malignant neoplasm of other and unspecified parts of mouth
146 Malignant neoplasm of oropharynx
147 Malignant neoplasm of nasopharynx
148 Malignant neoplasm of hypopharynx
149 Malignant neoplasm of other and ill-defined sites within the lip, oral cavity, and pharynx

Malignant neoplasm of digestive organs and peritoneum (150-159)
150 Malignant neoplasm of esophagus
151 Malignant neoplasm of stomach
152 Malignant neoplasm of small intestine, including duodenum
153 Malignant neoplasm of colon
154 Malignant neoplasm of rectum, rectosigmoid junction, and anus
155 Malignant neoplasm of liver and intrahepatic bile ducts
156 Malignant neoplasm of gallbladder and extrahepatic bile ducts
157 Malignant neoplasm of pancreas
158 Malignant neoplasm of retroperitoneum and peritoneum
159 Malignant neoplasm of other and ill-defined sites within the digestive organs and peritoneum

Malignant neoplasm of respiratory and intrathoracic organs (160-165)
160 Malignant neoplasm of nasal cavities, middle ear, and accessory sinuses
161 Malignant neoplasm of larynx
162 Malignant neoplasm of trachea, bronchus, and lung
163 Malignant neoplasm of pleura
164 Malignant neoplasm of thymus, heart, and mediastinum
165 Malignant neoplasm of other and ill-defined sites within the respiratory system and intrathoracic organs

Malignant neoplasm of bone, connective tissue, skin, and breast (170-176)
170 Malignant neoplasm of bone and articular cartilage
171 Malignant neoplasm of connective and other soft tissue
172 Malignant melanoma of skin
173 Other malignant neoplasm of skin
174 Malignant neoplasm of female breast
175 Malignant neoplasm of male breast

Kaposi's sarcoma (176)
176 Kaposi's sarcoma

Malignant neoplasm of genitourinary organs (179-189)
179 Malignant neoplasm of uterus, part unspecified
180 Malignant neoplasm of cervix uteri
181 Malignant neoplasm of placenta
182 Malignant neoplasm of body of uterus
183 Malignant neoplasm of ovary and other uterine adnexa
184 Malignant neoplasm of other and unspecified female genital organs
185 Malignant neoplasm of prostate
186 Malignant neoplasm of testis
187 Malignant neoplasm of penis and other male genital organs
188 Malignant neoplasm of bladder
189 Malignant neoplasm of kidney and other unspecified urinary organs

Malignant neoplasm of other and unspecified sites (190-199)
190 Malignant neoplasm of eye
191 Malignant neoplasm of brain
192 Malignant neoplasm of other and unspecified parts of nervous system
193 Malignant neoplasm of thyroid gland
194 Malignant neoplasm of other endocrine glands and related structures
195 Malignant neoplasm of other and ill-defined sites
196 Secondary and unspecified malignant neoplasm of lymph nodes
197 Secondary malignant neoplasm of respiratory and digestive systems
198 Secondary malignant neoplasm of other specified sites
199 Malignant neoplasm without specification of site

Malignant neoplasm of lymphatic and hematopoietic tissue (200-208)
200 Lymphosarcoma and reticulosarcoma
201 Hodgkin's disease
202 Other malignant neoplasm of lymphoid and histiocytic tissue
203 Multiple myeloma and immunoproliferative neoplasms
204 Lymphoid leukemia
205 Myeloid leukemia
206 Monocytic leukemia
207 Other specified leukemia
208 Leukemia of unspecified cell type

Benign neoplasms (210-229)
210 Benign neoplasm of lip, oral cavity, and pharynx
211 Benign neoplasm of other parts of digestive system
212 Benign neoplasm of respiratory and intrathoracic organs
213 Benign neoplasm of bone and articular cartilage
214 Lipoma
215 Other benign neoplasm of connective and other soft tissue
216 Benign neoplasm of skin
217 Benign neoplasm of breast
218 Uterine leiomyoma
219 Other benign neoplasm of uterus
220 Benign neoplasm of ovary
221 Benign neoplasm of other female genital organs
222 Benign neoplasm of male genital organs
223 Benign neoplasm of kidney and other urinary organs
224 Benign neoplasm of eye
225 Benign neoplasm of brain and other parts of nervous system
226 Benign neoplasm of thyroid gland
227 Benign neoplasm of other endocrine glands and related structures
228 Hemangioma and lymphangioma, any site
229 Benign neoplasm of other and unspecified sites

Carcinoma in situ (230-234)
230 Carcinoma in situ of digestive organs
231 Carcinoma in situ of respiratory system
232 Carcinoma in situ of skin
233 Carcinoma in situ of breast and genitourinary system
234 Carcinoma in situ of other and unspecified sites

Neoplasms of uncertain behavior (235-238)
235 Neoplasm of uncertain behavior of digestive and respiratory systems
236 Neoplasm of uncertain behavior of genitourinary organs
237 Neoplasm of uncertain behavior of endocrine glands and nervous system
238 Neoplasm of uncertain behavior of other and unspecified sites and tissues

Neoplasms of unspecified nature (239)
239 Neoplasm of unspecified nature

3. ENDOCRINE, NUTRITIONAL AND METABOLIC DISEASES, AND IMMUNITY DISORDERS

Disorders of thyroid gland (240-246)
240 Simple and unspecified goiter
241 Nontoxic nodular goiter
242 Thyrotoxicosis with or without goiter
243 Congenital hypothyroidism
244 Acquired hypothyroidism
245 Thyroiditis
246 Other disorders of thyroid

Diseases of other endocrine glands (250-259)
250 Diabetes mellitus
251 Other disorders of pancreatic internal secretion
252 Disorders of parathyroid gland
253 Disorders of the pituitary gland and its hypothalamic control
254 Diseases of thymus gland
255 Disorders of adrenal glands
256 Ovarian dysfunction
257 Testicular dysfunction
258 Polyglandular dysfunction and related disorders
259 Other endocrine disorders

Nutritional deficiencies (260-269)
260 Kwashiorkor
261 Nutritional marasmus
262 Other severe protein-calorie malnutrition
263 Other and unspecified protein-calorie malnutrition
264 Vitamin A deficiency
265 Thiamine and niacin deficiency states
266 Deficiency of B-complex components
267 Ascorbic acid deficiency
268 Vitamin D deficiency
269 Other nutritional deficiencies

Other metabolic disorders and immunity disorders (270-279)
270 Disorders of amino-acid transport and metabolism
271 Disorders of carbohydrate transport and metabolism
272 Disorders of lipoid metabolism
273 Disorders of plasma protein metabolism
274 Gout
275 Disorders of mineral metabolism
276 Disorders of fluid, electrolyte, and acid-base balance
277 Other and unspecified disorders of metabolism
278 Obesity and other hyperalimentation
279 Disorders involving the immune mechanism

Diseases of blood and blood-forming organs (280-289)
280 Iron deficiency anemias
281 Other deficiency anemias
282 Hereditary hemolytic anemias
283 Acquired hemolytic anemias
284 Aplastic anemia
285 Other and unspecified anemias
286 Coagulation defects
287 Purpura and other hemorrhagic conditions
288 Diseases of white blood cells
289 Other diseases of blood and blood-forming organs

5. MENTAL DISORDERS

Organic psychotic conditions (290-294)
290 Senile and presenile organic psychotic conditions
291 Alcoholic psychoses
292 Drug psychoses
293 Transient organic psychotic conditions
294 Other organic psychotic conditions (chronic)

Other psychoses (295-299)
295 Schizophrenic psychoses
296 Affective psychoses
297 Paranoid states
298 Other nonorganic psychoses
299 Psychoses with origin specific to childhood

Neurotic disorders, personality disorders, and other nonpsychotic mental disorders (300-316)
300 Neurotic disorders
301 Personality disorders
302 Sexual deviations and disorders
303 Alcohol dependence syndrome
304 Drug dependence
305 Nondependent abuse of drugs
306 Physiological malfunction arising from mental factors

307 Special symptoms or syndromes, not elsewhere classified
308 Acute reaction to stress
309 Adjustment reaction
310 Specific nonpsychotic mental disorders following organic brain damage
311 Depressive disorder, not elsewhere classified
312 Disturbance of conduct, not elsewhere classified
313 Disturbance of emotions specific to childhood and adolescence
314 Hyperkinetic syndrome of childhood
315 Specific delays in development
316 Psychic factors associated with diseases classified elsewhere

Mental retardation (317-319)
317 Mild mental retardation
318 Other specified mental retardation
319 Unspecified mental retardation

6. DISEASES OF THE NERVOUS SYSTEM AND SENSE ORGANS

Inflammatory diseases of the central nervous system (320-326)
320 Bacterial meningitis
321 Meningitis due to other organisms
322 Meningitis of unspecified cause
323 Encephalitis, myelitis, and encephalomyelitis
324 Intracranial and intraspinal abscess
325 Phlebitis and thrombophlebitis of intracranial venous sinuses
326 Late effects of intracranial abscess or pyogenic infection

Hereditary and degenerative diseases of the central nervous system (330-337)
330 Cerebral degenerations usually manifest in childhood
331 Other cerebral degenerations
332 Parkinson's disease
333 Other extrapyramidal diseases and abnormal movement disorders
334 Spinocerebellar disease
335 Anterior horn cell disease
336 Other diseases of spinal cord
337 Disorders of the autonomic nervous system

Other disorders of the central nervous system (340-349)
340 Multiple sclerosis
341 Other demyelinating diseases of central nervous system
342 Hemiplegia and hemiparesis
343 Infantile cerebral palsy
344 Other paralytic syndromes
345 Epilepsy
346 Migraine
347 Cataplexy and narcolepsy
348 Other conditions of brain
349 Other and unspecified disorders of the nervous system

Disorders of the peripheral nervous system (350-359)
350 Trigeminal nerve disorders
351 Facial nerve disorders
352 Disorders of other cranial nerves
353 Nerve root and plexus disorders
354 Mononeuritis of upper limb and mononeuritis multiplex
355 Mononeuritis of lower limb
356 Hereditary and idiopathic peripheral neuropathy
357 Inflammatory and toxic neuropathy
358 Myoneural disorders

359 Muscular dystrophies and other myopathies

Disorders of the eye and adnexa (360-379)
360 Disorders of the globe
361 Retinal detachments and defects
362 Other retinal disorders
363 Chorioretinal inflammations and scars and other disorders of choroid
364 Disorders of iris and ciliary body
365 Glaucoma
366 Cataract
367 Disorders of refraction and accommodation
368 Visual disturbances
369 Blindness and low vision
370 Keratitis
371 Corneal opacity and other disorders of cornea
372 Disorders of conjunctiva
373 Inflammation of eyelids
374 Other disorders of eyelids
375 Disorders of lacrimal system
376 Disorders of the orbit
377 Disorders of optic nerve and visual pathways
378 Strabismus and other disorders of binocular eye movements
379 Other disorders of eye

Diseases of the ear and mastoid process (380-389)
380 Disorders of external ear
381 Nonsuppurative otitis media and Eustachian tube disorders
382 Suppurative and unspecified otitis media
383 Mastoiditis and related conditions
384 Other disorders of tympanic membrane
385 Other disorders of middle ear and mastoid
386 Vertiginous syndromes and other disorders of vestibular system
387 Otosclerosis
388 Other disorders of ear
389 Hearing loss

7. DISEASES OF THE CIRCULATORY SYSTEM

Acute rheumatic fever (390-392)
390 Rheumatic fever without mention of heart involvement
391 Rheumatic fever with heart involvement
392 Rheumatic chorea

Chronic rheumatic heart disease (393-398)
393 Chronic rheumatic pericarditis
394 Diseases of mitral valve
395 Diseases of aortic valve
396 Diseases of mitral and aortic valves
397 Diseases of other endocardial structures
398 Other rheumatic heart disease

Hypertensive disease (401-405)
401 Essential hypertension
402 Hypertensive heart disease
403 Hypertensive renal disease
404 Hypertensive heart and renal disease
405 Secondary hypertension

Ischemic heart disease (410-414)
410 Acute myocardial infarction
411 Other acute and subacute form of ischemic heart disease

412 Old myocardial infarction
413 Angina pectoris
414 Other forms of chronic ischemic heart disease

Diseases of pulmonary circulation (415-417)
415 Acute pulmonary heart disease
416 Chronic pulmonary heart disease
417 Other diseases of pulmonary circulation

Other forms of heart disease (420-429)
420 Acute pericarditis
421 Acute and subacute endocarditis
422 Acute myocarditis
423 Other diseases of pericardium
424 Other diseases of endocardium
425 Cardiomyopathy
426 Conduction disorders
427 Cardiac dysrhythmias
428 Heart failure
429 Ill-defined descriptions and complications of heart disease

Cerebrovascular disease (430-438)
430 Subarachnoid hemorrhage
431 Intracerebral hemorrhage
432 Other and unspecified intracranial hemorrhage
433 Occlusion and stenosis of precerebral arteries
434 Occlusion of cerebral arteries
435 Transient cerebral ischemia
436 Acute but ill-defined cerebrovascular disease
437 Other and ill-defined cerebrovascular disease
438 Late effects of cerebrovascular disease

Diseases of arteries, arterioles, and capillaries (440-448)
440 Atherosclerosis
441 Aortic aneurysm and dissection
442 Other aneurysm
443 Other peripheral vascular disease
444 Arterial embolism and thrombosis
445 Atheroembolism
446 Polyarteritis nodosa and allied conditions
447 Other disorders of arteries and arterioles
448 Diseases of capillaries

Diseases of veins and lymphatics, and other diseases of circulatory system (451-459)
451 Phlebitis and thrombophlebitis
452 Portal vein thrombosis
453 Other venous embolism and thrombosis
454 Varicose veins of lower extremities
455 Hemorrhoids
456 Varicose veins of other sites
457 Noninfective disorders of lymphatic channels
458 Hypotension
459 Other disorders of circulatory system

8. DISEASES OF THE RESPIRATORY SYSTEM

Acute respiratory infections (460-466)
460 Acute nasopharyngitis [common cold]
461 Acute sinusitis
462 Acute pharyngitis
463 Acute tonsillitis
464 Acute laryngitis and tracheitis

465 Acute upper respiratory infections of multiple or unspecified sites
466 Acute bronchitis and bronchiolitis

Other diseases of upper respiratory tract (470-478)
470 Deviated nasal septum
471 Nasal polyps
472 Chronic pharyngitis and nasopharyngitis
473 Chronic sinusitis
474 Chronic disease of tonsils and adenoids
475 Peritonsillar abscess
476 Chronic laryngitis and laryngotracheitis
477 Allergic rhinitis
478 Other diseases of upper respiratory tract

Pneumonia and influenza (480-487)
480 Viral pneumonia
481 Pneumococcal pneumonia [Streptococcus pneumoniae pneumonia]
482 Other bacterial pneumonia
483 Pneumonia due to other specified organism
484 Pneumonia in infectious diseases classified elsewhere
485 Bronchopneumonia, organism unspecified
486 Pneumonia, organism unspecified
487 Influenza

Chronic obstructive pulmonary disease and allied conditions (490-496)
490 Bronchitis, not specified as acute or chronic
491 Chronic bronchitis
492 Emphysema
493 Asthma
494 Bronchiectasis
495 Extrinsic allergic alveolitis
496 Chronic airways obstruction, not elsewhere classified

Pneumoconioses and other lung diseases due to external agents (500-508)
500 Coal workers' pneumoconiosis
501 Asbestosis
502 Pneumoconiosis due to other silica or silicates
503 Pneumoconiosis due to other inorganic dust
504 Pneumopathy due to inhalation of other dust
505 Pneumoconiosis, unspecified
506 Respiratory conditions due to chemical fumes and vapors
507 Pneumonitis due to solids and liquids
508 Respiratory conditions due to other and unspecified external agents

Other diseases of respiratory system (510-519)
510 Empyema
511 Pleurisy
512 Pneumothorax
513 Abscess of lung and mediastinum
514 Pulmonary congestion and hypostasis
515 Postinflammatory pulmonary fibrosis
516 Other alveolar and parietoalveolar pneumopathy
517 Lung involvement in conditions classified elsewhere
518 Other diseases of lung

519 Other diseases of respiratory system

9. DISEASES OF THE DIGESTIVE SYSTEM

Diseases of oral cavity, salivary glands, and jaws (520-529)
520 Disorders of tooth development and eruption
521 Diseases of hard tissues of teeth
522 Diseases of pulp and periapical tissues
523 Gingival and periodontal diseases
524 Dentofacial anomalies, including malocclusion
525 Other diseases and conditions of the teeth and supporting structures
526 Diseases of the jaws
527 Diseases of the salivary glands
528 Diseases of the oral soft tissues, excluding lesions specific for gingiva and tongue
529 Diseases and other conditions of the tongue

Diseases of esophagus, stomach, and duodenum (530-537)
530 Diseases of esophagus
531 Gastric ulcer
532 Duodenal ulcer
533 Peptic ulcer, site unspecified
534 Gastrojejunal ulcer
535 Gastritis and duodenitis
536 Disorders of function of stomach
537 Other disorders of stomach and duodenum

Appendicitis (540-543)
540 Acute appendicitis
541 Appendicitis, unqualified
542 Other appendicitis
543 Other diseases of appendix

Hernia of abdominal cavity (550-553)
550 Inguinal hernia
551 Other hernia of abdominal cavity, with gangrene
552 Other hernia of abdominal cavity, with obstruction, but without mention of gangrene
553 Other hernia of abdominal cavity without mention of obstruction or gangrene

Noninfective enteritis and colitis (555-558)
555 Regional enteritis
556 Ulcerative colitis
557 Vascular insufficiency of intestine
558 Other noninfective gastroenteritis and colitis

Other diseases of intestines and peritoneum (560-569)
560 Intestinal obstruction without mention of hernia
562 Diverticula of intestine
564 Functional digestive disorders, not elsewhere classified
565 Anal fissure and fistula
566 Abscess of anal and rectal regions
567 Peritonitis
568 Other disorders of peritoneum
569 Other disorders of intestine

Other diseases of digestive system (570-579)
570 Acute and subacute necrosis of liver
571 Chronic liver disease and cirrhosis
572 Liver abscess and sequelae of chronic liver disease

573 Other disorders of liver
574 Cholelithiasis
575 Other disorders of gallbladder
576 Other disorders of biliary tract
577 Diseases of pancreas
578 Gastrointestinal hemorrhage
579 Intestinal malabsorption

10. DISEASES OF THE GENITOURINARY SYSTEM

Nephritis, nephrotic syndrome, and nephrosis (580-589)
580 Acute glomerulonephritis
581 Nephrotic syndrome
582 Chronic glomerulonephritis
583 Nephritis and nephropathy, not specified as acute or chronic
584 Acute renal failure
585 Chronic renal failure
586 Renal failure, unspecified
587 Renal sclerosis, unspecified
588 Disorders resulting from impaired renal function
589 Small kidney of unknown cause

Other diseases of urinary system (590-599)
590 Infections of kidney
591 Hydronephrosis
592 Calculus of kidney and ureter
593 Other disorders of kidney and ureter
594 Calculus of lower urinary tract
595 Cystitis
596 Other disorders of bladder
597 Urethritis, not sexually transmitted, and urethral syndrome
598 Urethral stricture
599 Other disorders of urethra and urinary tract

Diseases of male genital organs (600-608)
600 Hyperplasia of prostate
601 Inflammatory diseases of prostate
602 Other disorders of prostate
603 Hydrocele
604 Orchitis and epididymitis
605 Redundant prepuce and phimosis
606 Infertility, male
607 Disorders of penis
608 Other disorders of male genital organs

Disorders of breast (610-611)
610 Benign mammary dysplasias
611 Other disorders of breast

Inflammatory disease of female pelvic organs (614-616)
614 Inflammatory disease of ovary, fallopian tube, pelvic cellular tissue, and peritoneum
615 Inflammatory diseases of uterus, except cervix
616 Inflammatory disease of cervix, vagina, and vulva

Other disorders of female genital tract (617-629)
617 Endometriosis
618 Genital prolapse
619 Fistula involving female genital tract
620 Noninflammatory disorders of ovary, fallopian tube, and broad ligament
621 Disorders of uterus, not elsewhere classified
622 Noninflammatory disorders of cervix
623 Noninflammatory disorders of vagina
624 Noninflammatory disorders of vulva and perineum

Appendix E: List of Three-Digit Categories

625 Pain and other symptoms associated with female genital organs
626 Disorders of menstruation and other abnormal bleeding from female genital tract
627 Menopausal and postmenopausal disorders
628 Infertility, female
629 Other disorders of female genital organs

11. COMPLICATIONS OF PREGNANCY, CHILDBIRTH AND THE PUERPERIUM

Ectopic and molar pregnancy and other pregnancy with abortive outcome (630-639)

630 Hydatidiform mole
631 Other abnormal product of conception
632 Missed abortion
633 Ectopic pregnancy
634 Spontaneous abortion
635 Legally induced abortion
636 Illegally induced abortion
637 Unspecified abortion
638 Failed attempted abortion
639 Complications following abortion and ectopic and molar pregnancies

Complications mainly related to pregnancy (640-648)

640 Hemorrhage in early pregnancy
641 Antepartum hemorrhage, abruptio placentae, and placenta previa
642 Hypertension complicating pregnancy, childbirth, and the puerperium
643 Excessive vomiting in pregnancy
644 Early or threatened labor
645 Prolonged pregnancy
646 Other complications of pregnancy, not elsewhere classified
647 Infective and parasitic conditions in the mother classifiable elsewhere but complicating pregnancy, childbirth, and the puerperium
648 Other current conditions in the mother classifiable elsewhere but complicating pregnancy, childbirth, and the puerperium

Normal delivery, and other indications for care in pregnancy, labor, and delivery (650-659)

650 Normal delivery
651 Multiple gestation
652 Malposition and malpresentation of fetus
653 Disproportion
654 Abnormality of organs and soft tissues of pelvis
655 Known or suspected fetal abnormality affecting management of mother
656 Other fetal and placental problems affecting management of mother
657 Polyhydramnios
658 Other problems associated with amniotic cavity and membranes
659 Other indications for care or intervention related to labor and delivery and not elsewhere classified

Complications occurring mainly in the course of labor and delivery (660-669)

660 Obstructed labor
661 Abnormality of forces of labor
662 Long labor
663 Umbilical cord complications
664 Trauma to perineum and vulva during delivery

665 Other obstetrical trauma
666 Postpartum hemorrhage
667 Retained placenta or membranes, without hemorrhage
668 Complications of the administration of anesthetic or other sedation in labor and delivery
669 Other complications of labor and delivery, not elsewhere classified

Complications of the puerperium (670-677)

670 Major puerperal infection
671 Venous complications in pregnancy and the puerperium
672 Pyrexia of unknown origin during the puerperium
673 Obstetrical pulmonary embolism
674 Other and unspecified complications of the puerperium, not elsewhere classified
675 Infections of the breast and nipple associated with childbirth
676 Other disorders of the breast associated with childbirth, and disorders of lactation
677 Late effect of complication of pregnancy, childbirth, and the puerperium

12. DISEASES OF THE SKIN AND SUBCUTANEOUS TISSUE

Infections of skin and subcutaneous tissue (680-686)

680 Carbuncle and furuncle
681 Cellulitis and abscess of finger and toe
682 Other cellulitis and abscess
683 Acute lymphadenitis
684 Impetigo
685 Pilonidal cyst
686 Other local infections of skin and subcutaneous tissue

Other inflammatory conditions of skin and subcutaneous tissue (690-698)

690 Erythematosquamous dermatosis
691 Atopic dermatitis and related conditions
692 Contact dermatitis and other eczema
693 Dermatitis due to substances taken internally
694 Bullous dermatoses
695 Erythematous conditions
696 Psoriasis and similar disorders
697 Lichen
698 Pruritus and related conditions

Other diseases of skin and subcutaneous tissue (700-709)

700 Corns and callosities
701 Other hypertrophic and atrophic conditions of skin
702 Other dermatoses
703 Diseases of nail
704 Diseases of hair and hair follicles
705 Disorders of sweat glands
706 Diseases of sebaceous glands
707 Chronic ulcer of skin
708 Urticaria
709 Other disorders of skin and subcutaneous tissue

13. DISEASES OF THE MUSCULOSKELETAL SYSTEM AND CONNECTIVE TISSUE

Arthropathies and related disorders (710-719)

710 Diffuse diseases of connective tissue
711 Arthropathy associated with infections
712 Crystal arthropathies
713 Arthropathy associated with other disorders classified elsewhere
714 Rheumatoid arthritis and other inflammatory polyarthropathies
715 Osteoarthrosis and allied disorders
716 Other and unspecified arthropathies
717 Internal derangement of knee
718 Other derangement of joint
719 Other and unspecified disorder of joint

Dorsopathies (720-724)

720 Ankylosing spondylitis and other inflammatory spondylopathies
721 Spondylosis and allied disorders
722 Intervertebral disc disorders
723 Other disorders of cervical region
724 Other and unspecified disorders of back

Rheumatism, excluding the back (725-729)

725 Polymyalgia rheumatica
726 Peripheral enthesopathies and allied syndromes
727 Other disorders of synovium, tendon, and bursa
728 Disorders of muscle, ligament, and fascia
729 Other disorders of soft tissues

Osteopathies, chondropathies, and acquired musculoskeletal deformities (730-739)

730 Osteomyelitis, periostitis, and other infections involving bone
731 Osteitis deformans and osteopathies associated with other disorders classified elsewhere
732 Osteochondropathies
733 Other disorders of bone and cartilage
734 Flat foot
735 Acquired deformities of toe
736 Other acquired deformities of limbs
737 Curvature of spine
738 Other acquired deformity
739 Nonallopathic lesions, not elsewhere classified

14. CONGENITAL ANOMALIES

740 Anencephalus and similar anomalies
741 Spina bifida
742 Other congenital anomalies of nervous system
743 Congenital anomalies of eye
744 Congenital anomalies of ear, face, and neck
745 Bulbus cordis anomalies and anomalies of cardiac septal closure
746 Other congenital anomalies of heart
747 Other congenital anomalies of circulatory system
748 Congenital anomalies of respiratory system
749 Cleft palate and cleft lip
750 Other congenital anomalies of upper alimentary tract
751 Other congenital anomalies of digestive system

752　Congenital anomalies of genital organs
753　Congenital anomalies of urinary system
754　Certain congenital musculoskeletal deformities
755　Other congenital anomalies of limbs
756　Other congenital musculoskeletal anomalies
757　Congenital anomalies of the integument
758　Chromosomal anomalies
759　Other and unspecified congenital anomalies

15. CERTAIN CONDITIONS ORIGINATING IN THE PERINATAL PERIOD

Maternal causes of perinatal morbidity and mortality (760-763)
760　Fetus or newborn affected by maternal conditions which may be unrelated to present pregnancy
761　Fetus or newborn affected by maternal complications of pregnancy
762　Fetus or newborn affected by complications of placenta, cord, and membranes
763　Fetus or newborn affected by other complications of labor and delivery

Other conditions originating in the perinatal period (764-779)
764　Slow fetal growth and fetal malnutrition
765　Disorders relating to short gestation and unspecified low birthweight
766　Disorders relating to long gestation and high birthweight
767　Birth trauma
768　Intrauterine hypoxia and birth asphyxia
769　Respiratory distress syndrome
770　Other respiratory conditions of fetus and newborn
771　Infections specific to the perinatal period
772　Fetal and neonatal hemorrhage
773　Hemolytic disease of fetus or newborn, due to isoimmunization
774　Other perinatal jaundice
775　Endocrine and metabolic disturbances specific to the fetus and newborn
776　Hematological disorders of fetus and newborn
777　Perinatal disorders of digestive system
778　Conditions involving the integument and temperature regulation of fetus and newborn
779　Other and ill-defined conditions originating in the perinatal period

16. SYMPTOMS, SIGNS, AND ILL-DEFINED CONDITIONS

Symptoms (780-789)
780　General symptoms
781　Symptoms involving nervous and musculoskeletal systems
782　Symptoms involving skin and other integumentary tissue
783　Symptoms concerning nutrition, metabolism, and development
784　Symptoms involving head and neck
785　Symptoms involving cardiovascular system
786　Symptoms involving respiratory system and other chest symptoms
787　Symptoms involving digestive system
788　Symptoms involving urinary system
789　Other symptoms involving abdomen and pelvis

Nonspecific abnormal findings (790-796)
790　Nonspecific findings on examination of blood
791　Nonspecific findings on examination of urine
792　Nonspecific abnormal findings in other body substances
793　Nonspecific abnormal findings on radiological and other examination of body structure
794　Nonspecific abnormal results of function studies
795　Nonspecific abnormal histological and immunological findings
796　Other nonspecific abnormal findings

Ill-defined and unknown causes of morbidity and mortality (797-799)
797　Senility without mention of psychosis
798　Sudden death, cause unknown
799　Other ill-defined and unknown causes of morbidity and mortality

17. INJURY AND POISONING

Fracture of skull (800-804)
800　Fracture of vault of skull
801　Fracture of base of skull
802　Fracture of face bones
803　Other and unqualified skull fractures
804　Multiple fractures involving skull or face with other bones

Fracture of spine and trunk (805-809)
805　Fracture of vertebral column without mention of spinal cord lesion
806　Fracture of vertebral column with spinal cord lesion
807　Fracture of rib(s), sternum, larynx, and trachea
808　Fracture of pelvis
809　Ill-defined fractures of bones of trunk

Fracture of upper limb (810-819)
810　Fracture of clavicle
811　Fracture of scapula
812　Fracture of humerus
813　Fracture of radius and ulna
814　Fracture of carpal bone(s)
815　Fracture of metacarpal bone(s)
816　Fracture of one or more phalanges of hand
817　Multiple fractures of hand bones
818　Ill-defined fractures of upper limb
819　Multiple fractures involving both upper limbs, and upper limb with rib(s) and sternum

Fracture of lower limb (820-829)
820　Fracture of neck of femur
821　Fracture of other and unspecified parts of femur
822　Fracture of patella
823　Fracture of tibia and fibula
824　Fracture of ankle
825　Fracture of one or more tarsal and metatarsal bones
826　Fracture of one or more phalanges of foot
827　Other, multiple, and ill-defined fractures of lower limb
828　Multiple fractures involving both lower limbs, lower with upper limb, and lower limb(s) with rib(s) and sternum
829　Fracture of unspecified bones

Dislocation (830-839)
830　Dislocation of jaw
831　Dislocation of shoulder
832　Dislocation of elbow
833　Dislocation of wrist
834　Dislocation of finger
835　Dislocation of hip
836　Dislocation of knee
837　Dislocation of ankle
838　Dislocation of foot
839　Other, multiple, and ill-defined dislocations

Sprains and strains of joints and adjacent muscles (840-848)
840　Sprains and strains of shoulder and upper arm
841　Sprains and strains of elbow and forearm
842　Sprains and strains of wrist and hand
843　Sprains and strains of hip and thigh
844　Sprains and strains of knee and leg
845　Sprains and strains of ankle and foot
846　Sprains and strains of sacroiliac region
847　Sprains and strains of other and unspecified parts of back
848　Other and ill-defined sprains and strains

Intracranial injury, excluding those with skull fracture (850-854)
850　Concussion
851　Cerebral laceration and contusion
852　Subarachnoid, subdural, and extradural hemorrhage, following injury
853　Other and unspecified intracranial hemorrhage following injury
854　Intracranial injury of other and unspecified nature

Internal injury of chest, abdomen, and pelvis (860-869)
860　Traumatic pneumothorax and hemothorax
861　Injury to heart and lung
862　Injury to other and unspecified intrathoracic organs
863　Injury to gastrointestinal tract
864　Injury to liver
865　Injury to spleen
866　Injury to kidney
867　Injury to pelvic organs
868　Injury to other intra-abdominal organs
869　Internal injury to unspecified or ill-defined organs

Open wound of head, neck, and trunk (870-879)
870　Open wound of ocular adnexa
871　Open wound of eyeball
872　Open wound of ear
873　Other open wound of head
874　Open wound of neck
875　Open wound of chest (wall)
876　Open wound of back
877　Open wound of buttock

878 Open wound of genital organs (external), including traumatic amputation
879 Open wound of other and unspecified sites, except limbs

Open wound of upper limb (880-887)
880 Open wound of shoulder and upper arm
881 Open wound of elbow, forearm, and wrist
882 Open wound of hand except finger(s) alone
883 Open wound of finger(s)
884 Multiple and unspecified open wound of upper limb
885 Traumatic amputation of thumb (complete) (partial)
886 Traumatic amputation of other finger(s) (complete) (partial)
887 Traumatic amputation of arm and hand (complete) (partial)

Open wound of lower limb (890-897)
890 Open wound of hip and thigh
891 Open wound of knee, leg [except thigh], and ankle
892 Open wound of foot except toe(s) alone
893 Open wound of toe(s)
894 Multiple and unspecified open wound of lower limb
895 Traumatic amputation of toe(s) (complete) (partial)
896 Traumatic amputation of foot (complete) (partial)
897 Traumatic amputation of leg(s) (complete) (partial)

Injury to blood vessels (900-904)
900 Injury to blood vessels of head and neck
901 Injury to blood vessels of thorax
902 Injury to blood vessels of abdomen and pelvis
903 Injury to blood vessels of upper extremity
904 Injury to blood vessels of lower extremity and unspecified sites

Late effects of injuries, poisonings, toxic effects, and other external causes (905-909)
905 Late effects of musculoskeletal and connective tissue injuries
906 Late effects of injuries to skin and subcutaneous tissues
907 Late effects of injuries to the nervous system
908 Late effects of other and unspecified injuries
909 Late effects of other and unspecified external causes

Superficial injury (910-919)
910 Superficial injury of face, neck, and scalp except eye
911 Superficial injury of trunk
912 Superficial injury of shoulder and upper arm
913 Superficial injury of elbow, forearm, and wrist
914 Superficial injury of hand(s) except finger(s) alone
915 Superficial injury of finger(s)
916 Superficial injury of hip, thigh, leg, and ankle
917 Superficial injury of foot and toe(s)
918 Superficial injury of eye and adnexa

919 Superficial injury of other, multiple, and unspecified sites

Contusion with intact skin surface (920-924)
920 Contusion of face, scalp, and neck except eye(s)
921 Contusion of eye and adnexa
922 Contusion of trunk
923 Contusion of upper limb
924 Contusion of lower limb and of other and unspecified sites

Crushing injury (925-929)
925 Crushing injury of face, scalp, and neck
926 Crushing injury of trunk
927 Crushing injury of upper limb
928 Crushing injury of lower limb
929 Crushing injury of multiple and unspecified sites

Effects of foreign body entering through orifice (930-939)
930 Foreign body on external eye
931 Foreign body in ear
932 Foreign body in nose
933 Foreign body in pharynx and larynx
934 Foreign body in trachea, bronchus, and lung
935 Foreign body in mouth, esophagus, and stomach
936 Foreign body in intestine and colon
937 Foreign body in anus and rectum
938 Foreign body in digestive system, unspecified
939 Foreign body in genitourinary tract

Burns (940-949)
940 Burn confined to eye and adnexa
941 Burn of face, head, and neck
942 Burn of trunk
943 Burn of upper limb, except wrist and hand
944 Burn of wrist(s) and hand(s)
945 Burn of lower limb(s)
946 Burns of multiple specified sites
947 Burn of internal organs
948 Burns classified according to extent of body surface involved
949 Burn, unspecified

Injury to nerves and spinal cord (950-957)
950 Injury to optic nerve and pathways
951 Injury to other cranial nerve(s)
952 Spinal cord injury without evidence of spinal bone injury
953 Injury to nerve roots and spinal plexus
954 Injury to other nerve(s) of trunk excluding shoulder and pelvic girdles
955 Injury to peripheral nerve(s) of shoulder girdle and upper limb
956 Injury to peripheral nerve(s) of pelvic girdle and lower limb
957 Injury to other and unspecified nerves

Certain traumatic complications and unspecified injuries (958-959)
958 Certain early complications of trauma
959 Injury, other and unspecified

Poisoning by drugs, medicinals and biological substances (960-979)
960 Poisoning by antibiotics
961 Poisoning by other anti-infectives

962 Poisoning by hormones and synthetic substitutes
963 Poisoning by primarily systemic agents
964 Poisoning by agents primarily affecting blood constituents
965 Poisoning by analgesics, antipyretics, and antirheumatics
966 Poisoning by anticonvulsants and anti-Parkinsonism drugs
967 Poisoning by sedatives and hypnotics
968 Poisoning by other central nervous system depressants and anesthetics
969 Poisoning by psychotropic agents
970 Poisoning by central nervous system stimulants
971 Poisoning by drugs primarily affecting the autonomic nervous system
972 Poisoning by agents primarily affecting the cardiovascular system
973 Poisoning by agents primarily affecting the gastrointestinal system
974 Poisoning by water, mineral, and uric acid metabolism drugs
975 Poisoning by agents primarily acting on the smooth and skeletal muscles and respiratory system
976 Poisoning by agents primarily affecting skin and mucous membrane, ophthalmological, otorhinolaryngological, and dental drugs
977 Poisoning by other and unspecified drugs and medicinals
978 Poisoning by bacterial vaccines
979 Poisoning by other vaccines and biological substances

Toxic effects of substances chiefly non-medicinal as to source (980-989)
980 Toxic effect of alcohol
981 Toxic effect of petroleum products
982 Toxic effect of solvents other than petroleum-based
983 Toxic effect of corrosive aromatics, acids, and caustic alkalis
984 Toxic effect of lead and its compounds (including fumes)
985 Toxic effect of other metals
986 Toxic effect of carbon monoxide
987 Toxic effect of other gases, fumes, or vapors
988 Toxic effect of noxious substances eaten as food
989 Toxic effect of other substances, chiefly nonmedicinal as to source

Other and unspecified effects of external causes (990-995)
990 Effects of radiation, unspecified
991 Effects of reduced temperature
992 Effects of heat and light
993 Effects of air pressure
994 Effects of other external causes
995 Certain adverse effects, not elsewhere classified

Complications of surgical and medical care, not elsewhere classified (996-999)
996 Complications peculiar to certain specified procedures
997 Complications affecting specified body systems, not elsewhere classified
998 Other complications of procedures, not elsewhere classified
999 Complications of medical care, not elsewhere classified

SUPPLEMENTARY CLASSIFICATION OF FACTORS INFLUENCING HEALTH STATUS AND CONTACT WITH HEALTH SERVICES

Persons with potential health hazards related to communicable diseases (V01-V09)

V01 Contact with or exposure to communicable diseases
V02 Carrier or suspected carrier of infectious diseases
V03 Need for prophylactic vaccination and inoculation against bacterial diseases
V04 Need for prophylactic vaccination and inoculation against certain viral diseases
V05 Need for other prophylactic vaccination and inoculation against single diseases
V06 Need for prophylactic vaccination and inoculation against combinations of diseases
V07 Need for isolation and other prophylactic measures
V08 Asymptomatic human immunodeficiency virus [HIV] infection status
V09 Infection with drug-resistant microorganisms

Persons with potential health hazards related to personal and family history (V10-V19)

V10 Personal history of malignant neoplasm
V11 Personal history of mental disorder
V12 Personal history of certain other diseases
V13 Personal history of other diseases
V14 Personal history of allergy to medicinal agents
V15 Other personal history presenting hazards to health
V16 Family history of malignant neoplasm
V17 Family history of certain chronic disabling diseases
V18 Family history of certain other specific conditions
V19 Family history of other conditions

Persons encountering health services in circumstances related to reproduction and development (V20-V29)

V20 Health supervision of infant or child
V21 Constitutional states in development
V22 Normal pregnancy
V23 Supervision of high-risk pregnancy
V24 Postpartum care and examination
V25 Encounter for contraceptive management
V26 Procreative management
V27 Outcome of delivery
V28 Antenatal screening
V29 Observation and evaluation of newborns and infants for suspected condition not found

Liveborn infants according to type of birth (V30-V39)

V30 Single liveborn
V31 Twin, mate liveborn
V32 Twin, mate stillborn
V33 Twin, unspecified
V34 Other multiple, mates all liveborn
V35 Other multiple, mates all stillborn
V36 Other multiple, mates live- and stillborn
V37 Other multiple, unspecified
V39 Unspecified

Persons with a condition influencing their health status (V40-V49)

V40 Mental and behavioral problems
V41 Problems with special senses and other special functions
V42 Organ or tissue replaced by transplant
V43 Organ or tissue replaced by other means
V44 Artificial opening status
V45 Other postsurgical states
V46 Other dependence on machines
V47 Other problems with internal organs
V48 Problems with head, neck, and trunk
V49 Problems with limbs and other problems

Persons encountering health services for specific procedures and aftercare (V50-V59)

V50 Elective surgery for purposes other than remedying health states
V51 Aftercare involving the use of plastic surgery
V52 Fitting and adjustment of prosthetic device
V53 Fitting and adjustment of other device
V54 Other orthopedic aftercare
V55 Attention to artificial openings
V56 Encounter for dialysis and dialysis catheter care
V57 Care involving use of rehabilitation procedures
V58 Encounter for other and unspecified procedures and aftercare
V59 Donors

Persons encountering health services in other circumstances (V60-V69)

V60 Housing, household, and economic circumstances
V61 Other family circumstances
V62 Other psychosocial circumstances
V63 Unavailability of other medical facilities for care
V64 Persons encountering health services for specific procedures, not carried out
V65 Other persons seeking consultation without complaint or sickness
V66 Convalescence and palliative care
V67 Follow-up examination
V68 Encounters for administrative purposes
V69 Problems related to lifestyle

Persons without reported diagnosis encountered during examination and investigation of individuals and populations (V70-V83)

V70 General medical examination
V71 Observation and evaluation for suspected conditions not found
V72 Special investigations and examinations
V73 Special screening examination for viral and chlamydial diseases
V74 Special screening examination for bacterial and spirochetal diseases
V75 Special screening examination for other infectious diseases
V76 Special screening for malignant neoplasms
V77 Special screening for endocrine, nutritional, metabolic, and immunity disorders
V78 Special screening for disorders of blood and blood-forming organs
V79 Special screening for mental disorders and developmental handicaps
V80 Special screening for neurological, eye, and ear diseases
V81 Special screening for cardiovascular, respiratory, and genitourinary diseases
V82 Special screening for other conditions
V83 Genetic carrier status

SUPPLEMENTARY CLASSIFICATION OF EXTERNAL CAUSES OF INJURY AND POISONING

Railway accidents (E800-E807)

E800 Railway accident involving collision with rolling stock
E801 Railway accident involving collision with other object
E802 Railway accident involving derailment without antecedent collision
E803 Railway accident involving explosion, fire, or burning
E804 Fall in, on, or from railway train
E805 Hit by rolling stock
E806 Other specified railway accident
E807 Railway accident of unspecified nature

Motor vehicle traffic accidents (E810-E819)

E810 Motor vehicle traffic accident involving collision with train
E811 Motor vehicle traffic accident involving re-entrant collision with another motor vehicle
E812 Other motor vehicle traffic accident involving collision with another motor vehicle
E813 Motor vehicle traffic accident involving collision with other vehicle
E814 Motor vehicle traffic accident involving collision with pedestrian
E815 Other motor vehicle traffic accident involving collision on the highway
E816 Motor vehicle traffic accident due to loss of control, without collision on the highway
E817 Noncollision motor vehicle traffic accident while boarding or alighting
E818 Other noncollision motor vehicle traffic accident
E819 Motor vehicle traffic accident of unspecified nature

Motor vehicle nontraffic accidents (E820-E825)

E820 Nontraffic accident involving motor-driven snow vehicle
E821 Nontraffic accident involving other off-road motor vehicle
E822 Other motor vehicle nontraffic accident involving collision with moving object
E823 Other motor vehicle nontraffic accident involving collision with stationary object
E824 Other motor vehicle nontraffic accident while boarding and alighting
E825 Other motor vehicle nontraffic accident of other and unspecified nature

Other road vehicle accidents (E826-E829)

E826 Pedal cycle accident
E827 Animal-drawn vehicle accident

E828 Accident involving animal being ridden

E829 Other road vehicle accidents

Water transport accidents (E830-E838)

E830 Accident to watercraft causing submersion

E831 Accident to watercraft causing other injury

E832 Other accidental submersion or drowning in water transport accident

E833 Fall on stairs or ladders in water transport

E834 Other fall from one level to another in water transport

E835 Other and unspecified fall in water transport

E836 Machinery accident in water transport

E837 Explosion, fire, or burning in watercraft

E838 Other and unspecified water transport accident

Air and space transport accidents (E840-E845)

E840 Accident to powered aircraft at take-off or landing

E841 Accident to powered aircraft, other and unspecified

E842 Accident to unpowered aircraft

E843 Fall in, on, or from aircraft

E844 Other specified air transport accidents

E845 Accident involving spacecraft

Vehicle accidents, not elsewhere classifiable (E846-E849)

E846 Accidents involving powered vehicles used solely within the buildings and premises of an industrial or commercial establishment

E847 Accidents involving cable cars not running on rails

E848 Accidents involving other vehicles, not elsewhere classifiable

E849 Place of occurrence

Accidental poisoning by drugs, medicinal substances, and biologicals (E850-E858)

E850 Accidental poisoning by analgesics, antipyretics, and antirheumatics

E851 Accidental poisoning by barbiturates

E852 Accidental poisoning by other sedatives and hypnotics

E853 Accidental poisoning by tranquilizers

E854 Accidental poisoning by other psychotropic agents

E855 Accidental poisoning by other drugs acting on central and autonomic nervous systems

E856 Accidental poisoning by antibiotics

E857 Accidental poisoning by anti-infectives

E858 Accidental poisoning by other drugs

Accidental poisoning by other solid and liquid substances, gases, and vapors (E860-E869)

E860 Accidental poisoning by alcohol, not elsewhere classified

E861 Accidental poisoning by cleansing and polishing agents, disinfectants, paints, and varnishes

E862 Accidental poisoning by petroleum products, other solvents and their vapors, not elsewhere classified

E863 Accidental poisoning by agricultural and horticultural chemical and pharmaceutical preparations other than plant foods and fertilizers

E864 Accidental poisoning by corrosives and caustics, not elsewhere classified

E865 Accidental poisoning from poisonous foodstuffs and poisonous plants

E866 Accidental poisoning by other and unspecified solid and liquid substances

E867 Accidental poisoning by gas distributed by pipeline

E868 Accidental poisoning by other utility gas and other carbon monoxide

E869 Accidental poisoning by other gases and vapors

Misadventures to patients during surgical and medical care (E870-E876)

E870 Accidental cut, puncture, perforation, or hemorrhage during medical care

E871 Foreign object left in body during procedure

E872 Failure of sterile precautions during procedure

E873 Failure in dosage

E874 Mechanical failure of instrument or apparatus during procedure

E875 Contaminated or infected blood, other fluid, drug, or biological substance

E876 Other and unspecified misadventures during medical care

Surgical and medical procedures as the cause of abnormal reaction of patient or later complication, without mention of misadventure at the time of procedure (E878-E879)

E878 Surgical operation and other surgical procedures as the cause of abnormal reaction of patient, or of later complication, without mention of misadventure at the time of operation

E879 Other procedures, without mention of misadventure at the time of procedure, as the cause of abnormal reaction of patient, or of later complication

Accidental falls (E880-E888)

E880 Fall on or from stairs or steps

E881 Fall on or from ladders or scaffolding

E882 Fall from or out of building or other structure

E883 Fall into hole or other opening in surface

E884 Other fall from one level to another

E885 Fall on same level from slipping, tripping, or stumbling

E886 Fall on same level from collision, pushing or shoving, by or with other person

E887 Fracture, cause unspecified

E888 Other and unspecified fall

Accidents caused by fire and flames (E890-E899)

E890 Conflagration in private dwelling

E891 Conflagration in other and unspecified building or structure

E892 Conflagration not in building or structure

E893 Accident caused by ignition of clothing

E894 Ignition of highly inflammable material

E895 Accident caused by controlled fire in private dwelling

E896 Accident caused by controlled fire in other and unspecified building or structure

E897 Accident caused by controlled fire not in building or structure

E898 Accident caused by other specified fire and flames

E899 Accident caused by unspecified fire

Accidents due to natural and environmental factors (E900-E909)

E900 Excessive heat

E901 Excessive cold

E902 High and low air pressure and changes in air pressure

E903 Travel and motion

E904 Hunger, thirst, exposure, and neglect

E905 Venomous animals and plants as the cause of poisoning and toxic reactions

E906 Other injury caused by animals

E907 Lightning

E908 Cataclysmic storms, and floods resulting from storms

E909 Cataclysmic earth surface movements and eruptions

Accidents caused by submersion, suffocation, and foreign bodies (E910-E915)

E910 Accidental drowning and submersion

E911 Inhalation and ingestion of food causing obstruction of respiratory tract or suffocation

E912 Inhalation and ingestion of other object causing obstruction of respiratory tract or suffocation

E913 Accidental mechanical suffocation

E914 Foreign body accidentally entering eye and adnexa

E915 Foreign body accidentally entering other orifice

Other accidents (E916-E928)

E916 Struck accidentally by falling object

E917 Striking against or struck accidentally by objects or persons

E918 Caught accidentally in or between objects

E919 Accidents caused by machinery

E920 Accidents caused by cutting and piercing instruments or objects

E921 Accident caused by explosion of pressure vessel

E922 Accident caused by firearm missile

E923 Accident caused by explosive material

E924 Accident caused by hot substance or object, caustic or corrosive material, and steam

E925 Accident caused by electric current

E926 Exposure to radiation

E927 Overexertion and strenuous movements

E928   Other and unspecified environmental and accidental causes

Late effects of accidental injury (E929)
E929   Late effects of accidental injury

Drugs, medicinal and biological substances causing adverse effects in therapeutic use (E930-E949)
E930   Antibiotics
E931   Other anti-infectives
E932   Hormones and synthetic substitutes
E933   Primarily systemic agents
E934   Agents primarily affecting blood constituents
E935   Analgesics, antipyretics, and antirheumatics
E936   Anticonvulsants and anti-Parkinsonism drugs
E937   Sedatives and hypnotics
E938   Other central nervous system depressants and anesthetics
E939   Psychotropic agents
E940   Central nervous system stimulants
E941   Drugs primarily affecting the autonomic nervous system
E942   Agents primarily affecting the cardiovascular system
E943   Agents primarily affecting gastrointestinal system
E944   Water, mineral, and uric acid metabolism drugs
E945   Agents primarily acting on the smooth and skeletal muscles and respiratory system
E946   Agents primarily affecting skin and mucous membrane, ophthalmological, otorhinolaryngological, and dental drugs
E947   Other and unspecified drugs and medicinal substances
E948   Bacterial vaccines
E949   Other vaccines and biological substances

Suicide and self-inflicted injury (E950-E959)
E950   Suicide and self-inflicted poisoning by solid or liquid substances
E951   Suicide and self-inflicted poisoning by gases in domestic use
E952   Suicide and self-inflicted poisoning by other gases and vapors
E953   Suicide and self-inflicted injury by hanging, strangulation, and suffocation
E954   Suicide and self-inflicted injury by submersion [drowning]
E955   Suicide and self-inflicted injury by firearms and explosives
E956   Suicide and self-inflicted injury by cutting and piercing instruments
E957   Suicide and self-inflicted injuries by jumping from high place
E958   Suicide and self-inflicted injury by other and unspecified means
E959   Late effects of self-inflicted injury

Homicide and injury purposely inflicted by other persons (E960-E969)
E960   Fight, brawl, and rape
E961   Assault by corrosive or caustic substance, except poisoning
E962   Assault by poisoning
E963   Assault by hanging and strangulation
E964   Assault by submersion [drowning]
E965   Assault by firearms and explosives
E966   Assault by cutting and piercing instrument
E967   Child and adult battering and other maltreatment
E968   Assault by other and unspecified means
E969   Late effects of injury purposely inflicted by other person

Legal intervention (E970-E978)
E970   Injury due to legal intervention by firearms
E971   Injury due to legal intervention by explosives
E972   Injury due to legal intervention by gas
E973   Injury due to legal intervention by blunt object
E974   Injury due to legal intervention by cutting and piercing instruments
E975   Injury due to legal intervention by other specified means
E976   Injury due to legal intervention by unspecified means
E977   Late effects of injuries due to legal intervention
E978   Legal execution

Terrorism (E979)
E979   Terrorism

Injury undetermined whether accidentally or purposely inflicted (E980-E989)
E980   Poisoning by solid or liquid substances, undetermined whether accidentally or purposely inflicted
E981   Poisoning by gases in domestic use, undetermined whether accidentally or purposely inflicted
E982   Poisoning by other gases, undetermined whether accidentally or purposely inflicted
E983   Hanging, strangulation, or suffocation, undetermined whether accidentally or purposely inflicted
E984   Submersion [drowning], undetermined whether accidentally or purposely inflicted
E985   Injury by firearms and explosives, undetermined whether accidentally or purposely inflicted
E986   Injury by cutting and piercing instruments, undetermined whether accidentally or purposely inflicted
E987   Falling from high place, undetermined whether accidentally or purposely inflicted
E988   Injury by other and unspecified means, undetermined whether accidentally or purposely inflicted
E989   Late effects of injury, undetermined whether accidentally or purposely inflicted

Injury resulting from operations of war (E990-E999)
E990   Injury due to war operations by fires and conflagrations
E991   Injury due to war operations by bullets and fragments
E992   Injury due to war operations by explosion of marine weapons
E993   Injury due to war operations by other explosion
E994   Injury due to war operations by destruction of aircraft
E995   Injury due to war operations by other and unspecified forms of conventional warfare
E996   Injury due to war operations by nuclear weapons
E997   Injury due to war operations by other forms of unconventional warfare
E998   Injury due to war operations but occurring after cessation of hostilities
E999   Late effects of injury due to war operations